PHYSICAL THERAPY
for Children

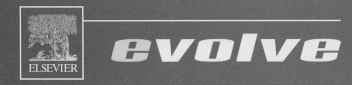

∴ *To access your Student Learning Resources, visit:*

http://evolve.elsevier.com/Campbell/PTchildren/

Evolve® Student Learning Resources for *Campbell/Vander Linden/Palisano: Physical Therapy for Children,* **Third Edition,** offers the following features:

- **Critical thinking questions**
  Helps reinforce what you learn.

- **DVD clips**
  List of video clips on DVD with their running times.

- **WebLinks**
  Links to APTA, vendors, and other websites specific to your needs.

- **Pediatric Clinical Specialist Examination Questions and Answers**
  Sample test questions and answers modeled after the pediatric specialty exam.

- **And more**
  Additional resources and activities.

PHYSICAL THERAPY
for Children

SUZANN K. CAMPBELL, PT, PhD, FAPTA
Professor and Head, Department of Physical Therapy
College of Applied Health Sciences
University of Illinois at Chicago
Chicago, Illinois

Associate Editors

DARL W. VANDER LINDEN, PT, PhD
Professor, Department of Physical Therapy
Eastern Washington University
Spokane, Washington

ROBERT J. PALISANO, PT, ScD
Professor, Programs in Rehabilitation Sciences
Drexel University
Philadelphia, Pennsylvania

SAUNDERS

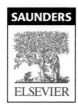

ELSEVIER

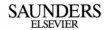

SAUNDERS
ELSEVIER

11830 Westline Industrial Drive
St. Louis, Missouri 63146

PHYSICAL THERAPY FOR CHILDREN, THIRD EDITION

ISBN 13: 978-0-7216-0378-0
ISBN 10: 0-7216-0378-5

Notice

ISBN 13: 978-0-7216-0378-0
ISBN 10: 0-7216-0378-5

Acquisitions Editor: Marion Waldman
Developmental Editor: Teri Zak
Publishing Services Manager: Patricia Tannian
Project Manager: John Casey
Designer: Jyotika Shroff

Printed in United States of America

Last digit is the print number: 9 8 7 6 5 4 3

CONTRIBUTORS

JENNIFER L. AGNEW, BScPT, BHK
Physiotherapist, Hospital for Sick Children
Rehabilitation Services, Chest and Cystic Fibrosis Clinic
Toronto, Ontario
Chapter 27: Cystic Fibrosis

JO A. ASHWELL, BScPT
Physiotherapist
Comcare Health Services, Pediatric Division
Niagara Falls, Ontario
Chapter 27: Cystic Fibrosis

DONNA BERNHARDT BAINBRIDGE, PT, EdD, ATC
Research Project Director
The University of Montana Rural Institute
Missoula, Montana;
Special Olympics Global Advisor for FUNfitness and
    Fitness Programming
Chapter 18: Sports Injuries in Children

DEBRA BLEAKNEY, PT
President, OPT Therapy Services, Ltd.
Wilmington, Delaware
Chapter 14: Osteogenesis Imperfecta

NINA S. BRADLEY, PT, PhD
Associate Professor, Department of Biokinesiology and
    Physical Therapy
University of Southern California
Los Angeles, California
*Chapter 3: Motor Control: Developmental Aspects of
    Motor Control in Skill Acquisition*

SUZANN K. CAMPBELL, PT, PhD, FAPTA
Professor and Head, Department of Physical Therapy
College of Applied Health Sciences
University of Illinois at Chicago
Chicago, Illinois
*Chapter 1: Evidence-Based Decision Making in Pediatric
    Physical Therapy*
*Chapter 2: The Child's Development of Functional
    Movement*

SHIRLEY J. CARLSON, PT, MS, PCS
Physical Therapist
The Spokane Guilds' School
Spokane, Washington
Chapter 33: Assistive Technology

LISA ANN CHIARELLO, PT, PhD, PCS
Associate Professor, Drexel University
Programs in Rehabilitation Sciences
Philadelphia, Pennsylvania
Chapter 31: Early Intervention Services

KATHRYN STEYER DAVID, PT, MS, PCS
Physical Therapist
Heartland Area Education Agency
Johnston, Iowa
Chapter 19: Developmental Coordination Disorders

MAUREEN DONOHOE, PT, PCS
Senior Staff Physical Therapist
Alfred I. DuPont Hospital for Children
Wilmington, Delaware
Chapter 13: Arthrogryposis Multiplex Congenita;
Chapter 14: Osteogenesis Imperfecta

HELENE DUMAS, PT, MS
Manager, Research Center for Children with Special
Health Care Needs
Franciscan Hospital for Children
Boston, Massachusetts
*Chapter 26: Children Requiring Long-Term Ventilator
    Assistance*

SUSAN K. EFFGEN, PT, PhD
Joseph Hamburg Professorship in Rehabilitation Sciences
Director, Rehabilitation Sciences Doctoral Program
College of Health Sciences
University of Kentucky
Lexington, Kentucky
Chapter 32: The Educational Environment

CARRIE G. GAJDOSIK, PT, MS
Associate Professor, Physical Therapy Department
School of Physical Therapy and Rehabilitation Science
College of Health Professions and Biomedical Sciences
The University of Montana
Missoula, Montana
Chapter 6: Musculoskeletal Development and Adaptation

RICHARD L. GAJDOSIK, PT, PhD
Professor, Physical Therapy Department
School of Physical Therapy and Rehabilitation Science
College of Health Professions and Biomedical Sciences
The University of Montana
Missoula, Montana
Chapter 6: Musculoskeletal Development and Adaptation

LAURA H. HANSEN, PT, MS
Physical Therapist
Preschool Program, J. Iverson Riddle Development
Center
Morganton, North Carolina
Chapter 20: Children with Motor and Cognitive Impairments

SUSAN R. HARRIS, PT, PhD, FAPTA
Professor, School of Rehabilitation Sciences
Faculty of Medicine
University of British Columbia
Vancouver, British Columbia
Chapter 1: Evidence-Based Decision Making in Pediatric Physical Therapy

PATRICIA REYNOLDS HILL, PT, MA
Director, Physical Therapist Assistant Program
Washtenaw Community College
Ann Arbor, Michigan
Chapter 29: Thoracic Surgery

KATHLEEN A. HINDERER, PT, PhD
Physical Therapy Consultant
Ann Arbor, Michigan
Chapter 25: Myelodysplasia

STEVEN R. HINDERER, PT, MD
Associate Professor
Department of Physical Medicine and Rehabilitation
Wayne State University School of Medicine
Director, Center for Spinal Cord Injury and Recovery
Rehabilitation Institute of Michigan
Detroit Medical Center
Detroit, Michigan
Chapter 25: Myelodysplasia

BETSY A. HOWELL, PT, MS
Physical Therapist
C. S. Mott Children's Hospital
University of Michigan Health Systems
Ann Arbor, Michigan
Chapter 29: Thoracic Surgery

LINDA KAHN-D'ANGELO, PT, ScD
Professor of Physical Therapy
University of Massachusetts
Lowell, Massachusetts
Chapter 35: The Special Care Nursery

KAREN KARMEL-ROSS, PT, PCS, LMT
Pediatric Clinical Specialist
University Hospitals of Cleveland
Rainbow Babies and Children's Hospital
Cleveland, Ohio;
Owner, Straight Ahead Pediatric Physical Therapy
Mayfield Village, Ohio
Chapter 12: Congenital Muscular Torticollis

M. KATHLEEN KELLY, PT, PhD
Assistant Professor and Vice-Chair, Department of Physical Therapy
School of Health & Rehabilitation Sciences
University of Pittsburgh
Pittsburgh, Pennsylvania
Chapter 26: Children Requiring Long-Term Ventilator Assistance

GINETTE KERKERING, PT
Physical Therapist, St. Luke's Rehabilitation at
Sacred Heart Children's Hospital
Spokane, Washington
Chapter 24: Brain Injuries: Traumatic Brain Injuries, Near-Drowning, and Brain Tumors

SUSAN E. KLEPPER, PT, PhD
Assistant Professor of Clinical Physical Therapy
Program in Physical Therapy
Columbia University
New York, New York
Chapter 9: Juvenile Rheumatoid Arthritis

THUBI H. A. KOLOBE, PT, PhD
Associate Professor, Department of Rehabilitation
Science
College of Allied Health
University of Oklahoma Health Sciences Center
Oklahoma City, Oklahoma
Chapter 30: The Environment of Intervention
Chapter 31: Early Intervention Services

HÉLÈNE M. LARIN, PT, PhD
Associate Professor, Department of Physical Therapy
Ithaca College
Ithaca, New York
Chapter 4: Motor Learning: Theories and Strategies for the Practitioner

JUDY LEACH, PT
Physical Therapy Consultant
Kopoho, Hawaii
Chapter 17: Orthopedic Conditions

BENJAMIN R. LOVELACE-CHANDLER, PT, PhD, PCS
Kids' SPOT
Orange, California
Chapter 36: Private Practice Pediatric Physical Therapy: A Quest for Independence and Success

VENITA S. LOVELACE-CHANDLER, PT, PhD, PCS
Department of Physical Therapy
Chapman University
Orange, California
Chapter 36: Private Practice Pediatric Physical Therapy: A Quest for Independence and Success

CYNTHIA L. MAGEE, PT, MS
Private Pediatric Practitioner
Medford, New Jersey
Chapter 28: Asthma: Multi-System Implications

TERESA L. MASSAGLI, MD
Associate Professor of Rehabilitation Medicine and Pediatrics
University of Washington and Children's Hospital and Regional Medical Center
Seattle, Washington
Chapter 23: Spinal Cord Injury

MARY MASSERY, PT, DPT
Owner, Massery Physical Therapy
Glenview, Illinois
Chapter 28: Asthma: Multi-System Implications

IRENE R. MCEWEN, PT, PhD
George Lynn Cross Research Professor
College of Allied Health
University of Oklahoma Department of Rehabilitation Sciences
Oklahoma City, Oklahoma
Chapter 20: Children with Motor and Cognitive Impairments

SANDRA M. MCGEE, PT, PCS
Physical Therapist III
Children's Hospital of Philadelphia
Philadelphia, Pennsylvania
Chapter 10: Hemophilia

MERILYN L. MOORE, PT
OT/PT/TR Supervisor
Harborview Medical Center
Seattle, Washington
Chapter 34: The Burn Unit

ELLEN STAMOS NORTON, PT, PCS
Owner, Pediatric Private Practice
Poway, California
Chapter 22: Brachial Plexus Injury

JOAN A. O'KEEFE, PT, PhD
Private Pediatric Practitioner and Consultant
Chicago, Illinois
Chapter 7: Genomics and Genetic Syndromes Affecting Movement

SANDRA J. OLNEY, BSc (PT&OT) MEd, PhD
Professor and Director, School of Rehabilitation Therapy
Associate Dean (Health Sciences), Queen's University
Kingston, Ontario
Chapter 21: Cerebral Palsy

ROBERTA KUCHLER O'SHEA, PT, PhD
Assistant Professor
Department of Physical Therapy
Governors State University
University Park, Illinois
Chapter 33: Assistive Technology

ROBERT J. PALISANO, PT, ScD
Professor
Programs in Rehabilitation Sciences
Drexel University
Philadelphia, Pennsylvania
Chapter 1: Evidence-Based Decision Making in Pediatric Physical Therapy

CHERYL PATRICK, PT
Senior Physical Therapist
Children's Memorial Hospital
Chicago, Illinois
Chapter 11: Spinal Conditions

WENDY E. PHILLIPS, PT, MS, PhD
Physical Therapist and Developmental Consultant in
Private Practice
Atlanta, Georgia
Chapter 37: Medicolegal Issues in the United States

CAROLE RAMSEY, OTR/L, ATP
Supervisor of Occupational Therapy
University Hospital School, University of Iowa
Iowa City, Iowa
Chapter 33: Assistive Technology

SHARI L. RENAUD, BHScPT, BKIN
Physiotherapist, Hospital for Sick Children
Rehabilitation Services
Toronto, Ontario
Chapter 27: Cystic Fibrosis

CYNTHIA A. ROBINSON, PT, MS
Department of Rehabilitation Medicine
University of Washington
Seattle, Washington
Chapter 34: Special Settings and Special Considerations

RACHEL A. UNANUE ROSE, PT, PhD, PCS
Assistant Professor, Department of Physical Therapy
School of Health Related Professions
University of Alabama at Birmingham
Birmingham, Alabama
Chapter 35: The Special Care Nursery

KRISTINE A. SHAKHAZIZIAN, PT
Physical Therapist
Jennersville Regional Hospital
West Grove, Pennsylvania
Chapter 23: Spinal Cord Injury

DAVID B. SHURTLEFF, MD
Professor, Department of Pediatrics
University of Washington
Seattle, Washington
Chapter 25: Myelodysplasia

MICHAEL L. SPOTTS, JD
Attorney in Private Practice
Atlanta, Georgia
Chapter 37: Medicolegal Issues in the United States

MEG STANGER, PT, MS, PCS
Director of Occupational and Physical Therapy
Children's Hospital of Pittsburgh
Pittsburgh, Pennsylvania
Chapter 16: Limb Deficiencies and Amputations

JEAN L. STOUT, PT, MS
Research Physical Therapist
Center for Gait and Motion Analysis
Gillette Children's Specialty Healthcare
St. Paul, Minnesota
Chapter 5: Gait: Development and Analysis
*Chapter 8: Physical Fitness During Childhood and
    Adolescence*

WAYNE A. STUBERG, PT, PhD, PCS
Professor and Director
Physical Therapy and Motion Analysis Lab
Munroe-Meyer Institute
University of Nebraska Medical Center
Omaha, Nebraska
*Chapter 15: Muscular Dystrophy and Spinal Muscular
    Atrophy*

ANN TAYLOR
Nichols, Oklahoma
Chapter 30: The Environment of Intervention

DARL W. VANDER LINDEN, PT, PhD
Professor of Physical Therapy
Eastern Washington University
Spokane, Washington
Chapter 22: Brachial Plexus Injury

SARAH L. WESTCOTT, PT, PhD
Clinical Associate Professor
Physical Therapy Department
University of Puget Sound
Tacoma, Washington
*Chapter 3: Motor Control: Developmental Aspects of
    Motor Control in Skill Acquisition*

MARILYN J. WRIGHT, BScPT, MEd
Clinical Specialist
McMaster Children's Hospital
Assistant Clinical Professor
McMaster University
Hamilton, Ontario
Chapter 21: Cerebral Palsy

*To Martin and Virginia Reetz, Shirley Carlson, and Linda, Joseph, and Lena Palisano
and to all the children who have enriched our personal and professional lives,
but especially to*

**Dianne and Debbie
Abby and Mitchell
Christina, Joey, and Michael**

PREFACE

As Cherry[1] said in a description of philosophy and science in pediatric physical therapy, specialty practice in pediatrics derives from the general philosophy of physical therapy but must address additional concerns that are different from those of physical therapy for adults. For example, clinical decision making must be guided by the knowledge that the natural development of children interacts with disability. As a result, physical therapists must anticipate and provide for children's changing needs. In addition, interventions must address the issues and problems identified by children and their caregivers. To the extent possible, children and caregivers must be intimately involved in both developing the plan of care and in its implementation in natural settings for children —the home, school, and community. The philosophy of family-centered care continues to guide the editors of this book, and, to this end, the third edition of *Physical Therapy for Children* includes an exciting new chapter, The Environment of Intervention.

In the third edition of *Physical Therapy for Children*, the editors have used two additional conceptual models to guide the updating and revision of existing chapters and the development of both new chapters and new technological information resources such as a DVD and a dedicated website organized by the contents of each chapter. The conceptual models that guided our work include the International Classification of Function, Disability and Health (ICF)[2] of the World Health Organization and the Guide to Physical Therapist Practice[3] of the American Physical Therapy Association. Descriptions of these conceptual models can be found in the opening chapter on the evidence-based practice of pediatric physical therapy. We recommend that readers commence using this book with Chapter 1 as a guide to our philosophy, terminology, and conceptual framework for *Physical Therapy for Children*.

The Guide to Physical Therapist Practice should, of course, be used by all pediatric physical therapists in developing plans of care. We have, however, chosen to use the ICF as our model of the disabling process, rather than the model used in the Guide, because the ICF presents the dimensions of disability in a positive light, emphasizing activity rather than functional limitations, and participation rather than disability. The editors believe that all interventions provided by physical therapists should have as their goal the promotion of activity and participation as defined in the ICF model. Use of this model is helpful in directing attention to the ultimate purpose of providing intervention for children and education for their parents; therefore, this book focuses on prevention of disability throughout childhood and during the transition to living successfully as an adult.

The goal of our book continues to be the provision of a comprehensive reference for pediatric practice. To accomplish this goal, the remaining chapters in Section I of *Physical Therapy for Children* provide foundational knowledge in development, motor control, and motor learning. The eight chapters in this section should lead to understanding motor performance in children. These chapters provide information on the development of functional motor skills, gait, and the musculoskeletal structures; motor control and learning; research-based clinical decision making; and health-related physical fitness. A new chapter on genomics reviews the biology of genetic conditions and describes a number of these conditions that are common in clinical practice.

Sections II through IV of the book describe the impairments of body function and structure and the physical therapy management of activity and participation limitations common in pediatric musculoskeletal, neurologic, and cardiopulmonary conditions, respectively. Each chapter has been updated for the new edition, and application of the content is illustrated with evidence-based case studies from the authors' practices. Finally,

---

[1]Cherry DB. Pediatric physical therapy: Philosophy, science, and techniques. Pediatric Physical Therapy, 3:70-75, 1991.
[2] World Health Organization. International Classification of Function, Disability and Health. Geneva: World Health Organization, 2001.
[3] American Physical Therapy Association. Guide to physical therapist practice, 2nd ed. Physical Therapy, 81(1):2001.

Section V addresses special settings and special considerations, including the burn unit, the special care nursery, early intervention, the educational environment, private practice, and medicolegal issues, such as child abuse and neglect, and public laws addressing disabilities in childhood. An addition to this section is the new chapter on the environment of intervention.

The editors of the third edition of *Physical Therapy for Children* are especially proud of the application of new technologies to expand the horizons of the reader. New in this edition are case studies for several chapters that capture the activities, functional limitations, examination and evaluation, and physical therapy management of children with disabilities in moving pictures on the DVD that accompanies this book. Case studies and other topics that are accompanied by video clips have a DVD icon in the margin of the text, as shown on the thumb margin of this page. Numerous video clips can also be found on the DVD to accompany the descriptions of typical motor development in Chapter 2. The second new feature is the dedicated Evolve website for the book. Here instructors will find downloadable images from the text that can be used to enhance their teaching. Addresses for other websites will be useful for students, instructors, and clinicians to link to organizations serving families of children with disabilities, research laboratories, and many other useful Internet sites. Students and clinicians preparing for pediatric specialist certification will find questions and educational exercises on the website to reinforce their learning.

The editors are grateful to the authors of this new edition and to the editorial and media consultants at Elsevier for creating the new features that bring this book alive and connect pediatric physical therapists to the world at large through the resources of the Internet. I would also like to thank University of Illinois at Chicago Doctor of Physical Therapy student Jennifer Mitol for her excellent work producing the introduction to the DVD and my co-editors, Darl Vander Linden and Robert Palisano, for their valuable contributions to all aspects of the work.

Suzann K. Campbell
Senior Editor
Chicago, Illinois
February 22, 2005

CONTENTS

SECTION I

UNDERSTANDING MOTOR PERFORMANCE IN CHILDREN

Section Editor
Suzann K. Campbell
PT, PhD, FAPTA

Chapter 1

EVIDENCE-BASED DECISION MAKING IN PEDIATRIC PHYSICAL THERAPY

ROBERT J. PALISANO
PT, ScD

SUZANN K. CAMPBELL
PT, PhD, FAPTA

SUSAN R. HARRIS
PT, PhD, FAPTA

Every day, pediatric physical therapists must make decisions that affect the lives of children and their families. On what basis do we make these important decisions? Physical therapy has long used the empirical base of collective experience in clinical practice that is passed down from clinicians and educators to successive generations of new practitioners. Although this knowledge has served clinicians and their clients well throughout the brief history of our discipline, today's health care climate requires more. Increasingly, physicians and other health professionals, third-party payers, and the public expect that physical therapists will use scientific evidence and more valid and reliable decision-making methods as the basis for their practice. In managed care settings, cost efficiency and client satisfaction measures are expected as guides to what will be approved and reimbursed. Care principles enunciated by clients have entered the picture, too, as consumers became active advocates for best practice (Harrison, 1993), a trend that is consistent with family-centered services.

Pediatric physical therapists make several types of decisions: (1) who needs intervention and why; (2) what are the expected outcomes of intervention and how should they be documented; (3) how children in need of intervention should be served, for example, which procedural interventions should be applied, what types of information and instruction should be provided, how should services be coordinated; (4) the number of visits required to achieve expected outcomes; and (5) how the overall clinical program should be evaluated for effectiveness and efficiency in meeting the needs of children and families, achieving functional outcomes, promoting health, and preventing secondary impairments and participation restrictions. The overall objective of this chapter is to enable pediatric physical therapists to (1) apply processes and strategies of evidence-based practice and decision making and (2) reflect on the assumptions and rationale for their clinical decisions. The chapter is written from the perspective of the pediatric physical therapist attempting to provide "best practice" and is a resource for other chapters in this textbook.

EVIDENCE-BASED PRACTICE

Evidence-based practice refers to the use of current knowledge and research to guide clinical decision making within the context of the individual client (Sackett et al., 1996). During the past decade, the concept of evidence-based practice has become a "benchmark" for best practice.

WHAT IS EVIDENCE-BASED PRACTICE?

In 1992, the Evidence-Based Medicine Working Group described evidence-based practice as an emerging paradigm. In this paradigm, evidence from clinical research is emphasized in decision making while intuition, unsystematic clinical experience, and pathophysiologic rationale are de-emphasized. Evidence-based practitioners must critically appraise research and translate evidence to practice. These competencies reflect the perspective that health care providers have the responsibility to document the effectiveness of interventions, including the ability to provide quality care and a desirable cost/benefit ratio (Lansky et al., 1992).

Evidence-based practice involves "integration of best research evidence with clinical expertise and patient values" (Sackett et al., 2000, page 1). Decision making is the process by which evidence is (or is not) applied to practice. The statement "evidence alone does not make decisions, people do" (Haynes et al., 2002) reflects the integral role of the therapist in translation of evidence to practice. Evidence is applied within the context of values and preferences of individual patients, clinical expertise of the practitioner, and health care resources (Guyatt et al., 2000). Child and family preferences, therapist perspectives, and environmental factors are likely to influence decision making. Therapists must apply evidence in ways that address the needs of children and families. Interventions must be acceptable to children and families and meaningful to their daily lives. Clearly, evidence-based practice is a process that involves more than knowledge of current research; this may explain why in health care, transfer of evidence to practice is slow and sometimes does not occur (Chassin & Galvin, 1998).

To what extent do pediatric physical therapists base their clinical decisions on the best available knowledge and research evidence? Therapists make decisions on complex issues related to examination, prognosis, expected outcomes, the plan of care, and coordination of care on a daily basis. Yet the information on which decisions are based is of variable quality. Peer-reviewed research provides the strongest evidence. Often, however, research is limited or lacking. Other sources of evidence that inform decision making include expert consensus, information from textbooks and continuing education courses, advice from a colleague, and personal experience (Thomson-O'Brien & Moreland, 1998).

FINDING EVIDENCE

The need for evidence often begins with a question about prognosis, intervention, or expected outcomes. Families frequently ask questions such as: Will my child walk? How often should my child receive therapy? What can I do to help my child to walk? The most comprehensive and systematic method for finding research evidence is through a literature search of peer-reviewed journals. The ability to express a gap in knowledge as a clear and concise question is an important first step in finding evidence (Lou, 2002). This section provides an overview for searching electronic databases for published research articles on a focused clinical question.

Research is first reported in peer-reviewed journals. Peer-reviewed journals also publish systematic reviews that synthesize the results of several original research studies in an effort to summarize the overall evidence for an intervention. Peer review involves appraisal of articles submitted for publication by reviewers selected for their content expertise. The decision on whether to publish a manuscript is based on the recommendations of the reviewers and the editor. To minimize the potential for reviewer bias, many journals do not disclose the names or affiliations of authors to reviewers. This type of peer review is referred to as a masked or blinded review. Similarly, names of the reviewers are not disclosed to authors. Information on editorial policy is included in a journal and often on a journal website. Textbooks are a secondary source of research. Book chapters generally are not peer-reviewed. Authors of textbooks cite published research and thus are a secondary source, but they may interpret findings based on personal perspectives. Similarly, newsletters, magazines, and reports published by health care, professional, and consumer organizations are generally secondary sources and information is not peer-reviewed.

Electronic databases are the most efficient method for searching the literature. Electronic databases provide bibliographic references to thousands of peer-reviewed journals and can be searched from a personal computer via the Internet. In addition to the complete reference, databases provide links to the abstract and in some cases the full text. An increasing number of journals provide electronic versions of full-text articles that can be downloaded from a personal computer and printed. There is often no cost for individual and institutional subscribers. On-line retrieval of journal articles is a valuable resource for evidence-based practice. *Physical Therapy*, *Developmental Medicine and Child Neurology*, *Pediatric Physical Therapy*, and *Physical & Occupational Therapy in Pediatrics* are journals read by pediatric physical therapists that are available on-line.

MEDLINE, published by the National Library of Medicine with bibliographic references to over 4600 biomedical journals and over 12 million citations, is the largest database. MEDLINE is available on the Internet at no cost through the National Library of Medicine Gateway and PubMed. Introduced in 2000, Gateway is a web-based system that allows users to search simultaneously in multiple retrieval systems at the U.S. National Library of Medicine. In addition to journal citations, users can search monographs, serials, audiovisual materials, and several other databases maintained by the National Library of Medicine. PubMed was developed by the National Center for Biotechnology at the National Library of Medicine in conjunction with publishers of medical literature. PubMed provides full text articles of participating journals (some publishers require a fee or subscription).

Other electronic bibliographic databases that are relevant to pediatric physical therapy are the Cumulative Index to Nursing and Allied Health Literature (CINAHL), Educational Resources Information Center (ERIC), and PsycINFO (Psychological Abstracts). CINAHL indexes more than 1200 journals, books, and dissertations in nursing and allied health areas including physical therapy, occupational therapy, and medical technology. ERIC is a database of annotated citations for education-related research, technical reports, and journal articles. ERIC contains annotated references to educational materials issued in the monthly Resources in Education and to journal articles issued in the monthly Current Index to Journals in Education. PsycINFO (Psychological Abstracts) indexes and abstracts books, dissertations, and journal articles in the psychologic and behavioral sciences.

Ovid and PubMed are systems that search the MEDLINE database; each has advantages and disadvantages. PubMed is a government-sponsored system that is free to anyone who can access the Internet. Ovid is a privately owned system developed by Ovid Technologies. Ovid provides access to health and medical databases including MEDLINE, CINAHL, and PsycINFO, enabling the user to search multiple databases at the same time. Identification of key words or phrases that will identify the articles related to a clinical question is essential for a successful literature search. In MEDLINE, terms to describe the content of an article come from a standardized list of vocabulary and definitions called MeSH, or Medical Subject Headings. Additional strategies for combining keywords, limiting and expanding the scope of the search, are used depending on the topic and purpose of the search. When reporting the results of a systematic review, authors should describe how a search was conducted, including the date of the search, databases searched, keywords and search strategies (e.g., years searched, combinations of key words), and the full references for relevant articles. Therapists are encouraged to document the strategies used to search for literature. Regular literature searches by a clinical program or therapy staff are excellent for quality assurance and efforts to provide best practice.

There are several specialized electronic databases of interest to pediatric physical therapists. PEDro: The Physiotherapy Evidence is an initiative of the Centre for Evidence-Based Physiotherapy located at the University of Sydney in Australia. PEDro was developed to provide rapid access to bibliographic details and abstracts of randomized controlled trials and systematic reviews in physiotherapy. It also contains a tutorial for reviewing evidence. The Cochrane Database of Systematic Reviews is a collection of regularly updated systematic reviews of the effects of health care. The reviews are concentrated on controlled trials and are highly structured. Many are meta-analyses, statistically combining data from multiple reviews. Hooked on Evidence, sponsored by the American Physical Therapy Association, is a database of research reports that is available to members. Therapists who contribute to the database follow a standardized format to review current research. To date over 1200 extractions of articles from 250 journals have been entered into the database. The National Guideline Clearinghouse is a public resource for evidence-based clinical practice guidelines sponsored by the Agency for Healthcare Research and Quality in partnership with the American Medical Association and the American Association of Health Insurance Plans.

Appraisal of Evidence

Evidence-based decision making is predicated on the physical therapist's ability to analyze and apply information. This process involves access to current research, appraisal of evidence, and determination of how findings apply to individual children and their families. Harris (1996) and Golden (1980) pose several thought-provoking questions for professionals to ask themselves when analyzing the scientific merit of an intervention:

1. Is the theory on which the intervention is based consistent with current knowledge?
2. Is the population for whom the intervention is intended identified?
3. Are the goals and outcomes of intervention consistent with the needs of the intended population?
4. Are potential adverse effects of the intervention identified?
5. Is the overall evidence critiqued?
6. Are advocates of the intervention open to discussing its limitations?

A negative response to one or more of these questions is a warning sign that an intervention is not evidence-based.

Sackett (1986) proposed a five-level system that relates the experimental design to levels of evidence and grades of recommendation. The results of a randomized controlled trial (RCT) provide the strongest evidence (levels I and II). An RCT is an experimental design in which subjects are randomly assigned to an experimental or control group permitting the strongest inferences about cause and effect. (Did the experimental intervention cause the documented changes?) Inferences on cause and effect are more limited for quasi-experimental designs in which group assignment is not randomized (levels III and IV) or there is no control group (level V). Sackett also specified three grades of recommendations for systematic reviews. A grade A recommendation indicates that outcomes are supported by at least one level I study. A grade B recommendation indicates outcomes are supported by at least one level II study. A grade C recommendation indicates that outcomes are supported by level III, IV, or V studies. The Oxford Centre for Evidence-Based Medicine has elaborated on Sackett's levels of evidence.

Awareness of the distinction between *efficacy* and *effectiveness* is important for therapists attempting to translate evidence to practice. Efficacy refers to outcomes of interventions provided in a controlled setting under experimental conditions. The RCT provides evidence of efficacy, that is, whether an intervention is effective when applied to a selective sample under controlled conditions. Although the RCT provides the strongest evidence of a cause-effect relationship between the intervention and outcomes, trials are costly and often difficult to implement with children with developmental disabilities. To adhere to the rigor of an experimental design, the intervention is often provided under conditions that are not representative of many practice settings. Consequently, when attempting to apply the results of an efficacy study, therapists must consider whether subject characteristics and the manner in which intervention was provided generalize to children on their caseloads and how to adapt the intervention to constraints within their practice settings.

Effectiveness refers to outcomes of interventions provided within the scope of clinical practice. Effectiveness studies typically involve quasi-experimental and nonexperimental designs that provide lower levels of evidence of causal relationships. In contrast to efficacy studies, interventions are examined within the context of typical practice settings. Rather than attempting to control for potential extraneous or confounding variables, researchers collect data on variables that potentially mediate or moderate the direct effect of the intervention and use multivariate statistical analyses. Examples of factors that may mediate the direct effect of an intervention include child characteristics (age, severity of condition, interests, and motivation), family characteristics (family dynamics, resources, supports), and features of the physical and social environment. Effectiveness research includes observational designs that describe current practice and predictive designs for identifying child, family, and environmental factors that are determinants of intervention outcomes. Although nonexperimental research designs do not permit cause-and-effect inferences, they can provide valuable information for understanding factors that are determinants of outcomes in clinical practice.

Qualitative research is an emerging method of inquiry about clinical practice (Hammell & Carpenter, 2004; Ritchie, 1999). The experiences and values of consumers (e.g., children and families) are an integral component of health services research that is too often missing in clinical research. Qualitative research methods for interviewing and observing children, families, and therapists are useful in understanding processes associated with effective communication, coordination of care, and instruction. By including children and their families as participants or co-researchers, rather than as subjects to be studied by others, qualitative research directly encompasses consumer values into the design and execution of those studies. Participatory action research is a methodology that links experts/researchers, practitioners, and consumers as a team to address specific questions or issues. Mentoring is provided by expert /researcher team members; providers and consumers provide guidance about content—the questions or issues to address, feasibility of proposed practices, and dissemination of information in usable formats. Participatory action research has been used by individuals working with families of children with disabilities (Singer et al., 1999). Law (2002a) and the CanChild Centre for Childhood Disability Research website provide guidelines for critical review of quantitative and qualitative studies.

The *critically appraised topic (CAT)* provides a format for therapists to summarize the research evidence from a literature search conducted as part of clinical practice (Fetters et al., 2004; Law, 2002b). A critically appraised topic is a 1- to 2-page summary of research related to a focused clinical question that includes implications for practice. The format is intended to facilitate transfer of evidence to practice.

SYSTEMATIC REVIEW

A recently published systematic review is an efficient way for therapists to inform themselves of current evidence. A systematic review is a "study of studies"! All relevant research is analyzed in an effort to determine the overall evidence for an intervention. In a well-conducted systematic review, the author(s) define a focused clinical question, identify criteria for inclusion of a study in the review, perform a comprehensive literature search, present criteria used to critique the internal validity of each study, indicate how results are analyzed, and interpret findings in a manner that enhances application to clinical practice (Cook et al., 1997). Just like a research report, therapists must critique a systematic review. A systematic review is only as good as the quality of each study.

Meta-analysis is a mathematical synthesis of the results of two or more research reports. A meta-analysis can be performed on studies that used reliable and valid measures and report some type of inferential statistic (e.g., t-test, ANOVA). Effect size and odds ratio are two statistics used for meta-analysis. An effect size is the mean difference on the outcomes of interest between subjects in experimental and control groups. The most basic method of measuring effect size is the d-index. The d-index is the mean difference between groups in terms of common standard deviation. Cohen (1988) provided the following guidelines for interpretation of the d-index: d = 0.2 represents a small intervention effect, d = 0.5 represents a medium intervention effect, and d = 0.8 represents a large intervention effect.

The odds ratio has mathematical properties that allow data from several studies to be combined to determine the overall effect. Figure 1-1 illustrates the odds ratio from a meta-analysis of four randomized controlled trials. The odds ratio is presented on a scale of 0.10 to 10.0; 1.00 is the line of no effect. Each study is represented on the graph by a horizontal line. The vertical mark in the middle of the line is the odds ratio and the diamonds at the far left and right indicate the boundaries of the 95% confidence interval. If a horizontal line crosses the line of no effect, the odds ratio is *not* significantly greater than 1 ($p > 0.05$). When the horizontal line is to the right of the line of no effect, the odds ratio is significantly greater than 1 ($p < 0.05$). In Figure 1-1, the odds ratio for only one study is significantly greater than 1 (top study). The horizontal lines for the remaining three studies cross the line of no effect, indicating the odds ratio is not significantly greater than 1. The thicker horizontal line at the bottom is the overall odds ratio for the four studies. The overall odds ratio is 0.90 ($p > 0.05$) indicating that subjects who received the experimental intervention were not more likely to improve compared to subjects who did not receive the experimental intervention (control group). Miser (2000) suggests an odds ratio of 2.0 or greater represents a strong intervention effect. An odds ratio of 2.0 indicates that subjects who received the intervention are two times more likely to have improved on the outcomes measured compared with subjects who did not receive the intervention.

Examples of published systematic reviews of interest to pediatric physical therapists include the effectiveness of dorsal rhizotomy surgery and physical therapy compared to physical therapy alone (McLaughlin et al., 2002), strength training programs for children with cerebral palsy (Dodd et al., 2002), neurodevelopmental treatment (Butler & Darrah, 2001), sensory integration compared with other intervention strategies (Vargas & Camilli, 1999), and conductive education (Darrah et al., 2004). When searching MEDLINE, the scope of a literature search can be limited to systematic reviews. This is a good strategy for determining whether a systematic review has been published on the clinical question of interest.

PRACTICE GUIDELINES AND PATHWAYS

Practice guidelines are systematically developed statements to assist patient and practitioner decisions about management of a health condition. The emergence of practice guidelines within the U.S. health care system was precipitated by large variation among health care providers in the type and amount of services for patients with similar conditions. Practice guidelines are intended to provide current standards for quality practice in order to improve effectiveness and efficiency of health care. The focus is generally on people with a particular condition or disorder (e.g., preterm infants at risk for developmental

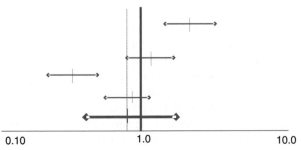

• **Figure 1-1**   Graph of meta-analysis using the odds ratio.

0.10   1.0   10.0

disabilities), and many guidelines are discipline-specific (e.g., guide for physical therapist intervention in the neonatal intensive care unit). In general, practice guidelines include recommendations for the following:

- Who should receive intervention
- Expected outcomes
- Documentation including selection of reliable and valid tests and measures
- Utilization of services (frequency and duration, number of visits)
- Procedural interventions
- Coordination of care
- Discharge planning

Recommendations in practice guidelines should be derived from systematic review of peer-reviewed research and, when research is limited or lacking, consensus statements based on expert opinion. Systems such as the one proposed by Sackett (1986) are used to grade recommendations. A procedure for discussion among a knowledgeable target group and objective criteria for consensus are used to generate statements. The Guide to Post-Stroke Rehabilitation (U.S. Department of Health and Human Services, 1995) is an example of a clinical practice guideline in which recommendations are based on research evidence and, when research was not available, expert consensus. Strong consensus was defined as agreement with a recommendation by 90% or more of the experts. Consensus was defined as agreement by 75% to 89% of the experts. In 1990, the Section on Pediatrics of the American Physical Therapy Association sponsored a consensus conference on the effectiveness of physical therapy in the management of children with cerebral palsy (Campbell, 1990). The summary statements described interventions supported by some research evidence, interventions that lack supporting research, and interventions that lack supporting research but, based on the clinical opinion of conference participants, were judged to warrant investigation.

Here are three examples of practice guidelines relevant to pediatric physical therapy:

- Competencies for Physical Therapists in Early Intervention (Effgen et al., 1991)
- Practice Guidelines for the Physical Therapist in the Neonatal Intensive Care Unit (Sweeney et al., 1999)
- Providing Physical Therapy Services Under Parts B & C of the Individuals with Disabilities Education Act (IDEA) (McEwen, 2000).

These guidelines are primarily based on expert opinion (as opposed to expert consensus).

A *clinical pathway* is a type of practice guideline that is developed by a provider organization to standardize patient episodes of care for specific conditions. A clinical pathway is a multidisciplinary tool that indicates the usual interventions and expected outcomes in a definitive length of time for management of a patient population in a specific setting. Clinical pathways are most common for high incidence conditions and the acute and subacute settings. The impetus for clinical pathways is to increase the efficiency of health care (favorable outcomes that are cost efficient) by reducing unexplained variation in type and intensity of intervention and improving coordination of care. Typically, a pathway specifies the sequence and components of care for each day, the discipline responsible for each component of care, and the expected goals and outcomes. Critical pathway and care paths are other terms used to describe a standard care plan. The evidence to support published clinical pathways varies considerably, and for many pathways the effectiveness has not been evaluated. Methods of evaluation include the impact of the clinical pathway on the following:

- Intensity of service
- Quality assurance
- Patient satisfaction with how care is provided
- Patient outcomes

Campbell (1999) has developed a clinical pathway for follow-up examination of infants at risk for developmental disabilities during the first year of life. Readers are referred to Scalzitti (2001) for an overview of application of evidenced-based guidelines to physical therapy practice.

Evaluation of Practice Guidelines and Pathways

In 1998 an international group of researchers and policy makers formed the AGREE collaboration in order to improve the quality and effectiveness of clinical practice guidelines. AGREE stands for Appraisal of Guidelines for Research and Evaluation. The collaboration includes members from Denmark, Finland, France, Germany, Italy, the Netherlands, Spain, Switzerland, the United Kingdom, Canada, New Zealand, and the United States. An instrument was designed to assess clinical practice guidelines developed by local, regional, national, or international groups and government organizations. The AGREE instrument is a useful resource for physical therapists deciding whether to implement recommendations in a practice guideline or pathway. The instrument provides guiding questions and a response scale to assess the scope and purpose of a guideline, the people involved in development, rigor of development, clarity and presentation of recommendations, applicability, and editorial independence. The instrument and training manual are available on the AGREE website.

CHILD AND FAMILY PERSPECTIVES

Evidence-based decision making encompasses the perspectives of the child and family. Presentation of information to families in useful and acceptable formats encourages their active participation in decision making. By presenting evidence in family-friendly format, pediatric therapists can enhance informed shared decision making on the part of their young clients (Weston, 2001). In fact, research has shown that patients who are more informed and more involved in their own decision making are more likely to adhere to their treatment regimens, and experience better health outcomes (Simpson et al., 1991; Stewart et al., 1999).

Parents of children with disabilities have also become active providers of information by using the power of the Internet. It is not uncommon for a parent to ask a question about information from the Internet that is unfamiliar to the therapist. Because the quality and accuracy of information available on websites vary greatly, the physical therapist can assist a family to critique information and determine its relevance to the child and family. Examples of websites for families of children with disabilities are as follows:

a. *Family Voices* is a national grassroots network of families and professionals who are advocates for health care services for all children and youth with special health care needs; the services are family-centered, community-based, comprehensive, coordinated, and culturally competent.

b. *Pathways Awareness Foundation* is a national nonprofit organization dedicated to raising awareness about the benefit of early detection and early therapy for children with physical movement differences.

c. *KidPower* is an on-line resource and support network for families whose children have cerebral palsy or other disabilities.

d. *Bright Foundation* (<u>BR</u>ain <u>I</u>njury <u>G</u>roup - <u>H</u>ope through <u>T</u>reatment) is a nonprofit parent group with involvement of clinical and research professionals whose focus is infants and children with acquired brain injury. The website includes current research reviews, therapy effectiveness reviews, advocacy information, and a practical advice and support forum.

A consumer's guide to therapeutic services for families of children with disabilities was developed through the combined efforts of several professional and parent organizations (Human Services Research Unit, 1995). Included in the guide is a consumer checklist that consists of the following six questions:

1. Will achievement of goals make a real difference in the lives of the child and family?

2. Is there a formal process to discontinue or change the course of intervention if there is no progress?

3. Are interventions as much a part of the child's day-to-day life as possible?

4. Are parents, teachers, and other individuals present in the child's daily life as involved in the planning and provision of intervention as they could be?

5. Are the professionals involved in assessing the child and planning intervention experienced in serving children with similar disabilities?

6. Are sources of financial support sufficient for the cost of the planned intervention?

From the perspective of the child and family, the answer to all six questions should be yes.

RESPONSIBILITY TO PROVIDE EVIDENCE-BASED INTERVENTIONS

Traditionally, physical therapists have assumed that it is the responsibility of the researchers in our profession to determine the effectiveness of interventions. We disagree with this perspective and support the viewpoint of Harris (1996) that "the responsibility to deliver evidence-based treatment rests with all members of a profession." Objective documentation of goals and outcomes (Randall & McEwen, 2000) and consideration of the factors that may have contributed to change provide therapists a basis for determining need for service, deciding on the most appropriate interventions, and evaluating outcomes. Such an approach was modeled very successfully in a goals-oriented study by Ketelaar and colleagues (2001) to determine whether the motor abilities of children with cerebral palsy who were receiving functional physical therapy improved more than the motor abilities of children in a reference group whose intervention was based on normalization of the quality of movement. Collaboration between children, families, clinicians, and researchers is important to identify the most relevant questions. Physical therapists are strongly encouraged to consider the levels of evidence that form the basis for their clinical decisions. In particular, the impact of decisions based on expert opinion and personal experience should be carefully monitored and alternatives considered should the outcome of the decision be less than desirable.

CLINICAL REASONING AND DECISION MAKING

Physical therapists must have a strong knowledge base and the abilities to problem solve and make sound clinical judgments in order to effectively transfer research to practice. Research on problem solving has repeatedly confirmed that skill in problem solving is problem-specific, indicating that one can solve problems better with a comprehensive base of knowledge about the problem. Clinical reasoning refers to the many ways a practitioner thinks about and interprets an idea or phenomenon and incorporates knowledge, experience, problem solving, judgment, and decision making (Fleming, 1991). Watts (1985) described decision making as both an art and a science. She suggested that many decisions are made with a degree of uncertainty and reflect intuitive thought processes. Magistro (1989) proposed that clinical decisions in physical therapy are derived from both knowledge and practice experiences that intelligently influence our courses of action. He discussed the role of intuition and suggested that practice decisions are not always apparent as rational thought processes. Magistro's perspective is consistent with Brenner's (1984) conceptualization of professional development. Brenner described the transition from novice to expert as a shift from the use of explicit, verbally based theoretic knowledge to the use of highly implicit and embodied practical knowledge.

Mattingly (1991) has proposed an interpretive or meaning-centered model of clinical reasoning in occupational therapy that emphasizes implicit and embodied knowledge. She conceptualized clinical reasoning as the process of deciding on the appropriate action for an individual patient at a particular time. Knowledge is viewed as a starting point but not as a strict plan for action. As part of the process of individualizing intervention, the therapist makes judgments and improvises in moving from general practice guidelines to the requirements of a specific situation. Mattingly suggested that the knowledge that guides judgment and improvisation is often embodied in the therapist's hands or eyes. Part of the therapist's expertise, therefore, is reflected in implicit thought processes that are translated into habitual ways of observing and interacting with patients. The perspective that clinical reasoning involves more than the ability to apply theory and learned technical skill may explain the frustration of physical therapy students when they first attempt to apply classroom material to the clinical setting.

Mattingly (1991) proposed that, through experience, therapists develop the implicit knowledge that is integral to clinical reasoning. The therapist learns to attend to relevant cues and modify therapeutic interventions in response to these cues. Furthermore, therapists are often not completely aware of how they use implicit knowledge to identify problems, develop intervention plans, and engage the patient in the therapeutic process. Based on results of a study in which occupational therapists de-

scribed their assessment practices (Rogers & Masagatani, 1982), Mattingly suggested that pediatric therapists incorporate a minimum of five domains of knowledge into their thought processes: (1) understanding of the child's motivation, commitments, and tolerances; (2) assessment of the environment in which the task is taking place; (3) knowledge of the child's physical and cognitive deficits and capacities; (4) perception of the therapeutic relationship; and (5) immediate and long-term goals. Effective clinical reasoning enables the pediatric therapist to individualize interventions and address the unique meaning of health and disability as it relates to a particular child.

Embrey and associates (Embrey & Adams, 1996; Embrey & Hylton, 1996; Embrey & Nirider, 1996; Embrey et al., 1996) used qualitative research methodology to describe the thought processes of three experienced (greater than 10 years of pediatric experience) and three novice (less than 2 years of pediatric experience) pediatric physical therapists while providing direct intervention to children with cerebral palsy. Therapists watched videotapes of the intervention sessions and were encouraged to "verbalize whatever comes to mind" following predetermined guidelines. The therapists' comments were transcribed and coded to identify and describe their decision-making processes. The experienced therapists verbalized changing their procedures every 46 seconds compared with every 86 seconds for the novice therapists. Experienced therapists verbalized sensitivity to the emotional and social needs of the children every 2 minutes; novice therapists verbalized psychosocial sensitivity every 3 minutes. Both groups of therapists verbalized self-monitoring (reflection on some aspect of their performance) during intervention about every 3 minutes. When verbalizing self-monitoring, experienced therapists made positive comments 81% of the time as compared with novice therapists' only 36% of the time. Self-monitoring was verbalized in conjunction with other characteristics of decision making 84% of the time by experienced therapists and 57% of the time by novice therapists. The experienced therapists appeared to make procedural changes and respond to the emotional and social needs of children with less interruption of the therapeutic process, whereas the novice therapists appeared to be limited in their clinical options when they perceived that therapy goals were not being achieved. The investigators suggest that within a treatment session, therapists make rapid, on-the-spot, clinical decisions based on improvisation and intuition.

A great deal remains to be learned about clinical reasoning of pediatric physical therapists. The results of the studies by Embrey and co-workers (Embrey & Adams,

1996; Embrey & Hylton, 1996; Embrey & Nirider, 1996; Embrey et al., 1996) provide preliminary support for the concept that clinical reasoning involves the application not only of theory and psychomotor skill but also of intuitive or implicit thought processes. Pediatric physical therapists are encouraged to strive for better understanding of their thought processes not only to enhance their own professional development but also to serve their clients and educate physical therapy students more effectively. A better understanding of clinical reasoning is essential for the development of comprehensive decision models that reflect the broad scope of pediatric physical therapy.

CLINICAL DECISION THEORY

Clinical decision theory (Dowie & Elstein, 1988) assumes that clinical judgment encompasses such a complex set of tasks that mathematic algorithms and decision-making models, incorporating the results of research on important clinical problems, are likely to be more successful than is clinical judgment for making diagnostic and intervention decisions. In decision theory, probabilities of various outcomes are assessed based on variables such as previous historical events or assessments, potential negative results of various decisions, and patient or family judgments regarding the value of various potential positive and negative outcomes. In the diagnostic area, for example, risk for cerebral palsy or developmental motor delay could be estimated based on a combination of findings such as medical complications captured by cumulative risk scores, general movement assessment, and tests of postural control and motor milestone achievement at successive ages. Bayesian statistical models allow the degree of risk calculated at earlier points in time to be incorporated as factors in an equation using current test results, thus establishing a cumulative risk probability that takes into account prior history as well as current functioning (Slovick & Lichtenstein, 1971). Studies of decision equations based on variables such as these have almost universally found that diagnostic decisions made with such algorithms are much more reliable than those based on clinicians' judgments (Dawes et al., 1989).

Why have decision models proved to be better than experienced clinicians' judgments? As Goldberg (1991) suggested, rehabilitation specialists tend to base decisions on personal clinical experience, intuition, and hunches. Studies of clinical judgment suggest the many ways in which bias is introduced into the examination and decision-making process when operating in such a mode (Sackett et al., 1985). Practitioners are liable to make errors of both omission and commission in clinical

examinations, and evaluative judgments made from data collected tend to be overly affected by recent experiences with other clients. Furthermore, the sensory perception of clinicians varies from time to time, owing to fatigue and other factors, including assumptions made from client history and from biased expectations. Studies have also revealed that practitioners immediately formulate hypotheses regarding what is wrong (or right) and then collect data to rule out or rule in the various hypotheses entertained (Dowie & Elstein, 1988). Obviously, if the true situation is not one of the entertained hypotheses, judgment is likely to go awry. Experienced clinicians tend to have a broader base of knowledge from which to generate appropriate hypotheses than do novices (Embrey & Nirider, 1996; Embrey et al., 1996); nevertheless, their clinical decisions can still be limited by any of the various factors just mentioned. Use of standardized assessments, a systematic data-gathering protocol, and decision algorithms can guard against such unreliability in clinical judgment.

■ FRAMEWORKS FOR DECISION MAKING

After many years of development, the International Classification of Functioning, Disability and Health (ICF) was approved by the Executive Board of the World Health Organization in January 2001. The overall aim of the ICF is to provide a scientific basis for understanding and studying health and health-related states, outcomes, and determinants. The ICF also is intended to provide a common language for the description of health and health-related states in order to improve communication among health care providers, researchers, policy makers, and people with disabilities. The ICF emphasizes "components of health" rather than "consequences of disease" (i.e., participation rather than disability) and environmental and personal factors as important determinants of health. The ICF model is available to read and print (PDF file) on the World Health Organization website.

The diagram of the ICF model is presented in Figure 1-2. The ICF has two parts. Part 1: Functioning and Disability includes three components of health: body functions & structures, activities, and participation. Part 2: Contextual Factors includes environmental and personal factors. Contextual factors influence components of health. For example, the impact of activity (ability to walk) and participation (ability to travel with classmates at school when going to lunch) may be influenced by the environment (distance from classroom to cafeteria and time to travel this distance) and personal factors (the child's

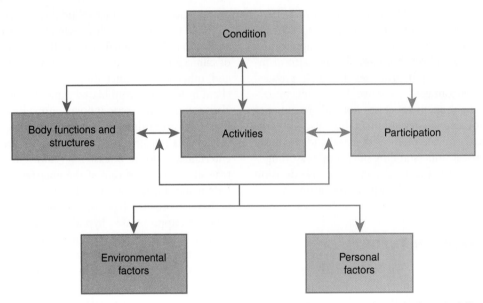

◆ **Figure 1-2** Interactions between the components of the International Classification of Functioning, Disability and Health. *(World Health Organization, 2001.)*

fitness and motivation to walk). The bidirectional arrows are inclusive of all possible relationships. The challenge when applying the ICF is to identify the relationships that are most relevant for an individual child and family.

Body functions are the physiologic and psychologic functions of body systems. Physiologic functions include respiration, vision, sensation, muscle performance, and movement. Psychologic functions include attention, memory, emotion, thought, and language. *Body structures* are the anatomic parts of the body such as organs, limbs, and their components. *Impairments* are problems in body functions or structures. Examples of impairments are lack of sensation, limited ability to process sensory information, muscle weakness, difficulties with balance, inadequate motor planning, reduced endurance, skeletal malalignment, and joint contracture. *Activity* is the performance of a task or action by an individual. Activities represent the integrated use of body functions and vary in complexity. Examples of activities are maintaining and changing body positions, walking and moving around, manipulation of objects, and self-care. *Activity limitations* are difficulties in performing age-appropriate tasks or actions. *Participation* is involvement in a life situation. Most children participate in home life, school, community activities and organizations, and social relationships with friends. Participation is highly individualized. What is important to one child may be of little consequence to another child. *Participation restrictions* are problems in involvement in life situations. *Environmental factors* make up the physical, social, and attitu-

dinal environment in which people live and conduct their lives. *Personal factors* are the particular background of the individual's life and living that *are not* part of a health condition or disorder. These factors may include gender, race/ethnicity, age, fitness, lifestyle, habits, coping styles, and past and current experiences.

The decision to adopt the ICF model for the third edition of *Physical Therapy for Children* was made because of the emphasis on components of health and on environmental and personal factors as important determinants of health. The *Guide to Physical Therapist Practice* (American Physical Therapy Association, 2001) is based on a similar disablement framework. The model Person with a Disability and the Rehabilitation Process (National Center for Medical Rehabilitation Research, National Institutes of Health, 1993) is referenced in the *Guide* and provided a conceptual framework for the first two editions of *Physical Therapy for Children*. Table 1-1 compares the differences in terminology between the two models.

An example of a child with spastic diplegia will be used to illustrate application of the ICF for clinical decision making (Fig. 1-3). The child's impairments in the neuromuscular and musculoskeletal systems include hamstring and gastrocnemius muscle hypoextensibility, reduced muscle force production, poor balance, and limited muscular endurance. The child's activity limitations include difficulty walking on a sloping surface, walking amid people, and climbing playground equipment. At school, the child occasionally falls when walking from the bus to the classroom. Although the child has

TABLE 1-1	Comparison of Terminology between a Disablement Model and the International Classification of Functioning, Disability and Health

LEVEL	DISABLEMENT MODEL	INTERNATIONAL CLASSIFICATION OF FUNCTIONING, DISABILITY, AND HEALTH
Systems level	Impairment	Body functions and structures
Person level	Functional limitation	Activity
Person-environment interaction level	Disability	Participation

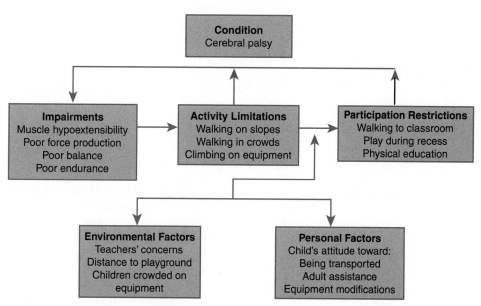

◆ Figure 1-3. Example of application of the International Classification of Functioning, Disability, and Health to clinical decision making. *(World Health Organization, 2001.)*

several friends and enjoys physical activity, participation in recess and physical education is restricted. Social and physical environmental factors that may contribute to restricted participation include the following: teachers are concerned that the child will get injured; the child's classroom is located at the end of the school most distant from the playground; the terrain of the school yard is uneven; and students are crowded on the playground equipment. In applying the ICF framework, the therapist must not only identify impairments, activity limitations, and participation restrictions but also hypothesize cause-effect relationships. What are the causes of restricted participation during recess and physical education? There is evidence that an exercise program to improve muscle strength and endurance will improve gait characteristics (Dodd et al., 2002). Is there evidence that instruction and practice in climbing on playground equipment (motor

learning) will improve participation? Collaboration with the teachers to discuss their safety concerns and the feasibility of providing additional space and time when the child attempts to climb on playground equipment are examples of environmental considerations. The child's feelings about energy conservation (e.g., being transported to the playground), modifications of playground equipment, and support from adults are examples of personal factors to consider in formulating an intervention plan. Note that in Figure 1-3, only the hypothesized interactions are depicted. The arrow from the participation restrictions and activity limitation to impairments represents a secondary impairment.

The ICF framework will be considered further when problems and processes for making diagnostic, prognostic, outcomes evaluation, and program evaluation decisions are discussed. The ICF will also be applied

---

Box 1-1 | **Considerations for Using the International Classification of Functioning, Disability, and Health as a Framework for Clinical Decision Making**

IMPAIRMENTS

- Not all impairments are modified by physical therapy
- Not all impairments cause activity limitations and participation restrictions
- Relate impairments to activity limitations and participation restrictions
- Impairments are identified from examination and evaluation of body functions and structures

ACTIVITIES

- Relate activity limitations to participation restrictions
- Activity limitations can cause secondary impairments
- Activities are measured by norm-referenced and criterion-referenced assessments

PARTICIPATION

- Reflects child and family perspectives
- Is context dependent (environmental and personal factors)
- Is one aspect of health-related quality of life
- Is measured by child and parent self-report
- Is measured by observations in natural environments

---

throughout the text. Box 1-1 lists considerations for applying the ICF to clinical decision making.

PHYSICAL THERAPY DIAGNOSIS AND PROGNOSIS

Historically, answers to the question "Who needs treatment by a physical therapist and what for?" were simple to obtain. Physicians identified the problem—the medical diagnosis—and referred children to physical therapists, sometimes with a specific prescription, at other times for "evaluation and treatment" at the therapist's discretion. For many of the disorders treated by pediatric physical therapists, physicians remain the primary diagnosticians at the level of identification of pathophysiologic processes. Unfortunately, standardized practice guidelines are not available to guide physicians in deciding who would benefit from therapy (and when) so physicians' practices vary widely. For example, research on physicians' decisions regarding referral for physical therapy of children with suspected cerebral motor dysfunction indicates that the decision to refer is related to the physician's diagnostic certainty, perceived severity of the child's involvement, and belief in the value of physical therapy (Campbell et al., 1995). The diagnostic certainty expressed by physicians in this study, who reviewed a series of standardized videotaped cases, varied widely. Furthermore, the probability

of referral varied with physician specialty. Orthopedists were less likely and physiatrists more likely to refer a child younger than 2 years of age for physical therapy than were pediatricians or neurologists.

Research also demonstrates that disclosure practices can be improved. Despite recommended guidelines for sharing diagnostic information which leave about 75% of families satisfied with the manner and structure of disclosure of diagnostic information, about half of parents remain dissatisfied with the information content delivered (Baird et al., 2000). It is recommended that information about the diagnosis present a balanced viewpoint rather than just a list of problems and that a follow-up appointment be scheduled not too far after the original disclosure to enable parents to continue to discuss the diagnosis. Parents should be sent written material soon after the initial disclosure as a back-up to the verbal information, and it is important that accurate information be provided at all stages of service delivery. Parents often have questions years after the initial diagnosis.

Under the current health care system and evolving state licensure laws, physical therapists increasingly serve as the point of entry into physical therapy services, either as independent practitioners, as part of a comprehensive diagnostic and intervention team, as related service providers in educational settings, or as practitioners in other venues. To be worthy of such a powerful role, physical therapists need valid and reliable decision-making procedures that result in the provision of truly necessary services in the most cost-effective manner. They also need skill in information sharing with families, especially during periods of uncertainty regarding the diagnosis and prognosis, because families often believe that their concerns are not heard (Knafl et al., 1995).

The diagnostic and prognostic decisions that physical therapists make are typically in the realm of impairments and activity limitations. In the *Guide to Physical Therapist Practice* (American Physical Therapy Association, 2001), a diagnosis is defined as a cluster of signs, symptoms, syndromes, or categories whose purpose is to guide the physical therapist in determining the most appropriate intervention for a child and family. Prognosis refers to the predicted level of improvement in function and the duration and frequency of intervention needed to achieve the expected outcomes. For example, therapists are best qualified to make decisions regarding whether a client has impairments of strength or passive range of motion, the presence of and degree to which a client has activity limitations because of mobility issues, and the presence of developmental gross motor delay and the types of impairments contributing to that delay. Only a few diagnostic tests, however, have adequate sensitivity and specificity to identify and define the impairments and functional limitations we hope to diagnose. Aylward (1997) described the need to evaluate tests further for both diagnostic classification accuracy and also relative risk, that is, the probability of a child later displaying a developmental problem if results of an earlier screening test were abnormal or suspect.

THE PROBLEM OF PREDICTABILITY

Most often, the decision regarding who needs treatment revolves around the diagnosis of developmental delay or the presence of signs of aberrant development, such as those seen in the motor control dysfunction associated with cerebral palsy. Recent research on the General Movement assessment suggests that the pathologic movement qualities characteristic of cerebral palsy can be reliably identified in the first few months of life with a sensitivity of 95% and specificity of 96% (Ferrari et al., 2002; Prechtl et al., 1997). More general use of this assessment in developmental follow-up of infants at risk for CNS dysfunction should facilitate earlier referral for intervention.

The most useful means for assessing delayed development are standardized developmental scales that have been normed on large populations. The positive predictive validity of those tests that currently exist, however, is often low because a proportion of children with delayed development in early infancy demonstrate recovery at older ages.

What do we know about prediction of outcomes from early developmental assessment? The bulk of the older literature on assessment in infancy suggests that little regarding outcome in later years can be successfully predicted for individual children (Harbst, 1990; Kopp, 1987; Piper et al., 1991; Rosenblith, 1992). For example, poor motor performance scores early in life have some capacity for identifying children at risk for developmental problems, but sometimes in a nonspecific way. Poor motor scores may later be associated with cerebral palsy, cognitive impairment, or even blindness and behavioral problems (Campbell & Wilhelm, 1985; Ferrari et al., 1990; Nelson & Ellenberg, 1982). The process of recovery from early medical complications and the environment that a family provides for optimal recovery and facilitation of development also contribute to the difficulty in predicting developmental outcomes.

Unfortunately, test scores at any single point in time may be inadequate for making a decision regarding whether a child's development is permanently impaired until the time for maximally effecting important long-term outcomes has already passed. A conceptual framework that encompasses the complexity involved in early brain lesions or abnormal development is needed. Aylward and Kenny (1979) and Gordon and Jens (1988) have suggested models for early identification of developmental disabilities (Campbell, 1993), and Campbell (1999) recently suggested a critical pathway for follow-up examination of infants at risk for developmental disabilities in the first year of life. A test that showed promise in the prediction of poor motor outcome, the Alberta Infant Motor Scale (AIMS; Darrah et al., 1998), was included in the model for examination of infants under 10 months of age. Recently, however, Campbell and colleagues (2002) demonstrated that the Test of Infant Motor Performance (TIMP) has a sensitivity of 92% and specificity of 76% at 3 months for predicting 12-month AIMS performance. Furthermore, the TIMP performed better than the AIMS at 3 months for identifying the delay associated with a later diagnosis of cerebral palsy (Barbosa et al., 2003). Thus, the TIMP may be a more useful test in the period prior to 4 months of age, although this test, like others, has the problem of overidentification of at-risk infants (Campbell et al., 2002). Use of the TIMP in conjunction with the General Movement assessment might reduce the number of misidentifications.

CLASSIFICATION SYSTEMS

Use of taxonomic classification systems for describing impairments and functional limitations is a means to improve clinical decision making. All therapists know that no two children with the same disorder are exactly alike. Establishing taxonomies for the description of constellations of impairments or functional limitations occurring in children with particular conditions can lead to improved diagnosis and prognosis on which to base clinical decisions. Taxonomic classification is also useful in generating studies of differential intervention effects for subcategories of disability and studies of whether different types of interventions are most appropriate for children classified by severity of impairment or activity limitations. But are there ways to identify the underlying impairments at the systems level, and are there clinically practical means for classification of children based on either impairment or activity limitation?

Work on developing diagnostic systems for classifying patients with low back pain is already well under way in physical therapy (Binkley et al., 1993). Research on neonates and young infants also suggests that we may, indeed, have the means for identifying the primary impairments in cerebral palsy at an early age (Prechtl et al., 1997). All pediatric clinicians know that children with cerebral palsy are characterized by stereotypic movement patterns and lack of selective control. Prechtl and colleagues have developed an assessment of general movement that characterizes the movement pattern in cerebral palsy as being one of "cramped synchrony," with a paucity of selective joint movements, especially in the rotational components (Ferrari et al., 1990). Their work has also demonstrated that clinical examination of children with known signs of brain pathophysiologic impairment can identify the effects of such lesions on movement. These effects can then be qualitatively and quantitatively described longitudinally and used to predict recovery or nonrecovery from early nonoptimal medical conditions and events. The test is totally noninvasive because it involves observation of spontaneous movement from 15-minute to 1-hour videotapes (depending on age). Use of this general movement examination to diagnose high risk for cerebral palsy has the potential to eliminate the problem of late referral because of diagnostic uncertainty identified by Campbell et al. (1995). Westcott and Bradley (Chapter 3) review the research demonstrating the exceptionally strong predictive validity of this test.

Crenna and colleagues (1992) have demonstrated that cerebral palsy can also be described on the basis of a constellation of impairments, leading to a taxonomic classification system that differs greatly from traditional ways of classifying cerebral palsy by area of involvement and presence of spasticity or movement dysfunction. The impairments used for classification include spasticity, muscle coactivation, muscle hypoextensibility, and paresis.

Categories of the taxonomy have been related to functional performance capabilities in children with hemiplegia.

Palisano and associates (1997) have developed the Gross Motor Function Classification System (GMFCS) for children with cerebral palsy that is based on the concepts of functional abilities and limitations. The GMFCS was developed for children with cerebral palsy who are 12 years of age and younger and is analogous to the staging and grading systems used in medicine. A classification is made by determining which of five levels best represents the child's present abilities and limitations in gross motor function in home, school, and community settings. The authors propose that classification based on functional abilities and limitations should enhance communication among professionals and families with respect to (1) efficient utilization of medical and rehabilitation services, (2) the creation of databases describing the development of children with cerebral palsy, and (3) comparing and generalizing the results of program evaluations and outcomes research. The terms *functional related groups*, *severity of disability*, *case-mix complexity*, and *risk adjustment* have been used to describe methods of grouping patients for evaluating internal quality standards or for comparative analysis of intervention outcomes across sites (benchmarking).

The GMFCS is intended to be quick and easy to use. Classification is based on the child's self-initiated movement with emphasis on sitting and walking. The title for each level represents the highest level of mobility that a child is expected to achieve between 6 and 12 years of age (Box 1-2). The description for each level is broad and not intended to describe all aspects of the motor function of individual children. For each level, separate descriptions are provided for children in the following age bands: less than 2 years, 2 to 4 years, 4 to 6 years, and 6 to 12 years. Distinctions among levels of gross motor function are based on functional limitations, the need for assistive mobility devices (walkers, crutches, canes), wheeled mobility, and to a lesser extent quality of movement. The scale is ordinal with no intent that the distances between levels be considered equal or that children with cerebral palsy be equally distributed among the five levels. Evidence of inter-rater reliability, content, construct, and predictive validity has been reported (Palisano et al., 1997; Palisano et al., 2000; Wood & Rosenbaum, 2000). Morris and Bartlett (2004) performed a systematic review to describe the impact of the GMFCS. They concluded that the GMFCS has had a major impact on the health care of children with cerebral palsy with good uptake internationally and across the spectrum of health care professions for use in research design and clinical practice and to provide a system for clear communication.

Box 1-2	Summary of Level of Mobility That a Child Is Expected to Achieve between 6 and 12 Years of Age for Each of the Five Levels of the Gross Motor Function Classification System

Level	Abilities and Limitations
I	Walks without restrictions; limitations in more advanced gross motor skills
II	Walks without assistive devices; limitations walking outdoors and in the community
III	Walks with assistive mobility devices; limitations walking outdoors and in the community
IV	Self-mobility with limitations; children are transported or use power mobility outdoors and in the community
V	Self-mobility is severely limited even with the use of assistive technology

MOTOR DEVELOPMENT CURVES

Guided by the perspective that knowledge of prognosis for gross motor function of children with cerebral palsy would assist in determining (1) goals and management plans that are consistent with a child's potential and (2) the extent interventions improve gross motor function beyond expectations based on age and severity of impairment, Rosenbaum and colleagues (2002) conducted a prospective longitudinal study of the development of gross motor function of 657 children with cerebral palsy. Children were stratified by age and GMFCS level and randomly selected from an accessible population of 2108 children in Ontario identified as having cerebral palsy. Motor function was measured using the 66-item version of the Gross Motor Function Measure (GMFM-66) (Russell et al., 2002). The assessments were performed by physical therapists and occupational therapists after achieving the criterion for inter-rater reliability. Children younger than 6 years of age were assessed every 6 months, and children 6 years of age and older were assessed every 9 to 12 months. Children were assessed an average of four times. Each child's classification level at the start of the study was used to create the five motor development curves. The model that provided the best "fit" of GMFM-66 scores was nonlinear and included two parameters: the *rate parameter*, an estimate of how fast children approach their limit of gross motor function, and the *limit parameter*, an estimate of maximum potential for gross motor function.

The gross motor development growth curves (Fig. 1-4) represent the average pattern of development for each of the five classification levels. The dotted vertical lines represent what has been operationally defined as the Age-90 value. The Age-90 value is the age in years by which children are expected to reach 90% of their motor development potential. The predicted average maximum GMFM-66 score differs significantly for each classification system level. On average, children at level I do not

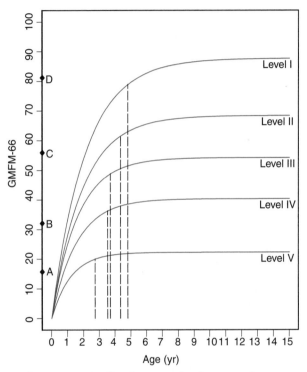

◆ **Figure 1-4**   Predicted average development of gross motor ability by Gross Motor Function Classification System category (Level I to Level V). Vertical dashed lines indicate average age-90, the age in years at which children are expected to achieve 90% of their potential for motor development. Diamonds on the vertical axis marked *A* to *D* indicate the Gross Motor Function Measure-66 score at which children are expected to have a 50% chance of successfully completing selected gross motor test items. *A* (item 21), therapist holds child sitting upright, child lifts head for 3 seconds. *B* (item 24), child maintains sitting, arms free, for 3 seconds. *C* (item 69), child walks forward 10 steps. *D* (item 87), child walks down 4 steps, alternating feet. *(Reprinted with permission from Rosenbaum, PL, Walter, SD, Hanna, SE, Palisano, RJ, Russell, DJ, & Raina, P. Prognosis for gross motor function in cerebral palsy: Creation of motor development curves. Journal of the American Medical Association, 288:1357–1363, 2002.)*

achieve the maximum score of 100. The predicted average Age-90 scores vary from 4.8 years (children in level I) to 2.7 years (children in level V). For levels I and II, 50% of children are expected to achieve 90% of their maximum predicted GMFM-66 score by 5.8 years of age. Children classified in levels III, IV, and V progress faster to their maximum GMFM-66 score compared to children classified in level I. The average Age-90 score does not differ between children in level I and level II.

How should the gross motor development curves be used in decision making? Rosenbaum and associates (2002) anticipate that the curves will help children and families understand the outlook for gross motor function. The curves should prove useful for planning interventions, enabling families and professionals to collaborate and make informed decisions about the most appropriate therapy goals for a child. The curves also provide an effective way to assess whether a child's motor progress is consistent with patterns of children of similar age and severity. Rosenbaum and associates (2002) believe that the gross motor development curves will have important implications for evaluation of interventions by providing evidence of the extent to which a particular intervention improves a child's gross motor function beyond what is predicted by the curves.

When sharing the gross motor curves with children, families, and other health care providers, therapists must clearly explain *what the curves do* and *do not measure*! The GMFM-66 measures (a) abilities that are usually achieved by age 5 in children without motor impairments and (b) capability, defined as what a child "can do" in a standard condition. The number of children below age 2 was small; therefore, the earliest part of the curves may not reflect actual development. The gross motor development curves do not measure many components of health that are important for children with cerebral palsy. These components include the following:

- Movement efficiency and endurance
- Adapted function (achieved with mobility aids)
- Wheeled mobility
- Performance of mobility during daily activities and routines (child-environment interaction)
- Wellness and physical fitness
- Prevention of secondary impairments (e.g., skeletal alignment, range of motion, pain)

Prognosis for goals and outcomes that are not measured by the GMFM-66 *should not* be inferred from the motor development curves! The *CanChild* research team also has constructed gross motor development curves for children with Down syndrome using a model similar to the one used for children with cerebral palsy (Palisano et al., 2001).

ESTABLISHING A PLAN OF CARE

Having identified the need for intervention, the therapist's next important decision is the plan of care. What are the goals and expected outcomes, what interventions should be implemented, how often, and for how long? Such decisions are frequently sources of professional conflict because members of each discipline view the child's needs from their unique perspectives and may identify entirely different outcomes and potential solutions for the same constellation of impairments, activity limitations, and participation restrictions. Even when clinicians agree on overall outcomes, priorities may differ (Butler, 1991). The resolution of such conflicts through the use of effective team consensus-building processes, however, can lead to elegant program plans that truly meet clients' needs. Both preventive and ameliorative approaches may be necessary; however, both stages of life and stages of the disease or condition affect the decision regarding which outcomes are the most important to attain in the limited time that is likely to be available (Campbell, 1997).

For example, if primary impairments can be limited by early therapy, some activity limitations that would otherwise result as a part of the natural history of a condition may be avoided. Thus, prevention involves attempts to limit impairment resulting from the lesion or disorder and to promote developmentally appropriate functional abilities. For example, most therapists believe that early intervention for children with spastic diplegia produces a more efficient later gait. Little research exists to document such effects, however. One of the few studies that suggests such a result is a comparison of early (before 9 months) versus late Vojta therapy that reported that children whose treatment began before 9 months of age walked earlier, on average, and with better postural alignment than did those treated later (Kanda et al., 1984). Theoretically, early intervention should also result in prevention or reduction of secondary impairments, such as contractures and skeletal deformities that are not generally present as primary impairments in early infancy. Rather, they develop later as a result of habitual movement using compensatory patterns or overactive muscles with paretic antagonists or as a result of overall poverty of movement and disuse. Barbosa and colleagues (2003) have also shown that infants who are later diagnosed as having cerebral palsy may show regression in lower extremity skills at 3 to 4 months of age. Research is needed to evaluate whether this loss of skills could be prevented. Until we develop tests that clearly separate elements of underlying impairment from activity limitations that may be primary or may result from use of compensatory strategies to enhance function, we will be unable to document the value of early or preventive intervention for cerebral palsy and other conditions present in early childhood. With appropriate measurement tools available, studies of the efficacy and effectiveness of early intervention at the impairment level will be possible. Until such time as this information is available, however, therapists will continue to come into conflict with physicians and other professionals (including other therapists) who believe that intervention does not need to begin early or can be carried out by parents, does not need to include procedural interventions by therapists, and should be aimed at provision of compensatory strategies to increase function rather than address underlying impairment.

When activity limitations persist for long periods and are not remediable or cannot be compensated for, children may fail to succeed in normal life roles, such as participation in school, play, or family activities. Therapy planning should start with interdisciplinary assessment of activity and participation in natural environments when a condition that impairs developmental progress and functional capabilities is already well established. This involves asking which roles and skills are needed and appropriate for a child at his or her particular stage of life and must involve the family and teachers as full participants in the examination process. In the case of our example of the child with spastic diplegia, walking in the community is a long-term goal but an important decision is whether the child should be transported at the moment to allow him or her greater participation in family outings. Other members of the rehabilitation team will have their own unique contributions to make to the solution of the problems of lack of mobility and other functional limitations. Giangreco (1995) emphasized that *all* professionals should have the same goals rather than separate disciplinary goals when intervention takes place in a school setting.

Environmental setting is an important consideration for deciding on mobility methods and interventions. Research suggests that children with cerebral palsy are more dependent on adult assistance and use wheeled mobility most often when outdoors or in the community (Palisano et al., 2003; Tieman et al., 2004). Therapy services for children in educational settings in the United States is, by law, aimed at improving participation in the education program in the least restrictive environment. Therapists, teachers, families, and other professionals must all be clear regarding these priorities and realize that decision making for school therapy may not address all the therapy needs of children with disabilities.

HYPOTHESIS-ORIENTED ALGORITHM FOR CLINICIANS II

The Hypothesis-Oriented Algorithm for Clinicians (HOAC) was developed by Rothstein and Echternach (1986) to provide physical therapists with a systematic method for clinical decision making and patient care that is independent of methods of examination and intervention philosophy. An algorithm uses a branching approach to decision making, involving several steps that are intended to narrow the focus of the problem and direct the practitioner to the appropriate plan of action. The Hypothesis-Oriented Algorithm for Clinicians II (HOAC II) (Rothstein et al., 2003) was designed to be more compatible with contemporary practice and to include the concept of prevention. HOAC II is not supported by a database, is not computer generated, and is not intended to provide specific guidelines for examination and intervention decisions. Rather, the HOAC II provides a format to guide the physical therapist through the decision-making process.

The focus of the HOAC II is on patient-centered outcomes. Existing and anticipated problems are identified by the patient or therapist. For each identified problem, the therapist generates hypotheses as to the cause(s), formulates an intervention plan that addresses the hypothesized cause(s), and documents outcomes. Children who receive physical therapy often have several primary and secondary impairments that can cause activity limitations and participation restrictions. When using the HOAC II, therefore, therapists are encouraged to consider all possible hypotheses, to prioritize multiple hypotheses, and to consider how each hypothesis relates to the others. Management of anticipated problems is a unique aspect of the HOAC II. For children with neuromuscular and musculoskeletal impairments who experience excessive or asymmetric weight-bearing forces while walking, anticipated problems might include skeletal deformity and joint contracture. For anticipated problems, intervention is aimed at eliminating risk factors. In this example, depending on the rationale for why the child is likely to have skeletal deformity and joint contracture, interventions might involve muscle strengthening, stretching, an orthosis, and reducing weight-bearing forces through use of wheeled mobility when traveling long distances. The HOAC II model is compatible with the elements of patient/client management in the *Guide to Physical Therapist Practice* (American Physical Therapy Association, 2001) described in the next section.

GUIDE TO PHYSICAL THERAPIST PRACTICE

The *Guide to Physical Therapist Practice* (American Physical Therapy Association, 2001) is a consensus document based on the opinions of more than 800 physical therapist clinicians. The *Guide* was developed by the American Physical Therapy Association between 1995 and 1997. The second edition was published in 2001. The purpose of the *Guide* is to (1) describe generally accepted physical therapist practice, (2) standardize terminology, and (3) delineate preferred practice patterns that describe common sets of management strategies used by physical therapists for selected patient/client diagnostic groups. The *Guide* represents a first step in the development of practice guidelines (which are usually based on a comprehensive search of peer-reviewed literature) in that it classifies patients/clients and identifies the range of current options for care. A patient is an individual who receives physical therapy and procedural intervention. A client is someone who is not necessarily sick or injured but could benefit from physical therapy. Clients are also businesses, school systems, and others to whom physical therapists offer services. The *Guide* is not based on clinical research but is intended to promote outcomes research. In addition to physical therapists, the guide was developed for use by health care policy makers, third-party payers, managed care providers, and other health care professionals.

The *Guide* incorporates the concepts of disablement, prevention, and wellness. Part One describes the elements of patient/client management and explains the tests, measures, and interventions performed by physical therapists. Part Two includes the preferred practice patterns grouped into four areas: musculoskeletal, neuromuscular, cardiovascular/pulmonary, and integumentary. As the *Guide* is presently constituted, the term "preferred practice pattern" is misleading. Practice patterns are broad in scope and inclusive of all procedural interventions that are justifiable. Interventions that are supported by research evidence are not distinguished. The *Guide* is intended to do the following:

1. Enhance the quality of physical therapy
2. Enhance coordination of care among health care providers
3. Improve patient/client satisfaction with physical therapy services
4. Promote appropriate utilization of physical therapy services
5. Increase efficiency of and reimbursement for physical therapy services
6. Promote cost reduction through prevention and wellness initiatives

Model of Patient/Client Management

The model of patient/client management is designed to maximize outcomes through a systematic and comprehensive approach to decision making. The model includes five elements: examination, evaluation, diagnosis, prognosis, and intervention leading to optimal outcomes (Fig. 1-5).

Examination

The physical therapist is required to perform an examination before conducting any intervention. The examination consists of the history, systems review, and selected tests and measures. The history is an account of the child's past and current health status, which is obtained through an interview with the child and caregivers and review of medical and educational records. As part of the history, the physical therapist identifies the child and family expectations and desired outcomes of physical therapy. A useful means for documenting and quantifying family expectations is the Canadian Occupational Performance Measure (Law et al., 1991). The physical therapist then considers whether these expectations and outcomes are realistic in the context of examination and evaluation data.

The systems review is a brief screening that is intended to help focus the subsequent examination and identify possible health problems that require consultation with or referral to another health care provider. A thorough systems review is critical for direct access to physical therapy services. After analyzing information from the history and systems review, the physical therapist examines the child more closely, selecting tests and measures to obtain sufficient data to make an evaluation, establish a diagnosis and a prognosis, and select appropriate interventions.

Evaluation

Evaluation refers to the physical therapist's analysis and synthesis of results of the examination and leads to a physical therapy diagnosis. Evaluation is a process in which the physical therapist makes judgments about the status of the child based on the information gathered from the examination. This step includes judgment of the severity of impairment, functional limitation, and disability; system involvement; the living environment; and social supports. The definition of evaluation in the *Guide* is more specific than what is common in clinical practice in which evaluation is used interchangeably with assessment and examination.

Diagnosis

The physical therapy diagnosis is a label encompassing a cluster of signs, syndromes, or categories. The diagnosis is reached through the evaluation process and is intended

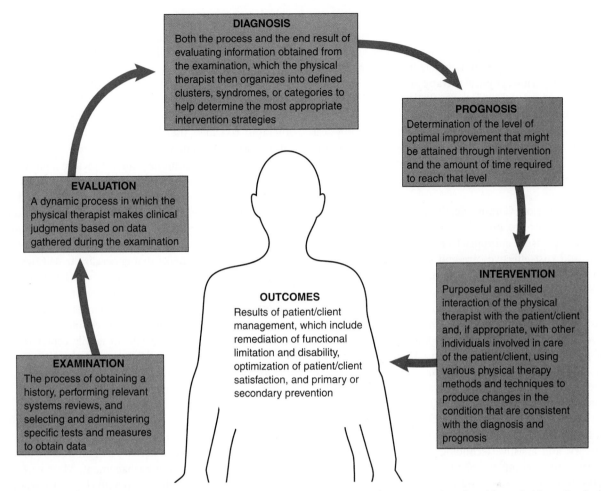

DIAGNOSIS
Both the process and the end result of evaluating information obtained from the examination, which the physical therapist then organizes into defined clusters, syndromes, or categories to help determine the most appropriate intervention strategies

PROGNOSIS
Determination of the level of optimal improvement that might be attained through intervention and the amount of time required to reach that level

EVALUATION
A dynamic process in which the physical therapist makes clinical judgments based on data gathered during the examination

INTERVENTION
Purposeful and skilled interaction of the physical therapist with the patient/client and, if appropriate, with other individuals involved in care of the patient/client, using various physical therapy methods and techniques to produce changes in the condition that are consistent with the diagnosis and prognosis

EXAMINATION
The process of obtaining a history, performing relevant systems reviews, and selecting and administering specific tests and measures to obtain data

OUTCOMES
Results of patient/client management, which include remediation of functional limitation and disability, optimization of patient/client satisfaction, and primary or secondary prevention

• **Figure 1-5** The elements of patient/client management leading to optimal outcomes. (*Reprinted from Guide to Physical Therapist Practice with the permission of the American Physical Therapy Association.*)

to guide the physical therapist in determining the most appropriate interventions for each child and family. Diagnosis as an element of physical therapy management does not refer to the medical diagnosis (disease or pathophysiology). Rather, the diagnosis involves patients/clients who are grouped by impairments of the musculoskeletal, neuromuscular, cardiopulmonary, or integumentary system. Diagnosis is associated with a preferred pattern of patient/client management that identifies the range of current options for care.

Prognosis
Perhaps the greatest challenge to patient/client management is determination of the likely outcomes of intervention. Prognosis refers to the predicted optimal level of improvement in function and the amount of service needed to reach that level (frequency and duration of intervention). A trend in managed health care is to use periodic and episodic intervals of therapy services based

on specific functional problems. This approach is a marked departure for children with developmental disabilities for whom ongoing services have traditionally been reimbursed based on medical diagnosis. Presently, therapists have limited evidence to guide decisions on level of service. At this point in the process of patient/client management, the physical therapist establishes a plan of care that includes the following:

1. Long-term and short-term goals and expected outcomes
2. Intervention procedures and techniques
3. Recommendations for duration and frequency of intervention
4. Discharge criteria

In the *Guide*, expected outcomes are the changes that are anticipated as a result of implementing the plan of care. Expected outcomes should be measurable and time limited. Outcomes of therapy include changes in health, wellness, and fitness, an emerging area of pediatric practice.

Intervention

Intervention is the purposeful and skilled interaction of the physical therapist with the patient/client and, when appropriate, with other individuals involved in patient/client care. Various physical therapy procedures and techniques are used during intervention to enable the child and family to achieve goals and outcomes that are consistent with the child's diagnosis and prognosis. Physical therapy intervention has three components: (1) coordination, communication, and documentation; (2) patient/client instruction; and (3) procedural interventions.

Coordination, Communication, and Documentation. These services are provided for all children and their families to ensure appropriate, coordinated, comprehensive, and cost-effective care and efficient integration or reintegration to home, community, and work (job/school/play). Services may include (1) case management, (2) coordination of care with family and other professionals, (3) discharge planning, (4) education plans, (5) case conferences, and (6) documentation of all elements of patient/client management. Based on our experience in tailoring continuing education experiences for the needs of physical therapists, this is an area of particular challenge. Children with disabilities are managed in a variety of settings, from public schools to private offices or rehabilitation facilities to specialty clinics for orthotics, surgery, and assistive technology. Therapists in each of these settings complain of the lack of coordination of services among settings and the paucity of effective and timely information sharing among health professionals, teachers, and families.

Patient/Client Instruction. These services are provided for all families to provide information about the child's current condition, the plan of care, and future transition to home, work, or community roles. Methods of instruction include demonstration; modeling; verbal, written, or pictorial instruction; and periodic reexamination and reassessment of the home program. The educational backgrounds, needs, and learning styles of family members must be considered during this process. As part of family-centered services, therapists collaborate with children and families to identify how to incorporate exercise and practice of functional movements in daily activities and routines.

Procedural Interventions. Procedural interventions provided by physical therapists include (1) therapeutic exercise; (2) functional training in self-care and home management; (3) functional training in the community and at work (job/school/play); (4) manual therapy techniques; (5) prescription, application, and fabrication of devices and equipment; (6) airway clearance techniques; and (7) physical agents and mechanical modalities. The first three interventions listed are included most often in the plan of care.

Outcomes

At each step of patient/client management, the physical therapist considers the possible outcomes. The therapist also engages in outcome data collection and analysis. Outcomes include minimization of functional limitation, optimization of health status, prevention of disability, and optimization of patient/client satisfaction. Horn and colleagues (1997) have introduced and tested an innovation in documenting outcomes of intervention, which therapists can use to show that treatment of impairments results in functional improvements that generalize to settings outside the immediate treatment environment. Three domains that appear repeatedly in the research on interpersonal aspects of care are information exchange; respectful and supportive care; and partnership and enabling (King et al., 1996). In a review of research on family-centered care, Rosenbaum and associates (1998) concluded that parents of children with physical disabilities have positive perceptions of how services are provided to their children but are not as satisfied with information exchange.

Preferred Practice Patterns

The preferred practice patterns are organized by the five elements of patient/client management. Most preferred practice patterns are applicable to both children and adults. The three patterns specific to children are Neuromuscular Pattern B: Impaired Neuromotor Development; Neuromuscular Pattern C: Impaired Motor Function and Sensory Integrity Associated with Congenital or Acquired Disorders of the Central Nervous System in Infancy, Childhood, and Adolescence; and Cardiovascular/Pulmonary Pattern G: Impaired Ventilation, Respiration/Gas Exchange, and Aerobic Capacity/Endurance associated with Respiratory Failure in the Neonate. The *Guide to Physical Therapist Practice* does not specifically address physical therapist practice in early intervention and in the public schools. Public laws and guidelines for physical therapist practice in these settings are presented in Chapters 31 and 32.

EVALUATING INTERVENTION OUTCOMES

Physical therapists typically evaluate the effectiveness of an intervention by comparing patient performance with preset short- and long-term goals and outcomes developed on the basis of patient testing and observation. How can we guarantee, however, that the outcomes we identify are really the result of our intervention and not the effect of other interventions, of natural development, or of recovery? And how can we be sure that our interventions do not result in unintended negative consequences?

A first step in assessing intervention outcomes (in a nonexperimental fashion) is to develop, conduct, and write a case report or series of case reports on one or more children in one's caseload. Although case reports do not employ the controls needed to establish cause-and-effect relationships, they *are* helpful in deriving clinical hypotheses or "hunches" about why a specific intervention may or may not be effective for a particular child (Backman & Harris, 1999). In her excellent manual for clinicians on how to write case reports, McEwen (2001) stated that a case report "refers to descriptions of practice that do not involve research methodology" (p 5). McEwen went on to point out that case reports provide an excellent mechanism to enable practicing therapists to integrate best research evidence with their own clinical expertise and patient values and choices. Case reports require that therapists review the relevant research literature, develop measurable therapy objectives for the children they plan to include, assess the reliability of those outcome measures, and describe the children's histories, previous treatments, examination results, and medical characteristics in rich detail. In the case reports manual, McEwen has outlined each of these steps, relating them to the *Guide to Physical Therapist Practice*. There are many diverse examples of case reports in the pediatric rehabilitation literature (e.g., Almeida et al., 1997; Carmick, 1997; Jones et al., 2003; Karman et al., 2003), but there is also a need for many more if we are to truly call ourselves evidence-based practitioners.

One clinical decision tool that has been used increasingly by pediatric physical therapists to assess the effectiveness of their interventions is the single-subject research design. The single-subject design is an experimental paradigm that is particularly useful for practicing clinicians who wish to study intensively the effects of intervention on individual patients within their caseload (Gonnella, 1989; Harris, 1993).

Nearly all pediatric physical therapists must develop individualized, measurable objectives for the children with whom they work as part of "best-practice" procedure, and the single-subject design represents a logical extension of this procedure. In developing individual behavioral objectives, therapists are required to specify patient outcomes that are expected to change as a result of introducing intervention. These behavioral objectives are analogous to outcome measures that are a form of

dependent variable, a term that is universal to all types of experimental research designs.

A second major component of experimental research is selection of the independent variable or, in the case of physical therapy, the specific treatment technique that is being applied in an effort to effect positive change in the outcome variable. Obviously, careful treatment planning for the pediatric patient involves not only the selection of the outcome or target behavior, as represented in the individualized therapy objective, but also selection of a specific treatment technique that is designed to enhance change or facilitate improvement in the outcome behavior. In comparing the single-subject research design to physical therapy as it is typically provided in a clinical setting, Gonnella (1989) stated that the first few steps are similar: the problem behavior is identified, baseline data are collected on the problem behavior, a treatment plan is developed and implemented, and changes in the problem behavior are assessed. However, several important differences exist between the single-subject design and the therapeutic model.

Whereas typically only one baseline assessment is taken in the therapeutic model, single-subject design mandates that a minimum of three data points be collected on the outcome behavior before treatment is introduced (Barlow et al., 1984). A second criterion of single-subject research is that a very specific design should be implemented that involves sequential application and withdrawal of the intervention. Finally, performance must be measured repeatedly (and frequently) throughout each phase of the design. For a visual comparison of these two models as described and depicted by Gonnella (1989), see Figure 1-6.

Other important criteria of single-subject research designs are that the data collection procedures are both replicable and reliable (Ottenbacher, 1986). Percent agreement is typically used to assess consistency of scoring the behavioral objectives or outcome measures between two or more independent raters.

In his excellent text on single-subject designs for occupational and physical therapists, Ottenbacher (1986) has outlined six important steps for setting up such designs: (1) determining the setting in which the behavior or performance will be observed and recorded; (2) deciding on the method to collect data; (3) determining the length of time that the behavior will be observed and measured; (4) observing and recording client behavior; (5) recording and plotting the data collected; and (6) continuing the measurement and recording procedures until requirements of the design have been satisfied. Pediatric physical therapists who wish to set up single-subject designs in their own clinical settings are advised to consult the

THERAPEUTIC MODEL	SINGLE-SUBJECT EXPERIMENTAL PARADIGM
1. Evaluate patient's status	Evaluate patient's status
One baseline measure (BL)	*Three or more BLs
Specify problem(s)	Same
Measure problem(s)	Same
Specify goal(s)	Same
Specify therapeutic intervention (TI)	Same
	*Specify design to assess efficacy
2. Apply TI	*Apply TI within design strategy
Adjust TI to patient's response	Same
3. Evaluate patient's response	Evaluate patient's response
	*Repeated measures

*Indicates absence or difference in approach from the current model.

◆ **Figure 1-6**   Comparison of therapeutic process with single-subject paradigm. *(From Gonnella, C. Single-subject experimental paradigm as a clinical decision tool. Physical Therapy, 69:603, 1989. Reprinted from* Physical Therapy *with the permission of the American Physical Therapy Association.)*

Ottenbacher text, as well as other references in the physical therapy literature that describe this important clinical decision tool (Gonnella, 1989; Harris, 1993).

Since the early 1980s, pediatric physical and occupational therapists have used single-subject designs to examine the effects of "tone-reducing" (inhibitive) casts and orthoses in improving gait and standing balance in children with cerebral palsy (Harris & Riffle, 1986; Hinderer et al., 1988); to evaluate the influence of some specific well-defined neurodevelopmental treatment techniques on increasing heel contact (Laskas et al., 1985) and decreasing knee flexion during gait (Embrey et al., 1990) in children with cerebral palsy; to assess the effects of two different treatment approaches (behavior modification and a neurophysiologic approach) in reducing tongue protrusion in young children with Down syndrome (Purdy et al., 1987); and to examine the effects of different modes of mobility on school performance of children with myelodysplasia (Franks et al., 1991). These are but a sampling of the published reports that have used single-subject designs to examine treatment effectiveness in children with developmental disabilities. A recent single-subject study examined the effect of passive range-of-motion (ROM) exercises on lower-extremity goniometric measurements of six adults with cerebral palsy, ranging in age from 20 to 44 years (Cadenhead et al., 2002).

In the following paragraphs, two published single-subject studies will be described—one involving two children with spastic diplegia and the other involving three children with myelodysplasia. Reference will be made to the ICF model in discussing the goals and outcomes of each of these studies.

In a single-subject study published in 1988, Hinderer and colleagues set out to evaluate the relative effects of tone-reducing casts and standard plaster casts on gait characteristics and functional locomotor activities in two young children with cerebral palsy. The first child (case 1) was a 3.5-year-old boy with mild spastic diplegia and mild mental retardation; spasticity was greater on the right. Some of the impairments noted in this child included gait deviations such as moderate in-toeing on the right, decreased stride length on the left, toe-dragging, forefoot weight bearing, limited trunk rotation, and high-guard posture of the upper extremities. Activity limitations included the inability to walk up and down stairs without support and the inability to squat or rise to standing without support.

The second child (case 2) was a girl, age 5 years 9 months, with asymmetric spastic diplegia (greater involvement on the left), moderate ataxia, and normal intelligence quotient (IQ). Impairments included poor static and dynamic balance and unsteady gait with frequent falling. Specific gait deviations consisted of mild in-toeing on the left and difficulty with left toe clearance, limited trunk rotation, and a wide base of support. Activity limitations that resulted from these impairments included the inability to walk backward and balance on one leg and the need for upper extremity support to climb stairs and to move from squatting to standing.

An A-B-A-C crossover single-subject design was used in this study to evaluate the effects of the two different types of casts (the independent variables or specific intervention techniques). Tone-reducing casts were defined as those that "maintain the ankle at zero degrees and stabilize the toes and foot in neutral alignment by incorporating a footplate which supports the toes and the metatarsal, peroneal and longitudinal arches of the foot" (Hinderer et al., 1988, p. 371). Standard plaster casts held the ankle in neutral alignment but did not include a footplate.

The study began with both children in a baseline (A1) phase (no casts). In the second phase of the study, case 1 wore tone-reducing casts (B) and case 2 wore standard casts (C). Then the baseline condition (A2) was reinstituted for both subjects, after which the crossover of treatments occurred so that the design for case 1 was A1-B-A2-C and the design for case 2 was A1-C-A2-B.

Outcome measures (target behaviors) included footprint data used to analyze various gait parameters, specific developmentally appropriate fine motor tasks, and videotaped ratings by an interdisciplinary panel of experts on gait and functional motor activities. Data were collected two or three times per week for 19 weeks. The number of data points per phase ranged from 5 to 12. Inter-rater percent agreement for the gait measures was 96.1% and for the fine motor measures was 97.4%. Subjective impressions were also obtained from parents of the two children and their treating therapists.

One of the benefits of sequential application and withdrawal of interventions, as occurs in single-subject designs, is the ability to control for natural history, developmental maturation, and practice effects. Analysis of the fine motor data for the children in this study revealed that their performance continued to improve even during the baseline (no-cast) phases—thus suggesting that practice of these tasks was contributing more to their improvement than were the specific interventions. In a typical therapeutic model as described by Gonnella (1989) (see Fig. 1-6), such control is not possible and the treating therapist might assume that the improvements are due to the intervention itself, whereas such improvements may, in fact, be due to practicing the task or to other intervening variables such as developmental maturation.

Another benefit of this particular crossover design is the opportunity to compare two different interventions. Greater increases in stride length were noted for both children during the tone-reducing cast phases as compared with the standard cast condition. Blinded videotape analysis by the panel of experts revealed mild gait improvements for case 2 during the tone-reducing cast phase and improvements in standing balance, ability to walk backward, and ability to squat and return to upright. Owing to poor compliance by case 1, a standardized sequence of gait and functional motor activities was not obtained.

Although this study provided some limited support for the relative benefits of tone-reducing casts as compared with standard casts, the authors concluded by making a plea for practitioners to document their own outcomes of tone-reducing casts and orthoses: "Single-subject research designs offer a clinically appropriate means for reliably studying their effectiveness, and are particularly indicated when studying a heterogeneous population, such as individuals with cerebral palsy, whose clinical presentation varies from day to day" (Hinderer et al., 1988, p. 375).

Another single-subject study compared the relative effects of assistive device ambulation (walker or crutches) and wheelchair mobility on three school performance measures for children with myelodysplasia (Franks et al., 1991). Subjects were students aged 9, 10, and 15 years with L4 or L5 level myelomeningocele, all of whom had a physiologic cost index (an indicator of energy efficiency) of greater than 1.00 beat per meter when ambulating with assistive devices. The independent variables or specific interventions in this study were the assistive ambulation devices and the wheelchair. Outcomes assessed were reading fluency, visuomotor accuracy, and manual dexterity. A convincing rationale for this study was the frequent encouragement of ambulation for children with lumbar-level lesions in spite of the high energy costs (Waters & Lunsford, 1985).

In the case of these children with lumbar-level lesions, the pathophysiologic condition (myelodysplasia) led to impairments, including lower extremity paralysis, which had then resulted in activity limitations in gait and upright mobility. Basically, this study sought to examine whether ambulation, when energy cost is high, had a negative effect on school performance (participation). To examine these questions, an alternating condition single-subject design was used in which phase 1 was wheelchair propulsion, phase 2 was ambulation with crutches or walker, and phase 3 was again wheelchair propulsion. Each phase was 1 week in length (5 school days), with data collected daily on the three outcome measures: correct words per minute of a 100- to 200-word reading passage (reading fluency); visuomotor accuracy as assessed by the Motor Accuracy Test, Revised (Ayres, 1972); and manual dexterity as assessed on the Purdue Pegboard Assembly subtest (Tiffin, 1968). Although reading fluency was unaffected by the method of mobility and manual dexterity varied across the three subjects and the two treatment conditions, visuomotor accuracy scores were significantly lower for all three subjects during the assistive ambulation phase.

In an accompanying commentary on this article, Haley concluded that "implications of this study may cause us to step back from our often aggressive posture toward functional ambulation at all costs. If assisted ambulation is not energy efficient, time efficient, or safe or leads to an interruption in social, emotional, or cognitive growth, then alternate means of mobility must be considered. Is not the aim of the physical therapist to promote overall development rather than to promote ambulation at a significant cost? Is not efficient, independent mobility the real functional goal for children and their families?" (Haley, 1991, p. 578).

It is exactly these types of questions that we face daily in our clinical decision making as pediatric physical therapists. Using single-subject studies to systematically examine effects of specific interventions and replicating these studies across other subjects in other clinical settings will assist in allowing us to answer such questions. Therapists are encouraged to consult three references (Backman et al., 1997; Backman & Harris, 1999; Portney & Watkins, 2000) that provide more information and examples of different types of single-subject designs commonly used in rehabilitation settings. It is the responsibility of all practicing therapists, be they clinicians, researchers, or educators, to provide ethically responsible and effective interventions for their clients. Systematic examination of intervention outcomes, through such strategies as the single-subject design, can assist us in attaining this goal.

PROGRAM EVALUATION

Although individual physical therapists frequently believe that they have done their professional jobs thoroughly when they have appropriately assessed outcomes in individual clients, professional practice requires additional evaluation of the overall impact and costs of physical therapy programs. Goldberg (1991), for example, suggested that therapeutic and surgical outcomes for children with cerebral palsy include technical outcomes of typical interventions, functional outcomes, parent and child satisfaction with both outcome and service delivery, and cost-effectiveness relative to other intervention approaches. Here, the tools include formal program evaluations and quality assurance strategies involving evaluation of record keeping; monitoring of therapist adherence to program policies; assessment of interactions with clients, other providers, and third-party payers; and evaluation of client satisfaction and long-term outcomes.

MONITORING SERVICES WITH A DATABASE

Developments in the area of monitoring services and tracking outcomes include computerized approaches to

creating a database on patients served that may also provide systematic, structured individual patient reports to guarantee uniform reporting of significant information across both therapists and types of patients (Jenkins, 1989; Lehmann et al., 1984; Shurtleff, 1991; Slagle & Gould, 1992). A database is a generalized set of computer programs that allows (1) entry of a variety of data by different authorized users; (2) organization of the data for storage; and (3) retrieval, updating, reorganization, and printing of output in the form of summary reports (Lehmann et al., 1984). Yearly statistics can be rapidly collated, care trends can be monitored across time, and data can be used for prospective or retrospective research (Slagle & Gould, 1992). Use of a database approach can guard against errors of both omission and commission by structuring therapists' reports and by automatically providing checks of entered data against a range of appropriate responses. Development of national databases on specific client populations can form the basis for improving practice through comparison of institutional or regional differences in management strategies, identifying infrequent negative outcomes, and studying low-incidence conditions.

Slagle and Gould (1992) emphasized that only 27% of tertiary care neonatal units, responding to a national survey of database use, monitored the accuracy of their data, an essential element of a high-quality plan. Users liked their system best if it generated patient records, such as discharge summaries. In addition to these critical issues, Jenkins (1989) suggested that database developers should consider what aspects of care are likely to change over time in order to develop a system that is flexible in meeting long-term needs. Developers should consider how to collect enough data to be maximally useful for meeting such diverse needs as preparing annual reports and answering important research questions, while eliminating large amounts of data that are easy to collect but unlikely to be used (Slagle & Gould, 1992). In addition, a specific plan for maintaining overall quality of the database should be developed (Slagle & Gould, 1992).

In response to the growing trend for health care accountability, the Joint Commission on Accreditation of Healthcare Organizations (JCAHO) has incorporated the use of outcomes and other performance measures into the accreditation process (Schyve, 1996). JCAHO requirements focus on clinical performance measures designed to evaluate both the processes and outcomes of care. Processes of care include measures of patient satisfaction. The Measure of Processes of Caregiving (King et al., 1996) is a parent report measure for use in programs serving children with developmental disabilities. Two pediatric outcome measures for which there is an external data system are the Functional Independence Measure for Children (Braun, 1998) through the Uniform Data System for Medical Rehabilitation, Buffalo, New York, and the Pediatric Evaluation of Disability Inventory (Haley et al., 1992) through the Center for Rehabilitation Effectiveness, Boston, Massachusetts.

FORMAL PROGRAM EVALUATION

A more comprehensive approach to assessing program effectiveness is formal program evaluation (Shadish et al., 1991). Although frequently using well-known social science methodology, formal evaluation practice since the 1960s has developed into a discipline in its own right. The explicit purpose of program evaluation is to assess the effects of programs in meeting their stated goals for the purpose of improving subsequent decision making about the program and, in a broader sense, for improving future program planning. Evaluation theory, although initially idealistic, has been expanded and revised based on the experience of program evaluators operating in the real world. These experiences have led to the recognition that (1) the achievement of stated goals may not be the only useful product of a social program; (2) there are many stakeholders involved in the typical program, some of whom are more concerned that the interests of their particular group are addressed than that program goals have been achieved; and (3) politics always act on programs in ways that may be difficult to identify but may mean that program evaluation results are not likely to change programs effectively in major ways. Because of these real-world complications, new evaluation theories have arisen, some complementary and some in more direct opposition to others.

"Theory connotes a body of knowledge that organizes, categorizes, describes, predicts, explains, and otherwise aids in understanding and controlling a topic" (Shadish et al., 1991, p. 30). Ideal evaluation theory describes and justifies why certain evaluation practices lead to particular types of results; clarifies the activities, processes, and goals of evaluation; explicates relationships among evaluative activities and the processes and goals they facilitate; and empirically tests propositions to identify and address those that conflict with research or other knowledge about evaluation (Shadish et al., 1991). The purpose of program evaluation theory is to specify the practices that are feasible for evaluators to use to garner evidence for the value of programs and to reduce identified problems of relevance to the program. Formulation of an appropriate methodology for evaluating a program depends on proper identification of the uses to which the evaluation results will be put. The prospective program evaluation planner needs to know who wants to know what and to what end.

The uses of evaluation results are usually considered to be of two major types: summative (outcomes or products) and formative (evaluation for the purpose of improving the program and understanding the processes by which the program operates). The former makes the supposition that an outcome of the evaluation itself might be abolition of the program; the latter generally assumes that the program will continue to exist and that better ways of improving the product or the provision of services are sought. Because studies of the uses to which evaluation results are put have generally shown that effects trickle down into new-generation programs, producing slow, incremental change rather than resulting in revolutions in thinking and implementation, recent theorists have emphasized that evaluation results may be most usefully thought of as being "enlightening," that is, having future use for program planners in thinking about issues, defining problems, and developing new perspectives and ideas. Those who formulate policy and implement programs seldom actively search for evidence, or if they do, they tend to use whatever fits with their current understanding of the problem under study. Information such as this has led to important studies of the uses of program evaluation and theoretic formulations regarding how information can be most usefully disseminated. Whatever the purpose, program evaluation must be conducted based on the identified needs for the program and how well it satisfies the needs identified, as well as meets the needs that might not have been previously identified but happen to be satisfied by the program. The best program evaluation designs also search for potential negative effects, such as those identified by the study of Franks and colleagues (1991) on mobility in children with myelodysplasia.

Arguments have arisen among program evaluation theorists regarding the value of quantitative versus qualitative evaluation methods. The randomized, controlled clinical trial remains, at least in medical arenas, the most highly valued summative assessment of intervention outcomes, and is especially valuable in studies of intervention with children because of the control needed to rule out the effects of maturation and other threats to internal validity (Norton & Strube, 1989; Shadish et al., 1991). Combined with causal modeling of the theoretically and empirically derived processes and factors influencing outcomes, clinical trials are most powerful in studies with large numbers of subjects or in studies seeking to identify low-incidence but potentially highly dangerous unintended negative effects. Qualitative methods, however, offer flexibility, a dynamic quality, and a unique ability to reflect the world from the perspective of multiple program stakeholders and participants. They are especially well suited for gathering answers to formative questions about the quality of program implementation and its meaning to participants. They may also be highly useful for studying the processes by which programs achieve useful outcomes in meeting needs of patients and society. Of most importance, however, are methods appropriate to the level of development of the program (e.g., early development stage program, innovative demonstration project, established ongoing program), the problematic issues of concern to program stakeholders of various types, decisions under the control of the program to be made at a time when evaluation results will be available, and the level of uncertainty regarding critical program features. Methods tailored to these factors are most likely to result in effective use of program evaluation results.

Methods of program evaluation that emphasize the process of service delivery are well suited for examining the overall effectiveness of therapy programs. Wang and Ellett (1982) used the term *program validation* to describe a form of evaluative research useful in the development and refinement of innovative educational programs. The major purposes of program validation are to (1) obtain empirical evidence of the effectiveness of an innovative program, (2) identify aspects of the program that require improvement in order to achieve the intended outcomes, and (3) evaluate the feasibility of implementing the innovative program. Wolery and Bailey (1984) have proposed that a comprehensive evaluation of early intervention programs addresses the following questions:

1. Does the method of service delivery represent the best educational practice?
2. Is the intervention being implemented accurately and consistently?
3. Is an attempt being made to verify the effectiveness of the intervention objectively?
4. Does the program carefully monitor patient progress and demonstrate a sensitivity to points at which changes in service need to be made?
5. Does a system exist for determining the adequacy of patient progress and service delivery?
6. Is the program accomplishing its goals and objectives?
7. Does the service delivery system meet the needs and values of the community and clients it serves?

The questions proposed by Wolery and Bailey offer a framework for program evaluation of physical therapy services provided in a variety of settings, including the school system, acute care and rehabilitation hospitals for children, and private practices.

Two studies serve to illustrate the scope of program evaluation and how questions are developed specific to particular programs. Haley and colleagues (1988) evaluated how physical therapy and occupational therapy services were implemented in six publicly funded early intervention programs in the greater Boston area. The authors examined the influences of infant, family, and program variables on the therapy services provided over a 6-month period. Dependent variables included intensity of individual therapy, intensity of group therapy, ratio of direct therapy to group therapy, ratio of home therapy to center therapy, and ratio of therapy time to total program time. Therapist availability predicted best whether an infant received individual therapy. Infants with more delayed motor development tended to receive more individual therapy and more total therapy. Infants received a higher proportion of therapy when (1) motor quotient was low and parent education was high, (2) infants were younger and therapist availability was high, and (3) infants were younger and parent education was high. Diagnostic risk factors and age did not predict type or intensity of therapy. Although the study was exploratory in nature and should not be generalized to other early intervention programs, the results contribute to the understanding of how infant characteristics and therapist availability influence the degree and types of intervention.

Palisano (1989) evaluated two methods of therapy service delivery provided to students with learning disabilities who attended public school during the 1986–1987 school year. To serve adequately approximately 500 students receiving occupational therapy and physical therapy, the therapy staff of the Delaware County, Pennsylvania, intermediate unit had instituted group and consultation methods for providing services to students with learning disabilities who met eligibility criteria. The therapists and teachers of students who participated in the study had worked together during the previous school year using the two methods of service delivery. Students in classrooms that received a combination of large group and small group therapy were compared with students in classrooms that received large group therapy and consultation. Methods of evaluation included student progress in motor, visuomotor, and visuoperceptual skills; the therapy needs of each group; teacher satisfaction; and use of available therapy resources. Both methods appeared to represent sound therapy practice. Interaction between the therapist and the teacher in establishing goals and planning group sessions was identified as integral to the success of both methods of service delivery. Recommendations for the following year included placing greater emphasis on achievement of functional goals, establishing group behavioral objectives, and examining similarities and differences between the services provided by occupational therapy and physical therapy.

SUMMARY

Evidence-based decision making is integral to determining who needs physical therapy and why, how cases should be managed, how outcomes should be documented, and what methods should be used for evaluating the effectiveness of interventions. Pediatric physical therapists are becoming increasingly aware of the need to base their clinical decisions on the best available knowledge and research evidence. This involves finding and appraising research reports, systematic reviews, clinical practice guidelines and pathways and applying evidence to practice. Translation of evidence to practice occurs within the context of child and family identified needs. Sharing information with children and families in useful and acceptable formats encourages their active participation in decision making. The statement by Guyatt and colleagues (2000) that "research is never enough" acknowledges the need for therapists to have a strong knowledge base, problem solve, and make sound judgments based on expert consensus and personal experience. Conceptual frameworks like the International Classification of Functioning, Disability and Health, the Hypothesis-Oriented Algorithm for Clinicians II, and the Elements of Patient/Client Management can improve clinical reasoning and the decision-making process.

Although physical therapists typically evaluate outcomes on the basis of whether children achieve short- and long-term goals or demonstrate improvement on standardized assessments of motor development and function, these methods do not indicate whether the outcomes were the result of intervention, because children are also expected to change as a result of maturational processes. Single-subject research designs provide one clinical decision tool that enables pediatric physical therapists to evaluate the effectiveness of their interventions for individual patients and to discover information of use in future research. In addition to evaluations of individual patient outcomes, professional practice requires evaluation of the overall effectiveness and costs of physical therapy programs. Monitoring of program inputs, implementation, and outputs is enhanced by computerized programs that allow the creation of databases on patient populations and provide a systematic, structured individual patient report. Formal methods of program evaluation provide information for assessing whether programs meet important consumer and societal needs, are properly implemented for maximal impact, and actually serve targeted populations. Given the changing and complex nature of health care, pediatric physical therapists are challenged to enhance their use of more scientific evidence and more valid and reliable decision methods as the basis for their practice.

ACKNOWLEDGMENTS

The work reported in this chapter was partially supported by grants to S.K. Campbell from the Agency for Health Care Policy and Research and the National Institute for Child Health and Human Development.

REFERENCES

Almeida, GL, Campbell, SK, Girolami, GL, Penn, RD, & Corcos, DM. Multi-dimensional assessment of motor function in a child with cerebral palsy following intrathecal administration of baclofen. Physical Therapy, 77:751–764, 1997.

American Physical Therapy Association. Guide to Physical Therapist Practice, 2nd ed. Physical Therapy, 81:9–744, 2001.

Aylward, GP. Conceptual issues in developmental screening and assessment. Developmental and Behavioral Pediatrics, 18:340–349, 1997.

Aylward, GP, & Kenny, TJ. Developmental follow-up: Inherent problems and a conceptual model. Journal of Pediatric Psychology, 4:331–343, 1979.

Ayres, AJ. Southern California Sensory Integration Tests. Los Angeles: Western Psychological Services, 1972.

Backman, CL, Harris, SR, Chisholm, JM, & Monette, AD. Single-subject research in rehabilitation: A review of studies using AB, withdrawal, multiple baseline, and alternating treatment designs. Archives of Physical Medicine and Rehabilitation, 78:1145–1153, 1997.

Backman, CL, & Harris, SR. Case studies, single subject research, and N of 1 randomized trials: Comparisons and contrasts. American Journal of Physical Medicine and Rehabilitation, 78:170–176, 1999.

Baird G, McConachie H, & Scrutton D. Parents' perceptions of disclosure of the diagnosis of cerebral palsy. Archives of Diseases in Childhood, 83:475–480, 2000.

Barbosa VM, Campbell SK, Sheftel D, Singh J, & Beligere N. Longitudinal performance of infants with cerebral palsy on the Test of Infant Motor Performance and on the Alberta Infant Motor Scale. Physical & Occupational Therapy in Pediatrics, 23(3):7–29, 2003.

Barlow, DH, Hayes, SC, & Nelson, RO. The Scientist Practitioner: Research and Accountability in Clinical and Educational Settings. Emsford, NY: Pergamon Press, 1984.

Binkley, J, Finch, E, Hall, J, Black, T, & Gowland, C. Diagnostic classification of patients with low back pain: Report on a survey of physical therapy experts. Physical Therapy, 73:138–155, 1993.

Braun S. Featured instrument. The Functional Independence Measure for Children (WeeFIM instrument): Gateway to the WeeFIM System. Journal of Rehabilitation Outcomes Measurement, 2:63–68, 1998.

Brenner, P. From Novice to Expert: Excellence and Power in Clinical Nursing Practice. Reading, MA: Addison-Wesley, 1984.

Butler, C. Augmentative mobility: Why do it? Physical Medicine and Rehabilitation Clinics of North America, 2:801–815, 1991.

Butler, C, & Darrah, J. Effects of neurodevelopmental treatment (NDT) for cerebral palsy: An AACPDM evidence report. Developmental Medicine and Child Neurology, 43:778–790, 2001.

Cadenhead, SL, McEwen, IR, & Thompson, DM. Effect of passive range of motion on lower-extremity goniometric measurements of adults with cerebral palsy: A single-subject design. Physical Therapy, 82:658–669, 2002.

Campbell, SK (Ed.). Proceedings of the consensus conference on the efficacy of physical therapy in the management of cerebral palsy. Pediatric Physical Therapy, 2(3):121–176, 1990.

Campbell, SK. Future directions for physical therapy assessment in early infancy. In Wilhelm, IJ (Ed.). Physical Therapy Assessment in Early Infancy. New York: Churchill Livingstone, 1993, pp. 293–308.

Campbell, SK. Therapy programs for children that last a lifetime. Physical and Occupational Therapy in Pediatrics, 17(1):1–15, 1997.

Campbell, SK. Models for decision making. In Campbell, SK (Ed.). Decision Making in Pediatric Neurologic Physical Therapy. Philadelphia: Churchill Livingstone, 1999, pp. 1–22.

Campbell, SK, Gardner, HG, & Ramakrishnan, V. Correlates of physicians' decisions to refer children with cerebral palsy for physical therapy. Developmental Medicine & Child Neurology, 37:1062–1074, 1995.

Campbell, SK, & Wilhelm, IJ. Development from birth to three years of fifteen children at high risk for central nervous system dysfunction. Physical Therapy, 65:463–469, 1985.

Campbell SK, Kolobe THA, Wright BD, & Linacre JM. Validity of the Test of Infant Motor Performance for prediction of 6-, 9-, and 12-month scores on the Alberta Infant Motor Scale. Developmental Medicine and Child Neurology, 44:263–272, 2002.

Carmick, J. Use of neuromuscular electrical stimulation and dorsal wrist splint to improve the hand function of a child with spastic hemiparesis. Physical Therapy, 77:661–671, 1997.

Chassin, MR, & Galvin, RW. The urgent need to improve health care quality: Institute of Medicine National Roundtable on Health Care Quality. Journal of the American Medical Association, 280:1000–1005, 1998.

Cohen J. Statistical Power Analysis for the Behavioral Sciences, 2nd ed. Hillsdale, NY: Lawrence Erlbaum Associates, 1988.

Cook, DJ, Mulrow, CD, & Haynes, RB. Systematic reviews: Synthesis of best evidence for clinical decisions. Annals of Internal Medicine, 126:376–380, 1997.

Crenna, P, Inverno, M, Frigo, C, Palmieri, R, & Fedrizzi, E. Pathophysiological profile of gait in children with cerebral palsy. In Forrsberg, H, & Hirschfeld, H (Eds.). Movement Disorders in Children. Basel, Switzerland: Karger, 1992, pp. 186–198.

Darrah, J, Piper, M, & Watt, MJ. Assessment of gross motor skills of at-risk infants: Predictive validity of the Alberta Infant Motor Scale. Developmental Medicine and Child Neurology, 40:485–491, 1998.

Darrah, J, Watkins, B, Chen, L, & Bonin C. Conductive education for children with cerebral palsy: an AACPDM evidence report. Developmental Medicine and Child Neurology, 46:187–203, 2004.

Dawes, RM, Faust, D, & Meehl, PE. Clinical versus actuarial judgment. Science, 243:1668–1674, 1989.

Dodd KJ, Taylor NF, & Damiano DL. A systematic review of the effectiveness of strength-training programs for people with cerebral palsy. Archives of Physical Medicine & Rehabilitation, 83(8):1157–1164, 2002

Dowie, J, & Elstein, A (Eds.). Professional Judgment: A Reader in Clinical Decision Making. New York: Cambridge University Press, 1988.

Echternach, JL, & Rothstein, JM. Hypothesis-oriented algorithms. Physical Therapy, 69:559–564, 1989.

Effgen, SK, Bjornson, K, Chiarello, L, Sinzer, L, & Phillips, W. Competencies for physical therapy in early intervention. Pediatric Physical Therapy, 3:77–80, 1991.

Embrey, DG, & Adams, LS. Clinical applications of procedural changes by experienced and novice pediatric physical therapists. Pediatric Physical Therapy, 8:122–132, 1996.

Embrey, DG, & Hylton, N. Clinical applications of movement scripts by experienced and novice pediatric physical therapists. Pediatric Physical Therapy, 8:3–14, 1996.

Embrey, DG, & Nirider, B. Clinical applications of psychosocial sensitivity by experienced and novice pediatric physical therapists. Pediatric Physical Therapy, 8:70–79, 1996.

Embrey, DG, Yates, L, & Mott, DH. Effects of neuro-developmental treatment and orthoses on knee flexion during gait: A single subject design. Physical Therapy, 70:626–637, 1990.

Embrey, DG, Yates, L, Nirider, B, Hylton, N, & Adams, LS. Recommendations for pediatric physical therapists: Making clinical decisions for children with cerebral palsy. Pediatric Physical Therapy, 8:165–170, 1996.

Evidence-Based Medicine Working Group. Evidence-based medicine: A new approach to teaching the practice of medicine. Journal of the American Medical Association, 268(17):2420–2425, 1992.

Ferrari, F, Cioni, G, & Prechtl, HFR. Qualitative changes of general movements in preterm infants with brain lesions. Early Human Development, 23:193–231, 1990.

Ferrari, F, Cioni, G, Einspieler, C, Roversi, F, Bos, AF, Paolicelli, PB, Ranzi, A, & Prechtl, HFR. Cramped synchronized General Movements in preterm infants as an early marker for cerebral palsy. Archives of Pediatric Adolescent Medicine, 156:460–467, 2002.

Fetters, L, Figueiredo, EM, Keane-Miller, D, McSweeney, DJ, & Tsao CC. Critically appraised topics. Pediatric Physical Therapy, 16:19–21, 2004.

Fleming, MH. Clinical reasoning in medicine compared to clinical reasoning in occupational therapy. American Journal of Occupational Therapy, 45:988–996, 1991.

Franks, CA, Palisano, RJ, & Darbee, JC. The effect of walking with an assistive device and using a wheelchair on school performance in students with myelomeningocele. Physical Therapy, 71:570–577, 1991.

Giangreco, MF. Related services decision-making: A foundational component of effective education for students with disabilities. Physical and Occupational Therapy in Pediatrics, 15(2):47–67, 1995.

Goldberg, MJ. Commentary: Measuring outcomes in cerebral palsy. Journal of Pediatric Orthopedics, 11:682–685, 1991.

Golden, GS. Nonstandard therapies in the developmental disabilities. American Journal of Diseases in Childhood, 134:487–491, 1980.

Gonnella, C. Single-subject experimental paradigm as a clinical decision tool. Physical Therapy, 69:601–609, 1989.

Gordon, BN, & Jens, KG. A conceptual model for tracking high-risk infants and making early service decisions. Journal of Developmental and Behavioral Pediatrics, 9(5):279–286, 1988.

Guyatt, GH, Haynes, RB, Jaeschke RZ, et al. Users' guides to the medical literature: XXV. Evidenced-based medicine: Principles for applying the users' guide to patient care. Journal of the American Medical Association, 284:1290–1296, 2000.

Haley, SM. Commentary on "The effect of walking with an assistive device and using a wheelchair on school performance in students with myelomeningocele." Physical Therapy, 71:577–578, 1991.

Haley, SM, Coster, WJ, Ludlow, IH, Haltiwanger, JT, & Andrellos, P. Pediatric Evaluation of Disability Inventory. Boston: PEDI Research Group, 1992.

Haley, SM, Stephens, TE, & Larsen, AM. Patterns of physical and occupational therapy implementation in early motor intervention. Topics in Early Childhood Special Education, 7(4):46–63, 1988.

Harbst, KB. Indicators of cerebral palsy 1985–1988. Physical and Occupational Therapy in Pediatrics, 10(3):85–107, 1990.

Hammell, KW, & Carpenter, C. Evidence-Based Practice in Rehabilitation: Informing Practice Through Qualitative Research. Edinburgh: Elsevier, 2004.

Harris, SR. Research techniques for the clinician. In Connolly, BH, & Montgomery, PC (Eds.). Therapeutic Exercise in Developmental Disabilities, 2nd ed. Hixson, TN: Chattanooga Group, 1993, pp. 211–220.

Harris, SR. How should treatments be critiqued for scientific merit? Physical Therapy, 76:175–181, 1996.

Harris, SR, & Riffle, K. Effects of inhibitive ankle-foot orthoses on standing balance in a child with cerebral palsy. Physical Therapy, 66:663–667, 1986.

Harrison, H. The principles for family-centered neonatal care. Pediatrics, 92:643–650, 1993.

Haynes, RB, Deveaux, PJ, & Guyatt, GH. Physician's and patients' choices in evidenced-based practice. British Medical Journal, 324:1350, 2002.

Hinderer, KA, Harris, SR, Purdy, AH, Chew, DE, Staheli, LT, McLaughlin, JF, & Jaffe, KM. Effects of "tone-reducing" vs. standard plaster casts on gait improvement of children with cerebral palsy. Developmental Medicine and Child Neurology, 30:370–377, 1988.

Horn, EM, Warren, SF, & Jones, HA. An experimental analysis of neurobehavioral motor intervention. Developmental Medicine and Child Neurology, 37:697–714, 1997.

Human Services Research Unit. Consumer's Guide: Therapeutic Services for Children with Disabilities. Cambridge, MA: Human Services Research Institute, 1995.

Jenkins, D. A practical introduction to databases: Part 2. Biomedical Instrumentation and Technology, 23:109–112, 1989.

Jones MA, McEwen IR, & Hansen L. Use of power mobility for a young child with spinal muscular atrophy. Physical Therapy, 83:253–262, 2003.

Kanda, T, Yuge, M, & Yamori, Y. Early physiotherapy in the treatment of spastic diplegia. Developmental Medicine and Child Neurology, 26:438–444, 1984.

Karman, N, Maryles, J, Baker, RW, Simpser, E, & Berger-Gross, P. Constraint-induced movement therapy for hemiplegic children with acquired brain injuries. Journal of Head Trauma & Rehabilitation, 18:259–267, 2003.

Ketelaar, M, Vermeer, A, t'Hart, H, van Petegem-van Beek, E, & Helders, PJM. Effects of a functional therapy program on motor abilities of children with cerebral palsy. Physical Therapy, 81:1534–1545, 2001.

King, GA, King, SM, & Rosenbaum, PL. Interpersonal aspects of caregiving and client outcomes: A review of the literature. Ambulatory and Child Health, 2:151–160, 1996.

Kopp, CB. Developmental risk: Historical reflections. In Osofsky, JD (Ed.). Handbook of Infant Development. New York: Wiley, 1987, pp. 881–912.

Knafl KA, Ayres L, Gallo AM, Zoeller LH, & Breitmayer BJ. Learning from stories: Parents' accounts of the pathway to diagnosis. Pediatric Nursing, 21:411–415, 1995.

Lansky, D, Butler, JBV, & Waller, FT. Using health status measures in the hospital setting: From acute care to outcome management. Medical Care, 30(5 suppl):MS57–MS73, 1992.

Laskas, SA, Mullen, SL, Nelson, DL, & Willson-Broyles, M. Enhancement of two motor functions of the lower extremity in a child with spastic quadriplegia. Physical Therapy, 65:11–16, 1985.

Law M (Ed.). Evidence-Based Rehabilitation: A Guide to Practice. Thorofare, NJ: Slack Inc., 2002a, pp. 305–338.

Law M (Ed.). Building evidence in practice. In Evidence-Based Rehabilitation: A Guide to Practice. Thorofare, NJ: Slack Inc., 2002b, pp. 185–194.

Law, M, Baptiste, S, Carswell-Opzoomer, A, McColl, MA, Polatajko, H, & Pollack, N. Canadian Occupational Performance Measure Manual. Toronto, CA: CAOT Publications, 1991.

Lehmann, JF, Warren, CG, Smith, W, & Larson, J. Computerized data management as an aid to clinical decision making in rehabilitation medicine. Archives of Physical Medicine and Rehabilitation, 65:260–262, 1984.

Lou, JQ. Searching for the evidence. In Law M (Ed.). Evidence-Based Rehabilitation: A Guide to Practice. Thorofare, NJ: Slack Inc., 2002, pp. 71–94.

Magistro, CM. Clinical decision making in physical therapy. Physical Therapy, 69:525–534, 1989.

Mattingly, C. What is clinical reasoning? American Journal of Occupational Therapy, 45:979–986, 1991.

McEwen, I. (Ed.) Writing Case Reports: A How-To Manual for Clinicians, 2nd ed. Alexandria, VA: American Physical Therapy Association, 2001.

McEwen, I. (Ed.). Providing Physical Therapy Services Under Parts B & C of the Individuals with Disabilities Education Act (IDEA). Fairfax, VA: Section on Pediatrics, American Physical Therapy Association, 2000.

McLaughlin J, Bjornson K, Temkin N, Steinbok P, Wright V, Reiner A, Roberts T, Drake J, O'Donnell M, Rosenbaum P, Barber T, & Ferrel A. Selective dorsal rhizotomy: Meta-analysis of three randomized controlled trials. Developmental Medicine and Child Neurology, 44(1):17–25, 2002.

Misor, WF. Applying a meta-analysis to daily clinical practice. In Geyman , JP, Deyo, RA, & Ramsey, SD (Eds.). Evidence-Based Clinical Practice: Concepts and Procedures. Woburn, MA: Butterworth-Heinemann, 2000, pp. 57–64.

Morris, C, & Bartlett, D. Gross Motor Function Classification System: Impact and utility. Developmental Medicine and Child Neurology, 46:60–65, 2004.

National Institutes of Health. Research Plan for the National Center for Medical Rehabilitation Research. NIH Publication No. 93-3509. Bethesda, MD: National Institutes of Health, 1993.

Nelson, KB, & Ellenberg, JH. Children who "outgrew" cerebral palsy. Pediatrics, 69:529–536, 1982.

Norton, BJ, & Strube, MJ. Making decisions based on group designs and meta-analysis. Physical Therapy, 69:594–600, 1989.

Ottenbacher, KJ. Evaluating Clinical Change: Strategies for Occupational and Physical Therapists. Baltimore: Williams & Wilkins, 1986.

Palisano, RJ. Comparison of two methods of service delivery for students with learning disabilities. Physical and Occupational Therapy in Pediatrics, 9(3):79–100, 1989.

Palisano, R, Rosenbaum, P, Walter, S, Russell, D, Wood, E, & Galuppi, B. Development and reliability of a system to classify gross motor function of children with cerebral palsy. Developmental Medicine and Child Neurology, 39:214–223, 1997.

Palisano, RJ, Hanna, S, Rosenbaum, P, et al. Validation of a model of motor development for children with cerebral palsy. Physical Therapy, 80:974–985, 2000.

Palisano, RJ, Walters, S, Russell, D, Rosenbaum, P, Gemus, M, Galuppi, B, & Cunningham, L. Gross motor function of children with Down syndrome: Creation of motor growth curves. Archives of Physical Medicine and Rehabilitation, 82:494–500, 2001.

Palisano, RJ, Tieman, BL, Walter, SD, et al. Effect of environmental setting on mobility methods of children with cerebral palsy. Developmental Medicine and Child Neurology, 45:113–120, 2003.

Piper, MC, Darrah, J, Pinnell, L, Watt, MJ, & Byrne, P. The consistency of sequential examinations in the early detection of neurological dysfunction. Physical and Occupational Therapy in Pediatrics, 11(3):27–44, 1991.

Portney, LG & Watkins, MP. Single subject designs. In Foundations of Clinical Research: Applications to Practice, 2nd ed. Philadelphia: W.B. Saunders, 2000, pp. 223–264.

Prechtl HFR, Einspieler C, Cioni G, Bos AF, Ferrari F, & Sontheimer D. An early marker for neurological deficits after perinatal brain lesions. Lancet, 349:1361–1363, 1997.

Purdy, AH, Deitz, JC, & Harris, SR. Efficacy of two treatment approaches to reduce tongue protrusion of children with Down syndrome. Developmental Medicine and Child Neurology, 29:469–476, 1987.

Randall, KE, & McEwen, IR. Writing patient-centered functional goals. Physical Therapy, 80:1197–1203, 2000.

Ritchie, JE. Using qualitative research to enhance the evidenced-based practice of health care providers. Australian Journal of Physiotherapy, 45:251–256, 1999.

Rogers, J, & Masagatani, G. Clinical reasoning of occupational therapists during the initial assessment of physically disabled patients. Occupational Therapy Journal of Research, 2:195–219, 1982.

Rosenbaum, PL, King, S, Law, M, King, G, & Evans, J. Family-centered service: A conceptual framework and research review. Physical and Occupational Therapy in Pediatrics, 18(1):1–20, 1998.

Rosenbaum, PL, Walter, SD, Hanna, SE, Palisano, RJ, Russell, DJ, & Raina, P. Prognosis for gross motor function in cerebral palsy: Creation of motor development curves. Journal of the American Medical Association, 288:1357–1363, 2002.

Rosenblith, JF. A singular career: Nancy Bayley. Developmental Psychology, 28:747–758, 1992.

Rothstein, JM, & Echternach, JL. Hypothesis-oriented algorithm for clinicians: A method for evaluation and treatment planning. Physical Therapy, 66:1388–1394, 1986.

Rothstein, JM, Echternach, JL, & Riddle DL. Hypothesis-oriented algorithm for clinicians II (HOAC II): A guide for patient management. Physical Therapy, 83:455–470, 2003.

Russell, D J, Rosenbaum, PL, Avery, L, & Lane, M. Gross Motor Function Measure (GMFM-66 & GMFM-88) User's Manual: Clinics in Developmental Medicine No 159. London, England: Mac Keith Press, 2002.

Sackett, DL, Haynes, RB, & Tugwell, P. Clinical Epidemiology: A Basic Science for Clinical Medicine. Boston: Little, Brown, 1985.

Sackett DL. Rules of evidence and clinical recommendations on use of antithrombotic agents. Chest, 89(2 suppl.):2S–3S, 1986.

Sackett, DL, Rosenberg, WMC, Gray, JAM, Haynes, RB, & Richardson, WS. Evidence based medicine: What it is and what it isn't. British Medical Journal, 312:71–72, 1996.

Sackett, DL, Strauss, SE, Richardson, WS, et al. Evidence-Based Medicine: How to Practice and Teach EBM, 2nd ed. New York, NY: Churchill Livingstone, 2000, p 1.

Scalzitti, DA. Evidence-based guidelines: Application to clinical practice. Physical Therapy, 81:1622–1628, 2001.

Schyve, PM. The evolving role of the Joint Commission for the Accreditation of Health Care Organizations. Joint Commission Journal on Quality Improvement, 11:S54–S57, 1996.

Shadish, WR, Jr, Cook, TD, & Leviton, LC. Foundations of Program Evaluation: Theories of Practice. Newbury Park, CA: Sage, 1991.

Shurtleff, DB. Computer databases for pediatric disability: Clinical and research applications. Physical Medicine and Rehabilitation Clinics of North America, 2:665–687, 1991.

Simpson, M, Buckman, R, Stewart, M, Magyar, P, Lipkin, M, Novak, D, & Till, J. Doctor-patient communication: The Toronto consensus statement. British Medical Journal, 303:1385–1387, 1991.

Singer, GHS, Marquis J, Powers, L, Blanchard, L, DiVenere, N, Santelli, B, & Sharp, M. A multi-site evaluation of parent to parent programs for parents of children with disabilities. Journal of Early Intervention, 22(3):217–229, 1999.

Slagle, TA, & Gould, JB. Database use in neonatal intensive care units: Success or failure. Pediatrics, 90:959–965, 1992.

Slovick, P, & Lichtenstein, S. Comparison of Bayesian and regression approaches to the study of information processing in judgment. Organizational Behavior and Human Performance, 6:649–744, 1971.

Stewart, M, Brown, JB, Boon, H, Galajda, J, Meredith, L, & Sangster, M. Evidence on doctor-patient communication. Cancer Prevention & Control, 3:25–30, 1999.

Sweeney, JK, Heriza, CB, Reilly, MA, Smith C, & VanSant AF. Practice guidelines for the physical therapist in the neonatal intensive care unit (NICU). Pediatric Physical Therapy, 11:119–132, 1999.

Thomson-O'Brien, MA, & Moreland, J. Evidence-based information circle. Physiotherapy Canada, Summer 1998, pp. 184–189.

Tieman, BL, Palisano, RJ, Gracely, EJ, & Rosenbaum, PL. Gross motor capability and performance of mobility in children with cerebral palsy: A comparison across home, school, and outdoors/community settings. Physical Therapy, 84:419–429, 2004.

Tiffin, J. Purdue Pegboard Examiner Manual. Chicago: Scientific Research Associates, 1968.

U.S. Department of Health and Human Services. Clinical Practice Guideline Number 16: Post-Stroke Rehabilitation, Rockville, MD: Agency for Health Care Policy and Research, 1995, pp. 18–21.

Vargas S, & Camilli G. A meta-analysis of research on sensory integration treatment. American Journal of Occupational Therapy, 53(2):189–198, 1999.

Wang, MC, & Ellet, CD. Program validation: The state of the art. Topics in Early Childhood Special Education, 1(4):35–49, 1982.

Waters, RL, & Lunsford, BR. Energy cost of paraplegic locomotion. Journal of Bone and Joint Surgery (American), 67:1245–1250, 1985.

Watts, N. Decision analysis: A tool for improving physical therapy practice and education. In Wolf, SL (Ed.). Clinical Decision Making in Physical Therapy. Philadelphia: FA Davis, 1985, pp. 7–23.

Weston, WW. Informed and shared decision-making: The crux of patient-centred care. Canadian Medical Association Journal, 165:438–439, 2001.

Wolery, M, & Bailey, DD. Alternatives to impact evaluation: Suggestions for program evaluation in early intervention. Journal of the Division for Early Childhood, 4:27–37, 1984.

Wood, E, & Rosenbaum, P. The gross motor function classification system for cerebral palsy: A study of reliability and stability over time. Developmental Medicine and Child Neurology, 42:292–296, 2000.

World Health Organization. International Classification of Function, Disability, and Health. Geneva: World Health Organization, 2001.

Chapter 2

The Child's Development of Functional Movement

Suzann K. Campbell
PT, PhD, FAPTA

Working knowledge of motor development is the very basis of the practice of pediatric physical therapy. It provides the norms for functioning of children at various ages that guide diagnosis and treatment planning through emphasis on selection of age-appropriate skills as functional outcomes. Development of effective plans of care for children also requires knowledge of the cognitive milestones that must be recognized in order to provide intervention in a stimulating and motivating environment and to take advantage of interactions among cognitive, perceptual, and motor development. Developing such an environment for the provision of intervention typically involves use of adapted play activities at a cognitive level appropriate for an individual child, regardless of the child's level of motor development. The challenge is perhaps greatest when motor and cognitive levels in a particular child are exceedingly different.

Movement, on the other hand, also promotes cognitive and perceptual development (Anderson et al., 2001; Bertenthal & Campos, 1987). The two go hand in hand to foster functional performance. Therapists must consider in their intervention planning how to structure therapy to facilitate best all aspects of their clients' development and to take advantage of the interactive nature of developmental subsystems, especially when activity limitations are present and likely to be lifelong. The *Guide to Physical Therapist Practice* (American Physical Therapy Association, 2001) suggests that goals of therapy should focus on treatment of impairments (e.g., strength, endurance, or range of motion), but anticipated outcomes of intervention should include minimization of functional and activity limitations, optimization of health status, prevention of disability in daily life, and consumer satisfaction (see Chapter 1). Nevertheless, when to emphasize treatment of physical impairments and activity limitations through exercise and other therapeutic modalities, when to concentrate on finding compensatory means to promote participation in a variety of social and developmental areas, and when to combine the two are important considerations in an ongoing debate among practitioners.

In order to contribute to this debate, the specific purposes of this chapter are to describe the important milestones in the development of functional movement in children and to introduce a discussion of the processes by which development occurs, which will be elaborated on in Chapter 3 on motor control. It seems appropriate first to define what is meant by functional movement and activity. Fisher (1992) has reviewed the various meanings of the term "function" that rehabilitation professionals have used in the design and evaluation of tests and measures. Function is variously described as having a definite end or purpose and as being goal directed and meaningful. A functional limitation represents a failure of the individual's performance to meet a standard expectation. In the language of the International Classification of Function, Disability and Health (ICF) functional limitations impair activity (World Health Organization, 2001). When permanent, functional or activity limitations result in a reduction in behavioral skills, task accomplishment, or fulfillment of appropriate social roles. The alleviation of effects of activity limitations on behavior or social roles is defined for the purposes of this volume as the promotion of participation (see Chapter 1 on clinical decision making for further elaboration of ICF definitions). In rehabilitation, impaired functional performance resulting in disabilities is frequently evaluated by examining the degree of assistance the client needs to perform activities of daily living (ADL). The use of technology to compensate for functional limitations and promote activity, however, means that participation in age-appropriate social roles can be achieved through alternative means to promote quality of life (Butler, 1991).

Certainly all therapists would agree that ADL should be considered under the rubric of "functional activity." But children engage in many meaningful movement activities that appear to lack a well-defined goal. Spinning, bouncing, and endless repetition of newly learned movements, such as going up and down steps and putting things into containers and taking them out, are just a few examples (Shirley, 1931). We would probably call this "play" or "practice," but regardless of terminology, therapists surely see these activities as important aspects of motor development, motor learning, and environmental mastery. In other words, they represent functional activities for the child's stage of development despite their lacking apparent goals. Repetition of motor behaviors might serve a variety of useful functions, such as muscle strengthening, trial of a variety of approaches to assembling effective task-related movements, testing the limits of balance, and learning to deal with the reactive forces produced elsewhere in the body by muscle contraction of

prime movers for a particular activity. Certainly, children demonstrate a remarkable intensity of purpose when practicing emerging skills. Vander Linden (personal communication, 1993) provides several examples of his daughter Abby's development. Abby played almost compulsively with nesting cups for about 2 weeks, and when she could nest all 10, she was no longer interested in them. Similarly, she repeatedly went up and down a 4-inch step onto a screened porch in their home, insisting that her parents open the porch door for her to access the porch for stepping practice and resisting enticements to play with toys instead.

Based on many observations such as these, the definition provided by Fisher (1992) that I prefer is that functional activity, or occupation, in the framework of occupational therapy theory and practice, is "what people do" (p. 184). These words imply that movements are self-chosen, self-directed, and, therefore, meaningful in the life of the individual at his or her particular place in the life cycle (Fisher, 1992; Oppenheim, 1981). Given this definition, our descriptive presentation will review information regarding what children do and the general order in which they do it, beginning with infants' spontaneously generated, that is, self-directed, movements and gradually incorporating information on tasks that are easier for adults to identify as purposeful and goal directed.

In keeping with the importance to pediatric physical therapists of knowledge of functional motor development, the main objectives of this chapter are to (1) briefly review the history of theories of motor development, (2) describe current information and hypotheses regarding general processes and principles of motor development, and (3) provide an overview of the developmental course of acquisition of upright posture and mobility and of object manipulation—the two most basic functions that underlie meaningful movement activities. Brief attention will be paid to issues in cognitive development, play, and the interaction of motor skill acquisition and perceptual-cognitive development, including memory for activities. The chapter concludes with an abbreviated review of tests of motor development and functional motor behavior of use to physical therapists from the point of view of the theoretic perspectives provided in earlier parts of the chapter.

MOTOR DEVELOPMENT THEORIES

Throughout the history of physical therapy, theories of child development have changed dramatically, eliciting successive revisions of intervention approaches to maximizing motor development and activity in children. Underlying the changes in developmental theory are differing conceptualizations of the respective roles of changing structure and function within the individual and of the influence of the environment on the developmental course. Thelen and colleagues (1987) summarized the major theoretic approaches as encompassing three theories: (1) neural-maturationist, (2) cognitive, and (3) dynamical systems. Each has an interesting history that in itself makes fascinating reading because of the strong role that changing biases and accumulation of new knowledge play in how research efforts are designed and how their results are interpreted and judged (Bergenn et al., 1992; Thelen, 1995; Thelen & Adolph, 1992). These theories are reviewed briefly in this chapter, and their major distinguishing features are summarized in Table 2-1. Further elaboration can be found in Chapter 3 on motor control.

NEURAL-MATURATIONIST THEORIES

The neural-maturationist point of view was pioneered by Gesell (1928a, 1928b, 1945; Gesell et al., 1934, 1940, 1975), Shirley (1931), and others. This view proposed that the ontogeny of behavior is "an intrinsic property of the organism, with maturation leading to an unfolding of predetermined patterns, supported, but not fundamentally altered by the environment" (Thelen et al., 1987, p. 40). According to this approach, functional behaviors appear as the nervous system matures, with more complex behaviors being based on the activity of progressively higher levels of the nervous system. This theory, therefore, depends on the assumption of hierarchic maturation of neural control structures.

Gesell's point of view and research findings resulted in the development of important tests of motor milestones

TABLE 2-1	**Comparison of Developmental Theories**			
	NEURAL-MATURATIONIST	**COGNITIVE: BEHAVIORAL**	**COGNITIVE: PIAGETIAN**	**DYNAMICAL SYSTEMS**
View on "stages"	Stages of motor development occur as a result of CNS maturation	Stages are merely empirical descriptions of behavior	Stages represent alternating periods of equilibrium and disequilibrium	Apparent stages of development are actually states of relative stability arising from the self-organizing, emergent properties of a multitude of systems, each developing at its own continuous rate
Driving forces for development	Development spirals with alternating periods of flexor vs. extensor dominance and symmetry vs. asymmetry based on maturation of the CNS	Development occurs through interaction of the individual with the environment	Development occurs through interaction between cognitive-neural structures and environmental opportunities for action	The individual develops as the organism recognizes the affordances of the environment and selects (self-organizes) the most appropriate available responses to tasks
Building blocks of development	Reflexes	Pavlovian and operant responses to environmental stimuli	First actions using reflexes and later from voluntary actions	Multiple cooperating systems with individual rates of development and self-motivated exploration of the environment

and other adaptive behaviors that have had, and continue to have, a monumental influence on practice in the area of diagnosis of developmental delay or deviance (Thelen & Adolph, 1992). Virtually all subsequent tests of development contained items derived from Gesell's work. Gesell emphatically believed in stages of development as biologic imperatives. Although he recognized that there are individual differences among children and was a strong believer in freedom of human action, he never resolved the paradox between these beliefs and his insistence on maturation as the predominant force driving development.

Thelen and Adolph (1992) pointed out, however, that among Gesell's less remembered contributions is the idea that the nature of development forms a spiraling function, with alternations between extremes in a variety of behavioral realms, including alternating dominance between flexor and extensor muscle activity. He believed in a principle of functional asymmetry in which the child must break free of symmetric movement patterns to achieve functional goals such as manipulation.

Pediatric physical therapy developed according to this theoretic model. As a result, emphasis was placed on examination of stages of reflex development and motor milestones as reflections of increasingly higher levels of neural maturation (Horak, 1991). Treatment of the child with central nervous system (CNS) dysfunction was organized around inhibition of primary reflexes that were believed to persist and produce activity limitations, along with facilitation of righting and equilibrium reactions that were supposedly the underlying coordinative structures for development of skilled voluntary motor behavior. It was generally assumed that functional outcomes would naturally follow.

COGNITIVE THEORIES

Cognitive theories of motor skill development are of two types. One is based on the approach of B.F. Skinner and the other on J. Piaget.

Behavioral Theory

Skinner (1972) developed a behavioral approach to development that emphasizes the importance of contingent learning and posits reinforcement from the environment as the motivator and shaper of both motor and cognitive development (see also Bijou, 1989; Catania & Harnad, 1988). In this theoretic approach, the environment is the site of developmental control.

In more contemporary developmental psychology, behavioral analysis theory was based on Skinner's later radical behaviorism and on the interbehaviorism of

Kantor, in which the developing individual is conceived of as a pattern of psychologic responses in interaction with the environment (Bijou, 1989). Progressions in development depend on opportunities and circumstances inherent in the individual's makeup and in his or her past and present physical and social environments. Developmental progress occurs through Pavlovian responses to previous stimulation and by operant processes in which responses are controlled by consequences. Operant responses are acquired and maintained by contingent stimuli with acquired or primary reinforcing functions, and the strength of these interactions is affected by conditions such as timing and frequency of reinforcements. Although sometimes misused, behavior modification approaches have greatly aided the training of specific skills for children with mental retardation (Bijou, 1989), and the knowledge base of the behavioral approach helped therapists to break down skills into component parts for easier learning by children with impaired neural control mechanisms. Angulo-Kinzler (2001) used a behavioral approach to demonstrate the ability of 3-month-old infants to discover and adopt specific solutions to a movement problem—kicking within an experimenter-specified range of motion. Clinical problems are approached based on the beliefs that each problem has its unique history and that the intervention program should be individually tailored to the specific problem behavior.

A frequently misunderstood aspect of behavioral analysis theory is the role of individuals in their own development. The individual is not perceived of as passive and responding only when stimulated. Rather, the individual is considered to be adjusting in continual interaction with the environment. The critical feature of this theory is that it is a psychology of the individual in interaction with the environment. Unlike Gesell's concept of development (Gesell, 1945), stages of development are considered to be merely empirical descriptions and not in any sense causal explanations of behavior. The research methodology of behavioral analysis is, therefore, one of single-subject designs or within-subject comparisons designed to demonstrate functional relationships rather than to test theories. The elaboration of such designs has been a significant contribution to clinical research science in physical therapy.

Piagetian Theory

A second cognitive theory based primarily on the work of Piaget (1952) emphasizes an interaction between maturation of cognitive-neural structures and environmental opportunities to promote action (Beilin, 1989; Flavell, 1963). Control functions are found in the development of higher-level plans based on biologic structures, termed schemata in Piagetian theory or motor programs or subroutines in motor control theory (Bruner, 1970; Connolly, 1970; see also Chapter 4). Cognitive mechanisms of all types are believed to derive from knowledge gained through action based at first on innate hereditary reflexes and instinctual capacities and later on experience forming concrete intelligent operations. Cognitive development culminates in abstract intelligence based on coordination of fundamental cognitive operations.

Piagetian theory had little effect on pediatric physical therapy from the perspective of planning the motor aspects of therapeutic programming because it was primarily a cognitive theory and because it continued to emphasize the evolution of functional behaviors from reflexive movements. These movements were believed to be practiced and coordinated with developing mental structures. Adaptive responses were thought to develop through psychologic processes interacting with maturation of neural structures. In this view, the most important processes are successive equilibrium, disequilibrium, and re-equilibration, resulting from the interaction of maturation and experience. An important aspect of Piagetian theory is the view of the individual as possessing a self-regulating system of psychologic processes that provides balance between assimilation of environmental experiences and accommodation of existing cognitive structures to that experience. The individual is a homeorrhetic system that, by virtue of its self-regulating characteristics, constantly adjusts itself to maintain equilibrium despite disturbances from the environment, thus driving developmental progress. Viewing the operation of these psychologic processes in children who were observed while solving interesting problems led to theories of the mental structures constructed by children as a result of their activity. Neo-Piagetian work has emphasized research on the functioning of these psychologic processes (Beilin, 1989).

The concept of stages played a major role in early Piagetian theory, although in his later conceptions of development, when faced with evidence contradicting some of his hypotheses, he realized that stage theory tended to lead one to think in terms of periods of rest or equilibrium, whereas development was, in fact, never static (Beilin, 1989). In later years, Piaget, like Gesell, tended to see development as a spiraling process, an important principle that we will return to later. Description of stages nonetheless forms the framework for discussions of development of cognitive systems in Piagetian theory.

Four main stages were posited, each with multiple substages. The first is the stage of sensorimotor intelligence from birth to about 18 to 24 months (Beilin, 1989). Repetition in action is a major factor in this stage, culminating in the major achievement of symbolic functioning.

The second period of representational thought, from 1.5 to 2 through 6 years of age, involves the development of language and of one-way mappings of logical thought that allow classifications to be developed. (Current work on classifications suggests that they can be performed perceptually much earlier than Piaget projected, probably as early as 3 months of age in a primitive form [Hayne et al., 1987].) Experiments detailing the errors of logical thought in this period were influential in revealing the lack of sophistication in children's mental constructions that was not previously obvious. In the third period of concrete operations, thought processes become reversible, allowing conservation of number, weight, and volume under transformation conditions. In the final period of cognitive development, formal operations beginning at about age 11 permit logical thinking in a hypothetico-deductive mode.

The impact of Piagetian theory on pediatric physical therapy was primarily on the inclusion of interesting spectacles and problem-solving activities in therapeutic programs to assist in the cognitive-motivational aspects of facilitating motor development. Therapists used problems such as the search for hidden objects (object permanence) and problems involving means-ends relationships and container-contained ideas as therapeutic media to motivate children to move and to examine and promote the perceptual-cognitive aspects of development and motor learning (Campbell & Wilson, 1976; Fetters, 1981).

DYNAMICAL SYSTEMS THEORY

Thelen and colleagues (Thelen, 1995; Thelen & Corbetta, 1994; Thelen & Ulrich, 1991; Thelen et al., 1987, 1989, 1993; Ulrich, 1989) have proposed a dynamical functional perspective on motor development that currently drives most research on motor development. Dynamical systems theory emphasizes process rather than product or hierarchically structured plans and places neural maturation on an equal plane with other structures and processes that interact to promote motor development. These "structures become progressively integrated with the self-organized properties of the system" (Thelen et al., 1987, p. 41) to gradually optimize skilled function. Cooperating systems include musculoskeletal components, sensory systems, central sensorimotor integrative mechanisms, and arousal and motivation (see Chapter 3) (Heriza, 1991; Horak, 1991; Shumway-Cook & Woollacott, 1985, 1993; Thelen et al., 1987). In this theoretic approach, both these internal components of the organism and the external context of the task are equivalent in determining the outcome of behavior because behavior is task-specific. In this model of infant motor development, therefore, the environment is as important as the organism. Because, however, the infant's cooperating systems, such as those involving strength and postural control, do not develop at the same rate, certain components are seen as rate limiting or constraining to the performance of any specific behavior.

In a seminal paper in the physical therapy literature, Heriza (1991) described the basic concepts of dynamical systems theory and suggested various approaches to testing its utility in planning and assessing the outcomes of therapeutic interventions. For example, eight subsystems are postulated to be involved in the development of infant locomotion:

1. Pattern generation of the coordinative structure leading to reciprocal lower extremity activity, consisting primarily of alternating flexor muscle activation
2. Development of reciprocal muscle activity of flexor and extensor muscles
3. Strength of extensor muscles needed for opposing the force of gravity
4. Changes in body size and composition
5. Antigravity control of upright posture of the head and trunk
6. Appropriate decoupling of the tight synchronization characteristic of early reciprocal lower extremity movements, such that the knee moves out of phase with the hip and ankle
7. Visual flow sensitivity required to maintain posture while moving through the environment
8. Ability to recognize the requirements of the task and be motivated to move toward a goal

This listing makes it clear that the development of a particular motor pattern, in this case upright locomotion, depends on a combination of mechanical, neurologic, cognitive, and perceptual factors in addition to environmental contributions specific to both the task and the context of the infant's action. Each of the subsystems develops at its own rate but is constrained or supported by physical and environmental factors, such as a nutritional diet, especially one that is adequate in iron (Lynch & Stoltzfus, 2003; Morbidity & Mortality Weekly Report, 2002) and experiences providing the opportunity to practice antigravity trunk extension while prone, standing upright, and stepping. For example, since the implementation of advice to encourage parents to have infants sleep on their back (American Academy of Pediatrics Task Force on Infant Positioning and SIDS, 1992), investigators have shown that back-sleeping infants are less likely to roll over at 4 months of age than infants who sleep in the prone position (Jantz et al., 1997) and have lower developmental scores at 6 months of age (Dewey et al., 1998), a difference that was no longer apparent at 18 months. Sleep position in a group of premature infants also affected ability to maintain the head elevated and lower it

with control at 56 weeks' postconceptional age, although global developmental was not affected (Ratliff-Schaub et al., 2001). Salls and colleagues (2002) reported that 2-month-old infants who spent 15 minutes or less awake time in the prone position differed significantly in gross motor milestone attainment from the normative population for the Denver II test. Changing the environment available to the infant for practicing movements as a result of medical recommendations to prevent sudden infant death syndrome (SIDS) appears to have altered the timing of motor development.

In the dynamical systems view of development, the movements of locomotion are conceived not as derived from a set of instructions from the nervous system nor as built from chains of reflexes but as self-organizing and emergent as a result of the interaction of the subsystems described. The locus of control for function shifts over time, depending on the dominance or constraints of various subsystems. Spontaneous exploration of movement possibilities and flexible selection of the most appropriate movement synergy for accomplishing goal-directed actions are key processes in development in the view of the proponents of dynamical systems theory (Thelen & Corbetta, 1994). Transitional periods, when movement patterns appear more variable, are thought to be sensitive periods in development when intervention might be particularly effective. Research is needed to identify these sensitive periods in the development of specific functional behaviors, thereby providing new knowledge to guide intervention by therapists.

Based on dynamical systems theory, developmental change is seen not as a series of discrete stages but as a series of states of stability, instability, and phase shifts in which new states become stable aspects of behavior (Thelen, 1995). Research involves the search for collective variables or patterns of behavior that reflect the action of the component parts involved in a particular environment or task context (Newell & Vaillancourt, 2001). An example of research designed to identify the collective variables that might show qualitative change as new movement patterns appear, as well as the control variables that limit or facilitate the transition between patterns, is the work on the developmental transition between walking and running of Whitall and Getchell (1995).

Although running has generally been described as differing from walking in having a flight phase, Whitall and Getchell (1995) did not find this to be the case in the early development of running. Nor could they find another variable that differed significantly between the two patterns of movement, suggesting that the transition was really one between two similar movements and not two qualitatively different patterns at all. These researchers recommended that the search for a collective variable for describing the qualitative difference between walking and running should be continued by assessing the possible role of arm movements. Young runners had difficulty generating both horizontal forces (reflected in a small increase in stride length over that used in walking) and vertical forces (reflected in little flight and little hip extension in running). Whitall and Getchell (1995) surmised that the ability to produce or regulate force by the ankle extensors was a key control parameter for emergence of running. They suggested that another control parameter might be ability to organize posture during high-velocity movement.

A dynamical systems approach to studying the transition from reaching without grasping to reaching with grasping was more successful in showing a sharp transition from predominant use of one pattern to predominant use of the other over a period of approximately 1 to 2 weeks (Wimmers et al., 1998a, 1998b). In keeping with the prediction of dynamical systems theory, in the weeks just before the shift from predominance of one mode of reaching to the other, infants showed instability of mode choice; that is, they frequently switched between types of reaching during a single session of reaching opportunities (Wimmers et al., 1998a). Individual infants demonstrated the phase shift at different ages (usually between 13 and 20 weeks of age), and a search for control parameters driving the change showed that arm weight and arm circumference (which increased with age in a continuous, linear fashion) were significantly related to the change in preferred mode of reaching (Wimmers et al., 1998b). Computer modeling of infant grasp learning is also revealing how the infant grasp reflex can be shaped to achieve a variety of arm movements leading to successful grasping without the need for visual guidance (Oztop et al., 2004), bringing back the old question of whether voluntary movements are derived from reflexes. The model proposes that two assumptions are sufficient for an infant to learn effective grasping: that infants can sense the effects of their motor activity and can use feedback to adjust movement planning parameters.

Although use of dynamical systems theory to drive therapeutic theory and practice in physical therapy is still in its infancy (Tscharnuter, 1993), it is already clear that this model focuses the attention of the therapist on a number of important aspects of the therapeutic process of facilitating functional activity and participation. These aspects include (1) search for the constraints in subsystems that limit motor behavior, such as contractures or weakness, leading to treatment goals related to reduction of impairments; (2) creation of an environment that supports or compensates for weaker or less mature (rate-limiting) components of the systems that contribute to

development of motor control so as to promote activity and participation; (3) attention to setting up a therapeutic environment that affords opportunities to practice tasks in a meaningful and functional context; (4) use of activities that promote exploration of a variety of movement patterns that might be appropriate for a task; and (5) search for control parameters, such as speed of movement or force production, that can be manipulated by intervention to facilitate the attainment of therapeutic goals, especially during sensitive periods of development during which behavior is less stable (Fetters, 1991a, 1991b; Heriza, 1991). Chapter 3 on motor control and Chapter 4 on motor learning explore these concepts as therapeutic guides in more detail.

Myrtle McGraw, although generally considered a member of the maturationist school, developed a theory of motor development in the 1930s that contained the rudiments of many of the components of the modern dynamical systems approach to understanding the development of motor skills (Bergenn et al., 1992; McGraw, 1935). McGraw was a psychologist who studied the effects of intensive intervention, beginning at 20 days of age, with Johnny, the weaker of twin boys named Johnny and Jimmy. Her research was conducted at the height of the nature-nurture controversy between maturationists and behaviorists. In summary, her work showed that providing up to 7 hours a day of exercise of newly emerging developmental skills in the first year of life did not increase the rate of motor development. Her anecdotal comments, however, indicated that the exercised twin had more relaxed muscle tone and better coordination of movement than the twin whose movements and exploration had been restricted to a crib for much of the day, with no interaction with people other than for needed care.

McGraw's work was interpreted at the time as supporting the maturationist theory that the environment had little effect on child development. In the second year of his life, however, McGraw provided Johnny with a stimulating environment and extensive practice opportunities (3 hours per day) for developing motor skills that were not otherwise likely to develop in a child younger than 2 years, such as roller skating, climbing inclines of 70°, and jumping off high pedestals. Under these conditions, Johnny excelled in physical growth, problem solving of difficult motor control situations, and attainment of skills that Jimmy refused even to try during the periodic testing sessions that occurred. McGraw also noted the remarkable persistence in tasks demonstrated by Johnny, as well as his extensive visual review of the situation before embarking on a task. Films of the twins at age 40 years, moreover, demonstrated that the twin who exercised intensively during the first 2 years had an impressive physique and elegantly coordinated movement compared with those of his twin. In recounting her life's work and its interpretation by herself and others, McGraw illustrated how the biases of the times are reflected in how research results are interpreted and received.

Although the results of an analysis of two individual cases cannot be accepted as providing fundamental laws of motor development, McGraw's study makes it clear that we have little idea of the possibilities inherent in the very young child who is seldom stimulated to achieve the full potential of early motor skill development. By analogy, we can assume that we have barely scratched the surface in our understanding of how therapeutic intervention might be used to mitigate the effects of motor dysfunction. Research on treadmill training of infants (Bodkin et al., 2003; Ulrich et al., 2001), behavioral shaping of movement exploration efforts (Angulo-Kinzler, 2001), and mathematical modeling of developmental processes (Oztop et al., 2004) show promise for dramatically altering our approaches to intervention for children with disabilities in the future.

DEVELOPMENTAL PROCESSES AND PRINCIPLES

Based on her study of Johnny and Jimmy, as well as 68 other babies studied longitudinally without special intervention, McGraw constructed a set of developmental principles, many of which remain current (or are once again current) today. She conceived of movements as behaviors within an action system in which objects in the environment are as important a part of the action system as the movements themselves. "Any activity is composed of many ingredients, some of which may for convenience be considered as external and others as internal with respect to the organism, but none of these factors can be considered as external to the behavior" (McGraw, 1935, p. 303). McGraw also recognized that multiple components are interwoven in the development of behavior patterns (McGraw, 1935, pp. 302–303):

> The growing of a behavior pattern is likened to a design in the process of being woven, composed as it is of various colored threads. All of the threads do not move forward at the same time or at the same rate. The weaver picks up the gold thread and weaves it back and forth, though at the same time steadily forward. Then he drops it in order to bring the blue thread forward a distance, until finally the two become united to make the pattern complete. The design is contingent upon the interrelation of the various threads. It is not the summation of the

blue and gold threads but their position with respect to each other and to the piece as a whole that determines the design.

McGraw also described the uneven nature of development, in which a given behavior pattern has a period of "inception, incubation, consummation, and decline" (1935, p. 305). The results of her longitudinal studies on the intratask course of development of important motor patterns were published in 1945 (McGraw, 1963) and remain highly informative today (although her description of brain development itself has long been out of date). Because of her daily observations, she often saw a movement pattern appear only once or twice (examples of beginner's luck) and then disappear before becoming a stable part of the infant's repertoire. When first becoming stable, the activity seems overworked and exaggerated. Furthermore, she noted that "as the child begins to get control over a pattern or an aspect of a pattern, the activity itself becomes the incentive for repetition" (McGraw, 1935, p. 307). Thus, early in life, movement for the sake of movement is a functional activity.

Therapists who perceive these evanescent periods of self-driven motivation to practice emerging movements and who follow the lead of children in the flow of therapy are likely to be among those whose clients are both happy and productive in intervention sessions. Because children with disabilities may have fewer options for exploration of movement opportunities, it is important to note that research supports the importance of caregiver guidance in assisting children with self-discovery efforts. For example, young children with developmental disabilities do have mastery motivation (i.e., persistent task-directed behavior in moderately challenging problem-solving situations) that is similar to that of other children, but their level of motivation is related to their mental, rather than chronologic, age and is improved in those who experience high levels of adaptive interaction with their mothers (Blasco et al., 1990; Hauser-Cram, 1996).

McGraw suggested that a stable movement pattern may seem to disappear as a part of the child's repertoire, becoming superseded by some rapidly developing new behavior, but ultimately the movement is restricted to its most specific and economic form. She was among the first to note the presence of normal regressions in motor behavior and has been credited as one of the first developmental psychologists to recognize the bidirectionality of neural and behavioral development (Bergenn et al., 1992; Bevor, 1982; Oppenheim, 1981; Provost, 1981). A behavior may also become integrated with other behaviors to form a complex activity; thus, McGraw noted that the developmental course of a behavior may look quite different during different stages of its maturation. A "second wind" for a behavioral pattern in decline as a part of the movement repertoire was also noted.

Because McGraw noted these various characteristics across many developing movement patterns, she believed that fits and starts, spurts and regressions, and overlapping of patterns undergoing emergence, development, and decline were firm developmental principles and that snapshots of development, such as motor milestone tests, could not adequately reflect the underlying processes of development (Bergenn et al., 1992). McGraw firmly believed that there were sensitive periods (she actually used the term "critical period" but later regretted it because of its "use it or lose it permanently" interpretation in biology) in which interventions could produce the most influence on developing behavioral patterns (Bailey et al., 2001). During a sensitive period, certain experiences have particularly influential effects on development, although these effects are not necessarily irreversible or nonmodifiable with subsequent experience (Bruer, 2001). McGraw believed that the period of greatest susceptibility to exercise was one in which a behavior pattern was entering its most rapid phase of development. Delay did not mean that intervention could no longer affect the behavior pattern (the concept of critical period), but rather that the interference of other ongoing developmental programs, including changes in anthropometric configuration of the body with growth, can decrease effectiveness. Unfortunately, we still have little idea of how these developmental principles might be systematically applied in a therapeutic milieu, but dynamical systems theory has brought them back to the forefront of scientific thinking about the processes of motor development. When research provides prescriptions for most effectively structuring therapy based on a child's current repertoire and presence of instability in selection of behavioral response modes, readiness level for learning new skills, constraints that limit the possibility of change, and task or environmental characteristics that will be influential in evoking developmental progress, we are likely to make great strides in the efficient packaging of therapeutic programs (Bower & McLellan, 1992). Even more important will be knowledge that helps therapists to coach parents in effectively assisting children in their own self-initiated attempts to drive developmental progress.

McGraw ended her monumental study of human development by foreseeing the development and potential of dynamical systems–based motion analysis. "Perhaps the time will come when the movements of growth can be expressed in mathematical formulas as precisely as the movements of celestial bodies, but until that time arrives we shall have to be content with cumbersome descriptive analyses" (McGraw, 1935, p. 312). The work by Wimmers and colleagues (1998b) on the developmental transition between two modes of reaching and Oztop and colleagues' (2004) computational modeling of learning to grasp are just two examples of elegant quantitative descriptions of the processes of change during motor development that McGraw predicted.

CONTEMPORARY ISSUES IN UNDERSTANDING PRINCIPLES OF MOTOR DEVELOPMENT

Despite a new theoretic perspective that models development as encompassing multiple organismic components in the creation of coordinative structures for posture and movement and emphasizes the crucial role of the environment and task characteristics in organizing emergent movements, certain principles of motor development have consistently appeared in the conceptual framework of various students of motor development. These principles include the notions that development of motor skills generally proceeds in a cephalocaudal and proximodistal direction, that neural maturation is an important component of unfolding skill development, and that motor development appears, at least on the surface, to be more stagelike than continuous, having a spiraling nature in which regressions, consolidations, and reappearances of underlying fundamental processes occur (Bevor, 1982).

What is becoming clear is that these long-standing theoretic concepts must be expanded to incorporate a new understanding of the underlying developmental processes. For example, new research on developmental processes discussed in Chapter 3 on motor control has revealed that certain factors are rate limiting to motor development, with strength, postural control, and perceptual analysis capabilities being among the most important. When compensations are provided experimentally to eliminate the effects of these rate-limiting factors, the developing motor system may display previously unrecognized potential. Patterns of movement appear that seem precocious because they were previously denied expression owing to immaturity of certain of the cooperating systems.

Dynamical systems theory has also demonstrated that stagelike external behavior, such as the switch from reaching without grasping to reaching with grasping (Wimmers et al., 1998a, 1998b) can emerge from continuously changing underlying processes. Here a new stage seems to appear de novo only because the continuous developments of a number of cooperating systems finally merge in a way that allows the new behavior to appear. The behavior appears to reflect an entirely novel stage of development when in fact the underlying processes in multiple systems were developing continuously in a gradually accretive fashion. We will use more information about the development of eye-hand coordination to illustrate these points.

Cephalocaudal and Proximodistal Developmental Direction

The processes involved in the advanced stages of development of functional reaching include (1) visual fixation to localize the object and choose a hand transport program, (2) foveal analysis for perceptual identification of the object needed for anticipatory adaptation of the action to fit the characteristics of the object, (3) manual capture, and (4) object manipulation (Hay, 1990). By the time of birth, a primitive body scheme has already developed that provides the infant with a hand transport program. Infants have been observed in utero during real-time ultrasound imaging to perform hand-to-mouth activities, touch other parts of their own bodies, and explore the uterine walls—all, of course, without visual guidance (Sparling, 1993). Shortly after birth, they are able to launch the hand toward an object, preferring one that is moving (von Hofsten, 1982). (This competence fits well with the known characteristics of early development of the retina, which is more mature in the movement-sensitive periphery than in the foveal area [Abramov et al., 1982].) The hand, although open, does not engage in actual grasping in most cases, and the coordination of the movement does not include corrections of direction or hand-shaping for the object's properties during the course of the reach (Vinter, 1990). In fact, the entire arm is launched as a single unit in a pattern that can best be described as a swipe, a coordinative strategy that is quite unlike the lift-project strategy typical of more mature reaching. Nevertheless, such reaches can sometimes result in use of precision-type grips very early in infancy. Oztop and colleagues (2004) used information in the literature to guide the development of a computer model of the early stages of learning to grasp which demonstrates that arm movements along with the infant grasp reflex and tactile search can be used to guide the development of a variety of grasping strategies without the need for visual guidance in the early months of life.

Because we know that further development will include gradual refinement of hand use as part of reaching and grasping, this sequence of development would appear to follow the proximodistal developmental rule. The course of development, however, is much more complicated. First, reaching at 1 to 2 months is typically done with a fisted hand, rather than the open hand of the newborn, and reaching under visual control with an open hand begins at 4 to 5 months (Vinter, 1990). Furthermore, successful reach-and-grasp can often occur in the period from 1 to 2 months if the head is supported to eliminate a major problem in developing a successful coordinative strategy. Thus, when external controls are provided for the posturally incompetent head, the infant may be able to coordinate a reach-and-grasp successfully, even though, as we have seen, consistent use of reaching with grasping is not present until 13 to 20 weeks of age (Wimmers et al., 1998a).

These and other observations have led to the suggestions that postural control is a rate-limiting factor in early motor development (Shumway-Cook & Woollacott, 1993) and that distal competence may be masked by deficiencies in postural control of the head and neck. Although it seems readily apparent that the ability to control the head to maintain stability of visual perception is an important competence in a general sequence of cephalocaudal progression of development, many aspects of proximal and distal control of the extremities are undergoing contemporaneous development that may not be overtly observable under normal conditions (see Fetters et al., 1989; Heriza, 1991; and Loria, 1980, for further examples). Many exceptions to a proximodistal progression of development have been found (Heriza, 1991).

An important consequence of understanding these new findings from research is that therapists should not conceive of individual body parts as developing independently, sequentially, or purely as a result of nervous system maturation when planning therapeutic intervention. Although various segments of the body may develop their patterns of control for any given task at different rates, any movement pattern is a composite, involving coordination of all the body subsystems. Furthermore, the apparent directionality of development does not appear to be inherent only in the genetic direction of nervous system development, but rather is a result of the interactive functioning of the multiple systems children bring to exploration of the problems and possibilities inherent in a particular task at a particular point in their development (Thelen, 1990). The characteristics and demands of the task are critical in organizing the response of the subsystems (Oztop et al., 2004), but each child's response is unique in its kinematics and time of appearance (Thelen et al., 1993; Wimmers et al., 1998a). In early infancy, for example, the enormous mass of the child's head relative to the size of the rest of the body places constraints on the functions that are possible. Lifting the head and sustaining its upright position while the body is prone therefore entails coordinating the trunk and extremities to create a stable base for head movement. Until the head can be adequately stabilized in space, other movement functions of the body in the prone position cannot be fully expressed.

What seems to play a major role, then, in the general observation of cephalocaudal progression of development are the infant's strength of key muscle groups and anthropometric characteristics, that is, the ability to control the large mass of the head relative to the rest of the body and cope with the high center of mass. Although cephalocaudal progression is a notion that seems to hold as an overall generalization regarding the postural control of the whole body, most movements used by infants entail the coordination of multiple body parts if they are to be effective. The coordination of a prone-on-elbows-with-head-turn strategy for responding to an interesting sound with visual fixation is a good example.

In developing items for the Test of Infant Motor Performance (Campbell et al., 1995), an interesting sequence of development was discovered in the organization of a response to a sound made behind an infant's head as the infant lay in the prone position (Liao & Campbell, 2004, unpublished data). An immature response involved dragging the face across the surface to turn the head toward the sound and visualize it. By 4 months of age, typically developing infants were able to support themselves on their elbows with head lifted and turn toward the sound. Over the course of weekly examinations, however, we noticed that some infants tended to alternate for several weeks between the mature response described and one in which they lifted the head and extended the upper trunk, but seemed unable to turn their head toward the sound source despite obvious interest in the stimulus. After several weeks in which the two modes of response alternated, the individual infant's response stabilized in its most mature form. What intrigued us was why an infant who could lift his head, but apparently could not organize his posture so as to turn it toward an interesting sound, would not choose to go back to an earlier, successful response, that is, putting his head down on the surface to turn it. It appears that once the infant has the ability to extend the neck and trunk in prone position, he would forgo successful task accomplishment (i.e., seeing the interesting sound source) in favor of an unsuccessful head lifting strategy that was used repeatedly over a period of a couple of weeks until he could consistently put together all the components of the most mature response strategy using prone-on-elbows as a base of support. Green and colleagues' (1995) description of the changes in load bearing with development show that body weight must be shifted caudally such that load bearing surfaces include the lateral thighs and lower abdomen before successful head turning with the head erect occurs. Based on our data, this development appears to occur over a short period of a couple of weeks and represents an ability to dissociate movement of the upper part of the body from the pelvis and lower extremities.

The examples given earlier illustrate the power of the dynamical systems perspective by pointing out that multiple systems and processes are developing at any given time, each at its own rate and instantaneous level of competence. What then appears to be a newly appearing "stage" may merely be the time at which one or more rate-limiting factors finally achieve a level of development in a continuous trajectory that supports the appearance of a new, stable form of behavior. The new behavior appears discontinuous with what went before only because the underlying continuous processes were not visible. In the example from research on the Test of Infant Motor Performance, it can be recommended that a treatment plan for helping a child with motor dysfunction to achieve the ability to freely use head and later hands in a prone position might profitably include learning to organize the load-bearing parts of the lower body. Further research to identify the critical processes and subsystems that contribute to qualitative changes in infant behavior should be productive in refining intervention strategies to promote motor development in children with disabilities.

NERVOUS SYSTEM MATURATION AS ONE DRIVING FORCE FOR DEVELOPMENT

Although McGraw (1963), Gesell (1928a, 1928b), and Shirley (1931) emphasized brain maturation as being the major force driving development (despite their own contrary evidence for the important role of external factors), dynamical systems theory has sometimes seemed to view neural maturation with less credence than I believe it deserves. The nervous system in dynamical systems theory is described as merely another system in its developmental contribution, no more important than any other system. In children with mental retardation or cerebral motor dysfunction, however, therapists are well aware of the serious limitations in adapting movement to functional purposes imposed by a compromised CNS. In this chapter development and functions of the nervous system in movement are described; Chapter 6 provides information on another important cooperating component, the musculoskeletal system.

Research suggests that about 30% of the entire genome is expressed only in the brain (Nowakowski, 1987). Although it is true that we now know that experience drives brain development in just as important a way as do genetic programs (Greenough et al., 1987), the notion that no hierarchy of important functions or no unique function of structures exists is simply not true, especially in the human brain, with its highly encephalized processes. What is true is that lower levels of the nervous system, such as the midbrain and the spinal cord, have been recognized to be capable of controlling many finely coordinated movements, not only simple reflexes, and that vast amounts of the CNS are involved in the production and control of even the most basic movements. For example, animal research described in Chapter 3 has revealed that well-coordinated stepping movements can be evoked from activation of spinal cord circuits. Involvement of higher levels of the nervous system, however, is necessary to control the body's overall equilibrium during gait and to express the intentionality of functional movements. Similarly, the modeling research of Oztop and colleagues (2004) suggests that spinal circuits involved in the primitive grasp reflex can be used to organize more sophisticated grasping strategies through use of feedback derived from reaching activity. The locus of control for a given movement varies, however, depending on task requirements and previous experience with similar tasks. Thus, environmental demands become a part of the neural ensemble for producing movement, and the infant's practice of exploratory movements creates inputs that drive brain development.

To return to the example of development of eye-hand coordination, humans display a major shift from subcortically organized movement in the first 3 to 4 months to increasing involvement of cortical circuits at 4 to 5 months (Paillard, 1990). Infants with later evidence of cortical blindness, for example, may be able to track an object visually in the newborn period, using brainstem processing mechanisms. Although the organism's own activity is influential in directing the early course of neural plasticity (Greenough et al., 1987), this example of deviant development reinforces the concept that the higher levels of the CNS are necessary (but not sufficient) for normal human development to occur. Visual functions involving binocularity seem particularly dependent on development of cortical visual circuits. For example, most infants can align their eyes appropriately in the first month of life, but only when visual cortex dominance columns have been refined do they gain control of both the sensory (optical fusion) and the motor (eye convergence) aspects of binocularity (Thorn et al., 1994).

Reaching, too, differs fundamentally in the newborn and the 6-month-old (Paillard, 1990). Reaching is a unitary action in the young infant; a differentiation among reach, grasp, manipulation, and release will later result from maturation of cortical systems in conjunction with anthropometric changes (Wimmers et al., 1998a, 1998b) and learning gained from experiences in the world of objects (Fentress, 1990). As seen in patients with a stroke

that affects fine hand function, cortical activity is necessary for the more delicate aspects of motor control of the hand, and it cannot develop adequately unless the encephalic structures are intact. No examples have been reported in the literature of a capability of higher primates to develop or regain fine finger control in the absence of the primary motor cortex.

Establishment of monosynaptic connections between the motor cortex and spinal cord motoneurons is associated with the appearance of selective control of digital movements in primates (Schoen, 1969); these connections are not present in neonatal monkeys and develop gradually during the first 8 months after birth. Improvement in monkeys' abilities to retrieve small pieces of food from indentations is seen when a wide range of rapid, small movements involving the forearm or shoulder joint appear to assist more efficient distal performance of the digits. This description is remarkably similar to descriptions of the development of fidgety movements in human infants at 2 to 3 months of age (Hadders-Algra & Prechtl, 1992). These movements herald the development of goal-directed movements, including the emergence of consistently effective reaching and grasping. These small synergistic movements in monkeys do not survive pyramidotomy, nor do selective digital movements.

At about the same time that fidgety movements develop, the appearance of ballistic movements (swipes and swats) heralds the switch from coactivation of muscle groups to the reciprocal coordination of muscle activity that characterizes more mature motor patterns (Hadders-Algra et al., 1992). Wimmers and colleagues (1998b) suggest that use of coactivation patterns may also be correlated with reaching with a fisted hand and that the ability to reciprocally activate muscles may be related to both changes in arm circumference and the switch to reaching with an open hand. Although we do not know what leads to the appearance of reciprocal patterns of muscle activity, it is notable that this development does not seem to appear in children with cerebral palsy (CP) (Leonard et al., 1990).

According to Paillard (1990), four features characterize the evolution of the primate nervous system, culminating in the human brain, and promote use of the hand as an elaborate tool for manipulating the environment. These features are (1) extension of the precentral cortex developed principally for fine sensory-guided steering and control of the hand and digits, which is included in the computer model of Oztop and colleagues (2004); (2) enlargement of the lateral cerebellum, again relating to control of forelimb segments and to timing and smoothing of movements; (3) specialization of the parietal association cortex for precise visual guidance of goal-directed arm and hand movements; and (4) prominent development of the frontal association areas that funnel information to motor control regions, mainly through basal ganglia loops. Here we see an example of multiple subsystems in the brain cooperating with the musculoskeletal structures characteristic of the human organism to produce functional movement.

The frontal areas process information related to goal-directed behavior and anticipated consequences of intended acts involving the basic capacity to guide response choice by stored information (Goldman-Rakic, 1987; Paillard, 1990). Major developments in this area in the human infant begin at about 8 months and reach a maximum at 2 years of age. Activity in frontal areas cooperates in motor functions through basal ganglia circuits (Hoover & Strick, 1993). The basal ganglia are involved in the internal generation of automatic movements, the predictive monitoring of head and arm activities (Fentress, 1990), and the acquisition and learning of motor skills through their five parallel pallidal-thalamo-cortical loops, including projections to primary motor cortex, where the dynamics of movement patterns are selected (Georgopoulos et al., 1992).

Eye-head-body orientation activities and target-reaching activities have been shown in lower vertebrates to be coordinated primarily by brainstem centers, prominently involving the superior colliculus (Paillard, 1990). In keeping with identification of these behaviors in very young infants, arm projection at that age is possible without cerebral cortical control. Functional manipulation, such as the fine digital control involved in food taking in experimental primates, however, depends on the additional coordinated action of cortical pathways from higher centers (Fentress, 1990). Elegant hand-grasping and manipulation movements of the primate are dependent on inputs from cerebral cortical levels that are coordinated with lower-level eye-hand-head activity. Overall, however, the primary role of higher-level CNS structures is to tune, guide, learn, and select, adapt, or inhibit execution of basic movements by lower levels of the nervous system. The therapist views this as increasing ability to control movements selectively and adapt them to functional purposes.

Motor control functions are not assumed at successively higher hierarchic levels, leaving behind previously used primitive behaviors and control centers; rather, many levels of the nervous system cooperate in the production of movement behaviors. Typically, no single active site for any particular behavior can be identified; behavior is, rather, an emergent property of the cooperation of various subsystems, with task characteristics organizing the response (Thelen et al., 1993). That is, the characteristics of the task lead the nervous system with its distributed functions to select from a variety of currently available options for assembling a task-related action. The next section of this chapter elaborates on a theory of nervous system development and function that provides an appropriate explanatory model for how the developing organism actively constructs its own operating system for functional behavior.

The Theory of Neuronal Group Selection

According to a popular summary by Edelman (1992) of current theories of nervous system functioning, previous psychologic theories have failed spectacularly in shedding light on how the human mind originates in the functioning of the physical brain because they have neglected the biology of the system. Popular models describing the brain as analogous to a computer with hardware (neurons) and software (motor programs) bear only superficial resemblance to the actual operation of the brain. Edelman's theory is based instead on facts that are garnered from biologic research but are also consistent with behavioral observations. Called the neuronal group selection theory, it has three basic tenets. These tenets describe how the anatomy of the brain is produced during development, how experience selects for strengthening certain patterns of responses from the anatomic structures, and how the resulting maps of the brain give rise to uniquely individual behavioral functions through a process called reentry. Sporns and Edelman (1993) further describe how such a system solves the problem of managing movement in an organism with multiple degrees of freedom, and Newell and Vaillancourt (2001) describe their new conceptualization of how changes in reorganization of the biomechanical degrees of freedom occur during motor learning.

The first tenet of Edelman's theory (1992) is concerned with developmental selection by which the characteristic neuroanatomy of a species is formed. The genetic code of the species does not specify the wiring diagram but instead inscribes the constraints of the process of formation of neural networks, resulting in a primary repertoire of species-specific behavior. In humans, for example, these behaviors appear to include rhythmic movements of the lower extremities, expressed in kicking and neonatal stepping (Thelen, 1990), mouth-to-hand behaviors, visual following of moving objects, and projection of the arm toward objects (von Hofsten, 1982). An overproduction of early synaptic connections formed by activity and cell death or retraction of unexercised connections may explain why individual wiring diagrams vary somewhat yet still maintain the same general form across members of the species.

The second tenet of Edelman's (1992) neuronal group selection theory involves the development of a secondary repertoire of functional circuits from the basic neuro-anatomic network through a process of selective activation that strengthens or weakens synaptic connections based on individual experience. The secondary repertoire includes mechanisms underlying skilled motor behavior, memory, and other important functions and is unique to the individual. In a movement system with multiple degrees of freedom, a variety of ways to accomplish the movements involved in functional tasks can arise (Sporns & Edelman, 1993), but to become incorporated into the secondary repertoire, the functional synergy selected must (1) accomplish the task and (2) allow for postural stability of the body during the task. Adolph (1997) showed that the first movement strategy selected for a risky task such as descending a steep slope is goal directed and may be highly inefficient, even foolhardy. During development, however, infants try out a variety of movement strategies that happen to occur to them, often accidentally, before readily selecting the most safe and economical one for the task at hand. Similarly, Oztop and colleagues' (2004) model of learning to grasp suggests that a variety of arm movements with differing coordinative structure among the joints of the arm are explored by the infant with feedback from tactile inputs shaping the selection of effective strategies.

Edelman's third tenet describes how the first two selectional processes interact to connect biology with psychology. The primary and secondary repertoires of species-typical and uniquely individual functional neural circuits must form maps connected by massively parallel and reciprocal connections. Edelman gives the example that the visual system of the monkey consists of more than 30 different maps, each with a unique degree of functional segregation for orientation, color, movement, and other functions and each linked to the others by parallel and reciprocal connections that can be accessed by the reentry process. By this process, a nervous system with distributed functions is formed.

Selection occurs over neuronal groups from various maps throughout the region and the nervous system as a whole to produce a particular behavior. The behavior is unique to the individual in whom it occurs because of variations in maps caused by the effects of individual experience on their development. The combination of neuronal groups from selected multiple maps of an area's function (for example, the hand motor area of primary cerebral motor cortex combined with selections from maps that are concerned with receipt of visual and tactile information and ones concerned with postural function of the neck and shoulder) allows the production of a movement that is precisely tuned to the environmental demands for functional performance yet unique to the

individual's capacity for processing sensory inputs and for combining selections of neuronal groups from his or her individual regional maps. A selectionist system with distributed functions requires a repertoire of variable actions in order to provide adaptability; that is, a variety of means for responding to environmental demands and internal changes such as growth must be available.

A selectionist model of the nervous system is consistent with the research of Keshner and colleagues (1989), demonstrating that when overtly similar movements are studied in a group of individuals, each person performs the movement with his or her own unique combination of synergistic muscle activation patterns. Thelen and colleagues (1993) have demonstrated similar findings in infants learning to reach. Although a group of infants tended to use a similar strategy of coactivating muscular antagonists when first learning to reach, each infant came at the task in a unique way based on preferred posture, movement, and energy level. Two quiet infants, for example, organized their reaches by lifting their arms and extending them slowly forward. Two other infants, who were highly active and frequently engaged in bilateral arm flapping, needed to damp down their oscillations to reach successfully. These infants used high-velocity swipes to orient their arms toward the toy. In testing infants on the Test of Infant Motor Performance, we also observed variations in how infants approached the orientation-to-sound task in the prone position. For example, one infant extended his neck and trunk when he heard the sound, but being unable to shift his load bearing caudally and support himself on his elbows in order to turn his head, he instead flapped his arms and legs, causing his trunk to rock forward and backward, and eventually negotiated a partial turn of his trunk toward the sound source by pivoting on his abdomen (Campbell, 1998, unpublished data).

In keeping with each individual's march to a personal internal drum, each phenotypic neuronal group has a combination of excitatory and inhibitory connections, allowing the final motor output to be assembled selectively based on current demands and past experience with the task that has strengthened or weakened the tendencies to select particular groups from particular maps (Edelman, 1992; Thelen, 1990). Essential to this development is exposure of the nervous system to a sufficient sample of coactivated sensory signals to permit the neuronal groups to respond differentially to various objects and events in the environment (Sporns, 1994). Obtaining such a sampling of experience occurs during development when an infant spontaneously explores the environment through movement. To have adaptive value, the responding neuronal groups must also contribute to functional activity in the organism. Resulting from these selections, higher-order dynamic structures called global maps are formed that link sensory and motor maps. Such correlated activity is essential to operation of a system based on variability in response units, which become strengthened through use and adaptive value. Such resulting global maps are able to interact with memory processes and other unmapped functions such as those of the basal ganglia and cerebellum. Global maps allow the connection between local maps and motor behavior, new sensory inputs, and further neural processing as important aspects of development and learning.

Neuronal group selection theory does not hold that programs are executed by the nervous system; rather, dynamic loops are created that continually match movements and postures to task-related sensory signals of multiple kinds. Functioning is based on statistical probabilities of signals, not coded signals or preformed programs. Georgopoulos and colleagues (1993), for example, have demonstrated that the precise directionality of a reaching movement can be specified by vectors calculated from the neural activity of large populations of cells in the motor cortex, each of which individually has a preferred directionality but also fires in relation to movements in multiple directions. Edelman (1992) further theorized that the system has biologic "values" that are species-specific and drive the selective strengthening of synaptic activities based on experience. These values influence adaptive processes by linkage between the global mappings and activity in hedonic centers and the limbic system of the brain in a way that fulfills homeostatic needs of the organism that have been set through evolution. For example, the computer model of Oztop and colleagues (2004) includes a variable labeled by the authors "joy of grasping" which models the sensory feedback received by the infant from achieving a successful stable grasp and that, in turn, strengthens the future selection of grasping strategies.

In a computer model of a visual system with a set "value" that prefers light to no-light conditions in the center of a "visual" field (similar to that produced in humans by evolution), initially nondirected movements of an "arm" have been shaped to target an object (Edelman, 1992; Thelen, 1995). If one appreciates that newborn infants possess a primary repertoire that includes moving the mouth to the hand, seeking light, and producing head turns or arm projections in response to moving objects in the visual field, it is not difficult to perceive of the theory of neuronal group selection as an explanation for the gradual process of learning to reach successfully to grasp an object and put it into the mouth. The research of Oztop and colleagues (2004) recently produced the first successful computational model of the process of learning to grasp.

With repeated experience in reaching and grasping as an "individual problem-solver working each day" (Thelen et al., 1993), infants modulate their intrinsic dynamics, discovering the most stable trajectory, joint coordination, and patterns of muscle activation (Thelen et al., 1993), thereby creating their own personal maps. For example, Strick and Preston (1982a, 1982b) have suggested that separate representations of hand motor patterns at cerebral cortical levels may reflect the modular organization of sensorimotor units underlying the distinctive uses of the hand for power gripping or as a palpatory sensory surface. Dynamical systems theory, however, emphasizes that the nervous system is only one subsystem infants use to self-organize exploration of the environment.

Map creation through an individual's use of movement to drive brain plasticity can go awry. Byl and colleagues (1997), for example, reported that when a monkey was trained and reinforced for performing a stereotyped movement thousands of times, the simultaneous activation of muscles and tactile-kinesthetic receptors resulted in degradation of the primary sensory cortex maps. Neurons in the cortical area related to hand function become responsive to stimulation almost anywhere on the hand (even the back of the hand), a condition Byl and colleagues describe as a dedifferentiation of the normally exquisitely organized response patterns of the sensory cortex. They believe that this animal model may reflect the process of repetitive strain injury with focal dystonia in humans and that the findings support use of a sensorimotor retraining approach to treating this disorder in order to redifferentiate sensory maps in the cerebral cortex. If we think of the constrained and repetitive movements used by infants with CNS dysfunction, it is not hard to conceive of the possibility that they also have a poorly differentiated sensory cortex. The key to understanding and treating this type of problem is recognition that maps are formed connecting various areas of the brain based on the simultaneous activity of sensory and motor systems. We learn (and train the brain to select) what we do. Stereotyped simultaneous activity leads to poorly differentiated brain maps, whereas learning to use a variety of flexible patterns to accomplish common tasks leads to rich, complex brain organization compatible with adaptability to environmental demands and the internal changes accompanying growth.

Experience-Expectant and Experience-Dependent Neural Maturation

Greenough and colleagues (1987) have also discussed the importance of environmental experience in driving development of the brain, and their work provides further elaboration on Edelman's theory of neuronal group selection in a maturational context. Although no scientific evidence exists to suggest that training or an enriched environment leads to development of new neurons, extensive evidence documents the effect of training and environment on numbers and properties of synaptic connections among neural cells. Greenough and colleagues (1987) suggested that genetically specified directions lead to initial synaptic connectivities through a process of overproduction of populations of cells that are pruned by exposure to experiences common to all members of a species, such as the array of visual inputs to which infants are typically exposed. The result is species-typical behaviors akin to the primary repertoire described by Edelman (1992).

Greenough and colleagues (1987) called this process experience-expectant development and suggested that it occurs through the death of cells that do not establish productive connections. It has been discovered, however, that the genetic code may actually program cell death (Barinaga, 1993). If neurons have access to particular nerve growth factors, they may be able to escape their programmed fate. By such genetic-environmental interactions, development occurs by a size-matching process whereby the appropriate number of neurons survives to serve peripheral needs. By one's own developmental processes, therefore, each individual obtains a personal, unique structure and functional movement.

A second process, akin to Edelman's secondary repertoire and called experience-dependent neural maturation, is proposed to be the process by which each individual achieves further uniqueness in structure and function through exposure to an individualized set of experiences that establishes strong connectivities among cells based on strengthening of neural synapses that are "exercised" through both sensory and motor experiences (Greenough et al., 1987). The specific structure and function of a person therefore depend on both species-typical connectivities and the amount and strength of other connections resulting from personal experiences specific to each individual and his or her life history. Of most importance, in both aspects of neural plasticity, synaptic connectivity is linked to the individual's own activity in conjunction with genetic programs and environmental opportunities. Thus, the individual in a very real sense is the creator of his or her own unique brain and, by extension, functional motor behavior (Thelen, 1990). Furthermore, Anderson and colleagues (2001) argue that the acquisition of motor skills through self-produced motor activity orchestrates psychologic changes that expose infants to patterns of information that can be used in the acquisition and control of skills in a variety of other domains.

SENSITIVE PERIODS IN DEVELOPMENT

Bertenthal and Campos (1987), in a commentary on Greenough and colleagues' theory, summarized research that may support the theory that experience-expectant and experience-dependent maturation of neural systems could be the basis of sensitive periods in development. They stressed that experience-dependent plasticity of the nervous system can initiate the generation of new synaptic connections and is available throughout the life span. The effects of experiences during a sensitive period, however, are expected to be qualitatively different from those at other points in the life span (Thompson, 2001). The theory also predicts that sensitive periods in experience-expectant development can be extended by various means, including deprivation of sensory inputs that allow synaptic competition for connections to persist longer than is usual.

Most of the animal research on the influence of environmental stimuli on neural plasticity has been on cerebral cortical areas, especially those devoted to visual function. Research has documented the existence of sensitive and in some cases critical periods for development of visual perceptual skills (Horton, 2001; Thorn et al., 1994), once again suggesting the superior benefits of intervention earlier, rather than later, in life. Some evidence also exists to suggest effects of interventions on the sensory cortex, the motor cortex, and the cerebellum (Greenough et al., 1987; Nudo et al., 1996). For example, extensive practice of specific finger activities by monkeys led to enlarged areas of the motor cortex devoted to activation of the exercised fingers (Nudo et al., 1996).

Several sensitive periods in cognitive development have been demonstrated to occur during infancy (Fischer, 1987). At 2 to 4 months, infants demonstrate the ability to vary activity within a single action sequence to reach a simple goal, such as grasping a toy within reach. At 7 to 8 months, several actions can be related in a single functional unit, such as a delayed-response task, using vision to guide a manual manipulation or compare multiple objects, and using a string to activate a toy. By 12 to 13 months, a number of actions can be coordinated to perform a function such as putting a ball into a small hole in a toy box. At 18 to 21 months, symbolic representation is achieved in which a memory of an object can activate an action without the object's being present. Various types of evidence, such as changes in rates of synaptogenesis and electroencephalographic changes, show discontinuities at related time periods.

Unfortunately, only few data are available on the subject of sensitive periods as they affect motor skill development, particularly in children with acquired or congenital disabilities. Zelazo and colleagues (1972,

1983), however, demonstrated the effect of early stepping experience in human infants on maintenance of stepping behavior and earlier age of walking. Heriza (1991) has proposed that sensitive periods exist in the development of locomotor behavior that can be identified through kinematic analysis of rhythmic alternating movements of the legs based on dynamical systems theory and hypothesized that these transitional periods are important points for intervention in children at risk for developmental disabilities. Piek and colleagues (2002) extended the analysis of development of limb coordination patterns to the upper extremities. Dynamical systems theory suggests that when children vary in their selection of a movement strategy in response to a particular task, this period of instability represents a special opportunity for directing development. Kanda and colleagues (1984, 2004) have also reported superior benefits on quality of movement and walking in children with CP of early, as opposed to later or less intense, exposure to Vojta therapy, and Scherzer and colleagues (1976) suggested that children with CP who were treated at an earlier age than others also demonstrated greater benefits. These preliminary suggestions that intervention to promote motor development may vary in effectiveness based on timing of therapy are tantalizing, and further research on this topic is direly needed for improving the scheduling of intervention for maximizing outcomes. To be successful, however, research designs must be tailored specifically to the search for answers to the sensitive period question (Bruer, 2001; Thompson, 2001). Specifically, research to demonstrate a sensitive period requires that the same type, intensity, and duration of intervention be delivered at different stages of development.

PERIODIC EQUILIBRATION IN A SPIRALING PATTERN OF DEVELOPMENT

Piaget (1952) suggested that the experience of acting on the world (assimilation) with whatever sensorimotor schema is currently dominant was frequently met with resistance because the objects of interest were not easily adapted to the current schema (e.g., handling a soft cookie when the motor activity of crumpling or shaking was currently popular). This misfit between the child's current sensorimotor functioning and the response of handled objects leads to disequilibrium, which drives developmental progress through the child's persistence in gradually accommodating to the properties of objects eliciting interest. In so doing, the child eventually develops a different approach to handling the cookie and thereby alters the cognitive structure as well. I would suggest that our infants' alternation over several weeks

between symmetric head and trunk extension versus supporting themselves on their elbows in response to a sound stimulus is an example of children learning to accommodate to new physical capabilities (head and trunk extension) while attempting to accomplish a task, in other words, flexible problem solving.

Ames and colleagues (1979), following from Gesell's earlier observations, posited a similar process of alternating equilibrium and disequilibrium in behavioral characteristics that they believed cycled periodically. For example, toddlers at 18 months are likely to be trying to their parents because they have definite wants but few words with which to express them; they may communicate with crying and tantrums instead. (The reader should note that in this and other sections of the chapter, ages given are normative or average times of appearance of described behaviors; individual developmental rates may, of course, differ to some extent.) At 2 years, the child has developed more language and coordination and is emotionally on an even keel. Disequilibrium returns again at about 2.5 years, when this little person becomes more difficult to live with—bossy, rigid, and oppositional. Cooperation and sharing in play have not yet appeared, and the 2.5-year-old wants to hold onto any toy "he is playing with, has played with, or might in the future want to play with" (Ames et al., 1979, p. 28). The age of 3 years is again an easy time emotionally, whereas at 3.5 years children are insecure and anxious, yet determined and self-willed. At 3, children need their security blankets and thumbs a great deal. The 4-year-old is described as wild and wonderful. This child loves humor and is secure and self-confident, although going overboard in either enthusiasm or anger, even threatening to run away when upset. Five-year-olds are more inwardly directed, prefer to stay within known boundaries, and have less interest in novel experiences. These children are careful to attempt only what can most definitely be achieved but are, nonetheless, expansive intellectually, loving to talk and learn about things. "Why?" is the word of choice. By 5.5 years, however, another period of disequilibrium seems to occur, but it is one characterized by extremes—shy at one moment, extremely bold the next. The child may seem to be in a constant state of tension, chewing on pencils and fidgeting. By 6.5 years, however, a calmer, more even-tempered child again emerges, moving toward the inner-directed 7-year-old.

Gesell (Heriza, 1991), Rood (Stengel et al., 1984), Bly (1983), and others have suggested that motor development also consists of an alternation and recombination of patterns of flexion, extension, and symmetry versus asymmetry, leading ever onward toward improved mobility and stability in posture and movement in opposition to the force of gravity. At different times, various patterns predominate, but an alternation between stability and instability of functioning characterized also by switches between symmetry and asymmetry is thought to be characteristic of normal developmental progression. Heriza has summarized these principles based on Gesell's early work as viewing growth "not as a linear process but a spiral one where structure and function jointly mature leading to regression, asymmetries, and reorganization. Although Gesell is best known for his principles of direction of development and individuating maturation, his principle of reciprocal interweaving "foreshadows [a] contemporary systems view of motor development" (Heriza, 1991, p. 102). As we have seen, McGraw (1935) held a similar view, but she and other early developmental researchers lacked the contemporary ability to reveal the underlying systems changes that produce these overtly observed patterns of development and tended to stress nervous system maturation as the driving force.

To summarize, studies have suggested that development proceeds in a continuous spiral characterized by "paired-but-opposed types of responses that occur in repeated alternation" (Ames et al., 1979, p. 4) and with relative periods of stability and instability (Heriza, 1991) that may reflect underlying developmental continuity within multiple subsystems involved in maturation. Regressions are also normal aspects of developmental processes (Bevor, 1982; Corbetta & Bojczyk, 2002; Oppenheim, 1981; Provost, 1981). Ages 2, 5, 10, and 16 years are considered to be periods of emotional equilibrium; ages 3.5, 7, and 13 as periods of relative inwardness and withdrawal; and ages 4, 8, and 14 as periods of expansive behavior (Ames et al., 1979). Research has suggested that periods of rapid behavioral changes of many kinds occur at approximately 4, 6 to 7, 10 to 12, and 14 to 16 years (Fischer, 1987). Similarly, Shumway-Cook and Woollacott (1985) suggested that motor patterns in the development of postural stability undergo a period of disequilibrium between 4 and 6 years, when a physical growth spurt occurs. Changes in perceptual functions during this period offer an alternative, or possibly an additional, explanation (Kirshenbaum et al., 2001).

Whether these findings can be correlated with specific periods of brain growth is an interesting question. Overall brain growth stages have been correlated with mind growth, a process called "phrenoblysis" (Epstein, 1979). Although Greenough and colleagues (1987) cautioned that spurts in growth of the whole brain or in head circumference may not be reflective of relative differences in timing of growth rates in the various regions of the brain, Goldman-Rakic (1987) has shown that concurrent spurts of synaptogenesis take place in many regions of the cerebral cortex of rhesus monkeys during the period of rapid behavioral growth in ability to perform delayed-response tasks. In humans, this stage occurs beginning at about 8 months, with rapid developments in understanding of object permanence, and can be correlated with rapid synaptogenesis in the visual cortex (Fischer, 1987; Goldman-Rakic, 1987). In humans, however, the prefrontal cortex, the area of the brain that has been related to delayed-response tasks, has an extensive period of synaptogenic development, peaking at 1 to 2 years and remaining high until about 7 years.

During the second postnatal brain growth stage (2 to 4 years), there are striking developments in sensory function, including binocularity, hearing, and language. Evidence suggests that earlier-occurring defects in these functions can be remedied only during the growth stage. For example, the fact that children with strabismus leading to amblyopia will never have normal three-dimensional (3-D) depth perception if the strabismus is not corrected before 60 days of constant misalignment during the first 9 months of life is important evidence of a critical period in development (Tychsen, 2001).

In summary, significant principles of motor development include (1) the concept that an apparent cephalocaudal progression results not from genetically directed brain development but rather from a process of coordination of a variety of subsystems in response to the affordances of the environment for action, (2) spiraling development characterized by periods of relative stability and instability and sensitive periods in which development is especially responsive to environmental influences and therapeutic intervention, and (3) self-regulating active construction of developmental progress on the part of the child. Most developmentalists would now agree that the individual is formed through interaction among genetically determined processes, individual history, and environmental opportunities at least partially created by the organism itself. Seen in this light, the infant's actions structure the organization and complexity of her or his brain and psychologic development, not the other way around (Anderson et al., 2001).

"STAGES" OF MOTOR DEVELOPMENT

The next section will elaborate on the observable "stages" of gross and fine motor development that represent milestones of developmental progress toward achieving the goals of upright posture, mobility, and manipulation—essential elements of environmental mastery and control. As infants attain and perfect these major developmental motor skills, they are incorporated into functional activities such as self-care, feeding, and play. Important milestones of motor development in later years of childhood will also be briefly addressed.

The major gross motor milestones of the first 12 to 18 months include achieving an indefinitely maintained upright head posture, attaining prone-on-elbows position, rolling from supine to prone, independent sitting, attaining hands-and-knees position, moving from sitting to four-point position and prone, creeping on hands and knees, pulling to a stand, standing independently, and walking independently (van Blankenstein et al., 1962). As each position or skill is attained, further development will entail the perfecting of postural control in these positions and the ability to make rapid, effortless transitions from one position to another. These developments are discussed in Chapter 3.

Despite the greater complexity of our more recent view of the development of motor behavior, including the idea of underlying continuity of development in multiple systems, it is possible to summarize the perfection of use of various parts of the body in an overall schema of cephalocaudal direction. During the first quarter of the first year of life, infants develop the ability to control their heads in virtually all positions in space, although control will continue to be fine-tuned during successive months. The second quarter reveals major advances in control of the arms and upper trunk, although once again continued refinements occur later. Arm movements are aided by increasing ability to control the destabilizing effects of arm movements on other parts of the body. During the third quarter, initial stages involving mastery of control of the lower trunk and pelvis in the upright position occur, and the final quarter of the first year reveals the development of milestones in mobility and control of the lower parts of the legs in conjunction with upright stance and overall postural control.

INFANCY

Functional Head Control

At birth, infants already have the capacity to right the head from either full flexion or full extension when they are supported in an upright position. A stable vertical head position, however, cannot usually be sustained for more than a second or two, if at all. Supine, or with the head supported in a reclining position, head-turning to either side of midline can usually be elicited by attracting the infant's visual orientation to a moving object. At about 2 months, the infant can sustain the head in midline in the frontal plane during supported sitting but often appears to be looking down at his or her feet, so that

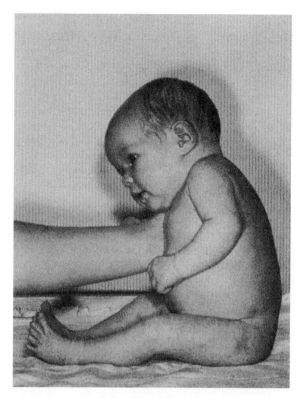

◆ **Figure 2-1**   Early head control in space is characterized by ability to stabilize the head in midline but with eyes angled downward from the vertical. *(From van Blankenstein, M, Welbergen, UR, & de Haas, JH. Le développement du nourrisson: Sa première année en 130 photographies. Paris: Presses Universitaires de France, 1962, p. 26.)*

the eyes are oriented about 30° below the horizontal plane as in Fig. 2-1 (Campbell, SK, Kolobe, TH, Osten, E, Girolami, G, & Lenke, M, unpublished research, 1992). Turning of the unsupported head in the upright position is not usually possible. If the child can be enticed to lift the head to the vertical position, oscillations are typically seen with inability to maintain a stable upright posture. Finer synergistic control of neck flexor and extensor muscles typically appears in the third month, when the head is indefinitely stable in a vertical position and can be freely turned to follow visual stimulation, although sometimes with brief oscillations and loss of control.

When stabilizing control of the head in the upright position has been attained, the infant can typically organize head and trunk activity so that when placed prone with the arms extended along the sides of the body, the prone-on-elbows position is rapidly assumed by lifting the head and extending the thoracic spine while simultaneously bringing both arms up to rest on the elbows (Fig. 2-2). Given the large weight of the head relative to

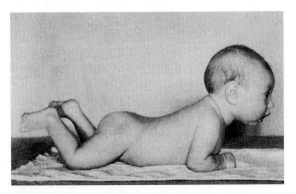

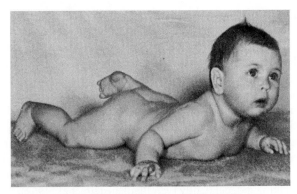

◆ **Figure 2-2** Early stage of prone-on-elbows posture with stable neck extension, elbows close to trunk, and flexed hips and knees. *(From van Blankenstein, M, Welbergen, UR, & de Haas, JH. Le développement du nourrisson: Sa première année en 130 photographies. Paris: Presses Universitaires de France, 1962, p. 25.)*

◆ **Figure 2-3** Advanced stage of prone-on-elbows posture, with free movement of head and arms and extended lower extremities. *(From van Blankenstein, M, Welbergen, UR, & de Haas, JH. Le développement du nourrisson: Sa première année en 130 photographies. Paris: Presses Universitaires de France, 1962, p. 34.)*

the rest of the body at this age, a stabilizing postural function of the legs and pelvis must provide a stable base of support for simultaneous neck and trunk extension with arm movement. Green and colleagues (1995) demonstrated that the developmental progression in both supine and prone positions involves a gradual shifting of the load-bearing surfaces in a caudal direction.

Turning the head to either side while prone on the elbows may still be difficult to coordinate at this stage, and lateral head-righting also remains imperfect. Nevertheless, by the end of the third or fourth postnatal month, the head, in conjunction with organized trunk and lower extremity extension, has largely perfected the maintenance of stable positioning in space appropriate for the further development of eye-head-hand control and of independent sitting to come (Fig. 2-3). Bushnell and Boudreau (1993) believe that a stable head is a prerequisite for initial ability to perceive depth cues from kinetic information (movement of an object relative to its surroundings or to self), which is present by 3 months of age. Once established by 4 or 5 months of age, binocular vision is used to identify depth cues.

Commensurate with acquisition of functional control of head positioning are important developments in control of the arms. During the second and third months, generalized movements of the arms and body have altered their earlier writhing quality (Cioni & Prechtl, 1990). Small fidgety movements appear throughout the body, the arms and legs may show oscillations during movement, and ballistic swipes and swats with legs or arms appear for the first time (Hadders-Algra & Prechtl, 1992). For example, if the legs are flexed up to the chest and then released while the infant is supine, the legs may extend so

that the heels pound the supporting surface, or when excited, the infant may make large arm-swiping movements in the air. As noted earlier, the first evidence of reciprocal activity of muscular antagonists about the shoulder underlies the ability to perform these ballistic movements (Hadders-Algra et al., 1992). Ferrari and colleagues (1990) suggested the importance of these developing qualitative changes in spontaneous movement by demonstrating that they herald the appearance of goal-directed reaching and by indicating that they do not appear in children destined to be diagnosed as having CP. Children with spastic CNS dysfunction also tend to move in tight ranges characterized by simultaneity of activity in multiple limbs, referred to as cramped synchrony, and general movements that tend to repeat monotonously. The characteristics of children with dyskinetic CP are different (Einspieler et al., 2002). Until the second post-term month, these infants displayed a poor repertoire of general movements, circling arm movements, and finger spreading. These movements remained until 5 months when they became associated with lack of arm and leg movements toward the midline.

Upright Trunk Control

The initial ability to maintain sitting independently on propped arms when placed is achieved after the infant is able to (1) extend the head and trunk in prone position so as to use the legs and pelvis as the load-bearing surfaces and (2) control the pelvis and lower extremities while using the arms or moving the head in supine position, that is, has developed anticipatory stabilizing responses to counteract internally generated forces caused by movement (Green et al., 1995). Midway through the first year,

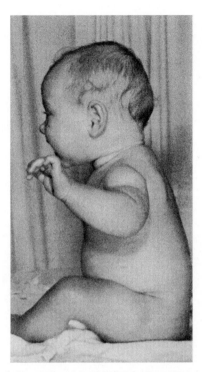

◆ **Figure 2-4**   Early stage of independent sitting, with arms used for balance. *(From van Blankenstein, M, Welbergen, UR, & de Haas, JH. Le développement du nourrisson: Sa première année en 130 photographies. Paris: Presses Universitaires de France, 1962, p. 39.)*

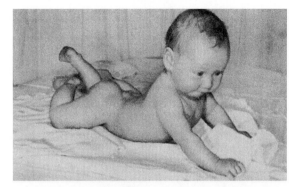

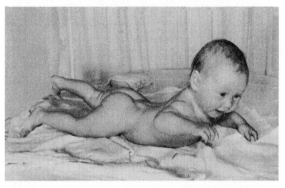

◆ **Figure 2-5**   In the most advanced stage of the prone posture, arms and legs move freely from a stable trunk. *(From van Blankenstein, M, Welbergen, UR, & de Haas, JH. Le développement du nourrisson: Sa première année en 130 photographies. Paris: Presses Universitaires de France, 1962, p. 37.)*

the average child has achieved the ability to sit alone (Fig. 2-4) and can successfully manipulate an object with one hand while the other hand holds it, although sitting and manipulating at once may still be a challenge. Poking fingers explore crevices and crumbs and herald the fine selective digital control that characterizes the human organism. Strong extension throughout the body in the prone position and caudal shift of the load bearing surfaces allows significant freedom of action for the arms and head (Fig. 2-5). Bushnell and Boudreau (1993) believe that ability to perceive the characteristics of objects through their manipulation now allows the child to use configural cues from objects in depth perception. Despite these developments in arm control, the child in sitting lacks the fine pelvic and lower extremity control needed for moving into and out of the position or for turning the trunk freely on a stable base. Pelvic control functions begin to be developed at this time, however, in rolling from supine to prone position (Fig. 2-6), pivoting while prone, and playing with the legs and feet while supine.

Lower Trunk Control in the Upright Position

During the third quarter of the first year, functional movements free the child from a spot on which she or he

is placed by others. Control of lower trunk and pelvis, combined with previously achieved upper body skills, provides new mobility when prone (Fig. 2-7), crawling and creeping (Fig. 2-8), pulling to a stand, moving from supine to four-point and sitting positions, and moving down to hands and knees or prone position from sitting (Fig. 2-9). Inherent in each activity are freedom from a strong midline symmetry that previously characterized postural control and the continued refinement of rotational abilities within the axis of the trunk.

The presence of oscillations also continues to herald new developments. Rocking on four limbs before launching into creeping (Adolph et al., 1998) and bouncing while standing before beginning to cruise along furniture are examples of self-induced actions that appear to be important precursors of functional skills.

Fine Lower Extremity Control in the Upright Position

Once the child has attained competence at standing and cruising along furniture, the legs and feet move toward perfection of selective control because the trunk and pelvis

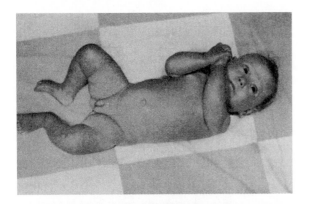

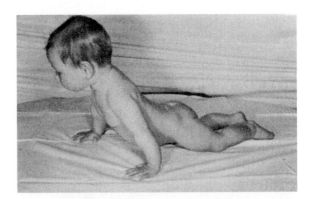

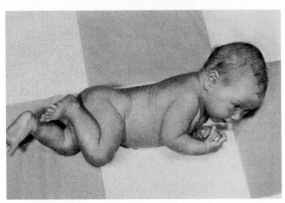

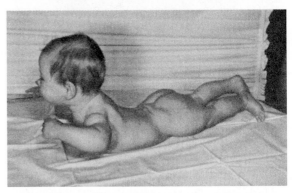

• **Figure 2-7**   Dynamic play in prone position includes push-ups on extended arms and "flying" with strong trunk extension and scapular retraction. *(From van Blankenstein, M, Welbergen, UR, & de Haas, JH. Le développement du nourrisson: Sa première année en 130 photographies. Paris: Presses Universitaires de France, 1962, p. 47.)*

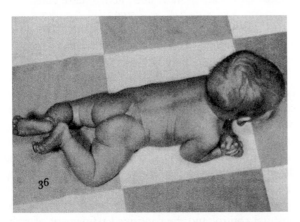

• **Figure 2-6**   Rolling from supine to prone with head-righting. *(From van Blankenstein, M, Welbergen, UR, & de Haas, JH. Le développement du nourrisson: Sa première année en 130 photographies. Paris: Presses Universitaires de France, 1962, p. 36.)*

are increasingly reliable supports that permit freedom of lower extremity activities. In creeping, pelvic swiveling motions give way to reciprocal hip flexion and extension activity, and creeping velocity increases because an arm and a leg on the same side of the body can be placed in simultaneous flight. The child can lower himself or herself from standing (Fig. 2-10); bear-walk with dorsiflexed ankles, flexed hips, and partially extended knees (Fig. 2-11); and finally, stand and walk independently at 9 to 15 months of age (Fig. 2-12). As an example of typical regressions in the course of development, the early stage of walking is accompanied by a return to two-handed reaching which declines again in frequency as balance control improves (Corbetta & Bojczyk, 2002).

The gradual refinement of gait is described by Stout in Chapter 5. In summary, during the first several months of walking experience, creeping is gradually abandoned and heel-strike in gait develops, allowing faster walking with longer strides. As children become bigger, older, and more experienced, steps become longer, narrower (reflecting a narrowing of the base of support), straighter (reflecting increasing control over the path of progression), and more consistent (Adolph et al., 2003). Walking practice is a stronger predictor of improvement in walking skill than age and duration of walking experience. Roberton and Halverson (1984) hypothesized the following temporal sequence of further development of foot locomotion patterns: walking; running; single leap, jumping down or

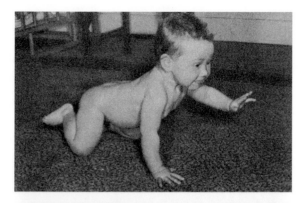

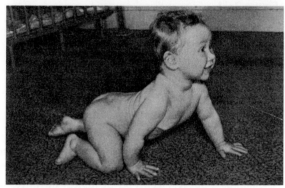

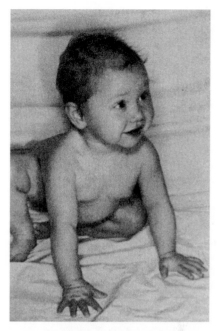

◆ **Figure 2-9** The infant moves from sitting to the four-point position over one leg. *(From van Blankenstein, M, Welbergen, UR, & de Haas, JH. Le développement du nourrisson: Sa première année en 130 photographies. Paris: Presses Universitaires de France, 1962, p. 57.)*

◆ **Figure 2-8** Creeping on hands and knees. *(From van Blankenstein, M, Welbergen, UR, & de Haas, JH. Le développement du nourrisson: Sa première année en 130 photographies. Paris: Presses Universitaires de France, 1962, p. 53.)*

bounce-jumping, and galloping (in uncertain order, but generally at about 2 to 2.5 years); hopping on dominant foot (seldom before age 3) and then nondominant foot; and skipping and sideways galloping or sliding. Although some children may manage a skip by age 4, many reach an early level of proficiency only by age 7. A rhythmic step-and-hop movement is even more difficult and does not appear until well into the primary school years, when it may be used in many dance forms. Before describing the further development of gross motor skills in preschoolers, however, the sequence of development of functional hand use in infancy will be described.

Object Manipulation

Development of fine motor function entails two major features: control of the hand as a terminal device for reaching and grasping and object manipulation and release. Postural control for reaching and grasping has been briefly described earlier in this chapter and is further discussed in Chapter 3; an excellent volume devoted to development of all aspects of the capacity to reach, grasp, and release, as well as the functional use of the hands, has been edited by

Bard and colleagues (1990). Oztop and colleagues (2004) describe the development of a computational model of the early phases of learning to grasp. This chapter, on the other hand, emphasizes development of the manipulative functions of the hand.

Karniol (1989) has documented the stages of object manipulation in the first year of life. These stages of spontaneous behaviors observed in daily life occur in a hierarchic form that progresses from rotation (angular displacement) to translation (movement parallel to the object itself) to vibration (rapid periodic movements of either translation or rotation). Later stages involve combinations of these actions and bimanual activities. The invariant sequence of spontaneous behaviors documented by Karniol (1989) is as follows:

Stage 1, rotation of held objects—by 2 months. With improvements in head stability and visual perception, holding objects becomes an intentional act. Objects are first held when they come directly into the infant's reach and are later (by 3 to 4 months) twisted while being held. Karniol (1989) indicated that through this action infants learn that objects can be held and their appearance transformed by rotation. Wallace and Whishaw (2003) showed that infants use four grasping patterns in the first 5 months, including fisted grasps, pre-precision

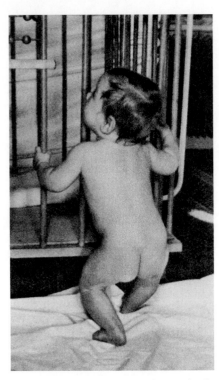

• **Figure 2-10** Lowering from standing to the floor with control. *(From van Blankenstein, M, Welbergen, UR, & de Haas, JH. Le développement du nourrisson: Sa première année en 130 photographies. Paris: Presses Universitaires de France, 1962, p. 57.)*

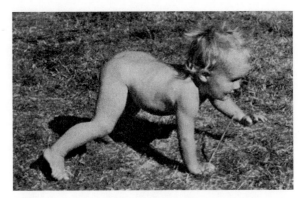

• **Figure 2-11** "Bear-walking" on hands and feet. *(From van Blankenstein, M, Welbergen, UR, & de Haas, JH. Le développement du nourrisson: Sa première année en 130 photographies. Paris: Presses Universitaires de France, 1962, p. 54.)*

grips (thumb to side of index or middle finger), precision grips of objects, and self-directed grasps of their own body or clothing.

Stage 2, translation of grasped objects—by 3 months. Typical of this stage is reaching for an object while in the prone position and bringing it to the mouth. The object may also be rotated. What the infant learns through these types of action is that he or she can translate objects in order to look at, or mouth, them and that it is not possible to reach objects further distant than the length of the arm.

Stage 3, vibration (shaking) of held objects—by 4 months. In this stage infants learn that they can make interesting noises by rapidly flexing and extending their arms and can make the noise stop by holding still. If the object does not produce a noise, it may be translated or rotated and examined before being dropped, but visual attention is not a dominant part of this activity.

Stage 4, bilateral hold of two objects—by 4.5 months. The infant may hold an object in one hand and shake an object held in the other, thereby learning that it is possible to do more than one thing at a time (Fig. 2-13).

Stage 5, two-handed hold of a single object—by 4.5 months. First use of bimanual holding is to hold an object, such as a bottle, steady, but it rapidly advances to holding (and often rotating) large objects that require the use of two hands. These actions allow the child to learn that two hands can steady and rotate objects better than can one hand, as well as permit the holding of large objects.

Stage 6, hand-to-hand transfer of an object—at 4.5 to 6 months. Transfer is usually followed by repeated actions on the object with the second hand, thereby learning that whatever can be done with the right hand can also be done with the left.

Stage 7, coordinated action with a single object in which one hand holds the object while the other manipulates or bangs it—at 5 to 6.5 months. A quintessential example of this type of activity is holding a toy in one hand while picking at it with the other (Fig. 2-14). Displacements of the object caused by handling are followed by rotational readjustments of the hand that holds it. These activities teach the infant that two hands can do more than can one hand alone and that noise can be produced from striking objects that do not respond to vibrating.

Stage 8, coordinated action with two objects, such as striking two blocks together—at 6 to 8.5 months. Through these actions, the infant learns to produce interesting effects by moving one object toward another.

Stage 9, deformation of objects—at 7 to 8.5 months. At this stage, the infant learns that it is possible to alter

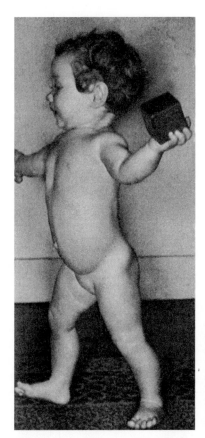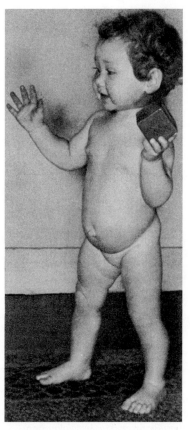

♦ **Figure 2-12**   The infant walks and carries a toy, with wide-based gait and hands in "guard" position. *(From van Blankenstein, M, Welbergen, UR, & de Haas, JH. Le développement du nourrisson: Sa première année en 130 photographies. Paris: Presses Universitaires de France, 1962, pp. 64–65.)*

the way things look or sound by ripping, bending, squeezing, or pulling them apart.

Stage 10, instrumental sequential actions—at 7.5 to 9.5 months. These activities involve the sequential use of two hands for goal-oriented functions, so that the infant learns that coordinated use of the hands leads to desired outcomes. The infant may, for example, open a box with one hand and take out its contents with the other.

The achievement of these stages completes the development of the essentials of manual manipulation. More complex actions follow that are related to the functional characteristics of objects or to imaginary play in which an object can be whatever one pretends it to be (Karniol, 1989). Manual manipulations become automatized, leaving attention to be directed more toward the functional use of objects.

Based on the previously discussed research of Edelman (1992), Thelen (1990), Thelen and colleagues (1993), Oztop and colleagues (2004), and Keshner and colleagues (1989), we can hypothesize that, although functional hand use develops in a regular, invariant sequence, it is likely that each infant uses unique coordinative patterns and kinetics to achieve manipulative goals that are circumscribed by individual variations in body structure, experiences, and rate of neural and physical maturation. Because the task characteristics structure the infant's unique response, parents play an important role in providing opportunities that support development.

Karniol (1989) suggested that parents and others who choose toys for infants have two important functions: (1) helping infants to master the abilities of each stage by providing objects that are appropriate for emerging skills and (2) facilitating infants' developing sense of capability to control their world by providing objects that are responsive to current manipulative abilities. Thus, Karniol and others believed that mastery of controlling objects in the environment is influential in development of the infant's general sense of competence and in providing initial sensorimotor knowledge of the permanence of objects and of cause-effect relationships. Karniol reviewed research demonstrating the influence on persistence at tasks and

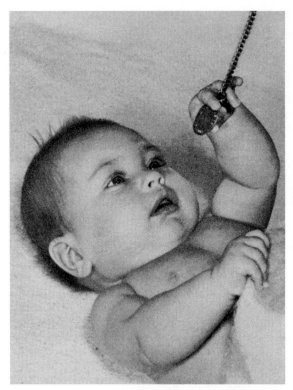

⬩ **Figure 2-13**   Bilateral hold of two objects: One hand holds the blanket, the other reaches for a keychain (stage 4 of Karniol, 1989). *(From van Blankenstein, M, Welbergen, UR, & de Haas, JH. Le développement du nourrisson: Sa première année en 130 photographies. Paris: Presses Universitaires de France, 1962, p. 91.)*

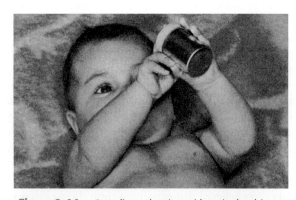

⬩ **Figure 2-14**   Coordinated action with a single object: holding a toy with one hand while poking at it with another (stage 7 of Karniol, 1989). *(From van Blankenstein, M, Welbergen, UR, & de Haas, JH. Le développement du nourrisson: Sa première année en 130 photographies. Paris: Presses Universitaires de France, 1962, p. 93.)*

IQ at age 3 of play with objects that provide contingent feedback and are appropriate for the infant's manual manipulative competencies. Similarly, in a search for the correlates of performance of infants in descending slopes that varied in riskiness, Adolph (1997) found that experience in dealing with steps and backing off furniture at home was related to superior ability to negotiate risky slopes. Furthermore, use of teaching strategies by Mexican-American mothers was found to be correlated with their infants' motor development (Kolobe, 2004).

As each stage is attained, the presentation of any object results in action appropriate to the motor stage, whether or not the object lends itself well to that action. Thus, in stage 3, all objects are considered shakeable whether or not they make noise when shaken. Infants who could crawl plunged recklessly down slopes too steep to negotiate safely in order to get to their mothers at the landing (Adolph, 1997). With more experience in crawling and walking, failures on risky slopes frequently led to accidental use of a different pattern (one that an infant already knew from previous activities) that was successful, such as sliding down the slope backward or in sitting. The alternative mode then became one that children purposely selected for descending slopes they perceived to be risky. These facts are not well explained by developmental theories that suggest that children perceive the affordances of the environment and act on them (Fetters, 1991a, 1991b; Pick, 1992; Thelen, 1990), but this type of function was recognized by Piaget (Flavell, 1963) and included in his principle of assimilation. This principle states that when cognitive structures develop a particular schema, it is applied indiscriminately to objects in the environment, assimilating them to the existing cognitive structure. Piaget also posited that repeated experiences with attempted assimilations of inappropriate objects results in gradual accommodation to their properties and the appearance of both new behaviors and new cognitive structures.

On the other hand, a selectionist theory of motor development suggests that children must use on-line decision making to choose the appropriate motor synergy for use in a given situation (Adolph, 1997). Case-Smith and colleagues (1998) have shown that the characteristics of objects, such as differences in size and presence of moveable parts, lead to immediate use of distinct actions when grasping that are appropriate to the object's characteristics. For example, a given infant might display more mature patterns of grasp when handling a toy with moveable parts than when handling a pellet, so even infants do seem to have some capability to recognize the affordances for manipulation offered by different objects despite having preferred modes of operating on items in the environment. A surprising finding of Adolph's research on slope descent was that infants who had, week after week, practiced crawling down slopes that ranged from easy to hard, nevertheless did not transfer their experience with deciding which slopes were too risky to attempt to making the decision whether or not to traverse a risky slope once they learned to walk. Experienced crawlers, when faced as new walkers with slopes they had done over and over again for weeks on hands and knees, heedlessly plunged down slopes that were too risky for their immature walking skills. These infants did no better than control group subjects with no previous experience with slope descent. Only with more experience walking did infants become more cautious and choose to use an alternative mode of locomotion for difficult slopes. Because infants did make judgments indicating that they found some slopes too risky to attempt, Adolph surmised that children (1) used vision first to decide whether a slope was negotiable with just a quick glance, (2) then decided either to go or to take a longer look, and (3) then decided either to go or to use haptic exploration of the surface with actions such as a hand or foot pat, followed by (4) going using preferred current mode of locomotion (crawling or walking). With more experience, they became able to select an alternative, safer mode, such as sliding down backward. In a later study in which Adolph and Avolio (2000) added lead weights to infants' bodies during slope traversal, infants recognized that slopes that were safe without weights were risky with added loads and those infants who engaged in exploratory activity on the starting platform displayed greater ability to produce adaptive responses to risky slopes rather than failed attempts to descend.

Because Adolph (1997) did not find that previous extensive experience with slopes of varying riskiness was useful when the means of preferred locomotion changed from crawling to walking, she believes that a selectionist view of what infants learn from experience with everyday problem-solving challenges is appropriate to describe what children have learned from the slope experiments. Each new presentation of a slope presented a choice: to go with the currently preferred mode of locomotion, to choose an alternative (presumably safer) mode of locomotion, or to avoid the situation, using a detour attempt or simply sitting down and waiting for the caretaker to come to the rescue. Notably, the latter was seldom selected with slopes that were moderately risky; it seemed that infants were goal oriented rather than safety oriented. Their choice was made based on, first, visual information, and then if still uncertain, tactile and proprioceptive information. The choice was usually their preferred mode of locomotion until they had many weeks of experience and had, usually accidentally, discovered an already familiar motor

strategy that appeared to be safer or more successful. As they gained experience crawling or walking, their choice was made more and more quickly; after many weeks of practice, a short glance was enough for making a decision. Near their ability boundary (slopes that generated less than predictable success in descending without falling), they appeared to have less than adequate knowledge of their own motor capabilities and instead made the decision based on desire to achieve the goal of returning to their caregiver and a quick judgment of whether or not to go based on visual or haptic information. Failure (i.e., falling) did not predict whether infants would choose to go on a subsequent trial, so they appeared to learn little between trials based on successful or unsuccessful outcomes. Adolph concludes that infants have extensive capability to use sensory inputs to make decisions about choice of motor actions although they are not always right about their motor capabilities for solving the problem at hand. They choose to act rather than avoid a challenging situation, do not engage in trial-and-error learning, but rather continue to rely on their visual-haptic analysis of whether or not to engage in risky behavior. When useful motor synergies happened serendipitously, however, they seemed to recognize the adaptability of such patterns and used them on subsequent trials as alternatives to generally preferred modes of locomotion that were riskier to use in a given situation. Goldfield (1997) summarizes Adolph's (1997) findings by indicating that "inexperienced infants tend to be drawn inexorably toward the goal, rather than stopping at a choice point, and apparently do not notice the available affordances.... Conversely, the experienced infant who has explored the available affordances may be overly conservative because the affordance information about slopes is inherently inhibitory; that is, it specifies ways for slowing, stopping, and changing direction" (p. 157). Thus, it seems that infants generate information visually, use their preferred mode of locomotion if the choice is to go, and then over time learn, accidentally or through a general wealth of experience with variable-level surfaces, to select from a variety of possible choices the most efficacious method of traversing risky terrain. One must conclude that adaptive locomotion (i.e., selecting the most appropriate method for the task at hand) requires exploratory movements to obtain information and a repertoire of available movement synergies from which to select (Adolph, 1997). This research once again emphasizes that advances in motor behavior depend on having a variety of movement patterns from which to choose when faced with challenging new opportunities for action. As a result, children with disabilities, who generally have a limited vocabulary of movement synergies, are constrained in their motor development by a lack of experience with a variety of movement patterns and may also have limited perceptual capabilities for making on-line judgments about the likelihood of successfully accomplishing a motor task even when they have an intense interest in the goal.

THE PRESCHOOL AND EARLY SCHOOL YEARS

Functional Motor Skills in Preschoolers

We turn now to a description of the functional skills of preschool children, combining information on both gross and fine motor function in practical use. Toddlers operate with different anthropometric characteristics than infants. Toddlers gain about 5 pounds in weight and 2.5 inches in height each year, the latter resulting mostly from growth of the lower extremities (Colson & Dworkin, 1997). Fifty percent of adult height is reached between the ages of 2 and 2.5 years. Children now walk well (although steps are still short and constrained) and enjoy the sheer pleasure of movement through running, climbing up and down stairs independently, and jumping off the bottom step (Ames et al., 1979). The 2-year-old child can kick a ball and steer a push-toy, and by 2.5 years the child can walk on tiptoes, jump with both feet, stand on one foot, and throw and catch a ball using arms and body together. Galloping may appear, but only leading with the preferred foot (Roberton & Halverson, 1984). The more practical pleasures of dressing independently (pulling on a simple garment at 2 years and pulling off pants and socks by 2.5 years) and eating with a spoon with little spilling also develop (Ames et al., 1979). Food preferences can become a touchy subject by around 2.5 years; nevertheless, the toddler is gradually developing impulse control (Colson & Dworkin, 1997).

The 3-year-old child can alternate feet easily when ascending stairs, can control speed of movement well, and takes pleasure in riding a tricycle (Ames et al., 1979). Hopping may emerge, although it is often a momentary, single hop on the preferred foot (Roberton & Halverson, 1984). Surprisingly, however, by 3.5 years, the child may seem less secure and physically coordinated, stumbling frequently and showing a fear of falling (Ames et al., 1979). Hands may show excessive dysmetria during block stacking. Nevertheless, typical 3-year-olds feed themselves well and can hold a glass with only one hand. At 3.5 years, mealtime may again become trying because the food must be put on the plate in a certain way and the sandwich has to be cut just so. The same may be true of the dressing process, with special objection being expressed against clothing that goes over the head. The

typical 3-year-old can put on pants, socks, and shoes, but buttoning may be difficult. Nearly all 3-year-olds are consistently dry during the daytime, and bowel training is well established as the physical skills and the emotional willingness to participate in toilet training come together (Colson & Dworkin, 1997). The ability to delay gratification is developing, and toddlers strive for autonomy while continuing to intermittently seek reassurance from caregivers to whom they are securely attached.

Despite these generalizations, preschoolers exhibit a variety of individual behavioral styles (Colson & Dworkin, 1997). About 10% of children are considered "difficult" because of increased levels of activity, emotional negativity, and low adaptability. Another 15% of children are described as "slow to warm up" because they take a long time to adapt to new situations.

Typical 4-year-olds have been described by Ames and colleagues (1979) as characteristically out-of-bounds in their exuberance. Behavior in all spheres is frequently wild, and self-confidence and bragging seem endless. The 4-year-old can walk downstairs with one foot per step, catch with hands only, and learn to use roller skates or a small bicycle. (But remember McGraw's experiments demonstrating that learning these skills is possible much earlier.) Athletic activities are particularly enjoyed, especially running, jumping, and climbing. Four-year-olds can button large buttons and lace shoelaces, feed themselves independently except for cutting, and talk and eat at the same time. The average Chinese child can use chopsticks to finish more than half the meal at 4.6 years (Wong et al., 2002). Most can take responsibility for washing hands and face and brushing teeth as well as dressing and undressing without help except for tying their shoes or differentiating front from back of some garments (Ames et al., 1979).

Five-year-olds tend to be more conforming than the exuberant 4-year-old (Ames et al., 1979). Children begin to learn to dodge well at 5 years (Roberton & Halverson, 1984) and can skip, long jump about 2 feet, climb with sureness, jump rope, and do acrobatic tricks. Handedness is well established, and overhand throwing is accomplished (Ames et al., 1979). (Current research suggests that hand preference is already stable by 12 to 13 months in most children [Fagard, 1990].) The 5-year-old likes to help with household tasks, play with blocks, and build houses. Eating is independent, including using a knife except for cutting meat, although dawdling and wriggling in the chair may be trying to parents. The challenge of dressing oneself is past, so children age 5 may ask for more help than they need (usually only for tying shoes or buttoning difficult buttons), and overall, undressing is generally easier than dressing.

At age 6, children are constantly on the go, "lugging, tugging, digging, dancing, climbing, pushing, pulling" (Ames et al., 1979, p. 49). Six-year-olds seem to be consciously practicing body balance in climbing, crawling over and under things, and dancing about the room. They swing too high, build too tall, and try activities exceeding their ability. Indoors, awkwardness may cause accidents, and the child seems less coordinated than during the previous year. Despite excellent eating skills, falling out of the chair or knocking over full glasses is not uncommon.

STEPS IN MOTOR SKILL DEVELOPMENT

In the various motor skills developed in the preschool and elementary school years, each body segment has its own developmental trajectory within the overall coordinative structure; one part can be at a different level of skill than another, although all parts tend to be at a primitive level early or at an advanced level when skills are well learned (Roberton & Halverson, 1984). Furthermore, when demands of the task change (increased height, distance, or accuracy requirements), or when fatigue sets in, one body component may regress in its action while another continues to perform at an advanced level of skill. Thus, task requirements are once again seen to be influential in determining the characteristics of motor responses. For hopping and other skills, such as catching, throwing, and jumping, Roberton and Halverson (1984) provided detailed analyses and photographs of the intra-task developmental steps for each critical body component, instruction in how to make detailed observations to categorize the level of skill of body segments, and advice for guiding the learning of these childhood skills.

Physical therapists would find this information useful in planning intervention for children with mild physical disabilities or clumsiness. For example, as children learn to throw, the trunk goes through similar stages of development as those found in early developmental motor activities. The trunk is initially passive, then increasingly a stabilizer for the function of the extremities, and finally a participant in actively imparting force to the flight of the ball. Jumping changes from a functional activity characterized best as falling and catching to one of projection, flight, and landing, each with components that add force and speed or shock absorption to lend elegance and style to the activity.

Although many tests of motor development include assessment of hopping skills, most therapists probably would not view this as a particularly functional activity because children seldom hop spontaneously (Roberton & Halverson, 1984). Physical educators, however, believe that hopping is an important developmental skill because

a hop is often required in situations such as controlling momentum during sudden stops and in handling unexpected perturbations to balance, as well as for pleasurable play activities such as skipping. Hopping is also an excellent activity for describing the development of various strategies leading, finally, to skillful action.

Skillful hopping requires projected flight off the supporting leg and a pumping action of the swinging leg that assists in force production. Initial prehop attempts involve extension of the supporting leg as the child tries to lift off with the nonsupporting leg raised high. The first successful strategy, however, is usually a quick hip-and-knee flexion that pulls the supporting leg off the floor and into momentary flight (actually falling off balance and flexing the leg) while the swing leg remains inactive. At the next level of skill, the supporting leg again extends but with limited range and early timing relative to the point of takeoff. In skillful hopping, the swinging leg leads the takeoff, and extension of the supporting leg occurs late; thus the action becomes one of "land, ride, and extend" (Roberton & Halverson, 1984, p. 62). Just as with infants learning to descend risky slopes (Adolph, 1997), children learn through practice how to control their intrinsic dynamics to produce efficient movements that accomplish intended goals.

Sports and playground games become increasingly important parts of children's motor activities when they enter school and when complex feats of coordination become possible. Children have, however, individual rates of development of the components of motor skill, some undoubtedly innate, some based on cultural characteristics and family interest in development of physical skills. McGraw's (1935) work demonstrates, for example, that toddlers can develop motor skills that are usually considered inappropriate, primarily because of safety issues. Furthermore, research has generally supported the belief that African-American children have superior motor skills, especially those involving speed and agility, relative to white children (Cintas, 1988; Lee, 1980; Plimpton & Regimbal, 1992). Most authors have explained these differences on the basis of socioeconomic status and differences in permissiveness of child rearing (Williams & Scott, 1953).

INTERACTIONS BETWEEN PERCEPTUAL-COGNITIVE DEVELOPMENT AND MOTOR DEVELOPMENT

The work of Bertenthal and Campos (1987) is significant in demonstrating that experience, not maturation alone, drives perceptual-cognitive development and that self-induced movement is critical in evoking advancements in a number of important cognitive processes. Through ingenious studies that varied locomotor experience levels by studying natural differences, such as length of time infants had been creeping, and unusual childhood events, such as being confined to a cast for a long period or being given a walker to induce locomotion before it occurred independently, Bertenthal and Campos have shown that self-induced locomotion is a critical ingredient in the development of depth perception that mediates avoidance of heights when a child is placed on a visual cliff. This behavior normally develops between 7 and 9 months of age but is related more to degree of locomotor experience than to age at locomotion. Bertenthal and Campos also reviewed other evidence that self-produced locomotion promotes developmental progress in functions such as memory for locations and ability to localize objects objectively with reference to external landmarks rather than egocentrically. Children who did not creep have also been demonstrated to be cognitively delayed when compared with children with creeping experience (McEwan et al., 1991). Adolph (1997) found that only 2 of 24 infants in her study of slope descent were able to transfer what they had learned from crawling on slopes to the choice of whether to traverse risky slopes as new walkers. Those infants were younger and smaller at crawling onset but older and more maturely proportioned at walking onset than infants who did not show transfer of learning from crawling on slopes to the decision regarding traversal by walking. These infants therefore had more experience with crawling than other infants. Infants who spent a long time as bellycrawlers also were able to descend steeper slopes than other infants. Two infants in the study who were consistently reckless (i.e., traversed hopelessly risky slopes despite repeated experiences of falling) were infants who spent little time as crawlers and walked very early. Adolph and colleagues (1998) have also demonstrated that, although not all children go through a belly crawling stage, duration of experience with belly crawling is correlated with speed and efficiency at onset of creeping on hands and knees. These findings call into question the previous assumption that varying patterns of development of locomotion are merely that, variations without developmental significance for learning and future motor performance.

In general, therapists must take into account in treatment planning not only the precocity of an infant's abilities to perceive the basic affordances of the environment in terms of action possibilities but also the long period of development of motor skills and spatial-cognitive and other perceptual functions for fine-tuning choices regarding how to act on objects. For example, infants can adapt their reaching to the actual distance of an object at 3.5 to 5.5 months (Vinter, 1990). Depth perception is based on kinetic information at 3 months, binocular information at 5 months, and pictorial information at 7 to 9 months. Children preform the hand for the anticipated shape of an object at about 9 to 10 months and can adapt for anticipated weight by 14 to 16 months (Corbetta & Mounoud, 1990). At 18 to 30 months, children sometimes fail to take into account object size, attempting impossible actions on miniature objects such as sitting in a dollhouse chair (DeLoache et al., 2004). Children under the approximate age of 6 are not able to conserve the amount of a substance when the shape of its container is altered (Beilin, 1989). By 7 or 8 years of age, however, they recognize that pouring water from a wide container to one that is narrower has not increased the amount of water (Roberton & Halverson, 1984). Weight, however, is not conserved until 9 or 10 years, and volume not until 11 or 12. As mentioned earlier, Bushnell and Boudreau (1993) propose that motor development is a rate-limiting factor in many of these perceptual-cognitive skills because movements make available information needed for the acquisition of related perceptual abilities. Although they believe that self-generated movements are the typical means for acquiring these abilities, they think that assistance with the necessary movements may also help infants to learn, an obvious area for research on intervention with children with disabilities.

Gibson used the term differentiation to describe the improvements that occur in perception over the course of development (Pick, 1992). According to Pick, Gibson stated that "progressive differentiation occurs with respect to information specifying the meaningful properties of the world" (Pick, 1992, p. 789). Gibson believed that perception involves an active effort to make sense of the world, but the action is exploratory, not executive in the sense of using physical manipulation. Perception improves because we detect more of the aspects, features, and nuances that convey the meaning of objects and events, such as how risky it might be to descend a steep slope. It seems likely that the alternations in apparent self-confidence, coordination, and other characteristics of children reported by Ames and colleagues (1979) and Adolph (1997) are related to their best attempts to make sense of the world as physical characteristics and control over intrinsic dynamics of the body, neural maturation, perceptual abilities, and other developmental subsystems change with growth and experience.

Although the importance of motor experience in the longitudinal development of many of the perceptual functions described earlier has not, to my knowledge, been explored by researchers aside from Adolph's inquiry regarding decisions about traversible slopes (1997), the finding that self-directed activity is influential in some spatial-cognitive functions suggests the need to pay attention to providing compensations for functional limitations that may hinder children's development when physical disabilities are present. Bertenthal and Campos (1987), for example, have shown that use of a walker before endogenously produced locomotion was present positively affected performance on the visual cliff problem. Thus, maneuvering under self-control appears to be more important than does locomotor movement per se. Although a review of the literature on the influence of baby walker use on age of walking suggests that walking onset may be delayed by 11 to 26 days when a walker is used (Burrows & Griffiths, 2002), perhaps therapists should reconsider prohibitions regarding the use of walkers for children with developmental disabilities if safety during usage can be assured.

Bushnell and Boudreau (1993) propose that if infants are unable to engage in motor activities necessary to the acquisition or practice of specific perceptual or cognitive skills, the motor problem may block mental development. An example is that lack of self-generated mobility may lead to failure to begin to code spatial location based on environmental landmarks rather than in relation to self. In their review of the development of haptic perception (ability to acquire information about objects with the hands and to discriminate and recognize objects from handling them as opposed to looking at them), Bushnell and Boudreau (1993) noticed a developmental timetable suggesting that infants under 7 months of age can already distinguish objects by characteristics such as temperature and hardness, that from 6 months on they can distinguish textures, and that ability to perceive weight emerges at about 9 months of age. Finally, distinguishing objects by configurational shape emerges sometime after 12 to 15 months. These authors believe that this timetable is explained by constraints placed on infants by their motor development, specifically the exploratory procedures or hand movements they are capable of making at various ages. Rubbing with the fingers, for example, is typically used to assess the texture of an object, and repeatedly lifting and lowering an object is used to gauge weight. Until an infant can use the property most appropriate for gaining knowledge about an object's multiple characteristics, such perceptual knowledge cannot be gained or used. Temperature and hardness can be appraised by static contact or pressure; thus these properties of objects would logically be among the first to be recognized by an infant. In Adolph's (1997) study of slope behavior, it may be that infants used their vision and patting abilities only to decide that a risky slope provided a stable continuous path toward a landing below but were unable to consider whether their physical capabilities included sufficient balance to control gravitational and inertial forces that would result from their attempts to descend until they had sufficient experience with a variety of other movement patterns to help them learn about controlling intrinsic dynamics.

GROSS MOTOR ACTIVITY IN A FUNCTIONAL CONTEXT: PLAY

Research on childrens' activity memory, or ability to explicitly recall activities they observe or create, is helpful in considering how to structure therapeutic exercise to promote memory regarding what has been experienced. Ratner and Foley (1994) reviewed the literature on activity memory and suggest that children remember activities better if (1) there was a clear outcome of the activity, (2) actions within the activity were logically sequenced such that cause and effect were obvious throughout the activity, and (3) the child engaged in planning of the actions involved in the activity in advance of carrying it out (not just mental imaging of it) or were asked to plan to remember what happened. Young children do not always profit from external memory cues, at least not until 3 years of age or older, depending on the type of cue. Nevertheless, childrens' behaviors show that they both consciously and verbally anticipate the unfolding and outcomes of activities by at least 2 years of age, even telling themselves "no, no" when about to perform some forbidden action (Ratner & Foley, 1994). At this point, imaginary play with objects that are not present appears, and children express surprise when outcomes of actions are not what they expected. Play then provides the opportunity for children to voluntarily act out intentions and to learn the difference between plans and outcomes. By 20 months of age, children are able to work toward a concrete goal, such as building a house from blocks, exhibit checking behaviors, correct mistakes, and acknowledge successful achievement of the goal. Repetition of an activity typically enhances memory of it when recall support is provided, and even infants 4 to 6 months of age can be shown to have some retrospective processing of events in that experiments demonstrate that they actively notice properties of an activity that were previously not noticed. Preschoolers allowed to demonstrate what happened will recall far more of an activity than if only verbal recall is elicited. Therapists should consider the mental ages of the children they treat with a mind toward creating therapeutic activities that provide children with disabilities the opportunity to develop cognitive skills such as planning and activity memory as they engage in exercise to reduce impairments.

When seen in its functional context as a learning device, motor activity can also be seen to have a stagelike character. Physical activity play (i.e., play with a vigorous physical component) has three developmental stages (Pellegrini & Smith, 1998). In infancy, babies engage in what Thelen (1995) has called rhythmic stereotypies or repetitive gross motor activities without any obvious purpose, including body rocking, foot kicking, and leg waving. Whole-body, self-motion play is also called peragration, and Adolph (1997) suggests that such activities are the most direct route to knowledge—infants plunge in and obtain important information as a result. These behaviors peak around the midpoint of the first year of life with as much as 40% of a 1-hour observation at 6 months being composed of such play (Pellegrini & Smith, 1998).

A second stage called exercise play begins at the end of the first year (Pellegrini & Smith, 1998). Such play can be solitary or with others, increases from the toddler to the preschool periods, and then declines during the primary school years. It accounts for about 7% of behavior observed in child care settings. Activities included in exercise play include running, chasing, and climbing. Children with physical disabilities may need alternatives for participating in such play, particularly with other children.

The third phase of physical activity play is rough-and-tumble play such as wrestling, kicking, and tumbling in a social context. Often this type of play appears first in interaction with a parent, typically a father. Rough-and-tumble play increases through the preschool and primary school years and peaks just before early adolescence. No gender differences are noted in peragration activities, but males engage in more exercise play and rough-and-tumble play than females.

The functional benefits of physical activity play may be deferred or immediate. Pellegrini and Smith (1998) suggest that the benefits of rhythmic play in infants is immediate in improving control of specific motor patterns, that is, the primary repertoire in Edelman's terms. Through active self-generated body movement, infants create perturbations to balance for which they gradually learn to accommodate or plan; such play also provides interesting visual and perhaps auditory spectacles for development of perceptual systems. Strength and endurance are also developed through such activities. Pellegrini and Smith (1998) posit that the function of exercise play is specifically to promote muscle differentiation, strength, and endurance. Chapter 8 provides further information on health-related physical fitness, which may have its roots in early play behavior. Pellegrini and Smith (1998) describe animal research on the juvenile period suggesting that it is a sensitive period for such development (recall McGraw's experiment with Johnny and Jimmy and their respective adult physiques). Play may also have

cognitive benefits in terms of providing a break from attention-demanding activities, thus leading to distributed practice and creating an enhanced arousal level of benefit to subsequent engagement in mental activities. Seen in this light, recess becomes something more than a meaningless break in the routine.

Pellegrini & Smith (1998) hypothesize that rough-and-tumble play serves a social function, especially for boys, related to establishing and maintaining dominance in social groups (girls are believed to use verbal skills more than boys in establishing dominance hierarchies). As a by-product, children also may use rough-and-tumble play as a way to code and decode social signals. For example, in early rough-and-tumble play with parents, children learn that this is "play" and not aggression. Rosenbaum (1998) suggests that this view of motor activity raises the question of what goals we should pursue in therapeutic interventions. Is it more important to provide opportunities to "travel" than to concentrate on improving gait? Do children with disabilities benefit from adapted recreational activities such as horseback riding in terms of social skills and cognitive function, as well as in motor skills per se? What is lost in terms of self-esteem or ability to decode social signals in children with disabilities if they are "protected" from rough-and-tumble play?

USING DEVELOPMENTAL SEQUENCES AS A THERAPEUTIC FRAMEWORK

Most of our contemporary clinical approaches to developing intervention plans for children with disabilities were originally based on use of the developmental sequence as the primary framework for planning intervention. New theoretic models for understanding the achievement of functional motor skills suggest that this framework, as a rigid structure for approaching intervention, is inadequate. Atwater (1991), for example, suggested that a number of issues must be considered when deciding whether to follow a normal developmental sequence in planning treatment. These issues include the knowledge that (1) multiple underlying processes involving both distal and proximal function develop contemporaneously; (2) motor milestones and their components develop in overlapping sequences, with spurts and regressions being common; (3) many variations in the development of motor milestones occur in typically developing children, and thus motor milestones cannot be considered to be an invariant sequence leading to skill; (4) development in multiple domains must be considered; (5) the age of the child and the extent and type of disability are important considerations in determining which skills will be most functional for a child at any given time; and (6) child and family involvement in decisions regarding the goals of therapy must be considered. The discussion earlier in the chapter regarding contemporary theories of development and neural plasticity provides additional information in support of Atwater's suggestion (1991). She aptly quotes Bobath and Bobath (1984) in stating that

> treatment should not attempt to follow the sequence of development... regardless of the age and physical condition of the individual child. Rather, it should be decided what each child needs most urgently at any one stage or age, and what is absolutely necessary for him to participate for future functional skills, or for improving the skills he has but performs abnormally (Atwater, 1991, p. 91).

I would add the suggestion that an emphasis on processes underlying developmental progress, such as the role of self-induced exploratory movement in both motor learning and in perceptual and cognitive development, and the motivation on the part of children to engage in repetitive, apparently goal-less, practice of activities during sensitive periods of development, should be considered in treatment planning. Further information on sensitive periods of development for basic motor functions will be needed to target times appropriately for most effective intervention, especially for children with disabilities.

Also of great importance is identification of the most effective strategies for promoting the attainment of functional goals involving motor activity. Based on research on facilitation of cognitive development in disadvantaged children, early learning environments, and basic learning strategies, Ramey and Ramey (1992) have identified the following essential daily ingredients to promote intellectual development in children: (1) encouragement of exploration; (2) mentoring in basic skills such as labeling, sequencing, and noting means-ends relations; (3) celebration of developmental advances; (4) guided rehearsal and extension of new skills; (5) protection from inappropriate disapproval, teasing, or punishment; and (6) provision of a rich and responsive language environment. Many of these ingredients are likely to be equally important in promoting motor development in children with physically challenging conditions; research on the design of specific teaching and learning strategies for such children is direly needed. Chapter 4 reviews what is known.

Atwater (1991) recommended that treatment planning should focus on encouragement of functional independence to prevent cognitive retardation and learned helplessness that will be highly disabling in adolescence and adulthood, even when this means giving up goals for improving movement quality. Fetters (1991c) and Harris

(1990) agree, suggesting that ecologically valid treatment programs have as their goals the movements that are necessary and useful to humans as they move about in their environment. Fetters (1991c), however, emphasized that there may be trade-offs inherent in working for function of which therapists should be cognizant. Independence in ambulation may be accomplished only with high physiologic cost; the achievement of faster reaching may result in poorer trunk control.

Although I agree wholeheartedly with the recommendations and observations of these three thoughtful scientific practitioners, I have also argued that therapists must choose wisely when making decisions regarding use of compensatory patterns or assistive devices to facilitate functioning of children with CNS dysfunction. Wise decision making involves giving due consideration to whether use of compensatory patterns may lead to later secondary impairments of a musculoskeletal nature that could also be severely disabling in the future (Campbell, 1991). It is not acceptable to include in a treatment plan a goal for functional movement that does not also meet a requirement that working toward such an objective will not be likely to contribute to potential future deformity, skin breakdown, osteoporosis (Henderson et al., 2002), or other preventable secondary impairment (Campbell, 1997). A focus on health promotion and disease prevention, in addition to a focus on functional improvement to promote current and future activity and participation, is important, indeed, required as physical therapists assume responsibility for direct access care without physician referral. Box 2-1 provides a sampling of health promotion concerns and resources that should be considered to be a part of the armamentarium of every pediatric physical therapist.

Research presented here on the processes of motor development also suggests that children (1) should have the opportunity to make decisions about choosing how to act (rather than being assisted or guided) when a task is presented so that they can exercise their perceptual capabilities, (2) need to engage in exploration through movement in order to develop their appreciation for the affordances of objects and the environment and for whether they possess the motor skill for successful action, and (3) benefit from having a variety of movement synergies available from which to select the most appropriate adaptive strategy in an on-line process of making decisions about how to achieve immediate task goals.

To accomplish these objectives and provide children with a variety of movement strategies with which they can approach the world of infinite possibilities for meaningful activity, we need both our extensive knowledge of biomechanics and more information on the natural history of conditions we treat. Indeed, I believe that the com-

| Box 2-1 | Examples of Health Promotion Concerns and Resources |

1. Injury prevention education, including use of car seats and helmets and safe (or no) use of baby walkers (Burrows & Griffiths, 2002), swings and other play equipment, and toys. A useful reference on typical injuries in children is Agran, PH, Anderson, C, Winn, D, Trent, R, Walton-Haynes, L, & Thayer, S. Rates of pediatric injuries by 3-month intervals for children 0-3 years of age. Pediatrics, 111:e683-e692, 2003, accessed at http://www.pediatrics.org/cgi/content/full/111/6/e683. Falls are the leading cause of injury in this age group.
2. "Back-to-sleep" to prevent SIDS (sudden infant death syndrome) and awake play in the prone position to promote motor development (see American Academy of Pediatrics Task Force on Infant Positioning and SIDS, 1992).
3. Effects of second-hand smoke.
4. Nutrition, including the value of breast-feeding through at least 6 months of age and need for a diet adequate in essential nutrients. A useful reference is de Onis, M, Garza, D, Victora, CG, Onyango, AW, Frongillo, EA, & Martines, J. The WHO multicentre growth reference study: Planning, study design, and methodology. Food and Nutrition Bulletin, 25(1):S15-26, 2004. Encourage an active lifestyle to prevent obesity.
5. Clarifying myths regarding ill effects of immunizations. A useful reference is Wolfe, RM, Sharp, LK, & Lipsky, MS. Content and design attributes of antivaccination web sites. JAMA, 287:3245–3248, 2002.
6. Promote mental health. Two useful references are Thomasgard, M, & Metz, WP. Promoting child social-emotional growth in primary care settings: Using a developmental approach. Clin Pediatrics, 43:119–127, 2004; Petterson, SM, & Albers, AB. Effects of poverty and maternal depression in early child development. Child Development, 72:1794–1813, 2001.

bination of attention to assisting persons with disabilities to improve their functional capabilities through promoting achievement of useful, meaningful activities performed as efficiently as possible, along with prevention of musculoskeletal and other complications, constitutes the unique features of physical therapy. In Chapter 1 and throughout this book, we therefore recommend that therapists use the framework for describing the disabling process developed by the National Center for Medical Rehabilitation Research and used in the *Guide to Physical Therapist Practice* (American Physical Therapy Association, 2001) that approaches disability from the perspective of the multiple, interacting dimensions of the human organism, from the cellular to the societal (National Advisory Board on Medical Rehabilitation Research, 1993), but, preferably, move toward use of the International Classification of Function, Disability and Health of the World Health Organization (World Health Organization, 2001) because of its positive outlook on disability and global acceptability.

Such a comprehensive approach to clinical decision making requires the use of appropriate assessments on which to base treatment planning and outcome evaluation. Tests of motor development and functional skills that meet appropriate psychometric standards and are useful in clinical settings are discussed in the next section. Other tests are described in Chapters 3 and 8 as well as in chapters throughout the book on examination and treatment of children with specific disabilities.

TESTS OF MOTOR DEVELOPMENT AND FUNCTIONAL PERFORMANCE

Physical therapists use motor milestone and functional performance tests to document children's developmental level in relation to age-related standards and to observe the activity abilities and limitations that may be present. Tests of specific functional skills, such as dressing and feeding, are also used to assess current levels of functioning and to document developmental progress and achievement of expected intervention and family education outcomes. Constraints causing functional limitations can be assessed with various tests of impairment. Those related to postural control and musculoskeletal impairment are described in Chapters 3 and 6. In conjunction with family interviews and home or school observations, therapists can examine competencies in fulfilling age-appropriate roles and identify areas of disability that should be addressed with a therapeutic program in consultation with other professionals and the family.

Although all tests to be described in this chapter are standardized scales with acceptable psychometric properties according to the American Physical Therapy Association's Standards for Tests and Measurements in Physical Therapy (Task Force on Standards for Measurement in Physical Therapy, 1991), some tests remain under development, so complete information is not available. Those selected for brief discussion include the Test of Infant Motor Performance (TIMP), Harris Infant Neuromotor Test, Miller First Step, Bayley II, Peabody Developmental Motor Scales, Bruininks-Oseretsky Test of Motor Proficiency, Gross Motor Function Measure, Pediatric Evaluation of Disability Inventory, and Functional Independence Measure for Children. Tests selected for discussion were limited by space, and commonly used tests such as the Denver II (Frankenburg et al., 1990, 1992) and the Gesell Revised Developmental Schedules (Knobloch et al., 1980) are not included because of poor specificity (43%) with high overreferral rates (Glascoe et al., 1992) and out-of-date norms, respectively. The reader may consult Palisano (1993) or Stengel (1991) for more information on these and other tests. Finally, the Pediatric Clinical Test of Sensory Interaction for Balance is briefly described as an example of a test of children's capability to use perception to control movement responses.

Although the tests described are at various stages of development, none is a test of participation in daily life in which observations take place in an ecologically valid setting. Those that purport to assess disability do so through report of a knowledgeable informant, such as the parent, guardian, or teacher. Some tests are more useful for individual treatment planning, others for comparing global performance to age standards for diagnostic and classification purposes or for programmatic assessment of overall rehabilitation outcomes. Use of a combination of the tests would provide comprehensive assessment of functional skills in children with physical disabilities, although improved tests and well-thought-out, comprehensive protocols are still needed (Campbell, 1989, 1996; Fetters, 1991c; Haley et al., 1993; Long & Tieman, 1998).

SCREENING TESTS

The Harris Infant Neuromotor Test (HINT) (Harris & Daniels, 1996) is a 22-item screening test to identify developmental delay in infants from 3 to 12 months of age. The test includes items to assess neuromotor milestones, active and passive muscle tone, head circumference, stereotypic movement patterns, behavioral interactions, and the caregiver's assessment of the infant's development. Rather than reflecting a specific developmental theme, items were selected specifically because of research evidence suggesting sensitivity to delayed development. In a study of 54 high-risk infants (Harris & Daniels, 2001), concurrent validity with the Bayley II motor scale in the first year of life was −0.89 (high scores on the HINT indicate poorer performance, accounting for the negative correlation). The predictive validity of the HINT in the first year to Bayley

II motor scale scores at 17 to 22 months was −0.49, accounting for 24% of the variance in Bayley II scores. Correlations with the Bayley II mental scale were lower. Age standards for the test are under development in a sample of 400 full-term infants in four Canadian provinces (Harris et al., 2003). A classification analysis for diagnostic purposes (sensitivity and specificity) has not yet been reported for the full test, but caregiver impressions concur highly with motor development measured concurrently with the Bayley scales. The test takes less than 30 minutes to administer and score, is primarily observational, and can be used by a variety of health care professionals.

The Miller First Step Screening Test for Evaluating Preschoolers (Miller, 1992) is a screening test to identify children at risk for developmental delays. The test is appropriate for assessing cognitive, communicative, physical, social-emotional, and adaptive function in children from 2 years 9 months to 6 years 2 months of age. Function is defined as performance on games using toys that are entertaining and exciting for children in this age group. The test was normed on a U.S. sample of 100 boys and 100 girls in each 6-month age grouping. It takes 17 minutes to administer and score performance on the 18 games.

COMPREHENSIVE DEVELOPMENTAL ASSESSMENT

The Bayley II (Bayley, 1993) is a revised and renormed version of the Bayley Scales of Infant Development (BSID) (Bayley, 1969), necessitated by changes in infants' developmental rate since 1969 (Campbell et al., 1986). The scales contain norm-referenced (based on a sample of 1700 U.S. children) motor and mental scales for children from birth to 42 months of age and a criterion-referenced behavioral scale for examining such areas as affect, attention, exploration, and fearfulness. Use of the latter has revealed the problems with self-regulation of very low birth weight preterm infants, supporting the need for neurobehavioral intervention in the first 6 months of life (Wolf et al., 2002). Functions on the mental scale include object permanence, memory, problem solving, and complex language. The motor scale assesses both fine and gross motor function, including fine manipulative skills, coordination of large muscle groups, dynamic movement, postural imitation, and stereognosis. A strength of the test is that items have been carefully evaluated for bias based on cultural factors.

Scores of infants tested longitudinally in the first year with the 1969 motor scale have not been demonstrated to be stable (Coryell et al., 1989), and Bayley herself recommended that three consecutive tests be used to estimate performance during the first 15 months of life

(Rosenblith, 1992). The small amount of research on various aspects of the validity of the Bayley II is reviewed by Koseck (1999), including potential scoring problems of which users should be aware. Harris and Daniels (2001) reported the correlation between Bayley II motor scale scores in the first year of life with scores at 17 to 22 months of age to be only 0.34. As a result, therapists are advised to be conservative in assuming predictive capabilities of the new test until further research is available. The Bayley II takes about 45 to 60 minutes to administer.

MOTOR ASSESSMENTS

The TIMP (Campbell et al., 1995) is a test for infants younger than age 4 months, including prematurely born infants as young as 32 weeks of postconceptional age. Function on this scale is defined as the postural and selective control needed for functional movements in early infancy, including head and trunk control in prone, supine, and upright positions. Version 5.1 of the TIMP has 13 items scored pass-fail on the basis of observations of spontaneous activity and 29 scaled items administered by the examiner according to a standardized format. Elicited items present the infant with problems to solve that require organization of head and trunk posture in space to orient to interesting spectacles, interact with the tester, or regain a preferred postural configuration. Scores are correlated with age (0.83), are sensitive to degree of medical complications experienced in the newborn period ($R^2 = 0.72$, $p < 0.00001$, when age and risk are used to predict test performance; Campbell et al., 1995), and discriminate among infants with varying risk for poor developmental outcome (Campbell & Hedeker, 2001). Rasch psychometric assessment of test results indicates that the test forms an interval-level scale (Campbell et al., 2002b). Test-retest reliability over a 3-day period for infants across the age range of the test was 0.89 (Campbell, 1999), and at 3 months of age scores above and below 0.50 standard deviation below the mean on the TIMP identified 80% of the same children identified as above or below the 10th percentile on the AIMS at the same age (Campbell & Kolobe, 2000). The predictive validity of TIMP scores at 3 months to 12-month Alberta Infant Motor Scale percentile ranks was sensitivity 0.92 and specificity 0.76 (Campbell et al., 2002a). TIMP scores at 3 months have a sensitivity of 0.72 and specificity of 0.91 for predicting Peabody Developmental Gross Motor Scale scores at preschool age (Kolobe et al., 2004). TIMP scores in infancy are correlated with Bruininks-Oseretsky scores at school age (partial correlation = 0.36; Flegel & Kolobe, 2002). Ecologic validity of the TIMP has been demonstrated by research indicating that 98% of TIMP item-

handling procedures are similar to demands for movement placed on infants by their caregivers in dressing, bathing, and play interactions (Murney & Campbell, 1998). The test is sensitive to changes in motor performance of preterm infants in the weeks prior to term age (Unanue & Westcott, 2003) and to developmental differences in infants who will later be diagnosed as having CP (Barbosa et al., 2003). Two studies have demonstrated that the test is sensitive to the effects of physical therapy in the form of neurodevelopmental treatment in the special care nursery (Girolami & Campbell, 1994) and in the form of a home program following nursery discharge (Lekschulchai & Cole, 2001). New age standards for the TIMP are under development in a sample of approximately 1000 U.S. infants of all ethnicities; a 10-minute screening version is also under development. A self-instructional CD is available for use in learning to score the test (Liao & Campbell, 2002).

The Peabody Developmental Motor Scales (PDMS) (Folio & Fewell, 2000; Hinderer et al., 1989) contain separate scales for gross and fine motor assessment for children from birth to 71 months of age. Functions examined by the gross motor scale include reflexes, balance, nonlocomotor and locomotor activities, and receipt and propulsion of objects. The fine motor scale examines grasp, hand functions, eye-hand coordination, and manual dexterity. The PDMS was renormed in 1997–1998 on 2003 children (Folio & Fewell, 2000). Fine motor ratings were reported to be more reliable for children with delays (0.96) than for those without delays (0.76), but these results were related more to the statistical effect created by the greater variability of the delayed group than to actual disagreements between raters (Stokes et al., 1990). Goyen and Lui (2002) used the Peabody scales to demonstrate differences in gross and fine motor performance over time in "apparently normal" high-risk infants and reported that the presence of gross motor deficiencies increased over the period from 18 months to 5 years, but Darrah and colleagues (2003) showed that serial assessments of motor function did not show stability over time, which could be a result of nonlinear development in children *or* because of the psychometric properties of test items themselves. Kolobe and colleagues (1998) examined the sensitivity to change in children with motor delay or CP of the gross motor scale and found it to be as sensitive to change over a 6-month period as the Gross Motor Function Measure (Russell et al., 1989) described in the next section. The test takes 45 to 60 minutes to administer.

The Bruininks-Oseretsky Test of Motor Proficiency is a test of gross and fine motor function for children from 4.5 to 14.5 years of age (Bruininks, 1978). The test has subscales for running speed and agility, balance, bilateral coordination, strength, upper limb coordination, response speed, visual-motor control, and upper limb speed and dexterity. Although the test is largely one of coordination and balance (Krus et al., 1981), several subtests have items that are clearly related to functional demands for school-age children, such as cutting within lines and ball activities and physical education skills such as sit-ups, shuttle-runs, and long jumping. Bruininks-Oseretsky scores were sensitive to the differences in motor development of 8-year-old children with a history of bronchopulmonary dysplasia when compared with other preterm infants or full-term infants; furthermore, test scores were even poorer in those who had been treated with steroids than in those who had not (Short et al., 2003). The test was normed on 765 U.S. subjects. The test takes 45 to 60 minutes to administer (a 15- to 20-minute short form is available).

ASSESSMENTS DESIGNED FOR CHILDREN WITH DISABILITIES

The Gross Motor Function Measure (GMFM) (Rosenbaum et al., 1990; Russell et al., 1989) is a test specifically designed and validated for measuring change over time in gross motor function in children with CP. The test has also been validated as useful in children with Down syndrome (Gemus et al., 2001). Function in this test is defined as the child's degree of achievement of a motor behavior (regardless of quality) when instructed to perform or when placed in a particular position. Spontaneously chosen movements are not assessed. The test's items are distributed over five dimensions to measure how much children can do, not the quality with which they do it. These dimensions include lying and rolling; sitting; crawling and kneeling; standing; and walking, running, and jumping. The test was validated for sensitivity to change over a 6-month period in children with CP from 5 months to 16 years of age. Change judged from blind evaluation of videotapes was correlated with GMFM test scores at 0.82. Kolobe and colleagues (1998) found that, as would be expected, children with motor delay changed more on the GMFM over a 6-month period than did children with CP. The test has not been normed on a sample of able-bodied children, but generally all items are achievable by 5-year-olds with normal motor function. Rasch analysis of test items to create an interval-level test resulted in the formation of a new 66-item version called the GMFM-66 (Avery et al., 2003). A computer program is available for scoring the GMFM-66. The full 88-item version of the test requires 45 to 60 minutes to administer.

The GMFM has been extensively used in research on interventions such as intensive physical therapy and selective dorsal rhizotomy, documenting its value for use in clinical practice and decision making (for a summary, see Bjornson et al., 1998a). Because children with CP are generally considered to be highly variable in performance from day to day, Bjornson and colleagues (1998b) studied test-retest reliability over a 1-week period and found intraclass correlations for all subsections to be at least 0.80. Russell and colleagues (1998) assessed the responsivity of the GMFM to change in children with Down syndrome below age 6. They found that, although children showed significant changes in scores over a 6-month period that were also greater for the youngest children than those demonstrated by the Bayley II, the correlation between GMFM scores and parents' or therapists' judgments of change was poor and lower than that obtained in studies of change responsivity in children with CP. Correlations were improved if raters accepted parents' reports of item achievement when the child did not demonstrate the behavior during testing. Finally, scores on the total GMFM and on the subsections using predominantly the legs are correlated with independently obtained assessments of leg strength, accounting for 55 to 65% of the common variance, but are not correlated with aerobic power or with arm strength (Parker et al., 1993). The Gross Motor Performance Measure, a companion test of postural control in items from the GMFM (Boyce et al., 1991), is described in Chapter 3. A gross motor disability classification system for grouping children by level of disability, similar in nature to a disease staging system, which was recently developed by the same research group (Palisano et al., 1997), is described in Chapter 1 on clinical decision making. The validity of the classification system for predicting developmental growth curves in children with CP has been demonstrated (Rosenbaum et al., 2002).

The Pediatric Evaluation of Disability Inventory (PEDI) is a discriminative device for detecting functional limitations and participation in terms of age-appropriate independence and is also a tool for program evaluation in tracking progress in individual children with disabilities (Feldman et al., 1990; Haley et al., 1991, 1992). Function in this scale is defined as ability to perform ADL with or without modifications or assistance as reported by a knowledgeable informant. On the PEDI, 197 items measure functional skills in self-care, mobility, and social function, and 20 items assess the extent of caregiver assistance and modifications needed to reduce or eliminate disabilities in each domain. The test was normed on 412 U.S. children without disabilities, and initial validity for discriminating function and assistance needed was derived from a clinical sample of 102 children with various disabilities (Feldman et al., 1990). Both normative standard scores and scaled scores are provided for each of its three domains. The test takes 20 to 30 minutes to complete by therapists or teachers and 45 to 60 minutes by structured parent interview. Hey and colleagues at Boston Children's Hospital have developed a parent self-administered version of the PEDI that took an average of 35 minutes to complete in a sample of 110 parents (Hey, LA, Kasser, J, Rosenthal, R, Ramsing, N, & Katz, J, unpublished data, 1992). Scoring software to obtain Rasch logit measures is available. Direct testing of children's performance in an ecologically valid setting is not specified but could be done.

The Functional Independence Measure for Children (WeeFIM) is a discipline-free test of disability for assessing functions in self-care, sphincter control, mobility, locomotion, and communication and social cognition (Granger et al., 1989; Msall et al., 1992a). Function in this scale is defined as caregiver assistance needed to accomplish daily tasks. The WeeFIM is descriptive of caretaker and special resources required because of functional limitations and is useful in tracking outcomes over time across health, developmental, and community settings. Although insufficient detail is provided to be useful in making treatment decisions, it is an excellent tool for description of overall rehabilitation outcomes, for use in program evaluation, and for cross-disciplinary communication. The test has 18 items measured on a 7-point ordinal scale for use with children with developmental disabilities from 6 months to 12 years of age. Pilot normative work on a sample of 222 U.S. children demonstrated significant correlations between total WeeFIM scores and age ($r = 0.80$) (Msall et al., 1992b). The test has been used with children with extreme prematurity, CP, Down syndrome, congenital limb disorders, myelodysplasia, and traumatic brain injury (Msall, ME, personal communication, 1992). The test requires 20 to 30 minutes to complete.

Finally, given the evidence from studies such as Adolph's (1997), which illustrates how children use their perception of the affordances of the environment, one test that assesses childrens' ability to use their multiple senses to solve problems involving conflicting information for control of upright posture will be briefly mentioned; information on test findings in children with different disabilities is discussed in Chapter 3. Deitz and colleagues (1996) developed the Pediatric Clinical Test of Sensory Interaction for Balance in order to assess children's standing stability under varying sensory conditions, including standing on stable versus foam surfaces, with and without vision, and with information from body sway relative to the surround occluded. Children must "select"

the right sensory inputs to interpret their stability situation correctly, and these researchers have shown that children with learning disabilities and motor delays perform more poorly on the test than typically developing children. Tests of impairment such as this should be useful clinically to differentiate movement problems caused by sensory processing difficulties from problems with coordination of the motor ensemble.

In summary, a number of well-designed tests are available for screening and examining functional motor performance in children, and several tests assess specific motor constructs, activity, and functional limitations of children with disabilities. Some of these tests require further validation in clinical practice, but early results are promising. No standardized tests have yet emerged from the new interest in contemporary theories of motor development and motor control, perhaps because dynamical systems theory emphasizes the process rather than products of development. Measures derived from dynamical systems theory should (1) include examination of a variety of subsystems related to the motor ensemble, such as the musculoskeletal system, perception, and movement patterns; and (2) use age-appropriate tasks and variation in the environment (Heriza, 1991). Measurement of periods of instability in patterns of movement selected by the child in response to tasks in varying contexts is deemed to be important. Long and Tieman (1998) recently reviewed tests for conformity to the challenges of a dynamical systems perspective as outlined by Heriza (1991). They found that some tests examine age-appropriate tasks and subsystems performance but do not specifically address contextual variations or search for instability of selection of movement patterns just before systematic appearance of a qualitatively new motor behavior. The latter is a key issue in assessment of motor development from a dynamical systems perspective because such periods of instability are believed to be sensitive periods for effective intervention.

Evaluation of the results of tests of function and disability gives the therapist knowledge of what the child can do, with or without assistance from technology or caregivers. These results are important in diagnosis of developmental delay or deviance and for providing basic information regarding the child's motor competencies for accomplishing the important tasks of childhood play and for experiencing the joy of activity used for pleasure and for purposeful exploration of the world. More information, however, is needed for planning intervention when functional limitations are identified. Roberton and Halverson (1984) have described, in a beautifully succinct way, the process of developing a plan for helping a child to learn movement. Once having observed in what way and how the child responds to a movement task believed to be developmentally appropriate, the prospective coach must consider what the environment demands for the child to succeed at the task and also must interpret the child's response. "What is the meaning of a child's solution to a particular movement problem? Does it indicate a more advanced form of movement? Does it suggest improved perceptual functioning? Is the solution a cognitive attempt to avoid a balance-threatening position? Does the child's response suggest that the task is too stressful, too complex at that particular moment—that the child is not 'ready' for it?" (Roberton & Halverson, 1984, p. 3). According to dynamical systems theory, we would also ask what constraints in a variety of cooperating subsystems might be limiting performance and whether the child's selected movement strategy is stable or in transition. Based on task analysis and an interpretation of the child's solution, the teacher must decide whether to intervene or to leave the child and the environment alone. If the decision is to intervene, the teacher must decide whether to redesign the physical environment, verbally or physically coach the child, or show the child a possible solution. After implementing the decision, reexamination is used to evaluate the effectiveness of the intervention.

SUMMARY

Theories of motor development have evolved over time, but current thinking suggests that development is a complex outcome of the maturation of multiple physiologic systems in combination with demands placed on children by the environment and task-related experiences. In keeping with this idea, pediatric physical therapists use examination and interview processes to identify activity and participation needs of children along with impairments and environmental conditions that may present barriers to satisfying and efficient performance. Planning of intervention based on these results incorporates goals of parents and children. The other chapters in this foundational section provide further information to aid the physical therapist with these basic processes of examination, clinical instruction, and decision making. The information provided in these chapters will enable pediatric physical therapists to apply current concepts and research for the benefit of our clients-children with disabilities and their families.

ACKNOWLEDGMENT

Partial support for work described in this chapter was provided by the Foundation for Physical Therapy and the National Center for Medical Rehabilitation Research of the U.S. National Institutes of Health.

REFERENCES

Abramov, I, Gordon, J, Hendrickson, A, Hainline, L, Dobson, V, & LaBossiere, E. The retina of the human infant. Science, 217:265–267, 1982.

Adolph, KE. Learning in the development of infant locomotion. Monographs of the Society for Research in Child Development, 62(3):1–140, 1997.

Adolph, KE, & Avolio, AM. Walking infants adapt locomotion to changing body dimensions. Journal of Experimental Psychology, 26:1148–1166, 2000.

Adolph, KE, Vereijken, B, & Denny, MA. Learning to crawl. Child Development, 69:1299–1312, 1998.

Adolph, KE, Vereijken, B, & Shrout, PE. What changes in infant walking and why. Child Development, 74:475–497, 2003.

American Academy of Pediatrics Task Force on Infant Positioning and SIDS. Positioning and SIDS. Pediatrics, 89:1120–1126, 1992.

American Physical Therapy Association. Guide to Physical Therapist Practice, 2nd ed. Physical Therapy, 81:9–746, 2001.

Ames, LB, Gillespie, C, Haines, J, & Ilg, FL. The Gesell Institute's Child from One to Six: Evaluating the Behavior of the Preschool Child. New York: Harper & Row, 1979.

Anderson, DI, Campos, JJ, Anderson, DE, Thomas, TD, Witherington, DC, Uchiyama, I, & Barbu-Roth, MA. The flip side of perception-action coupling: Locomotor experience and the ontogeny of visual-postural coupling. Human Movement Science, 20:461–487, 2001.

Angulo-Kinzler, RM. Exploration and selection of intralimb coordination patterns in 3-month-old infants. Journal of Motor Behavior, 33:363–376, 2001.

Atwater, SW. Should the normal motor developmental sequence be used as a theoretical model in pediatric physical therapy? In Lister, MJ (Ed.). Contemporary Management of Motor Control Problems: Proceedings of the II STEP Conference. Alexandria, VA: Foundation for Physical Therapy, 1991, pp. 89–93.

Avery, LM, Russell, DJ, Raina, PS, Walter, SD, & Rosenbaum, PL. Rasch analysis of the Gross Motor Function Measure: Validating the assumptions of the Rasch model to create an interval-level measure. Archives of Physical Medicine & Rehabilitation, 84:697–705, 2003.

Bailey, DB, Jr, Bruer, JT, Symons, FJ, & Lichtman, JW. Critical Thinking About Critical Periods. Baltimore: Paul H. Brookes Publishing Co., 2001.

Barbosa, VM, Campbell, SK, Sheftel, D, Singh, J, & Beligere, N. Longitudinal performance of infants with cerebral palsy on the Test of Infant Motor Performance and on the Alberta Infant Motor Scale. Physical & Occupational Therapy in Pediatrics, 23(3):7–29, 2003.

Bard, C, Fleury, M, & Hay, L (Eds.). Development of Eye-Hand Coordination across the Life Span. Columbia, SC: University of South Carolina Press, 1990.

Barinaga, M. Death gives birth to the nervous system. But how? Science, 259:762–763, 1993.

Bayley, N. Manual for the Bayley Scales of Infant Development. New York: Psychological Corporation, 1969.

Bayley, N. Bayley II. San Antonio: Psychological Corporation, 1993.

Beilin, H. Piagetian theory. In Vasta, R (Ed.). Annals of Child Development, Vol. 6. Greenwich, CT: JAI Press, 1989, pp. 85–131.

Bergenn, VW, Dalton, TC, & Lipsitt, LP. Myrtle B. McGraw: A growth scientist. Developmental Psychology, 28:381–395, 1992.

Bertenthal, BI, & Campos, JJ. New directions in the study of early experience. Child Development, 58:560–567, 1987.

Bevor, TG. Regressions in Mental Development: Basic Phenomena and Theories. Hillsdale, NJ: Lawrence Erlbaum Associates, 1982.

Bijou, SW. Behavior analysis. In Vasta, R (Ed.). Annals of Child Development, Vol. 6. Greenwich, CT: JAI Press, 1989, pp. 61–83.

Bjornson, KF, Graubert, CS, Buford, VL, & McLaughlin, J. Validity of the Gross Motor Function Measure. Pediatric Physical Therapy, 10:43–47, 1998a.

Bjornson, KF, Graubert, CS, McLaughlin, JF, Kerfeld, CI, & Clark, EM. Test-retest reliability of the Gross Motor Function Measure in children with cerebral palsy. Physical and Occupational Therapy in Pediatrics, 18(2):51–61, 1998b.

Blasco, PM, Hrncir, EJ, & Blasco, PA. The contribution of maternal involvement to mastery performance in infants with cerebral palsy. Journal of Early Intervention, 14:161–174, 1990.

Bly, L. The Components of Normal Movement during the First Year of Life and Abnormal Motor Development. Oak Park, IL: Neuro-Developmental Treatment Association, 1983.

Bobath, B, & Bobath, K. The neuro-developmental treatment. In Scrutton, D (Ed.). Management of the Motor Disorders of Children with Cerebral Palsy. London: Spastics International Medical Publications, 1984, pp. 6–18.

Bodkin, AW, Baxter, RS, & Heriza, CB. Treadmill training for an infant born preterm with a grade III intraventricular hemorrhage. Physical Therapy, 12:1107–1118, 2003.

Bower, E, & McLellan, DL. Effect of increased exposure to physiotherapy on skill acquisition of children with cerebral palsy. Developmental Medicine and Child Neurology, 34:25–39, 1992.

Boyce, W, Gowland, C, Hardy, S, Rosenbaum, P, Lane, M, Plews, N, Goldsmith, C, & Russell, D. Development of a quality of movement measure for children with cerebral palsy. Physical Therapy, 71:820–832, 1991.

Bruer, JT. A critical and sensitive period primer. In Bailey, DB, Jr, Bruer, JT, Symons, FJ, & Lichtman, JW, Critical Thinking About Critical Periods. Baltimore, MD: Paul H. Brookes Publishing Co., 2001, pp. 3–26.

Bruininks, RH. Bruininks-Oseretsky Test of Motor Proficiency: Examiner's Manual. Circle Pines, MN: American Guidance Service, 1978.

Bruner, JS. The growth and structure of skill. In Connolly, K (Ed.). Mechanisms of Motor Skill Development. New York: Academic Press, 1970, pp. 63–94.

Burrows, P, & Griffiths, P. Do baby walkers delay onset of walking in young children? British Journal of Community Nursing, 7:581–586, 2002.

Bushnell, EW, & Boudreau, JP. Motor development and the mind: The potential role of motor abilities as a determinant of aspects of perceptual development. Child Development, 64:1005–1021, 1993.

Butler, C. Augmentative mobility: Why do it? Physical Medicine and Rehabilitation Clinics of North America, 2(4):801–815, 1991.

Byl, NN, Merzenich, MM, Cheung, S, Bedenbaugh, P, Nagarajan, SS, & Jenkins, WM. A primate model for studying focal dystonia and repetitive strain injury: Effects on the primary somatosensory cortex. Physical Therapy, 77:269–284, 1997.

Campbell, SK. Measurement in developmental therapy: Past, present, and future. In Miller, LJ (Ed.). Developing Norm Referenced Standardized Tests. Binghamton, NY: Haworth Press, 1989, pp. 1–13.

Campbell, SK. Framework for the measurement of neurologic impairment and disability. In Lister, MJ (Ed.). Contemporary Management of Motor Control Problems: Proceedings of the II STEP Conference. Alexandria, VA: Foundation for Physical Therapy, 1991, pp. 143–153.

Campbell, SK. Quantifying the effects of interventions for movement disorders resulting from cerebral palsy. Journal of Child Neurology, 11(suppl 1):S61-S70, 1996.

Campbell, SK. Therapy programs for children that last a lifetime. Physical and Occupational Therapy in Pediatrics 17(1):1–15, 1997.

Campbell, SK. Test-retest reliability of the Test of Infant Motor Performance. Pediatric Physical Therapy, 11:60–66, 1999.

Campbell, SK, & Hedeker, D. Validity of the Test of Infant Motor Performance for discriminating among infants with varying risk for poor motor outcome. Journal of Pediatrics, 139:546–551, 2001.

Campbell, SK, & Kolobe, THA. Concurrent validity of the Test of Infant Motor Performance with the Alberta Infant Motor Scale. Pediatric Physical Therapy, 12:1–8, 2000.

Campbell, SK, Kolobe, THA, Osten, E, Lenke, M, & Girolami, GL. Construct validity of the Test of Infant Motor Performance. Physical Therapy, 75:585–596, 1995.

Campbell, SK, Kolobe, THA, Wright, B, & Linacre, JM. Validity of the Test of Infant Motor Performance for prediction of 6-, 9-, and 12-month scores on the Alberta Infant Motor Scale. Developmental Medicine & Child Neurology, 44:263–272, 2002a.

Campbell, SK, Siegel, E, Parr, CA, & Ramey, CT. Evidence for the need to renorm the Bayley Scales of Infant Development based on the performance of a population-based sample of twelve-month-old infants. Topics in Early Childhood Special Education, 6(2):83–96, 1986.

Campbell, SK, & Wilson, JM. Planning infant learning programs. Physical Therapy, 56:1347–1357, 1976.

Campbell, SK, Wright, BD, & Linacre, JM. Development of a functional movement scale for infants. Journal of Applied Measurement, 3(2):191–204, 2002b.

Case-Smith, J, Bigsby, R, & Clutter, J. Perceptual-motor coupling in the development of grasp. American Journal of Occupational Therapy, 52:102–110, 1998.

Catania, A, & Harnad, S (Eds.). The Selection of Behavior—The Operant Behaviorism of B.F. Skinner: Comments and Consequences. New York: Cambridge University Press, 1988.

Cintas, HM. Cross-cultural variation in infant motor development. Physical and Occupational Therapy in Pediatrics, 8(4):1–20, 1988.

Cioni, G, & Prechtl, HFR. Preterm and early postterm behaviour in low-risk premature infants. Early Human Development, 23:159–191, 1990.

Colson, ER, & Dworkin, PH. Toddler development. Pediatrics in Review, 18:255–259, 1997.

Connolly, K. Skill development: Problems and plans. In Connolly, K (Ed.). Mechanisms of Motor Skill Development. New York: Academic Press, 1970, pp. 3–21.

Corbetta, D, & Bojczyk, KE. Infants return to two-handed reaching when they are learning to walk. Journal of Motor Behavior, 34:83–95, 2002.

Corbetta, D, & Mounoud, P. Early development of grasping and manipulation. In Bard, C, Fleury, M, & Hay, L (Eds.). Development of Eye-Hand Coordination across the Life Span. Columbia, SC: University of South Carolina Press, 1990, pp. 188–213.

Coryell, J, Provost, BM, Wilhelm, IJ, & Campbell, SK. Stability of Bayley Motor Scale scores in the first two years. Physical Therapy, 69:834–841, 1989.

Darrah, J, Hodge, M, Magill-Evans, J, & Kembhavi, G. Stability of serial assessments of motor and communication abilities in typically developing infants—Implications for screening. Early Human Development, 72:97–110, 2003.

Deitz, JC, Richardson, P, Crowe, TK, & Westcott, SL. Performance of children with learning disabilities and motor delays on the Pediatric Clinical Test of Sensory Interaction for Balance (P-CTSIB). Physical and Occupational Therapy in Pediatrics, 16(3):1–21, 1996.

DeLoache, JS, Uttal, DH, & Rosengren, KS. Scale errors offer evidence for a perception-action dissociation early in life. Science, 304:1027–1029, 2004.

Dewey, C, Fleming, P, & Golding, J. Does the supine sleeping position have any adverse effects on the child? II. Development in the first 18 months. Pediatrics (CZE), 101:E5, 1998.

Edelman, GM. Bright Air, Brilliant Fire: On the Matter of the Mind. New York: Basic Books, 1992.

Einspieler, C, Cioni, G, Paolicelli, PB, Bos, AF, Dressler, A, Ferrari, F, Roversi, MF, & Prechtl, HF. The early markers for later dyskinetic cerebral palsy are different from those for spastic cerebral palsy. Neuropediatrics, 33:73–78, 2002.

Epstein, HT. Correlated brain and intelligence development in humans. In Hahn, ME, Jensen, C, & Dudek, BC (Eds.). Development and Evolution of Brain Size: Behavioral Implications. New York: Academic Press, 1979, pp. 111–131.

Fagard, J. The development of bimanual coordination. In Bard, C, Fleury, M, & Hay, L (Eds.). Development of Eye-Hand Coordination across the Life Span. Columbia, SC: University of South Carolina Press, 1990, pp. 262–282.

Feldman, AB, Haley, SM, & Coryell, J. Concurrent and construct validity of the Pediatric Evaluation of Disability Inventory. Physical Therapy, 70:602–610, 1990.

Fentress, JC. Animal and human models of coordination development. In Bard, C, Fleury, M, & Hay, L (Eds.). Development of Eye-Hand Coordination across the Life Span. Columbia, SC: University of South Carolina Press, 1990, pp. 3–25.

Ferrari, F, Cioni, G, & Prechtl, HRF. Qualitative changes of general movements in preterm infants with brain lesions. Early Human Development, 23:193–231, 1990.

Fetters, L. Object permanence development in infants with motor handicaps. Physical Therapy, 61:327–333, 1981.

Fetters, L. Foundations for therapeutic intervention. In Campbell, SK (Ed.). Pediatric Neurologic Physical Therapy. New York: Churchill Livingstone, 1991a, pp. 19–32.

Fetters, L. Cerebral palsy: Contemporary treatment concepts. In Lister, MJ (Ed.). Contemporary Management of Motor Control Problems: Proceedings of the II STEP Conference. Alexandria, VA: Foundation for Physical Therapy, 1991b, pp. 219–224.

Fetters, L. Measurement and treatment in cerebral palsy: An argument for a new approach. Physical Therapy, 71:244–247, 1991c.

Fetters, L, Fernandez, B, & Cermak, S. The relationship of proximal and distal components in the development of reaching. Journal of Human Movement Studies, 17:283–297, 1989.

Fischer, KW. Relations between brain and cognitive development. Child Development, 58:623–632, 1987.

Fisher, AG. Functional measures, Part 1: What is function, what should we measure, and how should we measure it? American Journal of Occupational Therapy, 46:183–185, 1992.

Flavell, JH. The Developmental Psychology of Jean Piaget. Princeton, NJ: Van Nostrand, 1963.

Flegel, J, & Kolobe, THA. Predictive validity of the Test of Infant Motor Performance as measured by the Bruininks-Oseretsky Test of Motor Proficiency at school age. Physical Therapy, 82:762–771, 2002.

Folio, MR, & Fewell, RR. Peabody Developmental Motor Scales 2nd ed. Austin, TX: Pro-Ed, Inc., 2000.

Frankenburg, WK, Dodds, J, Archer, P, Bresnick, B, Maschka, P, Edelman, N, & Shapiro, H. Denver II. Denver: Denver Developmental Materials, 1990.

Frankenburg, WK, Dodds, J, Archer, P, Shapiro, H, & Bresnick, B. The Denver II. A major revision and restandardization of the DDST. Pediatrics, 89:91–97, 1992.

Gemus, M, Palisano, R, Russell, D, Rosenbaum, P, Walter, SD, Galuppi, B, & Lane, M. Using the Gross Motor Function Measure to evaluate motor development in children with Down syndrome. Physical & Occupational Therapy in Pediatrics, 21(2–3):69–79, 2001.

Georgopoulos, AP, Ashe, J, Smyrnis, M, & Taira, M. The motor cortex and the coding of force. Science, 256:1692–1695, 1992.

Georgopoulos, AP, Taira, M, & Lukashin, A. Cognitive neurophysiology of the motor cortex. Science, 260:47–52, 1993.

Gesell, A. Infancy and Human Growth. New York: Macmillan, 1928a.

Gesell, A. The Mental Growth of the Pre-school Child: A Psychological Outline of Normal Development from Birth to the Sixth Year, Including a System of Developmental Diagnosis. New York: Macmillan, 1928b.

Gesell, A. The Embryology of Behavior. New York: Harper & Row, 1945.

Gesell, A, Amatruda, CS, Castner, BM, & Thompson, H. Biographies of Child Development: The Mental Growth Careers of Eighty-four Infants and Children. New York: Arno Press, 1975.

Gesell, A, Halverson, HM, Thompson, H, Ilg, FL, Castner, BM, Ames, LB, & Amatruda, CS. The First Five Years of Life. New York: Harper & Row, 1940.

Gesell, A, Thompson, H, & Amatruda, CS. Infant Behavior: Its Genesis and Growth. New York: McGraw-Hill, 1934.

Girolami, G, & Campbell, SK. Efficacy of a neuro-developmental treatment program to improve motor control of preterm infants. Pediatric Physical Therapy, 6:175–184, 1994.

Glascoe, FP, Byrne, KE, Ashford, LG, Johnson, KL, Chang, B, & Strickland, B. Accuracy of the Denver-II in developmental screening. Pediatrics, 89:1221–1225, 1992.

Goldfield, EC. Toward a developmental ecological psychology. Monographs of the Society for Research in Child Development, 62(3):152–158, 1997.

Goldman-Rakic, PS. Development of cortical circuitry and cognitive function. Child Development, 58:601–622, 1987.

Goyen, T-A, & Lui, K. Longitudinal motor development of "apparently normal" high-risk infants at 18 months, 3 and 5 years. Early Human Development, 70:103–115, 2002.

Granger, CV, Hamilton, BB, & Kayton, R. Guide for the Use of the Functional Independence Measure (WeeFIM) of the Uniform Data Set for Medical Rehabilitation. Buffalo, NY: Research Foundation, State University of New York, 1989.

Green, EM, Mulcahy, CM, & Pountney, TE. An investigation into the development of early postural control. Developmental Medicine and Child Neurology, 37:437–448, 1995.

Greenough, WT, Black, JE, & Wallace, CS. Experience and brain development. Child Development, 58:539–559, 1987.

Hadders-Algra, M, & Prechtl, HFR. Developmental course of general movements in early infancy. I. Descriptive analysis of change in form. Early Human Development, 28:201–213, 1992.

Hadders-Algra, M, Van Eykern, LA, Klip-van den Nieuwendijk, AWJ, & Prechtl, HFR. Developmental course of general movements in early infancy. II. EMG correlates. Early Human Development, 28:231–253, 1992.

Haley, SM, Baryza, MJ, & Blanchard, Y. Functional and naturalistic frameworks in assessing physical and motor disablement. In Wilhelm, IJ (Ed.). Physical Therapy Assessment in Early Infancy. New York: Churchill Livingstone, 1993, pp. 225–256.

Haley, SM, Coster, WJ, & Faas, RM. A content validity study of the Pediatric Evaluation of Disability Inventory. Pediatric Physical Therapy, 3:177–184, 1991.

Haley, SM, Coster, WJ, Ludlow, LH, Haltiwanger, JT, & Andrellos, PJ. The Pediatric Evaluation of Disability Inventory: Development Standardization and Administration Manual. Boston: New England Medical Center Publications, 1992.

Harris, SR. Efficacy of physical therapy in promoting family functioning and functional independence for children with cerebral palsy. Pediatric Physical Therapy, 2:160–164, 1990.

Harris, SR, & Daniels, LE. Content validity of the Harris Infant Neuromotor Test. Physical Therapy, 76:727–737, 1996.

Harris, SR, & Daniels, LE. Reliability and validity of the Harris Infant Neuromotor Test. Journal of Pediatrics, *139*:249–253, 2001.

Harris, SR, Megens, AM, Backman, CL, & Hayes, V. Development and standardization of the Harris Infant Neuromotor Test. Infants and Young Children, *16*:143–151, 2003.

Hauser-Cram, P. Mastery motivation in toddlers with developmental disabilities. Child Development, *67*:236–248, 1996.

Hay, L. Developmental changes in eye-hand coordination behaviors: Preprogramming versus feedback control. In Bard, C, Fleury, M, & Hay, L (Eds.). Development of Eye-Hand Coordination across the Life Span. Columbia, SC: University of South Carolina Press, 1990, pp. 217–244.

Hayne, H, Rovee-Collier, C, & Perris, EE. Categorization and memory retrieval by three-month-olds. Child Development, *58*:750–767,1987.

Henderson, RC, Lark, RK, Gurka, MJ, et al. Bone density and metabolism in children and adolescents with moderate to severe cerebral palsy. Pediatrics, *110*:e5, 2002.

Heriza, C. Motor development: Traditional and contemporary theories. In Lister, MJ (Ed.). Contemporary Management of Motor Control Problems: Proceedings of the II STEP Conference. Alexandria, VA: Foundation for Physical Therapy, 1991, pp. 99–126.

Hinderer, KA, Richardson, PK, & Atwater, SW. Clinical implications of the Peabody Developmental Motor Scales: A constructive review. Physical and Occupational Therapy in Pediatrics, *9*(2):81–106, 1989.

Hoover, JE, & Strick, PL. Multiple output channels in the basal ganglia. Science, *259*:819–821, 1993.

Horak, FB. Assumptions underlying motor control for neurologic rehabilitation. In Lister, MJ (Ed.). Contemporary Management of Motor Control Problems: Proceedings of the II STEP Conference. Alexandria, VA: Foundation for Physical Therapy, 1991, pp. 11–27.

Horton, JC. Critical periods in the development of the visual system. In Bailey, DB, Jr, Bruer, JT, Symons, FJ, & Lichtman, JW (Eds.). Critical Thinking About Critical Periods. Baltimore, MD: Paul H. Brookes Publishing Co, 2001, pp. 45–65.

Jantz, JW, Blosser, CD, & Fruechting, LA. A motor milestone change noted with a change in sleep position. Archives of Pediatrics and Adolescent Medicine, *151*:565–568, 1997.

Kanda, T, Pidcock, FS, Hayakawa, K, Yamori, Y, & Shikata, Y. Motor outcome differences between two groups of children with spastic diplegia who received different intensities of early onset physiotherapy followed for 5 years. Brain Development, *26*:118–126, 2004.

Kanda, T, Yuge, M, Yamori, Y, Suzuki, J, & Fukase, H. Early physiotherapy in the treatment of spastic diplegia. Developmental Medicine and Child Neurology, *26*:438–444, 1984.

Karniol, R. The role of manual manipulative stages in the infant's acquisition of perceived control over objects. Developmental Review, *9*:205–233, 1989.

Keshner, EA, Campbell, D, Katz, R, & Peterson, BW. Neck muscle activation patterns in humans during isometric head stabilization. Experimental Brain Research, *75*:335–364, 1989.

Kirshenbaum, N, Riach, CL, & Starkes, JL. Non-linear development of postural control and strategy use in young children: A longitudinal study. Experimental Brain Research, *140*:420–431, 2001.

Knobloch, H, Stevens, F, & Malone, AF. Manual of Developmental Diagnosis, rev. ed. New York: Harper & Row, 1980.

Kolobe, TH. Childrearing practices and developmental expectations for Mexican-American mothers and the developmental status of their infants. Physical Therapy, *84*:439–453, 2004.

Kolobe, THA, Bulanda, M, & Susman, L. Predicting motor outcome at preschool age for infants tested at 7, 30, 60, and 90 days after term age using the Test of Infant Motor Performance. Physical Therapy, *84*:1144–1156, 2004.

Kolobe, THA, Palisano, RJ, & Stratford, PW. Comparison of two outcome measures for infants with cerebral palsy and infants with motor delays. Physical Therapy, *78*:1062–1072, 1998.

Koseck, K. Review and valuation of psychometric properties of the Revised Bayley Scales of Infant Development. Pediatric Physical Therapy, *11*:198–204, 1999.

Krus, PH, Bruininks, RH, & Robertson, G. Structure of motor abilities in children. Perceptual and Motor Skills, *52*:119–129, 1981.

Lee, AM. Child-rearing practices and motor performance of black and white children. Research Quarterly for Exercise and Sport, *51*:494–500, 1980.

Lekskulchai, R, & Cole, J. Effect of a developmental program on motor performance in infants born preterm. Australian Journal of Physiotherapy, *47*:169–176, 2001.

Leonard, CT, Moritani, T, Hirschfeld, H, & Forssberg, H. Deficits in reciprocal inhibition of children with cerebral palsy as revealed by H reflex testing. Developmental Medicine and Child Neurology, *32*:974–984, 1990.

Liao, P-jM, & Campbell, SK. Comparison of two methods for teaching therapists to score the Test of Infant Motor Performance. Pediatric Physical Therapy, *14*:191–198, 2002.

Long, TM, & Tieman, B. Review of two recently published measurement tools: The AIMS and the TIME. Pediatric Physical Therapy, *10*:62–66, 1998.

Loria, C. Relationship of proximal and distal function in motor development. Physical Therapy, *60*:167–172, 1980.

Lynch, SR, & Stoltzfus, RJ. Iron and ascorbic acid: Proposed fortification levels and recommended iron compounds. Journal of Nutrition, *133*(9):2978S–2984S, 2003.

McEwan, MH, Dihoff, RE, & Brosvic, GM. Early infant crawling experience is reflected in later motor skill development. Perceptual and Motor Skills, *72*:75–79, 1991.

McGraw, MB. Growth: A Study of Johnny and Jimmy. New York: Appleton-Century, 1935.

McGraw, MB. The Neuromuscular Maturation of the Human Infant. New York: Hafner, 1963. (Original work published by Columbia University Press, 1945.)

Miller, LJ. The Miller First Step (Screening Test for Evaluating Preschoolers). New York: Psychological Corporation, 1992.

Morbidity & Mortality Weekly Report. Iron deficiency – United States, 1999–2000. Morbidity & Mortality Weekly Report, *51*(40):897–899, 2002.

Msall, ME, Braun, S, Duffy, L, DiGaudio, K, LaForest, S, & Granger, C. Normative sample of the Pediatric Functional Independence Measure: A uniform data set for tracking disability (Abstract). Developmental Medicine and Child Neurology, *34*(suppl 66):19, 1992a.

Msall, ME, Braun, S, Granger, C, DiGaudio, K, & Duffy, L. The Functional Independence Measure for Children (WeeFIM), Developmental Edition (Version 1.5). Buffalo, NY: Uniform Data Set for Medical Rehabilitation, 1992b.

Murney, ME, & Campbell, SK. The ecological relevance of the Test of Infant Motor Performance Elicited Scale items. Physical Therapy, *78*:479–489, 1998.

National Advisory Board on Medical Rehabilitation Research. Research Plan for the National Center for Medical Rehabilitation Research. NIH Publication No. 93-3509. Bethesda, MD: National Institutes of Health, 1993.

Newell, KM, & Vaillancourt, DE. Dimensional change in motor learning. Human Movement Science, *20*:695–715, 2001.

Nowakowski, RS. Basic concepts of CNS development. Child Development, *58*:568–595, 1987.

Nudo, RJ, Milliken, GW, Jenkins, WM, & Merzenich, MM. Use-dependent alterations of movement representations in primary motor cortex of adult squirrel monkeys. Journal of Neuroscience, 16:785–807, 1996.

Oppenheim, RW. Ontogenetic adaptations and retrogressive processes in the development of the nervous system and behavior: A neuro-embryological perspective. In Connolly, K, & Prechtl, HFR (Eds.). Maturation and Development: Biological and Psychological Perspectives. Philadelphia: JB Lippincott, 1981, pp. 73–109.

Oztop, E, Bradley, NS, & Arbib, MA. Infant grasp learning: A computational model. Experimental Brain Research, 180:480–503, 2004.

Paillard, J. Basic neurophysiological structures of eye-hand coordination. In Bard, C, Fleury, M, & Hay, L (Eds.). Development of Eye-Hand Coordination across the Life Span. Columbia, SC: University of South Carolina Press, 1990, pp. 26–74.

Palisano, RJ. Neuromotor and developmental assessment. In Wilhelm, IJ (Ed.). Physical Therapy Assessment in Early Infancy. New York: Churchill Livingstone, 1993, pp. 173–224.

Palisano, R, Rosenbaum, P, Walter, S, Russell, D, Wood, E, & Galuppi, B. Development and reliability of a system to classify gross motor function in children with cerebral palsy. Developmental Medicine and Child Neurology, 39:214–223, 1997.

Parker, DF, Carriere, L, Hebestreit, H, Salsberg, A, & Bar-Or, O. Muscle performance and gross motor function of children with spastic cerebral palsy. Developmental Medicine and Child Neurology, 35:17–23, 1993.

Pellegrini, AD, & Smith, PK. Physical activity play: The nature and function of a neglected aspect of play. Child Development, 69:577–598, 1998.

Piaget, J. The Origins of Intelligence in Children. New York: International Universities Press, 1952.

Pick, HL, Jr. Eleanor J. Gibson. Learning to perceive and perceiving to learn. Developmental Psychology, 28:787–794, 1992.

Piek, JP, Gasson, N, Barrett, N, & Case, I. Limb and gender differences in the development of coordination in early infancy. Human Movement Science, 21:621–639, 2002.

Plimpton, CE, & Regimbal, C. Differences in motor proficiency according to gender and race. Perceptual and Motor Skills, 74:399–402, 1992.

Provost, B. Normal development from birth to 4 months: Extended use of the NBAS-K. Part II. Physical and Occupational Therapy in Pediatrics, 1(3):19–34, 1981.

Ramey, CT, & Ramey, SL. Effective early intervention. Mental Retardation, 30(6):337-345, 1992.

Ratliff-Schaub, K, Hunt, CE, Crowell, D, Golub, H, Smok-Pearsall, S, Palmer, P, Schafer, S, Bak, S, Cantey-Kiser, J, O'Bell, R, & the CHIME Study Group. Relationship between infant sleep position and motor development in preterm infants. Developmental and Behavioral Pediatrics, 22:293–299, 2001.

Ratner, HH, & Foley, MA. A unifying framework for the development of children's activity memory. Advances in Child Development and Behavior, 25:33–105, 1994.

Roberton, MA, & Halverson, LE. Developing Children—Their Changing Movement. A Guide for Teachers. Philadelphia: Lea & Febiger, 1984.

Rosenbaum, P. Physical activity play in children with disabilities: A neglected opportunity for research? Child Development, 69:607–608, 1998.

Rosenbaum, P, Russell, D, Cadman, D, Gowland, C, Jarvis, S, & Hardy, S. Issues in measuring change in motor function in children with cerebral palsy: A special communication. Physical Therapy, 70:125–131, 1990.

Rosenbaum, PL, Walter, SD, Hanna, SE, Palisano, RJ, Russell, DJ, & Raina, P. Prognosis for gross motor function in cerebral palsy: Creation of motor development curves. Journal of the American Medical Association, 288:1357–1363, 2002.

Rosenblith, JF. A singular career: Nancy Bayley. Developmental Psychology, 28:747–758, 1992.

Russell, D, Palisano, R, Walter, S, Rosenbaum, P, Gemus, M, Gowland, C, Galuppi, B, & Lane, M. Evaluating motor function in children with Down syndrome: Validity of the GMFM. Developmental Medicine and Child Neurology, 40:693–701, 1998.

Russell, D, Rosenbaum, P, Cadman, D, Gowland, C, Hardy, S, & Jarvis, S. The Gross Motor Function Measure: A means to evaluate the effects of physical therapy. Developmental Medicine and Child Neurology, 31:341–352, 1989.

Salls, JS, Silverman, LN, & Gatty, CM. The relationship of infant sleep and play positioning to motor milestone achievement. American Journal of Occupational Therapy, 56:577–580, 2002.

Scherzer, AL, Mike, V, & Ilson, J. Physical therapy as a determinant of change in the cerebral palsied infant. Pediatrics, 58:47–52, 1976.

Schoen, JHR. The corticofugal projection to the brain stem and spinal cord in man. Psychiatry, Neurology and Neurosurgery, 72:121–128, 1969.

Shirley, MM. The First Two Years: A Study of Twenty-five Babies. Vol. I. Postural and Locomotor Development. Minneapolis, MN: University of Minnesota Press, 1931.

Short, EJ, Klein, NK, Lewis, BA, Fulton, S, Eisengart, S, Kercsmar, C, Bale, J, & Singer, LT. Cognitive and academic consequences of bronchopulmonary dysplasia and very low birth weight: 8-year-old outcomes. Pediatrics, 112:e359, 2003.

Shumway-Cook, A, & Woollacott, M. The growth of stability: Postural control from a developmental perspective. Journal of Motor Behavior, 17:131–147, 1985.

Shumway-Cook, A, & Woollacott, M. Theoretical issues in assessing postural control. In Wilhelm, IJ (Ed.), Physical Therapy Assessment in Early Infancy. New York: Churchill Livingstone, 1993, pp. 161–171.

Skinner, BF. Cumulative Record: A Selection of Papers, 3rd ed. New York: Meredith, 1972.

Sparling, JW (Ed.). Concepts in Fetal Movement Research. New York: Haworth Press, 1993.

Sporns, O. Selectionist and instructionist ideas in neuroscience. International Review of Neurobiology, 37:3–26, 1994.

Sporns, O, & Edelman, GM. Solving Bernstein's problem: A proposal for the development of coordinated movement by selection. Child Development, 64:960–981, 1993.

Stengel, TJ. Assessing motor development in children. In Campbell, SK (Ed.). Pediatric Neurologic Physical Therapy, 2nd ed. New York: Churchill Livingstone, 1991, pp. 33–65.

Stengel, TJ, Attermeier, SM, Bly, L, & Heriza, CB. Evaluation of senso-rimotor dysfunction. In Campbell, SK (Ed.). Pediatric Neurologic Physical Therapy. New York: Churchill Livingstone, 1984, pp. 13–87.

Stokes, NA, Deitz, JL, & Crowe, TK. The Peabody Developmental Fine Motor Scale: An interrater reliability study. American Journal of Occupational Therapy, 44:334–340, 1990.

Strick, PL, & Preston, JB. Two representations of the hand in area 4 of a primate. I. Motor output organization. Journal of Neurophysiology, 48:139–149, 1982a.

Strick, PL, & Preston, JB. Two representations of the hand in area 4 of a primate. II. Somatosensory input organization. Journal of Neuro-physiology, 48:150–159, 1982b.

Task Force on Standards for Measurement in Physical Therapy. Standards for tests and measurements in physical therapy practice. Physical Therapy, 71:589–622, 1991.

Thelen, E. Coupling perception and action in the development of skill: A dynamic approach. In Bloch, H, & Bertenthal, BI (Eds.). Sensory-Motor Organization and Development in Infancy and Early Child-hood. Dordrecht, Netherlands: Kluwer Academic, 1990, pp. 39–56.

Thelen, E. Motor development. A new synthesis. American Psychologist, *50*:79–95, 1995.

Thelen, E, & Adolph, KE. Arnold L. Gesell: The paradox of nature and nurture. Developmental Psychology, *28*:368–380, 1992.

Thelen, E, & Corbetta, D. Exploration and selection in the early acquisition of skill. International Review of Neurobiology, *37*:75–102, 1994.

Thelen, E, Corbetta, D, Kamm, K, Spencer, JP, Schneider, K, & Zernicke, R. The transition to reaching: Mapping intention and intrinsic dynamics. Child Development, *64*:1058–1098, 1993.

Thelen, E, Kelso, JAS, & Fogel, A. Self-organizing systems and infant motor development. Developmental Review, *7*:39–65, 1987.

Thelen, E, & Ulrich, BD. Hidden skills: A dynamic systems analysis of treadmill stepping during the first year. Monographs of the Society for Research in Child Development. Serial No. 223, Vol. 56, No. 1. Chicago: University of Chicago Press, 1991.

Thelen, E, Ulrich, BD, & Jensen, JL. The developmental origins of locomotion. In Woollacott, MH, & Shumway-Cook, A (Eds.). Development of Posture and Gait across the Life Span. Columbia, SC: University of South Carolina Press, 1989, pp. 23–47.

Thompson, RA. Sensitive periods in attachment? In Bailey, DB, Jr, Bruer, JT, Symons, FJ, & Lichtman, JW (Eds.). Critical Thinking About Critical Periods. Baltimore, MD: Paul H. Brookes Publishing Co, 2001, pp. 83–106.

Thorn, F, Gwiazda, J, Cruz, AA, Bauer, JA, & Held, R. The development of eye alignment, convergence, and sensory binocularity in young infants. Investigative Ophthalmology and Visual Science, *35*:544–553, 1994.

Tscharnuter, I. A new therapy approach to movement organization. Physical and Occupational Therapy in Pediatrics, *13*(2):19–40, 1993.

Tychsen, L. Critical periods for development of visual acuity, depth perception, and eye tracking. In Bailey, DB, Jr, Bruer, JT, Symons, FJ, & Lichtman, JW (Eds.). Critical Thinking About Critical Periods. Baltimore, MD: Paul H. Brookes Publishing Co, 2001, pp. 67–80.

Ulrich, BD. Development of stepping patterns in human infants: A dynamical systems perspective. Journal of Motor Behavior, *21*:329–408, 1989.

Ulrich, DA, Ulrich, BD, Angulo-Kinzler, RM, & Yun, J. Treadmill training of infants with Down syndrome: Evidence-based developmental outcomes. Pediatrics, 108:E84, 2001. Accessed at http://www.pediatrics.org/cgi/content/full/108/5/384.

Unanue, RA, & Westcott, SL. The responsiveness of the Test of Infant Motor Performance (TIMP) in preterm infants (abstract). Pediatric Physical Therapy, *15*:64, 2003.

van Blankenstein, M, Welbergen, UR, & de Haas, JH. Le développement du nourrisson: Sa première anné en 130 photographies. Paris: Presses Universitaires de France, 1962.

Vinter, A. Manual imitations and reaching behaviors: An illustration of action control in infancy. In Bard, C, Fleury, M, & Hay, L (Eds.). Development of Eye-Hand Coordination across the Life Span. Columbia, SC: University of South Carolina Press, 1990, pp. 157–187.

von Hofsten, C. Eye-hand coordination in the newborn. Developmental Psychology, *18*:450–461, 1982.

Wallace, PS, & Whishaw, IQ. Independent digit movements and precision grip patterns in 1-5-month-old human infants: Hand babbling, including vacuous then self-directed hand and digit movements, precedes targeted reaching. Neuropsychologia, *41*:1912–1918, 2003.

Whitall, J, & Getchell, N. From walking to running: Applying a dynamical systems approach to the development of locomotor skills. Child Development, *66*:1541–1553, 1995.

Williams, JR, & Scott, RB. Growth and development of Negro infants: Motor development and its relationship to child-rearing practices in two groups of Negro infants. Child Development, *24*:103–121, 1953.

Wimmers, RH, Savelsbergh, GJP, Beek, PJ, & Hopkins, B. Evidence for a phase transition in the early development of prehension. Developmental Psychobiology, *32*:235–248, 1998a.

Wimmers, RH, Savelsbergh, GJP, van der Kamp, J, & Hartelman, P. A developmental transition in prehension modeled as a cusp catastrophe. Developmental Psychobiology, *32*:23–35, 1998b.

Wolf, MJ, Koldewijn, K, Beelen, A, Smit, B, Hedlund, R, & de Groot, IJ. Neurobehavioral and developmental profile of very low birthweight preterm infants in early infancy. Acta Paediatrica, *91*:930–938, 2002.

Wong, S, Chan, K, Wong, V, & Wong, W. Use of chopsticks in Chinese children. Child Care, Health & Development, *28*:157–161, 2002.

World Health Organization. International Classification of Function, Disability and Health. Geneva: World Health Organization, 2001.

Zelazo, PR. The development of walking: New findings and old assumptions. Journal of Motor Behavior, *15*:99–137, 1983.

Zelazo, PR, Zelazo, NA, & Kolb, S. "Walking" in the newborn. Science, *176*:314–315, 1972.

MOTOR CONTROL: DEVELOPMENTAL ASPECTS OF MOTOR CONTROL IN SKILL ACQUISITION

NINA S. BRADLEY
PT, PhD

SARAH L. WESTCOTT
PT, PhD

The term "motor control" is now commonly used in both research and clinical arenas of physical therapy, perhaps so commonly as to erode a clear understanding of its meaning. This chapter seeks to familiarize the clinician with the research field of motor control and, more specifically, how motor control applies to issues of motor development by addressing four objectives. The first objective of this chapter is to provide a brief discussion of some theories, hypotheses, and models that have shaped the direction of research and current views on motor control. Research conducted to test theories, hypotheses, and models of motor control, in turn, have led scientists to propose that physiologic, psychologic, and mechanical mechanisms or processes play select roles in the control of movement and can be studied under conditions of controlled observation. Thus the second objective of this chapter is to describe some of the processes that may control movement initiation or execution. The third objective and emphasis of this chapter is to present the work of researchers that both describes motor skill acquisition and attempts to reveal the processes that drive or permit acquisition of skills such as posture, gait, reaching, and grasping. The fourth objective is to explore how a physical therapist might examine a child's movement problems employing current knowledge of motor control. If the four objectives are adequately addressed, the reader should ultimately understand how evidence about motor control can assist and guide physical therapy examination, evaluation, and intervention.

THEORIES, HYPOTHESES, AND MODELS

Defining the term *motor control* and describing many of the theoretic constructs common to the field are not easy tasks, in part because motor control is a multidisciplinary field of study drawing from a broad range of disciplines including anatomy, physiology, psychology, kinesiology, engineering, and physical therapy. Historically, theories of motor control typically emerged from within a field such as anatomy or psychology, whereas hypotheses and models often emerged from the integration of ideas across fields. One consequence of this cross-pollination is that theoretic constructs and terminology have taken on slightly different definitions from one disciplinary view to the next, often leaving resolution of the discrepancy in definitions to the persevering student. In this section we will briefly review some of the more well-known theories, hypotheses, and models of motor control to gain an understanding of the ideas commonly embraced or challenged.

Theories of motor control attempt to unite various observations and laws that emerge from scientific study to explain why they exist or how they relate to one another. Theories also provide the foundation for development of hypotheses, models, and new theories. Three distinctly different theoretic perspectives are currently encountered in motor control literature: maturational, learning, and dynamic-based views. In the discussion to follow, we will briefly consider each view. Hypotheses, in contrast, attempt to predict the relationship between observations and defined (or experimental) conditions. For example, the maturational-based theory of motor control proposes that emergence of behavior is primarily attributable to maturational changes in the nervous system. A hypothesis based on this theory is that independent finger movements emerge at 7 months of age because of specific physiologic changes occurring in the primary motor cortex, the corticospinal tract, or both just before 7 months. When experiments by a large number of scientists testing a hypothesis produce consistent findings, the hypothesis becomes a law. Thus, laws define highly predictable relationships between variables, and in some instances these relationships can be mathematically specified. Fitts' law, for example, states that accuracy requirements and the distance over which a movement occurs can be used to predict movement time (Fitts, 1954). Models, in contrast to laws, are idealized constructs that incorporate a few select variables believed to be most powerful in explaining relationships between events and are used by scientists to both visualize and test theories. A basic understanding of hypotheses and models is useful because they provide the rationale for most research designs and views currently found in motor control literature, as well as guidance for examination and intervention in physical therapy. For further elaboration on these topics, the reader is referred to discussions by Schmidt and Lee (1998) and Shumway-Cook and Woollacott (2001).

HISTORICAL PERSPECTIVE

In the late 1800s the neurologist Ramón y Cajal discovered that Golgi silver stain could selectively label individual nerve cells. This advance led to the neuron doctrine and set the course for neurobiologic research and thinking in the twentieth century (Shepherd, 1991). The notion of "structure-function" and the maturational-based theory of motor control are two theoretic products of the neuron doctrine. Using silver stain, anatomists found that structural features distinguish subpopulations of neurons within and between regions of the nervous system and that morphologic changes occur during development. The array of morphologic findings led to the view that structural organization of the nervous system determines behavioral function (structure-function). Physiologists provided evidence for structure-function control of behavior by isolating portions of the nervous system (reduced preparations) that produced stereotypic movements such as the stretch reflex, the brisk contraction of a muscle in response to a quick elongation of the muscle stimulating its proprioceptors. Based on his many studies of reflex function in the spinal cord of cats, dogs, and monkeys, Sherrington (1947 [original work published 1906]) espoused the view that behavior is hierarchically organized and the simple reflex (composed of a receptor, conductor, and effector organ) is the fundamental unit of neural integration. Furthermore, he proposed that motor behavior is the composite coordination of simple reflexes (e.g., reflex chaining) as excitatory and inhibitory actions are summated at the synapse.

Maturational-Based Theories

Sherrington's notion of reflex chaining so dominated the study of physiology in the first half of the twentieth century that physiologists gave little attention to other views of motor control in explanations of behavior (Gallistel, 1980). Structure-function organization and reflex chaining were commonly employed rationales in studies of motor development as evidenced by the temporal correlations commonly drawn between emerging stimulus-evoked behavior and anatomic changes in neural pathways (e.g., Humphrey, 1964). Thus early studies identified the neuroanatomic changes occurring around the time a new behavior emerged without considering whether other variables contributed to the behavioral change. Consequently, scientists proposed that certain predictable changes during neural maturation are the causal determinants of behavioral development (Hooker, 1958; McGraw, 1945), establishing the foundation for maturational theories. Concurrent with these developments, hierarchic reflex chaining evolved to include the notion that reflex behaviors are expressions of an animal's phylogenetic origins (Humphrey, 1970). Such views merged into the notions that earliest movements are primitive behaviors controlled by phylogenetically older neural structures and earliest movements eventually disappear as older neural structures are inhibited by later differentiating neural structures that are phylogenetically more recent (Touwen, 1984). It appears there was little or no scientific challenge of these neuromaturational views, perhaps because students of development took little notice of other directions in neurobiologic research that were emerging at the time (Gallistel, 1980).

Learning-Based Theories

During this same time period, psychologists were also attempting to form theories of development. Behaviorism looked to the role of the environment in shaping behavior and sought to determine what attributes of the environment trigger or shape behavior. Response chaining, for example, proposed that feedback becomes more strongly associated with action over practice, automating the sequences of action executed by the nervous system (Rosenbaum, 1991). According to response chaining, the environment is the controller of the automating process. Response chaining, like reflex chaining, explains the ordering of movements as the consequence of feedback from one movement that in turn activates the next movement. Thorndike extended the notion of response chaining to address how motor skills are learned, and in the law of effect he proposed that skills emerge as we repeat actions that are rewarded (Schmidt & Lee, 1998).

The law of effect and emphasis on feedback can also be identified in contemporary theories and models of motor learning such as Adams' closed-loop theory (Adams, 1971) and more recently in a theoretic construct put forward by Sporns and Edelman (1993). Adams proposed that we develop a perceptual memory trace for what a correct movement should feel like (expected sensory consequences) based on intrinsic feedback generated during movement implementation. The perceptual trace evaluates the actual sensory consequences (feedback) of a movement each time it is executed and selects the movement attributes that are compatible with the perceptual memory trace to establish a memory trace for movement execution parameters. According to Adam's learning-based theory, feedback during movement is required to learn a movement, but subsequent research indicated that we do not need to monitor ongoing movements in order to reinforce desirable movement parameters (Taub & Berman, 1968). This inconsistency between experimental results and theoretic prediction was subsequently addressed by Schmidt's schema theory (Schmidt, 1975), discussed later in this chapter.

As theories are tested, the outcomes reveal their shortcomings, clarify the boundaries of our understanding, and raise a new generation of questions. For example, tests of response chaining raised questions such as how do we learn or execute movements when we cannot constantly monitor movement-dependent feedback, or how do we manage to execute an apparently endless variety of new and varied movements with minimal difficulty. Cognitive and developmental psychologists sought to explain the development of new skills as either the determinants or the consequences of increasing cognitive abilities. For example, Piaget proposed that early motor skill acquisition is the outcome of preverbal learning processes incorporating sensorimotor experiences to form early notions of causation that are stored to later serve as an internal reference during the development of language and concrete cognitive operations. According to Piagetian theory, preverbal learning and motor skill acquisition are maturational processes that permit concrete and abstract learning to take place (Keogh & Sugden, 1985). Furthermore, a recent theoretic proposal suggests that over evolutionary time, observed actions such as reaching to grasp may have driven language specialization in the human brain (Oztop & Arbib, 2002; Rizzolatti & Arbib, 1998). In contrast to maturationist theories, learning-based theories suggest that development of motor skill is the consequence of learning by trial and error to master and sequence units of action that in their rudimentary form are genetically determined. Connolly (1977) proposed, for example, that genetics endow the infant with the equivalent of computer hardware (neurologic and biomechanical features) and the infant's cognitive activities, equivalent to computer software, function to modify and adapt rudimentary units of movement into skilled action.

One of the most widely embraced of the learning theories, schema theory, proposes that motor development is a function of learning rules to evaluate, correct, and update memory traces for a given class of movements (Schmidt, 1975). Schema theory assumes the presence of three constructs: general motor programs and two types of memory traces, recall schema, and recognition schema. In schema theory, general motor programs are loosely defined as sets of instructions that are responsible for organizing the invariant or fundamental components of a movement. Recall schemas are defined as memories of relationships between past movement parameters, past initial conditions, and the movement outcomes they produced. Recognition schemas are defined as memories of relationships between past movement parameters, past initial conditions, and the sensory consequences they produced. It is theorized that recall schemas function to establish rules regarding the relationship between movement parameters of a general motor program, such as force or velocity, and movement outcome for a given set of initial conditions that can be used to plan similar movements under anticipated conditions. Recognition schema, in turn, are proposed to compare sensory consequences with movement outcome in light of initial conditions to form a second set of rules that can be used to predict the expected sensory consequences for similar movement outcomes during anticipated initial conditions. The expected sensory consequences are proposed to serve as a perceptual memory trace for evaluating new movements. When movements are generated too quickly (ballistically) to be corrected by feedback as they are executed (i.e., open loop), it is theorized that intrinsic feedback, an efferent copy of the motor command, can be compared with the expected sensory consequences to evaluate the movements during execution or after they are completed. It is theorized that the schema are established and refined as a function of practice. New research suggests that there may be an interdependence between parameters such as time and force during schema development. Motor learning related to manipulation of one parameter may have a negative effect on learning the other parameter (Whitacre & Shea, 2000). See Chapter 4 by Larin for further discussion of motor learning theories.

Schema theory does not attempt to explain the establishment of motor programs, nor does it attempt to ascribe them to specific neural structures. The term "motor program" is employed in a variety of ways by researchers from a variety of disciplinary backgrounds, which may help explain why there is no consensus as to what constitutes a motor program (Rosenbaum, 1991). In motor learning literature, motor programs are commonly invoked to explain the stereotypic attributes of a complex movement pattern that persist as movement parameters or context is altered. For example, it has been suggested that we have a general motor program for writing our name and its instructions are recognized in the features common to signing our name under different conditions with different tools, different parameters of movement, even different sets of muscles (Raibert, 1977). Motor learning literature also ascribes to motor programs the ability to generate complex movements without benefit of concurrent feedback, such as reaching for a target after administration of a local anesthetic or tourniquet, as well as ballistic movements that may be completed before feedback can contribute to the movement (Schmidt & Lee, 1998). In each of these instances, motor programs are viewed as learned sets of instructions. In neurobiology, however, motor programs are also called pattern generators and are viewed as genetically inherited sets of instructions that control the stereotypic features of innate behaviors such as mating, defense, and locomotion (Kupfermann, 1991). Some of the strongest arguments in neurobiology for the existence of general motor programs refer to the many examples of an animal's ability to execute functional movements in the absence of feedback (Lashley, 1917; Polit & Bizzi, 1979; Taub & Berman,

1968). Where the movement instructions are stored is yet to be determined, but some investigators implicate the sensorimotor cortex (Asanuma & Keller, 1991), primary motor cortex (Holdefer & Miller, 2002), and cerebellum (Sanes et al., 1990) in motor learning or the prefrontal association cortex in motor memory and planning (Fuster, 2000; Kupfermann, 1991; Seitz et al., 2000).

Dynamic-Based Theories

A more recent theory receiving broad interest in recent years, established to explain the development of motor control, is the dynamic systems theory proposed by Thelen and her colleagues (Thelen & Smith, 1994; Thelen & Ulrich, 1991; Smith & Thelen, 2003). The theory seeks to address what drives skill acquisition and a particular problem poorly handled by previous theories: how does a child move from one developmental stage of skill to another? A fundamental hypothesis of the theory is that there are multiple identifiable variables, such as muscle power, body mass, arousal, neural networks, motivation, and environmental forces (e.g., gravity and friction), that establish a context for movement initiation and execution. A second fundamental hypothesis is that the relationship (interaction) among these variables is in constant flux and therefore shapes the features of a movement as it unfolds. Thus dynamic systems theory proposes that developmental changes in motor behavior and skill performance can be explained in terms of dynamics common to physical, biologic, and computational systems. Developmental stages are viewed as attractor states that are governed by a set of variables, and transitions in behavior are viewed as flips between attractor states powered by change in one or more of the variables. For example, an animal may be capable of producing coordinated limb movements for stepping but incapable of locomoting until related postural skills are sufficient (Bradley, 1992). Or the pattern of limb movements may abruptly vary with changes in movement parameters such as velocity (Thelen & Smith, 1994). Behavioral solutions are thus the composite solution of neural, biomechanical, and environmental forces acting in concert (Swinnen et al., 1994). Variability in motor behavior as opposed to deterministic movement is thus a part of the development or learning process. In fact it has been suggested recently that variability is a crucial feature of learning optimal motor behavior (Riley & Turvey, 2002) and can be argued to be part of the generalized motor program for rhythmic interlimb coordination (Amazeen, 2002).

Theoretic work by Sporns and Edelman (1993) has extended dynamic theory by developing the notion of dynamic selection. Rather than assuming the existence of genetically predetermined motor programs, they hypothesize that motor skills emerge from an interaction between development-related changes in movement dynamics and brain structure-function. Given that musculoskeletal anatomy and related biomechanics change dramatically over the course of development, the theory is primarily concerned with how the brain's circuitry can readily change to match or accommodate these changes. The theory incorporates three key hypotheses: a developing organism is genetically endowed with spontaneously generated behaviors that make up the basic movement repertoire; it is also endowed with a sensory system capable of detecting and recognizing movements having adaptive value; and the developing organism can select movements having adaptive value by varying synaptic strengths within and between brain circuits such that successive event selections will progressively modify the movement repertoire. In essence the theory proposes that there is a "handshaking" relationship between evolving movement mechanics and ongoing maturation of brain circuits, all of which is edited or biased by the adaptive value of a movement experienced. Recognizing the value of a movement experience will strengthen the probability of repetition, strengthening a behavior; failure to recognize its value will reduce the probability of repetition, thereby weakening the behavior. Thus this latter theory embraces attributes of maturational, learning, and dynamic theories to explain motor control development. This theoretical perspective has been supported recently by Hadders-Algra (2000, 2001a) based on the typical development of postural control and abnormalities that occur with this development in infants and children with cerebral palsy (CP) and developmental coordination disorder (DCD).

CURRENT HYPOTHESES OF MOTOR CONTROL

Rather than proposing some unifying theory, many current hypotheses of motor control attempt to identify controlling variables for specific types of movement. Central pattern generators (CPGs) are proposed to account for the basic neural organization and function required to execute coordinated, rhythmic movements, such as locomotion, chewing, grooming (e.g., scratching), and respiration. CPGs are commonly defined as interneuronal networks, located in either the spinal cord or brainstem, that can order the selection and sequencing of motoneurons independent of descending or peripheral afferent neural input. Neural input from select supraspinal regions, such as the brainstem reticular nuclei, activate CPGs, and peripheral afferents, propriospinal regions, and other supraspinal regions modulate the

output of CPGs and adapt the behavior to the movement context. Work in invertebrate species suggests that pattern generators can even alter their own configurations (i.e., intrinsic modulation) to produce more than one pattern associated with the same or different behaviors (Katz & Frost, 1996). CPGs can also modulate the inputs they receive, gating potentially disruptive reflex actions such as nociceptive activation of the flexor withdrawal reflex when a limb is fully loaded during the stance phase of locomotion (for further review of pattern generators, see Grillner, 1996; Levitan & Kaczmarek, 1997; Rossignol, 1996). Until recently, the early presence of orderly or coordinated motor patterns at the onset of embryonic movement appeared to suggest that CPGs, including those for locomotion, are established during initial differentiation of the nervous system (Bradley & Bekoff, 1989). However, more recent cellular studies appear to indicate that embryonic behaviors are the product of transient neural networks (discussed later in this chapter) that may have little or no participation in mature pattern-generating networks (O'Donovan & Chub, 1997). Nonetheless, a growing body of literature examining the continuum of stepping behaviors in fetuses, premature infants, term infants, and young infants is beginning to make a strong case for the view that human locomotion is also governed by CPGs (Bradley, 2003). Promising research in humans to substantiate the presence of CPGs for locomotion has centered around locomotor recovery studies in adults with spinal cord lesions and hemiplegia, (reviewed by MacKay-Lyons, 2002). Research on infants and children with CP (Bodkin et al., 2003; McNevin et al., 2000; Schindl et al., 2000) and Down syndrome (Ulrich et al., 2001) who train on treadmills with partial body weight support have also shown positive outcomes.

A number of hypotheses of motor control specifically attempt to explain how we control discrete arm movements. According to the equilibrium-point hypothesis, also called the mass-spring hypothesis, the nervous system strives to control joint position in space, and every position can be defined by a unique combination of agonist and antagonist muscle forces that result in a net stiffness (Feldman, 1986). It is argued that muscles function like springs, and once a motor program is sufficiently established, it activates the appropriate muscles to contract and move a limb segment until the segment reaches the point in space where all active and passive muscle forces are in equilibrium. The equilibrium points composing a trajectory or end point of movement are achieved as a function of neural commands that regulate coactivation of alpha and gamma motoneurons (Feldman, 1986). Experimental evidence for the latter point is found in studies of spinal-transected frogs indicating that spinal neurons code for spatial equilibrium points of the leg during grooming (Bizzi et al., 1991); however, recent experimental studies using human subjects suggest that end point knowledge is insufficient and that the brain must also have some knowledge of the movement dynamic (Gomi & Kawato, 1996, 1997; Mah, 2001). Proponents of the equilibrium-point hypothesis, however, argue that alternative interpretations of the data demonstrate support for the hypothesis (Feldman et al., 1998). Other hypotheses attempt to distinguish whether we learn to control movement with respect to intrinsic body coordinates of joint position, referred to as joint space, or with respect to extrinsic coordinates, referred to as hand space in the case of reaching (Kalaska & Crammond, 1992; Scott & Kalaska, 1995). Finally, some hypotheses attempt to determine which parameters, such as time, distance, or force, are controlled during movement initiation before correction. Most notable among these, the impulse-variability model proposes that the nervous system controls movement by planning the phasing and duration of muscle contractions (for a review see Meyer et al., 1990). For further discussions on hypotheses of motor control, the reader is referred to additional sources (Jeannerod, 1990; Schmidt & Lee, 1998; Shumway-Cook & Woollacott, 2001; Swinnen et al., 1994).

Researchers are also investigating the use of models for motor control based on developments in the fields of robotics and neural networks. Both approaches seek to incorporate perception and action to explain control of movement. Robotic models are based on the physics of perception and movement, assigning mathematic values to known neural and biomechanical relationships to explain movement outcome. Currently, in the area of autonomous robotics there is interest in simulating principles of dynamic systems using a new method called computational neuroethology. The method attempts to account not only for the neural and biomechanical elements of a robot but also for environmental context and the new phenomena that may emerge during action within that environment (Chiel & Beer, 1997; Stringer et al., 2003; van Heijst et al., 1998). Neural network models are based on the assumption that no simplistic, predictable relationship exists among nerve cells to explain movement, but rather it is the phenomenon of their complex interactions that is believed to explain the movement outcome. Thus neural networks focus primarily on specifying the array of cellular and network properties that may govern how a population of neurons will self-assemble under a given set of conditions. For example, CPGs are typically modeled as discrete populations of neurons, but more recent studies examining rhythmic behaviors in invertebrates (Levitan & Kaczmarek, 1997)

and chick embryos (O'Donovan & Chub, 1997) suggest that at least in some systems, the behavior emerges from the populational dynamics of neural interactions. In a neural network model, rhythmicity is attributed to reiterative functions as a consequence of recurrent connectivity within the neuron population, and populational behavior is chiefly attributed to various inhibitory relays (i.e., reciprocal inhibition) and select intracellular mechanisms (i.e., inhibitory rebound). During development, populational behavior may vary as a function of changing cellular properties; for example, some immature neurons have excessively negative resting membrane potentials such that inhibitory transmitters induce transient depolarizations and potentiate immature excitatory connections within a neural network producing spontaneous activity. Furthermore, the populational behavior of neural networks may flip between two or more stable states as a consequence of either intrinsic or extrinsic transmitter regulation (Katz & Frost, 1996). Models of motor control are in a sense an end point, the assimilation of data from experiments testing hypotheses derived from theories. Models can then, in turn, be used to test the extent to which we can generalize the findings of studies testing hypotheses and theories. As ideas are put through these tests, we can become more confident in estimating how they may be effectively applied in addressing practical and clinical problems of motor control.

■ MOTOR CONTROL VARIABLES

Characteristic of contemporary motor control research is the notion that multiple variables contribute to the initiation and execution of a movement. Thus it is generally assumed that to understand how movements are controlled, one must be able to identify which variables are important and determine how they interact during movement. In this section we will identify some possible variables and consider how investigators currently think these variables contribute to motor control. Borrowing from the ideas of Bernstein (1967), some investigators speak of motor control variables as systems or subsystems of control composed of many intrapersonal and extrapersonal variables (Thelen & Ulrich, 1991). In more eclectic terms, variables may be anything, be it physical, physiologic, or psychologic, that has an impact on movement planning or execution. Thus to identify the underlying processes that determine skill acquisition during development, one must know not only which variables are important at a given age, but also how each variable changes during development and the impact of that change on all the other variables involved. To successfully accomplish such a task requires an experimentalist's approach that controls as many variables as possible while methodically manipulating the one in question, a task that is rarely feasible in human studies. Furthermore, if a variable is dynamically context specific, even the experimental approach may be too artificial to truly understand its impact on motor control. Nonetheless, researchers are attempting to identify variables that are critical to motor skill acquisition. By nature, these variables are interactive, but for convenience we will refer to them here as being sensorimotor variables, mechanical variables, cognitive variables, and task requirements.

SENSORIMOTOR VARIABLES

Sensorimotor variables are those physiologic mechanisms or processes that reside within the nervous system. CPGs are an example of a sensorimotor variable. By selecting and timing the activity of motoneurons, they play a key role in determining the pattern of muscle activity during movement (Grillner, 1996; Rossignol, 1996). For example, in the case of locomotion, CPGs determine which muscles are active in the stance phase of gait and which are active in swing. CPGs can produce motor patterns or synergies similar to those produced during normal behavior even when deprived of afferent (sensory) information, but pattern generators are not the only determinants of the synergies that characterize rhythmic movements. When a cat rapidly shakes a paw to dislodge an irritant, for example, a novel combination of flexor and extensor activity is produced, referred to as a mixed synergy. The mixed synergy is partially determined by a spinal CPG and partially determined by motion-dependent feedback from the leg (Koshland & Smith, 1989).

Movement synergies and neural mechanisms that alter or regulate them can also be viewed as sensorimotor variables controlling movement. A common view is that the formation of synergies for movement is the nervous system's solution to controlling the multiple degrees of freedom inherent in coordinating a multisegmented body (Bernstein, 1967). Recent research has supported this hypothesis as relatively few (1 to 3) synergies have been identified in frogs' unrestrained kicking (d' Avella et al., 2003) and in human movements such as squats, walking, and going up and down a step (St-Onge & Feldman, 2003). Although synergies, such as flexor and extensor synergies, have long been viewed as the stereotypic motoneuron patterns inherent in spinal neural circuitry, current views suggest that movement synergies can be context specific and highly individualistic (Keshner, 1990) and can change during the acquisition of coordina-

tion (Carsen & Riek, 2001). Supporting this view, anatomic and physiologic data in cats suggest that motoneuron pools for biarticular muscles of the leg are actually a collection of smaller pools that can be separately recruited in a task-specific manner (Pratt & Loeb, 1991). For example, portions or all of these pools may be recruited depending on movement parameters such as velocity or acceleration (Zernicke & Smith, 1996). Other studies suggest that synergies characterizing voluntary movement, particularly of the upper extremity, may be controlled by premotor cortical areas because specific patterns of corticoneuronal activity in these areas can be recorded before the onset of practiced movements (Georgopolous, 1990; Ghez, 1991, Seitz et al., 2000). Sensorimotor variables that may contribute to regulation of muscle synergies to enhance performance include mechanisms controlling joint stiffness (Hasan, 1986; Mah, 2001), joint net torque (Horak & Macpherson, 1996; Young & Marteniuk, 1998), visuomotor and visuospatial processes (Abbruzzese & Berardelli, 2003; Lee et al., 1990; Schmidt & Lee, 1998), and in essence, all other perceptuomotor processes tuned to participate in planning or executing a movement (Todorov & Jordan, 2002). Developmental aspects of sensorimotor variables also include processes of change such as differentiation and refinement of neural networks, changes in sensory perception, neural conduction characteristics, changing motor unit properties, and force-producing capabilities. The latter two topics are considered more fully with respect to musculoskeletal development in Chapter 6.

MECHANICAL VARIABLES

Mechanical contributions to motor control are of particular interest in many disciplinary areas of research. Changes in total body mass and relative distribution of mass during development are accompanied by changes in length and center of mass per body segment. These changes, in turn, alter inertial forces due to gravity and friction during movement (Zernicke & Smith, 1996). In some instances these inertial forces may assist movement. In other instances they may oppose movement (Jensen et al., 1997). Together with other variables, they help shape movement (Chiel & Beer, 1997; Zernicke & Smith, 1996). Studies in animals and humans have demonstrated that motor skills are greatly affected by inertial forces (Hoy et al., 1985; Schneider et al., 1990) and that part of learning to perfect a skill is learning to anticipate and use these forces to execute a movement more efficiently (Schneider et al., 1989). The viscoelastic properties of musculoskeletal tissues are also an important mechanical variable in the control of movement (Tardieu et al.,

1989). The passive elastic attributes of these tissues contribute to action by absorbing and releasing energy and have been suggested to reduce neural programming requirements for movement execution (Mah, 2001; Schneider et al., 1989; Zernicke & Smith, 1996).

COGNITIVE VARIABLES

Cognitive variables may include variables that are dependent on conscious and subconscious processes such as reasoning, memory, or judgment to optimize performance. Such variables might include arousal, motivation, anticipatory or feedforward strategies, the selective use of feedback, practice, and memory. Variations in arousal can probably modify any other control variable, such as pattern generation (Thelen et al., 1982), or even whether a behavior is demonstrated (Bradley, 1992). Motivation may make multiple contributions to the control of movement. In some instances it may serve primarily to trigger activity, and in other instances motivation may determine the form of the consequent movement. For example, it has been suggested that hand path is straighter during reaches for a moving target than for a stationary one because the infant is more motivated to reach and make contact with a moving target (Hofsten, 1991). Cognitive-related variables likely emerge with and assist in skill mastery; toddlers as young as 13 to 14 months of age having only a few weeks of standing experience can selectively determine when to use manual assistance for maintaining postural control while standing on an array of support surfaces (Stoffregen et al., 1997). Cognitive processes associated with action are also important for acquiring spatial maps (memories) of the movement environment (McComas et al., 1997), are apparent in earliest anticipatory behaviors during infancy (such as the anticipatory head and eye turning during games of peekaboo), and may be delayed or differently configured in children with Down syndrome (Aruin & Almeida, 1997).

Anticipatory strategies, also called feedforward strategies, are a select form of anticipatory behavior characterized by movement adjustments time locked to voluntary movements (Massion, 1992). In the control of posture, anticipatory strategies minimize equilibrium disturbance and/or assist in completing the desired movement. In other acts, anticipatory strategies minimize the amount of attention dedicated to monitoring feedback and making corrections after initial movement execution. Although anticipatory strategies are not usually conscious cognitive processes, they involve subconscious forecasting processes (Massion, 1992) that are essential for minimizing movement errors during perceptuomotor tasks (Viviani

& Mounoud, 1990) and sometimes require considerable training such as the anticipatory postural adjustments observed in dancers (Mouchnino et al., 1990). Indeed, it is argued that anticipatory strategies are learned, that they are relatively fixed under stable conditions, but are adapted in less fixed situations only by learning from past movement experiences (Massion, 1992). Anticipatory strategies are observed in postural adjustments before the onset of whole body movements (Nashner & Forssberg, 1986), postural adjustments prior to onset of arm movements (Horak et al., 1984), shaping and orientation of the hand before contact with an object to be grasped (Jeannerod, 1984), and strategies to time body movements with timing demands of the environment (Viviani & Mounoud, 1990).

Children, like adults, demonstrate anticipatory postural adjustments in trunk muscles before lifting the arm in a sitting position as early as 6 to 8 months of age (van der Fits et al., 1999). In the standing position, the presence of anticipatory postural adjustments depend on the time the child has practiced in standing and walking, becoming more consistently observed at approximately 16 to 17 months of age (Assaiante et al., 2000; Witherington et al., 2002). Anticipatory postural adjustments in the trunk and leg muscles before other behaviors such as lifting the arms (Hay & Redon, 2001; Riach & Hayes, 1990) or rising onto tiptoe (Haas et al., 1989) can be recognized as early as 4 years of age, but may go through a period of increased variability between 6 and 8 years of age, before showing consistency at 9 to 12 years of age (Westcott & Zaino, 1997). Anticipatory postural adjustments related to the initiation of gait appear after 1 to 17 months of walking experience and are not fully mature until around 6 to 8 years of age (Assaiante et al., 2000; Ledebt et al., 1998; Malouin & Richards, 2000). Anticipatory strategies during preparation to grasp can also be observed as early as 9 months of age (Forssberg et al., 1991; Hofsten & Rönnqvist, 1988) and appear to be present by 4 postnatal months, as evidenced by postural adjustments in neck and trunk musculature when infants are about to be pulled to sit or picked up from supine (Bayley, 1969) and adjustments in gaze as they anticipate an object's trajectory (van der Meer et al., 1994).

Whether all of these anticipatory strategies share some fundamental means of regulation has not been addressed experimentally, to our knowledge, but it is speculated that similarities may exist between feedforward strategies in postural and arm trajectory control (Massion, 1992). Nor is there any clear locus of control for any of the identified anticipatory strategies. It is generally thought that anticipatory postural adjustments are controlled by local spinal cord and brainstem networks, as well as by transcortical loops, including the motor and premotor cortices (Massion, 1992). Models of feedforward control hypothesize that the controller is likely to be a network that receives and compares afferent feedback and information about the desired movement (efferent copy) to set gain adjustments for modifying movement commands as they are executed (Massion, 1992). They may also function to reprogram postural responses (Burleigh & Horak, 1996; Horak & Nashner, 1986) or delay initiation of the voluntary command (Massion, 1992) when the command is destabilizing. Evidence to date suggests that feedforward strategies emerge subsequent to feedback strategies during development of a skill such as postural control in stance (Haas et al., 1989; Ledebt et al., 1998; Witherington et al., 2002), that they are disrupted in children with CP (Liu, 2001; Nashner et al., 1983; Westcott et al., 1998; Zaino, 1999), and that they are delayed or inadequate in children and young adults with Down syndrome (Aruin & Almeida, 1997; Sugden & Keogh, 1990).

The amount of attention dedicated to monitoring a movement is also viewed as a variable that can be modified to perfect a motor skill. It has been suggested that during development, children initially execute new movements in a ballistic manner, ignoring feedback, then swing to the opposite extreme attempting to process excessive amounts of feedback, before finally learning to selectively attend to feedback. An example of this transition proposed by Hay (1979) is described under "Reaching" later in this chapter. It is generally thought that once the child (or adult) learns to selectively attend to feedback, more attention (or mental processing) can be assigned to reading the environment and predicting the environmental changes and movement outcome as the movement is executed (Keogh & Sugden, 1985). Other cognitive variables related to learning, such as form and quantity of practice and the role of memory, are addressed within the context of motor learning in Chapter 4.

TASK REQUIREMENTS

Task requirements can also be considered distinct motor control variables. Task requirements may include any variable that can contribute to or in some way alter movement, including biomechanical requirements, meaningfulness, predictability, or any other variable associated with a given movement context. Physiologic recordings from several sensorimotor centers of the brain indicate that their participation in a task is context specific (Crutcher & Alexander, 1990; Ghez, 1991; Lemon, 1988). Task requirements shape motor strategies such as the response selection to postural perturbations, for example, recover a posture, step into a new posture, or execute

protective extension (Burleigh & Horak, 1996; Horak & Nashner, 1986). Task requirements can also result in the gating of reflexes, for example, a noxious stimulus applied to the foot may produce a flexor withdrawal response if the leg is in the swing phase of gait, but an extensor "contact" response if the leg is in the stance phase (Rossignol & Drew, 1986). Similarly, task requirements may alter the strategy a child uses to reach for an object (Hofsten, 1991), and evidence suggests that the meaningfulness of the task may enhance or mask performance (van der Weel et al., 1991). The role of meaningfulness is demonstrated by comparing performance when a child is asked to perform a relatively abstract task (e.g., instructed to repetitively pronate and supinate as far as possible) versus a concrete task (e.g., instructed to strike a tambourine, a task requiring repetitive pronation and supination). Children with CP generate larger movement excursions following the concrete instructions than after the abstract instructions (van der Weel et al., 1991). In summary, task requirements, like all other variables we have considered, appear to play a crucial role in the control of movement. Control variables may add to or subtract from movement such that there may be multiple possible behavioral outcomes for a given set of centrally generated movement instructions.

For therapists interested in learning- or dynamic-based theories, thoughtful analyses of task requirements can generate both a deeper understanding of the minimal requirements for completing a task and an array of hypotheses as to why a client cannot complete the task. Analysis can also assist in determining how to modify and reduce task requirements so that a client can successfully complete the modified version of the task. For example, if biomechanical variables are rate limiting (i.e., the task requires more muscle force or rate of change in force than a patient can currently generate), the therapist may look for ways of scaling the amount of force required. If leg extensor muscles are too weak for a patient to rise from regular-height chairs, treatment may consist of standing from chairs of greater height, from chairs with armrests of varying height, or from an array of surfaces under varying degrees of buoyancy (in a pool). If cognitive variables are rate limiting and the task requires analysis of the environment or anticipatory planning, the therapist may try to simplify the environment by reducing the number of distracting stimuli or range of possible choices that can be made and identify ways to enhance the interest in and focus on an essential cue for motor planning. For example, while initially working on eye-hand coordination, distracting stimuli may be removed from the room, the amount of effort (i.e., strength, coordination, or postural context) required to reach may be reduced, and the amount of spatiotemporal uncertainty may be minimal to none. The task would include elements known to be of significant interest to the child (e.g., favorite toys, cartoon characters, colors, textures, sounds). As success is achieved, the competing stimuli may be gradually returned, the amount of spatiotemporal uncertainty may be increased, the amount of effort required may be increased (strength, coordination, postural context), and effort may be made to expand the child's interests or attention. Applying learning-based theories, the objective would be to provide an array of movement conditions associated with an array of possible movement consequences from which the child can formulate rules of association. Applying dynamic-based theories, the objective would be to provide an array of movement contexts that would allow the child to discover his or her own movement solutions (see also discussions by Aruin & Almeida, 1997; Latash & Anson, 1996; Newell & Valvano, 1998).

MOTOR SKILL ACQUISITION IN CHILDREN

This section examines specific areas of motor development in children and the variables currently viewed as critical to the process of skill acquisition. As will be demonstrated, many of the apparently key sensorimotor variables for control of a skill are already present in the earliest phases of postnatal development, suggesting that the basic neural substrate for orderly generation of skilled movement may be in place months to years before maturation of the nervous system is complete and adult behaviors are observed. Although neural maturation of sensorimotor variables for motor control is necessary to attain adult levels of skill, it is not sufficient to fully account for how or when skilled movement is achieved. Here we will consider some of the variables identified by researchers and how these variables may contribute to the control of four specific skill areas—postural control, locomotion, reaching, and grasping—during development.

POSTURAL CONTROL

Postural control is achieved via the cooperative interaction of neural sensory (e.g., visual, vestibular, and somatosensory systems) and motor systems and cooperating musculoskeletal systems so as to meet the behavioral goals of postural orientation and stability (Horak & MacPherson, 1996). Although each of the three systems is considered essential to optimal control of both static and dynamic posture, each system can compensate to some extent for the other two (Horak et al., 1990), and the relative importance of each system appears to vary with contextual demands (Horak et al., 1989; Horak & MacPherson, 1996). As we will see, acquiring skill to process and use the ensemble of sensory information in selecting a motor strategy may more fully account for the postnatal development of postural control than indices of physiologic maturation of any given system. Achievement of postural control is often described in terms that emphasize the closed loop or sensory feedback aspects of balance correction or reactive postural adjustments. Adaptive postural control, however, also employs open loop or anticipatory postural adjustments. These anticipatory strategies function to minimize potential postural perturbations arising with movement initiation and to assist in achieving the desired movement. Thus the process of establishing effective anticipatory strategies may also more fully account for the development of postural control than indices of postnatal changes in the closed loop attributes of any given sensory or motor system or its impairment during development (Horak et al., 1988). In this section we will consider the contribution of sensory, motor, and musculoskeletal system variables, contributing to the acquisition of postural control.

Sensory System Variables
Vision
Vision is perhaps the most powerful sensory system functioning to regulate posture, both for feedback correction and for selection of anticipatory postural strategies (Butterworth & Hicks, 1977; Hatzitaki et al., 2002; Lee & Aronson, 1974; Sundermier & Woollacott, 1998). The first to ascribe a proprioceptive function to vision, Gibson (1966) suggested that as light from the visual field strikes the retina, changes in light associated with movement create "optical flow patterns" interpreted by the brain to determine the position of the head and body with respect to the surrounding environment. It is argued that the large-amplitude postural sway observed in blind individuals is due to the absence of this optical flow information (Lee, 1980). Optical flow patterns can evoke dramatic postural responses in both children and adults. In a now classic set of studies, Lee and Lishman (1975) demonstrated that when an adult stands inside a closed space formed by three walls and a ceiling, a forward or backward movement of the wall facing the person (center wall, Fig. 3-1) will trigger a larger sway amplitude (S) than under static visual conditions; the effect is greater if the postural task is made more difficult (e.g., standing on one leg). The effect of this visual stimulus is greatest if the visual stimulus moves along the anterior-posterior axis of vision (referred to as a looming visual stimulus, A) and least

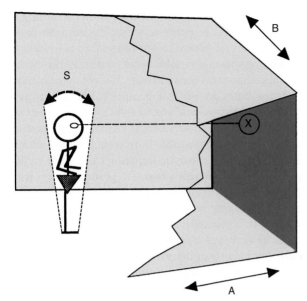

♦ **Figure 3-1**   The subject is placed in the center of a partial room formed by three walls and a ceiling that can be slid along in direction *A* or *B*. When the subject is facing wall *X*, room motion in direction *A* creates a looming visual stimulus and triggers an increase in the magnitude of sway (*S*) in the anterior-posterior plane. Younger children are likely to sway closer to their limits of stability (noted by the dashed lines forming an inverted cone) when presented with a looming visual stimulus, but not when the visual stimulus moves side to side (direction *B*). *(Adapted from Lee, DN, & Aronson, E. Visual proprioceptive control of standing in human infants. Perception & Psychophysics, 15:529–532, 1974.)*

effective if it moves tangential (side to side, B) to the visual axis. In the latter case, extraocular muscle activity during visual tracking is thought to provide proprioceptive information used to discriminate between environment and body movements (Butterworth & Hicks, 1977; Lee & Lishman, 1975). In general, if the subject faces the center wall as it is slowly moved toward the subject, the subject will sway backward; if the wall is moved away from the subject, the subject will lean forward. If the entire enclosure is moved sideways from the subject's left to right (or vice versa), however, little or no change in posture is detected.

Children begin to demonstrate distinct postural responses to optical flow patterns early in development (Butterworth & Hicks, 1977; Lee & Aronson, 1974; Sundermier & Woollacott, 1998). When placed in the moving room, children 13 to 17 months of age with 0.5 to 6.5 months of walking experience sway excessively and are apt to fall in response to a looming visual stimulus (Butterworth & Hicks, 1977). Postural responses to looming visual stimuli can be detected during stance as

early as 5 months of age, preceding onset of independent stance (Foster et al., 1996). Forward-backward sway responses to looming visual stimuli are also observed during independent sitting in infants at 11 and 16 months of age (Butterworth & Hicks, 1977). The potential for visually triggered responses appears to be present by 2 postnatal months and perhaps as early as 6 postnatal days. For example, when a looming visual stimulus is presented to the infant supported in an infant seat, directionally appropriate neck muscle activity is observed; namely, approaching stimuli trigger neck extensor activity, and withdrawing stimuli trigger neck flexor activity (Yonas et al., 1977). Visual proprioception appears to play a dominant role in postural control during early childhood; if the eyes are closed during postural displacements in the anterior-posterior plane on a movable platform under conditions of normal vestibular and somatosensory information, the magnitude of sway for children 4 to 6 years of age is significantly greater than for children 7 to 10 years of age (Shumway-Cook & Woollacott, 1985a). By 7 to 10 years of age, children demonstrate responses similar to those in adults. Vision in the older child continues to have a powerful influence on postural control. Better visual perceptual and processing ability has been shown to be highly correlated to ability to balance on one foot in 11- to 13-year-old children (Hatzitaki et al., 2002). Furthermore, it appears that if children lack visual information during development, they do not learn to minimize their postural sway to the same degree with increasing age as sighted children (Portfors-Yeomans & Riach, 1995; Prechtl et al., 2001). Prechtl and colleagues (2001) suggest that the visual system exerts a calibrating effect on the proprioceptive and vestibular systems, which, when missing in children who are blind from birth, causes prolonged ataxia-like movements during postural control. Researchers studying adults have categorized individuals into those that appear visual field dependent and those that demonstrate visual field independence (Isableu et al., 2003). Based on the visual categorization, adults demonstrate different choices in motor responses to perturbations. When visual information is eliminated, individuals with visual field dependence utilize whole trunk stabilization responses (co-contractions), whereas those who are visual field independent show more variable, flexible balancing ability.

Vestibular and Somatosensory System Variables
The vestibular system is activated and drives postural activity to regulate head control and to reference gravitational forces in order to prevent slow drift of the trunk during complicated postural control tasks (Horak et al., 2002). The somatosensory system primarily triggers postural

activity related to body positioning and righting. Recent evidence from study of adults suggests that the somatosensory and vestibular systems interact at premotoneuronal levels via common circuitry to influence the overall outcome of motoneuron activation (Horak et al., 2001). When both head and body movement occur, as is common in many functional movements, the two sensory systems appropriately influence the motor outcome based on the various head/body configurations. The location of somatosensory input (i.e., the weight-supporting structure and the use or not of hands to support or balance the body) also greatly influences the postural muscle activity in reaction to or in anticipation of perturbations (Jeka & Lackner, 1994).

The vestibular and somatosensory systems are capable of generating directionally appropriate responses in the trunk and legs following anterior-posterior displacements in infants and toddlers in sitting (Harbourne et al., 1993; Hirschfeld & Forssberg, 1994) and in stance (Sveistrup & Woollacott, 1996). Commonly used testing methods and leg responses are illustrated in Figure 3-2. It is likely that vestibular and somatosensory systems participate in these postural tests during infancy because directionally appropriate muscle responses are generated even when infants are blindfolded (Woollacott et al., 1987). Directionally appropriate muscle responses are occasionally present during tests in sitting by 4 to 5 months of age (Hadders-Algra et al., 1996: Harbourne et al., 1993). As children master pull to stand and independent stance, directionally appropriate leg muscle responses are occasionally present following the onset of mechanically induced sway by 7 to 9 months of age. Some infants can regain upright posture independently after the perturbation in stance and demonstrate directionally appropriate responses by 14 to 15 months of age, as they master independent walking (Haas et al., 1989; Shumway-Cook & Woollacott, 1985a; Sveistrup & Woollacott, 1996; Woollacott et al., 1987).

During the earliest phases of skill acquisition in sit and stance, reactive muscle responses tend to be slower and more variable than at subsequent phases of skill acquisition (Hadders-Algra et al., 1996; Shumway-Cook & Woollacott, 1985a; Sveistrup & Woollacott, 1996). As expected, latencies and consistency of response to tests of postural skill gradually approach adult levels of performance over childhood. It has been suggested that postural responses in infants and adults during sit and stance are produced by a CPG (Hirschfeld & Forssberg, 1994). Argument for this view is that directionally appropriate responses to perturbations in sitting are generated as early as 4 to 5 months of age and before acquisition of independent sitting (Harbourne et al., 1993), suggesting that the response patterns are not acquired by learning

(Hadders-Algra et al., 1996). Furthermore, according to this view, correct response selections are available in established central networks, but retrieval or activation of possible responses is variable because afferent and efferent neural components are immature. It is also possible that early responses are variable because young infants have not yet experienced and stored associations between the nuances of intertrial mechanical variability and best response. It is equally possible, borrowing from Sporns and Edelman's (1993) theoretic framework discussed earlier, that infants are inherently biased to produce a great array of responses so as to acquire sufficient memories for solving more challenging tasks at later ages. Variable responses also may be attributed to the availability of vision, for when vision is occluded infants produce more reliable vestibular and somatosensory-evoked neck responses following anterior-posterior displacements in sitting than when vision is available (Woollacott et al., 1987).

Intersensory Conflicts

Perhaps a more powerful account of initial limitations in postural control and progressive skill acquisition is set forth in studies that test a child's ability to manage intersensory conflict situations. Younger children find it nearly impossible to ignore visual information, even when it is grossly incorrect, as underscored by the tendency of children to sway and fall when confronted by a looming visual stimulus (Butterworth & Hicks, 1977; Lee & Aronson, 1974). The looming stimulus presents a sensory conflict for the child; visual proprioception indicates that the relationship between posture and environment has changed, while vestibular information regarding the relationship between posture and gravity and somatosensory information regarding the relationship between posture and support surface have not changed. Even in instances when visual and vestibular sensory information are reliable, conflicting somatosensory input, induced by rotation of the platform (see Fig. 3-2), will result in excessive sway or falls in 4- to 6-year-old children (Shumway-Cook & Woollacott, 1985a). However, a more recent study using the moving room test (see Fig. 3-1) suggests that infants may start learning to reduce dependence on unreliable visual information shortly after they begin walking; the incidence of steps, staggers, or falls in response to room movement progressively declines with age after 3 or more months of walking experience (Foster et al., 1996). When children are presented with conflicting sensory information using computerized posturography tests that manipulate visual or somatosensory information (sensory organization testing, SOT) during stance on a movable platform, they are generally able to resolve the conflict and remain standing, but the magnitude of sway is increased from

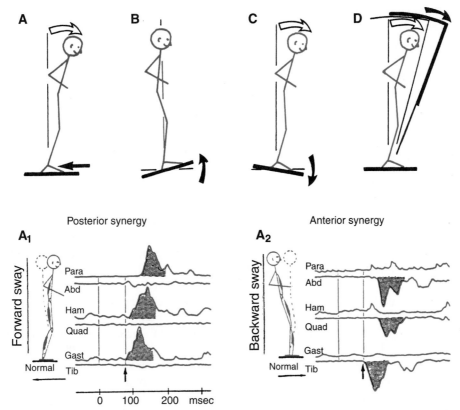

♦ Figure 3-2 When a child is placed standing on a movable platform that is then displaced in the posterior direction at a fixed rate and duration (computer driven), the child sways forward and the posterior synergy is activated in a distal to proximal sequence over time to realign the head and trunk over the base of support (A_1). Conversely, displacement of the platform in the anterior direction produces a posterior sway that is corrected by activation of the anterior muscle synergy, also in a distal to proximal sequence (A_2). In both conditions illustrated, normal visual, vestibular, and somatosensory inputs are available. If the platform is rapidly rotated to produce ankle dorsiflexion (*B*) or plantarflexion (not shown), visual and vestibular inputs remain relatively stable throughout the perturbation, whereas somatosensory receptors register displacement. If, however, the platform is rapidly rotated in the same direction and synchronous with normal sway (*C*), somatosensory input remains relatively stable because the ankle angle changes little during the perturbation, whereas vestibular and visual receptors register the postural sway. Visual information regarding sway can be altered during testing by closing the eyes or by placing a dome around the head to provide a stable visual field (*D*). If vision is stabilized during platform translations, as in *A*, visual inputs will be in conflict with normal vestibular and somatosensory information. If vision is stabilized during platform rotations, as in *B*, both visual and vestibular inputs will be in conflict with somatosensory information. Finally, if vision is stabilized during platform rotations synchronized to normal sway (*C*), visual and somatosensory inputs will be in conflict with normal vestibular information. *(Adapted from Nashner, LM, Shumway-Cook, A, & Marin, O. Stance posture control in select groups of children with cerebral palsy: Deficits in sensory organization and muscular coordination. Experimental Brain Research, 49:393–409, 1983, Fig. 1; and Horak, FB, & Nashner, LM. Central programming of postural movements: adaptation to altered support-surface configurations. Journal of Neurophysiology, 55:1369–1381, 1986, Fig. 2.)*

control levels, particularly in children 4 to 6 years of age. Examination of the coupling between somatosensory information and body sway suggests that children around age 6 years may have difficulty uncoupling the sensory information that is less relevant to the task, thus showing higher sway variability as compared to adults (Barela et al., 2003). Postural responses during SOT approach adult levels of performance between 7 and 10 years of age (Rine et al., 1998; Shumway-Cook & Woollacott, 1985a).

Research on the SOT and a clinical version of this test, the Pediatric Clinical Test of Sensory Interaction for Balance (Deitz et al., 1996), has demonstrated that there are differences between children with disabilities in the development, use, and the ability to coordinate sensory information to trigger appropriate postural motor activity. Children with Down syndrome and general cognitive delays seem to continue to over-rely on the visual system (Shumway-Cook & Woollacott, 1985b; Westcott et al.,

1997b). Children with ataxic CP demonstrate difficulty triggering motor responses when sensory information is conflicting (Nashner et al., 1983). Children with DCDs tend to have problems with utilizing vestibular information and reacting to sensory conflicts (Deitz et al., 1996). Readers are directed to the review by Westcott and Burtner (2004) for more detailed findings related to children with different disabilities.

Motor System Variables

Reactive Postural Adjustments

During stance perturbations, infants generate appropriate muscle responses even before they can sit or stand independently. When infants 4 to 5 months of age are manually supported in sitting and then briefly released, the lumbar paraspinals and hamstrings are recruited if the pelvis collapses anteriorly, whereas the paraspinals and quadriceps muscles are recruited if the pelvis collapses posteriorly (Harbourne et al., 1993). When infants 7 to 9 months of age stand with assistance on a moving platform, directionally appropriate responses may be observed in only one or two leg muscles. Muscle onset latencies under these conditions are greater and more variable than during independent stance at later ages (Hadders-Algra et al., 1996; Hirschfeld & Forssberg, 1994; Sveistrup & Woollacott, 1996). Children 4 to 6 years of age often have muscle response latencies that are greater and more variable than children under 4 years of age. For example, when displaced in an anterior direction, children as young as 15 months of age sequentially activate the gastrocnemius and hamstrings, also referred to as the posterior synergy, at latencies within the ranges for children 7 to 10 years of age; however, the average and range in temporal values for these parameters are considerably greater in 4- to 6-year olds (Shumway-Cook & Woollacott, 1985a). It has been suggested that the greater variability observed in children 4 to 6 years of age may reflect a period of transition as vision becomes less important and somatosensory information becomes more important in the control of posture (Shumway-Cook & Woollacott, 1985a). During this transition, children may be trying to process excessive amounts of information rather than selectively attending to the most pertinent sensory information, as has been suggested for other types of motor skill acquisition (Hay, 1979). Children may attempt to process excessive amounts of information as a strategy for coping with limited ability to anticipate change in the environment (Keogh & Sugden, 1985). Yet another possible explanation for the variations in children's muscle response patterns may be found in variations in the biomechanics during testing (Harbourne et al., 1993; Hirschfeld & Forssberg, 1994).

Some mention should be made regarding the failure of researchers to find distinct sequences of development in postural motor responses (Perham et al., 1987). This probably reflects the fact that complex neuromuscular responses are available early in development, but that a child's ability to select the most favorable strategy and the immediate context in question are critical determinants. It is noteworthy that children with Down syndrome can produce correct neuromuscular patterns (i.e., posterior synergy with a distal to proximal activation of leg and thigh muscles) in response to postural perturbations in stance but the patterns are initiated at a greater latency than in other children of similar chronologic age (Shumway-Cook & Woollacott, 1985b). Thus, in children with Down syndrome, motor patterns for postural control appear to be available and similar to those in children who are typically developing, but may not be adequately timed to effectively regain upright posture before reaching the boundaries of stability in stance. Protective responses, however, appear to emerge before righting and equilibrium responses in children with Down syndrome (Haley, 1987), providing a highly effective strategy for limiting injury and a reasonably adaptive strategy if one cannot rely on other postural strategies. Later in development, children and young adults with Down syndrome learn to use co-contraction motor patterns to maintain postural control, another effective adaptive strategy for delayed triggering of the motor adjustments (Aruin & Almeda, 1997; Shumway-Cook & Woollacott, 1985b).

In children with CP, results of sitting perturbation studies (Brogen et al., 1998) suggest the presence of disordered muscle activations (reactive postural adjustment [RPA] reversals [cephalo-caudal muscle activation], simultaneous activation of ventral muscles, excessive co-contractions) for sitting postural control. In standing studies, children with spastic hemiplegia have poor timing and delayed muscle onset latencies as well as reversals in muscle activation (proximal to distal sequencing rather than the expected distal to proximal pattern of muscle activation) in the legs with spasticity (Nashner et al., 1983). Children with spastic diplegia showed nonselective activation of agonist and antagonist muscles with increased frequency of reversals (proximal to distal recruitment of leg and thigh muscles), increased recruitment of antagonist muscles, and decreased activation of trunk musculature in response to standing platform perturbations (Burtner et al., 1998; Nashner et al., 1983; Woollacott et al., 1998). Some children with CP also showed an increase in center of pressure (COP) displacement during standing, especially in a radial direction, and slowed frequencies of sway. A transverse rotation control contribution may be critical for postural stability in children with CP owing to their overall relatively poor ankle control as compared to children without CP (Ferdjallah et al., 2002).

Collectively, these findings and previous points of discussion suggest at least one possible hypothesis regarding the emergence of postural skills. Namely, children may possess the potential to produce a particular postural response despite the inability to evoke it under given testing conditions, because the postural response may be masked or overridden by more reliable strategies for a given context. The context specificity of a response is further underscored by the gradual changes in strategy observed over repeated trials when the postural perturbation is modified (Forssberg & Nashner, 1982). When children 4 to 6 years of age are subjected to repeated mechanical rotations of the ankle (into dorsiflexion) in stance, the posterior synergy is gradually suppressed because, under this context, activation of the synergy is potentially destabilizing (Shumway-Cook & Woollacott, 1985a). Furthermore, it appears that children begin to either consciously or subconsciously select a postural strategy from an array of possibilities (e.g., step, squat, reach for support pole) based on context as early as 13 to 14 months of age (Stoffregen et al., 1997).

Anticipatory Postural Adjustments

Cognitive processes for predicting the postural requirements and selecting timely anticipatory strategies in a given environment and movement context are also potential rate-limiting variables in postural control development. Typically, as we become expert in a movement task, we learn to recognize those sensory cues most reliable for predicting how the environment may change during movement execution, and we learn to ignore less useful cues. Simultaneously, we learn to predict how our movements will change our relationship with respect to a more or less predictable environment and therefore determine the postural requirements for the task. In the adult, for example, when asked to rise onto tiptoes (from a plantigrade to digitigrade posture), ankle dorsiflexors are activated nearly 200 ms before ankle plantar flexors, apparently to shift the COP at the foot-floor interface a sufficient amount forward before onset of postural elevation (Haas et al., 1989).

Anticipatory activity can be observed in infants when reaching from various lying and sitting positions (van der Fits et al., 1999). Interestingly, these anticipatory postural adjustments appear primarily during goal-directed arm movements, as compared to spontaneous movements. As early as one year of age, children have been shown to activate postural muscles in anticipation of destabilizing upper extremity movements (Forssberg & Nashner, 1982). Recently, this finding has been replicated by examining infants between 10 and 17 months of age who are developing independent standing and walking behaviors (Witherington et al., 2002). While standing, the infants were enticed to pull open a drawer to retrieve toys. Through electromyography (EMG) measurement, the authors demonstrated that anticipatory postural adjustment (APA) activity in the gastrocnemius muscles (to counteract the reach and pull movement of the arm) showed a progressive developmental change across the age levels tested, with occasional APAs seen in the 10- to 13-month-old infants and more consistent and temporally specific APAs in the 16- to 17-month-olds. Adaptation of the APAs to different resistances of the drawer appeared related to the experience of the infant with pulling drawers open, as well as the amount of time they had been able to stand or walk alone.

Given the preceding findings in infants, recent examination of APAs during a sit and reach in typical children 2 to 11 years of age has shown surprising findings (van der Heide et al., 2003). The development of anticipatory postural adjustments *in sitting* appeared variable and incomplete by age 11 years when compared to adults. The authors report that APAs, which were consistent in adults tested, were absent in all the children. In contrast, 3- to 4-year-old children *in standing* and voluntarily releasing a load demonstrate an APA response seen via kinematic and EMG recording. But the APAs are variable, with the child demonstrating immature as well as adultlike activity (Schmitz et al., 2002). At age 4 to 5 years, children are reported to show adultlike APAs (forward COP shift) when an armload weight is removed voluntarily (Hay & Redon, 1999) and when asked to stand digitigrade (Haas et al., 1989). However, some children are unable to achieve digitigrade stance even by 10 years of age. The latter children exhibit insufficient anticipatory forward shifts in COP before onset of postural elevation, with dorsiflexor to plantar flexor muscle onset latencies of less than 60 ms (Haas et al., 1989). Similar anterior shifts in COP are present before raising an arm while standing at 3 to 5 years, but these are less well coordinated (Hay & Redon, 2001; Riach & Hayes, 1990). Children of this age were found to actually increase their postural perturbation with arm movement by use of anterior COP shift. The corresponding feedback response to balance this forward movement was late to activate, thus causing a delayed stop of the forward shift, a delayed backward shift, and difficulty returning to stability. In children 6 to 8 years of age, the anticipatory COP shift and the feedback reaction to maintain balance during the reaching movement were reported to be more continuous, systematic, and harmonious. In 9- to 10-year-olds, the anticipatory compensation was shown only when the postural control disturbance was reaching "perilous" limits (Hay & Redon,

2001). During a stand and reach activity, children 6 to 8 years of age have been shown to have APAs, but they demonstrate greater variability of muscle coordination patterns than 9- to 12-year-olds during the same activity (Westcott & Zaino, 1997). Overall, these studies suggest that there is a developmental progression and refinement or modulation of APAs that improves with experience in movement. The absence of APAs documented with reaching from sitting may relate to the lack of need for the activity during the specific reach measured in the study (i.e., not reaching the "perilous" limits suggested to be critical by Hay and Redon [2001] in relationship to APAs in standing).

APAs have also been examined during the gait initiation process. Ledebt and associates (1998) demonstrated that APAs (posterior COP shift) were present in children as young as 2.5 years of age, but not coordinated with the velocity of the step forward, as is seen in adults, until 6 to 8 years of age. Other researchers have suggested that typically developing children, age 4 to 6 years, will demonstrate adultlike patterns of anterior tibialis activity and posterior COP shifts during gait initiation (Malouin & Richards, 2000). Some of this discrepancy may be due to the experience each child had with walking. Using walking experience rather than age to divide a group of children, Assaiante and co-workers (2000) examined children with 1 to 17 months of *walking experience* versus children 4 to 5 years of age. Their findings suggest that inexperienced walkers use gait initiation APAs involving lateral rather than posterior COP shifts and use both the upper and lower body to make the shifts. Infants learning to walk have also been monitored for the amount of forces they apply to the contact surface. The infants who are almost walking independently will use the applied force to the contact surface in anticipation of body sway control for walking. As children acquire more walking experience, they show less activation of the more proximal muscle groups and more activation of the ankle musculature, which is more adultlike (Assaiante et al., 2000). Children from 1 to 5 years of age have been shown to be able to activate postural adjustments in reaction to a perturbation (holding the limb back) during gait initiation (Woollacott & Assaiante, 2002). Variable responses are seen in the younger children, but the 4- to 5-year-olds showed a shift in the response (decrease in latency and increase in amplitude of muscles for push-off) as measured by both kinematics and EMG.

The overlap in refinements of feedback (perturbation-triggered corrections) and feedforward postural control in children between 1 and 10 years of age suggests that they are two distinct processes that emerge in parallel during development. Furthermore, it is suggested that children begin to learn anticipatory postural strategies to coordinate posture and locomotion with the onset of voluntary movements to sit, crawl, and walk (Haas et al., 1989; Witherington et al., 2002). APA developmental differences in children with disabilities have been demonstrated in children with CP, Down syndrome, and DCD. Hadders-Algra and colleagues (1999) suggest that infants and children with CP demonstrate variable APAs. Seemingly, these children cannot choose appropriate APA to use. As a result, they keep trying different strategies or falling back to use of immature strategies such as co-contractions (Hadders-Algra et al., 1999). A study of rapid arm raising in stance suggests that anticipatory activation of trunk muscles is appropriate but very delayed in individuals with Down syndrome when compared with age-matched control subjects (Aruin & Almeida, 1997), underscoring the potential importance of cognitive-related processes in postural control. To cope with the large COP shifts of the feet, these individuals appear to adopt more immature co-contraction strategies to maintain postural control. Children with dyslexia were recently shown to have difficulty with fast walking over uneven ground, suggesting problems with APA development and use (Moe-Nilssen et al., 2003).

Musculoskeletal System Variables

In children under 4 years of age, some key rate-limiting variables are biomechanical in nature. Most notably, in the first postnatal year, the center of mass is proportionally higher than at any other age because of the combination of a large head and short limbs, requiring large force generation and regulation by neck and upper trunk musculature to counter the inertial forces created by displacements of the head. Second, in young walkers, the actual distance between floor contact and the center of mass is very small and results in much higher frequencies of postural sway with relatively larger arcs of motion than at later ages (Hayes & Riach, 1989; Usui et al., 1995). Consequently, younger children sway faster and closer to their limits of stability than older children and adults. Also, COP along the anterior-posterior axis of the foot is more posterior at younger ages (Usui et al., 1995). Although younger children can produce adultlike muscle synergies for postural correction at latencies similar to adult values, given the aforementioned biomechanical constraints, adultlike responses may be too slow for regaining upright posture. Some developmental studies have also reported that the biomechanics associated with head position and pelvic rotation during perturbation trials can be notably variable (Harbourne et al., 1993; Hirschfeld & Forssberg, 1994). Thus it is likely that some trends in available postural data, such as the greater variability observed at younger ages, may be the consequence of small variations in postural alignment at onset of data collection trials rather than solely the consequence of an immature neural control system. That is to say, variable responses also may be the consequences of postural variations associated with behavioral variables such as restlessness, fatigue, apprehension, and novelty during laboratory testing.

Changes in the biomechanical alignment of the body prior to a motor action can affect the postural activity, both RPAs and APAs (Latash et al., 2003). For example, Aruin (2003) demonstrated that when adults made fast bilateral shoulder extension movements from several different trunk alignment positions (erect and with forward upper body bend of 15° to 60°), the APA activity of individual muscles within muscle pairs varied to accommodate both the change in the postural muscle lengths and the altered stability of the person due to the forward bend. Biomechanical alignment changes have also been examined in some children with disabilities. When children with mild to moderate CP (children who were able to ambulate independently either with or without adaptive equipment) were perturbed in erect (crossed legs position or tailor-sit position, mean pelvic angle 89°) and crouched (legs positioned forward, mean pelvic angle 135°) sitting postures, the mechanical configuration of the crouched posture provided a solution to instability in sitting. These children were shown to be able to modulate their RPA EMG activity in the crouch position, whereas they could not do this in the erect position. Thus the atypical musculoskeletal positioning used by these children improved their RPA postural responses (Brogen et al., 2001). The question remains, however, whether the children performed better in the crouch position because the position offered something specific relative to the children's disability or if this is just the most practiced sitting position of children with mild to moderate CP. If the latter, the child may have learned the most adaptability in the crouch position.

In standing, when children with spastic diplegia or with typical development adopt a crouched position (hips and knees flexed and ankles dorsiflexed) (Burtner et al., 1999; Woollacott et al., 1998), or when solid ankle-foot orthoses are worn (Burtner et al., 1999), the musculoskeletal constraints (different starting position, as well as the presence of spasticity) affect RPA muscle recruitment during balance perturbation in both groups. The motor coordination patterns used by the typically developing children became more like those of age- and gender-matched children with CP who were in a crouched position or wore the solid ankle-foot orthoses. A similar effect is found in APAs of children with typical development when asked to reach forward from a crouched standing position (Thorpe

et al., 1998). These studies support the hypothesis that musculoskeletal differences that lead to altered biomechanical resting postures contribute to postural control dysfunction.

LOCOMOTION

The locomotor capabilities of the neonate and young infant have been vigorously explored. The theoretic bases and experimental designs for these studies were drawn from more than three decades of study into the control of locomotion in animals. Studies of locomotion and other rhythmic behaviors in animals have been important because they enabled investigations of motor control to move from a focus on classic reflex paradigms to the broader domain of natural, spontaneous motor behavior and the development of new research methods to study both naturally occurring behavior and corresponding physiologic systems under behaviorally restricted conditions. In particular, because locomotion is a rhythmic behavior with many kinematic and EMG features that are repeated across cycles in predictable patterns under stable conditions, studies typically focus on the production of these features to test specific hypotheses of locomotor control and theories of motor control more generally. Because animal studies have contributed significantly to both the knowledge of and methods used to study locomotion in humans, and because they continue to influence clinical studies, such as the assisted weight support paradigms for treadmill locomotion training, some animal studies on the control of locomotion will be considered briefly (for more details see Bonnot et al., 2002; Rossignol, 1996). Detailed discussion on the refinement of locomotion during childhood is presented in Chapter 5.

Development of Locomotion in Animals

Animal studies demonstrate the potential to produce either locomotion or potentially related forms of rhythmic limb movements during embryonic or neonatal development (Bradley & Bekoff, 1989). Newborn kittens, when separated from their mothers during feeding, take a few very hypermetric and awkward steps to return to their mother's teats, often falling in the process (Bradley & Smith, 1988). During these efforts, steps are occasionally characterized by the stereotypic features of reciprocal flexor-extensor EMG patterns similar to those occurring during adult locomotion. Adultlike muscle patterns are most readily apparent, however, when kittens are posturally supported while stepping on the moving belt of a treadmill or making stepping motions midair (air-stepping). Typically, steps over ground are accompanied by extensive coactivation of antagonists at the ankle, suggesting that coactivation may be a functional strategy for increasing joint stiffness to compensate for limitations in postural control or muscle force production (Bradley & Smith, 1988). The appearance of adult features for locomotion in muscle activity of newborn kittens, alternating flexor-extensor muscle synergies (Bradley & Bekoff, 1990) and limb kinematics in chick embryos (Chambers et al., 1995) and cellular studies of spinal cord activity in neonatal mice (Bonnot et al., 2002; Branchereau et al., 2000; Whelen, 2003) and rats (Kjaerulff & Kiehn, 1996) suggest that the neural networks for locomotion are established during embryogenesis.

Parallels between Developing Animals and Humans

The presence of stepping movements in human fetus, early onset of infant stepping in premature infants, and rhythmic leg movements of infant kicking provide argument for development of basic stepping circuitry for locomotion in humans during embryogenesis as in other animals (Bradley, 2003). The presence of some potential for locomotion at birth raises the question of whether that potential is established early in fetal development. Here again a parallel may be drawn with animal studies. Ultrasound studies of human fetal movement indicate that isolated kicks are initiated during the ninth embryonic week and alternating leg movements, reported to resemble neonatal stepping, are initiated with postural changes ("backward somersaults") in utero during the fourteenth embryonic week (de Vries et al., 1982). Thus human fetuses appear to exhibit stepping during the first half of the gestational period, about the same portion of the embryonic period when chicks exhibit organized EMG and kinematic features during spontaneous motility (Bradley & Bekoff, 1990; Chambers et al., 1995). Given that low-risk preterm infants born at 34 weeks of gestational age demonstrate orderly kinematic patterns similar to those of full-term newborns, and that those features differing from full-term infants appear to be attributable to dynamic interactions emerging during movement (Heriza, 1988; Geerdink et al., 1996; Jeng et al., 2002), the parallel between human fetuses and chick embryos appears reasonable (Fig. 3-3). In other words, the neural foundations for locomotion in humans may be assembled during neurogenesis, as they appear to be in other animals (Bradley & Bekoff, 1989; Butt et al., 2002).

Several parallels can also be drawn between studies of neonatal animals and rhythmic, locomotor-like leg movements in human infants. When supported on the treadmill, infants perform repetitive leg movements characterized by several kinematic features similar to adult locomotor behavior (Thelen & Ulrich, 1991; Ulrich et al., 1994; Yang

et al., 1998b). Although infants 6 to 12 months of age become more reliable in producing a sustained pattern of alternating steps that is timed to the treadmill belt speed, even infants as young as 10 days of age occasionally demonstrate these features (Yang et al., 1998b). Neonatal infant stepping shares many features with early treadmill stepping. Most notably, hip, knee, and ankle joints are synchronously flexed during the swing phase and synchronously extended during the extensor phase; the excursions are accompanied by nonspecific EMG patterns; and there is an absence of both heel strike and push-off at the transitions between swing and stance (Forssberg, 1985). These features are also characteristic of infant kicking within the first 1 to 3 postnatal months (Jensen et al., 1994, 1995), further suggesting that some of the mechanisms controlling treadmill stepping, and therefore locomotion, are already functional at birth.

Development of Locomotor Muscle Patterns in Humans

Until recently, it was believed that infant locomotion lacked adultlike features typically observed in EMG recordings. Failure to observe adultlike EMG patterns was often attributed to late myelinization of descending paths at caudal spinal levels (Sutherland et al., 1980), late maturation of cortical structures (Forssberg, 1992), or late myelination of peripheral nerves (Sutherland et al., 1988). However, in a study of treadmill locomotion, infants as young as 10 days of age occasionally produced steps characterized by alternating activation of antagonist muscles, and the extent of coactivation decreased with practice (Yang et al., 1998b). The relative duration of flexor and extensor burst durations also varied with treadmill speed in a manner similar to that in adults. Furthermore, it has been demonstrated that prewalking infants, age 4 to 12 months, can respond with adultlike interlimb coordinated responses when given unilateral leg perturbations while supported to walk on a treadmill (Pang & Yang, 2002, 2003). The failure to observe adultlike EMG patterns for locomotion in previous studies of prewalkers and early walkers may have been the result of adaptive strategies that masked this potential. For example, infants may have coactivated antagonist muscles to increase joint stiffness and stabilize limb posture as a compensation for insufficient postural control or control of force generation for supporting and transporting body mass (Bradley & Smith, 1988; Okamoto & Okamoto, 2001). Also, testing conditions may have masked the potential to generate adultlike locomotor EMG patterns; that is, support in stance or movement against gravity in supine likely altered the task requirements (Ulrich et al., 1994), necessitating a different EMG pattern. Conversely, the testing conditions

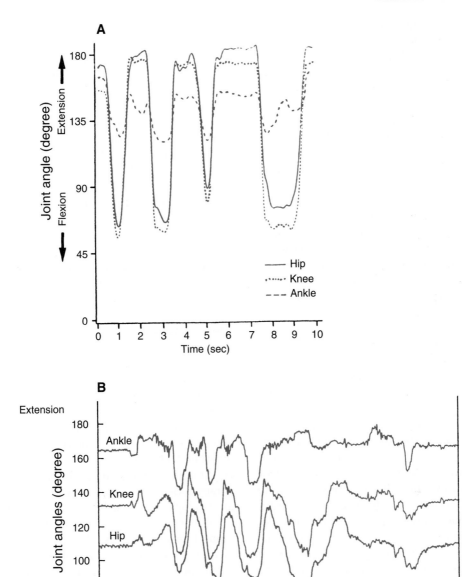

• **Figure 3-3**   Kinematic analyses indicate that lower extremity movements are organized very early in development. When preterm infants initiate a sequence of several kicks at 40 weeks of gestational age, the alternation of flexion and extension at the hip is synchronous with motions of the knee and ankle in the same direction (**A**) and is similar to kicking movements during spontaneous motility in chick embryos in ovo at 9 embryonic days of age (**B**). (*A adapted from Heriza, CB. Comparison of leg movements in preterm infants at term with healthy full-term infants. Physical Therapy, 68:1687–1693, 1988, Fig. 2.*)

may have lacked key features for expressing locomotor EMG patterns. For instance, in cats, the velocity of limb movements contributes to the generation of certain EMG patterns (Zernike & Smith, 1996).

Although there is wide support for the view that basic features of locomotion are spinally mediated (Butt et al., 2002), some argue that uniquely human features of gait emerge as spinal neural networks are transformed with maturation of higher neural centers (Forssberg, 1992). Specifically, it is argued that the basic patterns of alternating flexion and extension observed during neonatal stepping persist with development of locomotion, but that maturing sensorimotor input suppresses activation of ankle extensor motoneurons to permit heel contact at the onset of stance. As further support for this view, it is argued that the absence of heel strike in children with CP occurs because cerebral injury impairs development of higher-center control over spinal neural networks for locomotion (Forssberg, 1985). Conversely, some researchers speculate that attributes of gait, such as heel strike, need not be specifically dictated by higher neural centers because they may emerge from the inertial interactions and associated feedback between body segments during movement (Cheron et al., 2001; Thelen & Ulrich, 1991; Zernicke & Smith, 1996). For example, when cats walk at relatively fast speeds, the sartorius muscle produces a two-burst pattern, one during late stance and one during late swing, but the second burst does not consistently occur at slower walking speeds. Kinematic and kinetic analyses suggest that the burst in late swing functions to counteract extensor forces at the knee during faster walking speeds, but it is not required and therefore not recruited at slower speeds because viscoelastic properties of knee flexors are sufficient to counter these forces. In adult humans, examination of muscle actions during the walk-to-run transition demonstrates lower swing-related ankle, knee, and hip flexor activation and higher stance-related activation of the ankle and knee extensors during running than walking (Prilutsky & Gregor, 2001). It is suggested that the exaggerated sense of effort in lower extremity flexors during swing of a fast walk may trigger the locomotor pattern to change from the walk to run pattern. Whether the muscle activity associated with heel strike or other attributes of gait is due to centrally organized commands or is the result of motion-dependent feedback has yet to be determined in infants.

An interesting case study of a premature infant who sustained a left grade III/IV intraventricular hemorrhage presented data on changes in right and left initial foot contact from 6 to 16 months corrected age (Bodkin et al., 2003). The researchers initially noted a definite asymmetry between the left and right foot at initial contact during supported walking on a treadmill, hypothesized to be due to the central nervous system (CNS) insult. However, with practice on the treadmill over 4 months, this asymmetry decreased and either a foot flat or heel strike contact was observed with both feet. This motor pattern continued for a time after the treadmill training ended, then reverted to the previous asymmetric pattern. This finding might suggest that the absolute velocities or rate of change in velocity typically achieved during early over-ground locomotion are insufficient to express adultlike ankle control in the step cycle. However, when given the higher velocities of the treadmill to stimulate the walking pattern, the appropriate heel-strike pattern emerges even though the infant suffered early brain damage. Although this is a study of just one infant, the resultant gait patterns, with and without treadmill training, suggest an influence of both the CNS and the peripheral environment.

Biomechanical Variables

The emergence of locomotion during development is determined by the interactive aspects of anatomy and environment during movement. Typically, infant stepping is not readily elicited beyond the first to second postnatal month under standard testing conditions, and it was long argued that the behavior disappears as a consequence of encephalization processes (the taking over of control) by maturing higher motor centers (McGraw, 1940). However, the postnatal decreases in rate of stepping temporally correlate with rapid weight gain, suggesting that morphologic changes in body mass may contribute to the "disappearance" of infant stepping. Two lines of evidence support this hypothesis. One, when infants are submerged in water up to chest level, both stepping rate and amplitude increase in comparison with stepping out of water (Thelen et al., 1984). Two, if weights equivalent to the weight gains at 5 and 6 postnatal weeks are added to the ankles of infants at 4 postnatal weeks, both stepping rate and amplitude decrease in comparison with stepping without ankle weights (Thelen et al., 1984). Thus buoyancy appears to diminish the dampening effect of body mass and gravitational interactions, whereas added weight appears to augment the effect of these interactions. Results of animal studies underscore the notion that morphologic features of the organism interact with the environment to either express or mask potential abilities. Fetal rat pups, for example, exhibit interlimb coordination during spontaneous movements under buoyant conditions several days before testing under nonbuoyant conditions (Bekoff & Lau, 1980). Frog tadpoles exhibit coordinated leg movements several stages earlier in development if they can push off a mesh surface placed in an aquatic tank

(Stehouwer & Farel, 1984). The latter point invites reconsideration of the discussion regarding heel contact in gait: heel strike may not be observed until independent walking is established because of immature morphologic characteristics of the infant foot interacting with a support surface. Given the considerable structural change the foot undergoes during the first postnatal year or more, it is conceivable that initial biomechanical features of the foot do not readily afford initiation of heel strike or push-off in the young infant.

Variables under Investigation

There is a growing interest in the relative contributions of mechanical and neural variables underlying control of leg movements in infants as methods for study of kinematic and kinetic methods have become more affordable and less labor intensive. A collection of studies, for example, suggests that intersegmental dynamics are the critical determinants of leg coordination during kicking (Jensen et al., 1994, 1995; Schneider et al., 1990), treadmill locomotion (Ulrich et al., 1994), and the development of walking (Cheron et al., 2001; Marques-Bruna & Grimshaw, 2000). During both kicking and supported treadmill locomotion, active muscle forces are used to initiate hip flexion against gravity, but it appears that gravity and passive (inertial) forces largely determine the spatiotemporal patterns of corresponding knee and ankle excursions. Furthermore, the extent of synchrony between leg joint rotations during kicking varies with the infant's posture and appears to be greater when the infant is supported upright than when supine. The greater synchrony between leg joints in an upright posture may be due to the greater gravitation-related forces and therefore muscle force (and recruitment effort) required to overcome gravitational forces (Jensen et al., 1994). Conversely, the lesser synchrony between leg joints during supine kicking may be due to the more variable effects of gravity on the hip and ankle during the supine kick cycle. When the hip and ankle are positioned between 0° and 90°, gravity assists extension, whereas gravity assists flexion as joint position exceeds 90° (Schneider et al., 1990). During both kicking and treadmill locomotion, the swing phase appears attributable to active flexor (muscle) forces at the hip, whereas the extensor phase is primarily attributable to gravity and passive (inertial) forces and, to a lesser extent, active flexor (muscle) forces as hip flexor muscles lengthen (Fig. 3-4). During the first 8 months of walking, phase shifts have been recorded with lower extremity range of motion showing decreases, hip-knee-ankle relationships beginning to resemble mature gait patterns, time to peak angular velocity shortening, and stability of ankle angular velocity phasing improving (Marques-Braun &

Grimshaw, 2000). Examining the intersegmental dynamics differently, the extent to which the covariation of thigh, shank, and foot angles were constrained on a plane in three-dimensional space was shown to improve rapidly (within <6 months from the onset of unsupported walking) (Cheron et al., 2001). This was followed by slower changes that were hypothesized to be related to maturation of anthropometric parameters.

Paradigms developed to study spinal control of interlimb coordination have also been adapted to determine whether similar neural mechanisms control stepping in human infants. For example, when infants are supported on a treadmill and one leg is blocked during swing phase, the stance phase of the contralateral leg is lengthened, as in adult cats and humans (Yang et al., 1998a). Responses vary with extent of loading in the stance limb (e.g., increases in load result in lengthening of extensor burst duration and delay in onset of swing), which indicates that human infants as young as 3 months of age possess mechanisms for adaptive stepping observed in cats and kittens and attributed to spinal circuitry (Pang & Yang, 2001; Yang et al., 1998a). Nonetheless, studies in cats show that cortical centers normally play an important role in these adjustments, indicating that perception and planning are important neural contributions to control of locomotion (Drew, 1993). Animal studies also indicate that experience-based learning is important for refining rudimentary locomotor skills. For example, findings from a kinetic study of locomotion in neonatal chicks suggest that practice is required to acquire efficient energy absorption strategies for yield in stance (Muir et al., 1996). Experience-based learning for refinement of locomotor skills appears to be under way before the onset of independent locomotion. In a recent study of infants 9 months of age or older, perturbation of two or more consecutive steps resulted in aftereffects characterized by increased vertical clearance of the toe for one to two steps after the perturbation was removed (Pang et al., 2003).

REACHING

The past 25 years have seen dramatic demonstrations and reappraisals of the reaching abilities of newborn and young infants. In commonly employed static testing situations with the infant placed supine, reaching for a dangling, stationary target, such as a red ring, is initiated at approximately 3 to 4 postnatal months. Yet investigators have demonstrated that if newborns are adequately supported in an inclined posture and presented with a moving target, rudimentary eye-hand coordination can be distinguished from random hand movements within days after birth. By 3 months of age, infants exhi-

A

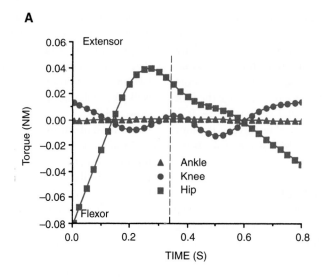

B

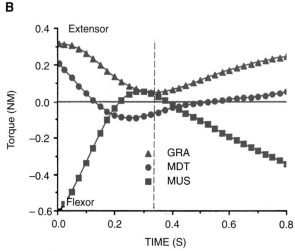

◆ **Figure 3-4** Motions of adjacent limb segments during kicking may arise from active forces due to muscle activity and passive forces due to gravity and inertia of the limb segments. For example, in the data presented here, an infant initiates a kick cycle starting from a semiextended position of 125° and achieves a peak flexion of 80° at 0.32 second (vertical dashed line) before the hip returns to the extended position. The motion into flexion is attributable primarily to an initial hip flexor force or torque that is maximal at the outset (0.0 s) and begins to drop off as the hip moves into flexion (**A**). The hip flexor force is due to active muscle force (MUS) during the first 0.2 second (**B**). An extensor force develops between 0.2 and 0.3 second (**A**) as active hip flexor force decreases to 0 newton-meter (**B**) and serves to slow and reverse the hip motion into extension (0.32 s). Throughout the extension of the hip, there are small passive extensor forces due to gravity (GRA) and inertia (MDT) and a growing active hip flexor force (MUS) to lower the leg (**B**). *(Adapted from Schneider, K, Zernicke, RF, Ulrich, BD, Jensen, JL, & Thelen, E. Understanding movement control in infants through the analysis of limb intersegmental dynamics. Journal of Motor Behavior, 22:493–520, 1990, Fig. 3; reprinted with permission of the Helen Dwight Reid Educational Foundation. Published by Heldref Publications, 1319 Eighteenth St., NW, Washington, DC 20036-1802. Copyright © 1990.)*

bit eye-foot coordination as demonstrated by ability to learn to kick a mobile (Angulo-Kinzler et al., 2002). The infants achieved this by either increasing their kicking frequency or by altering their posture dependent on where the mobile was placed. By 4 months of age, infants are adept at contacting a moving object with their hands, and by 9 months they demonstrate adultlike reaching patterns as they catch a moving object. In this section, features characterizing the development of reaching and tracking skills will be described. For additional discussion on the control of reaching, the reader may wish to refer to more comprehensive texts (Swinnen et al., 1994; Thelen & Smith, 1994).

Rudimentary Reaching Skills

A growing body of work suggests that arm movements of the neonate, like kicking movements, are rudimentary expressions of skilled reaching that emerges during the first postnatal year. Even arm movements of newborns appear to be purposeful (van der Meer et al., 1995) and spatiotemporally structured (Hofsten & Rönnqvist, 1993). It is generally held that reaching in the neonatal period is visually triggered and that hand trajectories are directed actions. For example, the number of arm movements is significantly greater when 3-day-old infants visually fixate on an object than when they do not (Hofsten, 1982). Similarly, when presented with a ball, a picture of a ball, or a blank card, infants 8 to 16 days old make more directed arm movements when presented with the ball or picture than the blank card (Rader & Stern, 1982). The directness of neonatal reaches was quantified in a study of 3-day-old newborns supported in a reclining infant seat and presented with a stimulus moving in an arc 12 cm from the eyes (Hofsten, 1982). Measurements for every hand movement exceeding 5 cm indicated that forward-extending arm movements were aimed much closer to the target (32° off target) while infants visually fixated on the target than while they looked elsewhere (52° off target) or closed their eyes (54° off target). Presentation of an object in the visual field elicited longer horizontal and vertical hand paths during arm movements than when no stimulus was present (Bergmeier, 1992). The directness of early reaching may indicate that there is a genetically established neural coordinate system that links the trajectories of the hand with the face and visually fixated objects within reach (Hofsten, 1982). Furthermore, ultrasound evidence of hand-to-face contact by 10 weeks of gestation (de Vries et al., 1982) suggests that there is a basic, genetically scripted neural network linking hand space with body space by the end of the first trimester of fetal development. Alternatively, early hand trajectory may be an emergent product of biomechanical variables rather than the product of detailed neural commands (Corbetta & Thelen, 1994; Fetters & Todd, 1987).

Infants 1 to 19 weeks of age, when presented with a slowly moving object, continue to display interest in the object, but during the weeks that neonatal reaching is transformed into functional reaching, the role of vision appears to change somewhat, and there are periods when reaching is less readily observed. Age-dependent declines in reaching responses are reported to occur between 8 and 16 postnatal days (Rader & Stern, 1982) and in the seventh postnatal week (Hofsten, 1984). Because neonatal reaching was initially viewed as a primitive, reflex-like behavior, the age-dependent decline was attributed to maturation of descending neural inputs, an argument similar to that for the "disappearance" of infant stepping (Connolly, 1977). It has also been suggested that the decline in reaching may occur because object contact, and therefore behavioral reinforcement, is rare, or because the infant does not have sufficient optimal opportunities (e.g., postural context) to practice during this time period (Bower, 1979). Alternatively, as infants become more interested in looking at objects, visual attention may inadvertently extinguish neonatal reaching efforts (Bergmeier, 1992). In the neonatal period, the hand is typically open during forward extension of the arm (Hofsten, 1982), but around the seventh postnatal week, when the rate of reaching briefly decreases, infants seem more interested in looking at the object and the hand posture is more likely to be fisted (Hofsten, 1984). Around 12 postnatal weeks, however, the frequency of reaching increases, and the hand resumes an open posture during reaches (Hofsten, 1984). During this time period, infants appear to acquire some ability to visually determine realistic reaching distances because they rarely initiate effort to contact objects out of reach (Field, 1977). Between 12 and 16 weeks, infants acquire considerable skill in aiming their reaches (Hofsten & Rönnqvist, 1988). By 15 weeks, infants can contact a moving object in as much as 90% of trials, and between 15 and 18 weeks, contact shifts from just touching to catching the moving object (Hofsten, 1979). Vision functions to elicit reaching throughout the transition from neonatal to functional reaching, but it is not used to guide hand trajectory (Lasky, 1977; Wishart et al., 1978) or to orient the hand toward the object before initial contact during this transitional period in skill level (Lockman et al., 1984). In fact, infants do not appear to require vision of their hands for initiating reaching or contact and grasp of an object (Clifton et al., 1993). These findings seem to suggest that younger infants initiate reaching using a ballistic strategy to aim the hand toward the target and then switch to a feedback strategy (vision, proprioception, or both) to make corrective movements for grasping once the object is contacted (Clifton et al., 1993). At 4 to 5 months of age, reaches are as good with vision available during the reach as when vision is removed after onset of the reach (Clifton et al., 1993; Wishart et al., 1978), and infants begin to adjust their gaze, anticipating the future trajectory of an object (van der Meer et al., 1994).

Infant Reaching Strategies

During the period from 12 to 36 postnatal weeks, several major changes occur in the form of reaching that suggest the development of a new control strategy (Hofsten, 1991). To determine how reaching is perfected and to investigate strategies used to control reaching during development, the velocity and distance paths of hand transport are measured from video records of infant performances. Based on standard research methods used in studies of adult behavior, trajectories are dissected into movement units, each containing one acceleration phase and one deceleration phase. Adult reaches are characterized by 1 to 2 movement units; the first unit functions to transport the hand 70 to 80% of the distance to the target,

and is relatively long in duration, and the second unit functions to home in on the object and is relatively short in duration (Jeannerod, 1981). Between 19 and 31 postnatal weeks, infants progressively restructure reaches for a moving object from an average of 4 movement units per reach to 2 movement units (Hofsten, 1991); yet even at 19 weeks, 22% of reaches contain only 1 or 2 movement units. The sequencing of movement units is also modified; the transport unit is the first movement unit in half of the reaches at 19 weeks, extending an average distance of 80 cm, whereas at 31 weeks, it is the first unit in 84% of reaches and extends 137 cm. Finally, the hand path trajectory straightens with age (Fig. 3-5), suggesting that, by 31 weeks, improved spatial planning contributes to advances in aiming skill as the hand is now transported closer to the target in a more efficient manner during the first movement unit, requiring fewer subsequent units to correct for errors (Hofsten, 1991). Another possible component of the improvements in typical infants' reaching may be related to improvements in postural control. As postural control improves in supine between 12 and 24 weeks of age, a decreased number of reaching move-

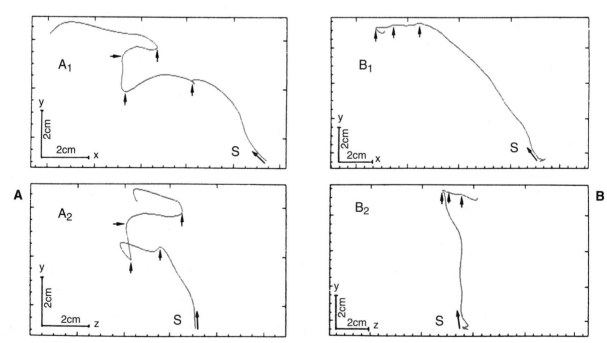

◆ **Figure 3-5**   Hand paths become straighter and contain fewer movement units during the first postnatal year when reaching for a moving target. During a reach at 19 weeks of age (**A**), 4 movement units are identified (by arrows) in views from the front (A_1) and the side (A_2). Note that these movement units are similar in length. During a reach at 31 weeks of age in the same infant (**B**), only 3 movement units are identified from the front (B_1) and side (B_2). Note that most of the reaching distance is covered in the first movement unit. *(Adapted from Hofsten, C von. Structuring of early reaching movements: A longitudinal study. Journal of Motor Behavior, 23:280–292, 1991, Figs. 3 and 4; reprinted with permission of the Helen Dwight Reid Educational Foundation. Published by Heldref Publications, 1319 Eighteenth St., NW, Washington, DC 20036-1802. Copyright © 1991.)*

ment units, a decreased length of the displacement path of the hand, and an increase in the length and duration of the first movement unit have been shown to be correlated (Fallang et al., 2000). Given that there is this pattern of control in young infants, the kinematic quality of reaching movements in preterm infants has been suggested as a possible construct to be examined to predict later motor coordination problems. Fallang and colleagues (2003) have shown in a group of preterm and full-term infants without diagnosed motor disorders that the high-risk preterm group of infants performs nonoptimal reaching behavior at age 6 months, which differs from the low-risk preterm and full-term group.

Infants 5 to 9 months of age do not appear to use the adult pattern of control when seated and reaching to grasp a stationary object placed on a horizontal (table) surface (Fetters & Todd, 1987). Under these conditions, movement units tend to be similar in duration (200 ms) for all ages, reaching distances, and positions (or order) within a reach (Fig. 3-6). Furthermore, there may not be a decrease in the number of movement units within the

path or a change in the straightness of hand path under these conditions between 5 and 9 months of age. Both hand path distance (equivalent to twice the shortest possible distance) and mean reaching duration (800 ms) also appear to be stable across ages and within adult limits, only more variable. These findings suggest that the movement speed and curvature of early functional reaching observed under stationary reaching conditions may be fundamental properties of both skilled and unskilled reaching controlled by biologic or physical constraints emerging from body-environment interactions (Fetters & Todd, 1987). These findings also point to the effect of task context on measurements used to explore control variables and the likelihood that control strategies vary with context (Hofsten, 1991). It has been suggested, for example, that hand path is straighter when reaching for a moving object than when reaching for a stationary one (Hofsten, 1979).

During the period from 5 to 9 months, infants begin to use visual information at the end of the reach as the hand approaches the target to correct for errors in hand path trajectory (Hofsten, 1979). Before 5 months of age,

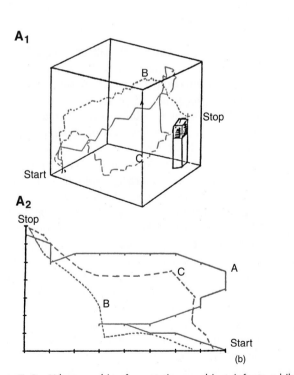

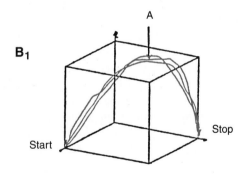

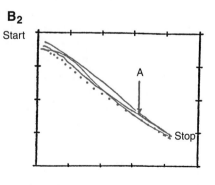

(b)

◆ **Figure 3-6**   When reaching for a stationary object, infants exhibit reaches containing multiple movement units similar in duration. Three reaches are shown for a 9-month-old infant from a side view (A_1) and an overhead view (A_2). Note the irregularities both within and between reaches as compared with adult performance from the side view (B_1) and overhead view (B_2). *(Adapted from Fetters, L, & Todd, J. Quantitative assessment of infant reaching movements. Journal of Motor Behavior, 19:147–166, 1987, Figs. 4 and 5; reprinted with permission of the Helen Dwight Reid Educational Foundation. Published by Heldref Publications, 1319 Eighteenth St., NW, Washington, DC 20036-1802. Copyright © 1987.)*

they take little notice of the hand during flight, but thereafter, if vision of the hand is blocked, as when infants reach for a virtual (mirror image) object, performance is frequently disrupted (Lasky, 1977). Although infants continue to use a ballistic reaching strategy well into childhood, withdrawal of visual feedback begins to impair reaching skill at 6 to 7 months of age (Lasky, 1977; Wishart et al., 1978). To determine how reaching movements are controlled, investigators have explored parameters that characterize the straightness of the hand trajectory. In adults, the curved hand path during reaching is composed of straight line segments linked sequentially. The end of one segment and beginning of the next corresponds to a speed valley (deceleration and reacceleration) and a change in direction of the hand (Jeannerod, 1981). It is thought that each movement segment is ballistically generated and that corrections are made at these junctions between movement segments. To test whether path corrections are necessarily restricted to these speed valleys, Mathew and Cook (1990) examined the curved hand path in reaching trials of infants between 4 and 8 months of age who were presented with a suspended object having some motion. Three-dimensional analyses of hand trajectories indicated that the initial movement segment is directed toward the object at all ages tested and that changes in the path after reach onset tend to curve the hand toward the target to correct for error (Fig. 3-7). Also, measures of hand speed within a movement segment correlate with veering of the hand toward the target within the movement segment, suggesting that error correction occurs continuously rather than only at discrete intervals in hand transport. The relationship between veering within a movement unit and target location may indicate that when vision is available, reaching is not executed using a ballistic strategy. On the other hand, continuous veering within a movement unit may be the biomechanical consequence of projecting the arm through space, a notion that is consistent with the equilibrium point hypothesis for joint position in the mass-spring model of arm control (Hofsten, 1991; Polit & Bizzi, 1979).

During the first postnatal year, interlimb coordination of the arms and hands during reaching is characteristically variable. It has long been argued that early unilateral reaching is a consequence of asymmetric tonic neck reflexes, and bilateral reaching emerges as these reflex influences lessen (Fagard, 1994). Other possible explanations for variability in reaching strategies may be postural context during the reach and the characteristics of the target object (Diedrich et al., 2001; Fagard, 1994). In a longitudinal case study of one infant from 3 to 52 weeks of age, instances of bimanual reaching appeared to correlate with more variable kinetics, greater limb stiffness, and greater

reaching velocities in the following arm as compared with the leading arm. These findings led the investigators to conclude that bimanual reaching predominates until infants learn to differentially control the following arm at approximately 6 to 7 months of age (Corbetta & Thelen, 1994). The degree of coupling between arms during reaching also appears to depend on the complexity of bimanual cooperation required, that is, whether one hand can remain relatively passive or must produce complementary movement patterns such as when holding a box lid up with one hand while extracting a toy with the other. Complementary bilateral reaching skill emerges at 9 to 10 months of age (Fagard & Pezé, 1997).

A recent study comparing adults with Down syndrome to typical adults and children found that the individuals with Down syndrome were able to demonstrate stable bimanual coordination during a circle drawing task that appeared adultlike (Robertson et al., 2002). In contrast, their unimanual ability was less coordinated and similar to the children examined in the study. This suggests that the individuals with Down syndrome have more mature bilateral reach and fine motor skill and less mature unilateral ability. This may be due to improved postural control via using both sides of the body during the bimanual activity, but this is yet to be examined experimentally.

Reaching Strategies in School-Age Children

Studies in older children suggest that reaching strategies change very little from 9 months until approximately 7 years of age, at which time there appears to be a transitional period leading to an adult reaching strategy. When the visual field is displaced by a prism, children 5 years of age reach out to the apparent target location in 1 or 2 movement units before making corrective movements to move the hand to the actual target location (Hay, 1979). In contrast, 7-year-olds execute multiple small movement units (referred to as early braking), producing hand paths that begin to veer toward the actual target location early in the path, and 9- to 11-year-olds execute an initial movement unit that approaches the virtual target location but is then followed by a second, corrective unit (referred to as smooth braking) that alters the path before the hand reaches the virtual target location (Fig. 3-8). These findings suggest that 5-year-olds continue to use ballistic strategies much like those of older infants, whereas 7-year-olds constantly monitor their movements in a closed loop strategy to control their reaches. Between 9 and 11 years of age, children begin to combine these strategies to increase the efficiency of their movements and to reduce the amount of attention required (Hay, 1979; Keogh & Sugden, 1985). These changes in reach strategy appear to coincide with developmental changes in how children

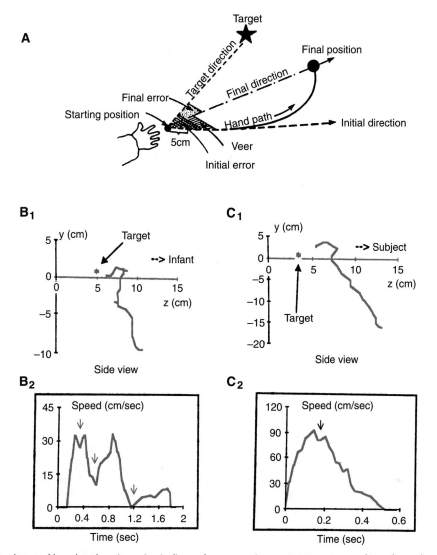

♦ Figure 3-7 Analyses of hand path trajectories indicate that corrective movements occur throughout the reach even in young infants. Measurements of veering within a movement unit (*A*) indicate that initial hand trajectory is oriented toward the target and that correction in hand path is not limited exclusively to speed valleys (arrows in B_2 and C_2) adjoining consecutive movement units. Speed valleys, characteristic of adult reaching (C_2), are also characteristic of infant reaching at as early as 6 postnatal months (B_2), but are more numerous and greater in relative magnitude due to the greater number of irregularities in hand path (B_1 versus C_1). *(Adapted from Mathew, A, & Cook, M. The control of reaching movements by young infants. Child Development, 61:1238–1258, 1990, Figs. 1 and 2.)*

utilize sensory information for guiding and adjusting arm position during reach. Hay and colleagues (1994) examined perceptual skill during an arm positioning task and found that, in the absence of vision, 8-year-olds produced greater errors in movement amplitude than both 6- and 10-year-olds, yet at the end of a trial, using kinesthetic information, they were able to detect and reduce the magnitude of their end point error. Specific study of typical children's ability to correct forearm position when perturbed found that 4- to 9-year-old

children gradually learn to master fine timing adjustments to perturbations (Schmitz et al., 2002). Furthermore, in study of 4- to 11-year-old typical children in a goal-directed reaching protocol in which forearm movements reacted to externally applied forces, it was shown that as age increased, the children showed less variability in their movements to the target and they adapted to external perturbations more quickly (Konczak et al., 2003). But even the 11-year-old children were not showing precision similar to the adults. Based on these

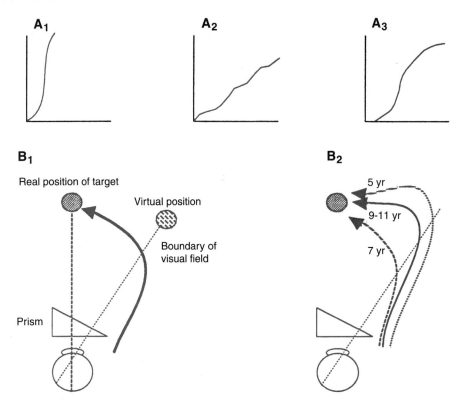

• **Figure 3-8** Hand paths during reaching to a stationary target correspond to the use of visual information to plan and control reaching. Ballistic reaches exhibit smooth trajectories with no distinct points of path correction, suggesting that they are preplanned and executed open loop (A_1), whereas early braking reaches are executed closed loop, using vision to continuously monitor and correct error (A_2). Late-braking reaches, in contrast, combine open loop and closed loop strategies to maximize reaching efficiency by preplanning 70% to 80% of the trajectory and then correcting trajectory error in the final approach to the target (A_3). The use of these three strategies can be demonstrated by using a prism to displace the visual field (B_1). Under these conditions, it is apparent that children 5 years of age use a ballistic reaching strategy, because they correct their hand path only after they have reached or surpassed the target's virtual position (B_2). In contrast, 7-year-olds, using an early braking strategy, identify the discrepancy between real and virtual target position as soon as the hand enters the visual field, and 9- and 11-year-olds, using a late-braking strategy, almost reach the virtual target position before detecting the discrepancy. *(Adapted from Hay, L. Spatial-temporal analysis of movements in children: Motor programs versus feedback in the development of reaching. Journal of Motor Behavior, 11:188–200, 1979, Figs. 1 and 4; reprinted with permission of the Helen Dwight Reid Educational Foundation. Published by Heldref Publications, 1319 Eighteenth St., NW, Washington, DC 20036-1802. Copyright © 1979.)*

studies, the child's ability to understand and utilize sensory information for reach correction continues to develop through at least the first 11 years.

In a related vein, one current view of the clumsiness seen in children with mild to moderate movement dysfunction is that a sensory or attention problem hinders the ability of these children to identify or selectively attend to the most pertinent information during a reach (Estil et al., 2002; Mandich et al., 2003; Schellekens et al., 1983). For example, study of hand paths during movement between two buttons in a repetitive tapping task in 8- to 10-year-olds with minimal neurologic dysfunction suggests that these children must constantly monitor and correct their actions. It is believed that using

this closed loop strategy leaves little opportunity to attend to information for executing anticipatory adjustments and minimizing the amount of error correction required. In comparison with age-matched controls, children with minimal neurologic dysfunction appear to execute more movement units per reach. The first movement unit is less likely to be the longest unit or to achieve the greatest acceleration, and each unit tends to contain more acceleration irregularities (Schellekens et al., 1983). Not surprisingly, these children tend to have more difficulty maintaining task orientation. When asked to reach from a starting point to a stationary target, 8- to 10-year-old children with DCD were less accurate than typical peers due to spending less time in the deceleration phase of the reach (Smyth et al., 2001). When the visual conditions were manipulated (vision removed after reach began, or only target or target and hand visible), the DCD group did not seem to take advantage of the visual information available. In a different task, manual tracking of a continuously moving stimulus (a coincident-timing task) with a predictable path, children with motor coordination dysfunction (ages 6 and 11) were slower than age-matched controls (van der Meulen et al., 1991a). Their movement distance during an acceleration phase was more variable than that of control children, their tracking motions were more delayed, and they performed more trials with apparently suboptimal attention. However, 7-year-olds with minimal brain dysfunction gave themselves more time to cope with less efficient reaching skills by planning a hand trajectory that would intercept a moving target further along its trajectory (Forsström & Hofsten, 1982). When these children were presented with an unpredictable tracking task, they had greater difficulty attending to the task than age-matched controls, perhaps because they could not identify a compensatory strategy (Estil et al., 2002; van der Meulen et al., 1991b). For more discussion on the establishment of coincident-timing strategies, the reader is referred to a review by Goodgold-Edwards (1991).

As was suggested for the infant during development, postural control may also be affecting the reaching behavior of children with DCD. Johnston and colleagues (2002) have documented differences in the APA of shoulder and trunk muscles in 8- to 10-year-old children with and without DCD during a goal-directed reaching movement. The children with DCD demonstrated longer reaction times and movement times of their reach as compared to children who were typically developing. From a postural muscle perspective, the DCD group used earlier onsets of shoulder and posterior trunk muscles and later than typical activations of the anterior trunk muscles. Johnston and colleagues (2002) hypothesize that the altered timing of postural muscle activation influences the speed and quality of the reach movement. Whether the altered postural movements are part of the primary problem or a compensation for difficulty with necessary sensory integration to complete the task is yet to be determined.

In summary, the variables and processes that contribute to an emerging control of reaching skills during infancy and childhood are similar to variables contributing to those for posture and locomotion. In each instance, rudimentary aspects of control can be observed in very young infants if optimal conditions are provided, suggesting that some neural contributions to control of these skills are established in the fetal or neonatal period of development. In each instance, early skills appear to be more or less automatic; that is, they appear to be activated by relevant stimuli and

shaped by contextual variables, such as the biomechanical interactions of moving body segments in space. Feedback does not appear to play an important role in controlling these early skills. Each of these early skills, however, undergoes important transformations as children learn to monitor their movements, predict the potential consequences of their actions for a given context, and develop anticipatory strategies for efficient movement execution. As shown in the following section, these variables also contribute to the development of grasp control.

Grasping

Hand function has long been viewed as one of the key responsibilities of the motor cortex. Study of monkeys suggests that there are two cortical areas of importance to the grasping movement, the ventral premotor cortex containing the visuomotor neurons that respond to the location and components of the object, and the hand field of the primary motor cortex containing the neurons for finger muscle activation (Fogassi et al., 2001). Classical studies linked onset of fine motor milestones with myelination of the lateral precentral gyrus (Lawrence & Hopkins, 1976). Based originally on pyramidal lesion studies in monkeys (Lawrence & Kuypers, 1968), it is generally accepted that reaching and grasping are also controlled by separate subcortical neural systems. Following lesion of the lateral brainstem, monkeys cannot control hand movements independently of arm movements, yet they can use the limbs for walking and climbing. After lesion of the ventrolateral path, in contrast, monkeys can no longer control the posture of the limb, but they can pick up food with their hands. Studies suggest that the potential for coordinated hand movements may be present earlier than previously appreciated and that anatomic changes in descending neural paths, although necessary, may not be sufficient to account for development of hand control. For example, ultrasound recordings indicate that human fetuses begin extending their fingers during isolated arm movements by 12 weeks of gestation (de Vries et al., 1982, 2001), long before myelination of the corticospinal tract can account for these rudimentary actions. Furthermore, observation of spontaneous hand movements in neonates indicates that the hand is not always in a stereotypic posture of flexion (closed fist) or extension (open). The hands continuously move between these extremes and, in so doing, they exhibit considerable variability, suggesting that the potential for independent finger control is present at birth. This potential is underscored by recent neuroanatomic and neurophysiologic studies in infants indicating that monosynaptic corticospinal connections are present at birth (Eyre et al., 2000, 2001). By 3 months, index finger forces can be clearly differentiated from those of other fingers during grasping (Lantz et al., 1996). If there is sufficient neural substrate to produce motor commands for independent finger actions at birth, why do fine motor milestones typically emerge several months later? In this section, the acquisition of grasp control and studies identifying variables that may account for acquisition are reviewed.

Rudimentary Perceptual Control of Grasping

Although reaching and grasping skills are intimately related in a functional sense, control of grasping is distinguished from control of reaching by the different roles ascribed to the anatomic structures discussed previously and by apparent differences in perceptuomotor control of these two skills (Hofsten, 1990). The initial trajectory of reaching (phase 1 reaching) is based on visual definition of the object's location in space and executed using a ballistic or open loop strategy, processes that do not appear to be linked with control of grasping. During execution of the reach (phase 2 reaching), visual feedback (Jeannerod, 1981) or proprioceptive feedback (Prablanc & Pélisson, 1990) may be used to define arm position as part of a closed loop strategy to correct for initial errors in trajectory. At the onset of phase 2 reaching, the hand is open maximally and then begins to close just before target contact, suggesting that anticipatory preparation for grasping is integrated with phase 2 reaching (Jeannerod, 1981).

Data indicate that before 2 months of age, infants execute only the ballistic phase of reaching, and activity of the hand is not separately controlled from that of the limb to attempt grasping. The hand is typically open during neonatal reaching; however, hand posture is independent of the reach trajectory and does not vary with or without visual fixation of the target (Hofsten, 1984). Thus the prevailing view is that during reaching in the neonatal period, the arm and hand are synergistically coupled (Hofsten, 1990). This synergistic link between arm and hand is said to be functionally disconnected at approximately 2 postnatal months when the hand is more frequently fisted during arm movements into extension. By 3 months of age, the hand begins to open once again during reaching, but only when the infant visually fixates on the target (Hofsten, 1984). Such gains are typically attributed to anatomic changes in corticomotoneuronal connections (Lawrence & Hopkins, 1976), but another variable to consider at this age is the development of binocular coordination for depth perception (Hofsten, 1990). Acquisition of grasp control at this particular period of development may be primarily attributable to the emergence of adequate visual processing for learning how to implement closed loop (visually dominated) con-

trol of hand movements. By 4 months of age, infants can use vision to correct hand trajectory when it is displaced by a prism (McDonnell, 1975). By 5 to 6 months of age, infants expect to see their hand during a reach, and if vision of the hand is blocked, their performance is disturbed (Lasky, 1977). Furthermore, infants 5 to 6 months of age use visual information for adjusting grip configuration relative to object size (Newell et al., 1993). Around 6 postnatal months, infants can occasionally execute an adultlike (phase 1 and 2) reach-to-grasp movement pattern, and by 9 months of age, they can execute the pattern reliably (Hofsten, 1979). To briefly return to an earlier question regarding control of independent finger movements, we might hypothesize that independent finger movements and grasping skills emerge in the middle of the first year because the visual system is now sufficiently operational to employ and sculpture available corticomotoneuronal networks or because infants at this age have finally acquired a sufficient amount of initial visual experience of the hand to master control of the fingers. The extent of these visual experiences of the hands, in turn, may be limited initially by postural requirements (e.g., stabilizing both head and hand position to visualize the effects of self-initiated finger actions) such that postural control may be another rate-limiting variable in acquisition of independent finger movements.

The overall effects of postural requirements and initial position of the fingers, hand and arm have been examined using computer modeling. Two models to predict grasping have been developed, an end-effector model (based simply on the movements of the thumb and index finger) (Smeets & Brenner, 2002) and a posture model (based on complex movements of all joints involved in the reach and grasp) (Meulenbroek et al., 2001a). Smeets and Brenner (2002), based on comparing the two models' predictions to actual reach and grasp in typical adults, suggest that a model which includes postural constraints on the movement and one that just describes the movement of the fingers equally account for many aspects of the grasping pattern most accurately when the movement starts with the fingers in contact. Neither model, however, adequately reflects what is seen in the mature adult when reaching to grasp an item. Smeets and Brenner (2002) conclude that the addition of postural constraints to a model of grasping are not responsible for the main characteristics of the reach and grasp movement. Meulenbroek and associates (2001b) argue that the postural components are crucial to grasping prediction especially when analyzing the altered reach and grasp patterns of individuals with movement dysfunction. Using the posture model, these researchers suggest that they can predict the altered reach and grasp patterns observed in individuals with spastic hemiparesis. As suggested by others, the essential constraints on development and control of grasp have yet to be determined (Newell et al., 1993).

Emergence of Anticipatory Control

With the onset of functional reaching, infants begin to develop perceptual abilities for reading the environment in such a way as to shape reaching and grasping skills. At the onset of functional reaching, they are not inclined to reach for objects that are placed at the perimeter of their reach (Fetters & Todd, 1987). At 5 months of age, they begin to orient their hand toward the object, either just before or at the beginning of the reach (Hofsten & Fazel-Zandy, 1984; McCarty et al., 2001), as well as shape the hand in anticipation of object size constraints during manipulation (Newell et al., 1993). At this age, infants primarily rely on contact with the object to orient and successfully grasp the object, but over the next 3 months, infants begin to use visual information to both anticipate contact and orient their hand with respect to the object (Lockman et al., 1984). When adults reach to grasp an object, the distance between index finger and thumb is set with respect to object size at the onset of reaching (Jakobson & Goodale, 1991; Jeannerod, 1981). Anticipation of object size is similarly observed in the hand posture of 9- to 13-month-old infants during reaching (Hofsten & Rönnqvist, 1988), suggesting that young infants quickly learn to preprogram reaches for object size, location, and distance on the basis of visual information. The grasp of infants older than 9 months continues to exhibit some immature features, one being the relatively constrained range in hand opening when infants are presented with an assortment of objects varying in size. The hand may open in exaggerated postures, often considered residual retention of more primitive or yet undifferentiated manual behaviors due to corticomotoneuronal immaturity (Twitchell, 1970). Alternatively, infants may open the hand widely as a strategy to compensate for limited ability to estimate the task requirements for grasping an object (Hofsten, 1990); adults exhibit similar exaggerated hand postures when visual feedback is withdrawn or unpredictable (Jakobson & Goodale, 1991), or intermittent (Bennett et al., 2003). Finally this exaggerated hand opening in the infant could be due to the small size of the hand in relation to the object. A body-scaled relation of the grip configuration, based on an equation including the size and mass of the object to be grasped and the length and mass of the grasping hand, has been demonstrated to be invariant across young children (6 to 12 years of age) and adults (Cesari & Newell, 1999, 2000). The force applied during grasp and the duration of the grasp and

displacement phases of prehension have also recently been shown to adhere to the same body-scaled relationship (Cesari & Newell, 2002). These findings support the idea that mature grasp and displacement are ultimately controlled within a single action that relates to body size and object perception. Anticipatory strategies apparent in control of precision grip and load forces are discussed next.

Maturation of Precision Grip and Load Force Control

Once contact is initiated, the infant must coordinate normal (grip) and frictional (load) forces to grasp and lift an object (Johansson & Westling, 1988). Adults coordinate these forces synchronously, whereas infants and young children coordinate them sequentially (Forssberg et al., 1991). To quantitatively examine grip control, infants are encouraged to pick up a toy that is equipped with force transducers to measure the grip forces of the opposing thumb and index finger and the load force necessary to lift the object off the table (Fig. 3-9). During the preload phase (initial contact with the object), infants as young as 8 months of age contact the object with one finger before the other, creating a latency to onset of grip force that is significantly greater than in infants 18 months of age or older. Infants and young children also tend to press down on the object, creating a negative load force before reversing the direction of force to successfully lift the object off the table. Infants and young children generate a significant portion of the total grip force (often twice the magnitude of adult grasps) for grasping before initiating the load force, and during the load phase they typically exhibit multiple peaks in records for both of these forces. Adults, in contrast, scale the increases in grip and load forces in an economic, synchronous, and nearly linear manner with only a single peak near the middle of the load phase (Forssberg et al., 1991). These findings suggest that the smooth execution of an adult grasp is the consequence of anticipating the object's weight so as to select an appropriate target force magnitude and scaling over time (Johansson & Westling, 1988). This anticipation of necessary grip-force adjustments for precision grip to lift, hold, and replace an object has been shown in adults to be related to experience with a predictable stimulus (Winstein et al., 2000). This collective experience, called central set, appears to affect the response gain of both voluntary and triggered rapid grip force adjustments to be set to a certain extent prior to perturbation onset in a similar manner as the effects of central set on lower extremity reactive postural adjustments to platform perturbations. This suggests that in motor control there may be a general rule governing anticipatory processes.

The studies on control of grasp (Forssberg et al., 1991,

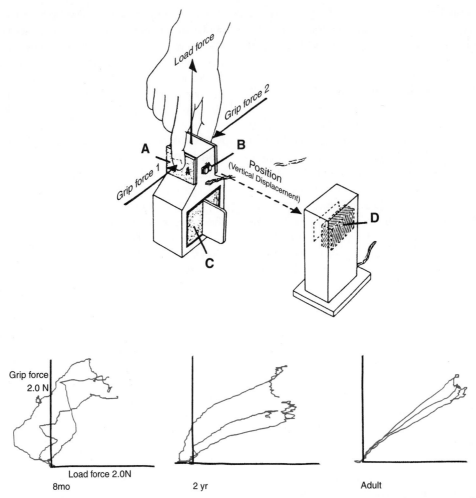

♦ Figure 3-9 One method for quantitatively describing grasping skills and examining aspects of motor control is to measure the combination of grip and load forces over time. Precision grip force is the net normal force exerted by the index finger (Grip Force 1) and thumb (Grip Force 2), and load force is the tangential or friction force exerted when lifting the object against gravity (positive values) or pushing the object down into the table (negative force). The mass of the object can be varied by exchanging weights (*C*), and displacement of the object can be detected by infrared diodes (*B*) and a sensor (*D*). By 8 months of age, infants first press down on the object (negative *X* values), then increase grip force (positive *Y* values) before initiating a load (positive *X* values) to lift the object. By 2 years of age, positive load and grip forces are scaled in a synchronous, more linear fashion similar to that in adults, and negative loading force is less apparent. *(Adapted from Forssberg, H, Eliasson, AC, Kinoshita, H, Johansson, RS, & Westling, G. Development of human precision grip. I. Basic coordination of force. Experimental Brain Research, 85:451–457, 1991, Figs. 1 and 4.)*

1992, 1995) are consistent with a reoccurring theme of this chapter: infants appear to possess the neural substrate to execute skilled motor patterns early in development, but demonstration of this potential is unreliable. First, these studies indicate that by 6 to 8 months of age infants can produce each of the actions required for a precision grip, and by 12 months of age infants can occasionally assemble all the components to produce adultlike force patterns, but there is considerable variability in performance across trials (Butterworth et al., 1997). These studies also indicate that infants and young children use

far more force than required, a common finding in studies of motor development (Keogh & Sugden, 1985). It has been suggested that the variability and excessive forces used in their strategies may be the consequence of immature corticospinal pathways or motor units (Forssberg et al., 1991). On the other hand, variable performance and use of excessive force may be compensatory strategies to cope with limited experience leading to limited stored anticipatory or central set and one or more limited perceptuomotor abilities, such as the ability to extract sufficient information from visual input. Children as young as

2 years of age are able to adjust grip and load forces with respect to the degree of friction or potential slip during repeated lifts of the same object, but when the coefficient of friction is randomized over trials, they cannot adapt grip and load forces effectively. Thus with sufficient practice they can formulate rules for more adultlike performance, but if confronted with uncertainty, they do not know how to draw from limited previous experience.

Because it was assumed that the nervous system is hierarchically organized, it was widely held in the developmental literature that cortical control over reflexes determines when various forms of grasping emerge or disappear by dominating or inhibiting an action, or failing to accomplish either because of immature neural transmission (Twitchell, 1970). Such assumptions do not appear to be compatible, however, with current electrophysiologic studies of the motor cortex. Although motor cortex and corticospinal inputs function to recruit hand muscles (Lemon & Mantel, 1989), motor cortex activity does not exhibit a consistent relationship with respect to either a movement or a movement-related activity in other areas of the brain. Such inconsistencies have led investigators to support a heterarchic rather than hierarchic view of motor control (Kalaska & Crammond, 1992). Recent studies on the control of the precision grasp in children with CP also challenge these assumptions and demonstrate that maturation of the motor cortex and corticomotoneuronal pathways, although necessary, are not sufficient to account for the development of either typical or atypical motor control (see also Newell et al., 1993). Variables such as anticipatory control and effective use of feedback information also must be considered if control of movements is to be more fully understood. When typical children 6 to 8 years of age are asked to grasp and lift a 200-g object repeatedly, they initiate nearly synchronous, linear increases in grip and load forces with a single peak in magnitude, as do adults. Children with CP (diplegia or hemiplegia), in contrast, tend to initiate the forces sequentially, as do younger typical children (Eliasson et al., 1991). That is to say, at least some children with CP can produce the requisite forces, but they have difficulty selecting or executing efficient grasp strategies. Available data indicate that these children have difficulty regulating the timing and magnitude of force during both dynamic and static phases, and they tend to bear down on the object before lifting it (Fig. 3-10). When these children are asked to grasp and lift objects of two different weights, presented in blocked and randomized trials, they also have difficulty scaling forces with respect to object weight during both nonrandom and random presentation of the two weights (Eliasson et al., 1992), but if they are given a sufficient number of practice trials, they can

anticipate and scale grasp force parameters (Eliasson et al., 1995; Steenbergen et al., 1998) and learn better precision isometric grip force, but not to the same extent as children of the same age who are typically developing (Valvano & Newell, 1998). Children with CP may also have difficulty stabilizing their gaze so that they can effectively use the available visual information (Lee et al., 1990). Given that the normal acquisition of grasp control has a protracted period of development (Forssberg et al., 1991, 1992, 1995), it is also probable that these children do not experience sufficient amounts and variety of practice to use available information for developing efficient strategies, an issue previously raised by Goodgold-Edwards (1991).

Refinements in the control of grasping continue to occur well into late childhood. Examination of the fine details of grip force amplitude and timing control has suggested that children age 7 to 8 years still do not exhibit finger force components typical of adult skill (Inui & Katsura, 2002). By 12 years of age, children approximate adult patterns of control and accuracy of bimanual isometric finger force production for both inphase (both hands pinching a load cell device at the same time) and antiphase (one hand pinching, then the other) activation (Harabst et al., 2000). When coordinating grasp and lift of objects, young children execute grasps characterized by multipeaked variations in grip and load forces and do not execute the smooth, coincident increases and decreases in these forces characteristic of adult grasping until approximately 8 years of age (Forssberg et al., 1991). Transitions to smooth, single-peak force patterns may in part be due to gradual improvements in anticipatory strategies. To test the use of anticipatory strategies, children 1 to 15 years of age lifted each of two different weights over 6 consecutive trials and then over 25 trials with the weights randomly presented (Forssberg et al., 1992). Results suggested that children as young as 1 to 2 years of age scale grip and load force based on information from the preceding lift of the object, and by 2 to 3 years of age, they can use this information to adjust the rate of increase in grip and load force for each weight. Furthermore, 2- to 3-year-olds can transfer weight information from lifts with one hand to modulate lifts with the other hand (Gordon et al., 1994). It appears that the scaling of grip and load force rates continues to change until approximately 8 to 15 years of age, depending on the order of presentation of the weights, suggesting that anticipatory skills do not achieve adult levels until some point in this age range. Children begin to use visual information (size of object to estimate its weight) to anticipate task requirements and scale grip and load forces by 3 to 4 years of age (Gordon et al., 1992). Data seem to suggest that by 5 to 6 years of age children can make compensations for slip (Forssberg et al., 1995) and adjust lifts with one hand

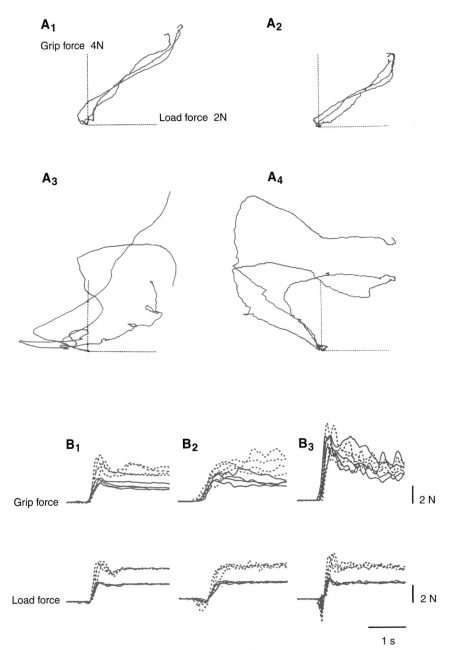

◆ Figure 3-10   Children with cerebral palsy demonstrate some of the same force patterns during grasping to lift as those observed in younger typically developing children. Although age-matched (6- to 8-year-olds) normal children (A_1) exhibit synchronous scaling of grip and load forces, some children with diplegia (A_3) or hemiplegia (A_4) exhibit marked negative load force at the onset of a grasp, serial ordering of grip and positive loading forces, and grip force magnitudes twice that of normal children. However, children with less severely disabling cerebral palsy, such as one child with mild diplegia (A_2), may exhibit more normal, age-appropriate grasp patterns. In addition to difficulty coordinating grip and load forces, children with hemiplegia (B_2) and diplegia (B_3) have greater difficulty scaling grip force with respect to object weight than normal children (B_1). During lifts of a 400-g weight (dashed lines), typically developing children apply larger grip forces than for a 200-g weight (solid lines), and grip force quickly peaks and then drops to a stable level. Grip forces in children with cerebral palsy, in contrast, are slow to reach peak magnitude, are unstable during the static phase of the lift, and are not scaled reliably with respect to object weight. (*A adapted from Eliasson, AC, Gordon, AM, & Forssberg, H. Basic co-ordination of manipulative forces of children with cerebral palsy. Developmental Medicine and Child Neurology, 33:661–670, 1991, Fig. 4. B adapted from Eliasson, AC, Gordon, AM, & Forssberg, H. Impaired anticipatory control of isometric forces during grasping by children with cerebral palsy. Developmental Medicine and Child Neurology, 34:216–225, 1992, Fig. 3.*)

based on lifts with the other hand (Gordon et al., 1994) with skill approaching adult levels of performance but require more practice than adults to do so.

Collectively, the studies described in this section demonstrate that grasping is a complex skill involving many different aspects of sensorimotor control. Innate or rudimentary skills, biomechanics, experience, and other context-dependent variables probably contribute to the rapid changes in motor control observed in the first year of life. Even during earliest exercise of skill, infants are probably building a database of information for transforming their skills as they become increasingly more intent on shaping their experiences. Probably one of the views enjoying the greatest consensus among researchers in the field of motor control today is the view that all aspects of movement execution, including the basic physiology, biomechanics, perceptual processing, and development of strategies, must be closely examined under varying movement conditions to better understand the acquisition of motor control during typical development and when it goes awry.

MOTOR CONTROL RESEARCH: CLINICAL IMPLICATIONS

The implied assumption of motor control research is that it will advance clinical interventions to improve or restore motor function limited as a consequence of disease or injury. This is indeed an exciting time for those researchers and clinicians interested in building links between movement science and clinical rehabilitation practice to improve examination and treatment of movement problems. New ideas and approaches are emerging as scientists and clinicians test the generality of theory-driven findings applied to various patient populations. It will take well-designed studies addressing specific links between science and practice, however, to know precisely the implications of motor control studies for specific problems encountered in rehabilitation practice. In this section, some possible implications of movement science for clinical practice are briefly discussed with respect to examination and intervention for motor control problems.

CLINICAL EXAMINATION TOOLS

The vast majority of tools currently available for examination of motor control are based on neural maturation or learning theories, but more recently developed tools appear to reflect changing views of development, such as that espoused by the dynamic systems theory. Maturational-based tools can be readily identified by an emphasis on

reflex testing (Palisano, 1993) or evoked behaviors because it is assumed that expression of these behaviors indicates the level of neural integration and function achieved (Touwen, 1984). In many of these tests, little or no consideration is given to other variables that may enhance, depress, or otherwise alter expression of the evoked behaviors. Even some maturational-based tools are beginning to consider broader views of motor development, however, as variables such as state behavior (e.g., level of arousal) are included in testing protocols or grading of responses. In many cases, the theoretic underpinnings of a given tool are not so clear. For instance, some motor assessment tools are composed of tests to determine milestone achievements and may be viewed as indicators of the extent of neural maturation and corticospinal control, as posed by McGraw (1940, 1945), or as behavioral indicators of cognitive maturation, as originally posed by Piaget (Keogh & Sugden, 1985). In other instances, examinations are composed of milestones solely because they appear to display statistical or diagnostic significance (Hopkins & Prechtl, 1984). Tools incorporating a dynamic-based view of development attempt to examine spontaneous, self-produced movements under more naturalistic conditions, recognizing that multiple variables contribute to movement (Hadders-Algra & Prechtl, 1992). All motor examinations provide some indication of ability or extent of control, but we have yet to realize tests that tell us precisely how and why control is limited or has broken down, and this is one of the greatest barriers in our efforts to bridge the gap between the research lab and the clinic. In this section, several tools that incorporate examination of self-produced movements that have been recently developed for use in identifying infants at risk for developmental disabilities will be reviewed, including the General Movement Assessment, Dubowitz Neurological Assessment, Movement Assessment of Infants, and Alberta Infant Motor Scale. Following this, several tests that attempt to tease out the multiple variables that contribute to movement and the quality of movement of older children will be highlighted, including motor coordination tests, such as the Toddler and Infant Motor Evaluation and the Gross Motor Performance Measure; sensory tests, such as the Miller Assessment for Preschoolers and the Sensory Integration and Praxis Tests; and functional activity skills tests, such as the Assessment of Motor and Process Skills.

Infant Examination

General Movement Assessment

Using the General Movement Assessment (GMA) requires examination of the spontaneous movements of preterm and term newborns and young infants (Einspieler et al.,

1997). The GMA has been broadly applied to term and preterm infants with an array of clinical diagnoses in recent years, and results suggest that it is an effective tool for predicting neurologic outcome at 2 years of age, in CP in particular (Prechtl, 1997). The examination consists of observation and classification of spontaneous movements while the infant lies in the supine position. Only movements generated while the infant is in an awake, noncrying state are analyzed and classified by movement quality. Classifications include writhing, fidgety, wiggling-oscillating, saccadic, and ballistic, and classification definitions distinguish frequency, amplitude, power, speed, flow, irregularity, and abruptness of the movements. Based on ethnologic methods, the design of the GMA reflects a theoretic view that maturation is not a fixed sequence of differentiation, but rather a continuous transformation of behavior (Hopkins & Prechtl, 1984). The theoretic framework of the GMA also incorporates the views that general spontaneous movement is a distinct, coordinated pattern of activity in the healthy newborn and that self-organizing neural networks, extrinsic factors, and endogenous maturational processes are likely contributors to the emergence of the different movement qualities (Hadders-Algra & Prechtl, 1992).

Recent applications of the GMA tool suggest that it has strong predictive potential for examining the neurologic status of a preterm, term, or young infant (Prechtl, 2001). Intertester agreement appears to be good to strong, sensitivity is strong across age groups from preterm to 3 months corrected age, and specificity is strong by 3 months of age (Einspieler et al., 1997). Low specificity at earlier ages is attributed to spontaneous resolution of early dysfunction. A recent review suggests that prediction to developmental outcome is best at 2 to 4 months, which is the age of "fidgety GM" (Hadders-Algra, 2001b). Definitely abnormal fidgety movement, meaning an absence of this type movement, is reported to predict CP accurately 85% to 98% of the time. More specific analysis of GM also has suggested that particular types of CP (e.g., dyskinetic and hemiplegia CP) can be detected early on the basis of certain qualities of the movement observed (Einspieler et al., 2002; Guzzetta et al., 2003). If the infant with definitely abnormal GM does not go on to have CP, there is some suggestion that other developmental problems such as DCD will occur. Also, mildly abnormal GMs are related to later development of DCD and attention deficit and hyperactivity disorders (Hadders-Algra, 2002; Hadders-Algra & Groothuis, 1999). The GMA appears to exhibit greater sensitivity and specificity than neurologic examination in brain-damaged preterm and term infants between 26 weeks of gestational age and 6 months corrected age (Cioni et al., 1997a, 1997b). Move-

ments that are disorganized, excessively monotonous, cramped, or stereotypic are highly correlated with neural malformations or severe brain lesions (Albers & Jorch, 1994; Bos et al., 1998; Ferrari et al., 1997). It is interesting to note that GMA scores do not appear to correlate with neurologic examinations consisting of commonly elicited reflexes and behaviors or muscle tone (Geerdink & Hopkins, 1993; Hadders-Algra & Prechtl, 1992).

Dubowitz Neurological Assessment

The Dubowitz Neurological Assessment of the Preterm and Full-Term Newborn Infant is an example of a tool based on traditional, neuromaturational views of development, designed to examine preterm and full-term infants soon after birth and during the neonatal period for the purpose of detecting deviations or resolutions of neurologic problems (Dubowitz & Dubowitz, 1981). It consists of 32 items evaluating four areas: response decrement to repeated stimuli, movement and tone, reflexes, and behavior. Using a five-point scale, scoring of each item is criterion-referenced and criteria are ordered according to expected changes with increasing postconceptional age. The infant's state of arousal is considered in the interpretation of findings. Selection and design of the test items for the Dubowitz Neurological Assessment were based on four criteria: expected findings for full-term infants at 3 days of age; good agreement between observers; some measure of higher neurologic function; and usefulness for examining ill infants. Test items are examiner-evoked responses with the exception of one item for describing the quality of spontaneous body movements and another for identifying the presence of specific abnormal movement or posture. The authors report that a cluster of abnormal scores, such as the presence of asymmetries or increased tone and diminished leg mobility, may indicate that an intraventricular hemorrhage has occurred (Dubowitz & Dubowitz, 1981) and motor abnormalities may eventually emerge (Dubowitz et al., 1984). They also suggest that an abnormal score during initial examination may be of less prognostic significance than milder but more persisting signs. From the findings, it may be suggested that these examiner-evoked movements provide very little information on the control of movement or its development, except when viewed collectively, and even then the primary information seems to be an indication of general neural intactness, not of the specific motor pathologic processes likely to unfold. Based on examination using the Dubowitz Neurological Assessment at term age in 130 consecutive graduates of a Neonatal Intensive Care Unit (NICU), followed by re-examination at 1 year of age with another age-appropriate assessment, the Dubowitz demonstrated high prediction of normal outcome (96% correct), but lower prediction of abnormal outcome (56%) (Molteno et al., 1999). The lack of sensitivity to specific motor dysfunction in these types of examinations may be because the test procedures only superficially screen brain function, but reasons for dysfunction can be varied and even multifactorial. Nonetheless, study of the tool suggests that scores differentiate between full-term and preterm infants, and correlate with perinatal risk rating, ultrasonography findings, and neurologic status at 1 year, leading investigators to suggest that the Dubowitz Neurological Assessment is a valid tool and may be used to develop management protocols in the NICU (Campbell, 1999; Mercuri et al., 2003; Molteno et al., 1995).

Movement Assessment of Infants

The Movement Assessment of Infants (MAI) is a tool designed for the purposes of identifying motor dysfunction, changes in the status of motor dysfunction, and establishment of an intervention program for infants from birth to 1 year of age (Chandler et al., 1980). The MAI is a criterion-referenced examination composed of 65 items selected to evaluate four areas: muscle tone, reflexes, automatic reactions, and volitional movement. Each item is scored on a scale of 0 to 4 or 0 to 6 points and checked for asymmetric or rostrocaudal variations to obtain an "at-risk score" for motor dysfunction. Like other maturational-based assessment tools, the current version of the MAI contains many examiner-evoked test procedures and it does not attempt to control for contextual variables such as state of arousal. It does include, however, items to examine spontaneous motor features such as self-initiated postures and behaviors commonly identified in milestone schedules of development that are scored for quality or level of proficiency. Theoretic justification for items of the MAI has not been specified, but it would appear that each is included for its statistical potential to discriminate abnormal deviations in motor development.

The psychometric properties of the MAI have been studied by several investigators and the findings reviewed (Palisano, 1993). In general, studies seem to indicate that rater reliability is weakest for items requiring handling of the infant by the examiner and greatest for those not requiring handling (Haley et al., 1986). Studies also appear to indicate that the MAI is sensitive, readily identifying deviations in motor development that may predict motor dysfunction at later ages, but that it exhibits poor specificity because it also identifies some normal infants (Schneider et al., 1988) and infants with transient medical problems as being at risk for later motor dysfunction (Harris, 1987; Swanson et al., 1992). It appears that the most consistently reliable and predictive portion of the

MAI is the section on volitional movement, because it is the only section to exhibit a strong relationship with outcome (at 18 months of age) at both the 4-month and 8-month examinations (Swanson et al., 1992). Most recently, the predictability of the MAI has been examined in infants with extremely low birth weight (Salokorpi et al., 2001). Adequate sensitivity and high specificity for predicting CP at 1 and 2 years age were documented. Lower sensitivity and specificity were noted for prediction of more minor motor disorders such as DCD.

Alberta Infant Motor Scale

The Alberta Infant Motor Scale (AIMS) was developed as a screening tool to identify infants at risk for motor dysfunction (Piper & Darrah, 1994; Piper et al., 1992). It is purely an observational scale, in which movement ability is documented in infants from birth to 18 months of age, with the infant in prone, supine, sitting, and standing positions. High reliability (intraclass correlation coefficient [ICC] > 0.90) has been demonstrated in trained and untrained raters (Blanchard et al., 2004; Piper et al., 1992). Normative information, based on 2022 infants from the Canadian province of Alberta, is also available for use of the test to document motor development delay (Piper & Darrah, 1994). This test is quick and easy to give and seems to estimate developmental levels most accurately between 4 and 10 months of age (Liao & Campbell, 2004). Discriminative validity for identifying infants with atypical movement as atypical was 89% (Darrah et al., 1998). Predictive validity of assessments at 4 and 8 months of age for identifying delayed motor development at 18 months of age revealed sensitivity and specificity of 77% and 82%, respectively, using cut-off scores below the 10th percentile at 4 months, and 86% and 93%, respectively, using cut-off scores below the 5th percentile at 8 months. The test is not designed to document why an infant may have difficulty with movement, but by asking the therapist to step back and observe the infant carefully across the different postures, the therapist can potentially focus on what the limiting factors may be. Then further testing of specific systems, such as force production capability, postural control, sensory acuity, cognitive capability, motivation, etc., can ensue.

Childhood Examination

Toddler and Infant Motor Evaluation

The Toddler and Infant Motor Evaluation (TIME) was developed to quantify the theoretical construct of quality of movement in infants and children 4 months to 3.5 years of age for discriminative purposes and potentially to monitor change across time or due to therapeutic intervention (Miller & Roid, 1994). Based on specific observation and quantification of quality of movement in children with motor delays, the authors developed the items for the test (Miller & Roid, 1993). The test consists of five subtests—Mobility, Motor Organization, Stability, Social/Emotional Abilities, and an optional Functional Performance subtest. Also, there are three clinical subtests—Quality Rating, Atypical Positions, and Component Analysis. The majority of the assessment is completed via observation of the child with the parent or caregiver assisting to place the child in different positions or to provoke various movements. The test can be scored in real time or videotaped for later scoring. The parent or caregiver is also interviewed to determine the Functional Performance score. The test is child- and family-friendly in terms of stress during testing, and the subtests potentially can direct the therapist to specific systems that may be affecting movement success. The reliability and validity of the test are reported to be high, but the responsiveness (ability to show clinically meaningful change across time or with intervention) has yet to be fully evaluated (Miller & Roid, 1993). A recent review of use of the test to monitor change across time in two children suggests that some changes in the test construction may improve the responsivity (Rahlin et al., 2003).

Gross Motor Performance Measure

The Gross Motor Function Measure (GMFM) (see Chapter 2) and its companion, the Gross Motor Performance Measure (GMPM), were specifically designed to examine the status and change in status of motor proficiency due to therapeutic interventions in children with CP (Boyce et al., 1991; Gowland et al., 1998; Russell et al., 1989). The theoretic basis for design of the GMFM was the measurement property of responsiveness, or ability to show change in motor function, in a population of children from 5 months to 12 years of age who have CP. Studies suggest that the GMFM is both a responsive (Russell et al., 1989) and valid (Bjornson et al., 1997) measurement tool. The GMPM consists of 20 motor skills commonly performed by children who are typically developing and younger than 5 years of age derived from the GMFM that measure proficiency in eight areas of motor function: activities in supine, prone, four-point, sitting, kneeling, and standing positions and during walking and climbing. Each item is scored for three attributes using a criterion-referenced scale to indicate the postural alignment, selective control and coordination, and stabilization of weight during the task. Most items involve either movements requiring a change in posture, such as during progression (crawling or walking) or action while maintaining a posture (extending an arm while in sitting or four-point position). The GMPM was designed to examine qualities

of movement believed by therapists to be problematic but amenable to intervention in children with CP. The use of physical aids or orthoses is noted on the score sheet, but use of these is not reflected in scoring and no other possible variables affecting motor control are considered. The GMPM does not examine qualities of performance such as speed, effort, or efficiency, nor can it specify the underlying cause of dysfunction in control. Studies of GMPM measurement properties by the authors suggest that inter-rater, intra-rater, and test-retest reliability are good to excellent (Gowland et al., 1995; Thomas et al., 2001). Construct validity was demonstrated via differences in scores between children with varied diagnoses, severities of motor disorder, and ages. There appears to be moderate agreement between GMPM and GMFM scores for children with CP and age-matched controls but lower agreement between GMPM scores and therapists' ratings of performance. Nevertheless, there appears to be good agreement between changes in GMPM scores and therapists' indications of improvement in children with CP, suggesting that the GMPM is a responsive motor performance examination (Boyce et al., 1995).

Miller Assessment for Preschoolers

The Miller Assessment for Preschoolers (MAP) was designed as a screening tool to identify mild or moderate delays in development of children between approximately 3 and 6 years of age at risk for future school-related problems and to refer them for more in-depth examinations (Miller, 1982). The current version of the MAP consists of 27 core items to address sensory, motor, cognitive, and combined abilities, drawn from previously existing tools based on statistical support, time required to execute an item, and extent of equipment required. Sensorimotor items include tests of position and movement sense, stereognosis, postural stability, mobility, and coordination (fine motor, gross motor, and oral motor). Unlike most available motor examinations, some sensorimotor items are specifically treated as cognitive dependent, such as the ability to sequence or imitate movements. The assessment also considers the role of behavior (e.g., concentration, need for reward, social interaction) in examining performance. To date there have been a few studies of limited scope evaluating MAP measurement properties and the test's usefulness (Daniels & Bressler, 1990; Miller, 1988; Schneider et al., 1995). Most recently construct and predictive validity has been assessed in Israeli children with positive findings for both types of validity (Parush et al., 2002a, 2002b, 2002c). As in other tests available, the MAP can describe motor abilities and limitations, but the examination results do not delineate precisely why or how motor control has broken down.

Sensory Integration and Praxis Tests

The Sensory Integration and Praxis Tests (SIPT), formerly known as the Southern California Sensory Integration Tests, are sensorimotor assessment tools for children between the ages of 4 and 9 years having mild to moderate learning impairment in the absence of frank organic disease, mental retardation, and primary sensory deficit (Ayres, 1989). Unlike many examinations, the theoretic basis for design, sensory integration theory, is precise and composed of three primary postulates: (1) learning is dependent on the intake and processing of sensory experiences from movement and the environment; (2) deficits in sensory processing can lead to deficits in motor planning and execution; and (3) active participation in meaningful tasks can improve sensory integrative processes and motor learning (Fisher & Bundy, 1992). The assessment tool consists of 17 tests. Initial portions of the SIPT examining balance, proprioceptive and tactile sensation, and control of specific movements are used to identify whether there is a sensory processing disorder in one of three areas—vestibular-proprioception, tactile discrimination, or sensory modulation—that may be indicative of integrative dysfunction. If a cluster of scores suggests dysfunction in one of these areas, subsequent portions of the SIPT are used to identify a disorder in bilateral integration and sequencing praxis, somatodyspraxia, or sensory modulation. Although the examiner using the SIPT seeks to identify only sensory processing problems, the tests examine motor performance across a broad range of tasks that includes tests for tactile discrimination, movement planning, tactile defensiveness, perception of form and space, and visuomotor coordination. Like most formalized examinations of sensorimotor abilities, the SIPT is standardized and can be scored by computer (at Western Psychological Services in the United States). Owing to the complexity of the test, specialized training is required to purchase and perform the test reliably. The available studies on measurement properties and test usefulness suggest that the SIPT has the ability to differentiate between children with and without motor disability (Cermack & Murray, 1991; Mulligan, 1996). The responsiveness (ability of a test to reflect meaningful change after intervention) was documented in a pilot study using a preliminary version of the test (Kimball, 1990). More recently, the SIPT was used to evaluate the effectiveness of sensory integration and a rhythm development program (Le Bon Depart) (Leemrijse et al., 2000). Changes in SIPT scores were demonstrated after the interventions. These studies together support the validity of the SIPT and suggest that it could be used as a responsive outcome measure for intervention studies.

Assessment of Motor and Process Skills

The Assessment of Motor and Process Skills (AMPS) was developed to evaluate motor skills and series of actions (called process skills) leading to completion of a task (Fisher, 1994). Design of the AMPS is based on sensory integration theory for the purpose of examining the behavioral manifestation of sensory integrative dysfunction in children (Bundy & Fisher, 1992) and adults (Fisher, 1994). Selection of specific items in the AMPS is based on the assumption that the items collectively represent the abilities underlying performance of common tasks and therefore can be used to estimate overall function and to identify specific deficits limiting function for use in planning therapeutic intervention. The AMPS contains 15 motor skills items to examine strength, posture, mobility, fine motor capabilities, and subtle postural adjustment capabilities, plus 20 process skills to measure attentional, conceptual, organizational, and adaptive capabilities. To evaluate these skills, the subject selects a common activity, such as fixing a sandwich, from a range of 30 possible activities listed in the AMPS manual. Each of the skills is then scored on a four-point scale describing levels of competence displayed while the subject completes the activity. Scores for each of the motor skills are then adjusted for the level of task difficulty so that performance can be related to a continuum of performance capacity to compare and predict performance for tasks of lesser or greater difficulty. Studies published thus far on adult populations suggest that AMPS is a valid tool across cultures (Goto et al., 1996) and gender (Duran & Fisher, 1996). Recently, the authors have developed a version for the school setting, the School AMPS scale (Fisher et al., 2000). Support for the rater reliability, scale validity, and person response validity has been demonstrated by one study (Fisher et al., 2000). More research needs to be completed on this school scale prior to general use in practice, but this test does incorporate the dynamic systems perspective through evaluation of components of movement for functional skill activities.

In summary, a number of motor examinations are currently available, and only a small representative sample of more general, comprehensive tools is reviewed here. As efforts continue to extend research in motor control to issues of assessment, development of specific measures consistent with current knowledge of the processes and mechanisms of motor control will continue. These new tools, which borrow directly from current research methods in motor control, will represent a new generation of standardized, selective motor control examinations for children, more akin to specific laboratory tests. Examples of this selective motor assessment approach attempting to evaluate components or systems affecting movement are the Melbourne Assessment of Unilateral Upper Limb Function (Johnson et al., 1994), measurement of prehensile movements (Steenbergen et al., 1998), and an array of postural assessments adapted to children (Westcott et al., 1997a).

IMPLICATIONS FOR TREATMENT

It seems reasonable to start from the acknowledged assumption that issues regarding application of contemporary research in motor control to clinical assessment also pertain to application of the same research to intervention. Conceptualization begins with understanding the theoretic basis for why a certain action is taken and specifying the expected consequences predicted by the theory enlisted. Excellent reviews of the theoretic bases and expected consequences enlisted by physical therapists during much of this century are available (Gordon, 1987; Horak, 1991, 1992) and will only be highlighted here. Some examples of possible implications for intervention drawn from motor control research will complete this section and chapter.

Evolving Bases for Treatment

Most neurotherapeutic approaches used in physical therapy were originally based on reflex and hierarchic models of motor control (Gordon, 1987; Horak, 1991). Intervention approaches based on maturational-based theory typically ascribed to a hierarchic model of motor skill acquisition and enlisted a facilitation model of treatment. In practical terms, it was assumed that motor development in the child progressed in a specific sequence of reflexes, movement patterns, and milestones, and that a child had to experience each facet of this sequence to acquire normal, age-appropriate motor control. Based on the facilitation model of treatment, it was assumed that externally driven sensory experience of these sequences, such as the passive and guided movements generated by a therapist or caregiver, could alter the damaged nervous system in such a way that the child with motor impairment might acquire more typically functioning motor pathways. Conversely, the facilitation model also assumed that abnormal or undesirable movement experiences could reinforce pathologic pathways, severely limiting ultimate gains in motor control. Such logic can be found in various forms of treatment adapted from theoretic neurorehabilitation models developed by (but not limited to) the Bobaths (Bobath & Bobath, 1984), Brunnstrom (1970), Knott (1966), and Vojta (Aufschnaiter, 1992). Typically, maturational-based treatment approaches have emphasized inhibiting abnormal postural muscle tone and primitive reflexes, breaking up abnormal movement patterns, and

providing movement experiences in prescribed sequences to acquire motor skills (e.g., proximal to distal progression of body control and hierarchically ordered motor milestones). Documented dissatisfactions with this approach include poor carryover to functional activities, insufficient active movement by the patient, lack of attention to movement-related variables that are extrinsic to the nervous system, and failure to produce the expected normal movement patterns once abnormal muscle tone or primitive reflexes were inhibited (Horak, 1991).

As dissatisfaction with maturational-based approaches to treatment and other related therapies grew, aspects of each were combined and modified to incorporate more recent motor control research. One approach, developed by Carr and Shepherd (1998), is organized around goal-directed, functional behaviors and considers the importance of both peripheral and central neural function as well as the environment in learning to accomplish specific functional goals. The goal-oriented approach is based on the systems model of motor control (Bernstein, 1967). According to this model, function of each contributing system and interaction among systems are dictated by the demands of task goals during a given movement (Fig. 3-11A). Thus, unlike other approaches, the goal-directed approach assumes that movement patterns will vary according to the goal and systems contributing to a given movement. Similarly, the goal-directed approach assumes that there may be multiple satisfactory movement pattern solutions for achieving a goal; therefore, a patient is encouraged to find multiple strategies for accomplishing a goal. Active, self-initiated movement is encouraged and principles of motor learning are used to enhance practice and learning of new movement strategies. Some aspects of this approach are yet undeveloped, such as methods for more precisely specifying the quality of movement and how to specifically enhance the motor learning processes, especially in children (Horak, 1991; Valvano, 2004). Nevertheless, this goal-directed treatment approach is the closest approximation to a dynamic theory-based (or systems) model of rehabilitation currently found in clinical practice.

Shumway-Cook & Woollacott (2001) have offered specific ideas re examination and intervention for using a goal- or task-oriented approach with reference to physical therapy for children as well as adults. They suggest that the examination procedures focus on three areas: (1) functional skill ability in the area of interest (such as postural stability, gait, reach and grasp movements, etc.); (2) strategies (organization of sensory and perceptual information and movement patterns) used to complete these functional skills; and (3) impairments constraining the strategies used to complete the functional skills. The im-

A

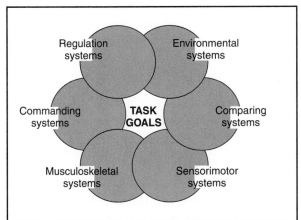

B

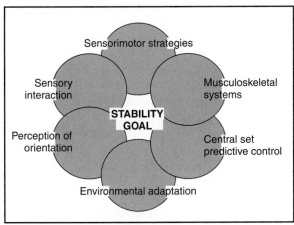

◆ **Figure 3-11**   The Systems Model of Motor Control (**A**) and Systems Model of Rehabilitation (**B**) specify a collection of systems as contributing to the control of movement. The organization of these systems is heterarchic rather than hierarchic, suggesting that control shifts among the contributing systems as a function of the goal for a given task. (**A** adapted from Horak, FB. Assumptions underlying motor control for neurologic rehabilitation. In Lister, MJ [Ed.]. Contemporary Management of Motor Control Problems, Proceedings of the II Step Conference. Alexandria, VA: Foundation for Physical Therapy, 1991, pp. 11–28, Fig. 4-7. **B** adapted from Horak, FB. Motor control models underlying neurologic rehabilitation. In Forssberg, H, & Hirschfeld, H [Eds.]. Movement Disorders in Children, Medicine and Sport Science, Vol. 36. Basel: Karger, 1992, pp. 21–30, Fig. 2.)

pairments constraining the strategies available to the client could come from any system, cognitive, sensory, or motor, involved in the control of the movements as depicted in Figure 3-11, A. To illustrate this for a specific class of goals, Horak (1992) hypothesized that the systems

involved in a postural stability goal would include those depicted in Figure 3-11, B. Starting from the upper right corner of the model, the musculoskeletal system contributes the net biomechanical forces for postural control resulting from active contractile forces, passive elastic forces, and displacements of multilinked body segments. The central set provides anticipatory strategies based on past experience to minimize the potential for postural instability as it emerges during movement. Environmental adaptation provides a means for using both feedforward and feedback control to adapt postural strategies to a particular task or environment. Based on somatosensory, vestibular, and visual information, perception of orientation determines the postural orientation goal for the task at hand. Sensory interaction provides a means for adjusting the relative dominance of all sensory inputs based on current postural context, previous postural experience, and postural expectations. Finally, sensorimotor strategies provide a collection of innate and learned movement strategies (that can be adapted by the actions of all other systems) to simplify planning of an action and effectively meet the postural goal. Intervention would then focus on three areas: (1) the resolution, reduction, or prevention of impairments affecting functional ability; (2) the development of effective (efficient) strategies to perform task-specific activities; and (3) the development of ability to utilize these strategies across changing task and environmental conditions (Shumway-Cook & Woollacott, 2001). Intervention strategies would be directed at changing the individual's constraining impairments, and manipulating the task and environment to promote motor learning. Manipulation of the task and environment would occur through alterations of feedback and patterns or locations of motor skill practice based on motor learning principles that are explained in detail in Chapter 4. Use of strategies such as these in programs to increase children's participation and reduce disability in daily life are described in Chapter 30.

Applications of Motor Control Research to New Interventions

Several specific applications of the theoretical positions and research findings presented in this chapter follow to demonstrate how research in motor control can influence pediatric physical therapy intervention. Most of the interventions described have a preliminary evidence base for use in clinical practice, but more research is necessary to truly define the appropriate populations, applications, doses, and benefits of the interventions. Treadmill and strength training for gait and functional mobility, constraint-induced movement therapy for upper extremity use, metronome training and cognitive interventions for improved coordination, and a discussion of the potential effects of the timing and intensity of intervention are briefly reviewed.

Improving gait and functional mobility are primary goals of many pediatric physical therapy interventions. Based on the motor control research centering around the hypothesis that our locomotor gait pattern is controlled via a CPG, partial weight bearing treadmill training as a way of triggering the gait CPG has emerged as a possible effective intervention. As was noted earlier in the chapter, the use of this intervention has been evaluated in children with CP (Richards et al., 1997; Schindl et al., 2000; Song et al., 2003) and children with Down syndrome (Ulrich et al., 2001). Positive effects in terms of improvements in gait speed, cadence, stride length, and functional skills such as standing and transferring were attained in the children with CP who ranged from 1.7 to 18 years of age with Gross Motor Function System Classification levels of II to IV. Infants with Down syndrome who used treadmill practice learned to walk on average approximately 3 to 4 months before a control group that did not have the practice (Ulrich et al., 2001). This earlier walking behavior could potentially impact the rate of development in cognitive and behavioral skills through earlier ability to explore the environment, but this has not been examined experimentally at this time.

On a somewhat different avenue to improve gait, researchers using a systems approach to examination have suggested that children with CP may have increased difficulty with gait owing in part to impaired force production capability of their lower extremity muscles. A series of studies by Damiano and colleagues documented that children with CP do have weakness in the majority of lower extremity muscles as compared to peers who are typically developing (Damiano et al., 2002). Children with CP were then shown to be able to improve their activation and strength in specific lower extremity muscles after a standard weight lifting protocol in a similar manner to children without disabilities and without any increase in spasticity (Damiano et al., 1995b; MacPhail & Kramer, 1995). Several studies have shown that the increase in muscle strength resulted in an improved gait pattern, less crouch, and faster speed (Damiano & Abel, 1998; Damiano et al., 1995a; Eagleton et al., 2004), and improved gross motor ability (standing, sit-to-stand, walking, running, jumping activities) (Blundell et al., 2003; Damiano & Abel, 1996; Kramer & MacPhail, 1994; MacPhail & Kramer, 1995).

Constraint-induced movement therapy was designed based on research with nonhuman primates and adults after stroke who demonstrated a learned nonuse phenomenon specifically of the involved upper extremity with a measurable reduction of cortical representation of the involved limb (DeLuca et al., 2003). This therapy has been applied to children with CP who have one upper extremity more involved than the other in single subject or case study research (Charles et al., 2001; Crocker et al., 1997; DeLuca et al., 2003; Michaud et al., 2003; Pierce et al., 2002) and two small group experimental studies (Taub et al., 2004; Willis et al., 2002). The therapy employs a restraint of the less involved upper extremity via use of slings or casts, and then actively engages the child to practice movement using the more involved upper extremity. The length of time for the restraint and practice has ranged from 2 to 3 weeks, 4 to 6 hours a day. Several outcome measures such as the fine motor section of the Peabody Developmental Motor Scales (PDMS) have been used to demonstrate improvement in amount of use and dexterity of the involved upper extremity for both fine and gross motor activities after the intervention. Both Willis and associates (2002) and Taub and associates (2004) compared groups of children with CP receiving constraint-induced therapy with control groups of children receiving regular physical therapy but no constraint-induced intervention and documented statistically and clinically significant improvement in upper extremity use when the intervention group was compared to the control group. Taub and associates (2004) also documented changes in upper extremity use at home via parent ratings, and maintenance of benefits 6 months after the intervention had ended were found in both studies. Further research is necessary to determine more specifically when, how long, and under what specific situations this intervention is successful as well as to identify any possible negative effects of using restraints (Siegert et al., 2004).

Changing coordination in children with less severe motor dysfunction such as DCD has been challenging. Motor control research has suggested that these children may have difficulty with utilizing and prioritizing sensory input to control motor output (Johnston et al., 2002; Mandich et al., 2003). Three types of intervention are currently being studied to determine effectiveness of improving coordination. Metronome training, based on capitalizing on the entrainment possibilities of the auditory system, has been examined in a randomized pre-test, post-test control group study in children with attention deficit disorder (Shaffer et al., 2001). The researchers documented significant positive outcomes in favor of the metronome group in attention, motor control, language, reading, and regulation of aggressive behaviors. A cognitive intervention, consisting of teaching problem-solving strategies and guided discovery of child- and task-specific strategies, is based on several of the theoretical positions on motor control presented earlier in this chapter. Teaching these strategies has been shown to be as effective and more long lasting than the standard contemporary intervention in improving motor goals (Miller et al., 2001). Another cognitive training technique, based on findings that children with DCD have difficulty with representation of visual-spatial coordinates of intended movement, focuses on imagery intervention designed to train the forward modeling of purposive actions and is delivered by an interactive CD-ROM (Wilson et al., 2002). A pre-test, post-test control and comparison group design with random assignment was used. The imagery protocol was found to be as effective as a standard perceptual-motor training protocol in improving the development of motor skill. All these techniques for changing coordination need a larger evidence base to support widespread use in clinical practice.

Research concerning the timing, type, and intensity of therapeutic interventions is a final example of applications of motor control research to physical therapy. These issues of intervention are at a beginning level of theoretical research at this time. Based on the Neuronal Group Selection Theory, Hadders-Algra (2001a) has suggested that some infants with specific pre- or perinatal brain damage show stereotyped motor behavior produced theoretically by a limited repertoire of primary subcortical neuronal networks. Therefore, she suggests that these infants need to be assisted at an early age to enlarge the primary neuronal networks. At a later age, these infants begin to demonstrate a problem in selection of the most efficient neuronal activity, perhaps due to problems with sensory processing. Intervention focus should then change to provision of ample opportunities for active practice to improve sensory processing and motor coordination. In relation to older children, Bartlett & Palisano (2000) have suggested we examine the multivariate determinants of motor change for children with CP in order to anticipate what areas we should focus on. Use of motor development curves drawn for different severity levels as designated by the Gross Motor Function Classification System, based on follow-up of children with CP age 1 to 12 years, potentially could assist with determination of specific intervention issues that should be the focus of treatment (Rosenbaum et al., 2002). In terms of intensity of intervention, the standard intervention for children in the United States is one to three times per week, for 30 to 60 minutes per session with the therapy ongoing throughout childhood. Based on the motor control and motor learning literature, it can be hypothesized that a greater intensity of intervention from a therapist might be more beneficial during the early learning of a motor skill than while the skill is routinely practiced to consolidate the skill to refine coordination.

From this perspective, Trahan and Malouin (2002) examined the effects of an intensive intervention (four times/week for 4 weeks) alternating with 8-week periods without physical therapy over a total 6-month period. In their small sample of young (mean age 22.6 months) children with CP at Gross Motor Function Classification System levels IV and V, gains made during the intensive therapy were maintained over the longer periods without intervention. They hypothesize that this regimen may optimize motor training.

Application of Motor Control Theory to a Clinical Example

With the close of this chapter, an example of how the systems model for rehabilitation might be used from a clinical perspective is provided for the reader to ponder. Consider a 20-month-old child with mild spastic diplegic CP, who is a new walker eagerly attempting to reach for a bright shiny toy with one hand while standing and holding on to a small piece of furniture with the other hand. Employing the model in Figure 3-11B, the goal is to remain standing while reaching for the toy. The systems can be reviewed first from a developmental perspective, based on the infant's age, size, and maturation of motor ability. The musculoskeletal system will contribute biomechanical variables such as a relatively high center of gravity resulting in a greater sway frequency (see the section on posture) and produce responses limited by a small and relatively undeveloped lever system at the leg-ankle-foot for generating force against the floor. Because the infant is a new walker and has little experience, the central set will have limited predictive capacity and few anticipatory strategies from which to generate a plan for minimizing a shift in center of mass as the reach is initiated. Thus the central set may be viewed as a limiting system in this task. Given limited predictive skills, environmental adaptations may only generate feedback strategies for correcting postural perturbations creating demands on attention that reduce the infant's attention to other tasks or interests. Because the infant has several months of experience in a gravitational environment, perception of orientation is not likely to be a limiting system in this task. The infant will likely rely almost exclusively on vision to control his or her posture because sensory interaction, also a limiting system, will not yet have determined how to adjust the relative dominance of each contributing sensory system. Because of biomechanical variables (faster sway and shorter distance to the limits of stability) and a dependence on feedback rather than feedforward correction strategies, the timing or sequencing of ankle (sensorimotor) strategies may not be sufficiently effective or reliable to correct posture before the infant sways to the limits of stability. In this case, sensorimotor strategies may select to stabilize posture by increasing stiffness about the ankle (e.g., co-contracting antagonist ankle muscles) or to prepare to break a fall by selecting a directionally appropriate protective extension response.

In contrast to hypothetical interpretations, immature motor skills or actions have typically been viewed as indicative of a nervous system not yet able to execute adaptive, coordinated motor commands. If one embraces multifactorial assumptions of motor control, however, immature motor actions may also be viewed as adaptive strategies to cope with inherent immaturity in one or more contributing systems. The failure to see a motor pattern associated with more mature responses need not mean that it cannot be produced by sensorimotor strategies; rather, the pattern may be potentially available, but not seen because other contributing systems cannot support it. Immature motor actions may also be the emergent consequences of biomechanical or other environmental constraints and affordances that contribute forces or cues and shape the movement differently as it is executed through a physical space or movement context. Studies by Thelen and colleagues provide a wide range of examples describing how infant kicking is altered with changes in biomechanics and environment (Thelen & Smith, 1994).

When the presence of the infant's neural lesion (spastic diplegia) is added to the systems model analysis, consideration must also be given to the various direct and indirect effects of the lesion, including disuse, on each contributing system. Attempting to reach for the toy, the infant rises up on his toes, the heels seldom in contact with the ground, reducing the effectiveness of an ankle strategy and increasing the likelihood of a hip strategy for correcting postural sway. In this instance, in addition to the contributions of normal rate-limiting systems, weakness and changes in compliance of leg muscles further diminish the effectiveness of the postural lever system. Given the state of other systems, sensorimotor strategies may select to activate extensor muscles excessively in an effort to control posture for a number of possible reasons. For example, the extensor posture may keep the center of mass forward within a new cone of stability that is biomechanically more advantageous than if the center of mass shifts posteriorly; if the center of mass shifts posteriorly, strength or timing of the anterior postural synergy may not be sufficient to make a correcting anterior adjustment in posture. Another possible reason for selection of the extensor synergy may be to reduce the number of degrees of freedom and enhance stiffness where phasing or force generation of muscle is insufficient. Because each system's

participation is viewed as being organized around a specific task, even atypical motor behaviors can be interpreted as being the patient's current solution for attempting to achieve a goal (see also Latash & Anson, 1996). According to the systems model, each contributing system is also influenced by the function of all other systems. Thus another implication of the model is that if function of one or more systems is altered by a pathologic process, other systems will be altered as well. Similarly, if these systems have not fully matured at the time a pathologic process occurs, maturational processes of any or all systems may be seriously altered. Another implication for intervention is the need to anticipate both the direct and indirect effects of a pathologic process on each contributing system. For example, a lesion affecting the musculoskeletal system may result in a significantly reduced level of activity, practice, and variety of experiences necessary for maturation of the central set or any other contributing systems.

Given the outcome of the analysis of this child's difficulty with postural stability, specific interventions could be applied to improve impairments in force production capability (strengthening exercises, movement practice, etc.), postural control (practice of recovery of postural control after perturbations or active movement under a variety of sensory conditions), hypertonicity (handling techniques, ankle-foot orthoses, drug therapies); potential development of contractures (positioning, stretching, ankle-foot orthoses, etc.); and to improve functional ability through movement practice (treadmill training, active practice of the actual skill in varied environments and tasks with varied feedback, etc.).

As one becomes discontent with the current state of knowledge, experience, or practice, it is difficult to not be somewhat frustrated and critical. Criticism of accepted practices may create the impression that the current state of affairs, in this case clinical practice, is not advancing fast enough. Such is not necessarily the case or necessarily the view of those generating the criticism. As discussed previously in this chapter, maturational-based views and approaches to practice have experienced considerable criticism. However, as research in motor control continues to advance, maturational-based approaches to treatment have also undergone modification by their creators (Bobath & Bobath, 1984), a point not always appreciated by either the practitioners or critics of maturational-based views (Mayston, 1992). Future motor control research and efforts to link it with practice may even lead to preservation of some treatment approaches currently under scrutiny, but advances in knowledge may also suggest different reasons or different expected outcomes from those previously proposed (Shumway-Cook & Woollacott, 2001).

A uniquely specified "motor control theory" does not exist, and thus it is illogical to say there is a motor control approach to examination or treatment. There is, however, a dynamic disciplinary field of motor control research that offers opportunities to develop, test, and thoughtfully critique assumptions underlying physical therapy practice.

■ SUMMARY

In this chapter, we describe motor control theoretical information and processes as related to development of motor behaviors in children with and without motor disabilities. Using current research findings, several specific motor behaviors, locomotion, postural control, reaching, and grasping, are highlighted. Applications of motor control principles to the physical therapy management of children with motor disabilities are suggested in terms of examination options and intervention strategies.

■ REFERENCES

Abbruzzese, G, & Berardelli, A. Sensorimotor intergration in movement disorders. Movement Disorders, 18:231–240, 2003.

Adams, JA. A closed-loop theory of motor learning. Journal of Motor Behavior, 3:111–149, 1971.

Albers, S, & Jorch, G. Prognostic significance of spontaneous motility in very immature preterm infants under intensive care treatment. Biology of the Neonate, 66:182–187, 1994.

Amazeen, PG. Is dynamics the content of a generalized motor program for rhythmic interlimb coordination? Journal of Motor Behavior, 34:233–251, 2002.

Angulo-Kinzler, RM, Ulrich, B, & Thelen, E. Three-month-old infants can select specific leg motor solutions. Motor Control, 6:52–68, 2002.

Aruin, AS. The effect of changes in the body configuration on anticipatory postural adjustments. Motor Control, 7:264–277, 2003.

Aruin, AS, & Almeida, GL. A coactivation strategy in anticipatory postural adjustments in persons with Down syndrome. Motor Control, 1:178–191, 1997.

Asanuma, H, & Keller, A. Neuronal mechanisms of motor learning in mammals. Neuroreport, 2:217–224, 1991.

Assaiante, C, Woollacott, M, & Amblard, B. Development of postural adjustment during gait initiation: kinematic and EMG analysis. Journal of Motor Behavior, 32:211–226, 2000.

Aufschnaiter, D von. Vojta: A neurophysiological treatment. In Forssberg, H, & Hirschfeld, H (Eds.). Movement Disorders in Children, Medicine and Sport Science, Vol. 36. Basel: Karger, 1992, pp. 7–15.

Ayres, AJ. Sensory Integration and Praxis Tests. Los Angeles: Western Psychological Services, 1989.

Barela, JA, Jeka, JJ, & Clark, JE. Postural control in children. Coupling to dynamic somatosensory information. Experimental Brain Research, 150:434–442, 2003.

Bartlett, DJ, & Palisano, RJ. A multivariate model of determinants of motor change for children with cerebral palsy. Physical Therapy, 80:598–614, 2000.

Bayley, N. Bayley Scales of Infant Development. New York: Psychological Corporation, 1969.

Bekoff, A, & Lau, B. Interlimb coordination in 20-day rat fetuses. Journal of Experimental Zoology, 214:173–175, 1980.

Bennett, SJ, Elliot, D, Weeks, DJ, & Keil, D. The effects of intermittent vision on prehension under binocular and monocular viewing. Motor Control, 7:46–56, 2003.

Bergmeier, SA. An investigation of reaching in the neonate. Pediatric Physical Therapy, 4:3–11, 1992.

Bernstein, N. The Coordination and Regulation of Movements. London: Pergamon, 1967.

Bizzi, E, Mussa-Ivaldi, FA, & Gisler, S. Computations underlying the execution of movement: A biological perspective. Science, 253:287–291, 1991.

Bjorson, KF, Graubert, CS, Buford, VL, & McLaughlin, J. Validity of the Gross Motor Function Measure. Pediatric Physical Therapy, 10:43–47, 1997.

Blanchard, Y, Neilan, E, Busanich, J, Garavuso, L, & Klimas, D. Interrater reliability of early intervention providers scoring the Alberta Infant Motor Scale. Pediatric Physical Therapy, 16:13–18, 2004.

Blundell, SW, Shepherd, RB, Dean, CM, Adams, RD, & Cahill, BM. Functional strength training in cerebral palsy: A pilot study of a group circuit training class for children aged 4–8 years. Clinical Rehabilitation, 17:48–57, 2003.

Bobath, K, & Bobath, B. The neuro-developmental treatment. Clinics in Developmental Medicine, 90:6–18, 1984.

Bodkin, AW, Baxter, RS, & Heriza, CB. Treadmill training for an infant born preterm with a grade III intraventricular hemorrhage. Physical Therapy, 83:1107–1118, 2003.

Bonnot A, Whelan PJ, Mentis GZ, & O'Donovan MJ. Locomotor-like activity generated by the neonatal mouse spinal cord. Brain Research Review, 40:141–151, 2002.

Bos, AF, Martijn, A, Okken, A, & Prechtl, HF. Quality of general movements in preterm infants with transient periventricular echodensities. Acta Paediatrica, 87:328–335, 1998.

Bower, TGR. Human Development. San Francisco: Freeman, 1979.

Boyce, W, Gowland, C, Hardy, S, Rosenbaum, P, Lane, M, Plews, N, Goldsmith, C, & Russell, D. Development of a quality of movement measure for children with cerebral palsy. Physical Therapy, 71:820–832, 1991.

Boyce, W, Gowland, C, Rosenbaum, PL, Lane, M, Plews, N, Goldsmith, CH, Russell, DJ, Wright, V, Potter, S, & Harding, D. The Gross Motor Performance Measure: Validity and responsiveness of a measure of quality of movement. Physical Therapy, 75:603–613, 1995.

Bradley, NS. What are the principles of motor development? In Forssberg, H, & Hirschfeld, H (Eds.). Movement Disorders in Children, Medicine and Sport Science, Vol. 36. Basel: Karger, 1992, pp. 41–49.

Bradley, NS. Connecting the dots between animal and human studies of locomotion. Focus on "Infants adapt their stepping to repeated trip-inducing stimuli." Journal of Neurophysiology, 90:2088–2089, 2003.

Bradley, NS, & Bekoff, A. Development of locomotion: animal models. In Woollacott, M, & Shumway-Cook, A (Eds.). The Development of Posture and Gait Across the Lifespan. Columbia: University of South Carolina Press, 1989, pp. 48–73.

Bradley, NS, & Bekoff, A. Development of coordinated movement in chicks: I. Temporal analysis of hindlimb muscle synergies at embryonic days 9 and 10. Developmental Psychobiology, 23:763–782, 1990.

Bradley, NS, & Smith, JL. Neuromuscular patterns of stereotypic hindlimb behaviors in the first two postnatal months. I. Stepping in normal kittens. Developmental Brain Research, 38:37–52, 1988.

Branchereau, P, Morin, D, Bonnot, A, Ballion, B, Chapron, J, & Viala, D. Development of lumbar rhythmic networks: from embryonic to neonate locomotor-like patterns in the mouse. Brain Research Bulletin, 53:711–718, 2000.

Brogen, E, Forssberg, H, & Hadders-Algra, M. Influence of two different sitting positions on postural adjustments in children with spastic diplegia. Developmental Medicine & Child Neurology, 43:534–546, 2001.

Brogen, E, Hadders-Algra, M. & Forssberg, H. Postural control in sitting children with cerebral palsy. Neuroscience and Biobehavioral Reviews, 22:591–596, 1998.

Brunnstrom, S. Movement Therapy in Hemiplegia. New York: Harper & Row, 1970.

Bundy, AC, & Fisher, AG. Evaluation of sensory integration dysfunction. In Forssberg, H, & Hirschfeld, H (Eds.). Movement Disorders in Children, Medicine and Sport Science, Vol. 36. Basel: Karger, 1992, pp. 272–277.

Burleigh, A, & Horak, F. Influence of instruction, prediction, and afferent sensory information on the postural organization of step initiation. Journal of Neurophysiology, 75:1619–1627, 1996.

Burtner, PA, Qualls, C, & Woollacott, MH. Muscle activation characteristics of stance balance control in children with spastic cerebral palsy. Gait and Posture, 8:163–174, 1998.

Burtner, PA, Woollacott, MH, & Qualls, C. Stance balance control with orthoses in a group of children with spastic cerebral palsy. Developmental Medicine and Child Neurology, 41:748–757, 1999.

Butt, SJ, Lebret, JM, & Kiehn, O. Organization of left-right coordination in the mammalian locomotor network. Brain Research and Brain Research Review, 40:107–117, 2002.

Butterworth, G, & Hicks, L. Visual proprioception and postural stability in infancy. A developmental study. Perception, 6:255–262, 1977.

Campbell, SK. Test-retest reliability of the Test of Infant Motor Performance. Pediatric Physical Therapy, 11:60–66, 1999.

Carr, JH, & Shepherd, RB. Neurologic Rehabilitation: Optimizing Motor Performance. Oxford: Butterworth and Heinemann, 1998.

Carson, RG, & Riek, S. Changes in muscle recruitment patterns during skill acquisition. Experimental Brain Research, 138:71–87, 2001.

Cermak, SA, & Murray, EA. The validity of the constructional subtests of the Sensory Integration and Praxis Tests. American Journal of Occupational Therapy, 45:539–543, 1991.

Cesari, P, & Newell, KM. The scaling of human grip configurations. Journal of Experimental Psychology: Human Perception and Performance, 25:927–935, 1999.

Cesari, P, & Newell, KM. The body scaling of grip configurations in children aged 6–12 years. Developmental Psychobiology, 36:301–310, 2000.

Cesari, P, & Newell, KM. Scaling the components of prehension. Motor Control, 6:347–365, 2002.

Chambers, SH, Bradley, NS, & Orosz, MD. Kinematic analysis of wing and leg movements for type I motility in E9 chick embryos. Experimental Brain Research, 103:218–226, 1995.

Chandler, LS, Andrews, MS, & Swanson, MW. Movement Assessment of Infants. Rolling Bay, WA: Chandler, Andrews, & Swanson, 1980.

Cheron, G, Bengoetxea, A, Bouillot, E, Lacquaniti, F, & Dan, B. Early emergence of temporal co-ordination of lower limb segments elevation angles in human locomotion. Neuroscience Letters, 308:123–127, 2001.

Chiel, H, & Beer, AR. The brain has a body: Adaptive behavior emerges from interactions of nervous system, body and environment. Trends in Neuroscience, 20:553–557, 1997.

Charles, J, Lavinder, G, & Gordan, A. Effects of constraint-induced therapy on hand function in children with hemiplegic cerebral palsy. Pediatric Physical Therapy, 13:68–76, 2001.

Cioni, G, Ferrari, F, Einspieler, C, Paolicelli, PB, Barbani, MT, & Prechtl, HF. Comparison between observation of spontaneous movements and neurological examination in preterm infants. Journal of Pediatrics, 130:704–711, 1997a.

Cioni, G, Prechtl, HF, Ferrari, F, Paolicelli, PB, Einspieler, C, & Roversi, MF. Which better predicts later outcome in full-term infants: Quality of general movements or neurological examination? Early Human Development, 50:71–85, 1997b.

Clifton, RK, Muir, DW, Ashmead, DH, & Clarkson, MG. Is visually guided reaching in early infancy a myth? Child Development, 64:1099–1110, 1993.

Connolly, K. The nature of motor skill development. Journal of Human Movement Studies, 3:128–143, 1977.

Corbetta, D, & Thelen, E. Shifting patterns of interlimb coordination in infants' reaching: A case study. In Swinnen, SP, Heuer, H, Massion, J, & Casaer, P (Eds.). Interlimb Coordination: Neural, Dynamical, and Cognitive Constraints. San Diego: Academic Press, 1994, pp. 413–438.

Crocker, MD, Mackay-Lyons, M, & McDonnell, E. Forced use of upper extremitiy in cerebral palsy: a single case design. American Journal of Occupational Therapy, 51:824–833, 1997.

Crutcher, MD, & Alexander, GE. Movement-related neuronal activity selectively coding either direction or muscle pattern in 3 motor areas of the monkey. Journal of Neurophysiology, 64:151–163, 1990.

d' Avella, A, Saltiel, P, & Bizzi, E. Combinations of muscle synergies in the construction of a natural motor behavior. Nature Neuroscience, 6:300–308, 2003.

Damiano, DL, & Abel, MF. Relation of gait analysis to gross motor function in cerebral palsy. Developmental Medicine and Child Neurology, 38:389–396, 1996.

Damiano, DL, & Abel, MF. Functional outcomes of strength training in spastic cerebral palsy. Archives of Physical Medicine and Rehabilitation, 79:119–125, 1998.

Damiano, DL, Dodd, K, & Taylor, NF. Should we be testing and training muscle strength in cerebral palsy? Developmental Medicine and Child Neurology, 44:68–72, 2002.

Damiano, DL, Kelly, LE, & Vaughan, CL. Effects of a quadriceps femoris strengthening program on crouch gait in children with cerebral palsy. Physical Therapy, 75:658–667, 1995a.

Damiano, DL, Vaughan, CL, & Abel, MF. Muscle response to heavy resistance exercise in children with spastic cerebral palsy. Developmental Medicine and Child Neurology, 37:731–739, 1995b.

Daniels, LE, & Bressler, S. The Miller Assessment for Preschoolers: Clinical use with children with developmental delay. American Journal of Occupational Therapy, 44:48–53, 1990.

Darrah, J, Piper, M, & Watt, MJ. Assessment of gross motor skills of at-risk infants: Predictive validity of the Alberta Infant Motor Scale. Developmental Medicine and Child Neurology, 40:485–491, 1998.

de Vries, JIP, Visser, GHA, & Prechtl, HFR. The emergence of fetal behavior: I. Qualitative aspects. Early Human Development, 7:301–322, 1982.

de Vries, JI, Wimmers, RH, Ververs, IA, Hopkins, B, Savelsbergh, GJ, & van Geijn, HP. Fetal handedness and head position preference: A developmental study. Developmental Psychobiology, 39:171–178, 2001.

Deitz, J, Richardson, PK, Westcott, SL, & Crowe, TK. Performance of children with learning disabilities on the Pediatric Clinical Test of Sensory Interaction for Balance. Physical & Occupational Therapy in Pediatrics, 16:1–21, 1996.

DeLuca, SC, Echols, K, Ramey, SL, & Taub, E. Pediatric constraint-induced movement therapy for a young child with cerebral palsy: Two episodes of care. Physical Therapy, 83:1003–1013, 2003.

Diedrich, FJ, Highlands, TM, Spahr, KA, Thelen, E, & Smith, LB. The role of target distinctiveness in infant perseverative reaching. Journal of Experimental Child Psychology, 78:263–290, 2001.

Dubowitz, L, & Dubowitz, V. The Neurological Assessment of the

Preterm and Full-term Newborn Infant. Clinics in Developmental Medicine, 79:1–103, 1981.

Dubowitz, LMS, Dubowitz, V, Palmer, PG, Miller, G, Fawer, CL, & Levine, MI. Correlation of neurologic assessment in the preterm newborn infant with outcome at 1 year. Journal of Pediatrics, 105:452–456, 1984.

Duran, LJ, & Fisher, AG. Male and female performance on the Assessment of Motor Process Skills. Archives of Physical Medicine and Rehabilitation, 77:1019–1024, 1996.

Eagleton, M, Iams, A, McDowell, J, Morrison, R, & Evans, CL. The effects of strength training on gait in adolescents with cerebral palsy. Pediatric Physical Therapy, 16:22–30, 2004.

Einspieler, C, Cioni, G, Paolicelli, PB, Bos, AF, Dressler, A, Ferrari, F, Roversi, MF, & Prechtl, HF. The early markers for later dyskinetic cerebral palsy are different from those for spastic cerebral palsy. Neuropediatrics, 33:73–78, 2002.

Einspieler, C, Prechtl, HF, Ferrari, F, Cioni, G, & Bos, AF. The qualitative assessment of general movements in preterm, term and young infants—Review of the methodology. Early Human Development, 50:47–60, 1997.

Eliasson, AC, Gordon, AM, & Forssberg, H. Basic co-ordination of manipulative forces of children with cerebral palsy. Developmental Medicine and Child Neurology, 33:661–670, 1991.

Eliasson, AC, Gordon, AM, & Forssberg, H. Impaired anticipatory control of isometric forces during grasping by children with cerebral palsy. Developmental Medicine and Child Neurology, 34:216–225, 1992.

Eliasson, AC, Gordon, AM, & Forssberg, H. Tactile control of isometric fingertip forces during grasping in children with cerebral palsy. Developmental Medicine and Child Neurology, 37:72–84, 1995.

Estil, LB, Ingvaldsen, RP, & Whiting, HT. Spatial and temporal constraints on performance in children with movement co-ordination problems. Experimental Brain Research, 147:153–161, 2002.

Eyre, JA, Miller, S, Clowry, GJ, Conway, EA, & Watts, C. Functional corticospinal projections are established prenatally in the human foetus permitting involvement in the development of spinal motor centres. Brain, 123:51–64, 2000.

Eyre, JA, Taylor, JP, Villagra, F, Smith, M, & Miller, S. Evidence of activity dependent withdrawal of corticospinal projections during human development. Neurology, 57:1543–1554, 2001.

Fagard, J. Manual strategies and interlimb coordination during reaching, grasping, and manipulating throughout the first year of life. In Swinnen, SP, Heuer, H, Massion, J, & Casaer, P (Eds.). Interlimb Coordination: Neural, Dynamical, and Cognitive Constraints. San Diego: Academic Press, 1994, pp. 439–460.

Fagard, J, & Pezé, A. Age changes in interlimb coupling and the development of bimanual coordination. Journal of Motor Behavior, 29:199–208, 1997.

Fallang, B, Saugstad, OD, Grogaard, J, & Hadders-Algra, M. Kinematic quality of reaching movements in preterm infants. Pediatric Research, 53:836–842, 2003.

Fallang, B, Saugstad, OD, & Hadders-Algra, M. Goal directed reaching and postural control in supine position in healthy infants. Behavioral Brain Research, 115:9–18, 2000.

Feldman, AG. Once more on the Equilibrium-Point Hypothesis (l model) for motor control. Journal of Motor Behavior, 18:17–54, 1986.

Feldman, AG, Ostry, DJ, Levin, MF, Gribble, PL, & Mitnitski, AB. Recent tests of the equilibrium-point hypothesis (lambda model). Motor Control, 2:189–205, 1998.

Ferdjallah, M, Harris, GF, Smith, P, & Wertsch, JJ. Analysis of postural control synergies during quiet standing in healthy children and children with cerebral palsy. Clinical Biomechanics, 17:203–210, 2002.

Ferrari, F, Prechtl, HF, Cioni, G, Roversi, MF, Einspieler, C, Gallo, C, Paolicelli, PB, & Cavazzuti, GB. Posture, spontaneous movements, and behavioral state organization in infants affected by brain malformations. Early Human Development, 50:87–113, 1997.

Fetters, L, & Todd, J. Quantitative assessment of infant reaching movements. Journal of Motor Behavior, 19:147–166, 1987.

Field, J. Coordination of vision and prehension in young infants. Child Development, 48:97–103, 1977.

Fisher, AG. Development of a functional assessment that adjusts ability measures for task simplicity and rater leniency. In Wilson M (Ed.). Objective Measurement: Theory Into Practice, Vol. 2. Norwood: Ablex, 1994, pp. 145–175.

Fisher, AG, Bryze, K, & Atchison, BT. Naturalistic assessment of functional performance in school settings: Reliability and validity of the school AMPS scales. Journal of Outcome Measurements, 4:491–512, 2000.

Fisher, AG, & Bundy, AC. (1992). Sensory integration theory. In Forssberg, H, & Hirschfeld, H (Eds.). Movement Disorders in Children, Medicine and Sport Science, Vol. 36. Basel: Karger, 1992, pp. 16–20.

Fitts, PM. The information capacity of the human motor system in controlling the amplitude of movement. Journal of Experimental Psychology, 47:381–391, 1954.

Fogassi, L, Gallese, V, Buccino, G, Craighero, L, Fadiga, L, & Rizzolatti, G. Cortical mechanism for the visual guidance of hand grasping movements in the monkey: A reversible inactivation study. Brain, 124:571–586, 2001.

Forssberg, H. Ontogeny of human locomotor control. I. Infant stepping, supported locomotion and transition to independent locomotion. Experimental Brain Research, 57:480–493, 1985.

Forssberg, H. Evolution of plantigrade gait: Is there a neuronal correlate? Developmental Medicine and Child Neurology, 34:920–925, 1992.

Forssberg, H, Eliasson, AC, Kinoshita, H, Johansson, RS, & Westling, G. Development of human precision grip. I. Basic coordination of force. Experimental Brain Research, 85:451–457, 1991.

Forssberg, H, Eliasson, AC, Kinoshita, H, Westling, G, & Johansson, RS. Development of human precision grip. IV. Tactile adaptation of isometric finger forces to the frictional condition. Experimental Brain Research, 104:323–330, 1995.

Forssberg, H, Kinoshita, H, Eliasson, AC, Johansson, RS, Westling, G, & Gordon, AM. Development of human precision grip. II. Anticipatory control of isometric forces targeted for object's weight. Experimental Brain Research, 90:393–398, 1992.

Forsström, A, & Hofsten, C von. Visually directed reaching of children with motor impairments. Developmental Medicine and Child Neurology, 24:653–661, 1982.

Foster, EC, Sveistrup, H, & Woollacott, MH. Transitions in visual proprioception: A cross-sectional developmental study of the effect of visual flow on postural control. Journal of Motor Behavior, 28:101–112, 1996.

Fuster, JM. Executive frontal functions. Experimental Brain Research, 133:66–70, 2000.

Gallistel, CR. The Organization of Action: A New Synthesis. Hillsdale, NJ: Lawrence Erlbaum Associates, 1980.

Geerdink, JJ, & Hopkins, B. Qualitative changes in general movements and their prognostic value in preterm infants. European Journal of Pediatrics, 152:362–367, 1993.

Geerdink, JJ, Hopkins, B, Beek, WJ, & Heriza, CB. The organization of leg movements in preterm and full-term infants after term age. Developmental Psychobiology, 29:335–351, 1996.

Georgopolous, AP. Neurophysiology of reaching. In Jeannerod, M (Ed.). Attention and Performance XIII. Hillsdale, NJ: Lawrence Erlbaum Associates, 1990, pp. 227–263.

Ghez, C. Voluntary movements. In Kandel, ER, Schwartz, JH, & Jessell,

TM (Eds.). Principles of Neuroscience, 3rd ed. New York: Elsevier, 1991, pp. 609–625.

Gibson, JJ. The Senses Considered as Perceptual Systems. Boston: Houghton Mifflin, 1966.

Gomi, H, & Kawato, M. Human arm stiffness and equilibrium-point trajectory during multi-joint movement. Biological Cybernetics, 76:163–171, 1997.

Gomi, H, & Kawato, M. Equilibrium-point control hypothesis examined by measured arm stiffness during multijoint movement. Science, 272:117–120, 1996.

Goodgold-Edwards, SA. Cognitive strategies during coincident timing tasks. Physical Therapy, 71:236–243, 1991.

Goto, S, Fisher, AG, & Mayberry, WL. The assessment of motor and process skills applied cross-culturally to the Japanese. American Journal of Occupational Therapy, 50:798–806, 1996.

Gordon, AM, Forssberg, H, & Iwasaki, N. Formation and lateralization of internal representations underlying motor commands during precision grip. Neuropsychologia, 32:555–568, 1994.

Gordon, AM, Forssberg, H, Johansson, RS, Eliasson, AC, & Westling, G. Development of human precision grip. III Integration of visual cues during the programming of isometric forces. Experimental Brain Research, 90:399–403, 1992.

Gordon, J. Assumptions underlying physical therapy intervention: theoretical and historical perspectives. In Carr, JH, & Shepherd, RB (Eds.). Movement Science Foundations for Physical Therapy in Rehabilitation. Rockville, MD: Aspen, 1987, pp. 1–30.

Gowland, C, Boyce, W, Wright, V, Russell, D, Goldsmith, C, & Rosenbaum, P. Reliability of the Gross Motor Performance Measure. Physical Therapy, 75:597–602, 1995.

Gowland, C, Rosenbaum, P, Hardy, S, Lane, M, Plews, N, Goldsmith, C, Russell, D, Wright, V, Potter, S, & Harding, D. Gross Motor Performance Measure Manual. Kingston: Queen's University, 1998.

Grillner, S. Neural networks for vertebrate locomotion. Scientific American, 274:64–69, 1996.

Guzzetta, A, Mercuri, E, Rapisardi, G, Ferrari, F, Roversi, MF, Cowan, F, Rutherford, M, Paolicelli, PB, Einspieler, C, Boldrini, A, Dubowitz, L, Prechtl, HF, & Cioni G. General movements detect early signs of hemiplegia in term infants with neonatal cerebral infarction. Neuropediatrics, 34:61–66, 2003.

Haas, G, Diener, HC, Rapp, H, & Dichgans, J. Development of feedback and feedforward control of upright stance. Developmental Medicine and Child Neurology, 31:481–488, 1989.

Hadders-Algra, M. Two distinct forms of minor neurological dysfunction: perspectives emerging from a review of data of the Groningen Perinatal Project. Developmental Medicine and Child Neurology, 44:561–571, 2002.

Hadders-Algra, M. Early brain damage and the development of motor behavior in children: Clues for therapeutic intervention? Neural Plasticity, 8:31–49, 2001a.

Hadders-Algra, M. Evaluation of motor function in young infants by means of assessment of general movements: A review. Pediatric Physical Therapy, 13:27–36, 2001b.

Hadders-Algra, M. The Neuronal Group Selection Theory: A framework to explain variation in normal motor development. Developmental Medicine and Child Neurology, 42:566–572, 2000.

Hadders-Algra, M, Brogren, E, & Forssberg, H. Ontogeny of postural adjustments during sitting in infancy: variation, selection and modulation. Journal of Physiology, 493:273–288, 1996.

Hadders-Algra, M, Groothuis, AMC. Quality of general movements in infancy is related to the development of neurological dysfunction, attention deficit hyperactivity disorder and aggressive behavior. Developmental Medicine and Child Neurology, 41:381–391, 1999.

Hadders-Algra, M, & Prechtl, HFR. Developmental course of general movements in early infancy. I. Descriptive analysis of change in form. Early Human Development, 28:201–213, 1992.

Hadders-Algra, M, van der Fits, IBM, Stremmelaar, EF, & Touwen, BCL. Development of postural adjustments during reaching in infants with CP. Developmental Medicine & Child Neurology, 41:766–776, 1999.

Haley, S. Sequence of development of postural reactions by infants with Down syndrome. Developmental Medicine and Child Neurology, 29:674–679, 1987.

Haley, SM, Harris, SR, Tada, WL, & Swanson MW. Item reliability of the Movement Assessment of Infants. Physical and Occupational Therapy in Pediatrics, 6(1):21–39, 1986.

Harabst, KB, Lazarus, JA, & Whitall, J. Accuracy of dynamic isometric force production: The influence of age and bimanual activation patterns. Motor Control, 4:232–256, 2000.

Harbourne, RT, Giuliani, C, & Mac Neela, J. A kinematic and electromyographic analysis of the development of sitting posture in infants. Developmental Psychobiology, 26:51–64, 1993.

Harris, SR. Early detection of cerebral palsy: sensitivity and specificity of two motor assessment tools. Journal of Perinatology, 7:11–15, 1987.

Hasan, Z. Optimized movement trajectories and joint stiffness in unperturbed, inertially loaded movements. Biological Cybernetics, 53:373–382, 1986.

Hatzitaki, V, Zisi, V, Kollias, I, & Kioumourtzoglou, E. Perceptual-motor contributions to static and dynamic balance control in children. Journal of Motor Behavior, 34:161–170, 2002.

Hay, L. Spatial-temporal analysis of movements in children: motor programs versus feedback in the development of reaching. Journal of Motor Behavior, 11:188–200, 1979.

Hay, L, Fleury, M, Bard, C, & Teasdale, N. Resolving power of the perceptual and sensorimotor systems in 6- to 10-year-old children. Journal of Motor Behavior, 26:36–42, 1994.

Hay, L, & Redon, C. Development of postural adaptation to arm raising. Experimental Brain Research, 139:224–232, 2001.

Heriza, CB. Comparison of leg movements in preterm infants at term with healthy full-term infants. Physical Therapy, 68:1687–1693, 1988.

Hirschfeld, H, & Forssberg, H. Epigenetic development of postural responses for sitting during infancy. Experimental Brain Research, 97:528–540, 1994.

Hofsten, C von. Development of visually guided reaching: The approach phase. Journal of Human Movement Studies, 5:160–178, 1979.

Hofsten, C von. Eye-hand coordination in the newborn. Developmental Psychology, 18:450–461, 1982.

Hofsten, C von. Developmental changes in the organization of prereaching movements. Developmental Psychology, 20:378–388, 1984.

Hofsten, C von. A perception-action perspective on the development of manual movements. In Jeannerod, M (Ed.). Attention and Performance XIII. Hillsdale, NJ: Lawerence Erlbaum Associates, 1990, pp. 739–762.

Hofsten, C von. Structuring of early reaching movements: A longitudinal study. Journal of Motor Behavior, 23:280–292, 1991.

Hofsten, C von, & Fazel-Zandy, S. Development of visually guided hand orientation in reaching. Journal of Experimental Child Psychology, 38:208–219, 1984.

Hofsten, C von, & Rönnqvist, L. Preparation for grasping an object: A developmental study. Journal of Experimental Psychology: Human Perception and Performance, 14:610–621, 1988.

Hofsten, C von, & Rönnqvist, L. The structuring of neonatal arm movements. Child Development, 64:1046–1057, 1993.

Holdefer, RN, & Miller, LE. Primary motor cortical neurons encode functional muscle synergies. Experimental Brain Research, 146:233–243, 2002.

Hooker, D. Evidence of prenatal function of the central nervous system in man. New York: American Museum of Natural History, 1958.

Hopkins, B, & Prechtl, HFR. A quantitative approach to the development of movements during early infancy. Clinics in Developmental Medicine, 94:179–197, 1984.

Horak, FB. Assumptions underlying motor control for neurologic rehabilitation. In Lister, MJ (Ed.). Contemporary Management of Motor Control Problems, Proceedings of the II Step Conference. Alexandria, VA: Foundation for Physical Therapy, 1991, pp. 11–28.

Horak, FB. Motor control models underlying neurologic rehabilitation. In Forssberg, H, & Hirschfeld, H (Eds.). Movement Disorders in Children, Medicine and Sport Science, Vol. 36. Basel: Karger, 1992, pp. 21–30.

Horak, FB, Buchanan, J, Creath, R, & Jeka, J. Vestibulospinal control of posture. Advances in Experimental Medicine and Biology, 508:139–145, 2002.

Horak, FB, Diener, HC, & Nashner, LM. Influence of central set on human postural responses. Journal of Neurophysiology, 62:841–853, 1989.

Horak, FB, Earhart, GM, & Dietz, V. Postural responses to combinations of head and body displacements: Vestibular-somatosensory interactions. Experimental Brain Research, 141:410–414, 2001.

Horak, FB, Esselman, P, Anderson ME, & Lynch, MK. The effects of movement velocity, mass displaced, and task certainty on associated postural adjustments made by normal and hemiplegic individuals. Journal of Neurology, Neurosurgery and Psychiatry, 47:1020–1028, 1984.

Horak, FB, & MacPherson, JM. Postural orientation and equilibrium. In Rowell, LB, & Sheperd, JT (Eds.). Handbook of Physiology, Section 12, Exercise: Regulation and Integration of Multiple Systems. New York: Oxford University Press, 1996, pp. 255–292.

Horak, FB, & Nashner, LM. Central programming of postural movements: adaptation to altered support-surface configurations. Journal of Neurophysiology, 55:1369–1381, 1986.

Horak, FB, Nashner, LM, & Diener, HC. Postural strategies associated with somatosensory and vestibular loss. Experimental Brain Research, 82:167–177, 1990.

Horak, FB, Shumway-Cook, A, Crowe, TK, & Black, FO. Vestibular function and motor proficiency of children with impaired hearing, or with learning disability and motor impairments. Developmental Medicine and Child Neurology, 30:64–79, 1988.

Hoy, MG, Zernicke, RF, & Smith, JL. Contrasting roles of inertial and muscle moments at the knee and ankle during paw-shake response. Journal of Neurophysiology, 54:1282–1294, 1985.

Humphrey, T. Some correlations between the appearance of human reflexes and the development of the nervous system. Progress in Brain Research, 4:93–135, 1964.

Humphrey, T. The development of human fetal activity and its relation to postnatal behavior. Advances in Child Development and Behavior, 5:1–57, 1970.

Inui, N, & Katsura, Y. Development of force control and timing in a finger-tapping sequence with an attenuated-force tap. Motor Control. 6:333–346, 2002.

Isableu, B, Ohlmann, T, Cremieux, J, & Amblard, B. Differential approach to strategies of segmental stabilisation in postural control. Experimental Brain Research, 150:208–221, 2003.

Jakobson, LS, & Goodale, MA. Factors affecting higher-order movement planning—A kinematic analysis of human prehension. Experimental Brain Research, 86:199–208, 1991.

Jeannerod, M. Intersegmental coordination during reaching at natural visual objects in infancy. In Long, J, & Baddeley, A (Eds.). Attention and Performance IX. Hillsdale, NJ: Lawrence Erlbaum Associates, 1981, pp. 153–168.

Jeannerod, M. The timing of natural prehension movement. Journal of Motor Behavior, 26:235–254, 1984.

Jeannerod, M (Ed.). Attention and Performance XIII: Motor Representation and Control. Hillsdale, NJ: Lawrence Erlbaum Associates, 1990.

Jeka, JJ, & Lackner, JR. Fingertip contact influences human postural control. Experimental Brain Research, 100:495–502, 1994.

Jeng, SF, Chen, LC, & Yau, KI. Kinematic analysis of kicking movements in preterm infants with very low birth weight and full-term infants. Physical Therapy, 82:148–159, 2002.

Jensen, JL, Ulrich, BD, Thelen, E, Schneider, K, & Zernicke, RF. Adaptive dynamics of the leg movement patterns of human infants: I. The effects of posture on spontaneous kicking. Journal of Motor Behavior, 26: 303–312, 1994.

Jensen, JL, Thelen, E, Ulrich, BD, Schneider, K, & Zernicke, RF. Adaptive dynamics of the leg movement patterns of human infants: III. Age-related differences in limb control. Journal of Motor Behavior, 27:366–374, 1995.

Jensen, RK, Sun, H, Treitz, T, & Parker, HE. Gravity constraints in infant motor development. Journal of Motor Behavior, 29:64–71, 1997.

Jiang, J, Shen, Y, & Neilson, PD. A simulation study of the degrees of freedom of movement in reaching and grasping. Human Movement Science, 21:881–904, 2002.

Johansson, RS, & Westling, G. Coordinated isometric muscle commands adequately and erroneously programmed for the weight during lifting task with precision grip. Experimental Brain Research, 71:59–71, 1988.

Johnson, LM, Randall, MJ, Reddihough, DS, Oke, LE, Byrt, TA, & Bach, TM. Development of a clinical assessment of quality of movement for unilateral upper-limb function. Developmental Medicine and Child Neurology, 36:965–973, 1994.

Johnston, LM, Burns, YR, Brauer, SG, & Richardson, CA. Differences in postural control and movement performance during goal directed reaching in children with developmental coordination disorder. Human Movement Science, 21:583–601, 2002.

Kalaska, JF, & Crammond, DJ. Cerebral cortical mechanisms of reaching movements. Science, 255:1517–1523, 1992.

Katz, PS, & Frost, WN. Intrinsic neuromodulation: Altering neuronal circuits from within. Trends in Neuroscience, 19:54–61, 1996.

Kawai, M, Savelsbergh, GJ, & Wimmers, RH. Newborns' spontaneous arm movements are influenced by the environment. Early Human Development, 54:15–27, 1999.

Keogh, J, & Sugden, D. Movement Skill Development. New York: Macmillan, 1985.

Keshner, EA. Equilibrium and automatic postural reactions as indicators and facilitators in the treatment of balance disorders. In Touch: Topics in Pediatrics (Lesson 4). Alexandria, VA: American Physical Therapy Association, 1990, pp. 1–17.

Kimball, JG. Using the Sensory Integration and Praxis Tests to measure change: A pilot study. American Journal of Occupational Therapy, 44:603–608, 1990.

Kjaerulff O, & Kiehn O. Distribution of networks generating and coordinating locomotor activity in the neonatal rat spinal cord in vitro: A lesion study. Journal of Neuroscience, 16:5777–5794, 1996.

Knott, M. Neuromuscular facilitation in the child with central nervous system deficit. Journal of the American Physical Therapy Association, 7:721–724, 1966.

Konczak, J, Jansen-Osmann, P, & Kalveram, KT. Development of force adaptation during childhood. Journal of Motor Behavior, 35:41–52, 2003.

Koshland, GF, & Smith, JL. Paw-shake responses with joint immobilization—EMG changes with atypical feedback. Experimental Brain Research, 77:361–373, 1989.

Kramer, JF & MacPhail, HEA. Relationships among measures of walking efficiency, gross motor ability, and isokinetic strength in adolescents with cerebral palsy. Pediatric Physical Therapy, 6:3–8, 1994.

Kupfermann, I. Localization of higher cognitive and affective functions: the association cortices. In Kandel, ER, Schwartz, JH, & Jessell, TM (Eds.). Principles of Neuroscience, 3rd ed. New York: Elsevier, 1991, pp. 823–838.

Lantz, C, Melén, K, & Forssberg, H. Early infant grasping involves radial fingers. Developmental Medicine and Child Neurology, 38:668–674, 1996.

Lashley, KS. The accuracy of movement in the absence of excitation from the moving organ. American Journal of Physiology, 43:169–194, 1917.

Lasky, RE. The effect of visual feedback of the hand on the reaching and retrieval behavior of young infants. Child Development, 48:112–117, 1977.

Latash, ML, & Anson, JG. What are normal movements in atypical populations? Behavioral and Brain Sciences, 19:55–106, 1996.

Latash, ML, Ferreira, SS, Wieczorek, SA, & Duarte, M. Movement sway: changes in postural sway during voluntary shifts of the center of pressure. Experimental Brain Research, 150:314–324, 2003.

Lawrence, DG, & Hopkins, DA. The development of the motor control in the rhesus monkey: evidence concerning the role of corticomotorneuronal connections. Brain, 99:235–254, 1976.

Lawrence, DG, & Kuypers, HGJ. The functional organization of the motor system in the monkey: I. The effects of bilateral pyramidal lesions. Brain, 91:1–14, 1968.

Ledebt, A, Blandine, B, & Breniere, Y. The build-up of anticipatory behavior. Experimental Brain Research, 120:9–17, 1998.

Lee, DN. The optic flow-field: The foundation of vision. Philosophical Transactions of the Royal Society of London B, 290:169–179, 1980.

Lee, DN, & Aronson, E. Visual proprioceptive control of standing in human infants. Perception & Psychophysics, 15:529–532, 1974.

Lee, DN, Daniel, BM, Turnbull, J, & Cook, ML. Basic perceptuo-motor dysfunctions in cerebral palsy. In Jeannerod, M (Ed.). Attention and Performance XIII. Hillsdale, NJ: Lawrence Erlbaum Associates, 1990, pp. 583–603.

Lee, DN, & Lishman, JR. Visual proprioceptive control of stance. Journal of Human Movement Studies, 1:87–95, 1975.

Leemrijse, C, Meijer, OG, Vermeer, A, Ader, HJ, & Diemel, S. The efficacy of Le Bon Depart and Sensory Integration treatment for children with developmental coordination disorder: A randomized study with six single cases. Clinical Rehabilitation, 14:247–259, 2000.

Lemon, R. The output map of the primate motor cortex. Trends in Neuroscience, 11:501–506, 1988.

Lemon, R, & Mantel, GWH. The influence of changes in discharge frequency of corticospinal neurones on hand muscles in the monkey. Journal of Physiology, 413:351–378, 1989.

Levitan, IB, & Kaczmarek, LK. Neural networks and behavior. In The Neuron. Cell and Molecular Biology. New York: Oxford, 1997, pp. 451–474.

Liao, PM, & Campbell, SK. Examination of the item structure of the Alberta Infant Motor Scale. Pediatric Physical Therapy, 16:31–38, 2004.

Liu, WY. Anticipatory postural adjustments in children with cerebral palsy and children with typical development during forward reach tasks in standing. Philadelphia, PA, MCP Hahnemann University, 2001, pp. 111–173 (dissertation).

Lockman, JJ, Ashmead, DH, & Bushnell, EW. The development of anticipatory hand orientation during infancy. Journal of Experimental Child Psychology, 37:176–186, 1984.

MacKay-Lyons, M. Central pattern generation of locomotion: A review of the evidence. Physical Therapy, 82:69–83, 2002.

MacPhail, HE, & Kramer, JF. Effect of isokinetic strength training on functional ability and walking efficiency in adolescents with cerebral palsy. Developmental Medicine and Child Neurology, 37:763–775, 1995.

Mah, CD. Spatial and temporal modulation of joint stiffness during multijoint movement. Experimental Brain Research, 136:492–506, 2001.

Malouin, F, & Richards, CL. Preparatory adjustments during gait initiation in 4-6-year-old children. Gait and Posture, 11:239–253, 2000.

Mandich A, Buckolz E, & Polatajko H. Children with developmental coordination disorder (DCD) and their ability to disengage ongoing attentional focus: more on inhibitory function. Brain and Cognition, 51(3):346–356, 2003.

Marques-Bruna, P, & Grimshaw, P. Changes in coordination during the first 8 months of independent walking. Perceptual Motor Skills, 91:855–869, 2000.

Massion, J. Movement, posture and equilibrium—Interaction and coordination. Progress in Neurobiology, 38:35–56, 1992.

Mathew, A, & Cook, M. The control of reaching movements by young infants. Child Development, 61:1238–1258, 1990.

Mayston, MJ. The Bobath concept—Evolution and application. In Forssberg, H, & Hirschfeld, H (Eds.). Movement Disorders in Children, Medicine and Sport Science, Vol. 36. Basel: Karger, 1992, pp. 1–6.

McCarty, ME, Clifton, RK, Ashmead, DH, Lee, P, & Goubet, N. How infants use vision for grasping objects. Child Development, 72:973–987, 2001.

McComas, J, Dulberg, C, & Latter, J. Children's memory for locations visited: Importance of movement and choice. Journal of Motor Behavior, 29:223–229, 1997.

McDonnell, P. The development of visually guided reaching. Perception & Psychophysics, 18:181–185, 1975.

McGraw, MB. Neuromuscular development of the human infant as exemplified in the achievement of erect locomotion. Journal of Pediatrics, 17:747–771, 1940.

McGraw, MB. The Neuromuscular Maturation of the Human Infant. New York: Hafner Press, 1945.

McNevin, NH, Coraci, L, & Schafer, J. Gait in adolescent cerebral palsy: the effect of partial unweighting. Archives of Physical Medicine and Rehabilitation, 81:525–528, 2000.

Mercuri, E, Guzzetta, A, Laroche, S, Ricci, D, vanHaastert , I, Simpson, A, Luciano, R, Bleakley, C, Frisone, MF, Haataja, L, Tortorolo, G, Guzzetta, F, de Vries, L, Cowan, F, & Dubowitz, L. Neurologic examination of preterm infants at term age: comparison with term infants. Journal of Pediatrics, 142:647–655, 2003.

Meulenbroek, RGJ, Rosenbaum, DA, Jansen, C, Vaughan, J, & Vogt, S. Simulated and observed effects of object location, object size, and initial aperture. Experimental Brain Research, 138:219–234, 2001a.

Meulenbroek, RG, Rosenbaum, DA, & Vaughan, J. Planning reaching and grasping movements: Simulating reduced movement capabilities in spastic hemiparesis. Motor Control, 5:136–150, 2001b.

Meyer, DE, Smith, JEK, Kornblum, S, Abrams, RA, & Wright, CE. Speed-accuracy tradeoffs in aimed movements: Toward a theory of rapid voluntary action. In Jeannerod, M (Ed.). Attention and Performance XIII. Hillsdale, NJ: Lawrence Erlbaum Associates, 1990, pp. 173–226.

Michaud, LJ, Klein, A, Hudson, P, Gehrke, K & Custis-Allen, L. Constraint-induced movement therapy in pediatric hemiplegia: A case series. Archives of Physical Medicine and Rehabilitation, 84:E2, 2003.

Miller, LJ. Miller Assessment of Preschoolers. Littleton, CO: Foundation for Knowledge in Development, 1982.

Miller, LJ. Longitudinal validity of the Miller Assessment for Preschoolers: Study II. Perceptual Motor Skills, 66:811–814, 1988.

Miller, LJ, & Roid, GH. Sequence comparison methodology for the analysis of movement patterns in infants and toddlers with and without motor delays. American Journal of Occupational Therapy, 47:339–347, 1993.

Miller, LJ, & Roid, GH. The T.I.M.E. Toddler and Infant Motor Evaluation, a standardized assessment. San Antonio, Texas: Therapy Skill Builders, 1994.

Miller, LT, Polatajko, HJ, Missiuna, C, Mandich, AD, & McNab, JJ. A pilot trial of a cognitive treatment for children with developmental coordination disorder. Human Movement Science, 20:183–210, 2001.

Moe-Nilssen, R, Helbostad, JL, Talcott, JB, & Toennessen, FG. Balance and gait in children with dyslexia. Experimental Brain Research, 150:237–244, 2003.

Molteno, C, Grosz, P, Wallace, P, & Jones, M. Neurological examination of the preterm and full-term infant at risk for developmental disabilities using the Dubowitz Neurological Assessment. Early Human Development, 41:167–176, 1995.

Molteno, CD, Thompson, MC, Buccimazza, SS, Magasiner, V, & Hann, FM. Evaluation of the infant at risk for neurodevelopmental disability. South African Medical Journal, 89:1084–1087, 1999.

Mouchnino, L, Aurenty, R, Massion, J, & Pedotti, A. Coordinated control of posture and equilibrium during leg movement. In Brandt, T, Paulus, W, Bles, W, Dieterich, M, Krafczyk, S, & Straube, A (Eds.). Disorders of Posture and Gait. Stuttgart: Georg Thieme, 1990, pp. 68–71.

Muir, GD, Gosline, JM, & Steeves, JD. Ontogeny of bipedal locomotion: Walking and running in the chick. Journal of Physiology, 493:589–601, 1996.

Mulligan, S. An analysis of score patterns of children with attention disorders on the Sensory Integration and Praxis Tests. American Journal of Occupational Therapy, 50:647–654, 1996.

Nashner, LM, & Forssberg, H. Phase-dependent organization of postural adjustments associated with arm movements while walking. Journal of Neurophysiology, 55:1382–1394, 1986.

Nashner, LM, Shumway-Cook, A, & Marin, O. Stance posture control in select groups of children with cerebral palsy: Deficits in sensory organization and muscular coordination. Experimental Brain Research, 49:393–409, 1983.

Newell, KM, McDonald, PV, & Baillargeon, R. Body scale and infant grip configurations. Developmental Psychobiology, 26:195–205, 1993.

Newell, KM, & Valvano, J. Therapeutic intervention as a constraint in learning and relearning movement skills. Scandiavian Journal of Occupational Therapy, 5:51–57, 1998.

O'Donovan, MJ, & Chub, N. Population behavior and self-organization in the genesis of spontaneous rhythmic activity by developing spinal networks. Seminars in Cell and Developmental Biology, 8:21–28, 1997.

Okamoto, T, & Okamoto, K. Electromyographic characteristics at the onset of independent walking in infancy. Electromyography and Clinical Neurophysiology, 41:33–41, 2001.

Oztop, E, & Arbib, MA. Schema design and implementation of the grasp-related mirror neuron system. Biological Cybernetics, 87:116–140, 2002.

Palisano, RJ. Neuromotor and developmental assessment. In Wilhelm, IJ (Ed.). Physical Therapy Assessment in Early Infancy. New York: Churchill Livingstone, 1993, pp. 173–224.

Pang, MY, Lam, T, & Yang, JF. Infants adapt their stepping to repeated trip-inducing stimuli. Journal of Neurophysiology, 90:2731–2740, 2003.

Pang, MY, & Yang, JF. Sensory gating for the initiation of the swing phase in different directions of human infant stepping. Journal of Neuroscience, 22:5734–5740, 2002.

Parush, S, Winokur, M, Goldstand, S, & Miller, LJ. Long-term predictive validity of the Miller assessment for preschoolers. Perceptual Motor Skills, 94:921–926, 2002a.

Parush, S, Winokur, M, Goldstand, S, & Miller, LJ. Prediction of school performance using the Miller Assessment for Preschoolers (MAP): A validation study. American Journal of Occupational Therapy, 56:547–555, 2002b.

Parush, S, Yochman, A, Jessel, AS, Shapiro, M, & Mazor-Karsenty, T. Construct validity of the Miller assessment for preschoolers and the pediatric examination of educational readiness for children. Physical and Occupational Therapy in Pediatrics, 22(2):7–27, 2002c.

Perham, H, Smick, JE, Hallum, A, & Nordstrom, T. Development of the lateral equilibrium reaction in stance. Developmental Medicine and Child Neurology, 29:758–765, 1987.

Pierce, S, Daly, K, Gallagher, KG, Gershkoff, AM, & Schaumburg, SW. Constraint-induced therapy for a child with hemiplegic cerebral palsy: A case report. Archives of Physical Medicine and Rehabilitation, 83:1462–1463, 2002.

Piper, MC, & Darrah, J. Motor Assessment of the Developing Infant. Philadelphia: W.B. Saunders, 1994.

Piper, MC, Pinnell, LE, Darrah, J, Maguire, T, & Byrne, PJ. Construction and validation of the Alberta Infant Motor Scale (AIMS). Canadian Journal of Public Health, 83(Suppl 2):S46–50, 1992.

Polit, A, & Bizzi, E. Characteristics of motor programs underlying arm movements in monkeys. Journal of Neurophysiology, 42:183–194, 1979.

Portfors-Yeomans, CV, & Riach, CL. Frequency characteristics of postural control of children with and without visual impairment. Developmental Medicine and Child Neurology, 37:456–463, 1995.

Prablanc, C, & Pélisson, D. Gaze saccade orienting and hand pointing are locked to their goal by quick internal loops. In Jeannerod, M. (Ed.). Attention and Performance XIII. Hillsdale, NJ: Lawrence Erlbaum Associates, 1990, pp. 653–676.

Pratt, CA, & Loeb, GE. Functionally complex muscles of the cat hindlimb. 1. Patterns of activation across sartorius. Experimental Brain Research, 85:243–256, 1991.

Prechtl, HF. General movement assessment as a method of developmental neurology: New paradigms and their consequences. Developmental Medicine and Child Neurology, 43:836–842, 2001.

Prechtl, HF. State of the art of a new functional assessment of the young nervous system. An early predictor of cerebral palsy. Early Human Development, 50:1–11, 1997.

Prechtl, HFR, Cioni, G, Einspieler, C, Bos, AF, & Ferrari, F. Role of vision on early motor development: Lessons from the blind. Developmental Medicine and Child Neurology, 43:198–201, 2001.

Prilutsky, BI, & Gregor, RJ. Swing- and support-related muscle actions differentially trigger human walk-run and run-walk transitions. Journal of Experimental Biology, 204:2277–2287, 2001.

Rader, N, & Stern, JD. Visually elicited reaching in neonates. Child Development, 53:1004–1007, 1982.

Rahlin, M, Rheault, W, & Cech, D. Evaluation of the primary subtest of Toddler and Infant Motor Evaluation: Implications for clinical practice in pediatric physical therapy. Pediatric Physical Therapy, 15:176–183, 2003.

Raibert, MH. Motor control and learning by the state-space. Tech. Rep. AI-TR-439. Cambridge, MA: Massachusetts Institute of Technology, Artificial Intelligence Laboratory, 1977.

Riach, CL, & Hayes, KC. Anticipatory postural control in children. Journal of Motor Behavior, 22:250–266, 1990.

Richards, C, Malouin, F, Dumas, F, Marcoux, S, LePage, C, & Menier, C. Early and intensive treadmill locomotor training for young children with cerebral palsy: A feasibility study. Pediatric Physical Therapy, 9:158–165, 1997.

Riley, MA, & Turvey, MT. Variability and determinism in motor behavior. Journal of Motor Behavior, 34:99–125, 2002.

Rine, RM, Rubish, K, & Feeney, C. Measurement of sensory system effectiveness and maturational changes in postural control in young children. Pediatric Physical Therapy, 10:16–22, 1998.

Rizzolatti, G, & Arbib, MA. Language within our grasp. Trends in Neuroscience, 21:188–194, 1998.

Robertson Ringenbach, SD, Chua R, Maraj, BK, Kao, JC, & Weeks, DJ. Bimanual coordination dynamics in adults with Down syndrome. Motor Control, 6:388–407, 2002.

Rosenbaum, DA. Human Motor Control. San Diego: Academic Press, 1991.

Rosenbaum, PL, Walter, SD, Hanna, SE, Palisano, RJ, Russell, DJ, Raina, P, Wood, E, Bartlett, DJ, & Galuppi, BE. Prognosis for gross motor function in cerebral palsy: Creation of motor development curves. Journal of the American Medical Association, 288:1357–1363, 2002.

Rossignol, S. Neural control of stereotypic limb movements. In Rowell, LB, & Sheperd, JT (Eds.). Handbook of Physiology, Section 12, Exercise: Regulation and Integration of Multiple Systems. New York: Oxford University Press, 1996, pp. 173–216.

Rossignol, S, & Drew, T. Phasic modulation of reflexes during rhythmic activity. In Grillner, S, Stein, PSG, Stuart, DG, Forssberg, H, & Herman, RM (Eds.). Neurobiology of Vertebrate Locomotion. London: Macmillan Press Ltd., 1986, pp. 517–534.

Russell, DJ, Rosenbaum, PL, Cadman, DT, Gowland, C, Hardy S, & Jarvis, S. The Gross Motor Function Measure: A means to evaluate the effects of physical therapy. Developmental Medicine and Child Neurology, 31:341–353, 1989.

Salokorpi, T, Rajantie, I, Kivikko, I, Haajanen, R, & Rajantie, J. Predicting neurological disorders in infants with extremely low birth weight using the Movement Assessment of Infants, 13:106–109, 2001.

Sanes, JN, Dimitrov, B, & Hallett, M. Motor learning in patients with cerebellar dysfunction. Brain, 113:103–120, 1990.

Schellekens, JMH, Scholten, CA, & Kalverboer, AF. Visually guided hand movements in children with minor neurological dysfunction: Response time and movement organization. Journal of Child Psychology and Psychiatry, 24:89–102, 1983.

Schindl, MR, Forstner C, Kern, H, & Hesse, S. Treadmill training with partial body weight support in nonambulatory patients with cerebral palsy. Archives of Physical Medicine and Rehabilitation, 81:301–306, 2000.

Schmidt, RA. A schema theory of discrete motor skill learning. Psychological Review, 82:225–260, 1975.

Schmidt, RA, & Lee, TD. Motor Control and Learning: A Behavioral Emphasis, 3rd ed. Champaign, IL: Human Kinetics, 1998.

Schmitz, C, Martin, N, & Assaiante C. Building anticipatory postural adjustment during childhood: A kinematic and electromyographic analysis of unloading in children from 4 to 8 years of age. Experimental Brain Research, 142:354–364, 2002.

Schneider, E, Parush, S, Katz, N, & Miller, LJ. Performance of Israeli versus U.S. preschool children on the Miller Assessment for Preschoolers. American Journal of Occupational Therapy, 49:19–23, 1995.

Schneider, JW, Lee, W, & Chasnoff, IJ. Field testing of the Movement Assessment of Infants. Physical Therapy, 68:321–327, 1988.

Schneider, K, Zernicke, RF, Schmidt, RA, & Hart, TJ. Changes in limb dynamics during the practice of rapid arm movements. Journal of Biomechanics, 22:805–817, 1989.

Schneider, K, Zernicke, RF, Ulrich, BD, Jensen, JL, & Thelen, E. Understanding movement control in infants through the analysis of limb intersegmental dynamics. Journal of Motor Behavior, 22:493–520, 1990.

Scott, SH, & Kalaska, JF. Changes in motor cortex activity during reaching movements with similar hand paths but different arm postures. Journal of Neurophysiology, 73:2563–2567, 1995.

Seitz, RJ, Stephan, KM, & Binkofski, F. Control of action as mediated by the human frontal lobe. Experimental Brain Research, 133:71–80, 2000.

Shaffer, RJ, Jacokes, LE, Cassily, JF, Greenspan, SI, Tuchman, RF, & Stemmer, PJ Jr. Effect of interactive metronome training on children with ADHD. American Journal of Occupational Therapy, 55:155–162, 2001.

Shepherd, GM. Foundations of the Neuron Doctrine. New York: Oxford University Press, 1991.

Sherrington, CS. The Integrative Action of the Nervous System. New Haven: Yale University Press, 1947. (Original work published 1906.)

Shumway-Cook, A, & Woollacott, M. The growth of stability: postural control from a development perspective. Journal of Motor Behavior, 17:131–147, 1985a.

Shumway-Cook, A, & Woollacott, M. Dynamics of postural control in the child with Down syndrome. Physical Therapy, 9:1315–1322, 1985b.

Shumway-Cook, A, & Woollacott, M. Motor Control Theory and Practical Applications. Baltimore: Lippincott Williams & Wilkins, 2001.

Siegert, RJ, Lord, S, & Porter, K. Constraint-induced movement therapy: Time for a little restraint? Clinical Rehabilitation, 18:110–114, 2004.

Smeets, JB, & Brenner, E. Does a complex model help understand grasping? Experimental Brain Research, 144:132–135, 2002.

Smith, LB, & Thelen, E. Development as a dynamic system. Trends in Cognitive Science, 7:343–348, 2003.

Smyth, MM, Anderson, HI, & Churchill, A. Visual information and the control of reaching in children: A comparison between children with and without developmental coordination disorder. Journal of Motor Behavior, 33:306–320, 2001.

Song WH, Sung, IY, Kim, YJ, & Yoo, JY. Treadmill training with partial body weight support in children with cerebral palsy. Archives of Physical Medicine and Rehabilitation, 84:E2, 2003

Sporns, O, & Edelman, GM. Solving Bernstein's problem: A proposal for the development of coordinated movement by selection. Child Development, 64:960–981, 1993.

St-Onge, N, & Feldman, AG. Interjoint coordination in lower limbs during different movements in humans. Experimental Brain Research, 148:139–149, 2003.

Steenbergen, B, Hulstijn, W, Lemmens, IHL, & Meulenbroek, RGJ. The timing of prehensile movements in subjects with cerebral palsy. Developmental Medicine and Child Neurology, 40:108–114, 1998.

Stehouwer, DJ, & Farel, PB. Development of hindlimb locomotor behavior in the frog. Developmental Psychobiology, 17:217–232, 1984.

Stoffregen, TA, Adolph, K, Thelen, E, Gorday, KM, & Sheng, YY. Toddlers' postural adaptations to different support surfaces. Motor Control, 1:119–137, 1997.

Stringer, SM, Rolls, ET, Trappenberg, TP, & de Araujo, LET. Self-organizing continuous attractor networks and motor function. Neural Networks, 16:161–182, 2003.

Sugden, DA, & Keogh, JF. Problems in Movement Skill Development. Columbia: University of South Carolina Press, 1990.

Sundermier, L, & Woollacott, MH. The influence of vision on the automatic postural muscle responses of newly standing and newly walking infants. Experimental Brain Research, 120:537–540, 1998.

Sutherland, DH, Olshen, RA, Biden, EN, & Wyatt, MP. The development of mature walking. Clinics in Developmental Medicine, *104/105*:1–227, 1988.

Sutherland, DH, Olshen, R, Cooper, L, & Woo, SL. The development of mature gait. Journal of Bone and Joint Surgery, *62*:336–353, 1980.

Sveistrup, H, & Woollacott, MH. Longitudinal development of the automatic postural response in infants. Journal of Motor Behavior, *28*:58–70, 1996.

Swanson, MW, Bennet, FC, Shy, KK, & Whitfield, MF. Identification of neurodevelopmental abnormality at four and eight months by the Movement Assessment of Infants. Developmental Medicine and Child Neurology, *34*:321–337, 1992.

Swinnen, SP, Heuer, H, Massion, J, & Casaer, P (Eds.). Interlimb Coordination: Neural, Dynamical, and Cognitive Constraints. San Diego: Academic Press, 1994.

Tardieu, C, Laspargot, A, Tabary, C, & Bret, M. Toe-walking in children with cerebral palsy: contributions of contracture and excessive contraction of triceps surae muscle. Physical Therapy, *69*:656–662, 1989.

Taub, E, & Berman, AJ. Movement and learning in the absence of sensory feedback. In Freedman, SJ (Ed.). The Neuropsychology of Spatially Oriented Behavior. Homewood, IL: Dorsey Press, 1968.

Taub, E, Ramey, SL, DeLuca, S, & Echols, K. Efficacy of constraint-induced movement therapy for children with cerebral palsy with asymmetric motor impairment. Pediatrics, *113*:305–312, 2004.

Thelen, E, Fisher, DM, & Ridley-Johnson, R. The relationship between physical growth and a newborn reflex. Infant Behavior and Development, *7*:479–493, 1984.

Thelen, E, Fisher, DM, Ridley-Johnson, R, & Griffin, NJ. Effects of body build and arousal on newborn infant stepping. Developmental Psychobiology, *15*:447–453, 1982.

Thelen, E, & Smith, LB. A Dynamic Systems Approach to the Development of Cognition and Action. Cambridge, MA: MIT Press, 1994.

Thelen, E, & Ulrich, BD. Hidden skills: A dynamic systems analysis of treadmill stepping during the first year. Monographs of the Society for Research in Child Development, *56*:1–98, 1991.

Thomas SS, Buckon CE, Philips, DS, Aiona, MD, & Sussman, MD. Interobserver reliability of the Gross Motor Performance Measure: Preliminary results. Developmental Medicine and Child Neurology, *43*:97–102, 2001.

Thorpe, D, Zaino, C, Westcott, S, & Valvano, J. Comparison of postural muscle coordination patterns during a functional reaching task in typically developing children and children with cerebral palsy. Physical Therapy, *78*:S80–81, 1998.

Todorov, E, & Jordan, MI. Optimal feedback control as a theory of motor coordination. Nature Neuroscience, *11*:1226–1235, 2002.

Touwen, BCL. Primitive reflexes—Conceptual or semantic problem? Clinics in Developmental Medicine, *94*:115–125, 1984.

Trahan, J & Malouin, F. Intermittent intensive physiotherapy in children with cerebral palsy: A pilot study. Developmental Medicine and Child Neurology, *44*:233–239, 2002.

Twitchell, TE. Reflex mechanisms and the development of prehension. In Connolly, K (Ed.). Mechanisms of Motor Skill Development. London: Academic Press, 1970, pp. 25–37.

Ulrich, BD, Jensen, JL, Thelen, E, Schneider, K, & Zernicke, RF. Adaptive dynamics of the leg movement patterns of human infants: II. Treadmill stepping in infants and adults. Journal of Motor Behavior, *26*:313–324, 1994.

Ulrich, DA, Ulrich, BD, Angulo-Kinzler, RM, & Yun, J. Treadmill training of infants with Down syndrome: Evidence-based developmental outcomes. Pediatrics, *108*:E84, 2001.

Usui, N, Maekawa, K, & Hirasawa, Y. Development of the upright pos-

tural sway of children. Developmental Medicine and Child Neurology, *37*:985–996, 1995.

Valvano, J. Activity-focused motor interventions for children with neurological conditions. Physical and Occupational Therapy in Pediatrics, *24*:79–107, 2004.

Valvano, J, & Newell, KM. Practice of a precision isometric grip-force task by children with spastic cerebral palsy. Developmental Medicine and Child Neurology, *40*:464–473, 1998.

van der Fits, IB, Klip, AW, van Eykern, LA, & Hadders-Algra, M. Postural adjustments during spontaneous and goal-directed arm movements in the first half year of life. Behavioral Brain Research, *106*:75–90, 1999.

van der Heide, JC, Otten, B, van Eykern, LA, & Hadders-Algra, M. Development of postural adjustments during reaching in sitting children. Experimental Brain Research, *151*:32–45, 2003.

van der Meer, ALH, van der Weel, FR, & Lee, DN. Prospective control in catching by infants. Perception, *23*:287–302, 1994.

van der Meer, ALH, van der Weel, FR, & Lee, DN. The functional significance of arm movements in neonates. Science, *267*:693–695, 1995.

van der Meulen, JHP, Vandergon, JJD, Gielen, CCA, Gooskens, RHJ, & Willemse, J. Visuomotor performance of normal and clumsy children. 1. Fast goal-directed arm-movements with and without visual feedback. Developmental Medicine and Child Neurology, *33*:40–54, 1991a.

van der Meulen, JHP, Vandergon, JJD, Gielen, CCA, Gooskens, RHJ, & Willemse, J. Visuomotor performance of normal and clumsy children. 2. Arm-tracking with and without visual feedback. Developmental Medicine and Child Neurology, *33*:118–129, 1991b.

van der Weel, FR, van der Meer, ALH, & Lee, DH. Effect of task on movement control in cerebral palsy: Implications for assessment and therapy. Developmental Medicine and Child Neurology, *33*:419–426, 1991.

van Heijst, JJ, Vos, JE, & Bullock, D. Development in a biologically inspired spinal neural network for movement control. Neural Networks, *11*:1305–1316, 1998.

Viviani, P, & Mounoud, P. Perceptuomotor compatibility in pursuit tracking of two-dimensional movements. Journal of Motor Behavior, *22*:407–443, 1990.

Westcott, SL & Burtner, P. Postural Control in Children: Implications for Pediatric Practice. Physical and Occupational Therapy in Pediatrics, *24*:5–55, 2004.

Westcott, SL, Lowes, LP, & Richardson, PK. Evaluation of postural stability in children: Current theories and assessment tools. Physical Therapy, *77*:629–645, 1997a.

Westcott, S.L., Lowes, L.P., Richardson, P.K., Crowe, T.K., & Deitz, J. Difference in the use of sensory information for maintenance of standing balance in children with different motor disabilities. Developmental Medicine & Child Neurology, *39*(suppl 75):32–33, 1997b.

Westcott, SL, & Zaino, CA. Comparison and development of postural muscle activity in children during stand and reach from firm and compliant surfaces. Society for Neuroscience Abstract, *23*:1565, 1997.

Westcott, SL, Zaino, CA, Miller, F, Thorpe, D, & Unanue, R. Anticipatory postural coordination and functional movement skills by degree of cerebral palsy in children age 6-12 years. Society for Neuroscience Abstracts, *24*:149, 1998.

Whelan PJ. Developmental aspects of spinal locomotor function: Insights from using the in vitro mouse spinal cord preparation. Journal of Physiology, *553*:695–706, 2003.

Whitacre, CA, & Shea, CH. Performance and learning of generalized motor programs: Relative (GMP) and absolute (parameter) errors. Journal of Motor Behavior, *32*:163–175, 2000.

Willis, JK, Morello, A, Davie, A, Rice, JC, & Bennett, JT. Forced use treatment of childhood hemiparesis. Pediatrics, *110*:94–97, 2002.

Wilson, PH, Thomas, PR, & Maruff, P. Motor imagery training ameliorates motor clumsiness in children. Journal of Child Neurology, *17*:491–498, 2002.

Wimmers, RH, Savelsbergh, GJ, Beek, PJ, & Hopkins, B. Evidence for a phase transition in the early development of prehension. Developmental Psychobiology, *32*:235–248, 1998.

Wimmers, RH, Savalsbergh, GJ, van der Kamp, J, & Hartelman, P. A developmental transition in prehension modeled as a cusp catastrophe. Developmental Psychobiology, *32*:22–35, 1998.

Winstein, CJ, Horak, FB, & Fisher, BE. Influence of central set on anticipatory and triggered grip-force adjustments. Experimental Brain Research, *130*:298–308, 2000.

Wishart, JG, Bower, TGR, & Dunked, J. Reaching in the dark. Perception, *7*:507–512, 1978.

Witherington, DC, von Hofsten, C, Rosander, K, Robinette, A, Woollacott, MH, & Bertenthal, BI. The development of anticipatory postural adjustments in infancy. Infancy, *3*:495–517, 2002.

Woollacott, M, & Assaiante, C. Developmental changes in compensatory responses to unexpected resistance of leg lift during gait initiation. Experimental Brain Research, *144*:385–396, 2002.

Woollacott, MH, Burtner, P, Jensen, J, Jasiewicz, J, Roncesvalles, N, & Sveistrup, H. Development of postural responses during standing in healthy children and children with spastic diplegia. Neuroscience & Biobehavioral Reviews, *22*:583–589, 1998.

Woollacott, M, Debu, B, & Mowatt, M. Neuromuscular control of posture in the infant and child. Journal of Motor Behavior, *19*:167–186, 1987.

Yang, JF, Stephens, MJ, & Vishram, R. Transient disturbances to one limb produce coordinated, bilateral responses during infant stepping. Journal of Neurophysiology, *79*:2329–2337, 1998a.

Yang, JF, Stephens, MJ, & Vishram, R. Infant stepping: A method to study the sensory control of human walking. Journal of Physiology, *507*:927–937, 1998b.

Yonas, A, Bechtold, AG, Frankel, D, Gordon, FR, McRoberts, G, Norcia, A, & Sternfels, S. Development of sensitivity to information for impending collision. Perception and Psychophysics, *21*:97–104, 1977.

Young, RP, & Marteniuk, RG. Stereotypic muscle-torque patterns are systematically adopted during acquisition of a multi-articular kicking task. Journal of Biomechanics, *31*:809–816, 1998.

Zaino, CA. Motor control of a functional reaching task in children with cerebral palsy and children with typical development: A comparison of electromyographic and kinetic measurements. Philadelphia, PA: Allegheny University of the Health Sciences, 1999, pp. 50–104 (dissertation).

Zernicke, RF, & Smith, JS. Biomechanical insights into neural control of movement. In Rowell, LB, & Sheperd, JT (Eds.). Handbook of Physiology, Section 12, Exercise: Regulation and Integration of Multiple Systems. New York: Oxford University Press, 1996, pp. 293–330.

Chapter 4

MOTOR LEARNING: THEORIES AND STRATEGIES FOR THE PRACTITIONER

HÉLÈNA M. LARIN
PT, PhD

Learning or relearning motor tasks is a significant element of the rehabilitation process for a child with a neurologic or orthopedic impairment. Physical therapists continue to search for a better understanding and application to rehabilitation of the phenomenon of motor learning. The recent development of models for analyzing tasks and structuring practice to promote motor learning may provide a helpful perspective for the pediatric physical therapist. Such models offer a means to systematically organize knowledge of movement, skill acquisition and performance, and development.

For over a century, researchers from various fields have investigated aspects of motor learning. At the cellular level, from animal studies, the "system [underlying learning is said] to consist of many parallel, redundant and possibly interacting components" (Newell & Corcos, 1993). Researchers conducted in vivo studies primarily with persons without disabilities, with adults more than with children, and in laboratories more than in naturalistic environments, and they addressed isolated performance or learning behaviors. Despite working in these somewhat restricted milieux, researchers developed theories and models representing the body of knowledge of their time and also proposed a series of related instructional strategies. Through the years and even more today, physical therapists have had the difficult task of integrating the latest findings from research on motor learning into their working knowledge, in both the educational (Heriza & Sweeney, 1994) and clinical setting (Hayes et al., 1999).

The review of videotapes of pediatric physical therapists during individual treatment sessions of preschool children with cerebral palsy (CP) (moderate spastic diplegia) revealed that they implemented most of the recognized strategies for motor learning and teaching (Larin, 1992). Throughout the sessions, therapists kept the children active, emphasized mobility over stability activities, and took periodic breaks. To a high degree, they maintained a stimulating environment related to the task at hand. The frequency of use for each instructional strategy, as assessed with the Motor Teaching Strategy Coding Instrument (MTSCI-1), however, varied among therapists; the level of experience with individuals with neurologic impairments was a factor in some cases. In a content analysis of recordings during two subsequent interviews, therapists demonstrated varying degrees of awareness or, sometimes, implicit knowledge of particular motor learning strategies. For example, the use of active mode, stimulating environmental conditions, waiting periods, assisted types of movements, and positive feedback received greater acknowledgment than the use of movement goals, specific task descriptions, or quantitative types of feedback.

The relationship between clinicians' practice and implicit professional knowledge presented a mixed pattern that appeared to vary according to the characteristics of the (self-selected) tasks performed and the therapists' cognition of the motor learning strategies (Larin, 1992). Overall, therapists were aware of scientific knowledge of diverse origins, including some in motor learning, but were particularly cognizant of ecologic, motivational, and developmental theories.

A decade later, research brings additional information and challenges to physical therapists. A greater awareness and understanding of the contemporary body of knowledge on motor learning may help practitioners to maximize therapeutic opportunities. It may help therapists to (1) engage in self-analysis of their practice and identification of new or less exploited strategies; (2) adapt the information to their individual needs; (3) plan and perform examination and intervention sessions from a new perspective; and (4) engage in research documenting the applicability of principles of motor learning to intervention with children with functional activity limitations.

To these ends, literature on concepts and strategies of motor learning and teaching is reviewed in the three main sections of this chapter; throughout, research findings on the learning process of children are highlighted. In the first section, a brief historical summary of the development of motor control and motor learning theories is presented. In the second, motor learning models from three authors who attempted to bridge the gap between theory and practice are briefly introduced. These models form the basis for the third section, in which a variety of instructional strategies are reviewed along with presentation of examples from pediatric clinical practice.

MOTOR CONTROL AND MOTOR LEARNING THEORIES: AN HISTORICAL PERSPECTIVE

How does a person learn to control a new movement? How does one account for the complexity and variety of motor behavior in the process? These are some of the major questions theorists in motor control and motor

learning have attempted to answer. The evolution of these concepts has gradually come to influence the body of knowledge, as well as the practice, of physical therapy.

THEORETIC GROUNDWORK

According to early views on the subject, motor learning was a process of "habit" formation (James, 1890); recently more sophisticated approaches have dealt with motor control and motor learning in terms of information processing theories and ecologic theories. The development of information processing theories can be related to the study of both slow and fast movements. The closed loop theories of movement control (Adams, 1971) emphasized the need for sensory input, sensory feedback, and rewards during repetition of movements that are slow and self-paced, the goal being to augment the intrinsic feedback and develop a perceptual memory trace of movements. These instructional strategies were considered necessary as event reinforcers.

In contrast, theorists who studied quickly executed movements discovered the existence of a structured, linear, hierarchic organization within the central nervous system (CNS) (Sheridan, 1984) and minimized the importance of the role of feedback. "Open loop" or "motor program" theories attributed skill acquisition to a central, executive motor program responsible for producing and executing selected, sequential subroutines in a top-down fashion for short, fixed, repeatable, automatic sequences of movements (Marteniuk, 1976). Consequently, step-by-step instructional strategies were promoted following systematic, developmental stages, with elicited movements prevailing over spontaneous movements and a preference for reflex activity over self-initiated activity. In a third point of view, McCulloch (1945), among others, proposed an "heterarchic" view of information processing: different levels of control interact, cooperate, and transfer control according to the need at hand rather than being subservient to an executive (Sheridan, 1984).

SCHEMA THEORIES AND SENSORIMOTOR THEORIES

Another concept, *schema*, was to become significant in our understanding of information processing. In 1899, Woodworth and followers had enunciated the concept of schema as a set of rules serving as instructions for producing unique sequences of motor commands applicable to a variety of similar actions, referred to as a movement class. In 1977, Schmidt revived and expanded this concept in a schema theory. Schmidt emphasized the role of memory in motor learning and proposed the notion of two states of memory: recall and recognition schemas "stored" or programmed in the CNS as sets of rules. In the case of rapid, ballistic movements, motor experiences and memories would activate the recall schema (rule for movement production) and recognition schema (rule for establishing the relation between knowledge of the initial conditions, the environmental outcomes, and the expected sensory consequences for the purpose of response evaluation), resulting in the formation of motor learning structures.

From the original schema theory of Schmidt, certain predictions relating to motor learning have emerged: (1) practice variability promotes the building of a schema, especially for children; (2) after varied practice, novel responses in open-skills situations can be produced about as accurately as they can be after repeated practice (more so in children); and (3) the capability for error detection should exist mostly after fast movement and not after slow movement. In the latter case the recognition schema is said to be used to govern the ongoing production of the movement, leaving no more error detection capability after a slow movement (Schmidt, 2005).

To account for the great adaptability of the CNS, theorists attempted to combine the previous positions to develop what may be referred to as sensorimotor theories (Abbs et al., 1984; Marteniuk et al., 1988; Schmidt & Wrisberg, 2004). They maintained the concepts of *heterarchy, schema,* a form of *motor program,* and added an *ecologic element* (from evolving behavioral theories mentioned later). Concepts such as *feedforward* and *feedback* processes within the CNS were also included.

Feedforward processes involve preparation of the system for anticipated consequences of movements that, in part, provide a postural set. Feedback regarding what is happening (or has happened) makes possible changes or midcourse correction of movement to bring about convergence to a goal. If the movement occurs too quickly for feedback to be used effectively for correction during the course of a movement, feedback information can be used as instructional information in the planning of a more refined set of commands the next time.

A sensorimotor integration termed *multimovement coordination* is also proposed (Abbs et al., 1984; Marteniuk et al., 1988). Sensory events are coded in efferent terms, specific to each learned task, and have the function of modifying the central storage of information. Among other issues, contemporary theorists have attempted to resolve the problem of storage of large amounts of information in the CNS and the problem of coping with the immense and complex variability of parameters in movement production, referred to as degrees of freedom. To solve this problem, Asatryan and Feldman (1965) advanced the mass-spring model, which hypothesizes that equilibrium points between the torques of agonist and antago-

nist muscles are programmed for efficiency. In 1967, Bernstein revived the original Ferrier concept of *synergy,* a phenomenon in which groups of muscles and joints are coupled with a common pool of afferent and efferent information to produce coordinated patterns of movement. See Chapter 3 for further discussion of these concepts.

The development of instructional strategies paralleled the expansion of these integrative theories of motor control and motor learning. Emphasis on the role of memory outlined the significance of the cognitive element in motor learning. The constructs of schema and motor program reinforced the need for repetition to enhance motor learning. Finally, the concepts of coordinating multiple degrees of freedom and synergy brought a greater focus on action specificity in practice.

ECOLOGIC APPROACHES

Parallel to these developments and in reaction to the "habit" theory and information processing motor theories, Gibson (1966) and others (e.g., Turvey & Carello, 1986) proposed action systems or environment-related theories of motor control. For example, the direct perception theory (Michaels & Carello, 1981), a pure ecologic approach, considers the learning environment as specific to the child who actively and continuously explores and "picks up" the information "afforded" by the environment. Information is not presumed to be "processed" through memory or cognitive representation. Instead, according to the measure of attraction to the child, the biologic systems are said to "resonate" with the information the environment "broadcasts." According to this theory, perception and action form a closed unity; functional and relevant contexts for movement are therefore essential to promote motor learning.

Another aspect of this approach proposes that muscle groups and joints act as units, termed *muscle collectives or coordinative structures*; consequently, movements are said to be closely connected to the dynamic, mechanical properties of coordinative structures (e.g., length-tension and force-velocity relations), as opposed to a central representation. The formulation of these concepts has pointed toward more specific intervention strategies, such as (1) choosing or adapting individual, attractive sensorimotor environments; (2) acknowledging the child's interest in the selection of functional activities; and (3) promoting opportunities for muscle strengthening in particular needed ranges of movement, use of varied speeds, or coordinated movement patterns.

DYNAMIC SYSTEMS APPROACH

In the past two decades, further "action systems" have been proposed, but the latest theory developed, elaborated, and promoted is the dynamic pattern theory of Kelso and colleagues (Kelso, 1991; Scholz, 1990; Thelen et al., 1987), also referred to as the dynamical systems approach (Kamm et al., 1990). According to this theory, motor behavior is said to emerge from the dynamic cooperation of all subsystems within the context of a specific task: CNS, biomechanical, psychologic, and social-environmental components. Each component is perceived as necessary but insufficient to explain movement changes. Patterns of movement are portrayed not as rigidly fixed or programmed in the CNS but as flexible, adaptable, and dynamic, yet having "preferred" paths. Functional movement synergies are self-assembled according to the interaction between the environment and the individual's intention. The dynamic systems approach assumes that control is autonomous (a function of current state), emphasizes purposeful context more than instruction (cognition) as the driving force for motor behavior (motor learning), and stresses the study of movement pattern transitions ("phasing" phenomena) rather than regular, repetitive occurrences. These transitions are attributed to the nonlinear interactions among the system components. The phenomenon of "equifinality" (i.e., the attainment of a goal state despite perturbations) is underlined (Walter, 1998; Walter et al., 1998).

The identification of critical variables leading to motor changes or motor learning becomes the focus of dynamic systems theory. The provision of specific instructional strategies (verbal and nonverbal) to the learner is dependent on a detailed assessment, which includes (1) observable collective variables called *order parameters*, such as temporal and spatial phasing between limbs and interjoint relationships; and (2) the dynamics of variables called *control parameters*, such as speed, loudness of voice, or surface (Heriza, 1991; Scholz, 1990). A task-oriented approach is emphasized.

Other theories have also been proposed. For example, Willingham (1998) described a neuropsychologic theory of motor skill learning as a direct outgrowth of the motor control processes called COBALT (control-based learning theory). Cognitive components are said to be anatomically distinct and utilize different forms of representations. Action may be executed either in conscious, effortful mode or in an unconscious, automatic mode. Seiler (2000) expanded on earlier East-European theorists and presented the psychological action theory that emphasizes the intentions, anticipations, and perceptions of the learner. Actions may be regulated by the cognitive, the emotional, and the automated regulation systems. Further work on these and other variables will continue to expand our knowledge of motor learning and guide, to some extent, our therapeutic interventions by providing instructional models. Yet, to date, the dynamic systems approach remains the

primary focus of research to explore the complexity of motor learning.

MOTOR LEARNING CONSTRUCTS

Learning or relearning motor skills and improving the performance of motor skills are two main effects of practice of particular interest to physical therapists. Learning occurs through an interaction of external and internal factors that influence the ability to process information (Toglia, 1991). Motor learning refers to the increasing spatial and temporal accuracy of movements with practice (Willingham, 1998). It is considered a set of processes associated with practice that lead to relatively permanent changes in performance capability (Schmidt & Lee, 2005). That is, temporarily improved *performance* (related to transitory, fast changes) observed immediately following practice does not automatically equate to motor *learning* (related to persistent slow changes) or necessarily imply that learning has occurred (Newell et al., 2001). Age has been found to affect motor performance and learning but not the level of fitness of the learner (Etnier & Landers, 1998). Motor learning may be measured by the degree of long-term retention of performance capability, or the amount of transfer to different settings (near transfer), or to some different activity (far transfer). In therapeutic intervention, therefore, a conscious choice must be made between promoting motor learning and promoting performance; this choice determines the selection of instructional strategies. Furthermore, motor learning may occur through explicit learning (with instructions) and may also occur through implicit learning (without instructions and awareness of learning) (Pohl et al., 2001). Systems for guidance in the selection and organization of relevant strategies in a comprehensive, coherent, and practical way have resulted from the development of models of motor teaching.

MOTOR TEACHING MODELS

Models of motor teaching based on models of motor learning are few and relatively recent. They aim at improving the impact of motor teaching on persons with and without disabilities. The models have followed earlier work in the cognitive, educational domain. Orme's General Model of Teacher Behavior in Instruction (1978), including his series of practical teaching strategies, is one such source. Within this teaching model, the "teaching act" is described in six phases that are held to be necessary to elicit learning: (1) motivation, (2) presentation, (3) response guidance, (4) practice, (5) feedback, and (6) transfer. To be effective, these phases must be combined with arresting stimuli, including surprise, novelty, conflict, complexity, intensity, uncertainty, duration, and repetition. A close relationship exists between these cognitive concepts and those of the psychomotor-teaching models proposed by Gentile (1972, 1987), Marteniuk (1976, 1979), and Schmidt & Wrisberg (2004).

The Gentile (1987) model for acquisition of motor skills is based on the proposition that skill learning takes place in two stages: initial and late. In the initial stage of learning of motor skills, the learner discovers a reasonably effective approach to desired movement patterns. In the later stage, the learner concentrates on achieving *skilled* performance (i.e., goal attainment and economy of effort). The latter processes are said to be task dependent, changing according to the environmental context and the function of the action. It follows that instructional interventions should be based on the structure of the task and on the environmental context in which it is to be performed while assisting the learner in moving from the initial stage of motor learning to the stage of skill acquisition.

The information processes involved in Gentile's initial stage are also reflected in the Marteniuk model of motor teaching based on his description of information processes of motor skill acquisition in the Human Perceptual-Motor Performance Model (Marteniuk, 1976). Marteniuk recognizes attention (alertness) and anticipation (expectation) as being of utmost importance for CNS preparation to receive and process perceptual information. Preparation includes potential factors affecting arousal for the therapeutic instruction such as stimulus intensity, variety, complexity, uncertainty, and meaningfulness; induced muscle tension; and physical exertion. Thus perception, decision, and action form the three basic components of the model. The perceptual mechanisms include information detection, comparison and recognition of kinesthetic information, selective attention (through meaningfulness) and short-term memory (assisted by knowledge of performance [KP]), knowledge of result (KR), noninterference, motor sequencing, coding and "chunking," and rehearsal, all concepts that are discussed later in this chapter. The second component, the decision mechanism, is influenced by certain information characteristics and measured by the reaction time (RT), which is the interval of time between the presentation of an unanticipated stimulus and the initiation of a motor response. RT decreases with increased anticipation and with decreased temporal and spatial (event) uncertainty, amount of information, number of possible alternative movements, movement precision demand (e.g., target size), and directional accuracy demand (Schmidt & Wrisberg, 2004; Sideway, 1991). Other influential factors in decreasing RT are increased level of cognitive processes in mediating environmental stimuli and action, increased consistent practice, increased compatibility of information, and successively presented signals. Finally, the effector mechanism is said to contain a large number of motor commands; it organizes these commands to produce movement by activating muscles in correct sequential and temporal order.

Finally, Schmidt's Conceptual Model of Human Performance forms the basis for a series of comprehensive instructional strategies offered as guidelines (for able-bodied individuals) (Schmidt & Wrisberg, 2004). Three main areas are proposed for consideration in composing instructional strategies: (1) preparation and design of practice, (2) organization and scheduling of practice, and (3) feedback for skill learning. Relevant instructional strategies should be adapted to the learner's stage of learning, in this case, as defined by Fitts and Posner (1967): verbal-cognitive, motor, and autonomous stages. Figure 4-1 depicts the main elements of a motor teaching model.

A concise survey follows of the suggested, theoretically based strategies that have been studied with different populations by various investigators. The applicability of these strategies to the pediatric population has been tested in some cases, but in other cases is assumed and remains to be verified. Overall, there is a high degree of consensus about the appropriate use of strategies of motor teaching among the promoters of these strategies; minor conflicts exist in certain instances. In most cases, strategies aim at *explicit* motor learning.

MOTOR LEARNING AND TEACHING STRATEGIES

During a therapeutic session, each activity trial of the child becomes a unit of potential motor learning for which the therapist must decide on appropriate strategies. The selection of instructional strategies should reflect the *stage of learning* of the child (earlier or verbal-cognitive, associative, or later or motor, autonomous) and should be adapted to the motor task practiced (simple or complex). In addition, the potentially dichotomous goals of practice should be clear to the therapist: to optimize the child's *motor learning* (long-term retention and transfer to other tasks or settings) or the child's *motor performance* (greater ability within a task) during the treatment session. The specific goal of practice must be clear because

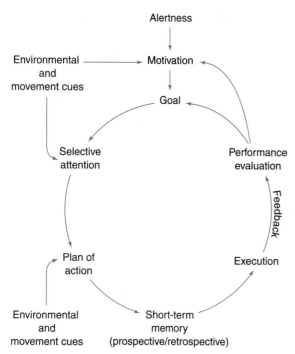

Alertness

Environmental and movement cues → Motivation

Goal

Selective attention

Performance evaluation

Plan of action

Feedback

Environmental and movement cues

Execution

Short-term memory (prospective/retrospective)

♦ **Figure 4-1**   Motor teaching model: information processes in motor learning.

instructional strategies effective in promoting retention of particular tasks, near transfer to a similar task, or far transfer to different activities will not necessarily lead to better performance during practice (Schmidt & Wrisberg, 2004). Furthermore, instructional strategies effective in promoting motor learning for simple tasks may greatly differ for complex tasks (Wulf & Shea, 2002). In addition, the therapist must consider three potential sensitive periods for instructional intervention: before, during, and after the execution of *each* activity trial, whether the activity is static or dynamic.

CONTEXT

Before and during a treatment session, the overall *context* must be set and remain adequate and conducive to the child's learning. To a high degree, therapists have been found to maintain a stimulating environment and to motivate the child through verbal and visual stimuli during a center-based treatment session (Carter, 1989; Larin, 1992).

The physical aspects of the environment must be considered. "Children learn more rapidly in stimulating and varied physical environments which meet basic human needs," including health and safety function, psychologic comfort, and aesthetic satisfaction, according to the "habitability" framework (Taylor & Gousie, 1988, p. 23). Because the physical aspects of the environment may be

potential stressors on the child, more or less noise, light, color, and space cannot be ignored and may exert a direct effect on the child's level of motivation during a treatment session. Understanding of the child's attentional abilities and level of sensory processing and organization, as well as the influence of the environmental changes on movement production, is also crucial in enabling the therapist to modify and adapt the environment appropriately and individually for each child (Cook Merrill et al., 1990). The fact that humans generally relate to surrounding environments in terms of their own body scales also needs to be considered (Warren, 1984).

Both children and adults have been found to respond positively to a multicontext treatment approach. In this approach, the individual is required to apply the newly learned skill to multiple situations (Toglia, 1991). Consequently, one goal is to bring the child to a "context-independent state," decreasing the likelihood of association between a particular piece of information and a particular context. However, children with disabilities have been found to demonstrate superior performance of skills in natural educational settings compared to an isolated therapy room (Karnish et al., 1995). Furthermore, children with developmental delay performed better in a one-to-one testing condition than in a structured game with peers (Doty et al., 1999). But individuals with severely limited physical and cognitive abilities who have demonstrated an increased level of goal attainment in a one-to-one therapy setting did not transfer the gains to their recess or home settings (Brown et al., 1998). An individual approach is warranted.

How to promote transfer from context-specific to context-independent function? In some clinical settings, an appropriate response has been the renovation of the traditional, contained treatment room with its standard equipment into various playground or household simulation contexts. Therapy may not begin and end at the threshold of a treatment room or even a treatment mat. The interaction milieu of home, school, and community remains the child's most functional context where varied practice and learning for transfer are most likely to occur.

Direct therapeutic intervention and program management ought to reflect this reality. For example, sitting in the waiting room, sitting for fine motor tasks or self-help, and sitting to pedal a tricycle become linked and provide real contexts for varied practice leading to motor learning of postural body control under a variety of conditions. Similarly, the same principle may be applied to climbing a bed, a chair, a step, or into someone's lap. Another aspect in using the "multicontext treatment approach" is to enhance movement that is of interest to the child. Engaging in social interaction with puppets, other children, or adults may modify a child's level of participation in an activity (positively or negatively, depending on interest level).

A combination of individual sessions and group of 2 (dyad) or more group treatment sessions may further increase motor learning of adult learners (McNevin et al., 2000). Group treatment sessions have been reported to be used by 68% of physical therapists in educational settings (Effgen & Klepper, 1994); 50% of therapists working with infants and young children provided combinations of individual and group treatment (Lawlor & Henderson, 1989). Yet limited information is available on the logistics and effectiveness of this approach in pediatrics.

Most therapy groups are informal—patients work on individual tasks or several patients are treated at the same time. Documentation is usually maintained on an individual rather than a group basis (Duncombe & Howe, 1995). Therapeutic factors that influence the outcome of group treatments have been identified in occupational therapy for patients with psychosocial disabilities (Falk-Kessler et al., 1991) but have not been fully investigated for clients with physical disabilities. Two small groups of preschool children with developmental delay demonstrated similar increases in both fine and gross motor skills from participating in either individual/direct therapy or group/consultation physical and occupational therapies (Davis & Gavin, 1994). School-age children with learning disabilities, however, were found to benefit significantly more from the large group and consultation intervention than from a combination of small and large group, therapist-directed intervention as measured by change on the Bruininks-Oseretsky Test of Motor Proficiency. Yet when the progress within each group was examined, both methods of service delivery were reported as effective for the particular group of students served (Palisano, 1989). In the adult population, the effectiveness of group education programs for low-back pain has yet to be demonstrated (Cohen et al., 1994), but group therapy has been found to be effective for individuals with hemiplegia, Parkinson disease, and multiple sclerosis (Duncombe & Howe, 1995). Clients in group therapy achieved their maximum goal earlier than individually treated clients and maintained their functional status; group therapy was also found to be more cost-effective (Duncombe & Howe, 1995; Trahey, 1991). Appropriate motor learning strategies must be considered in the delivery of group intervention design. Further investigations are needed on delivery models, functional outcomes, and cost-effectiveness of dyad and group therapy for children with physical disabilities.

The sociocultural-educational aspect of the context that pertains to the quality of the instructor-learner interaction also affects the child's learning with respect to the amount and type of information transmitted (Simpson & Galbo, 1986). Effective *learning contexts* are those that promote initiations by the learner, reciprocity and shared control over the interaction between the less skilled (child) and the more skilled (therapist) party, and provision of responsive or content feedback rather than simply corrective feedback to the learner. In such contexts, children, whether mildly or moderately disabled, may gain more control over their own learning and reduce their level of dependence on adult control (Glynn, 1985).

The therapist seeks an integration and a balance between the dichotomous roles of playmate and instructor in his or her therapeutic intervention with the child. The playmate's role must feel genuine and pleasing to the child, and the instructor's role denotes supportive, confident, and effective guidance/ assistance toward improved capabilities with a shared control of decision making. Therapeutic power is real and must be used with prudence. For example, the therapist may offer predetermined choices of activities to the child or take turns with the child in the decision-making process in an obvious, concrete, fair manner; above all, the therapist should address the child within the "higher-order thinking skills" of the child (Ritson, 1987) and incorporate risk-taking behaviors (Cintas, 1992) appropriate and relevant to the child. In a treatment session, this may translate into the therapist's setting a challenging game, verbalizing the action or movement goal, and/or providing some timely, explicit feedback to the child, in spite of the child's minimal or delayed verbal and nonverbal communication skills and while being acutely attentive to the child's level of active participation.

MOTIVATION AND PRIOR KNOWLEDGE

In the pretask execution period, the child should gain *motivation* and clear, purposeful *prior knowledge* of the activity through auditory, visual, or proprioceptive signals (Higgins, 1991). The instructional strategies that relate to motivation include, for instance, action goal setting, preferably by or in conjunction with the child; selective attention (e.g., instructions, demonstration-modeling, and interference); and rehearsal (e.g., mental practice or describing the actions to be done).

Motivated learning is intentional learning for improvement. The learner must have (1) the perception of a skill as meaningful, useful, desirable, and having personal implications; (2) the experience of satisfaction from executing a movement; and (3) encouragement toward higher, achievable goals after task execution. The therapist may indirectly but positively influence the child's personal goals, self-perceptions, and cognitive-affective experiences through verbal and nonverbal communication. For example, counting out loud (with a meaningful tone of voice) the seconds spent in stride-standing, moving back and forth to place a basketball in the basket, marking points, and raising the basket or stepping back a step are ways to further challenge the child. Such strategies, however, may not be successful in motivating all children in spite of similar cognitive levels.

Motivated learning is an individual process. According to Ratner and Foley (1994), to facilitate children's "activity memory" (an integrated part of learning), emphasis must be placed on the individual's goals within a person-based perspective. All four features of the activities should be considered: outcomes, relational structure (between the activity and the learner), prospective processes (characteristics of anticipation and planning), and retrospective activation (repetition). To optimize this process of motivation leading to activity memory and motor learning, further insight is necessary into the learner's individual motivational variables relevant to physical skills; movement behavior in different contexts; and personal strategies, thoughts, and emotional responses during the learning process (Pohl et al., 1992). Therapists need to assess patients' motivation efficiently. Yet, until a valid and reliable tool is developed, therapists will continue to rely on general discussion, observation of conduct and actions, and information from others to assess motivation (Carlson, 1997).

Creative Behavior

Besides altering context, encouraging creative behaviors is a powerful means of enhancing the child's motivation. These behaviors primarily include fluency (e.g., movement variability); flexibility (e.g., movement independence); originality (e.g., in movement sequences); and elaboration. To gain fluency, the child needs to solve the same movement problem or goal through a number of different organizational approaches (i.e., motor equivalence). For example, the practice of going up the stairs for a child who has not yet mastered this skill may involve supervised creeping on hands and knees, hands and feet, sideways cruising up while holding onto the rail, and forward walking up with assistance (a device or manually). Promoting flexibility in therapy could entail allowing and acknowledging a child's independent thinking and creative movement response. Providing some basic movement information to the child, such as "Let's find a way to twist your shoulders," may support this behavior as well as allow originality in the child's movement sequences and may result in the production of a completely novel response. Such an approach is supported by Gibson's (1988) concept of "exploration" described as an active process with a perceptual, cognitive, and motor aspect.

Asking appropriate questions that require the child to think at his or her cognitive level and to perform the results of that thought process may lead to the fourth factor of movement creativity—elaboration. Such motor instructional strategies that go beyond the command style and promote process-oriented rather than product-oriented approaches constitute in themselves sources of motivation and enhance the desired, perceived internal control of the child (Ritson, 1987).

Goal Setting

Setting goals is another major, motivational, and knowledge-based instructional strategy available for use during a therapy session. First the therapist must consider the child's social characteristics, such as gender, age, cultural background, and personal socialization experiences, because these factors have been found to modify the learning of fundamental motor skills in young children (Garcia, 1994). For example, knowing that children up to the age of approximately 11 tend to hold "mastery goals" may guide the therapist in providing self-referenced achievement tasks rather than social comparison. In addition, the therapist's assessment of the child's cognitive ability to understand the task or goal will have a direct impact on potential learning of motor skills. Realizing that immediate social environmental conditions can override some preexisting goals of the child, the therapist may choose to provide a goal. Two types of goals may be provided: the goal may be related to the action (e.g., "Let's go slide") or to the movement itself, in this case, climbing the steps leading to the slide (e.g., "Let's see you bring one foot up very high and quickly"). As observed in Larin's (1992) study, therapists offered a verbal goal in 44 to 88% (average, 75%) of the activity trials during treatment sessions; the action goal accounted for 43% and the movement goal made up 47% of the verbal goals.

It is recommended that either type of goal be specific, consistent, attainable, and short in duration and that the standards be high enough to foster improved performance but not so high as to provoke discouragement by repeated failure (Edwards, 1988; Jones & Cale, 1997). Error awareness is a necessary element of the learning process. To ensure a successful learning experience, however, the therapist should guide the learner to make a decision on (evaluate) the environmental goal or related movement in a systematic, comparative fashion. Gentile (1972) suggests such an approach:

- If a goal and movement are successful, use repetition.
- If a goal is unsuccessful in spite of apparent good movement, help the learner in identifying relevant environmental conditions.

- If a goal is successful but the movement produced a surprise success, describe the movement to the learner.
- If both the goal and the movement are unsuccessful, encourage the learner and analyze further the task at hand.

Overall, the therapist should continue to explore movement options with the learner until repeated success in both movement and goal attainment are achieved. The use of movement scripts (i.e., chunks of typical patterns associated with specific movement functions and dysfunctions) may assist physical therapists to focus the intervention and assist the learner to successfully reach the goals and learn the intended movements (Embrey & Hylton, 1996).

Another useful tactic of the therapist is to ask the learner to set the goal, supporting principles of client-centered practice. Children as young as 5 years old can accurately report perceived competence through the use of pictorial items. Children with neurodevelopmental problems are also able to use the information to set goals for therapy (although priorities may differ from their parents' reports) (Missiuna & Pollock, 2000).

Movements "preselected" by the child result in greater goal clarity, increased energy production, and success, as well as superior reproduction of movements as compared with "constrained" movements selected by the instructor (Lewthwaite, 1990; Runnings & Diewert, 1982; Sage, 1984; Schempp, 1983; Schmidt, 2005). Preselection by the child has been found to be especially effective for children with low ability (Goldberger & Gerney, 1990). Once again, the experience of personal "locus of control" during an instructional session is of great importance for motor learning (Coster & Jaffe, 1991).

INSTRUCTIONS

The therapist's instructions before practice are critical for motivational purposes but also as feedforward input to convey information about the task requirements, particularly if the task is complex (Wulf & Shea, 2002). This information may include a description of the task based on the learner's competencies, as well as on relevant environmental elements. The information may be verbally presented, nonverbally modeled, or both (Schmidt & Wrisberg, 2004). The therapist's verbal instructions have the potential to bring the child's *attention* to different levels of information about a movement task. This information is closely associated with feedback information and with the environment. Examples of different levels of information used to focus the child on reaching include the following (Newell et al., 1990):

1. Intrinsic, sensorimotor information may address precise muscle-response organization. Example: "Feel the muscles of your toes and legs pushing hard as you reach up" (*internal focus*).
2. Movement patterns or performance direction such as segmental body organization may be provided. Example: "Bring your arm up, elbow straight, and open your hands to reach up" (*internal focus*).
3. The end result in the form of the action goal may activate the desired pattern of movement (reaching up). Example: "Let's decorate the top of the mirror" (*external focus*).
4. Environmental information related to the action may guide the child's visual and auditory attentiveness. Example: "The mirror is taller than you and is on wheels; the decorations are sticky and a bit heavy" (*external focus*).

Appropriate instruction can enhance the child's selective attention and foster his or her ability to separate task-relevant information from task-irrelevant information, an integral part of the motor learning process based on Gibson's (1969) processes of perceptual learning: abstraction, filtering of irrelevant variables, and selective attention. With regard to the developmental, restrictive scanning strategies of younger children (Vurpillot, 1968), Stratton (1978) believes that lack of training and experience rather than processing capacity is the cause of children's deficits in information processing and attention capability. Children deserve to be given a chance to acquire strategies for improved selective attention.

Along with instruction, distractions may be provided. Interferences, such as people talking or walking or the therapist referring to other activities, may be presented to the child; these distractions simulate a real-world environment. Random practice, which will be discussed later, can also be considered as another source of contextual interference. Introducing this strategy early in the learning situation appears to produce the best results in improved ability to deal with irrelevant information (Stratton, 1978). Children with neurologic impairment, however, may display sensorivisual loss and cognitive deficits in the selective attentional system (Hood & Atkinson, 1990). Such a tactic, of course, must be used carefully with these children, for whom the addition of extraneous information may be overwhelming and counterproductive.

If explicit, verbal instructions are used about the motor activity (prior knowledge), first, instructions about the entire movement should be offered, describing the same speed and accuracy required in the desired skill (Gentile, 1987). According to the child's level of selective attention and capability of processing information, the therapist has the option to break down the verbal instructions, with an initial emphasis on only one or two essential/critical elements of the skill; brevity and meaningfulness are important in this case. Minimal guidance from research is available because only limited data have been gathered on individual needs and the complexity and distribution of instructions appropriate for different age groups.

A combination of distance and location information, however, has been found to allow greater accuracy of movement reproduction, whether the movement practiced is active or passive (Runnings & Diewert, 1982). Furthermore, initial, specific information can be long-lasting: emphasis on accuracy leads to improved accuracy, and emphasis on speed leads to improved speed (Schmidt & Lee, 2005). Allowing further trial-and-error (no prompting) attempts before providing feedback or further instructions has also been reported to be superior to use of a guiding stimulus (prompting) exclusively. Children with learning disorders (cognitive and motor) may benefit from the same opportunity.

Verbal prompting is a useful strategy but should not be provided in proportion to the learning difficulty (Koegel & Rincover, 1976). Adults can enhance their learning and performance if they use an external focus rather than an internal focus on their own movements (Wulf & Shea, 2002). Children with CP have been reported to respond with greater movement excursions (forearm pronation or supination) to concrete instructions (e.g., "Bang the drums"), rather than abstract instructions (e.g., "Turn the handle back and forth as far as possible") when compared with nondisabled children, who showed no difference between tasks (van der Weel et al., 1991). Consequently, instructions aimed at the learner's attention need to be carefully selected and adapted to the child's capabilities. Adolescents with severe intellectual limitations have been found to complete motor skills in lesser time when a constant-time delay (CTD) was introduced (i.e., insertion of a fixed amount of time between a cue to perform a skill and a prompt to assist the learner) (Zhang et al., 2000).

Nonverbal prompting should also be considered. Particularly for motor skill acquisition and retention of task processing occurring in the nondominant hemisphere, facilitating attention with a combination of verbal and nonverbal strategies to the skill has been found to bring higher outcomes. A rationale is proposed: interhemispherical transfer promotes motor learning (Fairweather & Sidaway, 1994).

OBSERVATIONAL LEARNING

Observational learning (demonstration or modeling) may complement or replace verbal instructions particularly for the learning of complex skills (Wulf & Shea, 2002). Children tend to be more visually dependent than adults, who rely more on a combination of proprioceptive and visual input (Shumway-Cook & Woollacott, 1985). Observational motor learning is thus an effective strategy for developing the perceptual skills necessary for children to selectively attend to environmental cues (Arend, 1980). In addition, observational motor learning is said to improve performance, learning, and self-confidence in young children (Weiss et al., 1998). Modeling is task-specific and may be enhanced by verbal labeling (including spatial and temporal information [Schmidt & Lee, 2005]), rehearsal, temporal spacing of demonstrations, and verbal pre-training (i.e., the child verbally cueing himself or herself about movement demands) (Gould & Roberts, 1982). With low-skilled subjects, however, peer modeling (i.e., watching an unskilled person learning a motor skill) has been found to be more effective than instructor modeling (Schmidt & Lee, 2005). Effective use of modeling is said to include an initial series of demonstrations (before practice) followed by further demonstrations in the early stage of practice (Weeks & Anderson, 2000).

Therapists were observed to use demonstrations minimally in the treatment of preschool children with a diagnosis of CP, although they claimed greater use with children 6 years of age and older (Larin, 1992). Coordinating therapy sessions among therapists with similar children to encourage reciprocal peer modeling is a potentially valuable tool for motor learning as discussed earlier under dyad and group therapy. Wulf and Shea (2002) also suggest combining observation and physical practice to further increase motor learning.

PURPOSEFUL TASKS

"Given appropriate tasks and sufficiently guided practice, gross motor skill learning in young children can be effectively enhanced through planned instruction" (Haubenstricker & Seefeldt, 1986, p. 65). Purposeful tasks are more appropriate than reflexive or passive behaviors (Bernstein, 1967). Purposeful tasks are active, voluntarily regulated (from initiation to termination), goal directed (Croce & DePaepe, 1989), and meaningful to the learner (Ratner & Foley, 1994; van der Weel et al., 1991). Heart rates and perceived exertion ratings are significantly lower during purposeful tasks than during nonpurposeful activities (Bakshi et al., 1991). In addition, the individual's freely chosen work rate (preferred rhythm) has been found to be the most efficient for performance across a variety of tasks (Fetters, 1991; Sparrow, 1983), particularly for 5-year-old children (Williams, 1985). Purposeful tasks of individuals with neuromotor disorders, however, do not necessarily lead to the same level of movement efficiency achieved by nondisabled individuals. Gait studies in children with CP, for example, have revealed reduced muscle activity, uneven kinetic energy patterns, and mechanical energy cost above normal values (Olney, 1989). Similar findings were also reported in a study of the kinematics and kinetics of running in children with CP (Davids et al., 1998). More recently, Valvano (2004) proposed a model of practice for children with neurologic conditions that integrates activity-focused and impairment-focused interventions. Fell (2004) also described a conceptual framework with parameters that can be used to adjust or progress interventions and include motor learning.

The "will to act" on the part of the learner builds up over a long time before a movement begins (120 ms); in fact it is longer than reaction time to a stimulus (30 to 80 ms) (Kelso, 1991). Hence, the pretask period is important for information processing, decision making, and response programming. The ability to rapidly process information increases progressively up to 18 years of age, reducing response latency (Clark, 1982); this phenomenon has been found to be more prevalent in males than females (Thomas et al., 1981). In addition, the speed of the reaction time is related to a series of factors, as previously mentioned. Both children's and adults' most accurate anticipations, when confronted with velocity problems, are made when they experience them in the context of their daily activities (Wade, 1980), a natural phenomenon referred to as stimulus-response compatibility (Schmidt & Wrisberg, 2004). Functional, ecologic, relevant goals elicit faster and smoother movements than nonfunctional goals (Lin et al., 1998). Certain biomechanical parameters have also been identified as decisive in achieving optimum anticipatory postural adjustments and motor outcome, for example, configuration of the base of support before moving (Brenière et al., 1987) or in regaining balance (Tarantola et al., 1997). Moreover, feedback anticipation seems to emerge from feedback experiences (Haas et al., 1989). The degree of anticipatory response increases with age. Ten-year-olds have shown more anticipatory responses than 7-year-olds, who show more than 4-year-olds (Thomas & Nelson, 2001). Individuals with motor coordination problems, however, take longer to organize and initiate movement sequences (Piek & Skinner, 1999) particularly when processing proprioceptive information (not visual information) (Smyth & Glencross, 1986). Children with CP show deficits in the sensorimotor organization and muscular coordination of their anticipatory activities (Duff & Gordon, 1998; Nashner et al., 1983); they tend to compensate with early onset of force production and overall high force outputs (Eliasson et al., 1991, 1992).

Based on this research, the therapist should promote practice of relevant, functional, purposeful tasks; use spatial and temporal anticipation strategies to increase the readiness of the child to respond (i.e., informing the child of what will occur [and when]); and use routine rather than random activities to influence reaction time and facilitate anticipation skills (Schmidt & Wrisberg, 2004) necessary for the development of activity memory (Ratner & Foley, 1994). Permitting information processing to occur requires a "waiting" period on the part of the therapist. Therapists have been observed waiting for the child's action or reaction in an average of 66% of activity trials in a treatment session (range, 48%–93%). Most therapists (85% of the sample) were aware of their use of this strategy, but various rationales were offered (Larin, 1992). This strategy may be applied in mental and physical practice.

KINESTHETIC MENTAL PRACTICE

Practice is usually thought of as being physical (i.e., execution of a task with one's body); however, both physical and mental practice are useful strategies of motor teaching. Both produce a similar, dynamic pattern of cortical activation when performed. Furthermore, a combination of mental and physical practice seems to be the most productive (Jackson et al., 2001). Mental practice is also called *cognitive rehearsal* or *imagery practice*. Kinesthetic mental practice is the act of repeating the imagined movements several times with the intention of learning a new ability or perfecting a known skill (Ravey, 1998); it is imagining one's correct performance of a motor task without any associated overt movement. This strategy has been mainly designated as an end result of practice, but it may be used in the pretask or post-task execution period, or between physical trials to enhance performance over motor learning. Using 3 to 5 minutes of mental practice, beginners and highly skilled performers have been reported to benefit from this type of practice, particularly in correcting errors in execution, increasing concentration, and strategy rehearsal. Random imagery practice has been found to facilitate kinesthetic retention better than blocked imagery (Gabriele et al., 1987). Alternating actual practice and imagery practice has also been found to facilitate motor learning more than alternating actual practice and rest (Kohl et al., 1992). Mental practice can also be left to the learner to use outside the coaching sessions.

Kinesthetic mental practice may also increase speed (Rawlings et al., 1972, in Maring, 1990), endurance (Lee, 1990), balance (Fansler et al., 1985), accuracy and efficiency (Maring, 1990), and potentially isometric muscle strength (Cornwall, 1991; Yue & Cole, 1992). A group of adolescents with mild cognitive impairments performed with significantly greater accuracy and less variability when combining physical practice with imagery rather than using physical practice alone (Poretta & Surburg, 1995; Surburg et al., 1995). Adults with Huntington's disease increased their performance after a 10-minute training period using motor imaging, but adults with Parkinson's disease did not (Yaguez et al., 1999). Individuals with cortical and subcortical damage may therefore have reduced ability to produce the appropriate imaginary process and need to be assessed before this strategy is implemented. Schmidt & Wrisberg (2004) indicated that prior experience might be necessary for effective use of mental practice. Despite the usefulness of mental practice, however, the emphasis should be on physical practice during a session (Feltz & Landers, 1983). The features of the activities (i.e., outcome, relation to learner, anticipation, and repetition) remain crucial to regulate and reflect the execution and interpretation of an act (Ratner & Foley, 1994) and to promote motor learning.

Therapists generally do not use much mental practice in intervention. Having a child anticipate a movement through mental practice is not considered a concrete enough activity for children younger than 5 years of age. When employed, however, therapists have reported using it occasionally with older children in practicing specific gross motor tasks, such as wheelchair transfers (Larin, 1992). Fazio (1992) presented an overview of "guided affective imagery" as an adjunct to a stimulating treatment approach. Given that planning a movement is, in itself, beneficial to motor learning, therapists may find that mental practice (adapted to the child's cognitive level) may be particularly effective in early practice. Findings with young adults (Schmidt & Lee, 2005) and with children 9 to 10 years old (Jarus & Ratzon, 2000) have pointed in this direction. For example, the therapist might say, "Let's think how it feels when you…, first you…, then you…," or "Try to imagine you watch yourself on television," or "Pretend you are doing it like in a dream, close your eyes…" Children should be given the opportunity to experience and learn from mental practice.

PHYSICAL PRACTICE: DETERMINANTS OF EFFECTIVENESS

Physical practice remains essential to motor learning. Information processing demands vary with the type of task, making task classification taxonomies useful as an adjunct to planning a developmentally appropriate motor learning program. Purposeful tasks have been classified as continuous, serial, or discrete; open or closed; and complex or simple (Schmidt, 2005; Schmidt & Wrisberg,

2004) (Table 4-1). In practice, based on the selected criterion (goal) and purposeful tasks, the therapist needs to address repetitions, task sequencing, scheduling of practice and fatigue effect, degrees of variability, physical guidance, and feedback.

Repetition

Repetitions lead to the acquisition of a motor skill if they occur under conditions that most closely resemble those normally encountered during the performance of that skill. Through repetition children have shown considerable improvement, as compared with older individuals, in learning a demanding movement (Nicolson, 1982). Three-month-old infants learned to kick and activate a mobile (Ohr et al., 1989) and infants 5 to 10 months old accelerated the development of their sitting postural responses with training (Hadders-Algra et al., 1996). Infants with Down syndrome learned to walk independently significantly faster following supported practice of stepping on a miniature treadmill (Ulrich et al., 2001). Children with motor delay and children with a diagnosis of CP have yielded similar findings from intensive, individual physical therapy sessions (Bower & McLellan, 1992; Mayo, 1991). Furthermore, in Horn and colleagues' (1999) study on the effects of a neurobehavioral intervention, young children with severe CP demonstrated gains in the acquisition of specific movement components of treated and untreated skills, as well as in the generalization of skills to a different environment. Repetitions, however, need to be sequenced and scheduled according to the child's capabilities.

Sequencing

The sequencing of tasks plays an important role in motor learning and teaching. Different paradigms exist for sequencing tasks and instructions effectively. Gentile's (1987, 1992) taxonomy of tasks is one guide for the examination of a child's functional abilities and response to task demands, for the selection of functionally appropriate activities, and for planning therapeutic interventions. Progression may require modifications of the activities in several directions on the taxonomy template. Table 4-2 provides a series of examples in which both body status and environmental context are considered. Knowledge of movement scripts (i.e., chunks of typical patterns of movement) may further assist physical therapists in performing these complex tasks (Embrey & Hylton, 1996). However, in sports, learners who self-selected the order in which they practiced the different versions of a task performed better than blocked and random groups (Titzer et al., 1993).

Other systems also exist to assist practitioners in the sequencing of motor skill learning. Bressan and Woollacott

TABLE 4-1   Task Classification: Types, Characteristics, and Implications

TYPE	CONTINUOUS	DISCRETE	SERIAL	OPEN	CLOSED	COMPLEX	SIMPLE
Characteristics	Series of ongoing modifications	Minimal feedback information effect	Combination of continuous and discrete	Constant, unpredictable, and uncertain environment	Stable predictable environment	Requires more coordination or more body parts	Requires less coordination and fewer body parts
	No recognizable beginning or end	Recognizable beginning and end		Need to adapt behavior to changing environment	Allow advance organization of movement	Requires longer time to initiate	Requires less time to initiate
	Longer movement time Fatiguing	Shorter movement time Minimal fatigue		Cannot effectively plan the response (on the spot decisions)	Can plan in advance Can learn with practice		
	Example: swim, run	Example: kick, write signature		Example: walk and step over obstacle	Example: put hat on		
Practical, instructional implications	Focus = sensory information and how to modify	Focus = pre-planning and production No attempt to modify during movement		Focus = nature of environment (try to learn irregularities)	Focus = generation of preprogrammed actions	Focus = keep arousal level fairly low	Focus = bring up arousal level
	More time for rest between trials	Less time for rest Increased number of trials		Variable practice Flexibility	Stability and consistency	More attention to describe and demonstrate Provide more feedback Budget more time	More direct practice repetitions Provide less feedback
	Error detection *during* movement	Develop error detection through own response-produced feedback *after* movement					

TABLE 4-2 **Gentile's Taxonomy of Tasks: Examples of Therapeutic Activities**

| | BODY STABILITY | | BODY IN MOTION | |
ENVIRONMENTAL CONTEXT	NO MANIPULATION	WITH MANIPULATION	NO MANIPULATION	WITH MANIPULATION
Stationary and no trial variability				
Stationary and trial variability				
Motion and no trial variability				
Motion and trial variability				

(1982) proposed a paradigm in which skill construction, stabilization, and differentiation represent phases in the progressive control of the muscle synergies' program for motor skill acquisition. Wickstrom (1977) and Roberton and Halverson (1977) broke down skills into components of movement (intratask) and determinants of movement sequences relevant to other tasks (intertask), the former leading to the latter. In 1991, Davis and Burton proposed an ecologic task analysis system based on the dynamic relationship between task environmental and performer factors. They suggested four instructional guidelines: (1) identify the task in terms of function (rather than perfection), (2) allow the learner choices and freedom to use movements, (3) identify and manipulate the relevant and critical task dimensions and performer's variables, and (4) provide direct instruction on the movement pattern using performer-scaled or intrinsic units of measure (e.g., ratio, rather than comparative, normative units).

Overall task sequencing has been considered according to various dimensions: general or specific, more or less complex, blocked or random, and part or whole. Schema theory supports the approach of developing a general base of motor activities before developing specific skilled activities (Kerr, 1978) for both open and closed skills.

More versus Less Complex

Referring to children with delayed development, Croce and DePaepe (1989) have suggested teaching sequentially less complex patterns before more complex skills. Winstein (1991b), however, has cautioned against reducing the difficulty of a task to the point at which the inherent nature of the task is altered. Such a practice could be detrimental to transfer of motor learning to the intended task. For example, emphasizing weight shift in standing as a subtask of locomotion did not achieve improved gait in adults with hemiparesis (Winstein et al., 1989), nor did a sitting activity heel-up heel-down rhythm task modify gait (Seitz & Wilson, 1987). In pediatrics, the use of infant walkers was not found to accelerate the onset or the quality of children's walking patterns (Kauffman & Ridenour, 1977).

One might extrapolate that children may not learn to kick in a standing position from practicing kicking in a sitting position or even performing pendular movements of the lower extremity in one-leg standing. Research results, however, are not entirely consistent with this view. Weight-bearing activities of the upper extremities have been reported to improve target-throwing skills in children 5 to 7 years of age with sensory integration disorders (Jarus & Gol, 1995). Using a specially designed tricycle to encourage hip extension resulted in improved gait in children with CP (King et al., 1993). Choosing and sequencing

tasks in a therapy session remains a complex yet important determinant of a child's motor learning. Clearly, more research is indicated.

In general, therapists have been reported to adhere, more or less consciously, to the concepts of general or specific and more or less complex task sequencing based on maturational and developmental theories (Larin, 1992). For example, a therapist may promote gross mobility before specific gait activities (e.g., initial heel contact), practice walking while holding onto a ball before free walking, or practice independent forward directional progression before changes of direction.

Blocked versus Random

The organization of task sequencing may be "blocked," that is, practiced in drill-type repetition in which all trials of a given task are completed before another task is undertaken (intratask processing), or in "random" sequence (i.e., mixed repetition of various tasks [intertask processing]). Random sequencing, however, has proved more beneficial than blocked sequencing for motor learning, as measured on retention tests of simple motor skills in adults. Random sequencing requires a greater number of trials than blocked practice, however, and typically degrades performance during the practice session; hence the acquisition-retention paradox known as the *contextual interference effect* (Fineman & Gentile, 1998; Schmidt & Lee, 2005; Shea & Morgan, 1979). The facilitative effect of high contextual interference has been related to an increase in task difficulty during practice that requires a higher level of attention (see earlier section on instructions) (Smith, 1997).

Blocked practice, however, is more effective than random practice in the early, verbal-cognitive stage of motor learning for novices, and for the learning of complex motor skills. Wulf and Shea (2002) reviewed a series of studies with children that indicated that random practice could be too demanding (attention, memory, motor) and less effective for learning complex skills, causing an "overload" of the system. Consequently, blocked practice was found more effective for this population.

One may conclude that, during a treatment session, it is important for the therapist to regard the sequencing of repetitions as a means to (1) explore movement options until there are one or more occurrences of total success (Gentile, 1987) and (2) practice several block or random skills accordingly. When random practice is used, the therapist should explain the paradoxic phenomenon to the adolescent or caregiver (i.e., the trade-off between poorer, immediate performance versus long-term learning and retention performance) as it is likely to affect motivation and motor learning. In general, however, therapists who stress the importance of repetition and claim to use this strategy have been observed to practice, on average, only four repetitions per activity, whether in a blocked or random sequencing (Larin, 1992). The principle of variety appears independent from and of higher order than the principle of repetition.

Part versus Whole

The sequence of the components of a task may also be presented in "parts" or as a "whole," depending on the nature of the skill. For rapid, discrete skills of short duration (less than 1 second), practice of the whole task from the outset leads to the best results. If the learner has the prerequisite skills to master the new skill in its entirety, or if the degree of cognitive processing is minimal, the "whole" method is reported to be far superior to one based on "parts" (Croce & DePaepe, 1989). The same approach applies to slower, serial, and continuous skills of long duration (more than 10 seconds). For very complex tasks, the most time-efficient approach is to first practice the most troublesome parts of the task. *Progressive part practice* follows to gradually integrate the parts as acquired into the whole task so as to minimize transfer problems between the two (Schmidt & Lee, 2005). According to the *specificity of learning hypothesis*, intertask transfer between two tasks does not happen or is very small even if the two tasks are different in only very minor ways. It is therefore essential to use correct techniques during practice to master a motor skill (Ashy et al., 1988). To do so, it seems imperative for the therapist to differentiate skill characteristics and adopt the use of a taxonomy to guide practice.

Scheduling

Scheduling of practice trials remains somewhat controversial. In general, "distributed" practice (i.e., when the amount of rest between trials equals or exceeds the amount of time in a trial) has been found to improve performance; and "massed" practice (i.e., when the amount of practice time in a trial is greater than the amount of rest between trials) enhances learning, in spite of fatigue (Gentile, 1987). Schmidt and Lee (2005), however, indicated that distributed practice facilitates both performance and learning more than massed practice for continuous tasks. More specifically, massed practice is advocated for discrete tasks, in which the skill level of the learner is higher and in which peak performance on a well-learned skill is needed. For continuous tasks, however, only slight negative effects of massed practice on learning are reported. In this case, distributed practice over a long time period is most beneficial because the tasks require greater energy expenditures. The same is true for complex tasks and in the presence of a lower level of motivation from the learner (Sage, 1984).

Realistically, motor activities are usually performed under gradually increasing amounts of fatigue; Schmidt & Wrisberg (2004) suggested that, to be effective, practice must be somewhat difficult and effortful. Studies to date offer mixed results with regard to the effect of fatigue on skill acquisition and transfer performance (Arnett et al., 2000). For children with CP, increased fatigue caused by repetition of activities has been found to be associated with progress toward certain motor goals (Bower & McLellan, 1992). One concludes that some degree of fatigue is a necessary element in motor learning and should be explained to the child and caregiver. Therapists must ensure (1) that the child's nutritional status, particularly the iron level, is adequate to sustain the physical performance and endurance required (Lozoff, 1989); (2) that treatment sessions contain sufficient rest to remain energizing and challenging for the child; (3) that treatment sessions are safe, avoiding accidents; and (4) that the child's post-training night sleep is optimal to ensure consolidation of motor learning (i.e., that stage 2 non–rapid eye movement sleep is obtained during the last quarter of the night) (Walker et al., 2002).

In therapy sessions as in sport training, practice periods tend to vary in length; no single, optimal practice/rest ratio has been determined to be most effective in maximizing learning in all types of tasks. Each task must therefore be analyzed, and the analysis used to guide decisions about practice scheduling. The issue of practice distribution and total practice involves *trade-off*. Distributed practice is said to result in the most learning per time in training while requiring the most total time to complete. Massed practice results in reduced benefits per time in training but requires the least total time (Schmidt & Lee, 1999, p. 297).

Variability

Another determinant of motor learning is the amount of variability—rehearsal of many variations of the same movement class. Actions within a movement class are said to share a particular relative timing and similar sequences of movements (Schmidt & Wrisberg, 2004): for example, clapping hands and making music, banging objects together, or altering a parameter or a part of an action such as throwing (e.g., higher, faster, longer). The conditions under which a task is learned affect the ability to navigate in error fields; the more "noise," the more rapid the learning of a new task with similar error structure (Newell & Corcos, 1993). There are two main purposes for using variability: first, to enhance generalizability and adaptability when one task-practice contributes to the performance of another in the same class of movement; and, second, to establish competence throughout a dimension (i.e., altering either distance, speed, direction, or timing) while maintaining the same fundamental pattern.

Use of variability as a teaching strategy has been more effective for children and female subjects than for male adults (Sage, 1984; Schmidt & Lee, 2005). Overall, low-variable practice (overlearning through practice of the same task) translates into greater performance on the practiced task; this outcome has also been found to apply to individuals with learning disabilities performing a serial-type motor skill (Heitman et al., 1997). High-variable practice yields high performance on task transfer within a similar movement class (Carson & Wiegand, 1979; Shea & Kohl, 1990) and better retention of learning when skill variations are from different classes of movement (Hall & Magill, 1995), as long as the tasks are similar to (and "surrounded by") the criterion task. However, there appears to be a point of threshold of the variability (Goodwin et al., 1998). High-variable practice leads to more generalizability, adaptability, and competence throughout a dimension (i.e., distance, speed, direction, or timing) while maintaining the same fundamental pattern. A caveat is that "similar" may mean different things at different ages (van Rossum, 1980); the breadth of a class of "similar" movements under a given motor program remains equivocal (Schmidt, 1977). For example, slowing down a movement too much might destroy its essential dynamics (Fetters, 1991; VanSant, 1990). Yet Horn and colleagues (1999) found that children 18 to 39 months old were able to generalize movement components to an untreated, related skill from a skill gained during sessions in which neurodevelopmental and behavioral approaches were used and skills practiced concurrently.

Optimum variability of practice for open or closed motor skills also differs. For open tasks, practice should be diversified, providing the learner with variations encountered in the habitual environment. However, Eidson and Stadulis (1991) reported no significant effect from the type of practice for an open skill in children with a moderate mental disability; variable practice, however, reduced error in a closed skill. Latash and colleagues (2002) also found that using variable tasks in practice was effective in improving finger coordination in a group of young adults with Down syndrome. In general, practice for closed tasks should be consistent, enabling the learner to refine the movement pattern (i.e., decrease the variability of the movement trajectory [Darling & Cooke, 1987]), particularly after the acquisition phase during the later stages of motor learning (Gentile, 1987). In early learning, for example, therapists may slow down the activity somewhat while practicing small blocks of several trials of an activity (open or closed). Soon after, one may introduce variation with two or more movement classes (Sage, 1984). Besides undertaking variable tasks, the learner needs to apply the newly learned skill to multiple situations or environments; both children and adults respond positively to a multicontext treatment approach (Toglia, 1991). To provide the optimal variability of practice, physical therapists should perform rapid procedural changes in harmony with the learner's motor behavior. Embrey and Adams (1996) revealed that experienced clinicians make smooth changes of procedures approximately every 46 seconds compared with the more abrupt changes of procedures by novices with a mean of every 86 seconds. Further insight into clinical decision making is necessary to assess fully the impact of procedure changes on the learner.

Guidance

Guidance from the instructor or from mechanical equipment (e.g., metronome) is an effective method to restrict movement errors during the performance of a task. Physical or verbal guidance techniques assist the learner, in varying degrees, through the proper movements of the task. The use of rhythmic auditory stimulation (RAS) was shown to improve the gait patterns of children with mild to moderate spastic diplegia (Thaut et al., 1998). Physical or verbal guidance or both, often referred to as "facilitation" in the therapeutic milieu, has traditionally been a major strategy used by therapists in neurorehabilitation. Carter's (1989) findings, however, indicated that therapists spend more time in handling behaviors (facilitation, stimulation, inhibition, passive movements, and other maneuvers) than in using verbal behaviors (instructions, praise, criticism). Therapists have also been observed to provide physical guidance during 78% of the activity trials in a treatment session while spending 11% on passive, task-related activities and 11% on allowing independent movements (Larin, 1992).

According to the "guidance hypothesis" (Salmoni et al., 1984), guidance has a considerable positive effect on performance during the trials of the practiced task (i.e., in the acquisition phase) but not on learning. It modifies the feel of the task, and the learner relies too strongly on it, developing a dependency (Salmoni and colleagues' guidance hypothesis, 1984). Continuous guidance alters the task, greatly reducing its specificity and transfer potential. Trial-and-error, or "discovery," procedures, however, result in learning (i.e., more effective retention and transfer performance). "Forced use" may be an adjunct strategy to promote such experience (Crocker et al., 1997).

Providing a relative frequency of guidance (i.e., for a certain percentage of trials during practice), however, is generally found to contribute more to learning than use of continuous input (Salmoni et al., 1984; Winstein, 1994), as will relative frequency rather than continuous feedback (Lee et al., 1990). Some guidance can be beneficial when interspersed with active practice trials. Moreover, with able-bodied individuals, guidance has been found most effective (1) in early practice of unfamiliar tasks, (2) for slower rather than rapid and ballistic tasks, and (3) in the prevention of injury and reduction of fear (Schmidt & Lee, 2005). For intervention with children with physical disabilities, Tscharnuter (1993) provides experiential guidelines in her approach on the grading and direction of therapeutic handling input (guidance) to provide proprioceptive, tactile, and kinesthetic experiential information relevant to tasks. These guidelines emphasize the stability aspect through activation from the support surface contact or base of support to achieve self-initiated movements. More recently, Wulf & Shea (2002) studied the role of physical assistance (use of pole with subjects on stabilometer) during a complex task. They concluded that physical assistance may be conducive to learning in this case (i.e., that it allows the learner to explore movement and to find an optimal solution to the motor problem).

Given that response time decreases with increasing age, the therapist should provide adequate time for a child to respond before intervening to initiate a motor sequence (Steyer David, 1985). The therapist should generally aim at reducing the use of guidance while increasing independent practice; this concept was noted to be predominant in therapists' current professional knowledge base (Larin, 1992). When needed, the therapist should explore a variety of ways to provide guidance. According to the age and stage of learning of the child, self-controlled practice (i.e., controlled by the child) needs also be considered (Wulf & Toole, 1999). A "relative frequency" of guidance should be provided rather than continuous input, alternating between trial and error, independent movements, and guided movements. Reduced guidance in therapy may progress from firm physical handling with verbal input to a lesser, modified physical contact and verbal input, to minimal verbal input with supervision, to nonverbal, nonphysical guidance, with the use of assistive devices from the environment throughout. Such characteristics of physical guidance are contained in the contemporary Neuro-Developmental Treatment (NDT)/ Bobath concept and in practice using facilitation techniques: guiding and grading physical, direct input toward and away from the base of support to facilitate stability and mobility, respectively. NDT emphasizes "gradual withdrawal of the therapist's direct input" and now promotes a "less hands-on" approach than was used in the past (Mayston, 1992; Howle, 2002).

Feedback

Some form of feedback is essential for motor learning. Feedback may occur before, during (concurrent), or after (terminal) and be immediate or delayed, with respect to the task execution. Terminal feedback has been studied the most and is the most frequently used in therapy (Larin, 1992).

Types of Feedback

Two types of feedback are recognized: intrinsic and extrinsic. Intrinsic feedback is related to the child's inherent, rich, and varied sensory channels involved in practicing a task, provided the CNS is intact. Intrinsic feedback may be augmented by information concerning the movement or the degree of goal attainment (Holding, 1965). Extrinsic feedback, also called augmented or enhanced feedback, speeds up the learning rate, whereas no feedback and irrelevant feedback conditions do not result in learning. Any feedback has the potential to generate rapid and permanent motor learning if it adds essential information to the task-intrinsic feedback of the learner, but it is not needed in all learning tasks. Certain skills provide sufficient task-intrinsic feedback to enable the learner to improve performance. In some cases, augmented feedback can even hinder skill learning (Magill, 1994).

Feedback may be provided verbally or nonverbally. The latter refers to sensory feedback, such as proprioceptive, auditory, visual, tactile, and electromyographic inputs, through the use of manual "handling" devices or media (Hartveld & Hegarty, 1996). Extrinsic feedback may be of several types: qualitative (e.g., "good," "right," "no") or quantitative feedback related to distance or magnitude of error (e.g., "three more steps"). It may trigger motivation and provide reinforcement. One purpose of extrinsic feedback is to give the child information (success or error) on the environmental outcome and on his or her movement patterns. Therapists, however, tend to provide primarily positive, qualitative verbal feedback (in Larin's study, 47% of activity trials compared with 6% of negative reinforcement and 9% of quantitative feedback). Furthermore, according to Carter's (1989) findings, therapists' "praise" may reinforce atypical as much as more appropriate movements and their "criticism" may act as punishment for atypical movements.

Outcome information is termed *knowledge of result* (KR) and refers to direction and magnitude (Schmidt & Wrisberg, 2004) or superficial movement features such as topology, timing (duration and speed), direction, amplitude or distance, or forcefulness (Gentile, 1987). Information on kinetics and kinematics is termed *knowledge of performance* (KP). Kinematic feedback is information on positions, time, velocities, patterns of coordination, or movement patterning; kinetic measures are descriptors of the forces that produce the kinematic variables (Schmidt, 2005). For Gentile (1987), kinematic feedback is mainly information on fundamental movement patterns such as timing or sequencing information.

There are inconsistencies between authors in their definitions of KR and KP, but they generally agree that KR information about goal achievement does not always ensure learning enhancement and that KP information about movement pattern is the most powerful form of feedback for motor learning and the most useful in motor teaching (Gentile, 1987; Schmidt & Lee, 2005) depending on the skill learned (Magill, 1994). Overall, a combination of KP and KR is superior to one or the other form of feedback alone for both open and closed skills. KP is particularly suggested for closed skills, and KR plus KP, including information on anticipatory functions, for open skills (Gentile, 1987). Thorpe and Valvano (2004) reported that some children with cerebral palsy (6 to 12 years old) may benefit from the use of KP alone or KP with cognitive strategies.

Accuracy of Feedback

The accuracy of augmented feedback is important. Erroneous feedback will diminish performance and learning, particularly when provided continuously. Periodic erroneous KR is less disruptive (Schmidt & Lee, 2005). Adolescents with a diagnosis of CP have shown improvement in the accuracy of their performance of a simple arm movement when provided with feedback on their actual time of movement, as have nondisabled individuals (Harbourne, 1991). Therefore, the therapist should (1) evaluate the skill (i.e., sensory-motor feedback, novelty, and difficulty level); (2) evaluate augmented feedback characteristics; and (3) evaluate the meaningfulness of the augmented feedback for the learner (Magill, 1994). At any time, feedback should focus on only one or two movement features, should be easily understood by the learner (e.g., "I like your quick reaching up above your head to catch the butterfly," or "It is good to push hard with your feet on the floor and keep a tall, straight back"), and be accompanied by nonverbal cueing.

Precision of Feedback

More precise, more frequent, and more immediate feedback during practice facilitates performance, but each has been found to be detrimental to learning and to produce dependency in the same way as physical guidance (see Salmoni and colleagues' guidance hypothesis, 1984). Increased precision of feedback content may lead to increased learning, but the precision level of the verbal feedback must be adapted to the learner's level (i.e., less

precision earlier, somewhat more precision later). An optimal level of precision has been hypothesized. If feedback is more or less precise than the optimum, subsequent performance is less accurate.

The optimal level of precision has been shown to increase with age. Young children naturally tend to ignore relevant information and respond immediately without using feedback (Barclay & Newell, 1980). Children, however, *can* use feedback to improve their learning, when required. Between the ages of 3.5 and 5 years, they have been reported to make fewer errors when provided with more precise feedback (Shapiro, 1977). Increasingly precise feedback, however, tends to result in more error for younger children (grade 2) but in more accuracy for older children (grade 4). The choice of wording and the format of presentation are critical. Verbal feedback should be presented in key words and short phrases whether it is about the environmental goal (e.g., "It is great that you put your hat on") or about the movement itself (e.g., "Your feet are nice and straight and no kissing knees," "It is very good holding your arms out with elbows straight like an airplane; let's count to 20 moving your wings up and down," "This was too fast and your chin was poking out").

Frequency of Feedback

Frequent feedback distracts and interferes with the information-processing activities leading to learning (retention). Frequent feedback produces excessive response variability in *simple* skill acquisition (Wulf & Schmidt, 1994) and increases the learner's dependency on the extrinsic feedback with neglect of intrinsic feedback. Concurrent feedback and terminal, continuous feedback (after each trial), although more effective for performance during practice and for guiding directly to the environmental goal, maximize dependency. The use of "relative" frequency is advocated over continuous feedback (Schmidt & Lee, 2005); for example, providing 50% relative feedback resulted in significantly better learning as measured by retention than providing 100% frequency feedback and concurrent feedback (Vander Linden et al., 1993; Wulf et al., 1994). In a one-to-one learning situation (such as a therapy session) of a simple task, reducing the relative frequency of feedback (i.e., increasing the number of no-feedback trials [blank trials]) may not only increase learning but may also help the learner to develop an error-detection mechanism and to become more active in problem solving. The optimal frequency appears to vary in direct proportion to the complexity of the task. In addition, asking the child to guess the performance *before* feedback is given helps him or her to focus attention on the task and its sensory qualities (Gentile, 1987).

Various methods exist to use a relative frequency of feedback in practice. Intermittent (occasional) feedback may be provided in several different, systematic ways. In *summary* feedback, feedback is withheld for a predetermined number of trials (e.g., 15 to 16 trials during a simple task or in the early part of practice or 5 trials during a complex task or as proficiency increases) (Gable et al., 1991). Then feedback is provided about each trial in a series of trials but only after the series is completed. In the practice of a complex perceptuomotor skill, however, adults have been found to learn equally well when summary feedback ranged between 1 and 20 trials (Christensen et al., 1992). In *average* feedback, an average score is provided after a series of trials is completed (e.g., "The last five times, you sat down slowly and gently all throughout with no flop"). Both summary and average feedback have been reported to promote similar acquisition and retention performance (Weeks & Sherwood, 1994).

More frequent feedback, however, might be required for the learning of *complex* skills, up to a certain level of experience. Studies of summary and average feedback in the learning of complex skills outline this finding. The same seems to be true for novices versus experienced learners. Concurrent feedback may also be of assistance in complex skill learning (Wulf & Shea, 2002).

In using feedback, the goals are improved learning and performance without feedback, with the child being capable of detecting his or her own errors. One approach consists of a *fading* procedure in which feedback usage is arbitrarily decreased, on an individual basis, from higher to lower relative frequency during the practice session, leading finally to a complete withdrawal. Still another approach is *bandwidth* corrective feedback, which is particularly useful in the earlier stage of learning. Informative feedback is provided only when the learner performs outside a preset band of accuracy (motivational feedback may be used within the bandwidth). For example, a therapist may decide to provide quantitative feedback (KR or KP) only when the child rotates the head less than 45° to look to the right and left sides. This procedure allows for a certain margin of error, and the absence of informative feedback helps reinforce the learner to execute repetitions. For movement tasks, bandwidth feedback has been reported to enhance accuracy and stability better than a pure, relative frequency condition (Winstein, 1991a). Bandwidth KR conditions facilitate learning regardless of the specificity of the movement goal (Lee & Maraj, 1994).

Recent studies on *learner-determined/self-controlled* presentation of feedback (KR) indicate that retention is facilitated for adult subjects who choose when to receive KR compared with subjects who received experimenter-determined KR. Learners chose relatively low feedback frequency and requested less and less feedback ("fading") over time (Schmidt & Lee, 2005; McNevin et al., 2000). In addition, less regularity of self-chosen KR-type of feedback has been associated with greater accuracy in performing tasks (Chen et al., 2001).

Timing of Feedback

Finally, the temporal aspect of extrinsic feedback is another factor influencing learning. Random KR is more beneficial than blocked KR (Schmidt & Lee, 2005). Delayed feedback plus the patient's estimation of outcome error have been reported to improve both performance and retention (motor learning) (Liu & Wrisberg, 1997). After a trial, three distinct periods of time may be considered: *feedback delay, postfeedback delay,* and *intertrial interval.* Extrinsic feedback provided immediately after a trial (a frequent schedule in physical therapy) is actually detrimental to learning, whereas feedback delayed by several seconds to several minutes has no significant negative effect on learning. Learning happens as long as competing events do not occur and interfere during the delay interval. Feedback delay allows the child to engage in the appropriate information processing and retention learning. The postfeedback delay interval (time between the provision of feedback and the next trial) does not appear as a powerful factor in learning as long as the interval is longer than approximately 5 seconds, allowing for planning the next movement. Extremely short (less than 5 seconds) or long (days or weeks) postfeedback delay intervals were reported to have a detrimental effect on performance accuracy, more so in children than in adults. A 12-second processing time, however, reduced performance variability, thereby increasing performance stability in children and adults (Schmidt & Lee, 2005). In addition, postresponse feedback tends to improve retention learning in young adults (Winstein et al., 1996). Other motor activities (interferences) performed during this interval also have a negative effect on the next performance but, in contrast to a feedback-delay interval, do not affect learning negatively and may even produce retention learning (Lee & Magill, 1985). This information has yet to be related to simple versus complex task learning.

The effects of the intertrial interval, that is, the time between two trials (the sum of the feedback delay and postfeedback delay intervals), have been the subject of controversy. If too short, inputs conducive to learning may not be processed; if too long, forgetting may occur. Practically, as long as the interval is not too short, this does not appear to affect motor learning adversely (Schmidt & Lee, 2005). Therapists, therefore, might optimally delay their intermittent feedback several seconds to several minutes and wait about 12 seconds before engaging the child in the next trial of activity.

Sequencing of Feedback

Feedback may be presented as a block (concentrating on one task component) or at random (frequent changes). Wulf & Shea (2002) provide initial findings on this topic that indicate that blocked feedback might be more beneficial for complex skill learning and random feedback for simple task learning in adult, healthy learners.

PRACTICE SESSION: LENGTH AND FREQUENCY

Some considerations are now presented regarding the length (duration) and frequency of the whole therapeutic (practice) session from a motor learning perspective. Length and frequency may vary for three main reasons: (1) the level of demands of the task and related fatigue of the child (i.e., physical, attention, processing, and performance in general); (2) the skill level of the child (i.e., beginner, intermediate, advanced); and (3) the nature of the skill. For beginners, sessions that are demanding should generally be short at first, gradually increasing with the skill level, but frequent and spaced over a long period of time. The intensity of intervention should be purposefully determined. Treatment goals should be functionally oriented and consequently require numerous hours of practice based on sound motor control and pedagogic principles (Croce & DePaepe, 1989; Singer, 1990).

Determining treatment intensity tends to be the privilege of institutional policy makers and individual therapists. In spite of tools such as the Pediatric Screening Manual (Taylor et al., 1983) to assist in this task, therapists stated rationales for intervention frequency and duration that appeared to be primarily based on economic, logistic, and experiential factors (Larin, 1992). Variations in the intensity of therapeutic intervention have been related to therapist availability and severity of infant motor delay; that is, infants with more delayed development tend to receive a greater amount of individual therapy time (Haley, 1988).

Recent meta-analyses have suggested that a high level of intensity and duration may have a positive effect on the efficacy of early intervention, particularly for populations with disabilities (Casto, 1985; Innocenti, 1991). More specifically, in neuropediatrics, Mayo (1991), Bower and McLellan (1992), Horn and colleagues (1999), and Bower and associates (1996) provided evidence that increasing the intensity, duration, and frequency of individual therapy sessions produced substantial change in children's motor development and accelerated acquisition of motor skills. In Mayo's study, infants younger than 18 months of age with delayed or atypical motor behavior who received weekly, individual, neurodevelopmental therapy for 1 hour over a period of 6 months showed greater changes in their motor development than those who received monthly, individual, 1-hour periods of intervention. In Bower and McLellan's study, children 2 to 12 years old with a diagnosis of CP of various types and learning difficulties were involved in individual, 1-hour therapy sessions each school day for 3 weeks; these children demonstrated accelerated acquisition of motor skills during the intervention period compared with before and after.

In a more recent study from Bower and associates (1996), 44 children of ages 3 to 11 years with spastic quadriplegia participated in four groups combining conventional versus intensive physical therapy, and generalized goals versus specific measurable goals. Over the 2-week period, intensive physical therapy produced a slightly greater effect as measured by the Gross Motor Function Measure (GMFM). However, the factor more strongly associated with increased motor skill acquisition was the use of specific measurable goals. Finally, in Horn and colleagues' (1999) study, children with severe CP, between 21 and 34 months old, who participated in a neurobehavioral intervention four times per week for 6 to 8 months demonstrated gains in the acquisition of specific movement components of a treated exemplar skill and of an untreated exemplar skill (requiring the targeted movement components). The children also demonstrated generalization of the trained exemplar skill by performing the skill in a different environment.

Individual intensive direct intervention cannot be excluded from a child's management program. Benefits and constraints must be carefully weighed in making decisions regarding the frequency and intensity of interventions to promote motor learning. Periods of time when movement patterns are in transition during the child's development may potentially emerge as sensitive periods for intervention (Heriza, 1991). Indicators of prognosis found in the "Guide to Physical Therapist Practice" (American Physical Therapy Association, 2001), however, "dictate" the extent of therapeutic sessions per episode of care and do not sufficiently consider the individual needs of the children from a motor-learning perspective. Such guidelines pose serious limitations on physical therapy practice and service delivery. Although the fewer, direct sessions may be optimized with a motor learning framework and specific goals attainment, therapists need to increasingly integrate dyad and group therapy, caregiver education and training, as well as virtual reality practice in their therapeutic intervention to meet the challenges.

CAREGIVER EDUCATION AND TRAINING

Type and frequency of intervention should never be limited to direct, individual, 30-minute to 1-hour treatment sessions or group sessions. The daily activities of the child offer numerous occasions for intervention and should be viewed as an indispensable part of the child's total plan of care. In these instances, the child's motor learning and motor performance may be enhanced or impaired. It is of utmost importance that the instructions provided to the parents or caregivers for addressing the child's functional motor activities reflect motor learning principles and employ relevant motor teaching strategies. The therapeutic and teaching process in caregiver education and training should include both behavioral and reflective orientations and aim at increased caregiver confidence. Behavioral, goal-directed, structured approaches appear most likely to produce change in skills, particularly when modeling, role-play, and feedback are used (van Hasselt et al., 1987). Approaches that include a broad range of relevant skills, such as problem-solving strategies, family interactions, and support, appear to be more effective (with the likelihood of maintenance and generalization) than those concentrating on a limited set of techniques or tasks (Cunningham, 1985).

The involvement of caregivers in planning and applying intervention is embodied in the notion of parent-professional partnership (Mittler & Mittler, 1983) and the family-centered approach (Rosenbaum et al., 1998), as well as in governmental mandates. Although no single approach can respond to the needs of all caregivers, guidelines on some specific strategies are available.

1. Responsiveness to caregiver needs is more important than the location or format of the program. Home and school- or center-based approaches should be considered (Gardner & Chapman, 1993).
2. Educational and training programs should lead to long-lasting intrinsic motivation rather than short-lasting extrinsic motivation. Caregiver education should focus on observation, recognition, and acceptance of subtle displays of improvement in the child's development because these have been found to be effective in motivating caregivers to participate in the implementation of home programs for their children (Moxley-Haegert & Serbin, 1983).
3. Mothers benefit from observing and interacting with therapists, often adopting and extrapolating some of the therapeutic activities into their daily routine (Hinjosa & Anderson, 1991).
4. Caregivers are not simply a vehicle for professionals' well-intentioned programs. What we ask of caregivers must make sense in terms of their individual goals, energies, living style, and philosophy (McConachie, 1991).

CONCLUSION

FUTURE RESEARCH

Clinical and laboratory research is required to further document the factors of critical importance to motor performance and motor learning of children involved in simple versus complex, functional activities. Normative data are greatly needed on information processing, particularly during the early stage of skill acquisition in young children. Comparative and single-subject data banks on the motor learning processes of children with motor impairment would assist the practitioner and researcher in their respective and collaborative activities. Instructional strategies for motor learning and performance must be tested on large populations of children at varied ages with different motor, cognitive, and social levels of functioning to ascertain their effectiveness.

Clinical research is also required to further understand therapists' practice and knowledge (explicit and implicit) of the motor learning framework. The study of groups of therapists treating various populations of children with neurologic and orthopedic impairment would reveal a more comprehensive picture of motor teaching patterns used in pediatric physical therapy. More specifically, investigation may address how therapists formulate goals (action or movement) for treatment sessions as a whole, as well as for each task practiced, with regard to emphasis on performance versus motor learning, function, or neuromuscular needs. Further insight into the therapists' taxonomy of tasks is necessary to ascertain the appropriateness and sequencing of strategies and optimal types of scheduling practice. Through research with series of single case studies and with control and experimental groups studies, the optimal proportions of strategies for different populations and skills could be determined.

IMPLICATIONS

The motor learning framework has direct implications for the physical therapist as clinical educator interacting with the child, the child's parents or caregivers, colleagues, and students. In the learning-teaching relationship, guidelines from models are useful to provide sound principles for adapting tested strategies to the learner. A motor learning approach is pertinent to each of these interactions.

Motor learning theories have been transposed into motor teaching models, and numerous instructional strategies, sometimes contradictory, have been suggested. Therapists already use many of the strategies with varying degrees of conscious selection and competency. Their professional working knowledge gradually incorporates the important elements of the theoretic motor learning framework. The professional challenge is to continuously relate new theories to knowledge-in-practice and consciously adapt one's practice accordingly. This chapter on motor learning provides pediatric physical therapists with information for such a process. It may also offer a means to guide therapists' systematic reflection on their practice and to foster renewed energy in therapy.

SUMMARY

Motor learning remains an important aspect of physical rehabilitation, and motor learning theories continue to guide the practice of physical therapy. Ecologic and dynamic systems approaches are currently at the forefront, yet in constant evolution. From motor learning constructs and models, a series of motor learning and teaching strategies have evolved. Therapists need to assess the context required and the level of motivation and prior learning of the learner, to provide targeted instructions, to select with the learner the types of tasks, to include and combine mental and physical practice considering their determinants, and provide strategic feedback. Length and frequency of practice vary according to task, fatigue, learner skill level, and nature of the skill. Caregiver education and training are essential to maximize motor learning.

CLINICAL EXAMPLE: PERFORMANCE VERSUS LEARNING

In an attempt to unify the various theoretic and instructional concepts presented in this chapter, clinical scenarios intended to foster motor learning and motor performance are now presented. Therapists are encouraged to develop other scenarios based on their clinical experience, reinforcing certain aspects of their professional knowledge and practice and modifying and improving others.

Two pediatric physical therapists are engaged in a 1-hour, direct intervention session, each therapist with a 5-year-old child of average cognitive ability who has a movement dysfunction (diagnosis: moderate spastic diplegia). The sessions include individual work and some intermittent interaction between the children (dyad

mode). Without underestimating potential biomechanical, physiologic, and other needs pertinent to the management of the children, and through discussion with each child (encouraging self-selected goals), the following functional goals are selected for their potentially broad application in daily activities. They are to be achieved after 6 months of intensive therapy and management.

A. *Improved performance goal*: Child wishes to walk along with peers. The child, wearing hinged ankle-foot orthoses, will be able to walk with a posterior walker the length of the corridor from the classroom to the gym (approximately 50 feet) together with other classmates without disabilities, with improved efficiency as measured by a 25% increase in step length and speed (distance per minute), a 25% decrease in cadence (steps per minute), and a decreased heart rate (beats per minute).

B. *New learning goal*: Child wishes to climb up stairs to avoid requesting assistance or using the elevator. The child will be able to walk up two-step staircase (10 cm) with an alternate pattern, holding onto one handrail, within 10 seconds.

The therapist's associated, movement-oriented therapeutic goal, in this case, is to obtain greater selective control (dissociation) of the lower extremities during gait as related to (1) range of movement (i.e., hip and knee flexion and extension); (2) muscle activity (i.e., stability and mobility; stance and swing); and (3) compensatory movement patterns (i.e., upper trunk, upper extremity excess assistance). Improved endurance is also targeted.

Walking and climbing stairs are dynamic, continuous, *complex*, open-type, functional activities. One child is functioning at the early stage or verbal-cognitive to motor stages of motor learning in which she needs to discover a reasonable, effective approach to stair climbing (learning) while the other child is in the associative to autonomous stage working at improving gait with the walker (performance). First, the similarities of therapeutic, instructional strategies used in the two scenarios are presented, followed by their respective differences.

SIMILARITIES

In both scenarios, the therapist pays attention to the physical aspect of intervention, planning and preparing the different functional areas to ensure security, fun, and appropriateness for the child's motivational level, attentional abilities, and sensory processing status. To this end, the playroom (treatment room) is organized into three ecologically valid stations entailing use of upright movement: cafeteria, library, and gym. The corridor leading to the washroom and classroom is also selected as a therapeutic environment.

In a friendly, respectful, and "partnership" manner, the therapist presents in an exciting and genuine way (verbal and nonverbal) the various predetermined, novel play areas. First, the therapist asks the child what he or she would like to do in each area, with more rather than fewer details (promoting preselected activities). Upon the child's response and according to the child's capacities, the therapist encourages the child through verbal guidance, for about 3 to 5 minutes, to imagine himself or herself doing the chosen activity. The activity may be repeated before moving to the next station (mixing actual and imaginary practice). Then the child is asked to observe the other child and the child or therapist may describe some of the possible movements (using peer-modeling with some verbal labeling) as necessary. The therapist adds his choice to the list, incorporating certain risk-taking behaviors, negotiates, takes turns in the decision making, and gradually fades out the instructions to the child.

The therapist's instructions to the child throughout the session incorporate elements of arresting stimuli (e.g., surprise or uncertainty) and are often presented in "chunks." These instructions relate primarily to the child's preselected environmental goals but may also relate to increasing the child's awareness of certain aspects of the movement pattern. The therapist may then question the child on the activity.

Alternating with questions, the therapist also provides relevant information directly about the skill of walking to increase the child's selective attention to critical features and to increase motor performance. At times this information is about aspects of the environment that affect gait (e.g., "The floor is hard, let's walk on the carpet, it feels soft," or "Watch for the door, which may open quickly; walk more to the side"). At other times, it is about the whole movement (e.g., "Let's walk nice and straight") and, as necessary, about one or two aspects of the movement practiced (e.g., "Keep your feet straight pointing toward … with a little space between," or "Arms down and knees up straight"). To target motor learning of stair climbing, the information is directed at the end result (e.g., reaching the book higher on the shelf). Apart from providing these forms of information (environmental, movement, and/or end result), the therapist fosters the child's self-correction in different ways. The therapist asks the child: "Tell me what you need to remember and pay attention to before you begin walking/climbing" (verbal pretraining).

In addition, functional selective attention is enhanced by introducing distractions randomly in the treatment session, according, of course, to the child's response (level of confusion and attentiveness) and also to the objective of the practice session (i.e., performance or learning). These might be people walking by, talking, playing, or singing (opened window or door or shared playroom) or using a combination of activities, such as entertaining a conversation or singing while walking. First distractions are gradually introduced (i.e., the child can anticipate them), but as soon as possible they are randomly presented (i.e., unanticipated) to promote greater adaptability and function.

To begin, the activity-goal may be practiced in block (for learning or performance). However, there is a benefit to having different activities practiced in a random fashion, each one repeated several times to maintain a reasonably high level of complexity. Because the child may not be performing optimally during the session, the paradox of performance and learning is explained (in age-appropriate terms) and encouragement given to the child and caregivers.

Most activities are generated voluntarily with particular attention to the initiation of the movements for the purpose of attaining shorter reaction times and decreased use of compensatory synergies. In addition to setting relative daily-living contexts, the therapist instructs the child (with and without the use of modeling) on how to prepare for movement, with an emphasis on adequate base of support and postural, biomechanical alignment and may ask "Are you ready?" Acknowledging the latency period of the child's reactions, the therapist waits for the child's voluntary initiation of movement. Then the therapist gradually reduces the anticipatory input to the child (fading process) and requests more accuracy and speed in performing the activities, increasing the child's adaptability through use of a greater level of uncertainty (random activities).

Walking and stair climbing are *complex* skills to learn and practice. In spite of this, when possible, each activity sequence is practiced in its entirety from the beginning. However, if the activity is too complex for the child and totally unsuccessful (end result and movement), the most troublesome parts of the activity are practiced individually, alternating regularly with practice of the whole activity (with physical guidance/assistance) for gradual integration and function (progressive part practice). For example, working toward climbing up could involve practicing sustaining weight transfer on one leg for short periods of time, maintaining an erect trunk while bringing the other leg up and down at different heights, transferring weight onto the other leg while placing a foot on the stool and swinging back and forth, and trunk leaning forward over a leg using momentum to climb up.

DIFFERENCES

The practice of walking and stair climbing for the alternative purposes of performance or learning requires different practice scheduling, degrees of variability, application of physical guidance, and provision of feedback to the child. The differences particular to the two motor-teaching scenarios follow.

In the scenario aiming at performance, the therapist chooses a distributed scheduling of practice in which the amount of rest between trials equals or exceeds the amount of time in a trial; hence, fatigue building to the point of impairing performance during the treatment session is avoided. Overlearning an activity becomes the goal; therefore, the therapist does not vary greatly among activities, and in this case, the time spent walking predominates in the treatment session.

In the early stage of motor performance, the therapist uses a higher degree of verbal and physical guidance/assistance to correct most of the child's movement errors and to obtain an immediate increase of performance. Precise, extrinsic feedback is offered frequently and immediately to the child during (concurrent) and after (continuous terminal) activity trials. The therapist praises the child's success, referring to the goal or movement, and indicates mistakes in a corrective and encouraging manner. In addition, the therapist supplies KR and KP focused on one or two movement features (including anticipatory function) easily understood by the child. Another tactic increasingly encouraged is to ask the child to "evaluate" the level of his or her performance before providing feedback. The feedback is not offered immediately after the performance but rather is delayed several seconds to several minutes and the next trial initiated another 5 to 12 seconds after the feedback. Yet another tactic is to ask the child when he or she wants to obtain feedback. At all times interferences (distractions) are minimized to strengthen the performance. In the later stage of refined motor performance, however, practice is associated primarily with intrinsic feedback and minimal therapist input.

On the other hand, in the scenario aiming at learning stair climbing, the therapist first chooses a massed scheduling of practice in which the amount of practice time in a trial is greater than the amount of rest between trials, in spite of fatigue building up and the likelihood that performance will deteriorate during the treatment session. The therapist then introduces a distributed practice schedule and gradually increases the intensity of practice with repetitions; the practice remains somewhat difficult and effortful and generates some level of fatigue.

High-variable practice leads to learning for retention and transfer, particularly in the case of open skills such as walking or stair climbing. The therapist diversifies the activities in two ways: (1) the practice of different but similar actions (intertask with the same movement class, e.g., marching, standing up from half kneeling [if one concedes that they all require various types of dissociation]); and (2) the practice of the same task altering one characteristic such as distance, speed, direction, or timing of the movement pattern (intratask, e.g., stair climbing sideways at moderate and fast speeds not too slow, and on varied heights of steps). In the early learning of an activity, the therapist reduces somewhat the speed and sequence of practice into blocks of several trials; afterward, the therapist shifts to random, variable practice, using the same speed and accuracy of the entire, desired, age-appropriate skill and practicing in different situations and environments. Block practice may be reintroduced as needed.

In practice for learning, the therapist uses the least possible amount of verbal and physical guidance/assistance (relative frequency) in a fading manner. A combination of trial-and-error, guided, and independent movements is incorporated in the child's practice session. When guidance/assistance is used, the degree and the timing are adjusted to the child's needs at the different periods of a task practice (i.e., preset anticipatory postural adjustments, movement initiation, sustained control, or termination) and to the child's need to gain stability and mobility. In the early stage of practice, however, when movements are somewhat slower and activities unfamiliar and the child is more fearful and at risk of injury, the therapist employs a greater amount of guidance/assistance while attempting to gradually reduce it as much as possible. This is achieved by offering less manual support, more distal assistance, or by using a medium between the therapist and the child (e.g., baton, ball, book).

Extrinsic feedback provided for learning purposes is of the same types as for performance, i.e., qualitative and quantitative (KR + KP); the level of precision and frequency, however, differs. Earlier in practice, the precision of the feedback is minimal, offered in key words or short sentences, and then increased as the child progresses. The therapist presents feedback in a relative frequency during the treatment session; the higher the task complexity for the child, the more feedback is provided unless the child indicates otherwise. The therapist chooses among five ways to determine this relative frequency: (1) fading (i.e., gradually reducing to no feedback); (2) average (e.g., after every fifth trial, giving feedback about that trial); (3) summary (e.g., after a predetermined number of five trials, giving feedback about all the previous trials); (4) bandwidth technique (i.e., only after trials in which performance is outside a predetermined acceptable range, allowing for a margin of error); or (5) learner/self-determined presentation of feedback (in age-appropriate terms). The timing of the feedback for learning remains the same as for performance purposes (i.e., several seconds to several minutes after a trial with a delay of 5 to 12 seconds before the next trial). Finally, to heighten learning, the therapist introduces other motor activities or distractors (interferences) at a higher rate than in the performance scenario, according to the child's cognitive and behavioral status.

REFERENCES

Abbs, JH, Gracco, VL, & Cole, KJ. Control of multimovement coordination: Sensorimotor mechanisms in speech motor programming. Journal of Motor Behavior, 16:195–231, 1984.

Adams, JA. A closed-loop theory of motor learning. Journal of Motor Behavior, 3:111–149, 1971.

American Physical Therapy Association. Guide to Physical Therapist Practice, 2nd ed. Physical Therapy, 81(1): 2001.

Arend, S. Developing perceptual skills prior to motor performance. Motor Skills: Theory into Practice, 4:11–17, 1980.

Arnett, MG, DeLuccia, D, & Gilmartin, K. Male and female differences and the specificity of fatigue on skill acquisition and transfer performance. Research Quarterly for Exercise and Sport, 71(2):201–205, 2000.

Asatryan, DG, & Feldman, AG. Biophysics of complex systems and mathematical models. Biophysics, 10:925–935, 1965.

Ashy, MH, Lee, AM, & Landin, DK. Relationship of practice using correct technique to achievement in a motor skill. Journal of Teaching in Physical Education, 7:115–120, 1988.

Bakshi, R, Bhambhani, Y, & Madill, H. The effects of task preference during purposeful and nonpurposeful activities. American Journal of Occupational Therapy, 45:912–916, 1991.

Barclay, C, & Newell, K. Children's processing of information in motor skill acquisition. Journal of Experimental Child Psychology, 30:98–108, 1980.

Bernstein, N. The Co-ordination and Regulation of Movements. Oxford: Pergamon Press, 1967.

Bower, E, & McLellan, DL. Effect of increased exposure to physiotherapy on skill acquisition of children with cerebral palsy. Developmental Medicine and Child Neurology, 34:25–39, 1992.

Bower E, McLellan, DL, Arney, J, & Campbell, MJ. A randomised controlled trial of different intensities of physiotherapy and different goal-setting procedures in 44 children with cerebral palsy. Developmental Medicine and Child Neurology, 38:226–237, 1996.

Brenière, Y, Cuong Do, M, & Bouisset, S. Are dynamic phenomena prior to stepping essential to walking? Journal of Motor Behavior, 19:62–76, 1987.

Bressan, ES, & Woollacott, MH. A prescriptive paradigm for sequencing instruction in physical education. Human Movement Science, 1:155–175, 1982.

Brown, DA, Effgen, SK, & Palisano, RJ. Performance following ability-focussed physical therapy intervention in individuals with severely limited physical and cognitive abilities. Physical Therapy, 78:934–950, 1998.

Carlson, JL. Evaluating patient motivation in physical disabilities practice settings. The American Journal of Occupational Therapy, 51:347–351, 1997.

Carson, LM, & Wiegand, RL. Motor schema formation and retention in young children: A test of Schmidt's schema theory. Journal of Motor Behavior, 11:247–251, 1979.

Carter, RE. A Behavioral Analysis of Interactions between Physical Therapists and Children with Cerebral Palsy during Treatment. Unpublished doctoral dissertation, Northern Illinois University, 1989.

Casto, G. The Relationships between Program Intensity and Efficacy in Early Intervention. Unpublished manuscript, Utah State University, Early Intervention Research Institute, Logan, Utah, 1985.

Chen, DD, Kaufman, D, & Chung, MW. Emergent patterns of feedback strategies in performing a closed motor skill. Perceptual and Motor Skills, 93:197–204, 2001.

Christensen, S, Fitch, N, & Winstein, C. Acquisition and retention of a partial weight bearing skill: Effect of practice with summary knowledge of results (Abstract). Physical Therapy, 72(suppl 6):S51–S52, 1992.

Cintas, HM. The relationship of motor skill level and risk-taking during exploration in toddlers. Pediatric Physical Therapy, 4:165–170, 1992.

Clark, JE. Developmental differences in response processing. Journal of Motor Behavior, 14:247–254, 1982.

Cohen, JE, Goel, V, Frank, JW, Bombardier, C, Peloso, P, & Guillemin, F. Group education interventions for people with low back pain. Spine, 19:1214–1222, 1994.

Cook Merrill, S, Slavik, B, Holloway, E, Richter, E, & David, S. Environment: Implications for Occupational Therapy Practice. Rockville, MD: American Occupational Therapy Association, 1990.

Cornwall, MW, Bruscato, MP, & Barry, S. Effect of mental practice on isometric muscle strength. Journal of Sports Physical Therapy, 13:231–234, 1991.

Coster, WJ, & Jaffe, LE. Current concepts of children's perceptions of control. American Journal of Occupational Therapy, 45:19–25, 1991.

Croce, R, & DePaepe, J. A critique of therapeutic intervention programming with reference to an alternative approach based on motor learning theory. Physical and Occupational Therapy in Pediatrics, 9(3):5–33, 1989.

Crocker, MD, MacKay-Lyons, M, & McDonnell, E. Forced use of the upper extremity in cerebral palsy: A single-case design. The American Journal of Occupational Therapy, 51:824–833, 1997.

Cunningham, C. Training and education approaches for parents of children with special needs. British Journal of Medical Psychology, 58:285–305, 1985.

Darling, WG, & Cooke, JD. Changes in the variability of movement trajectories with practice. Journal of Motor Behavior, 19:291–309, 1987.

Davids, JR, Bagley, AM, & Bryan, M. Kinematic and kinetic analysis of running in children with cerebral palsy. Developmental Medicine and Child Neurology, 40:528–535, 1998.

Davis, PL, & Gavin, WJ. Comparison of individual group/consultation treatment methods for preschool children with developmental delays. American Journal of Occupational Therapy, 48:155–161, 1994.

Davis, WE, & Burton, AW. Ecological task analysis: Translating movement behavior theory into practice. Adapted Physical Activity Quarterly, 8:154–177, 1991.

Doty, AK, McEwen, IR, Parker, D, & Laskin, J. Effects of testing context on ball skill performance in 5-year old children with and without developmental delay. Physical Therapy, 79(9):818–826, 1999.

Duff, SV, & Gordon, AM. Sensorimotor control of the hand in children with hemiplegic cerebral palsy: Use of tactile and proprioceptive information (Abstract). Physical Therapy, 78:S37, 1998.

Duncombe, LW, & Howe, MC. Group treatment: Goals, tasks, and economic implications. American Journal of Occupational Therapy, 49:199–205, 1995.

Edwards, R. The effects of performance standards on behavior patterns and motor skill achievement in children. Journal of Teaching in Physical Education, 7:90–102, 1988.

Effgen, SK, & Klepper, SE. Survey of physical therapy practice in educational settings. Pediatric Physical Therapy, 6:15–21, 1994.

Eidson, TA, & Stadulis, RE. Effects of variability of practice on the transfer and performance of open and closed motor skills. Adapted Physical Activity Quarterly, 8:342–356, 1991.

Eliasson, A, Gordon, AM, & Forssberg, H. Basic co-ordination of manipulative forces of children with cerebral palsy. Developmental Medicine and Child Neurology, 33:661–670, 1991.

Eliasson, A, Gordon, AM, & Forssberg, H. Impaired anticipatory control of isometric forces during grasping by children with cerebral palsy. Developmental Medicine and Child Neurology, 34:216–225, 1992.

Embrey, DG, & Adams, LS. Clinical applications of procedural changes by experienced and novice pediatric physical therapists. Pediatric Physical Therapy, 8:122–132, 1996.

Embrey, DG, & Hylton, N. Clinical applications of movement scripts by experienced and novice pediatric physical therapists. Pediatric Physical Therapy, 8:3–14, 1996.

Etnier, JL & Landers, DM. Motor performance and motor learning as a function of age and fitness. Research Quarterly for Exercise and Sport, 69(2):136–146, 1998.

Fairweather, MM, & Sidaway, B. Hemispheric teaching strategies in the acquisition and retention of a motor skill. Research Quarterly for Exercise and Sport, 65:40–47, 1994.

Falk-Kessler, J, Momich, C, and Perel, S. Therapeutic factors in occupational therapy groups. American Journal of Occupational Therapy, 45:59–66, 1991.

Fansler, CL, Poff, CL, & Shepard, KF. Effects of mental practice on balance in elderly women. Physical Therapy, 65:1332–1338, 1985.

Fazio, LS. Tell me a story: The therapeutic metaphor in the practice of pediatric occupational therapy. American Journal of Occupational Therapy, 46:112–119, 1992.

Fell, DW. Progressing therapeutic intervention in patients with neurologic disorders: A framework to assist clinical decision making. Journal of Neurologic Physical Therapy, 28(1):35–46, 2004.

Feltz, DL, & Landers, DM. The effects of mental practice on motor skill learning and performance: A meta-analysis. Journal of Sport Psychology, 5:25–57, 1983.

Fetters, L: Cerebral palsy: Contemporary treatment concepts. In Lister, MJ (Ed.). Contemporary Management of Motor Control Problems: Proceedings of the II Step Conference. Alexandria, VA: Foundation for Physical Therapy, 1991, pp. 219–224.

Fineman, JB, & Gentile, AM. Variability of practice and transfer of training (Abstract). Physical Therapy, 78:S42, 1998.

Fitts, PM, & Posner, MI. Human Performance. Belmont, CA: Brooks/Cole, 1967.

Gable, CD, Shea, CH, & Wright, DL. Summary knowledge of results. Research Quarterly for Exercise and Sport, 62:285–292, 1991.

Gabriele, TE, Hall, CR, & Buckolz, EE. Practice schedule effects on the acquisition and retention of a motor skill. Human Movement Science, 6:1–16, 1987.

Garcia, C. Gender differences in young children's interactions when learning fundamental motor skills. Research Quarterly for Exercise and Sport, 65:213–225, 1994.

Gardner, JF, & Chapman, MS. Developing Staff Competence for Supporting People with Developmental Disabilities. Baltimore: Paul H. Brookes, 1993.

Gentile, AM. A working model of skill acquisition with application to teaching. Quest, 44:3–23, 1972.

Gentile, AM. Skill acquisition: Action, movement, and neuromotor processes. In Carr, JA, & Shepherd, RB (Eds.). Movement Science:

Foundations for Physical Therapy in Rehabilitation. Rockville, MD: Aspen, 1987, pp. 93–154.

Gentile, AM. The nature of skill acquisition: Therapeutic implications for children with movement disorders. Medicine and Sport Science, 36:31–40, 1992.

Gibson, EJ. Principles of Perceptual Learning and Development. New York: Appleton-Century-Crofts, 1969.

Gibson, EJ. Exploratory behavior in the development of perceiving, acting, and the acquiring of knowledge. Annual Review of Psychology, 39:1–41, 1988.

Gibson, JJ. The senses considered as perceptual systems. Boston: Houghton-Miffin, 1966.

Glynn, T. Contexts for learning: Implications for mildly and moderately handicapped children. Australian and New Zealand Journal of Developmental Disabilities, 10:257–263, 1985.

Goldberger, M, & Gerney, P. Effects of learner use of practice time on skill acquisition of fifth grade children. Journal of Teaching in Physical Education, 10:84–95, 1990.

Goodwin, JE, Eckerson, JM, Grimes, CR, & Gordon, PM. Effect of different quantities of variable practice on acquisition, retention, and transfer of an applied motor skill. Perceptual and Motor Skills, 87:147–151, 1998.

Gould, DR, & Roberts, GC. Modeling and motor skill acquisition. Quest, 33:214–230, 1982.

Haas, G, Diener, HC, Rapp, H, & Dichgans, J. Development of feedback and feedforward control of upright stance. Developmental Medicine and Child Neurology, 31:481–488, 1989.

Hadders-Algra, M, Brogen, E, & Forssberg, H. Training affects the development of postural adjustments in sitting infants. Journal of Physiology, 493:289–298, 1996.

Haley, SM. Patterns of physical and occupational therapy implementation in early motor intervention. Topics in Early Childhood Special Education, 7:46–63, 1988.

Hall, KG, & Magill, RA. Variability of practice and contextual interference in motor skill learning. Journal of Motor Behavior, 27:299–309, 1995.

Harbourne, RT. Error detection skills in cerebral palsy (Abstract). Physical Therapy, 71(suppl 6):S9, 1991.

Hartveld, A, & Hegarty, JR. Augmented feedback and physiotherapy practice. Physiotherapy, 82:480–490, 1996.

Haubenstricker, J, & Seefeldt, V. Acquisition of motor skills during childhood. In Seefeldt, V. (Ed.). Physical Activity and Well Being. Reston, VA: American Alliance for Health, Physical Education, Recreation and Dance, 1986, pp. 41–104.

Hayes, MS, McEwen, IR, Lovett, D, Sheldon, MM, & Smith, D. Next step: Survey of pediatric physical therapists' educational needs and perceptions of motor control, motor development and motor learning as they relate to services for children with developmental disabilities. Pediatric Physical Therapy, 11:164–182. 1999.

Heitman, R, Erdmann, J, Gurchiek, L, Kovaleski, J, & Gilley, W. From the field. Constant versus variable practice in learning a motor task using individuals with learning disabilities. Clinical Kinesiology, 51:62–65, 1997.

Heriza, CB. Implications of a dynamical systems approach to understanding infant kicking behavior. Physical Therapy, 71:222–235, 1991.

Heriza, CB, & Sweeney, JK. Pediatric physical therapy: Part 1. Practice, scope, scientific basis, and theoretical foundation. Infants and Young Children, 7:20–32, 1994.

Higgins, S. Motor skill acquisition. Physical Therapy, 71:123–139, 1991.

Hinjosa, J, & Anderson, J. Mother's perceptions of home treatment programs for their preschool children with cerebral palsy. American Journal of Occupational Therapy, 45:273–279, 1991.

Holding, DH. Principles of Training. Oxford, England: Pergamon Press, 1965.

Hood, B, & Atkinson, J. Sensory visual loss and cognitive deficits in the selective attentional system of normal infants and neurologically impaired children. Developmental Medicine and Child Neurology, 32:1067–1077, 1990.

Horn, EM, Jones, HA, & Warren, SF. The effects of a neurobehavioral intervention on motor skill acquisition and generalization. Journal of Early Intervention, 22(1):1–18, 1999.

Howle, JM. Neuro-Developmental Treatment Approach: Theoretical Foundations and Principles of Clinical Practice. Laguna Beach: Neuro-Developmental Treatment Association (NDTA), 2002.

Innocenti, MS. More or less: A review of intensity as a program variable in early intervention. Paper presented at the meeting of the Society for Research in Child Development, Seattle, WA, April 1991.

Jackson, PL, Lafleur, MF, Malouin, F, Richards, C, & Doyon, J. Potential role of mental practice using motor imagery in neurologic rehabilitation. Archives of Physical Medicine and Rehabilitation, 82: 1133–1141, 2001.

James, W. The Principles of Psychology, Vol. 1. New York: Holt, 1890.

Jarus T, & Ratzon, NZ. Can you imagine? The effect of mental practice on the acquisition and retention of a motor skill as a function of age. The Occupational Therapy Journal of Research, 20(3):163–178, 2000.

Jarus, T, & Gol, D. The effect of kinesthetic stimulation on the acquisition and retention of a gross motor skill by children with and without sensory integration disorders. Physical and Occupational Therapy in Pediatrics, 14(3/4):59–73, 1995.

Jones, G, & Cale, A. Goal difficulty, anxiety and performance. Ergonomics, 40:319–333, 1997.

Kamm, K, Thelen, E, & Jensen, JL. A dynamical systems approach to motor development. Physical Therapy, 70:763–775, 1990.

Karnish, K, Bruder, MB, & Rainforth, B. A comparison of physical therapy in two school based treatment contexts...an isolated therapy room or a natural educational setting. Physical and Occupational Therapy in Pediatrics, 15(4):1–25, 1995.

Kauffman, IB, & Ridenour, M. Influence of an infant walker on onset and quality of walking pattern of locomotion: An electromyographic investigation. Perceptual and Motor Skills, 45:1323–1329, 1977.

Kelso, JAS. Anticipatory dynamical systems, intrinsic pattern dynamics and skill learning. Human Movement Science, 10:93–111, 1991.

Kerr, R. Schema theory applied to skill acquisition. Motor Skills: Theory into Practice, 3:15–20, 1978.

King, EM, Gooch, JE, Howell, GH, Peters, ML, Bloswick, DS, & Brown, DR. Evaluation of the hip-extensor tricycle in improving gait in children with cerebral palsy. Developmental Medicine and Child Neurology, 35:1048–1054, 1993.

Koegel, RL, & Rincover, A. Some detrimental effects of using extra stimuli to guide learning in normal and autistic children. Journal of Abnormal Child Psychology, 4:59–71, 1976.

Kohl, RM, Ellis, SD, & Roenker, DL. Alternating actual and imagery practice: Preliminary theoretical considerations. Research Quarterly for Exercise and Sport, 63:162–170, 1992.

Larin, H. Knowledge in Practice: Motor Learning Theories in Pediatric Physiotherapy. Unpublished doctoral dissertation, University of Toronto, 1992.

Latash, ML, Kang, N, & Patterson, D. Finger coordination in persons with Down syndrome: Atypical patterns of coordination and the effects of practice. Experimental Brain Research, 146:345–355, 2002.

Lawlor, MC, & Henderson, A. A descriptive study of the clinical patterns of occupational therapy working with infants and young children. American Journal of Occupational Therapy, 43:755–764, 1989.

Lee, TD, & Magill, RA. Can forgetting facilitate acquisition? In Goodman, D, Wilberg, RB, & Franks, IM (Eds.). Differing Perspec-

tives in Motor Learning, Memory, and Control. North Holland: Elsevier Science, 1985, pp. 3–22.

Lee, TD, & Maraj, BK. Effects of bandwidth goals and bandwidth knowledge of results on motor learning. Research Quarterly for Exercise and Sport, 65:244–249, 1994.

Lee, TD, White, MA, & Carnaham, H. On the role of knowledge of results in motor learning: Exploring the guidance hypothesis. Journal of Motor Behavior, 22:191–208, 1990.

Lewthwaite, R. Motivational considerations in physical activity involvement. Physical Therapy, 70:808–819, 1990.

Lin, K, Wu, C, & Trombly, CA. Effects of task goal on movement kinematics and line bisection performance in adults without disabilities. American Journal of Occupational Therapy, 52:179–187, 1998.

Liu, J, & Wrisberg, CA. The effect of knowledge of results delay and the subjective estimation of movement on the acquisition and retention of a motor skill. Research Quarterly for Exercise and Sport, 68:145–151, 1997.

Lozoff, B. Iron and learning potential in childhood. Bulletin of the New York Academy of Medicine, 65:1050–1066, 1989.

Magill, RA. The influence of augmented feedback on skill learning depends on characteristics of the skill and the learner. Quest, 46:314–327, 1994.

Maring, JR. Effects of mental practice on rate of skill acquisition. Physical Therapy, 70:165–172, 1990.

Marteniuk, RG. Information Processing in Motor Skills. New York: Holt, Rinehart & Winston, 1976.

Marteniuk, RG. Motor skill performance and learning: Considerations for rehabilitation. Physiotherapy Canada, 31:187–202, 1979.

Marteniuk, RG, Mackenzie, CL, & Leavitt, JL. Representational and physical accounts of motor and learning: Can they account for the data? In Colley, AM, & Beech, JR (Eds.). Cognition and Action in Skilled Behavior. North Holland: Elsevier Science, 1988, pp. 173–190.

Mayo, NE. The effect of physical therapy for children with motor delay and cerebral palsy. American Journal of Physical Medicine and Rehabilitation, 70:258–267, 1991.

Mayston, MJ. The Bobath concept: Evolution and application. Medicine and Sport Science, 36:1–6, 1992.

McConachie, HR. Home-based teaching: What are we asking parents? Child: Care, Health and Development, 17:123–136, 1991.

McCulloch, WS. A heterarchy of values determined by the topology of nervous nets. Bulletin of Mathematical Biophysics, 7:89–95, 1945.

McNevin, NH, Wulf, G, & Carlson, C. Effects of attentional focus, self-control, and dyad training on motor learning: Implications for physical rehabilitation. Physical Therapy, 80:373–385, 2000.

Michaels, CF, & Carello, C. Direct Perception. Englewood Cliffs, NJ: Prentice-Hall, 1981.

Missiuna, C, & Pollock, N. Perceived efficacy and goal setting in young children. Canadian Journal of Occupational Therapy, 67(2):101–109, 2000.

Mittler, PJ, & Mittler, H. Partnership with parents: An overview. In Mittler, P, & McConachie, H (Eds.). Parents, Professionals and Mentally Handicapped People: Approaches to Partnership. Beckenham: Croom Helm, 1983.

Moxley-Haegert, L, & Serbin, LA. Developmental education for parents of delayed infants: Effects on parental motivation and children's development. Child Development, 54:1324–1331, 1983.

Nashner, LM, Shumway-Cook, A, & Marin, O. Stance posture control in select groups of children with cerebral palsy: Deficits in sensory organization and muscular coordination. Experimental Brain Research, 49:393–409, 1983.

Newell, KM, Carlton, MJ, & Antoniou, A. The interaction of criterion and feedback information in learning a drawing task. Journal of Motor Behavior, 22:536–552, 1990.

Newell, KM, & Corcos, DM. Variability and Motor Control. Champaign, IL: Human Kinetics, 1993.

Newell, KM, Yeou-The, L, & Gottfried, MK. Time scales in motor learning and development. Psychological Review, 108(1):57–82, 2001.

Nicolson, RI. Cognitive factors in simple reactions: A developmental study. Journal of Motor Behavior, 14:69–80, 1982.

Ohr, PS, Fagen, JW, Rovee-Collier, C, Hayne, H, & Vander Linde, E. Amount of training and retention by infants. Developmental Psychobiology, 22:69–80, 1989.

Olney, S. New developments in the biomechanics of gait in children with cerebral palsy. In Topics in Pediatrics: Lesson 1. Alexandria, VA: American Physical Therapy Association, 1989.

Orme, M. Teaching Strategies Kit. Toronto, Ontario: Ontario Institute for Studies in Education, 1978.

Palisano, RJ. Comparison of two methods of service delivery for students with learning disabilities. Physical and Occupational Therapy in Pediatrics, 9(3):79–100, 1989.

Piek, JP, & Skinner, RA. Timing and force control during a sequential tapping task in children with and without motor coordination problems. Journal of the International Neuropsychological Society, 5:320–329, 1999.

Pohl, PS, McDowd, JM, Filion, DL, Richards, LG, & Stiers, W. Implicit learning of a perceptual-motor skill after stroke. Physical Therapy, 81:1780–1789, 2001.

Pohl, PS, Winstein, C, & Lewthwaite, R. Processes underlying motor learning: A methodological perspective (Abstract). Physical Therapy, 72(suppl 6):S10, 1992.

Poretta, DL, & Surburg, PR. Imagery and physical practice in the acquisition of gross motor timing of coincidence by adolescents with mild mental retardation. Perceptual and Motor Skills, 80:1171–1183, 1995.

Ratner, HH, & Foley, MA. A unifying framework for the development of children's activity memory. Advances in Child Development, 25:33–105, 1994.

Ravey, J. In response to mental practice and imagery: a potential role in stroke rehabilitation. Physical Therapy Review, 3:53–54, 1998.

Ritson, RJ. Psychomotor skill teaching: Beyond the command style. Journal of Physical Education, Recreation, and Dance, 58:36–37, 1987.

Roberton, MA, & Halverson, LE. The developing child—His changing movement. In London, B (Ed.). Physical Education for Children: A Focus on the Teaching Process. Philadelphia: Lea & Febiger, 1977.

Rosenbaum, P, King, S, Law, M, King, G, & Evans J. Family-centered service: A conceptual framework and research review. Physical and Occupational Therapy in Pediatrics, 18(1):1–20, 1998.

Runnings, DW, & Diewert, GL. Movement cue reproduction under preselection. Journal of Motor Behavior, 14:213–227, 1982.

Sage, GH. Motor Learning and Control: A Neuropsychological Approach. Dubuque, IA: William C. Brown, 1984.

Salmoni, AW, Schmidt, RA, & Walter, CB. Knowledge of results and motor learning: A review and critical reappraisal. Psychological Bulletin, 95:355–386, 1984.

Schempp, PG. Enhancing creative thinking: A study of children making decisions in human movement programs. Human Movement Science, 2:91–104, 1983.

Schmidt, RA. Schema theory: Implications for movement education. Motor Skills: Theory into Practice, 2:36–48, 1977.

Schmidt, RA, & Wrisberg, CA. Motor Learning and Performance. Champaign, IL: Human Kinetics Publishers, 2004.

Schmidt, RA, & Lee, TD. Motor Control and Learning: A Behavioral Emphasis. Champaign, IL: Human Kinetics, 2005.

Scholz, JP. Dynamic pattern theory: Some implications for therapeutics. Physical Therapy, 70:827–843, 1990.

Seiler, R. The intentional link between environment and action in the acquisition of skills. International Journal of Sport Psychology, 31:496–514, 2000.

Seitz, RH, & Wilson, CL. Effect on gait of motor task learning acquired in a sitting position. Physical Therapy, 67:1089–1094, 1987.

Shapiro, DC. Knowledge of results and motor learning in preschool children. Research Quarterly for Exercise and Sport, 48:154–158, 1977.

Shea, CH, & Kohl, RM. Specificity and variability of practice. Research Quarterly for Exercise and Sport, 61:169–177, 1990.

Sheridan, MR. Planning and controlling simple movements. In Smyth, MM, & Wing, AM (Eds.). The Psychology of Human Movement. London: Academic Press, 1984, pp. 47–82.

Sherwood, DE. The benefits of random variable practice for spatial accuracy and error detection in a rapid aiming task. Research Quarterly for Exercise and Sport, 67:35–43, 1996.

Shumway-Cook, A, & Woollacott, MH. The growth of stability: Postural control from a developmental perspective. Journal of Motor Behavior, 17:131–147, 1985.

Sideway, B. Motor programming as a function of constraints on movement initiation. Journal of Motor Behavior, 23:120–130, 1991.

Simpson, RL, & Galbo, JJ. Interaction and learning: Theorizing on the art of teaching. Interchange, 17:37–51, 1986.

Singer, RN. Motor learning research: Meaningful ways for physical educators or waste of time? Quest, 42:114–125, 1990.

Smith, PJ. Attention and the contextual interference effect for a continuous task. Perceptual and Motor Skills, 84:83–92, 1997.

Smyth, TR, & Glencross, DJ. Information processing deficits in clumsy children. Australian Journal of Psychology, 38:13–22, 1986.

Sparrow, WA. The efficiency of skilled performance. Journal of Motor Behavior, 15:237–261, 1983.

Steyer David, K. Motor sequencing strategies in school-aged children. Physical Therapy, 65:883–889, 1985.

Stratton, RK. Information processing deficits in children's motor performance: Implications for instruction. Motor Skills: Theory into Practice, 3:49–55, 1978.

Surburg, PR, Poretta, DL, & Sutlive, V. Use of imagery practice for improving a motor skill. Adapted Physical Activity Quarterly, 12:217–227, 1995.

Tarantola, J, Nardone, A, Tacchini, E, & Schieppati, M. Human stance stability improves with the repetition of the task: Effect of foot position and visual condition. Neuroscience Letters, 228:75–78, 1997.

Taylor, A, & Gousie, G. The ecology of learning environments for children. CEFP Journal, July-August:23–28, 1988.

Taylor, D, Christopher, M, & Freshman, S. Pediatric Screening: A Tool for Occupational and Physical Therapists. Seattle: University of Washington, 1983.

Thaut, MH, Hurt, CP, Dragon, D, & McIntosh, GC. Rhythmic entrainment of gait patterns in children with cerebral palsy. AACPDM Abstracts, 40:15, 1998.

Thelen, E, Kelso, JAS, & Fogel, A. Self-organizing systems and infant motor development. Developmental Reviews, 7:39–65, 1987.

Thomas, JR, Gallagher, JD, & Purvis, GJ. Reaction time and anticipation time: Effects of development. Research Quarterly for Exercise and Sport, 52:359–367, 1981.

Thomas, KM, & Nelson, CA. Serial reaction time learning in pre-school- and school-age children. Journal of Experimental Child Psychology, 79:364–387, 2001.

Thorpe, DE, & Valvano, J. The effects of knowledge of performance and cognitive strategies on motor skill learning in children with cerebral palsy. Pediatric Physical Therapy, 14(1):2–15, 2002.

Titzer, R, Shea, JB, & Romack, J. The effect of learner control on the acquisition and retention of a motor task. Journal of Sport and Exercise Psychology, 15(suppl):S84, 1993.

Toglia, JP. Generalization of treatment: A multicontext approach to cognitive perceptual impairment in adults with brain injury. American Journal of Occupational Therapy, 45:505–516, 1991.

Trahey PH. A comparison of cost-effectiveness of two types of occupational therapy services. American Journal of Occupational Therapy, 45:397–400, 1991.

Tscharnuter, I. A new therapy approach to movement organization. Physical and Occupational Therapy in Pediatrics, 13(2):19–40, 1993.

Turvey, MT, & Carello, C. The ecological approach to perceiving-acting: A pictorial essay. Acta Psychologica, 63:133–155, 1986.

Ulrich, DA, Ulrich, BD, Angulo-Kinzler, RM, & Yun, J. Treadmill training of infants with Down syndrome: Evidence-based developmental outcomes. Pediatrics 108(5):E84, 2001. Accessed at http://www.pediatrics.org/cgi/content/full/108/5/384.

Valvano, J. Activity-focused motor interventions for children with neurological conditions. Physical & Occupational Therapy in Pediatrics, 24(1,2):79–107, 2004.

Vander Linden, DW, Cauraugh, JH, & Green, TA. The effect of frequency of kinetic feedback on learning an isometric motor force production task in nondisabled subjects. Physical Therapy, 73:79–87, 1993.

van der Weel, FR, van der Meer, ALH, & Lee, DN. Effect of task on movement control in cerebral palsy: Implications for assessment and therapy. Developmental Medicine and Child Neurology, 33:419–426, 1991.

Van Hasselt, VB, Sisson, LA, & Aach, SR. Parent training to increase compliance in a young multihandicapped child. Journal of Behavior Therapy and Experimental Psychiatry, 18:275–283, 1987.

van Rossum, JHA. The level of organization of the motor schema. Journal of Motor Behavior, 12:145–148, 1980.

VanSant, AF. Life-span development in functional tasks. Physical Therapy, 70:788–798, 1990.

Vurpillot, E. The development of scanning strategies and their relation to visual differentiation. Journal of Experimental Child Psychology, 6:632–650, 1968.

Wade, MG. Coincidence anticipation of young normal and handicapped children. Journal of Motor Behavior, 12:103–112, 1980.

Walker, MP, Brakefield, T, Morgan, A, Hobson, JA, & Stickgold, R. Practice with sleep makes perfect: Sleep-dependent motor skill learning. Neuron, 35:205–211, 2002.

Walter, C. An alternative view of dynamical systems concepts in motor control and learning. Research Quarterly for Exercise and Sport, 69(4):326–333, 1998.

Walter, C, Lee, T, & Sternad, D. The dynamic systems approach to motor control and learning: Promises, potential limitations, and future directions. Research Quarterly for Exercise and Sport, 69(4):316–318, 1998.

Warren, W. Perceived affordance: visual guidance of stair climbing. Journal of Experimental Psychology: Human Perception and Performance, 10:683–703, 1984.

Weeks, DL, & Anderson, LP. The interaction of observational learning with overt practice: effects on motor skill learning. Acta Psychologica, 104:259-271, 2000.

Weeks, DL, & Sherwood, DE. A comparison of knowledge of results scheduling methods for promoting motor skill acquisition and retention. Research Quarterly for Exercise and Sport, 65:136–142, 1994.

Weiss, MR, McCullagh, P, Smith, AL, & Berlant, AR. Observational learning and the fearful child: Influence of peer models on swimming skill performance and psychological responses. Research Quarterly for Exercise and Sport, 69(4):380–394, 1998.

Wickstrom, RL. Fundamental Motor Patterns. Philadelphia: Lea & Febiger, 1977.

Williams, K. Age difference on a coincident anticipation task: Influence of stereotypic or "preferred" movement speed. Journal of Motor Behavior, 17:389–410, 1985.

Willingham, DB. A neuropsychological theory of motor skill learning. Psychological Review, 105(3):558–584, 1998.

Winstein, CJ. Knowledge of results and motor learning: Implications for physical therapy. Physical Therapy, 71:140–149, 1991a.

Winstein, CJ. Designing practice for motor learning: Clinical implications. In Lister, MJ (Ed.). Contemporary Management of Motor Control Problems. Proceedings of the II Step Conference. Alexandria, VA: Foundation for Physical Therapy, 1991b, pp. 65–76.

Winstein, CJ. Effects of physical guidance and knowledge of results on motor learning: Support for the guidance hypothesis. Research Quarterly for Exercise and Sport, 65:316–323, 1994.

Winstein, CJ, Gardner, ER, McNeal, DR, Barto, PT, & Nicholson, DE. Standing balance training: Effect on balance and locomotion in hemiparetic adults. Archives of Physical Medicine and Rehabilitation, 70:755–762, 1989.

Winstein, CJ, Pohl, PS, Cardinale, C, Green, A, Scholtz, L, & Sauber Waters, C. Learning a partial-weight-bearing skill: Effectiveness of two forms of feedback. Physical Therapy, 76:985–993, 1996.

Woodworth, RS. The accuracy of voluntary movement. Psychological Review, 3(suppl 2), 1899.

Wulf, G, Lee, TD, & Schmidt, RA. Reducing knowledge of results about relative versus absolute timing: Differential effects on learning. Journal of Motor Behavior, 26:362–369, 1994.

Wulf, G, & Schmidt, RA. Feedback-induced variability and the learning of generalized motor programs. Journal of Motor Behavior, 26:348–361, 1994.

Wulf, G, & Toole, T. Physical assistance devices in complex motor skill learning: Benefits of a self-controlled practice schedule. Research Quarterly for Exercise and Sport, 70:265–272, 1999.

Wulf, G, & Shea, CH. Principles derived from the study of simple skills do not generalize to complex skill learning. Psychonomic Bulletin & Review, 9(2);185–211, 2002.

Yaguez, L, Canavan, AG, Lange, HW, & Homberg, V. Motor learning by imagery is differentially affected in Parkinson's and Huntington's diseases. Behavior and Brain Research, 102:115–127, 1999.

Yue, G, & Cole, KJ. Strength increases from the motor program: Comparison of training with maximal voluntary and imagined muscle contractions. J Neurophysiology, 67:1114–1123, 1992.

Zhang, J, Gast, DL, Horvat, M, & Dattilo, J. Effect of a constant time delay procedure on motor skill completion durations. Education and Training in Mental Retardation and Developmental Disabilities, 35(3):317–325, 2000.

Chapter 5

GAIT: DEVELOPMENT AND ANALYSIS

JEAN L. STOUT
PT, MS

One of the first questions asked by many parents whose child has recently been diagnosed as having a motor impairment, or whose child has experienced an injury that affects movement is, "Will my child walk?" or "Will my child walk again?" The reason for emphasis on the task of walking apart from many other abilities (which are sometimes more functional), I believe, is the measure of independence and social acceptance with which the task of walking is associated. The ultimate goal for families, and sometimes pediatric therapists as well, becomes independent walking for the child. Although the variables that contribute to this important ability are numerous and complex, a child is usually able to stand and walk by 9 to 15 months of age (see Chapter 2). Normative data from the Alberta Infant Motor Scale (AIMS) indicate that 50% of infants will achieve independent standing by the age of 10.5 months, take first steps by 11 months, and walk independently by the age of 11.5 months (Piper & Darrah, 1994). Furthermore, the pattern is mature by the age of 3.5 years (Sutherland et al., 1980), all without instruction. The complexity of the task has been studied extensively since the days of Saunders (1953) and Murray (1964), and study continues today. Improved computerized techniques and new theories of motor control and balance contribute to better understanding of the components of walking. Understanding how we walk was once required only for those in the fields of child development and rehabilitation. Today walking is studied by many disciplines, including engineering. The extent and duration of the research in the area is a statement of its continued importance.

The purpose of this chapter is to provide an overview of the aspects of gait important to physical therapists treating children. These include the development of gait and its refinement in childhood, the typical components of walking as identified by gait analysis, and a description of some of the common gait deviations found in children with physical disabilities. Guidelines for when a computerized gait analysis is desirable will also be addressed. Those interested in more extensive information are referred to a number of excellent resources on the topic (Gage, 1991; Gage, 2004, Inman et al., 1981; Ounpuu et al., 1991; Perry, 1992; Rose et al., 1991; Stout et al., 1993, 1994; Sutherland, 1984; Sutherland et al., 1980, 1988; Winter, 1979, 1983, 1987, 1990).

DEVELOPMENT OF GAIT

Gage (1991) suggests that typical walking has five major attributes: (1) stability in stance, (2) sufficient foot clearance in swing, (3) appropriate pre-positioning of the foot for initial contact, (4) adequate step length, and (5) energy conservation. When independent ambulation begins in the toddler only the prerequisites for these attributes are present. The prerequisites, however, are likely to be more important to the attainment of walking than the attributes themselves. The attributes develop over time with typical growth, maturation, and refinement of the skill. Scales of motor development illustrate that even during the time period between first steps and independent walking important balance abilities are achieved (Bly, 1994; Piper & Darrah, 1994). This includes rudimentary anticipatory postural adjustments for gait initiation (Adolph et al., 2003; Assaiante et al., 2000). Loss of the five attributes occurs in atypical gait because of a loss or failure to achieve the prerequisites. The prerequisites related to the development and skill of locomotion have already been suggested in Chapter 2 during the review of the eight subsystems proposed on the basis of the dynamic systems theory (Heriza, 1991). These include adequate motor control and central nervous system (CNS) maturation (implying an intact neurologic system), adequate range of motion (ROM), strength, appropriate bone structure and composition, and intact sensation (proprioception). New research suggests that muscle activation patterns for pelvis stabilization may also be a prerequisite (Assaiante et al., 2000). As suggested by Campbell (Chapter 2), the development of a motor pattern (in this case walking) "depends on a combination of mechanical [including structural], neurologic, cognitive, and perceptual factors." When other factors are controlled, chronologic age is less significant than previously thought (Adolph et al., 2003). A brief description of the neurologic and biomechanical factors that contribute to the development and refinement of walking follows.

NEUROLOGIC FACTORS

Campbell (Chapter 2) and Bradley & Westcott (Chapter 3) have discussed the primary neurologic factors related to walking and other motor tasks. To briefly review, the basic neural organization and function used to execute locomotion is thought to be controlled by a central pattern generator located either in the spinal cord or in the brainstem (Connelly & Forssberg, 1997; Grillner, 1981). Descending neural input activates the central pattern generator (Jordan, 1986), and descending and peripheral input (Armstrong, 1986; Loeb, 1986) modify the output to adapt the execution to stability requirements and the demands of the specific task and environment. The central pattern generator is believed to organize the activation and firing sequence of muscles during gait. The parallels between developing animals and humans, and

the parallels between the sequencing and timing of infant stepping, kicking, and locomotion in infants with and without disabilities (Forssberg, 1985; Thelen, 1986; Thelen & Cooke, 1987; Thelen & Ulrich, 1991; Ulrich & Ulrich, 1995; Zelazo, 1983) have led individuals to suggest that the neural foundations for locomotion are present at a very early stage in prenatal development (Bradley & Bekoff, 1989). Postnatally, the major periods of accelerated brain growth in relation to body growth occur between 3 and 10 months of age (Epstein, 1979), and the myelination that develops during this time probably contributes to the neural organization required for independent locomotion. Sufficient maturation of information processing capabilities of the CNS for both internal and external stimuli is also believed to play a role (Assaiante et al., 2000; Zelazo, 1998).

BIOMECHANICAL FACTORS

Adequate ROM, strength, appropriate bone structure and composition, and body composition also affect the emergence of locomotion and its refinement. These variables have significant ramifications as mechanical factors in the development of walking. ROM, strength, bony structure, and the ability to manage gravitational and inertial forces of the lower extremities affect the early patterns of walking. In the presence of typical motor control and maturation, constraints in any of these mechanical variables change patterns; as the constraints change, so do the movement and the muscle activity involved in motor control. Kugler and colleagues (1982) suggest that changes seen in the development of many skills may be the result of critical dimension changes in the body of the growing child. Thelen and colleagues described how simple physical growth could be an explanation for the disappearance of the stepping reflex. This study was recently republished in 2002 (Thelen et al., 1984, 2002).

More recent work also corroborates the importance of mechanical factors, suggesting that infants often have to physically grow into the body dimensions needed for optimal functioning and develop adequate conduction time for activation of central pattern generators (Connelly & Forssberg, 1997; Jensen & Bothner, 1998, Jensen et al., 1997; Sun & Jensen, 1994). Gajdosik and Gajdosik present an extensive review of musculoskeletal development and adaptation in Chapter 6.

DETERMINANTS OF WALKING

Sutherland and colleagues (1980) identified five important determinants of mature walking. The determinants distinguish walking that is considered "mature" (age 3 years and older) from walking that is "immature" (age 2.5 years and younger). The most important of the 13 variables analyzed were the duration of single-limb stance, walking velocity, cadence, step length, and the ratio of pelvic span to ankle spread. The variable with the least discriminating power was the presence or absence of a heel strike at initial contact.

The duration of single-limb stance is, as the name implies, the length of time during which only one foot is on the ground during stance phase. As a child's walking pattern matures the duration of single-limb stance increases, implying a measure of increasing stability and increasing control. The most rapid change occurs between ages 1.5 and 3.5 years.

The remaining variables (with the exception of pelvic span to ankle spread) are temporal distance parameters that are influenced by growth. A linear relationship between step length and leg length is present from age 1 to age 7. A linear relationship between step length and age exists from age 1 to age 4. Walking velocity also increases with age up to age 7, although the rate of change decreases from age 4 to age 7. Cadence gradually decreases with age throughout childhood. The most rapid reduction in cadence occurs between the ages of 1 and 2 years. Because of this strong correlation with age, leg length, and stature, methods of normalization have been explored and endorsed to better understand their influence on these and other temporal distance parameters (Hof, 1996; O'Malley, 1996; Stansfield et al., 2001). Using a geometric normalization technique on Sutherland's data, it was demonstrated that preferred stride length and

cadence increase and decrease, respectively, up to age 3.5 and remain essentially constant into adulthood (Hof & Zylstra, 1997). The non-normalized changes with respect to age in these and other determinants are outlined in Table 5-1. These determinants will be discussed as the refinement of walking is described at various ages.

REFINEMENT OF GAIT BY AGE

Birth to Age 9 Months

The disproportionate contribution of fat content to overall increases in body mass over the first 8 months of postnatal life causes infants to be relatively weak during a time when they are developing the motor control and coordination skills to progress toward independent ambulation (Thelen et al., 1982, 1984). Studies suggest that bigger, fatter infants achieve locomotor milestones later than their smaller peers for this reason (Adolph, 1997). From birth to 6 months of age, the body fat of the infant rises from 12% to 25% of body mass (Spady, 1989). Adipose tissue is a major component of weight gain during the first 4 months of postnatal life, with increases in lipids accounting for more than 40% of total weight gain during this time (Fomon, 1967). Between 4 and 12 months of age increased lipid content accounts for approximately 20% of increased weight. With increasing age and mobility, fat content drops and muscle mass increases.

Not only mass but also body proportions change as infants grow. During the first few months of life, the fastest rate of growth occurs in the extremities as opposed to the head and trunk. Inertial characteristics of body segments

| TABLE 5-1 | Changes in Typical Time and Distance Parameters at Selected Ages from the Onset of Walking through Age 7 |

	AGE			
TIME AND DISTANCE PARAMETERS	**1 YEAR**	**1.5 YEARS**	**3 YEARS**	**7 YEARS**
Opposite toe-off (% cycle)	17	18	16	12
Opposite foot-strike (% cycle)	49	50	50	50
Single stance (% cycle)	32	32	35	38
Toe-off (% cycle)	67	68	66	62
Step length (cm)	22	25	33	48
Stride length (cm)	43	50	67	97
Cycle time (s)	0.68	0.70	0.77	0.83
Cadence (steps/min)	176	171	154	144
Walking velocity (cm/s)	64	71	86	114
Walking velocity (m/min)	38.4	42.6	51.6	68.4

Modified from Sutherland, DH, Olshen, RA, Biden, EN, & Wyatt, MP. The Development of Mature Walking. London: Mac Keith Press, 1988.

change with growth and the effects of gravity. It has been demonstrated that the resistance to motion in limb segments (segment moments of inertia) more than doubles and triples during the first 6 months of life (Jensen & Bothner, 1998; Sun & Jensen, 1994). The rate of change in gravitational moments appears to decrease relative to the rate of change in the developing extensor muscle moment in a cephalocaudal progression, which also influences the ability to move against gravity (Jensen et al., 1997).

The body structure of infants as they develop the ability to stand upright with support and to cruise independently affects their posture and movement patterns. Flexion "contractures" are present at the hips, and range of hip external rotation is slightly greater than range of internal rotation. Range of hip abduction is slightly increased at 8 to 9 months of age but has been slowly decreasing since birth (Coon et al., 1975; Haas et al., 1973; Phelps et al., 1985; Sutherland et al., 1988; Walker, 1991). Femoral anteversion* (a forward or anterior orientation of the head and neck with respect to the frontal plane) and femoral antetorsion (a twist of the bone in its longitudinal axis) of the hips are both present (Bleck, 1982, 1987; Cusick & Stuberg, 1992; Engel & Staheli, 1974; Fabray et al., 1973). The magnitude of the femoral torsion is 40° to 50°.

Structurally, the knees in the frontal plane exhibit genu varum, or bowing in the tibiofemoral angle (Fig. 5-1) (Salenius & Vankka, 1975; Tachdjian, 1990). The tibia and fibula exhibit neutral alignment about the longitudinal axis, which represents slight internal torsion relative to adult values (Staheli & Engel, 1972; Staheli et al., 1985). A medial inclination of the talotibial articulation is present in the infant, producing an everted talocrural mortise (Bernhardt, 1988; Root et al., 1971; Tachdjian, 1985; Valmassy, 1984). The medial inclination of the joint is manifested in an everted heel position in weight bearing. Supported walking at this age is characterized by wide abduction, external rotation, and flexion at the hips (Bly, 1994), bowed legs, and an everted heel position.

The postural control, development of antigravity muscle strength, and control of gravitational moments that are gained over the first 9 months of life are important precursors to the development of independent ambulation. Standing balance is also a necessary precursor to upright motor skill. The frequency and the amount of practice of activities such as kicking have been shown to affect the age of onset of ambulation, in infants with and without

---

*Femoral anteversion and femoral antetorsion are often used as synonymous terms in orthopedic literature to refer to the torsion or the medial twist between the axis of the head and neck of the femur and the axis of the femoral condyles.

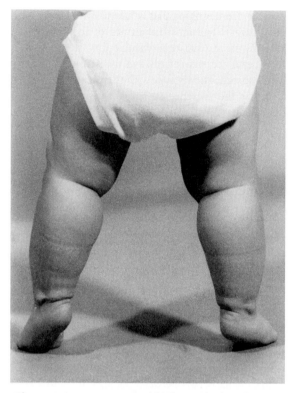

◆ **Figure 5-1**   An 8-month-old infant with physiologic varus in the tibiofemoral angle.

disabilities (Adolph, 1997; Ulrich & Ulrich, 1995). Antigravity strength of the hip flexors in the lower extremities is built early on in the developmental process by kicking from the supine position. Hip extensor strength in both concentric and eccentric types of muscle contractions similar to those used in ambulation begins from activities in the prone position but gradually builds as the infant begins creeping and kneeling activities. Bly describes infants of 8 months of age exhibiting the ability to rise from a kneeling to standing position, which requires closed chain hip and knee extension. Control of gravitational moments at the hip by the hip flexor and extensor muscles has typically occurred by 8 to 9 months of age (Jensen et al., 1997). Cruising along furniture builds strength of the hip abductors (Bly, 1994).

By 8 months of age, the visual, proprioceptive, and vestibular systems work together to consistently bring the center of mass back to a stable position after perturbation in a seated position (Woollacott et al., 1989). Needed postural corrections in response to visual flow for a particular skill often predate the development of that skill (Adolph, 1997; Butterworth & Hicks, 1977; Hirschfield & Forssberg, 1994; Woollacott et al., 1989). For example, Butterworth and Hicks (1977) demonstrated that infants who could sit alone but could not stand independently exhibited the same appropriate postural adjustments to visual information that simulated movement as did infants who were able to walk independently.

Age 9 to 15 Months

Lower extremity alignment and body structure at the onset of ambulation are characterized by a standing posture with a wide base of support and the hips in abduction, flexion, and slight external rotation. The tibias display mild internal torsion, and varus is still present in the tibiofemoral angle; the heel position in weight bearing remains everted because of the inclination of the mortise joint. The child's center of mass is proportionately closer to the head and upper trunk (at the lower thoracic level) than in an older child, whose center of mass is located at midlumbar level, or in an adult, whose center of mass is located at the sacral level (Palmer, 1944). Although differential growth rates are allowing the head to become relatively smaller than the rest of the body, the head is still proportionately large. The ratio of body fat to muscle mass is still high, contributing to weakness relative to the demands of upright posture. Coming upright against the force of gravity puts new demands on muscle strength. Muscles (particularly the abdominals, hip flexors, knee extensors, and ankle dorsiflexors) must work in new antigravity positions, which further increases functional weakness. Despite the structural limitations, infants exhibit the necessary postural responses to compensate for visual and support-surface perturbations that are inherent in the task of upright locomotion (Berger et al., 1985; Butterworth & Hicks, 1977; Shumway-Cook & Woollacott, 1985; Thelen et al., 1989; Woollacott et al., 1989).

The rate-limiting factors associated with the ability to demonstrate upright locomotion are (1) sufficient extensor muscle strength to support the body's weight on a single-limb base of support, (2) dynamic balance, and (3) postural control in the form of anticipatory and integrative postural adjustments (Assaiante et al., 2000; Connelly & Forssberg, 1997; Thelen et al., 1989). The critical dimension of the body to be controlled is the head within the limits of stability of the base of support. The base of support in an infant at the onset of ambulation is wide for both structural and stability reasons. Mediolateral (side to side) stability is achieved, but anteroposterior stability is limited. Progression takes place in the sagittal plane; if the head moves outside the limits of stability at the base of support, balance is lost.

Initial anticipatory postural adjustments used for gait initiation during the postural phase (mainly the lateral shift of body weight toward the stance limb) are present at the onset of walking, but those required during the locomotor phase (control of the swing side pelvic drop)

are not (Assaiante et al., 2000). Because the hip is the interface between the locomotor movements of the legs and head-arms-trunk postural control, strength and control at the hip is very important. Studies have shown that at the onset of ambulation, hip strength is inadequate to control the gravitational forces during gait and maintain balance. Infants actually "walk by falling" (Breniere & Bril, 1998). If balance is perturbed, control is regained by rudimentary mechanisms requiring torque adjustments at multiple joints (Roncesvalles et al., 2001).

The pattern displayed by a beginning walker is similar to that of an experienced walker on a slippery surface (i.e., small steps, a widened base of support, and maintenance of the body and limbs very upright in an extended, stiff position). Postural adjustments are made using movements of the entire body. The work of Sutherland and colleagues (1988) characterizes infant ambulation as consisting of a wide base of support, increased hip and knee flexion, full foot initial contact in plantar flexion, a short stride, increased cadence, and a relative footdrop in swing phase.

Motorically, the initial pattern and execution of the first steps are thought to be related to the patterns used in stepping and kicking during early infancy (Thelen & Cooke, 1987) and may be constrained by this pattern. That is, just as the structural makeup of the body drives the initial posture, so may the primitive generator for kicking and stepping drive the muscle activity for early walking. The reduced frequency of kicking in children with Down syndrome has been shown to be correlated with a later age of walking than in typically developing infants (Ulrich & Ulrich, 1995). Both kicking and stepping are alternating reciprocal patterns of movement between the limbs. Each has a flexion phase (in gait, analogous to swing) and an extension phase (in gait, analogous to stance). Thelen and colleagues (1989) suggest that the ability to generate steplike patterns is continuous from the newborn period through independent locomotion and that the pattern demonstrated in beginning upright ambulation is a modified, more flexible version of the earlier pattern that has been modified by changes in strength, neurologic maturation, and the mechanics of upright posture.

The electromyographic (EMG) patterns of activity at the onset of independent ambulation demonstrate significant co-contraction across antagonistic muscle groups—the anterior tibialis and gastrocnemius during swing phase and the quadriceps and hamstrings muscles during stance phase (Kazai et al., 1976; Okamoto & Kumamoto, 1972; Sutherland et al., 1980, 1988; Thelen & Cooke, 1987). Coactivation patterns result from the need for stability.

As stated previously, Thelen and colleagues suggest that it is not the pattern-generating capabilities or motor control postural abilities that constrain the onset of independent locomotion. Development of sufficient extensor strength is believed to be the critical variable (Thelen et al., 1989). This belief is consistent with other views for the requirements of walking, including stance phase stability (Gage, 1991), the need to maintain a net extensor muscle support moment as described by Winter (1987, 1990), and the inability of the hip to completely control the gravitational forces for balance (Breniere & Bril, 1998).

Age 18 to 24 Months

As the child grows, body structure changes, increases in strength, neurologic maturation, and walking experience all play a part in altering the walking pattern. By 18 months of age, the varus angulation of the tibiofemoral angle in the frontal plane has resolved and the limb is straight (Fig. 5-2) (Tachdjian, 1990; see also Chapter 6). No change is noted in excessive femoral antetorsion, although limitation in hip extension ROM is reduced to an average of 4°, indicating that remodeling is under way (Fabray et al.,

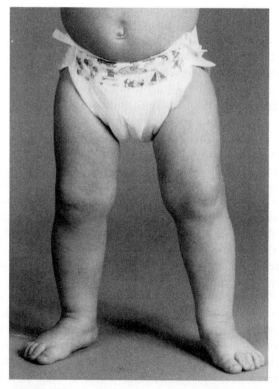

◆ **Figure 5-2** Standing posture of an 18-month-old toddler. The varus in the tibiofemoral angle has resolved, and the limb is straight.

1973; Phelps et al., 1985). Range of hip abduction is no longer excessive. Because of decreased abduction and improved stability, the base of support has decreased. Dynamic balance and strength have also improved. A heel strike has not consistently emerged in the 18-month-old child (Sutherland et al., 1980, 1988), but the lessened base of support allows for more anterior-posterior movement over the planted foot. Heel position remains everted (Root et al., 1971; Valmassy, 1984). The viscoelastic and inertial properties of the stretched stance limb begin to be exploited to propel the leg in swing (Thelen & Cooke, 1987). A knee flexion wave begins to emerge during initial stance phase as a heel strike develops and knee extensor contraction absorbs some of the impact of floor contact (Sutherland et al., 1980, 1988). The duration of stance phase remains prolonged, and cadence is increased relative to mature gait (see Table 5-1).

The efficiency of locomotion slowly improves during the period from 18 to 24 months of age as the center of mass descends from a position high above the lower extremities to one in close proximity to the chief motor power in the legs. Stability of any body is inversely related to the distance of its center of mass from its base of support. Between the first and second years of life, the legs are growing proportionately longer, becoming the most rapidly increasing dimension of the body. These events bring the center of mass closer to the proximal end of the lower limbs (Palmer, 1944).

Controversy exists over whether heel strike develops as a result of neurologic maturation or gradual changes in body structure, base of support, improved strength, and improved stability (Forssberg, 1985, 1992; Thelen & Cooke, 1987; Thelen et al., 1989). It is likely that each variable is important. A consistent heel strike develops by 24 months of age (Sutherland et al., 1980, 1988). Requirements include refined motor control, strength, and dynamic balance to sustain stability on a small area of contact (the heel). Children with impaired walking ability lack a heel strike at initial contact. This may be caused by either lack of motor control or the inherent choice of maintaining stability by use of a larger area of initial contact (Gage, 1991).

With 6 to 12 months of walking experience new strategies are employed for balance and postural control. Walking experience also plays a role. Decreases in peak head and trunk oscillations are noted during the first weeks and months of independent walking (Ledebt & Bril, 2000). A backward inclination of the trunk is noted at this age rather than the anticipatory forward inclination noted in older children and adults (Assaiante et al., 2000). Velocity normalized for height is increasing during this time. The deficit between muscular strength at the hip and vertical acceleration of the center of mass diminishes, which improves the control of the gravitational forces and the postural capacity of the musculoskeletal system as a whole (Breniere & Bril, 1998). As a result, single limb stance is more stable.

The role of walking experience cannot be overestimated. Adolph and colleagues have shown that after controlling for body dimensions and testing age, walking experience explained an additional 19% to 26% of variance in improvement in walking skill in a group of 210 infants of differing ages. Previous diary studies have demonstrated that infants may take as many as 9000 steps in a given day and travel the equivalent of 29 football fields (Adolph, 2002; Adolph et al., 2003).

The EMG patterns at this age show decreasing co-contraction in antagonistic muscle groups, implying increased control and stability. The primary changes occur in the duration of stance phase activity (Okamoto & Kumamoto, 1972; Sutherland et al., 1980, 1988). The durations of stance phase quadriceps, medial hamstring, and anterior tibialis muscle activity are all decreased in the 18- to 24-month-old as compared with those seen in the 12-month-old. By age 2, the late swing phase–early stance phase EMG activity monitored in the gastrocnemius-soleus complex of the 12- to 18-month-old child has disappeared (Sutherland et al., 1980, 1988).

Age 3 to 3.5 Years

Between the ages of 3 and 3.5 years, the joint angles associated with walking mature into the adult pattern (Sutherland et al., 1980, 1988). Structurally, the tibiofemoral angle, which was neutral at 18 months of age, now shows maximum valgus alignment (Salenius & Vankka, 1975) (Fig. 5-3). Femoral antetorsion of the hip is decreasing but remains increased in relation to that measured in an adult. The center of mass is closer to the extremities as the rate of lower extremity growth stabilizes (Palmer, 1944). Heel eversion in weight bearing can still be observed but is decreasing. Measurement by motion analysis demonstrates that a heel strike is consistently present in conjunction with a knee flexion wave in early stance (Sutherland et al., 1980, 1988). EMG activity has a mature pattern by this age.

Balance mechanisms continue to be refined during this period. Torque profiles of perturbation responses demonstrate that children in this age range continue to exhibit an immature pattern, but the pattern is clearly different from children with less walking experience (Roncesvalles et al., 2001). The vertical acceleration of the center of mass at foot contact also demonstrates a deficit in the capacity of the stance leg muscles to control balance. However, walking velocity normalized

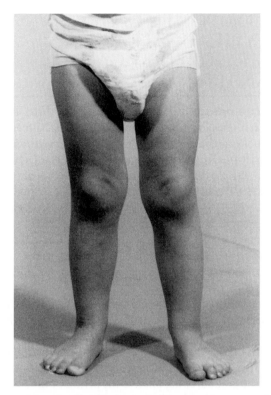

◆ **Figure 5-3** The tibiofemoral alignment of a 3-year-old showing maximum physiologic valgus.

for height is consistent with that of adults (Breniere & Bril, 1998).

Age 6 to 7 Years

By age 7, the gait patterns by standards of movement or motion are fully mature. Minimal changes are noted when compared with the adult pattern, although time and distance variables continue to vary with age and stature (Sutherland et al., 1980, 1988). Balance and postural control demonstrate renewed stability after a period of disequilibrium often seen between ages 4 and 6 years, and reach maturity (Breniere & Bril, 1998; Roncesvalles et al., 2001; Shumway-Cook & Woollacott, 1985; Woollacott et al., 1989). Structurally, the tibiofemoral angle has returned to neutral (Tachdjian, 1990), and femoral antetorsion is largely resolved but still slightly higher than that measured in the adult (Bleck, 1987; Fabray et al., 1973). The inclination of the talotibial joint is no longer present, and heel position is neutral by age 7 (Valmassy, 1984). A period of disproportionate growth with respect to body dimensions has also passed. The center of mass is still slightly higher than in the adult, at the level of the third lumbar vertebra (Palmer, 1944).

COMPONENTS OF TYPICAL GAIT AS MEASURED BY GAIT ANALYSIS

As stated previously, extensive research has been done and continues to be done in the area of gait. Numerous textbooks and basic research articles have been written on the topic (Gage, 1991, 2004; Inman et al., 1981; Ounpuu et al., 1991; Perry, 1992; Rose et al., 1991, 1993; Sepulveda et al., 1993; Stout et al., 1993; Sutherland, 1984; Sutherland et al., 1980, 1988; Winter, 1979, 1983, 1987, 1990; Zajac & Gordon, 1989). This section describes the typical components of mature walking as identified by three-dimensional computerized analysis of movement and forces, electromyography, and energy expenditure in a functional context.

One complete gait cycle refers to a single stride that begins when one foot strikes the ground and ends when the same foot strikes the ground again. The gait cycle is divided into two major phases—stance and swing. Stance phase is associated with the period of time when the foot is on the ground; swing phase is the period of time when the foot is in the air. The stance phase of the gait cycle occupies approximately 60% of the cycle, and the swing phase occupies approximately 40%.

Perry (1992) developed a generic terminology for the functional phases of gait that further divided the gait cycle into eight subphases. Each subphase has a functional objective that assists in the accomplishment of one of three basic tasks of the walking cycle: weight acceptance, single-limb support, and limb advancement (Rancho Los Amigos Medical Center, 1989). The basic tasks that Perry's group described are similar to the "attributes" discussed by Gage (1991): weight acceptance and single-limb support (stability in stance and pre-positioning of the foot for initial contact) and limb advancement (foot clearance in swing, pre-positioning of the foot for initial contact, and adequate step length).

Stance phase is divided into five subphases or instantaneous events (Fig. 5-4):

1. Initial contact (0%–2% of the cycle)
2. Loading response (0%–10% of the cycle)
3. Midstance (10%–30% of the cycle)
4. Terminal stance (30%–50% of the cycle)
5. Preswing (50%–60% of the cycle)

Opposite leg toe-off and opposite initial contact occur at 10% and 50% of the gait cycle, respectively. Thus there are two periods of double support during the walking cycle when both feet are on the ground. These occur during loading response (just after initial contact) and

preswing (just before toe-off). Each occupies approximately 10% of the gait cycle.

Swing phase begins at toe-off and occurs during the period of single support of the stance limb. Three subphases are identified (see Fig. 5-4):

1. Initial swing (60%–73% of the cycle)
2. Midswing (73%–87% of the cycle)
3. Terminal swing (87%–100% of the cycle)

TEMPORAL MEASUREMENT DEFINITIONS AND COMMON TERMS

The following definitions will be helpful in the description of walking as used in gait analysis:

Cadence: The frequency of steps taken in a given amount of time, usually measured in steps per minute.

Concentric muscle contraction: A shortening contraction that produces acceleration. Positive work results and power generation occurs.

Eccentric muscle contraction: A lengthening contraction that produces deceleration. Negative work results and power absorption occurs. The efficiency of negative work or power absorption by a muscle is three to nine times higher than that of positive work (Inman et al., 1981).

External load: Ground reaction forces, inertial forces, and gravitational forces that affect joint motion.

Isometric muscle contraction: A stabilizing contraction that produces no net power. Force is produced without length change in the muscle.

Joint moment: A force acting at a distance from an axis causing a rotation about that axis is called a torque or moment (moment equals force times perpendicular distance). In the body, moments are produced external to the body by ground reaction forces, forces related to gravity, and inertial forces. Moments internal to the body are produced by muscle forces, ligamentous forces, or forces produced by joint capsules. Joint moments in this chapter will represent the physiologic response of the body generated in response to an external load in accordance with the definition used by Ounpuu and colleagues (Ounpuu et al., 1991).

Joint power: The net rate of energy absorption or generation. *Mechanical power* is defined as the work performed per unit of time. *Joint power* is defined as the product of the net joint moment and the joint angular velocity. Muscles are the primary internal power producers in the body. Muscles can also be internal power absorbers. Ligaments usually absorb power.

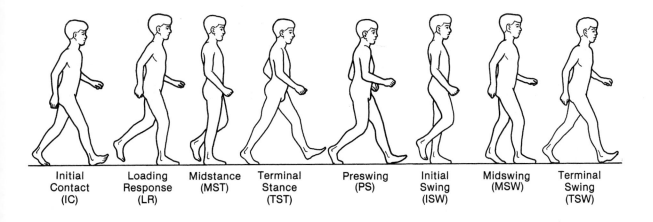

| Initial Contact (IC) | Loading Response (LR) | Midstance (MST) | Terminal Stance (TST) | Preswing (PS) | Initial Swing (ISW) | Midswing (MSW) | Terminal Swing (TSW) |

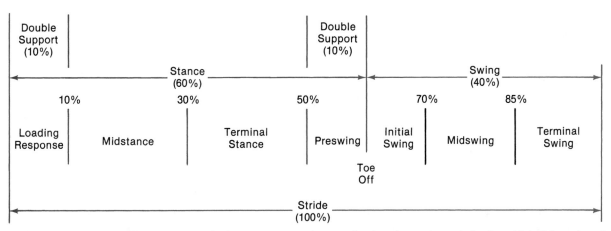

• **Figure 5-4** One complete four gait cycle depicting stance phase and swing phase. The cycle begins with initial contact of the right foot. Stance phase has four subphases after initial contact; swing phase has three subphases. Initial contact and toe-off are instantaneous events. *(Adapted from Gage, JR. An overview of normal walking. In Greene, WB [Ed.]. Instructional Course Lectures, Vol. 39. Park Ridge, IL: American Academy of Orthopaedic Surgeons, 1990.)*

Kinematics: The parameters used to describe motion without regard to forces. These include linear or angular displacements, velocities, and accelerations.

Kinetics: The parameters that describe the causes of the movement. These include external and internal forces such as gravitational forces, ground reaction forces, inertial forces, muscle or ligament forces, joint moments, and joint powers.

Step length: The longitudinal distance between the two feet. Right step length is measured from the first point of contact of the left foot to the first point of contact of the right foot.

Stride length: The longitudinal distance between the initial contact of one foot and the next initial contact of the same foot. It is the sum of the right and

left step lengths and represents the distance traversed in one complete gait cycle.

Walking velocity: The rate of walking or the distance traversed in a specified length of time. Velocity can be expressed as stride length divided by cycle time or the product of step length and cadence. Because of the correlation with leg length and therefore age, methods of normalization are used to evaluate comparisons of different velocities.

KINEMATICS

Kinematics in gait analysis can be collected in either two or three dimensions. Common to all types of computerized motion analysis is a reference system such as the use of external markers or targets placed on the body and aligned with respect to specific anatomic landmarks. Two-dimensional motion systems provide joint angles that are a direct measure of the motion of the marker set placed on the skin. Three-dimensional systems reference the marker coordinate system to an internal coordinate system based on an estimation of the locations of the anatomic joint centers. The outputs, regardless of two- or three-dimensional technique, are typically displayed as a series of graphs of a single gait cycle for each joint in a given plane of motion. Figure 5-5 gives an example of three-dimensional motion data from the Center for Gait and Motion Analysis of Gillette Children's Specialty Healthcare.

KINETICS

Kinetics represent the parameters that describe the causes of the movement. These include external and internal forces such as gravitational forces, ground reaction forces, inertial forces, muscle or ligament forces, joint moments, and joint powers. Kinetic data as part of two- or three-dimensional gait analysis are obtained from a combination of force plate and kinematic information. They are displayed as joint moments and joint powers. The force plate provides information regarding the ground reaction force, and the kinematics provide information regarding the joint angular velocities. Anthropometric measurements of the body are also required. The method commonly used to calculate joint moments and powers is called "inverse dynamics" and is based on a linked segment model approach (Winter, 1990). A ground reaction force method is another method sometimes used (Winter, 1990).

A moment or torque is a force acting at a distance that causes an object to rotate. A joint moment represents the physiologic response of the body generated in response to an external load (Ounpuu et al., 1991). At Gillette Children's, what is displayed on the graphs is the net joint moment, which represents the sum of all internal joint moments in a particular plane at a particular joint. The moments refer primarily to the muscle forces that are acting to control segment rotation, but internal joint moments can be generated by ligaments, joint capsules, and fascia as well. The net joint moment depicts which muscle group is dominant but does not denote the relative contributions of muscle groups on either side of the joint. For example, in the sagittal plane, a net extensor moment at the hip during stance phase implies that the hip extensors are dominant. Hip flexors may or may not contribute, but the overall moment is an extensor moment. The hip extensor muscles are active to counteract an external moment created by the ground reaction force that is tending to flex the hip (Fig. 5-6). The ground

reaction force tends to flex the hip because it is anterior to the joint center.

Power, in mechanical terms, is defined as the rate of doing work. *Joint power* is defined as the product of the net joint moment and the joint angular velocity. Muscles are the primary internal power producers in the body. A muscle's ability to produce power is affected by its cross-sectional area. Other factors that affect power include muscle fiber type, the length-tension ratio, and the degree of fatigue (see Chapter 6). Muscles can also be internal power absorbers. Ligaments usually absorb power. The power graphs display whether power is generated (positive work) or absorbed (negative work). Concentric muscle action is associated with power generation, and eccentric muscle action is associated with power absorption. In the previous example of the hip, the hip is extending in the presence of a net extensor moment; therefore, power generation occurs (Fig. 5-7). Typical sagittal plane kinematics and kinetics can be found in Figure 5-8.

ELECTROMYOGRAPHY

The electrical signal associated with the neuromuscular activation of a muscle is measured by electromyography (Basmajian & DeLuca, 1985; Winter, 1990). It represents the pattern of motor unit activation. Electromyographic data can provide information about the timing of muscle activity and, in some cases, about the intensity of muscle contraction. Under some conditions EMG amplitude has been shown to be related to force (Komi, 1973; Vredenbregt & Rau, 1973), but the usefulness of this aspect for assessment of walking is limited because the relationship is valid only under isometric conditions and when no coactivation is occurring.

The amplitude of an EMG signal is affected by the rate of motor unit firing and the number of motor units active at any given time. The type of motor units firing and the proportion of different motor units firing also affect amplitude. In addition, many external factors, including electrode location, type of electrode used, interelectrode distance, skin temperature, and amount of subcutaneous fat, also affect the amplitude of the signal (Basmajian & DeLuca, 1985). Comparing EMG amplitudes across muscles, or within or between subjects, should be done with caution and adequate understanding of the complexity involved in interpretation. Current research focuses on understanding the relationship of muscle activity and force with joint kinematics and kinetics using engineering principles (Zajac & Gordon, 1989). Combining engineering principles with neural network representations is advancing the understanding of the effects of EMG activity even further (Sepulveda et al., 1993).

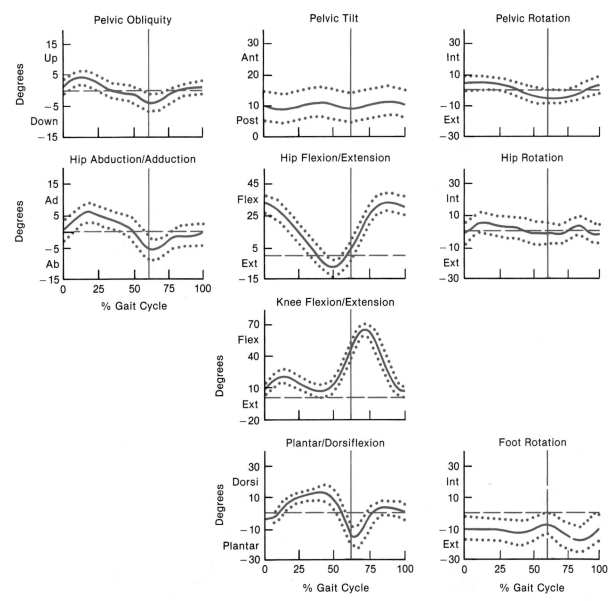

◆ **Figure 5-5**   Representative typical three-dimensional motion data from the Center for Gait and Motion Analysis of Gillette Children's Specialty Healthcare. In this and subsequent figures, one complete gait cycle is depicted and is normalized to 100% of the stride. The mean (*solid line*) and one standard deviation (*dashed line*) of composite data collected from children ages 4 to 19 years are displayed. Stance phase is separated from swing phase in each graph by the vertical line. Each graph represents the same walking cycle. Each row displays a different joint: from top to bottom are pelvis, hip, knee, and ankle. Each column displays the movements of a different joint in the same plane of motion; from left to right are the coronal plane (front view), sagittal plane (side view), and transverse plane (rotational view). *Note:* The pelvis is measured with respect to laboratory coordinates, the hip with respect to the pelvis, and the knee with respect to the thigh. Foot rotation graph represents foot progression angle, not rotation of the foot with respect to the tibia.

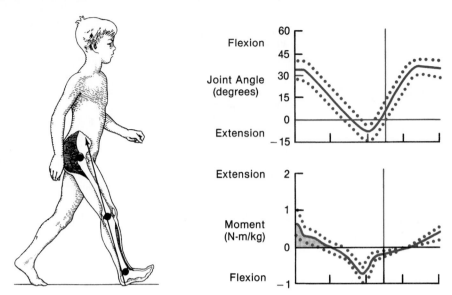

• **Figure 5-6** An example of an internal joint moment produced at the right hip. Because the ground reaction force falls anterior to the hip joint, the joint would flex without internally produced resistance. The joint moment graph demonstrates a net extensor moment at the hip (*shaded*) as the body's internal resistance to the external force. The internal moment is produced by dominant action of the hip extensor muscles. (*Adapted in part from Gage, JR. Gait Analysis in Cerebral Palsy. London: Mac Keith Press, 1991.*)

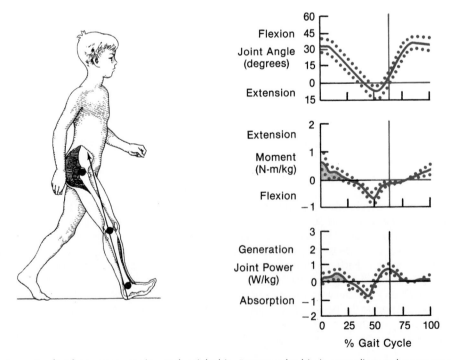

• **Figure 5-7** An example of power generation at the right hip. Because the hip is extending and a net extensor moment is present, power generation (*shaded*) occurs. The units for power are watts per kilogram. By convention, power generation is represented by positive deflection on the graph; power absorption is negative. (*Adapted in part from Gage, JR. Gait Analysis in Cerebral Palsy. London: Mac Keith Press, 1991.*)

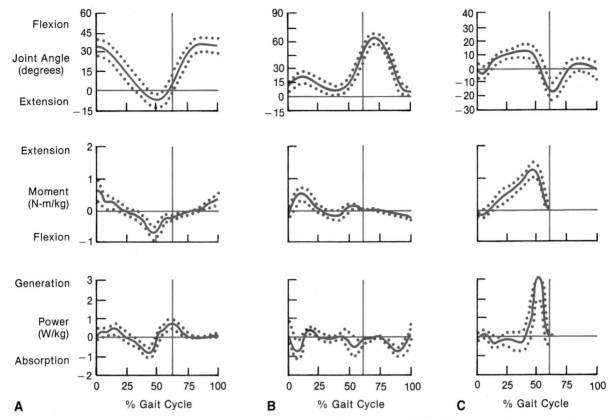

◆ **Figure 5-8**   Sagittal plane kinematics and kinetics of the hip (**A**), knee (**B**), and ankle (**C**). Each graph represents the same walking cycle, with the mean (*solid line*) and one standard deviation (*dashed line*). The top row shows the kinematic graphs; the middle row, the joint moments; and the bottom row, the joint powers. Units for the kinematics are degrees. The units for joint moments (newton-meters/kilogram) and powers (watts/kilogram) are standardized for body weight.

Each muscle has a particular time during the walking cycle when activity is present or absent and a particular pattern of increasing or decreasing motor unit activity. These timings have been documented for both children and adults (Ounpuu et al., 1991; Perry, 1992; Sutherland et al., 1988; Winter & Yack, 1987). An example can be found in Figure 5-9. EMG data can be collected using surface or fine wire (indwelling) electrodes. Reviews on the advantages and disadvantages of each have been published (Kadaba et al., 1985).

KINEMATICS, KINETICS, AND ELECTROMYOGRAPHY IN NORMAL GAIT

A detailed description of activity in the lower extremities during each phase of the gait cycle is presented in this section, including a summary of hip, knee, and ankle kinematics and kinetics with associated muscle activity. Sagittal

plane events are emphasized. The reader should refer to the kinematic and kinetic plots associated with each description.

SAGITTAL PLANE

At *initial contact* (0% of the gait cycle) the ankle is in a position of neutral dorsiflexion, the knee is in minimal flexion, and the hip is in approximately 35° of flexion. The objective of this event is appropriate pre-positioning of the foot to begin the gait cycle. The ground reaction force at initial contact is passing through the heel and is anterior to both the knee and the hip. The gluteus maximus and hamstrings muscles are active to control the external flexor moment at the hip. The hamstrings also assist in preventing knee hyperextension. Anterior tibialis and quadriceps activity initiates the loading response (Fig. 5-10).

Loading response (Fig. 5-11) is a period of acceptance of body weight while maintaining stability and progression. The purpose of loading response is to cushion or absorb the impact of the body's moment of inertia. It is the first

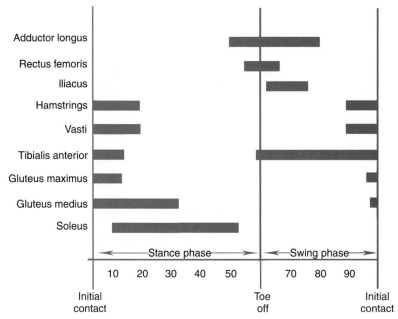

⬧ **Figure 5-9**   The phasic (on/off) EMG activity of the major muscles used during walking. *(Based on data from the Center for Gait and Motion Analysis, Gillette Children's Specialty Healthcare.)*

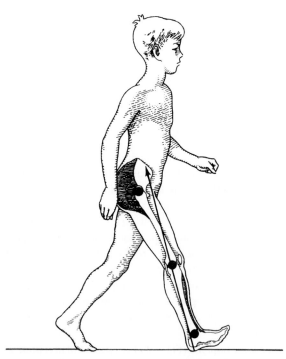

⬧ **Figure 5-10**   Initial contact of the gait cycle. *(From Gage, JR. Gait Analysis in Cerebral Palsy. London: Mac Keith Press, 1991.)*

period of double support and occurs between 0% and 10% of the gait cycle, beginning after initial contact and ending when the entire foot is in contact with the floor. The ankle is plantar flexing at this time under controlled eccentric contraction of the anterior tibialis muscle. The internal moment at the ankle is a net dorsiflexor moment because the dorsiflexor muscles are dominant. The power curve depicts absorption because the anterior tibialis muscle is contracting eccentrically. Gage (1991, 2004) and Perry (1992) refer to loading response as the first "rocker" of ankle stance phase.

During loading response, the knee undergoes an initial phase of flexion to approximately 15° (average value). Both hamstring activity and quadriceps muscle activity are present. Because the quadriceps muscles are acting eccentrically to decelerate knee flexion, the power graph depicts absorption. Whenever the joint movement and the joint moment are opposite each other, power absorption is occurring.

Concentric action of the gluteus maximus, gluteus minimus, and hamstrings are extending the hip. The hamstrings are able to work as hip extensors because knee motion is stabilized by the single joint muscles of the quadriceps. The net internal joint moment is extensor, and the power graph depicts generation. Because the external ground reaction force falls anterior to the hip joint, with-

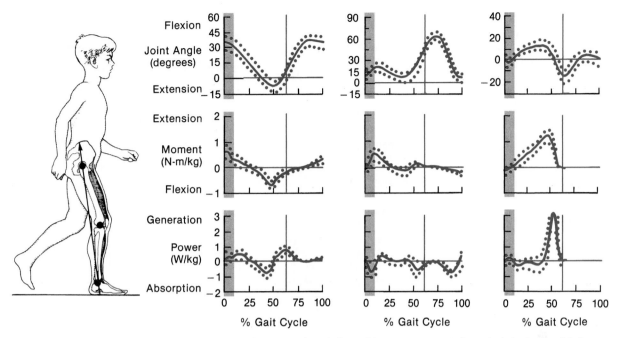

• **Figure 5-11**   Loading response (0%–10% of the gait cycle). *(Adapted from Gage, JR. Gait Analysis in Cerebral Palsy. London: Mac Keith Press, 1991.)*

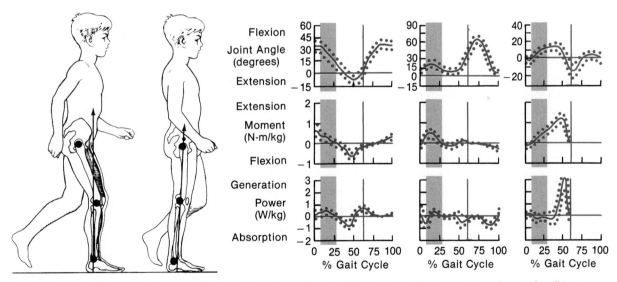

• **Figure 5-12**   Midstance (at 10%–30% of the gait cycle). *(Adapted from Gage, JR. An overview of normal walking. In Greene, WB [Ed.]. Instructional Course Lectures, Vol. 39. Park Ridge, IL: American Academy of Orthopaedic Surgeons, 1990.)*

out the action of the hip extensors the joint would collapse into flexion.

Midstance (Fig. 5-12) is the beginning of the single-support phase of the gait cycle and extends from the period of 10% to 30% of the cycle. The goal during midstance is to maintain trunk and limb stability and allow smooth progression over a stationary foot when the entire plantar surface is in contact with the floor. The ankle is in a period of increasing dorsiflexion that is controlled by eccentric contraction of the soleus muscle. The moment graph demonstrates a dominant plantar flexor moment and the power graph a period of absorption. The second rocker of ankle stance phase occurs during midstance (Gage, 1991, 2004).

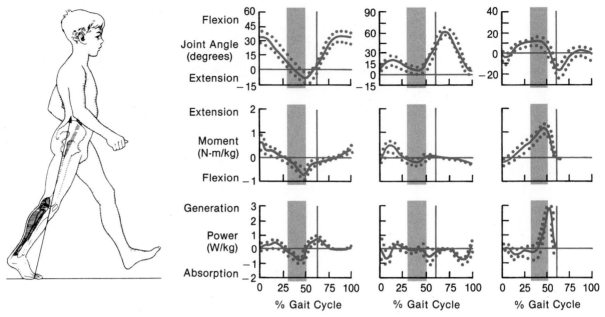

♦ **Figure 5-13**   Terminal stance (at 30%–50% of the gait cycle). *(Adapted from Gage, JR. Gait Analysis in Cerebral Palsy. London: Mac Keith Press, 1991.)*

The knee extends during midstance. The vastus medialis, vastus intermedius, and vastus lateralis muscles work initially to stabilize the knee until the ground reaction force passes anterior to the knee joint. Once the ground reaction force is anterior to the knee, extension is passive. The joint moment at the knee is an extensor moment. The power graph shows initial decreasing absorption followed by generation. This period of power generation is the only one produced at the knee during the entire gait cycle.

The hip continues to extend during midstance. The joint moment is extensor, and power is generated, implicating concentric action of the hip extensor muscles. The internal extension moment, however, is decreasing during this time. When the ground reaction force becomes posterior to the hip joint, a transition occurs from a concentric (power generation) extensor moment to an eccentric (power absorption) flexor moment.

Terminal stance (Fig. 5-13) is the second half of the single-support phase and occurs from 30% to 50% of the gait cycle. This period begins when the ground reaction force passes anterior to the knee and posterior to the hip and often occurs with heel rise. During this phase of the gait cycle, forward progression of the tibia is arrested and further increase in dorsiflexion is limited. The ankle begins a period of decreasing dorsiflexion by concentric contraction of the gastrocnemius and soleus muscles, producing power generation. One of the primary power productions that propels an individual through the walking cycle is generated at the ankle during terminal stance

(36% of the total power generation produced during the walking cycle) (Ounpuu et al., 1991; Winter, 1987). Heel rise marks the period of the third rocker of ankle stance phase (Gage, 1991, 2004).

The knee moves from relative extension to increasing flexion during terminal stance. An internal net flexor moment is dominant because the ground reaction force falls in front of the knee. Power is absorbed. The internal flexor moment is produced by a combination of ligamentous resistance and flexor activity of the gastrocnemius muscle.

The hip continues to extend during terminal stance. Because the ground reaction force is posterior to the joint center, extension is resisted by an internal flexor moment. Power is absorbed, suggesting that the flexor moment is produced by tension force of the iliofemoral ligament.

Preswing (Fig. 5-14) is the second period of double support during the walking cycle and occurs at 50% to 60% of the cycle. The function of preswing is to advance the limb into swing; preswing ends at toe-off. The stance phase extremity is unweighted as weight is accepted on the opposite limb. The ankle is now in true plantar flexion, and the plantar flexor moment remains dominant. The magnitude of the moment is rapidly decreasing, however, and power generation falls rapidly to zero.

The knee joint is flexing during preswing and reaches approximately 45° (average value) at toe-off. The internal muscle moment is extensor, and power is absorbed. Activity of the rectus femoris muscle is probably responsible

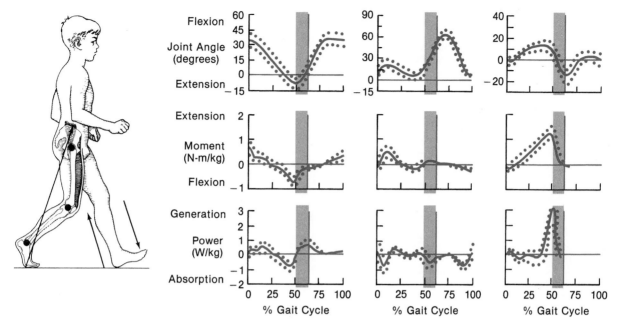

◆ **Figure 5-14**   Preswing (at 50%–60% of the gait cycle). *(Adapted from Gage, JR. Gait Analysis in Cerebral Palsy. London: Mac Keith Press, 1991.)*

for this activity and assists the deceleration of the moment of inertia of the shank.

The hip begins to flex in preswing. The dominant moment is a flexor moment, and power is generated. Concentric action of the hip flexor muscles, primarily the iliopsoas, produces the activity. Occasionally the rectus femoris muscle is active to augment hip flexion. This usually occurs at faster walking speeds. Peak flexor power of the hip is generated at toe-off. Hip musculature (both extensors and flexors) is responsible for the majority of positive work performed during the walking cycle (56%), with most being produced during stance phase (Ounpuu et al., 1991).

The objective of *initial swing* (Fig. 5-15) is foot clearance and limb advancement. Initial swing occurs from 60% to 73% of the gait cycle. Maximum plantar flexion occurs at the ankle in initial swing. At the same time, peak knee flexion occurs, uniquely timed for optimal clearance of the foot. The ankle then begins to dorsiflex by activity of the anterior tibialis muscle. The dominant muscle moment is a dorsiflexor moment. Power output is negligible. The hip flexes during initial swing, which also assists foot clearance. A flexor moment remains dominant, and power generation is occurring by concentric activity of the hip flexors.

The goals of *midswing* (Fig. 5-16) remain foot clearance and limb advancement, and it occurs between 73% and 87% of the gait cycle. The ankle is dorsiflexing during this time by concentric action of the anterior tibialis muscle. The knee is extending by inertial forces without muscle activity. The hip is flexing.

The primary purpose of *terminal swing* (Fig. 5-17) is pre-positioning of the limb for weight acceptance. This phase occupies the period between 87% and 100% of the gait cycle. The ankle begins to plantar flex by eccentric action of the anterior tibialis muscle to position the ankle in neutral. A flexor moment is dominant at the knee with power absorption as knee extension is controlled by eccentric action of the hamstrings to decelerate the forward swing of the thigh. The quadriceps muscles also become active to assist with control of the knee. Minimal movement is noted at the hip at this time.

CORONAL PLANE

The function of hip and pelvis motion in the coronal plane is to optimize the vertical excursion of the center of mass (Figs. 5-5 and 5-18). At initial contact the pelvis in the coronal plane is level and the hip is in neutral abduction and adduction. The stance side of the pelvis rises 5° at the beginning of loading response in conjunction with adduction of the stance limb. The dropping of the pelvis on the unsupported limb is caused by the ground reaction force on the supported limb, which produces an external adduction moment at hip, knee, and ankle. The external adduction moment is resisted by eccentric control of the hip abductors. This allows the stance side of the pelvis to rise and the unsupported side to drop.

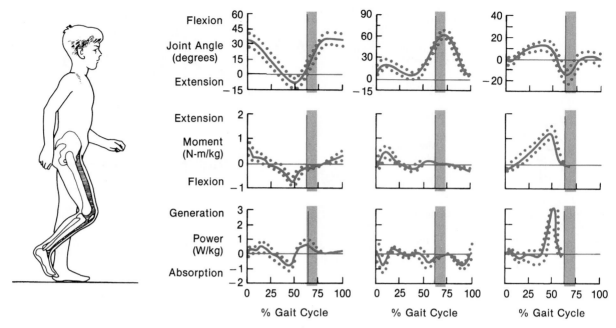

◆ **Figure 5-15** Initial swing (at 60%–73% of the gait cycle). *(Adapted from Gage, JR. An overview of normal walking. In Greene, WB [Ed.]. Instructional Course Lectures, Vol. 39. Park Ridge, IL: American Academy of Orthopaedic Surgeons, 1990.)*

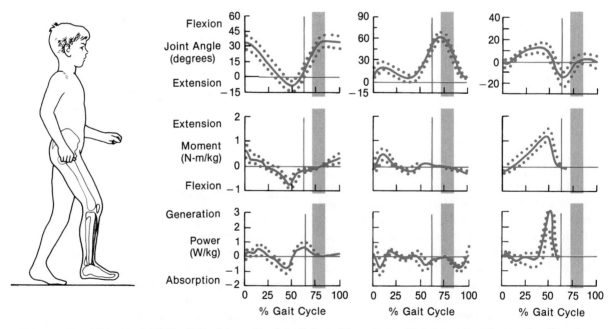

◆ **Figure 5-16** Midswing (at 73%–87% of the gait cycle). *(Adapted from Gage, JR. An overview of normal walking. In Greene, WB [Ed.]. Instructional Course Lectures, Vol. 39. Park Ridge, IL: American Academy of Orthopaedic Surgeons, 1990.)*

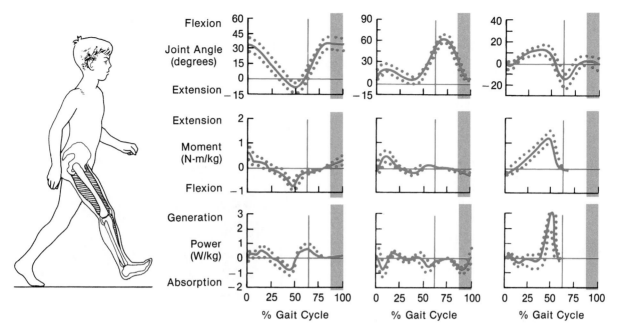

Figure 5-17 Terminal swing (at 87%–100% of the gait cycle). *(Adapted from Gage, JR. An overview of normal walking. In Greene, WB [Ed.]. Instructional Course Lectures, Vol. 39. Park Ridge, IL: American Academy of Orthopaedic Surgeons, 1990.)*

The pelvis and hip motion reverses in midstance as concentric control by the hip abductors of the stance limb acts to raise the pelvis. This action assists clearance on the swing side. During preswing the hip on the stance side goes into abduction in preparation for toe-off.

Ankle and foot motion in the coronal plane is complex, but it is also very important to efficient gait. It is not routinely measured during full body gait analysis because of inadequate multisegment foot models appropriate for the pediatric client with neuromuscular issues. The literature is confusing because of variations in the terms used to describe motions occurring in the foot. The following description is consistent with nomenclature used by Perry (1992).

At initial contact, as stated earlier, an external adduction moment is present at the ankle and foot. The position of the anatomic body of the calcaneus, which accepts floor contact, is lateral to the tibia, which transmits body weight onto the talus from above. This causes the calcaneus to evert on the talus and reduces the support the calcaneus provides the talus (Fig. 5-19A). The eversion of the calcaneus on the talus occurs during the initial part of the gait cycle (loading response and early midstance). It is controlled by ligaments surrounding the subtalar joint, as well as eccentric muscle action of the anterior tibialis and posterior tibialis muscles. Maximum eversion occurs at the onset of single-leg stance (15% of the gait cycle).

Motion reverses during the remainder of midstance under muscular action of the posterior tibialis and the soleus and the gradual shift of weight bearing to the forefoot. Subtalar joint neutral is reached by 40% of the gait cycle—the midpoint of terminal stance. Inversion locks the midtarsal joint and provides increased stability of the foot during weight bearing on the forefoot. It also moves the calcaneus back under the talus (see Fig. 5-19B). Peak inversion occurs at the end of terminal stance when ankle power generation is at its peak. Excessive inversion is avoided by co-contraction of the peroneal muscles (peroneus longus and peroneus brevis) during terminal stance and preswing. The subtalar joint is typically in a neutral position during swing phase until slight inversion begins again during the last 20% of the gait cycle.

TRANSVERSE PLANE

The end result of transverse plane motion is stride elongation (see Fig. 5-5). This is accomplished by internal pelvis and hip rotation under the control of the adductor magnus muscle. During the first half of stance phase internal rotation occurs at the pelvis and hip that reverses in the last half of stance. The pelvis is at its maximum posterior position at toe-off. The foot is positioned 5° to 10° (average value) external to the line of progression throughout the entire walking cycle. Subtalar joint action

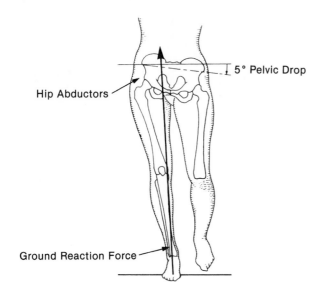

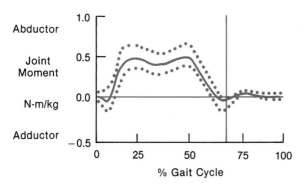

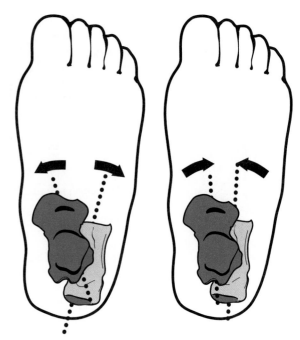

◆ **Figure 5-19** Subtalar action during stance phase. **A,** The offset in alignment between the body of the calcaneus, which accepts floor contact, and the tibia, which transmits body weight, causes the calcaneus to evert on the talus. The long axis of the calcaneus and the long axis of the talus diverge from each other as the talus rotates inward. **B,** Subtalar joint inversion during terminal stance repositions the calcaneus under the talus, and the long axis of the bones converge but are not parallel.

◆ **Figure 5-18** Coronal plane hip joint kinetics. *(From Gage, JR. Gait Analysis in Cerebral Palsy. London: Mac Keith Press, 1991.)*

produces rotation of the tibia as part of the closed chain mortise joint. The reader is referred to other texts for explanation of the transverse plane motions at the ankle and knee (Inman et al., 1981; Perry, 1992).

ENERGY EXPENDITURE

The purpose of many of the events in the walking cycle in all three planes of motion is to optimize energy expenditure or reduce the vertical translation of the center of mass. Gage (1991, 2004) includes energy conservation as one of the five attributes of normal gait and states that variation in this attribute encompasses the deviations of the other four attributes.

The mechanisms that the body uses to conserve energy are optimizing the excursion of the center of mass, control of momentum, and active or passive transfer of energy between body segments. The vertical and hori-

zontal displacements of the center of mass are almost sinusoidal and are equal and opposite during typical walking (Winter, 1987). The body accomplishes this through the three pelvic rotations (rotation, tilt, and obliquity) and coordinated knee and ankle motion. Inman and colleagues (1981) demonstrated that without pelvic rotation and with stiff limbs, the center of mass of the body would be lifted approximately 9.5 cm with each step. Normal vertical excursion of the body averages approximately 4.5 cm.

Determination of energy expenditure in gait has been a topic of research since the 1950s (Coates & Meade, 1960; Passmore & Durnin, 1955; Ralston, 1958). Various estimates are used to measure energy. Ralston (1958) hypothesized that individuals naturally select a speed of walking that allows a minimum of energy expenditure. More recent studies also support this hypothesis (Cavangna et al., 1983; DeJaeger et al., 2001). This has direct implications for the child with a motor impairment.

Research in energy expenditure specifically in children has revealed that younger children consume more energy than teenagers and adults (mass-specific gross rate of oxygen consumption, mL/min-kg) (DeJaeger et al., 2001; Koop et al., 2003; Waters et al., 1988). Despite the fact that children and adults walk in geometrically similar ways, size, changes in morphology, muscular efficiency, and motor skill during growth potentially have an effect on the expense of locomotion. Smaller children perform a greater amount of work per unit mass and per unit time to maintain a given walking speed than larger children. Additionally, children under the age of 5 years have more lean body mass and a greater surface area to body mass ratio, which results in a higher resting energy expenditure. Because of this, a given walking speed is not functionally equivalent at different ages. However, when alternative normalization methods are used to eliminate effects of body size, differences between children of different ages and adults disappear (Alexander, 1989; DeJaeger et al., 2001; Schwartz et al., 2004). This suggests that changes in the neuromuscular system play a relatively minor role in energy expenditure differences after 3 years of age. A comparison between mass normalized gross rate of oxygen consumption and net rate of oxygen consumption with a nondimensional normalization scheme is found in Figure 5-20.

An alternative to the use of measuring oxygen consumption to estimate energy expenditure involves calculation of the mechanical work required for walking. Kinematic measurements, anthropometric measurements, and kinetic analyses of internal and external loads are required for use of this method (Olney et al., 1990; Winter, 1990). The advantage of mechanical energy estimation is

that the energy requirements of individual joints can be calculated. One of the disadvantages, particularly in the assessment of atypical gait, is that the use of external loads to judge the work associated with walking does not measure the body's ability to efficiently respond to the external loads. Co-contraction associated with spasticity is unaccounted for (Rose et al., 1991). A review of mechanical and metabolic estimations of energy expenditure can be found elsewhere (Stout & Koop, 2004).

Heart rate is often used as a substitute clinical measure for oxygen uptake and therefore metabolic energy expenditure because of the linear relationship of heart rate to oxygen uptake (Rose et al., 1989, 1990). Low mechanical efficiency, however, creates disproportionately high submaximal heart rates in individuals with cerebral palsy (CP), making submaximal heart rate a poor predictor of aerobic capacity in this group (Bar-Or, 1983). I have observed high and inconsistent heart rate in relation to oxygen uptake in various clinical populations including CP. Caution should be taken if consideration is being given to this method of estimation of energy expenditure. See Chapter 8 for more information on aerobic capacity.

USE OF GAIT ANALYSIS IN ASSESSING IMPAIRMENTS

Gait analysis is a useful tool in examining walking impairments in children with physical disabilities because it provides objective measurement of the magnitude of deviations. It also allows the interpreter to analyze data

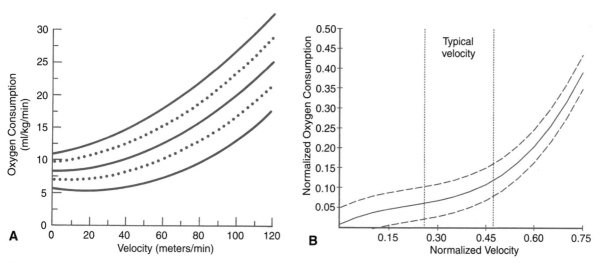

• **Figure 5-20** **A**, Typical values of the rate of metabolic oxygen consumption versus velocity for 150 children 2 to 19 years of age. The units for oxygen consumption are normalized by body weight. No normalization of velocity is used. The mean and 2 standard deviations are displayed. **B**, The same data presented normalized using nondimensional variables for both rate of oxygen consumption and velocity.

from all planes of motion for a single gait cycle. Just as computed tomography has improved on radiography, gait analysis improves on the evaluator's clinical examination and visual observation. Gait analysis data in the hands of a critical evaluator will never be used in isolation. Clinical examination by a physician, physical therapist, or trained kinesiologist and x-rays are vital aspects of the evaluation. The family's goals for treatment are important as well.

GUIDELINES FOR REFERRAL

Guidelines for determining when formal gait analysis should be recommended in the plan of care for a child with a walking disability depend on many factors. The child's age, diagnosis, progress in physical therapy, and goals of intervention are all taken into consideration. Analysis is best when the child's gait pattern is mature, but waiting for a mature walking pattern is not always possible. One key to remember is that current gait analysis techniques provide a single "snapshot" in time. Even if a gait pattern is consistent from cycle to cycle on a given day, if it is not consistent from one week or one month to the next, the value of that single snapshot for decision making is more limited. The utility of a gait analysis for children, adolescents, or adults who are making rapid progress in rehabilitation is more limited in scope for this reason.

Typically, the impetus for referral for gait analysis is a change in treatment. That change in treatment may or may not be surgical in nature. Bracing or prosthetic changes, or medication changes that may affect balance or walking, can be indicators as well. A three-dimensional gait analysis may not be the best measurement tool for assessing results of changes in a physical therapy program unless the treatment program specifically affects the child's walking.

Children under age 3 are not candidates for three-dimensional gait analysis because of their small physical size, their reluctance to cooperate for the duration of the required testing, and their immature gait patterns. Children between 3 and 5 years of age can be tested in the laboratory if their size, behavior, and walking are adequate for the testing process. Because their age and maturity of gait pattern are not ideal, analysis is usually reserved for use as a baseline before surgical intervention. In this age range, interventions such as selective dorsal rhizotomy have increased the number of children who have a gait analysis before the age of 5 years.

The optimal age for a formal three-dimensional gait analysis is typically from age 6 onward. Changes in treatment, whether they are bracing or prosthetic changes, medication changes, or surgical interventions, can all be evaluated. Analysis before a treatment change provides a baseline to assist in the decision-making process. Sometimes no specific treatment changes are recommended. Analysis after treatment provides evaluation of the effects of that treatment. Many people do not appreciate the importance of post-treatment assessment. What they fail to realize is that effective change and improvements in treatment techniques cannot occur without post-treatment assessment. The combined knowledge of previous post-treatment examinations plays an important part in the ability to accurately identify problems and solutions to pretreatment problems.

ASSESSING GAIT IMPAIRMENTS

A gait analysis laboratory should be considered a measurement tool. Information from a gait laboratory can assist in differentiation of primary impairments from secondary compensations. Primary impairments are those abnormalities that are a direct result of CNS injury; secondary compensations refer to the mechanisms used by the individual to circumvent the primary abnormalities. In addition to use in treatment of conditions such as CP and myelomeningocele, gait data can also be used to assess the effects of orthotic devices in various populations or of different prosthetic devices in individuals with amputations. Gait analysis at repetitive intervals can assist in the examination of the progression of a particular deformity or condition or the effects of a particular controlled treatment regimen (including surgery, medication, and physical therapy).

Specific physical therapy recommendations are often difficult to determine with gait laboratory data alone. Assessment during a gait analysis typically includes only a limited documentation of physical findings and is not a complete physical therapy examination. The EMG information from most gait laboratories does not provide information about strength of muscle contraction and cannot be used to determine which muscles are to be strengthened and how. A thorough knowledge of muscle mechanics and typical gait combined with manual muscle testing allows the therapist to answer these questions. EMG activity can, however, determine whether muscle activity is present or absent and the timing of that muscle activity, which can be useful to determine whether a particular muscle is available for strengthening and to conjecture about what the consequences of that strengthening might be. Kinetic analysis provides joint moment and power information that is sometimes useful for this purpose. In summary, the gait laboratory can be an objective measuring tool for the physical therapist.

Returning to the prerequisites for development of any skill, gait deviations can be created by abnormal motor control, spasticity, loss of ROM, decreased strength, loss of sensation, and bony deformity. Each can result in primary impairments and secondary compensatory mechanisms used to produce or to maintain useful function. Gait analysis can be used to distinguish between the two. It can be used to identify areas of bony abnormality and loss of functional ROM and to document areas of relative weakness or spasticity. The information is always used in conjunction with a clinical examination. The use of gait analysis in assessment of impairments in CP is discussed here as an example of how information is used and interpreted. Limitations of gait analysis are also discussed. Gait analysis is in no way limited to examination of CP or any one gait pathology.

COMMON GAIT DEVIATIONS IN CEREBRAL PALSY

Bony Deformity

Bony deformities are assessed best by clinical examination and radiography. Gait analysis data measure the functional effect of the bony deformity on the child's walking. Bony deformities are examples of secondary impairments because they are not caused directly by the CNS lesion. They can result from failure of physiologic bone remodeling, the effects of spasticity and muscle imbalance, disuse, attempts to function, or any combination of these factors. These deformities (except for leg length discrepancies) are best assessed in the transverse plane data. Once they have occurred they become a primary focus for orthopedic treatment because they cannot be corrected by conservative management. True bony deformity cannot be corrected by physical therapy. Three common bony abnormalities seen in children with CP are internal femoral torsion, external tibial torsion, and subtalar joint subluxation.

Internal Femoral Torsion (Femoral Antetorsion)

Visually, internal femoral torsion appears as internal rotation of the femurs during walking and is measured as such on kinematic analysis. Antetorsion (forward torsion) is a true structural twist deformity of the long axis of the femur. The cause is a combination of (1) persistent physiologic antetorsion in the infant because of delayed weight bearing and (2) abnormal muscle forces created by spasticity (Bleck, 1987; Gage, 1991). Femoral antetorsion is not synonymous with valgus angulation of the femoral neck-shaft angle (coxa valga) or the anterior or forward position of the head and neck of the femur relative to the frontal plane (anteversion). Antetorsion can be clinically measured as the degree of internal femoral rotation in the prone position required to position the greater trochanter

most "lateral" or parallel to the supporting surface (Ryder & Crane, 1953). Usually, in the presence of internal femoral torsion there is loss of passive external rotation range and the range of internal rotation is excessive. Often the ratio of internal to external rotation is equal to or greater than 3:1 (Fig. 5-21). Femoral antetorsion and the degree of internal rotation measured on kinematic data are correlated, but they are different measurements.

External Tibial Torsion

External tibial torsion is an external rotation or torsion of the long axis of the tibia. It is measured most appropriately by physical examination of the transmalleolar axis or thigh-foot axis and not by gait analysis, unless the system used measures the rotation of the foot with respect to the tibia. External tibial torsion is a true bony deformity that often develops as a secondary impairment to internal femoral torsion. Limited knee motion that results in repetitive dragging of the foot in an externally rotated posture for clearance can also result in the deformity. In the presence of femoral antetorsion, external tibial torsion is difficult to observe visually because the foot progression angle may not appear abnormal. The knee sometimes has a valgus appearance, but it is not a coronal plane abnormality (Fig. 5-22). The internal torsion of the femur is compensated by external torsion of the tibia so that the foot remains in the direction of progression (see Figs. 5-21 and 5-22).

Pes Valgus (Subtalar Joint Subluxation)

Pes valgus is most common in children with spastic diplegic or spastic quadriplegic types of CP and less often occurs in children with spastic hemiplegia. Caused by a relative subluxation of the talus on the os calcis, it usually develops because of muscle imbalance and a combination of tightness and weakness. Visually, the calcaneus is everted. Kinematic data do not identify subtalar joint subluxation. The effect of the deformity is measured in the plantar flexion-dorsiflexion and foot rotation graphs. Physical and radiographic examination is required.

Inadequate Range of Motion and Spasticity

Gage (1991) often refers to CP as a condition that preferentially affects two-joint muscles because it is primarily in the two-joint muscles that spasticity contributes to the abnormalities associated with walking. Most two-joint muscles are predominantly fast-twitch muscles used for rapid force production. Loss of ROM creates static contracture; spasticity imposes loss of ROM in dynamic situations because of resistance to stretch (Kruger & Gage, 1986; Rose et al., 1993). The effects of inadequate ROM and spasticity can be measured in all three planes of

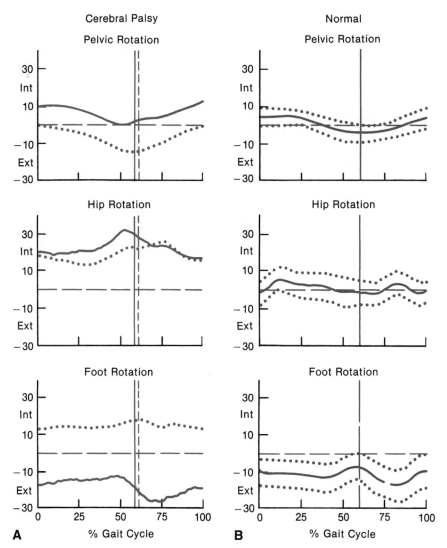

◆ Figure 5-21   An example of kinematic graphs from a 10-year-old child with spastic diplegic cerebral palsy (**A**) compared with normative data for pelvic and hip rotation and foot progression (**B**). Results of bony deformity are often seen in the transverse or rotational plane. Graphs for the child with cerebral palsy depict the right side (*solid line*) and the left side (*dashed line*) for a representative gait cycle. The normative graphs display the mean (*solid line*) and one standard deviation (*dashed line*). The hip rotation graph in the child with cerebral palsy shows bilateral internal hip rotation. The foot rotation graph displays an appropriate external foot progression on the right side (*solid line*) despite internal hip rotation on the right side. This could result from either subtalar joint subluxation or external tibial torsion, or a combination of both. By physical examination this child has bilateral femoral antetorsion and a right external tibial torsion.

motion but are most prevalently seen in the sagittal plane. Examples measured by gait analysis are an abnormal plantar flexion–knee extension couple, crouch gait, and limited swing-phase knee motion.

Abnormal Plantar Flexion–Knee Extension Couple

During normal walking, the plantar flexion-knee extension couple is a force couple whereby the soleus and the gastrocnemius muscles control forward momentum and the forward progression of the ground reaction force by

eccentric contraction. Children with CP often enter the walking cycle with a footflat initial contact, which rapidly places the gastrocnemius under premature tension at both ends of the muscle. Gage (1991) postulated that in response to the stretch, spasticity is elicited that can restrict tibial advancement, produce knee extension (hyperextension), and reduce the extent of dorsiflexion (plantar flexion). The spastic response is revealed in a biphasic pattern during stance phase of increasing dorsiflexion and then decreasing dorsiflexion in the kinematics and by an abnormal plantar

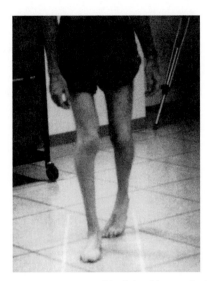

• **Figure 5-22** A 30-year-old adult with spastic diplegic cerebral palsy. Note the internal hip position on the right side (knee in) and the foot progression angle that is neutral to the line of progression. This individual has an external tibial torsion on the right side.

flexor power generation coincident in time with the first decrease of dorsiflexion in the cycle in the kinetics. Occasionally, the EMG activity is biphasic as well (Fig. 5-23). The abnormal power generation elevates the body's center of mass and functionally increases energy expenditure.

Crouched Posture

Caused by hip flexion contractures or tightness, knee flexion contractures or tightness, excessive plantar flexor muscle weakness, or any combination of these conditions, increased flexion is seen at all joints in the sagittal plane in crouched gait (Fig. 5-24).

Limited Swing-Phase Knee Motion

Limitation of motion at the knee in swing phase usually begins in preswing, when motion is also inadequate. Momentum for swing phase in normal gait is generated by the acceleration force of the gastrocnemius muscle that drives the ground reaction force behind the knee. When the gastrocnemius force generation is reduced, as is often the case in CP, the hip flexors supply the momentum to clear the extremity. The rectus femoris is often recruited as a hip flexor. If this muscle is spastic, it maintains its action as a knee extensor. The already diminished knee flexion in preswing is further inhibited by spastic restraint that does not allow further knee flexion (see Fig. 5-24).

Weakness

Weakness cannot be measured directly by gait analysis. The type of electromyography used does not provide infor-

mation regarding strength. Kinematic data measure only the effects; it is up to the clinician to interpret whether the pattern is present as the result of weakness or tightness. Kinetic data do provide a limited measure of weakness if full ROM is available at the joint. Power can be produced only if joint movement is present. The best measure of strength is by physical examination, although this is complicated by the presence of spasticity.

Hip Abductor Weakness

Weakness of the hip abductor muscles in CP, as in any other type of gait disorder, produces an uncontrolled pelvic drop on the swing side and lateral trunk shift over the stance limb. The ground reaction force in the coronal plane produces an external adduction moment at all joints of the stance limb. If abductor strength is insufficient, the lateral trunk shift positions the ground reaction force through the hip joint center so no abductor moment is needed. Hip abductor muscle weakness is frequently (but not necessarily) seen in children with femoral antetorsion because the torsion creates an inadequate lever arm over which the gluteus medius muscle is able to act, imposing functional weakness. On kinematic graphs hip abductor weakness is displayed as increased adduction. Differentiation between hip abductor muscle weakness and hip adductor tightness cannot be done solely using kinematic data.

Gastrocnemius-Soleus Weakness

Plantar flexor muscle weakness primarily affects terminal stance and preswing phases of the gait cycle, but midstance is also affected. During midstance, the soleus is not able to control the progression of the ground reaction force that is anterior to the ankle, and excessive dorsiflexion results. Heel rise is delayed in terminal stance because gastrocnemius power may also be insufficient. Excessive dorsiflexion can drive the knees into flexion as well. Quadriceps muscle activity may be required to maintain an upright posture if the trunk is vertical, resulting in increased energy expense. Clearance is achieved by the proximal hip flexors because the plantar flexor muscles alone are insufficient. This results in an insufficient acceleration force in terminal stance and imposes a slower gait velocity.

SUMMARY

The prerequisites for any motor function, including gait, develop as the CNS matures and the body grows, producing physiologic changes in the mechanics and the neurophysiology of the system. The attributes of typical gait are lost in pathologic conditions such as CP because of the primary impairments of loss of selective motor control and balance,

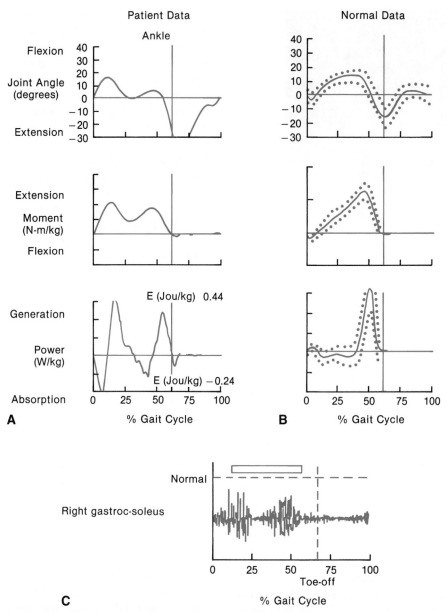

◆ **Figure 5-23** Kinematics and kinetics at the ankle joint demonstrating an abnormal plantar flexion–knee extension couple in a child with cerebral palsy (**A**) compared with normal (**B**). The ankle kinematics of the patient display a biphasic pattern in stance phase—increasing dorsiflexion–decreasing dorsiflexion—that repeats itself. This results in a biphasic plantar flexor moment as well, and an inappropriate midstance power generation. **C**, Surface EMG record from the gastrocnemius-soleus complex also exhibits two bursts of activity coinciding with the power generation.

abnormal tone and sensation, muscle weakness, and secondary impairments such as bony deformity and loss of ROM.

This chapter was designed to provide an overview of the refinement of gait in childhood, the components of typical gait as measured by gait analysis, and a brief introduction to the use of gait analysis in examination of impaired gait. A gait laboratory is only a measuring tool

and is a supplement, not a substitute, for other tools used to assess gait deviations.

Research in the area of gait continues to be a topic of great interest. As measurement techniques improve, our knowledge of walking and its development becomes more refined. With a clear understanding of typical gait, we can better understand the mechanisms of pathologic gait.

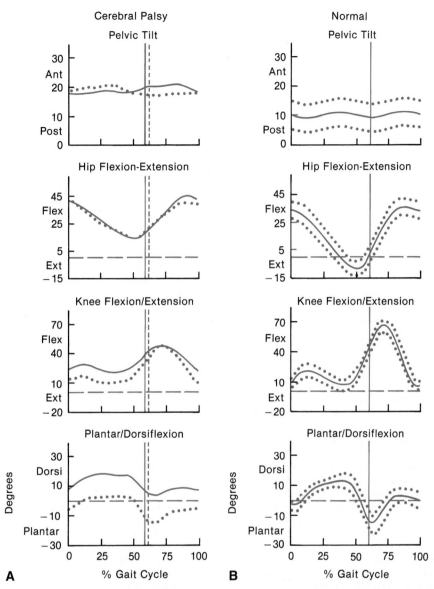

◆ **Figure 5-24**   Example of a crouched posture of increased hip and knee flexion in the sagittal plane of a 10-year-old child with cerebral palsy (**A**) as compared with normal (**B**). Patient data compare the child's right side (*solid line*) with the left (*dashed line*). The posture at the knee is asymmetric, with increased knee flexion during stance phase on the right side. Swing-phase knee flexion is also decreased.

Here the science of physical therapy melds into the art of physical therapy practice for the children we treat.

ACKNOWLEDGMENTS

I would like to thank Dr. Jim Gage and Dr. Steven Koop, whose philosophy and understanding of normal gait and treatment of children with gait pathologies are significant contributions to this chapter. I am privileged to work with both of them.

REFERENCES

Adolph, KE. Learning in the development of infant locomotion. Monographs of the Society for Research in Child Development. Serial #251, Vol. 62:3. Chicago: University of Chicago Press, 1997.

Adolph KE. Learning to keep balance. In Kail, R (Ed.). Advances in Child Development and Behavior. *30*:1–40, 2002.

Adolph, KE, Vereijken, B, & Shrout, PE. What changes in infant walking and why. Child Development, *74*:475–497, 2003.

Alexander, RM. Optimization and gaits in the locomotion of vertebrates. Physiology Reviews, 69:1199–1227, 1989.

Armstrong, DM. The motor cortex and locomotion in the cat. In Grillner, S, Stein, PSG, Stuart, DG, Forssberg H, Herman, RM, &

Wallen, P (Eds.). Neurobiology of Vertebrate Locomotion. London: Macmillan, 1986, pp. 121–137.

Assaiante, C, Woollacott M, & Amblard, B. Development of postural adjustment during gait initiation: Kinematic and EMG analysis. Journal of Motor Behavior, 32:211–226, 2000.

Bar-Or, O. Neuromuscular diseases. In Bar-Or, O. Pediatric Sports Medicine for the Practitioner. New York: Springer-Verlag, 1983, pp. 227–249.

Basmajian, JV, & DeLuca, CJ. Muscles Alive: Their Functions Revealed by Electromyography, 5th ed. Baltimore: Williams & Wilkins, 1985.

Berger, W, Quintern, J, & Dietz, V. Stance and gait perturbations in children: Developmental aspects of compensatory mechanisms. Electroencephalography and Clinical Neurophysiology, 61:385–395, 1985.

Bernhardt, DB. Prenatal and postnatal growth and development of the foot and ankle. Physical Therapy, 68:1831–1839, 1988.

Bleck, EE. Developmental orthopaedics: III. Toddlers. Developmental Medicine and Child Neurology, 24:533–555, 1982.

Bleck, EE. Orthopaedic Management in Cerebral Palsy. London: Mac Keith Press, 1987, pp. 323–328.

Bly, L. Motor Skills Acquisition in the First Year: An Illustrated Guide to Normal Development. Tucson, AZ: Therapy Skill Builders, 1994.

Bradley, NS, & Bekoff, A. Development of locomotion: Animal models. In Woollacott, MH, & Shumway-Cook, A (Eds.). Development of Posture and Gait Across the Lifespan. Columbia, SC: University of South Carolina Press, 1989, pp. 48–73.

Breniere, Y, & Bril, B. Development of postural control of gravity forces in children during the first 5 years of walking. Experimental Brain Research, 121:255–262, 1998.

Butterworth, G, & Hicks, L. Visual proprioception and postural stability in infancy: A developmental study. Perception, 6:255–262, 1977.

Cavagna, GA, Franzetti, P, & Fuchimoto, T. The mechanics of walking in children. Journal of Physiology, 343:323–339, 1983.

Coates, JE, & Meade, F. The energy demand and mechanical energy demand in walking. Ergonomics, 3:97–119, 1960.

Coon, V, Donato, G, Houser, C, & Bleck, EE. Normal ranges of hip motion in infants six weeks, three months, and six months of age. Clinical Orthopaedics and Related Research, 110:256–260, 1975.

Connelly, KJ, & Forssberg, H (Eds.). Neurophysiology and Neuropsychology of Motor Development. London: Mac Keith Press, 1997.

Cusick, BD, & Stuberg, WA. Assessment of lower-extremity alignment in the transverse plane: Implications for management of children with neuromotor dysfunction. Physical Therapy, 72:3–15, 1992.

DeJaeger, D, Willems, PA, & Heglund, NC. The energy cost of walking in children. Pflugers Archives, 441:538–543, 2001.

Engel, GM, & Staheli, LT. The natural history of torsion and other factors influencing gait in childhood: A study of the angle of gait, tibial torsion, knee angle, hip rotation, and the development of the arch in normal children. Clinical Orthopaedics, 99:12–17, 1974.

Epstein, HT. Correlated brain and intelligence development in humans. In Hahn, ME, Jensen, C, & Dudek, BC (Eds.). Development and Evolution of Brain Size: Behavioral Implications. New York: Academic Press, 1979, pp. 111–131.

Fabray, G, MacEwen, GD, & Shands, AR. Torsion of the femur: A study in normal and pathological conditions. Journal of Bone and Joint Surgery (American), 55:1726–1738, 1973.

Fomon, SJ. Body composition of the male referenced infant during the first year of life. Pediatrics, 40:863–867, 1967.

Forssberg, H. Ontogeny of human locomotor control: I. Infant stepping, supported locomotion and transition to independent locomotion. Experimental Brain Research, 57:480–493, 1985.

Forssberg, H. Evolution of plantigrade gait: Is there a neuronal correlate? Developmental Medicine and Child Neurology, 34:916–925, 1992.

Gage, JR. Gait Analysis in Cerebral Palsy. London: Mac Keith Press, 1991.

Gage, JR. A qualitative description of normal gait. In Gage, JR (Ed.). The Treatment of Gait Problems in Cerebral Palsy. London: Mac Keith Press, 2004, pp.42–70.

Grillner, S. Control of locomotion in bipeds, tetrapods, and fish. In Geiger, SR (Ed.). Handbook of Physiology, Vol. 2. Bethesda, MD: American Physiological Society, 1981, pp. 1179–1236.

Haas, SS, Epps, CH, Jr, & Adams, JP. Normal ranges of hip motion in the newborn. Clinical Orthopaedics, 91:114–118, 1973.

Heriza, C. Motor development: Traditional and contemporary theories. In Lister, MJ (Ed.). Contemporary Management of Motor Control Problems: Proceedings of the II STEP Conference. Alexandria, VA: Foundation for Physical Therapy, 1991, pp. 99–126.

Hirschfield, H, & Forssberg, H. Epigenetic development of postural responses for sitting during infancy. Experimental Brain Research, 97:528–540, 1994.

Hof, AL. Scaling gait data to body size. Gait & Posture, 4:222–223, 1996.

Hof, AL, & Zijlstra, W. Comment on "Normalization of temporal-distance parameters in pediatric gait." Journal of Biomechanics, 30:299, 1997.

Inman, VT, Ralston, HJ, & Todd, F. Human Walking. Baltimore: Williams & Wilkins, 1981.

Jensen, JL, & Bothner, KA. Infant motor development: The biomechanics of change. In van Praagh, E (Ed.). Pediatric Anaerobic Performance. Champaign, IL: Human Kinetics, 1998, pp. 23–43.

Jensen RK, Sun, H, Treitz, T, & Parker HE. Gravity constraints in infant motor development. Journal of Motor Behavior, 29:64–71, 1997.

Jordan, LM. Initiation of locomotion from the mammalian brainstem. In Grillner, S, Stein, PSG, Stuart, DG, Forssberg, H, Herman, RM, & Wallen, P (Eds.). Neurobiology of Vertebrate Locomotion. London: Macmillan Press, 1986, pp. 21–37.

Kadaba, MP, Wooten, ME, & Gainery, J. Repeatability of phasic muscle activity: Performance of surface and intramuscular electrodes. Journal of Orthopedic Research, 3:350–359, 1985.

Kazai, N, Okamoto, T, & Kumamoto, M. Electromyographic study of supported walking of infants in the initial period of learning to walk. In Komi, PV (Ed.). Biomechanics V: Proceedings of the Fifth International Congress on Biomechanics. Baltimore: University Park Press, 1976, pp. 311–318.

Komi, PV. Relationship between muscle tension, EMG, and velocity of contraction under concentric and eccentric work. In Desmedt, JE (Ed.). New Developments in Electromyography and Clinical Neurophysiology. Basel, Switzerland: S Karger AG, Medical and Scientific Publishers, 1973, pp. 596–606.

Koop, SE, Stout, JL, & Luxenberg, M. Energy expenditure in cerebral palsy during level walking. Gait and Posture, 18(suppl 2): S77–S78, 2003.

Kruger, MP, & Gage, JR. Stance phase foot rocker problems in spastic diplegia. Developmental Medicine and Child Neurology, 28(suppl 53):4, 1986.

Kugler, PN, Kelso, JA, & Turvey, MT. On the control and coordination of naturally developing systems. In Kelso, JAS, & Clark, JE (Eds.). The Development of Movement Control and Coordination. New York: John Wiley & Sons, 1982, pp. 79–93.

Ledebt, A, & Bril, B. Acquisition of uppper body stability during walking in toddlers. Developmental Psychobiology, 36:311–324, 2000.

Loeb, GE. Kinematic factors in the generation and role of sensory feedback during locomotion. In Grillner, S, Stein, PSG, Stuart, DG, Forssberg, H, Herman, RM, & Wallen, P (Eds.). Neurobiology of Vertebrate Locomotion. London: Macmillan Press, 1986, pp. 547–561.

Murray, MP, Drought, AB, & Kory, RC. Walking patterns of normal men. Journal of Bone and Joint Surgery (American), 46:355–360, 1964.

Okamoto, T, & Kumamoto, M. Electromyographic study of the learning process of walking in infants. Electromyography, *12*:149–158, 1972.

Olney, SJ, MacPhail, HEA, Hedden, DM, & Boyce, WF. Work and power in hemiplegic cerebral palsy gait. Physical Therapy, *70*:431–438, 1990.

O'Malley, M. Normalization of temporal-distance parameters in pediatric gait. Journal of Biomechanics, *29*:619–625, 1996.

Ounpuu, S, Gage, JR, & Davis, RB, III. Three-dimensional lower extremity joint kinetics in normal pediatric gait. Journal of Pediatric Orthopedics, *11*:341–349, 1991.

Palmer, CE. Studies of the center of gravity in the human body. Child Development, *15*:99–180, 1944.

Passmore, R, & Durnin, GA. Human energy expenditure. Physiological Reviews, *35*:801–839, 1955.

Perry, J. Gait Analysis: Normal and Pathological Function. Thorofare, NJ: Slack, 1992.

Phelps, E, Smith, LJ, & Hallum, A. Normal ranges of hip motion of infants between 9 and 24 months of age. Developmental Medicine and Child Neurology, *27*:785–793, 1985.

Piper, MC, & Darrah, J: Motor Assessment of the Developing Infant. Philadelphia: WB Saunders, 1994.

Ralston, HJ. Energy-speed relation and optimal speed during level walking. Internationale Zeitschrift fur Angewandte Physiologie, *17*:277–283, 1958.

Rancho Los Amigos Medical Center, Pathokinesiology Department, Physical Therapy Department. Observational Gait Analysis Handbook. Downey, CA: The Professional Staff Association of Rancho Los Amigos Medical Center, 1989.

Roncesvalles, MNC, Woollacott, MH, & Jensen, JL. Development of lower extremity kinetics for balance control in infants and young children. Journal of Motor Behavior, *33*:180–192, 2001.

Root, ML, Orien, WP, Weed, JH, & Hughes, RJ. Biomechanical Examination of the Foot, Vol. 1. Los Angeles: Clinical Biomechanics, 1971.

Rose, J, Gamble, JG, Burgos, A, Medeiros, J, & Haskell, WL. Energy expenditure index of walking for normal children and children with cerebral palsy. Developmental Medicine and Child Neurology, *32*:333–340, 1990.

Rose, J, Gamble, JG, Medeiros, J, Burgos, A, & Haskell, WL. Energy cost of walking in normal children and in those with cerebral palsy: Comparison of heart rate and oxygen uptake. Pediatric Orthopedics, *9*:276–279, 1989.

Rose, SA, DeLuca, PA, Davis, RB, III, Ounpuu, S, & Gage, JR. Kinematic and kinetic evaluation of the ankle following lengthening of the gastrocnemius fascia in children with cerebral palsy. Journal of Pediatric Orthopedics, *13*:727–732, 1993.

Rose, SA, Ounpuu, S, & DeLuca, PA. Strategies for the assessment of pediatric gait in the clinical setting. Physical Therapy, *71*:961–980, 1991.

Ryder, CT, & Crane, L: Measuring femoral anteversion: The problem and a method. Journal of Bone and Joint Surgery (American), *35*: 321–328, 1953.

Salenius, P, & Vankka, E. The development of the tibiofemoral angle in children. Journal of Bone and Joint Surgery (American), *57*:259–261, 1975.

Saunders, JB, Inman, VT, & Eberhart, HD. The major determinants in normal and pathological gait. Journal of Bone and Joint Surgery (American), *35*:543–559, 1953.

Sepulveda, F, Wells, DM, & Vaughan, CL. A neural network representation of electromyography and joint dynamics in human gait. Journal of Biomechanics, *26*:101–109, 1993.

Schwartz, M, Koop, S, Bourke, J, & Baker, R. A new normalization scheme for oxygen consumption data using non-dimensional gait variables. Proceedings of the 9th Annual Gait and Clinical Movement Analysis Society. Lexington, KY, 2004.

Shumway-Cook, A, & Woollacott, MH. The growth of stability: Postural control from a developmental perspective. Journal of Motor Behavior, *17*:131–147, 1985.

Spady, DW. Normal body composition of infants and children. Ross Conference on Pediatric Research, Ross Laboratories, Columbus, Ohio, *98*:67–73, 1989.

Staheli, LT, Corbett, M, Wyss, C, & King, H. Lower extremity rotational problems in children. Journal of Bone and Joint Surgery (American), *67*:39–47, 1985.

Staheli, LT, & Engel, GM. Tibial torsion: A method of assessment and a survey of normal children. Clinical Orthopaedics, *86*:183–186, 1972.

Stansfield, BW, Hillman, SJ, Hazelwood, E, Lawson, AA, Mann, AM, Loudon, IR, & Robb, JE. Sagittal joint kinematics, moments, and powers are predominantly characterized by speed of progression, not age, in normal children. Journal of Pediatric Orthopaedics, *21*: 403–411, 2001.

Stout, JL, Hagen, BT, & Gage, JR. Normal Walking: An Overview Based on Gait Analysis. Hagen, BT, & Stout, JL (Producers). St. Paul, MN: Gillette Children's Specialty Healthcare and Meditech Communications, 1993 (videotape).

Stout, JL, Hagen, BT, & Gage, JR. Principles of Pathologic Gait in Cerebral Palsy. Hagen, BT, & Stout, JL (Producers). St. Paul, MN: Gillette Children's Specialty Healthcare and Meditech Communications, 1994 (videotape).

Stout, JL & Koop, SE. Energy expenditure in cerebral palsy. In Gage, JR (Ed.). The Treatment of Gait Problems in Cerebral Palsy. London: Mac Keith Press, 2004, pp.146–164.

Sun, H, & Jensen, R. Body segment growth during infancy. Journal of Biomechanics, *27*:265–275, 1994.

Sutherland, DH. Gait Disorders in Childhood and Adolescence. Baltimore: Williams & Wilkins, 1984.

Sutherland, DH, Olshen, RA, Biden, EN, & Wyatt, MP. The Development of Mature Walking. London: Mac Keith Press, 1988.

Sutherland, DH, Olshen, RA, Cooper, L, & Woo, S. The development of mature gait. Journal of Bone and Joint Surgery (American), *62*:336–353, 1980.

Tachdjian, MO. The Child's Foot. Philadelphia: WB Saunders, 1985.

Tachdjian, MO. Pediatric Orthopaedics, Vol. 4, 2nd ed. Philadelphia: WB Saunders, 1990, pp. 2820–2835.

Thelen, E. Treadmill elicited stepping in seven-month-old infants. Child Development, *57*:1498–1506, 1986.

Thelen, E, & Cooke, DW. Relationship between newborn stepping and later walking: A new interpretation. Developmental Medicine and Child Neurology, *29*:380–393, 1987.

Thelen, E, Fisher, DM, & Ridley-Johnson, R. The relationship between physical growth and a newborn reflex. Infant Behavior and Development, *7*:479–493, 1984; republished as *25*:72–85, 2002.

Thelen, E, Fisher, DM, Ridley-Johnson, R, & Griffin, NJ. Effects of body build and arousal on newborn infant stepping. Developmental Psychobiology, *15*:447–453, 1982.

Thelen, E, & Ulrich, BD. Hidden skills: A dynamic systems analysis of treadmill stepping during the first year. Monographs of the Society for Research in Child Development, *56*:1–98, 1991.

Thelen, E, Ulrich, BD, & Jensen, JL. The developmental origins of locomotion. In Woollacott, MH, & Shumway-Cook, A (Eds.). Development of Posture and Gait Across the Lifespan. Columbia, SC: University of South Carolina Press, 1989, pp. 25–47.

Ulrich, BD, & Ulrich, DA. Spontaneous leg movements of infants with Down syndrome and nondisabled infants. Child Development, *66*:1844–1849, 1995.

Valmassy, RL. Biomechanical evaluation of child. In Ganley, JV (Ed.). Symposium on Podopediatrics. Philadelphia: WB Saunders, 1984, pp. 563–579.

Vredenbregt, J, & Rau, G. Surface electromyography in relation to force, muscle length, and endurance. In Desmedt, JE (Ed.). New Developments in Electromyography and Clinical Neurophysiology. Basel, Switzerland: S Karger AG, Medical and Scientific Publishers, 1973, pp. 607–622.

Walker, JM. Musculoskeletal development: A review. Physical Therapy, 71:878–889, 1991.

Waters, RL, Lunsford, BR, Perry, J, & Byrd, R. Energy-speed relationship of walking: Standard tables. Journal of Orthopaedic Research, 6:215–222, 1988.

Winter, DA. The Biomechanics of Human Movement. New York: John Wiley & Sons, 1979.

Winter, DA. Biomechanical motor patterns in normal walking. Journal of Motor Behavior, 15:302–330, 1983.

Winter, DA. The Biomechanics of Motor Control and Human Gait. Waterloo, Ontario: University of Waterloo Press, 1987.

Winter, DA. Biomechanics and Motor Control of Normal Human Movement, 2nd ed. New York: John Wiley & Sons, 1990.

Winter, DA, & Yack, HJ. EMG profiles during normal human walking: Stride to stride and intersubject variability. Electroencephalography and Clinical Neurophysiology, 67:402–411, 1987.

Woollacott, MH, Shumway-Cook, A, & Williams, HG. The development of posture and balance control in children. In Woollacott, MH, & Shumway-Cook, A (Eds.). Development of Posture and Gait Across the Lifespan. Columbia, SC: University of South Carolina Press, 1989, pp. 77–96.

Zajac, FE, & Gordon, ME. Determining muscle's force and action in multiarticular movement. Exercise Science and Sports Sciences Reviews, 17:187–231, 1989.

Zelazo, PR. The development of walking: New findings and old assumptions. Journal of Motor Behavior, 15:99–137, 1983.

Zelazo, PR. McGraw and the development of unaided walking. Developmental Review, 18:449–471, 1998.

Chapter 6

MUSCULOSKELETAL DEVELOPMENT AND ADAPTATION

CARRIE G. GAJDOSIK
PT, MS
RICHARD L. GAJDOSIK
PT, PhD

Pediatric physical therapists routinely address clinical conditions that influence the growth and development of the musculoskeletal system, either directly or indirectly. Therapeutic interventions are often designed to promote musculoskeletal adaptations in an effort to prevent or correct physical impairments with the hope of enhancing function and participation in daily life activities. Accordingly, knowledge of normal growth and development and of the principles of adaptation of the musculoskeletal system is essential for understanding the efficacy of interventions. The purposes of this chapter are to describe (1) the growth and development of muscle and bone and (2) the adaptation of muscle and bone, including the effects of various interventions designed to promote desired adaptations.

MUSCULOSKELETAL DEVELOPMENT

The embryologic development of muscle has been well described in many texts and articles, and few controversies exist regarding the sequence of gross anatomic changes during the embryologic period (Davis & Dobbing, 1974; Moore, 1988; Owen et al., 1980).

MUSCLE TISSUE

Embryonic myoblasts arise from mesodermal cells and eventually differentiate to form myotubes. These immature, multinucleate tubular structures, which develop from two distinct lineages, are labeled either "primary" or "secondary." The primary myotubes are first observed at approximately 5 weeks of gestational age and are known to develop and differentiate without neural influence. The secondary myotubes are seen several weeks later. The growth and development of these myotubes are more heavily dependent on neural input, without which they may be smaller, fewer in number, or malformed (Grove, 1989; Mastaglia, 1974; Miller, 1991; Sanes, 1987). By 20 weeks of gestational age, most myotubes have fused to form muscle fibers and many of the fibers have a microscopic content similar to that of adult fibers.

The motor unit, which consists of a motoneuron and the muscle fibers it innervates, begins its formation with the development of the neuromuscular junction. By 8 weeks of gestation, acetylcholine receptors are dispersed within the myotubular membrane (Hesselmans et al., 1993). This timing corresponds to the earliest fetal movement, which is observed in the intercostal muscles. The presence of motor activity indicates that a viable connection between the neuromuscular junction and the motor axon has occurred. Multiple motor axons originating from different somites innervate the developing end plates. This polyneuronal innervation results in motor units that are much larger than those found in adults. From 18 weeks' gestational age until several months post term synaptic elimination occurs gradually until each neuromuscular junction is innervated by only one axon (Gramsbergen et al., 1997: Lichtman & Colman, 2000). This adult pattern of one axon per muscle fiber permits a reproducible and predictable increase of force during performance of a task (Purves & Lichtman, 1980; Thompson, 1986). Why fetal muscles are innervated initially by several axons and later undergo the elimination of all but one axon is not well established. It does not appear that the reason is to ensure that every muscle fiber is innervated. In partially denervated muscles of animals, the few remaining muscle fibers still undergo synaptic elimination, thus reducing the size of the motor unit (Brown et al., 1976; Thompson & Jansen, 1977). During the last half of gestational growth, the number and size of muscle fibers increase rapidly so that most of the skeletal muscle has developed by birth. Through the first year of life, muscle fibers continue to increase in number from either the division of existing cells or the differentiation of myoblasts into secondary myotubes (Mastaglia, 1974). During the growing years, muscle fibers increase in length and cross-sectional area by the addition of sarcomeres (Kitiyakara & Angevine, 1963). Their final size is dependent on many factors, including blood supply, innervation, nutrition, gender, genetics, and exercise.

During fetal development, differentiation of the myotubes into the different types of muscle fibers (type I [slow twitch] and type II [fast twitch]) is directed by intrinsic genetic programs (Miller, 1991; Slaton, 1981). Muscle fibers develop from two distinct lineages. Muscle tissue derived from primary myotubes differentiates into the two basic fiber types predominantly without the influence of the motoneuron, whereas muscle tissue derived from the secondary myotubes is mostly dependent on innervation for differentiation into muscle fiber types (Butler et al., 1982; Grinnell, 1995; Grove, 1989; Miller, 1991). When the muscle tissue is initially innervated, most of the motor axons innervate the primary myotubes before the secondary. Because most primary myotubes eventually differentiate into type I fibers, these fibers are the first to appear in the fetus. Type II fibers, which mostly develop from the secondary myotubes, are observed at

about 30 weeks of gestation (Colling-Saltin, 1978; Grinnell, 1995). In some congenital myopathies, such as myotonic muscular dystrophy, differentiation of the myotubes into the various fiber types can be delayed (Farkas-Bargeton et al., 1988). In adults, the expression of muscle fiber types is dependent on neuronal input, regardless of whether the muscle was derived from primary or secondary myotubes. Fiber type preference is also strongly influenced by disease, the function of the muscle, type of physical activity, and electrical stimulation.

SKELETAL AND ARTICULAR STRUCTURES

Like muscle tissue, both the skeletal and articular tissues arise from the mesodermal layer of the embryo. Mesenchymal cells condense to form templates of the skeleton. From this point, two distinct processes of bone formation take place: (1) endochondral ossification and (2) intramembranous ossification. All bones, with the exception of the clavicle, mandible, and skull, are formed by endochondral ossification (also called intracartilaginous ossification) (Moore, 1988; Royer, 1974; Walker, 1991). During the early embryonic period, collagenous and elastic fibers are deposited on the mesenchymal models and form cartilaginous models. Bone minerals are deposited on these new models and gradually replace the cartilage via the process of ossification. Intramembranous ossification occurs directly in the mesenchymal model. Mesenchymal cells differentiate into osteoblasts that deposit a matrix called osteoid tissue. This tissue is organized into bone as calcium phosphate is deposited.

Ossification at the primary ossification centers, typically in the center of the diaphysis or body of the bone, commences at the end of the embryonic period (eighth fetal week). By the time of birth, the diaphyses are almost ossified, whereas the epiphyses, or distal ends of the bone, remain cartilaginous. During early childhood, the secondary ossification centers appear in the epiphyses, and ossification proceeds in this section of the bone. The timing of complete ossification varies with each particular bone. Most bones are fully ossified by 20 years of age, but for a few bones the process can continue into adulthood (Moore, 1988). After birth, long bones grow in length at the epiphyseal plate, which is between the diaphysis and the epiphysis. This cartilaginous plate rapidly proliferates on the diaphyseal side of the bone. The resultant chondrocytes, arranged in parallel columns, become enlarged and are then converted into bone by endochondral ossification (McKibbin, 1980; Rodriguez et al., 1992). Eventually the epiphyseal plate is ossified, the diaphyses and epiphyses are joined, and the growth of the bone in length is considered complete.

Bone also increases in size through appositional growth, which is the accumulation of new bone on the bone surfaces. This results in an increase in thickness and density of the diaphysis. The most rapid period of bone growth is prenatal. A marked decrease in the rate of growth is noted at birth, but throughout childhood the decline is more gradual. A midgrowth spurt occurs at age 7 and again at puberty (Gasser et al., 1991).

Joint formation begins about the time that the cartilaginous models are formed. In a specialized area between these models, the interzonal mesenchyma differentiates to form the joint. The basic structures of the joint are formed during the sixth to eighth weeks of gestation, but the final shape develops throughout early childhood under the influence of the forces of movement and compression (Drachman & Sokoloff, 1966). The hip is a good example of how a joint changes shape during the fetal period. At 12 weeks of gestational age, the acetabulum is extremely deep and the head of the femur, which is quite round, is well covered (Fig. 6-1) (Ralis & McKibbin, 1973). As the fetus increases in age, the relative depth of

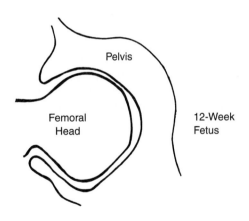

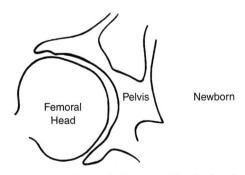

• **Figure 6-1**   A schematic diagram of the fetal and newborn hip joint illustrating the change in acetabular coverage of the femoral head. The coverage is extensive in the 12-week fetus, but reduced in the newborn.

the acetabulum decreases as the head of the femur becomes more hemispheric. At birth, the acetabulum is so shallow that it covers less than one half of the femoral head, and this results in a relatively unstable hip. This change is thought to allow for easier passage through the vaginal canal. During postnatal growth, the forces of compression and movement contribute to an increase in the depth of the acetabulum. The head of the femur becomes rounder, but it never achieves the roundness that it had during the early fetal period.

ADAPTATIONS OF MUSCLE AND BONE

The musculoskeletal system demonstrates a remarkable ability to adapt to the physical demands, or lack of physical demands, placed on the system. The presence of a pathologic condition may adversely influence the structure and function of any component of the system, and this process may result in impairments. For example, congenital deformities, disease processes, or abnormal growth of bone may lead to strength and length adaptations that cause impairments of the muscle-tendon unit (MTU). Congenital or acquired central nervous system deficits, such as cerebral palsy (CP), bring about sensorimotor changes that may promote unwanted shortening adaptations and length impairments of the MTU. These changes may ultimately compromise the structural and functional integrity of the joints and bone, leading to secondary impairments. Pathologic conditions of the MTU itself, for example, muscular dystrophies, may also lead to secondary, unwanted adaptations and impairments of the joints and bone. The normal process of adaptation can either enhance function or lead to impairment, activity restriction, and participation limitation.

CHANGES IN MUSCLE FIBER TYPES

Muscle fiber types are susceptible to both internal and external influences. In normal muscle, fiber types are randomly distributed to form a mosaic pattern and there is little variation in fiber size. In the presence of disease or dysfunction, this pattern is altered. When a muscle is reinnervated following denervation, one fiber type can become predominant and clump together, resulting in loss of the mosaic pattern. In addition, fiber size can change due to hypertrophy or atrophy. These changes have been useful in the diagnosis of certain pathologic conditions of muscle. Denervated muscles show atrophy of both major types of fibers, but type II fibers show more atrophy than type I fibers. Selective atrophy of type II fibers is common when muscle strength is compromised by disuse. Adults with steroid-induced strength deficits have selective type II atrophy (Rothstein & Rose, 1982). This same pattern may be observed in children who receive steroids to treat such diseases as juvenile rheumatoid arthritis. Malnourished children are at risk for a loss of type II fibers, which are thought to be converted to type I fibers (Ward & Stickland, 1991). Selective atrophy of type I fibers has been documented in an array of childhood neuromuscular disorders, such as hypotonia (Argov et al., 1984), congenital myotonic dystrophy (Farkas-Bargeton et al., 1988), and other congenital myopathies (Imoto & Nonaka, 2001). However, these finding are not consistent. Brooke and Engle (1969) reported excessive variability in fiber size in children with Duchenne muscular dystrophy (DMD), yet Imoto and Nonaka (2001) found type I atrophy in only 2 of 280 children with DMD. Children with Prader-Willi syndrome have been shown to have atrophy of type II fibers (Sone, 1994).

In children with spastic CP, a consistent picture of muscle histopathology has not been described in the literature. Varying degrees of atrophy and hypertrophy of type I and type II fibers have been reported and appear to be dependent on muscle group, severity of CP, and age of the child (Brooke & Engel, 1969; Castle et al., 1979; Ito et al., 1996; Romanini et al., 1989; Rose et al., 1994). Ito and colleagues (1996) reported a type I fiber predominance and a type IIB fiber deficiency in the gastrocnemius muscles of children with diplegic or hemiplegic CP. They also noted a greater variation in fiber size, particularly in type I fibers, in the older children or the more severely involved limb. In contrast, Rose and associates (1994) reported no difference in the distribution of type I fibers in children with spastic CP when compared with a control group of typically developing children. Unfortunately, the biopsies from the control group and the CP group were not from the same muscles. In this same study, 6 of the 10 children with CP had no evidence of atrophied fibers. Of the remaining 4 subjects, 2 had marked atrophy of type II fibers and 2 had significant atrophy of type I fibers.

Why do pediatric physical therapists need to know about muscle fiber types and their responses to outside influences? This question is difficult to answer because the clinical significance is not well understood. Rose and colleagues (1994) found that children with CP-spastic diplegia who had a predominance of type I fibers (in total area when compared with type II) expended more energy and had more prolonged electromyograph (EMG) activity during walking than children with CP and a predominance of type II fibers. Researchers speculate that spasticity may produce structural changes within the developing muscle (Friden & Lieber 2003; Ito et al., 1996; Rose et al., 1994). If so, controlling the spasticity in the very young child may be a method for promoting more normal muscle development, which in turn may allow for more efficient expenditure of energy and better participation in daily activities. Further studies of atypic fiber type distribution and its effect on activity level are needed. In the meantime, physical therapists should be aware that the two basic types of muscle fibers are influenced by exercise differently; that is, the effects of exercise on muscle fibers are training specific. Endurance training enhances the performance of type I fibers, whereas strength training enhances performance of type II fibers.

STRUCTURE AND FUNCTION OF THE NORMAL MUSCLE-TENDON UNIT

The normal MTU comprises skeletal muscle tissue proper (muscle fibers with actin and myosin protein filaments); two cytoskeletal systems within the muscle fibers (exosarcomeric and endosarcomeric); the supportive connective tissues within and around the muscle belly (endomysium, perimysium, and epimysium); and the dense regular connective tissues of the tendons that secure the MTU to bone. The total muscle force production is influenced by many factors, including the size of the muscle fibers, the firing rate of motor unit action potentials, the recruitment and derecruitment patterns, the muscle's architecture, the angle of pull, the lever arm, and the changes in the muscle's length.

The total muscle force is produced by the active and passive components of the MTU (Fig. 6-2), both of which are influenced by the MTU's length. To determine the active force produced by the MTU, the passive force is subtracted from the total force (see Fig. 6-2). The force produced by the active component depends primarily on the amount of overlap of the actin and myosin filaments. The maximum isometric force is produced near the resting length of an isolated muscle, and the isometric force decreases as the muscle is either lengthened or shortened relative to the resting length. This change in force in relation to the change in length forms the basis of the sliding filament theory of muscle contraction (Gordon et al., 1966; Huxley & Peachey, 1961). The isometric force is nearly maximal at the resting length because the actin and myosin filaments are in a position of optimal overlap (Figs. 6-3 and 6-4). The force generated by the active component of the MTU depends on the integrity of the central and peripheral nervous systems, the excitation-contraction coupling mechanism, and the cross-sectional area of the skeletal muscle tissues. In a completely relaxed skeletal muscle (i.e., when the central nervous system is not intact or when there is no artificial stimulation), no active tension exists.

When resting muscle is passively stretched, the force produced by the passive component of the MTU is thought to be brought about by three mechanisms: (1) by stretching stable cross-links between the actin and myosin filaments, (2) by stretching proteins within the exosarcomeric and endosarcomeric cytoskeleton (series elastic component), and (3) by deformation of the connective tissues of the muscle (parallel elastic component). The passive component accounts for the resistance felt during passive stretch of a fully relaxed muscle. The passive

tension that arises from the stretching of the stable interactions or cross-links between the actin and myosin filaments is the basis of the so-called filamentary resting tension hypothesis of passive tension (Hill, 1968, 1970a, 1970b). The stable bonds were believed to impart a stiffness because the actin-myosin cross-bridges stretch a short distance from the stable position before the contacts slip and reattach at other binding sites. Based on the results of more recent research methodologies, however, this theory is being revised. Recent studies have indicated that much of the stiffness of a stretched relaxed muscle actually comes from filamentous connections between the thick myosin filaments and the Z-disks of the sarcomere (Magid & Law, 1985), particularly when the sarcomere is stretched beyond the actin and myosin overlap (Granzier & Pollack, 1985) (Fig. 6-5). These filamentous connections consist of large, thin filaments of a giant protein that has been named "titin" (also called "connectin"). The titin protein attaches into the M-line region, or center of the myosin filament, courses longitudinally, and attaches into the Z-disks at the ends of the sarcomere. The titin protein forms a major component of the endosarcomeric cytoskeleton. This protein is now believed to be the major subcellular component that resists passive lengthening of a relaxed muscle, thus contributing to passive stiffness (Linke et al., 1996; Trombitas et al., 1998; Wang et al., 1993; Waterman-Storer, 1991). Nebulin is another giant protein that forms part of the endosarcomeric cytoskeleton. Nebulin is associated only with actin filaments within the I-band and is thought to provide structural support to actin's lattice array (see Fig. 6-5) (Waterman-Storer, 1991). Nebulin, however, is not thought to contribute to passive muscle stiffness.

In addition to titin's contribution to passive muscle stiffness, an intermediate-sized protein of the exosarcomeric cytoskeleton also is thought to contribute to passive

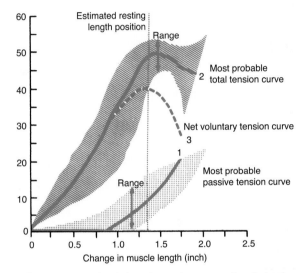

◆ **Figure 6-2**   Classic length-tension curves for skeletal muscle. Net voluntary active tension is predicted by subtracting passive tension from total tension. *(From Astrand, P, & Rodahl, K. Textbook of Work Physiology, 2nd ed. New York: McGraw-Hill, 1977, p. 102.)*

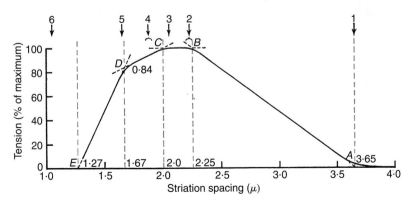

◆ **Figure 6-3**   Schematic summary of tension changes in relation to sarcomere length changes. Arrows along the top are placed opposite the striation spacings for critical stages of actin and myosin filament overlap (see Fig. 6-4). *(From Gordon, AM, Huxley, AF, & Julian, FJ. The variation in isometric tension with sarcomere length in vertebrate muscle fibers. Journal of Physiology, 184:185, 1966.)*

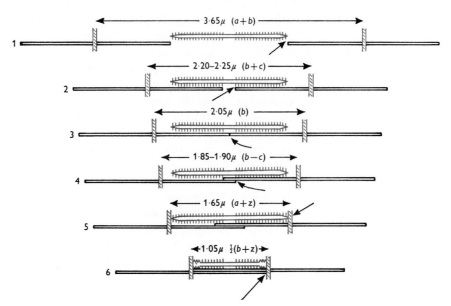

♦ **Figure 6-4** Critical stages in the increase of overlap between actin and myosin filaments as a sarcomere shortens. Numbers correspond to numbers in Figure 6-3. *(From Gordon, AM, Huxley, AF, & Julian, FJ. The variation in isometric tension with sarcomere length in vertebrate muscle fibers. Journal of Physiology, 184:186, 1966.)*

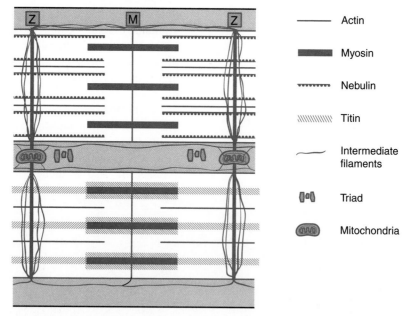

♦ **Figure 6-5** A schematic diagram of the proposed arrangement of cytoskeletal elements in and around the sarcomere. Both sarcomeres show the arrangement of intermediate filaments, composed mainly of the protein desmin, linking neighboring myofibrils both transversely and longitudinally at the Z-disk, and encircling the Z-disk. The upper sarcomere shows the arrangement of nebulin, running parallel to actin within the I-band. The lower sarcomere depicts titin's proposed location, stretching the full length of the half sarcomere, and attaching to myosin within the A-band. *(Modified from Waterman-Storer CM. The cytoskeleton of skeletal muscle: Is it affected by exercise? A brief review. Medicine and Science in Sports and Exercise, 23[11]:1243, 1991.)*

muscle stiffness. This protein is known as "desmin" (also called "skeletin") (Tokuyasu et al., 1983; Wang & Ramirez-Mitchell, 1983). Desmin is the major subunit of the intermediate protein filaments forming the Z-disks (Wang & Ramirez-Mitchell, 1983). It serves to interconnect Z-disks transversely and to connect Z-disks with organelles (e.g., mitochondria), but not with the T-tubule system (Tokuyasu et al., 1983) (see Fig. 6-5). Moreover, desmin extends longitudinally from Z-disk to Z-disk outside the sarcomere (Wang & Ramirez-Mitchell, 1983). Because of this longitudinal orientation between Z-disks outside the sarcomere, the protein will lengthen as the sarcomere is stretched. Thus, desmin's elasticity is also thought to contribute to the passive stiffness of a stretched muscle. In summary, research on the potential contribution of the "resting filamentary tension" and the titin and desmin proteins indicates that multiple subcellular components contained within the muscle fibers contribute to the passive resistance one feels when stretching a relaxed, nonactivated muscle.

In addition to the subcellular components that contribute to this exponential increase in resistance, increased passive resistance is also influenced by lengthening of the connective tissues of the endomysium, perimysium, and epimysium of the muscle belly. Support for the influence of the connective tissues of skeletal muscles on resistance to passive stretch has been provided by studies of the normal structure of these tissues. The perimysium has a well-ordered crisscross array of crimped collagen fibers (Rowe, 1974, 1981). Because of this organization, the perimysium is considered tissue that is a major contributor to extracellular passive resistance (Borg & Caulfield, 1980). Examination of the perimysium with light microscopy (Rowe, 1974) and scanning electron microscopy (EM) (Williams & Goldspink, 1984) revealed that the orientation of the crimped collagen changes as the length of the muscle changes. The crimped arrangement of the perimysium, a system of sheets with a three-dimensional weave surrounding muscle fasciculi, becomes uncrimped as the muscle is lengthened. This change, combined with mechanical realignment of the perimysium, contributes to the exponentially increased resistance, particularly near the end of maximal passive muscle lengthening. In contrast, tendons, which are composed of dense regular connective tissues, present very high stiffness (low passive compliance). Thus, the length of tendons can generally be considered constant and noncontributory to the overall passive length-tension relationships of the stretched MTU (Halar et al., 1978; Stolov & Weilepp, 1966; Tardieu et al., 1982b).

Knowledge of the basic structures contributing to passive length-tension relationships of muscles is important clinically. The increasing resistance that a therapist feels as a normal relaxed muscle is stretched stems from lengthening subcellular proteins and extracellular connective tissues. The resistance a pediatric therapist feels at the end of the range of a lengthened muscle with spasticity may result from the resistance borne by these subcellular proteins and the extracellular connective tissues, and not from an activation of spasticity.

Although some resistance to passive lengthening is probably present at most functional muscle lengths, passive resistance increases exponentially (curvilinearly) as the muscle is lengthened beyond its resting length; passive resistance is the equivalent of resting muscle tone. As stated earlier, passive stiffness is the resistance one feels when passively stretching a relaxed muscle. Passive compliance is the reciprocal of passive stiffness; thus, passive compliance is the "ease" with which the muscle lengthens. Although passive compliance can be represented as the ratio of change in muscle length to change in muscle force (Botelho et al., 1954), and passive stiffness can be represented as its reciprocal, to arrive at these measurements normally requires invasive research methods that are usually not possible in humans. Instead, passive compliance in humans is usually measured by the ratio of the change in the size of the joint angle to the change in the amount of passive torque (Gajdosik, 1991a; Gajdosik et al., 1990; Tardieu et al., 1982a; Tardieu et al., 1982). Passive stiffness can be represented by the ratio of the change in passive torque to a change in the joint angle.

FORCE AND LENGTH ADAPTATIONS IN THE MUSCLE-TENDON UNIT

Experiments with numerous animal models have shown that anatomic and physiologic length adaptations of the MTU can be induced by immobilization, denervation, local contraction produced by artificial stimulation, or a combination of these methods. Researchers have used the length-tension curves to provide information about changes in the length and passive compliance of muscles in light of histologic and histochemical changes in the muscles. A passive length-tension curve is developed based on muscle tension that is produced as the muscle is stretched from its resting length to its maximal length. The initial take-up part of the curve (left part of the curve) represents the resting length, and the end point of the curve (right part of the curve) represents the maximal length. Following intervention, the position and steepness of the curve may change, indicating a change in muscle length or stiffness. For example, a shift of the curve to the left indicates a shorter muscle, and a shift to the right indicates a longer muscle. A steeper curve indicates that the muscle is less compliant (stiffer).

When muscles were immobilized in shortened positions they showed a decrease in total force production, resulting from decreases in both the active force and the passive force (Alder et al., 1959; Williams & Goldspink, 1978). Muscle length also decreases (Alder et al., 1959; Stolov et al., 1971), a change brought about by a reduction in the number of sarcomeres (Goldspink et al., 1974; Tabary et al., 1972; Williams & Goldspink, 1978). The soleus muscles of young mice immobilized in the shortened position demonstrated a decrease in the postnatal addition of sarcomeres (Williams & Goldspink, 1973). Protein synthesis and protein breakdown studies have demonstrated that muscles immobilized in shortened positions showed significant loss of tissue protein because of decreased synthesis and increased degradation (Williams & Goldspink, 1971), primarily at the ends of the muscle fibers. Muscles immobilized in the shortened position also presented a decreased resting length (Goldspink et al., 1974) and a reduced maximal length with decreased passive compliance (increased stiffness) (Tabary et al., 1972; Tardieu et al., 1982b; Williams & Goldspink, 1978). The sarcomeres adapt in length to maintain optimal actin and myosin overlap in response to the loss in number of sarcomeres. When the immobilization is discontinued, the muscles readapt to gain their original sarcomere number and length characteristics.

Although changes in the resting lengths have been attributed to a loss of sarcomeres, the changes in passive compliance, demonstrated by changes in the steepness of the length-tension curves, have been attributed to changes in the connective tissues of the muscles (Tabary et al., 1972; Williams & Goldspink, 1978). Muscles immobilized in the shortened position demonstrated a greater abundance (Tabary et al., 1972; Williams & Goldspink, 1984) and remodeling (Williams & Goldspink, 1984) of connective tissues in the early stages of immobilization when compared to nonimmobilized controls. Greater abundance of connective tissue has been assessed by determining the relative concentration of hydroxyproline in relation to the total volume of the muscle (Williams & Goldspink, 1984). In the presence of immobilization, however, muscle fibers atrophy without a decrease in their number (Cardenas et al., 1977); thus, whether the absolute amount of connective tissue increases remains controversial. Evidence for remodeling was provided by scanning EM of the soleus muscles of mice immobilized in the shortened position for 2 weeks (Williams & Goldspink, 1984). The collagen fibers of the perimysium were oriented at more acute angles to the muscle fiber axis than were the collagen fibers of nonimmobilized muscles fixed in the same position. This collagen fiber arrangement at the immobilized shortened length resembled the arrangement found in nonimmobilized muscles held in lengthened positions (Fig. 6-6). As a result of the remodeling, greater tension per unit of passive elongation produced decreased passive compliance (increased stiffness). The passive length-tension curves were shifted to the left and appeared steeper, indicating that the muscles were shorter and stiffer after immobilization in the shortened position. The length-tension curves for young muscles (Fig. 6-7) and adult muscles were similar. Although the increased steepness of the curves for the muscles immobilized in the shortened position was explained by changes in the connective tissues, the decrease in the maximal passive force was probably influenced by a decrease in muscle mass because of muscle atrophy. Decreased muscle mass would result in the loss of subcellular proteins (myosin, actin, titin, and desmin), and this change would decrease both the maximal active and passive forces. The interrelationship of changes in the connective tissues and muscle proteins in light of changes in the form and position of length-tension curves is worthy of further study. Furthermore, applying the results of these studies with animals to explain the changes observed in human muscles must be done cautiously because the experimental conditions in the animal studies are usually not possible in humans.

Immobilization of muscles in lengthened positions has caused an increase in muscle length because of increases in the number of sarcomeres (Tabary et al., 1972; Williams & Goldspink, 1973, 1978), particularly at the ends of the muscle fibers. Similar results have been reported during normal postnatal growth of skeletal muscle fibers in young animals (Kitiyakara & Angevine, 1963; Williams & Goldspink, 1971). The addition of sarcomeres was accompanied by weight gain and increased protein synthesis after immobilization (Goldspink, 1977). The increased number of sarcomeres was not so great (19% increase) as the loss of sarcomeres in muscles immobilized in the shortened position (40% loss) (Tabary et al., 1972).

The active and passive length-tension curves for adult muscles that were immobilized in the lengthened position were shifted to the right (indicating that they were lengthened) compared with those of adult controls (i.e., nonimmobilized muscle). In young muscles immobilized in the lengthened position, however, the muscle belly length was decreased, so the curves of the experimental muscles were shifted to the left (Williams & Goldspink, 1978) (Fig. 6-8). Evidence suggests that a tendon elongates more readily in young, growing animals than in adult animals. In young mice with muscles immobilized in either the shortened or lengthened position, the overall muscle length was decreased, with a concomitant increase

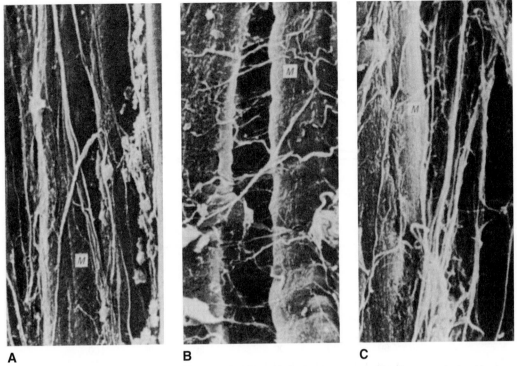

A   **B**   **C**

♦ **Figure 6-6**   Scanning electron micrographs of collagen fibers in the perimysium. **A**, Normal muscle fixed in the lengthened position. **B**, Normal muscle fixed in the shortened position. **C**, Muscle immobilized for 2 weeks in the shortened position and then fixed in the same position. M = muscle fiber, ×1300. *(From Williams, PE, & Goldspink, G. Connective tissue changes in immobilized muscle. Journal of Anatomy [London], 138[2]:347, 1984. Reprinted with the permission of Cambridge University Press.)*

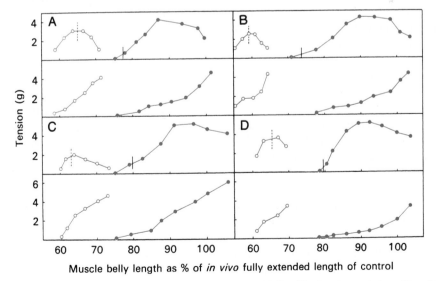

♦ **Figure 6-7**   Length-tension curves for young muscles (*A* to *D*) immobilized in the shortened position (o) and their controls (•). *(From Williams, PE, & Goldspink, G. Changes in sarcomere length and physiological properties in immobilized muscle. Journal of Anatomy [London], 127[3]:464, 1978. Reprinted with the permission of Cambridge University Press.)*

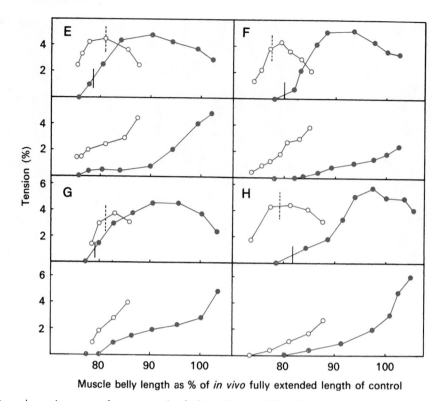

◆ **Figure 6-8**   Length-tension curves for young animals (*E* to *H*) immobilized in the lengthened position (o) and their controls (•). *(From Williams, PE, & Goldspink, G. Changes in sarcomere length and physiological properties in immobilized muscle. Journal of Anatomy [London], 127[3]:464, 1978. Reprinted with the permission of Cambridge University Press.)*

in tendon length (Williams & Goldspink, 1978). Thus, in young animals a shorter muscle belly may result in strength deficits that are independent of the length of the MTU during immobilization. As with muscles immobilized in the shortened position, the sarcomere length adapts to maintain optimal actin and myosin overlap. Muscles immobilized in the lengthened position readapted to their original lengths when the immobilization was discontinued.

Studies of peripheral denervation of skeletal muscles have revealed obvious loss of the ability of the animal to generate voluntary active tension. After denervation, the passive length-tension relationship showed gradual changes over a period of weeks, with steeper length-tension curves and limited extensibility between their resting lengths and their maximal lengths compared with those of controls (Stolov et al., 1970; Thomson, 1955). Studies have also revealed that length adaptations may result from myogenic—but not neurogenic—responses to the immobilized length of muscles. In adult rats, denervated muscles immobilized in shortened positions showed muscle belly shortening after 8 weeks (Stolov et al., 1971), and a similar change was observed in adult cats after 4 weeks, with loss of up to 35% of the sarcomeres

(Goldspink et al., 1974). The muscle belly shortening and decreased passive compliance were essentially the same as those observed in innervated muscles immobilized in shortened positions.

The reports that muscle length and associated physiologic changes may be independent of neuronal control were supported by studies of muscles stimulated with tetanus toxin (Huet de la Tour et al., 1979a, 1979b) or electrical stimulation (Tabary et al., 1981). Local injection of tetanus toxin into the soleus muscles of guinea pigs produced a shift in the passive length-tension curve toward the left, indicating a decrease in passive compliance (increased stiffness), and a 45% decrease in sarcomere number (Huet de la Tour et al., 1979b). The shortening adaptations were similar to those found after the muscles of cats were immobilized in shortened positions (Tabary et al., 1972). Analysis of the changes in sarcomere numbers in the soleus muscles of guinea pigs after length and tension were varied independently indicated that the length of muscles, not the tension, appeared to be the determining factor in sarcomere regulation (Huet de la Tour et al., 1979a). Contraction of a shortened muscle, however, may hasten sarcomere loss: electric stimulation of the sciatic nerve induced a 25% decrease in sarcomere numbers and decreased passive compliance within 12 hours (Tabary et al., 1981), whereas 5 days of shortening by immobilization in plaster casts alone was required to produce similar changes (Huet de la Tour et al., 1979b). The longitudinal growth rate of young, hypertonic muscles is also decreased. Spastic gastrocnemius muscles in very young mice have been shown to grow in length at only 55% of the rate of growing bone, whereas the rate of growth of normal gastrocnemius muscles was 100% of the rate of growing bone (Ziv et al., 1984).

Human Studies and Clinical Evidence

Studies of the length and passive compliance adaptations of the MTU in humans are less common than such studies in animals. Limited attempts to investigate the length and passive compliance responses to imposed changes in muscle length of children with neurologic impairments have been reported. Studies of children with CP and hypoextensible triceps surae muscles showed that they have muscle shortening and decreased passive compliance (increased stiffness) compared with findings in children with typical development (Tardieu et al., 1982a). In another study, nine children with hypoextensible triceps surae muscles were casted for 3 weeks with these muscles placed in the lengthened position (Tardieu et al., 1979). Four children showed passive length-tension curves that were shifted to the right with decreased slopes, indicating longer muscles with increased passive compliance, whereas five children had curves that were shifted to the right without a change in steepness (no change in passive compliance). In the same study, five children with hyperextensible triceps surae muscles were casted in a shortened position. The passive length-tension curves shifted to the left with increased slopes, indicating decreased passive compliance, in four of the five children.

In a follow-up study, children with CP and hypoextensible triceps surae muscles but no evidence of prolonged sustained contractions (group 1) were compared with children with CP and hypoextensible triceps surae muscles caused by an imbalance between triceps surae and dorsiflexion contractions (group 2) (Tardieu et al., 1982). Both groups were treated with progressive casting to lengthen the muscles. Group 1 showed a shift to the right of the passive length-tension curve without a change in the slope of the curve. Group 2 presented curves that were shifted to the right with decreased slopes, showing increased passive compliance (decreased stiffness) (Fig. 6-9). The authors suggested that the children in group 2 showed normal muscle adaptation because of the passive compliance adaptation. These findings suggest that human muscles undergo adaptations that may be similar to those that have been reported for animals. This assumption is

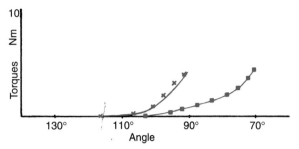

◆ **Figure 6-9**   Results of successful progressive casting in child from group 2. × = passive torque curve before treatment, ■ = passive torque curve after treatment. The curve shifted to the right with increased passive compliance. *(From Tardieu, G, Tardieu, C, Colbeau-Justin, P, & Lespargot, A. Muscle hypoextensibility in children with cerebral palsy: II. Therapeutic implications. Archives of Physical Medicine and Rehabilitation, 63:106, 1982.)*

based on the association of the passive curves of animal and of human muscles, measured by noninvasive methods, with the histologic and histochemical adaptations in animal muscles. The results of the study also elucidate the variability that can be expected in humans, particularly with regard to the possibility of different pathologic mechanisms underlying the adaptability of hypoextensible muscles in selected patient populations, such as children with CP (Tardieu et al., 1982).

Clinical observations clearly provide evidence that the musculoskeletal system of humans undergoes adaptations in response to immobilization, disuse, postural disturbances, and muscle imbalances in relation to specific pathologic disorders. It is well known that the skeletal muscles of a limb that is immobilized and not used will atrophy as a result of protein degradation (Sargeant et al., 1977). It is equally well known that normal muscle fibers respond to increased force and endurance demands by adaptive responses in structural, physiologic, and biochemical characteristics (Salmons & Hendriksson, 1981). The presence of pathologic conditions that alter skeletal muscles directly (e.g., muscular dystrophy) or indirectly from changes in the neurologic activity to the skeletal muscles (e.g., hypotonia or hypertonia) may lead to postural contractures and deformities from muscle imbalances and chronic positioning (Bunch, 1977; Sharrard, 1967; Tardieu et al., 1982a; Tardieu et al., 1982).

Many of the clinical manifestations of musculoskeletal disorders correlate well with the pathophysiologic conditions of the MTU described from experimental animal models. Abnormal shape in the structures of the vertebral column (e.g., hemivertebra) are associated with adaptations of the MTU and other soft tissues of the back. If the lower limbs of a child with flaccid paralysis are held in a specific posture for an extended period (e.g., hip flexion, abduction, and lateral rotation), the limbs adopt the characteristic position of the posture (Sharrard, 1967). Recent evidence suggests that children with CP and spasticity may have increased collagen accumulation within the endomysium of muscle that may contribute to increased muscular stiffness (Booth et al., 2001). Moreover, muscle fibers from upper extremity muscles of children with spastic CP have been shown to have shorter resting sarcomere lengths than normal muscle fibers (Friden & Lieber, 2003). This study provides support for intracellular and extracellular collagen remodeling that may contribute to increased resistance to passive stretch of muscles with spasticity.

Long-term conservative interventions, such as stretching and casting, may facilitate desired adaptations of the MTU and enhance activity, but much research is needed to examine these possibilities objectively. By contrast, surgical lengthening of the tendons of the triceps surae muscle group (Reimers, 1990a) and the hamstring muscle group (Damron et al., 1991; Lespargot et al., 1989; Reimers, 1990b) in children with CP has demonstrated enhanced activity. Studies that examine the combined influence of both conservative and surgical interventions are clearly needed to determine the most efficacious methods of improving participation in daily activities.

Bone deformities and alterations in the MTU may result from abnormal skeletal growth, or both MTU and bone adaptations may be associated with abnormalities in muscle tonicity and muscle imbalances found with conditions such as CP. Numerous developmental changes in the musculoskeletal system have been associated with CP, and the changes correlate well with the presence of spasticity and imbalances in muscle force and muscle length. These include changes in the femur and acetabulum resulting in medial femoral torsion and hip disorders (Beals, 1969; Lewis et al., 1964), hip adduction contractures and knee flexion contractures in spastic adductor and hamstring muscles (Reimers, 1974), and severe equinus deformity because of spasticity and shortening adaptations of the calf musculature (Tardieu et al., 1982).

SKELETAL ADAPTATIONS

The growth and resultant shape of the skeleton are affected by genetic coding, nutrition, and the combination of various mechanical forces that are imposed over time. The mass, girth, thickness, curvature, and trabecular arrangement of bone change as the forces of heredity and the environment play their roles. When examining skeletal adaptation, mechanical forces, such as muscle pull and weight bearing, are of interest to the pediatric physical

therapist. Martin and McCulloch (1987) reported a case study of a child with congenital absence of a left tibia. At birth the left fibula was larger than the right fibula. This was thought to result from the forces of movement in utero. When the child reached 2 years of age, the fibula was surgically centered in relation to the femur to act as a tibia. Sixteen months later, the fibula looked like a tibia in shape, size, and strength. The authors believed that the mechanical stresses delivered in a functional weight-bearing manner induced the changes in the bone. Mechanical forces affect the shape of the maturing skeleton, which in turn affects the biomechanical function of the musculoskeletal system. Deformations of the skeletal system can lead to abnormalities in movement and impedance of participation in activities.

Effects of Forces on Skeletal Growth

From the time the cartilaginous template is formed, the basic shape of the skeletal system does not change. Each bone grows in length, width, and girth, but its relative form remains unchanged. Natural and atypic angular changes occur from compressive, tension, and shear forces at the epiphyseal plate. Normal intermittent forces, such as those produced by weight bearing or muscle pull, stimulate lengthening of bone (Arkin & Katz, 1956). If these forces are too great or too small, the rate of growth is diminished.

Forces applied to the bone affect its shape by stimulating growth in areas of tension while inhibiting bone development in areas of compression (Arkin & Katz, 1956). Surgical techniques for correcting unequal leg lengths use compression and tension forces to affect bone growth. For children with leg length differences, surgical staples are applied to both sides of the epiphyseal plate of the longer leg to slow its growth until the shorter leg catches up (Edmonson & Crenshaw, 1980). The Ilizarov technique for limb lengthening uses tension to facilitate bone growth (Simard et al., 1992). With this technique, the cortex of the bone of the shorter leg is cut, and "gradual incremental distraction" is applied across the cut ends of the bone (Stanitski et al., 1996). Osteogenesis occurs in the space between the two ends of the cut bone. If forces are applied asymmetrically to the epiphyseal plate, the bone appears to bend; however, it is actually growing asymmetrically as the epiphyseal plate realigns to the direction of the force. Asymmetric compression on the epiphyseal plate is exemplified by surgical stapling of the medial aspect of the epiphyseal plate of the proximal tibia to retard growth on that side to correct a genu valgum deformity (Mielke & Stevens, 1996). Asymmetric proliferation of one or more epiphyseal growth plates located within a single bone can also lead to bone deformation. The spinal neural arch has six growth centers, three within each half of the arch. Chandraraj and Briggs (1991) speculated that uneven growth of either half of the neural arch may be a significant factor in the later development of idiopathic scoliosis.

Shear forces, which run parallel to the epiphyseal plate, can lead to torsional or twisting changes in the bone. The columns of chondrocytes around the periphery of the plate veer away from the shear forces in a twisting pattern (LeVeau & Bernhardt, 1984). The normal pull of muscles around a joint contributes to the shear forces, resulting in normal torsional changes in the long bones. For example, at birth, the tibia has 5° of medial torsion (Bernhardt, 1988). By maturity, the longitudinal orientation of the tibia has changed to 18° to 47° of lateral torsion (Kristiansen et al., 2001). The combination of atypic shear and com-

pressive forces can lead to skeletal deformities, such as vertebral wedging, femoral anteversion, femoral or tibial-fibular torsion, genu valgum or varum, and pes plano-valgus. Abnormalities of the skeletal system can lead to secondary problems of pain and dysfunction.

The typically developing child demonstrates interesting changes in the position of the knee in the frontal plane (Cheng et al., 1991; Heath & Staheli, 1993; Salenius & Vankka, 1975). At birth, the infant's knees are bowlegged (genu varum), but they gradually straighten until they reach a neutral alignment between the first and second years. The knee angulation then progresses toward genu valgum, reaching its peak between the ages of 2 and 4 years. After this time, the angle of genu valgum gradually decreases (Fig. 6-10). The final knee angle may differ

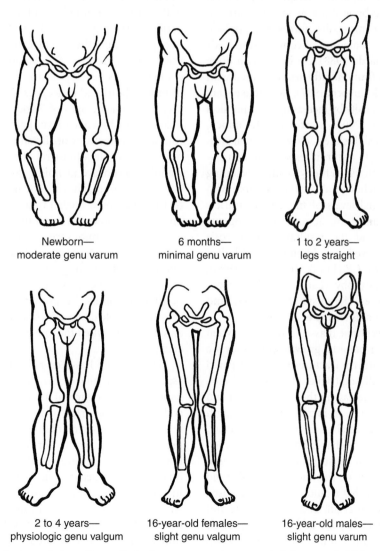

Newborn— moderate genu varum

6 months— minimal genu varum

1 to 2 years— legs straight

2 to 4 years— physiologic genu valgum

16-year-old females— slight genu valgum

16-year-old males— slight genu varum

♦ **Figure 6-10**   Physiologic evolution of lower limb alignment at various ages in infancy and childhood. *(Redrawn from Tachdjian, MO. Pediatric Orthopedics, 2nd ed. Philadelphia: WB Saunders, 1972, p. 1463.)*

according to race and gender. Heath and Staheli (1993) reported that by the age of 11 years the mean knee angle of white boys and girls was 5.8° of valgus, and no child demonstrated genu varus. In contrast, Cheng and associates (1991) found that Chinese children of both genders progressed to genu varus of less than 5° in the preteen years. Cahuzac and co-workers (1995) studied European children and determined that by the age of 16 years girls maintained a valgus knee position and boys had developed a genu varus of 4.4°. The pediatric therapist should be aware that the presence of genu varus between the ages of 2 and 11 years may be considered atypical in white children (Heath & Staheli, 1993), but caution should be used when interpreting this finding in children of other races.

The level of compressive forces also affects the thickness and density of the bone shaft (Martin & McCulloch, 1987; Royer, 1974). The bone thickens via appositional growth when normal compressive forces are applied, whereas a less than normal amount of compression leads to bone atrophy (Bernhardt, 1988). An increase in bone thickness and density is found in athletes compared with nonathletes (Martin & McCulloch, 1987). Nonathletes can, however, increase bone density by increasing their physical activity (Fuchs & Snow, 2002; Martin & McCulloch, 1987). Increases in cortical thickness, cross-sectional area, and resulting bone strength occur in response to increasing muscular strength and use in the typically developing child (Schönau, 1998; Nichols et al., 2001). Children who do not experience normal levels of movement, muscle strength, or weight bearing are at risk for osteopenia (reduced bone mass) and the resultant osteoporosis (Apkon, 2002), as is observed in children with myelodysplasia (Quan et al., 1998), CP (Lin & Henderson, 1996), Duchenne muscular dystrophy (Larson & Henderson, 2000), spinal cord injuries, (Kannisto et al., 1998), and juvenile rheumatoid arthritis (Hopp et al., 1991).

Age and diet also affect bone mass and strength. When children go through their pubertal growth spurt, they are most at risk for distal forearm fractures when compared to any other time of childhood (Bailey et al., 1989; Rauch et al., 2001). The rate of increase in the child's height and weight is greater than the rate of increase in the strength of the cortical bone at the radial metaphysis (Rauch et al., 2001). Thus, the bone is at a mechanical disadvantage when an adolescent falls onto an outstretched arm. Children who are obese show an increase in bone mass density and size, but not to the extent that would be predicted based on their weight (Goulding et al., 2000b). They are not adding bone as quickly as they are adding weight. Their incidence of upper extremity fractures is higher when compared to their lighter-weight peers (Goulding et al., 2000a; Whiting, 2002). The overall incidence of forearm

fractures in childhood has increased over the past 30 years and is postulated to result from the combination of vulnerable bone tissue with change in diet (i.e., higher soft drink consumption and lower calcium intake) and increase in risky physical activity, such as skate boarding and inline skating (Khosla et al., 2003).

The formation, growth, and integrity of articular cartilage are stimulated by compressive forces and movement between the bone surfaces (Ralis & McKibbin, 1973). Intermittent joint loading leads to healthy, thick cartilage, but constant loading interrupts normal nutrition, and the cartilage can eventually degenerate, leading to degenerative joint disease (Carter et al., 1987; Trueta, 1974). The role of movement in the development of joint shape and articular cartilage integrity is not clearly understood. In embryonic chicks, early joint formation occurred in the absence of mobility, but toward the end of the fetal period, cartilaginous bonds between the joint surfaces were present, and the articular surfaces were flattened and misshaped (Drachman & Sokoloff, 1966). Abnormal joint configurations develop also in children with movement disorders. Pearl and colleagues (2003) examined 84 children between the ages of 7 months and $13\frac{1}{2}$ years who had obstetric brachial plexus palsy that resulted in medial rotation contractures of the shoulder. Sixty-one percent had extreme glenohumeral deformities, including flat glenoids, biconcave glenoids, pseudoglenoids, and flattened, oval humeral heads. The mechanical forces created by the unopposed medial rotators had a profound effect on the development of this joint.

Skeletal deformities are common in children with muscle imbalances, spasticity, contractures, hypokinesis, and obesity, all of which apply abnormal mechanical forces to the growing skeleton. Although these deformities can occur throughout the growing period, the skeleton is most vulnerable during the first few years of life (prenatal and postnatal) when the rate of growth is greatest (Carter et al., 1987).

Fetal position has been related to various deformities, especially those that occur toward the end of the pregnancy. The incidence of tibial rotation and metatarsus adductus was reported to increase as the gestational age increased in preterm infants (Katz et al., 1990). Thus, preterm infants born closer to term were more likely to have rotational deformities than were younger preterm infants. Many factors can cause prenatal deformities, including decreased amniotic fluid, the limited space in which the fetus can move in utero, multiple births, and external forces from tightly stretched uterine and abdominal walls. Some associated deformities are congenital torticollis, plagiocephaly (asymmetric head), and pelvic obliquity (Fulford & Brown, 1977; LeVeau & Bernhardt,

1984; Sherk et al., 1981). During the third trimester, the hip is especially vulnerable to dislocating forces because of its shallow acetabulum (Ralis & McKibbin, 1973; Sherk et al., 1981). Suzuki and Yamamuro (1986) reported that infants delivered in the single-breech position (i.e., hips flexed and knees extended) had a higher incidence of congenital hip dysplasia (CHD) than did infants born in cephalic, double-breech (i.e., both hips and knees flexed), or footling positions. It was postulated that, with extreme hip flexion combined with knee extension, the hamstrings pulled the head of the femur downward, thus stretching the compliant hip capsule. After birth, the femur was dislocated by the upward pull of the iliopsoas muscle when the infants were diapered and wrapped with the hips extended. This theory may explain why the incidence of CHD is increased among those Native American populations in which newborns are strapped onto cradle boards or wrapped with the legs in adduction and extension (Coleman, 1968; Weinstein, 1987).

Although the acetabulum is shallow, children have more coverage of the femoral head by the acetabular labrum than adults (Horii et al., 2002). Labrum coverage provides some stability to the hip joint that the bony acetabulum cannot. During normal postnatal growth, the depth of the acetabulum increases, progressively covering more of the femoral head until the age of 8 years, when the adult level of femoral head coverage is reached (Beals, 1969). Normal compressive forces through the hip help to form the acetabulum and the femoral head into their appropriate shapes. Atypic pressures, such as those seen in children with obesity or spasticity, can deform the femur and component parts of the hip. Children with obesity are at increased risk for developing a flattened femoral head and slipped capital epiphysis due to the excessive weight on the developing femoral head (Chung et al., 1976; Loder & Greenfield, 2001). Children with spasticity are at risk for subluxation or dislocation from the asymmetric pull by spastic muscles around the hip (Gudjonsdottir & Mercer, 1997; Heinrich et al., 1991; Young et al., 1998).

Atypic changes in the shape of the acetabulum and femoral head have been reported in children with unstable or dislocated hips, such as children with congenitally dislocated hips, CP, or myelodysplasia. Buckley and colleagues (1991) examined 33 unstable hips in children with these disabilities and found that all had significantly more shallow acetabulae compared with those of a control group; the hip was most shallow in children with CP. The percentage of coverage of the head of the femur also was less for these children compared with that of control groups of children without disabilities. The children with disabilities had thinly developed articular surfaces and small, shallow acetabulae with poorly defined margins.

Beals (1969) reported that the acetabulae of children with CP in his study had appeared normal after birth, but that they did not increase in depth as expected by the age of 2 years. Nevertheless, acetabular depth was comparable with that of the typically developing population when the children were 8 years old. All but 1 of the 40 children included in this study were walking at this age, suggesting that the dynamic compressive forces of walking contributed to increased depth of the acetabulum. This relationship between hip stability and ambulation has been further supported in the literature by other studies (Abel et al., 1994; Vidal et al., 1985). Beals (1969) also supported use of a standing program to increase the depth of the hip joint.

The torsional changes of the bone observed in children with muscle imbalances or spasticity about the hip joint are good examples of the influence of the muscular system on the skeletal system. Femoral anteversion, or femoral torsion, is present when the proximal femur (i.e., head and neck) is rotated anteriorly in relation to the transcondylar axis of the femur. The greater trochanter is rotated to a more posterior location. At birth, the femur is in a position of about 30° of femoral anteversion (Fabry et al., 1973). The femoral head, neck, and greater trochanteric areas are made of pliable cartilage and attached to the rigid osseus diaphysis. As the infant develops, normal torsional forces about this point of fixation cause a decrease in femoral anteversion. Bleck (1987) speculated that these forces are created by active lateral hip rotation and extension, and Fabeck and colleagues (2002) calculated that forces created during walking have a major impact on the developmental changes in femoral anteversion. If active hip motions are minimal or walking is delayed, as is frequently observed in children with CP, the infantile femoral anteversion does not decrease as it should. Excessive femoral anteversion has been associated with the in-toed gait of children with and without disabilities. Merchant (1965) explained this association by an alteration of gluteus medius muscle function in the presence of excessive femoral anteversion. The gluteus medius muscle is most effective in stabilizing the pelvis during the stance phase of gait when its insertion on the greater trochanter is in direct alignment with its origin. In excessive femoral anteversion, the greater trochanter is posterior to the midpoint of the ilium. To achieve maximal efficiency, the femur is rotated medially to align the insertion with the origin. The end result is an in-toed posture.

Changes in either the muscular or skeletal systems because of internal or external forces often have interactive effects. Understanding the influences of these two systems on the development and final outcome of each system and recognizing the period when these systems are most mutable assist the therapist in designing effective treatment programs, as well as in knowing when to discontinue treatment procedures.

LONG-TERM EFFECTS OF ATYPICAL MUSCULOSKELETAL DEVELOPMENT

Many pathologic conditions of the musculoskeletal system have been identified in adults with developmental disabilities. Most commonly, these conditions develop during childhood but worsen during adulthood. One of the most common complaints by adults with CP is joint pain, especially in the lower extremities and the spine (Murphy et al., 1995; Schwartz & Engle, 1999; Turk et al., 1997). Other conditions observed in adults with CP include scoliosis, hip dislocation, cervical neck dislocations, contractures, arthritis, patella alta, overuse syndromes, nerve entrapments, and fractures (Gajdosik & Cicirello, 2001). Adults with Down syndrome are at risk for developing hip disorders, such as subluxation, dislocation, and osteoarthritis (Hresko et al., 1993).

Further study into the causes and prevention of secondary conditions is greatly needed to help guide the treatment of children with developmental disabilities. Pediatric therapists are appropriate professionals to educate parents and children about the lifelong attention that will need to be given to musculoskeletal problems, such as decreased strength and range of motion (ROM). When appropriate, adolescents should be taught to be responsible for their physical and cardiopulmonary needs. Another role for pediatric therapists is educating their fellow orthopedic physical therapists who treat adults about the orthopedic problems in this neglected population of adults with CP, myelodsyplasia, and other developmental disabilities. Campbell (1997) has written an excellent article on the issues surrounding secondary disabilities and how they can be addressed by pediatric therapists.

MEASUREMENT AND EFFECTS OF INTERVENTION

Fundamental goals of therapeutic intervention for physical disabilities include enhancing participation in daily activities and life roles by preventing or correcting the impairments that result from the underlying pathologic condition, or from the normal physiologic adaptations superimposed on the pathologic condition. Presumably activity and participation will be enhanced if impairments are prevented or corrected. Impairments of the ROM available about a joint or multiple joints and of the strength of the MTU are generally believed to contribute to activity

limitations and participation restrictions. Achieving maximal ROM by increasing the MTU length and achieving maximal strength are two fundamental goals of therapeutic intervention. Accurate assessments of ROM and strength are therefore important components of the physical therapy examination process.

RANGE-OF-MOTION EXAMINATION

A wide range of methods and instruments has been reported for examining the ROM about a joint or multiple joints, including simple visual estimation, use of various protractors and goniometers, measurements made from still photographs, and complex methods using computerized motion analysis systems. To most physical therapists, however, the universal goniometer (i.e., full-circle manual goniometer) remains the most versatile and widely used instrument in clinical practice. The design of the universal goniometer and the procedures for its use have been described in detail in numerous publications. The articles by M.L. Moore (1949a, 1949b) and the book by Norkin and White (1985) are particularly comprehensive and should be consulted for complete descriptions.

The reliability of goniometry is based on the reproducibility or stability of ROM measurements in relation to (1) the time intervals between comparable measurements or (2) the use of more than one rater. The ROM measurements must be reliable to be considered valid. Many factors influence the reliability and validity of goniometric measurements. These factors include consistency of the procedures applied, differences among joint actions and among the structure and function of body regions, passive versus active measurements, intrarater measurements (multiple measurements by one examiner) versus interrater measurements (multiple measurements by two or more examiners), normal day-to-day variations in ROM, and day-to-day variations in different pathologic conditions (Gajdosik & Bohannon, 1987).

Numerous studies have been reported on the ROM characteristics and the reliability of goniometry on adults, but reports on infants and children are more limited in number. Studies have demonstrated that full-term newborns present a limited range of hip and knee extension and greater dorsiflexion compared with measurements in adults (Drews et al., 1984; Waugh et al., 1983). These findings were attributed to the effects of intrauterine position and newborn flexor muscle tone. Consequently, clinicians should not use adult ROM values for comparisons with limb ROM measurements of the newborn. Studies with normal healthy children have indicated that ROM can probably be measured reliably (Haley et al., 1986), but studies of children with various pathologic conditions have shown that reliability varies with the number of raters and the pathologic problem. Pandya and colleagues (1985) studied seven upper and lower extremity joint limitations in 150 children with Duchenne muscular dystrophy and reported that intrarater reliability was high (intraclass correlation coefficient [ICC] range, .81-.91), but interrater reliability was lower, with a wide variation from joint to joint (ICC range, .25-.91). Stuberg and colleagues (1988) reported similar findings for children with CP.

Ashton and colleagues (1978) examined the day-to-day interrater reliability of measuring ROM of the hip in four children with spastic diplegia and found that the reliability tended to be lower for the two children with a moderate condition than for children with a mild condition. Harris and colleagues (1985) examined the goniometric reliability for a child with spastic quadriplegic CP and found that intrarater reliability exceeded interrater reliability, but both showed wide daily variations. Based on the extensive variability seen in children with CP, several groups of researchers have concluded that variances of ± 10° to 15° (Bartlett et al., 1985; Harris et al., 1985; Stuberg & Metcalf, 1988), ± 15° to 20° (Kilgour et al., 2003), and ± 18° to 28° (McDowell et al., 2000) in ROM over time do not signify a meaningful change in children with spastic CP.

Bartlett and colleagues (1985) compared four methods of measuring hip extension (by prone extension, Thomas test, Mundale method, and pelvic-femoral angle) in 45 children, of whom 15 had spastic diplegia, 15 had meningomyelocele, and 15 had no known pathologic condition. They reported that the Thomas test was particularly difficult to apply to patients with spastic diplegia and that improved reliability for these children would most likely result by using one of the other methods. The least reliable test in the group with meningomyelocele was that of Mundale, probably because of difficulty in identifying bony landmarks in the presence of obesity and deformities.

The results of these few studies clearly indicate that the reliability of ROM measurements is influenced by the specific patient problem. Additional research is needed to clarify the goniometric reliability among the many different types of patients treated by pediatric physical therapists. Moreover, studies are clearly needed to examine the effects of changes in ROM on activity. In other words, can improved ROM predict improved activity level? In the meantime, therapists are encouraged to do their own reliability studies to establish confidence intervals for recognizing changes in ROM that are clinically significant. Because intrarater reliability has generally been shown to be acceptable, another alternative

would be to have one therapist with demonstrated rating consistency perform all the goniometric measurements on one child.

STRENGTH EXAMINATION

Accurate measurement of strength is important for identifying strength deficits and in documenting changes in strength as a result of interventions. Numerous methods of measuring strength are available, including the traditional procedures of manual muscle testing (Kendall & McCreary, 1983), use of various handheld force dynamometers (Bohannon & Andrews, 1987), and computerized isokinetic testing systems (Rothstein et al., 1987). Although manual muscle testing is probably the most versatile and widely used method, evidence indicates that handheld dynamometers may yield more precise measurements and are more sensitive to small changes in strength (Bohannon, 1995). Isokinetic systems are constructed primarily for use with adults, but they can be used with children who are large enough to fit the various components. The components could be modified, or smaller isokinetic devices could be developed to meet the special size requirements of children. Although strength deficits are a common impairment in pediatric disabilities, the therapist must consider the reliability of the methods of measuring strength. Children with typical development and as young as 2 years old have produced consistent force with a handheld dynamometer (Gajdosik, 2003), and 6-year-olds have produced consistent force on isokinetic machines (Backman & Oberg, 1989; Merlini et al., 1995). Children must be able to understand the instructions and follow commands to produce accurate and reliable strength measurements. The reliability of the strength measurements may also vary with the time of day, particularly for patients who are fatigued by the end of the day; with the level of the child's enthusiasm; with the testing environment; and with the testing clinician's rapport with the child. As with goniometry, standardization of testing procedures should improve the reliability of strength measurements.

Several authors have reported good consistency when testing the strength of children ranging in age from 5 years to 15 years who had muscular dystrophy (e.g., Duchenne, limb-girdle, facioscapulohumeral, or myotonic muscular dystrophy). Strength was measured by manual muscle testing (Florence et al., 1984), isokinetic dynamometers (Sockolov et al., 1977), a handheld dynamometer (Stuberg & Metcalf, 1988), and an electronic strain gauge (Brussock et al., 1992). When strength was measured with a handheld dynamometer, children with meningomyelocele (9–17 years) (Effgen & Brown, 1992) or with Down syndrome (7–15 years) (Mercer & Lewis, 2001) yielded highly reliable results. The reliability of measurement of strength in children with CP appears to be more variable than in other patient populations. Van der Berg-Emons and associates (1996) examined the intraday reliability of isokinetic muscle strength in 12 children with spastic CP and 39 children with typical development between the ages of 6 and 12 years. Using an isokinetic device, they measured quadriceps and hamstring muscle strength at three different speeds. The children with CP had lower levels of reliability than the comparison group, and as the speed increased, the reliability decreased. The authors concluded that at 30°/s children with CP could produce consistent results, but at higher speeds the measurements were not repeatable. In contrast, Ayalon and associates (2000) reported excellent interday reliability when knee isokinetic strength was measured in 12 children with spastic CP. Several differences exist between the two studies. In the study by Ayalon and associates, strength was measured at a velocity of 90°/s and twice as many trials were used to find an average strength value. In addition, 50% of the children had hemiplegic CP, but in the study by van der Berg-Emons and associates (1996) the children had either a diplegic or quadriplegic distribution. Further study of the reliability of strength testing in children with CP is needed, especially with the variety of methods of measuring strength that are available to the pediatric therapist today.

The impact of spasticity on the strength of antagonist muscle groups also warrants consideration. The importance of considering strength measurements of antagonists to spastic muscles was demonstrated by examination of the strength changes of the dorsiflexor muscles after surgical lengthening of the triceps surae muscle group (Reimers, 1990a), and of the quadriceps muscles after surgical lengthening of the hamstring muscle group (Reimers, 1990b) of children with CP. The strength of the dorsiflexors increased by 50% 4 weeks after surgery and by more than 200% 14 months after surgery (Reimers, 1990a). The strength of the quadriceps muscle group decreased by 70% 4 weeks after surgery but was regained by 7 months, and by 13 months after surgery the strength had increased by more than 50% (Reimers, 1990b). Taken together, these studies confirm the idea that antagonist muscle strength improves when the spastic agonist muscle group is lengthened. We encourage clinicians to examine methods of objectively measuring muscle strength in children with CP to study the changes in muscle strength resulting from both conservative and surgical interventions.

In addition to the possibility of objectively measuring the voluntary force produced in spastic muscles, a combination of technologies may now permit objective assessments of the degree of underlying hypertonicity. Isokinetic passive movements at different velocities, combined with the recording of EMG activity of the agonist and antagonist muscles, could permit quantification of hypertonicity because muscles with spasticity present a markedly increased velocity-dependent neuromuscular response to passive lengthening (Damiano et al., 2001; Price et al., 1991). Rapid passive lengthening of spastic calf muscles through a dorsiflexion ROM can yield an increase in the amount of passive resistance and EMG activity. For example, Boiteau and colleagues (1995) passively stretched the calf muscles of 10 children with spastic CP at 10°/s and at 190°/s. They measured the resistance to the stretch at 10° of dorsiflexion and attributed the passive force at 10°/s stretch to nonreflex components. The force at the 190°/s stretch was much higher because it included reflex muscle activation from the spasticity (documented with EMG). The study demonstrated that the reflex and nonreflex components of spastic hypertonia can be measured reliably. If change in the passive resistive force caused by the reflex and the nonreflex components of spasticity can be assessed independently, the effects of specific therapeutic interventions that target each component can be determined and related to changes in activity and participation. These possibilities are particularly worthy of future study, and clinicians are encouraged to participate in research projects to help examine these possibilities.

EFFECTS OF INTERVENTION ON THE MUSCULOSKELETAL SYSTEM

Objective evidence of the effects of strengthening exercises for particular pediatric conditions is limited, but increasing. In the past, concerns about whether strengthening muscles of children with degenerative disorders would lead to a more rapid progression of the disorder have probably limited the application of strengthening programs. Some of the limited evidence available, however, indicates that active, submaximal exercise has no negative effect (de Lateur & Giaconi, 1979; Scott et al., 1981) and may be of limited value in increasing strength in Duchenne muscular dystrophy (de Lateur & Giaconi, 1979). Several studies with children and adults with CP have shown that after participating in a resistive exercise program, the values of their gait parameters improved (Andersson et al., 2003; Damiano & Abel, 1998; Damiano et al., 1995) and the scores on the Gross Motor Function Measure increased (Andersson et al., 2003; Damiano & Abel, 1998; Dodd et al., 2003; MacPhail & Kramer, 1995). In a study by O'Connell and Barnhart (1995), three children with CP and three with meningomyelocele participated in a progressive circuit muscular strength training program.

After 8 weeks, these children propelled their wheelchairs significantly farther during a 12-minute test period when compared with the pretraining test results. Their speed, however, did not increase during a 50-meter wheelchair dash. For individuals with CP, resistive strength training regimens have not been shown to adversely affect the level of spasticity (Andersson et al., 2003; MacPhail & Kramer, 1995), and a positive outcome has been noted by adults with CP who perceived a decrease in lower extremity spasticity lasting for several hours after training (Andersson et al., 2003). Concerns that children with CP would cocontract the antagonist during resistive strength training regimens have been allayed by recent literature that has shown neither an increase in the strength nor decrease in the ROM of the antagonist to the muscle being strengthened in individuals with CP (Andersson et al., 2003; Damiano et al., 1995; Damiano & Abel, 1998; Hovart, 1987). For example, Damiano and colleagues (1995) reported no change in hamstring strength or knee ROM following a 6-week progressive resistive exercise program for the quadriceps femoris of children with CP. Strength training should be an integral part of an intervention program for children with strength deficits, and we encourage clinicians to continue to document the relationship of strength changes to changes in the activity and participation levels of children.

Passive and active slow static stretching exercises are used routinely as accepted methods of addressing abnormally short MTUs. Static stretching is believed to promote lengthening adaptations of the MTU, represented clinically by increases in ROM. Given the difficulty of measuring the direct effects of stretching exercises on muscle and connective tissues in humans, the changes observed in the ROM in humans are assumed to be based on associated histologic, biochemical, anatomic, and physiologic changes similar to those observed directly in animal models. For example, evidence has indicated that static stretching of adult hamstring muscles brings about lengthening and passive resistance adaptations similar to the adaptations reported for animal muscles immobilized in the lengthened position (Gajdosik, 1991b). Even prolonged passive stretching of MTUs in a state of severe contracture from long-term hypertonicity and shortening may promote lengthening adaptations and increased ROM in children with CP (McPherson et al., 1984). Whether changes observed from the stretching regimens are brought about by decreased neurologic excitability (hypertonicity), by adaptations in the muscle and connective tissues of the MTU, or by both remains controversial and worthy of investigation.

Serial casting has also been used to promote lengthening adaptations of the MTU. Serial casting employs the principles of lengthening and shortening adaptations within the MTU. As discussed earlier in this chapter, investigators have demonstrated that when hypoextensible, abnormally short muscles of children with CP were serially casted in lengthened positions, increased length and passive compliance adaptations were enhanced (Tardieu et al., 1979, 1982a; Tardieu et al., 1982). In other words, the muscles were longer and more compliant. The researchers indicated that the adaptations resulted directly from changes in the MTU, but changes in the neurologic excitability of the muscles were not examined.

Given the possibility that connective tissue adaptations (i.e., proliferation and remodeling) may contribute to the adaptations observed in the MTU, procedures such as soft tissue, joint, and myofascial mobilization could also contribute to the desired adaptations. As a result of increased attention in continuing education offerings, treatment of the connective tissues in children is increasing. Case reports and systematic research on these approaches are direly needed.

The differences in effect between serial casting and inhibitive casting are difficult to identify. Whereas serial casting is the application of a series of casts with the purpose of lengthening the MTU, inhibitive casting entails the single application of a cast (typically bivalved for donning and doffing) that positions the joint in a neutral and normal position with the purpose of reducing or "inhibiting" tone. In a review of inhibitive casting principles and theories, Carlson (1984) indicated that proponents of inhibitive casting suggest that the casting procedures have a neurophysiologic influence on the motoneuron excitability that results in a reduction in spasticity. As stated earlier, the observed lengthening changes in the MTU may result from changes in the MTU directly or from changes in muscle activation patterns and not necessarily from changes in motoneuron excitability. The finding of enhanced strength and function of the antagonist muscle group after surgical lengthening of the agonist muscle groups (Reimers, 1990a, 1990b) supports the hypothesis that functional changes result from direct changes in muscle length, not from altered motoneuron excitability. This proposal was also supported by the finding that splinting spastic muscles of patients with brain damage changed ROM without altering the integrated EMG activity of the muscles when compared with the activity in muscles that were not splinted (Mills, 1984). Another study examined the effects of 3 weeks of dorsiflexion serial casting on the reflex characteristics of spastic calf muscles of seven children with CP (Brouwer et al., 1998). The authors reported that casting brought about increased dorsiflexion ROM and that the angle of reflex excitability elicited by a rapid dorsiflexion stretch also was shifted toward increased dorsiflexion. The soleus and tibialis anterior coactivation EMG tracings, however, did not change as a result of the casting. More recently, Brouwer and coworkers (2000) reported that 3 to 6 weeks of dorsiflexion serial casting for children with CP brought about decreased reflex excitability of the calf muscles when they were stretched rapidly. A major problem in interpreting the clinical reports of the effects of inhibitory casting is the confusing and variable definition of "tone." Is tone caused by central or peripheral influences or by both? Knowledge of the interrelationships among the length, tension, and passive compliance of the MTU and of the neurologic excitability of the muscles of children with neurologic impairment and how the interrelationships are influenced by therapeutic interventions remains sparse. Additional research is needed to explore the effects of many therapeutic methods on the active and passive characteristics of the MTU, including such methods as muscle strengthening and stretching, soft tissue mobilization, and casting. The application of passive isokinetic movements combined with recording of EMG, as described earlier in this chapter, could be used to examine the effects of these interventions on spastic muscles. In the meantime, clinicians should maintain objective records of strength and ROM and attempt to correlate these findings with specific therapeutic interventions and activity and participation outcomes.

The shape and size of the skeletal system are most susceptible to alteration during periods of rapid growth; hence undesirable forces, as well as appropriate corrective forces, are most influential during childhood. Many deformities that occur during the fetal or early postnatal period are more easily corrected in the infant than in the older child. For example, congenitally dislocated hips often readily respond to bracing during the first year of life (Sherk et al., 1981). If, however, the dislocated hip is not diagnosed until after 12 months, surgery is often necessary. Serial casting for wrist deformities in children with distal arthrogryposis was very effective when applied during infancy (Smith & Drennan, 2002). Bracing for idiopathic scoliosis is most effective for preventing worsening of the curve during the preteen and teenage years (Cassella & Hall, 1991). Once an individual has stopped growing, the external support is no longer needed.

The influence of orthoses on the growth of children has not been thoroughly investigated. Bleck (1987) reported that full-control hip-knee-ankle orthoses have not been successful in preventing structural deformities in children with CP. These children still developed dislocated hips or hip flexion contractures. In a study of 204 children, Lee (1982) reported that, regardless of the type of CP, the presence or absence of bracing did not influence the

development of deformities. Bracing did not diminish the need for surgery to correct deformities, nor did it prevent recurrences of deformities after the surgery. Lee and Bleck (1980) reported a 9% recurrence rate of shortening after Achilles tendon lengthening in children with CP who did not wear night splints to maintain tendon length. This rate, however, was comparable with that reported in other studies of children who did wear night splints (Bleck, 1987). Preventing deformities via bracing may be more difficult in children with abnormal tone than in those with normal tone or paralysis. Or, perhaps, results are related to the specific type of bracing that is employed. Plastic total contact orthoses may be more effective at preventing deformities than the traditional metal braces.

Orthoses can also lead to the development of secondary deformities. Lusskin (1966) reported two case studies of children with lower extremity paralysis resulting from poliomyelitis. Both children had marked tibial-fibular torsion and were braced in knee-ankle-foot orthoses with the knees and feet facing forward. As a result, a rotational force was placed at the ankle and foot, and these children developed severe metatarsus adductus and heel varus. Children who wear total contact ankle-foot orthoses for most of their growing years may be at risk for stunted growth of the foot and lower limb. The circumferential compressive forces and the restriction in active movement can interfere with normal musculoskeletal growth. Pediatric physical therapists have an important responsibility to understand and document the effects of external devices on the growing child. While trying to solve one problem, intervention may inadvertently create another.

Weight-bearing activities are thought to retard the loss of bone mass and help shape the joint. Mobile children with CP have greater bone mineral density when compared to their less mobile peers (Ihkkan & Yalcin, 2001; Wilmshurst et al., 1996). In a preliminary study, Stuberg (1992) found that 60 minutes of standing four or five times a week increased the bone mineral density of nonambulatory children with severe to profound CP. When the standing program was discontinued, bone mineral density decreased. Gudjonsdottir and Mercer (2002) reported an increase in bone mineral density in three of four children with CP who participated in an 8-week standing program. Standing programs may also help deepen the acetabulum. The contact between the femoral head and the acetabulum in weight bearing helps in the development of the normal shape of the acetabulum, which contributes to a stable hip socket (Beals, 1969; Harrison, 1961).

Movement has been reported to affect the formation and shape of joints in fetal animals (Drachman & Sokoloff,

1966; Murray & Drachman, 1969). Movement allows the compressive forces to be spread throughout the joint surface rather than be confined to a small area. Combining weight-bearing activities with movement would create more desirable forces for joint formation. Although no research has been reported on the effects on hip formation of stationary standing devices, such as prone boards or standing platforms, it appears reasonable to use caution when using these devices with very young children. Because remodeling of the bone and associated joints takes place most readily during the first few years of life and because the acetabular shape is fairly well defined by the age of 3 years (Ralis & McKibbin, 1973), early intervention with weight-bearing activities may have a substantial influence on the shape and function of the joint. To help shape the joint, chronologic age and not developmental age may be more important when determining when to begin weight-bearing activities. Although standing is important, the length of time the child stands during any one period needs to be controlled.

For the young child with severe delays in motor development in whom independent walking (with or without devices) is unlikely and hip dislocation is a risk, early and prolonged standing may be beneficial in developing a deeper hip joint. The shape of the acetabulum may not be appropriate for walking, but the hip may be more stable. Over time, this early standing may help prevent or decrease the severity of a dislocated hip. For children with milder delays, less stationary standing time and more weight bearing with movement may help develop a more normally shaped hip socket. This may contribute to an improved gait and a decrease in the risk of osteoarthritis in adulthood. More research in this area would give the pediatric physical therapist valuable information for designing intervention using programs with weight-bearing activities.

SUMMARY

This chapter reviewed the normal growth and development of the musculoskeletal system, with emphasis on the adaptations of muscle and bone associated with pathologic conditions encountered by pediatric physical therapists. The microscopic and macroscopic structure and function of the normal MTU and the force and length adaptations to imposed physical changes, such as immobilization and denervation, have been well documented in nonhuman studies using invasive methods of investigation. The results of human studies using noninvasive methods of investigation indicate that the human MTU undergoes adaptations similar to those reported for animals. The clinical evidence for the musculoskeletal adaptations supports these research findings.

In the developing child, atypic changes in the MTU can exert forces on the skeletal system, resulting in bone deformities. Pediatric physical therapists routinely measure physical impairments and develop therapeutic interventions designed to promote musculoskeletal adaptations. To document therapeutic efficacy in relation to specific pediatric disorders, therapists are encouraged to use objective measures of ROM and strength during specific interventions for correlating changes in musculoskeletal impairments with levels of activity and participation. Additional research is needed to examine the efficacy of therapeutic strengthening and stretching programs and their interrelation with other interventions, such as surgical procedures. The application of new research technologies, such as isokinetic dynamometry and EMG, now permits objective measurement of the impairments associated with neuromuscular disorders and the effects of interventions designed to influence these disorders. Further controlled studies will enhance the scientific basis for using physical therapy to promote participation in life activities.

REFERENCES

Abel, MF, Wenger, DR, Mubarak, SJ, & Sutherland, DH. Quantitative analysis of hip dysplasia in cerebral palsy: A study of radiographs and 3-D reformatted images. Journal of Pediatric Orthopedics, 14:283–289, 1994.

Alder, AB, Crawford, GNC, & Edwards, GR. The effect of limitation of movement on longitudinal muscle growth. Proceedings of the Royal Society of London. Series B: Biological Sciences, 150:554–562, 1959.

Andersson, C, Grooten, W, Hellsten, M, Kaping, K, & Mattsson, E. Adults with cerebral palsy: Walking ability after progressive strength training. Developmental Medicine and Child Neurology, 45:220–228, 2003.

Apkon, SK. Osteoporosis in children who have disabilities. Physical Medicine and Rehabilitation Clinic of North America, 13:839–855, 2002.

Argov, Z, Gardner-Medwin, D, Johnson, MA, & Mastaglia, FL. Patterns of muscle fiber-type disproportion in hypotonic infants. Archives of Neurology, 41:53–57, 1984.

Arkin, AM, & Katz, JF. The effects of pressure on epiphyseal growth. Journal of Bone and Joint Surgery (American), 38:1056–1076, 1956.

Ashton, BB, Pickles, B, & Roll, JW. Reliability of goniometric measurements of hip motion in spastic cerebral palsy. Developmental Medicine and Child Neurology, 20:87–94, 1978.

Ayalon, M, Ben-Sira, D, & Hutzler, Y. Reliability of isokinetic strength measurements of the knee in children with cerebral palsy. Developmental Medicine and Child Neurology, 42:396–402, 2000.

Backman, E, & Oberg, B. Isokinetic muscle torque in the dorsiflexors of the ankle of children 6-12 years of age. Scandinavian Journal of Rehabilitation Medicine, 21: 97–103, 1989.

Bailey, DA, Wedge, JH, McCulloch, RG, Martin, AD, & Bernhardson, SC. Epidemiology of fractures of the distal end of the radius in children as associated with growth. Journal of Bone and Joint Surgery (American), 71:1225–1230, 1989.

Bartlett, MD, Wolf, LS, Shurtleff, DB, & Staheli, LT. Hip flexion contractures: A comparison of measurement procedures. Archives of Physical Medicine and Rehabilitation, 66:620–625, 1985.

Beals, RK. Developmental changes in the femur and acetabulum in spastic paraplegia and diplegia. Developmental Medicine and Child Neurology, 11:303–313, 1969.

Bernhardt, DB. Prenatal and postnatal growth and development of the foot and ankle. Physical Therapy, 68:1831–1839, 1988.

Bleck, EE. Orthopedic Management in Cerebral Palsy. Philadelphia: JB Lippincott, 1987.

Bohannon, RW. Measurement, nature, and implications of skeletal muscle strength in patients with neurological disorders. Clinical Biomechanics, 10:283–292, 1995.

Bohannon, RW, & Andrews, AW. Inter-rater reliability of hand-held dynamometer. Physical Therapy, 67:931–933, 1987.

Boiteau, M, Malouin, F, & Richards, CL. Use of a hand-held dynamometer and the Kin-Com dynamometer for evaluating spastic hypertonia in children: A reliability study. Physical Therapy, 75:796–802, 1995.

Booth, CM, Cortina-Borja, MJF, Theologis, TN. Collagen accumulation in muscles of children with cerebral palsy and correlation with severity of spasticity. Developmental Medicine and Child Neurology, 43:314–320, 2001.

Borg, TK, & Caulfield, JB. Morphology of connective tissue in skeletal muscle. Tissue and Cell, 12:197–207, 1980.

Botelho, SY, Cander, L, & Guiti, N. Passive and active tension-length diagrams of intact skeletal muscle in normal women of different ages. Journal of Applied Physiology, 7:93–95, 1954.

Brooke, MH, & Engel, WK. The histographic analyses of human muscle biopsies with regard to fiber types: 4. Children's biopsies. Neurology, 19:591–605, 1969.

Brouwer, B, Wheeldon, RK, & Stradiotto-Parker, N. Reflex excitability and isometric force production in cerebral palsy: The effect of serial casting. Developmental Medicine and Child Neurology, 40:168–175, 1998.

Brouwer, B, Davidson, LK, & Olney, SJ. Serial casting in idiopathic toe-walkers and children with spastic cerebral palsy. Journal of Pediatric Orthopaedics, 20(2):221–225, 2000.

Brown, MC, Jansen, JKS, & Van Essen, D. Polyneuronal innervation of skeletal muscle in newborn rats and its elimination during maturation. Journal of Physiology, 261:387–422, 1976.

Brussock, CM, Haley, SH, Munsat, TL, & Bernhardt, DB. Measurement of isometric force in children with and without Duchenne's muscular dystrophy. Physical Therapy, 72:105–114, 1992.

Buckley, SL, Sponseller, PD, & Maged, D. The acetabulum in congenital and neuromuscular hip instability. Journal of Pediatric Orthopedics, 11:498–501, 1991.

Bunch, W. Origin and mechanism of postnatal deformities. Pediatric Clinics of North America, 24:679–684, 1977.

Butler, J, Cosmos, E, & Brienley, J. Differentiation of muscle fiber types in aneurogenic muscles of the chick embryo. Journal of Experimental Zoology, 224:65–80, 1982.

Cahuzac, J, Vardon, D, & Sales de Gauzy, J. Development of the clinical tibiofemoral angle in normal adolescents. Journal of Bone and Joint Surgery (British), 77:729–732, 1995.

Campbell, SK. Therapy programs for children that last a lifetime. Physical and Occupational Therapy in Pediatrics, 17(1):1–15, 1997.

Cardenas, DD, Stolov, WC, & Hardy, R. Muscle fiber number in immobilization atrophy. Archives of Physical Medicine and Rehabilitation, 58:423–426, 1977.

Carlson, SJ. A neurophysiological analysis of inhibitive casting. Physical and Occupational Therapy in Pediatrics, 4(4):31–42, 1984.

Carter, DR, Orr, TE, Fyhrie, DP, & Schurman, DJ. Influences of mechanical stress on prenatal and postnatal skeletal development. Clinical Orthopedics and Related Research, 219:237–250, 1987.

Cassella, MC, & Hall, JE. Current treatment approaches in the nonoperative and operative management of adolescent idiopathic scoliosis. Physical Therapy, 71:897–909, 1991.

Castle, ME, Reyman, TA, & Schneider, M. Pathology of spastic muscle in cerebral palsy. Clinical Orthopedics, 142:223–232, 1979.

Chandraraj, S, & Briggs, CA. Multiple growth cartilages in the neural arch. Anatomical Record, 230(1):114–120, 1991.

Cheng, JCY, Chan, PS, Chiang, SC, & Hui, PW. Angular and rotational profile of the lower limb in 2,630 Chinese children. Journal of Pediatric Orthopedics, 11:154–161, 1991.

Chung, SMK, Batterman, SC, & Brighton CT. Shear strength of the human femoral capital epiphyseal plate. Journal of Bone and Joint Surgery (American), 58:94–105, 1976.

Coleman, SS. Congenital dysplasia of the hip in the Navajo infant. Clinical Orthopedics and Related Research, 56:179–193, 1968.

Colling-Saltin, A. Enzyme histochemisty on skeletal muscle of the human fetus. Journal of Neurological Science, 39:169–185, 1978.

Damiano, DL, & Abel, MF. Functional outcomes of strength training in spastic cerebral palsy. Archives of Physical Medicine and Rehabilitation, 79:119–125, 1998.

Damiano, DL, Kelly, LE, & Vaughn, CL. Effects of quadriceps femoris muscle strengthening on crouch gait in children with spastic diplegia. Physical Therapy, 75:658–667, 1995.

Damiano, DL, Quinlivan, BF, Owen, BF, Shaffrey, M, & Abel, MF. Spasticity versus strength in cerebral palsy: Relationships among involuntary resistance, voluntary torque, and motor function. European Journal of Neurology, 8(Suppl. 5):40–49, 2001.

Damron, T, Breed, AL, & Roecker, E. Hamstring tenotomies in cerebral palsy: Long-term retrospective analysis. Journal of Pediatric Orthopedics, 11:514–519, 1991.

Davis, JA, & Dobbing, J (Eds.). Scientific Foundations of Paediatrics. Philadelphia: WB Saunders, 1974.

de Lateur, BJ, & Giaconi, RM. Effect on maximal strength of submaximal exercise in Duchenne muscular dystrophy. American Journal of Physical Medicine, 58:26–36, 1979.

Dodd, JK, Taylor, NF, & Graham, HK. A randomized clinical trial of strength training in young people with cerebral palsy. Developmental Medicine and Child Neurology, 45:652–657, 2003.

Drachman, DB, & Sokoloff, L. The role of movement in embryonic joint development. Developmental Biology, 14:401–420, 1966.

Drews, JE, Vraciu, JK, & Pellino, G. Range of motion of the joints of the lower extremities of newborns. Physical and Occupational Therapy in Pediatrics, 4(2):49–62, 1984.

Edmonson, AD, & Crenshaw, AH (Eds.). Campbell's Operative Orthopaedics, Vol. 2. St. Louis: Mosby, 1980.

Effgen, SK, & Brown, DA. Long-term stability of hand-held dynamometric measurements in children who have myelomeningocele. Physical Therapy, 72:458–465, 1992.

Fabeck, L, Tolley, M, Rooze, M, & Burny, F. Theoretical study of the decrease in the femoral neck anteversion during growth. Cells Tissues Organs, 171:269–275, 2002.

Fabry, G, Belguim, L, MacEwen, GD, & Shands, AR. Torsion of the femur. The Journal of Bone and Joint Surgery (American), 55:1726–1738, 1973.

Farkas-Bargeton, E, Barbet, JP, Dancea, S, Wehrle, R, Checouri, A, & Dulac, O. Immaturity of muscle fibers in the congenital form of myotonic dystrophy: Its consequences and its origin. Journal of the Neurological Sciences, 83(2–3):145–159, 1988.

Florence, JM, Pandya, S, King, WM, Robison, JD, Signore, LC, Wentzell, M, & Province, MA. Clinical trials in Duchenne dystrophy:

Standardization and reliability of evaluation procedures. Physical Therapy, 64:41–45, 1984.

Friden, J, & Lieber, RL. Spastic muscle cells are shorter and stiffer than normal cells. Muscle and Nerve, 26:157–164, 2003.

Fuchs, RK, & Snow, CM. Gains in hip bone mass from high-impact training are maintained: A randomized controlled trial in children. Journal of Pediatrics, 141:357–362, 2002.

Fulford, G, & Brown, J. Position as a cause of deformity in children with cerebral palsy. Developmental Medicine and Child Neurology, 18:305–314, 1977.

Gajdosik, CG. Ability of very young children to produce reliable isometric strength measurements. Abstract. World Congress of Physical Therapy, June 2003.

Gajdosik, CG, & Cicirello, N. Secondary conditions of the musculoskeletal system in adolescents and adults with cerebral palsy. Physical and Occupational Therapy in Pediatrics, 21:49–68, 2001.

Gajdosik, RL. Passive compliance and length of clinically short hamstring muscles of healthy men. Clinical Biomechanics, 6:239–244, 1991a.

Gajdosik, RL. Effects of static stretching on the maximal length and resistance to passive stretch of short hamstring muscles. Journal of Orthopedic Sports and Physical Therapy, 14:250–255, 1991b.

Gajdosik, RL, & Bohannon, RW. Clinical measurement of range of motion: Review of goniometry emphasizing reliability and validity. Physical Therapy, 67:1867–1872, 1987.

Gajdosik, RL, Guiliani, CA, & Bohannon, RW. Passive compliance of the hamstring muscles of healthy men and women. Clinical Biomechanics, 5:23–29, 1990.

Gasser, T, Kneip, A, Ziegler, P, Largo, R, Molinari, L, & Prader, A. The dynamics of growth of width in distance, velocity and acceleration. Annals of Human Biology, 18(5):449–461, 1991.

Goldspink, DF. The influence of immobilization and stretch on protein turnover of rat skeletal muscle. Journal of Physiology, 64:267–282, 1977.

Goldspink, G, Tabary, C, Tabary, JC, Tardieu, C, & Tardieu, G. Effect of denervation on the adaptation of sarcomere number and muscle extensibility to the functional length of the muscle. Journal of Physiology, 236:733–742, 1974.

Goulding, A, Jones, IE, Taylor, RW, Manning, PJ, & Williams, SM. More broken bones: A 4-year double cohort study of young girls with and without distal forearm fractures. Journal of Bone and Mineral Research, 15(10):2011–2018, 2000a.

Goulding, A, Taylor, RW, Jones, IE, McAuley, KA, Manning, PJ, & Williams, SM. Overweight and obese children have low bone mass and area for their weight. International Journal of Obesity, 24:627–632, 2000b.

Gordon, AM, Huxley, AF, & Julian, FJ. The variation in isometric tension with sarcomere length in vertebrate muscle fibers. Journal of Physiology, 184:170–192, 1966.

Gramsbergen, A, Ijkema-Paassen, J, Nikkels, PGJ, & Hadders-Algra, M. Regression of polyneural innervation in the human psoas muscle. Early Human Development, 49:49–61, 1997.

Granzier, HLM, & Pollack, GH. Stepwise shortening in unstimulated frog skeletal muscle fibers. Journal of Physiology, 362:173–188, 1985.

Grinnell, AD. Dynamics of nerve-muscle interaction in developing and mature neuromuscular junctions. Physiological Reviews, 75:789–834, 1995.

Grove, BK. Muscle differentiation and the origin of muscle fiber diversity. CRC Critical Reviews of Neurobiology, 4(3):201–234, 1989.

Gudjonsdottir, B, & Mercer, VS. Effects of a dynamic versus a static prone stander on bone mineral density and behavior in four children with severe cerebral palsy. Pediatric Physical Therapy, 14:38–46, 2002.

Gudjonsdottir, B, & Mercer, VS. Hip and spine in children with cerebral palsy: Musculoskeletal development and clinical implications. Pediatric Physical Therapy, 9:179-185, 1997.

Halar, EM, Stolov, WC, Venkatesh, B, Brozovivh, FV, & Harley, JD. Gastrocnemius muscle belly and tendon length in stroke patients and able-bodied persons. Archives of Physical Medicine and Rehabilitation, 59:467–484, 1978.

Haley, SM, Tada, WL, & Carmichael, EM. Spinal mobility in young children: A normative study. Physical Therapy, 66:1697–1703, 1986.

Harris, SR, Smith, LH, & Krukowski, L. Goniometric reliability for a child with spastic quadriplegia. Journal of Pediatric Orthopedics, 5:348–351, 1985.

Harrison, TJ. The influence of the femoral head on pelvic growth and acetabular form in the rat. Journal of Anatomy (British), 95:12–24, 1961.

Heath, CH, & Staheli, LT. Normal limits of knee angle in white children— Genu varum and genu valgum. Journal of Pediatric Orthopedics, 13:259–262, 1993.

Heinrich, SD, MacEwen, GD, & Zembo, MM. Hip dysplasia, subluxation, and dislocation in cerebral palsy: An arthrographic analysis. Journal of Pediatric Orthopedics, 11:488–493, 1991.

Hesselmans, LFGM, Jennekens, FGI, Van Den Oord, CJM, Veldman, H, & Vincent, A. Development of innervation of skeletal muscle fibers in man: Relation to acetylcholine receptors. Anatomical Record, 236:553–562, 1993.

Hill, DK. Tension due to interaction between sliding filaments in resting striated muscle: The effect of stimulation. Journal of Physiology, 199:637–684, 1968.

Hill, DK. The effect of temperature in the range of 0–35° C on the resting tension of frog's muscle. Journal of Physiology, 208:725–739, 1970a.

Hill, DK. The effect of temperature on the resting tension of frog's muscle in hypertonic solutions. Journal of Physiology, 208:741–756, 1970b.

Hopp, R, Degan, J, Gallager, JC, & Cassidy, JT. Estimation of bone mineral density in children with juvenile rheumatoid arthritis. Journal of Rheumatology, 18:1235–1239, 1991.

Horii, M, Toshikazu, K, Hachiya, Y, Nishimura, T, Hirasawa, Y. Development of the acetabulum and the acetabular labrum in the normal child: Analysis with radial-sequence magnetic resonance imaging. Journal of Pediatric Orthopaedics, 22:22–227, 2002.

Hovart, M. Effects of a progressive resistance training program on an individual with spastic cerebral palsy. American Corrective Therapy Journal, 41:7–11, 1987.

Hresko, MT, McCarthy, JC, & Goldberg, MJ. Hip disease in adults with Down syndrome. Journal of Bone and Joint Surgery (British), 75:604–607, 1993.

Huet de la Tour, E, Tabary, JC, Tabary, C, & Tardieu, C. The respective roles of muscle length and muscle tension in sarcomere number adaptation of guinea-pig soleus muscle. Journal de Physiologie, 75:589–592, 1979a.

Huet de la Tour, E, Tardieu, C, Tabary, JC, & Tabary, C. Decreased muscle extensibility and reduction of sarcomere number in soleus muscle following local injection of tetanus toxin. Journal of the Neurological Sciences, 40:123–131, 1979b.

Huxley, AF, & Peachey, LD. The maximum length for contraction in vertebrate striated muscle. Journal of Physiology, 156:150–165, 1961.

Ihkkan, KY, & Yalcin, E. Changes in skeletal maturation and mineralization in children with cerebral palsy and evaluation of related factors. Journal of Child Neurology, 16:425–430, 2001.

Imoto, C, & Nonaka, I. The significance of type 1 fiber atrophy (hypotrophy) in childhood neuromuscular disorders. Brain and Development, 23:298–302, 2001.

Ito, J, Araki, A, Tanaka, H, Tasaki, T, Cho, K, & Yamazaki, R. Muscle histopathology in spastic cerebral palsy. Brain and Development, 18:299–303, 1996.

Kannisto, M, Alaranta, H, Merikanto, J, Kroger, H, & Karkkainen, J. Bone mineral status after pediatric spinal cord injury. Spinal Cord, 36:641–646, 1998.

Katz, K, Naor, N, Merlob, P, & Wielunsky, E. Rotational deformities of the tibia and foot in preterm infants. Journal of Pediatric Orthopedics, 10:483–485, 1990.

Kendall, FP, & McCreary, EK. Muscles Testing and Function, 3rd ed. Baltimore: Williams & Wilkins, 1983.

Khosla, S, Melton, LJ, Dekutoski, MB, Achenback, SJ, Oberg, AL, & Riggs, BL. Incidence of childhood distal forearm fractures over 30 years: A population-based study. Journal of the American Medical Association, 290:1479–1485, 2003.

Kilgour, G, McNair, P, & Stott, NS. Intrarater reliability of lower limb sagittal range-of-motion measures in children with spastic diplegia. Developmental Medicine and Child Neurology, 45:391–399, 2003.

Kitiyakara, A, & Angevine, DM. A study of the pattern of post-embryonic growth of M. gracilis in mice. Developmental Biology, 8:322–340, 1963.

Kristiansen, LP, Gunderson, RB, Steen, H, & Reikeras, O. The normal development of tibial torsion. Skeletal Radiology, 30:519–522, 2001.

Larson, CM, & Henderson, RC. Bone mineral density and fractures in boys with Duchenne muscular dystrophy. Journal of Pediatric Orthopaedics, 20:71–74, 2000.

Lee, CL. Role of lower extremity bracing in cerebral palsy (Abstract). Developmental Medicine and Child Neurology, 24:250–251, 1982.

Lee, CL, & Bleck, EE. Surgical correction of equinus deformity in cerebral palsy. Developmental Medicine and Child Neurology, 22:287–292, 1980.

Lespargot, A, Tardieu, C, Bret, MD, Tabary, C, & Singh, B. Is tendon surgery for the knee flexors justified in cerebral palsy? French Journal of Orthopedic Surgery, 3(4):446–450, 1989.

LeVeau, BF, & Bernhardt, DB. Effects of forces on the growth, development, and maintenance of the human body. Physical Therapy, 64:1874–1882, 1984.

Lewis, FR, Samilson, RR, & Lucas, DB. Femoral torsion and coxa valga in cerebral palsy: A preliminary report. Developmental Medicine and Child Neurology, 6:591–597, 1964.

Lichtman, JW, & Colman, H. Synapse elimination and indelible memory. Neuron, 25:269–278, 2000.

Lin, PP, & Henderson, RC. Bone mineralization in the affected extremities of children with spastic hemiplegia. Developmental Medicine and Child Neurology, 38:782–786, 1996.

Linke, WA, Ivemeyer, M, Olivieri, N, Lolmerer, B, Ruegg, JC, & Labeit, S. Towards a molecular understanding of the elasticity of titin. Journal of Molecular Biology, 261:62–71, 1996.

Loder, RT, & Greenfiled, MVH. Clinical characteristics of children with atypical and idiopathic slipped capital femoral epiphysis: Description of the age-weight test and implications for further diagnostic investigation. Journal of Pediatric Orthopaedics, 21:481–487, 2001.

Lusskin, R. The influence of errors in bracing upon deformity of the lower extremity. Archives of Physical Medicine and Rehabilitation, 47:520–525, 1966.

MacPhail, HEA, & Kramer, JF. Effect of isokinetic strength-training on functional ability and walking efficiency in adolescents with cerebral palsy. Developmental Medicine and Child Neurology, 38:763–775, 1995.

Magid, A, & Law, DJ. Myofibrils bear most of the resting tension in frog skeletal muscle. Science, 230:1280–1282, 1985.

Martin, AD, & McCulloch, RG. Bone dynamics: Stress, strain, and fracture. Journal of Sports Sciences, 5:155–163, 1987.

Mastaglia, FL. The growth and development of the skeletal muscles. In Davis, JA, & Dobbing, J (Eds.). Scientific Foundations of Paediatrics. Philadelphia: WB Saunders, 1974, pp. 348–375.

McDowell, BC, Hewitt, V, Nurse, A, Weston, T, & Baker, R. The variability of goniometric measurements in ambulatory children with spastic cerebral palsy. Gait and Posture, 12:114–121, 2000.

McKibbin, B. The structure of the epiphysis. In Owen, R, Goodfellow, J, & Bullough, P (Eds.). Scientific Foundations of Orthopaedics and Traumatology. Philadelphia: WB Saunders, 1980.

McPherson, JJ, Arends, TG, Michaels, MJ, & Trettin, K. The range of motion of long term knee contractures of four spastic cerebral palsied children: A pilot study. Physical and Occupational Therapy in Pediatrics, 4(1):17–34, 1984.

Mercer, VS, & Lewis, CL. Hip abductor and knee extensor muscle strength of children with and without Down syndrome. Pediatric Physical Therapy, 13:18–26, 2001.

Merchant, AJ. Hip abduction muscle force. Journal of Bone and Joint Surgery (American), 47:462–475, 1965.

Merlini, L, Dell'Accio, D, & Granata, C. Reliability of dynamic strength knee muscle testing in children. Journal of Sports Physical Therapy, 22:73–76, 1995.

Mielke, CH, & Stevens, PM. Hemiepiphyseal stapling for knee deformities in children younger than 10 years: A preliminary report. Journal of Pediatric Orthopaedics, 16:423–429, 1996.

Miller, JB. Review article: Myoblasts, myosins, MyoDs, and the diversification of muscle fibers. Neuromuscular Disorders, 1:7–17, 1991.

Mills, VM. Electromyographic results of inhibitory splinting. Physical Therapy, 64:190–193, 1984.

Moore, KL. The Developing Human: Clinically Oriented Embryology, 4th ed. Philadelphia: WB Saunders, 1988.

Moore, ML. The measurement of joint motion: Part I. Introductory review of the literature. Physical Therapy Review, 29:195–205, 1949a.

Moore, ML. The measurement of joint motion: Part II. The technique of goniometry. Physical Therapy Review, 29:256–264, 1949b.

Murphy, KP, Molnar, GE, & Lankasky, K. Medical and functional status of adults with cerebral palsy. Developmental Medicine and Child Neurology, 37:1075–1084, 1995.

Murray, PDF, & Drachman, DB. The role of movement in the development of joints and the related structures: The head and neck in the chick embryo. Journal of Embryology and Experimental Morphology, 22:349–371, 1969.

Nichols, DL, Sanborn, CF, & Love, AM. Resistance training and bone mineral density in adolescent females. Journal of Pediatrics, 139:494–500, 2001.

Norkin, CC, & White, DJ. Measurement of Joint Motion: A Guide to Goniometry. Philadelphia: FA Davis, 1985.

O'Connell, DG, & Barnhart, R. Improvement in wheelchair propulsion in pediatric wheelchair users through resistance training: A pilot study. Archives of Physical Medicine and Rehabilitation, 76:368–372, 1995.

Owen, R, Goodfellow, J, & Bullough, P (Eds.). Scientific Foundations of Orthopaedics and Traumatology. Philadelphia: WB Saunders, 1980.

Pandya, S, Florence, JM, King, WM, Robison, JD, Oxman, M, & Province, MA. Reliability of goniometric measurements in patients with Duchenne muscular dystrophy. Physical Therapy, 65:1339–1342, 1985.

Pearl, ML, Edgerton, BW, Kon, DS, Darakjian, AB, Kosco, AE, Kazimiroff, PB, & Burchette, RJ. Comparison of arthroscopic findings with magnetic resonance imaging and arthrography in children with glenohumeral deformities secondary to brachial plexus birth palsy. Journal of Bone and Joint Surgery (American), 85:890–898, 2003.

Price, R, Bjornson, KF, Lehmann, JF, McLaughlin, JF, & Hays, RM.

Quantitative measurement of spasticity in children with cerebral palsy. Developmental Medicine and Child Neurology, 33:585–595, 1991.

Purves, D, & Lichtman, JW. Elimination of synapses in the developing nervous system. Science, 210:153–157, 1980.

Quan, A, Adams, R, Ekmark, E, & Baum, M. Bone mineral density in children with myelomeningocele (Abstract). Pediatrics, 102:628, 1998.

Rauch, F, Neu, C, Manz, F, & Schoenau, E. The development of metaphyseal cortex – Implications for distal radius fractures during growth. Journal of Bone and Mineral Research, 16:1547–1555, 2001.

Ralis, Z, & McKibbin, B. Changes in shape of the human hip joint during its development and their relation to stability. Journal of Bone and Joint Surgery (British), 55:780–785, 1973.

Reimers, J. Contracture of the hamstrings in spastic cerebral palsy: A study of three methods of operative correction. Journal of Bone and Joint Surgery (British), 56:102–109, 1974.

Reimers, J. Functional changes in the antagonists after lengthening the agonists in cerebral palsy: I. Triceps surae lengthening. Clinical Orthopedics and Related Research, 253:30–34, 1990a.

Reimers, J. Functional changes in the antagonists after lengthening the agonists in cerebral palsy: II. Quadriceps strength before and after distal hamstring lengthening. Clinical Orthopedics and Related Research, 253:35–37, 1990b.

Rodriguez, TI, Razquin, S, Palacios, T, & Rubio, V. Human growth plate development in the fetal and neonatal period. Journal of Orthopaedic Research, 10(1):62–71, 1992.

Romanini, L, Villani, C, Meloni, C, & Calvisi, V. Histological and morphological aspects of muscle in infantile cerebral palsy. Italian Journal of Orthopaedics and Traumatology, 15:87–93, 1989.

Rose, J, Haskell, WL, Gamble, JG, Hamilton, RL, Brown, DA, & Rinsky, L. Muscle pathology and clinical measures of disability in children with cerebral palsy. Journal of Orthopaedic Research, 12:758–768, 1994.

Rothstein, JM, Lamb, RL, & Mayhew, TP. Clinical uses of isokinetic measurements: Critical issues. Physical Therapy, 67:1840–1844, 1987.

Rothstein, JM, & Rose, SJ. Muscle mutability. Part 2, Adaptation to drugs, metabolic factors, and aging. Physical Therapy, 62:1788–1798, 1982.

Rowe, RWD. Collagen fibre arrangement in intramuscular connective tissue. Changes associated with muscle shortening and their possible relevance to raw meat toughness measurements. Journal of Food Technology, 9:501–508, 1974.

Rowe, RWD. Morphology of perimysial and endomysial connective tissue in skeletal muscle. Tissue and Cell, 13:681–690, 1981.

Royer, P. Growth of bony tissue. In Davis, JA, & Dobbing, J (Eds.). Scientific Foundations of Paediatrics. Philadelphia: WB Saunders, 1974.

Salenius, P, & Vankka, E. The development of the tibiofemoral angle in children. Journal of Bone and Joint Surgery (American), 57:259–261, 1975.

Salmons, S, & Hendriksson, J. The adaptive response of skeletal muscle to increased use. Muscle and Nerve, 4:94–105, 1981.

Sanes, JR. Cell lineage and the origin of muscle fiber types. Trends in Neurosciences, 10(6):119–121, 1987.

Sargeant, AJ, Davies, CTM, Edwards, RHT, Maunder, C, & Young, A. Functional and structural changes after disuse of human muscle. Clinical Science and Molecular Medicine, 52:337–342, 1977.

Schönau, E. The development of the skeletal system in children and the influence of muscular strength. Hormone Research, 49:27–31, 1998.

Schwartz, L, Engle, JM, & Jensen, MP. Pain in persons with cerebral palsy. Archives of Physical Medicine and Rehabilitation, 80:1243–1246, 1999.

Scott, OM, Hyde, SA, Goddard, C, Jones, R, & Dubowitz, V. Effect of exercise in Duchenne muscular dystrophy. Physiotherapy, 67:174–176, 1981.

Sharrard, WJW. Paralytic deformity in the lower limb. Journal of Bone and Joint Surgery (British), 49:731–747, 1967.

Sherk, HH, Pasquariello, PS, & Watters, WC. Congenital dislocation of the hip. Clinical Pediatrics, 20(8):513–520, 1981.

Simard, S, Marchant, M, & Mencio G. The Ilizarov procedures: Limb lengthening and its implications. Physical Therapy, 72:25–34, 1992.

Slaton, D. Muscle fiber types and their development in the human fetus. Physical and Occupational Therapy in Pediatrics, 1(3):47–57, 1981.

Smith, DW, & Drennan, JC. Arthrogryposis wrist deformities: Results of infantile serial casting. Journal of Pediatric Orthopaedics, 22:44–47, 2002.

Sockolov, R, Irwin, B, Dressendorfer, RH, & Bernauer, EM. Exercise performance in 6- to 11-year-old boys with Duchenne muscular dystrophy. Archives of Physical Medicine and Rehabilitation, 58:195–200, 1977.

Sone, S. Muscle histochemistry in the Prader-Willi syndrome. Brain and Development, 16: 183–188, 1994.

Stanitski, D, Shahcheraghi, H, Nicker, D, & Armstrong, P. Results of tibial lengthening with the Ilizarov technique. Journal of Pediatric Orthopaedics, 16:168–172, 1996.

Stolov, WC, Riddell, WM, & Shrier, KP. Effect of electrical stimulation on contracture of immobilized, innervated and denervated muscle (Abstract). Archives in Physical Medicine and Rehabilitation, 52:589, 1971.

Stolov, WC, & Weilepp, TG. Passive length-tension relationship of intact muscle, epimysium, and tendon in normal and denervated gastrocnemius of the rat. Archives in Physical Medicine and Rehabilitation, 47:612–620, 1966.

Stolov, WC, Weilepp, TB, Jr, & Riddell, WM. Passive length-tension relationship and hydroxyproline content of chronically denervated skeletal muscle. Archives in Physical Medicine and Rehabilitation, 51:517–525, 1970.

Stuberg, WA. Considerations related to weight-bearing programs in children with developmental disabilities. Physical Therapy, 72:35–40, 1992.

Stuberg, WA, Fuchs, RH, & Miedaner, JA. Reliability of goniometric measurements of children with cerebral palsy. Developmental Medicine and Child Neurology, 30:657–666, 1988.

Stuberg, WA, Metcalf, WK. Reliability of quantitative muscle testing in healthy children and in children with Duchenne muscular dystrophy using a hand-held dynamometer. Physical Therapy, 68:977–982, 1988.

Suzuki, S, & Yamamuro, T. Correction of fetal posture and congenital dislocation of hip. Acta Orthopaedica Scandinavica, 57:81–84, 1986.

Tabary, JC, Tabary, C, Tardieu, C, Tardieu, G, & Goldspink, G. Physiological and structural changes in the cat's soleus muscle due to immobilization at different lengths by plaster casts. Journal of Physiology, 224:231–244, 1972.

Tabary, JC, Tardieu, C, Tardieu, G, & Tabary, C. Experimental rapid sarcomere loss with concomitant hypoextensibility. Muscle and Nerve, 4:198–203, 1981.

Tardieu, C, Huet de la Tour, E, Bret, MD, & Tardieu, G. Muscle hypoextensibility in children with cerebral palsy: I. Clinical and experimental observations. Archives of Physical Medicine and Rehabilitation, 63:97–102, 1982a.

Tardieu, C, Tabary, JC, Tabary, C, & Tardieu, G. Adaptation of connective tissue length to immobilization in the lengthened and shortened positions in the cat soleus muscle. Journal de Physiologie, 78:214–220, 1982b.

Tardieu, C, Tardieu, G, Colbeau-Justin, P, & Huet de la Tour, E. Trophic muscle regulation in children with congenital cerebral lesions. Journal of the Neurological Sciences, *42*:357–364, 1979.

Tardieu, G, Tardieu, C, Colbeau-Justin, P, & Lespargot, A. Muscle hypoextensibility in children with cerebral palsy: II. Therapeutic implications. Archives of Physical Medicine and Rehabilitation, *63*:103–107, 1982.

Thompson, WJ. Changes in the innervation of mammalian skeletal muscle fibers during postnatal development. Trends in Neurosciences, *9*:25–28, 1986.

Thompson, WJ, & Jansen, JKS. The extent of sprouting of remaining motor units in partly denervated immature and adult rat soleus muscle. Neuroscience, *2*:523–535, 1977.

Thomson, JD. Mechanical characteristics of skeletal muscle undergoing atrophy of degeneration. American Journal of Physical Medicine, *34*:606–611, 1955.

Tokuyasu, KT, Dutton, AH, & Singer, SJ. Immunoelectron microscopic studies of desmin (skeletin) localization and intermediate filament organization in chicken skeletal muscle. The Journal of Cell Biology, *96*:1727–1735, 1983.

Trombitas, K, Greaser, M, Labeit, S, Jin, JP, Kellermayer, M, Helmes, M, & Granzier, H. Titin extensibility in situ: Entropic elasticity of permanently folded and permanently unfolded molecular segments. The Journal of Cell Biology, *140*:853–859, 1998.

Trueta, T. The growth and development of bone and joints: Orthopedic aspects. In Davis, JA, & Dobbing, J (Eds.). Scientific Foundations of Paediatrics. Philadelphia: WB Saunders, 1974.

Turk, MA, Geremski, CA, & Rosenbaum, PF. Secondary Conditions of Adults with Cerebral Palsy: A Final Report. Syracuse, NY: State University of New York, 1997.

van der Berg-Emons, RJG, van Baak, MA, de Barbanson, DC, Speth, L, & Saris, WHM. Reliability of tests to determine peak aerobic power, anaerobic power and isokinetic muscle strength in children with spastic cerebral palsy. Developmental Medicine and Child Neurology, *38*:1117–1125, 1996.

Vidal, J, Deguillaume, P, & Vidal, M. The anatomy of the dysplastic hip in cerebral palsy related to prognosis and treatment. International Orthopaedics, *9*:105–110, 1985.

Walker, JM. Musculoskeletal development: A review. Physical Therapy, *71*:878–889, 1991.

Wang, K, & Ramirez-Mitchell, R. A network of transverse and longitudinal intermediate filaments is associated with sarcomeres of adult vertebrate skeletal muscle. The Journal of Cell Biology, *96*:562–570, 1983.

Wang, K, McCarter, R, Wright, J, Beverly, J, & Ramirez-Mitchell, R. Viscoelasticity of the sarcomere matrix of skeletal muscles: The titin-myosin composite filament is a dual-stage molecular spring. Biophysical Journal, *64*:1161–1177, 1993.

Ward, SS, & Stickland, NC. Why are slow and fast muscles differentially affected during prenatal under-nutrition? Muscle and Nerve, *14*(3):259–267, 1991.

Waterman-Storer, CM. The cytoskeleton of skeletal muscle: Is it affected by exercise? A brief review. Medicine and Science in Sports and Exercise, *23*(11):1240–1249, 1991.

Waugh, KG, Minkel, JL, Parker, R, & Coon, VA. Measurement of selected hip, knee, and ankle joint motions in newborns. Physical Therapy, *63*:1616–1621, 1983.

Weinstein, SL. Natural history of congenital hip dislocation (CHD) and hip dysplasia. Clinical Orthopedics and Related Research, *225*:62–75, 1987.

Whiting, SJ. Obesity is not protective for bones in childhood and adolescence. Nutrition Reviews, *60*:27–36, 2002.

Williams, PE, & Goldspink, G. Longitudinal growth of striated muscle fibers. Journal of Cell Science, *9*:751–767, 1971.

Williams, PE, & Goldspink, G. The effect of immobilization on the longitudinal growth of striated muscle fibers. Journal of Anatomy (London), *116*:45–55, 1973.

Williams, PE, & Goldspink, G. Changes in sarcomere length and physiological properties in immobilized muscle. Journal of Anatomy (London), *127*:459–468, 1978.

Williams, PE, & Goldspink, G. Connective tissue changes in immobilized muscle. Journal of Anatomy (London), *138*:342–350, 1984.

Wilmshurst, S, Ward, K, Adams, JE, Langton, CM, & Mughal, MZ. Mobility status and bone density in cerebral palsy. Archives of Disease in Childhood, *75*:164–165, 1996.

Young, NL, Wright, JG, Lam, TP, Rajaratnam, K, Stephens, D, & Wedge, JH. Windswept hip deformity in spastic quadriplegic cerebral palsy. Pediatric Physical Therapy, *10*:94–100, 1998.

Ziv, I, Blackburn, N, Rang, M, & Koreska, J. Muscle growth in normal and spastic mice. Developmental Medicine and Child Neurology, *26*:94–99, 1984.

Chapter 7

❧

GENOMICS AND GENETIC SYNDROMES AFFECTING MOVEMENT

JOAN A. O'KEEFE
PT, PhD

Knowledge in the field of molecular genetics has exploded over the past 20 years, creating a revolution in the diagnosis and categorization of genetic disorders. The Human Genome Project (HGP), a national endeavor seeking to identify all human genes and their functions, has been instrumental in this process. These advances have led to the confirmation of new syndromes that were previously undefined and to the genetic reclassification of many congenital malformations. In many cases the precise molecular genetic defect has been characterized and the aberrant type or amount of gene products has been identified. Research is avidly investigating the role of these gene products in normal development. The future holds great promise for further identification of genetic disorders and development of therapeutic strategies. This chapter will discuss (1) suggested core competencies in genetics for physical therapists, (2) dysmorphology, (3) brief overviews of normal gene structure and function, DNA mutations, and developmental biology, (4) specific genetic disorders common in pediatric physical therapy practice, and (5) anticipated future advances in genomic medicine.

■ CORE COMPETENCIES IN GENETICS

Pediatric physical therapists frequently work with clients who have a genetic disorder. It is imperative for those working in this field to have the detailed genetics knowledge base necessary to function as an independent and skilled practitioner in this new era of genomics and developmental biology. This understanding is pertinent to diagnostic identification, disease etiology and pathogenesis, prognostic indicators, treatment ramifications, neurologic outcomes, and lifespan issues. The advances in genomics will also allow practitioners to share information about treatment effectiveness with children, having clear diagnostic classifications instead of global diagnoses such as dysmorphic features, developmental delay, and cognitive impairments, including mental retardation (MR). In addition, individuals with specific genetic disorders may have a predisposition to developing certain musculoskeletal impairments or conditions that may be preventable; clear diagnostic categories enable development of more precise clinical guidelines. Genetic disorder identification will enable researchers to perform studies of motor and other types of behavioral development in infants and children with a specific diagnosis or syndrome. Although there is some research examining motor development in well-known genetic disorders, such as Down syndrome, there is a paucity of such data for the majority of genetic disorders. In addition, publishing case studies on children with a constellation of clinical features constituting an unrecognized syndrome or condition might allow physical therapists to contribute to future advances in genetic diagnosis and classification. In summary, correct and more precise genetic diagnostics allow the therapist and family to establish realistic outcome goals, appropriate health care management, and prevention or management of certain secondary problems such as scoliosis or obesity.

Frequently the pediatric physical therapist is one of the first team members performing initial assessments in early intervention and as such should be capable of identifying signs or symptoms of a genetic syndrome (specific or not). After identification of suspicious phenotypic features, it is the therapist's responsibility to recommend a medical genetics evaluation and s/he should thus be aware of the avenues families might take in obtaining such services. Unfortunately, many physical therapists have had little or no genetics education in their professional training and few feel confident in referring individuals for genetic testing or counseling (Long et al., 2001). Core competencies in genetics for all health care professionals have been established by the National Coalition of Health Care Professionals in Genetics (NCHPEG). The minimum competencies include knowing when and how to make a referral to a genetics professional, understanding the psychosocial and ethical implications of genetic services, and appreciating one's limitations in genetic expertise. The entire list of competencies can be found at the NCHPEG website www.nchpeg.org/. This site also contains links to educational materials, programs, and other resources.

Physical therapy clinicians need established guidelines for eliciting genetic information from families; legal, privacy, and confidentiality considerations; and appropriate genetic professional referral procedures. Sanger and colleagues have delineated the role of the physical therapist in the referral and genetic disease identification process (Sanger et al., 2001). Family history taking might elucidate an inherited genetic disorder, although not those that arise from a de novo mutation. The pediatric physical therapist should be well versed in family history taking so that occurrence of disorders in multiple family members would alert one to a possible genetic diagnosis (Schaefer, 2001). Dysmorphic features (atypical physical anatomy/development) may be discovered or observed by the physical therapist during the physical examination. See Box 7-1 for an overview of dysmorphology and Box 7-2 for a list (some with definitions) of common anatomic anomalies. The physical therapist should also note any additional anatomic or physiologic abnormalities, such as brain malformations or epilepsy, that have been previously detected by medical testing (magnetic resonance imaging, computed tomographic scan, electroencephalogram). The neuromotor assessment will identify muscle weakness or tone abnormalities, motor control or dyscoordination problems, motor developmental delay, and sensory integration problems. Combining results from assessments by other members of the early intervention or interdisciplinary team may suggest global developmental delays, learning and behavioral difficulties, apraxias, language deficits, or behaviors suggesting an autistic spectrum disorder. These assessments may collectively be pertinent to the ultimate genetic diagnosis.

Clinical guidelines for referring a child for a genetics assessment are not universal. However, some common indications for a genetics referral include a cognitive or global developmental delay, a question of dysmorphic features, the presence of birth defects or congenital malformations (single or more), and cognitive impairment. The Texas Department of Health has developed clinical guidelines suggesting that a child might need genetic services or a referral to a geneticist. See Table 7-1 for a partial list of these guidelines.

It has been suggested that children with global developmental delay, even in the absence of dysmorphisms or other physical features suggesting a particular syndrome, should be referred to a geneticist for cytogenetic and molecular testing (Shevell et al., 2003). The rationale is that testing, especially with recent advances in technology, has a significantly high yield of accurate diagnostic identification. Early genetic testing is also extremely important to a family's reproductive planning. An accurate genetic diagnosis has been found to alter future childbearing decisions (Meryash & Abuelo, 1988) and may offer the possibility of preimplantation genetic testing to screen for known genetic defects.

Box 7-1   Dysmorphology and Common Clinical Malformations

Dysmorphology is the study of atypical anatomic development or morphogenesis resulting in abnormal physical features. Key clinical definitions in dysmorphology are based on the specific pathogenesis of physical defects (Jones, 1997, 2004), but terms are frequently used interchangeably in clinical practice, and this can be confusing. A malformation is a structural defect in an organ or body part because of an abnormal developmental process. Examples include cleft lip/palate and polydactyly. A dysplasia is an abnormal organization of cells into tissues and the structural consequences (e.g., hemangioma or a limb defect). A deformation is an alteration in the form, shape, or position of a normally formed body part by mechanical forces (e.g., plagiocephaly; internal tibial torsion); this typically occurs in the fetal period and not during embryogenesis. The cause can be intrinsic, such as weakness associated with a muscle disease, or extrinsic, such as intrauterine constraint or reduced amniotic fluid (oligohydramnios). A disruption is an abnormal breakdown of tissue in the normal fetus causing an anatomic defect of an organ or segment of the body; this may be infectious, vascular, or mechanical in origin. Examples include porencephaly due to cerebral infarction and limb defects caused by amniotic bands (see Chapter 16). A sequence is any of the above four primary defects which then causes a pattern of multiple secondary structural anomalies (e.g., torticollis with secondary positional plagiocephaly, facial asymmetry, and scoliosis). A syndrome is a pattern of multiple malformations due to a single cause (genetic or environmental) such as that caused by the teratogen, alcohol, or the absence of genetic material, as in the deletion syndromes. In clinical genetics it is important to distinguish between an isolated congenital anomaly and one that is part of a syndrome with a pattern of malformations. The physical therapist should perform a complete physical examination when assessing children for developmental delay or other neuromotor problems in order to determine whether any dysmorphisms exist. Positive findings would then assist in determining whether a child should be referred for a genetics evaluation

Presently, an identified genetic defect accounts for only about one third of all congenital malformations (Nelson & Holmes, 1989). Of stillbirths only 25% have been linked to specific chromosomal, mendelian, or biochemical causes (Wapner & Lewis, 2002). This number may be artificially low because many families are not given the option or choose not to perform testing. In addition, insurance companies do not usually pay for such tests on spontaneously aborted fetuses and routine cytogenetic testing (i.e., a karyotype) may be normal and will not detect subtle chromosomal rearrangements or deletions. Further technologic advances in genomic research with more efficient and cost-effective tests will undoubtedly identify the precise genetic defect in a greater percentage of birth defects.

INTERNET GENETIC RESOURCES

An abundance of genetic information is now available to professionals and families online. The Online Mendelian Inheritance in Man (OMIM) database is a comprehensive catalogue that provides health professionals and the scientific community with current information about most genetic disorders (McKusick, 1998, 2000). Each entry contains a detailed description of the disorder including clinical/phenotypic features, molecular and population genetics, inheritance patterns, cytogenetic tests, animal models when available, and an extensive literature review. Gene Tests is another useful online resource that contains a superb Gene Reviews section for health care professionals with clinical descriptions, differential diagnosis, molecular genetic testing, clinical management, references, and links to national foundations for specific genetic conditions. It also lists regional facilities that perform genetic testing and have multidisciplinary team clinics for certain disorders. All health care professionals should be knowledgeable about Medline/PubMed to search for and directly access research articles in biomedical science. In addition, most individual chromosomal or mendelian genetic conditions also have their own websites with varying information about diagnostic testing, clinical descriptions and normative data, therapeutic management, and research.

OVERVIEW OF NORMAL GENE STRUCTURE AND FUNCTION

Human somatic cells contain 23 pairs of different chromosomes in their nuclei; 22 of these pairs are autosomes, and 1 pair are the sex chromosomes (X,Y).

Box 7-2   List and Selected Definitions of Common Clinical Dysmorphisms

STRUCTURAL BRAIN ANOMALIES

Anencephaly
Myelomeningocele (see Chapter 25)
Encephalocele
Holoprosencephaly—failure of forebrain separation (variable severities)
Porencephalic cysts—cysts or cavities within brain from infarction or developmental migration defects
Lissencephaly—smooth brain lacking convolutions
Dandy-Walker malformation or cyst—expansion of fourth ventricle in the posterior fossa with variable cerebellar or callosal agenesis
Agenesis of corpus callosum
Hydrocephalus
Microcephaly (head circumference >3 SD below mean)
Macrencephaly (also called megalencephaly; may be seen unilaterally and is then called hemimegalencephaly)—an unusually large, heavy, and malfunctioning brain from defect in neuronal proliferation

CRANIAL ANOMALIES

Craniosynostosis or plagiocephaly—asymmetric head shape in coronal or sagittal plane (may be from asymmetric/premature suture closure, asymmetric brain growth, or fetal/infant positioning)
Delayed closure of fontanels
Flat or prominent occiput
Frontal bossing or prominent central forehead

ABNORMAL PATTERN OF SCALP AND FACIAL HAIR

Anterior upsweep
Posterior midline defects
Posterior parietal hair whorl—abnormal location or shape results from early defect in brain development
Widow's peak

ABNORMAL FACIAL FEATURES

Flat
Round
Broad
Triangular
Coarse

EYE/ORBIT ABNORMALITIES

Hypotelorism (eyes close together)
Hypertelorism (eyes wide apart)
Short palpebral fissure (decreased horizontal distance of the eye)
Slanted palpebral fissure (from asymmetric brain growth relative to facial growth)
Inner epicanthal folds (redundant skin of inner eyelid)
Shallow orbital ridge
Prominent supraorbital ridge
Synophrys (midline eyebrow)
Blepharophimosis (ptosis of eyelid)
Lacrimal gland defects
Strabismus
Nystagmus
Myopia
Blue sclera
Microphthalmos
Colobomata of iris
Unusual patterning or color of iris (e.g., Brushfield's spots are speckled white rings in periphery of iris)
Glaucoma
Large or small cornea, corneal opacity
Cataracts
Retinal pigmentation

NASAL ABNORMALITIES

Low nasal bridge
Prominent nasal bridge
Broad nasal bridge
Broad nasal root
Small or short nose, anteverted nostrils
Prominent nose

MAXILLARY/MANDIBULAR ABNORMALITIES

Maxillary or mandibular hypoplasia
High arched palate
Cleft palate/lip
Micrognathia (small mandible)
Prognathism

MOUTH AND ORAL REGION

Cleft lip/palate
Bifid uvula
Abnormal philtrum
Prominent /full lips
Macro- or microstomia (large or small mouth opening)
Cleft tongue
Micro or macroglossia (small or large tongue)
Laryngeal abnormalities
Dental anomalies: aplasia (missing teeth), hypodontia (small or conical teeth), irregular placement, late tooth eruption, neonatal teeth

EXTERNAL EARS

Low set (helix meets skull below plane extending through inner eye canthi)

Box 7-2 — List and Selected Definitions of Common Clinical Dysmorphisms—cont'd

Malformed auricles (lobes)
Preauricular tags or pits

NECK

Webbed
Redundant skin
Short

OTHER SKELETAL ANOMALIES

Pectus excavatum (funnel chest)
Pectus carinatum (pigeon breast)
Short sternum or thoracic cage
Ribs (rib fusions, hypo- or hyperplasia, abnormal
    number, cervical ribs)
Scoliosis (see Chapter 11)
Vertebral defects (may be associated with general
    bone disorder)—hemivertebrae, flat, wedged,
    gibbus, lack of segmentation, odontoid hypoplasia
    with cervical spine instability

LIMB AND JOINT ANOMALIES

Arachnodactyly
Brachymelia (short limbs)
Brachydactyly (short digits)
Small hands/ feet
Clinodactyly (medial or lateral curving of fingers/toes;
    typically fifth digit)

Camptodactyly (permanent flexion of one or more
    digits with missing inner phalangeal creases
    indicating lack of finger movement from before 8th
    week of gestation)
Limb reduction (Chapter 16)
Triphalangeal thumb
Aplasia/hypoplasia (thumb, radius, metacarpals,
    metatarsals)
Polydactyly (extra digits; medial side is termed
    preaxial, lateral side is postaxial)
Broad thumb, toe
Syndactyly (incomplete finger or toe separation; may
    be cutaneous)

HEMATOLOGY/ ONCOLOGY

Anemia
Thrombocytopenia
Leukocytosis
Various tumors/carcinomas
Immunoglobulin or cell-mediated (T-cell)
    immunodeficiencies

GROWTH ABNORMALITIES

Obesity
Craniofacial or segmental hypertrophies/ asymmetries

From Jones, KL (Ed.). Smith's Recognizable Patterns of Human Malformation, 5th ed. Philadelphia: W.B. Saunders Co., 1997, pp. 1–7 and 771–844 and Jones, KL. Dysmorphology. In Behrman, RE, Kliegman, RM, & Jenson HB (Eds.). Nelson Textbook of Pediatrics, 17th ed. Philadelphia: W.B. Saunders Co., 2004, pp. 616–623.

TABLE 7-1 — Indications for Genetic Services

BIRTH DEFECTS	CHRONIC DISEASES	DEVELOPMENTAL PROBLEMS	SENSORY DEFICITS
Cataracts	Bleeding disorder	Autism/ PDD	Extreme farsightedness
Cleft lip/palate	Childhood cancer	Attention deficits/hyperactivity	Extreme nearsightedness
Congenital heart disease	Kidney or urinary tract disease	Developmental delay	Hearing loss/ impairment
Contractures	Slow growth or short stature	Failure to thrive	Retinal problems
Diaphragmatic hernia	Cystic fibrosis	Learning disability	
Genital malformations	Sickle cell disease	Low muscle tone	
Glaucoma	Thalassemia	Mental illness	
Misshapen skull		Cognitive impairment	
Missing or extra fingers/toes		Regression in development	
		Speech problems	
Other congenital anomalies			

Modified from the Texas Department of Health (www.genetests.org/ and TEXGENE).

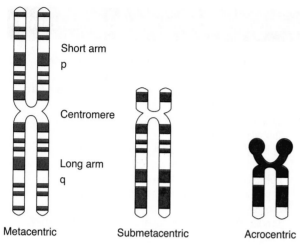

Short arm
p

Centromere

Long arm
q

Metacentric   Submetacentric   Acrocentric

◆ **Figure 7-1**   Centromere location classifies metacentric, submetacentric, and acrocentric chromosomes. Note the short arm is labeled p and the long arm is q.

The members of each pair of autosomes are homologs, one derived from the mother and the other from one's father. Chromosomes are also classified by the position of their centromeres; metacentric ones are centrally located, acrocentric ones are near the tip, and submetacentric chromosomes have centromeres between these two (Fig. 7-1). The chromosomes are composed of DNA coiled around a histone protein core. The DNA contains the genetic code for manufacturing all the proteins necessary for cellular structure and enzymatic reactions. The specific triplet sequence of the nucleotides cytosine, thymine, adenine, or guanine (CTAG) is known as a codon; each codon dictates which specific amino acid is inserted into a protein. A gene is a length of DNA that codes for a specific protein. Protein synthesis occurs via a two-step process, transcription and translation. Nuclear transcription of mRNA occurs on a DNA template via RNA polymerase enzymes and various transcription factors including activators, enhancers, and silencers (Fig. 7-2). Transcription factors serve both general functions common to all cells and specific ones that only initiate gene transcription in certain cell types. Transcription factors also depend on specific DNA-binding motifs, which are proteins configured in unique ways to allow gene specificity in transcription factor binding. All genes also contain a 5′ untranslated region to which certain promoters may attach to regulate gene activity. The same genes are contained in every cell type in one's body but only certain ones are transcriptionally active or turned on; this allows specificity for differentiated cellular functions and cell-specific protein manufacture. Following transcription of the primary mRNA, genetic splicing

normally occurs to splice out introns (noncoding regions), leaving the exons (or protein coding sequences). Splicing is controlled by DNA sequences on either side of the exon. The mature mRNA then moves into the cytoplasm where protein translation occurs on ribosomes. Further post-translational modifications of proteins may occur such as addition of carbohydrate side chains that might be important for mature protein folding or configuration.

A gene's specific location on a chromosome is called a *locus. Alleles* are different DNA sequences for a particular gene. If a person has the same allele on both chromosome pairs, that person is homozygous for that gene. Heterozygotes have different alleles. A genotype refers to an individual's alleles and precise genetic make-up at a specific locus. One's phenotype is the physical or physiologic manifestation of the genotype, and the two do not always coincide, for a variety of reasons.

TYPES OF DNA

Only about 1% to 2% of our DNA actually encodes proteins and the function of the remaining noncoding sequences remains poorly understood (Collins et al., 2003; Jorde et al., 2003). There are approximately 30,000 human genes, a number found to be surprisingly lower than earlier estimates of 50,000 to 140,000. Single copy DNA is seen only once or a few times in the genome, and it makes up roughly 45% of our DNA. This is the DNA that makes up introns, exons, and the sequences interspersed between genes whose function is largely unknown. Approximately 55% of genomic DNA is repetitive in that sequences are repeated hundreds to thousands of times over again. In this category are both dispersed and satellite DNA sequences. Dispersed DNA includes the common so-called *Alu* repeats; these are important from a clinical genetics standpoint because they can generate copies of themselves, insert into other copies of the genome, and thus cause a genetic disorder if a protein-coding gene sequence is disrupted. Repeat elements may also promote unequal crossover during meiosis, resulting in deletions or duplications of gene sequences between these repeats. Some of the microdeletion syndromes, such as Williams and Prader-Willi/Angelman syndromes, may be secondary to this phenomenon (see section on chromosomal microdeletions). Satellite DNA is clustered in specific chromosomal locations, and some types vary in length among individuals; this type of DNA is thus extremely important for human genetic mapping studies (Jorde et al., 2003).

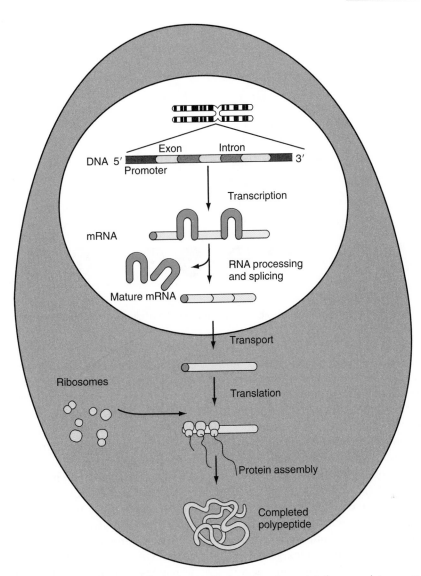

◆ **Figure 7-2**   Process of DNA transcription and protein translation. Gene inset details exons, introns, and the 5′ promoter region to which transcription factors may bind.

▌ MUTATION

Mutations or alterations in DNA sequences bring about our incredible genetic variation and may also cause genetic disorders. Mutations in one's germline cells are able to be transmitted from one generation to the next and are thus inherited. There are many types of mutations that have potential health consequences. In *single-point mutation*, a base pair is substituted or replaced by another. This might result in an amino acid change within the protein, a premature termination of transcription (and thus translation), or an abnormal long polypeptide. Any of these scenarios can have significant consequences for genetic disorders and development. A

mutation causing a deletion or insertion of a base pair(s) can result in extra or missing amino acids, changes in all downstream amino acids, or a truncated protein. Most cases of cystic fibrosis (see Chapter 27) are caused by a three base pair deletion in the gene for an epithelial chloride ion channel.

A dosage-sensitive gene is one that is adversely affected by reductions or increases in its protein product. "Gain of function" mutations are typically characterized by gene overexpression producing a dominant disease (see later discussion). For example, duplication of entire genes can occur, resulting in increased copies of the gene products. This occurs in Charcot-Marie-Tooth disease, a peripheral neuron disease with progressive distal muscular

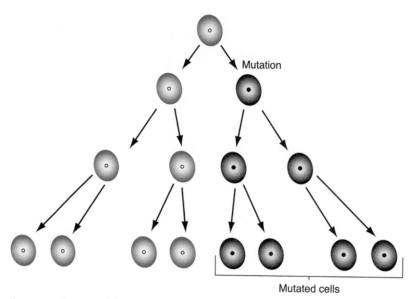

Mutation

Mutated cells

♦ **Figure 7-3** Somatic or germline mosaicism results when mutations occur during cell proliferation in either somatic cells or gametes, respectively.

atrophy, in which an extra copy of contiguous genes on chromosome 17 including one encoding a peripheral myelin protein causes the movement disorder (Jorde et al., 2003). "Loss of function" mutations are a consequence of reduced gene expression and hence protein quantities. A mutation in a gene's promoter region frequently causes a reduction in the encoded protein. A dominant disease results from a single copy of a mutation so that heterozygotes will be affected. *Haploinsufficiency* occurs in dominant disorders when there is a 50% reduction in a protein that then causes a loss of function disease. Recessive genetic disorders require both copies of the allele to be mutated so that only homozygotes are affected. Frequently there is a 50% reduction in a gene's product in the heterozygote or carrier condition that fortunately is sufficient for normal function. An example of this would be the thalassemias, blood disorders resulting from mutations and subsequent reductions in the hemoglobin chains (Jorde et al., 2003).

Certain DNA sequences are called transposons or mobile elements because they are able to duplicate themselves and then insert into abnormal sites on chromosomes. Transposons have been found to cause some cases of neurofibromatosis (see section on single gene disorders) and hemophilia (see Chapter 10). A type of mutation recently discovered is the expansion of copies of tandem repeated DNA sequences during meiosis, causing altered gene transcription and thereby genetic disease. This occurs in fragile X syndrome (see section on sex-linked diseases).

When a mutation occurs during embryonic development only certain body cells are affected; this is termed *somatic mosaicism* (Fig. 7-3). Because the genetic defect exists in a limited population of somatic cells the phenotypic expression is milder. In tissue-specific mosaicism only certain tissues display the genetic abnormality complicating the diagnosis because not all tissues can be sampled for karyotyping. *Germline mosaicism* occurs when an individual's germline either partially or entirely contains a genetic mutation but the somatic cells do not. The individual does not express the disease but can transmit the mutation to offspring. This phenomenon has been described for osteogenesis imperfecta type II, achondroplasia, neurofibromatosis type I, Duchenne muscular dystrophy (MD), and hemophilia A (Jorde et al., 2003).

Mutations may be naturally occurring, spontaneous events or secondary to mutagens such as radiation or chemicals. Mutation rates do not occur equally throughout the genome. Larger genes are in general more likely to undergo mutations simply based on their size. Examples of large genes frequently affected by mutations include the dystrophin gene in muscular dystrophy (see Chapter 15) and the neurofibromin gene in neurofibromatosis 1 (see single gene disorder section). In addition, mutation "hot spots" exist in which nucleotide sequences are more prone to mutagenesis. Mutation rates may also be increased with either advanced maternal or paternal age. Some single gene disorders such as Marfan syndrome and achondroplasia increase with advanced paternal age (Rolf & Nieschlag, 2001).

Notwithstanding the myriad of potential mechanisms for mutations to occur, DNA replication is usually surprisingly accurate. This is because DNA repair mechanisms exist to identify an error and excise and replace the altered bases with correct ones. Certain genetic diseases result when DNA repair is deficient, especially mutations occurring in the genes encoding repair enzymes. The autosomal recessive disorder ataxia telangiectasia, for example, is characterized by progressive cerebellar ataxia beginning in early childhood, oculomotor apraxia, vascular skin lesions or telangiectases, increased malignancy rates, immunodeficiency, and chromosome instability and breakage (especially due to ionizing radiation). It is due to a deficit in cell surveillance and halting of the cell cycle following DNA damage (Berneburg & Lehmannn, 2001); this normally occurs to allow repair before cell replication when the damage would be perpetuated and when breaks would result in loss of genomic DNA.

GENETICS AND DEVELOPMENT

Many of the instructions for normal development are encoded by genes. Embryogenesis involves the complex processes of axis specification (i.e., dorsal/ventral, anterior/posterior, medial/lateral, left/right), pattern formation (the spatial arrangement of cells to form tissues and organs), and organ/limb development. Numerous birth defects are caused by mutations in genes encoding proteins that provide signals or form structures necessary for normal embryo development (Epstein, 1995).

Nonhuman models are frequently used to study the genetics of developmental biology (Veraska et al., 2000). This is possible because most genes are conserved across a wide range of species. In addition, many of the regulatory signaling pathways are used repeatedly in development to control various patterning and developmental events. Most of the genetic mediators involved in development are growth factors or paracrine signaling molecules and their receptors, DNA transcription factors, or extracellular matrix proteins such as the collagens, fibrillins, or elastin. These are all expressed in a unique spatial and temporal pattern that drives the correct development of body structures.

Paracrine molecules are secreted by cells and diffuse over short distances to act locally at specific targets. Presently, four major families of paracrine signaling molecules have been identified: (1) the fibroblast growth factor (FGF) family (McIntosh et al., 2000), (2) the hedgehog family, (3) the wingless (Wnt) family (Miller, 2001), and (4) the transforming growth factor-beta (TGF-β) family (Ducy & Karsenty, 2000). The sonic hedgehog (Shh) protein is one such molecule and is important in axis specification and in patterning the neural tube, somites, and limbs (McMahon, 2000). Mutations in the *Shh* gene encoding this protein can cause holoprosencephaly, an abnormality in the formation of the dorsal/ventral axis so that the forebrain fails to completely separate. Interestingly, attachment of the Shh protein to cholesterol is necessary for correct patterning of hedgehog signaling. Thus, environmental factors that influence cholesterol metabolism could easily interact with the *Shh* gene in a multifactorial fashion (see section on multifactorial disorders). Mutations in the FGF receptor family genes have been implicated in craniosynostosis and achondroplasia (see Chapter 17).

DNA transcription factors activate, enhance, repress, silence, or modify transcription of other genes. They do so by containing DNA-binding domains that allow them to interact with specific DNA sequences. In certain cases they bend DNA so that other factors are then able to make contact with promoter regions of genes. Frequently they regulate transcription of many genes so that mutations in these have numerous developmental consequences, possibly resulting in multiple congenital malformations. Examples of DNA transcription factors include the 39 *HOX* genes, all of which contain a highly conserved DNA binding region termed the homeodomain. Mutation or disruption of the *HOX* genes typically result in organ, body, or limb patterning defects (Mark et al., 1997).

CRANIOSYNOSTOSIS

Craniosynostosis is an example of a genetic developmental disorder that has been found to occur because of mutations in either paracrine molecule receptors or DNA transcription factors. Craniofacial development is directly related to morphogenesis of the underlying central nervous system (CNS) structures so that craniofacial anomalies are frequently associated with structural brain defects (Francis-West et al., 2003; Jorde et al, 2003; Wilkie & Morriss-Kay, 2001). Molecular diagnostic tests are now beginning to identify the specific gene(s) involved in these cranial and neural defects. Although it is beyond the scope of this chapter to discuss the genetic developmental biology in detail, some general pertinent information will be provided. Many craniofacial structures are derived from neural crest cells. These cells migrate from their specific forebrain, midbrain, hindbrain, or cervical areas and differentiate into mesenchymal (connective) tissue of their respective pharyngeal arch. The ultimate fate of each group of neural crest cells is determined by the so-called homeobox (*HOX*) containing genes that play a crucial role in embryonic development. A homeobox is a highly conserved DNA segment within an array of developmental genes first discovered in *Drosophila*.

Craniosynostosis is a congenital anomaly involving premature fusion or synostosis of the cranial sutures and is frequently associated with multiple CNS manifestations (Flores-Sarnat, 2002). The head is typically misshapen (called synostotic or nonpositional plagiocephaly) and underlying brain structures can be inhibited from growing properly. It is important for the pediatric physical therapist to recognize positional versus synostotic plagiocephaly; determination of this will involve obtaining an accurate birth and postnatal history. In synostotic plagiocephaly the child should be referred to a craniofacial clinic or geneticist, and in this case cranial banding or other techniques should not be prescribed until an accurate diagnosis is established.

The new era of molecular genetics has dramatically altered our understanding of the underlying mechanism causing craniosynostosis. Now almost 100 syndromes associated with craniosynostosis have been described, 10% of which have a defined molecular defect (Flores-Sarnat, 2002). The majority of these syndromes such as Apert, Crouzon, Pfeiffer, and Saethre-Chotzen syndromes, have autosomal dominance inheritance patterns and are frequently associated with additional congenital anomalies, especially limb defects. In certain cases causative genes such as the FGF family of receptors and homeobox genes including *MSX2* (Jabs et al., 1993) have been demonstrated. FGF receptors bind one of at least 12 FGFs and are involved in cell migration, growth, and differentiation during embryonic and postnatal development. They are abundantly expressed in developing bone and many skeletal dysplasias are caused by mutations in *FGFR* genes. For example, achondroplasia, an autosomal dominant disorder, is caused by a single amino acid substitution in the FGF receptor 3 molecule, thereby altering its activation (see Chapter 17). Mutations in at least four of the FGF receptors can cause a craniosynostosis syndrome. Both Crouzon and Pfeiffer syndromes are caused by a single amino acid substitution in the FGFR2 molecule. *MSX2* is a transcription factor encoded on chromosome 5q that is thought to play a role in programmed neural crest cell death in the skull.

CHROMOSOMAL DISORDERS

Chromosomal abnormalities occur when chromosome number or structure is altered. They cause a significant number of genetic disorders and are quite common (10%–15%) occurrences in human conceptions

(Carpenter, 2001; Hsu, 1998). Chromosomal disorders occur in 1 per 160 live births, and they are the leading cause of pregnancy loss, accounting for at least 50% of first trimester miscarriages and 20% of second trimester miscarriages. Numeric disorders result when an extra chromosome is present or when an entire chromosome is missing. These defects are typically due to a nondisjunction error during gametogenesis (Fig. 7-4); in general, these are not hereditary conditions, so the risk of recurrence may be low. Exceptions do occur, and accurate genetic counseling is indicated. Structural defects occur when there are deletions, inversions, duplications, translocations, or other types of rearrangements of chromosomes.

CHROMOSOME NUMBER ABNORMALITIES

Polyploidy is the presence of a complete extra set of chromosomes in a cell. In humans, the types of polyploidy that have been observed are triploidy with 69 chromosomes inside the cell nucleus and tetraploidy with 92 (Hsu, 1998). Most fetuses with polyploid conditions are spontaneously aborted and all are lethal. Triploidy is estimated to cause 15% of all chromosomal abnormalities occurring at conception and it is commonly caused by the fertilization of an egg with two sperm cells (Jorde et al., 2003).

Aneuploidy is the absence or duplication of a chromosome in a cell; usually only one chromosome is affected. The cells thus do not contain a multiple of 23 chromosomes in their nucleus. The most common cause of aneuploidy is the failure of chromosomes to disjoin during meiosis (see Fig. 7-4). These abnormalities are therefore genetic in origin but generally are not hereditary. Monosomy is the presence of only one copy of a chromosome in a diploid cell and trisomy is the presence of three copies. Fetuses with autosomal monosomies rarely survive to term but some trisomies are seen in appreciable numbers among live births. Mosaicism for a trisomy can also occur and is most typically due to a full trisomy conception followed by loss of the extra chromosome in some cells during mitosis in the embryo. The clinical manifestations in children with a mosaic disorder will then be milder.

STRUCTURAL CHROMOSOMAL DISORDERS

A *deletion* is caused by a chromosomal break and may occur interstitially or terminally on the chromosome (Fig. 7-5, *A*). Autosomal deletions are the next most common type of clinically significant chromosomal disorders after the autosomal aneuplodies (i.e., trisomy

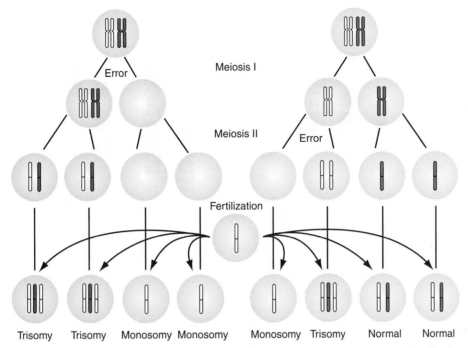

• **Figure 7-4**   Nondisjunction errors during meiosis cause monosomy or trisomy in offspring.

13, 18, and 21). A *translocation* is the interchange of genetic material between nonhomologous chromosomes; this is fairly common and occurs in at least 1 in 200 persons (Jacobs et al., 1992). *Reciprocal translocations* occur when there are two breaks on different chromosomes with equal exchange of genetic material between them (Fig. 7-5, *B*). Carriers usually have a normal phenotype because there is no loss or gain of genetic material. A carrier's offspring, however, might have a partial trisomy or monosomy and an abnormal phenotype. In a *Robertsonian translocation* the short arms of two acrocentric homologous chromosomes are lost and the long arms fuse at the centromere (Fig. 7-5, *C*). This only occurs with chromosomes 13, 14, 15, 21, and 22 because their short arms are very short and do not contain essential genetic material. The carriers have only 45 chromosomes in each cell but are normal because no genetic material is lost. Their children, however, may have a monosomy or trisomy (Fig. 7-5, *D*). A common Robertsonian translocation is between the long arms of 21 and 14; carriers are at risk of having children with monosomy or trisomy 14 or 21 (see Fig. 7-5, *D*, and later discussion). Unbalanced translocations are frequently associated with an atypical phenotype and recently have been identified in the gene-rich telomeric regions of chromosomes in clients with otherwise unexplained global developmental delay or cognitive impairment (Knight et al., 1999; Knight & Flint, 2000) (Fig. 7-6).

GENERAL CLINICAL PHENOTYPES SEEN IN CHROMOSOMAL ABNORMALITIES

Most chromosomal abnormalities are associated with developmental delay and cognitive impairment. This is due to the fact that a large percentage of our genes are involved with CNS development (Jorde et al., 2003). In addition, characteristic craniofacial features are typically seen because of altered facial, cranial, and possibly brain morphogenesis. Syndromes involving the autosomes are commonly associated with growth delay including poor prenatal and postnatal weight gain and short stature. Most autosomal genetic defects are also associated with congenital malformations, especially cardiac ones. The individual congenital malformations or anomalies may be nonspecific and therefore seen in numerous syndromes as well as in isolation (such as agenesis of the corpus callosum, microcephaly, etc.) or may be more precisely linked to a specific chromosomal problem (e.g., supravalvular or pulmonary artery stenosis in Williams syndrome).

MOLECULAR CHROMOSOME STUDIES

Cytogenetics is the study of chromosomes and their abnormalities. A karyotype is a chromosomal display ordered according to length; it is usually obtained from lymphocytes in blood samples. A normal karyotype

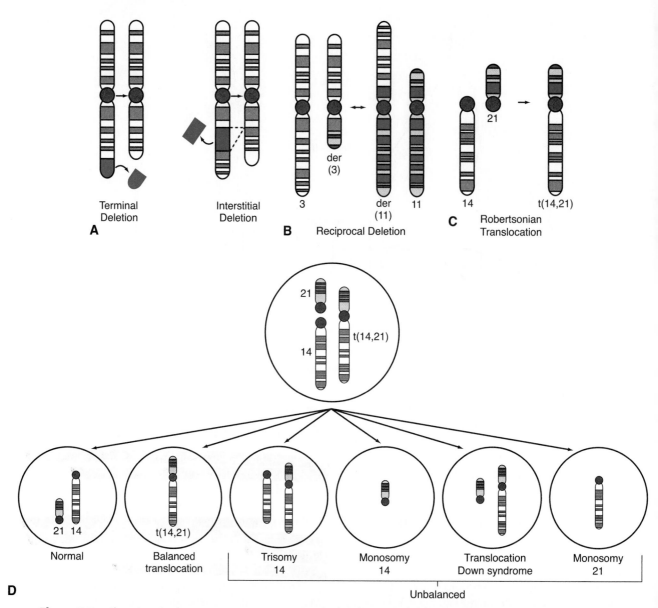

◆ **Figure 7-5** Alterations in chromosome structure. **A**, Terminal and interstitial deletions. **B**, Reciprocal translocations. **C**, Possible chromosome patterns of gametes and conception results from carriers of a Robertsonian translocation between chromosomes 14 and 21. **D**, Unequal crossing-over during meiosis causing insertions or deletions.

contains 22 pairs of autosomes and 2 sex chromosomes (X,Y). The normal female karyotype is 46,XX and the normal male is 46,XY. The short arm of a chromosome is labeled *p* for petite and the long arm is labeled *q* (Fig. 7-1). Chromosomes are most highly condensed during metaphase of mitosis when the chromosomes are lined up at the equatorial plane; hence, standard karyotyping is done during this phase when microscopic

examination is easiest. Several chromosomal banding techniques exist that allow greater resolution and detection of deletions, duplications, and other structural abnormalities. The major bands on each chromosome are numbered; thus, 5p21 refers to the second band in the first region of the short arm of chromosome 5. High-resolution banding involves using prophase or early metaphase chromosomes which are more distended

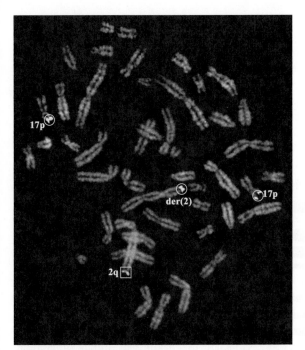

• **Figure 7-6**   FISH (fluorescence in situ hybridization) analysis showing an unbalanced telomere rearrangement between the short arm of chromosome 17 and the long arm of chromosome 2. The DNA probe for the 17p telomere region is shown within the circled areas, and the DNA probe for the 2q telomere region is shown within the boxed area. There are two normal chromosomes 17 (indicated by 17p) and one normal chromosome 2 (indicated by 2q). A derivative chromosome 2 is deleted for the 2q telomere probe and contains the 17p telomere probe (indicated by der(2)). Therefore, this individual has trisomy for the 17p telomere region and monosomy for the 2q telomere region. *(Courtesy of Dr. Christa Lese Martin, University of Chicago.)*

and therefore reveal more banding and even greater resolution than metaphase ones (Fig. 7-7).

FISH (fluorescence in situ hybridization) is the use of a chemically tagged chromosome-specific DNA probe to label a chromosomal sequence and then visualize it under a fluorescence microscope. FISH can thus be used to demonstrate chromosomal deletions, additions, and translocations. This technique can be extended with multiple color probes to detect several possible chromosomal alterations simultaneously (multicolor or M-FISH) (see Fig. 7-6). Additional sophisticated cytogenetic techniques exist such as spectral karyotyping (SKY) in which each chromosome is colored differently and can thus easily demonstrate rearrangements. A subtelomeric FISH screen may be useful diagnostically because subtle rearrangements of telomeric regions have been shown to account for 5% to 10% of idiopathic mental retardation (MR) (Flint & Knight, 2003). The telomere is a gene-rich area at the end of chromosomes. Molecular probes have been developed for every human telomere and the use of multicolor FISH to screen many chromosomes simultaneously has been shown to be a useful diagnostic measure in clients with global developmental delay or unexplained MR (see Fig. 7-6) (Knight et al., 1999, 2000). It is thought that shared telomere sequence homologies between non-homologous chromosomes mediate unbalanced chromosomal rearrangements.

COMMON AUTOSOMAL TRISOMIES

Nearly all autosomal trisomies are associated with advanced maternal age and occur because of a non-disjunction error in meiosis (Antonarakis et al., 1992;

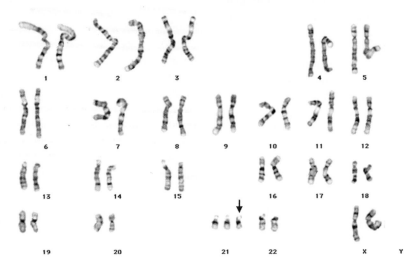

• **Figure 7-7**   Down syndrome karyotype. G-banding analysis showing trisomy for chromosome 21 is consistent with a clinical diagnosis of Down syndrome. *(Courtesy of Dr. Christa Lese Martin, University of Chicago.)*

Jorde et al., 2003) (see Fig. 7-4). The thought is that the long period of time oocytes are held in "suspension" in the first meiotic division (from a mother's embryonic development until her age at conception) is responsible for nondisjunction errors. Paternal age is not thought to be a factor because spermatocytes are continuously generated throughout life.

Down Syndrome (Trisomy 21)

Down syndrome, or trisomy 21, is the most common aneuploid condition compatible with survival. The karyotype of a female with trisomy 21 is 47,XX + 21 (Fig. 7-7). The typical phenotypic features seen in individuals with Down syndrome are included in Table 7-2. In 90% to 95% of children with Down syndrome the extra chromosome 21 is contributed by the mother, and advanced maternal age is a strong risk factor (Antonarakis, 1993; Antonarakis et al., 1992). Mean maternal age is 32 years. About 5% of individuals with Down syndrome have an inherited Robertsonian translocation (Thuline & Peuschel, 1982) with one copy of 21 translocated to another acrocentric chromosome (typically 14 or 21); the risk for recurrence is higher than in the typical nondisjunction type trisomy 21. From 2% to 4% of individuals with Down syndrome have mosaicism with some normal somatic cells and some with trisomy 21, resulting in a milder clinical expression (Mikkelsen, 1977). The karyotype of a female mosaic for Down syndrome is 47,XX, +21/46XX.

Studies have suggested that a critical region on the distal tip of the long arm of chromosome 21 is responsible for the phenotypic expression of Down syndrome (Delabar et al., 1993), but a single region theory has been debated (Korenberg et al., 1994). Current molecular studies are attempting to target the specific genes on chromosome 21 responsible for the Down syndrome phenotype, especially those causing the cognitive impairments. One popular theory suggests that gene overdosage causes the syndrome. The gene *DYRK* is a possible candidate for the CNS deficits given that overexpression in mouse models causes learning, memory, and neuromotor deficits (Altafaj et al., 2001). Superoxide dismutase, a free radical scavenger (Gulesserian et al., 2001; Netto et al., 2004), and amyloid precursor protein (*APP*) (Turrens, 2001) are additional chromosome 21 gene products hypothesized to be related to the neurologic symptoms of Down syndrome including premature aging and early onset Alzheimer's dementia. The gene overdosage theory has recently been challenged by studies failing to find overexpression of several proteins that are encoded by genes on chromosome 21 in the prenatal CNS of embryos with Down syndrome (Cheon et al., 2003a, 2003b).

Parents are often left with uncertainties regarding popular but not yet scientifically proved interventions for genetic disorders such as Down syndrome. For example, a nutrient-based therapy (*Nutrivene*) contains free radical scavengers; its use is based on the theory that overexpression of the enzyme, superoxide dismutase, causes excessive oxidative stress in brains (and other tissues) of individuals with Down syndrome which can be prevented by the supplement (Ani et al., 2000; Pastore et al., 2003).

Trisomy 18 (Edwards Syndrome)

Trisomy 18, or Edwards syndrome, is the second most common trisomy observed in term babies (1 in 6000 births). The majority (>90%) of trisomy 18 conceptions result in spontaneous abortion. There are over 100 associated typical malformations, and they include those of the cardiovascular, gastrointestinal, urogenital, and skeletal systems (Baty et al., 1994a). A distinctive hand deformity with flexion contractures of fingers which are overlapping (typically index finger overlying third) often helps the clinician in making an initial differential diagnosis. Ninety percent of infants die within 1 year, and the median age of survival is 2 weeks (Rasmusson et al., 2003). Girls and nonwhites appear to have longer survival times, but the reason for this is unknown. Typically, death is due to aspiration pneumonia, congenital heart defects, increased susceptibility to infections, and apnea. Children surviving past 1 year have significant developmental problems, and few are able to walk (Baty et al., 1994b; Carey, 1992). Neuromotor impairments include hypertonia following the initial hypotonia seen at birth.

Trisomy 13 (Patau Syndrome)

Trisomy 13, or Patau syndrome, is found in approximately 1 in 5000 births, but the median survival time is 1 week and only 5% of infants survive past 6 months (Rasmusson et al., 2003). It is estimated that 95% of trisomy 13 conceptions are lost. Clinical features of babies with this genotype include holoprosencephaly (incomplete development of forebrain), microcephaly, deafness, microphthalmia (small, abnormally shaped eyes), cleft lip/palate, congenital heart defects (80%), postaxial polydactyly, and severe to profound cognitive impairment (Baty et al., 1994a).

SEX CHROMOSOME ANEUPLOIDY

Disorders with abnormal numbers of sex chromosomes are less severe than those involving the autosomes because of X inactivation, a process whereby genes from one X chromosome are typically rendered transcriptionally in-

TABLE 7-2 Phenotypic Features In Down Syndrome

CRANIOFACIAL	MUSCULOSKELETAL/ CONNECTIVE TISSUE	EYES/VISION, EARS/HEARING	CARDIOVASCULAR	GASTROINTESTINAL	NEUROLOGIC	IMMUNOLOGIC
Inner epicanthal folds	Diastasis recti	Iris speckling (Brushfield's spots)	Ventricular septal defect	Duodenal stenosis/atresia	Mild microcephaly	Leukemia
Upward slanting palpebral fissures	Hypoplasia of middle phalanx, of fifth with clinodactyly (50–60%)	Myopia (70%)	Patent ductus arteriosus	Imperforate anus	Hypotonia	Chronic rhinitis and conjunctivitis
Flat facial profile	Joint hypermobility	Nystagmus (35%)	Tetralogy of Fallot	Hirschprung's disease	Mental retardation	Fluid in middle ear (60–80%)
Late fontanel closure	Hypoplastic pelvis with shallow acetabular angle	Strabismus (45%)			Developmental delay	
Aplasia/hypoplasia of frontal sinuses	Atlantoaxial instability (12%) with risk of spinal cord compression (rare)	Tear duct blockage (20%)			Early onset Alzheimer's disease	
Anomalous ears	Wide gap between toes 1 and 2	Conductive hearing loss (80%)			Small cerebellum and brainstem	
Low nasal bridge	Simian creases	Sensorineural or mixed hearing loss (10-20%)				
Shortened palate; maxillary and dental hypoplasia; irregular tooth placement						

From Epstein, CJ. Down syndrome, trisomy 21. In Scriver, CR, Beaudet, AL, Sly, WS, Valle, D (Eds.). Metabolic Basis of Inherited Disease. New York: McGraw-Hill, 1989, pp. 291-326; Jones, KL (Ed.). Smith's Recognizable Patterns of Human Malformation, 5th ed. Philadelphia: W.B. Saunders Co., 1997, pp. 8–14; Fong, CT, & Brodeur, GM. Down's syndrome and leukemia: Epidemiology, genetics, cytogenetics and mechanisms of leukemogenesis. Cancer Genetics and Cytogenetics, 28:55–76, 1987; Mazzoni, DS, Ackley, RS, & Nash, DJ. Abnormal pinna type and hearing loss correlations in Down's syndrome. Journal of Intellectual Disabilities Research, 38:549–560, 1994; Wisniewski, KE, Wisniewski, HM, & Wen, GY. Occurrence of neuropathological changes and dementia of Alzheimer's disease in Down's syndrome. Annals of Neurology, 17:278–282, 1985.

active in females (Jorde et al., 2003; Willard, 2000). The X chromosome is large and encodes more than 500 gene products. The Y chromosome in contrast is small and only encodes a few genes, most of which are involved with male differentiation and spermatogenesis. In order to ensure that females (with two copies of the X chromosome) and males produce equivalent quantities of X chromosome-derived gene products (a term called dosage compensation), one X chromosome in each female cell is inactivated early in embryonic development. This X inactivation is random so that it can be a paternally or maternally derived X chromosome, but it is fixed so that once inactive, always inactive (Fig. 7-8). X inactivation, however, is incomplete in that it does not cover the entire X chromosome. Genes located on the tips of X (which are highly homologous to those on the tips of the short arm of Y) are not inactivated and the numbers of these may be as high as 20% of the entire X genome. This is why females with Turner syndrome (XO) or other individuals with abnormal numbers of sex chromosomes have an atypical phenotype.

Turner Syndrome

Turner syndrome (45,XO; Fig. 7-9) is less severe than some of the autosomes because of typical X inactivation. The incidence of this disorder is 1 in 2500 live births. Individuals are female and characteristically have short stature, a wide neck or neck webbing, a broad trunk, heart defects, lack of breast development, dysplastic ovaries, osteoporosis later in life due to estrogen deficiency, and deficits in spatial tasks or visual memory (Ranke

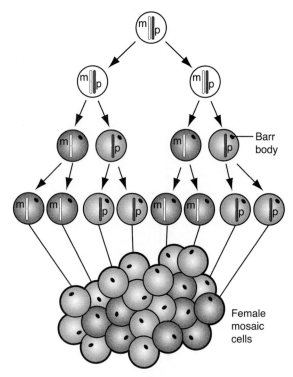

• Figure 7-8   Random X chromosome inactivation in female somatic cells.

& Saenger, 2001; Ross, 2001). Intelligence, however, is normal. There is much phenotypic variation because of mosaicism or partial deletion of the short arm of the X chromosome; 80% of cases are caused by a meiotic error

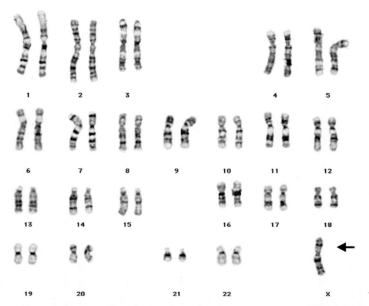

• Figure 7-9   Turner syndrome karyotype G-banding analysis showing monosomy for the X chromosome is consistent with a clinical diagnosis of Turner syndrome. *(Courtesy of Dr. Christa Lese Martin, University of Chicago.)*

in the father and thus Turner syndrome is not typically associated with advanced maternal age. The karyote is fairly common, accounting for 15% to 20% of spontaneous abortions, but the majority (99% or greater) are lost prenatally (Hsu, 1998).

Molecular studies have identified several genes involved in the Turner phenotype. The *SHOX* gene is located on the distal tip of X and Y; it encodes a transcription factor which when mutated causes reductions in long bone growth. In Turner syndrome, only one active copy of the gene is present; the haploinsufficiency or reduced gene dosage then causes short stature (Ogata, 2002; Zinn & Ross, 1998). It also probably explains some of the other skeletal features found in Turner syndrome, such as short metacarpals, cubitus valgus, short neck, and a high arched palate. Long bone growth is attenuated in utero, and statural growth lags during childhood and adolescence, resulting in adult heights averaging 4 feet 8 inches. Growth hormone treatment early in childhood has been used to increase ultimate adult height but not all individuals have a good growth response (Batch, 2002). Other phenotypic features may include a low hairline at the back of the neck and low-set ears. The hands and feet of affected individuals may be swollen at birth with soft nails because of lymphatic obstruction. Another cosmetic feature is the presence of multiple pigmented nevi or colored spots on the skin.

It is possible that factors other than estrogen deficiency might contribute to the severity of osteoporosis in Turner syndrome (Ross, 2001). For example, there may be defects in bone structure or strength related to the loss of unknown X chromosome genes. This is an area of major medical significance, which demands further study to help prevent osteoporosis and fractures in women with Turner syndrome. Girls and women with Turner syndrome often have difficulty with specific visual-spatial tasks, memory, motor coordination, and mathematical abilities. These deficits may also be due to loss of estrogen or as yet unidentified X chromosome genes important for the neural substrates mediating these behaviors. Many of these skills have been found to improve with estrogen administration.

Kleinfelter Syndrome

The most common karyotype of individuals with this syndrome is XXY; it occurs in 1 in 1000 male births and, surprisingly, even though the phenotypic features are mild, at least 50% of these conceptions are spontaneously aborted (Hsu, 1998). Usually there is no apparent abnormality until puberty when the testes fail to enlarge and gynecomastia may occur (Smyth, 1999). These males may have increased stature, sterility, slight IQ reduction (10–15 points below siblings), and learning disabilities but not MR. This syndrome is associated with advanced maternal age (Jorde et al., 2003).

CHROMOSOMAL DELETIONS

Typically, chromosome deletions observable under the microscope with a standard karyotype involve a large number of different genes and have a recognizable phenotype (for example, see cri-du-chat syndrome). The advent of high resolution banding and in particular FISH technologies has allowed the detection of smaller deletions and subtle chromosomal rearrangements. These techniques have also allowed more precision in defining a "critical region" of the chromosome that must be deleted in order to produce a given syndrome and the contiguous adjacent genes involved. Further subclassification has allowed identification of subsets of individuals with only certain phenotypic characteristics of a syndrome reflecting absence of an isolated gene or genes. Some of the microdeletion syndromes, including Prader-Willi, Angelman, and Williams syndromes, often involve deletion of regions flanked by multiple repeat elements (Vogels & Fryns, 2002). The presence of these repeats promotes unequal crossing-over events during meiosis resulting in deletions and duplications.

Cri-du-chat Syndrome

Cri-du-chat syndrome (46,XX, del [5p]: deletion 5p-syndrome; chromosome 5 short arm deletion) (Fig. 7-10) gets its name from the hallmark catlike cry infants typically display. Cri-du-chat syndrome was first described in 1963 by Lejeune and colleagues (Lejeune et al., 1963), and its prevalence is estimated to be 1 in 37,000 births (Higurashi et al., 1990). Eighty-five percent of the cases of cri-du-chat syndrome are due to spontaneous, de novo deletions and in most of these the deletion is paternally derived. Unequal segregation of a parental translocation is responsible for the remaining 15% and is thus familial. This deletion syndrome is not associated with advanced maternal age.

The characteristic features of children with cri-du-chat syndrome (Fig. 7-11) other than the catlike cry include low birth weight, hypotonia, feeding difficulties with failure to thrive, microcephaly, micrognathia, macrostomia, hypertelorism with downward sloping palpebral fissures, epicanthal folds, strabismus, low set ears, a broad nasal ridge, and a structural laryngeal abnormality. Information on neuromotor function is scarce but includes clumsiness and hyperactivity with repetitive body movements (Cornish & Pigrim, 1996; Dykens & Clark, 1997). Children may have chronic sleep

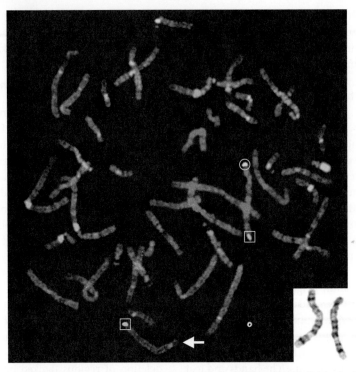

✦ Figure 7-10 G-banding and FISH (fluorescence in situ hybridization) analysis of an individual with cri-du-chat syndrome. As shown in the inset, G-banding analysis revealed a deletion of the short arm of chromosome 5 at band p14. FISH analysis using a DNA probe for the 5p telomere region, shown within the circled area, demonstrated that the deletion was terminal, because a hybridization signal was observed only on the normal chromosome 5 and not on the deleted homolog (indicated by an arrow). A control probe for the 5q telomere probe is shown within boxed areas. *(Courtesy of Dr. Christa Lese Martin, University of Chicago.)*

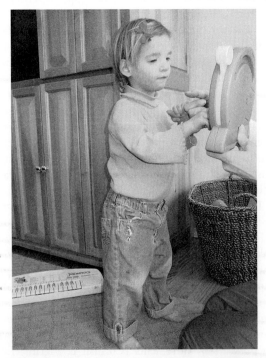

✦ Figure 7-11 Two-year-old girl with cri-du-chat syndrome.

problems and restlessness. Children tend to have IQs in the moderate to severe learning disability range, but studies have found significantly better receptive versus expressive language (Cornish et al., 1999). Many children are able to use basic sign or gestural language (Wilkins et al., 1980). Self-injurious behavior is common, including head banging and self-biting, but the occurrence of these behaviors appears to plateau in late childhood (Collins & Cornish, 2002; Dykens & Clarke, 1997). Individuals may have an obsessive attachment to objects as well as hypersensitivity to sound (Cornish & Pigrim, 1996). Studies indicate that more than 50% of children 10 years of age or older have expressive language capabilities adequate for communication (Wilkins et al., 1980).

Genes located in the deleted region include delta-catenin, a neuronal protein involved in cell motility and early neuronal development and thought to be associated with the cognitive dysfunction in cri-du-chat syndrome (Medina et al., 2000). The semaphorin F (*SEMAF*) gene encoding a protein implicated in neuronal migration and axonal pathfinding is also found within the deleted region. The haploinsufficiency (reduced gene dosage) for these two genes may disrupt normal brain development and lead to some of the neurologic manifestations of cri-du-chat syndrome (Simmons et al., 1998).

Wolf-Hirschhorn Syndrome

Wolf-Hirschhorn syndrome (46,XX, del [4p]) results from the deletion of the distal short arm of chromosome 4 resulting in craniofacial anomalies, ocular malformations, cleft lip/palate, congenital heart defects, microcephaly, and severe growth retardation (Jones, 1997). One third of all infants die within the first 2 years of life.

18p-Syndrome

In 18p-syndrome (or deletion of the short arm of 18) there are usually subtle phenotypic features with a diagnosis only after genetics testing subsequent to examination for developmental delay (Jorde et al., 2003). Children with 18p-syndrome may have mild to moderate growth deficits, hypotonia, mild microcephaly (29%), epicanthal folds (40%), hypertelorism (41%), ptosis (38%), micrognathia (25%), downturning mouth corners, and variable degrees of cognitive impairment (Jones, 1997). Typically there is better motor performance compared to language function. Twelve percent of individuals have holoprosencephaly and therefore a poor prognosis.

CHROMOSOMAL MICRODELETIONS

Prader-Willi syndrome and Angelman syndrome (PWS/AS) provide an example of genomic imprinting or the differential activation/inactivation of genes, depending on the parent from whom they are inherited (Jorde et al., 2003). The genetic defect in both of these syndromes is the deletion of 3-4 Mb on the long arm of chromosome 15 (q11q13) (Fig. 7-12). When inherited from the mother, the children develop Angelman syndrome and when inherited from the father they develop Prader-Willi syndrome. These syndromes have very different phenotypes because within the "critical" region of this deletion there are several genes that are transcriptionally active (i.e., turned on and therefore encode proteins) only on the chromosome inherited from the father (and inactive on the chromosome inherited from the mother). The same is true of different genes that are active only when located on the chromosome inherited from the mother. When the single active copy of these critical genes is lost through deletion, then the gene products are not manufactured and the syndrome results.

We now know that there are several genetic mechanisms responsible for PWS/AS (Cassidy & Schwartz, 1998, 2003). Deletions account for 70% to 80% of PWS/AS; the majority are interstitial deletions, many of which can be visualized by prometaphase banding examination. It is

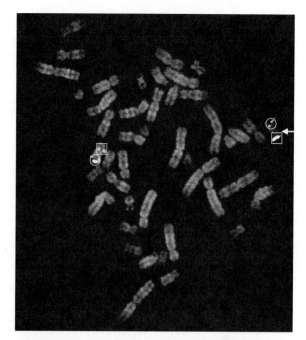

◆ **Figure 7-12**   Representative FISH (fluorescence in situ hybridization) analysis showing a deletion of the Prader-Willi/Angelman region on chromosome 15. The DNA probe shown within circled areas corresponds to the centromere region of chromosome 15. The DNA probe shown within boxed area just below the centromere probe corresponds to the *SNRPN* gene within the Prader-Willi/Angelman region; the arrow points to the deleted homolog. The second DNA probe shown within boxed area and located near the bottom of the long arm of chromosome 15 is a control probe. *(Courtesy of Dr. Christa Lese Martin, University of Chicago.)*

thought that low copy repeat gene clusters known to flank the deletion site predispose the area to unequal crossing-over events, resulting in the q11q13 microdeletion (Vogels & Fryns, 2002). A minority consist of unbalanced de novo translocations, which are easily detected by routine chromosome examination. In 25% of cases of PWS/AS the cause is uniparental disomy; this is when an individual receives two copies of a chromosome from one parent and none from the other (Fig. 7-13). If two copies of chromosome 15 are inherited from the mother, Prader-Willi syndrome results because there are no transcriptionally active paternal genes. Conversely, Angelman syndrome occurs with two paternal copies of chromosome 15. Point mutations in the "Angelman genes" or microdeletions in an imprinting center on 15 that effectively do not allow the downstream genes to be imprinted or turned on can also cause Prader-Willi syndrome, but these are rare events. Ongoing and future studies are investigating whether the phenotypic

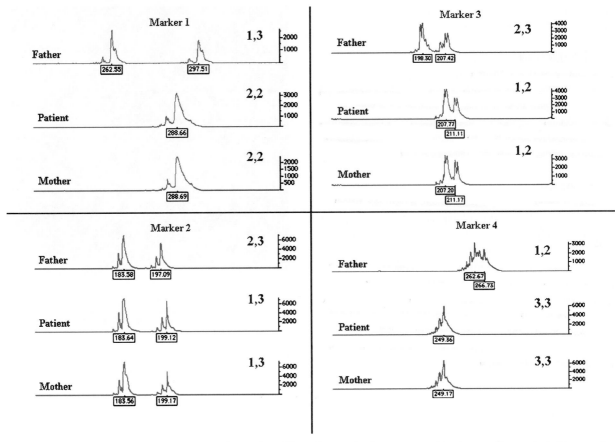

• **Figure 7-13** Uniparental disomy testing for Prader-Willi syndrome via chromosome 15 microsatellite analysis. The results of 4 microsatellite markers on chromosome 15 are depicted. For each marker the patient's, father's, and mother's samples are shown. The sizes of the alleles for each marker are indicated below each peak, and the genotype in each case is indicated to the right. Markers 1 and 4 are fully informative for maternal uniparental disomy of chromosome 15 in this patient, indicative of this patient having Prader-Willi syndrome. *(Courtesy of Dr. Soma Das, University of Chicago.)*

variation in PWS/AS may be secondary to the precise molecular defect. There are several types of genetic tests to confirm PWS/AS and distinguish between the molecular causes; this is extremely important for family counseling. FISH analysis will detect deletions (see Fig. 7-12) but cannot distinguish among the various genetic mechanisms. DNA-based methylation tests for detection of the imprinting pattern in the region of 15q11-q13 (Fig. 7-14) and uniparental disomy testing (Fig. 7-13) can then be done to determine the exact cause. The vast majority of PWS/AS cases occur sporadically no matter what the precise genetic defect. However, imprinting center mutations can be passed to offspring. In uniparental disomy, there may be an advanced maternal age effect especially if the embryo began with a trisomy and then lost the paternal chromosome 15. Otherwise, there is no parental age effect in these syndromes.

Prader-Willi Syndrome

Prader-Willi syndrome is characterized by diminished fetal activity, respiratory and feeding difficulties in infancy (frequently necessitating tube feeding), hypotonia, globally delayed developmental milestones, strabismus, decreased skin and eye pigmentation, small genitalia, hypogonadotropic hypogonadism, short stature, and small hands and feet (Cassidy & Schwartz, 2003). Minor criteria for a diagnosis also include thick, viscous saliva, speech articulation deficits, sleep apnea or a sleep disturbance, strabismus, and myopia. Molecular testing for the PWS deletion is now recommended for any infant or child with hypotonia, poor suck (or history of), and global developmental delay (Gunay-Aygun et al., 2001). In early childhood (12 months onward) there is excessive eating with gradual development of obesity with increasing age unless externally controlled. This hyperphagia is probably due to a hypothalamic disturbance in

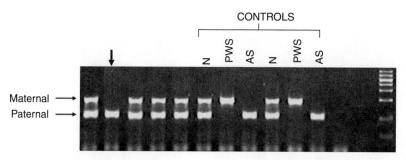

CONTROLS

◆ **Figure 7-14**   SNRPN methylation-PCR (polymerase chain reaction) to differentiate between Prader-Willi and Angelman syndromes. Bands labeled "maternal" and "paternal" correspond to methylated SNRPN and unmethylated SNRPN amplification products, respectively. The presence of both maternal and paternal bands is indicative of biparental inheritance of the *SNRPN* gene, the presence of only the maternal band is indicative of Prader-Willi syndrome and the presence of only the paternal band is indicative of Angelman syndrome. The results of 6 control samples and 5 patient samples are shown. Of the control samples, N = normal control, PWS = Prader-Willi syndrome control, and AS = Angelman syndrome control. The patient sample indicated with an arrow demonstrates a patient positive for Angelman syndrome. *(Courtesy of Dr. Soma Das, University of Chicago.)*

the satiety center. Cognitive impairments exist but ranges of intelligence are from low normal to moderate MR Behavioral problems in childhood may include temper tantrums, stubbornness, manipulative behavior, and obsessive-compulsive characteristics (Boer et al., 2002; Clarke et al., 2002). Average motor milestones have been reported to be about twice the typical average age with walking by about 2 years. Scoliosis can occur in all age groups.

Multiple genes (20 plus) are strongly suspected in the etiology of Prader-Willi syndrome, and traditional positional cloning techniques as well as animal models are being used to identify the genes most likely to cause PWS. One such gene is called small nuclear ribonucleoprotein N (*SNRPN*); it is involved in alternative mRNA splicing and is not expressed in any patient with PWS regardless of the underlying genetic mechanism (Wevrick & Francke, 1996).

Angelman Syndrome

Angelman syndrome (AS) is a neurodevelopmental disorder characterized by severe learning difficulties, ataxia with jerky movements and a puppet-like gait, a seizure disorder with a characteristic electroencephalogram (EEG), subtle dysmorphic facial features, a sleep disorder, and frequent and sometimes inappropriate laughter (Boyd et al., 1988; Buntinx et al., 1995; Clayton-Smith, 1993; Robb et al., 1989). The movement and laughing behaviors led to the early coining of the disorder as "happy puppet syndrome," but this term is now rarely used because of its potentially derogatory connotation. The facial features in individuals with Angelman syndrome are subtle and include a wide, smiling mouth, the appearance of a prominent chin due to maxillary

hypoplasia, and deep set eyes. The majority of persons have pale blue eyes due to decreased pigmentation of the iris. Most children have a delay in developmental milestones and slowing of head growth during the first year of life. Expressive speech rarely occurs but receptive language is at a higher level, so the use of sign language is recommended for communication in the majority of individuals.

Genes that have been implicated in the etiology of AS include a receptor subunit of the inhibitory neurotransmitter GABA and the E6-associated protein ubiquitin-protein ligase (*UBE3A*) gene (Burger et al., 2002; Matsuura et al., 1997). Knockout mice with the GABA receptor subunit disruption demonstrate learning and memory deficits, motor deficits, hyperactivity, and a disturbed sleep-wake cycle (DeLorey et al., 1998), behaviors that are all common in individuals with AS. *UBE3A* is an imprinted gene with silencing of the paternal allele in the hippocampus and cerebellum of mice. Mutant mice with a maternal deficiency of *UBE3A* show some similarities to human AS including motor dysfunction, inducible seizures, learning deficits, and severely impaired long-term potentiation (LTP), the neurophysiologic basis for learning and memory (Jiang et al., 1998). Interestingly, recent reports have demonstrated cases of AS following intracytoplasmic sperm injection (ICSI) as part of in vitro fertilization. This may indicate that environmental influences with ICSI could possibly interfere with establishing the maternal imprint in the oocyte (Cox et al., 2002; Orstavik et al., 2003).

Williams Syndrome

Williams syndrome has been identified as a contiguous gene syndrome with deletion of a critical region

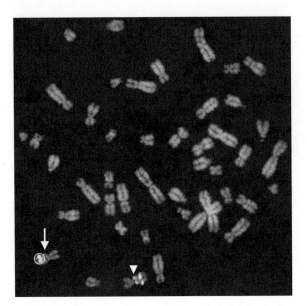

◆ **Figure 7-15** FISH (fluorescence in situ hybridization) analysis showing a deletion of the Williams syndrome region on chromosome 7. The DNA probe (*arrowhead*) corresponds to the Elastin (*ELN*) gene within the Williams syndrome critical region; the arrow points to the deleted homolog. The DNA probe within circled areas is a control probe and shows two normal copies. (*Courtesy of Dr. Christa Lese Martin, University of Chicago.*)

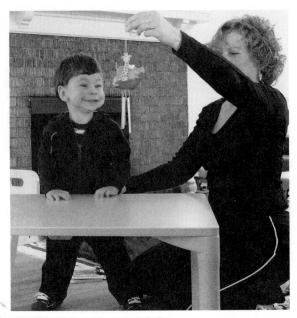

◆ **Figure 7-16** A boy with Williams syndrome.

encompassing the elastin gene on the long arm of chromosome 7 (7q1) (Fig. 7-15) (Ewart et al., 1993). The vast majority of cases result from de novo deletions in either parent and therefore the risk to future offspring is extremely low (Morris, 2003). A primary feature of Williams syndrome is cardiovascular disease secondary to elastin arteriopathy; elastin is normally present in high concentrations in the arterial walls of elastic arteries, such as the aorta. Supravalvular aortic stenosis and multiple peripheral pulmonary arterial stenoses are common, although any artery may be narrowed. The characteristics of individuals with Williams syndrome (Fig. 7-16) are variable but frequently include an "elfin"-like face with a wide mouth and full lips, a stellate pattern to the iris, strabismus, short stature, potential learning difficulties (ranging from mild cognitive impairment to attention deficit hyperactivity disorder [ADHD] to normal IQ), dental malformations, and infantile hypercalcemia (Morris et al., 1988). The unique cognitive profile includes significant weakness in visuospatial skills while language development typically displays strengths in the quantity and quality of vocabulary, auditory memory, and social use of language (Gosch et al., 1994; Mervis et al., 1998; Mervis & Klein-Tasman, 2000). Many children sing or play musical instruments with considerable expertise

and they rarely forget a name. Children with Williams syndrome have engaging personalities and tend to be very talkative. The cognitive impairments may be due to loss of the gene for LIM1-kinase, a brain specific enzyme that phosphorylates proteins frequently increasing their activation (Frangiskakis et al., 1996). Gastrointestinal problems causing pain may be significant in children with Williams syndrome and include gastroesophageal reflux (GER), hernias, chronic constipation, peptic ulcers, and diverticulitis. The traits that may be pertinent for the physical therapist include radioulnar synostosis, poor visual-motor integration, ADHD, joint laxity in infancy and later compensatory limitations, hypotonia, and auditory, oral and tactile sensory defensiveness (Cassidy & Morris, 2002; Kaplan et al., 1989; Morris et al., 1988; Pankau et al., 1993). Children with Williams syndrome usually walk by 2 years of age.

SINGLE GENE DISORDERS

Genetic defects in a single gene are often called mendelian conditions because they generally follow mendelian inheritance patterns. They result from a mutation at the single gene level in either the heterozygous or homozygous state. As of June 2005, 15,200 monogeneic defined traits have been identified in humans. Of these, 15,071 are located on autosomes, 903 are on the X chromosome, 62 are mitochondrial, and 56 are Y-linked. Many of these mutations (10,183) have been mapped to a specific chromosomal location, cloned, and sequenced.

Single gene disorders may be autosomal dominant, autosomal recessive, sex-linked, or mitochondrial, but many genetic disorders do not fit into rigid categories. Factors complicating inheritance patterns are the presence of de novo mutations (especially in cases of autosomal dominance), germline mosaicism, reduced penetrance, and variable disease expression (Jorde et al., 2003). *Germline mosaicism* occurs when the parent's germ cells (in part or whole) have the mutation but somatic cells do not (see Fig. 7-3). The parent does not express the disease but can transmit the mutation to offspring. This phenomenon has been described for osteogenesis imperfecta type II, achondroplasia, neurofibromatosis type I, Duchenne muscular dystrophy, and hemophilia A. In somatic mosaicism a mutation occurs during embryonic development, and therefore, only some of the somatic cells are affected, resulting in a milder phenotypic expression. Genetic disorders in which an individual may have the disease genotype but not the phenotype are said to have reduced *penetrance* (this is observed in fragile X syndrome, for example). *Variable expression patterns* are seen in genetic disorders in which penetrance may be complete but the severity of the disease can vary significantly. This is seen in neurofibromatosis type 1 and osteogenesis imperfecta (see Chapter 14). Explanations for variable expression rates are not always known but may be due to modifier gene interactions, environmental factors, and different types of mutations in the disease gene (also known as *allelic heterogeneity*).

Pleiotropic genes are those that affect multiple body systems. There are numerous pleiotropic genes, and their deletion or interruption will then have multisystem ramifications. For example, the neurofibromin gene is widely expressed in neurocutaneous and connective tissues and when mutated, as in neurofibromatosis I, there are multiple defects in neurologic, skeletal, and integumentary system functions (see later discussion).

A genetic disease with a single phenotype may also be caused by mutations at different locations. This is called *locus heterogeneity* and frequently results when one of two or more gene products necessary for a specific cellular function is mutated. As an example, the procollagen subunit chains are encoded by genes on two different chromosomes and osteogenesis imperfecta results with a mutation in either of these genes (see Chapter 14). In addition, a mutation in either one of two tumor suppressor genes results in tuberous sclerosis (see later discussion).

Advances in molecular genetics have elucidated mechanism(s) responsible for a phenomenon called *anticipation*, whereby certain neurologic diseases have a more severe expression or earlier onset in more recent generations (Jorde et al., 2003). Disease mutations have been found to be due to expansion of trinucleotide repeats with succeeding generations and thereby increased disease severity. There are generally two categories or patterns of repeat expansion diseases. One type is caused by a repeat CAG in a protein coding or exon region of a gene with larger expansions when transmitted paternally and a gain of function effect. This is seen in some of the spinocerebellar ataxias, Huntington disease, certain cases of syndactyly and polydactyly, and spinal and bulbar muscular atrophy. The second category includes much larger repeat expansions in the noncoding region of genes (within 3' or 5' untranslated regions or introns), especially when carried by the mother, and generate a loss of function effect (i.e., loss of gene transcription). Examples of this type include fragile X syndrome (see section on X-linked disorders), myotonic dystrophy (see Chapter 15), and Friedreich ataxia.

AUTOSOMAL DOMINANT DISORDERS

Autosomal dominant disorders occur when a single mutated gene inherited from one parent is dominant and therefore overrides the normal allele from the other parent. Most affected offspring are produced by the union of a normal parent with a heterozygous person. Each child of a parent with an autosomal trait has a 50% chance of being heterozygous and thus expressing the disease. Because of transmission in autosomes, males and females are *usually* equally affected and because of dominance generations are not *typically* skipped. A large proportion, however, of the cases of autosomal dominant disorders result from new mutations. Examples of autosomal dominant conditions include neurofibromatosis, tuberous sclerosis, achondroplasia (see Chapter 17), osteogenesis imperfecta (see Chapter 14), Marfan syndrome, and Huntington disease. Autosomal conditions account for over 90% of all genetic disorders.

Neurofibromatosis 1

Neurofibromatosis 1 (NF1) is a phenotypically heterogeneous multisystem disorder characterized by multiple café au lait spots, freckling in the axillary and inguinal region, and dermal or plexiform neurofibromas (Friedman and Birch, 1997; Friedman and Riccardi, 1999; Huson, 1994). It has a wide variance in expression and hence disease manifestation. Other serious but less common characteristics include CNS, optic, peripheral nerve sheath, and skeletal tumors. Tumors may be benign or malignant. The most serious skeletal complications are scoliosis, pseudarthrosis, vertebral dysplasia, and bony overgrowth. The frequency of the more serious complications in NF1 increases with advancing age and the disease characteristics have typical timelines for appearance. For example, cortical thinning is seen congenitally, café au lait spots and optic gliomas develop between 0 and 4 years, dysplastic scoliosis occurs between 6 and 10 years, and skin neurofibromas occur from puberty on.

A broad range of both nonverbal and verbal learning disabilities is evident in approximately 30% to 65% of children with NF1 (Kayl & Moore, 2000; North 1999). Deficits in IQ, executive function, attention, and motor skills have also been documented (Rosser & Packer, 2003). Studies suggest that the learning disorders may be caused by a cascade of neuronal biochemical abnormalities beginning with increased Ras activity, excessive inhibition of the GABA neurotransmitter, decreased LTP, and hence learning and memory deficits (Costa and Silva, 2002). Neuroimaging studies have demonstrated that macrocephaly may exist with greater gray matter volume; this finding has been positively correlated to the degree of learning disability. In addition, a larger corpus callosum is seen in some individuals with NF1, a finding correlated with reduced academic achievement, visual-spatial skills, and motor performance (Moore et al., 2000).

The *NF1* gene is located on chromosome 17 and its product is neurofibromin, a protein that controls cell proliferation and acts as a tumor suppressor (Cichowski & Jacks, 2001; Dasgupta & Gutman, 2003; Zhu & Parada, 2001), hence explaining tumor formation in affected individuals. Neurofibromin has several biochemical functions, such as modulating Ras-guanosine triphosphatase (GTPase) activity, adenylate cyclase, and microtubule binding, all of which could be critical for brain function (Costa & Silva, 2002). Many different types of mutations have been reported including stop mutations, deletions, substitutions, and insertions, most of which cause truncation of neurofibromin (Shen et al., 1996). NF1 knockout mice have learning and memory difficulties similar to those seen in humans (Rosser & Packer, 2003). Fifty percent of affected individuals have NF1 as a result of a new gene mutation. The risk for offspring inheriting the disease is 50% because of autosomal dominance inheritance. NF1 is one of the most common autosomal dominant inherited disorders with a frequency at birth of 1 in 3000 (Friedman & Riccardi, 1999). The mutation rate for the large NF1 gene is extremely high, but the cause of this is not yet known. Molecular genetic testing for the *NF1* gene is available but is rarely necessary because the clinical diagnosis is clear in most clients (Friedman, 2003).

Tuberous Sclerosis Complex

Tuberous sclerosis complex, which includes both tuberous sclerosis 1 and 2 (TSC 1 and TSC 2), is a multiorgan systemic disorder involving abnormalities of the brain, skin, kidney, and heart. TSC 1 and TSC 2 are two tumor suppressor genes encoding the proteins hamartin and tuberin on chromosomes 9 and 16, respectively. Seventy percent of individuals have TSC as a result of a new mutation in either TSC 1 or 2; there is a high mutation rate in these large genes (Sampson et al., 1989). The disorder is thought to have 100% penetrance but highly variable expression partially due to a high rate (10%–25%) of somatic mosaicism (Verhoef et al., 1999). The prevalence of tuberous sclerosis is 1 per 5800 births (Osborne et al., 1991). Table 7-3 delineates the clinical

TABLE 7-3	Tuberous Sclerosis Complex

MAJOR CLINICAL FEATURES	MINOR CLINICAL FEATURES
Facial angiofibromas or forehead plaques (47–90%)	Rectal polyps
Ungual or periungual fibromas (17–87%)	Bone cysts
Hypomelanotic skin macules (87–100%)	Multiple renal cysts
Connective tissue nevus (20–80%)	Gingival fibromas
Subependymal glial nodules (90%) or giant cell astrocytoma (6–14%)	Confetti-like skin lesions
Cortical or subcortical tubers (70%)	Cerebral white matter radial migration lines
Lung lymphangiomyomatosis (1–6%; primarily females age 20–40 years)	Pits in dental enamel
Renal angiomyolipoma (70%)	
Cardiac rhabdomyoma (47–67%)	

From Northrup, H, & Au, KS. Tuberous sclerosis complex. Gene Clinics, 2002; accessed at http//www.geneclinics.org/; Roach, ES, Gomez, MR, & Northrup, H. Tuberous sclerosis complex consensus conference: Revised clinical diagnostic criteria. Journal of Child Neurology, *13*:624–628, 1998.

features found in individuals with TSC. Criteria for a clinical diagnosis are two major features or one major feature and two minor features (Roach et al., 1998).

Greater than 80% of individuals with TSC have a seizure disorder including infantile spasms which may be intractable; some have benefited from epilepsy surgery (Avellino et al., 1997; Weiner et al., 1998). Neurodevelopmental and neurobehavioral disorders are common and include developmental delay (in >50%), cognitive impairment, pervasive developmental disorder (PDD), ADHD, and aggression (Curatolo et al., 1991; Gutierrez et al., 1998; Hunt & Dennis, 1987). The giant cell astrocytomas can enlarge causing increased intracranial pressure and cerebrospinal fluid obstruction and are associated with such high morbidity and mortality rates that timely removal is important (Weiner et al., 1998). Status epilepticus, bronchopneumonia, and renal disease are primary causes of premature death (Shepherd et al., 1991).

AUTOSOMAL RECESSIVE DISORDERS

In autosomal recessive inheritance both parents are typically heterozygous for the recessive mutated gene. There is a 25% recurrence rate with each pregnancy and consanguinity (mating of related individuals) is present more often than in other genetic disorders. Examples of the more common autosomal recessive disorders that physical therapists are likely to encounter are cystic fibrosis (see Chapter 27), spinal muscular atrophy (see Chapter 15), and sickle cell disease.

Biochemical Disorders

Many biochemical or inborn errors of metabolism are caused by metabolic enzyme deficiencies. The majority of these are inherited in an autosomal recessive manner. The incidence of metabolic disorders is estimated collectively to be 1 in 2500 births or about 10% of all single gene disorders in children (Jorde et al., 2003; Scriver et al., 2000). Although individually rare in frequency, they contribute a significant proportion of the morbidity and mortality rates for known childhood genetic disorders. The carrier or heterozygous condition is not typically associated with a disease. There are several classification systems for biochemical disorders, but in general most are caused by enzyme or cofactor deficits in the body's various metabolic pathways. Newborn screening programs typically test for elevated levels of metabolites for some of the more common genetic disorders such as phenylketonuria and galactosemia. Technologies such as mass spectroscopy linked with automated tissue sample handling and computerized analysis are making the identification of these rare disorders more efficient and

cost effective (Tobin & Boughton, 2000). Table 7-4 lists some of the metabolic disorders that cause neuromotor or musculoskeletal deficits and would thus be more common for physical therapists to encounter in clinical practice.

Classical *phenylketonuria* (PKU) results from a mutation in the phenylalanine hydroxylase gene encoded on chromosome 12. This enzyme participates in the breakdown of the essential amino acid, phenylalanine. Elevated phenylalanine then disrupts many neural processes including myelination, and cognitive impairment results if not treated. Treatment is dietary restriction of phenylalanine-containing foods. PKU has a wide variance in incidence depending on ethnicity with a much higher incidence in whites (1/10,000) than in Africans (1/90,000), for example. *Galactosemia* is an inherited disorder of carbohydrate metabolism typically caused by mutations in the galactose-1-phosphate uridyl transferase gene. If it is untreated, the child develops liver disease, growth retardation, and cognitive deficits. Early clinical signs include failure to thrive, cataracts, liver insufficiency, and developmental delay. The *lysosomal storage disorders* result from accumulation of undegraded substrate in lysosomes, most typically because of enzyme deficiencies. Examples include the mucopolysaccharidoses in which there is inability to break down glycosaminoglycans resulting in progressive deterioration in neurologic, cardiovascular, joint, hearing, and visual functions. Some biochemical disorders may be treated by dietary restriction or alteration, supplying the missing enzyme, or bone marrow transplantation/gene therapy to restore endogenous production of the missing gene product. For example, bone marrow transplantation has resulted in reduced neurologic deterioration and prolonged survival in children with Hurler syndrome (Peters et al., 1998).

SEX-LINKED DISORDERS

Because few genes are located on the Y chromosome, the majority of gender-linked genetic disorders are associated with the X chromosome (Jorde et al., 2003). It is important to remember that X chromosome inactivation occurs when discussing sex-linked disorders. X chromosome inactivation occurs early in female embryonic development and is a random event such that there will be approximately equal numbers of paternally derived and maternally derived X chromosomes that are inactivated in the cells of females (see Fig. 7-8). In addition, once an X chromosome is inactivated, it remains so for the life of the cell *and* all the descendents of that cell. Therefore, females are mosaics with 50% of their cells having

| TABLE 7-4 | **Selected Inborn Errors of Metabolism** | | |

SYNDROME/DISEASE	MUTATED GENE	INHERITANCE	CLINICAL FEATURES
Tay–Sachs disease	Beta-hexosaminidase	Autosomal recessive; 1/10,000–15,000 (Northern European)	Slowed development, hypotonia followed by hypertonia, mental retardation, tremors, seizures, blindness
Niemann-Pick disease 1A	Sphingomyelinase	Autosomal recessive	Brain deterioration with mental retardation, corneal opacities, hepatomegaly
Hurler syndrome or mucopolysaccharidoses I (MPS 1)	Alpha-L-iduronidase	X-linked recessive	Normal appearance at birth with progressive deterioration starting at about 6 months resulting in coarse facial features, hepatosplenomegaly, corneal clouding, dysostosis multiplex,* severe physical and cognitive decline with mental retardation, deafness, cardiac disease
Hunter syndrome or mucopolysaccharidoses II (MPS II)	Iduronate sulfatase	X-linked recessive	Coarse face, joint stiffness, skeletal deformities, mental retardation
Sanfilippo syndrome (A-D)	Heparan-N-sulfamidase Alpha-N-acetyl-glucosamidase N-acetylglucosamine-6-sulfatase	Autosomal recessive	Behavioral disorders, mental retardation, dysostosis multiplex*
Krabbe disease	Beta-galactosidase	Autosomal recessive	Hypertonicity, blindness, deafness, seizures, brain atrophy
Lesch-Nyhan disease	Hypoxanthine phosphoribosyl-transferase (HPRT)	X-linked recessive	Early gross motor delay /hypotonia; later hyperkinesis/spasticity; gouty arthritis
Classic galactosemia	Galactose-1-phosphate uridyl transferase	Autosomal recessive	Developmental delay, failure to thrive with poor growth, cataracts, hepatic insufficiency, mental retardation
Phenylketonuria (PKU)	Phenylalanine hydroxylase	Autosomal recessive	Normal at birth with delayed development by 12 months; if untreated hypertonicity, tremors, seizures, and mental retardation
Wilson's disease	ATP7B (involved in copper transport)	Autosomal recessive	Excess copper accumulation causes liver disease, neurologic problems (dysarthria, dyscoordination), arthropathy, cardiomyopathy

*Dysostosis multiplex: bony changes include thickened skull, long bones, and anterior ribs, short long bones, vertebral abnormalities.
From Jorde, LB, Carey, JC, Bamshad, MJ, White, RL (Eds.). Biochemical Genetics: Disorders of Metabolism in Medical Genetics, 3rd ed. St. Louis: Mosby, 2003, pp. 136–159.

maternally derived and 50% paternally derived X chromosomes. This mechanism ensures appropriate and equal gene dosing for males and females.

X-Linked Recessive Disorders

The majority of X-linked diseases are recessive. The inheritance patterns include lack of father to son transmission, skipped generations during which the heterozygous females are carriers, and a majority of males affected because females have two X chromosomes.

Duchenne Muscular Dystrophy. Duchenne muscular dystrophy is the most common X-linked disorder known (1/3500 live male births). It involves a mutation in the dystrophin gene and is extensively discussed in Chapter 15 along with Becker muscular dystrophy, another X-linked recessive disorder involving a dystrophin gene mutation.

Hemophilia A. Hemophilia A (see Chapter 10) is the well-characterized "typical" form of hemophilia caused by defective or complete lack of clotting factor VIII. Cloning and sequencing of the factor VIII gene helped to explain why there is variability in the severity of the disease (Jorde et al., 2003; Nussbaum et al., 2001). Individuals with nonsense mutations produce a truncated protein and a more severe clinical outcome, and those with a missense mutation result in a single amino acid substitution and a milder form of the disease. Interestingly, 50% of those with severe hemophilia have a chromosomal inversion that deletes the carboxy terminus of factor VIII. Recombinant DNA technology is now used to produce human factor VIII (versus a donor-derived form) with the advantage of lack of viral contamination. Gene therapy trials are promising, but no curative treatments are currently available.

Lesch-Nyhan Syndrome. Lesch-Nyhan syndrome is an inborn error of purine metabolism with a mutation in the hypoxanthine phosphoribosyltransferase (*HPRT*) gene (Jinnah & Friedmann, 2001). Excessive uric acid production results with renal, neurologic, and rheumatologic consequences. A gross motor delay is seen between 3 and 6 months with initial hypotonia; later there are hyperkinetic movements (chorea, ataxia, athetosis of hands/feet), and spasticity is ultimately observed. The child exhibits growth retardation and frequent vomiting. Self-injurious behavior beginning by lip biting and progressing to biting of fingertips and hands and head banging is common. Dysarthria and moderate cognitive impairment are the norm. The baby typically presents with orange uric acid crystals in the diaper and obstructive nephropathy. An acute gouty arthritis is seen with tophi (accumulation of sodium urate crystals) in subcutaneous tissues, especially the extensor surfaces of elbows, knees, fingers, and toes.

This disease can be detected prenatally by the absence of HPRT enzyme activity in cultured amniocytes or chorionic villi. The medical treatment for this disorder presently consists of allopurinol to inhibit xanthine oxidase activity and thereby reduce uric acid levels. This may alleviate or prevent the renal and musculoskeletal symptoms but does not affect the neurologic ones. It is hypothesized that the CNS symptoms are linked to abnormal dopaminergic function.

X- Linked Dominant Disorders

Fragile X Syndrome. Fragile X syndrome is the most common type of inherited cognitive impairment (Hagerman, 1996; Hammond et al., 1997; Opitz & Sutherland, 1984; Tarleton & Saul, 1993; Warren & Sherman, 2001). Other features of individuals with this syndrome include hypotonia, joint hypermobility, delayed motor milestones, autistic spectrum disorder and a somewhat characteristic face with elongated facies, large ears, and a prominent mandible. The term "fragile X" was coined based on the typical breaks and gaps in structure of the long arm of the X chromosome when it is cultured in a folic acid–deficient medium. This constriction was originally used for diagnostic purposes but has been replaced by more accurate and sophisticated molecular tests.

New molecular research and cloning of the defective gene (*FMR1*) in fragile X syndrome have helped to explain a perplexing pattern of inheritance called the Sherman paradox (Fu et al., 1991; Jorde et al., 2003). Males who carry the fragile X mutation but do not express the disease are called normal transmitting males. Only 9% of the brothers of transmitting males have fragile X, while 40% of their grandsons and 50% of their great-grandsons have the syndrome (Nolin et al., 1996). In addition, daughters of a normal transmitting male never have the syndrome, but their sons can inherit the disease. This "Sherman paradox" is not consistent with classic rules of X-linked inheritance that predict equal penetrance in males who inherit the disease. We now know that it is an X-linked dominant disorder with differential penetrance in males (80%) and females (30%) and variable expression, both of which are thought to be secondary to X chromosome inactivation. The degree of cognitive impairment is therefore mild in affected females (who are mosaics) and moderate in affected males (Riddle et al., 1998). In addition, the genetic defect is one of trinucleotide repeat expansion, and this explains the increased severity with successive generations.

The fragile X gene product is an RNA binding protein called FMRP, which is important in synaptic development, neuronal plasticity, and learning and memory (Oostra & Chiurazzi, 2001). It has been suggested that FMRP may be required for normal dendritic spine maturation and elimination in the cerebral cortex (Greenough et al., 2001). The 5' untranslated region of FMR1 contains a variable number (from 5 to 60) of CGG repeat units in normal individuals (Fu et al., 1991). Persons with fragile X syndrome have an expanded number (230 to >1000) of repeats, and this is considered a full mutation. Transmitting males and their daughters have what is called a "premutation" with an intermediate number of CGG repeats (52–200). The premutation expands to a full mutation only when transmitted by a female; this occurs during oogenesis and is due to meiotic instability. Therefore, daughters of normal transmitting males *only* have the premutation, never the full mutation, and they never have cognitive impairment. Also, daughters of affected males do not express the fragile X syndrome at either the clinical or the cytogenetic level.

Children inheriting the premutation, however, may have learning disabilities (Franke et al., 1996; Steyaert et al., 2003). Individuals with the premutation have normal expression of *FMRP* while those with the full mutation completely lack transcription of *FMRP* mRNA, probably due to aberrant methylation of the DNA repeats. Methylation state is positively correlated with the severity of expression of fragile X syndrome (Rousseau et al., 1994). Neuroimaging studies have revealed an abnormally small cerebellar vermis, an increased volume of the hippocampus, and a reduction in size of the superior temporal gyrus in persons with fragile X syndrome (Reiss et al., 1991a, 1991b, 1994).

Behavioral studies in children with fragile X syndrome have described abnormal gaze behavior, approach and avoidance conflict, and a high incidence of autistic spectrum disorder (Kau et al., 2002; Tarleton & Saul, 1993; Warren & Sherman, 2001). Pervasive deficits in conversational speech, early motor developmental delay, and severe delays in language have been reported. Surprisingly, adaptive behavior was not significantly associated with the levels of FMRP in boys or girls with fragile X (Glaser et al., 2003). However, testing of the gene product later in childhood may not reflect what is needed during a critical period of brain development.

The pediatric physical therapist may be instrumental in referring children for genetic testing and thus establishing an appropriate diagnosis in conditions such as fragile X syndrome, in which physical features are subtle or absent and do not allow accurate classification (Lachiewicz et al., 2000). Appropriate early diagnosis has significant ramifications for the entire extended family and has been shown to significantly adjust a carrier family's reproductive plans (Meryash & Abuelo, 1988). Molecular testing for fragile X can be done by antibody testing for the FMRP protein in hair roots, or by analysis of blood cells with molecular techniques for expanded repeats (Fig. 7-17). In addition, methylation state may be determined by sensitive restriction enzymes that cut DNA in specific locations.

Rett Syndrome. The molecular revolution in genetics has certainly been instrumental in advancing our understanding of Rett syndrome, a progressive neurodevelopmental disorder seen almost exclusively in females. "Classic" Rett syndrome is seen only in females; males with the specific genetic defect either are lost prenatally or are born with a severe congenital encephalopathy and die before age 2. Originally it was hypothesized that the mutations were always lethal in male embryos. The incidence of Rett syndrome is estimated to be between 1 in 10,000 and 1 in 15,000 (Brandt & Zoghbi, 2001).

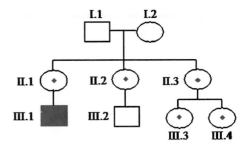

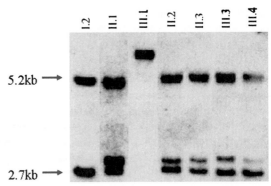

+ **Figure 7-17** Southern blot analysis of a family with fragile X syndrome. The Southern blot analysis is performed by digestion with EcoR1 and Eag1 restriction enzymes and probed with an FMR1-specific probe. The Southern blot analysis shows that individual III.1 is affected with fragile X syndrome and carries the full expansion of the *FMR1* gene. Individuals II.1, II.2, II.3, III.3, and III.4 are all carriers of a premutation of the *FMR1* gene. Individual I.2 is not a premutation carrier, indicating that individuals II.1, II.2, and II.3 have inherited the premutation allele from their father, I.1. *(Courtesy of Dr. Soma Das, University of Chicago.)*

Knowledge of the striking clinical features in Rett syndrome, especially the motor aspects, is important for a pediatric therapist to be aware of in order to refer appropriately for advanced medical/genetic work-up. The clinical manifestations of classic Rett syndrome are an apparently typical prenatal and perinatal period with normal development up until approximately 6 to 18 months of age (Hagberg et al., 1983; Witt-Engerstrom, 1992). More recent reports suggest that babies under 6 months with Rett syndrome may have mild hypotonia, a placid personality, and a weak suck and cry (Kerr, 1995). Head circumference is normal at birth but then growth decelerates anywhere from 3 to 48 months with eventual microcephaly. Then there is a short period during which advances in development are not seen, followed by a rapid regression in motor, language, and psychosocial functions. The loss of purposeful hand skills such as self-feeding and replacement with stereotyped repetitive hand motions such as wringing is a hallmark behavioral characteristic of the disease. Other problems include gait and trunk ataxia, tremors, apraxia, intermittent esotropia, autistic-like behavior, bruxism, breathing irregularities (hyperventilation or episodic apnea), GER, impaired bowel mobility, and vasomotor changes in the lower extremities. Fits of screaming and crying are common by 18 to 24 months (Coleman et al., 1988). There is a severe impairment in both expressive and receptive language with severe cognitive impairment. After the rapid deterioration/regression phase the disease becomes somewhat stable, although seizures then become more common and are seen in 50% of girls with Rett syndrome (Dunn & Macleod, 2001; Witt-Engerstrom, 1992). Kyphoscoliosis and hand and foot deformities resulting from dystonia are commonly seen and need to be aggressively managed because they are frequently unresponsive to conservative therapy (Budden, 1997; Tanguy, 1993). Osteoporosis occurs frequently, even in younger girls, which increases fracture risk (Budden & Gunness, 2001). Walking abilities are quite varied and range from complete inability to walk to independent walking without devices (Tanguy, 1993).

Although Rett syndrome was first identified by the Viennese pediatrician Rett in 1963 (Rett, 1966, 1986), Hagberg and colleagues (1983) were the first to extensively describe the behavioral characteristics seen in girls with Rett syndrome. They delineated four clinical stages seen after an apparently normal first 6 months or so of life: (I) early onset developmental stagnation at 6 to 18 months, (II) the rapid destructive stage at 1 to 3 years, (III) the pseudo-stationary stage from preschool to school age years, and (IV) the late motor deterioration stage. Some clinicians still use this staging system as a reference.

In 1999 the genetic basis of Rett syndrome was identified (Amir et al., 1999). Mutations in the *MECP2* gene encoding an X-linked methyl cytosine-binding protein, a presumed gene transcription regulator by DNA methylation, were identified in a significant number of girls with Rett syndrome (Fig. 7-18). Mutations in this gene account for the majority (80%) of cases of typical Rett syndrome. The overwhelming number (99.5%) of mutations are either new ones or are caused by mosaicism in the parent. Girls with Rett syndrome are mosaics for the *MECP2* mutation because of random X chromosome inactivation so that 50% of cells express the normal *MECP2* gene and 50% express the mutated one. There are rare instances of carrier females with a *MECP2* mutation who are unaffected or mildly affected because of nonrandom X chromosome inactivation and the favorably skewed preferential inactivation of the mutated *MECP2* allele (Amir et al., 2000; Wan et al., 1999). Nonrandom patterns of X chromosome inactivation may also contribute to the clinical variability often seen in girls with Rett syndrome. The type of mutation (missense versus truncating mutation) also plays a role in the phenotypic variability in Rett syndrome (Cheadle et al., 2000).

Atypical forms of Rett syndrome are either the more severe variant with congenital hypotonia and infantile spasms and milder forms with less severe, later onset developmental regression and milder cognitive impairment (Hagberg, 1995; Zappella et al., 1998). In addition, a

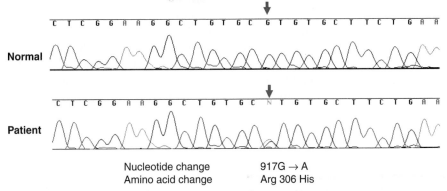

| Nucleotide change | 917G → A |
| Amino acid change | Arg 306 His |

• **Figure 7-18** Mutation analysis for *MECP2* gene in Rett syndrome via DNA sequencing. The figure depicts a portion of the MECP2 sequence in a normal control subject and in a patient with Rett syndrome. The position depicted with an arrow shows the presence of a mutation in the patient with Rett syndrome, where a guanosine nucleotide has been changed to an adenosine nucleotide. Both an adenosine and guanosine nucleotide is present in the patient, instead of only the guanosine nucleotide as seen in the normal control subject. The mutation in this patient is at nucleotide position 917 (917G >A) and results in the change of an arginine to histidine amino acid at residue 306 (Arg306His). (*Courtesy of Dr. Soma Das, University of Chicago.*)

broader phenotypic spectrum in disorders genetically related to Rett syndrome has been suggested by examples of *MECP2* mutations in babies with severe neonatal encephalopathy, children previously diagnosed with autism, females with mild learning disabilities, and the male population with cognitive impairment (Amir et al., 2000; Schanen et al., 1998; Wan et al., 1999). The frequency of *MECP2* mutations in the population with cognitive impairment is now being appreciated with appropriate genetic testing. In certain males the clinical picture is different from girls with classic Rett syndrome such that males never have a period of apparently normal development. They typically have moderate to severe cognitive impairment, significantly impaired communication, and motor control difficulties such as spasticity and tremors (Couvert et al., 2001; Orrico et al., 2000). Interestingly, several of the *MECP2* mutations found in males have not been seen in females with Rett syndrome.

PEDIATRIC NEUROLOGIC DISORDERS WITH VARIABLE INHERITANCE PATTERNS

Physical therapists frequently work with children who have structural brain anomalies identified from neural imaging techniques, such as magnetic resonance imaging (MRI) and computed tomographic (CT) scan. These neural defects may be isolated or they may be part of a syndrome with additional congenital anomalies. Examples include lissencephaly, callosal agenesis or dysgenesis, Dandy-Walker syndrome, holoprosencephaly, anencephaly, encephalocele, meningocele, hydrocephalus, microcephaly, megalencephaly (hemimegalencephaly), and macrocephaly (see Box 7-2 for definitions). Many of these CNS disorders are now known to have a genetic basis but the inheritance patterns can vary within each condition. In addition, certain childhood movement disorders, such as some forms of dystonia, are now known to be inherited. This section will cover the known genetic basis for lissencephaly, agenesis of the corpus callosum, Dandy-Walker malformation, microcephaly, and childhood dystonias.

Lissencephaly

Lissencephaly is a neuronal migration disorder characterized by a smooth cerebral cortex lacking its characteristic convolutions and often includes widespread neuronal heterotopias and agenesis or malformation of the corpus callosum (Fig. 7-19). Classic lissencephaly (type 1) is caused by abnormal neuronal migration between the 9th and 13th weeks of gestation resulting in a poorly organized cerebral cortex with four primitive layers instead of six, diffuse neuronal heterotopias, enlarged

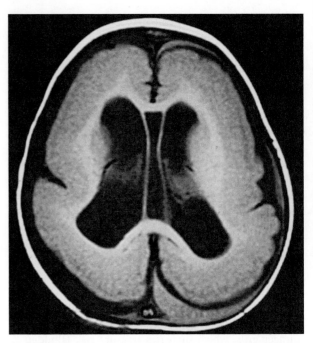

◆ **Figure 7-19**   MRI of an infant with lissencephaly. Note the absence of cerebral sulci and the maldeveloped sylvian fissures associated with enlarged ventricles. *(Reprinted with permission from Behrman, RE, Kliegman, RM, & Jenson, HB (Eds.). Nelson Textbook of Pediatrics, 17th ed. Philadelphia: W.B. Saunders Co., 2004, Fig. 585, p.1987.)*

ventricles, and frequently hypoplasia of the corpus callosum (Dobyns & Truwit, 2001). Children with lissencephaly may have global developmental delay, mild to severe psychomotor retardation, seizure disorder, and muscle tone abnormalities ranging from hypotonia to spasticity (Johnston & Kinsman, 2004). Technical advances in neuroradiology have helped to describe a number of syndromes involving lissencephaly. Several genetic causes have been characterized including mutations in the lissencephaly 1 (*LIS1*, also known as *PAFAH1B1*) gene, X-linked forms involving mutation in the doublecortin (*DCX*) gene, and deletions of 17p13.3 in Miller-Dieker syndrome (this region contains the *LIS1* gene as well as more than 10 other genes) (des Portes et al., 1998; Dobyns et al., 1992; Dobyns & Truwit, 2001; Lo Nigro et al., 1997). *LIS1* and *DCX* are involved in cortical neuronal migration and process growth, respectively (Friocourt et al., 2003). Recent mapping studies have delineated critical regions on chromosome 17 that differentiate the more severe form of lissencephaly seen in Miller-Dieker syndrome from isolated lissencephaly sequence (Cardoso et al., 2002, 2003). Not surprisingly, less involved clinical presentations were found in those with smaller deletions or missense mutations. Thus, the genomic revolution is helping to explain the behavioral variability therapists and other clinicians have observed in children with the same diagnosis.

Agenesis of the Corpus Callosum

Agenesis of the corpus callosum is a heterogeneous disorder with variable expression and a wide spectrum of clinical features and developmental outcomes (Johnston & Kinsman, 2004; Shevell, 2002). Behavioral characteristics therefore range from severe cognitive impairment and significant neurologic abnormalities to the apparently asymptomatic adult with normal intelligence. Agenesis of the corpus callosum (ACC) without lissencephaly can result from several mechanisms and variable inheritance patterns including autosomal dominant, autosomal recessive, and X-linked recessive inheritance (Dobyns, 1996; Dobyns & Truwit, 2001). A primary mechanism is when the large callosal axons form but fail to cross midline because of absence of the massa commissuralis; this leaves large bundles called Probst bundles along the medial hemispheric walls. In other types of defects the commissural axons or their cell bodies fail to form in the cerebral cortex. This latter type is seen in Walker-Warburg syndrome, and in X-linked hydrocephalus and the MASA syndrome (mental retardation, adducted thumbs, shuffling gait, and aphasia), both of which are caused by mutations in the L1 cell adhesion molecule (L1CAM), which is involved in neuronal migration and axonal growth. In certain syndromes the corpus callosum is present but atrophied and therefore thin. ACC is associated with chromosomal rearrangements or deletions such as the chromosome 4p16 deletion in Wolf-Hirschhorn syndrome, and there are at least 17 X-linked malformation syndromes with callosal agenesis as a phenotypic feature (Jones, 2004).

Dandy-Walker Malformation

A Dandy-Walker malformation or cyst results from failure of the roof of the fourth ventricle to form during embryonic development with expansion of the fourth ventricle into the posterior fossa (Johnston & Kinsman, 2004). Children may have hydrocephalus requiring shunting, and some have agenesis of the cerebellar vermis or corpus callosum. Most children have delays in motor development, but 50% have typical intellectual development (Boddaert et al., 2003). There are a great variety of malformations under the classification of Dandy-Walker, many of which do not have a common known etiology. However, autosomal recessive, autosomal dominant, and X-linked recessive forms of inheritance for syndromes including the Dandy-Walker malformation have been described.

Microcephaly

Microcephaly has both genetic and environmental etiologies. Primary microcephaly refers to conditions in which there are no other brain anomalies, and these typically are due to autosomal recessive or dominant inheritance patterns or are associated with chromosomal syndromes such as trisomy 18 and 21 and cri-di-chat syndrome (Johnston & Kinsman, 2004). It frequently results from abnormalities in neuronal migration with neuronal heterotopias and architectural aberrations. Many children have cognitive impairment (see Chapter 20) and have a seizure disorder.

Dystonia

The childhood dystonias are a heterogenous group of disorders, but most have a genetic etiology (Johnston, 2004; Uc & Rodnitzky, 2003). Dystonia is a type of sustained muscle contraction, frequently at end ranges of joint motion with a rotational component that causes abnormal postures and poor ability to grade movement. Several classification systems for dystonia exist, but a group of genetic disorders with progressive dystonia beginning in childhood is known as primary inherited dystonia or torsion dystonia. More than 10 different gene loci have been identified for this group of movement disorders including the *DYSi* gene that encodes torsion A, an ATP-binding protein. Idiopathic torsional dystonia, dopa-responsive dystonia, and myoclonus dystonia are caused by mutations in the ATP-binding protein torsin A, in the tyrosine hydroxylase enzyme, or the epsilon-sarcoglycan gene, respectively.

MITOCHONDRIAL DISORDERS

The energy or ATP-generating factories of cells have their own unique DNA, and mutations in mitochondrial DNA (mt DNA) cause a small but significant number of genetic diseases (Jorde et al., 2003; Nussbaum et al., 2001). mt DNA encodes some of the polypeptides involved in oxidative phosphorylation as well as certain ribosomal and transfer RNAs involved in protein manufacture. Mutations in mt DNA result in strictly maternal inheritance patterns. This is because mt DNA is located in the cytoplasm and the ovum supplies the zygote with all of its mitochondria. Therefore, a mother carrying a mutation in her mt DNA will pass it to all her offspring, while a father will transmit none of his mt DNA mutations. mt DNA has a 10-fold higher mutation rate than nuclear DNA because of lack of DNA repair enzymes and free radical damage generated by the process of oxidative phosphorylation.

Great phenotypic variability is found in mitochondrial disorders because of the "mosaicism" possible in cell populations; some mitochondria might contain a mutation while another in the same cell may not; this is called heteroplasmy. Tissues with large populations of mitochondria due to high energy requirements such as the CNS and muscle tend to be the ones most affected by mitochondrial diseases. Clinical features therefore frequently include myopathy, encephalopathy, and retinal degeneration. Examples of mitochondrial disorders that pediatric physical therapists might encounter include myoclonic epilepsy with ragged-red fiber disease (MERRF) and mitochondrial encephalomyopathy and stroke-like episodes (MELAS).

MULTIFACTORIAL INHERITANCE

Disorders that are due to a complex mixture of genetic and environmental factors are said to have a multifactorial inheritance pattern. Many isolated congenital malformations (i.e., non-syndromic birth defects) have a multifactorial etiology. Those that pediatric physical therapists commonly encounter include neural tube defects (NTDs), hydrocephalus, congenital hip dislocation, clubfoot (Barker et al., 2003; Dietz, 2002), cleft lip and/or palate, and congenital heart defects. Additionally, neurologic conditions such as the autistic spectrum disorders (Bailey et al., 1995) and idiopathic epilepsy are thought to result from both genetic and epigenetic factors. Although the precise nature of the genes and multiple factors that interact to bring about these disorders is far from completely understood, research is uncovering chromosomal locations and candidate genes at a rapid pace. The evidence for a genetic contribution to multifactorial disorders has come from comparing monozygotic versus dizygotic twins, familial aggregation studies, positioning cloning of "risk" genes, and clinical family descriptions (Jorde et al., 2003). Some of the developmental genes that can interact with the environment to cause congenital malformations include the cell adhesion molecule L-CAM1 in hydrocephalus (Sztriha et al., 2002), the transcription factor MSX1 and the growth factors TGF-alpha and TGF-beta 3 in orofacial clefts (Jugessur et al., 2003), SOX transcription factors in polydactyly/syndactyly, and the FGF receptor family in craniosynostosis and skeletal dysplasias (Flores-Sarnat, 2002). Definite gene-environmental interaction has been demonstrated by increased risk of limb deficiencies with maternal cigarette smoking and mutations in the *MSX1* gene (Hwang et al., 1998).

Many candidate genes and chromosomal locations have been identified for the various types of childhood and adult epilepsy, including myoclonic, absence, partial, and febrile seizures (Crunelli & Leresche, 2002; Hirose et al., 2003; Minassian et al., 1996; Ottman, 2001). Some types of epilepsy have classic mendelian inheritance patterns, and others are clearly multifactorial with genetic predispositions that interact with environmental factors to bring about the condition. A clearer understanding of the pathogenesis of seizure disorders and possible pharmacologic interventions has been greatly enhanced by molecular studies identifying specific mutations in membrane ion channels and neurotransmitter receptors.

The association between periconceptional folic acid intake and the prevention of NTDs is well described (see Chapter 25). It is not thought that a folic acid deficiency causes an NTD but that aberrant homocysteine metabolism in pregnant women may be corrected by folic acid supplementation (Botto et al., 1999). Specific causative genes have not yet been identified for NTDs, but putative ones are those involving vitamin B_{12}–dependent enzymes for homocysteine metabolism.

THE FUTURE

The Human Genome Project's initial goal was met via the successful sequencing and mapping of the entire human genome in April 2003. However, this was only the foundation for genomics research, and the future holds great potential for expanding upon this goal and to revolutionize medical diagnosis, treatment, and prevention of disease (Collins et al., 2003). Future work of the HGP will hopefully glean more information about structural and functional elements encoded in the human genome, identify more genes and their regulatory elements, and ultimately classify proteins and their role in human development and physiology.

Besides more accurate molecular characterization of disorders with a genetic component, advances catalyzed by the HGP have entered the clinical realm. Treatment specifically geared to an individual's genetic make-up is already being realized in cancer patients and will undoubtedly be expanded to more genetic conditions. Clinical opportunities from the HGP have been achieved in terms of gene-based identification of those with adverse response to drugs and presymptomatic prediction of diseases such as Alzheimer's disease, familial hypercholesteremia, breast and hereditary colorectal cancers, and rheumatologic conditions (Collins et al., 2003; Guttmacher & Collins, 2002).

Technologic advances in automation and computational analysis are occurring rapidly with the HGP. DNA microarray or chip technology has allowed research laboratories to progress from studying single genes over the course of months or years to investigating thousands of genes in a single day (The Chipping Forecast II, 2002; Tobin & Boughton, 2000). It is also one method to determine the DNA sequences of many individuals in an automated, cost effective, and efficient manner. These technologies will further accelerate the pace of DNA sequencing for clinical genetic diagnostics and prediction of disease.

Transgenic mice have been instrumental in understanding the roles that various genes play in normal development, physiology, and behavior (Jorde et al., 2003; Tobin & Boughton, 2000). Over 90% of human genes are represented in the mouse genome, and therefore the mouse is a critical animal model for understanding human genomics. Creating a transgenic mouse involves introducing a specific cloned DNA sequence into embryonic stem cells (cells that have the capability of developing into any of the tissues of the body) that are then placed into mouse embryos. A knockout model is created when a target gene is made nonfunctional, typically by inserting another DNA sequence within it. A multitude of studies can then be done to look at the effects of a gene's absence. Thousands of specific transgenic mouse strains have been created and have been instrumental for investigation of cancer and immunology, neural development and function, body weight regulation, arthritis, and addiction as well as numerous human genetic diseases (NF1, fragile X syndrome, cystic fibrosis, muscular dystrophy, achondroplasia, most of the lysosomal storage disorders, etc.) (Gieselmann et al., 2003). Newer so-called "knock-down" approaches to analyzing gene expression and function consist of introducing RNA inhibitor molecules and other small molecular ligands that inhibit expression of specific genes (Hannon, 2002; Stockwell, 2000). These methods have also entered into human clinical trials (see following discussion) and may have great therapeutic potential.

GENE THERAPY AND GENOMIC MEDICINE

The ultimate goal of the HGP is to translate genomic information or advances into therapeutic health benefits (Collins et al., 2003). Currently, there are numerous active clinical gene therapy trials in the United States, but the majority of these are for noninherited forms of cancer and 10% are for HIV-AIDS. Although gene therapy has been performed experimentally for over 15 years, the technique has met with tremendous challenges such that therapeutic gene therapy is not yet standard medical treatment for any genetic disorder. The obstacles have mainly been in delivery of an effective gene into appropriate target cells, the long-term production of the desired gene product, and the toxicity resulting from certain approaches. In somatic gene therapy or gene transfer, functional genes are inserted into the DNA of somatic cells through the use of a vector delivery system (usually a retrovirus).

In the hemophilias there have been six clinical trials using various gene transfer technologies and all have resulted in limited efficacy albeit low toxicity (Nathwani et al., 2003). Many expected gene therapy to have the most success in the hemophilias given that they result from a single circulating blood protein necessary in only minute amounts. In animal models for the muscular dystrophies, intramuscular injection of viral vectors carrying the normal dystrophin gene has shown the best results in terms of muscle pathology, but total body approaches without a significant immune response have not yet been achieved (Gregorevic & Chamberlain, 2003). The trials and tribulations of clinical gene therapy are illustrated most dramatically in children with sex-linked combined immune deficiency (SCID). Infants with SCID typically die within a year of their first infection unless treated. Conventional gene therapy of infants with SCID resulted in impressive levels of normal immune function in a majority of patients. (The approach involves hematopoietic stem cell isolation from the infant's bone marrow, incubation with retroviral vectors containing the normal version of the gene that causes the disease, and transfusion of cells back into the infant.). This medical breakthrough was later overshadowed by the development of leukemia in two patients, a finding that prompted the Food and Drug Administration to halt 27 clinical gene therapy trials (Kohn et al., 2003). Challenges that lie ahead are calculating the risk/benefit ratios for gene therapy-based interventions.

A novel and potentially powerful treatment approach for genetic disorders is via inhibiting expression from the mutant dominant gene through selective small interfering RNAs (siRNA). This strategy has been shown to be effective in allele-specific silencing of targeted mutant genes in mammalian cell model systems for neurologic disorders such as dystonia, spinocerebellar ataxia type 3, and frontotemporal dementia (Gonzalez-Alegre et al., 2003; Miller et al., 2003). In utero gene therapy approaches are now being investigated in animal models for disorders such as inborn errors of metabolism (Meertens et al., 2002) with goals of gene transfer to multiple tissues and sustained in vivo gene expression during embryonic development and throughout the lifespan. These and other techniques may have clinical ramifications for disorders detected during genetic screening, especially ones that require in utero treatment to prevent dysfunction. Additional genomic therapy strategies consist of genetically engineered biopharmaceuticals such as growth factors and immunologic agents. In multiple sclerosis, in which the blood-brain barrier inhibits the passage of many peripherally delivered drugs, the intracerebral introduction of genes coding for anti-inflammatory and neurotrophic molecules inhibits the destructive immunologic cascade and promotes growth and development of myelin-producing cells (Furlan et al., 2003). Germline gene therapy involves introduction or modification of germ cells so that the altered genome has the potential to be inherited or carried into the next generation. This approach, although not yet utilized in human reproductive medicine, has numerous ethical, legal, and societal implications.

▋ SUMMARY

This is an exciting time for clinicians and researchers working with children with genetic disorders. Our core knowledge of genetic disease etiology has expanded exponentially, and we are charged to keep up with this genomic revolution. Physical therapists are urged to expand their competencies in genetics so that we are able to add to the body of knowledge in diagnostic identification, prognosis, medical management, treatment outcomes, and lifespan issues associated with the various pediatric genetic disorders. Significant research on behavioral and physical development by physical therapy researchers in most of the newly identified genetic disorders is necessary as a foundation for both genetic classification and effective clinical practice. In addition, physical therapists might serve important roles as members of the research teams investigating the potential therapeutic health benefits of future gene therapy trials. Through this integrated approach, our mission of providing best practices for children with genetic disorders will be realized.

▋ REFERENCES

Altafaj, X, Dierssen, M, Baamonde, C, Marti, E, Visa, J, Guimera, J, Oset, M, Gonzalez, JR, Florez, J, Fillat ,C, & Estivill, X. Neurodevelopmental delay, motor abnormalities and cognitive deficits in transgenic mice overexpressing Dyrk1A (minibrain), a murine model of Down's syndrome. Human Molecular Genetics, 10:1915–1923, 2001.

Amir, RE, Van den Veyver, IB, Wan, M, Tran, CQ, Francke, U, & Zoghbi, HY. Rett syndrome is caused by mutations in X-linked MECP2, encoding methyl-CpG-binding protein 2. Nature Genetics, 23:185–188, 1999.

Amir, RE, Van den Veyver, IB, Schultz, R, Malicki, DM, Tran, CQ, Dahle, EJ, Philippi, A, Timar, L, Percy, AK, Motil, KJ, Lichtarge, O, Smith, EO, Glaze, DG, & Zoghbi, HY. Influence of mutation type and X chromosome inactivation on Rett syndrome phenotypes. Annals of Neurology, 47:670–679, 2000.

Ani, C, Grantham-McGregor, S, & Muller, D. Nutritional supplementation in Down syndrome: Theoretical considerations and current status. Developmental Medicine and Child Neurology, 42:207–213, 2000.

Antonarakis, SE. Human chromosome 21: Genome mapping and exploration circa 1993. Trends in Genetics, 9:142–148, 1993.

Antonarakis, SE, Petersen, MB, McInnis, MG, Adelsberger, PA, Schinzel, AA, Binkert, F, Pangalos C, Raoul, O, Slaugenhaupt, SA, Hafez, M, Cohen, MM, Roulson, D, Schwartz, S, Mikkelsen, M, Tranebjaerg, L, Greenberg, F, Hoar, DI, Rudd, NL, Warren, AC, Metaxotou C, Bartsocas, C, & Chakravarti, A. The meiotic stage of nondisjunction in trisomy 21: Determination using DNA polymorphisms. American Journal of Human Genetics, 50:544–550, 1992.

Avellino, AM, Berger, MS, Rostomily, RC, Shaw, CM, & Ojemann, GA. Surgical management and seizure outcome in patients with tuberous sclerosis. Journal of Neurosurgery, 87:391–396, 1997.

Bailey, A, Le Couteur, A, Gottesman, I, Bolton, P, Simonoff, E, Yuzda, E, & Rutter, M. Autism as a strongly genetic disorder: Evidence from a British twin study. Psychological Medicine, 25:63–77, 1995.

Barker, S, Chesney, D, Miedzybrodzka, Z, & Maffulli, N. Genetics and epidemiology in idiopathic congenital talipes equinovarus. Journal of Pediatric Orthopedics, 23:265–272, 2003.

Batch, J. Turner syndrome in childhood and adolescence. Best Practice and Research in Clinical Endocrinology and Metabolism, 16:465–482, 2002.

Baty, BJ, Jorde, LB, Blackburn, BL, & Carey, JC. Natural history of trisomy 18 and trisomy 13: I. Growth, physical assessment, medical histories, survival and recurrence risk. American Journal of Medical Genetics, 49:175–188, 1994a.

Baty, BJ, Jorde, LB, Blackburn, BL, & Carey, JC. Natural history of trisomy 18 and trisomy 13: II. Psychomotor development. American Journal of Medical Genetics, 49:189–194, 1994b.

Berneburg, M, & Lehmann, AR. Xeroderma pigmentosum and related disorders: Defects in DNA repair and transcription. Advances in Genetics, 43:71–102,2001.

Boddaert, N, Klein, O, Ferguson, N, Sonigo, P, Parisot, D, Hertz-Pannier, L, Baraton, J, Emond, S, Simon, I, Chigot, V, Schmit, P, Pierre-Kahn, A, & Brunelle, F. Intellectual prognosis of the Dandy-Walker malformation in children: The importance of vermian lobulation. Neuroradiology, 45:320–324, 2003 (e-pub).

Boer, H, Holland, A, Whittington, J, Butler, J, Webb, T, & Clarke, D. Psychotic illness in people with Prader Willi syndrome due to chromosome 15 maternal uniparental disomy. Lancet 359:135–136, 2002.

Botto, LD, Moore, CA, Khoury, MJ, & Erikson, JD. Neural tube defects. New England Journal of Medicine, 341:1509–1519, 1999.

Boyd, SG, Hardenc, A, & Patton, MA. The EEG in early diagnosis of the Angelman (happy puppet) syndrome. European Journal of Pediatrics, 147:508–513, 1988.

Brandt, VL, & Zoghbi, HY. Rett Syndrome. Gene Reviews, 2001; accessed at www.genetest.org.

Budden, SS. Rett syndrome: Habilitation and management reviewed. European Child and Adolescent Psychiatry, 6(Suppl 1):103–107, 1997.

Budden, SS, & Gunness, ME. Bone histomorphometry in three females with Rett syndrome. Brain Development, 23:S133–137, 2001.

Buntinx, IM, Hennekam, RCM, Brouwer, O, Stroink, H, Beuten, J, Mangelschots, K, & Fryns JP. Clinical profile of Angelman syndrome at different ages. American Journal of Medical Genetics, 56:176–183, 1995.

Burger, J, Horn, D, Tonnies, H, Neitzel, H, & Reis, A. Familial interstitial 570 kbp deletion of the UBE3A gene region causing Angelman syndrome but not Prader-Willi syndrome. American Journal of Medical Genetics, 111:233–237, 2002.

Butler, MG. Prader-Willi syndrome: Current understanding of cause and diagnosis. American Journal of Medical Genetics, 35: 319–332, 1990.

Cardoso, C, Leventer, RJ, Dowling, JJ,& Ledbetter, DH. Clinical and molecular basis of classical lissencephaly: Mutations in the LIS1 gene (PAFAH1B1). Human Mutation, 19:4–15, 2002.

Cardoso, C, Leventer, RJ, Ward, HL, Toyo-Oka, K, Chung, J, Gross, A, Martin, CL, Allanson, J, Pilz, DT, Olney, AH, Mutchinick, OM, Hirotsune, S, Wynshaw-Boris, A, Dobyns, WB, & Ledbetter, DH. Refinement of a 400-kb critical region allows genotypic differentiation between isolated lissencephaly, Miller-Dieker syndrome, and other phenotypes secondary to deletions of 17p13.3. American Journal of Human Genetics, 72:918–930, 2003 (e-pub).

Carey, JC. Health supervision and anticipatory guidance for children with genetic disorders (including specific recommendations for trisomy 21, trisomy 18, and neurofibromatosis I). Pediatric Clinics of North America, 39:25–53, 1992.

Carpenter, NJ. Molecular cytogenetics. Seminars in Pediatric Neurology, 8:135–146, 2001.

Cassidy, SB, & Schwartz, S. Prader-Willi and Angelman syndromes: Disorders of genomic imprinting. Medicine, 77:140–151, 1998.

Cassidy, SB. Genetics of Prader-Willi syndrome. In Greenswag and Alexander (Eds.). Management of Prader-Willi Syndrome, 2nd ed. New York: Springer-Verlag, 1995.

Cassidy, SB, & Morris, CA. Behavioral phenotypes in genetic syndromes: Genetic clues to human behavior. Advances in Pediatrics, 49:59–86, 2002.

Cassidy, SB, & Schwartz, S. Prader-Willi syndrome. In Gene Reviews, 2003; accessed at www.genetests.org.

Cheadle, JP, Gill, H, Fleming, N, Maynard, J, Kerr, A, Leonard, H, Krawczak, M, Cooper, DN, Lynch, S, Thomas, N, Hughes, H, Hulten, M, Ravine, D, Sampson, JR, & Clarke, A. Long-read sequence analysis of the MECP2 gene in Rett syndrome patients: Correlation of disease severity with mutation type and location. Human Molecular Genetics, 9:1119–1129, 2000.

Cheon, MS, Kim, SH, Yaspo, ML, Blasi, F, Aoki, Y, Melen, K, & Lubec, G. Protein levels of genes encoded on chromosome 21 in fetal Down syndrome brain: Challenging the gene dosage effect hypothesis (Part I). Amino Acids, 24:111–117, 2003a.

Cheon, MS, Kim, SH, Ovod, V, Kopitar Jerala, N, Morgan, JI, Hatefi, Y, Ijuin, T, Takenawa, T, & Lubec, G. Protein levels of genes encoded on chromosome 21 in fetal Down syndrome brain: Challenging the gene dosage effect hypothesis (Part III). Amino Acids, 24:127–134, 2003b.

Chichowski, K & Jacks, T. NF1 tumor suppressor in the nervous system. Experimental Cell Research, 264:19–28, 2001.

Clarke, DJ, Boer, H, Whittington, J, Holland, A, Butler, J, & Webb, T. Prader-Willi syndrome, compulsive and ritualistic behaviors: The first population-based survey. British Journal of Psychiatry, 180:358–362, 2002.

Clayton-Smith, J. Clinical research on Angelman syndrome in the United Kingdom: Observations on 82 affected individuals. American Journal of Medical Genetics, 46:12–15, 1993.

Coleman, M, Brubaker, J, Hunter, K, & Smith, G. Rett syndrome: A survey of North American patients. Journal of Mental Deficiency Research, 32:117–124, 1988.

Collins, MS, & Cornish, K. A survey of the prevalence of stereotypy, self-injury and aggression in children and young adults with cri du chat syndrome. Journal of Intellectual Disabilities Research, 46:133–140, 2002.

Collins, FS, Green, ED, Guttmacher, AE, & Guyer, MS. A vision for the future of genomics research. Nature, 422:1–13, 2003.

Cornish, KM, & Pigram, J. Developmental and behavioural characteristics of cri du chat syndrome. Archives of Diseases in Childhood, 75:448–450, 1996.

Cornish, KM, Bramble, D, Munir, F, & Pigram, J. Cognitive functioning in children with typical cri du chat (5p-) syndrome. Developmental Medicine and Child Neurology, 41:263–266, 1999.

Costa, RM, & Silva, AJ. Molecular and cellular mechanisms underlying the cognitive deficits associated with neurofibromatosis. Journal of Child Neurology, 8:27–29, 622–626, 646–651, 2002.

Couvert, P, Bienvenu, T, Aquaviva, C, Poirier, K, Moraine, C, Gendrot, C, Verloes, A, Andres, C, Le Fevre, AC, Souville, I, Steffann, J, des Portes, V, Ropers, HH, Yntema, HG, Fryns, JP, Briault, S, Chelly, J, & Cherif, B. MECP2 is highly mutated in X-linked mental retardation. Human Molecular Genetics, 10:941–946, 2001.

Cox, GF, Burger, J, Lip, V, Mau, UA, Sperling, K, Wu, BL, & Horsthemke, B. Intracytoplasmic sperm injection may increase the risk of imprinting defects. American Journal of Human Genetics 71:162–164, 2002.

Crunnelli, V, & Leresche, N. Childhood absence epilepsy: Genes, channels, neurons and networks. Nat Rev Neuroscience, 3:371–381, 2002.

Curatolo, P, Cusmai, R, Cortesi, F, Chiron, C, Jambaque, I, & Dulac, O. Neuropsychiatric aspects of tuberous sclerosis. Annals of the New York Academy of Science, 615:8–16, 1991.

Dasgupta, B, & Gutmann, DH. Neurofibromatosis 1: Closing the GAP between mice and men. Current Opinions in Genetic Development, 13:20–27, 2003.

Delabar, JM, Theophile, D, Rahmani, Z, Chettouh, Z, Blouin, JL, Prieur, M, Noel, B, & Sinet, PM. Molecular mapping of twenty-four features of Down syndrome on chromosome 21. European Journal of Human Genetics, 1:114–124, 1993.

DeLorey, TM, Handforth, A, Anagnostaras, SG, Homanics, GE, Minassian, BA, Asatourian, A, Fanselow, MS, Delgado-Escueta, A, Ellison, GD, & Olsen, RW. Mice lacking the beta3 subunit of the GABAA receptor have the epilepsy phenotype and many of the behavioral characteristics of Angelman syndrome. Journal of Neurosciences, 18:8505–8514, 1998.

des Portes, V, Pinard, JM, Billuart, P, Vinet, MC, Koulakoff, A, Carrie, A, Gelot, A, Dupuis, E, Motte, J, Berwald-Netter, Y, Catala, M, Kahn, A, Beldjord, C, & Chelly, J. A novel CNS gene required for neuronal migration and involved in X-linked subcortical laminar heterotopia and lissencephaly syndrome. Cell, 92:51–61, 1998.

Dietz, F. The genetics of idiopathic clubfoot. Clinical Orthopedics, 401:39–48, 2002.

Dobyns, WB. Absence makes the search grow longer (editorial). American Journal of Human Genetics, 58:7–16, 1996.

Dobyns, WB, Elias, ER, Newlin, AC, Pagon, RA, & Ledbetter, DH. Causal heterogeneity in isolated lissencephaly. Neurology, 42:1375–1388, 1992.

Dobyns, WB, & Truwit, CL. Lissencephaly and other genetic neuronal migration disorders. From the Lissencephaly Network, Inc., Fort Wayne, Ind., 2001. epub accessed at www.lissencephaly.org

Ducy, P, & Karsenty, G. The family of bone morphogenetic proteins. Kidney International, 57:2207–2214, 2000.

Dunn, HG, & MacLeod, PM. Rett syndrome: review of biological abnormalities. Canadian Journal of Neurologic Science, 28:16–29, 2001.

Dykens, EM, & Clarke, DJ. Correlates of maladaptive behavior in individuals with 5p- (cri du chat) syndrome. Developmental Medicine and Child Neurology, 39:752–756, 1997.

Epstein, CJ. Down syndrome, trisomy 21. In Scriver, CR, Beaudet, AL, Sly, WS, Valle, D (Eds.). Metabolic Basis of Inherited Disease. New York: McGraw-Hill, 1989, pp. 291–326.

Epstein, CJ. The new dysmorphology: application of insights from basic developmental biology to the understanding of human birth defects. Proceedings of the National Academy of Sciences USA, 92:8566–8573, 1995.

Ewart, AK, Morris, CA, Ensing, GJ, Loker, J, Moore, C, Leppert, M, & Keating, M. A human vascular disorder, supravalvular aortic stenosis, maps to chromosome 7. Proceedings of the National Academy of Sciences USA, 90:3226–3320, 1993.

Flint, J, & Knight, S. The use of telomere probes to investigate submicroscopic rearrangements associated with mental retardation. Current Opinion in Genetic Development, 13:310–316, 2003.

Flores-Sarnat, L. New insights into craniosynostosis. Seminars in Pediatric Neurology, 9:274–291, 2002

Frangiskakis, JM, Ewart, AK, Morris, CA, Mervis, CB, Bertrand, J, Robinson, BF, Klein, BP, Ensing, GJ, Everett, LA, Green, ED, Proschel, C, Gutowski, NJ, Noble, M, Atkinson, DL, Odelberg, SJ, & Keating, MT. LIM-kinase1 hemizygosity implicated in impaired visuospatial constructive cognition. Cell, 86:59–69, 1996.

Francis-West, PH, Robson, L, & Evans, DJ. Craniofacial development: The tissue and molecular interactions that control development of the head. Advances in Anatomy, Embryology, and Cell Biology, 169:III–VI, 1–138, 2003.

Franke, P, Maier, W, Hautzinger, M, Weiffenbach, O, Gansicke, M, Iwers, B, Poustka, F, Schwab, SG, & Froster, U. Fragile-X carrier females: Evidence for a distinct psychopathological phenotype? American Journal of Medical Genetics 64:334–339, 1996.

Fong, CT, & Brodeur, GM. Down's syndrome and leukemia: Epidemiology, genetics, cytogenetics and mechanisms of leukemogenesis. Cancer Genetics and Cytogenetics, 28:55–76, 1987.

Friedman, JM. Neurofibromatosis 1. 2003. GeneReviews. http//www.genetests.org/

Friedman, JM, & Birch, PM. Type 1 Neurofibromatosis: a descriptive analysis of the disorder in 1,728 patients. American Journal of Medical Genetics, 70:138–143, 1997.

Friedman, JM, & Riccardi, VM. Clinical epidemiological features. In Friedman, JM, Gutman, DH, Mac Collin, M, & Riccardi, VM (Eds.). Neurofibromatosis: Phenotype, Natural History, and Pathogenesis. John Hopkins University Press, Baltimore, 1999, pp 29–86.

Friocourt, G, Koulakoff, A, & Chafey, P, Boucher, D, Fauchereau, F, Chelly, J, & Francis, F. Doublecortin functions at the extremities of growing neuronal processes. Cerebral Cortex, 13:620–626, 2003.

Fu, Y-H, Kuhl, DPA, Pizzuti, A, Pieretti, M, Sutcliffe, JS, Richards, S, Verkerk, AJMH, Holden, JJA, Fenwick, RG, Jr., Warren, ST, Oostra, BA, Nelson, DL, & Caskey, CT. Variation of the CGG repeat at the fragile X site results in genetic instability: Resolution of the Sherman paradox. Cell, 67:1047–1058, 1991.

Furlan, R, Pluchino, S, & Martino, G. The therapeutic use of gene therapy in inflammatory demyelinating diseases of the central nervous system. Current Opinion in Neurology, 16:385–392, 2003.

Gieselmann, V, Matzner, U, Klein, D, Mansson, JE, D'Hooge, R, DeDeyn, PD, Lullmann, Rauch, R, Hartmann, D, & Harzer, K. Gene therapy: Prospects for glycolipid storage diseases. Philosophical Transactions of the Royal Society of London Series B Biological Sciences, 358: 921–925, 2003.

Glaser, B, Hessl, D, Dyer-Friedman, J, Johnston, C, Wisbeck, J, Taylor, A, & Reiss, A. Biological and environmental contributions to adaptive behavior in fragile X syndrome. American Journal of Medical Genetics, 117:21–29, 2003.

Gonzalez-Alegre, P, Miller, VM, Davidson, BL, & Paulson, HL. Toward therapy for DYT1 dystonia: Allele-specific silencing of mutant TorsinA. Annals of Neurology, 53:781–787, 2003.

Gosch, A, Stading, G, & Pankau, R. Linguistic abilities in children with Williams-Beuren syndrome. American Journal of Medical Genetics, 52: 291–296, 1994.

Greenough, WT, Klintsova, AY, Irwin, SA, Galvez, R, Bates, KE, & Weiler, IJ. Synaptic regulation of protein synthesis and the fragile X protein. Proceedings of the National Academy of Sciences, 98: 7101–7106, 2001.

Gregorevic, P, & Chamberlain, JS. Gene therapy for muscular dystrophy—A review of promising progress. Expert Opinion in Biological Therapy, 3:803–814, 2003.

Gulesserian, T, Seidl, R, Hardmeier, R, Cairns, N, & Lubec, G. Superoxide dismutase SOD1, encoded on chromosome 21, but not SOD2 is overexpressed in brains of patients with Down syndrome. Journal of Investigative Medicine, 49:41–46, 2001

Gutierrez, GC, Smalley, SL, & Tanguay, PE. Autism in tuberous sclerosis complex. Journal of Autism Developmental Disorders, 28:97–103, 1998.

Gunay-Aygun, M, Schwartz, S, Heeger, S, O'Riordan, MA, & Cassidy, SB. The changing purpose of Prader-Willi syndrome clinical diagnostic criteria and proposed revised criteria. Pediatrics, 108:e92, 2001 (electronic article).

Guttmacher, AE, & Collins, FS. Genomic medicine—A primer. New England Journal of Medicine, 347:1512–1220, 2002.

Hagberg, B. Clinical delineation of Rett syndrome variants. Neuropediatrics, 26:62, 1995.

Hagberg, B, Aicardi, J, Dias, K, & Ramos, O. A progressive syndrome of autism, dementia, ataxia, and loss of purposeful hand use in girls: Rett's syndrome: Report of 35 cases. Annals of Neurology, 14: 471–479, 1983.

Hagerman, RJ. Physical and behavioral phenotype. In Hagerman, RJ, Cronister, A (Eds.). Fragile X Syndrome: Diagnosis, Treatment and Research, 2nd ed. Baltimore: The Johns Hopkins University Press, 1996, pp. 3–87.

Hammond, LS, Macias, MM, Tarleton, JC, & Shashidhar Pai, G. Fragile X syndrome and deletions in FMR1: New case and review of the literature. American Journal of Medical Genetics, 72:430–434, 1997.

Hannon, GJ. RNA interference. Nature, 418: 244–251, 2002.

Higurashi, M, Oda, M, Iijima, K, Iijima, S, Takeshita, T, Watanabe, N, &Yoneyama, K. Livebirth prevalence and follow-up of malformation syndromes in 27,472 newborns. Brain Development, 12:770–773, 1990.

Hirose, S, Mohney, RP, Okada, M, Kaneko, S, & Mitsudome, A. The genetics of febrile seizures and related epilepsy syndromes. Brain Development, 25:304–312, 2003.

Hsu, LYF. Prenatal diagnosis of chromosomal abnormalities through amniocentesis. In Milunsky, A (Ed.). Genetic Disorders and the Fetus, 4th ed. Baltimore: John Hopkins University Press, 1998, pp. 179–248.

Hunt, A, & Dennis, J. Psychiatric disorder among children with tuberous sclerosis. Developmental Medicine and Child Neurology, 29:190–198, 1987.

Huson, SM. Neurofibromatosis 1: A clinical and genetic overview. In Husob, SM, & Hughes, RAC (Eds.). The Neurofibromatoses: A Pathogenetic and Clinical Overview. London: Chapman and Hall Medical, 1994, pp. 160–203.

Hwang, SJ, Beaty, TH, McIntosh. I, Hefferon, T, & Panny, SR. Association between homeobox-containing gene MSX1 and the occurrence of limb deficiency. American Journal of Medical Genetics, 75:419–423, 1998.

Jabs, EW, Muller, U, Li, X, Ma, L, Luo, W, Haworth, IS, Klisak, I, Sparkes, R, Warman, ML, Mulliken, JB, Snead, ML, & Maxson, R. A mutation in the homeodomain of the human MSX2 gene in a family affected with autosomal dominant craniosynostosis. Cell, 75:443–450, 1993.

Jacobs, PA, Browne, C, Gregson, N, Joyce, C, & White, H. Estimates of the frequency of chromosome abnormalities detectable in unselected newborns using moderate levels of banding. Journal of Medical Genetics, 29:103–108, 1992.

Jiang, Y, Armstrong, D, Albrecht, U, Atkins, CM, Noebels, JL, Eichele, G, Sweatt, JD, & Beaudet, AL. Mutation of the Angelman ubiquitin ligase in mice causes increased cytoplasmic p53 and deficits of contextual learning and long-term potentiation. Neuron, 21:799–811, 1998.

Jinnah, HA, & Friedmann, T. Lesch-Nyhan disease and its variants. In Scriver, CR, Beaudet, AL, Sly, WS, & Valle, D. (Eds.). The Metabolic & Molecular Bases of Inherited Disease. Vol. II. 8th ed. New York: McGraw-Hill, 2001, p. 2537.

Johnston, MV. Movement disorders. In Behrman, RE, Kliegman, RM, & Jenson, HB (Eds.). Nelson Textbook of Pediatrics, 17th ed. Philadelphia: W.B. Saunders Co., 2004, pp. 2022–2023.

Johnston, MV, & Kinsman, S. Congenital anomalies of the central nervous system. In Behrman, RE, Kliegman, RM, & Jenson, HB (Eds.). Nelson Textbook of Pediatrics, 17th ed. Philadelphia: W.B. Saunders Co., 2004, pp. 1983–1993.

Jones, KL. (Ed.). Smith's Recognizable Patterns of Human Malformation, 5th ed. Philadelphia: W.B. Saunders Co., 1997, pp. 1–7, 8–14, 38–39, 64–65, 771–844.

Jones, KL. Dysmorphology. In Behrman, RE, Kliegman, RM, & Jenson, HB (Eds.). Nelson Textbook of Pediatrics, 17th ed. Philadelphia: W.B. Saunders Co., 2004, pp. 616–623.

Jorde, LB, Carey, JC, Bamshad, MJ, & White, RL. Medical Genetics, 3rd ed. St Louis: Mosby, 2003.

Jugessur, A, Lie, RT, Wilcox, AJ, Murray, JC, Taylor, JA, Saugstad, OD, Vindenes, HA, & Abyholm, F. Variants of developmental genes (TGFA, TGFB3, and MSX1) and their associations with orofacial clefts: A case-parent triad analysis. Genetics and Epidemiology, 24:230–239, 2003.

Kaplan, P, Kirschner, M, Watters, G, & Costa, MT. Contractures in patients with Williams syndrome. Pediatrics, 84:895–899, 1989.

Kau, AS, Meyer, WA, & Kaufmann, WE. Early development in males with fragile X syndrome: A review of the literature. Microscopy Research and Technology, 57:174–178, 2002.

Kayl, AE, & Moore, BD, 3rd. Behavioral phenotype of neurofibromatosis, type 1. Mental Retardation Developmental Disabilities Review, 6:117–124, 2000.

Kerr, AM. Early clinical signs in the Rett disorder. Neuropediatrics, 26:67–71, 1995.

Knight, SJ, & Flint, J. Perfect endings: A review of subtelomeric probes and their use in clinical diagnosis. Journal of Medical Genetics, 37:401–409, 2000.

Knight, SJ, Regan, R, Nicod, A, Horsley, SW, Kearney, L, Homfray, T, Winter, RM, Bolton, P, & Flint, J. Subtle chromosomal rearrangements in children with unexplained mental retardation. Lancet, 354:1676–1681, 1999.

Knight, SJL, Lese, CM, Precht, K, Kuc, J, Ning, Y, Lucas, S, Regan, R, Brenan, M, Nicod, A, Martin Lawrie, N, Cardy, DLN, Nguyen, H, Hudson, TJ, Riethman, H, Ledbetter, DH, & Flint, J. An optimized set of human telomere clones for studying telomere integrity and architecture. American Journal of Human Genetics, 67:320–332, 2000.

Kohn, DB, Sadelain, M, & Glorioso, JC. Occurrence of leukaemia following gene therapy of X-linked SCID. Nature Reviews Cancer, 3:477–488, 2003.

Korenberg, JR, Chen, XN, Schipper, R, Sun, Z, Gonsky, R, Gerwehr, S, Carpenter, N, Daumer, C, Dignan, P, Disteche, C, Graham, JM, Jr., Hugdins, L, McGillivray, B, Miyazaki, K, Ogasawara, N, Park, J P, Pagon, R, Pueschel, S, Sack, G, Say, B, Schuffenhauer, S, Soukup, S, & Yamanaka, T. Down syndrome phenotypes: The consequences of chromosomal imbalance. Proceedings of the National Academy of Sciences, 91:4997–5001, 1994.

Lachiewicz, AM, Dawson, DV, & Spiridigliozzi, GA. Physical characteristics of young boys with fragile X syndrome: Reasons for difficulties in making a diagnosis in young males. American Journal of Medical Genetics, 92:229–236, 2000.

Lejeune, J, Lafourcade, J, Berger, R, Vialatta, J, Boeswillwald, M, Seringe, P, & Turpin, R. Trois ca de deletion partielle du bras court d'un chromosome 5. Comptes Rendus de l'Academie des Sciences (Paris), 257:3098, 1963.

Long, TM, Brady, R, & Lapham, EV. A survey of genetics knowledge of health professionals: Implications for physical therapists. Pediatric Physical Therapy, 13:156–163, 2001.

Lo Nigro, C, Chong, SS, Smith, ACM, Dobyns, WB, Carrozzo, R, & Ledbetter, DH. Point mutations and an intragenic deletion in LIS1, the lissencephaly causative gene in isolated lissencephaly sequence and Miller-Dieker syndrome. Human Molecular Genetics, 6:157–164, 1997.

Mark, M, Rijli, FM, & Chambon, P. Homeobox genes in embryogenesis-pathogenesis. Pediatric Research, 42:421–429, 1997.

Matsuura, T, Sutcliffe, JS, Fang, P, Galjaard, RJ, Jiang, Y, Benton, CS, Rommens, JM, & Beaudet, AL. De novo truncating mutations in E6-AP ubiquitin-protein ligase gene (UBE3A) in Angelman syndrome. Nature Genetics, 15:74–77, 1997.

Mazzoni, DS, Ackley, RS, & Nash, DJ. Abnormal pinna type and hearing loss correlations in Down's syndrome. Journal of Intellectual Disabilities Research, 38:549–560, 1994.

McMahon, AP. More surprises in the Hedgehog signaling pathway. Cell, 100:185–188, 2000.

McIntosh, I, Bellus, GA, & Jabs, EW. The pleiotropic effects of fibroblast growth factor receptors in mammalian development. Cell Structure and Function, 25:85–96, 2000.

McKusick, VA. Mendelian Inheritance in Man. Catalogs of Human Genes and Genetic Disorders, 12th ed. Baltimore: Johns Hopkins University Press, 1998.

Medina, M, Marinescu, RC, Overhauser, J, & Kosik KS. Hemizygosity of delta-catenin (CTNND2) is associated with severe mental retardation in cri-du-chat syndrome. Genomics, 63:157–164, 2000.

Meertens, L, Zhao, Y, Rosic-Kablar, S, Li, L, Chan, K, Dobson, H, Gartley, C, Lutzko, C, Hopwood, J, Kohn, D, Kruth, S, Hough, MR, & Dube, ID. In utero injection of alpha-l-iduronidase-carrying retrovirus in canine mucopolysaccharidosis type I: Infection of multiple tissues and neonatal gene expression. Human Gene Therapy, 13:1809–1820, 2002.

Mervis, CB, & Klein-Tasman, BP. Williams syndrome: Cognition, personality, and adaptive behavior. Mental Retardation Developmental Disabilities Research Reviews, 6:148–158, 2000.

Mervis, CB, Morris, CA, & Bertrand, J. Williams syndrome: Findings from an integrated program of research. In Tager-Flusberg, H (Ed.). Neurodevelopmental Disorders. Cambridge, MA: MIT Press, 1998, pp. 65–110.

Meryash, DL, & Abuelo, D. Counseling needs and attitudes toward prenatal diagnosis and abortion in fragile X families. Clinical Genetics, 33:349–355, 1988.

Miller, JR. The Wnts. Genome Biology, *3*:1–15, 2001.

Miller, VM, Xia, H, Marrs, GL, Gouvion, CM, Lee, G, Davidson, BL, & Paulson, HL. Allele-specific silencing of dominant disease genes. Proceedings of the National Academy of Sciences USA, *100*:7195–7200, 2003.

Mikkelsen, M. Down's syndrome: Cytogenetic epidemiology. Hereditas, 86:45–59, 1977.

Minassian, BA, Sainz, J, & Delgado-Escueta, AV. Genetics of myoclonic and myoclonus epilepsies. Clinical Neuroscience, *3*:223–235, 1995–1996.

Moore, BD, 3rd, Slopis, JM, Jackson, EF, De Winter, AE, & Leeds, NE. Brain volume in children with neurofibromatosis type 1: Relation to neuropsychological status. Neurology, 54:914–920, 2000.

Morris, CA, Demsey, SA, Leonard, CO, Dilts, C, & Blackburn, BL. Natural history of Williams syndrome: Physical characteristics. Journal of Pediatrics, *113*:318–326, 1988.

Morris, CA. Williams syndrome. Gene Reviews, 2003; accessed at www.genetests.org.

Nance, MA. Clinical aspects of CAG repeat diseases. Brain Pathology, 7:881–900, 1997.

Nathwani, AC, Nienhuis, AW, & Davidoff, AM. Current status of gene therapy for hemophilia. Current Hematology Reports, *2*:319–327, 2003.

Nelson, K, & Holmes, LB. Malformations due to presumed spontaneous mutations in newborn infants. New England Journal of Medicine, *320*:19–23, 1989.

Netto, CB, Siqueira, IR, Fochesatto, C, Portela, LV, da Purificacao Tavares, M, Souza, DO, Giugliani, R, & Goncalves, CA. S100B content and SOD activity in amniotic fluid of pregnancies with Down syndrome. Clinical Biochemistry, *37*:134–137, 2004.

Nolin, SL, Lewis, FA, 3rd, Ye, LL, Houck, GE, Jr., Glicksman, AE, Limprasert, P, Li, SY, Zhong, N, Ashley, AE, Feingold, E, Sherman, SL, & Brown, WT. Familial transmission of the FMR1 CGG repeat. American Journal of Human Genetics, 59:1252–1261, 1996.

North, K. Cognitive function and academic performance. In Friedman, JM, Gutmna, DH, Mac Collin, & M, Riccardi, VM (Eds.). Neurofibromatosis: Phenotype, Natural History, and Pathogenesis. Baltimore: John Hopkins University Press, 1999, pp. 162–189.

Northrup, H, & Au, KS. Tuberous sclerosis complex. Gene Clinics, 2002; accessed at http//www.geneclinics.org/.

Nussbaum, RL, McInnes, RR, & Willard, HF. Genetics in Medicine, 6th ed. Philadelphia: W.B. Saunders Co., 2001.

Ogata, T. SHOX haploinsufficiency and its modifying factors. Journal of Pediatric Endocrinology and Metabolism, *15*(Suppl 5):1289–1294, 2002.

Online Mendelian Inheritance in Man, OMIM. McKusick-Nathans Institute for Genetic Medicine, Johns Hopkins University (Baltimore, MD) and National Center for Biotechnology Information, National Library of Medicine (Bethesda, MD), 2000. World Wide Web URL: http://www.ncbi.nlm.nih.gov/omim/.

Oostra, BA, & Chiurazzi, P. The fragile X gene and its function. Clinical Genetics, *60*:399–408, 2001.

Opitz, JM, & Sutherland, GR. International workshop on the fragile X and X-linked mental retardation. American Journal of Medical Genetics, *17*:5–94, 1984.

Orrico, A, Lam, C, Galli, L, Dotti, MT, Hayek, G, Tong, SF, Poon, PM, Zappella, M, Federico, A, & Sorrentino, V. MECP2 mutation in male patients with non-specific X-linked mental retardation. FEBS Letters, *481*:285–288, 2000.

Orstavik, KH, Eiklid, K, van der Hagen, CB, Spetalen, S, Kierulf, K, Skjeldal, O, & Buiting, K. Another case of imprinting defect in a girl with Angelman syndrome who was conceived by intracytoplasmic sperm injection (letter). American Journal of Human Genetics, *72*:218–219, 2003.

Osborne, JP, Fryer, A, & Webb, D. Epidemiology of tuberous sclerosis. Annals of the New York Academy of Sciences, *615*:125–127, 1991.

Ottman, R. Progress in the genetics of the partial epilepsies. Epilepsia, *42*(S5):24–30, 2001.

Pankau, R, Gosch, A, & Wessel, A. Radioulnar synostosis in Williams-Beuren syndrome: A component manifestation (letter). American Journal of Medical Genetics, *45*:783, 1993.

Pastore, A, Tozzi, G, Gaeta, LM, Giannotti, A, Bertini, E, Federici, G, Digilio, MC, & Piemonte, F. Glutathione metabolism and antioxidant enzymes in children with Down syndrome. Journal of Pediatrics, *142*:583–585, 2003.

Peters, C, Shapiro, EG, Anderson, J, Henslee-Downey, PJ, Klemperer, MR, Cowan, MJ, Saunders, EF, deAlarcon, PA, Twist, C, Nachman, JB, Hale, GA, Harris, RE, Rozans, MK, Kurtzberg, J, Grayson, GH, Williams, TE, Lenarsky, C, Wagner, JE, & Krivit, W. Hurler syndrome: II. Outcome of HLA-genotypically identical sibling and HLA-haploidentical related donor bone marrow transplantation in fifty-four children. The Storage Disease Collaborative Study Group. Blood, *91*:2601–2608, 1998.

Ranke, MB, & Saenger, P. Turner's syndrome. Lancet, *358*:309–314, 2001.

Rasmussen, SA, Wong, LY, Yang, Q, May, KM, & Friedman, JM. Population-based analyses of mortality in trisomy 13 and trisomy 18. Pediatrics, *111*:777–784, 2003.

Reiss, AL, Aylward, E, Freund, LS, Joshi, PK, & Bryan, RN. Neuroanatomy of fragile X syndrome: The posterior fossa. Annals of Neurology, *29*:26–32, 1991a.

Reiss, AL, Freund, L, Tseng, JE, & Joshi, PK. Neuroanatomy in fragile X females: The posterior fossa. American Journal of Human Genetics, *49*:279–288, 1991b.

Reiss, AL, Lee, J, & Freund, L. Neuroanatomy of fragile X syndrome: The temporal lobe. Neurology, *44*:1317–1324, 1994.

Rett, A. Ueber ein eigenartiges hirnatrophisches Syndrom bei Hyperammoniamie in Kindesalter. Wien Medizinische Wochenschrift, *116*:723–738, 1966.

Rett, A. Rett syndrome: History and general overview. American Journal of Medical Genetics, *1*:21–25, 1986.

Riddle, JE, Cheema, A, Sobesky, WE, Gardner, SC, Taylor, AK, Pennington, BF, & Hagerman, RJ. Phenotypic involvement in females with the FMR1 gene mutation. American Journal of Mental Retardation, *102*:590–601, 1998.

Roach, ES, Gomez, MR, & Northrup, H. Tuberous sclerosis complex consensus conference: Revised clinical diagnostic criteria. Journal of Child Neurology, *13*:624–628, 1998.

Robb, SA, Pohl, K, RE, Baraitser, M, Wilson, J, & Brett, EM. The 'happy puppet' syndrome of Angelman: Review of the clinical features. Archives of Disease in Childhood, *64*:83–86, 1989.

Rolf, C, & Nieschlag, E. Reproductive functions, fertility and genetic risks of ageing men. Experimental Clinical Endocrinology and Diabetes, *109*:68–74, 2001.

Ross, JL. The adult consequences of pediatric endocrine disease II. Turner syndrome. Growth, Genetics, and Hormones, *17*:1–8, 2001.

Rosser, TL, & Packer, RJ. Neurocognitive dysfunction in children with neurofibromatosis type 1. Current Neurology and Neuroscience Report, *3*:129–136, 2003.

Rousseau, F, Heitz, D, Tarleton, J, MacPherson, J, Malmgren, H, Dahl, N, Barnicoat, A, Mathew, C, Mornet, E, Tejada, I, Maddalena, A, Spiegel, R, Schinzel, A, Marcos, JAG, Schorderet, DF, Schaap, T, Maccioni, L, Russo, S, Jacobs, PA, Schwartz, C, Mandel, JL. A multicenter study on genotype-phenotype correlations in the fragile X syndrome, using direct diagnosis with probe StB12.3: The first 2,253 cases. American Journal of Human Genetics, *55*:225–237, 1994.

Sanger, WG, Dave, B, & Stuberg, W. Overview of genetics and role of the pediatric physical therapist in the diagnostic process. Pediatric Physical Therapy, *13*:164–168, 2001.

Sampson, JR, Scahill, SJ, Stephenson, JB, Mann, L, & Connor, JM. Genetic aspects of tuberous sclerosis in the west of Scotland. Journal of Medical Genetics, *26*:28–31, 1989.

Schaefer, GB. Clinical genetics in pediatric physical therapy practice? The future. Pediatric Physical Therapy, *13*:182–184, 2001.

Schanen, NC, Kurczynski, TW, Brunelle, D, Woodcock, MM, Dure, LS, 4th, & Percy, AK. Neonatal encephalopathy in two boys in families with recurrent Rett syndrome. Journal of Child Neurology, *13*:229–231, 1998.

Scriver, CR, Sly, WS, Childs, B, Beaudet, AL, Valle, D, Kinzler, KW, Vogelstein, B (Eds.). The Metabolic and Molecular Bases of Inherited Disease. New York: McGraw Hill,. 2000.

Shen, MH, Harper, PS, & Upadhyaya, M. Molecular genetics of neurofibromatosis type 1 (NF1). Journal of Medical Genetics, *33*:2–17, 1996.

Shepherd, CW, Gomez, MR, Lie, JT, & Crowson, CS. Causes of death in patients with tuberous sclerosis. Mayo Clinic Proceedings, *66*:792–796, 1991.

Shevell, MI. Clinical and diagnostic profile of agenesis of the corpus callosum. Journal of Child Neurology, *17*:896–900, 2002.

Shevell, M, Ashwall, S, Donley, D, Flint, J, Gingold, M, Hirtz, D, Majnemer, A, Noetxel, M, & Sheth, RD. Practice parameter: evaluation of the child with global developmental delay: Report of the Quality Standards Subcommittee of the American Academy of Neurology and the Practice Committee of the Child Neurology Society, Quality Standards Subcommittee of the American Academy of Neurology and the Practice Committee of the Child Neurology Society, 2003.

Simmons, AD, Puschel, AW, McPherson, JD, Overhauser, J, & Lovett, M. Molecular cloning and mapping of human semaphorin F from the cri-du-chat candidate interval. Biochemical and Biophysical Research Communications, *242*:685–691, 1998.

Smythe, CM. Diagnosis and treatment of Kleinfelter syndrome. Hospital Practice, *15*:111–120, 1999.

Steyaert, J, Legius, E, Borghgraef, M, & Fryns, JP. A distinct neurocognitive phenotype in female fragile-X premutation carriers assessed with visual attention tasks. American Journal of Medical Genetics, *116A*:44–51, 2003.

Stockwell, BR Chemical genetics: ligand-based discovery of gene function. Nature Review Genetics *1*:116–125, 2000.

Sztriha, L, Vos, YJ, Verlind, E, Johansen, J, & Berg, B. X-linked hydrocephalus: A novel missense mutation in the L1CAM gene. Pediatric Neurology, *27*:293–296, 2002.

Tanguy, A. Orthopedic aspects of Rett syndrome. Annals of Pediatrics (Paris), *40*:237–241, 1993.

Tarleton, JC, & Saul, RA. Molecular genetic advances in fragile X syndrome. Journal of Pediatrics, *122*:169–185, 1993.

The Chipping Forecast II. Nature Genetics, *32*:461–552, 2002.

Thuline, HC, & Pueschel, SM. Cytogenetics in Down syndrome. In Pueschel, SM, & Rynders, JE (Eds.). Down Syndrome. Advances in Biomedicine and the Behavioral Sciences. Cambridge: Ware Press, 1982, p. 133.

Tobin, SL, & Boughton, A. The New Genetics: Molecular Concepts, Applications and Ramifications. Twisted Ladder Media, 2000.

Turrens, JF. Increased superoxide dismutase and Down's syndrome. Medical Hypotheses, *56*:617–619, 2001.

Uc, EY, & Rodnitzky, RL. Childhood dystonia. Seminars in Pediatric Neurology, *10*:52–61, 2003.

Veraska, A, Del Campo, M, & McGinnis, W. Developmental patterning genes and their conserved functions: From model organisms to humans. Molecular Genetics and Metabolism, *69*:85–100, 2000.

Verhoef, S, Bakker, L, Tempelaars, AM, Hesseling-Janssen, AL, Mazurczak, T, Jozwiak, S, Fois, A, Bartalini, G, Zonnenberg, BA, van Essen, AJ, Lindhout, D, Halley, DJ, & van den Ouweland, AM. High rate of mosaicism in tuberous sclerosis complex. American Journal of Human Genetics, *64*:1632–1637, 1999.

Vogels, F, & Fryns, JP. The Prader-Willi syndrome and the Angelman syndrome. Genetic Counseling, *13*:385–396, 2002.

Wan, M, Lee, SS, Zhang, X, Houwink-Manville, I, Song, HR, Amir, RE, Budden, S, Naidu, S, Pereira, JL, Lo, IF, Zoghbi, HY, Schanen, NC, & Francke, U. Rett syndrome and beyond: Recurrent spontaneous and familial MECP2 mutations at CpG hotspots. American Journal of Human Genetics, *65*:1520–1529, 1999.

Wapner, RJ, & Lewis, D. Genetics and metabolic causes of stillbirth. Seminars in Perinatology, *26*:70–74, 2002.

Warren, ST, & Sherman, SL. The fragile X syndrome. In Scriver, CR, Sly, WS, Childs, B, Beaudet, AL, Valle, D, Kinzler, KW, & Vogelstein, B (Eds.). The Metabolic and Molecular Bases of Inherited Disease. New York: McGraw-Hill, 2001.

Weiner, DM, Ewalt, DH, Roach, ES, & Hensle, TW. The tuberous sclerosis complex: A comprehensive review. Journal of American College of Surgeons, *187*:548–561, 1998.

Wevrick, R, & Francke, U. Diagnostic test for the Prader-Willi syndrome by SNRPN expression in blood. Lancet, *348*:1068–1069, 1996.

Wilkie, AO, & Morriss-Kay, GM. Genetics of craniofacial development and malformation. National Review in Genetics, *2*:458–468, 2001.

Wilkins, LE, Brown, JA, & Wolf, B. Psychomotor development in 65 home-reared children with cri-du-chat syndrome. Journal of Pediatrics, *97*:401–405, 1980.

Willard, HF. The sex chromosome and X chromosome inactivation. In Scriver, CT, Beaudet, AL, Sly, WS, & Valle, D (Ed.). The Molecular Bases of Inherited Disease, 8th ed. New York: McGraw-Hill, 2000.

Wisniewski, KE, Wisniewski, HM, & Wen, GY. Occurrence of neuropathological changes and dementia of Alzheimer's disease in Down's syndrome. Annals of Neurology, *17*:278–282, 1985.

Witt-Engerstrom, I. Age-related occurrence of signs and symptoms in the Rett syndrome. Brain Development, *14*:S11–20, 1992.

Zinn, AR, & Ross, JL. Turner syndrome and haploinsufficiency. Current Opinion in Genetic Development, *8*:322–327, 1998.

Zappella, M, Gillberg, C, & Ehlers, S. The preserved speech variant: A subgroup of the Rett complex: A clinical report of 30 cases. Journal of Autism and Developmental Disorders, *28*:519–526, 1998.

Zhu, Y, & Parada, LF. Neurofibromin, a tumor suppressor in the nervous system. Experimental Cell Research, *264*:19–28, 2001.

&

Chapter 8

PHYSICAL FITNESS DURING CHILDHOOD AND ADOLESCENCE

JEAN L. STOUT
PT, MS

The International Classification of Functioning, Disability and Health (ICF) emphasizes components of health as important factors of participation in society (World Health Organization, 2001). According to the initial press release, using the ICF framework, the World Health Organization estimates that as many as 500 million healthy life years are lost each year because of disability associated with health conditions. This statistic includes children. Ensuring physical fitness is one aspect of primary prevention and health promotion upon which the practice of physical therapy is based (American Physical Therapy Association, 2001) and is a construct that fits appropriately within the ICF model. As clinicians who design exercise programs and treat children with disabilities, we have a unique responsibility to understand and promote physical fitness as an aspect of those programs. It is a unique responsibility because we can have a great impact on the exercise lifestyle that children develop and carry with them throughout their lives. It is a

unique responsibility because we care for a group of children who might otherwise be physically inactive. Many believe that promotion of lifelong habits of physical activity in childhood will have direct and indirect effects on health and prevention of disease in adulthood (Blair et al., 1989; Haskell et al., 1985; Simons-Morton et al., 1987; Strong, 1990).

What defines "physical fitness" for able-bodied children? Are the criteria for physical fitness different in children with disabilities? How do we help children with physical disabilities incorporate physical fitness into the limitations of their disability? This chapter is designed to answer those questions and to provide the reader with an understanding of (1) physical fitness and the cardiopulmonary response to exercise in children of different ages who do not have disabling conditions; (2) the components of physical fitness (cardiorespiratory endurance, muscular strength and endurance, flexibility, and body composition) (Table 8-1); (3) the standards of fitness components consistent with good health; (4) the effects of training and conditioning on overall physical fitness; (5) the components of fitness in various special populations; and (6) guides for program planning. The chapter also includes a review of current physical fitness tests.

HEALTH, PHYSICAL ACTIVITY, AND PHYSICAL FITNESS

Physical fitness is difficult to define because it cannot be measured directly. Physical fitness is generally viewed as having two facets—health-related fitness and the more traditional motor fitness. Motor fitness generally includes physical abilities that relate to athletic performance, whereas health-related fitness includes abilities related to daily function and health maintenance. Physical activity

| TABLE 8-1 | Health-Related Fitness Components and the Rationale for Importance to Health Promotion and Disease Prevention |

COMPONENT	RATIONALE
Cardiorespiratory endurance	Improved physical working capacity
	Reduced fatigue
	Reduced risk of coronary heart disease
	Optimal growth and development
Muscular strength and endurance	Improved functional capacity for lifting and carrying
	Reduced risk of lower back pain
	Optimal posture
	Optimal growth and development
Flexibility	Enhanced functional capacity for bending and twisting
	Reduced risk of lower back pain
	Optimal growth and development
Body composition	Reduced risk of hypertension
	Reduced risk of coronary heart disease
	Reduced risk of diabetes
	Optimal growth and development

Adapted from Pate, PR, & Shephard, RJ. Characteristics of physical fitness in youth. In Gisolfi, CV, & Lamb, DR (Eds.), Perspectives in Exercise Science and Sports Medicine, Vol. 2: Youth, Exercise, and Sport. Indianapolis, IN: Benchmark Press, 1989, pp. 1–45.

is thought to be the path both to physical fitness and to good health, but they are not synonymous terms. Physical activity refers to the amount of exercise in which an individual engages. Studies suggest that a positive correlation exists between activity and fitness, but at least 80% of the variability in fitness measures cannot be explained (Pate et al., 1990; Ross & Gilbert, 1985; Ross & Pate, 1987). Physical activity may improve physical fitness and health at the same time, but the improvement in health may be caused by biologic changes different from those responsible for improvement in physical fitness (Haskell et al., 1985). Corbin (1987) suggested that some of the benefits from physical activity that are important to health have no relationship to what is defined as physical fitness per se. One example is the importance of regular exercise to a reduced risk of osteoporosis; osteoporosis is related to health but not to the components of physical fitness. We do not know how much physical activity is necessary for health and fitness in children.

The premise that physical activity is the path to both physical fitness and good health has become a primary focus in programs instituted by the United States Department of Health and Human Services. As early as 1985, the Centers for Disease Control put forth a specific activity plan for youth through old age to attain specific health fitness goals and achieve optimal health benefits. Developing lifelong physical activity patterns was one of

the specific goals for children (Haskell et al., 1985). In 1990, *Healthy Children 2000* was introduced—a major federal planning document for health promotion and disease prevention for children (United States Department of Health and Human Services, 1990). Eight objectives were outlined to increase the physical activity and fitness levels of youth, with a target date of attainment by the year 2000 (Table 8-2). Revised targets were incorporated into the draft objectives of *Healthy People 2010* as early as 1998 (United States Department of Health and Human Services, 1998). Many of the targets proposed for year 2000 were retained for the 2010 objectives. Only one target (objective 4, Table 8-2) has been surpassed for youth in grades 9 through 12. Others (objectives 5, 6, and 7, Table 8-2) moved away from year 2000 targets. Another (objective 8, Table 8-2) no longer appears in the new objectives. Perhaps the greatest disappointment has been lack of data available for children younger than high school (grades K through 8) (United States Department of Health and Human Services, 1995). As a result, as early as 1998, targets directed toward elementary-age and junior high–age children were dropped from the 2010 objectives. Progress review of the remaining objectives in April 2004 indicates that little to no progress is noted over the last 6 years toward 2010 objectives as monitored in high school youth. They remain at baseline levels (United States Department of Health and Human Services, 2004).

TABLE 8-2	Objectives for Improved Physical Activity and Fitness

RISK REDUCTION OBJECTIVES

1. Increase to at least 30% the proportion of people age 6 and older who engage regularly, preferably daily, in light to moderate physical activity for at least 30 minutes daily
2. Increase to at least 20% the proportion of people age 18 and older and to at least 75% the proportion of children and adolescents age 6 through 17 who engage in vigorous physical activity that promotes the development and maintenance of cardiorespiratory fitness 3 or more days per week for 20 or more minutes per occasion
3. Reduced to no more than 15% the proportion of people age 6 and older who engage in no leisure time physical activity
4. Increase to at least 40% the proportion of people age 6 and older who regularly perform physical activities that enhance and maintain muscular strength, muscular endurance, and flexibility
5. Increase to at least 50% the proportion of overweight people age 12 and older who have adopted sound dietary practices combined with regular physical activity to attain an appropriate body weight

SERVICE AND PROTECTION OBJECTIVES

6. Increase to at least 50% the proportion of children and adolescents in first through twelfth grade who participate in daily school physical education
7. Increase to at least 50% the proportion of physical education class time that students spend being physically active, preferably engaged in lifetime physical activities

HEALTH STATUS OBJECTIVE

8. Reduce overweight to a prevalence of no more than 20% among people age 20 and older and no more than 15% among adolescents age 12 through 19

From United States Department of Health and Human Services. Healthy Children 2000: National Health Promotion and Disease Prevention Objectives Related to Mothers, Infants, Children, Adolescents, and Youth. Washington, DC: Public Health Service, 1990.

Physical activity as the path to physical fitness is no less surprising than the relationship of physical activity to improved health and disease prevention. The content of the current nationwide objectives has been guided in part by the concept of health-related fitness. What is different may be the intensity of physical activity required to be physically fit compared with what is necessary to receive benefits to health. Regardless of intensity, both physical fitness and improved health begin with physical activity. If promotion of lifelong habits of physical activity in childhood has direct and indirect effects on fitness, health, and prevention of disease in adulthood (Blair et al., 1989; Haskell et al., 1985; Malina, 2001, Simons-Morton et al., 1987; Strong, 1990), this should be no less true for children with physical disabilities. The concept of physical fitness becomes more important because as individuals become less active in adulthood, the decrease in activity level is more likely to result in loss of function, injury, or both.

DEFINITION OF PHYSICAL FITNESS

As defined previously, health-related fitness is a state characterized by (1) an ability to perform daily activities with vigor and (2) traits and capacities that are associated with low risk of premature development of hypokinetic disease (i.e., physical inactivity) (Pate, 1983). Physical fitness is multidimensional. A combination of traits and capacities contributes to physical fitness, and the interaction among them creates true fitness. Each facet is a unique, independent characteristic or ability that is not highly correlated with other components. As the concept of health-related fitness has gained acceptance, four basic components have been identified: cardiorespiratory endurance, muscular strength and endurance, flexibility, and body composition. The rationale for the importance of these parameters in day-to-day functional capacity, health promotion, and disease prevention, and therefore physical fitness, is presented in Table 8-1. The relative independence of the components from one another has been verified by low correlations between components. Of the 60 possible correlation coefficients among test items for these components, only 6 were greater than 0.35 (Ross & Gilbert, 1985; Ross & Pate, 1987).

Cardiopulmonary response to exercise in the growing child is reviewed next. The remainder of this chapter is directed toward reviewing the components of health-related fitness and current physical fitness tests.

CARDIOPULMONARY RESPONSE TO EXERCISE

As in adults, the response of a child to exercise (a single event or repeated exercise) includes physiologic changes in the cardiovascular and pulmonary systems, as well as metabolic effects. In children, however, differences in physiologic changes are seen as growth and development occur. Physiologic capacities depend on growth of the myocardium, skeleton, and skeletal muscle. Maturation and improved efficiency of the cardiovascular, pulmonary, metabolic, and musculoskeletal systems are also important. The physical work capacity of children increases approximately eightfold in absolute terms between the ages of 6 and 12 years, partially as a result of growth and maturation (Adams, 1973). The absolute exercise capacity of children may be less than that of adults, but relative exercise capacity is similar.

Any exercise, in a child or an adult, increases the energy expenditure of the body. The energy for muscle contraction and exercise depends on splitting of adenosine triphosphate (ATP) at the cellular level. ATP is available in small quantities in resting muscle, but once contraction starts, additional sources are required if contraction is to be maintained. Three sources of ATP are available: (1) creatine phosphate (CP), (2) glycolysis, and (3) the tricarboxylic acid or Krebs cycle. It is beyond the scope of this chapter to describe these mechanisms in detail. The reader is referred to a standard textbook of exercise physiology (Brooks et al., 2004).

CP and glycolysis as sources of ATP are referred to as anaerobic pathways because they do not require the presence of oxygen. CP is found in the sarcoplasm of the muscle cell. During breakdown it releases a high-energy phosphate bond that can be combined with adenosine diphosphate (ADP) to create ATP.

$$CP \rightarrow C + P_i + Energy \qquad [1]$$
$$ADP + P_i + Energy \rightarrow ATP \qquad [2]$$

CP breakdown together with ATP production provides enough energy for 10 to 15 seconds of exercise. Glycolysis, the other anaerobic pathway, breaks down glucose to produce pyruvic acid or lactic acid and ATP. This reaction takes place in the sarcoplasm of the cell. Together, glycolysis and CP breakdown are methods of anaerobic energy production that can sustain energy for muscle contraction for 40 to 50 seconds.

Energy production by the tricarboxylic acid cycle is called an aerobic pathway because it requires oxygen. A supply of oxygen is required for sustained exercise and depends on the aerobic pathway. Most, if not all, activities use both aerobic and anaerobic pathways for supply of ATP, but often tasks are more highly dependent on one type of pathway than the other.

Because aerobic pathways must be used to sustain exercise, an index of maximal aerobic power is used to reflect the highest metabolic rate made available by aerobic energy. The most common index is maximal oxygen uptake (VO_{2max}), or the highest volume of oxygen that can be consumed per unit time. Oxygen supply to muscle is described by the Fick equation: oxygen uptake (VO_2) is equal to cardiac output (CO) times the difference in oxygen content between arterial (CaO_2) and mixed venous (CvO_2) blood, or

$$VO_2 = CO \times (CaO_2 - CvO_2)$$

Because CO is the product of heart rate and stroke volume, the following relationship is also true:

$$VO_2 = Heart\ rate \times Stroke\ volume \times Arteriovenous\ O_2\ difference$$

For VO_2 to increase, one or more of these factors must increase. During exercise, CO is elevated by increases in both heart rate and stroke volume. Elevated blood flow to the muscles increases the difference in oxygen content between arterial and venous blood.

VO_{2max} increases throughout childhood from approximately 1 L/min at age 5 years to 3 to 4 L/min at puberty (Braden & Strong, 1990). These changes occur as a result of maturation of the cardiovascular, pulmonary, metabolic, and musculoskeletal systems. As a child grows, the cardiopulmonary and musculoskeletal systems are integrated so that oxygen flow during exercise optimally meets the energy demands of the muscle cells, regardless of body size (Cooper et al., 1984).

Cardiac Output

CO in children, as in adults, rises at the beginning of exercise or on transition from a lower to a higher level of exercise. CO increases by an increase in both stroke volume and heart rate. CO in children is similar to that in adults despite the fact that stroke volume in a 5-year-old is about 25% of the stroke volume in an adult (Godfrey, 1981). Stroke volume increases as total heart volume increases. At all levels of exercise, stroke volume in boys is somewhat higher than it is in girls (Bar-Or, 1983c). CO levels in children are similar to those in adults because of an increased heart rate throughout childhood. Maximal heart rates in children vary between 195 and 215 beats per minute (bpm) and decrease by 0.7 to 0.8 bpm per year after maturity (Braden & Strong, 1990).

Arteriovenous Difference and Hemoglobin Concentration

At rest, the difference between arterial and mixed venous blood oxygen content is the same in children as in adults (Sproul & Simpson, 1964). Research suggests, however, that children have a higher blood flow to muscles after exercise than do young adults, resulting in a higher arteriovenous oxygen difference (Koch, 1974). Greater muscle blood flow facilitates increased oxygen transport to exercising muscles and thus a decrease in the oxygen content of the mixed venous blood.

Hemoglobin concentration is lower in children than in the average adult and thus affects the oxygen transport capacity of the blood in children (Krahenbuhl et al., 1985). Studies suggest that total hemoglobin concentration in 11- and 12-year-olds is approximately 78% of that in adults (Krahenbuhl et al., 1985).

Arterial Blood Pressure

Lower exercise blood pressure is seen in children than in adults, a finding consistent with a lower CO and stroke volume. Blood pressure may also be reduced because of lower peripheral vascular resistance secondary to shorter blood vessels (Bar-Or, 1983c).

Ventilation

Ventilation is the rate of exchange of air between the lungs and ambient air, measured in liters per minute. In absolute terms, ventilation increases with age. Ventilation normalized by body weight is the same for children and adults at maximal activity (Bar-Or, 1983c). At submaximal exercise levels, ventilation is higher in children and decreases with age, suggesting that children have a lower ventilatory reserve than do adults. Studies suggest that children have less efficient ventilation than do adults (i.e., more air is needed to supply 1 L of oxygen in a child than in an adult) (Bar-Or, 1983c).

Vital Capacity

Vital capacity in a 5-year-old child is about 20% of that in an adult and increases with age. It is highly correlated with body size, particularly height (Godfrey, 1981), and generally has not been found to be a limiting factor of exercise performance.

Respiratory Rate

Children have a higher respiratory rate than do adults during both maximal and submaximal exercise. A high rate of respiration compensates for decreased lung volume; respiratory rate decreases as lung volume increases (Bar-Or, 1983c).

Blood Lactate

Blood and muscle lactate levels are lower in children than in adults (Astrand, 1952; Ericksson et al., 1971, 1973). It has been suggested but not confirmed that lactate production is related to testosterone production and therefore to sexual maturity in boys. Low lactate production in children could limit glycolytic capacity and thus contribute to reduced anaerobic capacity.

Table 8-3 summarizes comparisons between children and adults for various cardiopulmonary variables. Growth and maturation play a vital part in determining the values of these variables. Despite size differences between adults and children (which might lead one to believe that oxygen transport in children is less efficient because they are smaller), optimal oxygen transport is maintained by highly integrated functions between the cardiopulmonary and musculoskeletal systems.

REVIEW OF TESTS OF PHYSICAL FITNESS

Numerous physical fitness tests have been developed and are in use in physical education curricula across the country. Five tests are worthy of review because of their nationwide use and the likelihood that they will constitute the standards for future testing of youth and children. One of these tests, the National Children and Youth Fitness Study Tests I and II (Ross & Gilbert, 1985; Ross & Pate, 1987), was used as the basis for current levels of fitness across the country by the United States Department of Health and Human Services (1990) in drafting objectives for *Healthy Children 2000*. Each test reviewed in this chapter emphasizes health-related fitness components. Most tests provide some information regarding interrater reliability, but none specifically includes information on the validity of individual test items. Most information on the validity of individual test items has been provided by separate investigators or published separately subsequent to the development of the test batteries (Cureton & Warren, 1990; Going, 1988; Jackson & Coleman, 1976; Jackson & Baker, 1986; Safrit, 1990). A comparison of four tests and their components is presented in Table 8-4.

AAHPERD Physical Best Program

This program, originally designed to be both a physical fitness measure and an educational program to promote health and prevent disease, was developed by the American Alliance for Health, Physical Education, Recreation, and Dance (AAHPERD) (1988). In 1993, AAPHERD adopted the FITNESSGRAM (Morrow et al., 1993) to measure physical fitness status and no longer uses its original fitness battery. The Physical Best Program remains

TABLE 8-3	Cardiopulmonary Function Variables and Response to Exercise in Children	
FUNCTION	**CHILD VS. ADULT RESPONSE**	**SEX DIFFERENCES**
Heart rate (max, submax)	Higher	M = F (max); F > M (submax)
Stroke volume (max, submax)	Lower	M > F
Cardiac output (max, submax)	Lower, similar	
Arteriovenous difference (submax)	Similar	
Blood flow to active muscle	Higher	M = F
Blood pressure	Lower	
Hemoglobin concentration	Lower	
Ventilation/kg body wt (max)	Similar	
Ventilation/ kg body wt (submax)	Higher	
Respiratory rate (max, submax)	Higher	
Tidal volume and vital capacity (max)	Lower	
Tidal volume and vital capacity (submax)	Lower	
Blood lactate levels (max, submax)	Similar/ lower Lower	M > F after puberty

Adapted from Bar-Or. Pediatric Sports Medicine for the Practitioner. New York; Springer-Verlag, pp. 19,31,46.
max = maximal exercise; submax = submaximal exercise.

active in its educational component to promote youth fitness.

Chrysler Fund–Amateur Athletic Union Physical Fitness Program

The Physical Fitness Program by Chrysler Fund-Amateur Athletic Union (1987) consists of four required items and one optional item. Although the test battery is norm-referenced, it is referenced by test administrators. The sample therefore is not systematically representative of the nation. A critique of the test suggests that not all data are externally valid. Significant differences in mean values in test items were noted when compared with those of other tests and when compared with results among different test administrators (Safrit, 1990; Sodoma, 1986). The test items show some variation from other tests (see Table 8-4). The absence of a standard testing protocol among test administrators raises questions about the reliability and thus the validity of the test.

FITNESSGRAM Program

This test is a battery that uses criterion-referenced standards. The program was developed by the Cooper Institute for Aerobics Research (1987). Since its initial development, it has been revised twice, most recently in 1999 (Cooper

Institute for Aerobics Research, 1999). Limited information is available on the reliability and validity of the specific standards in the test manual. Research on the validity and reliability of the cardiorespiratory endurance standards has been published separately (Cureton & Warren, 1990; McSwegin et al., 1998). Development of the standards was based on determining (1) the lowest level of the laboratory standard for cardiorespiratory endurance (VO_{2max}) consistent with minimal risk of disease and adequate functional capacity; (2) the timing standards of the mile walk-run, consistent with the minimal VO_{2max}; and (3) a comparison of the standards with available national normative data to evaluate both consistency and accuracy. Standards using the FITNESSGRAM for individuals with disabilities are currently being developed (Seaman et al., 1995; Winnick & Short, 1999).

National Children, Youth, and Fitness Study I and II

These tests were national studies undertaken to assess current levels of physical fitness of children and youth in the United States. Initiated by the United States Office of Disease Prevention and Health Promotion (Pate et al., 1987; Ross et al., 1985), the results have been used to set appropriate targets for improved health and fitness. The

| TABLE 8-4 | Review of Current Physical Fitness Tests | | | |

TEST	COMPONENT OF FITNESS	TEST ITEMS	STANDARD	RELIABILITY/ VALIDITY
Chrysler-AAU Physical Fitness Program (1987)	Cardiorespiratory endurance Lower back flexibility Muscular strength/ endurance Upper body muscle strength/endurance	Endurance run V-sit and reach Bent knee sit-up Pull-up/ flexed arm hang	Normative (for ages 6–16 yr) (not nationwide)	Not all data externally valid
Prudential FITNESSGRAM (Cooper Institute for Aerobics Research, 1987, 1993)	Cardiorespiratory endurance Lower back flexibility Upper body strength Abdominal strength Body composition Agility (K-3)	1-mile run Sit and reach Pull-up/flexed arm hang Sits ups Skinfold measurement Shuttle run	Criterion	(Morrow et al., 1993) Partial work reported 1990 (Cureton & Warren, 1990)
National Child and Youth Fitness Study (Ross & Gilbert, 1985; Ross & Pate, 1987)	Cardiorespiratory endurance Lower back flexibility Upper body strength/ endurance Abdominal strength/ endurance Body composition	1-mile walk-run Half-mile walk-run Sit and reach Modified pull-up Bent knee sit-up Sum of skinfolds (triceps/ subscapular/calf)	U.S. norms (for ages 6–8 yr)	(Ross, Katz, & Gilbert, 1985) (Ross et al., 1987)
Presidential Physical Fitness Program (President's Council, 1987)	Cardiorespiratory endurance Lower back flexibility Upper body strength/ endurance Abdominal strength/ endurance Ability/power	1-mile walk-run Sit and reach Pull-up Bent knee sit-up/ curl-up Shuttle run	U.S norms (for ages 6–18 yr)	General terms of validity reported; no specifics

NCYFS I produced normative data by sex and age and sex and grade for children and youth age 10 to 18 years, and NCYFS II provided the same information for children age 6 to 9 years. Training procedures were developed for test administrators, and interrater reliability estimates were found to be 0.99 for body composition measurements. Concurrent validity for some test items had already been established (Jackson & Coleman, 1976).

Presidential Physical Fitness Program

This is a norm-referenced test created by the President's Council on Physical Fitness and Sports (1987). Validity is not addressed, but some reliability information is provided.

COMPARISON OF TESTS

All the tests measure similar components of health-related fitness. Each includes items for testing cardio-respiratory endurance, muscular strength and endurance, and flexibility. Only two of the four tests measure body composition. The tests differ in the reference standard used. Tests are either norm-referenced (performance is compared with that of a national U.S. sample of children taking the same test) or criterion-referenced (performance is compared with a preset standard consistent with fitness). The criterion for each item is independent of the performance of other children on the same test.

The FITNESSGRAM is the only criterion-referenced test.

Appropriate reliability and validity data are not available for any of the tests reviewed, and thus the tests do not meet standards for measurement required of scientific clinical tools (American Psychological Association, 1985). Users must be cautious in the interpretation of scores and their meaning. Strict and rigid interpretation of the test results would be incorrect and should be avoided until further evidence of reliability and validity is available. Procedures for evaluating reliability and validity of criterion-referenced tests are available (Safrit, 1989).

COMPONENTS OF PHYSICAL FITNESS

The components of health-related fitness, as mentioned earlier, are cardiorespiratory endurance, muscular strength and endurance, flexibility, and body composition. The following information will be reviewed for each component:

1. The criterion measure of the component
2. Laboratory measurement
3. Developmental aspects of the component and standards by age
4. Field measurement of the component and its validity in relation to the criterion measure
5. Standards by age as determined by the FITNESS-GRAM program, a computer-scored fitness test with a health-related focus
6. Physical activities with high correlation to the particular fitness component
7. Response to training
8. Assessment of the component in children with disabilities

CARDIORESPIRATORY ENDURANCE

Criterion Measure

The most widely used criterion measure for cardiorespiratory endurance is directly measured VO_{2max}, sometimes referred to as maximal aerobic power. This component measures the capabilities of the cardiovascular and pulmonary systems and is significant because oxygen supply to the tissues depends on the efficiency and capacity of these systems. VO_{2max} is the highest rate of oxygen consumed by the body in a given time period during exercise of a significant portion of body muscle mass (Krahenbuhl et al., 1985). Cardiorespiratory endurance is so important to overall fitness that many people view physical fitness as being synonymous with cardiorespiratory endurance (Simons-Morton et al., 1987).

Laboratory Measurement

Laboratory measurement techniques include measurement of VO_{2max} during progressive exercise to the point of exhaustion with the use of an ergometer. This method is referred to as direct determination of VO_{2max}. Indirect determination methods predict VO_{2max} from submaximal exercise.

Direct Determination

An ergometer is a device that measures the amount of work performed under controlled conditions. The two devices commonly available are a cycle ergometer and a treadmill. The cycle ergometer has the advantage of being relatively inexpensive and portable, but compared with the treadmill, it exercises a smaller total muscle mass. With the cycle ergometer, local fatigue develops (primarily in knee extensors), resulting in premature termination of the testing. Depending on the source, values of VO_{2max} are reported to be 5% to 30% lower on a cycle ergometer than on a treadmill (Bar-Or, 1983a; Braden & Strong, 1990; Krahenbuhl et al., 1985). For children, the coordination and rhythm, or cadence, required on a cycle ergometer are sometimes difficult to achieve. Both the treadmill and the cycle ergometers present problems when used to test populations with disabilities, in particular those with impairments of balance or coordination.

A variety of protocols for direct determination can be used with children. The most common protocol is one in which resistance, inclination, speed, or height is increased every 1 to 3 minutes without interruption until the child can no longer maintain the activity. In interrupted protocols, which are sometimes used, there is an interruption between each successive increment of exercise. Examples of some common direct determination protocols are given in Table 8-5. The main criterion for indicating that VO_{2max} has been achieved during a progressive protocol is that an increase in power load is not accompanied by an increased VO_2 (usually 2 mL/kg/min or higher) (Krahenbuhl et al., 1985). Astrand (1952), however, reported that 5% of all children tested failed to reach a plateau in VO_2, even though evidence from secondary criteria suggested that exhaustion had been reached.

Despite the difficulty of determining attainment of VO_{2max}, studies suggest that the reliability of direct determination testing with children is high. Coefficients of variation of 3%, 5%, and 8% for VO_{2max} determined by treadmill walk-jogging, running, and walking, respectively, have been reported (Paterson & Cunningham, 1978). A mean variation of 4.5% was reported for children exercising to exhaustion on a cycle ergometer on 12 different occasions (Cumming et al., 1967).

TABLE 8-5	Direct Determination All-out Protocols

BRUCE TREADMILL PROTOCOL

STAGE	SPEED (MPH)	GRADE (%)	DURATION (MIN)
1	1.7	10	3
2	2.5	12	3
3	3.4	14	3
4	4.2	16	3
5	5.0	18	3
6	5.5	20	3
7	6.0	22	3

McMASTER PROGRESSIVE CONTINUOUS CYCLING TEST

BODY HEIGHT(CM)	INITIAL LOAD (WATTS)	INCREMENTS (WATTS)	DURATIONS (MIN)
<119.9	12.5	12.5	2
120–139.9	12.5	25.0	2
140–159.9	25.0	25.0	2
>160	25.0	25.0 (F) 50.0 (M)	2

Adapted from Bar-Or, O. Appendix II: Procedures for exercise testing in children. In Bar-Or, O, Pediatric Sports Medicine for the Practitioner. New York: Springer-Verlag, 1983, pp. 315–341.

Watts = joules per second.

Indirect Determination

Indirect determination methods use submaximal exercise to indirectly predict VO_{2max}. The child is not taken to his or her self-imposed maximum. Heart rate during one or more stages is the variable most commonly used to derive the index of VO_{2max}. Step tests for children are usually submaximal tests, using recovery heart rate to predict VO_{2max}. Evidence suggests that height-specific step tests can be reliable predictors of VO_{2max} (Francis & Feinstein, 1991). Important limitations exist, however, in predicting VO_{2max} from submaximal exercise data, and these should always be kept in mind (Wyndham, 1976). Examples of test protocols are presented in Table 8-6.

The W_{170} is an index used to predict mechanical power in a submaximal test. Two or more measurements of heart rate are obtained at different power or workloads, and heart rate is then extrapolated to 170 bpm. The corresponding power is W_{170}. This index, originally described by Wahlund (1948), is based on the assumption that heart rate is linearly related to power at 170 bpm or less. To minimize error, more than two heart rate measurements are taken, one of which is as close as possible to 170 bpm.

Developmental Aspects of Cardiorespiratory Endurance

Absolute maximal aerobic power, or VO_{2max}, increases with age throughout childhood and is slightly higher in boys than in girls (Krahenbuhl et al., 1985; Rutenfranz et al., 1990; Shvartz & Reibold, 1990). Initial differences during early childhood are approximately 10%, increasing to 25% by age 14 years, and exceeding 50% by age 16 (Krahenbuhl et al., 1985). The development of a greater muscle mass in boys and increasing differences in the amount of time spent in vigorous physical exercise are the most commonly given explanations. Overall, the physical working capacity of children increases approximately eightfold between the ages of 6 and 12 years. Few data are available on VO_{2max} for children younger than age 6 (Adams, 1973).

Relative to body weight, only a 1% change in VO_{2max} is noted between the ages of 6 and 16 years for boys (52.8 mL/kg/min at age 6; 53.5 mL/kg/min at age 16), whereas girls display a 12% reduction between the same ages (52.0 mL/kg/min at age 6; 40.5 mL/kg/min at age 16) (Krahenbuhl et al., 1985; Shvartz & Reibold, 1990). VO_{2max} is highly correlated with lean body mass. The decline in VO_{2max} in girls begins around age 10, when changes in body composition occur as girls develop a relatively increased amount of subcutaneous fat. When VO_{2max} is measured with reference to lean body mass, the difference in values between the sexes disappears (Braden & Strong, 1990).

TABLE 8-6	Indirect Determination Protocols

ADAMS SUBMAXIMAL PROGRESSIVE CONTINUOUS CYCLING TEST*

BODY WEIGHT (KG)	STAGE (WATTS)	STAGES 2 (WATTS)	STAGES 3 (WATTS)
30	16.5	33.0	50.0
30–39.9	16.5	50.0	83.0
40–59.9	16.5	50.0	100.0
>60	16.5	83.0	133.0

Stage duration = 6 min
Performance by W_{170}

MODIFIED 3-MINUTES STEP TEST†

STAGE	DURATIONS (MINS)	ASCENT RATE (ASCENTS/MIN)
1	3	22
2	3	26
3	3	30

Step height dependent on height
Performance by recovery heart rate

*Adapted from Bar-Or, O. Appendix II: Procedures for exercise testing in children. In Bar-Or, O. Pediatric Sports Medicine for the Practitioner. New York: Springer-Verlag, 1983, pp. 315–341.
†Adapted and reprinted by permission from Francis, K, & Culpepper, M. Height adjusted, rate specific, single stage, step test for predicting maximal oxygen consumption. Southern Medical Journal, 82:602–606, 1989.

Increases in body dimensions, however, do not account for all changes in VO_{2max} that occur with growth. When comparing same-sex adolescents of different ages with identical body weight or body height, the positive relationship with age remains (Sprynarova & Reisenauer, 1978). Functional changes in cardiovascular, pulmonary, and musculoskeletal systems resulting in improved efficiency with maturity may play a role. Cooper and colleagues (1984), however, suggested that the functional components of body systems are integrated so that aerobic capacity is optimized throughout the growth process.

Measurement in the Field

The most common measure of cardiorespiratory fitness in the field is a long-distance run of various structures or lengths. All the physical fitness batteries reviewed previously have a distance run test, commonly a 1-mile run. Test-retest reliability of VO_{2max} during field testing has been shown to be between .60 and .95 (Cunningham et al., 1977; Safrit, 1990). Jackson and Coleman (1976) studied the construct validity of various distance run tests and the concurrent validity of the 9- and 12-minute run tests in elementary schoolchildren. Results suggested that both the 9- and 12-minute distance runs were valid measures of the construct and displayed concurrent validity with VO_{2max}. Safrit (1990) suggested that a 9-minute run is a distance of at least 1 mile. Both the 1200- and 1600-meter runs were significantly related to VO_{2max}, but only the 1600-meter run had correlation coefficients above .60, which is generally accepted as the lower limit for a useful fitness test (Krahenbuhl et al., 1978; Mathews, 1973). Validation values in the range of .40 to .80 between corresponding performance and weight-relative VO_{2max} have been reported (Safrit, 1990).

Standards by Age

Standards of performance are determined by ranking a child's performance in relation to the performance of a group of children tested on the same test (norm-referenced standard) or against an established criterion found to be consistent with good health (criterion-referenced standard). One advantage of criterion-referenced standards is that they are independent of the proportion of the population that meets the standards. A ranking by a norm-referenced standard does not necessarily represent a desirable level of fitness or performance. The limitation of criterion-referenced standards, however, is that they are somewhat arbitrary and that the criteria used in the current physical fitness tests differ from one another (Cureton & Warren, 1990). Establishing the validity of criterion-referenced standards for performance is in progress.

Cureton and Warren (1990) described the procedures for development of criterion standards for the FITNESSGRAM Program. Validity coefficients for the FITNESSGRAM Program range from .73 to 1.00 when compared with the criterion standard of VO_{2max}. The actual percentage of VO_{2max} that is used during the walk-run test, however, is unknown, which makes evaluation of any or all values difficult. A comparison of walk-run standards by age is provided in Table 8-7.

Physical Activities

Activities that are highly correlated with development of cardiorespiratory endurance are boxing, running, rowing, swimming, cross-country skiing, and bicycling. The common component among these activities is a prolonged, sustained demand on the cardiorespiratory system that requires general stamina.

TABLE 8-7	One-Mile Walk-Run Standards					
	CRITERION* STANDARD		FITNESSGRAM† FIELD STANDARD		NCYFS I, II‡ PERCENTILES	
AGE (YR)	M	F	M	F	M	F
5	42.0	40.0	16:00	17:00	–	–
6	42.0	40.0	15:00	16:00	–	–
7	42.0	40.0	14:00	15:00	–	–
8	42.0	40.0	13:00	14:30	15	15
9	42.0	40.0	12:00	13:00	20	20
10	42.0	39.0	11:00	12:00	25	35
11	42.0	38.0	11:00	12;00	20	40
12	42.0	37.0	10:00	11:30	30	30
13	42.0	36.0	9:30	10:30	20	35
14	42.0	35.0	8:30	10:30	35	50
15	42.0	35.0	8:30	10:30	25	55
16	42.0	35.0	8:30	10:30	20	50
17	42.0	35.0	8:30	10:30	30	50

Adapted from Cureton, KJ, & Warren, GL. Criterion-referenced standards for youth health related fitness tests: A tutorial. Research Quarterly for Exercise and Sport, *61*:7–19, 1990; Ross, JG, Dotson, CO, Gilbert, CG, & Katz, SJ. The national youth and fitness study I: New standards for fitness measurement. Journal of Physical Education, Recreation and Dance, *56*:62–66, 1985; Ross, JG, Delpy, LA, Christenson, GM, Gold, RS, & Damberg, CL. The national youth and fitness study II: Study procedures and quality control. Journal of Physical Education, Recreation and Dance, *58*:57–62,1987.

*Criterion standard as set by FITNESSGRAM in ml/kg/min of oxygen uptake.

† Minutes required to complete a 1-mile walk-run

‡Percentile rank of children performing this standard in National Children, Youth, and Fitness Study (NCYES) I, II.

Response to Training

Debate exists over whether maximal aerobic power of prepubescents is a component that can be affected by training. Research results are equivocal. Those studies that report improvement in aerobic power with training suggest that the principles of training of prepubescents, that is, frequency, intensity, and duration, are similar to those for adults (Simons-Morton et al., 1987). The functional results of conditioning on the cardiorespiratory system include decreased heart rate, increased stroke volume, improved respiratory muscular endurance, and decreased respiration rate (Bar-Or, 1983c; Braden & Strong, 1990). A more specific focus on conditioning and training will be found later in this chapter.

Assessment of Cardiorespiratory Endurance in Children with Disabilities

Children with disabilities often exhibit decreased or limited exercise capacity relative to their nondisabled peers. This can result from either their limited participation in exercise, which leads to deconditioning, or the specific pathologic factors of their disability that limit exercise-related functions. Regardless of the cause, children with disabilities often enter a cycle of decreased activity that precipitates a loss of fitness and further decreases in activity levels.

Pathophysiologic factors that may limit cardiorespiratory endurance can sometimes be separated by the specific component of the Fick equation that they affect. This provides a convenient way to categorize conditions or diseases by the fitness components they affect most (Bar-Or, 1983c, 1986) (Figure 8-1). Studies suggest that maximal aerobic uptake is limited not only by central mechanisms of the cardiopulmonary system but also by peripheral mechanisms controlling blood flow, excitation processes in the muscle fiber, local fatigue, and enzyme availability (Green & Patla, 1992; Saltin & Strange, 1992; Sutton, 1992). When considering the limitations or reductions in VO_{2max} in children with disabilities, both central and peripheral limitations must be considered.

Cerebral Palsy

Directly measured maximal aerobic capacity of children and adolescents with cerebral palsy (CP) is 10% to 30% less than that of control subjects (Bar-Or et al., 1976; Lundberg, 1978; Lundberg et al., 1967). It would seem

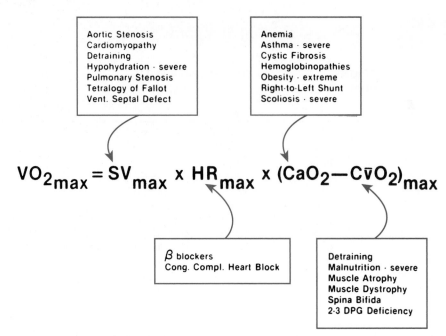

Figure 8-1   Maximal aerobic power (Vo$_{2max}$) and pathology. The Fick equation and specific pathologic conditions that affect its variables and reduce Vo$_{2max}$ are shown. *(From Bar-Or, O. Exercise as a diagnostic tool in pediatrics. In Bar-Or, O. Pediatric Sports Medicine for the Practitioner. New York: Springer-Verlag, 1983, p. 72.)*

that peripheral mechanisms related to the neuromuscular disorder itself are more likely to contribute to decreased capacity than are central cardiopulmonary mechanisms, although this has not been studied. When indirectly assessed from submaximal heart rate, aerobic capacity of adolescents was found to be reduced by 50% (Lundberg et al., 1967). Low mechanical efficiency creates disproportionately high submaximal heart rates in individuals with CP, making submaximal heart rate a poor predictor of maximal aerobic power (Bar-Or, 1983b). Submaximal exercise tests, in general, underestimate aerobic capacity in poorly trained individuals (Astrand & Rodahl, 1986; Wyndham, 1976). Numerous studies suggest that heart rate is a good predictor or an appropriate substitute clinical measure of VO$_2$ because of its linear relationship to heart rate (Rose et al., 1989, 1990). It is not a measure of maximal aerobic capacity, however, and therefore it is not an alternative measure of cardiorespiratory fitness.

An increase in blood flow to exercising muscles after conditioning is a response observed in children with CP but not seen in able-bodied children (Lundberg & Pernow, 1970). Spastic muscles of individuals with adult-onset brain damage exhibit subnormal blood flow during exercise (Landin et al., 1977). (Whether the rate of blood flow changes after conditioning in individuals with adult-onset brain injury is not known.) One hypothesis to

explain the increase in blood flow in conditioned individuals with CP is that it results from a decrease in spasticity. More rapid deterioration of maximal aerobic uptake is seen after discontinuation of training in children with CP than in able-bodied children (Bar-Or, 1983b).

Functional assessments that relate to the cardiorespiratory fitness of children with various disabilities are becoming more commonplace. The Pediatric Orthopedic Society of North America recently developed a functional outcomes questionnaire directed toward assessment of pediatric musculoskeletal conditions (Daltroy et al., 1998). Within this questionnaire are queries regarding a child's ability to complete a 1-mile and a 3-mile run. As more professionals caring for children with disabilities incorporate this assessment and others like it in daily practice, insight will be gained that may assist in determination of cardiorespiratory fitness. Standards for field testing aerobic capacity in individuals with CP using a long-distance run have been previously published for children age 10 to 17 years (Winnick & Short, 1985). The manual for the Brockport Physical Fitness Test (Winnick & Short, 1999) includes standards for children with a variety of disabilities. Seaman and colleagues (1995) present a review of alternative test items that can be used to assess aerobic capacity in children with various disabilities, including CP.

Juvenile Rheumatoid Arthritis

Maximal aerobic capacity measured by cycle ergometry in children with juvenile rheumatoid arthritis has been reported to be 15% to 30% lower than in their peers matched by age, sex, and body surface area (Giannini & Protas, 1991, 1992). No correlation was found between severity of articular disease and aerobic capacity, however. Children with juvenile rheumatoid arthritis have a shorter duration of exercise before exhaustion, which occurs at a lower than normal work rate with a lower peak heart rate. Deficient oxygen extraction from exercising muscles or low blood flow to exercising muscles has been postulated to occur in this population as a result of decreased activity levels (Bar-Or, 1983b, 1986).

Scoliosis

Chest deformity, decreased lung size, and decreased physical activity are believed to contribute to the lower maximal aerobic capacity of children with advanced scoliosis. No functional or exercise-related deficits are found in children with minor or moderate scoliosis (Bar-Or, 1983b). For those with advanced scoliosis, limitations of 50% to 70% in $\text{VO}_{2\text{max}}$ have been reported. VO_2 and minute ventilation are decreased and pulmonary artery pressure increased at maximal exercise relative to able-bodied standards. Some improvements are seen with conditioning.

Mental Retardation

Most studies indicate that individuals with mental retardation display lower $\text{VO}_{2\text{max}}$ scores than do their non-disabled peers (Lavay et al., 1990); however, significant variability has been reported among individuals with the same level of disability. Technical problems associated with testing individuals with mental retardation are encountered that create difficulties in establishing reliable and valid information. Treadmill testing appears to be the most reliable form of testing. Field test standards and alternative test items for aerobic capacity in individuals with both mild and moderate mental retardation are available (Seaman et al., 1995, Winnick & Short, 1999).

MUSCULAR STRENGTH AND ENDURANCE

The second component of physical fitness is muscular strength and endurance. Strength is required for movement and has a direct impact on effective performance. Strength is also important for optimal posture and reduced risk of lower back pain. Muscular strength, muscular endurance, and muscular power are not synonymous terms. Muscular strength refers to maximal contractile force. Muscular endurance is the ability of muscles to perform work and assumes some component of muscular strength. Muscular power refers to the ability to release maximal muscular force within a specified time. As velocity increases or time decreases (for maximal muscular force to be obtained), power increases. Because muscular endurance and muscular power have their basis in muscular strength, strength will be the primary focus of this discussion.

Laboratory Measurement

The laboratory standard for muscular strength is strength measured by dynamometry. Tests include isometric dynamometry, isokinetic dynamometry, and single-repetition maximal isotonic dynamometry. Most measurements are made on specific, selected muscles, and then results are extrapolated to give "whole body" strength. Unfortunately, a limitation for setting standards of strength is that force measurements depend on the type of dynamometer used (Blimkie, 1989). The most commonly selected measures are hand grip, elbow flexion and extension, knee flexion and extension, and plantar flexion strength.

Isokinetic strength testing during childhood and adolescence is a relatively new area of study. The reliability of isokinetic testing in children presents unique issues because of the variability of muscle coordination and neuromuscular maturation. Coefficients of variation from 5% to 11% have been reported (Blimkie, 1989). Children demonstrate the capacity to perform consistent maximal voluntary contraction under controlled conditions by age 6 to 7 years. The limited amount of research and available data do not allow definite conclusions on the effects of age and gender differences on isokinetic strength development. However, body weight and muscle cross-sectional area appear to correlate positively with isokinetic strength. Gender differences are minimal between ages 7 and 11. After age 13, boys tend to have greater isokinetic strength for the muscles tested (Baltzopoulos & Kellis, 1998; Gaul, 1996).

Developmental Aspects and Standards by Age

Grip Strength. Grip strength is the most commonly reported upper extremity strength measure in children. Absolute strength scores, however, are highly sensitive to the type of dynamometer used and to its positioning, making the results of studies difficult to compare. In general, single-hand grip strength increases from an average of approximately 5 kg for children at age 3 years to 45 kg for boys at age 17 and 30 kg for girls at age 17. Bilateral grip strength has been measured at a mean of 25 kg for children at age 7 years, increasing to an average of 95 kg for boys and 50 kg for girls by age 17 years (Blimkie, 1989). The rate of increase in strength for boys rises dramatically at puberty.

Elbow Flexion and Extension. Isometric elbow flexion strength is greater than isometric elbow extension strength throughout childhood and adolescence, and the difference between them increases with increasing age (Fowler & Gardner, 1967). The extension/flexion strength ratio for boys is approximately 0.76 at the age of 7.5 years and decreases to 0.57 during late adolescence. No data are available for girls.

Shoulder Flexion and Extension. A single study has addressed isokinetic strength values for shoulder flexion and extension in children (Brodie et al., 1986). Twenty-four untrained, prepubescent boys with an average age of 11.7 years were tested on a Cybex II (Ronkonkoma, NY) at six different velocities. Mean values for peak torque for shoulder extension were relatively constant at speeds of between 60°/s and 150°/s (13.2 and 13.7 newton-meters); mean values for shoulder flexion increased as speed increased (12.5–24.3 newton-meters).

Knee Flexion and Extension. Isokinetic knee flexion strength and knee extension strength also increase throughout childhood. Results from Alexander and Molnar (1973) and Molnar and Alexander (1973) indicated that knee extension strength exceeds knee flexion strength for both sexes at all ages. Average knee flexion strength varies from 30% to 50% of average knee extension strength for girls and 28% to 65% for boys. Boys have slightly greater strength than do girls before puberty but consistently greater strength from the age of 10 years onward.

Trunk Flexion and Extension. Few data are available for laboratory dynamometry standards for trunk strength in children. Clinical data have been collected for the ability of children to sustain isometric trunk flexion (actually a test of muscular endurance) between the ages of 3 and 7 years (Lefkof, 1986). An isotonic test of the number of hook-lying sit-ups performed was also included in the study. Both the endurance for isometric trunk flexion and the ability to perform sit-ups improved with age. The greatest improvement occurred between the ages of 5 and 6 years, when average performance at least doubled. These results are important because the typical field test for muscular strength and endurance is performance of sit-ups.

Composite Strength. Composite strength provides a measure of overall or general strength and consists of a total strength score from several muscle groups. Usually, grip strength, thrust strength (shoulder girdle), and shoulder pull measures are included in composite strength scores (Carron & Bailey, 1974; Faust, 1977). Unfortunately, I can find no measures of composite strength that include lower extremity or trunk strength. The pattern of increase in composite strength during childhood is similar to that of grip strength.

Evoked Responses

A second method for muscular function assessment in the laboratory is by evoked responses from electrical stimulation. Muscle contractile characteristics are studied with this methodology, including force production. Few data are available for children (Blimkie, 1989; Blimkie & Sale, 1998).

Developmental Aspects of Muscular Strength and Endurance

Gajdosik and Gajdosik describe the development of the musculoskeletal system in Chapter 6 of this volume. Development of strength depends on the development of force production and is influenced by numerous factors, for example, the muscle's cross-sectional area (Malina, 1986). Muscular strength in absolute terms increases linearly with chronologic age from early childhood in both sexes to approximately age 13 to 14 years. Increases in strength are closely related to increases in muscle mass during growth. Boys have greater strength than do girls at all ages (seen as early as age 3 years) and have larger absolute and relative amounts of muscle (kilogram of muscle per kilogram of body weight) (Blimkie, 1989; Malina, 1986). The sex difference in relative strength (per kilogram of body mass) before puberty is at least in part caused by a higher proportion of body fat in girls from midchildhood onward, a difference similar to the trend in cardiorespiratory endurance (Faust, 1977; Malina, 1986). Rarick and Thompson (1956) suggested that boys are 11% to 13% stronger than girls during childhood. This value reaches 20% by adulthood for strength per cross-sectional area of muscle (Maughan et al., 1983). Correlates and determinants of strength are thought to include age, body size, muscle size, muscle fiber type and size, muscle contractile properties, and biomechanical influences.

During adolescence, there is a marked acceleration in development of strength, particularly in boys. Boys between the ages of 10 and 16 years who were followed longitudinally showed a 23% increase in strength per year. Peak growth in muscle mass occurred during and after peak weight gain, but maximal strength development occurred after peak velocity of growth in height and weight, suggesting that muscle tissue increases first in mass and then in strength (Carron & Bailey, 1974; Malina, 1986). Girls generally show peak strength development before peak weight gain (Faust, 1977). Overall muscle mass increases more than 5 times in males from childhood to adulthood; the increase in females is 3.5 times.

Differentiation in strength between the sexes at puberty is, at least in part, caused by differences in hormonal concentrations, particularly testosterone. Hormones other than the male sex steroids also make an important contribution (Florini, 1987). Unfortunately, no pediatric studies to date have correlated age-associated changes in endocrinologic function with muscle size and muscular strength.

Measurement in the Field

Field measurements of muscular strength usually entail movement of part or all of the body mass against gravity. The two common tests for muscular strength are the flexed arm hang and the sit-up. All the fitness tests previously reviewed include a sit-up test and a pull-up or flexed arm hang test. The correlation between abdominal strength and endurance and shoulder girdle strength as measures of absolute strength for physical fitness is not well established. Although strength is considered an important part of physical fitness, the standards to meet minimal fitness requirements in this area are the least clear. This may result from lack of quantitative research in this area.

Sit-ups

The exact relationship between sit-up performance and abdominal strength and endurance is unclear. How abdominal strength is related to a given number of sit-ups is unknown. Test-retest reliability estimates for sit-ups measured for 11- to 14-year-olds range from 0.64 to 0.94 for both boys and girls (Safrit & Wood, 1987).

Standards of performance as determined by the FITNESSGRAM battery are listed in Table 8-8. The percentage of children who achieved criterion ranged from 80% at age 7 years to 62% at age 16 to 17 years (Blair et al., 1989). These results are slightly different from those attained on the NCYFS I and II (Ross & Gilbert, 1985; Ross & Pate, 1987).

Chin-ups and Flexed Arm Hang

The validity of chin-ups and the flexed arm hang as measures of upper body strength is questionable. Berger and Medlin (1969) suggested that the number of chin-ups as a measure of absolute strength is not valid because body weight is inversely related to the number of chin-ups performed. Considine (1973) demonstrated that pull-ups do not provide an indicator of shoulder girdle strength. The NCYFS II developed a modified pull-up test for 6- to 9-year-olds to overcome the problems associated with body weight (Pate et al., 1987).

Standards by Age

The standards of performance for the FITNESSGRAM Program are listed in Table 8-8. No data are available on the validity or reliability of these standards.

Branta and colleagues (1984) assessed the performance of children on the flexed arm hang as part of a longitudinal study of age changes in motor skills during childhood and adolescence. The minimum standards for fitness on the flexed arm hang set by the FITNESSGRAM Program are less than the measured performance for children at each age in this study. A general increase in the mean performance was noted throughout childhood in both sexes. The greatest gains occurred between the ages of 5 and 6 years and 12 and 13 years for girls and between 5 and 6, 7 and 8, and 13 and 14 years for boys. Both groups showed substantial improvements in performance at puberty. Sex differences were apparent by age 8 years. Relative gains across the age span were substantially higher for boys than for girls.

Physical Activities

Activities that have a high correlation with muscular strength are gymnastics, jumping, sprinting, weight lifting, and wrestling. Local muscular endurance is affected by cycling, figure skating, and middle-distance running.

Response to Training

Training-induced increases in strength can be influenced by numerous factors, including enhancement of motivation, improvement in coordination, increase in number of contractile proteins per cross-sectional area of muscle, and hypertrophy of muscle (Mersch & Stoboy, 1989). Gains in strength and muscle mass can be achieved by children with training at or after puberty. Prepubescent children also show improvements in force output with training but appear to have difficulty in increasing muscle mass (Bar-Or, 1983c; Sale, 1989). Strength improvements in prepubescent children have thus been attributed to neurologic adaptations to training and improved motor unit activation rather than to increased cross-sectional area of muscle (Blimkie et al., 1989; Komi, 1986; Weltman et al., 1986). Direct evidence for the role of neurologic adaptation during strength training has been documented by increases in integrated electromyograph amplitudes and maximal isokinetic strength following an 8-week strength program (Ozmun et al., 1994). Because the magnitude of changes in neuromuscular activation is generally smaller than the observed increases in strength, it has been postulated that improved movement coordination is a contributor to strength gains, particularly in complex multijoint exercises (Blimkie & Sale, 1998). Neuromuscular maturation in the prepubescent child is therefore an important contributor to strength and should not be underestimated.

TABLE 8-8	Field Standards for Strength							
	FITNESSGRAM* SIT-UPS		FITNESSGRAM PULL-UPS		FITNESSGRAM FLEXED ARM HANG		NCYFS I, II† SIT-UPS	
AGE(YR)	F	M	F	M	F	M	F	M
5	20	20	1	1	5	5	–	–
6	20	20	1	1	5	5	60	60
7	20	20	1	1	5	5	35–40	35–40
8	25	25	1	1	8	10	45–50	45–50
9	25	25	1	1	8	10	45–50	35–40
10	30	30	1	1	8	10	30–40	30–40
11	30	30	1	1	8	10	25–30	25–30
12	30	35	1	1	8	10	30	40
13	30	35	1	2	12	10	40	30
14	35	40	1	3	12	15	50	50
15	35	40	1	5	12	25	50	40
16	35	40	1	5	12	25	50	40

Data from Blair, SN, Clark, DG, Cureton, KJ, & Powell, KE. Exercise and fitness in childhood: Implications for a lifetime of health. In Gisolfi, CV, & Lamb, DR (Eds), Perspectives in Exercise Science and Sports Medicine, Vol. 2: Exercise, and Sport. Indianapolis, IN: Benchmark Press, 1989, pp. 401–430; Ross, JG, Delpy, LA, Cristenson, GM, Gold, RS, & Damberg, CL. The national youth and fitness study II: Study procedures and quality control. Journal of Physical Education, Recreation and Dance, 58:57–62, 1987; and Ross, JG, Dotson, CO, Gilbert, GG, & Katz, SJ. The national youth and fitness study I: New standards for fitness measurement. Journal of Physical Education, Recreation and Dance, 56:62–66, 1985.
*Number of sit-ups performed in 1 min.
†Percentile rank of children performing FITNESSGRAM standard from National Children, Youth, and Fitness Study (NCYFS) I, II.

Assessment of Muscular Strength and Endurance in Children with Disabilities

Muscular strength and endurance are crucial fitness components for walking, lifting, and performing most daily functions. Deficits of muscular strength in children with disabilities are a primary focus for the clinician in an attempt to improve (or maintain) maximum function. It is important to keep in mind, however, that strength as measured clinically is not simply the ability of a muscle to generate force. Strength as measured clinically is the effectiveness of the muscle force to produce movement of the joint. This encompasses both the ability of the muscle to generate force and appropriate skeletal alignment on which the muscles act. In children with disabilities, strength deficits result from either the muscles' inability to generate force or malalignment of the skeleton or a combination of both.

Muscular Dystrophy

Strength measurements by dynamometry in children with muscular dystrophy (MD) exhibit progressive deterioration as compared with healthy children (Fowler & Gardner, 1967). A failure of muscular strength to increase with growth is seen. The result is that the absolute strength in a child with MD at the age of 16 years is similar to that of a typical 5-year-old.

Serial longitudinal measurements indicate that muscle strength decreases linearly with age approximately 0.25 manual muscle testing units per year from ages 5 to 13 years. Typically, by the time strength declines to grade 4 (manual muscle testing units), isometric strength measures are 40% to 50% of normal control values (Kilmer et al., 1993; McDonald et al., 1995).

Muscular endurance, the ability to sustain static or rhythmic contraction for long periods, is also affected in children with MD. Ninety-two percent of the children tested by Hosking and colleagues (1976) scored below the 5th percentile for strength in holding the head 45° off the ground. Measurement on the Wingate anaerobic cycling test indicates that both peak muscular power and mean muscular power output are significantly less than is typical (Bar-Or, 1986). The test-retest reliability of this test for various neuromuscular and muscular disease conditions has been established (Tirosh et al., 1990).

Cerebral Palsy

Strength deficits in children with CP are common. Whether voluntary strength can be accurately measured in the presence of spasticity and abnormal motor control is controversial. Strength profiles for lower extremity muscle groups in children with spastic CP have recently become available (Wiley & Damiano, 1998). Children with spastic diplegia demonstrated strength values ranging from 16% to 71% of same-age peers depending on the muscle tested. The gluteus maximus and soleus muscles showed the greatest strength deficits. The involved side of children with hemiplegia exhibited values from 22% to 79% of strength values of same-age peers. The gluteus maximus and the anterior tibialis were the weakest muscles.

Inadequate joint moment and power production as measured by computerized gait analysis are seen in children with CP (Gage, 1991; Olney et al., 1988; Ounpuu, 2004). These measures provide indirect evidence in a functional context of decreased strength, because strength is a prerequisite for moment and power production. Power production by the ankle plantar flexor muscles in terminal stance phase provides a key source of power for forward motion during the typical walking cycle. Power production in terminal stance phase is often reduced in children with CP. Occasionally, inappropriately timed power production results in excessive, but nonproductive, energy expenditure during gait (Gage, 1991) (Fig. 8-2).

Muscular endurance is also decreased in CP. Performance on the Wingate anaerobic test in a group of children with CP resulted in averages that were 2 to 4 standard deviations below the mean (Bar-Or, 1986).

Little information is available regarding modification of lower extremity strength field test items in children with CP. Limited grip strength and flexed arm hang standards are available for upper extremity strength (Seaman et al., 1995). The United Cerebral Palsy Athletic Association uses functional abilities, including strength, to classify athletes for competition (United Cerebral Palsy Athletic Association, 1996).

FLEXIBILITY

The importance of flexibility as a component of health-related fitness is related to prevention of orthopedic impairments later in life, especially lower back pain (United States Department of Health and Human Services, 1990, 1998). Flexibility of the lower back, legs, and shoulders contributes to reduction of injury (Haskell et al., 1985). Limitations in spinal mobility can interfere with activities of daily living, such as dressing, turning, and driving. Restrictions in back mobility can also contribute to abnormalities in walking.

Criterion Measure

Joint range of motion (ROM) is the criterion used for standards of flexibility. Although the ROM measures for adults are well established and can be found in various textbooks (Norkin & White, 1985), ROM information for the pediatric population correlated with changes in stature is limited. Upper extremity ROM data for children are not well documented. The typical measurement tool is the universal goniometer. Gajdosik and Gajdosik review the reliability of goniometry in Chapter 6 of this text.

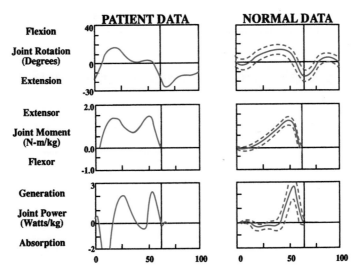

◆ **Figure 8-2** Sagittal plane joint rotation (kinematic), joint moment, and power (kinetics) of a child with cerebral palsy versus a normal child. The child's joint moment is biphasic, and the power graph indicates two distinct bursts of power generation instead of one. The first burst is abnormal and functions to drive the center of gravity upward, not forward, which is nonproductive energy expenditure. *(From Gage, JR. Gait Analysis in Cerebral Palsy. London: Mac Keith Press, 1991, p. 145.)*

Laboratory Measurement and Developmental Aspects of Flexibility

Extremity Range of Motion

Lower extremity passive ROM measurements have been described in the newborn, infant, and toddler (Drews et al., 1984; Phelps et al., 1985; Waugh et al., 1983). Newborn infants exhibit hypoextensibility of both hip and knee flexor muscles and increased popliteal angles consistent with the flexed posture in utero. Range increases in the first months of life. Ranges of hip abduction and rotations also differ from adult values.

Little to no information has been reported for ROM during childhood. Unpublished data from my laboratory on lower extremity ROM measurements in 140 children between the ages of 2 and 18 years suggest variation in some joints throughout childhood and relative stability in others (Stout JL, Phelps JA, Koop SE, unpublished data, 1991) (Table 8-9). Test-retest reliability is 0.95; interrater reliability is .90. Results suggested age and sex differences, with females exhibiting a trend toward more flexibility at all ages. Greater flexibility of the hamstring muscles in females is especially apparent during the teenage years in straight leg raising and popliteal angle measurements.

Posture and Spinal Mobility

Spinal mobility has been measured in both young children and adolescents (Haley et al., 1986; Moran et al., 1979). The technique of measurement of back mobility uses tape measure distance changes in bony landmark relationships before and after a standardized spinal movement. The concurrent validity of this measurement technique has been established (Moll & Wright, 1971; Moran et al., 1979). Anterior spinal flexion appears to remain relatively stable throughout childhood and adolescence, but lateral flexion increases linearly with age through adolescence and into early adulthood. Girls were significantly more flexible than boys in both anterior flexion and lateral flexion in the 5- to 9-year-old age group (Haley et al., 1986).

The relationship of posture to physical fitness is not often addressed in today's emphasis on health-related fitness. Previous research discussing the relationship of posture to fitness included the importance of posture to trunk strength and the potential for imbalance, back pain, headaches, foot pain, and orthopedic deformities (Clarke, 1979; Kendall & Kendall, 1952). Each aspect of posture may be important to mobility and cosmesis in children but becomes of greater importance in adulthood when impairment can lead to further deformity and loss of function.

The New York State Physical Fitness Test. This test includes a posture assessment method consisting of three profiles of 13 posture areas. The test is used for children in grades 4 through 12. The 13 areas include head, shoulder, spine, hips, feet, and arches in the coronal plane and neck, chest, shoulders, upper back, trunk, abdomen, and lower back in the sagittal plane. The 50th percentile requires good posture scores on more than half the posture items (Clarke & Clarke, 1987).

The Assessment of Behavioral Components. This scale, like the posture portion of the New York State Physical Fitness Test, includes a series of criterion-referenced postures in children. The scale rates the postures on degree of asymmetry and joint alignment (Hardy et al., 1988).

The Adams Forward Bending Test. This test is a commonly used screening test for scoliosis. The back is

TABLE 8-9	Selected Range-of-Motion Measurements During Childhood					
	2–5 YEARS		**6–12 YEARS**		**13–19 YEARS**	
RANGE-OF-MOTION MEASURE	M	F	M	F	M	F
Straight leg raise	70	75	65	75	60	70
Popliteal angle (unilateral)*	15	10	30	25	40	25
Abduction†	60	60	50	55	45	50
Internal rotation‡	45	50	50	55	45	45
Femoral antetorsion§	10	15	7	7	0	0

*Supine position.
†Measured with hip extension.
‡Prone position.
§Prone position by lateral placement of the greater trochanter.
Note: All measurement in degrees.

viewed as the individual bends the trunk forward to 90°. The classic sign of scoliosis is the presence of a posterior rib hump during this motion (Bleck, 1991). Although children with scoliosis often develop lack of spinal mobility if the scoliosis becomes severe, the Adams Forward Bending Test is not a test of trunk flexibility per se. Posture is often assessed in children with scoliosis for the presence of lordosis to assess hip flexibility; the presence of pelvic obliquity to assess flexibility of the hip adductors, abductors, and tensor fasciae latae; and the presence of a posterior pelvic tilt to assess hamstring muscle flexibility. For more information on scoliosis, see Chapter 11.

Gross Motor Performance Measure. This instrument, designed as a quality-of-movement companion instrument to the Gross Motor Function Measure, includes postural alignment as one of its performance attributes. A five-point scale of quality is used for assessment of the attribute. This instrument was developed specifically as an examination tool for children with CP (Boyce et al., 1991, 1995; Gowland et al., 1995).

Measurement in the Field

The field test for measurement of flexibility in tests of physical fitness is the sit and reach test, a measure of hamstring muscle and lower back flexibility. All physical fitness batteries used in the United States include a sit and reach test. The test-retest reliability of the sit and reach test has been found to be high; coefficients between .94 and .99 have been reported (Flint & Gudgell, 1966; Jackson & Baker, 1986; Macrae & Wright, 1969). Jackson and Baker (1986) assessed the criterion-related validity of the sit and reach test both for hamstring flexibility and for lower, upper, and total back flexibility. A moderate correlation was found with hamstring flexibility (0.64) and a low correlation with lower back flexibility (0.28). Upper back flexibility and total back flexibility were not correlated with the sit and reach scores.

Branta and colleagues (1984) found sex differences in the performance on the sit and reach test in children between 5 and 14 years of age, with girls showing better flexibility than boys at all ages. Girls showed little variability in flexibility from the ages of 5 to 11 years. Boys experienced a net loss of flexibility between the ages of 5 and 15. This is consistent with the goniometric measures of hamstring flexibility noted in my laboratory (Stout, JL, Phelps, JA, & Koop, SE, unpublished data, 1991).

Standards by Age

The criterion standard of performance on the FITNESSGRAM Program for the sit and reach test is 10 inches from the ages of 5 to 16 years. No variability with age or sex is allowed by the criterion. The FITNESSGRAM Program criterion is well below the average score obtained on the NCYFS I and II (Ross et al., 1985, 1987).

Physical Activities

Activities that require a high degree of flexibility include figure skating, gymnastics, jumping (track and field), and judo. Stretching is an important part of any exercise program for general warm-up before vigorous activity and to reduce the potential for injury. Possible physiologic mechanisms for the benefits of stretching include increased blood flow to muscles, increased mechanical efficiency of muscle and tendon, and reduction of viscosity within the muscle (Bar-Or, 1983c). Decreased resistance to extension of connective tissue leads to increased efficiency and power output by muscles. Much of this research has studied the adult population, but the same principles are believed to apply to children (Bar-Or, 1983c; Kuland & Tottossy, 1985; Yamashita et al., 1992).

Assessment of Flexibility in Children with Disabilities

For clinicians involved in the rehabilitation (or "habilitation") of children with musculoskeletal disorders, maintenance of flexibility or joint ROM is often a primary concern. Almost any musculoskeletal or neuromuscular disorder for which physical therapy is recommended includes treatment for loss of flexibility. Conditions such as CP, juvenile rheumatoid arthritis, MD, or long bone fracture are common examples.

In Chapter 6, Gajdosik and Gajdosik addressed both measurement and the effects of intervention on improving joint ROM in children. The interrater reliability of joint ROM measurements in children with spasticity has been found to be within the range of 0.50 to 0.85 (Ashton et al., 1978; Harris et al., 1985). Similar results have been found in adults (Boone et al., 1978; Ekstrand et al., 1982). Because maintenance of flexibility is an important component of most physical therapy programs for children with disabilities, methods for more reliable assessment of joint ROM are needed.

Field test standards for the sit and reach test and suggested modifications for test administration have been published for children with visual impairments, mental retardation, and Down syndrome (Seaman et al., 1995; Winnick & Short, 1985, 1999).

BODY COMPOSITION

The term "body composition" is understood to mean total body content of water, protein, fat, and minerals (Dell,

1989). In reference to health-related fitness, body composition is used as a measure of body fatness or obesity. Attainment of appropriate body weight for overweight individuals was an explicit objective of *Healthy Children 2000* that has actually moved away from its target (United States Department of Health and Human Services, 1990, 1995). *Healthy People 2010* has maintained objectives related to nutritional health of adolescents and youth as one of its focus areas (United States Department of Health and Human Services, 2000). Large discrepancies continue to exist between current nutrition practices and projected targets (Neumark-Sztainer et al., 2002). Because of the clustering effects of obesity with other risk factors for coronary artery disease, hypertension, and diabetes mellitus, the relevance of obesity to a child's present and future health cannot be overemphasized. The prevalence of childhood and youth obesity is increasing worldwide. In the United States alone, the prevalence of children classified as overweight has increased from 10% in 1988–1994 to 14.4% by 1999–2000 (Ogden et al., 2002, Vincent et al, 2003). Examination of the extent to which children exceed the overweight threshold indicates that the prevalence of overweight children getting heavier is increasing faster than the prevalence of children becoming overweight (Jolliffe, 2004). It has been suggested that regional distribution of abdominal fat is an important predictor of mortality, stroke, heart disease, and diabetes (Bray & Bouchard, 1988).

Laboratory Measurement

The purposes of body composition measurement, whether in the laboratory or in the field, is to obtain a measure of fat-free or lean body mass. Chemical analysis is the only direct method to measure body composition (Klish, 1989). Because this is expensive and impractical, even laboratory standards of measurement are from indirect assessment. Most standards rely on formulas and models of composition which assume that fat and lean body mass are constant. Because infants and children exhibit variable, not constant, body composition throughout childhood (Boileau et al., 1988; Haschke, 1989; Lohman, 1986; Spady, 1989), numerous problems in determining body composition in children are encountered. Use of adult standards leads to overestimation or underestimation of body fatness, depending on the technique (Boileau et al., 1988). All methods presented have some limitations for use with children, but all have been used. There is no one "gold standard" for children.

Densitometry

More commonly referred to as underwater or hydrostatic weighing, densitometry determines the density of an individual by dividing actual body weight by the decrease in weight when the person is completely submerged in water. The densities of fat and lean body mass are assumed to be constant and can be calculated for an individual when the density of the whole body is known. Although it is considered the gold standard for measurement of body composition in adults, it has limited applicability to young children.

Total Body Water

The measurement of total body water is used as a means of estimating the nonfat portion of the body because neutral fat does not bind water. Stable isotopes of hydrogen or oxygen are administered orally and then measured to determine the amount of dilution in a body fluid.

Bioelectric Impedance Analysis

This method is based on the principle that impedance to electrical flow varies in proportion to the amount of lean tissue present. A weak electric current is passed through the body, and its impedance is measured.

Developmental Aspects of Body Composition

From birth through adolescence, body composition is constantly changing. Part of this change is caused by chemical maturation as a result of increasing mineral mass and hydration of adipose tissue (Spady, 1989). Chemical maturation occurs after adolescence, when the constants relating one component of body composition to another stabilize, until the last decades of life (Boileau et al., 1984, 1988; Lohman, 1986; Slaughter et al., 1984).

The four major components of body composition are water, protein, fat, and mineral. Reference models describe the body composition of these components in the child at various ages (Fomon, 1967; Fomon et al., 1982; Haschke, 1989; Haschke et al., 1981; Ziegler et al., 1976). A composite of these reference models and changes with growth in males appears in Figure 8-3.

Fat is the most variable component of body composition during infancy and childhood. Increases begin in utero when fat content changes from 2.5% at 1 kg of body weight to 12% at term gestation (Spady, 1989). The proportion of body fat rises from 12% to an average of 25% from birth to 6 months of age. Fat content decreases during early childhood as muscle mass increases. Sex differences are noted early in childhood; girls exhibit a greater percentage of fat content than do boys. At 6 to 8 years of age, the average fat content for boys is 13% to 15%, and for girls it is 16% to 18% (Lohman, 1987). During adolescence, fat content increases in girls so that between the ages of 14 and 16 years the mean percentage of fat content is 21% to 23%.

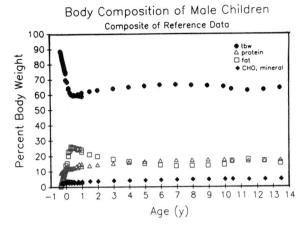

Body Composition of Male Children
Composite of Reference Data

• **Figure 8-3**   The normal body composition of male children as it changes with age. Data derived from data found in the descriptions of the reference fetus, infant, male child at 9 years, children from birth to 10 years, and the adolescent male. CHO = carbohydrate; tbw = total body water. *(From Spady, DW. Normal body composition of infants and children. 98th Ross Laboratories Conference on Pediatric Research, 98:67–73, 1989. Used with permission of Ross Products Division, Abbott Laboratories, Columbus, OH 43216. (c)1989 Ross Products Division, Abbott Laboratories.)*

Water content of the body is approximately 89% of body weight at 24 weeks of gestation and drops to 75% at 40 weeks (Spady, 1989). By 4 months of age, water content stabilizes at approximately 60% to 65% and remains at that level until puberty. Protein content as a proportion of body weight increases from approximately 13% at birth to 15% to 17% at age 10 years. Mineral content of the body rises from 3% at birth to 5% at age 18 years.

Differences between the sexes exist in each major component of body composition throughout childhood and are magnified at adolescence. The major changes during adolescence in both sexes are a decrease in the percentage of water and an increase in the percentage of osseous minerals (Haschke, 1989; Lohman et al., 1984).

Measurement in the Field

Examination of body composition in the field is by measurement of skinfold thickness. The validity of this measure is suspect, just as the validity of laboratory methods is in question. The major problem is that skinfold measurement is based on the assumption that body surface measures and body density relationships are stable throughout childhood (Lohman, 1982). Two other threats to the validity of this measurement are (1) that use of skinfold thickness implies that the subcutaneous fat layer reflects the total amount of fat in the body and (2) that selected measurement sites reflect average thickness.

These assumptions may not be true (Klish, 1989); however, Lohman and colleagues (1984) and Slaughter and colleagues (1984) did not find large deviations in skinfold distribution.

Despite this controversy, measurement of body composition is an important part of almost all health-related fitness tests. Concurrent validity has been demonstrated consistently with moderately high correlations of 0.70 to 0.85 between measurements of skinfolds and densitometry or potassium spectrometry (Going, 1988).

The typical sites for measurement of skinfold thickness are over the triceps brachii, subscapular area, and calf. Usually these areas are measured in some combination. Lohman (1987) has designed a series of charts for easy evaluation of skinfold thickness and percent body fatness based on either triceps and subscapular or triceps and calf skinfold measures. The method of estimation of percent body fatness from skinfold measurements involves estimating density from skinfold measurements and then converting density to percent body fatness. The reader is referred to other sources for more detailed information (Lohman, 1982, 1986; Slaughter et al., 1984). A 3% to 5% error is reported for adults when estimating body fatness from skinfold measurements (Lohman, 1982).

Standards by Age

The criterion values for ranges of body fatness conducive to optimal health in children are 10% to 25% for boys and 15% to 25% for girls (Lohman, 1987). Values higher than 25% in boys and 30% in girls are considered to place the child at risk for associated morbidity. This standard is consistent with the cutoffs at body composition of 32% for females and 25% for males set by the FITNESSGRAM Program (Blair et al., 1989). Results from the NCYFS I and II studies suggest that children within the 40th to 50th percentiles on the test items fall within the optimal ranges described earlier (Ross et al., 1985, 1987).

Response to Training

Conditioning and training programs may or may not affect body composition. If changes are to occur, the type of exercise must entail high-energy expenditure of high or intense effort. Appropriate activities include swimming, running, and weight training. Evidence of program effects on body composition is inconclusive in adults. Little information is available on children, but what is available indicates that percentage of body fatness can be reduced during training for specific sports but rises again when programs are discontinued (Parizkova, 1977; VonDobelin et al., 1972). General physical activity is associated with reduced body fatness as compared with physically inactive peers (Parizkova, 1974). Evidence is inconclusive as to whether obese children are less physically active than nonobese children.

Assessment of Body Composition in Children with Disabilities

Premature Infants

Clinicians treat many children with disabilities who were born prematurely. Premature birth has been shown to affect body composition (Spady et al., 1987). Compared with a "reference" fetus of similar weight, the premature infant has a higher total fat content and lower total body water content. These differences in composition are probably the result of living outside the womb and being faced with the necessity of increasing body fat for temperature regulation. The implications of this altered body composition during growth have not been studied, nor has body composition been studied in premature infants who experience neonatal complications. There may or may not be effects of premature birth on composition throughout childhood and into adulthood.

Cerebral Palsy

Few studies have been conducted on body composition of individuals with CP (Bandini et al., 1991; Berg & Isaksson, 1970; van den Berg-Emons et al., 1998). All reported that adolescents with CP are shorter and typically weigh less than their age-matched peers. Resting metabolic rate was found to be lower than the norm in all studies. However, contradictory findings were noted among the studies, which may or may not be related to differences in methodology. Results of the two older studies suggested that total body water as a percentage of body weight was higher in individuals with CP than in control subjects (Bandini et al., 1991; Berg & Isaksson, 1970). Findings in the later studies indicated the opposite, suggesting an increased percentage of body fat (van den Berg-Emons et al., 1998). Van den Berg-Emons and colleagues postulated that children with CP may have proportionately more subcutaneous fat in the lower extremity skinfold sites because of disuse. Thus using skinfold measurements as an estimation of body fat may not be appropriate in this population. The samples were relatively small and included children with a variety of types of CP and of functional levels. Both type of CP and functional level are likely to be important variables affecting body composition, but the conflicting results of the two studies cannot be resolved without further research.

Myelodysplasia

The study by Bandini and colleagues (1991) also included individuals with myelodysplasia. This group, on average, showed decreased stature, reduced fat-free mass, and increased percentage of body fat as compared with able-bodied peers. The percentage of body fat was above the 95th percentile for all subjects with myelodysplasia. A significant correlation was not found between skinfold thickness and body composition, which suggests that fat distribution may be altered because of the type of paralysis. A previous study had also suggested that skinfold measurements and fat distribution may be altered in myelodysplasia (Hayes-Allen & Tring, 1973). Both studies indicate that children with myelodysplasia are at risk for obesity.

CONDITIONING AND TRAINING

Whether the components of physical fitness can be affected by training programs is an important question, especially to clinicians who are designing programs for children with disabilities. Bar-Or (in 1983c) differentiated between the terms *conditioning* and *training*, which are often used interchangeably. *Physical conditioning* is defined as the process by which exercise, repeated over a specified duration, induces morphologic and functional changes in body systems and tissues. The tissues and systems can include skeletal muscles, the myocardium, adipose tissue, bones, tendons, ligaments, the central nervous system, and the endocrine system. Bar-Or (1983c) considered conditioning to consist of general exercise for overall physical fitness. *Training*, by contrast, is specific exercise designed to promote changes in performance of a particular type of activity. In the context of this chapter, training will be discussed in relation to specific fitness components, but overall conditioning will be discussed in reference to children with disabilities.

FITNESS COMPONENTS AND TRAINING IN CHILDREN

Many of the physiologic changes that result from training and conditioning in adults also take place during the process of growth and maturation in childhood. These naturally occurring changes make it difficult to study the specific effects of conditioning and training. The primary components of physical fitness of interest to trainers are cardiorespiratory endurance and physical strength.

Cardiorespiratory Endurance

Some controversy exists over whether maximal aerobic power or VO_{2max} can be increased by cardiorespiratory training in children (Bar-Or, 1983c; Krahenbuhl et al., 1985). Besides the improvements seen to occur naturally during growth and maturation, other problems in assessing the effects of training include seasonal differences in activity, difficulty in ensuring that a true VO_{2max} has been reached during the testing process, and the already high level of physical activity in young children.

Krahenbuhl and colleagues (1985), in a review of training programs, concluded that maximal aerobic power can be significantly increased after regular intensive training in children of 8 to 14 years of age. Endurance exercise appeared more effective than intermittent exercise. General physical education programs alone were not effective in improving VO_{2max}. Effective activities included running, cycle ergometry, and swimming. Increases of 8% to 10% were measured in effective programs. Some studies reported little or no change in VO_{2max} despite improved long-distance running performance after training programs lasting 1 to 9 weeks (Bar-Or, 1983c; Cumming et al., 1967).

Less controversy exists over whether training is effective in improving cardiorespiratory endurance in adolescence. The effects of training in adolescents appear to be similar to those in adults. The functional and morphologic changes of the cardiovascular and pulmonary systems that take place as a result of training are listed in Table 8-10. Training effects usually include increases in myocardial mass, stroke volume, ventilation, and respiratory muscular endurance.

Muscular Strength and Endurance

Muscular strength is a component of fitness that can be affected by training, especially in children at or after puberty. Resistance strength training refers to training for improved muscular strength by repeatedly overcoming heavy resistance. The practice of resistance strength training is problematic in preadolescent children because controversy exists regarding (1) whether children can make gains in strength and muscle mass, (2) whether gains improve athletic performance, and particularly (3) whether children are more susceptible to injury when participating in such training. Despite the controversy, resistance strength training has been shown to increase voluntary force production at all ages and may reduce the risk of injury during athletic participation (Blimkie & Sale, 1998; Sale, 1989).

In a review of strength training studies, Sale (1989) concluded that children can increase voluntary strength as a result of training, and furthermore, children show a greater increase in strength than do adults when training-induced strength improvements are expressed as a percentage of change. During maximal voluntary contraction, children can develop the same force per unit of muscle cross-sectional area as adults despite differences in absolute strength and muscle size.

TABLE 8-10	Cardiorespiratory Function Variables and Response to Training in Children
FUNCTION VARIABLE	**CHANGE WITH TRAINING**
Heart Volume	Increase
Blood Volume	Increase
Total hemoglobin	Slight increase
Stroke volume (max, submax)	Increase
Cardiac output (max, submax)	Increase, no change, or decrease
Arteriovenous difference (submax)	No change
Blood flow to active muscle	No change
Ventilation/kg body wt (max)	Increase
Ventilation/kg body wt (submax)	Decrease
Respiratory rate (submax)	Decrease
Tidal volume (max)	Increase
Respiratory muscle endurance	Increase

Adapted from Bar-Or, O. Physiologic responses to exercise in healthy children. In Bar-Or, O. Pediatric Sports Medicine for the Practitioner. New York: Springer-Verlag, 1983, p.49.

max = maximal exercise; submax = submaximal exercise.

As previously described, the strength increases associated with growth are closely related to increases in muscle mass, including an increase in the number of both sarcomeres and fibrils per muscle fiber (Malina, 1986). The enhancement of muscular strength caused by growth is estimated to be approximately 1.5 kg per year from the age of 6 to 14 years (Mersch & Stoboy, 1989). In conjunction with "muscular" adaptations, neural adaptations associated with improved coordination and motor learning may also play a role. For example, the increases in voluntary strength noted with training in prepubescent children have been found to be independent of increased muscle mass or hypertrophy such as that seen in postpubescent children or adults (Blimkie et al., 1989; Sale, 1989; Weltman et al., 1986). Improved motor unit activation and neural adaptations (including more appropriate co-contraction of synergist muscles and inhibition of antagonist muscles, as well as improvements in motor unit recruitment order and firing frequency within the prime movers) are believed to play a role in producing training effects in both adults and children (Komi, 1986; Moritani & DeVries, 1979). It has been suggested that, during the early stages of training, neural adaptation predominates in producing altered performance. Muscular adaptation contributes in the later stages of training (Blimkie & Sale, 1998; Sale, 1989) (Fig. 8-4).

PRINCIPLES OF TRAINING

The principles of an effective training program include specificity, as well as guidelines for intensity, frequency, and duration of exercise. Rules for children are essentially the same as those for adults.

Specificity

The changes that take place in the body as a result of training are specific to the type of exercise performed and to the tissue involved. Myocardial tissue, for example, is affected by long-distance running but not by resistance strength training. The type of contraction (concentric, eccentric, or isometric), the number of repetitions performed, the velocity of muscle contraction, and the particular muscles exercised all influence the results of a strength training program. Different sports develop different components of fitness.

Intensity

Activity at a certain intensity is required to achieve conditioning or training effects. Intensity should be determined as a percentage of the individual's maximum because the same amount of activity can represent two entirely different levels of intensity for two different individuals. For example, a child with CP who walks at the same velocity as an able-bodied child may consume twice as much oxygen, so walking as a form of exercise for the child with CP is more intense. Although VO_2 depends on the square of velocity, an average 6- to 12-year-old walking at an average velocity consumes about 25% of VO_{2max}; for a child with CP, VO_2 can be as high as 75% to 90% of VO_{2max} (personal observation, 1998).

Intensity threshold refers to the intensity of exercise below which few or no training or conditioning effects are observed (Bar-Or, 1983c). The intensity threshold of maximal aerobic power in adults required to produce a training effect is 60% to 70% of VO_{2max}. The threshold for strength is approximately 60% to 65% of maximal voluntary contraction. The principle of overload in strength training is in part related to the intensity threshold of exercise. Overload refers to a task that requires considerable voluntary effort to complete. No specific data are available for intensity thresholds for children, but they are thought to be at least equal to those of adults. Whether intensity thresholds for children with various disabilities are the same as those for able-bodied children is also unknown.

Frequency

The optimal frequency of training depends on the type of program, and frequency is interrelated with intensity and duration. Two or three times per week is a general rule of thumb (Bar-Or, 1983c).

Duration

Any program, whether a therapeutic program or a fitness program, requires a minimum implementation time before benefits are seen. Most effective conditioning programs

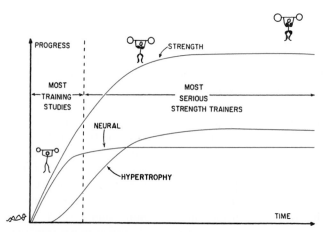

◆ **Figure 8-4**   Relative roles of neural and muscular adaptation in strength training. Neural adaptation plays the biggest role in the early phase of training, which can last up to several weeks. Muscular adaptation predominates later and is limited by the extent that muscles can hypertrophy. *(From Sale, DG. Strength training in children. In Gisolfi, CV, & Lamb, DR [Eds.]. Perspectives in Exercise Science and Sports Medicine, Vol. 2: Youth, Exercise, and Sport. Indianapolis, IN: Benchmark Press, 1989, p. 180.)*

last at least 6 to 8 weeks. The optimal duration of an exercise session depends on the type of program. In general, the session should consist of a warm-up phase of 10 minutes, an exercise phase above the exercise threshold for 15 to 30 minutes, and a 5- to 7-minute cool-down period. The warm-up phase has been shown to be important for increasing performance of both aerobic and anaerobic tasks in children (Bar-Or, 1983c). The warm-up period should include (1) activities to raise core body temperature, (2) stretching exercises, and (3) activities specific to the exercise task. The American Academy of Pediatrics (1983) recommends that strength-training regimens for children include activities to provide strength training for all parts of the body to ensure balanced development.

The duration of the exercise phase in strength training is sometimes associated with the goal of achieving maximal overload. This is usually done in one of two ways—either by repeating brief maximal contractions or by repeating submaximal contractions to the point of fatigue.

Progression

A conditioning or training program must be progressive in its demands for continued improvement. The intensity threshold, the duration of exercise sessions, the number of repetitions performed during a session, or the frequency of exercise sessions may need to be increased. All contribute individually and collectively to the progression of the exercise program.

CONDITIONING IN CHILDREN WITH DISABILITIES

Cerebral Palsy

As children with CP approach and move through adolescence, an important aspect of function is the ability to maintain ambulation. VO_2 during ambulation in preadolescent children with CP (ages 6 to 12 years) is more than twice that of able-bodied children walking at the same velocity (Koop et al., 1989, Stout & Koop, 2004). If body weight and adiposity increase in adolescence without an increase in muscular strength, maximal aerobic capacity decreases, and the task of walking becomes more and more difficult. Growth in mass is a cubic function (volume), and growth in strength is a function of the square (cross-sectional muscle area). As previously mentioned, muscles increase in mass first, then in strength (Malina, 1986). During the adolescent growth spurt, mass increases at a faster rate than does strength. For able-bodied children, this process occurs without noticeable deficit or loss of function, but for children with CP, loss of function sometimes occurs because the rate of increase in strength is inadequate to support the rate of increase in muscle mass. A major goal of physical therapy for adolescents with CP is maintenance of the ability to ambulate throughout the growth spurt. If a child has maximal strength and aerobic capacity on entering the growth spurt, function is also likely to be at maximal capacity. Conditioning in a child with CP could play a vital role in the process of maximizing the potential not only of the adolescent but of the preadolescent as well.

The ultimate goal of conditioning programs for children with CP is to retard or reverse the deterioration of capacity expected during adolescence. In a longitudinal study of adolescents with CP, Lundberg (1973) found that heart rate at a given power load increased an average of 10 bpm per year, implying decreasing efficiency. Studies have demonstrated that conditioning effects in the population of children and adolescents with CP are similar to those of children without disability (Bar-Or et al., 1976; Berg, 1970b; Lundberg & Pernow, 1970; Lundberg et al., 1967). Increased strength, ROM, and functional endurance have also been reported as a result of a strengthening program (Horvat, 1987). Greater attention is now given to the benefits of strengthening in both children and adolescents with CP. Damiano and colleagues report strength gains after a resistive exercise training program. Functional improvements in both gait and Gross Motor Function Measure scores are noted, as well as decreases in spasticity (Damiano & Abel, 1998; Damiano et al., 1995a, 1995b).

One study that addressed the issue of changes in body composition as a result of conditioning showed no change in the percentage of body fat after a 4-month program (Berg, 1970a). A conditioning response unique to individuals with CP is an increase in blood flow to exercising muscles (Lundberg & Pernow, 1970). This may reflect a physiologic mechanism in which conditioning and strengthening decrease the effects of spasticity.

Evidence suggests that neither regular physical education classes nor habitual activities are sufficient to induce conditioning changes in children with CP (Berg, 1970b; Dresen, 1985). The program must increase intensity beyond habitual exercise levels. The duration of the overall program should be longer than 6 weeks; results of 6-week training programs are equivocal (Ekblom & Lundberg, 1968). Target heart rate was typically maintained for 15 to 30 minutes in most studies. Activities in accordance with the child's ability were used; examples are cycle ergometry, swimming, running, and jogging. See Chapter 21 for more information on management of CP.

Cystic Fibrosis

Cystic fibrosis is a hereditary disease affecting the exocrine glands. The lungs, gastrointestinal tract, and sweat glands produce excessive secretion. Airway obstruction, infection, and respiratory failure result from excess viscous mucus in the respiratory tract. Results of studies emphasizing aerobic conditioning for 3 to 5 months suggest that VO_{2max}, endurance of respiratory muscles, and pulmonary function all show improvement (Jankowski, 1986; Orenstein et al., 1981; Zach et al., 1982). Jogging, cycling, swimming, weight lifting, and calisthenics of various durations and combinations were used.

In addition to the positive effects of conditioning on physical fitness, clinical benefits in the management of the disease are also reported (Bar-Or, 1985). Increased coughing and mucous clearance may reduce the need for chest therapy to manage secretions (Zach et al., 1982).

The effects of exercise on children with cystic fibrosis and other clinical populations must be closely monitored to reduce or avoid potential detrimental effects. Particular concerns in the population with cystic fibrosis are dehydration (especially in high heat) and oxygen desaturation (Bar-Or, 1985). See Chapter 27 for more information on management of cystic fibrosis.

Muscular Dystrophy

The effects of conditioning patients with MD have been evaluated in numerous studies, which produced equivocal results (Abrahamson & Rogoff, 1952; DeLateur & Giaconi, 1979; Fowler et al., 1965; Vignos & Watkins, 1966). Evaluation of the results must take into account that many of the studies were inadequately controlled for threats to internal validity. Results suggest that modest gains in strength can be made or the rate of deterioration retarded. In one study, DeLateur and Giaconi (1979) found no significant change in strength of the quadriceps femoris muscle after 6 weeks of a 6-month conditioning program of submaximal exercise. A modest, but not significant, increase in strength was found after 6 months. Each subject served as his or her own control. No deleterious effects of a strengthening program were found. Despite the lack of statistically significant effects, the increase in strength may be enough to deter future deterioration. See Chapter 15 for more information on management of MD.

▌ SUMMARY

This chapter was designed to provide information on physical fitness and conditioning in the able-bodied child for promoting health and preventing disease. The components of fitness, how they are tested, and how they contribute to health were reviewed. An understanding of physical fitness, physical activity, and conditioning is

valuable for appreciating the impact of disabling conditions on these variables. Health-related physical fitness is important for reducing future health risks in every child, regardless of the presence or absence of disability. Preadolescent fitness may be especially important to the child with a disability because of the effects the particular disability may have on the child as he or she enters puberty and adulthood. The design of exercise programs (their intensity, frequency, and duration) should encompass the minimal requirements for physical fitness, as well as incorporate therapeutic goals. Exercise programs should be designed so that the energy requirements for accomplishing day-to-day activities through the growth period are met. Meeting this goal is likely to require additional exercise beyond current therapy or physical education. One of our goals as pediatric therapists should be to ensure, to whatever extent possible, that our clients end their childhood with a fitness level suitable to a healthy adulthood. Research is needed to document the extent to which this goal can be met for specific populations and levels of disability.

Much research remains to be done in the able-bodied population as well. Reliability and validity studies must continue on criterion-based measures now being used to determine minimal fitness levels. Research must establish reliable, valid, and universal criteria, both in the laboratory and in the field. Continued identification of the relationship between childhood physical activity and fitness and health in adulthood is vital to our overall understanding of health-related fitness.

Research to benefit populations with disabilities or children with special needs has barely begun. With the inadequate base of research in children without disability, developing standards of fitness for specific disabled populations begins at a disadvantage. A question that remains to be answered is whether the fitness performance criteria for children without disabilities are valid for children with disabilities or special needs. Experience with development of testing and measurement tools for other purposes would suggest they are not. Are children with disabilities such as CP more fit because they expend in walking an amount of energy equivalent to that of an able-bodied person walking up and down stairs all day long? Are the thresholds and target zones for fitness improvement the same for children with a variety of disabilities as for able-bodied children? How are conditioning and training programs best designed for children with disabilities? Do conditioning programs initiated before the onset of puberty help maintain fitness during and after puberty? What are the physiologic and behavioral factors that limit a child's capacity to improve fitness variables or to exercise? How much exercise is detrimental? How do presurgical strengthening programs affect the recovery of strength after surgery? Questions such as these are only the beginning of our quest for understanding. The journey has just begun.

REFERENCES

Abrahamson, AS, & Rogoff, J. Physical treatment in muscular dystrophy (abstract). In Proceedings of the 2nd Medical Conference. Muscular Dystrophy Association, New York, 1952, pp. 123–124.

Adams, FH. Factors affecting the working capacity of children and adolescents. In Rarick, GL (Ed.). Physical Activity: Human Growth and Development. New York: Academic Press, 1973, pp. 89–90.

Alexander, J, & Molnar, GE. Muscular strength in children: Preliminary report on objective standards. Archives of Physical Medicine and Rehabilitation, 54:424–427, 1973.

American Academy of Pediatrics. Weight training and weightlifting: Information for the pediatrician. Physician and Sports Medicine, 11(3):157–161, 1983.

American Alliance for Health, Physical Education, Recreation, and Dance. The AAHPERD Physical Best Program. Reston, VA: American Alliance for Health Physical Education, Recreation, and Dance, 1988.

American Physical Therapy Association. Guide to physical therapist practice. Physical Therapy, 81:1–768, 2001.

American Psychological Association. Standards for Educational and Psychological Testing. Washington, DC: American Psychological Association, 1985.

Ashton BB, Pickles, B, & Roll, JW. Reliability of goniometric measurements of hip motion in spastic cerebral palsy. Developmental Medicine and Child Neurology, 20:87–94, 1978.

Astrand PO. Experimental Studies of Physical Working Capacity in Relation to Sex and Age. Copenhagen: Ejnar Munksgaard, 1952.

Baltzopoulos, V, & Kellis, E: Isokinetic strength during childhood and adolescence. In Van Praagh, E (Ed.). Pediatric Anaerobic Performance. Champaign, IL: Human Kinetics, 1998, pp. 225–240.

Bandini, LG, Schoeller, DA, Fukagawa, NK, Wykes, LJ, & Dietz, WH. Body composition and energy expenditure in adolescents with cerebral palsy or myelodysplasia. Pediatric Research, 29:70–77, 1991.

Bar-Or, O. Appendix II: Procedures for exercise testing in children. In Bar-Or, O. Pediatric Sports Medicine for the Practitioner. New York: Springer-Verlag, 1983a, pp. 315–341.

Bar-Or, O. Neuromuscular diseases. In Bar-Or, O. Pediatric Sports Medicine for the Practitioner. New York: Springer-Verlag, 1983b, pp. 227–249.

Bar-Or, O. Physiologic responses to exercise in healthy children. In Bar-Or, O. Pediatric Sports Medicine for the Practitioner. New York: Springer-Verlag, 1983c, pp. 1–65.

Bar-Or, O. Physical conditioning in children with cardiorespiratory disease. Exercise and Sport Sciences Reviews, 13:305–334, 1985.

Bar-Or, O. Pathophysiological factors which limit the exercise capacity of the sick child. Medicine and Science in Sports and Exercise, 18:276–282, 1986.

Bar-Or, O, Inbar, O, & Spira, R. Physiological effects of a sports rehabilitation program on cerebral palsied and poliomyelitic adolescents. Medicine and Science in Sports, 8:157–161, 1976.

Berg, K. Effect of physical activation and improved nutrition on the body composition of school children with cerebral palsy. Acta Paediatrica Supplement, 204:53–69, 1970a.

Berg, K. Effect of physical training of school children with cerebral palsy. Acta Paediatrica Supplement, 204:27–33, 1970b.

Berg, K, & Isaksson, B. Body composition and nutrition of school children with cerebral palsy. Acta Paediatrica Supplement, 204:41–52, 1970.

Berger, RA, & Medlin, RL. Evaluation of Berger's 1-RM chin test for junior high school mates. Research Quarterly, 40:460–463, 1969.

Blair, SN, Clark, DG, Cureton, KJ, & Powell, KE. Exercise and fitness in childhood: Implications for a lifetime of health. In Gisolfi, CV, & Lamb, DR (Eds.). Perspectives in Exercise Science and Sports Medicine, Vol. 2: Youth, Exercise, and Sport. Indianapolis, IN: Benchmark Press, 1989, pp. 401–430.

Bleck, E. Adolescent idiopathic scoliosis. Developmental Medicine and Child Neurology, 33:167–173, 1991.

Blimkie, CJR. Age and sex associated variation in strength during childhood: Anthropometric, morphologic, neurologic, biomechanical, endocrinologic, genetic, and physical activity correlates. In Gisolfi, CV, & Lamb, DR (Eds.). Perspectives in Exercise Science and Sports Medicine, Vol. 2: Youth, Exercise, and Sport. Indianapolis, IN: Benchmark Press, 1989, pp. 99–163.

Blimkie, CJR, Ramsay, J, Sale, D, MacDougall, D, Smith, K, & Garner, K. Effects of 10 weeks of resistance training on strength development in prepubertal boys. In Osteid, S, & Carlsen, KH (Eds.). Children and Exercise XIII. Champaign, IL: Human Kinetics, 1989, pp. 183–197.

Blimkie, CJR, & Sale, DG: Strength development and trainability during childhood. In Van Praagh, E (Ed.). Pediatric Anaerobic Performance. Champaign, IL: Human Kinetics, 1998, pp. 193–224.

Boileau, RA, Lohman, TG, & Slaughter, MH. Exercise and body composition in children and youth. Scandinavian Journal of Sport Sciences, 7:7–17, 1985.

Boileau, RA, Lohman, TG, Slaughter, MH, Ball, TE, Going, SB, & Hendrix, MK. Hydration of the fat-free body in children during maturation. Human Biology, 56:651–666, 1984.

Boileau, RA, Lohman, TG, Slaughter, MH, Horswill, CA, & Stillman, RJ. Problems associated with determining body composition in maturing youngsters. In Brown, EW, & Branta, CF (Eds.). Competitive Sports for Children and Youth: An Overview of Research and Issues. Champaign, IL: Human Kinetics, 1988, pp. 3–16.

Boone, DC, Azen, SP, Lin, CM, Spense, C, Baron, C, & Lee, L. Reliability of goniometric measurements. Physical Therapy, 58:1355–1360, 1978.

Boyce, WF, Gowland, C, Hardy, S, Rosenbaum, PL, Lane, M, Plews, N, Goldsmith C, & Russell, DJ. Development of a quality-of-movement measure for children with cerebral palsy. Physical Therapy, 71:820–828, 1991.

Boyce, WF, Gowland, C, Rosenbaum, PL, Lane, M, Plews, N, Goldsmith, CH, Russell, DJ, Wright, V, Potter, S, & Harding, D. The Gross Motor Performance Measure: Validity and responsiveness of a measure of quality of movement. Physical Therapy, 75:603–613, 1995.

Braden, DS, & Strong, WB. Cardiovascular responses to exercise in childhood. American Journal of Diseases of Children, 144:1255–1260, 1990.

Branta, C, Haubenstricker, J, & Seefeldt, V. Age changes in motor skills during childhood and adolescence. Exercise and Sport Sciences Reviews, 12:467–520, 1984.

Bray, GA, & Bouchard, C. Role of fat distribution during growth and its relationship to health. American Journal of Clinical Nutrition, 47:551–552, 1988.

Brodie, DA, Burnie, J, Eston, RG, & Royce, JA. Isokinetic strength and flexibility characteristics in preadolescent boys. In Rutenfranz, J, Mocellin, R, & Klimt, F (Eds.). Children and Exercise XII. Champaign, IL: Human Kinetics, 1986, pp. 309–319.

Brooks, GA, Fahey, TD, & Baldwin, K. Exercise Physiology: Human Bioenergetics and Its Applications, 4th ed. New York: McGraw-Hill, 2004.

Carron, AV, & Bailey, DA. Strength development in boys from 10–16 years. Monographs of the Society for Research in Child Development, 39:1–37, 1974.

Chrysler Fund–Amateur Athletic Union. Physical Fitness Program. Bloomington, IN: Chrysler Fund–Amateur Athletic Union, 1987.

Clarke, HH. Posture. Physical Fitness Research Digest, 9:1–23, 1979.

Clarke, HH, & Clarke, DH. Application of Measurement in Physical Education. Englewood Cliffs, NJ: Prentice-Hall, 1987, pp. 93–99.

Considine, WJ. An Analysis of Selected Upper Body Tasks as Measures of Strength (abstract). American Association of Health, Physical Education and Recreation, 25:74, 1973.

Cooper, DM, Weiler-Ravell, D, Whipp, BJ, & Wasserman, K. Growth-related changes in oxygen uptake and heart rate during progressive exercise in children. Pediatric Research, 18:845–851, 1984.

Cooper Institute for Aerobics Research. FITNESSGRAM Test Administration Manual. Champaign, IL: Human Kinetics, 1999.

Corbin CB. Youth fitness, exercise and health: There is much to be done. Research Quarterly for Exercise and Sport, 58:308–314, 1987.

Cumming, GR, Goodwin, A, Baggley, G, & Antel, J. Repeated measurements of aerobic capacity during a week of intensive training at a youth track camp. Canadian Journal of Physiology and Pharmacology, 45:805–811, 1967.

Cunningham, DA, MacFarlane-VanWaterschoot, B, Paterson, DH, Lefcoe, M, & Sangal, SP. Reliability and reproducibility of maximal oxygen uptake in children. Medicine and Science in Sports, 9:104–108, 1977.

Cureton, KJ, & Warren, GL. Criterion-referenced standards for youth health-related fitness tests: A tutorial. Research Quarterly for Exercise and Sport, 61:7–19, 1990.

Daltroy, LH, Liang, MH, & Fossel, AH. The POSNA pediatric musculoskeletal functional health questionnaire: Report on reliability, validity, and sensitivity to change. Journal of Pediatric Orthopaedics, 18:561–571, 1998.

Damiano, DL, & Abel, MF. Functional outcomes of strength training in spastic cerebral palsy. Archives of Physical Medicine and Rehabilitation, 79:119–125, 1998.

Damiano, DL, Kelly, LE, & Vaughan, CL. Effects of quadriceps muscle strengthening on crouch gait in children with spastic diplegia. Physical Therapy, 75:668–671, 1995a.

Damiano, DL, Vaughan, CL, & Abel, MF. Muscle response to heavy resistance exercise in children with spastic cerebral palsy. Developmental Medicine and Child Neurology, 37:731–739, 1995b.

DeLateur, BJ, & Giaconi, RM. Effect on maximal strength of submaximal exercise in Duchenne muscular dystrophy. American Journal of Physical Medicine, 58:26–36, 1979.

Dell, RB. Comparison of densitometric methods applicable to infants and small children for studying body composition. Ross Laboratories Conference on Pediatric Research, 98:22–30, 1989.

Dresen, MHW. Physical and psychological effects of training on handicapped children. In Binkhorst, RA, Kemper, HCG, & Saris, WHM (Eds.). Children and Exercise XI. Champaign, IL: Human Kinetics, 1985, pp. 203–209.

Drews, J, Vraciu, JK, & Pellino, G. Range of motion of the joints of the lower extremities of newborns. Physical and Occupational Therapy in Pediatrics, 4(2):49–62, 1984.

Ekblom, B, & Lundberg, A. Effect of training on adolescents with severe motor handicaps. Acta Paediatrica Scandinavica, 57:17–23, 1968.

Ekstrand, J, Wiktorsson, M, Oberg, B, & Gillquist, J. Lower extremity goniometric measurements: A study to determine their reliability. Archives of Physical Medicine and Rehabilitation, 63:171–175, 1982.

Ericksson, BO, Gollnick, PD, & Saltin, B. Muscle metabolism and enzyme activities after training in boys 11–13 years old. Acta Physiologica Scandinavica, 87:485–487, 1973.

Ericksson, BO, Karlsson, J, & Saltin, B. Muscle metabolites during exercise in pubertal boys. Acta Paediatrica Scandinavica Supplement, 217:154–157, 1971.

Faust, MS. Somatic development of adolescent girls. Society for Research in Child Development, 42:1–90, 1977.

Flint, MM, & Gudgell, J. Electromyographic study of abdominal muscular activity during exercise. Research Quarterly, 36:29–37, 1966.

Florini, JR. Hormonal control of muscle growth. Muscle and Nerve, 10:577–598, 1987.

Fomon, SJ. Body composition of the male reference infant during the first year of life. Pediatrics, 40:863–867, 1967.

Fomon, SJ, Haschke, F, Ziegler, EE, & Nelson, SE. Body composition of reference children from birth to age 10 years. American Journal of Clinical Nutrition, 35:1169–1173, 1982.

Fowler, WM, & Gardner, GW. Quantitative strength measurements in muscular dystrophy. Archives of Physical Medicine and Rehabilitation, 48:629–644, 1967.

Fowler, WM, Pearson, CM, Egstrom, GH, & Gardner, GW. Ineffective treatment of muscular dystrophy with an anabolic steroid and other measures. New England Journal of Medicine, 272:875–882, 1965.

Francis, K, & Feinstein, R. A simple height-specific and rate-specific step test for children. Southern Medical Journal, 84:169–174, 1991.

Gage, JR. Gait Analysis in Cerebral Palsy. London: Mac Keith Press, 1991.

Gaul, C. Muscular strength and endurance. In Docherty, D (Ed.). Measurement in Pediatric Exercise Science. Champaign, IL: Human Kinetics, 1996, pp. 225–228.

Giannini, MJ, & Protas, EJ. Aerobic capacity in juvenile rheumatoid arthritis patients and healthy children. Arthritis Care and Research, 4:131–135, 1991.

Giannini, MJ, & Protas, EJ. Exercise response in children with and without juvenile rheumatoid arthritis: A comparison study. Physical Therapy, 72:365–372, 1992.

Godfrey, S. Growth and development of the cardiopulmonary response to exercise. In Davis, JA, & Dobbing, J (Eds.). Scientific Foundations in Paediatrics. London: William Heinemann Medical Books, 1981, pp. 450–460.

Going, S. Physical best: Body composition in the assessment of youth fitness. Journal of Physical Education, Recreation and Dance, 59(9):32–36, 1988.

Gowland, C, Boyce, WF, Wright, V, Russell, DJ, Goldsmith, CH, & Rosenbaum, PL. Reliability of the Gross Motor Performance Measure. Physical Therapy, 75:597–602, 1995.

Green, HJ, & Patla, AE. Maximal aerobic power: Neuromuscular and metabolic considerations. Medicine and Science in Sports and Exercise, 24:38–46, 1992.

Haley, SM, Tada, WL, & Carmichael, EM. Spinal mobility in young children: A normative study. Physical Therapy, 66:1697–1703, 1986.

Harris, SR, Smith, LH, & Krukowski, L. Goniometric reliability for a child with spastic quadriplegia. Journal of Pediatric Orthopedics, 5:348–351, 1985.

Haschke, F. Body composition during adolescence. Ross Laboratories Conference on Pediatric Research, 98:76–82, 1989.

Haschke, F, Fomon, SJ, & Ziegler, EE. Body composition of a nine year old reference boy. Pediatric Research, 15:847–850, 1981.

Haskell, WL, Montoye, HJ, & Orenstein, D. Physical activity and exercise to achieve health-related fitness components. Public Health Reports, 100:202–212, 1985.

Hayes-Allen, MC, & Tring, FC. Obesity: Another hazard for spina bifida children. British Journal of Preventive and Social Medicine, 27:192–196, 1973.

Horvat, M. Effects of a progressive resistance training program on an individual with spastic cerebral palsy. American Corrective Therapy Journal, 41:7–10, 1987.

Hosking, GP, Bhat, US, Dubowitz, V, & Edwards, HT. Measurement of muscle strength and performance in children with normal and diseased muscle. Archives of Disease in Childhood, 51:957–963, 1976.

Institute for Aerobics Research. FITNESSGRAM Users Manual. Dallas, TX: Institute for Aerobics Research, 1987.

Jackson, AS, & Coleman, AE. Validation of distance run tests for elementary school children. Research Quarterly, 47:86–94, 1976.

Jackson, AW, & Baker, AA. The relationship of the sit and reach test to criterion measures of hamstring and back flexibility in young females. Research Quarterly for Exercise and Sport, 57:183–186, 1986.

Jankowski, JW. Exercise testing and exercise prescription for individuals with cystic fibrosis. In Skinner, JS (Ed.). Testing and Exercise Prescription for Special Cases. Philadelphia: Lea & Febiger, 1986.

Jolliffe, D. Extent of overweight among US children and adolescents from 1971-2000. International Journal of Obesity 28:4–9, 2004.

Kendall, HO, & Kendall, FP. Posture and Pain. Baltimore: Williams & Wilkins, 1952, p. 104.

Kilmer, DD, Abresch, RT, & Fowler, WM. Serial manual muscle testing in Duchenne muscular dystrophy. Archives of Physical Medicine and Rehabilitation, 74:1168–1171, 1993.

Klish, WJ. The "gold standard." Ross Laboratories Conference on Pediatric Research, 98:4–7, 1989.

Koch, G. Muscle blood flow after ischemic work during bicycle ergometer work in boys aged 12. Acta Pediatrica Belgica Supplement, 28:29–9, 1974.

Komi, PV. Training muscle strength and power: Interaction of neuromotoric, hypertrophic, and mechanical factors. International Journal of Sports Medicine, 7(suppl):10–15, 1986.

Koop, SE, Stout, JL, Drinken, WH, & Starr, RC. Energy cost of walking in children with cerebral palsy (abstract). Physical Therapy, 69:386, 1989.

Krahenbuhl, GS, Pangrazi, RP, Peterson, GW, Burkett, LN, & Schneider, MJ. Field testing of cardiorespiratory fitness in primary school children. Medicine and Science in Sports, 10:208–213, 1978.

Krahenbuhl, GS, Skinner, JS, & Kohrt, WM. Developmental aspects of maximal aerobic power in children. Exercise and Sport Sciences Reviews, 13:503–538, 1985.

Kuland, DN, & Tottossy, M. Warm-up strength and power. Clinics in Sports Medicine, 4:137–158, 1985.

Landin, S, Hagenfeldt, L, Saltin, B, & Wahren, J. Muscle metabolism during exercise in hemiparetic patients. Clinical Science and Molecular Medicine, 53:257–269, 1977.

Lavay, B, Reid, G, & Cressler-Chaviz, M. Measuring the cardiovascular endurance of persons with mental retardation: A critical review. Exercise and Sport Sciences Reviews, 18:263–290, 1990.

Lefkof, MB. Trunk flexion in healthy children aged 3 to 7 years. Physical Therapy, 66:39–44, 1986.

Lohman, TG. Measurement of body composition in children. Journal of Physical Education, Recreation and Dance, 53(7):67–70, 1982.

Lohman, TG. Applicability of body composition techniques and constants for children and youth. Exercise and Sport Sciences Reviews, 14:325–357, 1986.

Lohman, TG. The use of skinfold to estimate body fatness on children and youth. Journal of Physical Education, Recreation and Dance, 58(9):98–102, 1987.

Lohman, TG, Slaughter, MH, Boileau, RA, Bunt, J, & Lussier, L. Bone mineral measurements and their relation to body density in children, youth, and adults. Human Biology, 56:667–679, 1984.

Lundberg, A. Changes in the working pulse during the school year in

adolescents with cerebral palsy. Scandinavian Journal of Rehabilitation Medicine, 5:12–17, 1973.

Lundberg, A. Maximal aerobic capacity in young people with spastic cerebral palsy. Developmental Medicine and Child Neurology, 20:205–210, 1978.

Lundberg, A, Ovenfors, CO, & Saltin, B. The effect of physical training on school children with cerebral palsy. Acta Paediatrica Scandinavica, 56:182–188, 1967.

Lundberg, A, & Pernow, B. The effect of physical training on oxygen utilization and lactate formation in the exercising muscle of adolescents with motor handicaps. Scandinavian Journal of Clinical and Laboratory Investigation, 26:89–96, 1970.

Macrae, I, & Wright, V. Measurement of back movement. Annals of the Rheumatic Diseases, 52:584–589, 1969.

Malina, RM. Growth of muscle and muscle mass. In Falkner, F, & Tanner, JM (Eds.). Human Growth: A Comprehensive Treatise, Vol. 2: Postnatal Growth. New York: Plenum Press, 1986, pp. 77–99.

Malina, RM. Physical activity and fitness: pathways from childhood to adulthood. American Journal of Human Biology, 13:162–172, 2001.

Mathews, DK. Measurement in Physical Education, 4th ed. Philadelphia: WB Saunders, 1973, pp. 28–29.

Maughan, RJ, Watson, JS, & Weir, J. Strength and cross-sectional area of human skeletal muscle. Journal of Physiology, 338:37–49, 1983.

McDonald, CM, Abresch, RT, Carter, GT, Fowler, W, Jr., Johnson, ER, & Kilmer, DD. Profiles of neuromuscular diseases: Duchenne muscular dystrophy. American Journal of Physical Medicine and Rehabilitation, 74:S70–92, 1995.

McSwegin, PJ, Plowman, SA, Wolff, GM, & Guttenberg, GL. Validity of a one mile walk test for high school age individuals. Measurement in Physical Education and Exercise Science, 2:47–63, 1998.

Mersch, F, & Stoboy, H. Strength training and muscle hypertrophy in children. In Osteid, S, & Carlsen, KH (Eds.). Children and Exercise XIII. Champaign, IL: Human Kinetics, 1989, pp. 165–182.

Moll, JMH, & Wright, V. Normal range of spinal mobility: An objective clinical study. Annals of the Rheumatic Diseases, 30:381–386, 1971.

Molnar, GE, & Alexander, J. Objective, quantitative muscle testing in children: A pilot study. Archives of Physical Medicine and Rehabilitation, 54:224–228, 1973.

Moran, HM, Hall, MA, Barr, A, & Ansell, B. Spinal mobility of the adolescent. Rheumatology Rehabilitation, 18:181–185, 1979.

Moritani, T, & DeVries, HA. Neural factors versus hypertrophy in the time course of muscle strength gain. American Journal of Physical Medicine, 58:115–130, 1979.

Morris, JN, Heady, JA, Raffle, PAB, Roberts, CG, & Parks, JW. Coronary heart disease and physical activity of work. Lancet, 2:1053–1057, 1953.

Morrow, JR, Jr., Falls, HB, & Kohl, HW, III (Eds.). The Prudential FITNESSGRAM Technical Manual. Dallas, TX: The Cooper Institute for Aerobic Research, 1993.

Neumark-Sztainer, D, Story, M, Hannan, PJ, & Croll, J. Overweight status and eating patterns among adolescents: Where do youths stand in comparison with the Healthy People 2010 objectives? American Journal of Public Health, 92:844–851, 2002.

Norkin, CC, & White, DJ. Measurement of Joint Motion: A Guide to Goniometry. Philadelphia: FA Davis, 1985.

Ogden, CL, Flegal, KM, Carroll, MD, & Johnson, CL. Prevalence and trends in overweight among US children and adolescents, 1999-2000. Journal of the American Medical Association, 288:1728–1732, 2002.

Olney, SJ, Boyce, WF, & Wright, M. Lower extremity work patterns in gait of diplegic CP children (abstract). Physical Therapy, 68:847, 1988.

Orenstein, DM, Franklin, BA, Doershuk, HK, Hellerstein, KJ, Germann, KJ, Horowitz, JG, & Stern, RC. Exercise conditioning and cardiopulmonary physical fitness in cystic fibrosis. The effects of a three-month supervised running program. Chest, 80:392–398, 1981.

Ounpuu, S. Patterns of gait pathology. In Gage, JR (Ed.). The Treatment of Gait Problems in Cerebral Palsy. London: Mac Keith Press, 2004, pp. 217–237.

Ozmun, JC, Mikesky, AE, & Surburg, PR: Neuromuscular adaptations following prepubescent strength training. Medicine and Science in Sports and Exercise, 26:510–514, 1994.

Parizkova, J. Interrelationships between body size, body composition and function. Advances in Experimental Medicine and Biology, 49:119–123, 1974.

Parizkova, J. Body Fat and Physical Fitness: Body Composition and Lipid Metabolism in Different Regimens of Physical Activity. The Hague: Martinus Nijhoff, 1977, pp. 152–156.

Pate, RR. A new definition of youth fitness. Physician and Sports Medicine, 11:77–83, 1983.

Pate, RR, Dowda, MD, & Ross, JG. Associations between physical activity and physical fitness in American children. American Journal of Diseases of Children, 144:1123–1129, 1990.

Pate RR, Ross, JG, Baumgartner, TA, & Sparks, RE. The national children and youth fitness study II: The modified pull-up test. Journal of Physical Education, Recreation and Dance, 58:71–73, 1987.

Pate, RR, & Shephard, RJ. Characteristics of physical fitness in youth. In Gisolfi, CV, & Lamb, DR (Eds.). Perspectives in Exercise Science and Sports Medicine, Vol. 2: Youth, Exercise, and Sport. Indianapolis, IN: Benchmark Press, 1989, pp. 1–45.

Paterson, DH, & Cunningham, DA. Maximal oxygen uptake in children: Comparison of treadmill protocols at various speeds. Canadian Journal of Applied Sport Sciences, 3:188, 1978.

Phelps, E, Smith, LJ, & Hallum, A. Normal ranges of hip motion of infants between 9 and 24 months of age. Developmental Medicine and Child Neurology, 27:785–792, 1985.

President's Council on Physical Fitness and Sports. The Presidential Physical Fitness Program. Washington, DC: President's Council on Physical Fitness and Sports, 1987.

Rarick, GL, & Thompson, JAJ. Roentgenographic measures of leg size and ankle extensor strength of 7 year old children. Research Quarterly, 27:321–332, 1956.

Rose, J, Gamble, JG, Burgos, A, Medeiros, J, & Haskell, WL. Energy expenditure index of walking for normal children and children with cerebral palsy. Developmental Medicine and Child Neurology, 32:333–340, 1990.

Rose, J, Gamble, JG, Medeiros, J, Burgos, A, & Haskell, WL. Energy cost of walking in normal children and in those with cerebral palsy: Comparison of heart rate and oxygen uptake. Paediatric Orthopaedics, 9:276–279, 1989.

Ross, JG, Delpy, LA, Christenson, GM, Gold, RS, & Damberg, CL. The national youth and fitness study II: Study procedures and quality control. Journal of Physical Education, Recreation and Dance, 58:57–62, 1987.

Ross, JG, Dotson, CO, Gilbert, GG, & Katz, SJ. The national youth and fitness study I: New standards for fitness measurement. Journal of Physical Education, Recreation and Dance, 56:62–66, 1985.

Ross, JG, & Gilbert, GG. The national children and youth fitness study: A summary of findings. Journal of Physical Education, Recreation and Dance, 56:45–50, 1985.

Ross, JG, Katz, SJ, & Gilbert, GG: The national youth and fitness study I: Quality control. Journal of Physical Education, Recreation and Dance, 56:57–61, 1985.

Ross, JG, & Pate, RR. The national children and youth fitness study II: A summary of findings. Journal of Physical Education, Recreation and Dance, 58:51–56, 1987.

Ross, JG, Pate, RR, Delpy, LA, Gold, RS, & Svilar, M. The national children and youth fitness study II: New health related fitness norms. Journal of Physical Education, Recreation and Dance, 58:66–70, 1987.

Rutenfranz, J, Macek, M, Lange-Anderson, A, Bell, RD, Vavra, J, Radvansky, J, Klimmer, F, & Kylian, H. The relationship between changing body height and growth related changes in maximal aerobic power. European Journal of Applied Physiology, 60:282–287, 1990.

Safrit, MJ. Criterion-referenced measurement: Validity. In Safrit, MJ, & Wood, TM (Eds.). Measurement Concepts in Physical Education and Exercise Science. Champaign, IL: Human Kinetics, 1989, pp. 119–135.

Safrit, MJ. The validity and reliability of fitness tests for children: A review. Pediatric Exercise Science, 2:9-28, 1990.

Safrit, MJ, & Wood, TM: The test battery reliability of the health-related physical fitness test. Research Quarterly for Exercise and Sport, 58:160–167, 1987.

Sale, DG. Strength training in children. In Gisolfi, CV, & Lamb, DR (Eds.). Perspectives in Exercise Science and Sports Medicine, Vol. 2: Youth, Exercise, and Sport. Indianapolis IN: Benchmark Press, 1989, pp. 165–222.

Saltin, B, & Strange, S. Maximal oxygen uptake: Old and new arguments for a cardiovascular limitation. Medicine and Science in Sports and Exercise, 24:30–37, 1992.

Seaman, JA, & California Adapted Fitness Task Force. Test items and standards. In Seaman JA (Ed.). Physical Best and Individuals with Disabilities: A Handbook for Inclusion in Fitness Programs. Reston, VA: The American Alliance for Health, Physical Education, Recreation, and Dance, 1995, pp. 41–54.

Shvartz, E, & Reibold, RC. Aerobic fitness norms for males and females aged 6 to 75 years: A review. Aviation Space and Environmental Medicine, 61:3–11, 1990.

Simons-Morton, BG, O'Hara, NM, Simons-Morton, DG, & Parcel, GS. Children and fitness: A public health perspective. Research Quarterly for Exercise and Sport, 58:295–302, 1987.

Slaughter, MH, Lohman, TG, Boileau, RA, Stillman, RJ, VanLoan, M, Horswill, CA, & Wilmore, JH. Influence of maturation on relationship of skinfolds to body density: A cross-sectional study. Human Biology, 56:681–689, 1984.

Sodoma, CJ. Amateur Athlete Union physical fitness program validity for selected age group test results. Bloomington: Indiana University, 1986 (thesis).

Spady, DW. Normal body composition of infants and children. Ross Laboratories Conference on Pediatric Research, 98:67–73, 1989.

Spady, DW, Schiff, D, & Szymanski, WA. A description of the changing composition of the growing premature infant. Journal of Pediatric Gastroenterology and Nutrition, 6:730–738, 1987.

Sproul, A, & Simpson, E. Stroke volume and related hemodynamic data in normal children. Pediatrics, 33:912–916, 1964.

Sprynarova, S, & Reisenauer, R. Body dimensions and physiological indicators of physical fitness during adolescence. In Shephard, RJ, & Lavallee, H (Eds.). Physical Fitness Assessment. Springfield, IL: Charles C Thomas, 1978, pp. 32–37.

Stout, JL & Koop, SE. Energy expenditure in cerebral palsy. In Gage, JR (Ed.). The Treatment of Gait Problems in Cerebral Palsy. London: Mac Keith Press, 2004, pp.146–164.

Strong, WB. Physical activity and children. Circulation, 81:1697–1701, 1990.

Sutton, JR. $\dot{V}O_2$max—New concepts on an old theme. Medicine and Science in Sports and Exercise, 24:26–29, 1992.

Tirosh, E, Bar-Or, O, & Rosenbaum, P. New muscle power test in neuromuscular disease. American Journal of Diseases of Children, *144*:1083–1087, 1990.

United States Cerebral Palsy Athletic Association. Classification System for Athletes. Trenton, NJ, 1996, USCPAA.

United States Department of Health and Human Services. Healthy Children 2000: National Health Promotion and Disease Prevention Objectives Related to Mothers, Infants, Children, Adolescents, and Youth. Washington, DC: Public Health Service, 1990.

United States Department of Health and Human Services. Healthy People 2000: Progress Report for Physical Activity and Fitness. Washington, DC: Public Health Service, 1995.

United States Department of Health and Human Services. Healthy People 2010 Objectives: Draft for Public Comment. Washington, DC: United States Department of Health and Human Services, 1998.

United States Department of Health and Human Services. Healthy People 2010. Washington, DC: United States Department of Health and Human Services, 2000.

United States Department of Health and Human Services. Healthy People 2010: Physical Activity and Fitness Progress Review. Washington, DC: United States Department of Health and Human Services, 2004.

van den Berg-Emos, RJG, van Baak, MA, & Westerterp, KR. Are skinfold measurements suitable to compare body fat between children with spastic cerebral palsy and healthy controls? Developmental Medicine and Child Neurology, *40*:335–339, 1998.

Vignos, PJ, & Watkins, MP. The Emons et al 1998 effect of exercise in muscular dystrophy. Journal of the American Medical Association, *197*:843–848, 1966.

Vincent, SD, Pangrazi, RP, Raustorp, A, Michaud Tomson, L, & Cuddihy, TF. Activity levels and body mass index of children in the United States, Sweden, and Australia. Medicine and Science in Sports & Exercise, *35*;1367–1373, 2003.

VonDobelin, W, & Eriksson, BO. Physical training, maximal oxygen uptake and dimensions of the oxygen transporting and metabolizing organs in boys 11–13 years of age. Acta Paediatrica Scandinavica, *61*:653–657, 1972.

Wahlund, H. Determination of the physical working capacity. Acta Medica Scandinavica Supplement, *215*:5–108, 1948.

Waugh, KG, Minkel, JL, Parker, R, & Coon, VA. Measurement of hip, knee, and ankle joints in newborns. Physical Therapy, *63*:1616–1621, 1983.

Weltman, A, Janny, C, Rians, CB, Strand, K, Berg, B, Tippitt, S, Wise, J, Cahill, BR, & Katch, FI. The effects of hydraulic resistance strength training in pre-pubertal males. Medicine and Science in Sports and Exercise, *18*:629–638, 1986.

Wiley, ME, & Damiano, DL. Lower extremity strength profiles in spastic cerebral palsy. Developmental Medicine and Child Neurology, *40*:100–107, 1998.

Winnick, JP, & Short, FX. The Brockport Physical Fitness Test Manual. Champaign, IL: Human Kinetics, 1999.

Winnick, JP, & Short, FX: Physical Fitness Testing of the Disabled: Project UNIQUE. Champaign, IL: Human Kinetics, 1985, pp. 101–104.

World Health Organization. International Classification of Functioning, Disability and Health. Geneva: World Health Organization, 2001.

Wyndham, C. Submaximal test for estimating maximal oxygen intake. Canadian Medical Association Journal, *96*:736–742, 1976.

Yamashita, T, Seiichi, I, & Isao, O. Effect of muscle stretching on the activity of neuromuscular transmission. Medicine and Science in Sports and Exercise, *24*:80–84, 1992.

Zach, MS, Oberwalder, J, & Hausler, F. Cystic fibrosis: Physical exercise vs chest physiotherapy. Archives of Disease in Childhood, *57*:587–589, 1982.

Ziegler, EE, O'Donnell, AM, Nelson, SE, & Fomon, SJ. Body composition of the reference fetus. Growth, *40*:329–334, 1976.

MANAGEMENT OF MUSCULOSKELETAL IMPAIRMENT

Section Editor
Darl W. Vander Linden
PT, PhD

Chapter 9

JUVENILE RHEUMATOID ARTHRITIS

SUSAN E. KLEPPER
PT, PhD

Chronic arthritis in childhood can result from any one of a heterogeneous group of diseases, of which juvenile rheumatoid arthritis (JRA) is the most common. The disease causes joint swelling, pain, and limited mobility and can significantly restrict a child's activities. Table 9-1 lists the common clinical manifestations of JRA. Other conditions that may cause childhood arthritis include juvenile psoriatic arthritis (JPsA), juvenile ankylosing spondylitis (JAS), and other enthesitis-related arthritides. Arthritis may also be a feature of juvenile scleroderma, systemic lupus erythematosus, and dermatomyositis.

This chapter provides an overview of the impairments, activity limitations, and participation restrictions common to JRA and describes the role of the physical therapist as a member of the rheumatology team in the examination, evaluation, and intervention for the child with arthritis. Outcome instruments appropriate for use in JRA, issues related to school and recreational activities, surgical procedures, and adherence to therapeutic regimens are discussed. A case study illustrates the therapeutic management of a child with JRA.

ROLE OF THE THERAPIST

Physical therapists (PTs) are essential members of the pediatric rheumatology team that includes the rheumatologist, nurse, occupational therapist, ophthalmologist, orthopedist, and pediatrician. Other specialists, including dermatologists, cardiologists, orthopedists, orthotists, psychologists, and social workers provide occasional consultation as needed. The PT conducts a comprehensive examination to identify impairments caused by the disease and determine their relationship to observed or reported activity restrictions. Based on an evaluation of these findings, the PT develops a prioritized problem list and an intervention plan to reduce current impairments and prevent or minimize secondary problems. Therapists

TABLE 9-1	Common Clinical Manifestations of Juvenile Rheumatoid Arthritis (JRA)

Joint swelling, pain, stiffness
Limited joint motion; soft tissue contracture
Morning stiffness
Muscle atrophy; weakness; poor muscle endurance
Fatigue
Decreased aerobic capacity; reduced exercise tolerance
Growth abnormalities (local and general)
Acute or chronic uveitis (most common in pauciarticular JRA)
Systemic manifestations (may be severe in systemic JRA; mild to moderate in polyarticular JRA)
Osteopenia; osteoporosis (increased risk with long-term use of oral corticosteroids)
Gait deviations
Difficulties with activities of daily living
Possible activity / participation restrictions

work with parents to develop a home program that includes balanced rest and exercise, positioning, and joint protection techniques. They provide guidelines for choosing physical activities and consult with school personnel to ensure the child's full participation in educational activities.

The role of the therapist varies based on the care setting, and often more than one PT is involved in the child's care. PTs working in a specialized rheumatology center may perform the initial assessment, set treatment goals, plan a home program, and monitor the child's status at routine clinic visits. Therapists within the child's home, school, or community usually provide direct services. The frequency of therapy varies widely and depends on the child's physical status, reimbursement for therapy services, and the availability of therapists. A child with severe arthritis might receive intensive PT during a short inpatient rehabilitation stay. In contrast, many children with mild arthritis receive direct PT only during periods of disease exacerbation or when the arthritis limits mobility or function. For these children the PT often serves an important role as a consultant to provide education, monitor the child's functional status, and maintain communication with other members of the rheumatology team.

DIAGNOSIS AND CLASSIFICATION

Three systems are used to diagnose and classify childhood arthritis: the American College of Rheumatology (ACR) criteria for JRA (Brewer et al., 1977), the European

League Against Rheumatism (EULAR) criteria for juvenile chronic arthritis (JAC) (EULAR, 1977), and the International League of Associations for Rheumatology (ILAR) criteria for juvenile idiopathic arthritis (JIA) (Foeldvari & Bidde, 2000). The ACR criteria will be used in this chapter. JRA is defined as persistent arthritis, lasting at least 6 weeks, in one or more joints in a child younger than 16 years of age, when all other causes of arthritis have been excluded. Because there are no definitive laboratory tests for JRA, the diagnosis is primarily clinical and often delayed until a clear picture of the disease evolves. The child may exhibit mild anemia, elevated erythrocyte sedimentation rate (ESR), and radiographic evidence of periarticular swelling and osteopenia. These findings are not specific to JRA, but may be useful in ruling out other conditions, monitoring disease course, and guiding treatment. Table 9-2 shows the characteristics of three major disease onset types—systemic (sJRA), oligoarticular or pauciarticular (pauciJRA), and polyarticular (polyJRA) —defined by the clinical signs and symptoms observed during the first 6 months of the disease.

A pauciarticular onset occurs in 56% to 60% of children with JRA, mostly girls younger than 6 years of age (Cassidy & Petty, 2001). Disease signs include low-grade inflammation in four or fewer joints, most often the knee, followed in frequency by the ankles and elbows (Fig. 9-1). The hip and small joints of the hand are usually spared. The joint is swollen and may be warm, but not always painful. Systemic signs are unusual, but about 20% of children develop uveitis, an asymptomatic inflammation of the eye that may lead to functional blindness. These children must have their eyes examined by an ophthalmologist at diagnosis and at periodic intervals.

TABLE 9-2	Classification of Juvenile Rheumatoid Arthritis by Findings at Time of Onset		
CRITERION	**POLYARTHRITIS**	**OLIGOARTHRITIS (PAUCIARTICULAR DISEASE)**	**SYSTEMIC DISEASE**
Frequency of cases	40%	50%	10%
Number of joint involved	≥5	≤4	Variable
Age at onset	Throughout childhood; peak at 1–3 years	Early childhood; peak at 1–2 years	Throughout childhood; no peak
Sex ratio (F:M)	3:1	5:1	1:1
Systemic involvement	Moderate involvement	Not present	Prominent
Occurrence of chronic uveitis	5%	20%	Rare
FREQUENCY OF SEROPOSITIVITY			
Rheumatoid factors	10% (increase with age)	Rare	Rare
Antinuclear antibodies	40–50%	75–85%*	10%
Prognosis	Guarded to moderately good	Excellent except for eyesight	Moderate to poor

From Cassidy, JT, & Petty, RE. Textbook of Pediatric Rheumatology, 3rd ed. Philadelphia: WB Saunders, 1995.
*In girls with uveitis.

Systemic or topical corticosteroids are used to control the inflammation.

PolyJRA (Fig. 9-2), defined as arthritis in five or more joints, occurs in 25% to 28% of children with JRA, mostly girls (Cassidy & Petty, 2001). Onset is often insidious, with arthritis in progressively more joints. Arthritis is symmetric, affects both the large and small joints, and may include the cervical spine and temporomandibular joints. Joints are swollen and warm, but rarely red. Systemic symptoms are usually mild and include low-grade fever and mild to moderate hepatosplenomegaly and lymphadenopathy. About 19% develop chronic uveitis. One subgroup, mostly females with disease onset in late childhood or adolescence, are seropositive for the rheumatoid factor (RF+) and follow a disease course similar to that seen in adults with rheumatoid arthritis. They may have rheumatoid nodules on the elbows, tibial crests, and fingers and develop erosive synovitis early in the disease course. Nodules are less common in children with RF– disease, and fewer joints are affected. Persistent arthritis may occur, causing juxta-articular osteopenia, muscle atrophy, weakness, contractures, and growth disturbances (Cassidy & Petty, 2001).

Systemic JRA occurs in 10% to 12% of the cases. The diagnostic marker is a spiking fever of 39°C or higher that occurs once or twice daily (afternoon or evening), with a rapid return to normal or below between spikes. The fever is accompanied by a rash (discrete, erythematous macules) most often found on the trunk or limbs, but may be seen on the face, palms, and soles of the feet (Fig. 9-3). Other systemic signs include pleuritis, pericarditis, myocarditis, hepatosplenomegaly, and lymphadenopathy. Systemic disease may precede arthritis by several months or years. Fever, rash, and pericarditis often subside after the initial disease period, but may recur during periods of exacerbation of the arthritis (Cassidy & Petty, 2001).

INCIDENCE AND PREVALENCE

Studies using the ACR criteria, and reflecting mostly North American and European white populations, place the incidence of JRA between 2 and 20 per 100,000 at risk. Based on a Mayo Clinic study, the incidence in the United States decreased in recent years from 15 per 100,000 for the period from 1960 to 1969 to 7.8 per 100,000 for the years 1980 to 1993 (Peterson et al., 1996). The reported prevalence of JRA varies from 16 to 150 per 100,000. Age at onset and gender distribution vary by disease type. In a study of 300 children with JRA, Sullivan and colleagues (1975) reported the peak age at onset was between 1 and 3 years for the total group and for girls, primarily those with pauciJRA and polyJRA. Disease onset for boys showed two peaks, one at 2 years, representing mostly

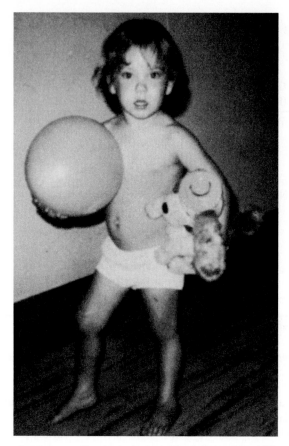

✦ **Figure 9-1** Pauciarticular juvenile rheumatoid arthritis causing swelling and flexion contracture of the right knee in a 3-year-old girl with disease duration of 1 year. *(From Cassidy, JT, & Petty, RE. Juvenile rheumatoid arthritis. In Cassidy, JT, & Petty, RE (Eds.). Textbook of Pediatric Rheumatology, 4th ed. Philadelphia: W.B. Saunders Co., 2001, Fig. 12-8, p. 231.)*

boys with polyJRA, and another between 8 and 10 years of age that may partly represent children with JAS. Almost twice as many females as males develop JRA. The ratio of girls to boys is 3:1 for pauciJRA (5:1 for those with uveitis) and 2.8:1 for polyJRA. There is no evidence of a peak age for onset or sex bias in sJRA (Cassidy & Petty, 2001).

ETIOLOGY AND PATHOGENESIS

The exact etiology of JRA is unclear, but the prevailing theory is that it is an autoimmune inflammatory disorder, activated by an external trigger, in a genetically predisposed host. A viral or bacterial infection often precedes disease onset. Physical trauma may be associated with onset, but may just draw attention to an already inflamed joint. The difference in onset types and disease course, higher prevalence of girls, narrow peak age periods of onset for all but sJRA, and the extensive immunologic abnormalities suggest JRA may not be a single disease. Different etiologic vectors may be responsible for each onset type, or a single pathogen may cause distinct clinical patterns as it interacts with the host.

The role of the immune system in the pathogenesis and persistence of inflammation is evident from the altered immunity, abnormal immunoregulation, and cytokine production. The T-cell abnormalities and pathology of the inflamed synovium suggest a cell-mediated pathogenesis. The presence of multiple autoantibodies, immune complexes, and complement activation indicate humoral abnormalities. The importance of genetic predisposition to JRA is not completely understood. Although there are few reports of familial or multigenerational cases of JRA, studies of over 3000 children with arthritis show concordance between siblings with JRA for age at onset, clinical manifestations, and disease course (Clemens et al., 1985). Many of the suspected genetic predispositions are within the major histocompatibility complex (MHC) region of chromosome 6, but the pathogenesis may involve the interactions of multiple genes. Recent studies indicate that correlations found between human leukocyte antigen (HLA) specificities and various types of JRA may have specific risk and protective effects that are age-related for each onset type and some course subtypes (Murray et al., 1999).

MEDICAL MANAGEMENT

The goals of pharmacologic therapy in JRA are to control the arthritis, prevent joint erosions, and manage extra-articular manifestations. Children with severe or persistent disease often require a carefully orchestrated combination of drug therapies started early in the disease course to control arthritis and prevent joint erosions. A core set of six outcome variables is often used in clinical trials to determine subjects' response to medical therapy (Giannini et al., 1997). These include physician global assessment of disease activity, parent/patient assessment of overall health status, functional ability, number of joints with active arthritis, number of joints with limited motion, and ESR. A positive clinical response is defined as improvement of at least 30% from baseline in at least three of the six variables, with no more than one of the other variables worsening by more than 30%.

Nonsteroidal anti-inflammatory drugs (NSAIDs) are the most widely used first line therapy. Naproxen, tolmetin, and ibuprofen are used most often, but other NSAIDs may be tried. The most common adverse effect is gastro-

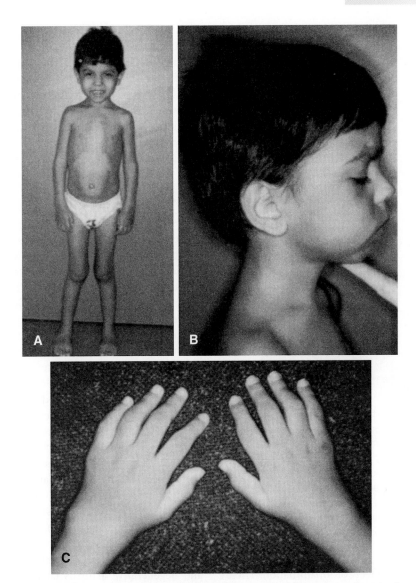

• **Figure 9-2**   The symmetric arthritis in large and small joints of the 6-year-old boy shown here is characteristic of polyarticular juvenile rheumatoid arthritis. **A**, Flexion contractures are seen at the elbows, hips, and knees, and a slight valgus deformity is noted at the knees. The wrists and proximal interphalangeal joints are held in flexion. **B**, Loss of extension of the cervical spine. **C**, Symmetric polyarthritis affects the metacarpophalangeal, proximal interphalangeal, and radiocarpal joints. *(From Cassidy, JT, & Petty, RE. Juvenile rheumatoid arthritis. In Cassidy, JT, & Petty, RE (Eds.). Textbook of Pediatric Rheumatology, 4th ed. Philadelphia: W.B. Saunders Co., 2001, Fig. 12-120, p. 234.)*

intestinal irritation, although NSAIDs that selectively inhibit the cyclooxygenase-2 (COX-2) enzyme may limit this problem. NSAIDs reduce fever, pain, and inflammation, but do not alter disease course. Methotrexate (MTX) is the most common disease-modifying antirheumatic drug (DMARD) prescribed for children with polyJRA and sJRA (Cron, 2002). The drug is usually administered orally once a week, although subcutaneous injection is given if the response is inadequate or the child experi-

ences adverse effects with the oral dose, including gastrointestinal upset. Although liver toxicity in children taking MTX appears to be rare, physicians check blood counts and liver enzymes every 4 to 8 weeks. Data on the health risks associated with long-term use of MTX in children are not yet available.

Patients with a poor prognosis who fail to respond to MTX are treated with one of the biologic reagents that target the tumor necrosis factor (TNF), a cytokine re-

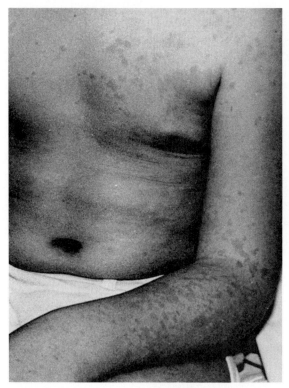

• **Figure 9-3** Typical rash of systemic-onset juvenile rheumatoid arthritis in a 3-year-old boy. The rash is salmon-colored, macular, and nonpruritic. Individual lesions are transient, occur in crops over the trunk and extremities, and may occur in a linear distribution (Koebner's phenomenon) after minor trauma such as a scratch. *(From Cassidy, JT, & Petty, RE. Juvenile rheumatoid arthritis. In Cassidy, JT, & Petty, RE (Eds.). Textbook of Pediatric Rheumatology, 4th ed. Philadelphia: W.B. Saunders Co., 2001, Fig. 12-13, p. 238.)*

sponsible for many of the effects of inflammation. These drugs include etanercept, infliximab, and adalimumab. In one clinical trial, children treated with etanercept showed significant improvement over a placebo on standard outcome measures (Lovell et al, 2000). Other biologic therapies being tested in adults with RA may prove useful in JRA. Sulfasalazine, another DMARD, has been shown to be effective in suppressing disease activity in some children, mostly in pauciJRA, but the risk for toxicity is high. Systemic glucocorticoid drugs are reserved for children, mostly those with sJRA, who do not respond to other therapies. Although steroids have a potent anti-inflammatory effect, they do not alter disease course or duration. Serious adverse effects of long-term oral steroids include iatrogenic Cushing's syndrome, growth disturbance, osteoporosis and fracture, diabetes mellitus, obesity, and increased susceptibility to infection. For children with refractory disease who are steroid-dependent, ag-

gressive therapy with cyclosporin A or cyclophosphamide may provide some benefit (Cron, 2002). Intra-articular injections of long-acting corticosteroids (Cron, 2002) are used successfully to treat severely inflamed and swollen joints. A recent study found that intra-articular steroid injections for lower extremity joints decreased the incidence of leg length discrepancies, a major cause of gait and postural abnormalities in children with JRA (Sherry et al., 1999).

PROGNOSIS

Most children do well with early and appropriate treatment, but many have persistent disease. A review of studies during the past several decades reported that 10 years after disease onset, 31% to 55% of children had persistent synovitis, 55% to 59% had radiographic evidence of joint erosions, and between one third and one half entered adulthood with active disease (Wallace & Levinson, 1991). Active disease was present in 21% to 71% of children with pauciJRA, 40% to 50% with polyJRA, and 25% to 58% with sJRA. Functional outcome in children with sJRA depends on disease course. About 50% follow a pauciarticular course, eventually recovering almost completely. The remaining group experience arthritis in progressively more joints, and may experience moderate to severe activity restrictions (Cassidy & Petty, 2001). Poor articular and functional outcomes in sJRA and polyJRA are linked to the presence of hip involvement and polyarthritis in the first year of disease activity (Spencer & Bernstein, 2002). Children with pauciJRA have the best prognosis for joint preservation and function, but may develop contractures during active disease and degenerative arthritis later. They also remain at a high risk for eye disease. About 5% to 10% follow an extended disease course, adding multiple joints after the first 6 months. Those who are RF+ often follow a course similar to children with RF+ polyJRA, with persistent disease and poor functional outcome. In contrast, outcome is usually good in boys with disease onset at 9 years of age or older, who are positive for the HLA-B27 gene, and have arthritis mostly in the hip and sacroiliac joints.

Reports of long-term functional outcomes in JRA vary, possibly because of differences in study methods. Ruperto and colleagues (1999) conducted a 15-year follow-up study of American and Italian patients with JRA. Subjects had favorable outcomes on measures of functional status, pain, overall well-being, and quality of life. However, in another study, adults with a history of JRA reported significantly greater pain, disability, and fatigue, and impaired physical function and perception of their health compared to age- and gender-matched controls (Peterson et al., 1997). The inconsistencies in these reports illustrate the importance of early and effective treatment of the disease to prevent or minimize adverse outcomes.

PHYSICAL THERAPY EXAMINATION

The approach to physical therapy examination in JRA must consider the child's age, motor development prior to disease onset, and cognitive and emotional development. By first gathering information about the child's activities and participation, the therapist is able to focus the physical examination on impairments that may contribute to the functional problems. However, the therapist must also closely monitor joint motion and integrity because loss of motion may be the first sign of joint damage and may signal an increased risk for functional decline. Appendix I lists standardized outcome instruments that provide quantitative data to guide intervention and evaluate change.

PARTICIPATION AND ACTIVITY RESTRICTIONS

The impact of JRA on a child's activities depends on the extent and duration of active disease, the child's resiliency and desire to be independent, and expectations placed on the child by parents and others. A child with pauciJRA may demonstrate few functional limitations, but one with severe polyJRA may need assistance with ADLs long past the time when other children are independent. They may have difficulty moving between standing and sitting on the floor, getting in and out of the bed or a bathtub, negotiating steps, and walking long distances. Even children with mild disease may be dependent for some self-care tasks if parents provide unnecessary assistance. Children may fail to develop gross motor proficiency if parents discourage them from typical childhood activities, such as riding a bike, climbing on playground equipment, or other active play (Morrison et al., 1991).

The child's participation will also be affected by the extent and quality of supportive services available and utilized by the child and family. Many children who report problems with some aspect of their educational program do not receive the related services recommended by the rheumatology team (Lovell et al., 1990; Lineker et al., 1996). Tardiness as a result of morning stiffness, and frequent absences due to illness or medical appointments may cause the child to miss academic time and social interactions with classmates. Children may feel different and somewhat isolated because they are unable to participate in the same activities as their classmates. Daily fluctuations in disease symptoms may also affect the child's mood and ability to cope (Schanberg et al., 2000). Adolescents with JRA may be unable to gain the same level of independence as their peers because of physical limitations and the need for continued medical care.

Several standardized instruments examine the child's activities. The Childhood Health Assessment Questionnaire (CHAQ), a measure of physical function designed for children age 1 to 19 years, includes 30 activities organized in eight categories (Fig. 9-4) (Singh et al., 1994). The respondent (parent or child 9 years and older) scores each item based on how much difficulty the child had performing the task during the past week (0 = without any difficulty; 1 = with some difficulty; 2 = with much difficulty; 3 = unable to do). An item is scored as "not applicable" if the child has difficulty because he/she is too young. The highest scored item in each section determines the score for that category. If the child needs an assistive device or help from another person to perform a task, the score for that category is at least 2. The Disability Index (DI), calculated as the average score for the eight categories, has a range of 0 to 3. Higher scores indicate greater disability. The CHAQ also includes a question about the presence and duration of morning stiffness and visual analog scales (VAS) to measure pain intensity and general health status.

Other questionnaires designed to measure physical function include the Juvenile Arthritis Functional Assessment Index (JASI) (Wright et al., 1996) and the Juvenile Arthritis Functional Assessment Report (JAFAR) (Howe et al., 1991). A school checklist can be used to examine school-related problems (Szer & Wright, 2000). The School Function Assessment may also be useful (Coster et al., 1998). Two other instruments measure both physical function and quality of life (QOL) in children with JRA. These are the Juvenile Arthritis Quality of Life Questionnaire (JAQQ) (Duffy et al., 1997) and the Pediatric Quality of Life Questionnaire (PedsQL) (Varni et al., 2002). The only instrument that measures the child's actual performance is the Juvenile Arthritis Functional Assessment Scale (JAFAS) (Fig. 9-5). The child is observed and timed while completing 10 tasks. The score is 0 if the time to complete the task is equal to or less than the criterion time, 1 if the time exceeds the criterion, and 2 if child cannot perform the task. The test takes 10 minutes and requires a minimum of simple equipment (Lovell et al., 1989).

JOINT STRUCTURE AND FUNCTION

The cardinal signs of inflammation are swelling, end-range stress pain, and stiffness. Swelling around a joint

In this section, we are interested in learning how your child's illness affects his/her ability to function in daily life. Please feel free to add any comments on the back of this page. In the following questions, please check the one response that best describes your child's usual activities (averaged over an entire day) *OVER THE PAST WEEK*. If your child has difficulty in doing a certain activity or is unable to do it because he/she is too young but NOT because he/she is RESTRICTED BY ARTHRITIS, please mark it as "Not Applicable." ONLY NOTE THOSE DIFFICULTIES OR LIMITATIONS THAT ARE DUE TO ARTHRITIS.

	Without ANY Difficulty	With SOME Difficulty	With MUCH Difficulty	UNABLE To Do	Not Applicable
DRESSING & GROOMING					
Is your child able to:					
• Dress, including tying shoelaces and doing buttons?	_____	_____	_____	_____	_____
• Shampoo his/her hair?	_____	_____	_____	_____	_____
• Remove socks?	_____	_____	_____	_____	_____
• Cut fingernails/toenails?	_____	_____	_____	_____	_____
ARISING					
Is your child able to:					
• Stand up from a low chair or floor?	_____	_____	_____	_____	_____
• Get in and out of bed or stand up in crib?	_____	_____	_____	_____	_____
EATING					
Is your child able to:					
• Cut his/her own meat?	_____	_____	_____	_____	_____
• Lift a cup or glass to mouth?	_____	_____	_____	_____	_____
• Open a new cereal box?	_____	_____	_____	_____	_____
WALKING					
Is your child able to:					
• Walk outdoors on flat ground?	_____	_____	_____	_____	_____
• Climb up five steps?	_____	_____	_____	_____	_____

*Please check any AIDS or DEVICES that your child usually uses for any of the above activities.

_____Cane   _____Devices used for dressing (button hook, zipper pull, long-handled shoe horn, etc.)
_____Walker   _____Built-up pencil or special utensils
_____Crutches _____Special or built-up chair
_____Wheelchair _____Other (Specify:_____)

*Please check any categories for which your child usually needs help from another person BECAUSE OF ARTHRITIS:

_____Dressing and Grooming   _____Eating
_____Arising   _____Walking

	Without ANY Difficulty	With SOME Difficulty	With MUCH Difficulty	UNABLE To Do	Not Applicable
HYGIENE					
Is your child able to:					
• Wash and dry entire body?	_____	_____	_____	_____	_____
• Take a tub bath (get in and out of tub)?	_____	_____	_____	_____	_____
• Get on and off the toilet or potty chair?	_____	_____	_____	_____	_____
• Brush teeth?	_____	_____	_____	_____	_____
• Comb/brush hair?	_____	_____	_____	_____	_____
REACH					
Is your child able to:					
• Reach and get down a heavy object such as a large game or books from just above his/her head?	_____	_____	_____	_____	_____
• Bend down to pick up clothing or a piece of paper from the floor?	_____	_____	_____	_____	_____
• Pull on a sweater over his/her head?	_____	_____	_____	_____	_____
• Turn neck to look back over shoulder?	_____	_____	_____	_____	_____
GRIP					
Is your child able to:					
• Write or scribble with pen or pencil?	_____	_____	_____	_____	_____

◆ **Figure 9-4** Childhood Health Assessment Questionnaire: Disability and Discomfort Sections. *(From Singh, G, Athreya, B, Fries, J, & Goldsmith, DP. Measurement of health status in children with juvenile rheumatoid arthritis. Arthritis and Rheumatism, 37:1762–1764, 1994.)*

	Without ANY Difficulty	With SOME Difficulty	With MUCH Difficulty	UNABLE To Do	Not Applicable
GRIP (*Continued*)					
• Open car doors?	_____	_____	_____	_____	_____
• Open jars that have been previously opened?	_____	_____	_____	_____	_____
• Turn faucets on and off?	_____	_____	_____	_____	_____
• Push open a door when he/she has to turn a door knob?	_____	_____	_____	_____	_____
ACTIVITIES					
Is your child able to:					
• Run errands and shop?	_____	_____	_____	_____	_____
• Get in and out of car or toy car or school bus?	_____	_____	_____	_____	_____
• Ride bike or tricycle?	_____	_____	_____	_____	_____
• Do household chores (e.g., wash dishes, take out trash, vacuuming, yardwork, make bed, clean room)?	_____	_____	_____	_____	_____
• Run and play?	_____	_____	_____	_____	_____

*Please check any AIDS or DEVICES that your child usually uses for any of the above activities:

_____Raised toilet seat   _____Bathtub bar
_____Bathtub seat   _____Long-handled appliances in reach
_____Jar opener (for jars opened previously)   _____Long-handled appliances in bathroom

*Please check any categories for which your child usually needs help from another person BECAUSE OF ARTHRITIS?

_____Hygiene   _____Gripping and Opening Things
_____Reach   _____Errands and Chores

We are also interested in learning whether your child has been affected by pain because of his or her illness.

*How much pain do you think your child has had because of his or her illness IN THE PAST WEEK?

Place a mark on the line below to indicate the severity of the pain.

No pain   Very severe pain
├───┤
0   100

HEALTH STATUS
1. Considering all the ways that arthritis affects your child, rate how your child is doing on the following scale by placing a mark on the line.

├───┤
0   100
Very well   Very poor

2. Is your child stiff in the morning?   _____Yes   _____No
   If YES, about how long does the stiffness usually last (in the past week)?
                              Hours/Minutes_____

◆ **Figure 9-4** (*con't*)

---

may be the result of intra-articular effusion, synovial hypertrophy, soft tissue edema, or periarticular tenosynovitis (Mier et al., 2000). The joint may also be enlarged as a result of bony overgrowth due to increased blood supply to the inflamed area. Swelling and protective muscle spasm contribute to pain. Inactivity stiffness, most noted upon awakening ("AM gel") and after periods of prolonged sitting is a common indicator of disease activity.

Chronic inflammation causes abnormalities in joint structure and function. Increased production of synovial fluid stretches and weakens the joint capsule and adjacent structures. Massive overgrowth of the synovium, called pannus, spreads over and invades the articular cartilage, releasing inflammatory enzymes into the synovial fluid.

Erosions in the articular cartilage and subchondral bone cause irregularities in the joint surface, compromising alignment, congruency, and stability (Cassidy & Petty, 2001). Early radiographs show periarticular swelling with widening of the joint space, juxta-articular osteopenia, and periosteal new bone (Reed & Wilmot, 1991). General demineralization, thinning and loss of articular cartilage, marginal erosions, and osteophytes occur with persistent disease (Cassidy & Petty, 2001). Nutritional deficiencies, low body weight, and decreased physical activity result in low bone density and risk for fracture (Kotaniemi et al., 1999). This is exacerbated by long-term use of systemic corticosteroids. Joint contractures result from intra-articular adhesions and fibrosis of adjacent tendons.

For each activity, please record how long the child took to perform the activity. If the activity was completed in less than or equal to the criterion time, then score the item as 0; if completed but requiring longer than the criterion time, score the item as 1; if unable to perform the activity, score the item as 2.

Activity	Criterion Time (seconds)	Observed Time (seconds)	Item Score		
			0	1	2
1. Button shirt/blouse	22.4	_____	____	____	____
2. Pull shirt or sweater over head	14.6	_____	____	____	____
3. Pull on both socks	27.2	_____	____	____	____
4. Cut food with knife and fork	12.8	_____	____	____	____
5. Get into bed	3.4	_____	____	____	____
6. Get out of bed	2.9	_____	____	____	____
7. Pick something up off of floor from standing position	2.4	_____	____	____	____
8. From standing position sit on floor, then stand up	4.0	_____	____	____	____
9. Walk 50 feet without assistance	15.1	_____	____	____	____
10. Walk up flight of 5 steps	3.7		____	____	____
		TOTAL SCORE	_____		

◆ **Figure 9-5**   Scoring for the Juvenile Arthritis Functional Assessment Scale. *(From Lovell, DJ, Howe, S, Shear, E, Hartner, S, McGirr, G, Schulte, M, & Levinson, J. Development of a disability measurement tool for juvenile rheumatoid arthritis: The Juvenile Arthritis Functional Assessment Scale. Arthritis and Rheumatism, 32:1393, 1989.)*

The therapist should be aware of the common patterns of joint restrictions in JRA and their potential effect on function (Appendix II). Arthritis may occur in any joint, but the large joints are affected most often. Hip arthritis occurs in 30% to 50% of children, mostly those with sJRA and polyJRA (Spencer & Bernstein, 2002). The early signs of hip disease may include pain in the groin, buttocks, medial thigh, or knee, or a gluteus medius limp. A child may compensate for a mild hip flexion contracture with increased lumbar lordosis. Children with pauciJRA may lose hip motion secondary to knee flexion contracture and leg length discrepancy. The knee is the joint most often affected in pauciJRA, but it is also involved in other disease types. Flexion contracture may result from joint immobility, spasm of the hamstrings, and shortening of the tensor fasciae latae. Chronic synovitis, with overgrowth of the medial femoral condyle, results in a valgus deformity that is exaggerated by tightness in the iliotibial band (ITB) (see Fig. 9-2). Ankle arthritis occurs in all disease types, but involvement of the small joints of the feet are more common in polyJRA. Problems include loss of ankle dorsiflexion, or less often of plantar flexion, metatarsalgia, subluxation of the metatarsophalangeal joints, hallux valgus, hallux rigidus, hammer toes, and overlapping toes. Arthritis of the subtalar joint may result in hindfoot valgus with forefoot pronation (Fig. 9-6) although some children develop calcaneal varus and a forefoot cavus deformity.

The cervical spine is frequently involved. Early signs include pain and stiffness in the back of the neck, with loss of extension and limitations in rotation and lateral flexion. Atlantoaxial subluxation may occur early in the disease, placing the child at risk for injury from trauma or

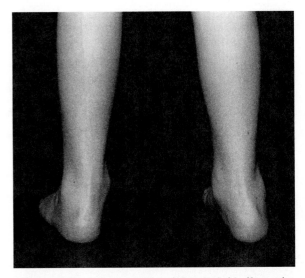

◆ **Figure 9-6**   A common foot deformity is hindfoot valgus with pronation.

during intubation for surgery. Cervical spine ankylosis is also common and causes similar problems during surgery. Restrictions in shoulder rotation, flexion, and abduction may occur with arthritis in the glenohumeral joint, as well as the acromioclavicular, sternoclavicular, and manubriosternal joints. Elbow flexion contractures occur early, and may be accompanied by loss of forearm supination. Arthritis in the wrist and small joints of the hands is most common in polyJRA. The pattern and extent of involvement are related to disease type, child's age, and maturation of the epiphyses at disease onset. Wrist malalignment associated with subluxation and undergrowth of the ulna, with ulnar deviation, occurs in children with disease onset at a young age. Those 12 years or older at onset have a pattern typical of adults, with radial deviation. The metacarpophalangeal (MCP) and proximal interphalangeal (PIP) joints are also involved, either directly by synovitis or indirectly as a result of inflammation in adjacent joints or tendon sheaths.

JOINT EXAMINATION

Joint counts for swelling (JC-S) and limitation of motion (JC-LOM) are recorded on a stick figure to document disease activity and joint restrictions (Fig. 9-7). Figure 9-8 shows two methods of verifying a joint effusion by observing fluctuations of fluid from one area of the joint to another, eliciting a bulge sign. To detect an effusion in the knee, the synovial pouch medial to the patella is emptied by stroking in an upward direction and then refilled by stroking along the lateral border in an upward or downward direction.

Active joint motion can be estimated by watching the child perform a series of movements during various games, such as "Simon Says," but goniometric measurement is necessary to document limited joint motion. Two standardized measures of the JC-LOM are the Articular Severity Score (ASS) and the Global Range of Motion Score (GROMS). The ASS scores global ROM for each joint, averaged for the right and left sides, on a 5-point scale (0 = no LOM; 1 = 25% LOM; 2 = 50% LOM; 3 = 75% LOM; 4 = fused) (Brewer & Giannini, 1982). In contrast, the GROMS (Epps et al., 2002) provides a single score for global joint function. Each joint movement is weighted from 0 (least important) to 5 (essential), based on experts' opinion of its functional importance. The examiner records the mean ROM in degrees for the right and left sides. The ratio of the measured value to the normative value is calculated to obtain the joint movement score. The total GROMS is calculated as the sum for all movements multiplied by 100 and divided by the number of movements (Table 9-3).

A reduced 10-joint version of the GROMS is also available that includes only those joint motions weighted as 5 (essential) on the original GROMS. The total score is calculated using the same method as the full scale. The Pediatric Escola Paulista de Medicina ROM Scale (pEPM-ROM) (Len et al., 1999) also includes 10 essential joint movements, but uses predetermined cut-off points for scoring (0 =full motion to 3 = severe limitation). The total score (0–3) for each side of the body is the sum of all joint scores divided by 10. Each scale demonstrates adequate concurrent validity with other measures of disease status and function in JRA (Epps et al., 2002; Len et al., 1999). Excellent test-retest and intertester agreement are reported for the pEPM-ROM (Len et al., 1999). Testing of the 10-joint GROMS continues. Although a reduced JC-LOM saves time during the examination, it may not be appropriate for patients whose arthritis is extensive or does not affect any of the 10 joints measured.

MUSCULAR STRUCTURE AND FUNCTION

Muscle atrophy and weakness are most severe near inflamed joints, but may also occur in distant areas and persist long after remission of the arthritis (Vostrejs et al., 1989; Dunn, 1993; Giannini & Protas, 1993; Oberg et al., 1994; Lindehammer & Backman, 1995; Lindehammar & Sandstedt, 1998; Hedrengren et al., 2001). Contributing

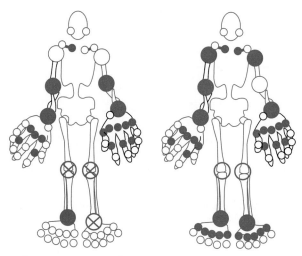

◆ **Figure 9-7**   Example of active joint count in a child with polyarticular disease. There are 38 active joints. The left figure shows 22 with effusion (•) or soft tissue swelling (X). The right figure shows joints with stress pain or tenderness (•). *(From Wright, FV, & Smith, E: Physical therapy management of the child and adolescent with juvenile rheumatoid arthritis. In Walker, JM, & Helewa, A (Eds.). Physical Therapy in Arthritis. Philadelphia: W.B. Saunders Co., 1996, p. 215.)*

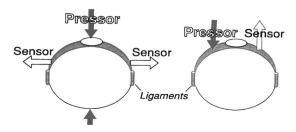

◆ **Figure 9-8**   Two ways of detecting joint effusions. *(From Smythe, HA, & Helewa, A: Assessment of joint disease. In Walker, JM, & Helewa, A (Eds.). Physical Therapy in Arthritis. Philadelphia: W.B. Saunders Co., 1996, p. 133.)*

| TABLE 9-3 | Calculating a GROMS Using All Joint Movements Except the Lumbar and Thoracic Spine* | | | | |

JOINT MOVEMENT	A MEASURED	B NORMATIVE	C A ÷ B	D MODE	E C × D
Cx spine extension	30	45	0.66	4	2.64
Cx spine rotation	60	80	0.75	4	3
Shoulder flexion	142.5	180	0.79	4	3.16
Shoulder abduction	180	180	1.00	4	4
Shoulder ER	85	85	1.00	3	3
Shoulder IR	70	70	1.00	3	3
Elbow extension	145	145	1.00	3	3
Elbow flexion	145	145	1.00	5	5
R/U supination	90	90	1.00	4	4
R/U pronation	90	90	1.00	4	4
Wrist flexion	67.5	90	0.75	3	2.25
Wrist extension	27.5	90	0.31	5	1.55
MCP (2-5)	68.75	90	0.76	5	3.8
PIP (2-5)	72.5	100	0.73	5	3.65
DIP (2-5)	47.5	90	0.53	4	2.12
Thumb flexion	20	70	0.29	5	1.45
Thumb abduction	30	50	0.60	5	3
Thumb DIP 1	30	90	0.33	2	0.66
Hip flexion	135	135	1.00	5	5
Hip extension	150	155	0.97	5	4.85
Hip abduction	50	50	1.00	4	4
Hip IR	15	45	0.33	2	0.66
Hip ER	40	45	0.88	4	3.52
Knee flexion	145	145	1.00	5	5
Knee extension	145	145	1.00	5	5
Ankle dorsiflexion	20	20	1.00	4	4
Ankle plantarflexion	50	55	0.91	4	3.64

From Epps, H, Hurley M, & Utley M. Development and evaluation of a single value score to assess global range of motion in juvenile idiopathic arthritis. Arthritis Care Research, *47*:398, 2002. Reprinted by permission of Wiley-Liss Inc., a subsidiary of John Wiley & Sons, Inc.
*GROMS = Global Range of Motion Scale; Mode = weighted value for joint movement based upon experts' opinion of its functional importance.
$$\text{GROMS} = \frac{\text{Sum of E} \times 100}{\text{Sum of D}} = \frac{88.95 \times 100}{110} = 80.86$$
Cx = cervical; DIP = distal interphalangeal; ER = external rotation; IR = internal rotation; MCP = metacarpophalangeal; PIP = proximal interphalangeal; R/U = radioulnar.

factors include alterations in anabolic hormones, production of inflammatory cytokines and high resting energy metabolism (Knops et al., 1999), abnormal protein metabolism (Henderson & Lovell, 1989), motor unit inhibition from pain and swelling, and disuse. Disease onset early in life and long periods of active arthritis may negatively impact muscle development (Vostrejs & Hollister, 1988). Common patterns include weakness in hip extension and abduction, knee extension, plantar flexion, shoulder abduction and flexion, elbow flexion and extension, wrist extension, and grip. Two studies suggested that muscle weakness may contribute to activity

restrictions in children with arthritis. Fan and colleagues (1998) found a significant relationship between 50-meter run times and lower extremity CHAQ scores in girls with JRA. Takken and associates (2003) also reported that muscle strength, measured by the Wingate anaerobic exercise test, was significantly correlated to CHAQ scores in 18 children with juvenile arthritis, ages 7 to 14 years.

Muscle bulk, strength, and endurance should be examined at disease onset and monitored regularly. Bilateral measurements of circumference quantify asymmetries in muscle bulk. Functional muscle strength can be estimated in young children by observing their performance of age-appropriate motor tasks or activities of daily living (ADLs). In older children, manual muscle testing can be done to measure isometric strength, especially if the child has pain while moving the limb against resistance. Instrumented measurements using a handheld or isokinetic dynamometer or modified sphygmomanometer (Wessel et al., 1999; Giannini & Protas, 1993; Dunn, 1993) provide consistent and reliable information in individuals with arthritis.

Dynamic muscle testing of functional muscle groups can be performed when there is no sign of joint inflammation or damage. The maximal weight the child can lift throughout the available ROM for 6 to 10 repetitions (6–10 RM) is usually sufficient to establish a baseline level of strength and monitor change (Kramer & Fleck, 1993). An alternative method for children who have pain on movement is to measure isometric strength at multiple angles throughout the ROM. Muscular endurance can be measured by having the child perform as many repetitions as possible at a specified percentage (60%–80%) of the 6 to 10 RM. A warm-up period of light activity should precede strength testing.

AEROBIC CAPACITY AND FUNCTION

Takken and colleagues (2002) examined five studies that directly measured peak oxygen consumption (VO_{2peak}) during progressive graded exercise tests in children with JRA. A meta-analysis of the pooled data showed that relative VO_{2peak} was 21.8% lower in children with JRA compared to healthy control subjects or reference values. Giannini and Protas (1991, 1992) also found that children with JRA had significantly lower peak workload, peak exercise heart rate (HR), and exercise time than healthy control subjects matched for age, gender, and body size. Mean HR and VO_{2peak} values during submaximal exercise were higher in subjects with JRA, suggesting they worked at a higher percentage of their aerobic capacity than control subjects during routine activities. Impaired aerobic fitness does not appear to be significantly related to the severity of joint disease, but may be due to hypoactivity secondary to disease symptoms, especially in children with long-standing arthritis (Henderson & Lovell, 1989; Giannini & Protas, 1991, 1992). Physiologic factors, including anemia, muscle atrophy, generalized weakness, and stiffness, resulting in poor mechanical efficiency may also limit the child's performance. Klepper and colleagues (1992) compared the performance of 20 children, ages 6 to 11 years, with polyJRA and 20 matched control subjects (age, gender, body mass index) on the 9-minute run-walk test. Subjects with JRA scored significantly below control subjects and were not able to maintain a steady running pace. The 6-minute walk test, used frequently in adults with arthritis, may provide a useful alternative to measure walking tolerance in children with JRA (Takken et al., 2001).

ASSESSMENT OF PAIN

Pain is a major cause of activity restrictions in JRA and a predictor of the child's adjustment to the disease. Acute pain may result from inflammation and some medical procedures. The cause of chronic pain is less clear, but may be at least partially due to abnormal joint loading during activity as a result of soft tissue restrictions and muscle imbalance. Older children, especially those with newly diagnosed JRA, report more pain than young children or those with long-standing disease, suggesting pain perception and report are more closely related to age than disease severity or duration (Hagglund et al., 1995). Assessment of pain should be ongoing and include a pain history, self-report for children over the age of 4 years, parent report, and behavioral observations. Validated pain behaviors in JRA include bracing, guarding, rubbing, rigidity, and flexing (Jaworski et al., 1995). Self-report tools for young children include the Wong-Baker Faces Rating Scale (Wong & Baker, 1988) and the Oucher (Beyer et al., 1992). The child can also complete a body map, using different colors to represent pain intensity (Fig. 9-9). Children over the age of 7 years can use a numeric rating scale, horizontal word graphic scale, or a visual analog scale (VAS). The Varni/Thompson Pediatric Pain Questionnaire (PPQ) (Thompson & Varni, 1986) provides a comprehensive assessment with both parent and child reports.

GROWTH DISTURBANCES AND POSTURAL ABNORMALITIES

Retardation of linear growth is associated with extended periods of active disease and is exacerbated by long-term use of systemic steroids. Accelerated growth may occur during remission if the epiphyses are still open. Puberty and the appearance of secondary sex characteristics may be delayed. Osteopenia, mainly in the appendicular skeleton, may be due to inadequate bone formation for age, low bone turnover, and depressed bone formation (Cassidy & Petty, 2001). Nutritional deficits are common and may exacerbate bone loss (Henderson & Lovell, 1989). Increased blood supply to the inflamed joint early in the disease may cause accelerated growth of the ossification centers, resulting in bony overgrowth. Leg length discrepancies often occur as a result of unilateral knee arthritis. Premature closure of the growth plates may also occur.

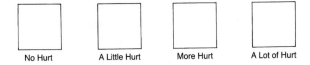

No Hurt   A Little Hurt   More Hurt   A Lot of Hurt

Pick the colors that mean *No Hurt, A Little Hurt, More Hurt,* and *A Lot of Hurt* to you and color in the boxes. Now, using those colors, color in the body to show how you feel. Where you have no hurt, use the *No Hurt* color to color in your body. If you have hurt or pain, use the color that tells how much hurt you have.

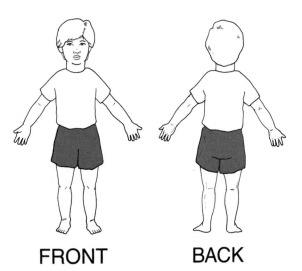

FRONT   BACK

+ **Figure 9-9** Pain may be assessed by allowing the child to color a body map. Intensity of pain is matched with four different colors.

This may be widespread and symmetric, as seen in the small hands and feet of some children with polyJRA, or isolated to a single digit (Cassidy & Petty, 2001). Micrognathia, or undergrowth of the mandible, may result from temporomandibular joint arthritis.

The therapist should observe the child's postural alignment in sitting and standing. Hip and knee flexion contractures, genu valgus, and foot deformities will affect the child's posture in standing. Children with asymmetric cervical spine arthritis may present with torticollis. Muscle imbalance may also occur from habitual postures adopted to relieve pain and pressure within the joints. Children with leg length differences may develop a functional scoliosis. Small lifts of known thickness placed under the shorter leg with the child standing will level the pelvis and confirm or rule out a scoliosis.

GAIT IMPAIRMENTS

Lechner and colleagues (1987) reported that children with JRA often demonstrate gait deviations, including decreased velocity, cadence, step and stride length compared with healthy control subjects or reference values. They also found that subjects had an increased anterior pelvic tilt through the entire gait cycle, and decreased hip extension and plantar flexion at terminal stance and push-off. These deficits may be secondary to weakness and loss of lower extremity ROM (Fan et al., 1998). Lower extremity pain and foot deformities described previously may also contribute to gait deviations. Gait analysis in the clinic is usually performed by observing the child's walking pattern while wearing shoes and while barefoot. Kinematic variables, including velocity and cadence, step length and width, stride length, and foot angle can be documented during a timed walk on an instrumented gait mat or pressure sensitive paper. The child is also observed walking up and down steps, on inclines, and while running. A videotape of the child's performance provides a permanent record and is useful in monitoring change.

■ INTERVENTION

The goals of physical therapy are to prevent or minimize impairments, maintain or improve function, and provide education and support to the child and family. Appendix III illustrates the physical therapy practice patterns in JRA. Treatment is geared to each child's physical, cognitive, and social development, and must also consider the family's cultural background. Physical activity and graded exercise are essential to manage the disease and maintain optimal health. Games and developmental play are useful to encourage young children to move, but joints with active disease or limited motion require direct attention. Exercise in a warm pool, where the heat and buoyancy of the water allow easier movement, is beneficial for children who have severe pain or limited mobility, or who have just had surgery. Most children with mild to moderate JRA can participate in land-based exercise.

Adherence to the therapeutic regimen is extremely important. Home exercise programs are necessary, but are often a source of conflict between the parent and child. The therapist can minimize the demands placed on the family, by suggesting ways to incorporate the treatment into the child's daily routine. Educational materials and other resources are available to help even young children understand the effect of arthritis on body structures. Giving the child some control over the exercise program, for example, choosing the time and place to exercise, may also improve adherence. Older children can collaborate with the parent and therapist to set goals and plan intervention.

Pain Management

Anti-inflammatory drugs used to control arthritis also provide analgesia, but take time to reach a therapeutic effect. Intra-articular steroid injections often induce disease remission in swollen and painful joints. Surgery may be necessary for children with damaged joints and unremitting pain. Physical measures used to treat pain include heat and cold, exercise, massage, and splinting. Rest, ice, compression, and elevation (RICE) reduces acute swelling and inflammation when applied immediately after an injury. Superficial heat, in the form of commercial hot packs or warm moist towels, applied for 20 minutes before exercise increases local blood flow, reduces muscle spasm, and improves tissue extensibility. Paraffin wax may reduce stiffness and pain in the hands before exercise. Young children prefer to "paint" the wax on their hands. Deep heat, including ultrasound and short-wave diathermy, is not used for pain control in JRA.

Balanced rest and exercise are important in managing pain. Children who participate in group aquatic or land-based exercise programs report decreased pain (Bacon et al., 1991; Klepper, 1999; Fisher et al., 2001; Takken et al., 2001). Restful sleep helps to reduce morning stiffness and pain. Resting splints support joints and may relieve pain during the night. A cervical pillow or soft collar may relieve neck pain. Using a sleeping bag at night maintains body warmth and reduces morning stiffness. Exercises performed at night after a warm bath may also decrease morning stiffness. One study found that children who received a massage by a parent before bed reported less pain and stress than those who did not (Field et al., 1997).

Cognitive behavioral therapy (CBT) techniques may also be effective. Walco and colleagues (1992) reported significant improvement in pain and function in 13 children immediately after eight sessions of progressive relaxation training (PRT), meditative breathing, and guided imagery. Effects remained 12 months later. Lavigne and associates (1992) found reductions in self-reported pain and pain behaviors in children with JRA who completed a program of PRT and electromyographic (EMG) biofeedback training. Distraction and imaginative play are useful in very young children. Some clinics offer a multidisciplinary program aimed at helping the child manage pain and disease symptoms.

Management of Joint Impairments

A daily regimen of ROM exercises and positioning is necessary to preserve joint motion and soft tissue extensibility. All joints with arthritis and adjacent joints should be moved through the available ROM once to twice a day. Active ROM is preferable, but gentle active-assisted ROM may be necessary when the child's movement is limited by pain and weakness. The Arthritis Foundation book "Raising a Child with Arthritis" provides an illustrated guide to ROM exercise and posture. The child can also be taught combination patterns cloaked in games that encourage motion in several joints at once. Prone positioning for about 30 minutes a day makes use of gravity to lengthen the flexor muscles in the lower limbs. The child can lie on a firm bed, keeping hips and knees extended and feet hanging off the edge. A sandbag weight placed over the buttocks will stabilize the pelvis. A rolled towel placed under the forehead can accommodate limited neck rotation or pain. Commercial or custom splints for the wrists, hands, elbows, knees, and ankles rest the joint and provide a prolonged static stretch.

Gentle manual stretching can begin when the arthritis is under control. Brief (60 seconds) stretching causes a temporary increase in tissue extensibility and is useful before placing the limb in a resting splint. Repeated bouts of stretching, with the joint held at the maximal possible range for several minutes each time, may achieve a more lasting increase in connective tissue length (Godges et al., 1993). Neuromuscular techniques, such as contract-relax, may improve joint motion. Several precautions are necessary during passive stretching. When stretching the hamstrings in a child with a knee flexion contracture, the stretching hand should be placed close to the joint to decrease the risk for posterior subluxation of the tibia. Pain during the stretch should be minimized to avoid reflex muscle spasm, which is counterproductive and may cause damage to the soft tissues and epiphyseal areas at the tendon-bone interface. Superficial heat applied before stretching and deep breathing performed during the stretch may facilitate relaxation. The child should perform active ROM exercise after stretching to use the muscle in its lengthened range.

Static progressive stretching (SPS), using serial splints or casts, extension orthoses, dynamic splints, or skin traction can be used to resolve contractures (Melvin & Wright, 2000). Serial splints can be molded and easily modified by the therapist as the child gains motion. One drawback is that the child can remove the splint, decreasing its effectiveness. In contrast, serial casts provide a continuous low load stretch, usually for about 72 hours, after which they are removed and bivalved. During the next 1 to 2 weeks the child wears the bivalved cast for 18 to 24 hours a day, removing it only for exercise sessions. A new cast is applied and the process repeated until optimal ROM is achieved (Wright & Smith, 1996). Dynamic splints can be ordered to fit the child. The tension is set to the child's tolerance, and increased gradually as ROM improves. The child wears the splint for several 1-hour intervals during the day. Use throughout the night provides continuous stretching. Skin traction applied at night has also been shown to be effective in reducing hip and knee flexion contractures, although it may cause disturbed sleep in some children. One study, using a single subject design, reported that a combination of nighttime skin traction, daytime use of an extension orthosis during weight-bearing activities, and physical therapy twice a week was effective in reducing active and passive ROM deficits in several children with JRA (Fredriksen & Mengshoel, 2000).

ORTHOPEDIC SURGERY AND THE ROLE OF THE PHYSICAL THERAPIST

Carefully planned orthopedic surgery in the young child is aimed at preserving joint health. In the older child with joint damage, reconstruction surgery may relieve pain and restore function. Staging the surgical procedures is important in a child with severe polyJRA. The first priority is to maintain or restore ambulation, followed by the need to improve the child's ability to perform ADLs. The choice of procedure depends on the child's age, disease activity, functional status, and condition of the joint.

Isolated soft tissue releases (STR) are performed to reduce pressure within the joint, relieve vascular congestion, improve joint nutrition, and promote repair of the cartilage with fibrocartilage (Clark et al., 1988). The most common procedures are adductor and psoas tenotomies to relieve hip flexion contractures, ITB fasciotomy, hamstring lengthening, and posterior capsulotomy to reduce knee flexion contractures. Initial postoperative care for the hip includes immobilization in an abduction and extension splint or brace. Major rotational problems require a full leg brace or positioning in a boot with a medial or lateral bar. Following STR at the knee, the leg is splinted in extension. ROM exercises begin within the first 48 hours unless there are problems with wound healing. Gait training begins as soon as possible. Prone positioning and avoidance of prolonged sitting are important during the postoperative period. Strengthening exercises begin when soft tissue inflammation resolves and ROM improves. Splints may be discontinued after about 8 weeks, but therapy continues for several months (Nestor et al., 2000).

Synovectomy is performed less frequently in children than adults, but may be done in conjunction with STR. The procedure may be useful in children with nearly normal ROM and minimal evidence of articular damage who have not responded to medical therapies. The major postoperative complication is soft tissue contracture, although this may occur less often with arthroscopic surgery (Nestor et al., 2000). ROM exercises begin soon after surgery to maintain preoperative joint motion. A

continuous passive motion (CPM) machine is used for the elbow or knee. After discharge and wound healing, dynamic splints may be prescribed to preserve ROM. Arthrodesis is useful in advanced arthritis of the ankle and hindfoot, wrist, and IP joints, especially if there is a risk for ankylosis in an abnormal position. Postoperative care includes immobilization in a cast, and exercise and positioning for adjacent joints. Protected weight bearing and ambulation with crutches or a walker follow lower limb surgery. Immobilization is maintained until there is radiographic evidence of successful fusion. Epiphysiodesis, or surgical arrest of the growth plate, may be used in some children with bony overgrowth. Osteotomy is considered when there is a severe valgus deformity at the knee if the articular cartilage is preserved and joint motion is normal. Postoperative care includes 4 to 6 weeks of immobilization (Nestor et al., 2000).

Total joint arthroplasty (TJA) is considered when there is irreversible joint damage, and the child has significant pain and functional limitation. The procedure is most frequently performed at the hip and knee, although prostheses are available for other joints. Several factors are considered in the decision, including the child's age, skeletal maturity, general physical status, upper extremity function, and ability of the child to successfully complete the lengthy and intensive postoperative rehabilitation regimen. Customized computer-designed prostheses may be necessary to accommodate changes in joint anatomy, small bone size, and osteoporosis. The longevity of the prosthesis must also be considered, especially when TJA is performed in young children. Procedures are staged if the child requires extensive surgery to ensure the best functional outcome. STRs may be done in conjunction with TJA to reduce contractures.

Preoperative therapy for lower extremity surgery includes general conditioning to improve ROM, strength, and stamina, as well as gait training with crutches or a walker, and instruction in postoperative precautions to protect the implant. Postoperative care for total hip arthroplasty (THA) is influenced by the surgical approach and type of implant (Nestor et al., 2001). Most surgeons require protected weight bearing for several weeks if an uncemented implant is used. With a posterior surgical approach, the child progresses from crutches or a walker to a cane. To protect the abductor muscle repair after an anterolateral approach, the child must use crutches or a walker for 6 to 8 weeks and avoid active hip abduction for 12 weeks (Nestor et al., 2000).

ROM exercises begin early, with precautions against hip flexion past 90°, hip adduction and internal rotation past neutral in order to avoid dislocation of the implant. A foam wedge placed between the legs maintains hip abduction when lying in bed or sitting; periods of prone positioning help stretch the hip flexors. A CPM machine may be used to improve joint mobility. Active exercise and walking in chest-deep water can begin once the wound is healed. The child also practices transfers, ambulation on level surfaces and stairs, and ADLs. Assistive equipment, including elevated toilet seats and dressing aids, are used to avoid excessive hip flexion. Precautions are usually maintained for the first 2 to 3 postoperative months, although some surgeons prefer a longer period. Activities that cause high impact loading on the joint, including running and jumping or carrying heavy objects, should be avoided.

Postoperative therapy following total knee arthroplasty begins on day 2, with active and passive ROM exercises. The goal is to achieve complete extension and flexion greater than 90°. A CPM machine can be used immediately, with an extension splint worn at other times. Therapy includes isometric exercises for the quadriceps and hamstrings, straight leg raises, and limited arc knee extension. The child can bear weight, wearing a knee immobilizer. Gait training with crutches or walker begins on day 2, and protected weight bearing with a cane continues for about 6 weeks until there is adequate healing of the extensor mechanism. Stationary cycling may be included in the regimen if the bike has a range limiter applied to the pedal that allows the therapist to control the degree of knee flexion required during cycling.

STRENGTHENING AND AEROBIC EXERCISE

Strengthening exercises target the muscles surrounding and supporting the joints with arthritis and adjacent areas. During acute joint inflammation, isometric exercise is recommended to maintain muscle bulk and strength. Resistance can be provided manually or by a stable external object, nonelastic webbing, or heavy elastic bands placed around the limb close to and proximal to the joint. Prolonged maximal isometric contractions should be avoided because they may increase intra-articular pressure and constrict blood flow through the muscles (James et al., 1994). The child is taught to perform and hold a submaximal contraction for approximately 6 seconds, exhaling during the contraction and inhaling during the relaxation phase. Five to 10 repetitions daily are sufficient (Minor & Westby, 2001). EMG biofeedback may be helpful in training the child to regulate the intensity of the contraction. Isometric exercises performed at multiple points within the ROM may prepare the joint for dynamic exercise after active disease resolves.

Dynamic exercise is added when joint inflammation subsides. Both concentric and eccentric exercises are in-

cluded. Functional movement patterns can be incorporated into the training, and variety introduced with programs such as Pilates, yoga, or tai chi. External resistance, in the form of light hand or cuff weights or elastic bands, can be safely added once the child is able to correctly perform 8 to 10 repetitions of motion against gravity without pain (Minor, 2001). Fisher and colleagues (2001) recently examined the effects of resistance exercise using isokinetic equipment in six children with JRA ages 6 to 14 years, who trained as a group three times a week for 8 weeks. Each child's program was individualized and progressed based on their initial test results and response to training. Subjects showed significant improvements in quadriceps and hamstring strength and endurance, contraction speed of the hamstrings, functional status, disability, and performance of timed tasks. Control subjects with JRA who did not exercise showed decreased muscle function during the same time period (Fisher et al., 2001).

Clear directions and illustrations of the exercises are necessary, and training sessions should be supervised. Children should use lighter weights and perform 2 to 3 sets of 10 to 15 repetitions. A good starting point is to use the amount of resistance the child was able to lift 6 to 10 times without discomfort. Progression is based on periodic reassessment. Each training session should begin with light aerobic and flexibility activities and end with cool-down and stretching activities. Resistance exercises should be performed twice a week, allowing time between sessions for rest and recovery (Faigenbaum et al., 2002).

Aerobic exercise is also important to improve the child's endurance for routine physical activities and play. A review of the available evidence for the benefits of aerobic exercise indicates that children with JRA who performed moderately vigorous (60%–85% HR_{max}) aerobic activity for at least 30 minutes twice a week for at least 6 weeks can improve their aerobic fitness (Klepper, 2003). The specific mode of exercise appears to be less important than the intensity, duration, and frequency. However, weight-bearing exercise is necessary to maintain optimal bone growth and density. Low impact activities to improve proprioceptive function, balance, and coordination can be incorporated into aerobic conditioning programs.

SELF-CARE ACTIVITIES

A primary goal for a child with JRA is to achieve independence in self-care within the home, school, and community. Expectations for independence differ at each age and stage of development. Treatment for an infant with JRA may include suggestions to parents for positioning to promote symmetry, prevent contractures, and facilitate function. A child with limited grasp may benefit from adapted toys. Toddlers or pre-school age children with JRA who are beginning to gain independence in ADLs may need extra time to practice these skills. Older children must master more complex tasks to achieve independence in school and community activities. For the adolescent or young adult, independence may revolve around the ability to drive, socialize with friends, hold a job, attend college, and formulate career plans.

Parents and children should receive instruction in the principles of joint conservation to reduce pain, fatigue, and deforming forces during activity. The child may be taught to carry objects on their forearms instead of grasping them with the hands, lift and carry objects close to the body, and use a backpack positioned close to the center of gravity or a rolling backpack to carry school items. Functional wrist and hand splints can support the joint during hand use, and assistive devices can compensate for a weak grip and reduce hand pain and fatigue. Dressing and hygiene aids include Velcro closures on clothing and shoes, elastic shoelaces, a long-handled shoehorn, dressing stick, buttonhook, zipper pull, and long-handled bath brush. Built-up handles on grooming items, eating utensils, and writing implements are often necessary for optimal function and independence.

Some modifications within the home may be beneficial, including replacing knobs and faucets with levers, using a jar opener or an electric can opener, adding a raised toilet seat, and installing safety bars in the bathtub. More substantial modifications, including widening doorways and adding a ramp to the entrance, are needed for a child who must use a wheelchair. The therapist must consider the financial, physical, and emotional impact of these changes on the family. The device or adaptation must be affordable, achieve the stated purpose, be easy to use, and be acceptable to the child and parent. Because training in ADLs can be time consuming and a source of conflict between the parent and child, consultation with a social worker or psychologist may help the parent manage stress and gain the child's cooperation.

FUNCTIONAL MOBILITY

Weight bearing and ambulation are vital for optimal bone growth and density, joint health, and muscle development. Standing, cruising, and walking should be encouraged at the expected age, although the use of infant walkers should be avoided because they may promote an abnormal gait pattern and carry a high risk for injury. Toddlers and pre-school age children should be encouraged to walk within the home and short distances outside. Shoes should support and cushion the joints of the feet and accommodate any deformities. Sneakers with a flexible sole, good arch support, and high heel cup are a good choice for most children. A wide, deep toe box may be necessary for a child with hallux valgus, hammer toes, or claw toes. A child with arthritis in the feet and toes should not wear high heels because of the excessive pressure on the metatarsophalangeal joints. A rocker-like addition to the sole of the shoe may provide a mechanical assist at toe-off for a child who has limited or painful toe hyperextension. A molded ankle-foot orthosis (AFO) may be necessary to support the ankle if pain and instability prevent weight bearing. Custom molded in-shoe orthoses can replace the standard insole to accommodate foot deformities and decrease pressure on those tender joints.

Few children with JRA require an assistive device for ambulation. However, if a child begins to show problems with weight bearing or difficulty walking, the cause should be determined and addressed immediately. Leg length differences can be accommodated by placing a lift on the sole of the shoe on the shorter side. A child with unilateral lower extremity pain or weakness can use a cane on the opposite side to unload the involved limb and increase stability during ambulation. A walker or crutches may be needed if problems are bilateral. Platform attachments can be added if the child has upper limb impairments.

Some children may need to use a form of wheeled mobility for long distances within the school or community environment. A wagon or stroller with a firm seat and back is appropriate for toddlers or pre-school age children. Older children can use a tricycle or bicycle with training wheels to get around the community. A powered scooter or lightweight wheelchair may be necessary for efficient mobility in school. Children with upper extremity arthritis often maneuver the wheelchair with their feet. Powered wheelchairs are usually reserved for the children with severe impairments, but may be necessary for a college student who must negotiate a large campus. Children who use a wheelchair should spend part of every day out of the chair, standing and walking to preserve bone health, prevent contractures, and maintain walking tolerance.

ISSUES RELATED TO SCHOOL

Children with JRA may need occasional modifications to their school program. These might include a second set of books for home, built-up or adapted writing tools, or an easel top for the desk in the classroom. Children with significant hand arthritis may need to record class notes on a tape recorder or word processor and take tests under untimed conditions. Modifications to the school schedule may include time out of the classroom to take medication or rest for brief periods during the day, extra time to travel between classes, or permission to use an elevator if the child is unable to negotiate stairs. Some schools provide these services voluntarily. In other situations, the child may need an individualized educational plan (IEP) or accommodations specified under Section 504 of the Vocational Rehabilitation Act. Vocational counseling is often necessary to prepare adolescents for the transition to higher education and work. Although most states mandate transition planning, Lovell and colleagues (1990) found that only 8% of children with JRA received vocational counseling.

Regular participation in physical education is encouraged. The instructor should be aware of the child's diagnosis and any activity restrictions or precautions. In general, the child should be allowed to monitor his/her own activity level, resting as needed. However, some activities are prohibited because of their potential for injury or joint damage. These prohibited activities include headstands and somersaults for a child with cervical spine disease; handstands, push-ups, cartwheels, and other similar activities in a child with wrist and hand arthritis; and high-impact running or jumping in a child with spinal or lower extremity arthritis. The therapist can consult with the physical education instructor to modify activities as necessary.

RECREATIONAL ACTIVITIES

Recreational activities provide physical and psychosocial benefits. The choice of activities depends on the child's preferences, physical status, motor skills, and fitness level. Participation on any given day must also be modified to accommodate disease symptoms. Scull and Athreya (1995) provided a useful guide to help parents and children choose activities for a child with JRA. Swimming, water or low-impact weight-bearing aerobics, and bicycling provide good cardiovascular exercise. Activities that cause high impact loading on inflamed or damaged joints should be avoided. Contact sports, including football, hockey, and boxing, and those with a high inherent potential for injury are discouraged. Competitive team sports may be physically and emotionally stressful, but each situation should be evaluated individually.

A physical conditioning program prior to participating in a sport prepares the child for the physical demands of the activity. Warm-up and stretching activities prior to each practice session or game and a cool-down period after the activity should be encouraged. Instruction in motor skills specific to the sport may be necessary. A sports orthosis or other adaptive equipment may improve joint alignment and stability.

▌SUMMARY

Juvenile rheumatoid arthritis (JRA) is an autoimmune inflammatory disorder and the most common rheumatic disease of childhood. Although the exact etiology is unclear, three distinct onset types are recognized—systemic, polyarticular, and pauciarticular. With advances in recognition and diagnosis of the disease and more effective medications to treat the joint inflammation, most children with JRA do well with early diagnosis and appropriate treatment. However, for many children, JRA results in both short- and long-term problems, including chronic joint swelling, pain, and limited motion, as well as muscle atrophy and weakness, poor aerobic function, and impaired exercise tolerance. General and localized growth disturbances, postural abnormalities, and gait deviations occur with persistent disease. Activity and participation restrictions that result from the arthritis and extra-articular manifestations can negatively impact the child's quality of life. The long-term prognosis depends upon the child's age at disease onset, onset type, severity and duration of active inflammation, and the quality and consistency of medical care and other resources available and utilized by the family. This chapter reviewed the most common characteristics of JRA, standardized examination and outcome measures developed for use in children with arthritis, and current research findings regarding the effects of exercise and physical activity in individuals with chronic inflammatory arthritis. Physical therapists are vital members of the pediatric rheumatology team, providing examination, evaluation, intervention, and monitoring of a child with JRA. Therapists also serve as an important resource to parents or caregivers and school and community personnel to adapt activities so the child with JRA can participate fully in the home, school, and community environments. As a result, physical therapists have the opportunity to add considerably to the quality of life of children with JRA.

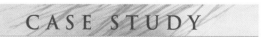

C A S E   S T U D Y

JASON

Client Description

Jason is a 13-year-old boy with polyarticular JRA of 8 years' duration. He lives in a single-family home with his parents and two siblings, an 18-year-old brother and a 16-year-old sister. He is in the 8th grade in a regional public junior high school and does well academically, but does not participate in any sports or other after-school activities. Jason's pediatrician provides routine medical care, and a pediatric rheumatology team at a specialized tertiary care center 2 hours from his home coordinates the care for his arthritis. His current medications include naproxen and methotrexate. He does not receive direct physical therapy, but has a home range of motion and strengthening exercise program prescribed by the rheumatology clinic PT. He also has wrist and hand splints fabricated by the clinic occupational therapist (OT). Jason sees both the OT and PT at periodic intervals of 3 to 6 months during his regular rheumatology clinic appointment.

Medical History

Jason's arthritis was diagnosed when he was 5 years old, after several months of joint swelling and pain, lethargy, and mild systemic symptoms. At the time of diagnosis, he had active joint inflammation in both knees, ankles, elbows, and wrists; more and more joints became involved over time. Jason had three STRs between the ages of 8 and 10 years to relieve tight plantar fascia and toe flexor tendons in both feet. However, the restrictions have recurred, and he continues to complain of foot pain.

Findings of Physical Therapy Examination

Primary Problems/Complaints

Jason's primary complaints during his clinic visit included morning stiffness lasting about 1 hour, low back pain during the day after sitting in his school desk for more than 20 minutes, neck pain when doing deskwork and riding in the school bus, foot pain, and general fatigue when walking around school and in the community. When asked about school and recreational activities, Jason stated his grades were good, but he had to work harder than other kids to make up material he misses when he is late or absent as a result of his arthritis. He stated that he feels different because he can't do some of the activities in physical education class and is not able to play any team sports at school or in the community. He missed a recent overnight school trip because his parents were afraid he would forget to take his medications and have problems getting up in the morning without their help. Jason also admitted to being concerned that his neck would hurt on the long bus ride. Jason's mother reported that he usually avoids family outings that involve hiking or other sports because he gets tired or his feet hurt. When asked about his home exercise program, Jason admitted that he did not do the prescribed exercises because they are boring. He also stated that his hand splints hurt and caused an itchy rash on his forearms.

Jason's Goals

Jason stated that he wanted to be like other kids his age. Next year, he will transfer to a large 4-year high school and is concerned about his ability to keep up with the other kids. Specifically he expressed a desire to have more energy, do the same physical activities as his classmates in gym, and play some type of recreational sport with his friends. He also stated that he would like to hike and cross-country ski with his family, when they take vacations in the mountains.

Results of Tests and Measures

Participation and Activity

Jason walks independently, but has trouble keeping pace with his friends. His gait pattern shows a shortened step length and lack of push-off. He bears weight mostly on the lateral borders of his feet. His standard scores on three gross motor subtests of the Bruininks-Oseretsky Test of Motor Proficiency (BOTMP) (running speed and agility, balance, bilateral coordination) are one standard deviation below the mean for his age. His CHAQ DI of 1.25 indicates moderate activity limitations. Specifically, he has difficulty tying his shoes, manipulating buttons, opening jars, taking notes in class, completing tests on time, getting to the floor and back up to standing in gym, and running. Jason's scores on the 10 cm Quality of My Life Scales, where higher scores indicate a better quality of life (QOL), were Overall QOL = 5 cm and Health Related QOL = 4. He rated his QOL as about the same as his last clinic visit, 3 months ago.

Impairments

Joint inflammation: Effusions are present in the wrists, MCPs and PIPs, ankles, and toes on both sides.

Passive range of motion (PROM): There are bilateral hip flexion contractures of 10°, limited abduction (0°–15°) and internal rotation (0°–30°) on the right side. Ankle dorsiflexion is 0° to 5° on both sides; plantar flexion is full. Hindfoot inversion is full; eversion is 0° bilaterally. Both feet show hallux valgus and hammer toe deformities. Cervical spine rotation and lateral flexion are limited by 50%; extension and flexion are WNL (within normal limits). Shoulder motion is full, but painful at end range. Jason has bilateral elbow flexion contractures of 20° and both wrists have limited extension (0°–45°).

Muscle function: Grip strength measured on a modified blood pressure cuff is 80/20 mm Hg (right) and 70/20 mm Hg (left). Smythe and Helewa (1996) reported a 20 mm Hg rise in pressure was equal to approximately 5 lb. Therefore, Jason's estimated grip strength values of 15 lb (right) and 7.5 lb (left) are considerably below the range reported for healthy children (Mathiowetz et al.,

1986). Leg strength is grossly 4/5 on MMT; arm strength is 3+/5. Jason's scores on the standardized curl-up (8) and upper trunk lift (5 inches) tests (Prudential Fitnessgram) are below the minimum health fitness standard for his age of 21 curl-ups and 9 inches, respectively.

Aerobic function: Jason's score on the 9-minute walk test was 1000 yards, which is below the health fitness standard of 1900 yards for his age.

Pain: He rates his overall pain intensity during the past week as 5 on a 10 cm VAS.

Prognosis

Plan of Care

Jason agreed to a 3-month contract with reevaluation at his next clinic visit. The contract included taking his full medication dose each week, performing ROM exercises at night, and taking a warm bath upon arising to decrease the morning stiffness that has resulted in tardiness for school. A schedule of aerobic exercise was developed, allowing Jason to choose among a number of activities. He also agreed to try wearing a soft cervical collar on the school bus to decrease neck pain. With the clinic's help, Jason's mother agreed to arrange for a 3-month trial of direct PT, with 45-minute sessions three times each week.

Expected Outcomes

Improved exercise tolerance and decreased foot pain when walking resulting in increased 9-minute walk distance; improved endurance for physical activity with friends and family; decreased difficulty with manipulative activities as measured by the CHAQ; improved ability to manage his own health care, including medications and exercise.

Interventions

Problem: Slow and Inefficient Gait

Goal 1: Jason will decrease the time he currently requires to walk between classes and other areas in his school by 50% (to be achieved in 3 months).

Goal 2: Jason will demonstrate increased step and stride length, improved heel to toe progression in stance, and increased push-off during gait (assessed by videotape of Jason's gait pattern).

Interventions for pain in the midfoot on loading and pain in MTP joints on push-off:

- Sneakers with a deep, wide toe box to accommodate toe deformities
- Evaluation for custom in-shoe orthoses to provide support for the cavus deformity and to reduce force on the metatarsophalangeal joints

Interventions for impaired PROM (hip flexion contracture, limited ankle dorsiflexion, subtalor eversion):

- Prone positioning for 30 minutes/day, placing rolled towel under forehead to accommodate limited neck rotation
- Daily self-stretching exercises for hip flexors and calf muscles
- PT to perform gentle mobilizations of subtalar joint to increase calcaneal eversion

Problem: Inability to Perform Activities in Physical Education Class and Participate in Recreational Sports

Goal 1: Jason will perform aerobic activity at an intensity of 75% of his maximum heart rate continuously for at least 15 minutes.

Goal 2: Jason will improve his BOTMP gross motor scores to age-appropriate levels.

Goal 3: Jason will participate in at least 80% of PE activities at each session within 3 months.

Interventions for poor lower extremity muscle strength and endurance:

- Strengthening regimen twice a week for hip abductors, extensors, external rotators, quadriceps, and hamstrings. Begin with dynamic exercise against gravity. Add resistance in the form of Theraband or light cuff weights when Jason can perform 15 repetitions of each exercise with good form.

Interventions for delayed gross motor skills and poor exercise tolerance:

- Develop general training program to improve Jason's balance, coordination, and speed, and lower extremity proprioceptive function
- Work on specific skills for the recreational sports Jason chooses to play

Interventions for poor exercise tolerance:

- Aerobic exercise three to four times a week (20–30 minutes); activities based on Jason's preferences

Problem: Difficulty with Manipulative Activities at Home and School

Goal: Jason will report decreased hand pain and difficulty performing manipulative activities (decreased CHAQ score for activities requiring hand use).

Interventions for weakness and pain in wrists and hands—consultation with OT:

- Revise resting splints; add liner to minimize skin irritation
- Make functional hand splint for use in school
- Recommend adaptive equipment (jar opener, built-up utensils; Velcro closures, or elastic shoelaces)

Interventions for hand and neck pain when working at school desk: Consult with school. Ask for evaluation and services under Section 504 of Rehabilitation Act.

- Use built-up writing tools, easel-top for desk, untimed conditions for tests.
- PT to consult with PE instructor to integrate Jason more fully into activities.

Problem: Poor Adaptation and Self-Efficacy in Managing the Diagnosis

Goal: Jason will assume increased responsibility for his own health care. The rheumatology team believes that poor adherence to the medical and therapeutic regimen contributes to Jason's problems. They agreed he should take a more active role in setting goals and planning intervention, including the following:

- Explore the services provided by the Arthritis Foundation and the American Juvenile Arthritis Organization (AJAO), including teen support groups and local, regional, and national family retreats.
- Work with the rheumatology clinic team to develop a contract with Jason to enlist his adherence to the medical and exercise routine.
- Participate in a short course of direct PT and OT to increase Jason's self-efficacy for managing his arthritis.

Outcomes

Jason's progress toward his goals was reevaluated at his regular 3-month rheumatology appointment. His mother reported that she contacted the school to ask that Jason be evaluated to determine if he is eligible for services and accommodations under Section 504 of the Rehabilitation Act. She was also able to find a PT to work with Jason in their home twice a week and to consult with the school PE instructor to modify some of the activities so that Jason can participate more fully in the class. Jason reports that, besides the exercises he performs during his therapy sessions, he does some type of aerobic physical activity for 15 minutes 2 to 3 days a week. His activity log, with each entry co-signed by a parent, verifies his statement. Jason also states that he has been more consistent in taking his medication and admits to feeling better, with less morning stiffness. His hand splints were modified by clinic OT, and he now wears them for at least 4 to 5 hours a night. His progress toward the goals established at his last visit is described below.

1. Jason states that he participates in about 50% of each PE class. He is not involved in any extracurricular sports at school, but plans to try out for the swim team at his community pool next summer.

2. Jason's score on the CHAQ DI is now 1.10, a decrease of 0.15. He reports less difficulty moving between standing and sitting on the floor, running, and performing some manipulative tasks.

3. Jason's performance on three of the BOTMP gross motor scales show improvement; his point score on the Running Speed & Agility Test increased from 9 to 11; his balance test point score increased from 23 to 26; the point score on the Bilateral Coordination Test increased from 11 to 13.

4. Jason's responses on the QOML scale show some improvement (overall QOL score is 7 cm and health-related QOL is 6 cm). He reports his health status since last visit is better.

Jason agreed to continue with his current therapy and physical activity program and take his full medication dose and wear his hand splints every night. He continues to resist using a cervical collar when riding the school bus because he does not want to look different from the other students.

▆ REFERENCES

American Physical Therapy Association. Guide to Physical Therapist Practice, 2nd edition. Fairfax, VA: APTA, 2001.

Ansell, BM, Rudge, S, & Schaller, JG. Color Atlas of Pediatric Rheumatology. London: Wolfe Publishing Limited, 1992, pp. 13–75.

Arthritis Foundation: Raising a Child with Arthritis. Atlanta: Arthritis Foundation, 1998.

Atwood, M. Developmental assessment and integration. In Melvin, J (Ed.). Rheumatic Disease in Adult and Child: Occupational Therapy and Rehabilitation, 3rd ed. Philadelphia: FA Davis, 1989, pp. 188–214.

Atwood, M. Treatment considerations. In Melvin, J (Ed.). Rheumatic Disease in Adult and Child: Occupational Therapy and Rehabilitation, 3rd ed. Philadelphia: FA Davis, 1989, pp. 215–234.

Bacon, M, Nicholson, C, Binder, H, & White, P. Juvenile rheumatoid arthritis: Aquatic exercise and lower extremity function. Arthritis Care and Research, 4:102–105, 1991.

Beyer, JE, Denyes, MJ, & Villarruel, AM: The creation, validation, and continuing development of the Oucher: A measure of pain intensity in children. Journal of Pediatric Nursing, 7:335–346, 1992.

Brewer, EJ, Bass, J, Baum, J, Cassidy, JT, Fink, C, Jacobs, J, Hanson, V, Levinson, JE, Schaller, J, & Stillman, JS. Current proposed revision of JRA criteria. Arthritis and Rheumatism, 20(suppl):195–202, 1977.

Cassidy, JT, & Petty, RE. Juvenile rheumatoid arthritis. In Cassidy, JT, & Petty, RE (Eds.). Textbook of Pediatric Rheumatology, 4th ed. Philadelphia: WB Saunders, 2001, pp. 218–321.

Cassidy, JT, & Petty, RE. Textbook of Pediatric Rheumatology, 2nd ed. New York: Churchill Livingstone, 1990.

Clark, DW, Ansell, BM, & Swan, M. Soft-tissue release of the knee in juvenile chronic arthritis. Journal of Bone & Joint Surgery, 70B:224, 1988.

Clemens, LE, Albert, E, & Ansell, BM. Sibling pairs affected by chronic arthritis of childhood: Evidence for a genetic predisposition. Journal of Rheumatology, 12:108–113, 1985.

Coster, W, Deeney, T, Haltiwanger, J, & Haley, S: School Function Assessment. Boston: Harcourt Brace & Co., 1998.

Cron, R: Current treatment for chronic arthritis in childhood. Current Opinions in Pediatrics, 14:684–687, 2000.

Duffy, CM, Arsenault, HL, Duffy, KN, Paquin, JD, & Strawczynski, H. The Juvenile Arthritis Quality of Life Questionnaire—Development of a new responsive index for juvenile rheumatoid arthritis and juvenile spondyloarthrytides. Journal of Rheumatology, 24:738–746, 1997.

Dunn, W. Grip strength of children aged 3 to 7 years using a modified sphygmomanometer: Comparison of typical children and children with rheumatic disease. American Journal of Occupational Therapy, 47:421–428, 1993.

Emery, HM. The rehabilitation of the child with juvenile chronic arthritis. Balliere's Clinical Pediatrics, 1:803–823, 1993.

Epps, H, Hurley, M, & Utley, M. Development and evaluation of a single score to assess global range of motion in juvenile rheumatoid arthritis. Arthritis Care and Research, 47:398–402, 2002.

European League Against Rheumatism. EULAR Bulletin No. 4: Nomenclature and Classification of Arthritis in Children. Basel: National Zeitung AG, 1977.

Faigenbaum, AD, Milliken, LA, Loud, RL, Burak, BT, Doherty, CL, & Westcott, WL. Comparison of 1 and 2 days per week of strength training in children. Research Quarterly for Exercise and Sport, 73:416–424, 2002.

Fan, J, Wessel, J, & Ellsworth, J: The relationship between strength and function in females with juvenile rheumatoid arthritis. Journal of Rheumatology, 3:1399–1405, 1998.

Field, T, Hernandez-Reif, M, Seligman, S, Krasnegor, J, Sunshine W, Rivas-Chacon, R, Schanberg, L, & Kuhn, C. Juvenile rheumatoid arthritis: Benefits from massage therapy. Journal of Pediatric Psychology, 22:607–617, 1997.

Fisher, NM, Venkatraman, JT, & O'Neil, K: The effects of resistance exercises on muscle function in juvenile arthritis. Arthritis and Rheumatism, 44:S276, 2001.

Foeldvari, I, & Bidde, M: Validation of the proposed ILAR classification criteria for juvenile idiopathic arthritis. Journal of Rheumatology, 27:1069–1072, 2000.

Fredriksen, B, & Mengshoel, AM. The effect of static traction and orthoses in the treatment of knee contractures in preschool children with juvenile chronic arthritis: A single subject design. Arthritis Care and Research, 13:352–359, 2000.

Giannini, EJ, Ruperto, N, Ravelli, A, Lovell, DJ, Felson, DT, & Martini, A. Preliminary definition of improvement in juvenile arthritis. Arthritis and Rheumatism, 40:1202–1209, 1997.

Giannini, MJ, & Protas, EJ: Aerobic capacity in juvenile rheumatoid arthritis patients and healthy children. Arthritis Care and Research 4:131–135, 1991.

Giannini, MJ, & Protas, EJ. Exercise response in children with and without juvenile rheumatoid arthritis: A case comparison study. Physical Therapy, 72:365–372, 1992.

Giannini, MJ, & Protas, EJ. Comparison of peak isometric knee extensor torque in children with and without juvenile arthritis. Arthritis Care and Research, 6:82–88, 1993.

Godges, JJ, MacRae, PG, & Engelke, KA: Effects of exercise on hip range of motion, trunk muscle performance, and gait economy. Physical Therapy, 73:468–477, 1993.

Guzman, J, Burgos-Vargas, R, Duarte-Salazar, C, & Gomez-Mora, P. Reliability of the articular examination in children with juvenile rheumatoid arthritis: Interobserver agreement and sources of disagreement. Journal of Rheumatology, 22:2331–2336, 1995.

Hagglund, KJ, Schopp, LM, Alberts, KR, Cassidy, JT, & Frank, RG. Predicting pain among children with juvenile rheumatoid arthritis. Arthritis Care and Research, 8:36–42, 1995.

Henderson, CJ, Lovell, DJ, Specker, BL, & Campaigne, BN. Physical activity in children with juvenile rheumatoid arthritis: Quantification and evaluation. Arthritis Care and Research, 8:114–119, 1995.

Henderson, CJ, & Lovell, DJ: Assessment of protein-energy malnutrition in children and adolescents with juvenile rheumatoid arthritis. Arthritis Care and Research, 2:108-113, 1989.

Hendrengren, E, Knutson, LM, Haglund-Akerlind, Y, & Hagelberg, S. Lower extremity isometric torque in children with juvenile chronic arthritis. Scandinavian Journal of Rheumatology, 30:69–76, 2001.

Hester, NO, Foster, R, & Kristensen, K. Measurement of pain in children: Generalizability and validity of the pain ladder and the poker-chip tool. In Tyler, DC, & Kane, EJ (Eds.). Advances in Pain Research and Therapy. New York: Raven Press, 1990, pp. 79–84.

Howe, S, Levinson, J, Shear, E, Hartner, S, McGirr, G, Schulte, M, & Lovell, D. Development of a disability measurement tool for juvenile rheumatoid arthritis: The Juvenile Arthritis Functional Assessment Report for children and their parents. Arthritis and Rheumatism, 34:873–880, 1991.

James, MJ, Cleland, LG, Gaffney, RD, Proudman, SM, & Gibson, RA. Effect of exercise on $_{99m}$Tc-STPA clearance from knees with effusions. Journal of Rheumatology, 21:501–504, 1994.

Jaworski, TM, Bradley, LA, Heck, LW, Roca, A, & Alarcon, GS. Development of an observation method for assessing pain behaviors in children with juvenile rheumatoid arthritis. Arthritis and Rheumatism, 38:1142–1151, 1995.

Klepper, S, Darbee, J, Effgen, S, & Singsen, B. Physical fitness levels in children with polyarticular juvenile rheumatoid arthritis. Arthritis Care and Research, 5:93–100, 1992.

Klepper, S. Effects of an eight-week physical conditioning program on disease signs and symptoms in children with chronic arthritis. Arthritis Care and Research, 12:52–60, 1999.

Klepper, S. Exercise and fitness in children with arthritis: Evidence of benefits for exercise and physical activity. Arthritis Care and Research, 49:435–443, 2003.

Knopps, K, Wulffraat, N, Lodder, S, Houwen, R, & de Meer, K: Resting energy expenditure and nutritional status in children with juvenile rheumatoid arthritis. Journal of Rheumatology, 26:2039–2043, 1999.

Kotaniemi, A, Savolainen, A, Kroger, H, Kautiainen, H, & Isomaki, H. Weight-bearing physical activity, calcium intake, systemic glucocorticoids. Chronic inflammation and body constitution as determinants of lumbar and femoral bone mineral density in juvenile chronic arthritis. Scandinavian Journal of Rheumatology, 28:19–26, 1999.

Kraemer, W, & Fleck, S. Strength Training for Young Athletes. Champaign, IL: Human Kinetics, 1993.

Lavigne, JV, Ross, CK, Barry, SL, Hayford, JR, & Pachman, LM. Evaluation of a psychological treatment package for treating pain in juvenile rheumatoid arthritis. Arthritis Care and Research, 5:101–110, 1992.

Lechner, DE, McCarthy, CF, & Holden, MK. Gait deviations in patients with juvenile rheumatoid arthritis. Physical Therapy, 67:1335–1341, 1987.

Len, C, Ferraz, M, Goldenberg, J, Oliveira, LM, Araujo, PP, Rodrigues, Q, Terreri, MT, & Hilario, MO. Pediatric Escola Paulista de Medicina range of motion scale: A reduced joint count score for general use in juvenile rheumatoid arthritis. Journal of Rheumatology, 26:909–913, 1999.

Libby, AK, Sherry, DD, & Dudgeon, BJ. Shoulder limitation in juvenile rheumatoid arthritis. Archives of Physical Medicine and Rehabilitation, 72:382–384, 1991.

Lindehammer, H, & Backman, E: Muscle function in juvenile chronic arthritis. Journal of Rheumatology, 22:1159–1165, 1995.

Lindehammer, H, & Sandstedt, P. Measurement of quadriceps muscle strength and bulk in juvenile chronic arthritis: A prospective, longitudinal 2-year survey. Journal of Rheumatology, 25:2240–2248, 1998.

Lineker, SC, Badley, EM, & Dalby, DM. Unmet service needs of children with rheumatic diseases and their parents in a metropolitan area. Journal of Rheumatology, 23:1054–1058, 1996.

Lovell, DJ, Giannini, EJ, Reiff, A, Cawkwell, GD, Silverman, ED, Nocton, JJ, Stein, LD, Gedalia, A, Ilowite, NT, Wallace, CA, Whitmore, J, & Finck, BK. Etanercept in children with polyarticular juvenile rheumatoid arthritis. Pediatric Rheumatology Collaborative Study Group. New England Journal of Medicine, 342:763–769, 2000.

Lovell, DJ, Athreya, B, Emery, HM, Gibbas, DL, Levinson, JE, Lindsley, CB, Spencer, CH, & White, PH. School attendance and patterns, special services, and special needs in pediatric patients with rheumatic disease. Arthritis Care and Research, 3:196–203, 1990.

Lovell, DJ, Howe, S, Shear, E, Hartner, S, McGirr, G, Schulte, M, & Levinson, J. Development of a disability measurement tool for juvenile rheumatoid arthritis: The Juvenile Arthritis Functional Assessment Scale. Arthritis and Rheumatism, 32:1390–1395, 1989.

Mathiowetz, V, Wiemer, DM, & Federman, SM. Grip and pinch strength norms for 6-19 year olds. American Journal of Occupational Therapy, 40:705–711, 1986.

Melvin, J, & Wright, FV. Procedure for serial casting of contractures from juvenile arthritis. In Melvin, J, & Wright, FV (Eds.). Rheumatologic Rehabilitation: Pediatric Rheumatic Diseases, Vol 3. Bethesda: American Occupational Therapy Association, 2000, pp. 295–297.

Mier, RJ, Wright, FV, & Bolding, DJ. Juvenile rheumatoid arthritis. In Melvin, J, & Wright, FV (Eds.). Rheumatologic Rehabilitation: Pediatric Rheumatic Diseases, Vol. 3. Bethesda: American Occupational Therapy Association, 2000, pp. 1–43.

Minor, M., & Westby, D. Rest and Exercise. In Robbins, L, Burckhardt, C, Hannan, M, & DeHoratius, R (Eds.). Clinical Care in the Rheumatic Diseases, 2nd ed. Atlanta: American College of Rheumatology, 2001, pp. 179–184.

Morrison, CD, Bundy, RC, & Fisher, AG. The contribution of motor skills and playfulness to the play performance of preschoolers. American Journal of Occupational Therapy, 45:687–694, 1991.

Murray, KJ, Moroldo, MB, Donnelly, P, Prahalad, S, Passo, MH, Giannini, EH, & Glass, DN. Age-specific effects of juvenile rheumatoid arthritis-associated HLA alleles. Arthritis and Rheumatism, 42:1843–1853, 1999.

Nestor, BJ, Figgie, MP, Wright, FV, & Melvin, J. Surgical treatment of juvenile rheumatoid arthritis. In Melvin, J, & Wright, FV (Eds.). Rheumatologic Rehabilitation: Pediatric Rheumatic Diseases, Vol. 3. Bethesda: American Occupational Therapy Association, 2000, pp. 249–266.

Oberg, T, Karsznia, B, Gare, A, & Lagerstrand, A. Physical training of children with juvenile chronic arthritis. Scandinavian Journal of Rheumatology, 23:92–95, 1994.

Petersen, LS, Mason, T, Nelson, AM, O'Fallon, WM, & Gabriel, SE. Juvenile rheumatoid arthritis in Rochester, Minnesota 1960–1993: Is the epidemiology changing? Arthritis and Rheumatism, 39:1385–1390, 1996.

Petersen, LS, Mason, T, Nelson, AM, O'Fallon, WM, & Gabriel, SE. Psychosocial outcomes and health status of adults who have had juvenile rheumatoid arthritis. Arthritis and Rheumatism, 40:2235–2290, 1997.

Reed, MH, & Wilmot, DM. The radiology of juvenile rheumatoid arthritis. A review of the English language literature. Journal of Rheumatology (Suppl) 31:2–22, 1991.

Rhodes, VJ. Physical therapy management of patients with juvenile rheumatoid arthritis. Physical Therapy, 71:910–919, 1991.

Ruperto, N, Ravelli, A, Migliavacca, D, Viola, S, Pistorio, A, & Duarte, C. Responsiveness of clinical measures in children with oligoarticular juvenile chronic arthritis. Journal of Rheumatology, 26:1827–1830, 1999.

Schanberg, LE, Sandstrom, MJ, Starr, K, Gil, KM, Lefebvre, JC, Keefe, FJ, Affleck, G, & Tennen, H. The relationship of daily mood and stressful events to symptoms in juvenile rheumatic disease. Arthritis Care and Research, 13:33–41, 2000.

Scull S, & Athreya, B. Childhood arthritis. In Goldberg B (Ed.). Sports and Exercise for Children with Chronic Health Conditions. Champaign: Human Kinetics, 1995, pp. 136–148.

Sherry, DD, Stein, LD, Reed, AM, Schanberg, LE, & Kredich, DW. Prevention of leg length discrepancy in young children with pauciarticular juvenile rheumatoid arthritis by treatment with intra-articular steroids. Arthritis and Rheumatism, 42:2330–2334, 1999.

Singh, G, Athreya, B, Fries, JF, & Goldsmith, DP. Measurement of health status in children with juvenile rheumatoid arthritis. Arthritis and Rheumatism, 37:1761–1769, 1994.

Smythe, HA, & Helewa, A: Assessment of joint disease. In Walker, JM, & Helewa, A (Eds.). Physical Therapy in Arthritis. Philadelphia: WB Saunders, 1996, pp. 129–148.

Spencer, CH, & Bernstein, BH. Hip disease in juvenile rheumatoid arthritis. Current Opinions in Rheumatology, 4:536–541, 2002.

Sullivan, DB, Cassidy, JT, & Petty, RE. Pathogenic implications of age of onset in juvenile rheumatoid arthritis. Arthritis and Rheumatism, 18:251–255, 1975.

Szer, IS, & Wright, FV: School integration. In Melvin, J, & Wright, FV (Eds.). Rheumatologic Rehabilitation: Pediatric Rheumatic Diseases, Vol. 3. Philadelphia: WB Saunders, 2000, pp. 223–230.

Takken, T, van der Net, J, & Helders, PJ. Relationship between functional ability and physical fitness in juvenile rheumatoid arthritis. Scandinavian Journal of Rheumatology, 32:174–178, 2003.

Takken, T, Hemel, A, van der Net, JJ, & Helders. PJ. Aerobic fitness in children with juvenile idiopathic arthritis: A systemic review. Journal of Rheumatology, 29:2643–2647, 2002.

Takken, T, van der Net, JJ, & Helders, PJ. Do juvenile idiopathic arthritis patients benefit from an exercise program? A pilot study. Arthritis Care and Research, 45:81–85, 2001.

Thompson, KL, & Varni, JW: A developmental cognitive-behavioral approach to pediatric pain assessment. Pain, 25:283–296, 1986.

Varni, JW, Waldron, SA, Gragg, RA, Rapoff, MA, Bernstein, BH, Lindsley, CB, & Newcomb, MD. Development of the Waldron/Varni pediatric pain coping inventory. Pain, 67:141–150, 1996.

Varni, J, Seid, M, Smith Knight, T, Burwinkle, T, Brown, J, & Szer, IS. The PedsQL in pediatric rheumatology: Reliability, validity, and responsiveness of the Pediatric Quality of Life Inventory generic core scales and rheumatology module. Arthritis and Rheumatism, 46:714–725, 2002.

Vostrejs, M, & Hollister, JR. Muscle atrophy and leg length discrepancies in pauciarticular juvenile rheumatoid arthritis. American Journal of Diseases of Childhood, 142:343-345, 1988.

Walco, GA, Varni, JW, & Ilowite, NT. Cognitive-behavioral pain management in children with juvenile rheumatoid arthritis. Pediatrics, 89:1075–1079, 1992.

Wallace, CA, & Levinson, JE. Juvenile rheumatoid arthritis: Outcome and treatment for the 1990's. In Athreya, B (Ed.). Rheumatic Disease Clinics of North America. Philadelphia: WB Saunders Co., 1991, pp. 891–905.

Wessel, J, Kaup, C, Fan, J, Ehalt R, Ellsworth, J, Speer C, Tenove, P, & Dombrosky, A. Isometric strength measurements in children with arthritis: Reliability and relation to function. Arthritis Care and Research, 12:238–246, 1999.

White, PH. Growth abnormalities in children with juvenile rheumatoid arthritis. Clinical Orthopedics and Related Research, *259*:46–50, 1990.

Wong, DL, & Baker, CM. Pain in children: comparison of assessment scales. Pediatric Nursing, *14*:9–17, 1998.

Wright, FV, Liu, G, & Milne, F. Reliability of the measurement of time-distance parameters of gait: A comparison in children with juvenile rheumatoid arthritis and children with cerebral palsy. Physiotherapy Canada, *51*:191–200, 1996.

Wright, FV, Longo Kimber, JL, Law, M, Goldsmith, CH, Crombie, V, & Dent, P. The Juvenile Arthritis Functional Status Index (JASI): A validation study. Journal of Rheumatology, *23*:1066–1079, 1996.

Wright, FV, & Smith, E. Physical therapy management of the child and adolescent with juvenile rheumatoid arthritis. In Walker, JM, & Helewa, A. (Eds.). Physical Therapy in Arthritis. Philadelphia: WB Saunders Co., 1996, pp. 211–244.

Wright, FV, Law, M, Crombie, V, Goldsmith, CH, & Dent, P. Development of a self-report functional status index for juvenile rheumatoid arthritis. Journal of Rheumatology, *21*:536–544, 1994.

APPENDIX I	Outcome Measurements in Juvenile Rheumatoid Arthritis

OUTCOME	LEVEL OF ICF	MEASUREMENT	REFERENCE
Disease Activity			
Active joint count	Impairment	ACR joint count	Guzman et al., 1995
Grip strength	Impairment	Modified sphygmomanometer or handheld dynamometer	Dunn, 1993
Morning stiffness	Impairment	Presence and duration of stiffness	Wright et al., 1996
Global ratings	Impairment	Physician rating on a VAS	Ruperto et al., 1999
Joint range of motion AAROM or PROM	Impairment	JC-LOM (ASS)	Klepper et al., 1992
		pEPM-ROM	Len et al., 1999
		GROMS / 10-joint GROMS	Epps et al., 2002
Muscle strength	Impairment	MMT	
		Modified sphygmomanometer	Dunn, 1993; Smythe & Helewa, 1996
		Handheld dynamometer	Wessel et al., 1999
		Isokinetic dynamometer	Giannini & Protas, 1993
Aerobic fitness	Impairment	Laboratory measures (VO$_{2peak}$)	Takken et al., 2002
		Standardized walk or run test	Klepper et al., 1992; Takken et al., 2001
	Impairment/activity	Physical activity monitoring	Henderson et al., 1995
Gait			
Characteristics of gait pattern	Impairment	Observation	
Time/distance parameters and kinetic parameters	Impairment	Footprint analysis	Wright et al., 1996
		Instrumented gait lab tests	Lechner et al., 1987
Gross and fine motor function	Activity	Developmental tests	Morrison et al., 1991
School function	Activity	School checklists	Szer & Wright, 2000
	Activity/participation	School function assessment	Coster et al., 1998
Pain behaviors	Activity	Observation	Jaworski et al., 1995
	Impairment	Child self-report	Beyer et al., 1992; Wong & Baker, 1988; Hester et al., 1990; Thompson & Varni, 1986
	Impairment/activity	Child self-report	Varni et al., 1996
Physical Function			
Parent/child report	Activity	CHAQ	Singh et al., 1994
		JAFAR	Howe et al., 1991
		JASI	Wright et al., 1992
Performance			
Quality of life	Activity	JAFAS	Lovell et al., 1989
Parent/child report	Impairment/activity	JAQQ	Duffy et al., 1997
	Participation	PedsQL	Varni et al., 2002
		QOML scale	

ICF, International Classification of Functioning, Disability, and Health; ACR, American College of Rheumatology; JC-LOM, (AS) Joint Count – Limitation of Motion, Articular Severity Score; pEPM-ROM, Paediatric Escola Paulista de Medicina-Range of Motion scale; GROMS, Global Range of Motion Scale; VO$_{2peak}$, peak oxygen uptake; VAS, visual analog scale; MMT, manual muscle test; CHAQ, Childhood Health Assessment Questionnaire; JAFAR, Juvenile Arthritis Functional Assessment Report; JASI, Juvenile Arthritis Functional Status Index; JAFAS, Juvenile Arthritis Functional Assessment Scale; JAQQ, Juvenile Arthritis Quality of Life Questionnaire; PedsQL, Pediatric Quality of Life Questionnaire; QOML, Quality of My Life.

APPENDIX II	Patterns of Joint and Soft Tissue Restrictions and Clinical Adaptations in Juvenile Rheumatoid Arthritis (JRA)*

CLINICAL MANIFESTATIONS	RESTRICTIONS/ADAPTATION
Cervical Spine	
In polyJRA and sJRA	Loss of EXT, rotation, side FLEX
Inflammation, narrowing, then fusion; observed first in C2-C3, but may progress to involve the entire cervical spine†	May develop torticollis if asymmetric Intubation for anesthesia†
Dysplasia of vertebral bodies	Eye movements or turning body compensate for ↓ neck ROM
Odontoid process instability (less common than in adult RA)	
Temporomandibular Joint	
Common in polyJRA; less common in pauciJRA; often associated with cervical spine disease	Restriction in opening mouth; pain on chewing; may need orthodontia
Mandibular asymmetry if unilateral involvement	Greater functional restrictions if cervical spine is involved and EXT is restricted
Undergrowth of the mandible (micrognathia); malocclusion of the teeth	
Shoulder Complex	
Most common in polyJRA†	Loss of active GL-H ABD and IR first limitations noted; limited FLEX, tightening of pectorals and scapular protractors; more dysfunction when elbow and wrist involved
Overgrowth of humeral head with irregular shape, shallow glenoid fossa	
Subluxation may occur	
Elbow	
Involved early in disease course†	EXT lost early; eventual limitation in FLEX and forearm rotation
Occurs in all types; symmetric in polyJRA and sJRA; asymmetric in pauciJRA†	Shoulder ROM initially compensates for ↓ supination; loss of > 45° EXT restricts ability to push-off from chair
Overgrowth of radial head restricts ROM	
Proximal radioulnar joint involved†	Wrist involvement accentuates loss of pronation and supination
Ulnar nerve entrapment possible	
Wrist	
All types; starts early; symmetric in polyJRA and sJRA; unilateral in pauciJRA†	Rapid loss of EXT; weakness of extensors; FLEX contracture and volar subluxation
Accelerated carpal maturation	Rests in flexion and ulnar deviation with spasm of wrist flexors
Undergrowth of ulna; ulnar shortening; may migrate dorsally	In older onset or RF+ polyJRA, tendency is toward radial deviation†
Radio- and intercarpal fusion	Distal radioulnar disease causes loss of pronation and supination
Flexor tenosynovitis; carpal tunnel syndrome is rare; may occur late in disease	
Hand	
Premature epiphyseal fusion and growth abnormalities	PIP (especially 4th) more common than DIP contractures
Flexor tenosynovitis may be dramatic	Loss of MCP FLEX (especially 2nd digit); loss of MCP hyperextension
	Marked decrease in grip strength
Involvement later in polyJRA and sJRA than in pauciJRA	Boutonniere < swan neck
MCP and CMP subluxation deformities	
Thoracolumbar Spine	
Unusual site in JRA	Kyphosis in association with neck and shoulder involvement
Steroid drug therapy may cause osteoporosis, wedging of vertebral bodies, small compression fractures	Lumbar lordosis 2° to hip flexion contractures; scoliosis 2° to lower limb asymmetries
	Pain with compression fractures†

(continued)

APPENDIX II Patterns of Joint and Soft Tissue Restrictions and Clinical Adaptations in Juvenile Rheumatoid Arthritis (JRA)*

CLINICAL MANIFESTATIONS	RESTRICTIONS/ADAPTATION
Hip	
Femoral head overgrowth	Flexion contractures, may be masked by lumbar lordosis
Osteoporosis	May present as pain in the groin, over buttocks, medial thigh, around knee[†]
Trochanteric growth changes	IR and ABD lost early 2° to pain and spasm of FLEXs and ADDs
Shallow acetabulum, ↓ femoral-neck angle, especially if weight bearing limited	
Lateral subluxation of femoral head aggravated by tight adductors	May have marked pain in standing
Potential for protrusio acetabuli, avascular necrosis	Gluteus medius weakness may cause Trendelenburg gait deviation[†]
Primary cause of ↓ ROM and dysfunction	Secondary deformities of the contralateral hip, knees, and lumbar spine
Occurs in polyJRA and sJRA after a few years	
Potential for regeneration of articular cartilage with fibrocartilage if remission of synovitis[†]	Mobility and weight bearing improve cartilage repair[†]
Knee	
Most common joint involved early in all types	Rapid development of flexion contracture
Overgrowth of distal femur may cause leg length discrepancy in unilateral disease	Rapid atrophy of quadriceps; loss of patellar mobility due to adhesions
Knee valgus aggravated by tight hamstrings and iliotibial band	Risk of femoral fracture associated with falling due to flexion and osteoporosis
Posterior tibial subluxation 2° to prolonged joint involvement or excessive correction of knee flexion contracture	Loss of flexion (often only to 90°) Secondary hip flexion contracture
Ankle/Foot	
Altered growth causes bony changes in tarsals with potential fusion	Early loss of inversion, eversion
Hindfoot valgus / varus due to ankle joint arthritis or 2° to knee valgus	Later loss of D-FL and PL- FL especially if ambulation is limited
MTP subluxation	Altered gait, loss of MTP hyperextension affects toe-off
Hallux valgus	Overlapping of IPs, especially with hallux valgus
IPs-growth changes due to premature epiphyseal closure	

* Data in this table are summarized from information published in Ansell 1992; Atwood 1989; Cassidy & Petty, 1990; Emery 1993; Libby et al., 1991; Reed & Wilmot, 1991; Rhodes, 1991; White, 1990; Cassidy, JT, & Petty, RE. Juvenile rheumatoid arthritis. In Cassidy, JT, & Petty, RE (Eds.). Textbook of Pediatric Rheumatology, 4th ed. Philadelphia: W.B. Saunders Co., 2001.

† The listing is not inclusive, but the features described are characteristic of juvenile arthritis.

ABD, abduction/abductors; ADD, adduction/adductors; CMP, carpometacarpal-phalangeal; D-FL, dorsiflexion; DIP, distal interphalangeal; EXT, extension; FLEX, flexion, flexors; GL-H, glenohumeral; IP, interphalangeal; IR, internal rotation; MCP, metacarpophalangeal; MTP, metatarsophalangeal; pauciJRA, pauciarticular JRA; polyJRA, polyarticular JRA; PL-FL, plantar flexion; ROM, range of motion; sJRA, systemic JRA. Adapted from Wright, FV, & Smith, E. Physical therapy management of the child and adolescent with juvenile rheumatoid arthritis. In Walker, JM, & Helewa, A. (Eds.). Physical Therapy in Arthritis. Philadelphia: W.B. Saunders Co., 1996, pp. 215, Table 12-6.

APPENDIX III   Interventions for Juvenile Rheumatoid Arthritis

Coordination, Communication, and Documentation
Anticipated goals
- Care is coordinated with child, family, school, and other professionals.
- Insurance payer understands needed rehabilitation services.
- Need for modifications in school is determined.
- Available resources are maximally utilized.
- Decision making is enhanced regarding child's health, wellness, and fitness needs.

Specific interventions
- Communication with community therapist, school personnel, and community resource providers
- Prescriptions and letters of medical necessity to support rehabilitation needs
- Individualized education plan (IEP); accommodations under Section 504 of Rehabilitation Act

Patient-Related Instruction
Anticipated goals
- Awareness and use of community resources are increased.
- Behaviors that protect joints from secondary impairments are enhanced.
- Functional independence in activities of daily living (ADL) is increased.
- Patient and family knowledge of the diagnosis, prognosis, interventions, and goals and outcomes is increased.

Specific interventions
- Home exercise program
- Instruction regarding joint protection principles
- Information from the Arthritis Foundation regarding disease
- Referrals to other community resources

Therapeutic Exercise
Anticipated goals
- Ability to perform physical tasks related to self-care, home management, community and school integration, and leisure activities is increased.
- Aerobic capacity is increased.
- Gait is improved.
- Joint and soft tissue swelling, inflammation, or restriction is reduced.
- Joint integrity and mobility are improved.
- Pain is decreased.
- Postural control is improved.
- Strength, power, and endurance are improved.

Specific interventions
- Aerobic conditioning
  - Aquatic exercise
  - Low impact weight-bearing exercise
- Gait and locomotor training
- Body mechanics training
- Postural training
- Strengthening, power, and endurance training
  - Active assistive, active, and resistive exercise
  - Task specific performance training

(continued)

APPENDIX III Interventions for Juvenile Rheumatoid Arthritis

- Flexibility exercise
  - Muscle lengthening
  - Range of motion
  - Gentle stretching/static progressive stretching
- Balance, coordination, and agility training

Functional Training in Self-Care and Home Management
Anticipated goals
- Ability to perform physical tasks related to self-care and home management is increased.
- Level of supervision required for task performance is decreased.
- Risk of secondary impairments is reduced

Specific interventions
- ADL training
- Assistive and adaptive device or equipment training
- Self-care or home management task adaptation
- Leisure and play recommendations
- Orthotic, protective, or supportive device or equipment training
- Injury prevention training

Functional Training in School, Play, Community, and Leisure Integration
Anticipated goals
- School attendance is improved
- Participation in peer groups for recreation and leisure activity is improved
- Architectural barriers to access home, school, and community resources are removed

Specific interventions
- Appropriate transportation plan to school identified on IEP
- Modifications to school instruction identified on IEP
- ADL training
- Assistive and adaptive device or equipment training
- Adaptation of equipment to allow inclusion in recreation and leisure activity
- Home and school site visit to plan for accommodation of any architectural barriers

Manual Therapy Techniques (Including Mobilization and Manipulation)
Anticipated goals
- Ability to perform motor skills is improved
- Joint integrity and mobility are improved

Specific interventions
- Connective tissue massage
- Passive range of motion
- Therapeutic massage

Prescription, Application, and Fabrication of Devices and Equipment
Anticipated goals
- Ability to perform physical tasks is increased
- Deformities are prevented
- Gait and locomotion are improved
- Joint stability is increased
- Optimal joint alignment is achieved
- Pain is decreased
- Protection of body parts is increased

(continued)

APPENDIX III   Interventions for Juvenile Rheumatoid Arthritis

Specific interventions
- Adaptive devices or equipment
- Assistive devices or equipment (ambulation aids, wheelchairs, ADL equipment)
- Splints and orthotic devices (shoe inserts, resting splints, dynamic splints, braces)
- Protective devices (splints, taping, elbow or knee pads)
- Supportive devices (compression garments, cervical collars)

Electrotherapeutic Modalities
Anticipated goals
- Muscle performance is increased
- Pain is decreased

Specific interventions
- Biofeedback

Physical Agents and Mechanical Modalities
Anticipated goals
- Pain is decreased
- Soft tissue swelling, inflammation, or restriction is reduced
- Tolerance to positions and activities is increased
- Joint integrity and mobility are improved

Specific interventions
- Cryotherapy (RICE—rest, ice, compression, elevation)
- Hydrotherapy (aquatic therapy, whirlpool tanks)
- Superficial thermal modalities (heat, paraffin baths, hot packs, fluidotherapy)
- Continuous passive motion devices

Modified from Scull, S. Juvenile rheumatoid arthritis. In Campbell, S, Vander Linden, D, & Palisano R (Eds.). Physical Therapy for Children, 2nd ed. Philadelphia: W.B. Saunders Co., 2000, p. 245.

Chapter 10

HEMOPHILIA

SANDRA M. MCGEE
PT, PCS

CLASSIFICATION

HEMOPHILIC ARTHROPATHY
Pathophysiology
Medical Management
Prognosis

FUNCTIONING AND DISABILITIES
Musculoskeletal Structure and Function
Activity Limitations
Participation and Disability

THE ROLE OF PHYSICAL THERAPY
Examination
Evaluation
Intervention

CASE STUDY

Hemophilia is the term used to collectively identify several X-linked disorders of blood coagulation. The most common of these disorders are factor VIII deficiency, or hemophilia A, found in 80% to 90% of the population with hemophilia, and factor IX deficiency, or hemophilia B. Hemophilia is present in approximately 1 in 10,000 males, and 60% to 65% of the patients will have a positive family history (Karayalcin, 1985).

Joint arthropathy from repeated hemarthroses is the most disabling consequence of the disorders. Recent advances in recombinant factor production and increased availability of factor replacement products in developed countries have resulted in more patients being treated prophylactically. This trend has greatly improved the quality of life of these patients and their families by reducing the incidence of joint hemorrhages and arthropathy. Unfortunately, easy access to factor replacement is not universally available and joint arthropathy continues to be the major cause of disability for thousands of people with hemophilia.

In this chapter the pathophysiology of hemarthrosis, medical management, primary impairments, activity limitations, and the role of physical therapy in examination and intervention are addressed. The case study presented at the conclusion of the chapter illustrates the physical therapy management (based on the American Physical Therapy Association's "Guide to Physical Therapist Practice") of one patient with hemophilia.

CLASSIFICATION

The severity of the disorder is determined by the amount of factor activity in the blood (Table 10-1). Over 60% of males with hemophilia A and 50% with hemophilia B have the severe form of the disorder. These patients are subject to recurrent hemorrhages that may occur spontaneously or as a result of minor trauma. Infants and toddlers may develop subcutaneous ecchymoses over bony prominences or large hematomas after intramuscular injections for vaccination against childhood diseases. By 3 to 4 years of age, bleeding into muscles and joints begins to present problems because of increased activity level, and it continues to be a major problem throughout childhood and adolescence.

In the moderate form of hemophilia A or B the patient may have spontaneous hemorrhages, but more frequently bleeding occurs as a result of trauma. The child with the mild form, however, will bleed only after severe trauma, and consequently hemophilia may not even be diagnosed in infancy or childhood (Buchanan, 1980).

Hemorrhages may occur anywhere in the body but most often are in the joint cavities. Muscles are the second most common site of bleeding, particularly in the iliopsoas, gastrocnemius, and forearm flexor muscle compartment. Hemorrhages within muscles can be dangerous owing to the risk of nerve compression from the hematoma. Patients with hemophilia may also be susceptible to

TABLE 10-1	**Relation of Factor Levels to Severity of Clinical Manifestations of Hemophilia A and B**	

TYPE	FACTOR LEVELS (VIII/IX) (PERCENT OF NORMAL)	TYPES OF HEMORRHAGE
Severe	<1	Spontaneous; hemarthroses and deep tissue hemorrhages
Moderate	1–5	Gross bleeding following mild to moderate trauma; some hemarthrosis; seldom spontaneous hemorrhage
Mild	5–25	Severe hemorrhage following moderate to severe trauma or surgery
High-risk carrier females	30–50	Gynecologic and obstetric hemorrhages

hematuria, mucous membrane hemorrhages, and central nervous system hemorrhages. Fortunately, central nervous system hemorrhages are uncommon, developing in approximately 3% of the hemophilic population, but they are the major cause of death from these bleeding disorders (Buchanan, 1980).

HEMOPHILIC ARTHROPATHY

PATHOPHYSIOLOGY

Hemarthrosis is the most clinically significant problem in hemophilia. It affects the hinge joints (knees, elbows, and ankles) most frequently because these joints have less muscular padding and a decreased ability to withstand lateral and rotary forces. When bleeding occurs into a joint, the joint becomes swollen, warm, and painful, and range of motion (ROM) is restricted (Corrigan, 1990). A single or infrequent bleeding episode will usually resolve without complication as the blood is resorbed. Recurrent hemarthroses, however, can lead to chronic synovitis and degenerative arthropathy. Although the mechanisms of recurrent bleeding leading to degenerative arthropathy are not completely understood, Joist and Ameri (1990) have outlined a reasonable hypothesis (Fig. 10-1). Recurrent hemarthroses cause synovial hypertrophy with formation of villi, as well as pannus formation on the joint cartilage. The hypertrophic, hyperemic synovium is more susceptible to mechanical trauma, leading to further bleeding. In addition, capsular stretching and muscle atrophy from immobilization and disuse increase joint instability, creating a vicious cycle that is difficult to break. The chronic synovitis and chemical reactions related to the

breakdown of the blood in the joint eventually lead to cartilage damage, bone erosion, and bone remodeling.

Arnold and Hilgartner (1977) classified hemophilic arthropathy into five stages based on roentgenographic findings (Fig. 10-2). In stage 1, no bony abnormalities are seen but soft tissue swelling is present. Stage 2 is characterized by osteoporosis and overgrowth of the epiphyses, but the joint integrity is maintained. In stage 3, subchondral cysts are visible, squaring of the patella is evident when the knee is involved, and the intercondylar notch of the knee and the trochlear notch of the elbow are widened. The articular cartilage, however, is still intact. By stage 4, the joint space has narrowed and there is damage to the cartilage. In stage 5, there is fibrous joint contracture, loss of joint space, extensive enlargement of the epiphyses, and total destruction of the articular cartilage.

All children with moderate or severe hemophilia are at risk for hemarthroses. The aim of intervention is to slow down or halt the progression of joint destruction.

MEDICAL MANAGEMENT

The primary treatment for hemophilia is replacement of the deficient factor. The goal of factor replacement is either to stop bleeding episodes that have already started (known as on-demand treatment) or to decrease or prevent bleeding episodes altogether (known as prophylactic treatment.)

In on-demand treatment, bleeding episodes are managed by intravenous factor replacement, extracted from normal plasma or manufactured from recombinant DNA. Factor replacement should occur as soon as the patient feels stiffness or discomfort in a joint. These "prodromal" sensations are believed to occur when bleeding is confined

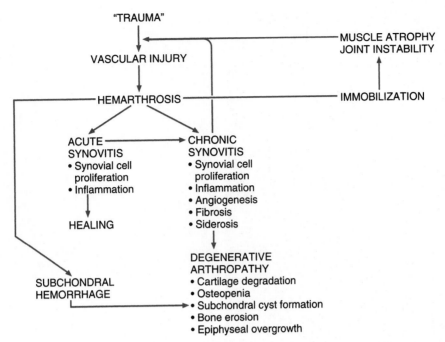

"TRAUMA"

VASCULAR INJURY

HEMARTHROSIS

MUSCLE ATROPHY
JOINT INSTABILITY

IMMOBILIZATION

ACUTE
SYNOVITIS
• Synovial cell
  proliferation
• Inflammation

HEALING

CHRONIC
SYNOVITIS
• Synovial cell
  proliferation
• Inflammation
• Angiogenesis
• Fibrosis
• Siderosis

DEGENERATIVE
ARTHROPATHY
• Cartilage degradation
• Osteopenia
• Subchondral cyst formation
• Bone erosion
• Epiphyseal overgrowth

SUBCHONDRAL
HEMORRHAGE

◆ **Figure 10-1**   Joist and Ameri's concept of the pathogenesis of hemophilic arthropathy. *(Redrawn from Joist, JH, & Ameri, A. Pathogenesis of hemophilic arthropathy. In Gilbert, MS, & Greene, WB [Eds.]. Musculoskeletal Problems in Hemophilia. New York: National Hemophilia Foundation, 1990, pp. 20–25.)*

to the synovium only and can precede objective signs of bleeding by 4 to 6 hours (Gilbert, 2000). In an effort to control the bleeding as quickly as possible, many families are taught to perform infusions at home. Factor replacement may also be given before vigorous exercise, such as participation in intramural sports or intensive physical therapy. Prophylactic treatment provides for replacement factor to be given on a regular basis, usually two or three times per week, depending on the factor (IX or VIII, respectively) being replaced. Prophylactic regimens are defined as primary when the prophylaxis is started before any joint bleeding episodes occur or secondary when prophylaxis is begun after a specific number of joint bleeds have occurred, usually no more than three. In 1994, the World Health Organization and the World Federation of Hemophilia jointly issued a statement recommending prophylaxis as the treatment of choice for children with severe hemophilia and many developed countries have adopted that recommendation (Mannucci et al., 2001).

In addition to factor replacement, hemarthroses are treated with rest, through immobilization and avoidance of weight bearing, until bleeding has resolved. Aspiration of the blood from the joints as a treatment modality has been reported in the literature after 1 to 2 decades of disuse (Corrigan, 1990; Gilbert, 2000).

Orthopedic surgery may be indicated in patients with chronic synovitis or severe joint destruction. Synovectomy, both open and by arthroscopy, is frequently performed on knees and elbows in an effort to reduce bleeding episodes when chronic synovitis has not responded to 3 to 6 months of conservative treatment (Gilbert, 2000). Radiosynoviorthesis by intra-articular injection of radioisotopes is also being performed to ablate the synovium and is a good alternative for children with high-titer inhibitors (Manco-Johnson et al., 2002). Arthrodeses, osteotomies, and arthroplasties have been used when severe joint destruction causes intractable pain and disability.

PROGNOSIS

Despite more aggressive and earlier home treatment of hemarthroses, severe joint arthropathy remains the major disabling consequence of hemophilia. Although the incidence of joint hemorrhages declines in late adolescence and early adulthood, joint destruction has already occurred in a large percentage of patients with severe hemophilia (Joist & Ameri, 1990).

The use of prophylaxis is changing this picture in developed countries. In Sweden and the Netherlands, boys with severe hemophilia have been treated with pro-

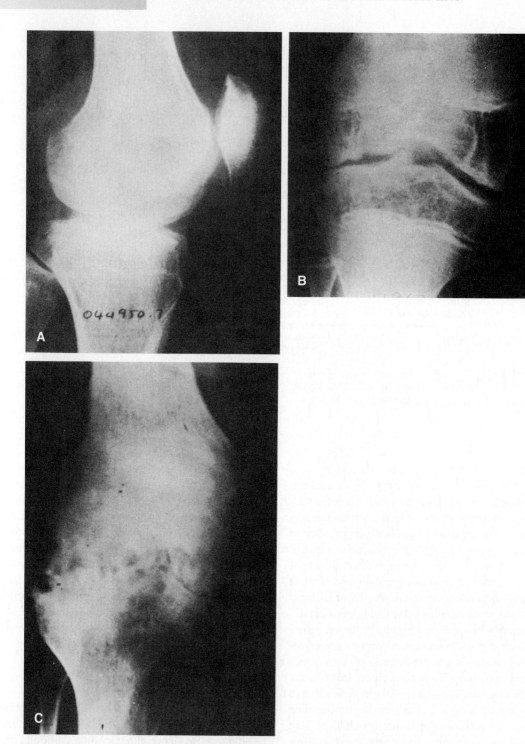

⬥ **Figure 10-2** Hemophilic arthropathy. In stage 1, soft tissue swelling occurs without bony changes. Stage 2 consists of early osteoporosis and epiphyseal overgrowth. **A** to **C** illustrate stages 3 to 5. **A**, Stage 3: Joint disorganization, with patellar squaring and subchondral cysts but intact articular cartilage. **B**, Stage 4: Narrowing of joint space and damage to cartilage. **C**, Stage 5: Loss of joint space, fibrous joint contracture, and total destruction of cartilage. *(From Arnold, WD, & Hilgartner, MW. Hemophilic arthropathy. Journal of Bone and Joint Surgery [American], 59:288–305, 1977.)*

phylaxis for more than 35 years and their experience has shown that hemophilic arthropathy can be prevented when prophylaxis is started before joint damage has occurred. Other European and North American countries have also published studies demonstrating reduced or eliminated joint bleeding episodes with prophylaxis (Van der Berg & Fischer, 2003). Unfortunately, factor supplies are not universally available and approximately 80% of the people with hemophilia worldwide have no replacement therapy available (Aledort, 2003). The practice of primary prophylaxis is a controversial issue. Some of the arguments against its use include continued concern over exposure to viruses in blood products, long-term cost-benefit ratio, and the difficulty in obtaining regular venous access in young patients (Liesner et al., 1996). There is also a lack of randomized, controlled trials comparing prophylaxis to aggressive on-demand treatment. One prospective study currently being conducted in the United States is measuring medical and orthopedic factors, as well as the costs, both financial and psychosocial, of both types of treatment (Aledort, 2003).

In addition, between 10% and 15% of patients with hemophilia A develop antibodies (inhibitors) that are directed against the activity of factor VIII. Hemostasis is more difficult to achieve in patients with inhibitors. Immune tolerance therapy that provides daily exposure to factor concentrate may eliminate the inhibitor over time (Shopnick & Brettler, 1996).

Over the past 2 decades, the hemophilic community has been devastated by the viral transmissions of HIV and hepatitis through blood products. From 80% to 90% of all persons with severe hemophilia A and 55% of those with severe hemophilia B who received factor replacement between 1979 and 1984 test positive for human immunodeficiency virus (HIV) (Hilgartner, 1991). Both the advent of a hepatitis B vaccine and the screening, heating, and pasteurization of blood products have diminished the incidence of hepatitis B, hepatitis C, and HIV infection as consequences of factor replacement therapy. No documented cases of HIV seroconversion in patients with hemophilia have been reported since 1985 (Corrigan, 1990). To further reduce the risks from factor replacement, factor VIII and factor IX concentrates have been made in culture by recombinant DNA techniques since the 1990s. Newly developed plasma/albumin-free recombinant factors should further reduce the risk of viral transmission.

Recent gene transfer trials have suggested that genetic correction of hemophilia is an attainable goal. Ongoing clinical trials are investigating a number of different viral vectors or ex vivo transfected skin fibroblasts for long-term factor production (Walsh, 2003).

FUNCTIONING AND DISABILITIES

MUSCULOSKELETAL STRUCTURE AND FUNCTION

Atkins and colleagues (1987) reported that the prevalence of joint contracture in patients with the severe form of hemophilia is between 50% and 95%. These contractures are the result of recurrent hemarthroses and intramuscular bleeding episodes and most frequently involve knee and elbow flexion and ankle plantar flexion. Although recurrent intramuscular hemorrhages are rare, a single large hematoma can cause permanent joint contracture because the large volume of blood will cause localized necrosis; as the blood is reabsorbed the dead muscle fibers are replaced by fibrous tissue in a shortened position. This occurs in about 10% of all muscle hemorrhages and is most common in the plantar flexor and forearm muscles.

Contractures secondary to recurrent hemarthroses are related to a number of factors. Acute bleeding episodes are painful, and the patient is placed in a splint in the position of comfort, which at the knee and elbow is typically in flexion. Multiple hemorrhages, with frequent immobilization, can result in muscle shortening around a joint. As hemarthroses recur, with synovial hypertrophy and eventual articular cartilage destruction, bony changes, such as genu valgus, posterior subluxation of the tibia, and osteophytes, may occur. These changes may restrict ROM in a more permanent manner.

Muscle weakness is usually found around affected joints. In a study by Pietri and associates (1992), 10 patients (from 8 to 23 years of age) with unilateral knee involvement were strength tested on a Cybex 340 (Cybex, Division of Lumex, Ronkonkoma, NY) for knee strength as measured by peak torque, total work, and average power output. The average number of knee hemarthroses per patient was seven, and minimal or no radiographic changes were seen in any patient. Peak torque at 60°/s, total work, and average power were all significantly lower in the involved knee. The decreased muscle function was attributed to immobilization resulting in muscle atrophy, as well as reflex inhibition of the alpha motoneuron pool of the quadriceps muscle and facilitation of the hamstrings from slowly adapting capsular receptors sensitive to pressure and distention.

Strickler and Greene (1984) studied isokinetic torque levels in the quadriceps and hamstring muscles of males with hemophilia, ages 7 through adult. All their subjects demonstrated knee flexor and extensor strength deficits when compared with age-matched healthy subjects.

Additionally, they found that as the degree of arthropathy and flexion deformities increased, muscle strength decreased, with a relatively greater decrease in extensor torque, resulting in a higher than normal flexor-extensor ratio. Normally, knee flexors are approximately 60% as strong as extensors. In the patients with hemophilia, flexor strength averaged 70% of extensors in those with no arthropathy and was greater than extensor strength in adolescents and adults with stage 4 arthropathy.

Hilberg and colleagues (2001) demonstrated that proprioception is impaired in persons with hemophilia. Static proprioceptive performance, as measured by single limb stance on hard or soft ground, with eyes open or closed, was significantly decreased in patients with severe hemophilia as compared to anthropomorphically matched healthy subjects. Angle reproduction was also impaired in persons with hemophilia at 20° and 100° of knee flexion.

Peripheral nerve lesions are a potential consequence of large intramuscular hemorrhages, owing to compression on the nerve from the rapidly expanding hemorrhage. The highest incidence of lesions is to the femoral nerve after iliacus muscle hemorrhages. Fortunately, in the majority of cases, nerve function returns to normal within a few weeks or months, but the affected limb must be protected until full function returns (Houghton & Duthie, 1979).

Postural deviations may also be seen in the child with hemophilia. Leg length discrepancies can occur with epiphyseal overgrowth from hyperemia. Mechanical, or apparent, discrepancy can occur from a pelvic obliquity caused by psoas shortening after one or more hemorrhages. Whether real or apparent, this discrepancy may result in a postural scoliosis (Fernandez-Palazzi et al., 1990).

Hemarthroses, intramuscular hemorrhages, and hemophilic arthropathy are all sources of pain. The pain of an acute hemorrhage is usually relieved shortly after hemostasis is achieved by factor replacement. The chronic pain associated with a severely damaged joint is much more difficult to alleviate. Analgesics that contain aspirin or antihistamines must be avoided because they inhibit platelet function necessary for clotting. Narcotics may be necessary for severe, chronic pain but must be prescribed cautiously. Drug abuse among adolescents and adult males with hemophilia is a recognized problem, with one study finding that 21% of older patients with severe hemophilia abused drugs, including alcohol and prescribed painkillers, as well as illegal drugs (Jonas, 1989). Transcutaneous electrical nerve stimulation, biofeedback, relaxation, and guided imagery may be used for pain relief. Orthopedic surgery may be necessary to reduce unremitting pain by fusing a painful joint or replacing it (Corrigan, 1990).

ACTIVITY LIMITATIONS

The activity limitations for the child with hemophilia are dependent on the number of joints involved and the severity of the joint arthropathy. Gait deviations are seen most often and result from frequent immobilizations with subsequent weakness, joint changes, muscle shortening, and pain. Even mild gait deviations can create additional stress on joints and contribute to perpetuating the cycle of vulnerability to stress, recurrent hemarthrosis, synovitis, and further joint destruction. Weight bearing on a flexed knee not only increases the stress on the tibiofemoral and patellofemoral surfaces but also increases the quadriceps force required to maintain available extension against gravity. Despite the greater force required, Strickler and Greene (1984) found that subjects with arthropathy and knee flexion contractures demonstrated significantly reduced knee extension torque values.

Wheelchairs are usually not needed for children with hemophilia, except when acute hemorrhages in more than one joint prohibit the use of assistive devices for ambulation. As the child progresses to adulthood, more orthoses or ambulation aids may be used; but even in the adult population, less than 4% of persons with severe hemophilia need wheelchairs for mobility (Globe, 2002).

Activities of daily living such as dressing, grooming, and hygiene may be problematic for the child with frequent elbow hemorrhages and decreased elbow extension and forearm pronation and supination. Carrying schoolbooks may stress the elbow joints and lead to bleeding. Although there are no functional assessment scales specific to the hemophilia population, evaluation using the Functional Independence Measure (FIM) or WeeFIM (for children younger than age 7) will provide a numerical score and an objective way to measure functional progress (State University of New York, 1991).

Cardiopulmonary endurance is frequently impaired in children with hemophilia. Koch and colleagues (1984) evaluated response to exercise in 11 boys with factor VIII deficiency, ranging in age from 8 to 15.5 years, according to a uniform bicycle protocol and compared their performances with data available for healthy children. All the boys had previously been encouraged to participate in the physical education program at school, as well as after-school activities. Although none of the patients had acute bleeding problems, pain, significant weakness, or orthopedic deformities, several had previously sustained lower extremity hemorrhages. Their performance on bicycle ergometry demonstrated that peak heart rate, minutes of exercise, physical working capacity (maximum workload per weight in kilograms), and mean power were all significantly lower than for a population of healthy children whose physical activities did not exceed age-appropriate recreation. The clinical implication stated by the authors was that physical education alone does not provide aerobic conditioning, so it is imperative to supplement physical education with an individualized exercise program for fitness. More recently, Falk and colleagues (2000) evaluated muscle strength and anaerobic power in boys between 8 and 18 years old with severe factor VIII deficiency. Leisure-time physical activities were also assessed by questionnaire. The boys with hemophilia had lower anaerobic power and dynamic strength than age-matched healthy peers. They also had a higher percentage of body fat and a significantly reduced level of reported physical activity than healthy peers.

The physical therapist may be involved in counseling the child and family about appropriate recreational activities to maintain cardiopulmonary and muscular fitness. Before beginning participation in any sport, a child should be evaluated for joint motion, muscle strength, flexibility, and ligament stability, with particular attention paid to those joints that are likely to be stressed by the chosen sport. Any deficiencies should be eliminated before participation in the sport begins. In addition, a sport-specific conditioning program should be implemented and appropriate protective wear discussed. See Chapter 18 on sports injuries for additional relevant information.

Participation in certain sports is contraindicated owing to the danger of traumatic hemorrhages. The National Hemophilia Foundation, in association with the American Red Cross, published a booklet in 1996 entitled *Hemophilia, Sports, and Exercise*. In this booklet, sports activities are divided into three categories: (1) recommended sports with minimal risks, such as swimming and cycling; (2) sports in which the physical, social, and psychological benefits usually outweigh the risks; and (3) sports in which the risks outweigh the benefits. Contact sports, such as boxing, football, hockey, racquetball, and rugby, are in the highest risk category and are not recommended for patients with hemophilia. Participation in most other sports can be considered, but the decision to participate should be made jointly by the child, his parents, and the members of a comprehensive hemophilia clinic team.

▌PARTICIPATION AND DISABILITY

For the child with hemophilia, the degree and type of participation restrictions are similar to those of the child with juvenile rheumatoid arthritis and are dependent on the age of the child, on the severity of the disease, ability to adhere to the prescribed treatment program, and often on the emotional support provided by the family.

The child with moderate or severe hemophilia is usually diagnosed shortly after birth or within the first few months of life. Parents are counseled to watch for signs of hemorrhages and to treat all head injuries as potentially life-threatening. As the child begins to pull to stand, a lightweight protective helmet is usually prescribed, and parents may be advised to use knee and elbow pads to protect the joints of children who are learning how to walk. Understandably, parents may become overprotective and discourage peer group activities and playground play, such as swinging and sliding, which helps develop balance and coordination.

For the young child who is on primary prophylaxis, a venous access device such as a Portocath, may be necessary for the frequent infusions. Although these devices make access much easier, they have adverse effects such as infection or thrombosis (Aledort, 2003).

The child with severe hemophilia will begin to have more frequent joint and muscle hemorrhages by 3 years of age, as his activity level increases and he becomes physically able to run and jump, which may increase the incidence of direct trauma. Pain and frequent visits to the emergency department for factor replacement therapy may become the norm for many of these children and their families. Varied responses to their pain may cause differing disabilities. Some children may use their pain to maintain dependency on their parents by refusing to participate in normal activities of daily living (ADL). Other children may deny their pain because they know it means they will receive an intravenous injection and be immobilized. The young child may not understand that prompt treatment will relieve the pain and limit the need for more infusions (Holdredge & Cotta, 1989).

The school-age child with frequent hemorrhages may have poor school attendance because of time spent in emergency departments and the need to immobilize the joint. With the advent of home replacement therapy, time lost from school has become less of a problem, although special arrangements may need to be made for transporting the child on crutches. In one investigation of academic achievement in school-aged children with severe factor VIII deficiency, Shapiro and colleagues (2001) found that children who had been on long-term prophylaxis and had less than 12 bleeding episodes a year had significantly higher scores on math, reading, and total achievement than children who had 12 or more bleeding episodes a year, regardless of the type of treatment received.

Participation in organized sports is an important aspect of the school-age child's and adolescent's social life that may not be available for the child with hemophilia. Certain sports are absolutely contraindicated, and participation in other sports must be carefully evaluated by the entire medical team and family. In a Dutch study investigating motor performance and disability in school-aged boys with hemophilia, 79% of the boys reported that their disease had an impact on their lives, especially related to sports activities (Schoenmakers et al., 2001).

By late adolescence, many young men with severe hemophilia may have at least one arthropathic joint that causes chronic pain and stiffness, which may be disabling, though no data exist to quantify the level of disability related to pain. The Musculoskeletal Committee of the World Federation of Hemophilia developed a scale for evaluating chronic pain using a 0 to 3 rating:

0 No pain; no functional deficit; no analgesic use needed (except for acute hemorrhage)

1 Mild pain; does not interfere with occupation or with ADL; may require occasional relief by a non-narcotic analgesic

2 Moderate pain; causes partial or occasional interference with occupation or ADL; may require occasional narcotics for relief

3 Severe pain; interferes with performing occupation or carrying out ADL; requires frequent use of non-narcotic or narcotic medication for relief (Holdredge & Cotta, 1989)

Published data on the degree of disability resulting from the musculoskeletal complications of hemophilia is limited, especially in children. Weissman (1977) reported on a study conducted by Ahlberg in 1966 on 250 boys and men with hemophilia. On a scale of 0 to 3, with 0 representing no disability and 3 representing severe arthropathy and wheelchair-dependent mobility, 50% scored 0 and less than 10% scored 3. As factor replacement products have become more available, the clinical impression is that the degree of disability has diminished. In a retrospective study by Globe and colleagues (2002), the health status of more than 300 patients treated at several hemophilia treatment centers (HTC) was assessed using two health-status scales. Using the Self-Care Measure, a 4-point single-item scale measuring a patient's ability to perform basic self-care, 88% of patients were independent in all self-care and only 1.2% were completely dependent on others for care.

The second scale, designed specifically for the study, is the Hemophilia Utilization Group Study (HUGS) Functional Status Measure, which uses a 4-item and 10-point scale to assess social interaction, overall well-being, work/school/usual activity status, and orthopedic status. For the 300 patients studied, the mean score for all items was 9.3 for children and 8.7 for adults (Globe et al., 2002).

THE ROLE OF PHYSICAL THERAPY

Physical therapy for the child with hemophilia is aimed at maintaining strength and ROM in all joints and at preventing or diminishing disability. The majority of this therapy will occur in a clinic or outpatient setting with adjunctive home exercise programs. Unless the child has neurologic involvement from a central nervous system hemorrhage, his limitations rarely affect his educational abilities, so school physical therapy is typically not indicated.

Kasper and Dietrich (1985) recommended that a daily exercise program be followed from early childhood and encouraged with as much enthusiasm as other medical care. Clinical observations would suggest that strong muscles help support joints and decrease the frequency of hemorrhages, and several studies have demonstrated that participation in strengthening programs resulted in reduced bleeding episodes (Greene & Strickler, 1983; Koch et al., 1984; Timmermans, 1990, Tiktinsky et al., 2002). The specific type of strengthening program appears to be less important than daily participation. In the studies cited here, a total of 69 patients participated in a wide variety of daily exercise programs for a period of 6 months to 11 years. In all these studies, strength improved in all patients, and bleeding frequency decreased in all but two patients in Timmerman's study.

EXAMINATION

Examination of the child with hemophilia should include gathering historical information about the location and frequency of bleeding episodes and the patient's normal activities. This information is essential in identifying the causative factors of hemorrhage and in designing a program to reduce the frequency and severity of hemorrhages. Objective data should include goniometric measurements of active and passive ROM and joint deformities, such as genu valgus. Valgus and varus stress tests and examination of calcaneal and subtalar mobility should be performed to determine ligamentous integrity. The Orthopedic Advisory Committee of the World Federation of Hemophilia has recommended using a physical joint examination scale that has been the gold standard worldwide for the past 20 years for evaluation of joint arthropathy. This scale assigns a score from 0 to 12 points for knees and ankles and 0 to 10 points for elbows, based on joint swelling, muscle atrophy, crepitus on motion, range of motion, joint contracture, and instability for all three joints, as well as axial deformity of the knee and ankle. With the more recent emphasis on preventing joint disease, this evaluation tool is not sensitive enough to detect early or subtle joint changes, nor is it designed to detect abnormalities in early childhood physical activities such as running, jumping, or hopping. Newer instruments are being developed to provide better information about early joint dysfunction and more age-specific activity limitations (Manco-Johnson et al., 2001).

Muscle strength is examined functionally in the child who is too young to participate in manual muscle testing; otherwise, manual muscle testing is performed. Isokinetic testing may be performed in the older child if more sensitive strength measures are desired, such as for postoperative rehabilitation or to determine readiness to participate in organized sports.

Leg lengths, both from the anterior-superior iliac spine to the medial malleolus and from the umbilicus to the medial malleolus, should be measured to rule out leg length discrepancy, either actual or apparent secondary to pelvic obliquity. Girth measurements at joints may reveal swelling, although they are more useful when done serially on one joint than in comparison with the contralateral limb, because repeated hemarthroses can cause bony overgrowth. Muscle girth measurements may be indicative of muscle atrophy.

In my clinic, gait is examined visually for gross abnormalities, including posture, stride length, stance time, and heel-toe progression. If a treadmill is available, increases in speed and elevation often reveal more subtle differences.

Balance and coordination can be screened quickly by observing stair climbing, single-limb stance, hopping, and skipping (if appropriate for age). Parental reports are usually accurate in identifying coordination problems, at which time more formal testing (e.g., with the Bruininks-Oseretsky Test of Motor Proficiency [Bruininks, 1978]) can be completed.

Gross motor development is examined annually in our clinic during early childhood using the Peabody Developmental Motor Scales-2 (Folio & Fewell, 2000) if developmental problems are suspected. Otherwise, a simple screening tool such as the Denver II (Frankenburg et al., 1992) will give information about development in gross motor, fine motor, cognitive, and ADL skills.

Pain assessment must include the nature and severity of pain. The pain of an acute bleeding episode must be distinguished from the chronic pain of arthropathy. In the very young child who cannot verbalize his pain, the parents are instructed to watch for decreased use of a limb or changes in activity patterns or personality as signs of an acute bleeding episode. The chronic pain of arthropathy will not be evident until joint destruction has progressed to stage 4 or 5, which usually does not occur before the end of the first decade or into the second decade of life. For these preadolescent and older boys, visual analogue or numerical (0 to 10) scales can be used to measure pain (see Chapter 9).

EVALUATION

Based on the examination findings and historical information provided by the patient, the physical therapist can determine the most appropriate intervention for the patient. Is this an acute or chronic problem? How does the patient's lifestyle affect his disease? How does the patient's disease affect his lifestyle? Goals and outcomes of treatment will be determined by the answers to these and other questions suggested by the examination findings.

INTERVENTION

When hemostasis has been achieved after an acute hemorrhage, the child and family should be instructed in active exercises for ROM and strengthening. Koch and colleagues (1982) describe a physical therapy program for the knee with the following rules:

1. Passive ROM is contraindicated.
2. The isometric technique of alternating muscle contraction and relaxation is beneficial.
3. When the quadriceps muscle strength is in the fair range, the patient is encouraged to achieve full active knee extension in supine and sitting positions.
4. Active resistive exercises may be initiated when available knee flexion is at least 90° and there is less than a 15° flexion contracture.

During this subacute phase, factor replacement therapy is usually given before participation in physical therapy to minimize the risk of rebleeding and may be continued at regular intervals until the hemorrhage resolves. The exercise program must be individualized to progress from isometric to active-assistive, active, and finally resistive mode as the pain and swelling diminish and ROM and strength increase. Modalities such as ice, transcutaneous electrical nerve stimulation, and splints may be used to decrease joint pain and swelling, and hydrotherapy will allow for ROM, strengthening, and gait training activities to be performed with minimal stress to the joints.

Contracture Management

If the patient has recurrent hemarthroses without achieving full ROM and strength between bleeding episodes, a contracture will develop. Exercise alone may not be able to overcome the muscle shortening and intracapsular adhesions that may have formed. Timmermans (1989) has described a program using manual traction and mobilization techniques to relax the joint capsule, increase ROM, and decrease painful movements. Her method, as described next, is one way of approaching contracture management, although it has not been shown to be more effective than other methods.

Manual traction is applied in the position of comfort, taking care that there are no angular movements. With traction maintained, gentle manipulations may be performed to facilitate the restricted motion (e.g., anterior shifting of the tibia facilitates knee extension). Such techniques should be used only when the patient has received factor replacement and the therapist is experienced in both mobilization and management of hemophilia. They should never be used in the presence of severe instability or synovitis.

If full ROM cannot be achieved through exercise, several nonsurgical options are available. Although purely passive manual stretching is rarely indicated, slow stretching of joint contractures over relatively long periods has been shown to be effective (Weissman, 1977). Dynamic splints can provide a low-intensity, prolonged stretch and can be used in the patient's normal environment without difficulty. To reduce the risk of inducing a bleeding episode, tension on the dynamic splint is started at 0 or 0.5 and increased very slowly. If joint hemorrhage should occur, the dynamic splint is discontinued until the hemorrhage has resolved and then reapplied at a reduced tension. In one study, seven patients with chronic knee flexion contractures of greater than 15° were fitted with dynamic splints (Lang, 1990). The patients wore the dynamic splints at night for several months (range: 4–10), and all demonstrated ROM increases of at least 5°. Although three of these patients experienced knee hemarthroses during the study, each was able to resume use of the splint without restrictions. Despite only modest increases in ROM, five of the seven patients reported decreased stiffness and subjective improvement in ambulation.

Dynamic sling traction has also been used to provide prolonged stretch but requires hospitalization and confinement to bed for an average of 2 weeks (Duthie, 1990). The Quengel cast-brace or Ilizarov device may be used when posterior subluxation of the tibia accompanies a knee flexion contracture. The cast brace has offset subluxation hinges that correct the subluxation while a toggle stick corrects the flexion contracture.

Serial casting and drop-out casts are another option for contracture management. My experience has been limited to use in patients who have severe gastrocnemius muscle hemorrhages with resultant decreased ROM. In one patient, a 70° knee flexion contracture present 1 month after hemorrhage was reduced to his prehemorrhage range of −15° of extension in 6 days by use of a drop-out cast and active knee extension exercises.

Orthotics

Splints and orthoses are commonly used in the management of joint and muscle hemorrhages, but their use must be carefully monitored to prevent overuse. The general rule is to use the least restrictive means necessary to protect the joint and to discontinue use when the joint is strong enough to be without the extra protection, which is usually when strength and joint stability are in the good range. Therapists may be involved in the fabrication of splints to provide rest to a joint after a bleeding episode or surgery; to prevent or decrease the number of hemorrhages in a chronic joint, prevent or correct joint deformity, or improve function; or to provide support for weak or unstable joints (Holdredge, 1989). The splints are used as an adjunct to therapy and should not be used without a comprehensive program of strengthening exercises and joint stability, gait, and functional training.

Strengthening

Strengthening can be achieved through isometric, isotonic, or isokinetic exercise. The choice of type of exercise depends on the patient's ability to move the joint without pain, particularly after an acute hemarthrosis, or if there is need for immobilization. Isometric exercises are prescribed immediately after an acute hemarthrosis and continued until the joint is no longer tensely swollen and hot and can be moved without pain. Concentric exercises are then begun and progressed through active-assistive, active, and resistive modes. If the equipment is available, isokinetic exercises can be initiated when muscle strength is in the good range. If the equipment is unavailable, Greene and Strickler (1983) have described a "modified isokinetic" knee strengthening program that consists of using simultaneous contraction of the flexors of one leg against the extensors of the other leg. The patient is instructed to push with as much force as tolerated while allowing the legs to fully extend over a 5- to 10-second period and then to switch position of the legs. The benefit of isokinetic exercise is that resistance is accommodated to maintain maximum muscle tension throughout the full arc of motion, regardless of the relative strength of the muscle at any point along the arc.

Exercises prescribed should not jeopardize an unstable joint by overly stressing it and thereby increasing the risk of bleeding. For that reason, slow-speed isokinetics (150°/s and below) should be used cautiously or avoided.

Progressive resistive exercise (isotonic or isokinetic) in the open chain provide both concentric and eccentric strengthening and are preferred initially to closed-chain eccentric exercise that could produce exercise-induced joint tissue damage from compressive forces. High repetition, low-load progressive resistance programs have been shown to be effective in increasing strength and decreasing bleeding frequency (Tiktinsky et al., 2002). All exercise programs should be advanced slowly to allow for monitoring of effects on the joints (Pietri et al., 1992). Any signs of bleeding, such as increased swelling or pain or decreased ROM, will necessitate reducing the intensity of the exercise program and possibly exercising only under cover of factor replacement until supporting muscles are stronger.

Gait and Proprioceptive Training

Gait training focuses on correct positioning of the lower extremities and appropriate use of all joints and muscle groups. The patient should be taught a springy way of moving by pushing with the ankle and forefoot to allow the shock absorption of walking to be transferred to the muscles rather than the joints. Temporary use of crutches will transfer some of the weight bearing to the arms, which will decrease the load and pain on an affected lower extremity joint and allow for a more normal gait pattern to be simulated. Orthoses, such as the University of California Biomechanical Laboratory (UCBL) foot orthosis, are helpful when ankle laxity leads to hindfoot valgus. Without the UCBL orthosis, weight bearing may cause abnormal stresses on all the joints of the lower extremity (Timmermans, 1990).

Proprioceptive training should be included in any rehabilitation program for patients with hemophilia. Exercises such as unilateral balance, balance on wobble boards, hopping side to side, lunging, and bouncing on a minitrampoline can be started as strength allows (Buzzard, 1998). In addition, Hilberg and colleagues (2003) have demonstrated that a program of core stabilization and lower extremity proprioceptive training can significantly improve performance on single limb stance tests.

Postsurgical Rehabilitation

Physical therapists in the pediatric setting will usually be involved in postsurgical rehabilitation only after synovectomy in the child with hemophilia. Osteotomies and arthrodeses are performed for severe chronic arthropathy with marked deformity, instability, and pain, but these procedures are not typically performed on children. Similarly, arthroplasties of the hip and knee are performed on adults with severe arthropathy but such procedures have not been reported in the pediatric literature.

CASE STUDY

JIMMY

Jimmy is a 12-year-old boy with severe factor VIII deficiency. Two years ago, with a stage 3 arthropathy and 6-month history of chronic synovitis, he had arthroscopic synovectomy of the right knee with excellent results: ROM of 0° to 130°; quadriceps and hamstring muscle strength both 4+/5; and only two right knee hemorrhages, 6 months and 10 months earlier. He has been able to resume his favorite sport of tennis in the past year. He has noticed an increase in the incidence of left knee hemarthroses, and in the past month has had five bleeding episodes in that knee. He has been put on every-other-day factor replacement and referred to physical therapy for intensive rehabilitation.

Current examination reveals a boggy, swollen, but cool left knee. ROM is –30° of extension to 70° of flexion in the left knee. Within the available range, quadriceps strength is 2/5 and hamstring strength is 3/5. Jimmy is ambulating with bilateral axillary crutches, with toe-touch weight bearing on the left. He scores a 6 of 7 (independent with assistive device) on all the mobility and transfer items on the FIM except tub transfers, which are scored a 4 (require moderate assistance). He denies resting pain but does have pain with motion.

Jimmy wants to be able to go to tennis camp in the summer, although his parents are not sure he should go because his left knee bleeding began when he started tennis lessons. They are afraid that the lessons three times per week may be causing too much stress on his knee joints.

Based on the history, the physical examination, Jimmy's goal of going to tennis camp, and his parent's concerns, the following intervention plan was established. For Jimmy to meet his goal and to address his parents' concerns, coordination with the hematology team regarding long-term prophylaxis and with the orthopedist regarding the extent of joint damage is imperative. If the orthopedist does not discourage tennis playing once both knees are rehabilitated, knee braces may need to be considered to reduce lateral stresses when Jimmy plays.

Jimmy also must agree to follow a conditioning program on a daily basis once his rehabilitation is completed as long as he is playing tennis. The conditioning program will include flexibility and strength training and aerobic conditioning to reduce the risk of injury.

Finally, the direct interventions chosen are aimed at first achieving full range of motion of both knees followed by strengthening, gait training, and conditioning.

Problem 1: 30° left knee flexion contracture

Goal: Improve ROM of both knees to 0° to 140°.

Plan:

1. Fabricate resting knee splint for hours of sleep to maintain maximum available extension at night. Revise splint as extension returns.
2. Use dynamic splinting during the day for prolonged stretch (Fig. 10-3).
3. Perform active ROM exercises.

Problem 2: decreased strength in both knees

Goal: Increase strength of quadriceps and hamstring muscles of both legs to normal.

Plan:

1. For left knee, begin with isometric exercises and contract and relax techniques for ROM and strengthening. Begin active-assistive and active exercises when pain abates. When ROM is 15° to 90°, begin resistive exercises and advance slowly using low weights and high repetitions (Fig. 10-4).
2. For right knee, begin isokinetic strengthening at 180°, 240°, and 300°/s and joint stability activities, such as progressive resistive straight leg raises and single-limb minisquats.
3. For both lower extremities, begin strengthening and joint stability activities for hips and ankles (e.g., straight leg raises in prone and side-lying positions, heel raises, and exercises using the Biomechanical Ankle Platform System [BAPS] board [Camp, Jackson, MI]).

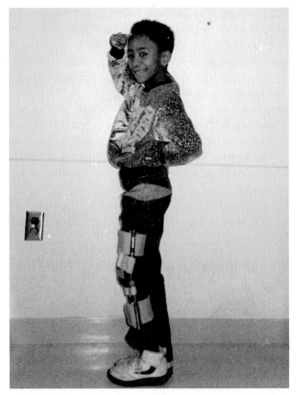

♦ **Figure 10-3** Dynamic splinting is used during the day to provide a prolonged stretch to the knee flexors.

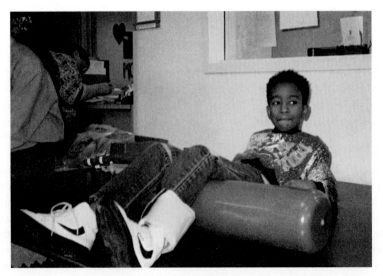

♦ **Figure 10-4** Resistive exercises with free weights are used for quadriceps strengthening. Later, isokinetic exercises will be added.

Problem 3: ambulation dysfunction: toe-touch weight bearing on left using bilateral axillary crutches

Outcome: Independent community ambulation without assistive devices.

Plan:

1. Maintain left weight bearing as tolerated in crutch ambulation until knee range is no less than 10° to 100° and quadriceps muscle strength is at least 3+/5.

2. Practice gait training on the treadmill at slow speeds to encourage heel-toe gait pattern and equal stride and step lengths.

3. Progress to independent household ambulation and then community ambulation as ROM and strength improve.

Problem 4: inability to participate in physical education classes and other athletic functions with friends

Outcome: Maintain cardiovascular fitness and resume tennis.

Plan:

1. Participate in aquatic therapy and swimming, three times per week for 20 to 30 minutes.

2. Contact school physical education teacher and discuss alternatives to regular physical education program.

3. Consider taping or knee cage for both knees to reduce rotary forces while playing tennis, when able.

Jimmy will be seen three times a week in physical therapy until his ROM and strength return to normal and he is ambulating without an assistive device. He will also be given a home exercise program to supplement his physical therapy sessions. Because Jimmy's left knee flexion contracture is an acute problem, his range is expected to return quickly and he should be off crutches in 2 to 3 weeks. His strength will return more slowly, but if he is compliant with his home program he can be cut back to once-a-week physical therapy for monitoring progress and adjusting the home program. Current radiographs will be reviewed with the orthopedist to determine if playing tennis is an appropriate expectation; if so, Jimmy should be able to resume playing tennis within 3 months.

REFERENCES

Aledort, LM. Orthopedic outcome studies and cost issues. Seminars in Thrombosis and Hemostasis, 29:55–60, 2003.

Arnold, WD, & Hilgartner, MW. Hemophilic arthropathy. Journal of Bone and Joint Surgery (American), 59:288–305, 1977.

Atkins, RM, Henderson, NJ, & Duthie, RB. Joint contractures in the hemophiliac. Clinical Orthopedics and Related Research, 219:97–105, 1987.

Bruininks, RH. Bruininks-Oseretsky Test of Motor Proficiency, Examiners Manual. Circle Pines, MN: American Guidance Service, 1978.

Buchanan, GR. Hemophilia. Pediatric Clinics of North America, 27:309–326, 1980.

Buzzard, BM. Proprioceptive training in haemophilia. Haemophilia, 4:528–531, 1998.

Corrigan, JJ. Coagulation disorders. In Miller, DR, & Bachner, RL (Eds.). Blood Disorders of Infancy and Childhood. St. Louis: Mosby, 1990, pp. 849–859.

Duthie, RB. Dynamic sling traction. In Gilbert, MS, & Greene, WB (Eds.). Musculoskeletal Problems in Hemophilia. New York: National Hemophilia Foundation, 1990, pp. 67–68.

Falk, B, Portal, S, Tiktinsky, R, Weinstein, Y, Constantini, N, & Martinowitz, U. Anaerobic power and muscle strength in young hemophilia patients. Medicine & Science in Sports & Exercise, 32:52–57, 2000.

Fernandez-Palazzi, F, Rupcich, M, Rivas, S, & Bosch, N. Biomechanical alterations that impair evolution and prognosis of haemophilic arthropathy. In Gilbert, MS, & Greene, WB (Eds.). Musculoskeletal Problems in Hemophilia. New York: National Hemophilia Foundation, 1990, pp. 34–44.

Folio, MR, & Fewell, RR. Peabody Developmental Motor Scales-2. Austin, TX: PRO-ED, 2000.

Frankenburg, WK, Dodds, JB, Archer, P, Bresnick, B, Maschka, P, Edelman, N, & Shapiro, H. Denver II Screening Manual. Denver: Denver Developmental Materials, 1992.

Gilbert, MS. Musculoskeletal complications of hemophilia: The joint. Haemophilia, 6(Suppl. 1):34-37, 2000.

Globe, DR, Cunningham, WE, Anderson, R, Dietrich, SL, Curtis, RG, Parish, KL, Miller, RT, Sanders, NL, & Kominski, G. Haemophilia Utilization Group Study: assessment of functional health status in haemophilia. Haemophilia, 8:121–128, 2002.

Greene, WB, & Strickler, EM. A modified isokinetic strengthening program for patients with severe hemophilia. Developmental Medicine and Child Neurology, 25:189–196, 1983.

Hilberg, T, Herbsleb, M, Gabriel, HHW, Jeschke, D, & Schramm, W. Proprioception and isometric muscular strength in haemophilic subjects. Haemophilia, 7:582–588, 2001.

Hilberg, T, Herbsleb, M, Puta, C, Gabriel, HHW, & Schramm, W. Physical training increases isometric muscular strength and proprioceptive performance in haemophilic subjects. Haemophilia, 9:86–93, 2003.

Hilgartner, MW. AIDS in the transfusion recipient. Pediatric Clinics of North America, 38:121–129, 1991.

Holdredge, S. Thermoplastic splints. In Funk, S (Ed.). Rehabilitation in Hemophilia: Proceedings of a Conference. New York: National Hemophilia Foundation, 1989, pp. 38–44.

Holdredge, S, & Cotta, S. Physical therapy and rehabilitation in the care of the adult and child with hemophilia. In Hilgartner, MW, & Pochedly, C (Eds.). Hemophilia in the Child and Adult. New York: Raven Press, 1989, pp. 235–262.

Houghton, GR, & Duthie, RB. Orthopedic problems in hemophilia. Clinical Orthopedics and Related Research, 138:197–216, 1979.

Joist, JH, & Ameri, A. Pathogenesis of hemophilic arthropathy. In Gilbert, MS, & Greene, WB (Eds.). Musculoskeletal Problems in Hemophilia. New York: National Hemophilia Foundation, 1990, pp. 20–25.

Jonas, DL. Drug abuse in hemophilia. In Hilgartner, MW, & Pochedly, C (Eds.). Hemophilia in the Child and Adult. New York: Raven Press, 1989, pp. 229–234.

Karayalcin, G. Current concepts in the management of hemophilia. Pediatric Annals, 14:640–655, 1985.

Kasper, CK, & Dietrich, SL. Comprehensive management of hemophilia. Clinics in Haematology, 14:491–492, 1985.

Koch, B, Cohen, S, Luban, NC, & Eng, G. Hemophiliac knee: Rehabilitation techniques. Archives of Physical Medicine and Rehabilitation, 63:379–382, 1982.

Koch, B, Galioto, FM, Jr, Kelleher, J, & Goldstein, D. Physical fitness in children with hemophilia. Archives of Physical Medicine and Rehabilitation, 65:324–326, 1984.

Lang, L. Dynasplint for knee flexion contractures in hemophilia. In Gilbert, MS, & Greene, WB (Eds.). Musculoskeletal Problems in Hemophilia. New York: National Hemophilia Foundation, 1990, pp. 83–86.

Liesner, RJ, Khair, K, & Hann, IM. The impact of prophylactic treatment on children with severe haemophilia. British Journal of Haematology, 92:973–978, 1996.

Manco-Johnson, MJ, Nuss, R, Funk, S, & Murphy, J. Joint evaluation instruments for children and adults with haemophilia. Haemophilia, 6:649–657, 2000.

Manco-Johnson, MJ, Nuss, R, Lear, J, Wiedel, J, Geraghty, SJ, Hacker, MR, Funk, S, Kilcoyne, RF, & Murphy, J. 32P radiosynoviorthesis in children with hemophilia. Journal of Pediatric Hematology/Oncology, 24:534–539, 2002.

Mannucci, PM, Mendolicchio, L, & Gringeri, A. Use of prophylaxis to prevent complications of hemophilia. In Monroe, D, Hedner, U, Hoffman, MR, Negrier, C, Savidge, GF, & White II, GC (Eds.). Hemophilia Care in the New Millennium. New York: Kluwer Academic/Plenum Publishers, 2001, pp. 59–64.

Pietri, MM, Frontera, WR, Pratts, IS, & Suarez, EL. Skeletal muscle function in patients with hemophilia A and unilateral hemarthroses of the knee. Archives of Physical Medicine and Rehabilitation, 73:22–26, 1992.

Schoenmakers, MA, Gulmans, VA, Helders, PJ, & van den Berg, HM. Motor performance and disability in Dutch children with haemophilia: A comparison with their healthy peers. Haemophilia, 7:293–298, 2001.

Shapiro, AD, Donfield, SM, Lynn, HS, Cool, VA, Stehbens, JA, Hunsberger, SL, Tonetta, S, & Gomperts, ED. Defining the impact of hemophilia: The Academic Achievement in Children with Hemophilia Study. Pediatrics, 108: E105, 2001.

Shopnick, RI, & Brettler, DB. Hemostasis. Clinical Orthopedics and Related Research, 328:34–38. 1996.

State University of New York at Buffalo, Center for Functional Assessment Research, Department of Rehabilitation Medicine. Guide for the Use of the Uniform Data Set for Medical Rehabilitation Including the Functional Independence Measure for Children (WeeFIM), 1991.

Strickler, EM, & Greene, WB. Isokinetic torque levels in hemophiliac knee musculature. Archives of Physical Medicine and Rehabilitation, 65:766–770, 1984.

Tiktinsky, R, Falk, B, Heim, M, & Martinovitz, U. The effect of resistance training on the frequency of bleeding in haemophilia patients, a pilot study. Haemophilia, 8:22–27, 2002.

Timmermans, H. Severe arthropathy of the hemophilic joint: A comprehensive rehabilitation program. In Funk, S (Ed.). Rehabilitation in Hemophilia: Proceedings of a Conference. New York: National Hemophilia Foundation, 1989, pp. 11–15.

Timmermans, H. The role of the physiotherapist. In Gilbert, MS, & Greene, WB (Eds.). Musculoskeletal Problems in Hemophilia. New York: National Hemophilia Foundation, 1990, pp. 115–121.

Van der Berg, HM, & Fischer, K. Prophylaxis for severe hemophilia: Experience from Europe and the United States. Seminars in Thrombosis and Hemostasis, 29:49–54, 2003.

Walsh, CE. Gene therapy progress and prospects: Gene therapy for the hemophilias. Gene Therapy, 10:999–1003, 2003.

Weissman, J. Rehabilitation medicine and the hemophilic patient. Mt. Sinai Journal of Medicine, 44:359–370, 1977.

∽

SPINAL CONDITIONS

CHERYL PATRICK
PT

The spine is the framework for our posture and our movement. It supports our cranium, extremities, and spinal cord; allows for trunk flexibility; acts as a shock absorber; and provides structural support for normal chest and respiratory development. Orthopedic concerns arise when spinal alignment is altered by congenital or progressive changes, producing scoliosis, kyphosis, or lordosis.

Each one or a combination of these conditions, if left untreated, may affect a child's pulmonary function, psychosocial well-being, potential for back pain, and life expectancy. We, as physical therapists, play a vital role in the detection and treatment of spinal conditions. Two to four percent of the population of school-age children (7–18 years) is at risk for adolescent idiopathic scoliosis, the most common form of scoliosis (Roach, 1999). The prevalence of other spinal conditions varies with the condition and underlying disease process (Bleck, 1991;

Weinstein, 1989). This chapter addresses the prevalence and natural history, identification, examination, and treatment of these spinal conditions. Specific case studies are presented to discuss impairments and restrictions in activity and participation of children with spinal conditions. Physical therapy intervention is emphasized, along with nonsurgical and surgical management of these spinal conditions.

DEVELOPMENT OF THE SPINE

Because pathologic spinal conditions are discussed in this chapter, it is necessary for the reader to have some knowledge of normal spinal development (Fig. 11-1). Therefore, a discussion of development in the embryologic, fetal, and childhood stages follows.

Fetal development is divided into three stages. The first 3 weeks after fertilization is termed the *pre-embryonic period*. The *embryonic period* is next, lasting from week 3 to week 8 of gestation; during this stage the organs of the body develop. The *fetal period* lasts from week 8 until term, and during this stage maturation and growth of all structures and organs occur (Moe et al., 1987).

Early development of the skeletal, muscular, and neural systems is related to the notochord. Cell proliferation occurs at approximately 3 weeks, forming a trilaminar structure with layers of ectoderm, mesoderm, and endoderm. Proliferation of the mesodermal tissue continues, forming 29 pairs of somites in the fourth week and the remainder (42–44 total) in the fifth week. Differentiation of the somites then occurs, producing 4 occipital, 8 cervical, 12 thoracic, 5 lumbar, 5 sacral, and 8 to 10 coccygeal somites. The occipital somites form a portion of the base of the skull and the articulation between the cranium and cervical vertebrae while the last 5 to 7 coccygeal somites disappear. Cervical, thoracic, lumbar, and sacral somites form the structures of the spine (Winter, 1983).

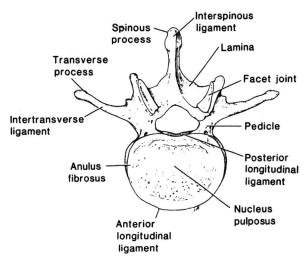

◆ **Figure 11-1**   The L2 vertebra viewed from above. *(From Moe, JH, Winter, RB, Bradford, DS, Ogilvie, JW, & Lonstein, JE. Scoliosis and Other Spinal Deformities, 2nd ed. Philadelphia: WB Saunders, 1987, p. 8.)*

Proliferation of the somites occurs, developing three distinct areas. Dorsally the cells become dermatome, giving rise to the skin. Medially to the dermatome, cells migrate deep to give rise to skeletal muscle. The ventral and medial cells migrate toward the notochord and neural tube to form the sclerotome (Moe et al., 1987; Winter, 1983).

The sclerotomal cells proliferate and differentiate, giving rise to rudimentary vertebral structures, including rib buds. Chondrification begins at the cervicothoracic level, extending cranially and caudally. Centers of chondrification allow for formation of the solid cartilage model of a vertebra with no line of demarcation between body, neural arch, or rib rudiments (Moe et al., 1987).

Ossification occurs at primary and secondary centers. Ossification begins during the late fetal period and continues after birth. Primary centers of ossification extend to the spinous, transverse, and articular processes. Secondary ossification centers develop at the upper and lower portions of the vertebral body, at the tip of the spinous processes, and at each transverse process. These centers expand in late adolescence. Secondary ossification centers also develop in the ribs—one at the head of the rib and two in the tubercle. Ossification of the axis, atlas, and sacrum differs slightly from that of the other vertebrae. The atlas has two primary centers and one secondary center of ossification, and the axis has five primary and two secondary centers of ossification. Ossification of the axis begins near the end of gestation with fusion of the two odontoid centers and is completed in the second decade of life with fusion of the odontoid and centrum. Fusion of the sacrum begins in adolescence

and is completed in the third decade of life (Moe et al., 1987).

Spinal growth occurs throughout adolescence. A knowledge of spinal growth is essential in nonsurgical and surgical treatment of spinal deformities. Spinal growth does not proceed in a uniform linear pattern (Tanner et al., 1966; Tanner & Whitehouse, 1976). Two periods of rapid spinal growth occur; the first from birth to age 3 years and the second during the adolescent growth spurt. Between 3 years and the onset of puberty, growth is linear.

The spinal pubertal growth spurts occur at different chronologic and Tanner ages for females and males. In females, the growth spurt coincides with Tanner 2 or a chronologic age of 8 to 14 years, with the maximum growth occurring at a mean of 12 years of age. The spurt lasts 2.5 to 3 years (Calvo, 1957). The growth spurt occurs later in males, at Tanner 3 or chronologic age 11 to 16 years, with the maximum growth at age 14 years. These values are average values based on white Anglo-Saxon populations (Duval-Beaupere, 1972).

A fused area of the spine does not grow longitudinally, as documented by Moe and colleagues (1964). The surgeon, therefore, considers the information on spinal growth potential for each individual case.

▉ SCOLIOSIS

DETECTION AND CLINICAL EXAMINATION

Detection of scoliosis is primarily by identification of trunk, shoulder, or pelvic asymmetries. Children with asymmetries should be referred to an orthopedic surgeon with an interest in and knowledge of scoliosis for a baseline evaluation. Ideally, the surgeon should specialize in pediatrics or pediatric spines, be affiliated with a reputable medical center, and be part of a team that includes an orthotist, a nurse, and a physical therapist.

An examination begins with a complete patient history to obtain information regarding curve detection, familial conditions, general health, and physical maturity. The physical examination includes assessment of spinal alignment by forward bending test, general alignment, shoulder and pelvic symmetry, trunk compensation using a plumb line, and leg length measurement. The magnitude of a rib hump is quantified using a scoliometer with the forward bending test (Moe et al., 1987). The scoliometer, an inclinometer designed by Bunnell (Bunnell, 1984), is placed over the spinous process at the apex of the curve to measure the angle of trunk rotation (ATR). The examiner also evaluates signs and symptoms of any underlying disease and neurologic status.

Radiographs (initially two views; lateral and anterior-posterior) are used to determine location, type, and magnitude of the curve, as well as skeletal age. Skeletal maturity is determined using the Risser sign, which quantifies the amount of ossification of the iliac crest, using grades 0 to 5. Grades 1 to 4 are excursions from 25% to 100%, starting at the anterior-superior iliac spine. Grade 5 categorizes fusion of the iliac crest with the ileum (Zaouss & James, 1958). Grade 0 represents absence of ossification. Grades 0, 1, and 2 correlate with skeletal immaturity, grade 3 with progressing skeletal maturity, grade 4 with cessation of spinal growth, and grade 5 with cessation of increase in height.

The spinal curvature is measured using the Cobb method. To complete the measurement, one must first identify the end vertebrae. The end vertebrae are described as the most cephalad vertebra of a curve whose upper surface maximally tilts toward the curve's concavity and the most caudal vertebra with maximal tilt toward the concavity. Lines are drawn as extensions of the end vertebra from either end plate or pedicles. The degree of curvature is measured as the angle formed by the intersection of lines perpendicular to these end vertebral lines (Dickson et al., 1984; Goldstein & Waugh, 1973). Minimal degree of curvature for diagnosis of scoliosis is 10° (Fig. 11-2). Magnetic resonance imaging, conventional tomography, myelography, and bone scans can be used to identify subtle central nervous system abnormalities and provide additional information as necessary to aid in diagnosis and detection of spinal conditions.

TERMINOLOGY

Spinal deformities are classified according to etiology, location, magnitude, and direction. Curvatures may be idiopathic, neuromuscular, or congenital and may further be classified by the area of the spine in which the apex of the curve is located: (1) cervical curve, between C1 and C6; (2) cervicothoracic curve, between C7 and T1; (3) thoracic curve, between T2 and T11; (4) thoracolumbar curve, between T12 and L1; (5) lumbar curve, between L2 and L4; and (6) lumbosacral curve, between L5 and S1. Magnitude is measured using the Cobb method as described previously.

Direction of the curve is designated right or left by the side of the convexity of the deformity (Herkowitz et al., 1999). Up to 90% of thoracic curves are right (Roach, 1999), and if a left thoracic curve is discovered, more extensive evaluation is required to rule out tumors or other neurologic problems (Roach, 1999; Rinsky & Gamble, 1988; Sarwark & Kramer, 1998).

There are two major types of curvatures; structural and nonstructural. A nonstructural curve fully corrects clinically and radiographically on lateral bend toward the apex

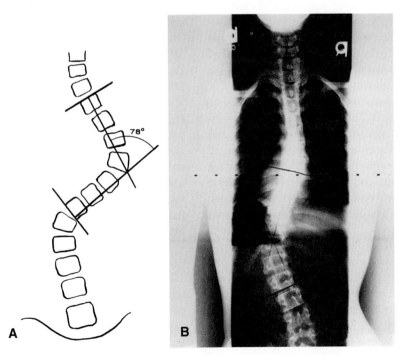

* **Figure 11-2**   **A**, Cobb's method of measuring the angle of the curve in scoliosis (see text). **B**, The Cobb method of measuring the curve angle of scoliosis as seen on a radiograph. *(A From Tachdjian, MO. Pediatric Orthopedics, 2nd ed. Philadelphia: WB Saunders, 1990, p. 2285.)*

of the curve and lacks vertebral rotation. A nonstructural curve is usually nonprogressive and is most often caused by a shortened lower extremity on the side of the apex of the curve. It is essential, however, to monitor nonstructural curves during growth because they may occasionally develop into structural deformities.

A structural curve cannot be voluntarily, passively, or forcibly fully corrected. Rotation of the vertebrae is toward the convexity of the curve. A fixed thoracic prominence or rib hump in a child with a thoracic deformity or a lumbar paraspinal prominence in a child with a lumbar curve is evidence of rotation when observed on clinical examination (Herkowitz et al., 1999).

IDIOPATHIC SCOLIOSIS

Idiopathic scoliosis denotes a lateral curvature of the spine of unknown cause and is the most common form of scoliosis in children.

Etiology, Incidence, and Pathophysiology

Infantile idiopathic scoliosis develops in children younger than age 3, usually manifesting shortly after birth. This form of scoliosis accounts for less than 1% of all cases (Miller, 1999). Infantile idiopathic scoliosis occurs more frequently in male infants and the majority of the curves are left. Eighty to ninety percent of these curves spontaneously resolve, but many of the remainder of cases will progress throughout childhood, resulting in severe deformity. Because infantile idiopathic scoliosis is common in England and northern Europe, but rare in the United States, environmental factors have been implicated in the development of the deformity (Herkowitz et al., 1999).

Juvenile idiopathic scoliosis develops between ages 3 and 9 years (Dobbs & Weinstein, 1999). The most common curve is right thoracic, occurring in males and females with equal frequency and most often recognized around 6 years of age. Juvenile idiopathic curves have a high rate of progression and result in severe deformity if untreated. A study by Wynne-Davies (1974) found the incidence of scoliosis in children younger than age 8 years to be 1.3%.

Adolescent idiopathic scoliosis (AIS) categorizes curves manifesting at or around the onset of puberty and accounts for approximately 80% of all cases of idiopathic scoliosis. The prevalence of idiopathic scoliosis is 2 to 4% of children ages 10 to skeletal maturity (Bleck, 1991; Roach, 1999). Three to nine percent of these children have curves greater than 10° and require intervention (Dickson et al., 1984; Weinstein, 1989). The overall female-to-male ratio for prevalence of AIS is 3.6:1. The female-to-male ratio is roughly equal (1.4:1) in curves of approximately 10°.

With curve magnitude of 20° or greater, the female-to-male ratio increases to 5:1 (Weinstein, 1989; Weinstein, 1994; Rogala et al., 1978). A greater percentage of curves will progress in the female patient, 19.3% compared with 1.2% of males. A large number of AIS curvatures are structural at the time of detection, although flexibility and the progression of these curves vary. Structural curves have a greater tendency to progress throughout adolescence at an average rate of 1° per month if untreated, whereas the nonstructural curves may remain flexible enough to avoid becoming problematic (Herkowitz et al., 1999).

An extensive amount of research has been devoted to discovering the cause of idiopathic scoliosis, but the mechanics and specific etiology are not clearly understood. A number of theories have been proposed that attempt to explain the mechanics of vertebral column failure and decompensation of the spine as seen in idiopathic scoliosis. These causes include insufficiency of the costovertebral ligaments, asymmetric weakness of the paraspinal musculature, unequal distribution of type I and type II muscle fibers, and collagen abnormalities. Clinical studies have focused on deviations in vibratory responses, proprioceptive deficits, and neurologic or vestibular dysfunction. Some authors proposed that some of the clinical changes such as vibratory and proprioceptive deficits are actually secondary to, rather than a cause of, the existing spinal deformity (Dickson et al., 1984; McInnes et al., 1991). A recent study on standing stability and body parameters compared able-bodied girls to those with AIS. The findings supported the concept of a primary or secondary dysfunction in the postural regulation system of the girls with AIS (Nault et al., 2002). Byl and Gray (1993) reported decreased performance of adolescents with idiopathic scoliosis, particularly those with severe curves, on complex balance activities especially when vision and proprioception were simultaneously challenged. The authors posed the question of whether balance changes are due to the structural impairment (scoliosis) or an underlying sensory impairment. They strongly suggested the need for longitudinal studies to determine if there is a predictive relationship between balance dysfunction and progressive scoliosis.

Although the specific etiology of idiopathic scoliosis is not known, data from studies by Wynne-Davies (1966, 1968) and Cowell and colleagues (1972) reflect the existence of a familial tendency. Familial prevalence of idiopathic scoliosis may reflect a growth pattern shared by families. The growth pattern and effects of biplanar spinal asymmetry during growth were discussed in a study by Dickson and associates (1984), which specifically examined the growth factors in the coronal and sagittal planes and their effect on progressive idiopathic scoliosis.

Structural changes vary with the degree of scoliosis and affect the anatomy and physiology of the spine, with the greatest change at the apex of the curve (Herring, 2002). Compression and distraction forces act on the growing spine to produce wedge-shaped vertebrae (larger on the convex side and smaller on the concave side). Associated changes are seen in the intraspinal canal and posterior arch, which may cause angulation and stretch on the spinal cord but rarely cause functional disturbances. Cord compression and functional changes occur most often secondary to an unusually tight dura mater, as seen in spines with marked dorsal kyphosis. Changes occurring on the concave side of the curvature include compression and degenerative changes of intravertebral disks and shortening of muscles and ligaments (Fig. 11-3). Changes in the thoracic spine directly affect the rib cage. The translatory shift of the spine causes an asymmetrically divided thorax, producing decreased pulmonary capacity on the convex side and increased pulmonary capacity on the concave side. Severe curves in the thoracic spine associated with increased angulation of the ribs posteriorly further reduce aeration of the lung on the convex side, potentially causing abnormal stresses on the heart and disturbed cardiac function (Dickson et al., 1984; Herring, 2002). Structural changes cause cosmetic deformity that, in turn, affects appearance and may affect psychosocial well-being.

Natural History

A progressive curve is defined by a sustained increase of 5° or more on two consecutive examinations occurring at 4- to 6-month intervals. An untreated progressive curve has the potential to increase in magnitude in adult life. The following are the main factors that influence the probability of progression in the skeletally immature patient (Weinstein, 1989):

1. The younger the patient at diagnosis, the greater the risk of progression.
2. Double-curve patterns have a greater risk for progression than single-curve patterns.
3. The lower the Risser sign, the greater the risk of progression.
4. Curves with greater magnitude are at a greater risk to progress.
5. Risk of progression in females is approximately 10 times that of males with curves of comparable magnitude.
6. Greater risk of progression is present when curves develop before menarche.

CONGENITAL SCOLIOSIS

Etiology, Incidence, and Pathophysiology

Congenital scoliosis curves are caused by anomalous vertebral development. Congenital anomalies of the vertebrae can be attributed to failure of vertebral segmentation or failure of vertebral formation. Both pathologic processes are frequently seen in the same spine and may occur either at the same or at different levels. Location of the pathologic process on the vertebrae (anterior, posterior, lateral, or a combination) determines the congenital deformity. Purely lateral deformity produces congenital scoliosis, and anterolateral and posterolateral deformities produce congenital kyphoscoliosis and lordoscoliosis, respectively (Winter, 1983, 1988).

A defect of segmentation is seen when adjacent vertebrae do not completely separate from one another, thereby producing an unsegmented bar, with no growth plate or disk between the adjacent vertebrae. A lateral, one-sided defect of segmentation produces severe progressive congenital scoliosis. Circumferential failure of segmentation produces en bloc vertebrae, an anomaly that results in loss of segmental motion and loss of longitudinal ver-

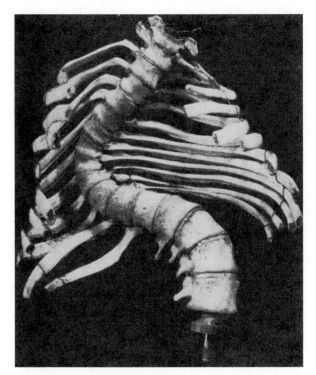

Figure 11-3 Anatomic specimen of the spine demonstrating structural changes of right thoracic scoliosis. Note vertebral wedging on the concave side and rotation of the vertebral bodies to the convexity of the curve. *(From James, JIP. Scoliosis. Baltimore: Williams & Wilkins, 1967, p. 13. © 1967, Williams & Wilkins Co., Baltimore.)*

tebral growth but no rotational or angular spinal deformity (Winter, 1983).

Defects of formation may be partial or complete. An anterior failure of formation of all or part of the vertebral body produces a kyphosis. A partial unilateral defect of formation of a vertebra produces a wedge-shaped hemivertebra (Fig. 11-4) with one pedicle and only one side with growth potential. A nonsegmented hemivertebra is completely fused to the adjacent proximal and distal vertebrae. A semisegmented hemivertebra is fused to only one adjacent vertebra and separated from the other by a normal end plate and disk. A segmented hemivertebra is separated from both the proximal and distal vertebrae by a normal end plate and disk. Hemivertebrae may be unbalanced, with the defect present on one side of the spine, or balanced, with different hemivertebrae present with defects on opposite sides of the spine compensating for any curves (Winter, 1983, 1988).

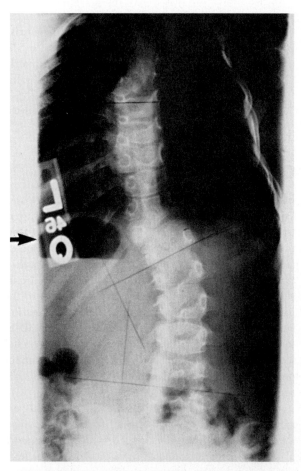

+ **Figure 11-4** Radiograph showing congenital scoliosis due to hemivertebrae of thoracic vertebrae. Compensatory scoliosis in the lumbar spine. (The arrow on the left indicates the hemivertebrae.)

The etiology of congenital scoliosis involves fetal environmental factors that affect development at 45 to 60 days after fertilization (Winter, 1988). A study by Wynne-Davies (1975) is a comprehensive review of 337 patients with congenital spinal anomalies and their families. She found that an isolated anomaly, such as a hemivertebra, was a sporadic lesion with no increased risk of spinal deformities for subsequent births or for children of parents who have the deformity. Multiple spinal anomalies, with or without the presence of spina bifida, are believed to be related etiologically to spina bifida and therefore carry a 5% to 10% risk to subsequent siblings for any one of the anomalies. A review by Winter (1983) of 1250 patients with congenital spinal anomalies, however, found few familial relationships (only 13 of 1250). Conclusions were drawn that hemivertebrae carry an approximately 1% chance of occurring in a first-degree relative of a patient with a hemivertebra. A relationship between multiple congenital anomalies and spina bifida was not noted.

Other spinal anomalies or other organ system anomalies may be associated with congenital spinal malformations. One of these anomalies is diastematomyelia, a congenital malformation of the neural axis in which there is sagittal division of the spinal cord. Diastematomyelia is often associated with an osseous, fibrous, or fibrocartilaginous spur attached to one or more vertebral bodies and the dura mater. Clinical signs of a spinal dysraphism include a hair patch, unequal foot size, various foot deformities (e.g., cavus feet), and asymmetric lower extremity circumference and strength. Other associated defects include urinary tract anomalies, hearing deficits, facial asymmetries, and Sprengel's deformity, which is a partially undescended scapula that may cause apparent webbing or shortening of the neck and limited shoulder range of motion (ROM) (Winter, 1983).

The risk of curve progression can be analyzed by examining the growth potential of the congenital anomaly. Many congenital curves become stable and do not progress. The highest risk of progression occurs when there is asymmetric growth in which the convexity outgrows the concavity. This discrepancy usually occurs when the anatomy of the convex side is relatively normal and the concave side is deficient. A shortened trunk may be the main deformity if both convex and concave growth deficiencies occur over multiple levels (Winter, 1988).

INTERVENTIONS FOR IDIOPATHIC AND CONGENITAL SCOLIOSIS

Treatment decisions are based on skeletal maturity of the child, growth potential of the child, and curve magnitude. In addition to surgical intervention, nonsurgical interventions include exercise, orthotic treatment, and electrical stimulation.

Nonsurgical Interventions

Idiopathic curves of less than 25°, curves of nonsurgical magnitude of any type in a skeletally mature patient, and nonprogressive congenital curves are evaluated by clinical examination every 4 to 6 months. Radiographs are obtained for congenital curves at each visit; however, unchanged results of a scoliometer examination may reduce the frequency of radiographs to every other visit, depending on individual physician and institution practice.

Exercise

A home exercise program designed to maintain or improve trunk and pelvic strength and flexibility is often prescribed for children with idiopathic or congenital scoliosis. Exercises include postural exercises (trunk extensor control, abdominal strengthening, gluteal strengthening), lateral flexion exercises, trunk shifts, stretching of pectorals and lower extremities, and respiratory exercises to increase chest capacity and maximize volume. In my clinical experience, compliance is often poor unless the child experienced back pain before diagnosis of scoliosis. Exercise as the sole treatment for prevention of progression of scoliotic curves has not been shown to be effective even if compliance is high (Lonstein & Renshaw, 1987). A 2003 study from Germany suggested that an intensive inpatient rehabilitative exercise program (6 hours/day for a minimum of 4–6 weeks, including both group and individual therapy) has the potential to reduce the incidence of progression in children with idiopathic scoliosis. The study does acknowledge the need for longer-term follow-up of the participants in order to evaluate the long-term effectiveness of the physical therapy program on the natural history of idiopathic scoliosis (Weiss et al., 2003).

Electrical Stimulation

Electrical stimulation is now rarely used as an intervention for idiopathic scoliosis. The theory of electrical stimulation use was to produce sufficient stimulation of muscles on the convex side of the curve to alter the direction of the deformity, decrease the pressure on the concave side of the curve, and allow for more normal vertebral growth. Studies have shown, however, that electrical stimulation had no effect on prevention of idiopathic curve progression, especially for patients with high-risk factors (Bertrand et al., 1992; Bylund et al., 1987).

Orthotic Management

The goal of orthotic management is to alter the natural history of curve progression in adolescent idiopathic scoliosis. The principles of orthotic management are based on the biomechanical hypothesis that spinal stability is directly proportional to the end support of the spine and inversely proportional to spinal flexibility and the approximate square of its length. Therefore, the amount of load that may be placed on the spine before collapse can be increased by firm support at the upper and lower ends. An orthosis provides this support at the lower end of the spine anteriorly and laterally on the abdomen, posteriorly and laterally on the buttocks, and by contour over the iliac crests, effectively decreasing the lumbar lordosis. The upper end is supported by neck, shoulder, and spinal musculature; by central nervous system reflexes; and possibly by a throat mold. These end supports result in a functional shortening of the spinal column, decreased spinal flexibility, and increased resistance to buckling. Indirect forces are applied laterally by pads, flanges, or slings, thus providing lateral and rotational correction (Kehl & Morrissy, 1988; Renshaw, 1985).

The indication for orthotic use depends on curve type, magnitude, and location. Orthoses are typically prescribed for children with idiopathic scoliosis who are skeletal immature (with a Risser sign of 0, 1, or 2) and have a curve from 25° to 45° (Green, 1986; Katz & Durrani, 2001; Renshaw, 1985). A curve with a greater magnitude at time of detection has an increased risk of progression. Similarly, the effect of an orthosis on prevention of curve progression decreases as the magnitude of the curve increases (Katz et al., 1997).

A Milwaukee brace or cervical-thoracic-lumbar-sacral orthosis (CTLSO) was the only spinal orthosis available until the 1970s, when the Boston bracing system was developed (Kehl & Morrissy, 1988; Renshaw, 1985). The Milwaukee brace is rarely used today. For curves with an apex of T8 or higher, a custom TLSO (thoracolumbosacral orthosis) with high axillary trim lines will be fabricated by an orthotist, rather than using a Milwaukee brace.

The Boston system was designed to decrease costs, improve the acceptability of orthotic wear, and simplify construction (Farady, 1983). A series of 24 prefabricated polypropylene pelvic molds lined with polyethylene foam constitute the Boston system (Fig. 11-5). An orthotist molds the brace to the patient, adding lumbar pads and relief areas. The rigid shell provides a firm support, and the foam lining allows for comfort. A Boston brace is an example of a TLSO and best treats a curve with an apex lower than T9 (Farady, 1983). A Boston brace may be modified by the addition of an extension on the concave side to achieve improved control of curves with an apex at T7 to T9 (Kehl & Morrissy, 1988).

Other TLSO types include the Wilmington and Charleston models. A Wilmington TLSO (Fig. 11-6) is

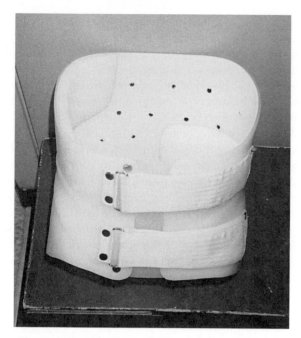

• **Figure 11-5** The Boston brace, underarm TLSO. Note pads for relief and pressure areas.

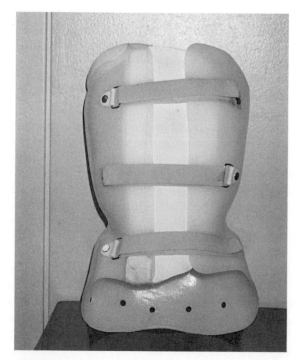

• **Figure 11-6** The Wilmington brace is a custom-molded, total-contact TLSO.

a total-contact, custom-molded orthosis that achieves maximal spinal correction by the tight contact and fit, not by pads and relief areas (Kehl & Morrissy, 1988). A Charleston orthosis is used for idiopathic curves and is worn only at night, because it is fabricated in the position of maximum side-bend correction (Price et al., 1990). A long-term follow-up by Price and colleagues (1997) found that 65 of 98 patients showed improvement or less than 5° change in curvature and only 17 patients progressed to the point of requiring surgery. The Charleston brace is most effective in the treatment of smaller, single thoracolumbar or lumbar curves (Katz et al., 1997).

The active theory of orthotics is that curve progression is prevented by muscle contractions responding to the brace wear. A study by Wynarsky and Schultz (1989), however, showed no statistical difference between myoelectrical activity during braced and unbraced states of female patients being treated with the Boston brace for idiopathic scoliosis. The passive theory is that curve progression is prevented through the external forces of the brace on the spine.

Exercises to be performed while wearing the brace, such as pelvic tilts, thoracic flexion, and lateral shifts, are often taught to patients to improve the active forces. Studies have shown no statistical difference in curve stability between those patients who comply with orthotic wear and exercises and those who comply only with orthotic wear (Carman et al., 1985). A physical therapist's main role is to encourage physical activity of the patient (e.g., during physical education class, aerobics, dance) while wearing the orthosis to maintain balance, coordination, and strength and to develop good habits of achieving and maintaining cardiorespiratory fitness. Specific trunk exercises, such as those for unbraced scoliosis, may be taught to the patient to perform while out of the brace and are designed to maintain trunk strength and flexibility.

Orthotic treatment continues until the curve is no longer controlled (usually 40° to 45° or higher) or skeletal maturity occurs, at which time weaning may begin. Twenty to twenty-six percent of orthotically treated curves will progress enough to require spinal fusion (Piazza & Basset, 1990; Katz & Durrani, 2001). High-risk factors include younger age at curve detection, higher magnitude, and low Risser sign, just as for untreated idiopathic scoliosis, although orthotic wear can positively influence the natural history of idiopathic scoliosis (Basset et al., 1986; Kehl & Morrissy, 1988; Katz & Durrani, 2001).

The weaning process takes about 12 months from the time of skeletal maturity and consists of gradually decreasing the amount of time wearing the brace. Studies by Carr and associates (1980), Basset and colleagues (1986), and Emans and co-workers (1986) have shown that a gradual loss of curve correction occurs over 2 to 5 years following successful orthotic management. An orthotic treatment is considered successful if the curve magnitude at the end of treatment is within 5° of the magnitude at the start of treatment.

Surgical Interventions

The major indication for spinal fusion is a documented progressive idiopathic curve that reaches 45° or greater. Curves greater than 40° are increasingly difficult to manage orthotically and also have significant risk of progression after skeletal maturity (Kostuik, 1990). The goals of spinal fusion are to halt the progression of the deformity to avoid the sequelae of pain and pulmonary dysfunction, achieve maximal correction in all three planes with minimal surgical risk, obtain a balanced trunk, and obtain a solid spinal arthrodesis (Drummond, 1991). The main objective of any scoliosis surgery is to obtain a solid arthrodesis because the fusion mass is ultimately what prevents further progression of the deformity (Drummond, 1991; Kostuik, 1990).

A posterior surgical approach is most often used for spinal fusion. Bone graft is packed into disk spaces and facet joints of the vertebrae after surgical exposure and preparation. The differences among posterior spinal fusion techniques lie with the instrumentation used to obtain correction and protect the fusion. The Harrington rod system is the standard for comparison with newer instrumentation, although this system is rarely used today because it does not allow for sagittal plane correction and produces a flattened lumbar lordosis secondary to the distraction forces.

The Luque instrumentation consists of two L-shaped rods attached with sublaminar wiring. This system allows for load sharing because multiple segments are wired and is therefore best suited to patients with poor bone quality, anomalies of the posterior spinal elements, or poor muscle or skin quality (Drummond, 1991; Kostuik, 1990). The Luque system (Fig. 11-7) can prevent loss of lumbar lordosis and provide stabilization to the pelvis. The disadvantage is a risk of neurologic damage (Herring, 2002). The Cotrel-Dubousset system (Fig. 11-8) uses two rods and compression or distraction hooks attached to either laminae or pedicles. The rods can be contoured to obtain sagittal plane correction, thus restoring lumbar lordosis and thoracic kyphosis (Drummond, 1991; Kostuik, 1990).

An anterior surgical approach includes opening of the thoracic cavity, resection of a rib, and excision through the diaphragm to expose the necessary vertebrae. To obtain correction and protect the spinal fusion, either Zielke or Dwyer screws are used on the vertebral bodies. Zielke screws are newer, provide control at each segment with a

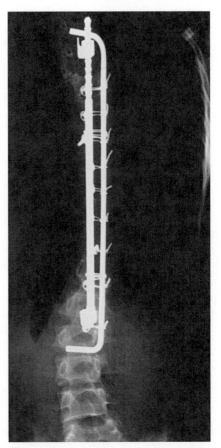

◆ **Figure 11-7**   Radiograph showing the Luque rod instrumentation system for corrective spinal surgery. Note the segmental wiring.

rod and screw, and prevent postinstrumentation kyphosis (Herring, 2002). An anterior approach may be used to fuse a thoracolumbar or lumbar idiopathic scoliosis.

A two-stage procedure is used for higher-magnitude curves or severe kyphoscoliotic curves. An anterior approach is used for the release of anterior spinal ligaments, a diskectomy, or a fusion with or without instrumentation. The procedure is completed by a posterior spinal fusion with instrumentation (Kostuik, 1990). Two procedures are necessary to gain range of the vertebral column for maximal correction of the curve and to provide stability from the fusion to prevent instrumentation failure or pseudarthrosis.

Anterior or posterior surgical approaches are used for fusion or congenital curves, depending on the area of the spine where the anomaly occurs. Surgical interventions for congenital scoliosis may include excision of the anomalous vertebrae, spinal fusion, or both. The fusion most often is performed in situ or without instrumentation on the convex side of the curve to prevent further curve

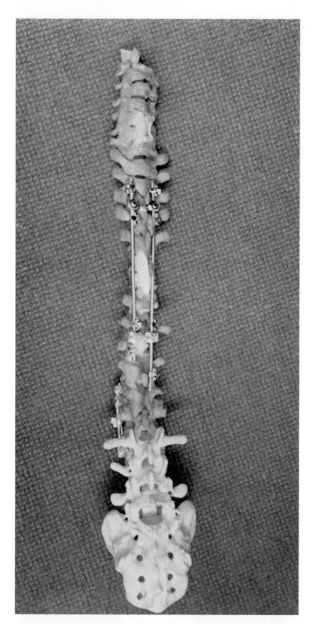

♦ **Figure 11-8** Cotrel-Dubousset instrumentation system implanted on a plastic spine.

progression because the goal of surgery is curve stabilization, not correction (Winter, 1983, 1988).

If a very young, skeletally immature patient has a significant curve that is not responsive to orthotic management, a procedure known as "rod without fusion" may be performed. A single, subcutaneous rod without compressive or distractive forces is placed along the scoliotic curve to control the direction of spinal growth. A fusion is not performed because this would cause a cessation of growth at the fused segments of spine. An orthosis is prescribed for the patient for full-time wear to protect the instrumentation and control any decompensation of the trunk (Herkowitz et al., 1999).

Postoperative Management

The postoperative use of an orthosis depends on the type of curve that was fused, the type of instrumentation used, and the postoperative alignment of the trunk. Postoperatively an orthosis is worn until the fusion is solid as determined by radiograph, typically for 9 to 12 months. Nearly all congenital scoliosis curves require postoperative orthotic or plaster cast treatment to protect the in situ fusion, to promote healing of the fusion, and to help correct any compensatory curves. Idiopathic scoliotic curves managed with a two-stage procedure, Luque rods, or an anterior spinal fusion with instrumentation require orthotic use until the fusion mass is well formed as determined by radiographs. Currently, a child with idiopathic scoliosis who is treated with posterior spinal fusion and Cotrel-Dubousset instrumentation does not require postoperative bracing if the trunk is compensated and the correction is satisfactory.

The average length of a hospital stay for a posterior spinal fusion (or a one-stage procedure) is 5 to 7 days, with physical therapy initiated on the second postoperative day. A physical therapist's role following any spinal fusion procedure includes patient instruction in body mechanics for bed mobility, transfers, dressing, and ambulation. Trunk rotation is contraindicated; therefore the therapist must instruct the patient in log-rolling and in coming from a supine position to sitting without rotation. Shoes and socks are donned or removed with the legs in tailor position, with negligible forward flexion. The therapist may also instruct the patient in donning or removing of the orthosis while in bed, while from a side-lying to a supine position, or while standing with assistance (if not contraindicated by physician's orders). For the acute stage, donning or removing of the orthosis in bed is preferable. The patient is instructed in general ROM and strengthening exercises (without resistance) for the extremities such as isometric quadriceps contractions, straight leg raises, supine abduction, and isometric gluteal sets. Because the patient's functional activities for the first 2 postoperative weeks are limited to showering and walking, the therapist's role is to encourage ambulation. Not only does this enable the patient to experience fewer side effects from bed rest, but it is also beneficial to the development of a strong, healthy fusion mass or arthrodesis.

On discharge from the hospital, the patient's postoperative activity remains restricted. In 1 month, the patient usually returns to school and can lift objects up to 5 pounds. At 3 months following surgery, bicycling, driving, swimming, and light jogging are allowed. The patient is able to lift objects weighing up to 10 pounds and also participate in noncontact sports (with physician approval) by 6 months postoperatively. By 1 year the patient may be involved in routine physical education classes, may lift more than 10 pounds, and may participate in other activities, such as skating, skiing, bowling, and amusement park rides. These guidelines are appropriate for the majority of patients with fusion of congenital and idiopathic curves regardless of which instrumentation is used.

OUTCOMES FOR PERSONS WITH IDIOPATHIC SCOLIOSIS

Most people with AIS live functional and normal lives with a mortality rate similar to that of the general population (Weinstein, 1981; Weinstein et al., 2003). The rate of intermittent back pain in people with curves of modest severity, 40° to 50°, is the same as in the general population (Roach, 1999). Weinstein and colleagues (2003) found that the reported incidence of chronic and acute back pain was significantly higher for persons with untreated idiopathic scoliosis. Large lumbar curves have been associated with increased incidence of low back pain, especially if there is development of lateral translation of the apical vertebrae (Weinstein, 1981).

Severe thoracic curves, greater than 100°, have been shown to decrease pulmonary vital capacity to below 70% to 80% of the normal value (Weinstein, 1981). Shortness of breath was reported by persons with a Cobb angle greater than 80° and a thoracic apex of the curve (Weinstein et al., 2003). Nachemson (1968) has suggested that the mortality rate is twice that of the general population for those with severe thoracic curves, with the risk increased by smoking.

The natural history of idiopathic scoliosis continues into adult life, because curves can progress after skeletal maturity. Risk of progression depends on curve magnitude and location (Lonstein & Winter, 1988). Curves of greater than 45° at the time of skeletal maturity have a higher risk of progressing and producing complications. Although thoracic and lumbar curves can both progress, progression in the thoracic region may cause significant complications because of the effects on the cardiopulmonary system. Complications of untreated scoliosis include severe cosmetic deformity and major disability, which may include pain, respiratory insufficiency, or right-sided heart failure (Herkowitz et al., 1999). Indications for adult treatment include back pain, compromised pulmonary function, psychosocial effects, and increased risk for premature death. The treatment plan is consistent with that for adolescent idiopathic scoliosis (Weinstein, 1989).

NEUROMUSCULAR SCOLIOSIS

The terms *neuromuscular scoliosis* and *myopathic scoliosis* describe curves that are due to neurologic or muscular disorders (Raimondi et al., 1989; McCarthy, 1999). The curve presentation and risk of progression of neuromuscular scoliosis differ from idiopathic or congenital curves in some cases. Curves may be secondary to pelvic obliquity (Lonstein & Renshaw, 1987), unilateral or asymmetric spasticity of trunk musculature, athetosis, or asymmetric movement patterns (Herring, 2002). Often a long "C-type" curve characterizes a neuromuscular curvature (Fig. 11-9), but as compensatory curves become structural, the pattern may change to an "S-type" curve. A neuromuscular curve typically develops at a young age and tends to be progressive (Fisk & Bunch, 1979). The prevalence of spinal deformities varies with the type of neuromuscular disease.

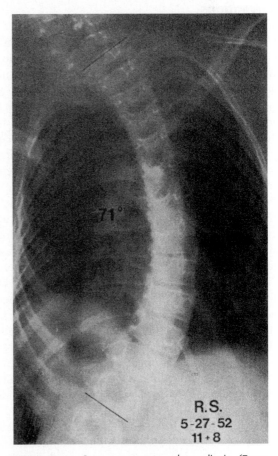

◆ **Figure 11-9**   Severe neuromuscular scoliosis. *(From Moe, JH, Winter, RB, Bradford, DS, Ogilvie, JW, & Lonstein, JE. Scoliosis and Other Spinal Deformities, 2nd ed. Philadelphia: WB Saunders, 1987, p. 277.)*

The highest prevalence of spinal deformities (90–100%) occurs with a dystrophy diagnosis, such as spinal muscular atrophy or muscular dystrophy, and in spinal cord injuries that result in quadriplegia in infants or young children. There is a 60% prevalence of spinal deformity in patients with myelomeningocele and a 25% prevalence in patients with cerebral palsy (Lonstein & Renshaw, 1987).

Etiology and Risk of Progression

The direct cause of neuromuscular scoliosis is unknown. One hypothesis is that spinal stability, which is directly proportional to the condition of the end support of the spine and inversely proportional to spinal flexibility and to the approximate square of spinal column length, is reduced in children with neuromuscular disease. Loss of muscle strength and loss of proprioception may also be factors in the development of scoliosis when it occurs in the relatively flexible and elongating spinal column of a child with a neuromuscular disease (Lonstein & Renshaw, 1987).

Interventions

Nonsurgical intervention of neuromuscular spinal curvatures includes clinical observation, radiographic examination, and orthotic management. Clinical observation allows a thorough assessment of the child's present and potential function, level of comprehension, and ability to cooperate (Fisk & Bunch, 1979). Although no research studies have shown that custom seating is effective in reducing or preventing progression of curves, it is an important part of clinical treatment in which the physical therapist plays a vital role. A good postural support system allows the child to interact with the environment. These children often have multiple disabilities, which are best addressed by the team approach of a physical therapist, an occupational therapist, a physician, an equipment vendor, and an orthotist. Please refer to Chapter 33 in this book regarding appropriate seating options for this population.

The child with a neuromuscular curvature managed by orthotics has special needs that must be considered when ordering or fabricating seating systems. The orthosis eliminates the normal flexibility of the spine, which potentially reduces the child's ability to adjust the footrests, operate the brakes, and propel the chair. A child with a neuromuscular curve may demonstrate pelvic obliquity requiring specialized custom-molded seating to provide adequate support and pressure relief. Because these children may also require lower extremity orthotics, adequate clearance in the seating device is necessary to accommodate orthoses.

Orthotic management might include the custom-molded, total-contact TLSO, underarm TLSO, or Milwaukee brace (Lonstein & Renshaw, 1987). Such orthoses are typically worn during all upright (i.e., sitting or standing) activities but are usually not worn at night.

The use of an orthosis must provide curve stabilization without limiting the child's functional abilities. For example, attempting to control the lordosis in an ambulating child with muscular dystrophy would eliminate compensatory functional posture and result in earlier use of a wheelchair. An orthosis may be used to support the trunk before any measurable deformity is present. For example, a young child with spinal muscular atrophy may be fitted with a TLSO that has the anterior rib portion relieved and covered with elastic material to provide support for use during therapy, during feeding, and while standing in a standing frame. The use of a TLSO can improve head and upper extremity control. An orthosis should also be used to maintain alignment and provide trunk support for children with quadriplegic paralysis secondary to birth injuries or acquired spinal cord injuries. In these children, the use of an orthosis allows for upright orientation and may provide the support necessary for the child to operate a head switch or sip-and-puff mechanism to control an electric wheelchair.

An experimental method, just beginning to be researched, is the use of botulinum toxin type A in the treatment of neuromuscular curves in patients with other severe complicating diseases that have caused delays in surgery. Nuzzo and colleagues (1997) treated 12 children with botulinum type A, as a supplement to other intervention strategies. Short-term results revealed no cases in which the scoliosis worsened. All children had some degree of curve reduction, with some reduction as much as 50°.

If a neuromuscular scoliosis continues to progress, hygiene, nursing care, functional abilities, pulmonary function, and life expectancy may be affected. Once again, a team approach is preferred for optimal management of children with neuromuscular disease.

Surgical Options

Surgical interventions for neuromuscular scoliosis are similar to those for idiopathic scoliosis. The curve may require both anterior and posterior fusion with instrumentation, posterior fusion with instrumentation, or fusion to the pelvis to correct obliquity and maintain symmetry. The goal of surgery is to achieve a stable and compensated spine.

An orthosis is almost always used postoperatively for support and immobilization of the fusion. Orthotic use is most often discontinued when a x-ray reveals adequate arthrodesis. Occasionally the patient may be placed in a body cast (Risser cast) in the operating room to protect against potential sheer stresses before the fabrication of a custom orthosis (Fisk & Bunch, 1979). The orthosis must be on the patient before initiation of out-of-bed mobility, unless otherwise specified by the physician.

The role of the physical therapist is similar to that for postoperative treatment of other curve types. The treatment may need to be modified to adjust to a patient's motor and cognitive abilities.

KYPHOSIS

A *kyphosis* is an abnormal posterior convexity of a segment of the spine. A spinal kyphosis may occur as a result of trauma, congenital conditions, or Scheuermann's disease or secondary to previous treatment of spinal tumors with laminectomy. Spinal kyphosis may also be found in children with osteochondrodystrophies, rickets, osteogenesis imperfecta, idiopathic juvenile osteoporosis, neurofibromatosis, myelomeningocele, and spondyloepiphyseal dysplasia. Spinal kyphosis should be differentiated from postural roundback (Herkowitz et al., 1999; Winter et al., 1973). The discussion in this section focuses on congenital kyphosis, Scheuermann's disease, and kyphosis in children with myelomeningocele.

CONGENITAL KYPHOSIS

Congenital kyphosis results when the anterior part of the vertebra is aplastic or hypoplastic and the posterior elements of the vertebra form normally. An anterior unsegmented failure of formation, or unsegmented bar, leads to progressive kyphosis. Congenital kyphoscoliosis or lordoscoliosis is the result when a combination of defective segmentation occurs at more than one location (Winter, 1983, 1988).

The natural history of congenital kyphosis includes progression, cosmetic deformity, back pain, and neurologic deficit. Congenital kyphosis is the most common cause of spinal cord compression caused by a spinal deformity (Winter et al., 1973). It is a potentially more debilitating deformity than congenital scoliosis without kyphosis. An anterior unsegmented bar at the thoracolumbar junction produces mild to moderate deformities but no reported paraplegia. Paraplegia is frequently noted with a progressive congenital kyphosis located in the upper thoracic spine when the posterior elements grow unaccompanied by anterior growth. The treatment of congenital kyphosis is surgery to prevent further progression (Winter, 1983).

SCHEUERMANN'S DISEASE

Scheuermann's disease is an often neglected deformity that develops during childhood and adolescence and is usually ascribed to poor posture. Diagnosis is made by these radiographic criteria: (1) irregular vertebral end plates, (2) narrowing of the intervertebral disk space, (3) anterior wedging of 5° or greater of one or more vertebrae, and (4) kyphosis greater than 40° that is uncorrected on active hyperextension. Scheuermann's disease can be found in the thoracic spine, producing an increased kyphosis; in the thoracolumbar and lumbar spine, producing a neutral appearance in the sagittal plane; and, more rarely, in the cervical spine (Herkowitz et al., 1999).

Little has been published on the pathophysiology of Scheuermann's disease; however, cadaver dissections have shown that the anterior longitudinal ligament is thickened and taut, as in other kyphoses, and that the vertebral bodies are wedged and the disk spaces narrowed. The spongiosa and bone are irregular and can show disruption where Schmorl's nodules have fractured the bony tubercle. Growth plates are disorderly as a result of this disruption (Herkowitz et al., 1999; Herring, 2002).

Clinical findings include tight pectorals and hamstrings. An increased thoracic kyphosis with a compensatory increased lumbar lordosis and forward head posture are seen. Associated scoliosis is present in 30% to 40% of children with Scheuermann's disease. The disease has also been reported to be transmitted as an autosomal dominant trait with an incidence of 0.4% to 8.3%. Males and females are affected equally. Radiographic findings are often not seen until age 11 (Herring, 2002). The chief complaint of patients is pain at the apex of the kyphosis.

Intervention

Treatment of Scheuermann's disease includes exercise, orthotic management, and surgical management. The prescribed exercises are specific for active trunk extensor strengthening, passive trunk stretching into extension, and general postural exercise (abdominals and gluteals). The child must be instructed to extend at the kyphotic section of the spine (usually thoracic) while maintaining a neutral or slightly flexed cervical and lumbar spine. Exercises addressing abdominal strengthening, especially of lower abdominal muscles, are important to help maintain an upright posture and decrease lumbar lordosis. A patient may have hip flexion contractures from increased lumbar lordosis and increased anterior pelvic tilt, and limited hamstring length as measured by straight leg raising due to kyphotic and crouched posture in sitting and standing. Stretching exercises are incorporated to improve overall alignment (Fig. 11-10). Exercise as the sole treatment has not been established as effective, although it has been shown to be beneficial in conjunction with other methods of treatment (Moe et al., 1987; Herring, 2002).

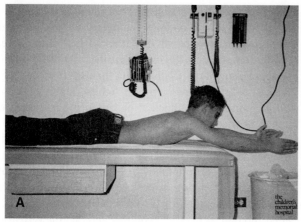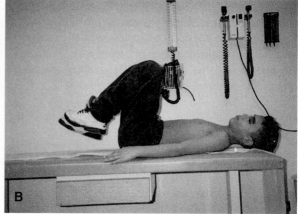

◆ **Figure 11-10** **A**, Active trunk extensor strengthening by prone lifts. **B**, Lower abdominal strengthening exercises.

Orthotic treatment is used when the kyphosis is greater than 50° to 60°. The use of a modified Milwaukee-type brace has a high reported success rate in the skeletally immature patient. The procedure is considered to be successful when the kyphosis decreases and vertebral bodies appear less wedge-shaped on radiographs (Moe et al., 1987).

Surgical management is often a two-stage procedure, with anterior diskectomy and intravertebral grafting coupled with a posterior compression arthrodesis. Posterior fusion alone in a child with a fixed kyphosis greater than 60° may be subject to significant complications and loss of correction of kyphosis with instrumentation failure (Herkowitz et al., 1999).

Postoperative treatment includes plaster casting, orthotic wear, or both. The orthosis of choice is usually a Milwaukee-type brace that can be modified to a TLSO after a 2- to 5-month postoperative period.

Postural Roundback

Postural roundback may often be confused with Scheuermann's disease; however, the kyphosis of postural roundback is not fixed and vertebrae show no end plate irregularity. Exercise alone, as described for treatment of Scheuermann's disease, is the treatment of choice for this condition. If the kyphosis progresses to more than 60°, it may be treated with a Milwaukee brace to prevent permanent structural changes (Moe et al., 1987).

KYPHOSIS AND MYELOMENINGOCELE

Spinal deformities are common in children with myelomeningocele. A congenital lumbar kyphosis, involving the portion of spine from the thoracolumbar junction to the sacrum, is unique to children with myelomeningocele.

Congenital kyphosis is easily recognized at birth because it is rigid and resistant to passive correction. Anatomically the pedicles are widely separated and protrude posterolaterally, accentuating the kyphotic appearance. The pedicles and laminae are splayed, pushing the deep back muscles to an anterior position. These deep back muscles may then serve as pathologic flexors of the lumbar spine (Fig. 11-11). Often, owing to the level of deficit, the psoas muscle is the only innervated muscle. The force of the psoas, coupled with activity in the quadratus lumborum and anterior abdominals, may cause progressive deformity (Herkowitz et al., 1999).

The congenital kyphosis may produce closure problems, caused by size and rigidity of the lesion. Orthopedic surgery, a kyphectomy or spinal osteotomy, may be done at the time of closure to help facilitate the procedure (Sharrad, 1968). Recurrent skin breakdown problems are common; therefore, special attention must be given to the use of adaptive equipment.

The kyphosis usually remains relatively stable until the child sits, using the hands for support. The child's sitting posture is marked by a forward trunk and sacral or lumbar sitting, instead of ischial weight bearing, and there may be a compensatory thoracic lordosis. These children often develop respiratory complications when the anterior rib cage lies on the pelvic brim, causing the abdominal contents to be forced against the diaphragm, restricting excursion and respiratory function (Herkowitz et al., 1999) (Fig. 11-12).

Treatment

Treatment of congenital kyphosis in children with myelomeningocele is limited. Bracing and stretching exercises are of no use because of the rigidity of the deformity and

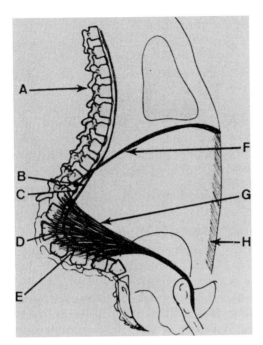

• **Figure 11-11**   Drawing illustrating the deforming forces found in congenital lumbar kyphosis. **A**, Compensatory dorsal lordosis. **B**, Contracted anterior longitudinal ligament. **C**, Contracted anulus fibrosus. **D**, Wedge-shaped vertebral bodies. **E**, Intervertebral disks narrowed anteriorly with the nucleus pulposus shifted posteriorly. **F**, Diaphragm attached to the apex of the deformity. **G**, Psoas muscle is hypertrophied and bowstrings across the curve. **H**, Anterior abdominal musculature. *(From Rothman, RH, & Simeone, FA. The Spine, 2nd ed. Philadelphia: WB Saunders, 1982, p. 252.)*

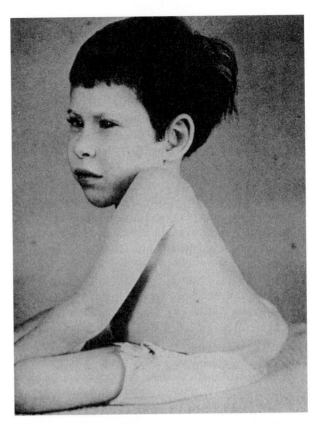

• **Figure 11-12**   Nine-year-old with a congenital lumbar kyphosis. Typical sitting posture serves to accentuate the kyphosis. The child is sitting directly on the sacrum and the lower portion of the lumbar spine. *(From Rothman, RH, & Simeone, FA. The Spine, 2nd ed. Philadelphia: WB Saunders, 1982, p. 252.)*

potential for skin breakdown. Exercises are useful in maintaining good ROM at the hips and shoulders. The surgical procedure, a kyphectomy, is controversial and may produce only limited correction. The procedure requires further research.

Postoperative treatment may include plaster casting or orthotic treatment to protect the fusion. Physical therapy is often involved to maximize endurance and mobility, as outlined in the earlier section on surgery for idiopathic scoliosis.

LORDOSIS

An anterior convexity (or a posterior concavity) of a segment of spine is termed a *lordosis.* Congenital lordosis is the result of bilateral posterior failure of segmentation (Winter, 1983). Lordosis, both fixed and flexible, may be found in children with a variety of diagnoses. Lordosis in children with myelomeningocele usually occurs in the

lumbar spine secondary to use of a tripod gait pattern. A lordosis may develop in the thoracic vertebrae to compensate for an increased lumbar kyphosis (Herkowitz et al., 1999).

Children without motor deficits may have an increased lumbar lordosis. Assessment includes testing of lower extremity ROM, spinal flexibility, trunk and lower extremity strength, posture, and gait. Interventions include abdominal strengthening (curls, crunches, and pelvic lifts), pelvic tilts in a supine position and standing, trunk extensor strengthening, and appropriate lower extremity stretching.

SPONDYLOLISTHESIS

Spondylolisthesis is the forward translatory displacement of one vertebra on another, usually occurring at the fifth lumbar vertebra. Five types of spondylolysis and spondylolisthesis have been classified by Wiltse and associates (1976) as follows:

1. *Dysplastic* malformations develop secondary to congenital malformations of the sacrum and posterior vertebral arch of L5. These malformations may include hypoplasia of the superior surface of the body of S1, hypoplasia-aplasia of the facets, elongation of the pars interarticularis, and spina bifida. The malformations decrease the efficiency of the posterior stabilizing system (Wiltse et al., 1976). The degree of slippage is usually severe and may produce neurologic deficits as the laminae of L5 are pulled against the dural sac (Herring, 2002).

2. *Isthmic* describes slippage occurring secondary to an elongation of the pars interarticularis, a break of the pars interarticularis, or a combination of both with the facets intact. A stress or fatigue fracture of the pars interarticularis is the basic pathologic occurrence. These pathogenic factors can cause elongation of the pars secondary to repeated microfractures that heal with the pars in an attenuated-elongated position. An isthmic spondylolisthesis may also be caused by an acute fracture of the pars (Herring, 2002).

3. A *degenerative* type occurs in adults older than age 50 years and is caused by the structural destruction of the capsule and ligaments of the posterior joints producing hypermobility of the segment.

4. A *traumatic* type, more correctly defined as a fracture, is caused by a sudden fracture of the posterior arch of a vertebral segment. The fracture may occur at the pedicle, laminae, or facet, leaving the pars interarticularis intact.

5. *Pathologic* spondylolisthesis occurs most often secondary to an infectious disease that destroys the posterior arch of the vertebra (Wiltse et al., 1976).

Dysplastic and isthmic spondylolisthesis types are the most common in the pediatric population. Spondylolisthesis is further described by degree of severity as characterized by percentage of slippage, grades I to IV. Grade I is the mildest slippage at less than 25%. Grade II is 25% to 50% slippage. Grade III is 50% to 75%, and grade IV is greater than 75% slippage (Herring, 2002; Wiltse et al., 1976).

Clinical Symptoms

A spondylolisthesis is often discovered on a radiograph taken for some other purpose. The clinical picture includes poor posture and increased lumbar lordosis in mild slippage. Higher-grade slippage may produce a flattened lumbar spine, a crease anteriorly at the umbilicus, and a prominent sacrum (Fig. 11-13). Symptoms may include low back pain relieved by rest, sciatic-type pain, local tenderness, hamstring spasm or tightness, and in severe cases, torso shortening (Herring, 2002).

Risk of Progression

The risk factors, clinically and radiographically, are similar to those for idiopathic scoliosis. Clinically, adolescents who are symptomatic are at a higher risk for increased slippage during their growth spurt. Females are at a greater risk than males, as are patients with increased ligament laxity, including persons with Down syndrome or Marfan syndrome. Radiographically, dysplastic types or patients with a 50% slippage, with a slip angle over 40° to 50°, or with bony instabilities or decreased anatomic stability of L5 and S1 are at greater risk for increased slippage (Moe et al., 1987; Herring, 2002).

Nonsurgical Intervention

Observation is the treatment of choice, with asymptomatic spondylolisthesis causing less than 50% slippage. These children are routinely followed two times per year with clinical and radiographic examinations. Normal activities are allowed if the degree of slippage is less than 25%. Activities such as weight lifting and contact sports are restricted in patients with a slippage greater than 25%. Patients also learn lumbar stabilization exercises in which they are taught to maintain pain-free, neutral alignment of the pelvis and lumbar spine while they vary their positions (O'Sullivan et al., 1997). Exercises include bridging, wall squats, abdominal strengthening, prone gluteal strengthening, and other stabilization exercises in supine. A therapeutic exercise ball may be incorporated into the exercise session to allow patients to achieve and maintain neutral lumbar spine stabilization on a mobile surface.

A lumbosacral orthosis is used to manage the symptomatic patient with a slippage percentage of less than 25%. Orthotic intervention may also be used to conservatively treat patients with a slippage of 25% to 50%. If symptoms persist, surgery is indicated.

Surgical Intervention

The indications for surgery are persistent back pain despite conservative measures including physical therapy, gait deviations, greater than 50% slippage, marked instability of the defect with slip progression, neurologic deficit/radiculopathy, or hamstring contracture (Herring, 2002). The goals of surgery are to prevent further slippage, immobilize the unstable segment, prevent further neurologic deficit and relieve any nerve root irritation, and correct clinical symptoms of poor posture, gait, and decreased hamstring length (Herring, 2002).

Surgical options are posterolateral arthrodesis, anterior arthrodesis, decompression, and reduction and instrumentation. The surgical procedure most often performed is a bilateral posterolateral arthrodesis in situ. The fusion usually extends from L4 to S1 and is performed with an

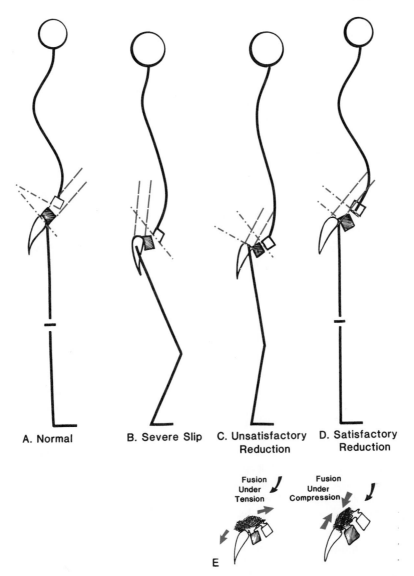

• **Figure 11-13**   **A**, Normal sagittal plane spinal alignment. **B**, Loss of alignment can be visualized following a severe L5 spondylolisthesis. The sacrum becomes vertical, and the resultant lumbosacral kyphosis "pushes" the lumbar spine forward. **C**, An unsatisfactory reduction occurs when L5 has little mobility and L4 lies anterior to the "anatomic zone" and is kyphotic in relationship to the sacrum. The fusion in this case will be under tension and less likely to hold. **D**, A satisfactory reduction occurs when L4 can be placed in the anatomic zone and oriented lordotic in relation to the sacrum. **E**, The more L4 can be positioned over the sacrum, the more posterior compressive forces will be directed across the fusion. In this position, sagittal plane alignment and hence deformity will be corrected. *(From Moe, JH, Winter, RB, Bradford, DS, Ogilvie, JW, & Lonstein, JE. Scoliosis and Other Spinal Deformities, 2nd ed. Philadelphia: WB Saunders, 1987, p. 418.)*

iliac bone graft (Grzegorzewski & Kumar, 2000). In severe cases, a combination of anterior and posterior arthrodesis may be used. The patients are immobilized in a TLSO brace with a thigh extension for 6 weeks to 3 months and then in a TLSO until the fusion is solid (VanRens & VanHorn, 1982; Verbeist, 1979). Physical therapy is indicated for bed mobility, gait training, and activities of daily living and may be initiated to regain normal hamstring flexibility.

A neurologic deficit is the most common reason to perform a decompression. A decompression consists of removal of the bony anatomy that is causing nerve root irritation. The segments are then fused posteriorly to prevent further slippage (VanRens & VanHorn, 1982; Verbeist, 1979).

A reduction of the spondylolisthesis is indicated in cases in which the sacrum is in a vertical position causing a severe lumbosacral kyphosis that displaces the lumbar spine anteriorly (see Fig. 11-13). The result is a marked compensatory lumbar lordosis. Closed and open reductions techniques are used currently. Closed reduction techniques include traction and casting with the goal being to stretch the soft tissue and realign the vertebrae. An open reduction technique can be anterior or posterior, with or without instrumentation, or a combination of surgical approaches may be used. An anterior fibular strut graft may be used for severe slips (Hu et al., 1996).

SUMMARY

Scoliosis, kyphosis, and lordosis are common pediatric orthopedic conditions of the spine. We, as pediatric physical therapists, often concentrate our therapy for many types of patients on the trunk for midline activities, symmetry, and stability for movement, and therefore we can play a vital role in early detection of spinal deformities. We encourage children to become active to improve their cardiorespiratory function, muscle strength, and endurance. We can provide a referral source for families, instruction in home exercises, input for selecting appropriate adaptive equipment and seating, and rehabilitative intervention following injury or surgery. We address issues concerning the spine on a daily basis and play an important role in achieving and maintaining good health through maximizing proper alignment and function.

CASE STUDIES

ANN

Examination

Ann, a 15-year-old girl with a diagnosis of idiopathic scoliosis (curves measuring 45° right thoracic and 42° left lumbar), was referred to physical therapy for assessment and intervention. Ann wished to increase her participation in extracurricular activities and improve her overall physical endurance. She wore a Lyon-type TLSO full time and knew that she would require a posterior spinal fusion in the future. The examination included testing of (1) lower extremity ROM; (2) lower extremity strength by manual muscle test; (3) trunk strength; (4) trunk flexibility; (5)

trunk symmetry, including levels of bony prominences (i.e., iliac crest, inferior border of scapulae); (6) activity level; (7) posture; and (8) gait.

Evaluation

The evaluation of the test findings revealed decreased trunk flexibility in all planes (forward flexion by one half, lateral flexion by one third, and extension by one fourth) and limited hamstring length (145° popliteal angle bilaterally). Cosmetically, she was well compensated in her trunk with curves of essentially equal magnitude. No formal cardiopulmonary testing was performed, but according to patient history, Ann was unable to walk more than 15 to 20 minutes without fatigue.

Diagnosis

Ann had general deconditioning of the cardiopulmonary and musculoskeletal systems. Impairments included primary anatomic changes of the vertebrae and surrounding structures; decreased spinal, trunk, and lower extremity ROM secondary to full-time orthotic wear; decreased trunk strength secondary to inactivity; and decreased endurance secondary to limited activity caused by orthotic wear. Because physical therapy cannot change the underlying pathophysiology of the spine in scoliosis, the impairments of trunk strength, decreased flexibility, and decreased cardiopulmonary endurance were addressed.

Prognosis and Plan of Care

Physical therapy intervention was recommended for a short duration. Outcomes and goals were set to address improvement in trunk flexibility, increased cardiopulmonary fitness, and improved participation in extracurricular activities.

Interventions

The primary intervention in this case was patient-related instruction. Ann was instructed in proper body mechanics to adjust to limited trunk mobility and in trunk strengthening and flexibility exercises to be performed daily when not wearing the orthosis. The exercises (knees to chest, pelvic tilts, four-point trunk extensor strengthening, curl-ups, oblique curl-ups, lateral flexion, and trunk shift) were specifically designed to address trunk flexion, trunk rotation, abdominal strength, and trunk extensor–hip extensor strength while avoiding hyperextension of the spine. Her physical therapy also addressed her cardiorespiratory status. She was started on a daily walk-run program with a goal of 45 minutes three to five times per week. She also rode a stationary bicycle for 20 to 30 minutes during each treatment session.

In most instances, Ann was allowed to participate in noncontact, organized sports activities. The physical therapist encouraged wearing the orthosis when possible during these activities. The physical therapist also played an important role in helping Ann understand the importance of maintaining flexibility and strength in preparation for a faster recovery following her anticipated posterior spinal fusion.

Outcomes

A checklist system was used to follow Ann's compliance with home exercises and orthotic wear. After initial sessions for evaluation and teaching of a home program, Ann was followed in the clinic at regular intervals (6–8 weeks) to reevaluate strength, flexibility, and ROM as additional indicators of compliance.

Ann was an active participant and very compliant with her flexibility and strengthening exercises. Her hamstring length improved to normal as measured by straight leg raise, her forward flexion was limited by one third, and she played on her school's basketball team. She was discharged from therapy after 3 months because she was continuing with a home program. She will undergo a posterior spinal fusion with Cotrel-Dubousset instrumentation in the future.

K A T I E

Examination

Katie, a 14-year-old girl with a diagnosis of athetoid cerebral palsy and a scoliosis measuring 54° (right thoracolumbar) out of her orthosis and 42° in her orthosis (custom-molded TLSO), was seen in a scoliosis clinic.

Katie received physical therapy twice weekly at her home. Her highest level of activity was limited household ambulation. She was a potential surgical candidate.

The physical therapy examination included testing of (1) posture in prone, supine, sitting, and standing positions; (2) lower extremity ROM; (3) lower extremity manual muscle strength, including cortical control and in-pattern grades; (4) balance in sitting and standing positions; (5) muscle tone; and (6) primitive reflexes.

Evaluation

Findings included bilateral hip flexion contracture of 15°; poor voluntary control of distal lower extremity musculature; ability to move from sitting to standing with minimal to moderate assistance by one person; athetoid/fluctuating tone; and present, but not obligatory, right asymmetric tonic neck reflex. Katie's activity limitations included (1) inability to perform independent self-care owing to decreased balance; (2) inability to efficiently propel her manual wheelchair owing to orthotic wear; and (3) inability to independently obtain and maintain proper postural alignment of the trunk because of the influence of primitive reflexes, trunk weakness, abnormal tone, and decreased proprioception.

Diagnosis

Katie had limitations of her neuromuscular systems. Impairments included (1) primary anatomic changes in the vertebrae, supporting structures, and musculature of the trunk; (2) decreased midline orientation abilities due to spinal deformity and cerebral palsy; (3) decreased spinal mobility due to orthotic wear; and (4) decreased ability to use compensations of the trunk during household ambulation due to orthotic restrictions.

Prognosis and Plan of Care

It was determined that intensive physical therapy services for a short duration would be indicated to address activity limitations. Physical therapy services addressed (1) assisted training in activities of daily living, (2) independent mobility with wheelchair modifications or change to an electric device, (3) balance, (4) endurance for facilitated ambulation, and (5) postural alignment and midline orientation in all positions.

Interventions

Katie and her family actively participated in direct physical therapy services as well as a home exercise program. Physical therapy addressed impairments through services two to three times per week, emphasizing trunk strengthening (abdominals, gluteals, extensors), active-assistive ROM of bilateral lower extremities, and facilitated weight bearing and ambulation to improve endurance and function.

Outcomes

Over 4 months, Katie progressed to require only minimal assistance for household ambulation. She started using a motorized wheelchair for community mobility in order to participate more fully in school and social activities.

The physical therapist plays a role in determining function, the effect of an orthosis on function, and the potential effect of surgical fusion on the child's function. To accomplish these objectives it is necessary to maintain verbal or written contact regarding the child's progress or regression with the child's orthopedic physician. In this particular case, surgery was postponed because the child was making improvements in independent household ambulation. Katie is expected to require surgery in the future, but her improved endurance and independence will give her an advantage for the procedure itself, as well as for recovery time.

ABBEY

Examination

Abbey, a 12-year-old girl with a diagnosis of grade III spondylolisthesis, was seen in a scoliosis clinic. A posture assessment, as well as ROM assessment, was completed.

Evaluation

Her clinical examination revealed (1) tight hamstrings with decreased ROM to 40° as measured by straight leg raising; (2) antalgic, crouch-type gait; (3) anterior abdominal crease at the level of the umbilicus; and (4) posterior pelvic tilt with prominent "heart-shaped" sacrum due to spasm of the hamstrings because of nerve root irritation. Surgery was recommended for reduction of the spondylolisthesis coupled with a fusion. Postoperatively this child wore a TLSO for immobilization.

Diagnosis and Prognosis

Her pathophysiologic features included (1) primary anatomic changes of the vertebrae and surrounding structures, (2) neurologic changes of the lower extremities secondary to nerve root pressure caused by the primary slippage of the vertebrae, and (3) potential for permanent neurologic changes of lower extremities and bowel and bladder if no intervention occurred. The associated impairments and activity limitations expected if there was no surgical intervention included (1) low back pain; (2) potential for decreased lower extremity function due to neurologic changes; (3) altered gait; and (4) altered alignment of spine and pelvis causing difficulties with clothing, sitting for long periods of time, and endurance. After surgery, activity limitations included decreased trunk strength and limited participation in extracurricular activities.

Interventions

Physical therapy included hamstring stretching, body mechanics instruction, and gait re-education. Physical therapy addressed the postsurgical issues through reha-

bilitation exercises once the fusion was stable. The child participated in pool activities, lumbar stabilization activities using the Swiss ball, and cardiovascular endurance activities after her fusion was stable. Proper surgical management and rehabilitation allowed this child to return to pain-free participation in desired activities.

▋ REFERENCES

Basset, GS, Burness, WP, & MacEwen, GD. Treatment of scoliosis with a Wilmington brace: Results in patients with 20–29 degree curves. Journal of Bone and Joint Surgery (American), 68:602–605, 1986.

Bertrand, SL, Drvaric, DM, Lange, N, Lucas, PR, Deutsch, SD, Herdon, JH, & Roberts, JM. Electrical stimulation for idiopathic scoliosis. Clinical Orthopedics and Related Research, 276:176–181, 1992.

Bleck, E. Annotation—Adolescent idiopathic scoliosis. Developmental Medicine and Child Neurology, 33:167–176, 1991.

Bunnell, W: An objective criterion for scoliosis screening. Journal of Bone and Joint Surgery (American), 66:1381–1387, 1984.

Byl, NN, & Gray, JM. Complex balance reactions in different sensory conditions: Adolescents with and without idiopathic scoliosis. Journal of Orthopaedic Research, 11:215–227, 1993.

Bylund, P, Aaro, S, Gottfries, B, & Jansson, E. Is lateral electric surface stimulation an effective treatment for scoliosis? Journal of Pediatric Orthopedics, 7:298–300, 1987.

Calvo, JJ. Observations on the growth of the female adolescent spine and its relationship to scoliosis. Clinical Orthopedics, 10:40–47, 1957.

Carman, D, Roach, JW, Speck, G, Wenger, DR, & Herring, JA. Role of exercises in the Milwaukee brace treatment of scoliosis. Journal of Pediatric Orthopedics, 11:65–68, 1985.

Carr, WA, Moe, JH, & Winter, RB. Treatment of idiopathic scoliosis in the Milwaukee brace, long term results. Journal of Bone and Joint Surgery (American), 62:8–15, 1980.

Cowell, HR, Hall, JN, & MacEwen, GD. Genetic aspects of idiopathic scoliosis. Clinical Orthopedics, 86:121–132, 1972.

Dickson, RA, Lawton, JD, Archer, JA, & Butt, WP. The pathogenesis of idiopathic scoliosis. Journal of Bone and Joint Surgery (British), 66:8–15, 1984.

Dobbs, MB, & Weinstein, SL. Infantile and juvenile scoliosis. Orthopedic Clinics of North America, 30:331–341, 1999.

Drummond, DS. A perspective on recent trends for scoliosis correction. Clinical Orthopedics and Related Research, 264:90–102, 1991.

Duval-Beaupere, G. The growth of scoliosis patients: hypothesis and preliminary study. Acta Orthopaedica Belgica, 38:365–376, 1972.

Emans, JB, Kaelin, A, Bancel, P, Hall, JE, & Miller, ME. The Boston bracing system for idiopathic scoliosis: Follow-up results in 295 patients. Spine, 11:792–801, 1986.

Farady, JA. Current principles in the non-operative management of structural adolescent idiopathic scoliosis. Physical Therapy, 63:512–523, 1983.

Fisk, JR, & Bunch, WH. Scoliosis in neuromuscular disease. Orthopedic Clinics of North America, 10:863–875, 1979.

Goldstein, LA, & Waugh, TR. Classification and terminology of scoliosis. Clinical Orthopedics, 93:10–22, 1973.

Green, N. Part-time bracing of adolescent idiopathic scoliosis. Journal of Bone and Joint Surgery (American), 68:738–742, 1986.

Grzegorzewski, A, & Kumar, SJ. In situ posterolateral spine arthrodesis for grades III, IV, and V spondylolisthesis in children and adolescents. Journal of Pediatric Orthopedics, 20:506–511, 2000.

Herkowitz, HN, Gardfin, SR, Balderson, RA, Eismont, FJ, Bell, GR, & Wiesel, SW. Rothman-Simeone: The Spine. Philadelphia: WB Saunders, 1999.

Herring, JA. Tachdjian's Pediatric Orthopedics, 3rd ed. Philadelphia: WB Saunders, 2002, pp. 213–312, 323–349, 1279–1291.

Hu, SS, Bradford, DS, Transfeldt, EE, & Cohen, M. Reduction of high-grade spondylolisthesis using Edwards instrumentation. Spine, 21:367–371, 1996.

Katz, DE, & Durrani, AA. Factors that influence outcome in bracing large curve in patients with adolescent idiopathic scoliosis. Spine, 26:2354–2361, 2001.

Katz, DE, Richards, S, Browne, RH, & Herring, JA. A comparison between the Boston brace and the Charleston bending brace in adolescent idiopathic scoliosis. Spine, 22:1302–1312, 1997.

Kehl, DK, & Morrissy, RT. Brace treatment in adolescent idiopathic scoliosis: An update on concepts and technique. Clinical Orthopedics and Related Research, 229:34–43, 1988.

Kostuik, JP. Current concepts review operative treatment of idiopathic scoliosis. Journal of Bone and Joint Surgery (American), 72:1108–1113, 1990.

Lonstein, JE, & Renshaw, TS. Neuromuscular Spine Deformities. Instructional Course Lectures, Vol. 36. St. Louis: Mosby, 1987, pp. 285–304.

Lonstein, JE, & Winter, RB. Adolescent idiopathic scoliosis. Orthopedic Clinics of North America, 19:239–246, 1988.

McCarthy, RE. Management of neuromuscular scoliosis. Orthopedic Clinics of North America, 30:435–449, 1999.

McInnes, E, Hill, DL, Raso, VJ, Chetner, B, Greenhill, BJ, & Moreau, MJ. Vibratory response in adolescents who have idiopathic scoliosis. Journal of Bone and Joint Surgery (American), 73:1208–1212, 1991.

Miller, NH. Cause and natural history of adolescent idiopathic scoliosis. Orthopedic Clinics of North America, 30:343–352, 1999.

Moe, JH, Sundberg, AB, & Gustlio, R. A clinical study of spine fusion in the growing child. Journal of Bone and Joint Surgery (British), 46:784–785, 1964.

Moe, JH, Winter, RB, Bradford, DS, Ogilvie, JW, & Lonstein, JE. Scoliosis and Other Spinal Deformities, 2nd ed. Philadelphia: WB Saunders, 1987, pp. 162–228, 237–261, 347–368, 403–434.

Nachemson, A. A long-term follow-up study of non-treated scoliosis. Acta Orthopaedica Scandinavica, 39:466–476, 1968.

Nault, ML, Allard, P, Hinse, S, LeBlanc, R, Caron, O, Labelle, H & Sadeghi, H. Relations between standing stability and body posture parameters in adolescent idiopathic scoliosis. Spine 27:1911–1917, 2002.

Nuzzo, RM, Walsh, S, Boucherit, T, & Massood, S. Counterparalysis for treatment of paralytic scoliosis with botulism toxin type A. American Journal of Orthopedics, 26:201–207, 1997.

O'Sullivan, PB, Phyty, GD, Twomey OT, & Allison, GT. Evaluation of specific stabilizing exercise in the treatment of chronic low back pain with radiologic diagnosis of spondylolysis or spondylolisthesis. Spine, 22:2259–2267, 1997.

Piazza, MR, & Basset, GS. Curve progression after treatment with the Wilmington brace for idiopathic scoliosis. Journal of Pediatric Orthopedics, 10:39–43, 1990.

Price, CT, Scott, DS, Reed, FR, Jr, & Riddick, MF. Nighttime bracing for adolescent idiopathic scoliosis with the Charleston bending brace: Preliminary report. Spine, 15:1294–1299, 1990.

Price, CT, Scott, DS, Reed, FR, Jr, & Riddick, MF. Nighttime bracing for adolescent idiopathic scoliosis with the Charleston bending brace: Long-term follow-up. Journal of Pediatric Orthopedics, 17:703–707, 1997.

Raimondi, AJ, Choux, M, & Dirocco, C. The Pediatric Spine: II. Developmental Anomalies. New York: Springer-Verlag, 1989, pp. 189–220.

Renshaw, TS. Orthotic Treatment of Idiopathic Scoliosis and Kyphosis. Instructional Course Lectures, Vol. 34. St. Louis: Mosby, 1985, pp. 110–118.

Rinsky, RA, & Gamble, JG. Adolescent idiopathic scoliosis. Western Journal of Medicine, 148:183–191, 1988.

Roach, JW. Adolescent idiopathic scoliosis. Orthopedic Clinics of North America, 30:353–365, 1999.

Rogala, E, Drummond, DS, & Gurr, J. Scoliosis: Incidence and natural history. Journal of Bone and Joint Surgery (American), 60:173–176, 1978.

Rothman, RH, & Simeone, FA. The Spine, 2nd ed. Philadelphia: WB Saunders, 1982, pp. 239–255, 263–282, 316–439.

Sarwark, JF, & Kramer, A. Pediatric spinal deformity. Current Opinions in Pediatrics, 101:82–86, 1998.

Sharrad, WJW. Spinal osteotomy for congenital kyphosis in myelomeningocele. Journal of Bone and Joint Surgery (British), 50:466–471, 1968.

Tachdjian, MO. Pediatric Orthopedics, 2nd ed. Philadelphia: WB Saunders, 1990, p. 2285.

Tanner, JM, & Whitehouse, RH. Clinical longitudinal standards for height, weight, height velocity and stages of puberty. Archives of Disease in Childhood, 51:170–179, 1976.

Tanner, JM, Whitehouse, RH, & Takaisni, M. Standards from birth to maturity for height, weight, height velocity and weight velocity: British children, 1965. Archives of Disease in Childhood, 47:454–471, 613–635, 1966.

van Rens, TG, & van Horn, JR. Long-term results in lumbosacral interbody fusion for spondylolisthesis. Acta Orthopaedica Scandinavica, 53:383–392, 1982.

Verbeist, H. The treatment of lumbar spondyloptosis or impending lumbar spondyloptosis accompanied by neurologic deficit and/or neurogenic intermittent claudication. Spine, 4:68–77, 1979.

Weinstein, SL. Adolescent idiopathic scoliosis: Prevalence and natural history. In Weinstein, SL (Ed.). The Pediatric Spine. New York: Raven Press, 1994, pp. 463–478.

Weinstein, SL. Adolescent idiopathic scoliosis: Prevalence and natural history. Instructional Course Lectures, Vol. 38, Chap. 6. St. Louis: Mosby, 1989.

Weinstein SL, Dolan, LA, Spratt, KF, Peterson, KK, Spoonamore, MJ, & Ponseti, IV. Health and function of patients with untreated idiopathic scoliosis: A 50-year natural history study. Journal of the American Medical Association, 289:559–567, 2003.

Weinstein, SL, Zavala, DC, & Ponseti, IV. Idiopathic scoliosis: Long-term follow-up and prognosis in untreated patients. Journal of Bone and Joint Surgery (American), 63:702–712, 1981.

Weiss, HR, Weiss, G, & Petermann, F. Incidence of curvature progression in idiopathic scoliosis patients treated with scoliosis inpatient rehabilitation (SIR): An age- and sex-matched controlled study. Pediatric Rehabilitation, 6:23–30, 2003.

Wiltse, LL, Newman, PH, & MacNab, I. Classification of spondylolysis and spondylolisthesis. Clinical Orthopedics, 117:23–29, 1976.

Winter, RB. Congenital Deformities of the Spine. New York: Thieme-Stratton, 1983, pp. 6–10, 43–49.

Winter, RB. Congenital scoliosis. Orthopedic Clinics of North America, 19:395–408, 1988.

Winter, RB, Moe, JH, & Wang, JF. Congenital kyphosis: Its natural history and treatment as observed in a study of one hundred and thirty patients. Journal of Bone and Joint Surgery (American), 55:223–256, 1973.

Wynarsky, GT, & Schultz, AB. Trunk muscle activities in braced scoliosis patients. Spine, 14:1283–1286, 1989.

Wynne-Davies, R. Familial (idiopathic) scoliosis. Journal of Bone and Joint Surgery (British), *50*:24–30, 1968.

Wynne-Davies, R. Infantile idiopathic scoliosis. Causative factors, particularly in the first six months of life. Journal of Bone and Joint Surgery (British), *57*:138–141, 1975.

Wynne-Davies, R. Congenital vertebral anomalies: Etiology and relationship to spina bifida cystica. Journal of Medical Genetics, *12*:280–288, 1975.

Zaouss, AL, & James, JIP. The iliac apophysis and the evolution of curves in scoliosis. Journal of Bone and Joint Surgery (British), *40*:442–453, 1958.

Chapter 12

CONGENITAL MUSCULAR TORTICOLLIS

KAREN KARMEL-ROSS
PT, PCS, LMT

Newborns may exhibit positional deformities at birth related to the intrauterine environment. One condition thought to be caused by in utero constraint that pediatric physical therapists need to have an understanding of is congenital muscular torticollis (CMT). CMT describes the posture of the head and neck from unilateral shortening of the sternocleidomastoid (SCM) muscle, causing the head to tilt toward and rotate away from the affected SCM muscle. In addition to the rotation and tilting, the infant may exhibit asymmetric neck extension and a forward head posture due to upper cervical extension. The muscular torticollis is named for the side of the involved SCM muscle.

If the muscular torticollis has developed secondary to gestational fetal constraint (versus trauma to the SCM during labor and delivery), characteristics noted at birth may also include deformation of the craniofacial skeleton on the same side as the affected SCM. These skeletal changes are caused by compression of the anterior chest and shoulder against the face and the resultant impact of mechanical forces on otherwise normal tissue, causing associated positional deformation (Chang et al., 1996; Cheng et al., 2000b; Clarren & Smith, 1977; Clarren, 1981; Davids et al., 1993; Dunn, 1974; Dunn, 1976; Graham, 1998; Graham, 2002; Ho et al., 1999; Yu et al., 2003).

The primary goal of intervention for CMT is to restore full neck movement as early as possible to help reverse or stop the progression of skull base deformity, to prevent cranial facial asymmetry, and to prevent bony and postural changes that may cause asymmetric motor development. The etiology and pathophysiology, examination, associated condition of deformational plagiocephaly, and intervention strategies and expected outcomes for CMT will be discussed in this chapter.

ETIOLOGY AND PATHOPHYSIOLOGY

There is little agreement on the etiology of congenital muscular torticollis. Theories include direct injury to the muscle, ischemic injury based on abnormal vascular patterns, rupture of the muscle, infective myositis, neurogenic injury, hereditary factors, and intrauterine compartment syndrome. The most often cited and most widely accepted theories are ischemia, birth trauma, and intrauterine malposition (Bredenkamp et al., 1990; Cooperman,

1997; Jones, 1968; McDaniel et al., 1984; Tom et al., 1987; Wei et al., 2001). Davids and colleagues (1993) postulated that head position in utero can selectively injure the SCM muscle, leading to the development of a perinatal compartment syndrome. In part, this theory may explain the upper extremity weakness one may observe on the same side as the involved SCM muscle. Position of the head and neck in utero or during labor and delivery of forward flexion, lateral bending, and rotation may cause a compression injury of the ipsilateral SCM muscle and brachial plexus, resulting in ischemia, reperfusion, edema, and neurologic injuries.

Muscular torticollis is the third most common congenital musculoskeletal anomaly after dislocated hip and clubfoot, with reports of incidence varying from 0.3% to 1.9% of newborns (Coventry & Harris, 1959; Cheng & Au, 1994; Cheng et al., 2001; Dunn, 1974; Jones, 1968; Ling, 1976). Associated with muscular torticollis at birth are ipsilateral mandibular asymmetry, ear displacement, plagiocephaly, scoliosis, pelvic asymmetry, congenital dislocated hip, and foot deformity (Cheng et al., 2000b; Dunn, 1974; Fulford & Brown, 1976; Graham, 2002; Hamanishi, 1994; Hollier et al., 2000; Hsieh et al., 2000; Jones, 1968; Smith, 1981; Tien et al., 2001; Watson, 1971).

The incidence of plagiocephaly has increased significantly since it was recommended that infants be placed on their backs to sleep to prevent sudden infant death syndrome (SIDS) in the 1992 "Back to Sleep" campaign (Argenta et al, 1996; Boere-Boonekamp & van der Linden-Kuiper, 2001; Huang et al., 1998, Huang et al., 1995; Kane et al., 1996; Najarian, 1999; Persing et al., 2003; Turk et al., 1996). Dunn (1974) reported the incidence of plagiocephaly and torticollis at 1 in 300 live births of prone sleeping infants. More recently, the incidence of plagiocephaly has been reported to have increased to as high as 1 in 60 live births, which may be partially explained by infants sleeping on their backs (Argenta et al., 1996; Boere-Boonekamp & van der Linden-Kuiper, 2001; Kane et al., 1996; Turk et al., 1996). Habal and colleagues (2003) have suggested in their research that a new syndrome, the "flathead" syndrome, is being introduced and may identify neurocognitive difference or delay disorders among patients who may have appeared normal prior to change in sleep position. It is hypothesized that infants born with torticollis are at risk for developing deformational plagiocephaly and this risk may be reduced if early intervention is initiated (Chang et al., 1996; Clarren, 1981; Graham, 2002; Graham et al., 2005a; Graham et al., 2005b).

If cranial deformation begins in utero, the deformational forces on the occiput may continue after birth if the infant sleeps supine and also spends time in supine or semisupine during waking hours. In this case, the cranial deformation may worsen after birth because the infant cannot yet move the head away from the supporting surface.

The risk factors for muscular torticollis and plagiocephaly are similar and include large birth weight, male gender, breech position, multiple birth, primiparous mother, difficult labor and delivery, use of vacuum or forceps assist, nuchal cord, and maternal uterine abnormalities (Boere-Boonekamp & van der Linden-Kuiper, 2001; Clarren, 1981; Dunn, 1974; Ho et al., 1999; Ling, 1976; Stellwagon et al., 2004; Smith, 1981).

The typical history of congenital muscular torticollis includes the appearance of a fibrous tumor (usually 1–3 cm in diameter and spindle shaped) in the SCM muscle between 14 and 21 days after birth (Fig. 12-1), although the first appearance can be as late as 3 months. The tumor will then disappear by 4 to 8 months of age. If the diagnosis is made within 2 to 6 weeks after birth, the term "pseudotumor of infancy" may be used (Jones, 1968; Wei et al., 2001).

Biopsy of the tumor reveals the histologic appearance of a fibroma. The tumor is characterized by a deposition of collagen and fibroblasts around the individual muscle fibers, with an absence of normal striated muscle. The severity and distribution of the fibrosis, its location within the muscle, individual growth patterns, and the amount of atrophy of normal muscle tissue will vary among patients. The nature of the fibrous tissue in the neonate suggests the disease may begin before birth and be related to in utero fetal positioning (Chan et al., 1992; Cheng et al., 2000b; Hsu et al., 1999; Jones, 1968; Lin & Chou, 1997; Simon et al., 2002; Tien et al., 2001). One may observe an associated head tilt because (1) the healthy myoblasts degenerate, (2) the remaining fibroblasts produce excess collagen, which results in a scar-like band and muscle contracture, or (3) the infant is unable to maintain a vertical head against gravity in static postures or during transitional movement.

Three subtypes of CMT have been identified:
- Sternomastoid tumor (SMT), in which a discrete mass is palpable within the SCM muscle and x-rays are normal
- Muscular torticollis (MT), in which there is tightness but no palpable mass within the SCM muscle and x-rays are normal
- Postural torticollis (POST), in which there is no SCM muscle tightness, no palpable mass, and x-rays are normal

The causes of postural torticollis may be benign paroxysmal torticollis (BPT), congenital absence of one or several cervical muscles or of the transverse ligament, or contracture of other neck muscles (Cheng et al., 2000b, Cheng et al., 2001; Cooperman, 1997).

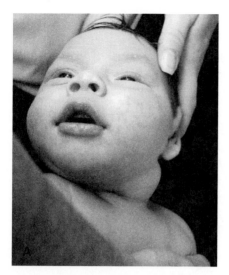
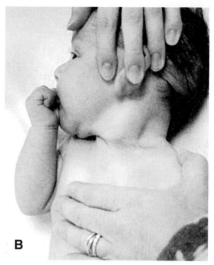

◆ **Figure 12-1**   **A**, Two-month-old infant with a fibrotic tumor in the left sternocleidomastoid (SCM) muscle involving the whole muscle. **B**, Same infant at 3 months of age.

ANATOMY OF THE STERNOCLEIDOMASTOID MUSCLE

The SCM muscle may be called the sternocleido-occipitomastoid, as it comprises four distinct bands (Fig. 12-2). A deep band, the cleidomastoid, runs from the medial third of the clavicle to the mastoid process, and three superficial bands form a "N" shape over the deep band. The three superficial bands are the (1) the cleido-occipital, which overlies the bulk of the cleidomastoid and inserts into the lateral third of the superior nuchal line of the occiput, (2) the sterno-occipital, and (3) the sternomastoid. Both of the latter two superficial bands arise from a common tendon attached to the superior margin of the sternum. The sterno-occipital inserts along with the cleido-occipital into the superior nuchal line, while the sternomastoid inserts into the superior and anterior borders of the mastoid. The SCM muscle is innervated by the second cervical nerve and the spinal portion of the accessory nerve, which also innervates the upper trapezius muscle. Infants with CMT as a result of uterine constraint often have involvement of the upper trapezius muscle on the same side as the involved SCM muscle. The trapezius is a synergist of the ipsilateral SCM muscle and has a similar action as the SCM muscle. The trapezius is also an important mover of the scapula. The contour of the lower part of the neck is formed by the fibers of the trapezius muscle and the contour of the upper part of the neck is formed by the fibers of the SCM muscle (Kapandji, 1974).

DIFFERENTIAL DIAGNOSIS

One in five children presenting with a torticollis posture has a nonmuscular etiology (Ballock & Song, 1996). Nonmuscular causes may include skeletal abnormalities such as Klippel-Feil syndrome or neurologic causes such as brachial plexus injury. Because many lesions can masquerade as congenital muscular torticollis, the initial examination should include a detailed history and a thorough physical examination to determine if the lesion is congenital or acquired. Acquired nontraumatic torticollis may be caused by ocular lesions, Sandifer syndrome, benign paroxysmal torticollis, dystonic syndromes, posterior fossa pathology, postencephalitis syndromes, Arnold-Chiari malformation, and syringomyelia (Cooperman, 1997; Coventry & Harris, 1959).

CHANGES IN BODY STRUCTURE AND FUNCTION (IMPAIRMENTS)

In infants with CMT, neck range of motion is decreased for ipsilateral rotation, contralateral lateral flexion, and contralateral asymmetric flexion and extension. The infant is not able to maintain a midline alignment of the head with the torso in static postures or during movement because of the neck muscle imbalance and muscle

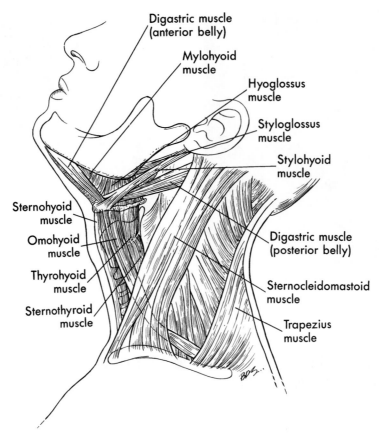

◆ **Figure 12- 2** Sternocleidomastoid muscle and other muscles of the neck. *(From Lingeman, RE. Surgical anatomy. In Cummings, CW, Fredrickson, FM, Harker, LA, Krause CJ, Schuller, DE, & Richardson, MA (Eds.). Otolaryngology: Head and Neck Surgery, Vol. 3, 3rd ed. St. Louis: Mosby, 1998, p. 1680.)*

contracture. Prolonged uncorrected head tilt caused by the underlying mechanism of imbalanced muscle pull acting on the growing spinal and craniofacial skeleton may worsen any scoliosis, skull and facial asymmetry, and influence compensatory movement patterns affecting motor control development (Ferguson, 1993; Karmel-Ross & Lepp, 1997; Shapiro, 1994; Slate et al., 1993; Yu et al., 2003).

Facial and cranial characteristics often observed in infants are shown in Figure 12-3 and include the following:
- Asymmetry of the craniofacial skeletal structures
- Asymmetry of the masticatory and tongue muscles
- Underdevelopment of the ipsilateral jaw; canting of the mandible and gum line; elevation of the temporomandibular joint; dental occlusional problems
- Inferiorly and posteriorly positioned ipsilateral ear; asymmetry of the ears with deformity of the ipsilateral ear, which may be cupped (bat ear)

- Asymmetry of the eyes with ipsilateral eye smaller; inferior orbital dystopia on the ipsilateral side
- Recessed eyebrow and zygoma on the ipsilateral side
- Deviation of the chin point and nasal tip
- Facial scoliosis (distorted craniofacial skeletal structures)
- Cranial base deformation, most prominent change occurring in the posterior cranial fossa

(Chang et al., 2001; Kondo & Aoba, 1999; Ferguson, 1993; Hidaka et al., 1996; Hollier et al., 2000; Shapiro, 1994; Watson, 1971; Yu et al., 2003).

Yu and colleagues (2003) found that cranial base deformity occurs as early as 1 month of age in infants with CMT. They also reported that gross facial deformity of jaw dysmorphology and occlusional tilting may worsen until 5 years of age and young adults with untreated CMT had asymmetric facial height and orbit size. Mandibular asymmetry was the most significant consistent finding of

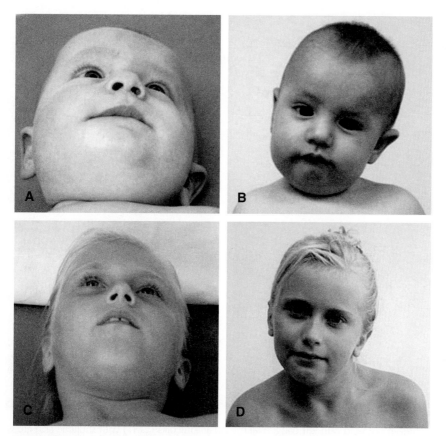

• **Figure 12-3   A,** Submental view of an 8-month-old infant with left congenital muscular torticollis (CMT) and frontal deformational plagiocephaly. Note recession of the frontal bone, eyebrow, and zygoma on the ipsilateral side and inferiorly and posteriorly positioned ipsilateral ear. **B,** En face view shows hemihypoplasia of the face, decreased vertical facial height on the left, asymmetry of the eyes with the ipsilateral eye smaller, inferior orbital dystopia, canting of the mandible, and deviation of chin and nasal tip. **C,** Submental view of an 8-year-old with untreated left CMT and frontal deformational plagiocephaly demonstrating the same facial asymmetries as the 8-month-old infant. **D,** En face view of same 8-year-old demonstrates similar cranial facial asymmetries and shortening of the left sternocleidomastoid muscle.

facial bone deformity. Ho and colleagues (1999) found that 60% (13 of 22 patients) with CMT had mandibular hypoplasia at birth. They identified mandibular hypoplasia as an early sign of CMT.

Slate and colleagues (1993) demonstrated a relationship between craniofacial asymmetry, congenital muscular torticollis, and cervical spine subluxation. They documented that 26 out of 30 patients with CMT had a C1–C2 subluxation with C1 rotated forward on C2. They suggested this finding may help explain the residual asymmetric head and neck tilt observed in children even after extensive physical therapy intervention for CMT.

Other neck muscles may be involved either secondary to the SCM muscle tightness or without SCM tightness if the in utero position of the infant's head and neck posture was one of lateral flexion and rotation to the same side. Often observed with CMT is anterior neck muscle tightness affecting the platysma, scalenus, hyoids, tongue, and facial muscles, contributing to difficulty in the development of oral motor skills and development of head extension in the prone position (Fig. 12-4).

Other musculoskeletal asymmetries may include trunk curvature toward the affected SCM, persistence of the asymmetric tonic neck reflex, and windswept hips with the hip joint markedly abducted on the facial side and adducted on the occipital side, causing the pelvis to tilt when the legs are brought together. When infants acquire the ability to sit, a double spinal curve may develop as the infant compensates for the head tilt and tries to bring the center of gravity over the base of support and compensate for contracture of the hip and pelvic tilt. Jones (1968) found that some children may elevate the shoulder, which

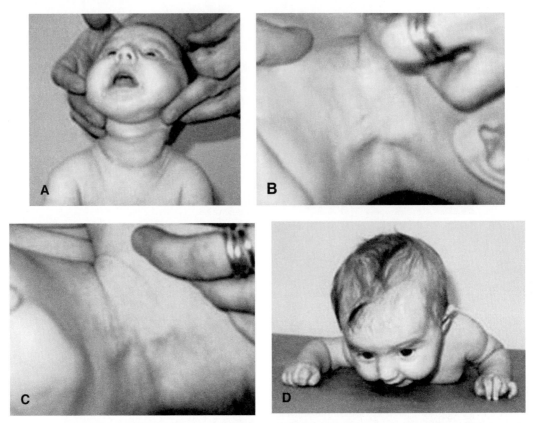

◆ **Figure 12-4** **A**, Three-month-old with left congenital muscular torticollis (CMT) with multiple skin creases indicating tightness of the skin and anterior neck muscles. **B**, Same infant illustrating the tightness of lateral and posterior skin and neck muscles. **C**, Same infant with stretch of the left sternocleidomastoid and upper trapezius muscles revealing tightness of the scalenes and the lateral triangle of the neck. **D**, Anterior neck muscle tightness makes it difficult for the infant to extend the head in prone to clear the airway and rotate the head to the left or right.

allows the head to be in midline. Other children present with level shoulders, but with a head tilt, which produces a lateral shift of the cervical spine leading to cervical spinal scoliosis.

TYPICAL ACTIVITY LIMITATIONS

The young infant with CMT is unable to have purposeful symmetric movement of the head because of the neck muscle contracture and neck muscle strength imbalances. Impaired mobility may lead to persistent asymmetry of early reflexes and reinforcement of an asymmetric postural preference. This is turn may cause neglect of the ipsilateral hand, decreased visual awareness of the ipsilateral visual field, interference of symmetric development of head and neck righting reactions, delayed propping and rolling over the involved side and limited vestibular, proprioceptive, and sensorimotor development. In the older child this may result in asymmetric weight bearing in sitting, crawling, walking, and transitional movement skills as well as incomplete development of automatic postural reactions. If not addressed, these persistent postural asymmetries may result in structural deformities such as pelvic obliquity and scoliosis (Fig. 12-5). Inability to turn the head and neck will cause the child to rotate the body to compensate and inability to recruit lateral neck flexion with automatic reactions will cause the child to compensate with overuse of the torso muscles. Often the child with CMT may appear similar to a child with hemiplegic cerebral palsy (Binder et al., 1987; Karmel-Ross & Lepp, 1997). Activity limitations include difficulty in sustaining midline head posture in an upright position, regaining head midline posture in vertical, prone, or supine with weight shifts, and maintaining midline head posture during movement. Both the infant and child will have difficulty with upper extremity weight bearing on the in-

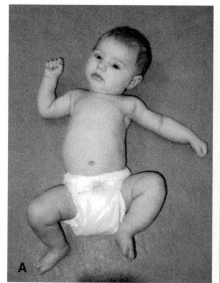
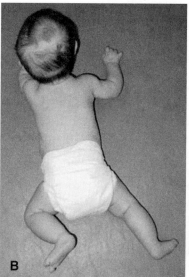
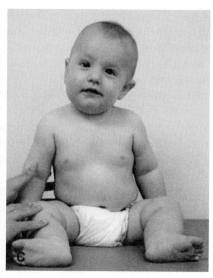
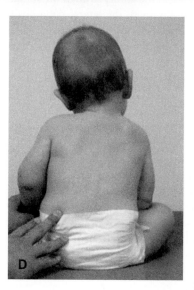
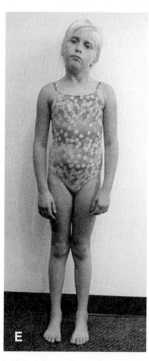
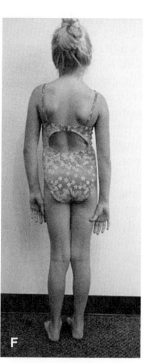

◆ **Figure 12-5**   Characteristic asymmetric postural deformities shown in a 3-month-old infant (**A** and **B**), an 8-month-old infant (**C** and **D**), and an untreated 8-year-old child (**E** and **F**). All have left congenital muscular torticollis and deformational plagiocephaly. **A**, Three-month-old in supine exhibiting characteristic asymmetric postural deformities including incurvation of the whole vertebral column, asymmetric tonic neck reflex, left arm abduction and internal rotation with forearm pronation, right hip abduction and external rotation, left hip adduction and internal rotation. **B**, Same 3-month-old infant in prone. Note that there is little change in the postural alignment. **C**, Anterior view of 8-month-old in sitting exhibiting scoliosis, internal rotation and extension of the upper extremity with scapular elevation, abduction, anterior tilt, and upward rotation. **D**, Posterior view of same 8-month-old in sitting, exhibiting ipsilateral shortening of the posterior cervical muscles, shoulder elevation, extension of the humerus, and rotation of the thorax. **E**, Anterior view of untreated 8-year-old in standing demonstrating characteristic asymmetric postural deformities including scoliosis. Long-standing shortening of the left sternocleidomastoid muscle has caused an unfavorable postural influence leading to spinal curvature, both upper extremity and lower extremity length differences, pelvic tilt with right hip joint abducted and left hip joint adducted. **F**, Posterior view of same 8-year-old.

volved side, reaching toward midline with forearm supination, shoulder external rotation and flexion, and full expression of upper extremity protective and equilibrium reactions. The infant will use compensatory maneuvers to be able to perform a task such as hand clapping by crossing midline to bring the uninvolved side upper extremity toward the involved arm. The systems contributing to these activity limitations include the musculoskeletal system (limited cervical range of motion and muscle strength) and the sensory systems of vision, vestibular function, and somatosensation needed to regulate posture. These systems also influence adaptive and anticipatory responses to help control head position and anticipate postural adjustments by adapting head positions during weight shifts and active exploration (Shumway-Cook & Woollacott, 1985).

The infant with CMT responds to these imposed restrictions with self-initiated movements that include a pattern of head tilting to the ipsilateral side and rotation to the contralateral side of SCM muscle involvement. The young infant with CMT is therefore unable to adapt appropriately to the supporting surface and has limited kinesthetic feedback, which affects the development of the sensorimotor systems, postural organization, orientation, and body schema. The infant may demonstrate difficulty participating in activities toward the involved SCM muscle side while developing appropriate postural, motor, and visual control of the uninvolved side. The infant may not exhibit organized midline behavior as a result of the foregoing asymmetries. Motor milestones may develop atypically because the various subsystems (visual, vestibular, somatosensory, and musculoskeletal) are developing asymmetrically and the infant is not experiencing normal interactions of each system as growth and development occur (Karmel-Ross & Lepp, 1997).

PHYSICAL THERAPY EXAMINATION

The physical therapy examination should include both the prenatal and birth history (vaginal or cesarean section delivery, use of vacuum or forceps assist, birth presentation, nuchal cord, birth order if multiple birth, birth weight, birth length), sex of the infant, side of SCM muscle involvement, other congenital anomalies, x-rays or other diagnostic testing, reports of previous subspecialists consulted, and age at diagnosis. The interview with the caregiver or parent should include questions about who provides care to the infant and amount of time the child spends in infant seats, car seats, swings, and other infant positioning devices as well as the amount of time spent prone and supine. Questions should also be asked about

sleeping position and head rotation preference when sleeping, sleeping surface, feeding problems, medications, previous physical therapy interventions, and present concerns regarding the torticollis and head shape.

FINDINGS IN CONGENITAL MUSCULAR TORTICOLLIS

The musculoskeletal system should be examined for restrictions in joint range of motion and muscle length with particular attention paid to ipsilateral neck rotation, contralateral lateral neck flexion, contralateral asymmetric flexion and extension, muscle and soft tissue extensibility, and skin creases about the neck (see Fig. 12-4**A** to **C**). Moving the head and neck passively through each motion allows the examiner to determine the infant's available range of motion. Gentle traction of the cervical spine may be used to assess the ability to align the spinal vertebrae in neutral and eliminate the lateral glide position induced by the shortened SCM muscle. Gentle traction between the shoulder complex and the occiput combined with specific head and neck motions may be used to assess the tightness of the upper trapezius, scalene, and posterior neck muscles of the ipsilateral side. The infant's active and passive neck range of motion (ROM) should be assessed in prone with the head and neck free of the supporting surface because the infant may not have enough ROM or strength to extend the head off of the supporting surface and clear the airway. Having both adequate ROM and active movement for this task is important for providing safe play time in prone (see Fig. 12-4**D**). Attention should also be directed toward the ipsilateral shoulder girdle and upper extremity to assess active movement toward midline with horizontal adduction and flexion, as well as ballistic shoulder movement. Movement of the forearm into supination and reach and grasp should also be examined. The trunk should be assessed for the ability to elongate with weight shifting. In addition, the pelvis and lower extremity on the ipsilateral side should be examined for ability to accept a weight-bearing load with proper biomechanical alignment.

Spinal motion should be assessed for restriction of extension, flexion, lateral flexion, and rotation (Greenman, 1989; Kautz & Skaggs, 1998). Resting head posture and passive and active ROM should be documented in supine, prone, and sitting postures. Active ROM of the head and neck can be documented by using body landmarks while having the infant follow an object or person's face and voice or measured using goniometry (Karmel-Ross & Lepp, 1997).

Examination of affected muscles should include palpation of the muscle for possible tumor and tonal quality.

The affected muscles should also be examined for extensibility as well as function in a variety of postures. Developmental reflexes may be used to elicit automatic responses. Elicited voluntary movement should be documented as a response against gravity or with gravity eliminated, and the range through which active movement progresses is noted. Understanding motivational strategies and cultural differences and encouraging participation of the caregiver or parent during the examination is important. Examiners can interview the caregiver or parent to determine prior movement experiences of the infant. The infant's behavioral state during testing should be documented.

Hip asymmetry may be assessed by comparing leg lengths, assessing the thighs for extra skin folds, and measuring hip abduction. The incidence of hip dysplasia associated with muscular torticollis has been reported to be between 8% and 20% in children with CMT, most often occurring on the same side as the involved SCM muscle (Hsieh et al., 2000; Tien et al., 2001; Watson, 1971). Infants with positive findings should be referred back to their primary care physician with a recommendation for an orthopedic consult.

PLAGIOCEPHALY AND FACIAL ASYMMETRY

Plagiocephaly (including head shapes of brachycephaly, scaphocephaly, and head shapes consistent with congenital syndromes) and facial asymmetry (facial scoliosis and hemihypoplasia) should be documented by photographs that include frontal, profile (left and right), posterior, vertex, and submental views that show head, shoulders, and torso. A tape measure is used to measure head circumference and spreading or sliding calipers are used to document head asymmetry. A narrative description of any noted asymmetries is used to document areas of occipital/parietal flattening, frontal/temporal flattening, head height differences, ear, orbit, and malar eminence alignment, bulging of parietal area, bossing of frontal area, eye size and alignment, canting of the mandible, narrowing of the temporal mandibular joint, alignment of the tongue and jaw with active movement or static posture, and any facial muscle asymmetry (Bruneteau & Mulliken, 1992; Farkas et al., 1992; Graham et al., 2004a; Huang et al., 1996; Huang et al., 1998; Hollier et al., 2000; Kreiborg et al., 1985; Littlefield et al., 1998; Littlefield et al., 2001).

In deformational plagiocephaly, the occiput and the frontal bone and the full face become deformed by molding forces induced by in utero constraint caused by compression of the fetal cranium between the maternal pelvic bone and lumbar sacral spine in the last trimester.

The most common vertex presentation is left occipital anterior, which correlates with left CMT and right occipital/left frontal flattening. Plagiocephaly may be concordant (same side) or discordant (opposite side) to the muscular torticollis at birth. Acquired deformational plagiocephaly, which develops in the first 3 months of life, is always concordant with CMT (Jones, 1968). The masticatory muscles are weaker on the affected SCM muscle side and may contribute to temporal mandibular joint dysfunction as it affects the formation of the joint (Captier et al., 2003; Chang et al., 2001; Ferguson, 1993; Kreiborg et al., 1985; Kondo & Aoba, 1999; Hidaka et al., 1996; Hollier et al., 2000; Shapiro, 1994; St. John et al., 2002; Watson, 1971; Yu et al., 2003).

Associated risk factors that may predispose the infant to deformational plagiocephaly include oligohydramnios, uterine malformations, cephalohematoma, complication of the birth process, postnatal positioning, primiparity, male gender, and muscular torticollis (Bredenkamp et al., 1990; Bruneteau & Mulliken, 1992; Danby, 1962, Graham, 2002; Graham et al., 2004a; Mulliken et al., 1999). In a cohort of 201 healthy infants, Peitsch and colleagues (2002) reported the incidence of "localized" occipital cranial flattening (defined as transcranial asymmetry >4 mm) at 24 to 72 hours after delivery to be 13% in singleton births and 56% in twins, with greater frequency of occipital flattening observed on the right side. A significant associated finding was auricular deformation on the side of occipital flattening.

The progression of deformational plagiocephaly seems to halt around 6 months of age when intrinsic brain growth slows down and the infant begins to sit independently. However, a number of studies have demonstrated that cranial facial asymmetry present at 6 months of age has a high probability of persisting into adolescence and adulthood (Argenta, 1996; Boere-Boonekamp & van der Linden-Kuiper, 2001; Chang et al., 2001; Clarren, 1981; Danby, 1962; Graham, 2004a; Leung & Leung, 1987; Littlefield et al., 1998; Yu et al., 2003). Bruneteau and Mulliken (1992) and Mulliken and colleagues (1999) reported muscular torticollis in 64% of infants with frontal deformational plagiocephaly and in 26% of infants with occipital deformational plagiocephaly.

Examination of infants with plagiocephaly should also include a screening assessment of vision, hearing, and infant vocalization. Automatic reactions, posture, and motor development should be thoroughly assessed using standardized tests. The Test of Infant Motor Performance (TIMP) is a good choice for infants from 32 weeks' gestational age through 4 to 5 months post term because a major construct assessed in this test is the infant's ability to independently control head position in a variety of spatial orientations (Campbell, 1995). The infant's primary behavior state during assessment, tolerance to stretching, and the ability to self-regulate should be documented as well. Finally, referrals to other professionals should be made when appropriate.

PHYSICAL THERAPY INTERVENTIONS

Intervention is directed toward resolving each impairment or activity limitation identified in the physical therapy examination. Currently, most authors advocate conservative, nonoperative treatment for CMT. This conservative intervention typically consists of passive neck ROM exercises (Fig. 12-6). It is equally important to include active assistive ROM, strengthening, and postural control exercises. Caregivers are instructed in how to carry and posi-

tion the infant to promote elongation of the involved SCM as well as how to promote active contraction of the contralateral SCM. Caregivers are also instructed in developmental exercises (Fig. 12-7) and how to reposition the child to prevent progression of deformational plagiocephaly (Fig. 12-8).

Correct postural alignment and education about maintaining correct postural alignment are an integral part of rehabilitation, with the overall goals being to restore full joint and muscle ROM, to prevent occurrence of irreversible contractures, and to restore full muscle strength. Performing daily therapeutic exercises will also promote motor development. The duration of physical therapy intervention and outcomes of intervention are dependent upon the cause of the torticollis, the initial deficit of passive neck rotation, and the age of the infant when intervention is initiated. Retrospective and prospective studies of passive neck ROM exercises have reported good to

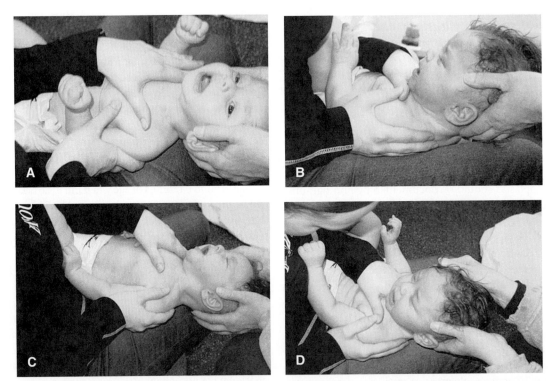

• **Figure 12-6** Two-person passive neck range of motion exercises for an infant with left congenital muscular torticollis. The shoulders are parallel to the pelvis, the pelvis is stabilized to prevent compensation during stretching by movement of the torso, and the shoulders are stabilized at the sternum, clavicle, ribs, and scapula by one person; the head and neck are free from the surface to allow for full neck motion; the second person holds under the occiput and applies a gentle traction to the cervical spine prior to performing neck motion to align the cervical spine in neutral and lengthen the muscles in the longitudinal axis. The holding hand on the left in the photos has been moved to show the tightness of the left sternocleidomastoid (SCM) muscle during the neck stretching exercises. **A**, Neck extension and asymmetric extension to the right to stretch the anterior neck muscles and left SCM muscle. **B**, Neck flexion and asymmetric flexion to the right to stretch the posterior cervical and left upper trapezius muscles. **C**, Neck lateral flexion right to stretch the left SCM muscle. **D**, Neck rotation left to stretch the left SCM muscle.

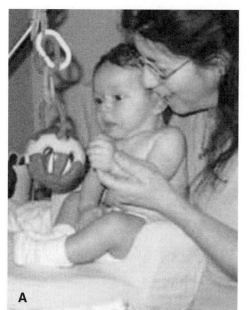
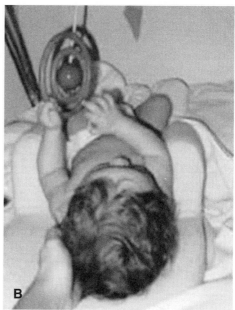

◆ **Figure 12-7**   Four-month-old infant with left congenital muscular torticollis. **A**, In a supported sitting position the infant's head is prevented from tilting to the left and toy placement directs visual gaze to the left, promoting head rotation to the left while manual guidance is given to the ipsilateral upper extremity for forward flexion, external rotation, and forearm supination during reach and grasp. **B**, In a supine position, the toys are placed slightly to the left to promote rotation of the head to the left while the central axis alignment of head to body is maintained with sustained light traction on the occiput or base of the skull. The infant is exercising in an open kinetic chain upper to actively strengthen left upper extremity flexion, external rotation, elbow extension, horizontal abduction, and adduction.

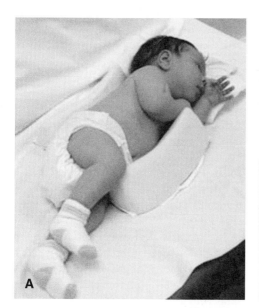
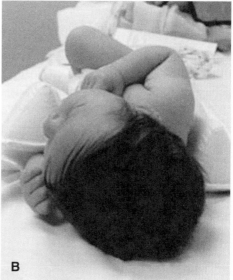

◆ **Figure 12-8**   Two-month-old infant with left congenital muscular torticollis and deformational plagiocephaly (left frontal region and the diagonal right occipital area are flattened, and the opposite areas are more full and bulging). **A**, Soft supports are placed anterior and posterior to the infant's trunk to allow the infant to be positioned in a three quarters side-lying position. **B**, A vertex view shows weight bearing of the calvarium on the fuller surface of the occiput while avoiding weight bearing on the already flattened area of the occiput.

excellent results, with success rates ranging from 61% to 99% when intervention was initiated before 1 year of age (Celayir, 2000; Chang et al., 1996; Cheng & Au, 1994; Cheng et al., 1999; Cheng et al., 2000a: Cheng et al., 2001; Demirbilek & Atayurt, 1999; Emery, 1994; Morrison & McEwen, 1982; Wei et al., 2001).

Published physical therapy intervention protocols for CMT vary considerably. They include neck stretching done twice daily, repeating each stretch five times with a 10-second hold (Emery, 1994); manual stretching by physiotherapists three times a week consisting of three repetitions of 15 manual stretches of the tight SCM, held for 1 second with a 10-second rest period combined with a prone sleeping home program (Cheng et al., 2000b, Cheng et al., 2001); two-person passive rotation neck stretching exercises carried out four to five times daily with at least 40 repetitions in each set (Demirbilek & Atayurt, 1999); and two-person neck stretching exercises of flexion, extension, rotation, and lateral flexion of 10 sets of each exercise with a 10 count hold for each repetition completed eight times each day (Celayir, 2000).

Contraindications for passive neck ROM include bony abnormalities, fracture, Down syndrome, myelomeningocele, a compromised circulatory or respiratory system, malignancy, osteomyelitis, tuberculosis, ruptured or lax ligaments, infection, shunt, or Arnold-Chiari malformation (Greenman, 1989). Caregivers providing ROM exercises should be instructed to observe for changes in vital signs, which may include color changes in the face, change in rate of breathing, eye rolling, perspiration, or nasal flaring and to stop exercises if any of these occur. Passive movement should be done slowly and stretching should not be done against an infant actively resisting the stretch. Infants exhibiting discomfort may exhibit avoidance behaviors including tense body posture, arching, facial grimacing, gaze aversion, crying, shutdown, or physiologic instability. Warm compresses, infant massage, and stretching after bath time may be helpful in reducing infant stress. The use of a toy and setting up the environment can facilitate the infant to visually look in the specific direction that promotes the desired neck muscle contraction and facilitate active stretch of the tight muscles.

BIOMECHANICS OF STRETCHING AND RECOMMENDED STRETCHING PROTOCOL

If one studies the origin and insertion of the SCM muscle and the biomechanics of this muscle, it will be clear that to properly stretch the SCM muscle, one should stabilize at the origin and insertion, moving the muscle into its elongated position. The elongated position can be attained with ipsilateral rotation, contralateral lateral flexion, and contralateral asymmetric extension from a starting point of neutral cervical spine alignment. The infant should be positioned supine with the head and neck free of the supporting surface and with both shoulders stabilized and held parallel to a stable pelvis. The best stretching routine is done with two persons, especially when working with an older infant or toddler, in which one person stabilizes the shoulders and the other person stretches the neck (see Fig. 12-6). Stretching should include all motions of the neck with particular attention to aligning the cervical spine with gentle traction prior to any motion. Anterior, posterior, and lateral neck muscles must all be stretched, and this can be done by including movements of rotation, lateral flexion, asymmetric flexion and extension, midline axial alignment rotation, lateral flexion, flexion, and extension. This stretching regimen should be done every 2 hours, if possible, for maximum benefit. Additional stretching exercises for the upper and lower extremities including the shoulder girdle and hip complex and the trunk should be included if impairments in shoulder and hip motion are present (Karmel-Ross & Lepp, 1997; Vandenburgh et al., 1989).

To maintain the ROM, the infant must develop strength and active use of muscles that are antagonists to the involved SCM muscle to help develop good midline control. For example, the infant must be able to place the contralateral ear to the shoulder, flex and extend head toward the uninvolved side, and rotate the head and neck toward the involved side. By 15 months of age the child can usually perform these movements with visual or verbal cueing if adequate passive neck ROM and strength are available.

ORTHOTIC DEVICES

Assistive devices that may be used to help obtain, maintain, or restrain motion include a fabricated to fit, soft neck collar or a "tubular orthosis for torticollis" (TOT) collar (Fig. 12-9). This collar was designed and developed at British Columbia's Children's Hospital. A contralateral torticollis postural positioning device may also be used (Fig. 12-10).

Use of these devices is indicated for those infants or children who are 4 months of age or older, have a constant head tilt of 5° or greater for more than 80% of awake time, and perform all movement transitions and motor skills with a constant head tilt. In addition to these indications, children must have adequate passive ROM of the neck (at least 10° of lateral flexion toward the noninvolved side) or have lateral head righting reactions that demonstrate the ability to lift the head away from the involved side (Jacques & Karmel-Ross, 1997).

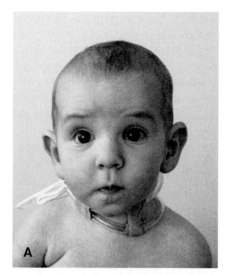
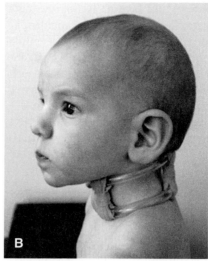

◆ **Figure 12-9**   Five-month-old infant with left congenital muscular torticollis concordant deformational plagiocephaly fitted with a tubular orthosis for torticollis (TOT Symmetric Designs Ltd., 125 Knott Place, Salt Spring Island, BC, Canada, V8K2M4). **A**, The anterior strut is shorter than the posterior strut and spans vertically from the anterior angle of the mandible to the midclavicle. **B**, The posterior strut is longer than the anterior strut and spans vertically from the occiput at the inferior nuchal line to the superior medial angle of the scapula where the levator scapulae muscle attaches.

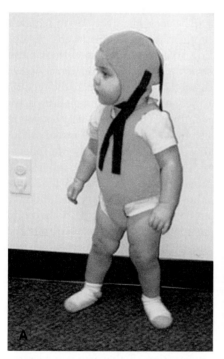
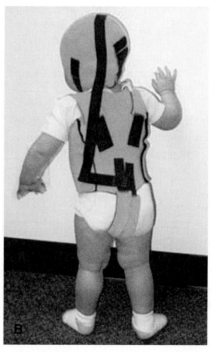

◆ **Figure 12-10**   Fifteen-month-old with right congenital muscular torticollis wearing a contralateral torticollis postural positioning device (CTPPD) consisting of a neoprene Velcro sensitive pediatric dynamic trunk orthosis and bathing cap (BENIK Corporation, 11871 Silverdale Way, NW, #107, Silverdale, Washington, 98383). Multiple strapping system designed by and added by author. **A**, The back strap simulates the pull of the contralateral upper trapezius muscle, and the front strap simulates the pull of the contralateral sternocleidomastoid muscle, preventing head tilt toward the side of the torticollis, and permits movement in the contralateral direction. **B**, The body vest provides stability to the shoulders and prevents ipsilateral shoulder elevation while the strapping system provides a pull toward the contralateral side. This dynamic system promotes normal postural alignment, strength, and sensory motor development.

The TOT collar should not be used as a passive support device. Possible complications include shoulder depression on the involved side, a shift in the shoulder girdle axis, and a lateral shift of the cervical spine. The infant should always be attended when using orthotic devices such as this and should never be allowed to wear these devices in a car seat or when sleeping. Vital signs should be observed at all times, and visual torticollis should be ruled out before these devices are used. The orthotics may be worn during awake time, and skin integrity should be checked when the orthosis is removed or at least every 2 hours.

INSTRUCTION TO CAREGIVERS

Reinforcing or improving neck ROM, strength, and postural control can be accomplished in any number of ways throughout the day. The caregiver should be taught how to carry and hold the infant, how to position the infant during sleep or nap time to create a prolonged stretch of the tight muscle and promote midline development, and how to present toys to the involved side to facilitate reaching in a horizontal and upward diagonal plane. The caregiver should also be taught to approach and feed the infant to promote looking toward the involved SCM muscle (Karmel-Ross & Lepp, 1997). Home exercise programs can include eliciting balance reactions for strength development. Once an adequate amount of neck muscle strength is obtained, the exercises should be task-specific so that the infant will use that strength to lift the head against gravity. This strengthening will promote development of transitional movements such as rolling and coming to sit from prone and supine.

▌MEDICAL MANAGEMENT

MANAGEMENT OF CONGENITAL MUSCULAR TORTICOLLIS

It is important for the physician, physical therapist, and family members all to understand how CMT may progress over time because physical therapy intervention must be carried out consistently on a daily basis until all therapy goals are achieved. These goals include full passive neck muscle ROM with no regression during growth spurts over a continuous 3-month period. Once a child is discharged from physical therapy services, the child's pediatrician should include CMT and deformational plagiocephaly assessment in well child follow-up visits to make sure there has been no regression of head tilt posture, loss of neck muscle ROM, changes in spinal align-

ment, or delay in motor skills (Persing, 2003). Because deformational plagiocephaly may be disguised by hair the pediatrician should palpate the head for volume asymmetries and note any abnormal dysplastic patterns of growth of the mandible as well as portions of the upper jaw and face related to mastication and occlusal disharmonies. Referral to an orthodontist or oral facial surgeon may be necessary.

Surgical intervention may be considered for children who do not improve after 6 months of conservative intervention that includes manual stretching of the SCM muscle. Indications for surgical consideration include a residual head tilt, deficits of passive rotation and of lateral flexion of the neck greater than 15°, a tight muscular band or tumor of the SCM, hemihypoplasia, or a poor outcome to correction of the deformational plagiocephaly. Ultrasound studies can identify the type and extent of muscle fibrosis revealing the pathologic characteristics of the affected SCM muscle and whether surgical intervention would be helpful in relieving the persistent symptoms (Cheng et al., 1999; Cheng et al., 2000b; Lin & Chou, 1997; Ling & Low, 1972; Maricevic et al., 1997; Minamitani et al., 1990; Simon et al., 2002).

The goals of surgery are to achieve a complete release of the shortened muscle and restore neck ROM and normal cervical spine mechanics, preserve neurovascular structures, and improve craniofacial asymmetry. Outcomes of surgical intervention are difficult to analyze due to the variety of surgical techniques used, the inconsistency in identifying homogeneous cohorts for type of SCM involvement (the site and extent of the disease within the muscle), and the variability in follow-up care including orthotics, physical therapy, and home exercise programs. Surgical procedures may include transection at one or more points of the SCM muscle body, total SCM excision, unipolar or bipolar releases at the tendinous attachments, functional SCM myoplasty, and more recently, endoscopic surgery. Common problems to each technique are damage to the facial, greater auricular, or spinal accessory nerves, visible scars, recurrent muscle band formation, loss of neck contour, and the recurrence of SCM contracture. Endoscopic surgery avoids many of these problems by allowing the surgeon to view the operative field directly with magnification, ensuring precise muscle fiber transection and preservation of the neurovascular structures. The best surgical outcomes have been reported in those children treated between 10 months and 5 years of age. Children who have releases before 1 year of age have the best chance of reversing their facial and skull deformities (Burstein & Cohen, 1998; Burstein, 2004; Cheng & Tang, 1999; Ling, 1976; Maricevic et al., 1997; Morrison & MacEwen, 1982).

PLAGIOCEPHALY

The key to successful management of deformational plagiocephaly associated with CMT is early diagnosis and intervention. Almost 80% of skull growth occurs before 12 months of age, affording only a small window of opportunity to provide nonsurgical treatment to correct the deformational plagiocephaly. A clinical pathway that includes the age of the infant at presentation, severity of the deformational plagiocephaly, resolution of the muscular torticollis, and response to conservative management (including an active repositioning program and neck exercises) will guide the practitioner in management of deformational plagiocephaly. These factors will also influence decisions regarding whether a cranial remodeling band may need to be prescribed (Clarren, 1979; Graham et al., 2004b; Kelly et al., 1999; Littlefield et al., 1998; Littlefield et al., 2001; Loveday & de Chalain, 2001; Persing et al., 2003; Raco et al., 1999; Ripley et al., 1994, Vles et al., 2000). To avoid postnatal progression of deformational plagiocephaly, Peitsch and colleagues (2002) recommended that infants identified at birth or shortly thereafter with greater than 4 mm of cranial vault asymmetry be closely monitored and placed on an early sleep positioning program and supervised awake tummy time.

Caregivers and parents will need instruction and encouragement to help keep the infant from lying on the flattened areas of the skull. The ideal time for this active repositioning is in the first 3 months of life when the skull is most malleable and there is rapid intrinsic brain growth (see Fig. 12-8). Repositioning may not be effective if the CMT persists, if the infant remains in a position of comfort that reinforces the plagiocephaly forces, or if the infant becomes too active during sleep to stay repositioned. Intrinsic brain growth slows at 5 to 6 months of age and if plagiocephaly is still quite obvious at that time, the remaining plagiocephaly is unlikely to resolve without cranial remodeling band treatment.

The infant with plagiocephaly should undergo a reassessment for head shape on a monthly basis by the child's pediatrician or physical therapist (if the infant is having ongoing physical therapy). Changes in deformational plagiocephaly should be documented by use of anthropometric measures, photographs, and a written description. The child's head shape should be observed from multiple angles including from above (vertex view) as part of the standard examination, since observing the baby's face from a frontal (en face) perspective often fails to reveal the asymmetry. From a vertex position the examiner can compare alignment of the orbits, zygoma, and ears in the frontal plane and assess the calvaria for frontal/temporal and contralateral occipital/parietal

flattening. The skeletal structures may have a greater degree of asymmetry than the soft tissue drape that partially masks the underlying imbalances along with hair, which will cover the calvaria as the infant becomes older (Kelly et al., 1999; Persing et al., 2003).

The Dynamic Orthotic Cranioplasty (DOC) Band was the first approved FDA class II neurology device generically known as a "cranial orthosis." It was developed as a proactive dynamic approach to treat deformational plagiocephaly in infants up to 24 months of age (Fig. 12-11). The DOC Band is designed to redirect growth and thus improve craniofacial symmetry of the cranial vault, face, and cranial base by (1) applying an immediate mild holding pressure to the most anterior and posterior prominences of the cranium where growth is not desired and (2) allowing room for growth in the adjacent, flattened regions. Infants must be seen on a weekly to biweekly basis to make adjustments to the inner foam liner of the

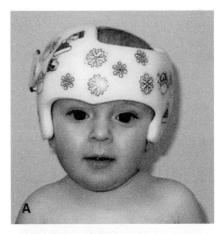

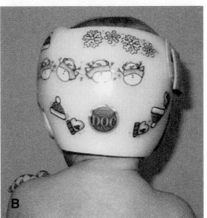

◆ **Figure 12-11**   Four-month-old infant with left congenital muscular torticollis and frontal deformational plagiocephaly wearing the DOC Band (Cranial Technologies, Inc., Phoenix, Arizona). **A,** En Face view. **B,** Posterior view.

band. It is this process of continuously modifying the band and resultant corrective pressures that make the DOC Band treatment dynamic (Fig. 12-12). This device offers a significant change from the original passive molding helmets in which the head grew into the helmet, taking on the shape of the helmet, with no change to the frontal deformation. The DOC Band is worn 23 out of every 24 hours, with the exception of 1 hour for skin care and passive neck ROM exercises. The length of the treat-ment and the number of cranial bands necessary for cor-rection will depend on the severity of the deformational plagiocephaly and the age at which treatment is begun. The use of a cranial remodeling band has been reported to have excellent results in reshaping the heads of infants with deformational plagiocephaly and has a more effec-tive outcome than repositioning (Clarren, 1981; Graham et al., 2004a; Graham et al., 2004b; Littlefield et al., 1998; Ripley et al., 1994; Vles et al., 2000).

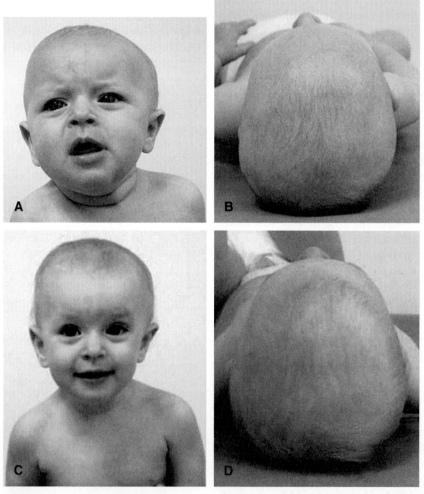

◆ **Figure 12-12** Four-month old infant with left congenital muscular torticollis and frontal deformational plagiocephaly. **A**, En face view prior to the start of DOC Band treatment. There is volume loss to the left frontal/temporal area and concordant right occipital/parietal area, recession of the left frontal and zygoma bones, posterior displacement of the ipsilateral ear, shortening of left vertical facial height, canting of the mandible, and developing hemihypoplasia. **B**, Vertex view prior to DOC Band treatment showing the frontal and maxillary horizons with concordant asymmetry and flattening of the right occipital area. **C**, Same infant at 12 months of age after DOC Band treatment and endoscopic surgery at 10 months of age to release the left sternomastoid muscle showing improved cranial facial symmetry and neck muscle length. **D**, Vertex view at 12 months of age after DOC Band treatment showing symmetric frontal and maxillary horizons and fullness to the right occipital area.

ANTICIPATED OUTCOMES OF PHYSICAL THERAPY INTERVENTION

Anticipated outcomes of physical therapy intervention are listed here in order of those more likely to be attained to those that are more difficult to attain:

- Full passive ROM of neck, trunk, and extremities (should be achieved before discharge from physical therapy)
- Active symmetric head rotation from midline to 80° left and right in supine, prone, sitting, and standing
- Active midline head-to-trunk alignment during static and dynamic play with only intermittent head tilts toward the involved side
- Normal antigravity trunk and neck strength with symmetry between uninvolved and involved sides
- Symmetry between left and right sides in righting and equilibrium reactions in both the horizontal and vertical planes
- Ability to assume head tilt toward the uninvolved side with or without rotation to the involved side during play activities involving either static or dynamic postures

Newborns are biologically constructed to develop symmetrically, although growth and development by design may cause different degrees of asymmetry to develop. This asymmetry may be partially compensated for or, conversely, made worse by activity, the environment, or internal structural restrictions. As an example, when the healthy full-term newborn infant is placed in the prone position with the elbows close to the trunk, with hips and knees flexed because of physiologic flexion, there is downward force on the shoulders, sternum, and clavicles, which actually helps to stabilize the attachment of the neck muscles anteriorly. As the infant lifts to extend and rotate the head to clear the airway, the infant is able to self-impose a stretch of anterior neck muscles, the SCM muscle, and the upper trapezius muscle. In the healthy infant this self-initiated activity self-treats any neck tightness and facilitates symmetric development of the pelvis, trunk, shoulder, upper extremities, and neck. Early reflexes such as the asymmetric tonic neck reflex (ATNR) and Gallant and arm passage reflex help to reinforce both stretching and strengthening of the neck, shoulder girdle, and trunk. In the child with CMT, however, where there is neck motion restriction, these early reflexes can work to reinforce postural asymmetries of the pelvis, trunk, shoulder, upper extremities, and neck.

Other factors that may contribute to the persistence of asymmetry in the child with CMT are delays in motor development, back-sleeping with no supervised tummy time to offset the constant supine positioning, and spending extended amounts of time semireclined in containment equipment such as car seats, infant seats, infant carriers, bouncy seats, or swings. Infants who do not spend time in prone and who spend too much time in containment equipment may have no opportunity to alter the surface against which their craniums lie, thus potentially perpetuating or imposing a deformational plagiocephaly as well as preventing development of neck strength and head control (Littlefield et al., 2003; Monson et al., 2003). Other factors that may cause an increase in the head tilt with or without actual SCM muscle contracture are excessive spontaneous muscle fiber discharge in the SCM muscle, teething, ear infections, acquisition of new motor skills, crying, fatigue, stress, and illness. Faulty central nervous system (CNS) motor programming related to muscle tone, joint function, learned motor programs or autonomic reactions may also cause an increase in the torticollis posture. When the torticollis posture is not corrected it may be due to unresolved SCM muscle contracture, rebound or sensory defensive positioning from overstretching, weakness of the antagonists, or abnormal muscle length-tension relationships (Karmel-Ross & Lepp, 1997).

Infants with CMT may have atypical motor planning and execution because of movement disturbances and musculoskeletal imbalances that developed in utero or during the first year of life. The anatomic and physiologic bases for variability common to motor learning in the first postnatal year are restricted, causing neuromotor patterns of asymmetry to develop which may cause motor delays in the infant (Shumway-Cook & Woollacott, 1985; Thelan, 1995; Tscharnuter, 1993). Understanding the relationship between movement disturbances and the associated effect of an abnormally shaped calvaria on the underlying cortex in children has been the focus of several recent studies (Balan et al., 2002; Binder et al., 1987; Habal et al., 2003; Miller & Clarren, 2000; Panchal et al., 2001).

SUMMARY

This chapter discussed the management of congenital muscular torticollis and deformational plagiocephaly. A fibrotic and shortened SCM muscle is the most typical finding in CMT along with a head tilt toward the involved SCM muscle. The etiology and pathogenesis of CMT is not completely understood but may be related to breech presentation, birth trauma, in utero constraint, nuchal cord, or use of suction and forceps at birth. Sonography and physical examination can confirm the pathology of CMT. Most cases of infants with CMT can be successfully managed with conservative treatment utilizing passive and active neck stretching exercises, active repositioning, neck strengthening, and postural control exercises to encourage the head to turn toward the involved SCM muscle side. The severity of the neck rotation restriction, the amount and distribution of fibrosis in the SCM muscle, and the age of the infant at initiation of physical therapy intervention will influence the success rate of conservative management. Surgical intervention may be indicated for those infants not responding to conservative treatment. A cranial remodeling band may be necessary to correct deformational plagiocephaly associated with CMT. Motor control and postural development as well as prevention and treatment of facial asymmetry and deformational plagiocephaly should be emphasized along with intervention of CMT.

CASE STUDY

Alex was referred to physical therapy at the age of 3 months for left CMT and deformational plagiocephaly. She was born by cesarean section at 38 weeks' gestation. She was vertex presentation and her mother remarked she had carried her low in her pelvis. Her parents became aware of their daughter's abnormal head shape a month after she was born and brought it to the attention of their pediatrician. Alex was a back sleeper with her head always rotated to her right. Her parents reported they tried to do as their pediatrician directed, to encourage her to look to her left. Alex would not stay repositioned and had no interest in looking to the left. When her parents felt the head shape and neck mobility were not improving, their pediatrician referred her for physical therapy.

Upon the initial examination, the clinical findings revealed a 65% loss of passive and active neck ROM for right lateral flexion, left rotation, and asymmetric flexion/extension to the right of midline. The torso had limited rotation to the left and lateral flexion to the right and the left upper extremity was limited in horizontal adduction, external rotation, shoulder flexion, forearm supination, and wrist extension. Alex was unable to maintain midline postural alignment in supine, prone, or sitting, and she did not demonstrate righting reactions of the head, neck, or trunk to her right side. She was unable to lift her head off the surface in prone to clear her airway. Alex's mother reported she did not like the prone position. Palpation of the neck muscles revealed she had

tightness throughout the left SCM muscle, hyoid muscles, left scalene muscles and left upper trapezius (Fig. 12-4). She had minimal reciprocal kicking, had truncal curvature with convexity to the right, windswept hips, and no left upper extremity ballistic shoulder movement or movements toward the midline. The left upper extremity was postured in internal rotation, shoulder elevation, and forearm pronation and the hand was fisted. She had a persistent asymmetric tonic reflex (see Fig. 12-5). She was not able to bear any weight on her upper extremities or grasp a toy. A pacifier was used to help calm her and her mother reported her as being "moody." She was being nursed and the mother reported she had more difficulty with nursing her on the right breast. She was unable to track a toy or her mother's face to the left of midline in supine.

Alex had a deformational plagiocephaly with right occipital/parietal flattening, right anterior ear shift, right anterior orbit shift, flattening of the left frontal/temporal area, increased posterior head height, and left narrowed fissure. The anterior fontanel was open to palpation and there was no suture ridging. Her cephalic index was 82.31% (1.92 standard deviations above the norm for her age and sex; the cephalic index is the relationship of the width of the head to the length of the head). She had 14 mm of cranial vault asymmetry, 3 mm of cranial base asymmetry, and 4 mm of facial asymmetry.

Physical therapy intervention began at 3 months of age and included passive and active neck ROM exercises, which were carried out by the parents on a daily basis. The parents were also instructed in how to position Alex during nap and sleep time to reduce the plagiocephaly. Her cranial vault asymmetry decreased by 4 mm with the positioning program by 5 months of age, but then no further decrease in asymmetry was measured. The frontal deformation was still apparent, and the family decided to pursue DOC Band treatment.

Alex was in the DOC Band for 4 months from age 6 to 10 months. She had excellent correction of the cranial vault asymmetry at the completion of the DOC Band treatment as shown in Figure 12-13.

The muscular torticollis required ongoing physical therapy with multiple visits each week when Alex was in growth spurts and losing neck ROM. Full passive neck ROM was achieved by 9 months of age, although this would regress with growth spurts. Alex still had an intermittent head tilt, poor sense of visual and postural midline, and weakness of the right neck muscles. Once Alex completed the DOC Band treatment, a TOT collar, a contralateral torticollis posture bracing system (CTPBS), and taping were used to assist her with developing neck strength, midline postural control, and automatic reac-

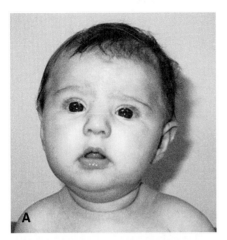
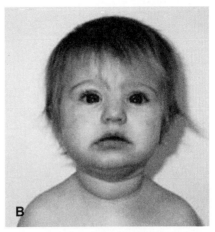

♦ **Figure 12-13**   **A**, Alex at 3 months of age. She has left congenital muscular torticollis (CMT) and frontal deformational plagiocephaly and exhibits characteristic cranial facial asymmetries, tilted head posture left, and contralateral head rotation right. **B**, Alex at 12 months of age after DOC Band treatment and physical therapy intervention for left CMT.

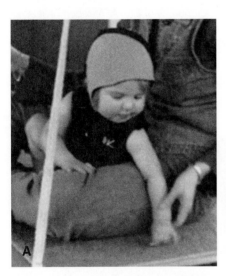
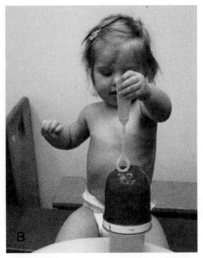

♦ **Figure 12-14**   **A**, Alex wears a contralateral torticollis postural positioning device (CTPPD), consisting of a neoprene Velcro-sensitive pediatric dynamic trunk orthosis and bathing cap with multiple strapping system. The CTPPD maintains the correct postural alignment as she bears weight on an extended arm to the ipsilateral side. **B**, This play activity promotes correct alignment of the scapula, humerus, forearm, and wrist during reach and grasp. Placement of the toy on a supporting surface promotes downward gaze, elongating the neck extensors, and strengthening the neck flexors in midline.

tions (Fig. 12-14). The CTPBS prevented the left head tilt from continuing to occur as she developed transitional skills of pull to stand, squat to stand, cruising, creeping, walking, and stair climbing.

The parents carried out a daily exercise routine that included neck ROM exercises every 2 hours with diaper changes, neck strengthening exercises (especially for the ability to lift the head off the surface using right neck muscles), and general ROM exercises with special attention to the left shoulder girdle, left upper extremity, torso for elongation of the left side, and ability to weight shift

over the left hip. Other home program exercises included activities to look to her left and to look left and upward with reach, making sure she tilted her head to the right with rotation to the left. In addition, activities to promote balance reactions were carried out, and the parents carried and positioned her to prevent a left head tilt and shortening of the left side of her torso.

At 15 months of age Alex could imitate and follow directions to put her right ear to her shoulder. She still had a mild strength difference in her neck muscles with the left slightly more responsive than the right. She was

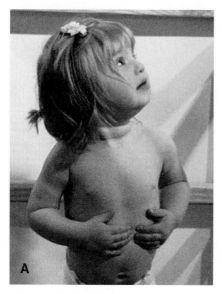 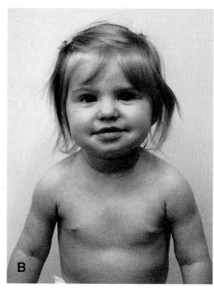

✦ **Figure 12-15** Alex was discharged from physical therapy at 15 months of age. **A,** Alex demonstrating ability to adopt posture opposite of congenital muscular torticollis (CMT) posture as she is able to look left and upward with head tilt right. **B,** Alex exhibiting no apparent plagiocephaly, cranial facial asymmetries, head tilt, or other postural deformities associated with CMT.

age appropriate with her motor skills and could maintain a midline head posture alignment. The timing and sequencing of her automatic reactions were appropriate except when she was fatigued. She was discharged from physical therapy at this time (Fig. 12-15).

The parents continue to carry out a home exercise program for Alex and will continue with physical therapy rechecks if any regression is observed in passive neck ROM.

▌ REFERENCES

Argenta, LC, David, LR, Wilson, JA, & Bell, WO. An increase in infant cranial deformity with supine sleeping position. Journal of Craniofacial Surgery, 7:5–11, 1996.

Balan, P, Kushnerenko, E, Sahlin, P, Huotilainen, M, Naatanen, R, & Hukki, J. Auditory ERPs reveal brain dysfunction in infants with plagiocephaly. Journal of Craniofacial Surgery, 13:520–525, 2002.

Ballock, RT, & Song, KM. The prevalence of nonmuscular causes of torticollis in children. Journal of Pediatric Orthopaedics, 16:500–504, 1996.

Binder, H, Eng, GB, Gaiser, JF, & Koch, B. Congenital muscular torticollis: Results of conservative management with long-term follow-up in 85 cases. Archives of Physical Medicine and Rehabilitation, 68:222–225, 1987.

Boere-Boonekamp, MM, & van der Linden-Kuiper, LT. Positional preference: Prevalence in infants and follow-up after two years. Pediatrics, 107:339–343, 2001.

Bredenkamp, JK, Hoover, LA, Berke, GS, & Shaw, A. Congenital muscular torticollis. Archives of Otolaryngology Head & Neck Surgery, 116:212–216, 1990.

Bruneteau, RJ, & Mulliken, JB. Frontal plagiocephaly: synostotic, compensational, or deformational. Plastic and Reconstructive Surgery, 89:21–33, 1992.

Burstein, FD, & Cohen, SR. Endoscopic surgical treatment for congenital muscular torticollis. Plastic and Reconstructive Surgery, 101:20–26, 1998.

Burstein, FD. Long term experience with endoscopic surgical treatment for congenital muscular torticollis in infants and children: A review of 85 cases. Plastic and Reconstructive Surgery, 114:491–493, 2004.

Campbell, SK, Kolobe, THA, Osten, ET, Lenke, M, & Girolami, GL. Construct validity of the Test of Infant Motor Performance. Physical Therapy, 75:585–596, 1995.

Captier, G, Leboucq, N, Bigorre, M, Canovas, F, Bonnel, F, Bonnafe, A, & Montoya, P. Plagiocephaly: Morphometry of skull base asymmetry. Surgery, Radiology and Anatomy, 25:226–233, 2003.

Celayir, AC. Congenital muscular torticollis: early and intensive treatment is critical, a prospective study. Pediatric International, 42:504–507, 2000.

Chan, YL, Cheng, JCY, & Metreweli, C. Ultrasonography of congenital muscular torticollis. Pediatric Radiology, 22:356–360, 1992.

Chang, PY, Tan, CK, Huang, YF, Sheu, JC, Wang, NL, Yeh, ML, & Chen, CC. Torticollis: A long term follow up study. Acta Paediatrica Taiwanica, 37:173–177, 1996.

Chang, PY, Chang, NC, Perng, DB, Chien, YW, & Huang, FY. Computer-aided measurement and grading of cranial asymmetry in children with and without torticollis. Clinical Orthodontics and Research, 4:200–205, 2001.

Cheng, JCY, Tang, SP, & Chen, TMK. Sternomastoid pseudotumor and congenital muscular torticollis in infants: A prospective study of 510 cases. Journal of Pediatrics, 134:712–716, 1999.

Cheng, JCY, & Au, AWY. Infantile torticollis: a review of 624 cases. Journal of Pediatric Orthopaedics, 14:802–808, 1994.

Cheng, JCY, Wong, MWN, Tang, SP, Chen, TMK, Shum, SLF, & Wong, EMC. Clinical determinants of the outcome of manual stretching in the treatment of congenital muscular torticollis in infants. Journal of Bone and Joint Surgery, 83:679–687, 2001.

Cheng, JCY, Tang, SP, Chen, TMK, Wong, MWN & Wong, EMC. The clinical presentation and outcome of treatment of congenital muscular torticollis in infants – A study of 1,086 cases. Journal of Pediatric Surgery, 35:1091-1096, 2000a.

Cheng, JCY, & Tang, SP. Outcome of surgical treatment of congenital muscular torticollis. Clinical Orthopaedics and Related Research, 362:190–200, 1999.

Cheng, JCY, Metreweli, C, Chen, TMK, & Tang, SP. Correlation of unltrasonographic imaging of congenital muscular torticollis with clinical assessment in infants. Ultrasound in Medicine & Biology, 26:1237–1241, 2000b.

Clarren, SK. Plagiocephaly and torticollis: Etiology, natural history, and helmet treatment. Journal of Pediatrics, 98:92–95, 1981.

Clarren, SK. Helmet treatment for plagiocephaly and congenital muscular torticollis. Journal of Pediatrics, 94:43–46, 1979.

Clarren, SK, & Smith, DW. Congenital deformities. Pediatric Clinics of North America, 24:665–677, 1977.

Cooperman, D. Differential diagnosis of torticollis in children. Physical and Occupational Therapy in Pediatrics. 17:1–11, 1997.

Coventry, MB, & Harris, LE. Congenital muscular torticollis in infancy. The Journal of Bone and Joint Surgery, 41:815–822, 1959.

Danby, PM. Plagiocephaly in some 10 year old children. Archives of Disease in Childhood, 37:500–504, 1962.

Davids, JR, Wenger, DR, & Mubarak, SJ. Congenital muscular torticollis: Sequela of intrauterine or perinatal compartment syndrome. Journal of Pediatric Orthopaedics, 13:141–147, 1993.

Demirbilek, S, & Atayurt, HF. Congenital muscular torticollis and sternomastoid tumor: Results of nonoperative treatment. Journal of Pediatric Surgery, 34:549–551, 1999.

Dunn, PM. Congenital postural deformities. British Medical Bulletin, 32:71–76, 1976.

Dunn, PM. Congenital sternomastoid torticollis: An intrauterine postural deformity. Archives of Disease in Childhood, 49:824–825, 1974.

Emery, C. The determinants of treatment duration for congenital muscular torticollis. Physical Therapy, 74:921–929, 1994.

Farkas, LG, Posnick, JC, & Hreczko. Anthropometric growth study of the head. Cleft Palate-Craniofacial Journal, 29:303–308, 1992.

Ferguson, JW. Surgical correction of the facial deformities secondary to untreated congenital muscular torticollis. Journal of Cranio-Maxillo-Facial Surgery, 21:137–142, 1993.

Fulford, GE, & Brown JK. Position as a cause of deformity in children with cerebral palsy. Developmental Medicine and Child Neurology, 18:305–314, 1976.

Graham, JM. Smith's Recognizable Pattern of Human Deformation, 2nd ed. Philadelphia: WB Saunders, 1988.

Graham, JM. Craniofacial deformation. Bailliere's Clinical Paediatrics, 6:293–316, 1998.

Graham, JM, Kreutzman, J, Earl, D, Halberg, A, Samayoa, C, & Guo, X. Deformational brachycephaly in supine-sleeping infants. Journal of Pediatrics, 146:253–257, 2005a.

Graham, JM, Gomez, M, Halberg, A, Earl, D, Kreutzman, J, Cui, J, & Guo, X. Management of deformational plagiocephaly: Repositioning versus orthotic therapy. Journal of Pediatrics, 146:258–262, 2005b.

Greenman, PE. Principles of Manual Medicine. Baltimore: Williams & Wilkins, 1989.

Habal, MB, Leimkuehler, TL, Chambers, C, Scheuerle, J, & Guilford, AM. Avoiding the sequela associated with deformational plagiocephaly. Journal of Craniofacial Surgery, 14:430–437, 2003.

Hamanishi, C, & Tanaka, S. Turned head-adducted hip-truncal curvature syndrome. Archives of Disease in Childhood, 70:515–519, 1994.

Ho, BCS, Lee, HE & Singh, K. Epidemiology, presentation and management of congenital muscular torticollis. Singapore Medical Journal, 40:675–679, 1999.

Hidaka, J, Morishita, T, & Nakata, S. The relationship between cranial-facial asymmetry and bilateral functional balance of the masticatory muscles. Journal of the Japanese Orthodontic Society, 55:329–336, 1996.

Hollier, L, Kim, J, Grayson, BH, & McCarthy, JG. Congenital muscular torticollis and associated craniofacial changes. Plastic and Reconstructive Surgery, 105:827–835, 2000.

Hsu, TC, Wang, CL, Wong, MK, Hsu, KH, Tang, FT, & Chen, HT. Correlation of clinical and ultrasonographic features in congenital muscular torticollis. Archives of Physical Medicine and Rehabilitation, 80:637–641, 1999.

Hsieh, YY, Tsai, FJ, Lin, CC, Chang, FCC, & Tsai, CH. Breech deformation complex in neonates. The Journal of Reproductive Medicine, 45:933–935, 2000.

Huang, MHS, Mouradian, WE, Cohen, SR, & Gruss, JS. The differential diagnosis of abnormal head shapes: separating craniosynostosis from positional deformities and normal variants. Cleft Palate-Craniofacial Journal, 35:204–211, 1998.

Huang, MHS, Gruss, JS, Clarren, SK, Mouradian, WE, Cunningham, ML, Roberts, TS, Loeser, JD, & Cornell, CJ. The differential diagnosis of posterior plagiocephaly: True lambdoid synostosis versus positional molding. Plastic and Reconstructive Surgery, 98:765–774, 1996.

Huang, CS, Cheng, HC, Lin, WY, Liou, JW, & Chen, YR. Skull morphology affected by different sleep positions in infancy. Cleft Palate-Craniofacial Journal, 32:413–419, 1995.

Jacques, C, & Karmel-Ross, K. The use of splinting in conservative and post-operative treatment of congenital muscular torticollis. Physical and Occupational Therapy in Pediatrics, 17:81–90, 1997.

Jones PG. Torticollis in Infancy and Childhood. Springfield, IL: Charles C Thomas Publisher; 1968.

Kane, AA, Mitchell, LE, Craven, KP ,& Marsh, JL. Observations on a recent increase in plagiocephaly without synostosis. Pediatrics, 97:877–885, 1996.

Kapandji, IA. The Physiology of the Joints, Vol 3. The Trunk and Vertebral Column, 2nd ed. London: Churchill Livingstone, 1974.

Karmel-Ross, K, & Lepp, M. Assessment and treatment of children with congenital muscular torticollis. Physical and Occupational Therapy in Pediatrics, 17:21–67, 1997.

Kautz, SM, & Skaggs, DL. Getting an angle on spinal deformities. Contemporary Pediatrics, 15:111–128, 1998.

Kelly, KM, Littlefield, TR, Pomatto, JK, Ripley, CE, Beals, SP, & Aoba, TJ. Importance of early recognition and treatment of deformational plagiocephaly with orthotic cranioplasty. Cleft Palate Craniofacial Journal, 36:127–130, 1999.

Kondo, E, & Aoba, T. Case report of malocclusion with abnormal head posture and TMJ symptoms. American Journal of Orthodontics and Dentofacial Orthopedics, 116:481–403, 1999.

Kreiborg, S, Moller, E, & Bjork, A. Skeletal and functional craniofacial adaptations in plagiocephaly. Journal of Craniofacial Genetics, 1:199–210, 1985.

Leung, YK, & Leung, PC. The efficacy of manipulative treatment for sternomastoid tumors. Journal of Bone and Joint Surgery, 69:473–478, 1987.

Lin, JN, & Chou, ML. Ultrasonographic study of sternocleidomastoid muscle in the management of congenital muscular torticollis. Journal of Pediatric Surgery, 32:1648–1651, 1997.

Ling, CM. The influence of age on the result of open sternomastoid tenotomy in muscular torticollis. Clinical Orthopaedics, 116:142–148, 1976.

Ling, CM, & Low, YS. Sternomastoid tumor and muscular torticollis. Clinical Orthopaedics, 86:144–150, 1972.

Lingeman, RE. Surgical anatomy. In Cummings, CW, Fredrickson, FM, Harker, LA, Krause CJ, Schuller, DE, & Richardson, MA (Eds.). Otolaryngology: Head and Neck Surgery, Vol. 3, 3rd ed. St. Louis: Mosby, 1998, p. 1680.

Littlefield, TR, Kelly, KM, Reiff, JL, & Pomatto, JK. Car seats, infant carriers, and swings: Their role in deformational plagiocephaly. Journal of Prothestics and Orthotics, 15:102–106, 2003.

Littlefield, TR, Reiff, JL, & Rekate, HL. Diagnosis and management of deformational plagiocephaly. BNI Quarterly, 17:18–25, 2001.

Littlefield, TR, Beals SP, Manwaring, KH, Pomatto JK, Joganic, EF, Golden, KA, & Ripley CE. Treatment of craniofacial asymmetry with DOC. Journal of Craniofacial Surgery, 9:11–7, 1998.

Loveday, BPT, & de Chalain, TB. Active counterpositioning or orthotic device to treat positional plagiocephaly. Journal of Craniofacial Surgery, 12:308–313, 2001.

Maricevic, A, & Erceg, M. Results of surgical treatment of CMT. Lijecnicki Vjesnik, 119:106–109, 1997.

Miller, RI, & Clarren, SK. Long term developmental outcomes in patients with deformational plagiocephaly. Pediatrics, 105:E26, 2000.

Minamitani, K, Inoue, A, & Okuno, T. Results of surgical treatment of muscular torticollis for patients 6 years of age. Journal of Pediatric Orthopaedics, 10:754–759, 1990.

McDaniel, A, Hirsch, BE, Kornblut, A, & Armbrustmacher, VM. Torticollis in infancy and adolescence. Ear, Nose and Throat Journal, 63:478–487, 1984.

Morrison, DL, & MacEwen, GD. Congenital muscular torticollis: Observations regarding clinical findings associated conditions and results of treatment. Journal of Pediatric Orthopaedics, 2:500–505, 1982.

Monson, RM, Deitz, J, & Kartin, D. The relationship between awake positioning and motor performance among infants who slept supine. Pediatric Physical Therapy, 15:196–203, 2003.

Mulliken, JB, Vander Woude, DL, Hansen, M LaBrie, RA, & Scott, RM. Analysis of posterior plagiocephaly: Deformational versus synostotic. Plastic and Reconstructive Surgery, 103:371–380, 1999.

Najarian, SP. Infant cranial molding and sleep position: Implications for primary care. Journal of Pediatric Health Care, 13:173–177, 1999.

Panchal, J, Amirsheybani, H, Gurwitch, R, Cook, V, Francel, P, Neas, B, & Levine, N. Neurodevelopment in children with single-suture craniosynostosis and plagiocephaly without synostosis. Plastic and Reconstructive Surgery, 108:1492–1498; discussion 1499–5000, 2001.

Peitsch, WK, Keefer, CH, LaBrie, RA. & Mulliken, J. Incidence of cranial asymmetry in healthy newborns. Pediatrics, 110:72–80, 2002.

Persing, J, James, H, Swanson, J, & Kattwinkel, J. Prevention and management of positional skull deformities in infants. Pediatrics, 112:199–202, 2003.

Raco, A, Raimondi, AJ, De Ponte, FS, Brunelli, A, Bristot, R, Bottini, DJ, & Ianetti, G. Congenital torticollis in association with craniosynostosis. Child's Nervous System, 15:163–168, 1999.

Rekate, HL. Occipital plagiocephaly: A critical review of the literature. Neurosurgical Focus, 2:1–11, 1997.

Ripley, LE, Pomatto, J, & Beals, SP. Treatment of positional plagiocephaly with dynamic orthotic cranioplasty. Journal of Craniofacial Surgery, 5:150–159, 1994.

Shapiro, JJ. Relationship between vertical facial asymmetry and postural changes of the spine and ancillary muscles. Optometry and Vision Science, 7:529–538, 1994.

Shumway-Cook, A, & Woollacott, M. The growth of stability; postural control from a development perspective. Journal of Motor Behavior, 17:131–147, 1985

Simon, FT, Tang, MD, Kuang-Hung, H, Wong, AMK, Hsu, CC, & Chang, CH. Longitudinal follow-up study of ultrasonography in congenital muscular torticollis. Clinical Orthopaedics and Related Research, 403:179–185, 2002.

Slate, RK, Posnick, JC, Armstrong, DC, & Buncic, R. Cervical spine subluxation associated with congenital muscular torticollis and craniofacial asymmetry. Plastic and Reconstructive Surgery, 91:1187–1195, 1993.

Smith, DW. Recognizable Patterns of Human Deformation. Philadelphia: WB Saunders, 1981.

Stellwagon, LM, Hubbard, E, & Vaux, K. Look for the "stuck baby" to identify congenital torticollis. Contemporary Pediatrics Archive, May: 1–14, 2004.

St. John, D, Mulliken, JB, Kaban, LB, & Padwa, B. Anthropometric analysis of mandibular asymmetry in infants with deformational posterior plagiocephaly. Journal of Oral and Maxillofacial Surgery, 60:873–877, 2002.

Thelen, E. Motor development, a new synthesis. American Psychologist, 50:79–5, 1995.

Tien, YC, Su, JY, Su, GT, Lin, GT, & Lin, SY. Ultrasonographic study of the coexistence of muscular torticollis and dysplasia of the hip. Journal of Pediatric Orthopaedics, 21:343–347, 2001.

Tom, LWC, Handler, SD, & Wetmore, RF. The sternocleidomastoid tumor of infancy. International Journal of Pediatric Otorhinolaryngology, 13:245–255, 1987.

Turk, AE, McCarthy, JG, Thorne, CHM, & Wisoff, JH. The "Back to Sleep Campaign" and deformational plagiocephaly: Is there cause for concern? Journal of Craniofacial Surgery, 7:12–18, 1996.

Tscharnuter, I. A new therapy approach to movement organization. Physical and Occupational Therapy in Pediatrics, 13:19–40, 1993.

Vandenburgh, HH, Hatfaludy, S, Karlisch, P & Shansky, J. Skeletal muscle growth is stimulated by intermittent stretch-relaxation in tissue culture. American Journal of Physiology, 256:C674–682, 1989.

Vles, JSH, Colla, C, Weber, JW, Beuls, E, Wilmink, J & Kingma, H. Helmet versus non-helmet treatment in nonsynostotic positional posterior plagiocephaly. Journal of Craniofacial Surgery, 11:572–574, 2000.

Watson, GH. Relationship between side of plagiocephaly, dislocation hip, scoliosis, bat ears and sternomastoid tumors. Archives of Disease in Childhood, 46:203–210, 1971.

Wei, JL, Schwartz, KM, Weaver, AL, & Orvidas, LJ. Pseudotumor of infancy and congenital muscular torticollis: 170 cases. Laryngoscope, 111:688–695, 2001.

Yu, CC, Wong, FH, Lo, LJ, & Chen, YR. Craniofacial deformity in patients with uncorrected congenital muscular torticollis: An assessment from three-dimensional computed tomography imaging. Plastic and Reconstructive Surgery, 113:24–33, 2003.

ARTHROGRYPOSIS MULTIPLEX CONGENITA

MAUREEN DONOHOE
PT, PCS

Arthrogryposis multiplex congenita (AMC) is a nonprogressive neuromuscular syndrome that is present at birth. AMC is characterized by severe joint contractures, muscle weakness, and fibrosis. Although the child's condition does not deteriorate as a result of the primary diagnosis, the long-term sequelae of AMC can be very disabling. Activity limitations occur in mobility and self-care skills that can lead to varying degrees of participation restriction.

Working with children with AMC presents the physical therapist with a variety of challenges. Many children who have AMC are bright and motivated. Physical therapists must use their knowledge of biomechanics and normal development to maximize functional skills. Proper timing for therapeutic and medical interventions helps maximize the child's opportunities for independence. Creativity is needed to adapt equipment and the environment to allow the child with AMC to be able to participate in life roles to the fullest extent possible.

In this chapter, we address the pathophysiology of AMC, its management from a medical and surgical perspective, physical therapy examination and evaluation, and specific physical therapy and team interventions used for children with AMC from infancy to adulthood.

INCIDENCE AND ETIOLOGY

Arthrogryposis, which is defined by the presence of contractures in two or more body areas, is diagnosed in 1 of every 3000 live births in the United States (Hall, 1997; Sells et al., 1996; Goodman & Gorlin, 1983). The etiology of AMC is unknown; however, the insult is believed to occur during the first trimester of pregnancy (Darrin et al., 2002; Hall, 1997; Wynne-Davies et al., 1981). Insults occurring early in the first trimester have the potential for creating more involvement of the child than those that occur late in the first trimester. The basic pathophysiologic mechanism for the multiple joint contractures appears to be the lack of fetal movement (Tachdjian, 1990).

The various forms of arthrogryposis include a neuromuscular syndrome (7%); congenital anomalies (6%);

chromosomal abnormalities (2%); contracture syndromes (35%); amyoplasia (43%), which is considered the "classic arthrogryposis"; and distal arthrogryposis (7%). Distal arthrogryposis, which affects primarily the hands and feet and is highly responsive to treatment, has a genetic basis and is inherited as an autosomal dominant trait (Hall et al., 1982). Gene mapping has been helpful in identifying those with arthrogryposis. Neuropathic arthrogryposis is found on chromosome 5 and can have survival moto-neuron gene deletion (Burglen et al., 1996; Shohat et al., 1997). Distal arthrogryposis type I maps to chromosome 9 (Bamshad et al., 1994; Bamshad et al., 1996).

AMC is associated with neurogenic and myopathic disorders in which motor weakness immobilizes the fetal joints, leading to joint contractures. It is not known whether all those with the neuropathic form of AMC have degeneration of the anterior horn cell, but of those studied post mortem, this is a consistent finding. A neurogenic disorder of the anterior horn cell is believed to cause muscle weakness with subsequent periarticular soft tissue fibrosis (Drummond et al., 1978; Goodman & Gorlin, 1983; Hall, 1989; Vanpaemel et al., 1997; Wynne-Davies et al., 1981). Because of the failure of the muscle to function, the joints in the developing fetus lack movement, which probably explains the stiffness and deformities of the newborn's joints. The fetus may have an imbalance in strength of oppositional muscle groups, creating the tendency toward a certain posture. For example, the fetus with good strength in the hamstrings and triceps brachii but weakness in the quadriceps and biceps brachii will have a flexed knee and extended elbow posture in utero. Decreased amniotic fluid throughout the pregnancy, but especially during the last trimester when the fetus is largest, may further inhibit freedom of movement in utero.

Although the etiology of AMC remains unknown, several factors have been implicated. Hyperthermia of the fetus is caused by a maternal fever greater than 37.8°C (100°F). Some mothers of children with AMC report having an illness with a fever for 1 to 2 days during the first trimester. Prenatal viral infection, vascular compromise of the blood supply between mother and fetus, uterine fibroid tumors, or a septum in the uterus have all been proposed as causes of AMC (Hall, 1997; Sells et al., 1996; Wynne-Davies et al., 1981).

PROGRESS IN PRIMARY PREVENTION

Arthrogryposis has been documented in artwork as early as the 1700s, although medical literature did not begin to address it until nearly the 1950s. Six major categories of

problems can occur during a pregnancy that could precipitate the lack of movement associated with congenital contractures: maternal illness, fetal crowding, neurologic deficits, vascular compromise, connective tissue/skeletal defects, and muscle defects (Hall, 1998). Given its nonspecific etiology, little progress has been made in the prevention of this rare disorder. However, significant improvements have been made in the management of children with AMC.

DIAGNOSIS

No definitive laboratory studies exist that can diagnose AMC prenatally. The majority of AMC cases are not genetically based, and therefore prenatal amniocentesis or chorionic villous sampling may be inconsequential. If a parent or physician suspects that something is amiss, a detailed level II ultrasound evaluation can be helpful in identifying anomalies and decreased fetal movements. Ultrasound studies in subsequent pregnancies would help relieve parental anxiety.

During the first 6 months of life an immunoglobulin study may identify evidence of a viral infection. After that time, an ophthalmologist can examine the eye for pigment clumps on the retina, called chorioretinitis. Chorioretinitis has no effect on vision but will establish whether the insult was the result of a prenatal viral process.

Muscle biopsy in AMC varies with the muscle under study. Histologic analysis reveals that relatively strong muscles appear virtually normal, and very weak muscles reveal fibrofatty changes but may have normal muscle spindles. Embryologically, the muscles are formed normally but are replaced by fibrous and fatty tissue during fetal development (Hall, 1997; Hall, 1981; Hall, 1985). Neuropathic and myopathic changes can be seen in different muscles in the same patient with electromyographic testing (Sarwark et al., 1990; Sodergard et al., 1997). Muscle biopsies along with blood tests and clinical findings rule out progressive and fatal disorders while providing evidence to support the diagnosis of AMC.

CLINICAL MANIFESTATIONS

Clinical manifestations of AMC demonstrate great variability but generally include severe joint contractures and lack of muscle development or amyoplasia. The typical severely affected body parts in the AMC population include, in decreasing order of prevalence, the foot (78%–95%), the hip (60%–82%), the wrist (43%–81%), the knee (41%–79%), the elbow (35%–92%), and the shoulder (20%–92%) (Scott & Nicholson, 2003; Sells et al., 1996). One may see these percentages vary in the literature based on how the cases have been diagnosed (i.e., care centers will see different mixes based on their specialty).

There are two commonly seen variations of AMC. In one type, the child has flexed and dislocated hips, extended knees, clubfeet (equinovarus), internally rotated shoulders, flexed elbows, and flexed and ulnarly deviated wrists (Fig. 13-1). In another type, the child has abducted and externally rotated hips, flexed knees, clubfeet, internally rotated shoulders, extended elbows, and flexed and ulnarly deviated wrists (Fig. 13-2). Parents often describe the legs in the first type as jackknifed and in the second type as froglike. Because of the stiffness of the joints, extremity movements are described as wooden or marionette-like. The position of the upper extremities in the second type is described as the "waiter's tip" position owing to the internally rotated shoulder, extended elbow, pronated forearm, and flexed wrist. Common to both types are clubfeet, flexed and ulnarly deviated wrists, and internally rotated shoulders. Other associated characteristics may include scoliosis, dimpling of skin over joints, hemangiomas, absent or decreased finger creases, congenital heart disease, facial abnormalities, respiratory problems, and abdominal hernias. Intelligence and speech are usually normal. Many arthrogrypotic syndromes occur that have the main characteristics of AMC but may also involve abnormal muscle tone, changes in cognition, seizure activity, feeding issues not related to muscle strength or jaw opening, and limited visual skills (Robinson, 1990; Vanpaemel et al., 1997).

MEDICAL MANAGEMENT

The main component of medical treatment includes well-timed surgical management (Hall, 1989; Palmer et al., 1985; St. Clair & Zimbler, 1985). Specific operations should be timed so that the child benefits optimally from the pro-

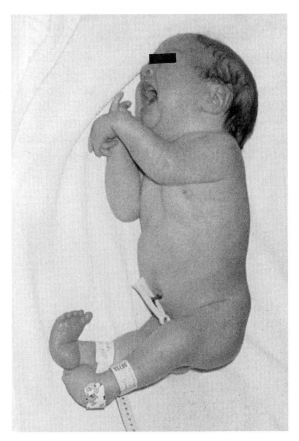

◆ **Figure 13-1** Infant with arthrogryposis multiplex congenita with flexed and dislocated hips, extended knees, clubfeet (equinovarus), internally rotated shoulders, flexed elbows, and flexed and ulnarly deviated wrists.

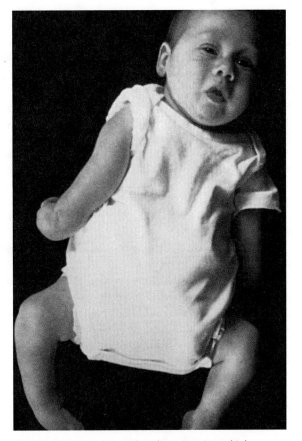

◆ **Figure 13-2** Infant with arthrogryposis multiplex congenita with abducted and externally rotated hips, flexed knees, clubfeet, internally rotated shoulders, extended elbows, and flexed and ulnarly deviated wrists.

cedure. For example, clubfoot surgery, performed to allow plantigrade feet, is often deferred until the child is able to pull to stand and is interested in standing. If surgical intervention is performed when a child is developmentally focusing on sitting and creeping, the foot is biased into plantar flexion and recurrence of the clubfoot is common prior to the child standing and walking. If the child is pulling to stand and beginning to walk, he or she can then easily self-stretch when standing and walking. One common clubfoot surgery is the posteromediolateral release (PMLR). The entire hindfoot is opened during surgery so as to shorten the lateral column, lengthen the medial column, and lengthen the tendo Achillis (Niki et al., 1997; Staheli et al., 1998). Occasionally, this procedure includes using wires to realign the talus and the calcaneus. If the clubfoot recurs, a second PMLR can be performed. The second procedure includes shortening the cuboid bone to help improve forefoot alignment. If the foot is tight just in the hindfoot and no forefoot adductus is noted, a distal tibial wedge osteotomy is done to realign the foot in reference to the floor. Later in life, when the child is near the end of growth, a triple arthrodesis can be performed prevent future inversion of the foot. This involves fusing the calcaneus to the cuboid, the talus to the navicular, and the talus to the calcaneus. Use of an external fixator such as an Ilizarov procedure to address recurrent clubfoot problems has had some promising results, although no long-term outcome studies are presently available (Brunner et al., 1997; Choi et al., 2001). Historically, in severe cases of equinovarus and in cases in which the Ilizarov procedure fails, a talectomy may be performed (Cassis & Capdevila, 2000; Letts & Davidson, 1999). Salvage procedures to correct recurrent problems are difficult, however, when a talectomy has been previously performed (Legspi et al., 2001; Niki et al., 1997; Staheli et al., 1998).

Children with AMC often have subluxed or dislocated hips. Dislocation is as frequently bilateral as unilateral. One dislocated hip is usually relocated to prevent secondary pelvic obliquity and scoliosis, unless the hip is extremely stiff (Sarwark et al., 1990; Staheli et al., 1987). Given that these hips tend to have poor acetabular development, if both hips are dislocated, they are not always surgically reduced because of the risk of continued unilateral dislocation even after open reduction. Those who advocate surgically reducing all dislocated hips most commonly use an anterolateral approach (MacEwen & Gale, 1983; Sarwark et al., 1990; Staheli et al., 1987; St. Clair & Zimbler, 1985; Szoke et al., 1996). Szoke and colleagues (1996) advocate early open reduction with a medial approach as resultant hip stiffness was greater for those who were older at the initial surgery. Yau and colleagues (2002) found that open reduction was necessary to have success in treating dislocated hips, as closed reduction in children with AMC was never successful. It may be more important to have mobile, painless, yet dislocated hips than to have very stiff but located ones. Prolonged immobilization following open or closed techniques can lead to the serious sequelae of fused or stiff hips.

Moderate to severe contractures of the knee joint can be addressed surgically, but in the conservative approach one waits until the child is ambulating comfortably before surgical correction. Knee flexion contractures are most commonly associated with capsular changes within the joint. Medial and lateral hamstring lengthening or sectioning (if the muscle is fibrosed) along with a posterior capsulotomy of the knee joint may be performed (Murray & Fixsen, 1997; Tachdjian, 1990). These contractures respond inconsistently to hamstring lengthenings and posterior capsulotomy because there is a subsequent loss of muscle strength and risk of scar tissue leading to further joint stiffness and recurrence of the contracture. A distal femoral osteotomy is more frequently successful in realigning the joint and changes the arc of motion without risk of increased scar tissue and loss of strength (DelBello & Watts, 1996; Jayakumar, 2004) (Fig. 13-3). Anterior epiphyseal stapling can be done on a growing child with moderate knee flexion contractures. This procedure allows the posterior aspect of the femur to continue to grow while the anterior aspect remains unchanged. The angle of the femur results in apparent knee straightening (Kramer & Stevens, 2001). Knee extension contractures are frequently addressed by quadriceps lengthening if there is at

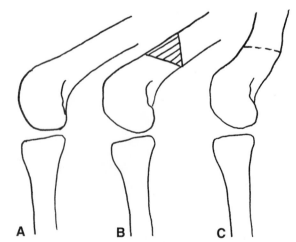

◆ **Figure 13-3** Diagram of a distal femoral wedge osteotomy performed to realign the contracted knee joint. **A,** Knee flexion contracture deformity before surgery. **B,** Distal femoral wedge osteotomy for reduction of the knee flexion deformity. **C,** Realignment after surgery.

least 25° of range of motion (ROM) in the knee. Intra-articular procedures such as a capsulotomy may be necessary if the knee is stiff. Some evidence suggests that surgery to address knee extension contractures results in better outcomes than surgery to address knee flexion contractures (Sodergard & Ryoppy, 1990). An important consideration before surgical intervention is determination of whether the limitation in ROM is creating problems with sitting or walking, and if so, if surgical intervention will likely improve the child's function. For example, if the legs extend straight out when sitting, this position may interfere with activities such as sitting at school desks or riding in a car, and as a result may decrease participation at school and in the community. The child should participate in decisions regarding surgical interventions as appropriate for his or her age.

Restrictions in shoulder movement are rarely addressed through surgical interventions such as capsular or soft tissue releases because the musculature is usually inappropriate for transfer. If adequate muscle strength and control are present, surgery may be indicated to place wrists and elbows in positions of optimal function. One scenario involves a child with symmetric weakness or severe contractures of the upper extremities. In this case, a dominant arm can be identified for feeding (postured in flexion) and the other arm for hygiene care (postured in extension) (Williams, 1973). If both arms were postured in extension, surgery would be necessary to position one arm in a functional flexion position. Such surgical considerations would include a pectoralis or triceps brachii transfer to give a child active elbow flexion with a posterior capsulotomy to allow for elbow flexion (Axt et al., 1997; Tachdjian, 1990). The muscle under consideration for transfer would need to be strong before transfer with adequate passive elbow flexion present. A consistent passive ROM and stretching program from birth is essential to maintain elbow motion for this type of surgery to be successful.

Wrists can be fused in positions for function if conservative splinting and stretching management have been unsuccessful. Wrists are fused in the dissimilar positions. Before a surgical wrist fusion, casting of the wrist for 1 week in the position of the potential fusion is suggested. During this time, the child's functional ADL (activities of daily living) skills are assessed while the child is wearing the cast to ascertain the appropriateness of this potential surgery. Surgical management through carpectomies or dorsal wedge osteotomies of the carpal bones should be considered only if finger function will be enhanced (Axt et al., 1997).

Scoliosis is frequently managed conservatively with bracing. In about one fifth of the children and adolescents with AMC, a long C-shaped thoracolumbar scoliosis develops (Tachdjian, 1990). If the curve continues to progress, surgical fusion should be considered. Most commonly, a posterior spinal fusion is performed. On large stiff curves, an anterior release of structures limiting spinal mobility may be necessary before the posterior spinal fusion to obtain satisfactory results (Yingsakmongkol & Kumar, 2000). The type of fixation used is based on the orthopedist's preference (see Chapter 11).

◼ BODY STRUCTURES AND FUNCTIONS

DIAGNOSIS AND PROBLEM IDENTIFICATION

The primary impairments in the child with AMC are limitations of joint movement and decreased muscle strength and bulk. Joint contractures are evident at birth, although a formal diagnosis of AMC may not be given at that time. In AMC, limitation of movement typically is seen in two or more joints in different body areas (Hall, 1989). No data are available to determine whether flexor or extensor musculature is most likely to be affected. From our experience, we have observed that approximately 65% of the children with AMC seen in our clinic have extended elbows; 35% have flexed elbows; 55% have extended knees; and 45% have flexed knees.

Contractures can develop from an imbalance in muscle pull of agonist and antagonist muscles but also when symmetric weakness is present on all sides of the joint, thus hindering movement. Theoretically, this may be indicative of the point in fetal development at which the insult occurs. For example, because flexors develop before extensors in the upper extremity, a child may develop elbow flexion contractures but does not develop the usual strength in either the biceps or triceps brachii subsequent to the time of insult.

Decreased muscle bulk is evidence of muscle weakness secondary to decreased functioning motor units in a muscle. Histologic analysis of muscles reveals nonspecific changes in the muscle such as fibrofatty scar tissue. Weakened muscles often have a fat layer around the muscle with dimpling of the skin. A muscle with a contracture but of normal strength through its available ROM may not have normal muscle bulk secondary to its inability to be active throughout the entire ROM.

PROBLEM IDENTIFICATION BY THE TEAM

The team evaluation establishes a baseline from which to set realistic and functional goals. In addition to physical therapists, the primary intervention team consists of patients and their families and such medical professionals as orthopedists and geneticists, occupational therapists, and orthotists. Occasionally, speech pathologists, dentists or oral surgeons, and ophthalmologists are consulted as well. One of the goals of the primary team is to educate the family about AMC. Families are taught that arthrogryposis is a nonprogressive disorder but that without positioning, stretching, and strengthening, or possible surgery, the child's impairments could lead to further activity limitations and participation restrictions in later life (Table 13-1).

During the initial examination by the team, photographs and videos are taken of the child, illustrating the child's position of comfort and specific contractures such as clubfeet. This is an objective way to document changes that occur during growth and throughout splinting procedures and should be repeated every 4 months for the first 2 years.

In physical therapy, baseline goniometry is performed, documenting passive ROM and the resting position of each joint. ROM can be measured with a standard goniometer cut down to pediatric size. Active ROM is measured

at the hips, knees, shoulders, elbows, and wrists. If possible, the same therapist consistently measures ROM for the child. Intratester and intertester reliability is determined for all therapists who evaluate children with AMC and should be checked annually. Functional active ROM is also assessed to assist with visualizing the whole composite of motions and evaluating functional abilities. For example, functional active ranges include assessment of the hand to the mouth, ear, forehead, top of head, and back of neck.

A formal manual muscle test is performed when appropriate. Ascertaining muscle grades for infants and very young children is performed by using palpation, observation of the ability of extremities to move against gravity, and evaluation of gross motor function. The strength of the extensor muscles of the lower extremities is especially important to determine the appropriate level of bracing. Less than fair (grade 3/5) muscle strength in hip extensors will require bracing above the hip. Less than fair (grade 3/5) strength in knee extensors requires bracing above the knee. Corrected clubfeet require molded braces during growth to minimize problems of recurrent clubfeet. Children with poor upper extremity function and

TABLE 13-1	**NCMRR Model of the Disabling Process for Children with AMC**			
PATHOPHYSIOLOGY	**IMPAIRMENTS**	**FUNCTIONAL LIMITATIONS**	**DISABILITY**	**SOCIETAL LIMITATIONS**
Prenatal damage to the anterior horn cell resulting in neurogenic and myopathic disorder Decreased number of motor units within a muscle	Multiple joint contractures that can be progressive with growth Fibrotic joint capsule Strength limitation with imbalance of oppositional muscles Stronger muscles are often shortened	Limited functional mobility skills, including rolling, creeping, transitional movements, and higher-level mobility skills Limited ability to transfer Limited ambulation Posture and limited strength of upper extremity determine alternative mobility options Decreased endurance	Limited independence in self-care skills, including dressing and feeding Dependence in transfers for ADL, including toileting Inability to manage uneven terrain Limited endurance for ambulation Limited independence in wheelchair mobility without costly adaptations Limited participation in physical activities due to endurance and safety	Limited opportunity for play with young peers Inability to live independently Limited access to educational and work opportunities Limited access to a wide range of environments Health insurance may not pay for adaptations necessary for least restrictive mobility device Social isolation

NCMRR, National Center for Medical Rehabilitation Research.

weak lower extremities may not be functional community ambulators as a result of decreased motor control and protective responses. Power mobility may be the most appropriate means of community locomotion.

Gross motor skills and functional levels of mobility and ADL are assessed. No current developmental tests have been designed for children with AMC, but these children usually score lower than average in formal gross motor tests secondary to inadequate strength and ROM in their extremities. Certain gross motor skills may never be attained owing to physical limitations. For example, some developmental milestones such as creeping may not be attained even though the child is able to stand and is beginning to walk. Cognitively, children with AMC tend to score average to above average in formal developmental tests (Sarwark et al., 1990; Sodergard et al., 1997; Williams, 1978).

The physical therapist assesses the child for current and potential modes of functional mobility. This may include ambulation with assistive devices or the use of manual or power wheelchair or mobility devices. The therapist evaluates movement patterns and muscle substitutions used to accomplish each motor task or ADL skill. Therapists should address a child with AMC from a biomechanical approach, because having limb segments aligned for mechanical advantage maximizes function and ultimately participation.

Following the examination, short-term and long-term goals are developed by the team related to splinting, stretching, developmental stimulation, surgical intervention, and bracing. Incorporating the family early on as part of the team is important to maximize the child's independence in ADL and mobility.

PHYSICAL THERAPY IN INFANCY

Physical limitations and deformities seen in infants with AMC include clubfeet, hip flexion contractures, knee extension contractures, shoulder tightness (especially internal rotation), and elbow and wrist flexion contractures. At birth these children are commonly breech presentations. In another type, common posturing includes abducted and externally rotated hips, flexed knees, internally rotated shoulders, extended and pronated elbows, and flexed wrists. There may be asymmetric posturing of the extremities, which is especially problematic at the hip when dislocation of only one hip is present. The resulting asymmetry makes surgical correction the treatment of choice to relocate the hip and secondarily prevent pelvic obliquity and scoliosis.

EXAMINATION

Formal assessment of an infant with AMC begins as soon as possible after birth. The assessment consists of goniometry of passive ROM with reevaluation of ROM done on a monthly basis during this period. The therapist also documents the presence and strength of muscles based on observation of the child's movements and palpation of muscle contractions. Muscles of the trunk and upper and lower extremities are evaluated. Formal developmental assessment tools are occasionally used but reflect poorly on a child with AMC because strength and ROM limitations preclude the achievement of many motor milestones. Delayed motor milestones may result in activity limitations and participation restrictions when children with AMC are compared to healthy peers on standardized developmental tests.

Motor milestones in these children are often delayed or skipped. For example, good trunk control and balance, coupled with upper extremities that are weak and in compromised positions, results in the development of the ability to scoot on the buttocks rather than creeping for early floor mobility. Functional mobility and the mechanism used in attaining this mobility are more important to evaluate than is assignment of a developmental level or score. The therapist assesses rolling, prone tolerance, sitting control, scooting, creeping, crawling, transitional movements, and standing tolerance and upright mobility. Occupational therapy (OT) plays a key role in assessing feeding, ADL skills, and manipulation of objects. Physical therapists also assess the fit of any supportive or assistive devices that may be used.

Although it is not imperative to use formal scales in assessing motor development, some useful tests include the Alberta Infant Motor Scale, the Bayley Scales of Infant Development, and the Peabody Developmental Motor Scales. The Pediatric Evaluation of Disability Inventory and the WeeFIM (Functional Independence Measure for Children) may be used to measure activity and participation (see Chapter 2 for more information on these measurement tools).

Physical therapy goals for very young children include maximizing strength, improving ROM, and enhancing general sensorimotor development. Education of the family emphasizes instruction in proper positioning, stretching techniques, and the avoidance of potentially harmful activities.

INTERVENTION STRATEGIES

Intervention strategies focus on reducing the joint contracture through stretching, thermoplastic serial splinting, positioning, and strengthening activities. Interventions address developmental skills, teaching compensatory strategies, especially in ADL and alternative modes of mobility, to maximize participation in age-appropriate activities.

Development, Strength, and Mobility

Infants with the first type of AMC described earlier begin life with limited positioning options as a result of hip flexion contractures. Consequently, stretching hip flexors and prone positioning are encouraged within the first 3 months of life. Developmentally, these infants learn to roll or scoot on their bottoms as their primary means of floor mobility, because it is nearly impossible to comfortably assume the quadruped position without reinforcing a flexed posture of the upper extremities. Although delayed in their ability to attain sitting independently, they are often able to do so by 15 months of age using trunk flexion and rotation. These children typically are able to stand when placed well before pulling to stand is initiated by the child. Usually, the child attempts walking after clubfoot surgery is completed and the child has lower extremity orthotics.

Clubfoot surgery performed early, using techniques which entail serial casting and a percutaneous tendo Achillis lengthening, often requires revisions by the time the child is developmentally ready to walk. Surgery after the first year of life when the child exhibits a readiness to walk allows the child to stand after clubfoot surgery and cast removal, which assists in stretching the feet into a plantigrade position and eliminates the need to perform multiple surgical revisions. Clubfoot surgery should be performed before 2 years of age when bony changes may occur that would necessitate more extensive osteotomy procedures rather than soft tissue releases. Also, most children begin some form of independent ambulation by the middle of their second year.

Infants with the second type of AMC posturing (hips externally rotated and flexed, knees flexed, elbows extended) have more positioning options. However, these children become frustrated with prone positioning secondary to their decreased ability to comfortably prop themselves up because of extended elbows. A towel roll or wedge under the infant's chest assists with increasing tolerance for this position. Positioning the hips in neutral rotation and neutral abduction is encouraged. Towel rolls can be placed along the lateral aspect of the thighs when the infant is sitting, and a wide Velcro band can be strapped around the thigh when the child is lying supine to keep the legs in more neutral alignment (Fig. 13-4). Developmentally, these children tend to be a little slower in attaining rolling but faster in attaining sitting and scooting than the children with the first type of posturing.

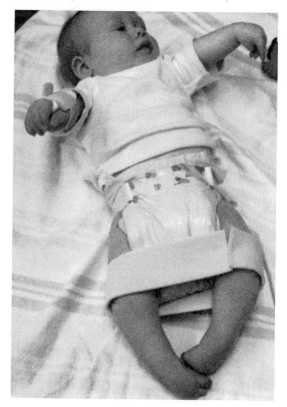

♦ **Figure 13-4**   This child with arthrogryposis multiplex congenita is wearing a wide Velcro band strapped around the thigh to keep the legs in more neutral alignment.

Although assuming the quadruped position and creeping are often feasible for this type of child, sitting and scooting are more energy efficient. Depending on muscle strength and the amount of bracing needed for standing, these children may never perform transitional movements from sitting on the floor to standing independently. They begin ambulating, as do their able-bodied counterparts, by the middle of their second year. Therapy focuses on addressing some key functional motor skills, such as rolling, sitting, hitching on the buttocks, standing, and strengthening those muscles that assist in maintaining posture. The goal is to maximize mobility to enhance participation in age-appropriate activities.

Strengthening during the first 2 to 3 years is most frequently addressed through developmental facilitation and play. Dynamic strengthening of the trunk can be achieved by having the child reach for, swipe at, or roll toys in the positions of sitting and static standing or while straddling the therapist's leg so that the child must rotate the trunk. These maneuvers incorporate stretching and strengthening into the therapeutic play activity. Aquatic therapy is often helpful for strengthening and developing functional mobility skills. If working on upright control in the pool, knee splints, specifically for use in the water, are helpful when bracing is needed on land, too. One way to determine whether functional training is having a strengthening effect is to ascertain the child's improved ability to perform the task.

Self-care skills, feeding, and manipulation of objects are dependent on hand function and elbow flexibility. Those children with limited upper extremity strength may have decreased ability to manipulate objects. Fortunately, these children tend to be resourceful in using other body parts, such as their feet or mouth, to manipulate objects when hands have inadequate strength and ROM. If the child has adequate ROM but inadequate strength, the child learns to support the arm on a leg or a table to assist in bringing the hand to the mouth. If the child is unable to get the hand to the mouth, adaptive equipment may make it possible to do some self-feeding. For example, if shoulder strength is absent, overhead arm slings are fashioned out of polyvinyl chloride piping and added to the high chair to permit finger feeding. If the upper extremities are postured in elbow extension, a typical and effective method of grasping an object is a hand cross-over maneuver, which affords some control and strength in holding or lifting an object. Electronic toys can be adapted so that the child can operate them via switches that can be activated by movement of the head, hand, or foot. These compensatory intervention strategies help to enhance skills needed for independence in ADL.

Standing is an important component of physical therapy during the first and second years. Families are encouraged to begin standing the child at approximately 6 months of age, as is normally done with able-bodied children. During standing, splints are used to maintain the lower extremities in adequate alignment. Shoes can be wedged to accommodate plantar flexion deformities and allow the child to bear weight throughout the plantar surface of the foot. Standing is initiated in a standing frame and progresses to independent static standing in the frame (Fig. 13-5). By 1 year of age, a child should be able to tolerate a total of 2 hours a day in the standing frame. This standing helps the child begin self-stretching of the feet and encourages the child to begin independent standing and walking. Use of a prone stander is usually avoided because this type of stander does not encourage dynamic trunk control, and therefore, the child is less likely to be working on the skills needed to stand outside the stander. Dynamic standing is encouraged through ball games such as kicking a soccer ball or batting a ball off a tee. Floor-to-stand activities usually do not begin to emerge until the child is ambulating securely, and sit-to-stand activities from a low chair usually begin to emerge

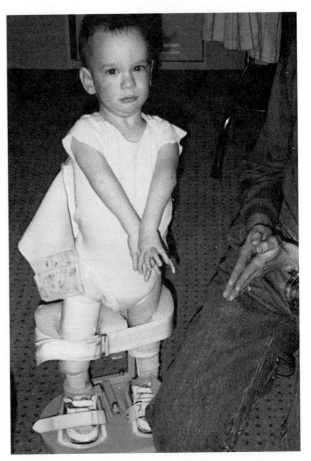

◆ Figure 13-5   Child who has arthrogryposis multiplex congenita in a standing frame.

when ambulation begins. Limitations in lower extremity strength and ROM can be addressed through splinting and bracing while the child is standing. Knee extension splints may be worn to compensate for weakness of knee extensors and mediolateral instability of the knees.

Stretching and Splinting

Because stretching programs for joint contractures are imperative, parents and caregivers are taught a stretching regimen from the time of the initial examination. This intervention strategy addresses one of the primary impairments of AMC. A stretching program is divided into three to five sets a day with three to five repetitions during each set. Each stretch is held for 20 to 30 seconds. With the realization that this is a significant time commitment, families are taught to incorporate stretching into times when the child would normally have one-on-one time with the caregiver, such as performing lower extremity stretches during diaper changes and upper extremity stretches during feeding. Dressing and bath times also provide good opportunities for stretching, especially once the child is self-feeding and out of diapers. Stretching must be a daily lifelong commitment for a person with arthrogryposis, but consistent stretching is most critical during the growing years and especially within the first 2 years of life.

To maintain the prolonged effect of the stretch, the extremity is maintained in a comfortable position of stretch with thermoplastic splints. Attempting to maintain the maximum stretch, rather than a comfortable position, over prolonged periods will cause skin breakdown and intolerance to splints. Splints are adjusted for growth and improvements in ROM, usually every 4 to 6 weeks during infancy. When fabricating ankle-foot orthoses (AFOs) for clubfeet, the calcaneus must be aligned in a neutral position because this will affect the entire foot's position. If the calcaneus is allowed to move medially with respect to the talus, the forefoot will fall into an undesirable varus position. When the hindfoot and forefoot are in a neutral position between varus and valgus, splinting can address insufficient dorsiflexion of the hindfoot rather than forefoot. This will prevent the potential problem of a midfoot break resulting in a rocker-bottom foot. To be maximally effective, AFOs are worn 22 hours per day.

Knee contractures are addressed early using splinting and stretching. For the first 3 to 4 months, anterior thermoplastic knee flexion splints for extension contractures or posterior knee extension splints for knee flexion contractures are worn up to 20 hours per day. For an older infant with knee extension contractures, it is advised that children not wear a knee flexion splint at greater than 50° of flexion for sleeping because this may encourage hip flexion contractures. Older babies with knee extension contractures should use the knee flexion splints for activities that require flexion such as sitting in the car seat or the high chair or when positioned in prone, utilizing the knee flexion the splint to enhance the quadruped position. Knee extension splints, which control knee flexion contractures or medial-lateral instability, are worn for standing activities and sleeping when a child is over 6 months of age. The splints encourage optimal lower extremity alignment during upright activity. Splints to control knee flexion contractures should be off 6 hours a day to allow floor mobility in a child with emerging skills. Knee extension splints for the management of knee flexion contractures must also be worn during sleep to be maximally effective.

Newborns are provided with cock-up wrist splints, but splints for hands are generally provided only after 3 months of age. This allows the child to integrate the normal physiologic flexion before placing a stimulus across the palm. Two sets of hand splints are fabricated. For day use, the child wears dorsal cock-up splints with a palmar arch in a position of neutral deviation and a slight stretch into extension as tolerated. This allows the child to have fingers available to manipulate toys. For night wear, the splint is a dorsal cock-up splint with a pan to allow finger stretching when the child is sleeping.

When considering elbow splinting, note that function and independence in ADL are improved when one elbow is able to flex adequately to reach the mouth and one elbow is in adequate extension to reach the perineum. Other factors to consider include available muscle strength and ROM, response to stretching, and potential future surgical procedures. Elbow extension splints are best worn while sleeping, but elbow flexion splints and elbow flexion-assist splints tend to be most functional when worn during the day. This allows the child to experiment with the hand in a more functional position for most play activities.

Young children respond most readily to conservative treatment using serial splinting, frequent stretching, and proper positioning. In Figure 13-6, *A*, the infant's posture is shown without leg splints. In Figure 13-6, *B*, the infant's lower leg is held out of the deforming postures through molded thermoplastic knee and AFO splints. The key to successful intervention for contractures is family education. Family education begins during the initial evaluation, as the caretakers not only are given general information about arthrogryposis but also receive information regarding their child's specific needs. Appropriate stretching exercises for involved joints are given with sketches or photographs to supplement the verbal instructions. Subsequent visits to the physical therapist allow work on splint fabrication and modification and positioning. Developmental play ideas are incorporated into the exercises to help the child progress developmentally. Physical therapists also work with the family to adapt age-appropriate toys to stimulate the child both physically and cognitively.

PHYSICAL THERAPY IN THE PRESCHOOL PERIOD

During the preschool period, the child's functional abilities and age appropriate participation vary based on the degree of involvement. Poor upper extremity function from the contractures and lack of muscle strength limit the child's independence in feeding, dressing, and playing at a time when typical peers are relishing their independence. This may be particularly distressing for the parents, who become more aware of the magnitude of their child's limitations when the child is no longer an infant in whom dependency is expected.

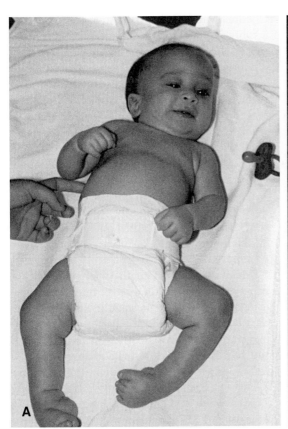
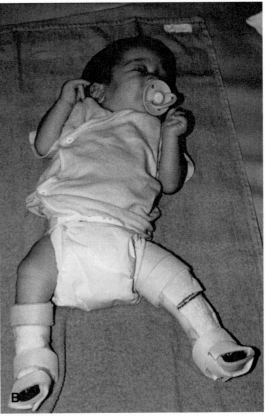

♦ **Figure 13-6**   **A**, A child who has arthrogryposis multiplex congenita without leg splints. **B**, The same child's lower extremity is held out of the deforming positions through use of molded thermoplastic knee splints and ankle-foot orthoses.

Structural limitations impeding participation in age-appropriate activities during this stage are similar to those found in the younger child. Restriction in joint ROM continues to be a problem secondary to rapid growth changes. Independent ambulation is often limited by poor protective responses of the upper extremities.

EXAMINATION

Passive and active ROM continue to be closely monitored by the physical therapist and caregivers. Proper fit of the splints is imperative in providing adequate stretch and positioning to impede the development of further deformities.

Functional muscle strength is an important component in the preschooler because it determines to a great degree the extent of bracing necessary and level of independence in self-care skills. Formal manual muscle testing (Kendall et al., 1993; Hislop & Montgomery, 2002) becomes more appropriate during this period because the child can comprehend verbal instructions. When testing

strength, it is important to grade the resistance throughout the arc of motion because the child with AMC will frequently be strong in the midrange but unable to move the extremity to the shortened end range. This finding is significant because the end range is where the child needs to work the muscle to maintain stretch of the antagonist muscles.

Gait assessment should include distance, use of assistive devices (includes braces and shoe adaptations, as well as upper extremity support), speed, symmetry of step length, gait deviations, and muscle activity. Some children ambulate as their primary means of locomotion; others rely on a stroller for community mobility. Despite research that supports powered mobility for the very young (Schiulli et al., 1988), mobility with wheelchairs is not usually addressed until school age when slow speed of ambulation, endurance, and safety concerns may preclude the child from interacting with peers. These children are bright and will often forgo ambulation for power mobility if it is presented too early. Forgoing ambulation early may limit standing for functional activities later in life.

GOALS

Ability rather than disability must be stressed, with a strong emphasis on assisting the child through problem solving rather than through physical assistance. The ultimate goals for this age are to reduce the disability and enhance independent ambulation and mobility with minimum bracing and use of assistive devices. Physical and environmental structural barriers may limit achievement of some fine and gross motor skills, but social skill attainment is paramount. Another goal is for the team to work together to improve the child's function in basic ADL skills.

INTERVENTION STRATEGIES

The team will work together during the preschool period to solve basic ADL challenges, such as independent feeding and toileting. For example, the use of a lightweight reacher may assist with dressing skills. Preschoolers usually can self-feed with adaptive equipment. These children are often toilet trained but lack the ability to perform the task independently.

Stretching

The need for stretching at this age continues to be addressed despite the preschooler's decreased tolerance to passive stretching three to five times a day. Two times a day for the stretching program is more realistic and appears to maintain ROM adequately in most cases. Families report that the best time for this is during dressing and bathing, which incorporates the program into an automatic part of the daily routine. Children can be taught how to assist with stretching through positioning. The child is also encouraged to verbally participate in the program, for example, by counting the number of repetitions. AFOs and positional splints continue to be worn to maintain the achieved positions.

Independent mobility in a safe and efficient manner is important for the preschooler to achieve and enhance social skills, as well as allow functional mobility. Independent ambulation with supportive bracing and with as few assistive devices as possible is stressed. Children with adequate strength and ROM who do not require bracing to walk generally need an AFO to prevent recurring clubfeet deformities. Older preschoolers with AMC are generally in the level of bracing that will be continued throughout school age.

Orthotics

Most orthotics are now fabricated from lightweight polypropylene and are more durable, less cumbersome, and more adjustable than the metal braces used previously.

Children with knee extension contractures tend to require less bracing than those with knee flexion contractures. If there is any question about the child's ability to maintain an upright position without hip support, the child's first set of long leg braces, a hip-knee-ankle-foot orthosis, will include a pelvic band. This type of orthosis is used for several reasons. The family may perceive that the child is regressing if initially unsuccessful ambulating without the pelvic band and later a band is added for ambulation success. The pelvic band encourages neutral rotation and abduction of the lower extremities. The pelvic band can also facilitate full available hip extension, and the hips can be locked in that position for prolonged standing. Once the child is ambulating with both hips unlocked, without jackknifing at the hips during stance, the pelvic band can be removed.

Maintaining hip strength, especially when the pelvic band is removed, continues to be important. One activity is to have the child begin static and dynamic standing on the tilt board. The child also begins taking steps forward, backward, and sideways. Strengthening, as with progressive resistive exercises, may be appropriate at this time. Clinical experience suggests that muscles may increase in strength by one half to a full muscle grade with exercise.

Ideally, the least amount of bracing is optimal, but if decreasing the bracing requires the child to use an assistive device that was previously unnecessary, the increased bracing may be more appropriate. A child with strong extensors such as the gluteus maximus and quadriceps is more functional than a child who requires bracing as a functional substitute for the extensors. The child with a good deal of bracing has difficulty donning and removing braces and is usually dependent for locking and unlocking hip and knee joints for standing and sitting.

Those children learning to walk may be limited in their independence if they do not have adequate strength and ROM to manipulate the assistive device, such as a walker, that is required to ambulate. Walkers are often heavy and cumbersome for the child, who may have inadequate protective responses in standing and upper extremity limitations. Thermoplastic material can be molded to the walker for forearm support when hand function is limited, affording the child added support and control (Fig. 13-7). Many children prefer to walk with someone rather than use a walker while they are gaining confidence in ambulatory skills. When learning to stand and walk, it is of utmost importance that the child learn how to use the head and trunk in order to stand and balance, and then weight shift for limb advancement. Those children who use ring- or gait-trainer walkers for ambulation often are delayed in learning these balance skills and are consequently limited in using upright control of balance for

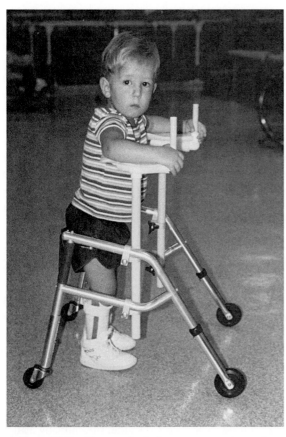

♦ **Figure 13-7**   Thermoplastic forearm supports can be customized to the walker.

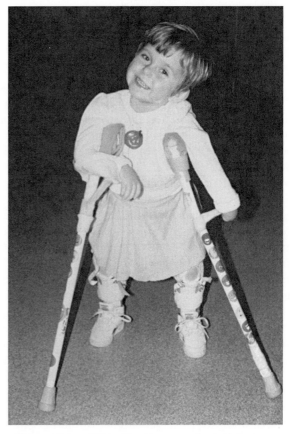

♦ **Figure 13-8**   Child with arthrogryposis multiplex congenita wearing polypropylene braces and using lightweight custom-made crutches constructed with polyvinyl chloride pipe.

transfers and ADL. Careful evaluation of ambulation potential is needed when deciding if a gait trainer is a good choice. These walkers will give children independence in walking for exercise but often do not translate into more independence in ambulation outside the walker.

Children with weak quadriceps and knee flexion contractures tend to ambulate with locked knee and ankle-foot orthoses. These braces can be fabricated with dial knee locks so that the knee position can be adjusted to coincide with the changing state of the knee flexion contracture. This will afford the ongoing opportunity to stretch out the contracture. Shoes may need external wedges to compensate for hip and knee flexion contractures that interfere with static standing. The child should be able to comfortably balance with the feet plantigrade without upper extremity support. For walking, assistive devices can be customized with thermoplastic material to allow for less awkward hand grips. Very lightweight crutches

can be custom-made of polyvinyl chloride pipe and thermoplastic material to give the child maximal independence (Fig. 13-8). Families may require assistance in identifying and removing environmental barriers that impede the child's independence both in the home and in the preschool environment.

Children in this age group are encouraged to participate in activities with children the same age in preschool, day care, swimming classes, and other peer group activities. They are encouraged to develop relationships with children who do not have disabilities, as well as with those who do. These early relationships help to enhance lifelong participation in integrated activities with peers. During the preschool period, many states mandate therapy services for children with special needs. Preschool services, as well as additional therapy services, are imperative for maximizing these children's skills for the demands they will encounter during school.

PHYSICAL THERAPY DURING THE SCHOOL-AGE AND ADOLESCENT PERIOD

The focus of physical therapy moves from the outpatient clinic into the classroom at this stage. The majority of children are enrolled in regular classrooms in their neighborhood schools, although they may have adaptive physical education, physical therapy, occupational therapy, and speech services to enhance the educational process.

Participation in school and classroom activities may be impeded by limitations in mobility. At school, children have increased demands to travel longer distances and move in groups under limited time frames. Alternative means of mobility may need to be addressed to enhance independence while managing materials (such as books and personal effects) with minimal outside assistance. Efficient and independent dressing, feeding, and toileting abilities take on a more compelling nature. Joint contractures continue to be problematic, especially through the last few growth spurts. This is a time when the adolescent is becoming more independent in self-care and adult monitoring of contractures tends to decrease. Unfortunately, appropriate interventions including exercise programs as well as surgical intervention often are postponed or ignored because of time and social considerations.

EXAMINATION

The school therapist acts as a team member, addressing goals of the child and family in regard to enhancing the child's educational experience. The physical therapy examination determines what types of training and adaptive equipment are needed to achieve educational objectives. Functional ADL skills are assessed to ascertain how efficiency and independence can be improved. The School Function Assessment (SFA) (Coster et al., 1998; Mancini et al., 2000) is a tool that is helpful in identifying functional skill levels in the school environment and in identifying activities for individualized educational plan (IEP) goals so that physical therapy's intervention can ultimately allow for greater participation of the child at school.

GOALS

During this period, the child with AMC must be responsible for self-care and for an exercise program to be performed to the best of the child's ability. If the child is physically unable to do these tasks, it is still important to be able to orchestrate care through verbal instructions to

a caregiver. The family must also become more responsible for expecting and allowing the child to be more independent. The goal of independence in mobility and keeping up with friends is important in the development of peer relationships. ROM continues to be a focus in management as the child with AMC will lose motion if he or she does not continue to stretch throughout the growing years. Teenagers who are going through their final growth spurt will often lose a significant amount of extension at the knees and the hips. If the teenager is not conscientious about night splint use and positioning for stretch, the ability to walk may be lost. Surgical intervention to regain ambulation skill during the second decade of life is not always an option.

INTERVENTION STRATEGIES

Dressing, toileting, and feeding may require adaptive equipment or setup for the child to be independent. Children with AMC require some selective pieces of adaptive equipment for achieving independence, but most are adaptable and innovative in using compensatory strategies rather than relying on assistive devices to achieve their goals. Frequently, classroom chairs and tables must be at custom-made heights to accommodate rising from a chair without manipulating brace knee locks. The desk top may need to be adjusted so that the child, by using a mouthstick or a wrist aid to hold writing implements, can maneuver items on the desk or write (Fig. 13-9). Implementation of ideas such as these limits disability by providing the child with successful compensatory strategies.

Continued compliance with the customized splinting and stretching program is expected. Children at this age may lose a few degrees of motion during growth, but further regression may result in loss of skills that were previously not a problem when more motion was available. Surgical intervention is sometimes helpful to improve joint position. A self-stretching program, utilizing assistive straps, braces, and positioning, can be incorporated into the child's routine to promote independence in attaining goals. The adolescent must be permitted to help plan his or her schedule, or compliance can be expected to be poor. Adaptive physical education in school, as well as adaptive sports programs outside school, can be adjuncts to physical therapy for promoting strength, endurance, and mobility. Vocational rehabilitation may be a helpful adjunct in assisting those with physical limitations to access future employment opportunities.

Speed and safety in independent mobility are important in the development of peer relationships. Families may be counseled during this time to consider powered mobility devices as an adjunct to manual mobility devices.

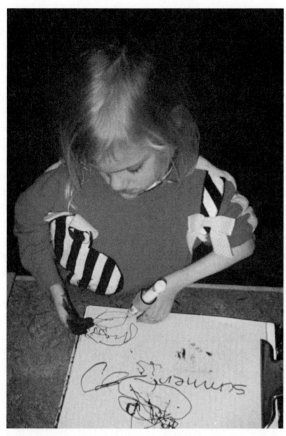

• **Figure 13-9** Child who has arthrogryposis multiplex congenita using a wrist aid to hold a crayon.

Cumbersome bracing, inefficient gait, and poor upper extremity function can limit a child's ability to participate in playground or social activities. Alternative modes of mobility may allow the child to participate safely. Use of alternative modes need not preclude ambulation but rather provides supplemental mobility for safety and energy conservation. Most children can achieve functional household ambulation but may require a wheelchair for efficient community mobility. The importance of standing and walking skills for maximal independence in the bathroom cannot be overstressed.

TRANSITION TO ADULTHOOD

Little has been published about the transition from childhood to adulthood for the person who has arthrogryposis. Sneddon (1999) published the results of a survey of 100 adults with AMC regarding issues related to aging. Limitations in activities during adulthood were related to

continued problems with ROM and strength that consequently limited independence in ADL, ambulation, and mobility. Those who required assistance with ADL during their school-age years continued to require assistance throughout their lifetime but were able to achieve a degree of independence with feeding, dressing, and grooming using selected assistive ADL devices. Those with severe joint involvement had long-term dependency on others for ADLs (Sodergard et al., 1997).

Pain appears to be a significant issue that occurs with aging. The majority of respondents reported difficulty with back and neck pain and increase in discomfort in other joints as well (Sneddon, 1999). Some specific problems that occur in adults are arthritic changes in weight-bearing joints and overuse syndromes in muscles and joints that are used for compensation or unique postures. Osteoarthritis, carpal tunnel problems, and neuropathies may develop as a result of prolonged joint constrictions and deformities. Increasing muscle weakness with increasing age has been found to occur, starting in early adulthood (Sneddon, 1999). Mobility problems emerging later in life may stem from secondary degenerative changes and muscle overuse syndromes (Hall, 1989). Manual or power wheelchairs may be more commonly used by adults than by adolescents and teenagers. Adults with AMC often use a wheelchair as their primary mode of mobility for long distances.

Advanced education is of utmost importance so that the adult with AMC becomes trained in a specialized skill or field. The type of work chosen will depend on the degree of activity limitations, education, and marketable skills. Computer-related work and other nonmanual occupations should be considered as employment options.

Many of the barriers that the adult with AMC will meet are physical barriers. The Americans with Disabilities Act has helped to reduce the presence of physical barriers. Transportation continues to limit access to vocational and avocational activities. Those who live near strong public transportation systems or have access to an automobile with proper adaptations have better opportunities for participation in activities outside the home. Advancements in technology allow those with arthrogryposis to have opportunities that enhance their freedom of mobility and their career options. Assistive technology can be of value in helping the patient safely and efficiently achieve work and leisure goals. Computers and voice-activated equipment may provide new freedoms for this population. Adult rehabilitation facilities, although probably unfamiliar with AMC owing to the small number of adults who have AMC, can provide services regarding assistive technology and orthotics as well as help in funding the equipment.

INTERVENTION STRATEGIES

Once skeletal growth has stopped, stretching is not as imperative, but maintaining flexibility and proper positioning is encouraged to impede the further development of deformities. Those with AMC who used orthoses during the school-age years typically continue to do so throughout adulthood. Those who used only ankle-foot orthoses for clubfoot control tend not to need these orthoses once growth is complete. One intervention required is joint conservation, which addresses the secondary impairments resulting from degenerative changes.

Information about the long-term sequelae of AMC in relation to degenerative changes, mobility levels, and use of adaptive ADL devices is critical to providing the most effective therapy to persons with AMC. However, there is a lack of research regarding the extent of independence of these children, adolescents, and adults in the area of ADL, use of manual or power wheelchairs, and ambulation ability. This lack of data may be because the children are followed early on within a medical model addressing their primary orthopedic concerns, but when they transfer to the educational setting and require less medical intervention, they are lost to follow-up. To meet the objective of providing the most appropriate therapy to these children, a nationwide database on functional outcomes, mobility, and associated long-term problems should be established.

▌SUMMARY

Arthrogryposis poses a variety of challenges for the health care team throughout the patient's lifetime. Although AMC is nonprogressive, its sequelae can limit participation in even basic ADLs. There is variability in clinical manifestations, but severe joint contractures and lack of muscle development are hallmarks of the disease. Each stage of development requires special attention for maximizing the child's function. An early goal of the team is to educate the family about AMC and to create the understanding that, without intervention, the child's body structure and functional skills could lead to further limitations in activity throughout a lifetime. Early medical and therapeutic management includes vigorous stretching, splinting, positioning, and strengthening, which will allow the child to develop optimal positions for functional ADL and enhance motor skill development. Timing of surgical procedures is critical to minimize intervention while maximizing benefits.

Each age has challenges physical therapy can have a positive impact on. During infancy, motor milestones are often delayed or skipped, and determining functional mobility is more important than ascribing a develop-

mental level. The intervention strategies focus on maximizing postural alignment through serial splinting and strengthening and on facilitating developmental activities. Ambulation is a preliminary primary goal, but once the child reaches school age, the focus shifts toward more independent, functional, and safe mobility. During the school-age years, the child must become more responsible for stretching exercises because stretching is an integral part of the program throughout the growing years. The team emphasizes assisting the child with problem solving and working toward independent mobility. Adaptive equipment is often necessary to allow the child with AMC to be independent in mobility and self-care. A comprehensive and integrated team approach is critical in developing strategies to meet these challenges. Ultimately, the goal is to have the child who has arthrogryposis grow to be an adult who is as independent as possible and an active participant in the community.

CASE STUDIES

WILL

Will was initially referred to physical therapy (PT) at 12 days of age by the orthopedic department. During the initial evaluation, photographs were taken to document postural alignment and position of his extremities. At the initial examination, the elbows were held in extension, the wrists were flexed and pronated, and the hips were in flexion, abduction, and external rotation (see Fig. 13-2). Plain films revealed that the right hip was dislocated. ROM was measured using a goniometer.

The family was instructed in passive ROM of the lower extremities during diaper changes and of the upper extremities during feeding. The following week, therapists fabricated customized low-temperature thermoplastic splints. These included AFOs, knee extension splints, and dorsal hand splints. As an infant, he was treated by medically based physical and occupational therapists every 3 to 4 weeks for splint adjustments and to monitor the home program. He also received weekly home-based early intervention services that emphasized developmental skills.

At 3 months of age, elbow flexion splints were fabricated and were worn 23 hours a day. To improve his hip alignment, his family used a wide Velcro strap to hold his legs in neutral alignment (see Fig. 13-4). Hip flexion contractures were reduced from 85° at birth to 25° at 3 months, and the hips could be adducted to neutral. Knee flexion contractures were 30° on the right and 25°

on the left. Forefoot abduction was 0° to 5° on the right and 0° to 10° on the left.

Muscle testing determined by palpation, and observation of active movement revealed active hip flexion, extension, and abduction. The hamstrings were active against gravity. The contractions of the quadriceps and plantar flexors were palpable. No biceps brachii contraction was palpable. There was, however, active shoulder flexion against gravity and at least fair strength of the pectoralis and triceps brachii.

At 6 months of age, he began a standing program in AFOs with wedged sneakers and knee extension splints in a standing frame. At 7 months of age he was able to sit independently when placed in sitting. At 10 months of age he developed rolling as a means of locomotion and could crawl on his belly for short distances. He was able to straddle sit on the floor and tolerate dynamic challenges to his balance. With his lower extremities stabilized he was able to move from supine to sitting.

Will entered a center-based early intervention program at 12 months of age. He received PT three times a week with the goals of independent mobility, improving ROM through stretching and positioning, and maximizing perambulation skills. He continued to be followed on a monthly basis in a medically based clinic to update the family's home program for Will and to adapt and progress his splints as appropriate. His family was performing a stretching program two to three times a day. At this point he began exploring the use overhead slings for antigravity upper extremity activities such as feeding and table top play.

At 14 months of age, Will had the ability to move from prone to sitting by widely abducting his hips and using his arms to raise and lower his trunk. By 16 months of age he could stand independently with knee splints, AFOs, and wedged sneakers but his hips were widely abducted so he relied on upper extremity support for success. Use of a figure eight strap on his thighs helped to control the excessive abduction of the hips allowing him to step but he required facilitation to weight shift.

By 20 months of age, Will was eager to stand and wanted to stand all the time. When supported through his axillae, he would walk. At 22 months of age, Will underwent bilateral posterior mediolateral releases for his clubfeet, which were subsequently placed in casts for 8 weeks. During that time, he used a cart for mobility. After cast removal, custom-made hip-knee-ankle-foot orthoses were fabricated and preambulation training began. He started standing with a posterior walker with the braces unlocked at the hips and rapidly progressed to taking two steps with the walker. During this period, Will received PT three times per week, with concentration on independent standing and walking. He also received adaptive aquatics two times per week. By 27 months of age, he was able to stand independently with both hips unlocked and could take two steps without upper extremity support.

At 30 months Will was able to walk 600 feet with a walker with unlocked hip joints. He could walk 6 feet without an assistive device. At that point gait training without a pelvic band was initiated, requiring verbal cues for Will to control excessive abduction.

At 5 years of age he had a triceps transfer and posterior elbow capsulotomy on the left upper extremity followed by a left wrist fusion into neutral to allow for greater independence in ADL. At 6 years of age, Will had distal femoral osteotomies for persistent knee flexion contractures. He had a wrist fusion with a tendon transfer on his left hand at age 10 to improve his hand function on the arm that now has better elbow flexion. He had knee extension osteotomies revised when he was 11 years old. He ambulates unlimited distances with knee-ankle-foot orthoses (KAFOs) and is able to walk limited household distances without braces. He is able to toilet, dress, and feed himself independently. He has received medically based PT services for a brief period postoperatively in order to get him back on his feet or to a higher level of function. Whenever he gets new braces and shoes, he consults his medically based therapist for the brace check out and shoe wedge measurement.

Will is now 13 and continues to receive weekly direct school-based therapy services. Emphasis of PT is on independent mobility within his educational environment. Stair ambulation continues to be challenging but necessary for fire drills. He is independently managing his braces, including donning, doffing, and locking. He actively works on a self-stretching program with emphasis on stretching his knees into extension. He continues to work on managing his books throughout the hallways and in the classroom. He received a power wheelchair when he was 10 years old but only uses it for independence in the community with his peers. At 13, he still walks the entire school day in his KAFOs with wedged sneakers. At this point his knees are again getting tight. He is unwilling to wear knee splints at night and is considering a partial distal femoral epiphyseodesis in the near future.

JOSEPH

Joseph is a 22-month-old male who is the third child in his family. His mother reported less activity during this pregnancy than during the previous two pregnancies but was not overly concerned. He was delivered by a planned cesarean section and presented in a frank breech position. He was diagnosed with AMC at birth and was subsequently transferred to a children's hospital for care.

PT was initiated when he was less than 2 days old. Posture was marked by hips so excessively flexed that his feet were positioned by his ears. He had hyperextended knees and his feet exhibited an equinovarus clubfoot deformity bilaterally. Torticollis with head rotation to the right was noted. The shoulders had what appeared to be normal passive range of motion. Joseph's elbows were flexed to 25°, his wrists were flexed and ulnarly deviated, and he had finger flexion contractures.

Photographs were taken to document posture and initial ROM. Goniometry was performed with a cut-down goniometer. Muscle strength was assessed through palpation and observation. Splinting of the feet and knees was initiated when he was 3 days old. Family and staff were educated on positioning to maximize hip extension. Joseph received passive ROM twice a day by a physical therapist, twice a day by nursing, and another one to two times a day by his dad, who stayed with him at the hospital. He was discharged from the hospital after 10 days. The extended stay was a result of feeding problems, which resolved before he was discharged. New splints were fabricated before discharge because of improvements made in ROM during his hospital stay. Home-based PT services were initiated when he returned home.

Joseph's health insurance plan had limited services for each lifetime condition. He qualified for 60 days of home-based PT services and 60 days of outpatient services. His family petitioned the insurance company, which agreed to pay for durable medical equipment past the 60 days but no therapy once his benefit was exhausted.

Medically related home-based services began at 14 days of age and focused on maximizing lower extremity alignment with emphasis on hip extension, knee flexion, and neutral foot alignment. A stretching program was initiated to address the torticollis (see Chapter 12 for additional information on interventions for torticollis). Positioning, handling, and developmental skills were addressed during this time as well. The home-based physical therapist was able to adjust Joseph's foot and knee splints for increased girth. By 1 month of age Joseph's hip flexions contractures had been reduced to 40°. Hips could be adducted to neutral and his knees could be flexed to 120°. The forefeet could be brought to neutral and the hindfeet corrected to –20° of dorsiflexion. Joseph exhibited a hypotonic trunk with poor head control, affecting prolonged positioning in his car seat and in prone. The car seat was padded with blanket rolls to allow neutral alignment of the head, trunk, and lower extremities. Adapted prone positions were addressed through football carries and prone positioning on mom's lap.

New foot splints were fabricated at 10 weeks of age. Knee splints were no longer needed at this time. Use of a strap to control excessive hip abduction was encouraged. He was seen every other week in a medically based PT clinic where the physical therapist worked with the family on the long-term therapy plan of stretching and strengthening to maximize developmental skills. The long-term goal was independent ambulation with AFOs without an assistive device within the next 3 years.

Joseph's home based PT benefit from his insurance was exhausted by the time he was 10 weeks old, but community-based early intervention (EI) services began at 14 weeks with weekly PT and occupational therapy. Emphasis of treatment was on trunk strengthening and head control activities as well as stretching.

He began a standing program in AFOs, wedged sneakers, and knee extension splints to help control his weak knees. This was initiated in a standing frame similar to the one shown in Figure 13-5. He progressed well with standing tolerance in the stander, and it was decided at 10 months to surgically correct his feet using posterior mediolateral releases. After 6 weeks of casting he received KAFOs for day use and Dennis Brown shoes with a bar for night wear. Physical therapy services were increased to two times a week at this point. After 3 months he was having difficulty with the Dennis Brown shoes and the bar, and they were replaced with AFOs for those times he was not in the KAFOs.

His EI physical therapist worked on standing and trunk strengthening for 5 months before it was decided that Joseph, at 15 months of age, would benefit from a pelvic band. He worked on standing and stepping with the HKAFOs for 6 weeks before starting postoperative medically based PT services at 17 months. In 8 weeks he went from standing in HKAFOs to walking limited community distances with a posterior walker and KAFOs.

At 21 months he is now able to walk in AFOs with a posterior walker but has a significant amount of internal rotation from tibial torsion, putting excessive force across his knees. He is able to walk up to 20 steps in KAFOs without upper extremity support and will retrieve toys from the floor and return to upright with close supervision. He is presently working on safe falling techniques.

He continues to receive weekly EI PT, which is focused on functional mobility skills. The family performs ROM exercises daily and is also working with Joseph on community ambulation with a walker.

REFERENCES

Axt, MW, Niethard, FU, Doderlein, L, & Weber, M. Principles of treatment of the upper extremity in arthrogryposis multiplex congenita type I. *Journal of Pediatric Orthopaedics Part B*, 6:179–185, 1997.

Bamshad, M, Bohnsack, JF, Jorde, LB, & Carey, JC. Distal arthrogryposis type 1: Clinical analysis of a large kindred. American Journal of Medical Genetics, 65:282–285, 1996.

Bamshad, M, Watkins, WS, Zenger, RK, Bohnsack, JF, Carey, JC, Otterud, B, Krakowiak, PA, Robertson, M, & Jorde, LB. A gene for distal arthrogryposis type I maps to the pericentromeric region of chromosome 9. American Journal of Genetics, 55:1153–1158, 1994.

Brunner, R, Hefti, F, & Tgetgel, JD. Arthrogrypotic joint contracture at the knee and the foot: correction with a circular frame. Journal of Pediatric Orthopaedics Part B, 6:192–197, 1997.

Burglen, L, Amiel, J, Viollet, L, Lefebura, S, Burlet, P, Clermont, O, Raclin, V, Landriau, P, Verloes, A, Munnich, A, & Melki, J. Survival motor neuron gene deletion in arthrogryposis multiplex congenita-spinal muscular atrophy association. Journal of Clinical Investigation, 98:1130–1132, 1996.

Cassis, N, & Capdevila, R. Talectomy for clubfoot in arthrogryposis. Journal of Pediatric Orthopaedics, 20:652–655, 2000.

Choi, IH, Yang, MS, Chung, CY, Cho, TJ, & Sohn, YJ. The treatment of recurrent arthrogrypotic club foot in children by the Ilizarov method. The Journal of Bone and Joint Surgery (Br), 83B:731–737, 2001.

Coster, WJ, Deeney, T, Haltiwanger, J, & Haley, SM. School Function Assessment. San Antonio, TX: The Psychological Corporation, 1998.

Darin, N, Kimber, E, Kroksmark, A, & Tulinius, M. Multiple congenital contractures: Birth prevalence, etiology, and outcome. Journal of Pediatrics, 140:61–67, 2002.

DelBello, DA, & Watts, HG. Distal femoral extension osteotomy for knee flexion contracture in patients with arthrogryposis. Journal of Pediatric Orthopedics, 16:122–126, 1996.

Drummond, DS, Siller, TN, & Cruess, RL. Management of arthrogryposis multiplex congenita. In AAOS Instructional Lectures, Montreal, Canada, 1978.

Goodman, RM, & Gorlin, RJ. Arthrogryposis. In Goodman, RM, & Gorlin, RJ (Eds.). The Malformed Infant and Child. New York: Oxford University Press, 1983, pp. 42–43.

Hall, JG. An approach to congenital contractures (arthrogryposis). Pediatric Annals, 10:249–257, 1981.

Hall, JG. Genetic aspects of arthrogryposis. Clinical Orthopedics, 194:44–53, 1985.

Hall, JG. Arthrogryposis. American Family Physician, 39:113–119, 1989.

Hall, JG. Arthrogryposis multiplex congenita: Etiology, genetics, classification, diagnostic approach, and general aspects. Journal of Pediatric Orthopaedics Part B, 6:157–166, 1997.

Hall, JG. Overview of arthrogryposis. In Staheli, LT, Hall, JG, Jaffe, KM, & Paholke, DO (Eds.). Arthrogryposis: A Text Atlas. New York: Cambridge Press, 1998, pp.1–25.

Hall, JG, Reed, SD, & Green, G. The distal arthrogryposis: Delineation of new entities—Review and nosologic discussion. American Journal of Medical Genetics, 1:185–239, 1982.

Hislop, HJ, & Montgomery, J (Eds.). Daniels & Worthingham's Muscle Testing: Techniques of Manual Examination, 7th ed. Philadelphia: WB Saunders, 2002.

Jayakumar, S. Personal communication. Alfred I. duPont Hospital for Children, Department of Orthopedics, Wilmington, DE, January, 2004.

Kendall, FP, McCreary, EK, & Provance, PG. Muscle Testing and Function, 4th ed. Baltimore: Williams & Wilkins, 1993.

Kramer, A, & Stevens, PM. Anterior femoral stapling. Journal of Pediatric Orthopedics, 21:804–807, 2001.

Legaspi, J, Li, YH, Chow, W, & Leong, JC. Talectomy in patients with recurrent deformity in clubfoot. Journal of Bone and Joint Surgery (Br), 83B:384–387, 2001.

Letts, M, & Davidson, D. The role of bilateral talectomy in the management of bilateral rigid clubfeet. The American Journal of Orthopedics, 28:106–110, 1999.

MacEwen, GD, & Gale, DI. Hip disorders in arthrogryposis multiplex congenita. In Katz, J, & Siffert, R (Eds.). Management of Hip Disorders in Children. Philadelphia: JB Lippincott, 1983, pp. 209–228.

Mancini, MC, Coster, W, Trombly, CA, & Heeren, TC. Predicting participation in elementary school of children with disabilities. Archives of Physical Medicine and Rehabilitation, 81:339–347, 2000.

Murray, C, & Fixsen, JA. Management of knee deformity in classical arthrogryposis multiplex congenita (amyoplasia congenita). Journal of Pediatric Orthopaedics Part B, 6:186–191, 1997.

Niki, H, Staheli, L, & Mosca, VS. Management of clubfoot deformity in amyoplasia. Journal of Pediatric Orthopedics, 17:803–807, 1997.

Palmer, PM, MacEwen, GD, Bowen, JR, & Matthews, PA. Passive motion therapy for infants with arthrogryposis. Clinical Orthopedics and Related Research, 194:54–59, 1985.

Robinson, RO. AMC: Feeding, language and other health problems. Neuropediatrics, 21:177–178, 1990.

Sarwark, JF, MacEwen, GD, & Scott, CI. Amyoplasia (a common form of arthrogryposis). Journal of Bone and Joint Surgery (American), 72:465–469, 1990.

Schiulli, C, Corradi-Scalise, D, & Donatelli-Schulthiss, ML. Powered mobility vehicles as aides in independent locomotion for very young children. Physical Therapy, 68:997–999, 1988.

Scott, CI, & Nicholson, L. Personal communication. Alfred I. duPont for Children, Genetics Department, Wilmington, DE, 2003.

Sells, JM, Jaffe, KM, & Hall, JG. Amyoplasia, the most common type of arthrogryposis: The potential for good outcome. Pediatrics, 97:225–231, 1996.

Shohat, M, Lotan, R, Magal, N, Shohat, T, Fishel-Ghodsian, N, Rotter, J, & Jaber, L. A gene for arthrogryposis multiplex congenita neuropathic type is linked to D5S394 on chromosome 5qter. American Journal of Human Genetics, 61:1139–1143, 1997.

Sneddon J. AMC & aging survey. Avenues, 10:1–3, 1999.

Sodergard, J, Hakamies-Blomqvist, L, Sainio, K, Ryoppy, S & Vuorinen, R. Arthrogryposis multiplex congenital: Perinatal and electromyographic findings, disability, and psychosocial outcome. Journal of Pediatric Orthopaedics Part B, 6:167–171, 1997.

Sodergard, J, & Ryoppy, S. The knee in arthrogryposis multiplex congenita. Journal of Pediatric Orthopedics, 10:177–182, 1990.

Staheli, LT, Chew, DE, Elliot, JS, & Mosca, VS. Management of hip dislocations in children with AMC. Journal of Pediatric Orthopedics, 7:681–685, 1987.

Staheli, LT, Hall, JG, Jaffe, KM, & Paholke, DO. Arthrogryposis: A Text Atlas. New York: Cambridge Press, 1998.

St.Clair, HS, & Zimbler, S. A plan of management and treatment results in the arthrogrypotic hip. Clinical Orthopedics and Related Research, 194:74–80, 1985.

Szoke, G, Staheli, LT, Jaffe, K, & Hall, J. Medial-approach open reduction of hip dislocation in amyoplasia-type arthrogryposis. Journal of Pediatric Orthopaedics, 16:127–130, 1996.

Tachdjian, MO. Arthrogryposis multiplex congenita (multiple congenital contractures). In Tachdjian, M (Ed.). Pediatric Orthopedics. Philadelphia: WB Saunders, 1990, pp. 2086–2114.

Vanpaelmel, L, Schoenmakers, M, van Nesselrooij, B, Pruijs, H, & Helders, P. Multiple congenital contractures. Journal of Pediatric Orthopaedics Part B, 6:172–178, 1997.

Williams, PF. The elbow in arthrogryposis. Journal of Bone and Joint Surgery (British), 55:834–840, 1973.

Williams, P. The management of arthrogryposis. Orthopedic Clinics of North America, 9:67–88, 1978.

Wynne-Davies, R, Williams, PF, & O'Conner, JCB. The 1960s epidemic of arthrogryposis multiplex congenita. Journal of Bone and Joint Surgery (British), 63:76–82, 1981.

Yau, PW, Chow, W, Li, YH, & Leong, JC. Twenty-year follow up of hip problems in arthrogryposis multiplex congenita. Journal of Pediatric Orthopaedics, 22:359–363, 2002.

Yingsakmongkol, W, & Kumar, SJ. Scoliosis in arthrogryposis multiplex congenita: Results after nonsurgical and surgical treatment. Journal of Pediatric Orthopaedics, 20:656-661, 2000.

Chapter 14

OSTEOGENESIS IMPERFECTA

DEBRA ANN BLEAKNEY
PT

MAUREEN DONOHOE
PT, PCS

Osteogenesis imperfecta (OI) is an inherited disorder of connective tissue. Other terms in the literature used to describe OI include fragilitas ossium and brittle bones. OI has an incidence of 1 in 20,000 live births, and its prevalence in the population is 16 per million (Wynne-Davies & Gormley, 1981). This disorder comprises a number of distinct syndromes and has great variability in its manifestations. The salient impairments of OI are lax joints, weak muscles, and diffuse osteoporosis, which results in multiple recurrent fractures. These recurring fractures, sustained from even minimal trauma, coupled with weak muscles and lax joints, result in major deformity. Additional impairments in OI with variable presentation include blue sclerae, dentinogenesis imperfecta, deafness, hernias, easy bruising, and excessive sweating. Without early and adequate intervention, these problems in children with OI may lead to irreversible deformities and disability. Physical therapy can have a positive impact on these children and their families. Therapists can accomplish this through strengthening exercises, adapting the environment, and educating the caregivers. Early physical therapy intervention helps prevent deformities and disability.

Too often children and adolescents with OI are overprotected as a result of the recurring fractures, leading to social isolation. This contributes to difficulty in interacting in peer play, adjusting to regular school, and achieving an independence level necessary to accomplish vocational goals. Because most children with OI have average or above-average intelligence, they may greatly benefit from a stimulating educational environment. These children become adults who are usually productive members of society. The management of their disabilities should therefore be directed toward obtaining optimal independence, social integration, and educational achievement. The overall prognosis of OI and its long-term sequelae depend on the severity of the disease, which ranges from very mild to severe. Likewise, the range of disability is from relatively mild with no deformities to extremely severe, with death occurring at birth or shortly thereafter.

In this chapter, we address the classification and pathophysiology of OI, medical and surgical interventions, physical therapy examination, evaluation, and interventions from infancy through adulthood. A case study of a child with OI is presented.

CLASSIFICATION

OI manifests as a group of impairments that vary in severity and that are marked by fragility of bone. It is not a single genetic disorder but is heterogeneous.

Because of the wide spectrum of this disease, there are many proposed classifications (Falvo et al., 1974; Sillence, 1981). Looser (1906) classified OI into two types: OI congenita and OI tarda. Seedorf (1949) further subclassified OI tarda into two types: tarda gravis and tarda levis. Historically, OI was classified based on clinical and descriptive characteristics (i.e., fracture healing and spinal deformities). The OI congenita and tarda classifications have clinical usefulness but do not reflect the scope of OI from a genetic or pathogenetic standpoint; however, the clinician will sometimes see these classifications referenced in the literature and in patients' medical records.

Osteogenesis imperfecta congenita (OIC), the most severe and disabling form, is characterized by numerous fractures at birth, dwarfism, bowing or deformities of the long bones, blue sclerae (80% of cases), and dentinogenesis imperfecta (80% of cases). Infants with OIC have a poor prognosis, with a high mortality rate resulting from either intracranial hemorrhage at birth or recurring respiratory tract infections during infancy (Tachdjian, 1990).

Osteogenesis imperfecta tarda (OIT), considered the milder form of OI in which fractures occur after birth, has been subclassified based on either the degree of bowing of the extremities or the number of fractures. Bowing correlates with the number of fractures and the severity of subsequent deformity (Tachdjian, 1990). The degree of bowing also indicates the potential need for surgical intervention.

The clinical characteristics of OIT type I include dentinogenesis imperfecta, short stature, and bowing of lower extremities, but the upper extremities are not bowed. Most children with OIT type I can ambulate but may need lower extremity orthotics. Surgery is often indicated for correction of the long bone deformity.

OIT type II is the least disabling form of OI in which fractures can occur in the first year of life or later, but in contrast to OIT type I, there is no bowing of the lower extremities. Most of these children approach average height and have excellent prognosis for ambulation.

Sillence and Danks (1978) have delineated four distinct genetic types of OI. This numerical classification system is based upon clinical presentation, radiologic criteria, and mode of inheritance and is generally well accepted by clinicians as well as basic scientists (Sillence, 1981). The Sillence classification uses a numerical system that correlates with morphologic and biochemical studies of OI (Sillence, 1981).

OI type I shows an autosomal dominant inheritance (Sillence, 1981; Sillence & Danks, 1978; Sillence et al., 1979). It is characterized by markedly blue sclerae throughout life, generalized osteoporosis with bone fragility, joint hyperlaxity, and presenile conductive hearing loss. These patients are generally short but are not as short as those with other forms of OI. At birth, weight and length are normal; short stature occurs postnatally. Dentinogenesis imperfecta is variably present. If dentinogenesis imperfecta is not present, this type of OI is further subclassified as OI type IA; if dentinogenesis imperfecta is present, the subclassification is OI type IB. Fractures may be present at birth (10%) or may appear at any time during infancy and childhood (Sillence, 1981). The frequency and development of skeletal deformity are also variable. The incidence of OI type I is 1 in 30,000.

Based on the Sillence classification, OI type II is either a common autosomal dominant form or a rare autosomal recessive form. OI type II is not compatible with life and infants either are stillborn or die within a few weeks. There is extreme bone fragility with minimal mineralization. Marked delay of ossification of the skull and facial bones is noted, and the long bones are crumbled (Tachdjian, 1990). The infants are small for their gestational age and have characteristic short, curved, and deformed limbs. The incidence as reported by Sillence is 1 in 62,487 live births.

According to the Sillence classification, OI type III can be autosomal dominant or recessive but is heterozygous. This form is severe, and there is progressive deformity of the long bones, skull, and spine, resulting in very short stature. Usually there is severe bone fragility, moderate bone deformity at birth, multiple fractures, and severe growth retardation. OI type III appears similar to OI type II except that the lack of skull ossification is not as marked and birth weight and length are within normal range. Sclerae have a variable hue, tending to be bluish at birth but becoming less so with age. Dentinogenesis imperfecta occurs in 45% of patients with OI type III. Hearing loss is common. As a result of the complications of severe kyphoscoliosis and resulting respiratory compromise, death occurs in childhood. OI type III is rare, and the exact incidence is not documented (Tachdjian, 1990).

OI type IV is rare and is inherited by autosomal dominant transmission. It is characterized by mild to moderate deformity and postnatal short stature. There is bone fragility and deformities of the long bones of variable severity. Sclerae tend to be normal, but dentinogenesis imperfecta is common. Hearing loss is variable. The prognosis for ambulation is excellent (Byers, 1988). The exact incidence of OI type IV is unknown (Tachdjian, 1990).

Sillence (1981) has compared his proposed nomenclature with the congenita or tarda classification. He relates type I to the congenita and tarda form of OI, type II to the congenita form (always), and types III and IV to both congenita and tarda forms. Sillence acknowledges that difficulty exists in this comparison because any syndromes accompanied by the onset of fractures at birth may be classified as congenita, whereas children with types I, III, or IV could have their first fracture at any time (Table 14-1).

TABLE 14-1   Classification of Osteogenesis Imperfecta

CLASSIFICATION*	INHERITANCE	FRACTURES	RADIOGRAPHIC FEATURES	STATURE	DENTIN	SCLERAE	HEARING	AMBULATION
Osteogenesis imperfecta congenita	Unknown	Extreme bone fragility at birth	Severe bowing of long bones	Dwarfism	Dentinogenesis imperfecta	Blue	Hearing loss	Nonambulatory
Osteogenesis imperfecta tarda type I	Unknown		Bowing of lower extremities	Short stature	Dentinogenesis imperfecta			Ambulation with braces
Osteogenesis imperfecta tarda type II	Unknown	Less disabling form	No bowing	Average height	Normal			Ambulatory
Osteogenesis imperfecta type IA	Autosomal dominant	Mild to severe bone fragility	Mildest form of OI	Short	Normal	Blue	Hearing loss	
Osteogenesis imperfecta type IB	Autosomal dominant	Mild to severe bone fragility	Mildest form of OI	Short	Dentinogenesis imperfecta	Blue	Hearing loss	
Osteogenesis imperfecta type IIA†	New autosomal mutation	Extreme bone fragility	Crumpled long bones, beaded ribs			Normal		
Osteogenesis imperfecta type IIB	New autosomal mutation	Extreme bone fragility	Crumpled long bones, normal ribs			Normal		
Osteogenesis imperfecta type IIC	New autosomal mutation	Extreme bone fragility	Long, thin fractured long bones, thin beaded ribs			Blue		
Osteogenesis imperfecta type III	Autosomal dominant (usual) Autosomal recessive (rare)	Variable bone fragility (often severe)	Progressive skeletal deformity (bowing)	Very short stature	Variable dentin abnormality	Variable; blue at birth	Hearing loss	
Osteogenesis imperfecta type IVA	Autosomal dominant	Bone fragility	Variable deformity	Short stature	Normal	Normal	Variable	Ambulatory
Osteogenesis imperfecta type IVB	Autosomal dominant	Bone fragility	Variable deformity	Short stature	Dentinogenesis imperfecta	Normal	Variable	Ambulatory

*Congenita and tarda are older forms of classification. OI types I through IV are based on the Sillence classification system.
†Osteogenesis imperfecta type II is lethal in the perinatal period.

PATHOPHYSIOLOGY

In all forms of OI, a defect in collagen synthesis results from an abnormality in processing procollagen to type I collagen, apparently causing the bones to be brittle. This defect affects the formation of both enchondral and intramembranous bone. The collagen fibers fail to mature beyond the reticular fiber stage. Studies show that osteoblasts have normal or increased activity but fail to produce and organize the collagen (Ramser & Frost, 1966). Histologically, there is variability among the different types of OI. In the more severe congenita form, the proportion of primitive osseous tissue with a woven matrix is markedly greater than in the tarda form (Bullough et al., 1981; Falvo & Bullough, 1973). A relative abundance of osteocytes is present, but intracellular matrix is deficient. In Sillence classification OI type I, morphologic findings include an increased amount of glycogen in osteoblasts, mild hypercellularity of bone (Albright et al., 1975), and no abnormality in collagen fiber diameter (Doty & Matthews, 1971). In OI type II, morphologic findings include poorly ossified cortical bone (Follis, 1952), abnormally thin corneal and skin collagen fibers (Bluemcke et al., 1972), hypercellularity of secondary bone trabeculae and cortical bone (Sillence & Danks, 1978), and deficient osteoid with deposition of argyrophilic material or primary trabeculae (Follis, 1952). In types III and IV, morphologic findings include an increased amount of woven bone, increased cellularity, increased number of resorption surfaces, and wide osteoid seams (Falvo & Bullough, 1973).

Those persons who have inherited OI tend to have a similar, if not the same, collagen defect as their parent. First-generation OI tends to be caused by a novel mutation of the gene. This specific gene mutation can then be passed to offspring. Genetic counseling when OI is found gives parents an accurate estimate of the risk of recurrence and an understanding of clinical variabilities in their family. The degree of severity in families is also variable. A mildly affected patient could give birth to a severely affected child. Describing to the parents the lifestyle of a child with OI may have more meaning than quoting risk figures (Solomons & Millar, 1973).

MEDICAL MANAGEMENT

No consistently effective medications are available to strengthen skeletal structures and prevent fractures. Improvements in medical care for the treatment of respiratory tract infections and in orthopedic management contribute to the improved outlook for a child with OI. Life expectancy appears to be increasing, but limited gains have been made in improving functional abilities (Albright, 1981).

New areas of research in OI are in the field of gene therapy (Niyibizi et al., 2000; Millington-Ward et al., 2002). Areas being investigated include cell replacement of the mutant gene, bone marrow transplants, and mutant allele suppression (Marini & Gerber, 1997).

Pharmacologic management for recurring fractures has included numerous medications and dietary supplements, some of dubious efficacy. Magnesium oxide, calcitonin, and fluoride have been administered in an attempt to decrease the frequency of fractures, but with inconsistent results (Granda et al., 1977). New research in postmenopausal women with osteoporosis has led to studies of children with OI using similar pharmacologic interventions. Bisphosphonates are having promising effects. Positive results such as reducing fractures and improving bone density have been reported from such pharmacologic agents as bisphosphonates (Batch et al., 2003; Landsmeer-Beker, 1997) including pamidronate and alendronate (Montpetit et al., 2003; Astrom & Soderhall, 1998, 2002; Falk et al., 2003; Lee et al., 2001). Sex hormones have been tried as a result of the clinical observation that fracture incidence diminishes after puberty. Although no dietary alterations have been shown to be effective, eating a well-balanced diet is highly recommended (Albright, 1981).

Once a fracture occurs, the bone is more susceptible to refracture. The already weakened structure predisposes the child to limb deformities from bowing of the long bones. Immobilization to assist in setting the bone in proper alignment can cause disuse osteoporosis, which, in turn, puts these fragile bones at greater risk of fracturing. Hence, a vicious circle is created: osteoporosis leads to fractures, and immobilization secondary to fracture creates disuse osteoporosis, which leads to further fractures. The goal, then, is to limit immobilization of the extremities as much as possible to prevent exacerbation of osteopenia and risk of more fractures.

Fractures in patients with OI generally heal within the normal healing time, although the resultant callus may be large but of poor quality. These fractures must be immobilized for pain relief and to promote healing in the correct alignment. Pseudarthrosis may occur when the fracture is not immobilized. Immobilization may be in the form of splinting with thermoplastic materials, orthoses, hip spica posterior shells, or casting. When there is malunion of fractures, angulation and bowing of the long bones occur, frequently accompanied by joint contractures. There may be disruption of the physis, resulting in asymmetric growth and deformity. When angulation occurs, mechanical forces tend to increase the deformity, thus aggravating the overall problem (Albright, 1981). The cartilaginous ends of the long bones are disproportionately large and have irregular articular surfaces. Fortunately, in nearly all patients with OI, the fracture rate diminishes near or after puberty.

The most successful means of fracture stabilization in long bones in OI is internal fixation with intramedullary rods (Jerosch et al., 1998). Although this method of stabilization is not without complications, the intramedullary rod can be helpful in preventing long bones from bowing after fractures and provides internal support to prevent further fractures. Indications for stabilization with rods include multiple recurring fractures and increasing long bone deformity that is interfering with orthotic fit and impairing function. The age of the patient and the size of the bone determine the type and timing of surgery. Intramedullary rod fixation of the femur is best done after 4 or 5 years of age when the thigh is not so short as to complicate surgery by compounding the technical difficulty. Surgical insertion of the rod in thin bones is also technically difficult.

The type of rod used depends on the type and severity of fracture. When a solid rod is used, bone growth may occur beyond the ends of the rods, necessitating subsequent surgery later for placement of a longer rod. Because children with severe OI are at greater than normal anesthetic risk from potential respiratory compromise, the number of operative procedures is best kept to a minimum. Special instrumentation has been designed that "elongates" with the child's growth, eliminating the need for multiple surgical revisions as the bone grows (Fig. 14-1). These extensible intramedullary fixation devices were first introduced by Bailey and Dubow (1965). They are used most frequently in the femur but may also be used in the humerus, tibia, and forearm. There is a high incidence of complications associated with using the intramedullary rods (Jerosch et al., 1998). Problems exist with the control of rotation and migration when using extensible rods; thus postoperative casting may be necessary. Orthoses may be needed after insertion of the rod for further external support. Early weight bearing with orthotic support is initiated as soon as possible. With internal fixation, there is a risk of osteopenia around the rod, especially with the telescoping rods.

Spinal deformities, including scoliosis and kyphosis, occur in 50% of patients with OI as a result of osteoporosis and vertebral compression fractures. Progressive spinal deformities such as scoliosis and pathologic kyphosis are more likely to occur in children with type III and IV OI than in those with type I OI (Engelbert et al., 1998). Kyphoscoliosis can be disabling and may be present in 20% to 40% of patients (Tachdjian, 1990). Unlike the

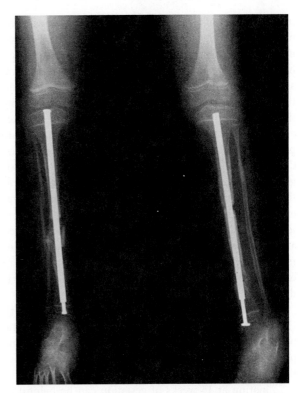

✦ **Figure 14-1**   Extensible intramedullary fixation rods that elongate as the bone grows in a child with osteogenesis imperfecta.

typical population, kyphoscoliosis in the OI population can be progressive over a lifetime, which further compounds the patient's short stature. The most common curve is that of thoracic scoliosis. Scoliotic and kyphotic curves in patients with OI are not usually amenable to conservative bracing. The bones in children with OI usually cannot withstand the forces of the brace, and the result is rib deformities rather than the intended effect on the spine (Albright, 1981). In adolescents and adults with severe OI, the incidence of scoliosis is 80% to 90%. Surgical stabilization is often advocated for the management of these deformities, but there is little documentation of long-term outcome (Engelbert et al., 1998; Hanscom et al., 1992).

IMPAIRMENT

DIAGNOSIS AND PROBLEM IDENTIFICATION

In the most severe forms of OI, the infant is born with multiple fractures sustained in utero or during the birth process. The prognosis of OI depends on its type. In the most severe forms, multiple fractures that have occurred in utero and during birth are associated with a high mortality rate. Prognostic indicators concerning survival and ambulation are the time of the initial fracture and the radiologic appearance of long bones and ribs at the time of the initial fracture. Spranger and associates (1982) devised a scoring system for providing an accurate prognosis for newborns with OI. This system coded the degree of skeletal changes based on clinical and radiographic findings in 47 cases. These investigators found that newborns who had marked bowing of their lower extremities but less severe changes in the skull, ribs, vertebrae, and arms and who had normal sclerae survived and had fewer fractures as they grew older. In the moderate and mild types, although the prognosis varies, there is a gradual tendency toward improvement when the incidence of fractures decreases after puberty.

If a family is known to be at risk of having a child with OI and the collagen defect has been identified in the parent, human chorionic villus biopsy can be done prenatally at 10 weeks of gestation to determine whether the child has the same defect. A prenatal ultrasound examination at 15 weeks of gestation can be helpful in identifying fractures, as well as possible mineralization problems (Byers, 1988).

The infant is usually of normal size at birth, but postnatal growth is impaired. Although no conclusive causative factors for this impaired growth are known, possible factors are the deformities themselves or abnormalities in the epiphyseal growth plates. The radiologic appearance of long bones associated with the most severe cases indicates bones with a thin radiolucent appearance. The malformed ribs affect respiratory function, which may lead to respiratory tract infections and reduced functional potential of the child.

Children with moderate OI are often identified after there have been several fractures from seemingly slight trauma. An example is a fractured humerus caused by the child holding onto a car seat while the caretaker is trying to get the child out of the car. Those children who begin having fractures of unknown origin at a young age can have collagen and biochemical studies done, usually from a skin biopsy. The tests can also be helpful in ruling out other disorders, such as idiopathic juvenile osteoporosis, leukemia, and congenital hypophosphatasia (which is fatal). No specific diagnostic abnormality indicating OI appears in laboratory tests; the diagnosis is made primarily from clinical and radiographic findings. In the infant, OI and achondroplasia are often confused because, in both conditions, children have large heads and short limbs. Radiographic reports, however, distinguish between the two.

DEXA (dual energy x-ray absorptiometry) is a helpful evaluation tool in the detection of low bone density. This is most useful in those children with milder forms of OI because it can detect changes more specifically than traditional radiographs (Moore et al., 1998). DEXA scans are also helpful in tracking drug efficacy in gaining bone density.

Collagen and biochemical studies can assist in differentiating a battered infant from an infant with OI. Radiographic studies are helpful because fractures at the epiphysis are rare in OI but common in child abuse, in which there is also evidence of soft tissue trauma. Bruising is common to both the infant with OI and the battered infant, but the bruising will disappear when the battered infant is in a safe environment. Three of the most helpful radiographic views in diagnosing OI are those of the skull (wormian bones), the lateral view of the spine (biconcave vertebrae or platyspondyly), and the pelvis (the beginnings of protrusio acetabuli) (Wynne-Davies & Gormley, 1981).

In the moderate to severe forms of OI, early childhood fractures lead to multiple recurring fractures because of the already weakened structure. The child develops limb deformities from bowing, which leads to impairment of mobility and of other functional skills. In the least severe forms of OI, because the first pathologic fractures occur later in childhood, there is less likelihood of recurring fractures with associated long bone deformities and therefore a better overall prognosis.

Engelbert and colleagues (1997), in a cross-sectional study of 54 children with OI, analyzed range of motion (ROM) and muscle strength for different types of OI. In OI type I, there was generalized hypermobility of the joints without a decrease in ROM. In type III, extremities, especially the lower extremities, were severely malaligned. In type IV, upper and lower extremities were equally malaligned. Muscle strength in OI type I was normal except for periarticular muscles at the hip joint. In OI type III, however, muscle strength was severely decreased, especially around the hip joint. In OI type IV, the proximal muscles of both the upper and lower extremity were weak.

Team members other than physical therapists who have an important role in the management of OI are orthopedists, orthotists, occupational therapists, audiologists, dentists, and geneticists. Little progress has been made in the primary prevention of this disorder, nor has there been much improvement in the medical management. With technologic enhancements and advances in neonatal care, more of these infants are surviving and presenting a management challenge to health care professionals.

EXAMINATION, EVALUATION, AND INTERVENTION

INFANCY

Typical participation restrictions for an infant with OI depend on the severity of the case. In severe cases, the most serious impairments are those of rib and skull fractures, which may compromise pulmonary status and neural status, respectively. Because of possible cardiopulmonary compromise, time may be spent in the neonatal intensive care unit, which could lead to decreased parental interaction and bonding. If OI is moderate to severe, parents have increased anxiety about holding the infant for fear of fracturing the infant's bones. This may result in minimal contact and may decrease the mutually nurturing interaction vital to both parent and child. Children with severe OI who have reduced mobility from skeletal deformities may be unable to achieve age-appropriate activities of daily living (ADL) or play in the normal peer environment.

Infants with OI are at a very delicate stage of life. They are completely dependent on their caregivers and have special needs regarding handling, positioning, and playing. During this stage, minimizing fractures, the development of further muscle weakness, and joint laxity is paramount. This is accomplished primarily through a physical therapy home program and parental education for proper positioning and handling.

At birth the infant may be of normal size, but postnatal growth is almost always stunted. Typical disabilities of the infant include a relatively large head, with a soft and membranous skull, and deformed limbs, which are usually short in the more severe forms of OI. Other features include a broad forehead and faciocranial disproportions, which give the face a triangular shape. Radiographically, fractures present at birth may be in varying stages of healing. The bones of infants with severe OI are short and wide with thin cortices, and the diaphyses are as wide as the metaphyses. Crepitation can be palpated at fracture sites.

The physical therapist should be aware of the infant's medical history of past and present fractures and know the types of immobilizations employed before beginning the examination. Pain is assessed using a tool such as the FLACC (face, legs, activity, cry, and consolability), which is an observational scale for assessing pain behaviors quantitatively with preverbal patients (Manworren & Hynan, 2003; Merkel et al., 2002). The caregiver's handling and positioning techniques during dressing, diapering,

and bathing are assessed. Assessing active, but not passive, ROM is essential. A standard goniometer can be used for measuring active ROM but may need to be cut down to a size suitable for the infant. As passive ROM testing is contraindicated in the majority of joints, active ROM is measured. Functional ROM may prove more useful because it will assist in visualizing the whole composite of motions needed in functional abilities. For example, functional active ranges would include the extent to which the child can bring the hand to the mouth or reach to the top of the head. If possible, the same therapist measures ROM during reevaluations. Intrarater and interrater reliability of goniometry should be determined for therapists and is checked annually if more than one therapist examines the child.

Assessing muscle strength is done through observation of the infant's movements and palpation of contracting muscles rather than by use of formal muscle tests. A gross motor developmental evaluation should also be performed because these children often have delayed development of gross motor skills secondary to fractures and muscular weakness. Delayed gross motor skills are manifested as activity limitations involving impaired achievement of motor milestones. Sitting by the age of 10 months is a good predictor of future walking ability (Daly et al., 1996). Some formal tests used include the Peabody Developmental Motor Scales (Folio & Fewell, 1983), which are normed and standardized; the Pediatric Evaluation of Disability Inventory (Haley et al., 1989), which is designed for tracking progress and assessing activity; the Bayley Scales of Infant Development II (Black and Matula, 1999) and the Brief Assessment of Motor Function for a quick description of gross, fine, and oral motor performance (Cintas et al., 2003). Finally, it is important to assess the appropriateness of equipment used for seating, transporting, and encouraging independent mobility of the infant.

Physical therapy includes early parent education in proper handling and positioning techniques. Bathing, dressing, and carrying the infant are critical times when the infant is at risk for fractures (Binder et al., 1984). When handling the infant, it is important that forces not be put across the long bones; instead the head and trunk should be supported with the arms and legs gently draped across the supporting arm. Some parents feel most comfortable supporting the infant on a standard-size bed pillow for carrying at home. It is important, however, to change the carrying position of the infant periodically because he or she develops strength by accommodating to postural changes. Dressing and undressing can be facilitated by using loose clothing and front or side Velcro closures. Overdressing should be avoided to reduce excessive sweating. Proper diapering includes a technique of rolling the infant off the diaper and supporting the buttocks with one hand with the infant's legs supported on the caregiver's forearm while the other hand positions the diaper. The infant should never be lifted by the ankles. Bathing is done in a padded, preferably plastic, basin. Infant carriers that are designed to safely support the head, trunk, and extremities are frequently used for household transporting. The carrier can be customized, such as a one-piece molded thoracolumbosacral orthosis, which can incorporate the legs so that they will not dangle and sustain injury. The carrier minimizes stresses to the fragile bones while positioning and transporting the infant. Physical therapy can be helpful in educating families in proper car seat use from an early age for this fragile population. Early on an infant can use a car bed or a rear-facing infant seat. Extra padding may need to be added on the transportation devices to snug up the fit and to pad the strap systems. Padding can be rearranged in the seat to accommodate the various devices the child may be in for immobilization of fracture sites. Given the low bone density and risk for fracture, the child should use a rear-facing car seat for as long as possible to maximize safety in the car.

Proper positioning of the infant is a critical component of the home program and management of the infant with OI. One supported position is side lying with towel rolls along the spine and extremities so that they are aligned and protected while the child is allowed active movement (Fig. 14-2). A prone position over a towel roll or with a soft wedge under the chest (if prone position is tolerated) is an alternative. When supine, the infant needs support for the arms, and the hips should be in neutral rotation with the knees over a roll (Fig. 14-3). Positions should be changed frequently and should not restrict active spontaneous movement, as spontaneous movement enhances muscle strengthening and bone mineralization (Binder et al., 1984). Positioning is useful not only for the purpose of protection from fracturing but also for minimizing joint malalignment and deformities. Figure 14-4 shows an infant's legs being poorly positioned in a baby carrier. The same infant seat is modified with lateral leg pads to keep the infant's hips and legs in neutral alignment, along with lower leg molded plastic splints (Fig. 14-5). Varying the position of the infant promotes the development of age-appropriate development skills.

Promotion of sensorimotor developmental skills is an ongoing component in the management of the infant and child. Identification of appropriate and safe toys for a child, as well as comfortable play positions that promote development, is often addressed jointly by the occupational therapist and physical therapist. For example, lying prone on a soft roll or over a parent's leg allows for weight-bearing use of the arms with co-contraction of shoulder musculature, which promotes active neck and back extensor muscle control (Fig. 14-6). Increasing muscle strength and support around the joint in activities such as this is especially important because the joint ligaments are lax. The prone-on-a-roll positioning also maintains good alignment of the extremities.

Developmental activities such as rolling and supported sitting should be encouraged as tolerated by the child. When encouraging rolling, the infant's arm is placed

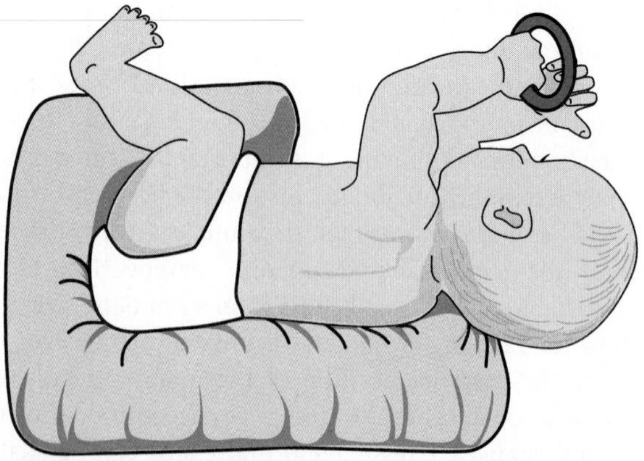

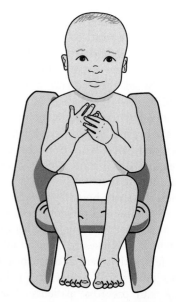

• **Figure 14-2**   Infant positioned lying on side using rolls. Emphasis is on maintaining trunk alignment while allowing for active and spontaneous but safe movement.

• **Figure 14-3**   Infant positioned supine with hips in neutral rotation, with knees flexed, and supported through the trunk.

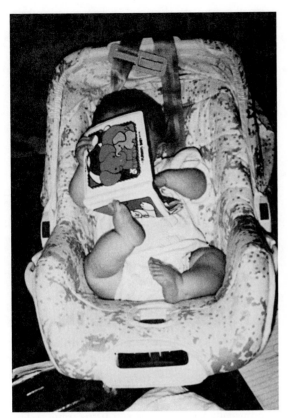

• **Figure 14-4**   Child positioned poorly in an infant seat.

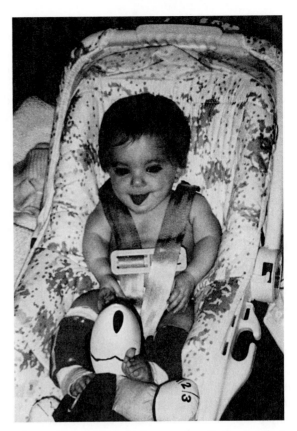

• **Figure 14-5**   Child with improved positioning in infant seat.

alongside his or her head, and then he or she attempts to roll over. Supported sitting is accomplished with seat inserts or corner chairs. Upright unsupported sitting can begin on the parent's lap with a pillow. When the child exhibits appropriate head control, short-sit and straddle activities can be done over the caregiver's leg or a roll but with avoidance of rotation across the lower extremity. These activities promote the development of protective and equilibrium responses and the beginning of protected weight bearing of the lower extremities. Many children with OI spend much time scooting on their buttocks before crawling is accomplished.

Awareness of proper handling while encouraging these developmental skills is of key importance. For instance, a pull-to-sit maneuver is contraindicated when using a distraction pull on the hands. Rather, this maneuver should be modified and facilitated by supporting the child around the shoulders while the child attempts to sit up. In working on trunk control over a ball, the therapist's hands are positioned on the pelvis and trunk rather than supporting or facilitating movement from the legs. Parents should be cautioned against using baby walkers and jumping seats because they do not foster proper positioning and weight

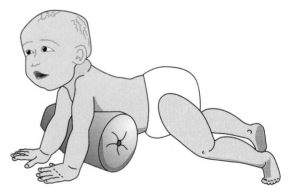

• **Figure 14-6**   Infant positioned prone on a roll encourages weight bearing, extremity and trunk alignment, and strengthening of extensor musculature during developmental play.

bearing. Baby walkers tend to give parents a false sense that the infant is protected. The child may have difficulty controlling these devices, resulting in unnecessary fractures. Active, spontaneous activity and exercise are encouraged in side-lying and supine positions, and in supported sitting, with the child reaching for, swiping at, rolling, and lifting lightweight toys of different textures. Pool exercises may begin as early as 6 months of age with the goals of promoting active exercise and weight bearing (Binder et al., 1984). Extremity movement may occur unobstructed in the water as the child is supported in a flotation device accompanied by a parent or the therapist. Long-sleeved clothing may be used to distribute the absorbed water weight evenly over the length of the limb, thus introducing a resistive component to the exercise.

At this stage, goals include teaching safe handling and positioning techniques to the caregivers and providing opportunities for development of age-appropriate skills. The intensity of treatment varies with the individual needs of the infant and family, but providing a home program and regular home visits by a physical therapist at least weekly is essential to ensuring that the environment is suitable for sensorimotor and cognitive development. The therapist can act as a resource and support for the caregivers as together they develop strategies to meet the challenges of safe caregiver handling, mobility, and developmental facilitation.

When fractures do occur, they may require splinting using a variety of materials such as perforated orthoplast or fiberglass. Ace wraps have been used to support and protect a limb in mild cases and in young infants. Fractures may heal within 2 weeks for the newborn and generally within the same time frame as other fractures in infancy (usually 6 weeks).

PRESCHOOL PERIOD

Bone fragility, joint laxity, and reduced muscle strength continue to be present in the preschool period but are now accompanied by secondary impairments of disuse atrophy and osteoporosis from fracture immobilization (Fig. 14-7). These structural changes and secondary impairments may limit mobility and subsequently restrict participation in play and socialization for the child with OI. This may affect the child's adjustment to regular school and hinder academic progress. The temperament of the child with OI may play a role in his ability to adjust to his activity limitations and participation restrictions. Cintas and colleagues (2003) demonstrated that the temperament of children with OI was comparable to those of nondisabled children except for having lower activity scores. Temperament was significantly and positively related with motor performance in persistence, approach, and activity.

At this stage, muscles are usually weak as a result of immobilization and relative disuse. Developmental motor skills may continue to lag because of frequent fractures and subsequent immobilizations, but cognitive skills should be appropriate for the child's age. When sustaining a fracture, children with OI typically complain little of

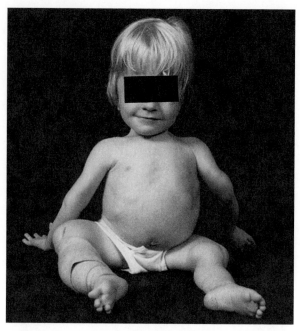

◆ **Figure 14-7** Child with osteogenesis imperfecta showing joint laxity and bony deformities: femoral anterolateral bowing and tibial anterior bowing.

pain and usually have minimal soft tissue trauma. There may be microfractures from repeated trauma at the epiphyseal plates, resulting in arrested growth and potential leg length discrepancy. In childhood, "popcorn calcifications" appear in the metaphyseal and epiphyseal areas of long bones (Goldman et al., 1980). It is postulated that these are fragmentations of the cartilaginous growth plate.

If the child begins to walk without adequate support, there is further bending of the long bones as a result of abnormal stress on the weakened structure. Bowing occurs in the anterolateral direction in the femur and anteriorly in the tibia. In those children who do not walk, lack of the normal weight-bearing stress leads to a honeycomb pattern of osteoporosis in the long bones.

Emphasis at this stage is on protected weight bearing and self-mobility for enhanced independence. Although proper positioning, handling, and transferring are still important, the emphasis shifts to the child's active participation in his or her care. During this period, the child with OI should have adequate upright control to begin bearing weight and at the very least, should be held in a standing position, as early weight bearing appears to have some beneficial effect (Gerber et al., 1990). When comparing radiographs of children with OI from the time of birth and several years later, the changing levels of bone density suggested that progressive osteoporosis had been superimposed on the basic bone defect (Bleck, 1981). Upper extremity bones were frequently more dense than those of the lower limbs and were less likely to fracture. This finding may be related to the use and stress put on upper extremity bones during self-care and play activities. A study by King and Bobechko (1971) concluded that limb immobilization caused osteoporosis; thus, to prevent the secondary impairment of osteoporosis in OI, supported weight bearing is advocated. The management principle used to implement appropriate weight bearing is to stress the lower limb bones while supporting the weakened structures through compression of the musculature around the bone. Contour-molded orthoses can be used to provide this compression and support.

For the preschool child, an evaluation of modes of mobility and adapted equipment is essential. An assessment of modification needs to promote supported sitting and mobility is also important. Equipment requires constant updating because of the changing positional needs related to mobilization-immobilization status. Splinting needs and adaptive ADL equipment are assessed for fit and usefulness. Developmental assessment tools that are appropriate include the Peabody Developmental Motor Scales, the Brief Assessment of Motor Function, and the Pediatric Evaluation of Disability Inventory to assess gross motor function and activity limitations in children with OI. Pain should continue to be assessed in the preschool-age child. Appropriate pain assessments include the self-report Numeric or Wong-Baker Faces Scale (Wong & Baker, 1988) or the FLACC Behavioral Scale (Manworren & Hynan, 2003).

Active exercise continues to be emphasized to increase muscle strength of the weakened muscles. Usually the hip extensor and abductor muscles are weak. Active exercise can be achieved primarily through developmental play. One developmental activity to increase weight bearing and maintain or increase strength in the quadriceps and hip extensor musculature involves having the child straddle a roll and come to stand with the therapist supporting the child's pelvis (Fig. 14-8). The therapist begins with the child sitting on a high roll that requires a small excursion of movement to go from sitting to standing and then gradually changes to using a lower roll. An active-resistive program graded for the patient's tolerance should be cautiously established. Use of light weights may be incrementally increased, but they should be attached close to large joints so as to avoid a long lever arm that increases the potential for fracture.

Early gym-related activities can be introduced at this age and include scooter board activities, riding tricycles, and playground games such as Simon Says, Red Light Green Light, and Follow the Leader. Activities that encourage overhead reaching are helpful in maximizing trunk

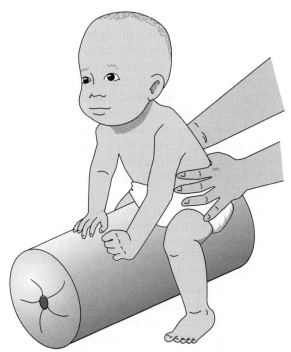

◆ **Figure 14-8** Straddle roll activity of supported sit-to-stand for lower extremity strengthening and weight bearing.

extension. These activities can include modified basketball activities when the ball is light and the child uses low speed passing. Racket sports using a tethered tennis ball help to build upper body strength. All activities should be closely monitored by a responsible adult to ensure safety. If the child is attending preschool, all members of the team should have a basic emergency plan if fractures should occur. This plan would include but is not limited to notification of family and splinting of involved extremities while awaiting supportive medical intervention.

An aquatic exercise program is an excellent therapeutic program for the child with OI. It can be started at an early age and can continue for a lifetime. There are many benefits to aquatic therapy, including the opportunity to socialize with peers in a safe environment, providing a safe method of strengthening muscles through resistance and assistance of the water, and the opportunity to improve cardiovascular fitness and to bear weight in a protected environment. The therapist can finely grade the progression of exercises in the pool by first using the buoyancy effect of the water to assist weak movements, then support the movements, and finally, use water to resist active movements. Exercises can be modified with floats by changing the length of the lever arm of the moving body part, through use of turbulence, and through altering the speed and direction of the movement (Duffield, 1983).

Pool exercises can also promote deep breathing to facilitate chest expansion and overall respiratory function, a goal that is especially important because chest deformities that compromise breathing capacity are common. Certain precautions should be taken when considering pool therapy for the child with OI. The heat of the water creates a rise in body temperature and increases metabolism, which is frequently already elevated in these children. It is suggested, therefore, that the time in the water, water temperature, and activity level be closely monitored for each child. Pool sessions are generally limited to 20 to 30 minutes.

Pool exercise therapy may interrupt the cycle of further disuse and secondary complications from immobilization. Aquatic therapy not only is an ideal therapeutic modality for the child with OI but also can be a therapeutic, lifelong avocational activity that can ameliorate the effects of the disabling process.

One key goal to be emphasized for the preschool child is safe, independent mobility, which is certainly a challenge if the child has frequent fractures. The aim is to prevent an activity limitation of reduced mobility resulting from the initial impairment. Researchers such as Perrin and Gerrity (1984) theorized that disabilities in intellectual development may occur when children have limited mobility. Opportunities for multiple safe modes of mobility should be explored to expand the child's repertoire of environmental experiences. A scooter for sitting propelled with legs or hands may be useful (Fig. 14-9).

The degree of ambulation attainable varies for preschool children with OI. Those children with limited ambulatory skills may need formal gait training, as well as instruction of family members. Interest in standing often occurs in the child's second year of life. Factors affecting the ability to stand and ambulate include the degree of bowing in the extremities and the muscle strength of the limbs. Ambulation is often introduced in the pool, for protected weight bearing. Because the buoyancy of water provides support for the body, weight bearing on weakened extremities and unstable joints can be gradually introduced without fear of causing trauma. Weight relief depends on the proportion of the body below the water level. For maximum weight relief for ambulation, the child begins standing in the pool where the water level is at the child's neck. Over time, the child gradually progresses to bearing more weight in shallow water. If the child with OI is recovering from a fracture, it is recommended that thermoplastic splints be used to further protect the extremity while in the pool. General guidelines for walking reeducation in water according to Duffield (1983) suggested that a patient start in parallel bars or a walking frame with the therapist initially supporting the

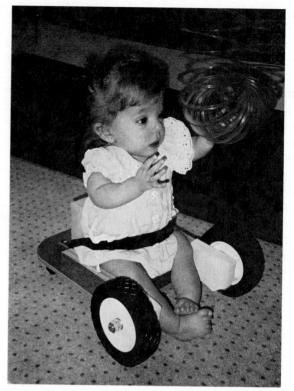

♦ **Figure 14-9** Scooter used for mobility that can be propelled by a child's legs or arms.

pelvis from the front. The patient practices weight shifts from side to side, forward, and backward and progresses to walking forward. The therapist cues the patient to lean slightly forward to counteract the upthrust of buoyancy, which tends to cause the child to overbalance backward. In this manner, protected walking for a child with OI can start much earlier than on a solid surface. Unsupported standing on solid ground is not recommended because it leads to rapid bowing of the long bones. When severe bowing of the extremities occurs, the child usually undergoes orthopedic surgery in the form of osteotomies. Age-appropriate lower extremity weight bearing is encouraged, although the child with moderate to severe OI needs external devices such as splints or braces to protect fragile long bones. Supported standing frames or orthoses such as hip-knee-ankle-foot orthoses (HKAFOs) may be used.

In moderate to severe OI, braces and splints are usually required to begin standing activities on solid surfaces. Use of orthotics provides the protected weight bearing needed to reduce the impact of stress on the osteoporotic bony deformities. Braces or splints are first used in conjunction with a standing frame. Prone standers with orthoses are used to grade the amount of weight borne on the lower extremities with progression from an inclined position to an upright position. The child may be fitted with a containment-type brace fabricated of lightweight thermoplastic material. These plastic orthoses can be fabricated to conform to the contours of the limb to provide support for the weakened structures around the bone. Often the first braces used during the toddler stage are made without knee joints and may have a pelvic band for maximal support. The pelvic band and locked hips minimize femoral rotation (Gerber et al., 1990). Knee joints can be added to the orthosis when the limb grows and strength increases (Fig. 14-10). Some braces use a lightweight plastic clamshell design and are contoured for ischial weight bearing. The child usually progresses from maximally supportive bracing to less cumbersome bracing as bony alignment and strength factors permit. HKAFOs can be beneficial in reducing tibial bowing and progressing in gross motor skills (Gerber et al., 1990). In a study of the effects of withdrawal of bracing in children with OI, when children used HKAFOs, they were less sedentary, more upright, and likely to be more independent than when not using the HKAFOs. A lower incidence of frac-

ture was also observed during periods of HKAFO use (Gerber et al., 1998).

Air splints have been used to prevent fractures and as a fracture management tool, either as a substitute for bracing or as a transition to bracing. Types of splinting include pneumatic trouser splints, which are used extensively in Europe. These air-filled trouser splints were introduced by Morel and Houghton (1982) for the support of the fragile long bones in OI. Morel has recommended that following the healing of the osteotomy for correction of long bone deformity these pneumatic splints be used for support. Letts and colleagues (1988) described pant orthoses called "vacuum pants" that were used in children with OI to enable weight bearing in a functional position during transition to knee-ankle-foot orthoses. Air splints such as the URIAS Pediatric C.P. Therapy Splints (J.A. Preston Corp., Jackson, MI) are readily available, need not be custom-made, and afford some flexibility when inflated to allow ambulation. Scott (1990) used these splints for instituting graded weight bearing and gait training in a child with OI. Drawbacks of the air splints are that they may be bulky and hot, so the child may not always tolerate them well.

The child graduates from using a standing frame with orthoses to ambulating in long leg braces with the knees locked in full extension. The preschooler may progress from parallel bars to various walkers or crutches as limb strength and ability improve. A walker that supports the majority of body weight through the trunk and pelvis is often used to assist in weight bearing during initial overland ambulation. This walker supports weight by means of a trunk support cuff and a padded pommel that is positioned between the child's legs. Rear-wheeled and four-point walkers followed by canes or crutches (depending on the type and severity of OI) may also be used (Fig. 14-11). Forearm attachments to walkers or crutches afford a degree of weight bearing distributed throughout the forearm to reduce stress on the arm and wrist, as well as to relieve some weight bearing on the lower extremities. Some children ambulate without braces when their fracture rate decreases in later years.

Customized mobility carts may be fabricated to encourage independent mobility when the child is immobilized, enabling the child to explore his or her environment, gain some independence, and maintain strength in the upper extremities. When there is good head and trunk control and the child can cognitively and safely handle a mobility device, power mobility may be an adjunct to preventing disability by allowing the child to keep up and interact with peers. These alternative mobility modes do not preclude ambulation but are useful additional mobility options. Regardless of the mode of mobility used, it is imperative

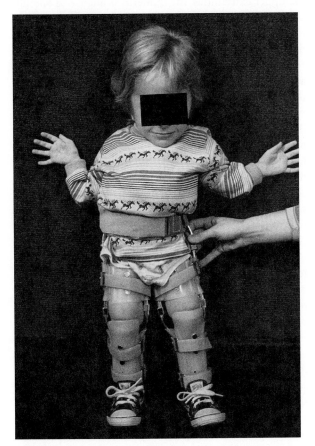

Figure 14-10   Child with osteogenesis imperfecta in plastic contoured hip-knee-ankle brace.

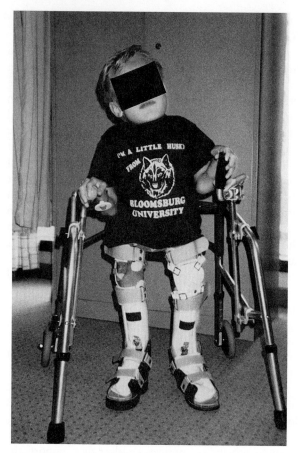

♦ **Figure 14-11** Child with osteogenesis imperfecta with long leg braces and reverse walker.

to provide the child with a degree of functional independence in the home and preschool environments that will promote participation in social activities.

Given that most states mandate car seats for children under the age of 6 years, it is important to assist families in proper seating choices once the child has outgrown the infant car seat. Children with the most severe forms of OI are safest in rear facing seating devices for as long as possible. A five point harness rather than a seat belt helps to distribute pressure from accidents more evenly. Booster seats should be used until the child meets the size restrictions for the seating rather than just focusing on the age restrictions of the law.

SCHOOL AGE AND ADOLESCENCE

Owing to reduced mobility and limited independence in ADL school-age children and adolescents often have limited ability to participate in peer related activities (Box 14-1). Social skill development may also be hampered if the

school-age child has been overprotected because of overwhelming fear and anxiety by caregivers regarding fractures. This may have an impact on the school-age child's scholastic endeavors and future vocational achievements. Studies have shown that children with OI tend to be intelligent and cheerful (Rezte, 1972). Parents and educators should encourage a positive attitude and excellence in school performance to prepare the child for a productive future.

At this age, the spine may exhibit varying degrees of deformity. Usually there is scoliosis, kyphosis, or both, resulting from compression fractures of the vertebrae, osteoporosis, and ligamentous laxity. The child with moderate to severe OI typically has marked bowing of the long bones from the multiple fractures and growth arrest at the epiphyseal plates. In the femur, the neck-shaft angle may be decreased with a coxa vara deformity and acetabular protrusion. The tibia is anteriorly angulated, which, in combination with the angulation of the femur, results in an apparent knee flexion contracture. The patellofemoral joint frequently dislocates, predisposing the patient to falls and fractures. Pes valgus frequently occurs at the ankle. In the upper extremities, the humerus is angulated laterally or anterolaterally and the forearms are limited in supination and pronation. The elbows often exhibit cubitus varus deformities, and elbow flexion contractures may be present.

Frequency of fractures tends to decrease markedly after puberty. Possible causes may be hormonal changes, increased awareness of how to prevent fractures, improvement in coordination, and increasing bone strength. Paradoxically, the adolescent who senses his or her increased stability and emerging independence may maximize involvement in activities, which increases the risk of more severe types of fractures. In an effort not to discourage these activities and independence, ongoing use of safe methods of mobility, caution, and responsible behavior should be stressed in patient instruction throughout childhood.

Physical therapy management at this stage involves other team members, including professionals in orthopedics, orthotics, occupational therapy, and rehabilitation engineering to maximize the child's independence in ADL, mobility, endurance, problem solving, and adjustment to the school environment.

Children and adolescents should be encouraged to do their share of the chores at home within their functional capacity. This allows the child to feel valued and lessens sibling rivalry (Thompson, 1990).

In this period, physical therapy may be helpful in returning the child to premorbid mobility status after a series of immobilizations from prepubertal fractures. The child may also require changes in bracing to accommo-

Box 14-1	International Classification of Functioning, Health, and Disability for Children with Osteogenesis Imperfecta		
CHANGES IN BODY STRUCTURE	**CHANGES IN BODY FUNCTIONS**	**ACTIVITY**	**PARTICIPATION**
Connective tissue disorder secondary to defect in collagen synthesis	Diffuse osteoporosis resulting in multiple recurrent fractures	Limited functional mobility skills, including rolling, creeping , transitional movements, and higher-level mobility skills	Limited participation in physical activities caused by endurance limitations and safety concerns
Brittle bones	Weak muscles Joint laxity Bowing of long bones	Limited ability to transfer Limited ambulation Decreased endurance	Limited peer play Infantilization Limited access to educational and work opportunities
	Scoliosis	Limited independence in self-care skills, including dressing and feeding	Limited access to wide range of environments
	Kyphosis	Limited ability for ambulation on uneven terrain	Limited independent living
		Limited independence in wheelchair mobility	Social isolation

date growth and body changes, such as increased or decreased mass. Lower extremity bracing continues to be of the lightweight plastic HKAFO or KAFO clamshell design, usually with joints.

Management of scoliosis and kyphosis is usually addressed by a spinal fusion, but the long-term results in maintaining alignment are questionable. Orthotic devices such as orthoplast jackets have been deemed ineffective in controlling scoliosis and kyphosis (Benson & Newman, 1981).

Along with occupational therapy, physical therapy can help maximize the child's independence by identifying safe, energy-efficient positions in which the child can work. Adaptive equipment is imperative for those with severe involvement. Occupational therapists, physical therapists, and rehabilitation engineers work together to adapt wheelchairs and seating and mobility devices to accommodate skeletal deformity, scoliosis, and kyphosis. A variety of lightweight and easily maneuverable manual wheelchairs can be adapted with seating inserts for trunk control and proper positioning. Vinyl upholstery is usually unsatisfactory for the child with OI because of the propensity for excessive perspiration. Proper wheelchair positioning is critical for prevention of further disabling deformities and for protection of the exposed extremities from trauma.

Physical therapy continues with the adolescent to work on ambulation, endurance, and strength. Household ambulation is usually achieved with assistive devices if adequate upper extremity strength is present. Walkers with progression to canes, or crutches may be used. In adolescence, ambulation without braces is less risky than before because the fracture rate decreases. Many children with OI who have primarily used the wheelchair for mobility are now able to ambulate about the house without any special change in their program. It is important to emphasize the maintenance of adequate skeletal alignment and maximal muscular strength throughout childhood to prepare for this improved function as an adolescent and adult. Community ambulation, however, is not practical, given the patient's short stature, the energy expenditure required, and the reduced muscle power. Most school-age and older children with OI use wheelchairs for community ambulation (Bleck, 1981). Independence in mobility is paramount because it has been shown to correlate with the degree of adaptation to the community environment. Bachman (1972) found that independence in travel away from home was the most important factor in an adolescent's ability to participate successfully outside the school environment.

Strengthening and endurance programs can be most successful when the child participates in developing a program that suits his or her interests and schedule. Programs can consist of progressive resistive exercises using incremental weights or adaptive sport activities. Enjoyable avocational activities that incorporate functional strengthening and mobility also must be stressed at this age. Although contact sports such as football, soccer, and baseball must be avoided, customized athletic and fitness programs are vital for youngsters with OI. These adaptive physical education activities can assist in improving physical health, finding a competitive outlet, helping to discover one's potential, and providing an opportunity to make friends (Patti, 1990). Sports and recreation activities should be encouraged as an adjunct to therapy. These activities will assist children to develop lifelong fitness interests. Some areas of adaptive sports that are available include swimming, challenger baseball, cycling, boating, noncontact martial arts, adaptive dance, billiards, golf, wheelchair sports, racket sports, and even sled hockey are available to the child who is interested. It is important to keep an open mind when helping a child develop fitness interests and to weigh the benefits against the risks when helping a child make choices. The physical therapist's role is to set appropriate parameters for participation, to provide precautions, and to upgrade the level of activity progressively. Volunteer jobs and social opportunities, such as the Boy Scouts and Girl Scouts, encourage emotional growth and develop leadership skills. Experience in a volunteer capacity can be helpful to the adolescent when applying for employment in the future (Fehribach, 1990).

In an 8-year cumulative management program, Gerber and colleagues (1990) found that a comprehensive rehabilitation program, long leg bracing, and surgical procedures on the femur resulted in a high level of functional activity for children with OI along with an acceptable level of risk for fractures. The three-part program consisted of early intervention emphasizing positioning and handling, muscle strengthening and aerobic conditioning, and protected ambulation. Included in the program were strengthening exercises for the pelvic girdle and lower extremity musculature, pool exercises, molded seating, long leg bracing, and gait training. Of the 12 children studied, 10 became functional ambulators, whereas 2 were household ambulators. Five children walked or took steps without braces, and 6 ambulated without gait aids. No child primarily used a wheelchair for mobility. All children of school age were enrolled in neighborhood schools. The physical activity of these children was high in that they participated in peer activities and some sports. Fractures were not eliminated through bracing, but the fracture rate was deemed acceptable.

TRANSITION TO ADULTHOOD

In the transition to adulthood, those who have OI are dealing with the secondary effects of disease because the fracture rate has declined or ceased by the late teen years. Some encounter problems with deafness in adult life. Scoliotic curves may be severe and may continue to progress. The incidence of scoliosis approaches 80% to 90% in teenagers and adults (Albright, 1981). Patients who have OI are especially susceptible to postmenopausal osteoporosis or the osteoporosis of immobilization (Sillence, 1981) when more fractures may occur (Paterson, 1995). Adults with OI also report problems with arthritic changes and back pain.

Emphasis of intervention during the transition to adulthood is on appropriate career placement, given the patient's intellectual capacity and consideration of the physical constraints. Because most patients with OI become productive members of society, optimal academic, social, and physical development will facilitate their opportunities to succeed in a competitive job market (Bleck, 1981). It is difficult to compete for jobs with physically healthy persons when life is complicated by repeated fractures, hospitalizations, and absences from work or school. Despite these problems, adults with OI tend to be ambitious and have low hostility levels. Half of adults with OI choose to marry and have children (Kiley et al., 1976). In a 1981 study by Bleck, 10 of 12 patients with OIC who had undergone early weight-bearing, orthotic, and mobility management programs attended regular educational facilities. The 12 patients with OIT who were managed by this program all attained complete independence in ADL, mobility, and ambulation (Bleck, 1981).

By the time these children reach adulthood, most use either manual or power wheelchairs for community mobility. Ambulation consists of household walking with an assistive device. Many of the children who previously relied on wheelchairs for household ambulation no longer needed them because they improved in functional mobility as adults.

CASE STUDY

JENNA

Jenna is a 5-year-old girl who has been diagnosed with type III/IV OI. Jenna presents clinically with type III characteristics (see Table 14-1), but a skin biopsy exhibited cellular and collagen characteristics more consistent with type IV OI. She is the fourth child in her family and no siblings have OI. At birth, she presented with five fractures despite delivery via cesarean section. Her family was initially trained in safe handling of their fragile child by the nursing staff in the newborn nursery. She was discharged on day 5 and referred to an OI clinic in the area. At 14 days of age Jenna was examined at the OI clinic by members of an interdisciplinary team, which included a physical therapist. She was transported to the clinic using a car bed in the family car. At this initial examination, her parents preferred to have Jenna rest supine on a bed pillow to reduce the risk of fractures her while moving and holding her.

The initial comprehensive examination included an assessment of handling by the parents, positioning of Jenna, and an assessment of the transportation device used to transport Jenna to medical appointments. Postural alignment and motor skills were also observed, but formal goniometry was deferred due to fractures.

Following the initial examination, the physical therapist worked with the family on a home program to promote proper positioning, handling, and facilitation of motor development within the context of daily activities. The parents were educated on how to safely change diapers and dress Jenna. They were shown how to safely hold Jenna in their arms rather than on a pillow with encouragement toward the prone position when being held by the parents. The car bed was padded with rolled receiving blankets to protect Jenna's fragile limbs while being transported in the family car. The family was taught to follow positioning guidelines to protect the limbs from fractures and also to facilitate proper skeletal alignment to minimize bony deformity. This included positioning the hips in a neutral position with extension whenever possible as her preferred position was flexion, abduction, and external rotation at the hips. The family was taught how to fabricate thermoplastic splints and use the splints to protect limb segments when fractures were suspected. They were provided thermoplastic splinting materials so they could fabricate and apply the splints at home.

Jenna's family was provided information on early intervention (EI) and began the process to get physical therapy services in her natural environment. EI physical therapy services began when Jenna was 4 months old. Jenna began participation in a clinical trial using pamidronate to reduce fracture frequency when she was 12 weeks of age. Jenna traveled every 8 to 10 weeks to a regional medical center for 3 days of intravenous pamidronate therapy until she was nearly a year old. At that point, she was old enough to receive the pamidronate therapy closer to home. Prior to starting pamidronate, Jenna was sustaining fractures about every other week. After beginning the pamidronate therapy, fracture frequency decreased to only a few a year.

Weekly early intervention physical therapy service initially concentrated on educating the family in how to safely handle and play with Jenna in her home environment. As Jenna's fracture frequency decreased and the family's comfort level increased, the emphasis of physical therapy then focused on strengthening the trunk and postural muscles. The physical therapist and family worked closely together to design appropriate activities to promote motor development and safe handling. They worked together on prone skills as well as rolling. As Jenna's trunk control improved, sitting skills were emphasized.

In addition to physical therapy services through the EI program, Jenna began an aquatic physical therapy program at 11 months of age. She was able to sit independently in waist deep water at 11 months of age, and was able to scoot in waist deep water at 18 months. She initiated walking in waist deep water with a walker at 18 months of age. After her family received a mobile hot tub, Jenna could swim year round at home several times a week.

During this time early intervention physical therapy services at home continued on a weekly basis as fractures allowed. Jenna began scooting on the floor in a sitting position at 20 months. At 30 months, she achieved supine to sit, and at 34 months she was able to crawl on her belly on the floor.

In addition, at 18 months, she began standing activities in knee extension splints and an upright stander. She underwent femoral intramedullary rodding at 20 months and was fitted with clam-shell HKAFOs at 23 months of age. At 28 months, she was walking with the HKAFOs and a walker. When she was 2.5 years old, Jenna gained the ability to move from supine to sitting independently. This skill was delayed due to her short arms, which made it difficult for her to push into an upright position. Once she attained this new skill, she practiced it so often in the first 48 hours that she sustained an upper extremity fracture and was unable to use this newly developed motor skill for another 4 weeks.

At 3 years of age, Jenna started preschool with her mother serving as a classroom aide. She received weekly school-based physical therapy services at the preschool where wheelchair mobility was emphasized. She initially used a manual wheelchair for temporary use until a power wheelchair was available when she was 3.5 years old. During this time she continued to progress with her ambulation and was able to sit to stand from a small bench with AFOs and a walker.

At 4 years of age, it was discovered that Jenna had a C-2 migration cranially with compression of foramen magnum and hydrocephalus. No medical intervention was indicated and this condition continues to be monitored.

Jenna has continued to progress in her mobility skills and when she was 4.5 years old, she participated in a Walk-a-Thon at school using a walker with a bench attached to it. This allowed Jenna to rest frequently and made it possible for her to participate in this school event with minimal adult assistance.

At 5 years of age, Jenna currently has a right tibia fracture and a suspected fracture of her left arm, which will prevent her walking with her walker for several weeks. She is still able to scoot on the floor for mobility and is able to use her power wheelchair for mobility as well. She continues to participate in an aquatics program with an emphasis on transitional mobility for prone and supine recovery in the water. She is able to walk 20 minutes in waist to chest deep water with a walker and can stand independently with close supervision. She currently requires adult assistance for wheelchair and toilet transfers due to the height of the transfer surfaces.

When the next school term begins, Jenna will enter a kindergarten classroom where her mother will continue to serve as a classroom aide. Physical therapy will be provided to Jenna by a school-based physical therapist. Physical therapy will be provided in the home if Jenna sustains a fracture and cannot attend school.

◾ REFERENCES

Albright, JA. Management overview of osteogenesis imperfecta. Clinical Orthopedics, *159*:80–87, 1981.

Albright, JP, Albright, JA, & Crelin, ES. Osteogenesis imperfecta tarda: The morphology of rib biopsies. Clinical Orthopedics, *108*:204–213, 1975.

Astrom, E, & Soderhall, S. Beneficial effect of bisphosphonate during five years of treatment of severe osteogenesis imperfecta. Acta Paediatrics, *87*:64–68, 1998.

Astrom, E, & Soderhall, S. Beneficial effect of long term intravenous bisphosphonate treatment of osteogenesis imperfecta. Archives of Disease in Childhood, *86*:356–364, 2002.

Batch, JA, Couper, JJ, Rodda, C, Cowell, CT, & Zacharin, M. Use of bisphosphonate therapy for osteogenesis in children and adolescents. Journal of Paediatrics and Child Health, *39*:88–92, 2003.

Bachman, WH. Variables affecting post school economic adaptation of orthopedically handicapped and other health-impaired students. Rehabilitation Literature, *3*:98, 1972.

Bailey, RW, & Dubow, HI. Experimental and clinical studies of longitudinal bone growth utilizing a new method of internal fixation crossing the epiphyseal plate. Journal of Bone and Joint Surgery (American), *47*:1669, 1965.

Benson, DR, & Newman, DC. The spine and surgical treatment in osteogenesis imperfecta. Clinical Orthopedics, *159*:147–153, 1981.

Binder, H, Hawkes, L, Graybill, G, Gerber, NL, & Weintrob, JC. Osteogenesis imperfecta: Rehabilitation approach with infants and young children. Archives of Physical Medicine and Rehabilitation, *65*:537–541, 1984.

Black, MM, & Matula, K. Essentials of Bayley Scales of Infant Development II Assessment. New York: John Wiley & Sons, 1999.

Bleck, EE. Nonoperative treatment of osteogenesis imperfecta: Orthotic and mobility management. Clinical Orthopedics, *159*:111–122, 1981.

Bluemcke, S, Niedorf, HR, Thiel, HJ, & Langness, U. Histochemical and fine structural studies on the cornea in osteogenesis imperfecta. Virchows Archives B, Cell Pathology, *11*:124–132, 1972.

Bullough, PG, Davidson, DD, & Lorenzo, JC. The morbid anatomy of the skeleton in osteogenesis imperfecta. Clinical Orthopedics, *159*:42–57, 1981.

Byers, PH. Osteogenesis Imperfecta: An Update: Growth, Genetics and Hormones, Vol. 4, Part 2. New York: McGraw-Hill, 1988.

Cintas, HL, Siegel, KL, Furst, GP, & Gerber, LH. Brief assessment of motor function: Reliability and concurrent validity of the Gross Motor Scale. American Journal of Physical Medicine and Rehabilitation, *82*:33–41, 2003.

Daly, K, Wisbeach, A, Sampera, I, Jr, & Fixsen, JA. The prognosis for walking in osteogenesis imperfecta. Journal of Bone and Joint Surgery (British), *78*:477–480, 1996.

Doty, SB, & Matthews, RS. Electronmicroscopic and histochemical investigation of osteogenesis imperfecta tarda. Clinical Orthopedics, *80*:191–201, 1971.

Duffield, MH. Physiological and therapeutic effects of exercise in warm water. In Skinner, AT, & Thomson, AM (Eds.). Duffield's Exercise in Water, 3rd ed. London: Bailliere Tindall, 1983.

Engelbert, RHH, Gerver, WJM, Breslau-Siderius, LJ, van der Graaf, Y, Pruijs, HEH, van Doorne, JM, Beemer, FA, & Helders, PJM. Spinal complication in osteogenesis imperfecta: 47 patients 1–16 years of age. Acta Orthopaedica Scandinavica, *69*:283–286, 1998.

Engelbert, RHH, van der Graaf, Y, van Empelen, MA, Beemer, A, & Helders, PJM. Osteogenesis imperfecta in childhood: Impairment and disability. Pediatrics, *99*:E3, 1997.

Falk, MJ, Heeger, S, Lynch, KA, DeCaro, KR, Bohach, D, Gibson, KS, & Warman, ML. Intravenous biophosphate therapy in children with osteogenesis imperfecta. Pediatrics, *111*:573–578, 2003.

Falvo, KA, & Bullough, PG. Osteogenesis imperfecta: A histometric analysis. Journal of Bone and Joint Surgery (American), *55*:275–286, 1973.

Falvo, KA, Root, L, & Bullough, PG. Osteogenesis imperfecta: A clinical evaluation and management. Journal of Bone and Joint Surgery (American), *56*:783–793, 1974.

Fehribach, G. Independent living. Presented before the Osteogenesis Imperfecta Foundation National Convention, Pittsburgh, 1990.

Folio, M, & Fewell, R. Peabody Developmental Motor Scales and Activity Cards. Allen, TX: DLM Teaching Resources, 1983.

Follis, RH, Jr. Osteogenesis imperfecta congenita: A connective tissue diathesis. Journal of Pediatrics, *41*:713–721, 1952.

Gerber, LH, Binder, H, Berry, R, Siegel, KL, Kim, HK, Weintrob, J, Lee, Y, Mizell, S, & Marini, J. Effects of withdrawal of bracing in matched pairs of children with osteogenesis imperfecta. Archives of Physical Medicine and Rehabilitation, *79*:46–51, 1998.

Gerber, LH, Binder, H, Weintrob, J, Grenge, DK, Shapiro, J, Fromherz, W, Berry, R, Conway, A, Nason, S, & Marini, J. Rehabilitation of children and infants with osteogenesis imperfecta: A program for ambulation. Clinical Orthopaedics and Related Research, *251*:254–262, 1990.

Goldman, AB, Davidson, D, Pavlov, H, & Bullough, PG. "Popcorn" calcifications: A prognostic sign in osteogenesis imperfecta. Radiology, *136*:351–358, 1980.

Granda, JL, Falvo, KA, & Bullough PG. Pyrophosphate levels and magnesium oxide therapy in osteogenesis imperfecta. Clinical Orthopedics, *126*:228–231, 1977.

Haley, SM, Faas, RM, Coster, WJ, Webster, H, & Gans, BM. Pediatric Evaluation of Disability Inventory. Boston: New England Medical Center, 1989.

Hanscom, DA, Winter, RB, Lutter, L, Lonstein, JE, Bloom, B, & Bradford, DS. Osteogenesis imperfecta. Journal of Bone and Joint Surgery (American), 74:598–616, 1992.

Jerosch, J, Mazzotti, I, & Tomasvic, M. Complications after treatment of patients with osteogenesis imperfecta with a Bailey-Dubow rod. Archives of Orthopaedic Trauma Surgery, 117:240–245, 1998.

Kiley, L, Sterne, R, & Witkop, CJ. Psychosocial factors in low-incidence genetic disease: The case of osteogenesis imperfecta. Social Work in Health Care, 1:409–420, 1976.

King, JD, & Bobechko, WP. Osteogenesis imperfecta: An orthopedic description and surgical review. Journal of Bone and Joint Surgery (British), 53:72–86, 1971.

Landsmeer-Beker, EA. Treatment of osteogenesis imperfecta with the bisphosphonate olpadronate (dimethylaminohydroxypropylidene bisphosphonate). European Journal of Pediatrics, 156:792–794, 1997.

Lee, YS, Low, SL, Lim, LAB, Loke, KY. Cyclic pamidronate infusion improves bone mineralization and reduces fracture incidence in osteogenesis imperfecta. European Journal of Pediatrics, 160:641–644, 2001.

Letts, M, Monson, R, & Weber, K. The prevention of recurrent fractures of the lower extremities in severe osteogenesis imperfecta using vacuum pants: A preliminary report in four patients. Journal of Pediatric Orthopedics, 8:454–457, 1988.

Looser, E. Zur Kenntnis der Osteogenesis imperfecta congenita und tarda (sogenannte idiopathische Osteopsathyrosis). Mitteilungen Grenzgebieten Medizin und Chirurgie, 15:161, 1906. (Translation: Toward an understanding of osteogenesis imperfecta and tarda [also known as idiopathic osteopsathyrosis]. Transactions of Frontiers of Medicine and Surgery.)

Manworren, RC, & Hynan, LS. Clinical validation of FLACC: Preverbal patient pain scale. Pediatric Nursing, 29:140–46, 2003.

Marini, JC, & Gerber, LH. Osteogenesis imperfecta: Rehabilitation and prospects for gene therapy. Journal of the American Medical Association, 277:746–750, 1997.

Merkel, S, Voepel-Lewis, T, & Malviya, S. Pain assessment in infants and young children: FLACC scale. American Journal of Nursing, 102:55–58, 2002.

Millington-Ward, S, Allers, C, Tuohy, G, Conget, P, Allen, D, McMahan, HP, Kenna, PF, Humphres, P, & Forrar, GJ. Validation in mesenchymal progenitor cells of a mutation-independent ex vivo approach in gene therapy for osteogenesis imperfecta. Human Molecular Genetics, 11:2201–2206, 2002.

Montpetit, K, Plotkin, H, Pauch, F, Bilodeau, N, Cloutier, S, Rabzel, M, & Glorieux, FH. Rapid increase in grip force after start of pamidronate therapy in children and adolescents with severe osteogenesis imperfecta. Pediatrics, 111:601–603, 2003.

Moore, MS, Minch, CM, Kruse, RW, Harke, HT, Jacobson, L, & Taylor, A. The role of dual energy x-ray absorptiometry in aiding the diagnosis of pediatric osteogenesis imperfecta. American Journal of Orthopedics, 27:797–801, 1998.

Morel, G, & Houghton, GR. Pneumatic trouser splints in the treatment of severe osteogenesis imperfecta. Acta Orthopaedica Scandinavica, 53:547–552, 1982.

Niyibizi, C, Smith, P, Mi,Z, Robbins, P, & Evans, C. Potential of gene therapy for treating osteogenesis imperfecta. Clinical Orthopedics, 379:S126–133, 2000.

Paterson, CR. Clinical variability and life expectancy in osteogenesis imperfecta. Clinical Rheumatology, 14:228, 1995.

Patti, G. Sports and OI. Presented before the Osteogenesis Imperfecta Foundation National Conference, Pittsburgh, 1990.

Perrin, EC, & Gerrity, PS. Development of children with a chronic illness. Pediatric Clinics of North America, 31:19–31, 1984.

Ramser, JR, & Frost, HM. The study of a rib biopsy from a patient with osteogenesis imperfecta: A method using in vivo tetracycline labeling. Acta Orthopaedica Scandinavica, 37:229–240, 1966.

Rezte, L. Osteogenesis imperfecta: Psychological function. American Journal of Psychiatry, 128:1446–1540, 1972.

Scott, EF. The use of air splints for mobility training in osteogenesis imperfecta. Clinical Suggestions, 2:52–53, 1990.

Seedorf, KS. Osteogenesis imperfecta: A study of clinical features and heredity based on 55 Danish families comprising 180 affected members. Opera ex Domo Biologiae Hereditariae Humanae Universitatis Hafniensis, Arhus: Universitetsforlaget, 20:1–229, 1949.

Sillence, DO. Osteogenesis imperfecta: Expanding panorama of variants. Clinical Orthopaedics and Related Research, 159:11–25, 1981.

Sillence, DO, & Danks, DM. The differentiation of genetically distinct varieties of osteogenesis imperfecta in the newborn period. Clinical Research, 26:178A, 1978.

Sillence, DO, Senn, A, & Danks, DM. Genetic heterogeneity in osteogenesis imperfecta. Journal of Medical Genetics, 16:101–116, 1979.

Solomons, CC, & Millar, EA. Osteogenesis imperfecta: New perspectives. Clinical Orthopaedics and Related Research, 96:299–303, 1973.

Spranger, J, Cremin, B, & Beighton, P. Osteogenesis imperfecta congenita. Pediatric Radiology, 12:21–27, 1982.

Tachdjian, MO (Ed.). Pediatric Orthopedics, Vol. 2, 2nd ed. Philadelphia: WB Saunders, 1990.

Thompson, CE. Raising a handicapped child. Presented before the Osteogenesis Imperfecta Foundation National Conference, Pittsburgh, 1990.

Wynne-Davies, R, & Gormley, J. Clinical and genetic patterns in osteogenesis imperfecta. Clinical Orthopaedics and Related Research, 159:26–35, 1981.

Wong, D, & Baker, C. Pain in children: Comparison of assessment scales. Pediatric Nursing, 14:9–17, 1988.

Chapter 15

MUSCULAR DYSTROPHY AND SPINAL MUSCULAR ATROPHY

WAYNE A. STUBERG
PT, PhD, PCS

Neuromuscular diseases include disorders of the motoneuron (anterior horn cells and peripheral nerves), neuromuscular junction, and muscle. Muscular dystrophy (MD) and spinal muscular atrophy (SMA) are two prevalent, progressive neuromuscular diseases that require physical therapy. Progressive weakness, muscle atrophy, contracture, deformity, and progressive disability characterize both diseases. No cure is available for either disease. "Incurable," however, is not synonymous with "untreatable," and the physical therapist can be influential in prevention of complications, preservation of function, and issues concerning quality of life.

The objective of this chapter is to present an overview of the childhood forms of MD and SMA, including the role of the physical therapist as a member of the management team. The clinical presentation of the diseases is reviewed, and examination procedures are presented to assist the clinician in identifying impairments, functional limitations, and disabilities associated with MD and SMA. Guidelines for physical therapy management are also outlined based on my clinical experience and review of related literature.

ROLE OF THE PHYSICAL THERAPIST

As a member of the management team in either the educational or medical setting, the physical therapist assists in the identification and amelioration of impairments, activity limitations, and participation restrictions for persons with MD or SMA. The team often includes physician(s) (neurologist, orthopedist, or physiatrist), physical therapist, occupational therapist, speech therapist, educator, social worker, genetic counselor, psychologist, and orthotist. Because therapists typically maintain a higher frequency of contact with families, referral to and ongoing communication with other team members become an important part of maintaining continuity of care.

The team approach should be family centered with a focus on collaborative goal setting among individuals with the disorder, family members, and professionals to ensure optimal care. By providing care using a family-centered philosophy, the pivotal role of the family is recognized and respected in the lives of persons with special health care needs.

Prevention is also an important role of the physical therapist. Stress on the child/individual and family can be reduced and coping facilitated through accurate prognostic information and recognizing signs that portend changing status and a resultant increase in disability. Examples of status change include the period before the loss of walking, before the need for architectural modifications to accommodate adaptive equipment for mobility, during transition from the educational to the vocational/avocational environment, or during the terminal stages of the disease when the decision to use mechanical ventilation will be a major issue for the family.

Providing information to family members, persons with MD or SMA, and other members of the team regarding physical limitations and expected participation restrictions is an important role for the physical therapist. Many resource materials are available online through the national Muscular Dystrophy Association (MDA) or through state chapter MDA offices.

PHYSICAL THERAPY EXAMINATION AND EVALUATION

Although the progression of MD and SMA is relatively well known, the clinician must carefully observe the child for changes that require intervention modifications. As stated by Thomas McCrae (1870–1935), "More is missed by not looking than by not knowing" (Siegel, 1986). Ongoing dialogue with families is invaluable in identifying family-centered goals and the need for program modification.

The physical therapy examination is the initial step in management of the child with MD or SMA and should include those components identified in the *Guide to Physical Therapist Practice* (American Physical Therapy Association [APTA], 2001). Specifically, the following must be carefully examined:

1. History with family concerns
2. Aerobic capacity and endurance
3. Assistive and adaptive devices
4. Community and work (job/school/play) integration
5. Environmental, home, and job/school/play barriers
6. Gait, locomotion, and balance
7. Integumentary status (when using orthoses, adaptive equipment, or wheelchair)
8. Muscle performance
9. Neuromotor development
10. Orthotic, protective, and supportive devices
11. Posture
12. Range of motion
13. Self-care and home management
14. Ventilation/respiration

Systematic documentation of disease progression is essential in timing of interventions during transitions from one functional status to another or during times of increased family need.

MUSCULAR DYSTROPHY

The etiology of MD is genetic inheritance. The pathophysiology underlying the disease is progressive loss of muscle contractility caused by the destruction of myofibrils. The specific cellular mechanism behind the destruction in Duchenne muscular dystrophy (DMD) and Becker muscular dystrophy (BMD) has been partially identified and is discussed later in the chapter. The rate of progression of myofibril destruction is variable among the various forms of MD, giving evidence for the possibility of more than one cellular mechanism in the destructive process.

The diagnosis of MD is confirmed by clinical examination and laboratory procedures, including electromyography, muscle biopsy, DNA analysis, and selected enzyme levels assayed from blood samples (Jones & North, 1997; Siegel, 1986). The criteria for classification of the various forms of MD include the mode of inheritance, age at onset, rate of progression, localization of involvement, muscle morphologic changes, and presence of a genetic marker if available. The MDA recognizes nine primary classifications of MD (Muscular Dystrophy Association, 2001). Table 15-1 lists the six most prevalent types that exhibit initial clinical signs in infancy, childhood, or adolescence. Emery-Dreifuss MD (humeroperoneal) is very rare and is discussed only briefly. Limb-girdle MD may exhibit signs in the teenage years, but the onset of symptoms is more typically in early adulthood, and therefore, along with the adult-onset forms of MD, it is not discussed in this chapter. The reader should refer to texts on neuromuscular diseases by Brooke (1986), Siegel (1986), and Harper (1989) for further information on clinical presentation and general management of MD.

The primary impairment in MD is insidious weakness secondary to progressive loss of myofibrils. In the case of the congenital forms of MD the weakness is pronounced at birth and easily recognizable. In DMD, the weakness becomes evident by age 3 to 5 years. In congenital and congenital myotonic MD, contractures present at birth also cause primary impairment. The incidence of mental retardation is highest in congenital myotonic MD, but it is less frequently reported in DMD or the other childhood forms.

Secondary impairments in all forms of MD include the development of contractures and postural malalignment. Postural malalignment is seen in antigravity positions of sitting and standing and often includes development of scoliosis. Other secondary impairments include decreased

| TABLE 15-1 | **Classification of Muscular Dystrophy** | | |

TYPE	ONSET	INHERITANCE	COURSE
Duchenne	1–4 years	X-linked	Rapidly progressive; loss of walking by 9 to 10 years; death in late teens
Becker	5–10 years	X-linked	Slowly progressive; maintain walking past early teens; life span into third decade
Congenital	Birth	Recessive	Typically slow but variable; shortened life span
Congenital myotonic	Birth	Dominant	Typically slow with significant intellectual impairment
Childhood-onset facioscapulohumeral	First decade	Dominant/recessive	Slowly progressive loss of walking in later life; variable life expectancy
Emery-Dreifus	Childhood to early teens	X-linked	Slowly progressive with cardiac abnormality and normal life span

respiratory capacity, easy fatigability, and occasionally obesity. Although significant intellectual impairment is not usual, IQ commonly averages 85, and consequently, 30% of boys with DMD have an IQ below 70 (Anderson et al., 2002). This finding has been related to a loss of dystrophin in the brain, and more specifically to a disruption in GABA receptors in the central nervous system (Anderson et al., 2002).

With the progression of muscle weakness, increasing caregiver assistance is required for persons with MD to carry out activities of daily living (ADL). Progressive disability is a hallmark of MD and requires multidisciplinary team management to maximize participation through the use of adaptive equipment and environmental adaptations.

Physical management in the treatment of MD is a key intervention because no drug or other therapy has been found to be curative (Brooke, 1986; Merlini et al., 2003). Physical therapy has been used to prolong the child's independence, slow the progression of complications, and improve the quality of life.

DYSTROPHIN-ASSOCIATED PROTEINS AND MUSCULAR DYSTROPHY

Within the past 15 years significant advances have been made in the molecular genetics and biology of the muscular dystrophies. These advances have followed the identification of the genetic defect behind DMD and the missing protein dystrophin. Many other proteins that are associated with dystrophin have been found to be defective or missing in other forms of MD. The proteins are termed *dystrophin-associated proteins* (DAPs) (Blake et al., 2002). The DAPs form a complex of extracellular, trans-

membrane, and intracellular proteins, which are represented in Figure 15-1.

Dystrophin acts as an anchor in the intracellular lattice to enhance tensile strength. The other proteins are thought to act as a physical pathway for transmembrane signaling. Absence of any transmembrane protein, however, would result in faulty mechanics of the cell membrane. For example, sarcoglycan defects are present in adult forms of MD (Emery, 2002).

DUCHENNE MUSCULAR DYSTROPHY

DMD is the most common X-linked disorder known, with an incidence of about 1 in 3500 live male births (Muscular Dystrophy Association, 2001). The prevalence of DMD in the general population is reported at about 3 cases per 100,000 (Emery, 1993; Muscular Dystrophy Association, 2001). Longevity is variable, from the late teens to early twenties up to the end of the third decade, depending on the rate of disease progression, presence of complications, and aggressiveness of respiratory care, including the use of assisted ventilation (Curran & Colbert, 1989).

Kunkel and associates (1985) identified the gene on the X chromosome (Xp21) that, when missing or defective, causes DMD and BMD, and Hoffman and associates (1987) then identified the protein (dystrophin) of the chromosome locus. Cloning of the dystrophin gene was the next major accomplishment, which provided a mechanism for prenatal or postnatal diagnosis and development of gene therapy (Koenig et al., 1987).

The etiology of muscle cell destruction in DMD and BMD is due to abnormal or missing dystrophin and its effect at the muscle cell membrane. Mechanical weakening

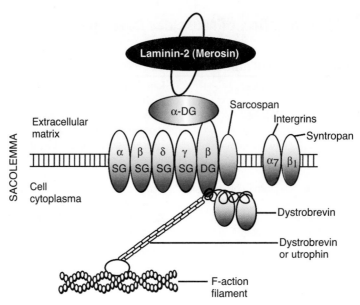

+ **Figure 15-1** Dystrophin-associated protein complex. Cross section through muscle membrane with intracellular, transcellular, and extracellular proteins. SG, sarcogylcan; DG, dystroglycan.

of the sarcolemma, inappropriate calcium influx, aberrant signaling, increased oxidative stress, and recurrent muscle ischemia are all hypothesized as mechanisms associated with myofibril damage (Petrof, 2002).

The focus of research for the treatment of DMD involves myoblast transfer therapy, gene and cell-based replacement therapy, attempts to increase production of other dystrophin-related sarcolemmal proteins (utropin), and use of drugs such as steroids. All therapies are in the experimental stage; myoblast transfer therapy is currently being evaluated in humans, the first human gene therapy trials for DMD using dystrophin are just beginning (Romero et al., 2002), but no trials have begun in humans on the use of utropin (Perkins & Davies, 2002). Evidence for the use of steroids and creatine is growing.

In myoblast transfer therapy the embryologic precursor cells of skeletal muscle (i.e., myoblasts) are obtained from a histocompatible donor. The cells are then injected into the muscle of the individual with DMD with the hope that the normal myoblasts will grow, mutate with the surrounding cells that are lacking dystrophin, and result in development of dystrophin. The results of the research in animals have shown that donor myoblast cells fuse with the dystrophic cells to form a hybrid multinucleated cell that produces dystrophin (Partridge et al., 1978). Myoblast transfer therapy is currently controversial, with the research by Law and colleagues (1997) supporting its efficacy, but others have reported disappointing results (Gussoni et al.,

1997; Karpati et al., 1992; Partridge, 2002) and lack of substantiation for the findings of Law and associates.

Gene therapy research involves the introduction of the dystrophin gene that is packaged in a modified adenovirus or retrovirus called a vector. Lee and colleagues (1991) produced an entire dystrophin gene, and more recently Amalfitano and associates (1998) developed the vector for delivering the gene. Minigenes, found to be effective in animal models of MD, have also been developed (Biggar et al., 2002). Human trials using gene therapy in limb-girdle MD (Stedman et al., 2000) and DMD/Becker MD are in progress (Romero et al., 2002).

Utropin is a muscle protein that has molecular similarity to dystrophin. Utropin levels in the muscle are high in the fetus and newborn but gradually diminish, until utropin is primarily found at the neuromuscular or musculotendinous junction in adults Courdier-Fruh and colleagues (2002) have demonstrated in vitro that utropin levels can be increased through upregulation. It is hypothesized that utropin might act as a substitute for abnormal or missing dystrophin.

Medical management of DMD has also included clinical trials of various drugs. Long-term steroid use (prednisone, deflazcacort, and oxandrolone) has been shown to improve outcomes, including prolonged independent and assisted walking by up to 3 years, improved isometric muscle strength by 60% in the arms and 85% in the legs when compared to untreated control subjects, as well as improved pulmonary function (Biggar et al., 2001; Merlini et al., 2003; Wong & Christopher, 2002). Reported side effects, however, include weight gain, particularly with prednisone, growth suppression, and osteoporosis. Strict dietary controls to offset the side effects are recommended (Wong & Christopher, 2002). The use of creatine in a randomized double-blind study of 15 boys with DMD has also demonstrated improved muscle strength and endurance and a reduction in joint stiffness (Louis et al., 2003). Louis and colleagues also reported improved bone mineral density in boys who were wheelchair users, suggesting that negative effect of steroids on bone mineral density might be offset with the use of creatine.

Although it is commonly agreed that the prevention of contractures and the preservation of independent mobility are primary goals of a physical management program (Vignos, 1983), the prolongation of ambulation through surgery or orthotics remains controversial. Some authors promote the use of surgery and lightweight bracing (Bach & McKeon, 1991; Bakker et al., 2000; Heckmatt et al., 1985; Hsu, 1995; Miller & Dunn, 1982; Taktak & Bowker, 1995); others express skepticism about prolonging the inevitable in a progressive disease when the financial and emotional costs to the family may be very high (Gardner-Medwin, 1979). A decreasing trend in the use of knee-ankle-foot orthoses (KAFOs) from 69% of the MDA clinics surveyed in 1989 to 27% in 2000 has been reported (Bach & Chaudhry, 2000) and would suggest a trend of less aggressive orthotic management in this population.

Surgical management has focused on the control of lower extremity contractures, use of orthoses in conjunction with surgery to prolong ambulation, and spinal stabilization for control of scoliosis. Achilles tendon lengthenings and fasciotomies of the tensor fasciae latae and iliotibial bands are two procedures commonly reported to be used in conjunction with orthotics and physical therapy to prolong ambulation (Bach & McKeon, 1991; Hsu, 1995). Posterior tibialis transfer into the third cuneiform to reverse equinovarus deformity has also been reported (Hsu, 1995). Surgical management of scoliosis typically includes the use of spinal instrumentation with Luque rods (Marchesi et al., 1997). Conservative management of scoliosis using orthoses remains prevalent (Bach, 2000), however, 85% of boys with DMD develop severe scoliosis (Rideau et al., 1984) and orthotic management has not been shown to stop the progression of the curve (Heller et al., 1997).

Impairments, Activity Limitations, and Participation Restrictions

Examination of the 4- to 5-year-old child demonstrates the onset of classical clinical features of DMD and the primary impairment of muscle weakness. The posterior calf is usually enlarged as a result of fatty and connective tissue infiltration, which corresponds to the term *pseudohypertrophic MD* that is used for the eponym DMD. The pseudohypertrophy can occasionally be seen to affect the deltoid, quadriceps, or forearm extensor muscle groups. Initial weakness of the neck flexor, abdominal, interscapular, and hip extensor musculature can be noted with a more generalized distribution with progression of the disease. Figure 15-2 demonstrates the trends of muscle strength decline up to age 16 years from a study by Brooke (1986). These data were obtained in a multiclinic study of 150 children with DMD over a follow-up period of 3 to 4 years. The data represent approximately 15 data points per boy as recorded during follow-up visits. Similar findings on anthropometric data, range of motion, spinal deformity, pulmonary function, and functional skills were reported by McDonald and colleagues (1995) in a cohort of 162 boys with DMD followed over a 3-year period.

Muscle strength can be documented using manual muscle testing (MMT), which has been reported to have acceptable intrarater reliability (Florence et al., 1992), although it is not as accurate as using specialized devices such as a dynamometer. Instruments such as a handheld dynamometer (Stuberg & Metcalf, 1988) or strain gauge devices (Brussock et al., 1992) can be used to obtain objective strength recordings in the older child to assist in prediction of disability, such as the loss of independent ambulation.

No limitations in range of motion (ROM) are typically noted before 5 years of age in DMD. Mild tightness of the gastrocnemius-soleus and tensor fasciae latae muscles usually occurs first. The normal lordotic standing posture is increased, and mild winging of the scapulae is then seen as a compensation to keep the center of mass behind the hip joint to promote standing stability (Fig. 15-3). Scoliosis typically develops just before or during adolescence.

Infancy to Preschool-Age Period

No significant impairments, activity limitations, or participation restrictions are typically seen in the infant or toddler with DMD, although Gardner-Medwin (1980) reported that half of the children fail to walk until 18 months of age. Delay in walking, however, rarely leads to the diagnosis of DMD. Symptoms are seldom noted before age 3 to 5 years, unless there is a positive family history and caregivers are looking for early signs. The mean age at diagnosis is usually reported to be around 5 years (Miller & Dunn, 1982).

Although there is no significant disability in early childhood, many disability-related issues must be addressed. The family will have questions regarding peer interaction,

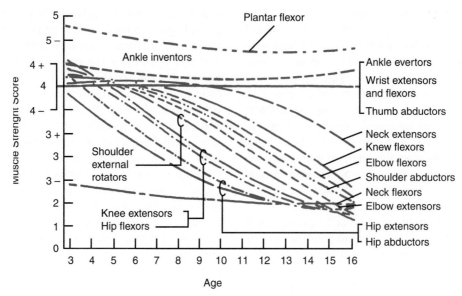

◆ **Figure 15-2** Muscle strength 50th percentile lines plotted against age of 150 children with Duchenne muscular dystrophy. *(Redrawn from Brooke, MH. A Clinician's View of Neuromuscular Diseases, 2nd ed. Baltimore: Williams & Wilkins, 1986.)*

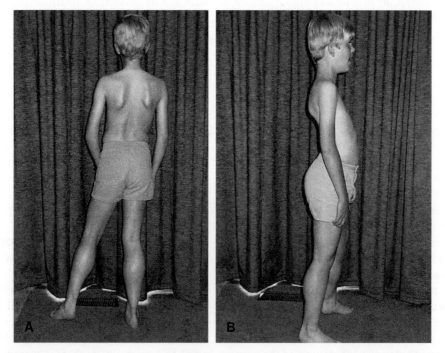

◆ **Figure 15-3** Typical standing posture of a 7-year-old boy with Duchenne muscular dystrophy. **A**, Posterior view; note the winging of the scapula, equinus contracture of the left ankle, and calf pseudohypertrophy. **B**, Lateral view; note increased lumbar lordosis.

routine activity level for the child, and the prognosis. The therapist must be aware of each family's coping response, goals, and needed supports to provide family-centered care. This is the appropriate time to discuss with the family the social aspects of the disability and to answer questions without portraying a future without hope.

Early School-Age Period

The initial disability in DMD typically occurs by age 5 years and includes clumsiness, falling, and inability to keep up with peers while playing. The young child's gait pattern is only slightly atypical, with an increased lateral trunk sway (waddling). Attempts at running, however, accentuate the waddling progression, and neither running nor jumping is attained. The Gowers sign (using the arms to push on the thighs to attain standing) is usually present after one or repeated trials of assuming standing position from sitting on the floor.

Stair climbing and arising to standing from the floor become progressively more difficult and signal the first significant functional limitation by age 6 to 8 years. Progressive changes in the gait pattern include the deviations of an increased base of support, pronounced lateral trunk sway (compensated Trendelenburg), toe-walking, and retraction of the shoulders with lack of reciprocal arm swing. Toe-walking initially may be a compensation for weakness of the abdominal and hip extensor muscles, resulting in lordosis and forward shift of the body's center of mass with later evidence of contracture of the posterior calf musculature.

Toe-walking caused by contracture of the posterior calf musculature, in-toeing with substitution of the tensor fasciae latae to compensate for weakness of the iliopsoas

muscles, falls resulting from progressive weakness, and complaints of fatigue while walking become increasingly frequent from age 8 to 10 years. A restrictive pattern of pulmonary impairment and progressive decline in maximal vital capacity also becomes increasingly evident (Galasko et al., 1995).

Examination Considerations

An examination to document functional impairment and disability progression is essential. Various formats have been reported (Brooke, 1986; Steffensen & Hyde, 2001; Vignos et al., 1996) that are variations of the guidelines initially published by Swinyard and associates (1957). A classification system published by Vignos and colleagues (1963) is outlined in Box 15-1. A more detailed examination format for DMD has been published by Brooke and associates (1981), which includes pulmonary function and timed performance of activities (see Appendix I). Normative data for DMD has been published using the clinical protocol by Brooke and associates (1989). Other functional assessment tools, such as the Pediatric Evaluation of Disability Inventory (PEDI) (Haley et al., 1992), School Function Assessment (SFA) (Coster et al., 1998), EK Scale (Steffensen & Hyde, 2001), or Barthel Index (Nair et al., 2001), should also be considered for use to give more specific information on the child's functional skills. The EK Scale was recently validated for DMD and SMA, and includes ordinal scoring of 10 categories including items on mobility, transfers, ability to cough/speak, and physical well-being. The PEDI, the SFA, or the Vignos (Brooke) functional testing format can be used for diagnosis of other types of MD or of SMA.

Box 15-1	**Vignos Functional Rating Scale for Duchenne Muscular Dystrophy**

1. Walks and climbs stairs without assistance
2. Walks and climbs stairs with aid of railing
3. Walks and climbs stairs slowly with aid of railing (over 25 seconds for eight standard steps)
4. Walks, but cannot climb stairs
5. Walks assisted, but cannot climb stairs or get out of chair
6. Walks only with assistance or with braces
7. In wheelchair: sits erect and can roll chair and perform bed and wheelchair ADL
8. In wheelchair: sits erect and is unable to perform bed and wheelchair ADL without assistance
9. In wheelchair: sits erect only with support and is able to do only minimal ADL
10. In bed: can do no ADL without assistance

Data from Vignos, PJ, Spencer, GE, & Archibald, KC. Management of progressive muscular dystrophy. Journal of the American Medical Association, *184*:103–112, 1963. Copyright © 1963, American Medical Association.

Muscle weakness is apparent in the school-age child by age 6 to 8 years and should be objectively documented using a handheld dynamometer (Stuberg & Metcalf, 1988), electrodynamometer (Saranti et al., 1980), isokinetic dynamometer (Molnar & Alexander, 1973; Scott et al., 1982), or other device. Use of a dynamometer in conjunction with manual muscle testing has been shown to provide reliable information on the progression of weakness in key muscle groups (Brussock et al., 1992; Fowler & Gardner, 1967; Stuberg & Metcalf, 1988). Contracture development should be documented using goniometry and a standardized protocol. Intrarater reliability of the measurements has been shown to be acceptable to provide objective information for program planning when a standardized measurement protocol is used (Pandya et al., 1985).

A clinical estimate of respiratory function can be obtained through measurement of respiratory rate and chest wall excursion (using a tape measure) and by noting the child's ability to cough and clear secretions. A portable spirometer is recommended to obtain a more direct and objective reading of expiratory capacity before the need for formal pulmonary function testing.

Physical therapy management typically begins when the child is initially diagnosed at age 3 to 5 years. Goals of the program are to provide family support and education, obtain baseline data on muscle strength and ROM, and monitor for the progression of muscle weakness that will lead to disability. Initial therapeutic input should not be burdensome to the child or family because the child is usually independent in all ADL before age 5 years. Information should be provided to the family pertaining to the therapist's role as a member of the management team. An appropriate activity level to avoid fatigue should be discussed with the family and school staff. Information on services through the local MDA office should be provided, including identification of support groups or contact families.

Intervention Considerations

The role of exercise in the treatment of MD is controversial (Ansved, 2001; Brooke, 1986; Fowler, 1982; Vignos, 1983). It is widely accepted that both overexertion (Johnson & Braddom, 1971; Vignos et al., 1963) and immobilization (Vignos et al., 1963) are detrimental. The use of graded resistive exercise has been reported to have a range of results from good (Vignos & Watkins, 1966) to limited (de Lateur & Giaconi, 1979) to adverse (Ansved, 2001). Resistive exercise would theoretically be indicated with the disproportionate loss of type II (fast-twitch) muscle fibers in DMD (Edwards, 1980). However, the use of resistive exercise in the young school-age child should not be universally prescribed. Prescribing a submaximal exer-

cise program early has been shown to have beneficial effects, but it should be offered only to families who have a specific desire to include it in the child's program. Consideration should be given to the fact that significant muscle weakness is not seen in the early stage of the disease and the use of an exercise program may be burdensome to the child and family.

If exercise is initiated early, the key muscle groups to be included are the abdominal, hip extensor and abductor, and knee extensor groups. Abdominal exercises should include trunk curls as opposed to sit-ups, which will primarily strengthen the hip flexors. Assistance may be required for neck flexor weakness, because the head typically cannot be flexed from a supine position. Cycling and swimming are excellent activities for overall conditioning and are often preferred over formal exercise programs (Gardner-Medwin, 1980; Vignos, 1983). Standing or walking for a minimum of 2 to 3 hours daily is highly recommended (Siegel, 1978; Ziter & Allsop, 1976). High resistance and eccentric exercise should be avoided (Ansved, 2001).

Breathing exercises have been shown to slow the loss of vital capacity and forced expiratory flow rate (Koessler et al., 2001; Rodillo et al., 1989). Game activities such as inflating balloons or using blow-bottles to maintain pulmonary function can easily be included in a home program and will decrease the severity of symptoms during episodes of colds or other pulmonary infections.

The use of electrical stimulation in DMD has also been suggested as a means of slowing the progression of weakness and improving function. Scott and co-workers (1986) studied the effect of low-frequency electrical stimulation on the tibialis anterior muscle of 16 children with DMD. A 47% increase in maximum voluntary contraction was observed in younger children following a stimulation protocol used for 8 weeks, with little change noted in older children. The authors concluded that the results were encouraging and that further study on muscle groups used for functional activities was needed.

One of the primary considerations in the early management program of the young school-age child is to retard the development of contractures. Contractures have not been shown to be preventable, but the progression can be slowed with positioning and an ROM program (Hyde et al., 2000; Scott et al., 1981; Seeger et al., 1985; Wong & Wade, 1995).

The initial ROM program should include stretching the gastrocnemius-soleus and tensor fasciae latae. Progressive contracture of the gastrocnemius-soleus and tensor fasciae latae corresponds to gait deviations of toe-walking and an increased base of support. Stretching for the gastrocnemius-soleus can be done using a standing runner's stretch. The child stands at a supportive surface, places one leg back at a time with the knee straight, and leans forward. The position also assists with maintenance of hip flexor flexibility; however, specific stretching for the hip flexors should be included when any limitation is noted. Having the child lie supine with one thigh off the edge of a mat or bed and the other held to the chest (Thomas test position) can be used to stretch the hip flexors initially. An alternative method is discussed later for use as progression of hip extensor weakness evolves. A standing stretch for the tensor is accomplished by having the child stand with one side toward the supportive surface with the feet away from the wall and with the knee kept straight while leaning sideways toward the supportive surface.

A home ROM program should be emphasized for the young child and the family instructed in the stretching exercises. There is lack of agreement as to the frequency and duration of the stretching program. Suggested frequency of the program varies from once daily (Gardner-Medwin, 1980; Miller & Dunn, 1982; Scott et al., 1981) to twice daily (Vignos et al., 1963; Ziter & Allsop, 1976), and duration from 1 repetition up to 10 (Vignos et al., 1963). Other authors have suggested a time frame of 10 (Ziter & Allsop, 1976) to 20 (Gardner-Medwin, 1980) minutes to complete the stretching exercises. As a general recommendation, each movement should be repeated for 5 to 10 repetitions with a 10-second hold in the stretched position. The stretch should be done slowly and should not be painful. Increased risk of injury with the loss of myofibrils and replacement by connective tissue is present because of decreased muscle elasticity, and caution in using excessive passive force is advised. Reassessment of the contracture progression should be used as the final guide to stretching frequency and duration.

The ROM program can often be supplemented as part of the physical education program at school. Special instruction should be provided to the physical education teacher to develop an adapted program, particularly if the teacher does not have an adapted physical education endorsement. General physical education activities will also require modification for the child's participation and should not be exhaustive. Physical fitness test activities such as push-ups, sit-ups, or timed running for long time periods should be modified or excluded to avoid fatigue or overwork weakness.

Night splints are helpful to slow the progression of ankle contractures. Scott and associates (1981) studied the efficacy of night splints and a home ROM program in a group of 59 boys diagnosed with MD ranging in age from 4 to 12 years. The subjects were categorized into three groups based on compliance with splint wear and use of stretching. The group that followed through on the daily passive stretching program and use of the below-knee splints over the 2 years of the study demonstrated significantly less progression of Achilles tendon contractures and less deterioration in functional skills, leading to a longer period of independent walking. Boys in the group that did not follow through on the stretching or splint program lost independent walking at a younger age. In a randomized study comparing the effect of ROM exercise with ROM and night splints, the combined intervention was found to be 23% more effective in slowing the progression of posterior calf contracture than ROM alone (Hyde et al., 2000). Similar findings were reported in a study by Seeger and colleagues (1985) that compared the use of night splints, stretching, and surgery.

The use of prone positioning at night to slow progression of the hip and knee flexion contractures may be possible if tolerated by the child. The recommendation to have the child sleep prone with the ankles off the edge of the bed has not been shown to affect the progression of the contractures but theoretically is sound.

Scoliosis is not common when the child is ambulatory, but the spine should be checked routinely (Wilkins & Gibson, 1976; Ziter & Allsop, 1976). Alignment of the spine should be closely monitored as weakness progresses to the stage of making walking difficult. Postural analysis using the forward bend test is recommended to monitor spinal alignment for scoliosis. Presence of a rib hump with the forward bend test verifies a structural versus functional curve of the spine. Amendt and colleagues (1990) have demonstrated that a rib hump measuring at least 5° of inclination with a scoliometer is a reliable method and correlated to radiographic assessment. The study by Amendt and colleagues (1990) was, however, not inclusive of children with DMD but demonstrates an objective method of noninvasive screening for scoliosis. Orthopedic referral is indicated if a rib hump is documented.

Falls and complaints of fatigue while walking become increasingly more frequent as the child reaches age 8 to 10 years. Guarding during stair climbing or during general walking should be considered to ensure safety as balance becomes tenuous. A manual wheelchair with appropriate fit and accessories will allow for limited mobility as walking becomes more difficult. As progression of weakness in the trunk and hip girdle begins to make walking difficult, a similar amount of weakness of the shoulder girdle musculature is also present, making propulsion of a manual wheelchair difficult except on level and smooth surfaces such as linoleum. A motorized scooter should be considered to provide the child with independence, provided that access is available in the home and school (Fig. 15-4).

Information should be made available to families concerning recreational activities provided through the local chapter of the MDA or other groups. Summer MDA camp

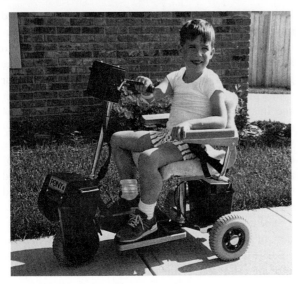

◆ **Figure 15-4**   Motorized three-wheeled scooter for independence in distance mobility as an adjunct to walking. *(OrthoKinetics, Inc., Waukesha, WI.)*

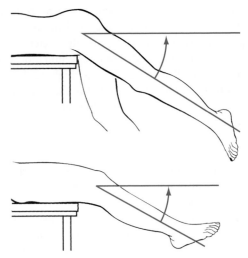

◆ **Figure 15-5**   Prognostic method used by Siegel to determine cessation of independent walking caused by lack of antigravity hip and knee extensor torque. *(Redrawn from Siegel, IM. Muscle and Its Diseases: An Outline Primer of Basic Science and Clinical Method. Chicago: Year Book Medical Publisher, 1986.)*

is a wonderful experience for most children, and a support group is often developed for the child or family through participation in MDA or other group activities that provide not only physical but also emotional support.

Adolescent Period

Adolescence marks a time of significant disability progression as a result of the combined impact of muscle weakness and development of contractures. Walking is lost as a means of mobility, and increasing difficulty in general mobility with transfers is seen. Use of a manual wheelchair or powered mobility becomes necessary during adolescence. If powered mobility is used, assistance with finances for purchase of equipment or home modifications for access is typically needed, with coordination through a social worker or MDA patient services coordinator. Changes in physical capacity such as muscle strength and pulmonary function using the EK Scale have been reported by Steffensen and colleagues (2002) for adolescents. Muscle weakness leads to increasing difficulty with ADL, including dressing, transfers, bathing, grooming, and feeding, and subsequent increasing involvement of the physical therapist and occupational therapist. Decisions regarding possible surgical intervention are also considered for the management of scoliosis or contractures or to prolong walking with the use of orthoses.

As muscle weakness becomes more pronounced in the trunk and hip musculature, and contractures of the hip flexors, tensor fasciae latae, and gastrocnemius-soleus progress, walking becomes increasingly difficult until

cessation of independent walking occurs, usually by age 10 to 12 (Brooke, 1986). If orthoses are used to maintain a standing or walking program, they should be initiated before the child reaches the stage of being nonambulatory.

Various methods to predict the termination of walking have been reported including 50% reduction in leg strength (Scott et al., 1982; Vignos & Archibald, 1960), manual muscle test grade below grade 3 for hip extensors or below grade 4 for ankle dorsiflexors (McDonald et al., 1995) or inability to climb steps. Brooke and colleagues (1989) reported the cessation of unassisted walking within 2.4 years (range of 1.2–4.1 years) when 5 to 12 seconds were required to climb four standard steps or within 1.5 years (range 0.6–2.2 years) when greater than 12 seconds were required. An alternative method, shown in Figure 15-5, has been suggested by Siegel (1977). The knee extension lag while sitting and the hip extension lag while prone are assessed to predict the cessation of independent walking. If the combined lag is greater than 90°, the termination of independent ambulation is within a few months. Monitoring and management of contractures becomes a key element in maintaining walking when the older child spends more time in a sitting position. Because the hip extensor musculature is significantly weak in the early stage of the disease and weakness of the quadriceps muscles becomes pronounced by age 8 to 10 years, inability to maintain the center of gravity behind the hip joint or in front of the knee joint during stance will lead to loss of the ability to stand.

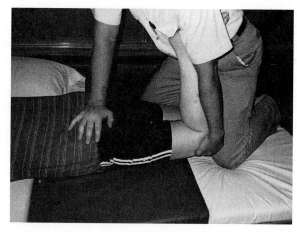

◆ **Figure 15-6**   Prone stretching of the hip flexor, iliotibial band, and tensor fasciae latae. The hip is first positioned in abduction and then moved into maximal hip extension and then hip adduction. The knee can be extended to provide greater stretch for the iliotibial band and tensor.

Manual stretching of the hip flexors, tensor fasciae latae, and heel cords is necessary because the older child demonstrates difficulty in carrying out the exercises without assistance. Prone lying will help retard the development of hip and knee flexor contractures, but stretching of the hip flexors and tensor using the method shown in Figure 15-6 is recommended. The leg is initially positioned in abduction, and then brought into the maximum allowable hip extension followed by hip adduction. A hamstring stretch can also be included in the exercise routine. However, a pattern of capsular tightness of the knee joint caused by prolonged sitting is more common than excessive hamstring contracture because use of the Gowers maneuver to assume standing maintains flexibility of the hamstrings during the period of independent ambulation. If a hamstring stretch is used, the leg should be slightly abducted to minimize the subluxing force placed across the hip joint that is present when the leg is in the sagittal plane during the maneuver.

Continuation of Standing or Walking

The use of orthoses for a standing program or continuation of supported walking is not appropriate for all individuals; in fact, it should be considered a personal rather than therapeutic decision. Although a standing program may be useful to slow the progression of contractures, a braced walking program has little long-term functional or practical application because the child will eventually use a wheelchair. Continuation of standing through use of a standing frame, knee immobilizers, or KAFOs is a goal at our facility to address the issue of decreased bone

mineral density (McDonald et al., 2002) and subsequent increased risk of fracture (Bianchi et al., 2003). Because surgery is often required in addition to orthotics for prolonged ambulation, both the parents and adolescent must agree in the management decision. Prolongation of ambulation through surgery and orthotics is not a common goal at our facility. Limited resources are more typically used for power mobility equipment, adaptive equipment, or environmental adaptations.

Prognostic factors for success that should be considered in making the decision to use orthoses to prolong walking include the residual muscle strength (approximately 50%) (Vignos, 1983); absence of severe contractures (Spencer & Vignos, 1962); timely application of the braces (Bach & McKeon, 1991; Spencer & Vignos, 1962); residual walking ability (Vignos & Archibald, 1960); and motivation of the child and family (Bowker & Halpin, 1978). The degree of mental impairment and obesity should also be considered. The timely use of orthoses has been shown to prolong walking (Bach & McKeon, 1991; Bowker & Halpin, 1978; Heckmatt et al., 1985) and to increase the child's longevity (Bach & McKeon, 1991; Miller & Dunn, 1982; Vignos et al., 1963).

If the decision to use orthoses to prolong standing or walking is made, KAFOs should be prescribed (Fig. 15-7) (Bakker et al., 2000; Bowker & Halpin, 1978; Siegel, 1975). Ankle-foot orthoses are appropriate for positioning but do not provide the knee stability required to avoid falls while walking. Although the use of AFOs to control equinus is common for other diagnoses such as cerebral palsy, with DMD the orthoses often interfere with the use of an ankle strategy and the preserved distal strength that is needed for standing balance and walking. A reciprocating or wheeled walker may be helpful when assistance for balance is needed. Assistive devices such as a standard walker, crutches, or canes are seldom functional because of the degree of proximal shoulder girdle and upper extremity muscle weakness. Standby assistance should be provided when KAFOs are used, owing to the risk of injury from falls. Closer guarding and increased assistance will be needed as the weakness progresses. Transfers to and from standing are dependent because the knee joints of the KAFO must be locked to provide stability. The KAFOs can be used for continuation of a standing program even after walking is no longer possible.

Surgical intervention is commonly needed in conjunction with the use of braced walking as contractures progress. Documented indications for surgery include ankle plantar flexion contractures of greater than 10°, iliotibial band contractures greater than 20°, or knee-hip flexion contractures greater than 20° but less than 45° (Bowker & Halpin, 1978). Subcutaneous tenotomy of the Achilles

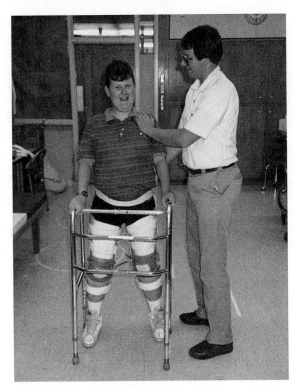

♦ **Figure 15-7** Polypropylene knee-ankle-foot orthosis and use of a reciprocating walker to promote walking for exercise in a 14-year-old boy with Duchenne muscular dystrophy. The reciprocating walker allows progression without picking up the device.

tendon and fasciotomy of the iliotibial bands are the most commonly reported surgical procedures (Bach & McKeon, 1991; Bowker & Halpin, 1978; Hsu, 1995; Siegel et al., 1972; Vignos, 1983). Transfer of the posterior tibialis tendon is occasionally used for correction of the equinovarus foot posture (Hsu, 1995; Scher & Mubarak, 2002).

An intensive postoperative management program is essential to retard the effects of immobilization (Siegel et al., 1986). Standing in the plaster casts can be done on the first or second postoperative day. Gait training is begun as tolerated, and general conditioning exercises for the hips, trunk, and upper extremities are recommended. Breathing exercises should also be stressed. A smooth transition from the casts to bracing is ensured by having the child fitted for the KAFOs before hospitalization for surgery.

Standing pivot transfers must eventually be replaced by one- or two-person lifts or use of equipment as a result of the development of knee and hip flexion contractures and pronounced weakness of the lower extremities. Transfers to and from the wheelchair, toilet, tub, car, and furniture usually become dependent by age 12 to 14. A sliding board, manual lift, or hydraulic lift can be used

during transfers. Proper instruction for transfers is needed because the degree of trunk muscle weakness makes sitting balance tenuous by this stage. If the caregiver is using manual lifting for transfers, he or she should be observed for and instructed in proper body mechanics and safety. A hydraulic lift can be used for transfers to and from the wheelchair, particularly when the adolescent is large or obese or when the caregiver cannot safely perform a manual lift. A U-style sling should be used with the lift to provide adequate head and trunk support during transfers. A tub lift or bath bench for bathing will be needed and a wheeled commode-shower chair should be considered depending on bathroom accessibility.

Mobility and Spinal Alignment

A power scooter as shown in Figure 15-4 should be considered as an initial power wheelchair prescription for the child who is hesitant to use a power wheelchair when walking is no longer possible. The scooter is often more easily accepted by the child and may be used for transition to a standard power wheelchair. If a power scooter is initially used, transition to a power wheelchair will be necessary when the adolescent is seen propping on the arm rests for trunk control. Asymmetric sitting postures must be aggressively managed owing to the correlation of increased sitting time and poor sitting posture with the onset of scoliosis. When limited resources are an issue, which is typically the case for children in managed care, a power wheelchair should be acquired without consideration for a scooter.

A manual wheelchair will be needed if nonaccessible areas for a powered wheelchair are encountered in the usual environment. Architectural barriers in the home or inability to transport a power wheelchair may also necessitate the use of a manual wheelchair.

Fit of the wheelchair must be closely monitored to provide adequate support. The reader should refer to Chapter 33 for information on wheelchairs and postural support systems. Special attention should be given to alignment of the spine and pelvis and to the need for customized accessories or modifications. Accessories to be considered for the manual or power wheelchair prescription should include a solid back and seat, lateral trunk supports, lumbar support, adductor pads, seat belt, and chest strap. The footrests should be modified to support the ankle in a neutral position. Additional items that may be appropriate include a tray; head support, if needed; or coated push rims, if the child has the strength to propel the wheelchair. A reclining back will allow a position change while sitting in the wheelchair and will help deter flexion contracture formation at the hip, or a tilt-in-space reclining option can be considered to allow for pressure relief. Midline placement of the control stick on a power wheelchair may be considered to assist in symmetric trunk alignment. If a cushion is required, it should maintain the pelvis in a level position.

Maintaining the spine in a neutral or slightly extended position is essential to retard the formation of a scoliosis. The spine should be in slight extension to increase weight bearing through the facet joints, minimize truncal rotation and lateral flexion, and slow the progression of scoliosis formation (Gibson et al., 1978; Wilkins & Gibson, 1976). Scoliosis is seen in approximately 15% to 25% of individuals before the cessation of walking (Miller et al., 1992; McDonald et al., 1995). Poor sitting posture, in addition to muscle weakness, has been shown to accelerate scoliosis formation and progression (Gibson & Wilkins, 1975). The prevalence of scoliosis (Cobb angle >10°) is 50% between the ages of 12 and 15 years and 90% by the age of 17 years (McDonald et al., 1995). Spinal orthoses may also retard the progression of scoliosis, although they have not been shown to prevent development of a significant scoliotic curve (Cambridge & Drennan, 1987; Colbert & Craig, 1987). Custom-molded seating inserts, corsets, and modular seating inserts are options to provide trunk support in an attempt to slow the progression of the scoliosis. Studies comparing the three methods of spinal control in DMD have concluded that the progression of the curvature was not significantly changed by any of the three methods (Colbert & Craig, 1987; Seeger et al., 1984).

Early surgical intervention is recommended for the control of scoliosis through the use of segmental spinal instrumentation with Luque rods or similar techniques (Marchesi et al., 1997; Miller et al., 1992; Sengupta et al., 2002). Miller and associates (1992) reported improved quality of life, attainment of a balanced sitting posture, and more normal alignment following surgical intervention for scoliosis. Pulmonary complications are reported as minimal if forced vital capacity is at least 35% of normal age-predicted values.

Exercise and Custom Equipment

With the cessation of walking in late childhood or early adolescence, the emphasis of an exercise program should shift from the lower extremities to active-assistive and active exercises of the upper extremities. More important, however, active exercise should be encouraged by having the adolescent assist as much as possible in ADL such as grooming, upper body dressing, and feeding through consultation with an occupational therapist. Key muscle groups for maintenance of strength for transfers include the shoulder depressors and triceps. The shoulder flexor and abductor and elbow flexor muscle groups are key

areas for exercises to maintain routine ADL such as self-feeding and hygiene. Weakness of the upper arm musculature by 16 years of age makes ADL such as dressing, feeding, or hygiene extremely difficult.

The ROM program will require further modification as the adolescent becomes nonambulatory. Stretching of the aforementioned lower extremity joints should be continued with stretching of the shoulder and elbow included. Limitation in shoulder flexion and abduction, elbow extension, forearm supination, and wrist extension are most common.

The family will need to consider additional equipment or home modifications as their child reaches adolescence. A van with a lift or ramp will be needed to transport a power wheelchair. Modification of the bathroom can significantly assist the family by using a wheeled commode chair for toileting and a bath chair and handheld shower for bathing. A tub lift is a second option for bathing. A urinal should be available at home and school to decrease the frequency of transfers to the toilet. Modifications of the bed are also frequently required because the adolescent is unable to change position. An airflow mattress, egg-crate foam cushion, or hospital bed are all possibilities to be considered. A positioning program to include position changes at night is necessary for adolescents who are thin to provide comfort and ensure against skin breakdown. Customized foam wedges fabricated by the therapist may also be helpful in positioning at night.

Transition to Adulthood

The transition to adulthood marks a time of continued progression of disability with greater reliance on assistive technology for environmental access and increased need for assistance to carry out routine ADL (Stuberg, 2001). Mobility using a power wheelchair is necessary because upper extremity and truncal weakness will typically not allow use of a motorized scooter. Assistance for ADL, including dressing, transfers, and bathing, is now required. Hygiene about the face and feeding become increasingly difficult but usually remain manageable. Many social issues also arise with the completion of educational programming and transition to a prevocational, vocational, or home environment on a more full-time basis. Another major issue that requires thoughtful consideration by the family, individual, and management team is the utilization of assisted ventilation with progressive respiratory involvement at the terminal stage of the disease.

All transfers require assistance during late adolescence and by adulthood typically require use of a hydraulic or other type of mechanical lift. A high-backed sling seat is indicated because head and trunk control is minimal with the progressive weakness.

A power recline feature on the power wheelchair may be desirable, depending on accessibility and family choice, if funding is available. If not, a regular schedule for pressure relief through lateral weight shifting with assistance is needed. A properly fitted and well-tolerated cushion to avoid skin breakdown becomes an important area of intervention with loss of the ability to weight shift in the wheelchair. Skin breakdown is not a typical problem in DMD, but a cushion should be considered. A Jay Medical cushion (Jay Medical, Boulder, CO) is often well tolerated and provides a firm base of support to control pelvic obliquity, yet the gel inserts can be adjusted to allow for adequate pressure distribution. A customized insert will be needed if deformity becomes severe (e.g., severe scoliosis without surgical stabilization).

A ball-bearing feeder may be required to assist arm movement when progression of upper extremity weakness makes independent feeding difficult (Chyatte et al., 1965). The device can also be used to assist with general use of the arms in conjunction with activities at a table, such as when using a computer. Coordination of planning with an occupational therapist to address feeding and dressing issues is needed to identify solutions to increased dependence in feeding, dressing, and hygiene.

To maintain independence in environmental access, consideration should be given for using environmental control devices. An environmental control unit included on the power wheelchair can be used to independently access the lights, telephone, television, motors on doors, or a computer, to name just a few applications. Computer access for vocational applications such as word processing or avocational activities such as games is available.

Breathing exercises, postural drainage, or intermittent pressure breathing treatments should be included in the management program based on results of pulmonary evaluation (Rodillo et al., 1989). Specific tests of pulmonary function that document respiratory status include forced vital capacity (FVC = amount of air expired following a maximal inspiration) and peak expiratory flow rate (highest flow rate sustained for 10 ms during maximal expiration). Continuous positive airway pressure (CPAP) is recommended when FVC is below 30% of age-adjusted norm values (Lyager et al., 1995; Steffensen et al., 2002). Assisted ventilation with tracheostomy is recommended when respiratory insufficiency is present with abnormal blood gas levels during the day or night (Steffensen et al., 2002). In addition to the breathing exercises and assisted coughing, the family and caregivers should be instructed in the technique of postural drainage.

Close monitoring of respiratory function should become routine with increasing age because respiratory failure or pulmonary infection is the major contributing factor to death in 75% of children with DMD (Gilroy & Holliday, 1982). Longevity in DMD can be significantly prolonged by assisted ventilation (Bach et al., 1987; Curran & Colbert, 1989; Eagle et al., 2002). A 1997 survey of MDA-sponsored clinics reported that 88% of clinic directors offered noninvasive ventilatory aid for acute respiratory failure (Bach & Chaudhry, 2000). Bach and Chaudhry (2000) stressed the need for health care professionals to explore attitudes toward mechanical ventilation because our perceived impression of patient desires may often be incorrect. The use of daytime intermittent positive-pressure ventilation via mask or nasal cannula, nocturnal bilevel positive airway pressure (BiPAP), CPAP, negative pressure ventilators, and suctioning should be considered for the chronic hypoventilation related to weakness of respiratory musculature (Bach & Chaudhry, 2000).

A power-controlled bed to allow elevation of the head for respiratory management should be considered. Use of a bed with elevating capability also allows for greater ease in transfers, and height adjustment promotes use of proper body mechanics by family members for activities that require assistance such as dressing. Mattress selection should also be reviewed with the family because an airflow mattress may be needed when increasing dependence for bed mobility is encountered. Use of an airflow mattress may decrease the frequency of need for turning and repositioning at night. If sitting in a wheelchair is no longer tolerated in the later stages of the disease, elevation of the head of the bed becomes beneficial for reading or watching television. An easel will be required for reading.

Although it may be assumed by care providers that the quality of life and therefore satisfaction are significantly reduced for severely disabled individuals with DMD, this notion may be incorrect. In a survey of 82 ventilator-assisted individuals with DMD, Bach and colleagues (1991) concluded that the vast majority of individuals had a positive affect and were satisfied with life despite the physical dependence. Furthermore, it was found in a survey of 273 physically intact health care professionals that they significantly underestimated patient life satisfaction scores, and therefore they may make patient management recommendations based on their attitudes rather than the patient's wishes. Bach and colleagues (1991) strongly recommended that we as professionals need to constantly inquire and objectively assess family and individual needs when interacting to provide therapeutic programs. Curran and Colbert (1989) have reported an average increase in longevity from 19 years 9 months to 25 years 9 months in individuals who use ventilatory assistance.

Respiratory insufficiency is a hallmark sign of the preterminal stage of DMD (Newsom-Davis, 1980). Progressive muscular weakness results in decreased ventilatory volumes caused by restriction of chest wall excursion. Coordination of care with the respiratory therapist is essential when clinical findings of respiratory muscle weakness, inability to cough, or chest wall restrictions are observed (Burke et al., 1971). Severe oxygen desaturation leading to a comatose state is evidence of the terminal stage of the disease.

Members of the team often become involved in answering questions regarding death. The physical therapist should be aware of the stages of disease progression and especially the preterminal signs to avoid making inappropriate comments concerning prognosis. Often little needs to be said, but rather a good listening ear is needed to help the family work through the crisis that is ever pending. It is often a comfort to individuals with DMD or family members that the end may come as a sleep without wakening. The person with DMD and his family members may indicate the need for additional support, but if issues are not being resolved adequately by the support that is available, consideration for involvement by a psychologist, counselor, clergy member, MDA support group, or other trained professional is indicated. Literature is available through the MDA to comfort family members, and texts are available if the family is interested (Charash, 1987; Ringel, 1987).

BECKER MUSCULAR DYSTROPHY

BMD, a more slowly progressive variant of DMD, has an incidence of about 1 in 20,000 births and a prevalence of 2 to 3 cases per 100,000 population (Emery, 1993). The impairments and participation restrictions of BMD closely resemble those of DMD; however, the progression is significantly slower, with a longevity into the forties (Emery & Skinner, 1976; Gilroy & Holliday, 1982). The genetic defect for BMD is located on the same gene as that for DMD only in a different area; therefore, dystrophin is present in reduced amounts or abnormal size rather than completely absent as in DMD, which may explain the slower progression of clinical symptoms (Liechti-Gallati et al., 1989).

Initial clinical symptoms are typically not identified in boys with BMD before late childhood or early adolescence. Emery and Skinner (1976) found the mean age at onset of symptoms to be 11 years, inability to walk at 27 years, and death at 42 years. The authors pointed out, however, that the range of walking cessation is very wide. Perhaps one of the best functional discriminators between BMD and DMD is that 97% of adolescents with DMD are using a wheelchair for mobility by age 11 years, whereas 97% of adolescents with BMD are still walking (Emery & Skinner, 1976). Another discriminator is the frequent complaint of muscle cramping in individuals with BMD that is rarely reported in DMD (Dubowitz, 1992).

The impairments of BMD are the same as in DMD, although less severe, and the initial clinical signs include frequent falls and clumsiness in the mid- to late teens. The pattern of weakness is the same as in DMD, and pseudohypertrophy of the calves may be present. The incidence of contracture, scoliosis, and other skeletal deformities is lower in BMD. Although not as severe as in DMD, hip, knee, and ankle plantar flexor muscle contractures can be present when walking is no longer possible. The use of night splints to maintain ankle dorsiflexion ROM is often indicated, along with a home program of heel cord stretching. Significant disability will develop by the midtwenties, requiring the use of power mobility and consideration for use of orthoses to maintain walking. KAFOs can also be used to prolong walking; however, braced ambulation will not be functional for community access but rather as a means of exercise. The general goals and management procedures outlined in the section on DMD are the same for BMD, including the progression from walking to use of power mobility.

Because the person with BMD lives much longer than someone with DMD, transition planning following school and assistance with living arrangements into adulthood become major issues. Vocational or avocational choices should be made with the disease progression and disability level in mind. Vocational rehabilitation services should be initiated before completion of high school to allow adequate time for evaluation. Governmental support through Medicaid, Social Security benefits, or other sources may be needed to offset expenses to allow for independent living because adaptive equipment and an attendant will be needed. Ongoing medical services are available through the MDA. No data are available regarding the number of individuals who go to college or become employed following high school, but with the assistive technology available to promote independence, either option can be explored.

CONGENITAL MUSCULAR DYSTROPHY

Congenital myopathies as a diagnostic category consist of many diseases, including congenital MD. Congenital MD is a heterogeneous group of muscle disorders with onset in utero or during the first year of life. Reported forms of congential MD are (1) congenital MD with central nervous system (CNS) disease (Fukuyama syndrome, Walker-Warburg disease, and muscle-eye-brain disease), (2) merosin-deficient congenital MD, (3) integrin-deficient congenital MD, and (4) congenital MD with normal merosin. Fukuyama, merosin-deficient, and normal merosin forms will be discussed. The reader should refer to the review article by Voit (1998) for additional information. Another valuable resource for information is the

Online Mendelian Inheritance of Man (OMIM) website of the National Center for Biotechnology. The mode of inheritance in congenital MD is reported as autosomal recessive (Emery, 2002; Muscular Dystrophy Association, 2000). Although all forms are rare, the range of severity and disability varies significantly among types.

In congenital MD with associated CNS disease (Fukuyama type), mental retardation and seizures are common along with moderate to severe hypotonia at birth and the presence of contractures (Fukuyama et al., 1981). Magnetic resonance imaging reveals nonspecific cerebral malformations and occasionally lissencephaly as pathologic features of the CNS disease. Contractures typically involve the lower extremities (hips and knees) and elbows. Other commonly reported dysmorphic features include congenital dislocation of the hips, pectus excavatum, pes cavus, kyphoscoliosis, and an unusually long face. Weakness of the extraocular muscles, optic atrophy, and nystagmus have been reported (Brooke, 1986). Children with this type of MD rarely attain the ability to walk (Emery, 2002). The genetic defect is at chromosome 9q31-q33 with speculation that the missing protein is "fukutin."

The early management program in children with congenital MD with nervous system disease should focus on family instruction, developmental activities to address delays in gross motor skill development, and aggressive management of contractures. Attention to positioning is necessary to guard against secondary deformity resulting from gravitational effects on the trunk with presence of moderate to severe hypotonia. Early intervention by an occupational therapist to address feeding and oral motor control issues is commonly coordinated with physical therapy. Impaired respiratory function and pulmonary complications are hallmark features of congenital MD. The family should be instructed in chest physical therapy, such as postural drainage, and consultation with a respiratory therapist may be needed on an ongoing basis.

Because many children with congenital MD and associated nervous system disease do not attain walking, maximizing functional skills in sitting becomes a primary goal of the physical therapy management program as the child ages. Therapeutic exercise to improve head and trunk control should be aggressively addressed with use of adaptive equipment to slow the progression of spinal deformity and contractures and to maximize access to the environment. Because mental retardation is common, power mobility may not be an option. Additional management issues for children with significant hypotonia are discussed later in the chapter in the section on acute SMA. In congenital MD with merosin deficiency, the typical clinical presentation includes hypotonia and weakness, contractures, normal intelligence, seizures (20%), and a delay

in acquisition of motor milestones. Infants demonstrate a delay in walking, with acquisition of walking ranging from 13 months to 6 years (North et al., 1996). Progressive contractures may be present, and in severe cases, the children may never walk. Longevity ranges from 15 to 30 years. Peporago and associates (1998) reported on a cohort of 22 children with merosin-deficient congenital MD. All children demonstrated severe floppiness at birth, normal intelligence, and delay in achievement of motor milestones. Merosin-deficient congenital MD is due to a defect at chromosome 6q22. Muscle weakness and contractures are the primary impairment in merosin-deficient congenital MD. Muscles innervated by the cranial nerves may be involved, requiring a feeding program that is coordinated with occupational therapy. Contractures must be managed aggressively with a home ROM program including manual stretching, positioning, and splinting. Because many of the children have a potential to develop walking, the ankle plantar flexion contractures may require orthopedic intervention if the contractures cannot be managed conservatively.

Activity limitations, such as delayed acquisition of gross motor skills, should not be managed by direct service therapy programs because a slower rate of skill progression is expected. Because these children vary in their rate of motor skill development, information can be provided to the family concerning probable rates of motor skill acquisition, but unrealistic therapeutic expectations should be avoided. Because there is a wide range of functional deficits in children with congenital MD, care must be taken in predicting functional gross motor outcomes or level of participation at home and school.

CHILDHOOD-ONSET FACIOSCAPULOHUMERAL MUSCULAR DYSTROPHY

Facioscapulohumeral MD is rare, with an incidence of 3 to 10 cases per million births (Stevenson et al., 1990). The disorder is inherited as autosomal dominant or recessive with the genetic defect on chromosome 4q35. The disorder affects males and females equally. Childhood-onset facioscapulohumeral MD typically results in the onset of clinical signs within the first 2 years but without significant impairment or disability until later in the first decade. Contractures are seldom a problem.

Infancy and Preschool-Age Period

The impairment of muscle weakness about the face and shoulder girdle is typically the only prominent feature of the disease during the infant and preschool-age period. Parents report that the child may sleep with the eyes partially open, and on physical examination weakness of the facial musculature is predominant. Children are frequently unable to whistle, and drinking with a straw may be difficult. When asked to purse the lips together and puff the cheeks out, the child is unable to maintain the cheeks out when even the slightest pressure is applied. The child's smile is also masked because of the weakness, thereby hindering communication as a result of inconsistency between what is spoken and the affect displayed.

Children with childhood-onset facioscapulohumeral MD typically develop independence in walking without significant delay. An excessive lordotic posture during walking is a classic clinical feature with progression of weakness. The scapulae are widely abducted and outwardly rotated, giving evidence of the degree of interscapular muscle weakness.

School-Age Period

Progressive disability occurs during the school-age period, with weakness becoming more generalized throughout the trunk, shoulder, and pelvic girdle musculature. Progression of childhood-onset facioscapulohumeral MD is more insidious than the adult form, and independent walking may be lost by the end of the first decade (Gardner-Medwin, 1980).

The severe winging of the scapula, a hallmark feature of the adult form of the disease, becomes more prominent with age in activities such as reaching overhead. Management should focus on instruction to the child and family on activities to avoid that may cause fatigue and on guarding against heavily resisted upper extremity activity. Studies of adults with facioscapulohumeral MD comparing dominant with nondominant arm strength have shown that overuse and perhaps just consistent use of the dominant arm play a significant role in progression of muscle weakness (Brouwer et al., 1992; Johnson & Braddom, 1971).

As weakness of the hip and knee extensors progresses, the use of KAFOs should be considered for assisted walking and transfers. When walking becomes increasingly difficult, power mobility using a scooter or power wheelchair should be considered because the degree of upper extremity weakness will not allow independence in propulsion of a manual wheelchair.

Transition to Adulthood

No specific prognostic information on the longevity of individuals with childhood-onset facioscapulohumeral MD is available, and therefore transition planning from the educational environment should be a goal of the therapy program. If severe weakness is present and significant assistance from the family is needed, individuals may not desire to plan for living outside the family home. If independent living is desired, coordination of planning with an attendant will be necessary and evaluation for accessibility issues will need to be completed. Assistance through vocational rehabilitation services should be coordinated with transition planning if vocational goals are identified.

CONGENITAL MYOTONIC MUSCULAR DYSTROPHY

Myotonic MD is the most common adult-onset neuromuscular disease, with an incidence of 1 in 8000 births (Harper, 1989). Congenital myotonic MD is rare and demonstrates severe clinical features of the adult-onset diagnosis. Inheritance is reported as autosomal dominant with genetic defect of chromosome 19q13.3 affecting males and females equally. More recently a second form of myotonic MD (proximal myotonic myopathy, or PROMM) has been reported and linked to chromosome 3q21 (Ricker, 2000).

Children with congenital myotonic MD are almost exclusively born to mothers with myotonic MD who have the chromosome 19 defect. Approximately 25% of children born to mothers with myotonic MD will have congenital myotonic MD (Harper, 1989). Most children demonstrate severe hypotonia and weakness at birth; however, a few children first have only signs of mental retardation by age 5 years and no significant motor impairment as infants. Because the children who initially have only mental impairment follow a progression of motor impairment similar to that of adult-onset myotonic MD, the infancy-onset form is discussed in this section of the chapter.

Mental retardation in congenital myotonic MD is common, with an average IQ of 65 typically reported (Harper, 1975; Roig et al., 1994). There is no evidence of progressive deterioration of mental function. A study by Rutherford and co-workers (1989) including 14 children provided prognostic information regarding survival and the relationship to mechanical ventilation at birth. No infant in the study survived who required mechanical ventilation for longer than 4 weeks.

Infancy

If the child survives the early weeks of life, the prognosis is one of steady improvement in motor function over the first decade, with most children developing independent walking (Harper, 1975, 1989; Roig et al., 1994). A follow-up study by O'Brien and Harper (1984) of 46 children reported only 4 children who died outside the neonatal period at ages 4, 18, 19, and 22 years. Four additional children demonstrated significant disability associated with a poor prognosis, and none was older than age 30 years. In a study of 115 children with congenital MD, Reardon and colleagues (1993) reported that 25% of the children lived to age 18 months, and of those who survived infancy, 50% lived into their mid-30s.

Severe weakness and partial paralysis of the diaphragm at birth are clinical features that often suggest the diagnosis of congenital myotonic MD. Myotonia (delay in relaxation after muscular contraction), a hallmark feature of adult myotonic MD, is typically not evident at birth in the congenital form but rather develops by 3 to 5 years of age (Brooke, 1986). Myotonia in congenital myotonic MD is typically not considered to be a significant impairment or a cause of functional limitations in comparison with the degree of weakness that is present. The symptoms of myotonia, however, are increased with fatigue, cold, or stress (Siegel, 1986). Typical facial features include a short median part of the upper lip, which gives the mouth an inverted-V shape. Facial movements are limited, with muscles innervated by the cranial nerves involved in the severe weakness pattern. Severe respiratory impairment is prominent in the newborn period, requiring resuscitation and assisted ventilation in most cases. Talipes equinovarus contractures are reported in over 50% of children, and a general pattern of arthrogryposis occurs in less than 5% (Harper, 1989).

Progressive improvement in gross motor skills can be expected if the child survives the newborn period. The presence and degree of intellectual impairment become a major factor in the progression of milestone acquisition. The development of hip abduction and external rotation contractures should be closely monitored if leg movement and habitual positioning favor the development of this secondary impairment.

Harper (1989), in a cohort of 70 children with congenital myotonic dystrophy, reported that hypotonia is rarely prominent beyond age 3 to 4 years. Children typically develop walking, but further motor impairment follows the clinical progression of adult-onset disease without definitive data being available into adulthood to document disease progression.

Consultation with a respiratory therapist on pulmonary care will be needed until the infant is weaned from assisted ventilation. Feeding may require the use of a nasogastric tube during the newborn period or early infancy, and initiation of a feeding program should be coordinated with an occupational therapist. A swallowing study may be indicated to evaluate potential for aspiration when the feeding program is initiated. If the newborn survives early respiratory difficulties, progressive improvement in pulmonary function is usually seen without need for ongoing intervention.

Talipes equinovarus contractures should be aggressively managed in infancy with casting, taping, and exercises but may ultimately require orthopedic intervention as they have been shown to significantly delay walking (Reardon et al., 1993). Ankle-foot orthoses or night splints may be indicated based on individual needs. In addition to home instruction for ROM activities to manage contractures, the family should be provided with a general program of activities to promote gross motor skill development. Because the natural progression of the disease is improvement of motor function, consultation rather than a direct service program is indicated, unless surgical intervention for contracture management is required.

School-Age Period

Consultation for development of adaptive physical education activities will be needed during the school-age period. Other physical therapy–related activities will depend on the use of orthoses and progression of gross motor skill development. Specific therapeutic exercise programs for strengthening have not been reported but may be indicated in addition to ROM activities.

Transition to Adulthood

The natural progression of myotonic MD is insidious weakness of the distal upper and lower extremity musculature and progressive increase in myotonia, leading to increasing disability. Children with congenital myotonic MD will demonstrate progression in the disease as described for adults, but typically at an earlier stage, usually by the middle of the second decade. The reader should refer to references on adult myotonic MD for further information on clinical course and management (Brooke, 1986; Harper, 1989; Siegel, 1986).

EMERY-DREIFUSS MUSCULAR DYSTROPHY

Emery-Dreifuss MD1 (EDMD1) is inherited as an X-linked recessive disorder at gene locus Xq28 resulting in the absence of the protein emerin. Emery-Dreifuss MD2 (EDMD2) is also inherited, but as an autosomal dominant or recessive disorder with a defect on chromosome 1q21.2 and defect of the protein lamin.

The clinical features of EDMD1 vary widely and include contracture of the posterior neck, elbow, and ankle joints. A humeroperoneal pattern of muscle weakness is observed with usual onset in the teen years, but ranging from neonatal to the third decade. Later progression of the weakness to the legs is reported. Contracture is typically seen before the onset of weakness. The onset of EDMD2 is most common in the first or second decade and a similar patter of contracture to EMMD1 is seen. The humeroperoneal weakness is more prominent, especially affecting the elbow flexors (Brooke, 1986). Cardiac abnormalities are more common in EDMD1, with sudden death (in persons ranging in age from 25 to 56 years) reported by Pinelli and colleagues (1987) in a large family cohort with bradyarrhythmias.

Physical therapy management is limited during the childhood period because disability is not common. Independent walking is typically maintained into adulthood without significant disability. A ROM program for contracture prevention is advised, but orthopedic intervention is common to correct the Achilles tendon contractures (Shapiro & Specht, 1991). Holter monitoring is advised when cardiac abnormalities are identified, and pacemakers are used to control rhythm.

SPINAL MUSCULAR ATROPHY

Classification of SMA into four groups is based on clinical presentation and progression (Table 15-2). Types I and II are commonly referred to as acute and chronic Werdnig-Hoffmann disease, respectively, type III as Kugelberg-Welander disease, and type IV as adult-onset SMA.

DIAGNOSIS AND PATHOPHYSIOLOGY

SMA comprises the second most common group of fatal recessive diseases after cystic fibrosis (Semprini, 2001). The pathologic feature of SMA is abnormality of the large anterior horn cells in the spinal cord. The number of cells is reduced, and progressive degeneration of the remaining cells is correlated with loss in function.

The diagnosis of SMA is confirmed by clinical examination and laboratory procedures, including electromyography, muscle biopsy, and genetic testing (Brooke, 1986; MacKenzie et al., 1994). Electromyographic findings include fibrillation and fasciculation potentials. Nerve conduction velocities are normal. Muscle biopsy demonstrates changes that are typical of a disease involving denervation (i.e., large groups of atrophic fibers are dispersed among groups of normal or hypertrophic fibers). The absence of fibrosis around the atrophic groups on the muscle biopsy helps delineate SMA from DMD.

SMA is typically inherited as autosomal recessive with the genetic defect on chromosome 5q11.2-13 (Semprini, 2001). The gene for SMA, termed *survival motor neuron* (SMN), was discovered in 1994 by MacKenzie and colleagues (1994) on chromosome 5q13 and is responsible for the production of a protein bearing the same name. The SMN protein is involved in maintenance of the anterior horn cell and when missing results in a lack of survival of the cell, leading to apoptosis (programmed cell death). In addition to the SMN gene, another defect of the gene in a near locus results in the lack of formation of neuronal apoptosis inhibitory protein (NAIP), which has also been shown to play a role in SMA. Variation in the amount of NAIP protein may explain the premature cell death seen in SMA, in association with the SMN gene defect (Robinson, 1995).

The incidence of Werdnig-Hoffmann disease is 1 in 10,000 live births (Semprini, 2001), and the incidence of Kugelberg-Welander disease is reported as 6 cases per 100,000 live births (Winsor et al., 1971). Reported incidence of the other forms is variable because of the inconsistency of applying classification criteria.

One criterion for classification of SMA is the level of functional ability (Dubowitz, 1989). The more typical classification criteria are multifactorial and involve age at onset of the first clinical signs, pattern of muscle involvement, age at death, and genetic evidence (Pearn, 1980).

SMA is a heterogeneous disorder containing several different clinical presentations and rates of progression. Progressive SMA of early childhood (type I) was first reported by Werdnig and Hoffmann in the late 1800s (Hoffmann, 1893; Werdnig, 1894). A more slowly progressive form of SMA (type III) with onset usually be-

| TABLE 15-2 | Classification of Spinal Muscle Atrophy |

TYPE	ONSET	INHERITANCE	COURSE
Childhood-onset, type I, Werdnig-Hoffmann (acute)	0–3 mo	Recessive	Rapidly progressive; severe hypotonia; death within first year
Childhood-onset, type II, Werdnig-Hoffmann (chronic)	3 mo–4 yr	Recessive	Rapid progression that stabilizes; moderate to severe hypotonia; shortened life span
Juvenile-onset, type III, Kugelberg-Welander	5–10 yr	Recessive	Slowly progressive; mild impairment

tween the ages of 2 and 9 years was reported by Kugelberg and Welander (1956) and also by Wohlfart and colleagues (1955). Werdnig-Hoffmann disease and Kugelberg-Welander disease have therefore become the eponyms for early-onset and juvenile-onset SMA, with many authors preferring to use the numeric classification system as outlined above in Table 15-2.

Pearn (1980), in a large multicenter study in England, reported SMA type II and III to be the most frequent, accounting for approximately 47% of the population. The next most prevalent forms were SMA type I at about 27% and adult-onset type IV at 8%; the other 18% had mixed classifications, including distal involvement, neurogenic SMA, SMA of adolescence with hypertrophied calf muscles, and childhood-onset SMA with cerebellar and optic atrophy.

No cure or treatment is available for SMA, but physical therapy is commonly advocated (Marshall, 1984; Watt & Greenhill, 1984). Poor prognosticators for long-term survival include early age at onset (before 4 months of age) that is often noted as weak fetal movement; fasciculations of the tongue in infancy; and severe, generalized weakness, particularly of the trunk and proximal musculature (Gamstorp, 1967). More recent evidence has shown that children with severe onset of symptoms may survive up to their fifth birthday (Borkowska et al., 2002).

ACUTE CHILDHOOD SPINAL MUSCULAR ATROPHY (TYPE I)

Impairments, Activity Limitations, and Participation Restrictions

The primary impairment in all forms of SMA is muscle weakness secondary to progressive loss of anterior horn cells in the spinal cord. Weakness is particularly pronounced in the acute and chronic childhood forms (types I and II) within the first 4 months. The cranial nerves are inconsistently involved in childhood-onset SMA, with rare involvement with juvenile onset. Contractures may be a primary impairment in acute-onset SMA, with reports of talipes equinovarus or other intrauterine deformities secondary to limited fetal movement. Muscle fasciculations, including fasciculations of the tongue, are most commonly reported in children with acute-onset SMA (Marshall, 1984). Unlike the faces of children with myotonic or facioscapulohumeral MD, children with acute childhood SMA appear alert and responsive. Respiratory distress is present early, and significant effort to augment breathing by use of the abdominal musculature is typical.

Secondary impairments in acute-onset SMA include the development of scoliosis and often contractures. It is widely reported in the literature that all children with SMA develop scoliosis, usually requiring surgical intervention (Granata et al., 1989c; Lonstein, 1989). Other secondary impairments include decreased respiratory capacity and easy fatigability. Because only the passage of time will allow differentiation of children with acute versus chronic childhood SMA, treatment should begin early with a focus on feeding, ROM, positioning, respiratory care, and selected developmental activities.

Infancy

In acute childhood SMA, weak or absent fetal movement during the last months of pregnancy is commonly reported by the mother. Significant weakness is present at birth or develops within the first 4 months, which manifests as inability to perform antigravity movements with the pelvic or shoulder girdle musculature and typical posturing in a gravity-dependent position (Fig. 15-8). The proximal musculature of the neck, trunk, and pelvic and shoulder girdles demonstrates the greatest weakness. Limited antigravity movement of distal upper and lower extremity musculature is present, and a positioning program in the newborn period or at the onset of symptoms is necessary. Use of wedges should be considered to avoid supine positioning in the presence of respiratory distress. If the supine position is used, rolled towels or bolsters are needed to keep the upper extremities positioned in midline and to prevent lower extremity abduction and external rotation. The side-lying position allows midline head and hand use for play without having to work against gravity. Prone positioning on wedges should be limited or not used, owing to the effort required for head righting to interact with the environment.

Respiratory care is a central focus of the habilitation program in acute childhood SMA. Children frequently require intubation for respiratory distress and tracheostomy. Coordination with nurses and respiratory therapists on a program that includes suctioning, assisted coughing, and postural drainage is necessary. The use of supported sitting should be closely monitored for spinal alignment and respiratory response. Use of an elastic binder around the abdomen in sitting may be useful for children who demonstrate a marked reduction in oxygen saturation when seated.

ROM exercises should be carried out to ensure maintenance of flexibility and comfort. Flexion contractures of the hips, knees and elbows, hip abductors, ankle plantar flexors, and positional torticollis are deformities that can be avoided with a comprehensive ROM and positioning program (Binder, 1989). The exercise program should also include limited activities for strengthening, such as lightweight toys or rattles with Velcro straps around the wrists or mobiles positioned close to the hands for easy access.

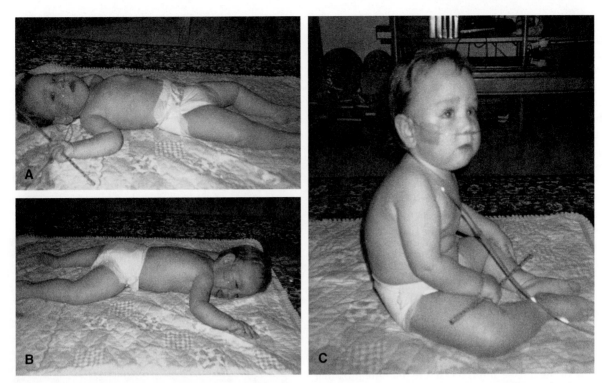

+ **Figure 15-8**   Typical postures seen in a young child with spinal muscular atrophy in supine (**A**), prone (**B**), and sitting (**C**) positions. Note the limited antigravity control and dependent posturing.

The use of hammocks has also been advocated to provide the child with the opportunity for movement with only slight movements of the body (Eng, 1989a, 1989b). Developmental activities such as the use of supported sitting for the development of head control should be of short duration to avoid fatigue.

Head control fails to develop or is significantly impaired in acute childhood SMA. The child is unable to lift the head from a prone position to clear the airway. Early developmental postures such as prone on elbows are not attained. The use of developmental exercise in acute childhood SMA is controversial but should be considered if the child tolerates the activities, because a few children with chronic childhood SMA exhibit clinical signs of weakness in the first year of life and as a result may be misdiagnosed as having acute SMA.

In conjunction with an occupational therapist, a feeding program that is safe and not excessively exhausting should be implemented. Small, frequent feedings may be necessary, and breast feeding may be difficult (Eng, 1989b). Special care with feeding is necessary to avoid aspiration and secondary respiratory problems.

Although death secondary to pneumonia or other respiratory complications is typical within a few months to a few years in acute childhood SMA, the child's death is usually not a struggle, owing to the degree of weakness and apnea (Eng, 1989b). The mean age of death is reported to be 6 months, with a range from 1 to 21 months reported by Merlini and associates (1989). However, with the use of ventilatory assistance, Bach and colleagues (2002) have reported survival up to 42 months. Counseling and support for the parents and family is an extremely important component in the management of these children.

CHRONIC CHILDHOOD SPINAL MUSCULAR ATROPHY (TYPE II)

Impairments, Activity Limitations, and Participation Restrictions

The onset of significant weakness in chronic childhood SMA usually appears within the first year, with the course of the disease widely variable. Pearn and colleagues (1978) reported that of a cohort of 141 children, 95% demonstrated clinical signs before age 3 years. Forty-six percent never walked (even with orthotics), 38% were able to walk unaided at some stage, and the median age at death exceeded 10 years.

Eng (1989b) has reported three separate subgroupings within type II based on the pattern of presentation and progression. In the most severely involved group, the children never developed the ability to sit alone and respiratory capacity was significantly reduced. In the intermediate group, the children sat alone but never developed the ability to walk and demonstrated a regression of forced vital capacity to 45% by age 10 years. In the final group, independent walking was attained but half of the children lost this ability toward the end of the first decade. Interestingly, in the group of patients who remained ambulatory in the study by Eng (1989b), forced vital capacity was maintained at 90% as compared with 65% for those who lost independent walking during the first decade. The results of the study led Eng to conclude that forced vital capacity may be a physiologic predictor of walking duration.

Contractures are infrequently an impairment in chronic SMA. The distribution of weakness is similar to acute childhood SMA with primary proximal involvement, but to a much less severe degree. Weakness is usually greatest in the hip and knee extensors and trunk musculature. Involvement of the distal musculature appears later in the course of the disease and is less severe than the proximal involvement. Involvement of the cranial nerves has been reported but is not considered to be a typical feature of SMA other than in the acute childhood form. Fasciculations of the tongue have been reported in approximately one half of the children.

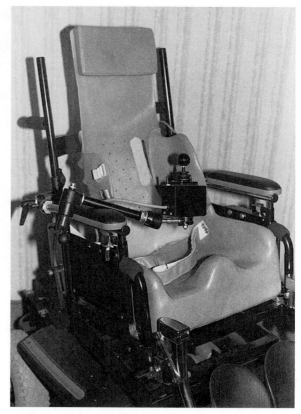

◆ **Figure 15-9**   Custom-molded sitting-support orthosis to provide trunk support in sitting.

Infancy

Because the clinical presentation and progression of chronic childhood SMA are highly variable, the management program must address the major impairments, activity limitations, and participation restrictions as they are manifested. Approximately 15% of children have impairments within the first 3 months, and the remaining children have impairments by 18 months of age (Merlini et al., 1989). The program for the newborn with chronic SMA should be similar to that for children with acute SMA. Some children may develop the ability to stand, but few are able to use walking as a primary means of mobility.

Sitting posture is an area of primary concern in the management program with children who demonstrate significant weakness, requiring external head and trunk support in antigravity positions. A molded sitting support orthosis as shown in Figure 15-9 provides optimal contouring of the torso for support in sitting, or a thoracolumbosacral orthosis (TLSO, or "body jacket") can also be used. Developmental activities provided on an ongoing basis are indicated to develop gross motor skills. Therapy sessions should be kept short to avoid fatigue and should emphasize selected developmental areas during each session because tolerance to handling in multiple positions is usually limited. Swimming has been reported to be beneficial in maintaining muscle strength and functional skills (Cunha, et al., 1996) Instruction to the family in the use of adaptive equipment for proper positioning is crucial in slowing the deforming effects of gravity on the spine when the child is sitting or standing.

If the child is not standing by the age of 16 to 18 months, adaptive equipment for standing should be considered. The rate of fracture in SMA has been reported to range from 12% to 15%, and weight bearing has been shown to decrease the frequency of lower extremity fractures (Ballestrazzi et al., 1989). A supine stander is recommended for children without adequate head control. Orthopedic consultation for a corset or TLSO should be considered for use in standing to maintain trunk alignment if the adaptive equipment does not provide adequate control.

Preschool-Age and School-Age Period

In the toddler, orthotics for standing might be considered (lightweight KAFOs); however, the progression of weakness may make walking an unrealistic goal. In a report of promotion of walking in 12 children with intermediate

SMA (ages 13 months to 3 years), Granata and associates (1989a) described success in attaining assisted ambulation, with 58% of the children using orthoses. Although only a small number of children were studied, these investigators also reported less severe scoliotic curves in the children who used the orthoses in comparison with a control group of children with SMA.

If a walking program is initiated, training in the parallel bars followed by use of a walker or other device to allow greater independence is desired. Close monitoring of safety with supported walking is necessary owing to the degree of weakness present and the potential for serious injury from a fall. The incidence of hip dislocation and contractures has also been reported as less when a supported walking program is used (Granata et al., 1989b).

Independence with mobility other than walking is a primary goal for the child who will not develop independence in walking or when walking is no longer possible (Jones et al., 2003). Because most power scooters do not provide adequate trunk control, use of a power wheelchair is indicated. If an orthopedic appliance is not used to support the trunk, close attention to fit is needed with use of lateral trunk supports and a trunk harness. Consideration should also be given to changing the side of the joystick every 6 months to avoid a pattern of leaning to one side. Prognosis for children with chronic childhood SMA is dependent on frequency and severity of pulmonary complications. Severe contractures as a result of prolonged sitting and progression of scoliosis are common, necessitating implementation of a consistent ROM program. Surgical intervention for spinal stabilization is an option if pulmonary function testing indicates a good prognosis for survival of the surgical intervention.

Transition to Adulthood

Survival into adulthood is extremely variable in chronic childhood SMA and depends on the progression of muscle weakness and secondary deformities. Because of the significant degree of muscle weakness, assistance is typically required for transfers and many ADL. An attendant or family member is needed to provide assistance for general ADL. Intelligence is rarely affected, and therefore vocational goals in areas of interest should be explored through vocational rehabilitation services.

An aggressive program of pulmonary care is required, including breathing exercises and postural drainage. Forced vital capacity has been shown to decrease about 1.1% per year, but mechanical ventilation is seldom needed (Steffensen et al., 2002). The ROM program should also be continued to control progression of the contractures unless a pattern of stability is recorded.

JUVENILE-ONSET SPINAL MUSCULAR ATROPHY (TYPE III)

Juvenile-onset SMA may demonstrate symptoms of weakness within the first year of life in the proximal hip and shoulder girdle musculature, but more typically the onset is later in the first decade. Rarely are bulbar signs seen with the disease. Calf pseudohypertrophy is reported in approximately 10% of the cases. Fasciculations are noted in about half of the patients, and minimyoclonus may be a primary impairment noted on examination but rarely interferes with function (Brooke, 1986; Dorscher et al., 1991).

Impairments, Activity Limitations, and Participation Restrictions

In a study by Dorscher and colleagues (1991) reviewing the status of 31 patients with Kugelberg-Welander disease, proximal lower extremity weakness was the most common impairment reported. Secondary impairments included postural compensations resulting from the muscle weakness, contractures, and occasionally scoliosis. An increased lumbar lordosis and compensated Trendelenburg gait pattern are common postural compensations for proximal muscle weakness of the lower extremities. Ankle plantar flexion contractures are occasionally reported but not with the frequency seen in DMD, which aids differentiation of the two diseases. Scoliosis was reported in about 20% of patients by Dorscher and colleagues (1991) but was reported in all patients by other researchers (Granata et al., 1989b). In adolescents with type III SMA the incidence of scoliosis and its severity are related to the degree of weakness and functional status. Individuals who maintain independent walking have a lower incidence of scoliosis and less severe curves if scoliosis develops.

School-Age Period

A similar clinical presentation to DMD is seen in juvenile-onset SMA. The initial disability usually becomes apparent within the first decade and includes difficulty in arising from the floor, climbing stairs, and keeping up with peers during play. A waddling gait, which becomes more pronounced with attempts at running, will also be observed. Unlike DMD, no significant disability of upper extremity function is usually noted and proximal upper extremity strength is well preserved. Walking can usually be maintained lifelong as the primary means of ambulation. In those cases when weakness is noted before 2 years of age, however, a wheelchair or scooter may ultimately be required for mobility over long distances.

Management for the adolescent with juvenile-onset SMA is consistent with the concepts previously presented in this chapter. ROM exercises should be prescribed as appropriate, and selected strengthening exercises may be indicated to maintain functional skills. Adaptive equipment for mobility is not usually indicated, but a power scooter for long-distance mobility may be needed in certain cases. If performance of ADL becomes a problem, collaboration with an occupational therapist to address concerns may also be needed.

Transition to Adulthood

Difficulty in ADL that requires lifting of moderately heavy objects overhead can be expected, and vocational activities that involve manual labor are not recommended. Because the life span is not significantly shortened, vocational planning is needed. No significant disability requiring adaptive equipment or environmental access is usually required until later in adulthood.

SUMMARY

Muscle weakness and contracture are hallmark features of the childhood forms of muscular dystrophy and spinal muscle atrophy. A background knowledge of therapeutic exercise, functional use of orthoses and adaptive equipment, and strategies to minimize disabilities secondary to these impairments allow the physical therapist to bring unique information and skills to the management team.

Many of the disorders significantly reduce longevity. Therefore, the patient's quality of life and attention to how the family copes with the stress should be included in the team's intervention program. Providing the children and families with support and realistic expectations is an ongoing challenge. Support groups or contact with another family that has had a similar experience can often help the family work through crisis periods, particularly when extended family support is not available.

Through the combined perspectives and innovative solutions of team members, a comprehensive program can be provided that takes into consideration the multifaceted demands of each individual and family. A philosophy of using a family-centered approach to care will help ensure that needs are met to the best of the team's ability.

CASE STUDIES

Each of the two cases that are presented began before development of the *Guide to Physical Therapist Practice* (APTA, 2001). However, the reports are presented with reference to the guide to assist the practitioner in application of the *Guide* to clinical practice.

DONALD

Donald is from a family with six siblings (three brothers and three sisters). Three of the four boys were diagnosed with DMD. No family history of neuromuscular disease had been reported previously, and diagnosis followed medical examination of Donald's older brother at age 5 years for clumsiness and frequent falls. Donald was 3 years of age at the time of diagnosis.

At the time of diagnosis Donald's management program would be included in Musculoskeletal Practice Pattern C: Impaired Muscle Performance of the *Guide to Physical Therapist Practice* (APTA, 2001). He exhibited no significant gait deviations but had mild shoulder girdle and trunk flexor muscle weakness, evidence of a Gowers sign after the third attempt to rise to standing from the floor, and pseudohypertrophy of the posterior calf musculature.

A physical therapy examination at age 8 years revealed a gait pattern typical for DMD as previously described. No significant participation restrictions were noted, and impairments were only minimal. Donald was independent on stairs using a handrail but demonstrated a two-foot-per-step progression. Functional status corresponded to grade 2 on the scale published by Vignos and associates (1963) (see Box 15-1). ROM was within normal limits, with the exception of mild limitation of ankle dorsiflexion with the knee in extension. Muscle strength was quantified with manual muscle testing and recorded as fair plus in the shoulder and hip girdle musculature, poor in the abdominals, and good minus in the intermediate and distal upper and lower extremities. A home program was provided that included daily ROM of the posterior calf musculature and instruction on general activities to avoid excessive fatigue. Services were coordinated by the local MDA clinic with a follow-up visit every 6 months.

Donald's initial disability was related to independent mobility with progressive loss of walking, which by age 12 involved inability to climb stairs and increased frequency of falls with attempts to walk on uneven surfaces. Furniture and walls were commonly used for balance. He was independent in scooting on the floor and used crawling for additional mobility at home. Although he was not able to stand from the middle of the floor, he was able to pull up to standing at a supportive surface. Night splints were initiated to augment the ROM program for the ankle plantar flexion contractures, and a manual wheelchair was provided for assistance with long-distance mobility. Muscle strength demonstrated progressive decline, with manual muscle testing measuring poor grades for the proximal hip and shoulder girdle musculature, fair plus grades for knee extension, and a Vignos scale rating of 5.

Mild tightness of the iliotibial band was present, and limitation of full hip and knee extension was noted. The ROM program was expanded to include the additional areas of tightness. With the progression of impairments beyond muscle function, a shift in Musculoskeletal Practice Pattern C to D: Impaired Joint Mobility, Muscle Function, Muscle Performance, and Range of Motion Associated with Capsular Restriction would be indicated.

By age 15, Donald was walking only short distances, and primarily for mobility within the home. A three-wheeled motorized scooter was provided for distance mobility, and Donald was independent in all transfers from the scooter. A raised toilet seat and tub bench were provided for the bathroom. He received adapted physical education and consultative physical therapy as a related service in the educational setting. He was followed through the MDA clinic, and Donald's home program was augmented by a school program, including standing using a prone stander, ROM exercises three times per week, and adaptive physical education activities for general mobility and upper and lower extremity strengthening.

Progressive weakness and flexion contractures at the hip and knee resulted in the loss of walking when Donald was 17. It should be noted that this is exceptionally late for the loss of walking because 10 to 11 years is more typically reported (Brooke, 1986). Because Donald's older brother had died following complications from a fracture resulting from a fall while wearing KAFOs, Donald and the family decided against continuation of a walking program using orthoses. A daily standing program at school was maintained until progression of the contractures resulted in a need to discontinue the program because orthopedic intervention was not desired by the family.

At age 26, Donald was at stage 8 on the Vignos Functional Rating Scale (see Box 15-1). He was living in an apartment with a full-time home health aide. The scoliosis that was documented 6 years earlier had not progressed, nor was any intervention required. Donald used a power wheelchair with joystick control as shown in Figure 15-10 owing to progression of upper extremity weakness and a need to provide greater trunk support in sitting. Assistance was required for all transfers, for bathing, and for dressing. A tub bench was used. Donald was independent with eating and personal hygiene such as brushing his teeth. He required assistance for bed mobility. The sliding board transfer demonstrated in Figure 15-11 became too difficult at age 23, requiring use of a manual lift or Hoyer for all transfers.

Donald assisted as an aide for an art teacher at a school for children with multiple disabilities (Fig. 15-12) until age 23, when his upper extremity weakness progressed to the point where he decided to stop working. He peace-

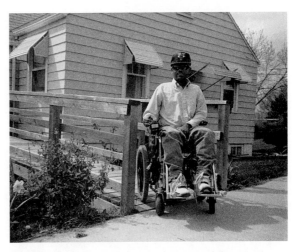

◆ **Figure 15-10**   Donald using power mobility.

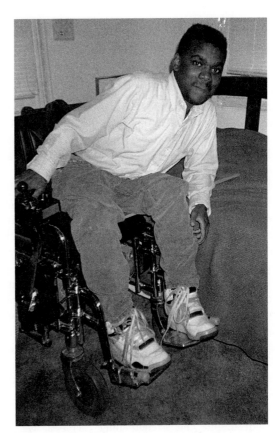

◆ **Figure 15-11**   Donald demonstrating sliding board transfer technique used for chair-to-bed transfers.

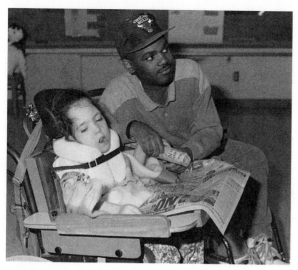

◆ **Figure 15-12** Donald assisting student in art class.

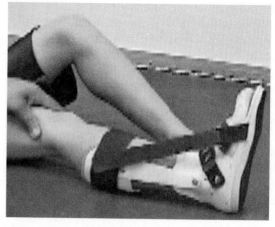

◆ **Figure 15-13** Night splints worn by Derek to maintain/improve ankle plantar flexor range of motion.

fully passed away at the age of 28 while sleeping at home following hospitalization for a bout of pneumonia.

DEREK

Derek is 9 years, 3 months of age, with diagnosis of a dystrophinopathy and probable Duchenne muscular dystrophy. History includes an unremarkable pregnancy and term birth. Derek weighed 8 lb 13 oz at birth and went home within 3 days. He has an older sister.

Derek's parents first began to have questions regarding his development at 17 months of age because of his delay in walking. His parents also reported what they perceived as clumsiness in his attempts to walk. Derek's pediatrician did not share the parents' concern regarding his delay or clumsiness in walking.

Following repeated expressions of concern by the family, Derek's pediatrician referred him for physical therapy services at age 5 because he was not able to keep up with peers, especially in activities that required running, jumping, or balance. He was seen by a physical therapist in a hospital setting for coordination and strengthening exercises. After almost 6 months of intervention, the physical therapist recommended further diagnostic testing as manual muscle test scores demonstrated a decline in strength despite the strengthening exercises. He was subsequently referred to the local MDA-sponsored neuromuscular clinic for further examination.

At Derek's initial visit to the neuromuscular clinic, his standing posture was found to be mildly lordotic, his gait exhibited increased lateral trunk sway toward the stance phase leg, he had difficulty hopping on one foot, he exhibited a positive Gowers sign when rising from the floor, and he needed to use a handrail when ascending or descending stairs. The physical examination found a pattern of mild proximal muscle weakness with most manual muscle test grades in the 4/5 range proximally and 5/5 distally. Creatine phosphate kinase testing resulted in a value of 20,009 IU/L (normal value 25–204 IU/L). DNA analysis found a deletion of exon 45 of the X chromosome, which resulted in a diagnosis of dystrophinopathy. A muscle biopsy to test for the presence or absence of dystrophin has not yet been done to definitively differentiate between Duchenne and Becker muscular dystrophy.

Prednisone was prescribed for Derek following the initial clinic visit with a dosage of 15 mg/day that was increased to 20 mg/day at the age of 9 years. Night splints (Fig. 15-13) and a home program for stretching of the posterior calf musculature were also initiated at the initial clinic visit with discontinuation of outpatient physical therapy services. His ankle dorsiflexion range of motion, which was at neutral at the initial visit, has improved to 10° with the knee extended and has remained stable through use of the night splints and stretching program. Improved muscle strength was recorded following the initiation of the prednisone regimen. Changes in muscle strength as documented with handheld dynamometry are shown in Table 15-3.

Currently, Derek is 9 years old and is in the fourth grade at his community elementary school. He receives consultative physical therapy at his school for input regarding his adapted physical education program and to address issues related to accessibility and fatigability during the school day. He is independently ambulatory with only mild gait deviations, which become more prominent when he attempts to run. He is independent in

| TABLE 15-3 | Handheld Dynamometry Scores Recorded with a Standardized Protocol with Isometric Contraction |

MEASUREMENT	POSITION	RIGHT (LB)		LEFT (LB)	
		7 yr – 2 mo	8 yr – 4 mo	7 yr – 2 mo	8 yr – 4 mo
Hip flexion	Supine, 90°	9	15	7	13
Hip extension	Supine, 90°	28	26	29	28
Hip abduction	Supine, 0°	9	17	8	16
Knee flexion	Sitting, 90°	13	16	11	16
Knee extension	Sitting, 90°	20	23	19	23
Ankle dorsiflexion	Supine, 90°	10	9	9	12
Ankle plantar flexion	Supine, 90°	52	54	50	56

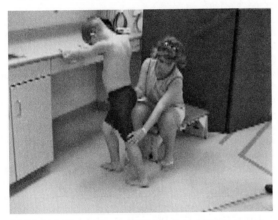

◆ **Figure 15-14** Runner's stretch used to stretch ankle plantar flexor muscles.

stair climbing using a handrail and is able to transfer from the floor to standing using a Gowers maneuver. His home program of heelcord stretching (five repetitions of a standing runner's stretch carried out daily (see Fig. 15-14), and night splint use are jointly monitored by the physical therapist at school and through the MDA clinic. At this point in time, he has no restriction on activity other than to avoid fatigue.

ACKNOWLEDGMENTS

My personal thanks goes to the children and their families who contributed to my knowledge of MD and SMA that made the writing of this chapter possible. Many challenges, accomplishments, disappointments, joys, and tears have paved the way. Special thanks to Donald and Derek and their families for sharing their stories, and to Becky, who first inspired me to take this path of clinical work.

REFERENCES

Amalfitano, A, Hauser, MA, Hu, H, Serra, D, Begy, CR, & Chamberlain, JS. Production and characterization of improved adenovirus vectors with the E1, E2b, and E3 genes deleted. Journal of Virology, 72:926–933, 1998.

Amendt, LE, Ause-Ellias, KL, Eybers, JL, Wadsworth, CT, Nielsen, DH, & Weinstein, SL. Validity and reliability testing of the scoliometer. Physical Therapy, 70:108–117, 1990.

American Physical Therapy Association (APTA). Guide to physical therapist practice. Physical Therapy 81:9–744, 2001.

Anderson, JL, Head, SI, Rae, C, & Morley JW. Brian function in Duchenne muscular dystrophy. Brain, 125:4–14, 2002.

Ansved T. Muscle training in muscular dystrophies. Acta Physiologica Scandinavica, 171:359–366, 2001.

Bach, JR. Ventilator use by Muscular Dystrophy Association patients. Archives of Physical Medicine and Rehabilitation, 73:179–183, 1992.

Bach, JR, Baird, JS, Plosky, D, Navado, J, & Weaver B. Spinal muscular atrophy 1: Management and outcomes. Pediatric Pulmonology, 34:16–22, 2002.

Bach, JR, Campagnolo, DI, & Hoeman, S. Life satisfaction of individuals with Duchenne muscular dystrophy using long-term mechanical ventilatory support. American Journal of Physical Medicine and Rehabilitation, 70:129–135, 1991.

Bach, JR, & Chaudhry, SS. Standards of care in MDA clinics. American Journal of Physical Medicine and Rehabilitation, 79:193–196, 2000.

Bach, JR, & McKeon, J. Orthopaedic surgery and rehabilitation for the prolongation of brace-free ambulation of patients with Duchenne muscular dystrophy. American Journal of Physical Medicine and Rehabilitation, 70:323–331, 1991.

Bach, JR, O'Brien, J, Krotenberg, R, & Alba, AS. Management of end stage respiratory failure in Duchenne muscular dystrophy. Muscle and Nerve, 10:177–182, 1987.

Backman, E, & Henriksson, KG. Low-dose prednisolone treatment in Duchenne and Becker muscular dystrophy. Neuromuscular Disorders, 5:233–241, 1995.

Bakker, JP, deGroot, IJ, Beckerman, H, deJong, BA & Lankhorst, GJ. The effects of knee-ankle-foot orthoses in the treatment of Duchenne muscular dystrophy: Review of the literature. Clinical Rehabilitation, 14:343–359, 2000.

Bakker, JP, deGroot, IJ, Beelen, A, & Lankhorst, GJ. Predictive factors of cessation of ambulation in patients with Duchenne muscular dystrophy. American Journal of Physical Medicine and Rehabilitation, 81:906–912, 2002.

Ballestrazzi, A, Gnudi, A, Magni, E, & Granata, C. Osteopenia in spinal muscular atrophy. In Merlini, L, Granata, C, & Dubowitz, V (Eds.). Current Concepts in Childhood Spinal Muscular Atrophy. New York: Springer-Verlag, 1989, pp. 215–219.

Bianchi, ML, Mazzanti, A, Galbiati, E, Saraifoger, S, Dubini, A, Cornelio, F, & Morandi, L. Bone mineral density and bone metabolism in Duchenne muscular dystrophy. Osteoporosis International, 14:761–767, 2003.

Biggar, WD, Gingras, M, Fehlings, DL, Harris, VA, & Steele, CA. Deflazacort treatment of Duchenne muscular dystrophy. Journal of Pediatrics, 138:45–50, 2001.

Biggar, WD, Klamut, HJ, Demacio, PC, Stevens, DJ & Ray, PN. Duchenne muscular dystrophy: Current knowledge, treatment, and future prospects, Clinical Orthopedics, 401:88–106, 2002.

Binder, H. New ideas in the rehabilitation of children with spinal muscular atrophy. In Merlini, L, Granata, C, & Dubowitz, V (Eds.). Current Concepts in Childhood Spinal Muscular Atrophy. New York: Springer-Verlag, 1989, pp. 117–128.

Blake, DS, Weir, A, Newey, SE, & Davis, KE. Function and genetics of dystrophia and dystrophia related proteins in muscle. Physiological Review, 82:291–329, 2002.

Bowker, JH, & Halpin, PJ. Factors determining success in reambulation of the child with progressive muscular dystrophy. Orthopedic Clinics of North America, 9:431–436, 1978.

Borkowska, J, Rudhik-Schoneborn, S, Hausmanowa-Petrusewicz, I & Zerre, K. Early infantile form of spinal muscle atrophy. Folia Neuropathologic, 40:19–26, 2002.

Brooke, MH. A Clinician's View of Neuromuscular Diseases, 2nd ed. Baltimore: Williams & Wilkins, 1986.

Brooke, MH, Fenichel, GM, Griggs, RC, Mendell, JR, Moxley, R, Florence, J, King, WM, Pandya, S, Robinson, J, Schierbecker, J, Singnor, L, Miller, JP, Gilder, BF, Kaiser, KK, Mandel, S, & Arfken, C. Duchenne muscular dystrophy: Patterns of clinical progression and effects of supportive therapy. Neurology, 39:475–481, 1989.

Brooke, MH, Griggs, RC, Mendell, JR, Fenichel, GM, Shumate, JB, & Pellegrino, RJ. Clinical trial in Duchenne dystrophy: I. The design of the protocol. Muscle and Nerve, 4:186–197, 1981.

Brouwer, OF, Paderg, GW, Van Der Ploeg, RJO, Ruys, CJM, & Brand, R. The influence of handedness on the distribution of muscular weakness of the arm in facioscapulohumeral muscular dystrophy. Brain, 115:1587–1598, 1992.

Brussock, CM, Haley, SM, Munsat, TL, & Bernhardt, DB. Measurement of isometric force in children with and without Duchenne's muscular dystrophy. Physical Therapy, 72:105–114, 1992.

Burke, SS, Grove, NM, & Houser, CR. Respiratory aspects of pseudohypertrophic muscular dystrophy. American Journal of Diseases of Children, 121:230–234, 1971.

Cambridge, W, & Drennan, JC. Scoliosis associated with Duchenne muscular dystrophy. Journal of Pediatric Orthopedics, 7:436–440, 1987.

Charash, LI, Lovelace, RE, Wolfe, SG, Kutscher, AH, Price, D, Leach, R, & Leach, CF. Realities in Coping with Progressive Neuromuscular Disease. Philadelphia: Charles Press Publishers, 1987.

Chyatte, SB, Long, C, & Vignos, PJ. Balanced forearm orthosis in muscular dystrophy. Archives of Physical Medicine and Rehabilitation, 46:633–636, 1965.

Colbert, AP, & Craig, C. Scoliosis management in Duchenne muscular dystrophy: Prospective study of modified Jewett hyperextension brace. Archives of Physical Medicine and Rehabilitation, 68:302–304, 1987.

Coster, W, Deeney, T, Haltiwanger, J, & Haley, S. School Function Assessment. San Antonio, TX: Therapy Skill Builders, 1998.

Courdier-Fruh, I, Barman, L, Briguet, A, & Meier, T, Glucocorticoid-mediated regulation of utrophin levels in human muscle fibers. Neuromuscular Disorders, 12(Suppl 1): S95–S104, 2002.

Cunha, MC, Oliveira, AS, Labronici, RH, & Gabbai, AA. Spinal muscular atrophy type II and III. Evolution of 50 patients with physiotherapy and hydrotherapy in a swimming pool. Arquivos Neuro-psiquiatria, 54:402–406, 1996.

Curran, FJ, & Colbert, AP. Ventilator management in Duchenne muscular dystrophy and postpoliomyelitis syndrome: Twelve years' experience. Archives of Physical Medicine and Rehabilitation, 70:180–185, 1989.

deLateur, BJ, & Giaconi, RM. Effect on maximal strength of submaximal exercise in Duchenne muscular dystrophy. American Journal of Physical Medicine, 58:26–36, 1979.

Dorscher, PT, Mehrsheed, S, Mulder, DW, Litchy, WJ, & Ilstrup, DM. Wohlfart-Kugelberg-Welander syndrome: Serum creatine kinase and functional outcome. Archives of Physical Medicine and Rehabilitation, 72:587–591, 1991.

Dubowitz, V. The clinical picture of spinal muscular atrophy. In Merlini, L, Granata, C, & Dubowitz, V (Eds.). Current Concepts in Childhood Spinal Muscular Atrophy. New York: Springer-Verlag, 1989, pp. 13–19.

Dubowitz, V. The muscular dystrophies. Postgraduate Medical Journal, 68:500–506, 1992.

Eagle, M, Baudouin, SV, Chandler, C, Giddings, DR, Bullock, R, & Bushby, K. Survival in Duchenne muscular dystrophy: improvements in life expectancy since 1967 and the impact of home nocturnal ventilation. Neuromuscular Disorders, 12:926–929, 2002.

Edwards, RHT. Studies of muscular performance in normal and dystrophic subjects. British Medical Bulletin, 36:159–164, 1980.

Emery, AEH. Duchenne muscular dystrophy. Oxford: Oxford University Press, 1993.

Emery, AEH. The muscular dystrophies. Lancet, 359:687–695, 2002.

Emery, AEH, & Skinner, R. Clinical studies in benign (Becker-type) X-linked muscular dystrophy. Clinical Genetics, 10:189–201, 1976.

Eng, GD. Therapy and rehabilitation of the floppy infant. Rhode Island Medical Journal, 72:367–370, 1989a.

Eng, GD. Rehabilitation of the child with a severe form of spinal muscular atrophy (type I, infantile or Werdnig-Hoffman disease). In Merlini, L, Granata, C, & Dubowitz, V (Eds.). Current Concepts in Childhood Spinal Muscular Atrophy. New York: Springer-Verlag, 1989b, pp. 113–115.

Florence, JM, Pandya, S, King, WM, Robinson, JD, Baty, J, Miller, JP, Schierbecker, J, & Signore, LC. Intrarater reliability of manual muscle test (Medical Research Council Scale) grades in Duchenne's muscular dystrophy. Physical Therapy, 72:115–122, 1992.

Fowler, WM. Rehabilitation management of muscular dystrophy and related disorders: I. The role of exercise. Archives of Physical Medicine and Rehabilitation, 63:208–210, 1982.

Fowler, WM, & Gardner, GW. Quantitative strength measurements in muscular dystrophy. Archives of Physical Medicine and Rehabilitation, 48:629–644, 1967.

Fukuyama, Y, Osaw, M, & Suzuki, H. Congenital muscular dystrophy of the Fukuyama type: Clinical, genetic and pathological considerations. Brain and Development, 3:1–29, 1981.

Galasko, CSB, Williamson, JB, & Delany, CM. Lung function in Duchenne muscular dystrophy. European Spine, 4:263–267, 1995.

Gamstorp, I. Progressive spinal muscular atrophy with onset in infancy or early childhood. Acta Paediatrica Scandinavica, 56:408–423, 1967.

Gardner-Medwin, D. Controversies about Duchenne muscular dystrophy: II. Bracing for ambulation. Developmental Medicine and Child Neurology, 21:659–662, 1979.

Gardner-Medwin, D. Clinical features and classification of the muscular dystrophies. British Medical Bulletin, 36:109–115, 1980.

Gibson, DA, Koreska, J, & Robertson, D. The management of spinal deformity in Duchenne's muscular dystrophy. Clinical Orthopedics, 9:437–450, 1978.

Gibson, DA, & Wilkins, KE. The management of spinal deformities in Duchenne's muscular dystrophy. Clinical Orthopedics, 108:41–51, 1975.

Gilroy, J, & Holliday, P. Basic Neurology. New York: Macmillan, 1982.

Granata, C, Magni, E, Sabattini, L, Colombo, C, & Merlini, L. Promotion of ambulation in intermediate spinal muscle atrophy. In Merlini, L, Granata, C, & Dubowitz, V (Eds.). Current Concepts in Childhood Spinal Muscular Atrophy. New York: Springer-Verlag, 1989a, pp. 127–132.

Granata, C, Marini, ML, Capelli, T, & Merlini, L. Natural history of scoliosis in spinal muscular atrophy and results of orthopaedic treatment. In Merlini, L, Granata, C, & Dubowitz, V (Eds.). Current Concepts in Childhood Spinal Muscular Atrophy. New York: Springer-Verlag, 1989b, pp. 153–164.

Granata, C, Merlini, L, Magni, E, Marini, ML, & Stagni, SB. Spinal muscular atrophy: Natural history and orthopaedic treatment of scoliosis. Spine, 14:760–762, 1989c.

Gussoni, E, Blau, HM, & Kunkel, LM. The fate of individual myoblasts after transplantation into muscles of DMD patients. Nature & Medicine, 3:970–977, 1997.

Haley, SM, Coster, WJ, Ludlow, LH, & Haltiwanger, JT. Pediatric Evaluation of Disability Inventory (PEDI): Development, Standardization and Administration Manual. Boston: New England Medical Center Hospital, 1992.

Harper, PS. Congenital myotonic muscular dystrophy in Britain: I. Clinical aspects. Archives of Disease in Childhood, 50:505–513, 1975.

Harper, PS. Myotonic Dystrophy, 2nd ed. Major Problems in Neurology, Vol. 21. Philadelphia: WB Saunders, 1989.

Heckmatt, JZ, Dubowitz, V, & Hyde, SA. Prolongation of walking in Duchenne muscular dystrophy with lightweight orthoses: Review of 57 cases. Developmental Medicine and Child Neurology, 27:149–154, 1985.

Heller, KD, Forst, R, Forst, J, & Hengstler, K. Scoliosis in Duchenne muscular dystrophy. Prosthetics and Orthotics International, 21:202–209, 1997.

Hoffman, EP, Brown, RH, & Kunkel, LM. Dystrophin: The protein product of the Duchenne muscular dystrophy locus. Cell, 51:919–928, 1987.

Hoffmann, J. Ueber chronische spinale Muskelatrophie im Kindesalter, auf familiar Basis. Deutsche Zeitschrift fur Nervenheilkunde, 3:427, 1893.

Hsu, JD. Orthopedic approaches for the treatment of lower extremity contractures in the Duchenne muscular dystrophy patient in the United States and Canada. Seminars in Neurology, 15:6–8, 1995.

Hyde, SA, Floytrup, I, Glent, S, Kroksmark, A, & Salling, B. A randomized comparative study using two methods for controlling tendo Achilles contracture in Duchenne muscular dystrophy. Neuromuscular Disorders, 10:257–263, 2000.

Johnson, EW, & Braddom, R. Over-work weakness in facioscapulohumeral muscular dystrophy. Archives of Physical Medicine and Rehabilitation, 52:333–336, 1971.

Jones, KJ, & North, KN. Recent advances in diagnosis of the childhood muscular dystrophies; Journal of Paediatric Child Health, 33:195–201, 1997.

Jones, MA, McEwen, IR, & Hansen, L. Use of power mobility for a young child with spinal muscular atrophy. Physical Therapy, 83:253–262, 2003.

Karpati, G, Holland, P, & Worton, RG. Myoblast transfer in DMD: Problems in the interpretation of efficiency (Letter). Muscle and Nerve, 15:1209–1210, 1992.

Koenig, M, Hoffmann, EP, & Pertelson, CK. Complete cloning of the Duchenne muscular dystrophy (DMD) cDNA and preliminary genomic organization of the DMD gene in mouse and affected individuals. Cell, 50:509–517, 1987.

Koessler, W, Wanke, T, Winkler, G, Nader, A, Toifl, K, Kurz, H, & Zwick, H. 2 years' experience with inspiratory muscle training in patients with neuromuscular disorders. Chest, 120:765–769, 2001.

Kugelberg, E, & Welander, L. Heredofamilial juvenile muscular atrophy simulating muscular dystrophy. Archives of Neurology and Psychiatry, 75:500, 1956.

Kunkel, LM, Monaco, AP, Middlesworth, W, Ochs, SD, & Latt, SA. Specific cloning of DNA fragments absent from the DNA of a male patient with an X chromosome deletion. Proceedings of the National Academy of Science USA, 82:4778–4782, 1985.

Law, PK, Goodwin, TG, Fang, Q, Quinley, T, Vastagh, G, Hall, T, Jackson, T, Deering, MB, Duggirala, V, Larkin, C, Florendo, JA, Li, LM, Yoo, TJ, Chase, N, Neel, M, Krahn, T, & Holcomb, RL. Human gene therapy with myoblast transfer. Transplantation Proceedings, 29:2234–2237, 1997.

Lee, CC, Pearlman, JA, Chamberlain, JS, & Caskey, CT. Expression of recombinant dystrophin and its localization to the cell membrane. Nature, 349:334–336, 1991.

Liechti-Gallati, S, Koenig, M, Kunkel, LM, Frey, D, Boltshauser, E, Schneider, V, Braga, S, & Moser, H. Molecular deletion patterns in Duchenne and Becker type muscular dystrophy. Human Genetics, 81:343–348, 1989.

Lonstein, JE. Management of spinal deformity in spinal muscular atrophy. In Merlini, L, Granata, C, & Dubowitz, V (Eds.). Current Concepts in Childhood Spinal Muscular Atrophy. New York: Springer-Verlag, 1989, pp. 165–173.

Louis, M, Lebacq, J, Poortmans, JR, Belpaire-Dethiou, MC, Devogelaer, J, Van Hecke, P, Goubel, F, & Francaux, M. Beneficial effects of creatine supplementation in dystrophic patients. Muscle and Nerve, 27:604–610, 2003.

Lyager, S, Steffensen, B, & Juhl, B. Indicators of need for mechanical ventilation in Duchenne muscular dystrophy and spinal muscular atrophy. Chest, 108:779–785, 1995.

MacKenzie, AE, Jacob, P, Surh, L, & Besner, A. Genetic heterogeneity in spinal muscle atrophy: A linkage analysis-based assessment. Neurology, 44:919–924, 1994.

Marchesi, D, Arlet, V, Stricker, U, & Aeibi, M. Modification of the original luque technique in the treatment of Duchenne's neuromuscular scoliosis. Journal of Pediatric Orthopaedics, 17:743–749, 1997.

Marshall, CR. Medical treatment of spinal muscular atrophy. In Gamstorp, I, & Sarnat, HB (Eds.). Progressive Spinal Muscular Atrophies. International Review of Child Neurology Series. New York: Raven Press, 1984, pp. 163–171.

McDonald, CM, Abresch, RT, Carter, GT, Fowler WM, Johnson, ER, Kilmer, DMD, & Sigford, BJ. Profiles of neuromuscular diseases: Duchenne muscular dystrophy. American Journal of Physical Medicine and Rehabilitation, 74(Suppl):S70–S92, 1995.

McDonald, DG, Kinali, M, Gallagher, AC, Mercuri, E, Muntoni, F, Roper, H, Jardine, P, Jones, DH, & Pike, MG. Fracture prevalence in Duchenne muscular dystrophy. Developmental Medicine and Child Neurology, 44:695–698, 2002.

Merlini, L, Granata, C, Capelli, T, Mattutini, P, & Colombo, C. Natural history of infantile and childhood spinal muscular atrophy. In Merlini, L, Granata, C, & Dubowitz, V (Eds.). Current Concepts in Childhood Spinal Muscular Atrophy. New York: Springer-Verlag, 1989, pp. 95–100.

Merlini, L, Cicognani, A, Malaspina, E, Gennari, M, Gnudi, S, Talim, B,

& Franzoni, E. Early prednisone treatment in Duchenne muscular dystrophy. Muscle and Nerve, 27:222–227, 2003.

Miller, F, Moseley, CF, & Koreska, J. Spinal fusion in Duchenne muscular dystrophy. Developmental Medicine and Child Neurology, 34:775–786, 1992.

Miller, G, & Dunn, N. An outline of the management and prognosis of Duchenne muscular dystrophy in Western Australia. Australian Pediatric Journal, 82:277–282, 1982.

Molnar, GE, & Alexander, J. Objective, quantitative muscle testing in children: A pilot study. Archives of Physical Medicine and Rehabilitation, 54:224–228, 1973.

Muscular Dystrophy Association. Facts About Muscular Dystrophy. Tucson, AZ: Muscular Dystrophy Association, 2001.

Nair, KP, Vasanth, A, Gourie-Devi, M, Taly, AB, Rao, S, Gayathri, N, & Murali, T. Disabilities in children with Duchenne muscular dystrophy: a profile. Journal of Rehabilitation Medicine, 33:147–149, 2001.

Newsom-Davis, J. The respiratory system in muscular dystrophy. British Medical Bulletin, 36:135–138, 1980.

North, KN, Specht, LA, Sethi, RK, Shapiro, F, & Beggs, AH. Congenital muscular dystrophy associated with merosin deficiency. Journal of Child Neurology, 11:291–295, 1996.

O'Brien, T, & Harper, PS. Course, prognosis and complications of childhood-onset myotonic dystrophy. Developmental Medicine and Child Neurology, 26:62–67, 1984.

OMIM. Accessed at http://www3.ncbi.nlm.nih.gov/Omim. December 23, 2003.

Pandya, A, Florence, JM, King, WM, Robinson, JD, Oxman, M, & Province, MA. Reliability of goniometric measurements in patients with Duchenne muscular dystrophy. Physical Therapy, 65:1339–1342, 1985.

Partridge, TA, Grounds, M, & Sloper, JC. Evidence of fusion between host and donor myoblasts in skeletal muscle grafts. Nature, 273:306–308, 1978.

Partridge, T. Myoblast transplantation. Neuromuscular Disorders, 12(Suppl):1S3–S6, 2002.

Pearn, JH. Autosomal dominant spinal muscular atrophy: A clinical and genetic study. Journal of Neurologic Science, 38:263–275, 1978.

Pearn, JH. Classification of spinal muscular atrophies. Lancet, 1:919–922, 1980.

Pearn, JH, Carter, CO, & Wilson, J. The genetic identity of acute spinal muscular atrophy. Brain, 96:463–470, 1973.

Pegoraro, E, Marks, H, Garcia, CA, Crawford, T, & Connolly, AM. Laminin alpha2 muscular dystrophy: Genotype/phenotype studies of 22 patients. Neurology, 51:101–110, 1998.

Perkins, KJ, & Davies, KE. The role of utrophin in the potential therapy of Duchenne muscular dystrophy. Neuromuscular Disorders, 12:S78–S89, 2002.

Petrof, BJ. Molecular pathophysiology of myofiber injury in deficiencies of the dystrophin–glycoprotein complex. American Journal of Physical Medicine and Rehabilitation, 81:S162–S174, 2002.

Pinelli, G, Dominici, P, Merlini, L, DiPasquale, G, Granata, C, & Bonfiglioli, S. Cardiologic evaluation in a family with Emery-Dreifus muscular dystrophy. Giornale Italiano di Cardiologia, 17:589–593, 1987.

Reardon, W, Newcombe, R, Fenton, I, Sibert, J, & Harper, PS. The natural history of congenital myotonic muscular dystrophy: Mortality and long term clinical aspects. Archives of Disease in Childood, 68:177–181, 1993.

Ricker, K. The expanding clinical and genetic spectrum of the myotonic dystrophies. Acta Neurologica Belgium, 100:151–155, 2000.

Rideau, Y, Glorion, B, Delaubier, A, Tarle, O, & Bach, J. The treatment of scoliosis in Duchenne muscular dystrophy. Muscle and Nerve, 7:281–286, 1984.

Ringel, SP. Neuromuscular Disorders: A Guide for Patient and Family. New York: Raven Press, 1987.

Robinson, A. Programmed cell death and the gene behind spinal muscle atrophy. Canadian Medical Association Journal, 153:1459–1462, 1995.

Rodillo, E, Noble-Jamieson, CM, Aber, V, Heckmatt, JZ, Muntoni, F, & Dubowitz, V. Respiratory muscle training in Duchenne muscular dystrophy. Archives of Disease in Childhood, 64:736–738, 1989.

Romero, NB, Benveniste, O, Payan, C, Braun, S, Squiban, P, Herson, S, & Fardeau, M. Current protocol of a research phase I clinical trial of full length dystrophin plasmid DNA in Duchenne/Becker muscular dystrophy. Part II. clinical protocol. Neuromuscular Disorders, 121:S45–S48, 2002.

Roig, M, Balliu, PR, Navarro, C, Brugera, R & Losada, M. Presentation, clinical course and outcome of the congenital form of myotonic dystrophy. Pediatric Neurology, 11:208–213, 1994.

Rutherford, MA, Heckmatt, JZ, & Dubowitz, V. Congenital myotonic dystrophy: Respiratory function at birth determines survival. Archives of Disease in Childhood, 64:191–195, 1989.

Saranti, AJ, Gleim, GW, & Melvin, M. The relationship between subjective and objective measurements of strength. Journal of Orthopedic Sports and Physical Therapy, 2:15–19, 1980.

Scher, DM, & Mubarak, SJ. Sugical prevention of foot deformity in patients with Duchenne muscular dystrophy. Journal of Pediatric Orthopedics, 22:348–391, 2002.

Scott, OM, Hyde, SA, Goddard, C, & Dubowitz, V. Prevention of deformity in Duchenne muscular dystrophy: A prospective study of passive stretching and splintage. Physiotherapy, 67:177–180, 1981.

Scott, OM, Hyde, SA, & Goddard, E. Quantification of muscle function in children: A prospective study in Duchenne muscular dystrophy. Muscle and Nerve, 5:291–301, 1982.

Scott, OM, Vrbova, G, Hyde, SA, & Dubowitz, V. Responses of muscles of patients with Duchenne muscular dystrophy to chronic electrical stimulation. Journal of Neurology, Neurosurgery and Psychiatry, 49:1427–1434, 1986.

Seeger, BR, Caudrey, DJ, & Little JD. Progression of equinus deformity in Duchenne muscular dystrophy. Archives of Physical Medicine and Rehabilitation, 66:286–288, 1985.

Seeger, BR, Sutherland, AD, & Clark, MS. Orthotic management of scoliosis in Duchenne muscular dystrophy. Archives of Physical Medicine and Rehabilitation, 65:83–86, 1984.

Semprini, L, Tacconelli, A, Capon, F, Brancati, F, Dallapiccola, B, & Novelli, C. A single strand conformation polymorphism-based carrier test for spinal muscle atrophy. Genetic Testing, 5:33–37, 2001.

Sengupta, SK, Mehdian, SH, McConnell, JR, Eisenstein, SM, & Webb, JK. Pelvic or lumbar fixation for the surgical management of scoliosis in Duchenne muscular dystrophy. Spine, 27:2072–2079, 2002.

Shapiro, F, & Specht, L. Orthopaedic deformities in Emery-Dreifus muscular dystrophy. Journal of Pediatric Orthopedics, 11:336–340, 1991.

Siegel, IM. Plastic-molded knee-ankle-foot orthosis in the management of Duchenne muscular dystrophy. Archives of Physical Medicine and Rehabilitation, 56:322–328, 1975.

Siegel, IM. The Clinical Management of Muscle Disease: A Practical Manual of Diagnosis and Treatment. Philadelphia: JB Lippincott, 1977.

Siegel, IM. The management of muscular dystrophy: A clinical review. Muscle and Nerve, 1:453–460, 1978.

Siegel, IM. Muscle and Its Diseases: An Outline Primer of Basic Science and Clinical Method. Chicago: Year Book Medical Publishers, 1986.

Siegel, IM, Miller, JE, & Ray, RD. Subcutaneous lower limb tenotomy in the treatment of pseudohypertrophic muscular dystrophy. Archives of Physical Medicine and Rehabilitation, 53:404–406, 1972.

Spencer, GE, & Vignos, PJ. Bracing for ambulation in childhood progressive muscular dystrophy. Journal of Bone and Joint Surgery (American), 44:234–242, 1962.

Stedman, H, Wilson, JM, Finke, R, Kleckner, AL, & Mendell, J. Phase I clinical trial utilizing gene therapy for limb girdle muscular dystrophy: alpha-, beta-, gamma-, or delta-sarcoglyca gene delivered with intramuscular instillations of adeno-associated vectors. Human Gene Therapy, 11:777–790, 2000.

Steffensen, B & Hyde, S. Validity of the EK scale: A functional assessment of non-ambulatory individuals with Duchenne muscular dystrophy. Physiotherapy Research International, 6:119–134, 2001.

Steffensen, BF, Lyager, S, Werge, B, Rahbek, J & Mattsson, E. Physical capacity in non-ambulatory people with Duchenne muscular dystrophy or spinal muscular atrophy: A longitudinal study. Developmental Medicine & Child Neurology, 44:623–632, 2002.

Stevenson, WG, Perloff, JK, Weiss, JN, & Anderson, TL. Facioscapulohumeral muscular dystrophy: Evidence for selective, genetic electrophysiologic cardiac involvement. Journal of the American College of Cardiology, 15:292–299, 1990.

Stuberg, WA, Home accessibility and adaptive equipment in Duchenne muscular dystrophy: A case report. Pediatric Physical Therapy, 13:169–174, 2001.

Stuberg, WA, & Metcalf, WM. Reliability of quantitative muscle testing in healthy children and in children with Duchenne muscular dystrophy using a hand-held dynamometer. Physical Therapy, 68:977–982, 1988.

Swinyard, CA, Deaver, GG, & Greenspan, L. Gradients of functional ability of importance in rehabilitation of patients with progressive muscular and neuromuscular diseases. Archives of Physical Medicine and Rehabilitation, 38:574–579, 1957.

Taktak, DM, & Bowker, P. Lightweight, modular knee-ankle-foot-orthosis for Duchenne muscular dystrophy: Design, development, and evaluation. Archives of Physical Medicine and Rehabilitation, 76:1156–1162, 1995.

Vignos, PJ. Physical models of rehabilitation in neuromuscular disease. Muscle and Nerve, 6:323–338, 1983.

Vignos, PJ, & Archibald, KC. Maintenance of ambulation in childhood muscular dystrophy. Journal of Chronic Diseases, 12:273–290, 1960.

Vignos, PJ, Spencer, GE, & Archibald, KC. Management of progressive muscular dystrophy. Journal of the American Medical Association, 184:103–112, 1963.

Vignos, PJ, & Watkins, MP. The effect of exercise in muscular dystrophy. Journal of the American Medical Association, 197:121–126, 1966.

Vignos, PJ, Wagner, MB, Karlinchak, B, & Katirji, B. Evaluation of a program for long-term treatment of Duchenne muscular dystrophy. The Journal of Bone and Joint Surgery, 78A:1844–1852,1996.

Voit, T. Congenital muscular dystrophies: 1997 update. Brain Development, 20:65–74, 1998.

Watt, JM, & Greenhill, B. Commentary: Rehabilitation and orthopaedic management of spinal muscle atrophy. In Gamstorp, I, & Sarnat, HB (Eds.). Progressive Spinal Muscular Atrophies. International Review of Child Neurology Series. New York: Raven Press, 1984.

Werdnig, G. Eine fruhinfantile progressive spinale Amyotrophie. Archives fur Psychiatrie Nervenkrankheiten, 26:706–744, 1894.

Wilkins, KE, & Gibson, DA. Patterns of spinal deformity in Duchenne muscular dystrophy. Journal of Bone and Joint Surgery (Am), 58:24–32, 1976.

Winsor, EJ, Murphy, EG, Thompson, MW, & Reed, TE. Genetics of childhood spinal muscular atrophy. Journal of Medical Genetics, 8:143–148, 1971.

Wohlfart, G, Fex, J, & Eliasson, S. Hereditary proximal spinal muscular atrophy: A clinical entity simulating progressive muscular dystrophy. Acta Psychiatrica Neurologica Scandinavica, 30:395–406, 1955.

Wong, LY & Christopher, C. Corticosteriods in Duchenne muscular dystrophy: a reappraisal. Journal of Child Neurology, 17:184–190, 2002.

Wong, CK, & Wade, CK. Reducing iliotibial band contractures in patients with muscular dystrophy using custom dry floatation cushions. Archives of Physical Medicine and Rehabilitation, 76:695–700, 1995.

Ziter, FA, & Allsop, KG. The diagnosis and management of childhood muscular dystrophy. Clinical Pediatrics, 15:540–548, 1976.

| **APPENDIX** | **Clinical Protocol for Functional Testing in Duchenne Muscular Dystrophy*** |

A. Pulmonary
   1. Forced vital capacity.
   2. Maximum voluntary ventilation.
B. Functional grade (arms and shoulders). Select one.
   1. Starting with arms at the sides, the patient can abduct the arms in a full circle until they touch above the head.
   2. Can raise arms above head only by flexing the elbow (i.e., shortening the circumference of the movement) or using accessory muscles.
If 1 or 2 is entered above, how many kilograms of weight can be placed on a shelf above eye level, using one hand?
   3. Cannot raise hands above head but can raise an 8 oz glass of water to mouth (using both hands if necessary).
   4. Can raise hands to mouth but cannot raise an 8 oz glass of water to mouth.
   5. Cannot raise hands to mouth but can use hands to hold pen or pick up pennies from the table.
   6. Cannot raise hands to mouth and has no useful function of hands.
C. Pulmonary.
   1. Maximum expiratory pressure.
D. Time to perform functions. Enter time in seconds. T = tried but failed to complete by time limit of 120 seconds.
   1. Standing from lying supine.
   2. Climbing four standard stairs (beginning and ending standing with arms at sides).
   3. Running or walking 30 feet (as fast as is compatible with safety).
   4. Standing from sitting on chair (chair height should allow feet to touch floor).
   5. Propelling a wheelchair 30 feet.
   6. Putting on a T-shirt (sitting in chair).
   7. Cutting a 3 × 3-inch premarked square from a piece of paper with safety scissors (lines do not need to be followed precisely).
E. Functional grade (hips and legs). Select one.
   1. Walks and climbs stairs without assistance.
   2. Walks and climbs stairs with aid of railing.
   3. Walks and climbs stairs slowly with aid of railing (over 12 seconds for four standard stairs).
   4. Walks unassisted and raises from chair but cannot climb stairs.
   5. Walks unassisted but cannot rise from chair or climb stairs.
   6. Walks only with assistance or walks independently with long leg braces.
   7. Walks in long leg braces but requires assistance for balance.
   8. Stands in long leg braces but is unable to walk even with assistance.
   9. Is in wheelchair.
   10. Is confined to bed.

*From Brooke, MH, Griggs, RC, Mendell, JR, Fenichel, GM, Shumate, JB, & Pellegrino, RJ. Clinical trial in Duchenne dystrophy: I. The design of the protocol. Muscle and Nerve, 4:186–197, 1981.

Chapter 16

LIMB DEFICIENCIES AND AMPUTATIONS

MEG STANGER
PT, MS, PCS

The child with an amputation is defined as a person with an amputation who is skeletally immature because the epiphyses of the long bones are still open (Aitken, 1963). Amputations can be classified as congenital or acquired. Annual surveys of child amputee clinics in the United States indicate that 60% of childhood amputations are congenital and 40% are acquired (Tooms, 1992). Krebs and Fishman's (1984) study of 4105 children with limb deficiencies supports these findings.

Many different factors must be considered in the management of children with a limb deficiency or amputation. These factors differ from those involved in the management of adults with a limb deficiency or amputation because as children grow their musculoskeletal systems continue to develop. Children also are emotionally immature and variably dependent on adults for care and decision making regarding surgical and prosthetic issues.

In this chapter the etiology of limb deficiencies and amputations in children, surgical management, physical therapy intervention relative to a child's age and developmental function, and pediatric prosthetic options are discussed. Emphasis is on the aspects of management that differ from those encountered by adults with amputations. The role of the physical therapist includes education to parents of infants and children with limb deficiencies, development and progression of postoperative exercise programs, training in mobility and self-care skills, and providing input to both parents and the child or adolescent regarding prosthetic options. Studies have shown that children with limb deficiencies who participated in extensive rehabilitation programs have vocational skills with high employment potential (Tebbi, 1993).

CONGENITAL LIMB DEFICIENCIES

CLASSIFICATION

Various classification systems of congenital limb deficiencies have been developed. Greek terminology has been used to describe various deficiencies but is often inaccurate and ambiguous (Day, 1991). Frantz and O'Rahilly (1961) developed a classification system based on embryologic considerations and the absent skeletal portions. Swanson and colleagues (1968) modified that system with a classification system of seven categories based on embryologic failure: (1) failure of formation of parts (arrest of development), (2) failure of differentiation (separation of parts), (3) duplication, (4) overgrowth, (5) undergrowth (hypoplasia), (6) congenital constriction band syndrome, and (7) generalized skeletal deformities. Further modifications were made by the International Society for Prosthetics and Orthotics (ISPO) in 1973 and 1989. The classification developed by the ISPO has now been accepted and published as an international standard, International Standards Organization (ISO) 8548-1:1989, "Method of Describing Limb Deficiencies Present at Birth" (Day, 1991).

The ISO/ISPO classification of congenital limb deficiency is restricted to skeletal deficiencies described on anatomic and radiologic bases only; Greek terminology,

such as hemimelia and phocomelia, is avoided because of its lack of precision and difficulty of translation into languages that are not related to Greek (Day, 1991). Deficiencies are described as either transverse or longitudinal. In transverse deficiencies the limb has developed normally to a particular level beyond which no skeletal elements exist, although digital buds may be present. A transverse deficiency is described by naming the segment in which the limb terminates and then describing the level within the segment beyond which no skeletal elements exist (Day, 1991) (Fig. 16-1).

In longitudinal deficiencies there is a reduction or absence of an element or elements within the long axis of a limb. Normal skeletal elements may be present distal to the affected bones. A longitudinal deficiency is described by naming the bones affected in a proximal-to-distal

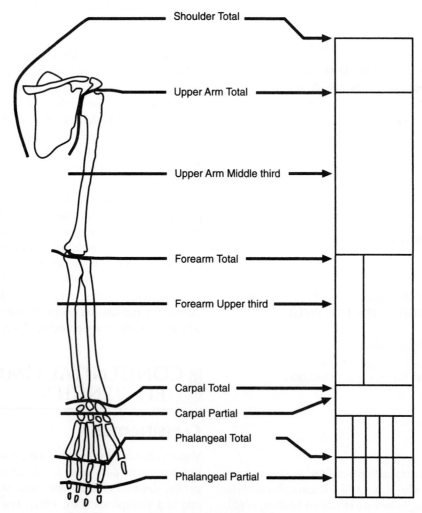

Shoulder Total

Upper Arm Total

Upper Arm Middle third

Forearm Total

Forearm Upper third

Carpal Total

Carpal Partial

Phalangeal Total

Phalangeal Partial

◆ **Figure 16-1**   Examples of transverse deficiencies at various levels of the upper extremity. *(From Day, HJ. The ISO/ISPO classification of congenital limb deficiency. In Bowker, JH, & Michael, JW [Eds.]. Atlas of Limb Prosthetics: Surgical, Prosthetic, and Rehabilitation Principles, 2nd ed. St. Louis: Mosby-Year Book, 1992, p. 747.)*

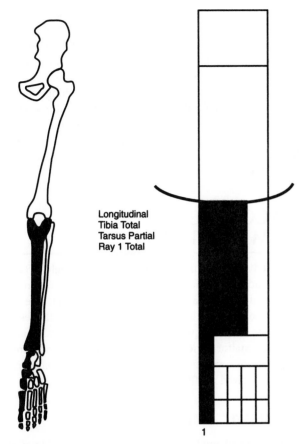

Longitudinal
Tibia Total
Tarsus Partial
Ray 1 Total

1

• **Figure 16-2**   Example of a longitudinal deficiency of the lower extremity. *(From Day, HJ. The ISO/ISPO classification of congenital limb deficiency. In Bowker, JH, & Michael, JW [Eds.]. Atlas of Limb Prosthetics: Surgical, Prosthetic, and Rehabilitation Principles, 2nd ed. St. Louis: Mosby-Year Book, 1992, p. 748.)*

sequence and stating whether each affected bone is totally or partially absent (Day, 1991) (Fig. 16-2).

ETIOLOGY

To fully understand the etiology of congenital limb deficiencies, a basic knowledge of embryonic skeletal development is necessary. Limb buds first appear at the end of the fourth week of embryonic development, arising from mesenchymal tissue. During the next 3 weeks the limb buds grow and differentiate into identifiable limb segments. Development of limb buds occurs in a proximodistal sequence, with upper limb development preceding lower limb development by several days. The mesenchymal tissue undergoes chondrification to become cartilaginous models of individual bones (Sadler, 1998). By the end of the seventh week a recognizable embryonic skeleton is present. Teratogenic factors must therefore be present at

some time between the third and seventh weeks of embryonic development to produce a limb deficiency.

The causative factor for most congenital limb deficiencies is unknown. A genetic link may be associated with a few limb anomalies but most limb deficiencies are the result of sporadic genetic mutation (Herring, 2002b). Several teratogenic factors have been identified (e.g., thalidomide, contraceptives, irradiation) as possible causative factors for congenital limb deficiencies. Limb deficiencies, especially of the upper extremity, may be associated with other congenital anomalies such as Holt-Oram, Fanconi, Poland, thrombocytopenia-absent radius, and VATER syndromes. This association has led to the theory that disruption of the blood supply in the subclavian artery during early embryonic development may be the cause of some congenital limb deficiencies (Weaver, 1998).

LEVELS OF LIMB DEFICIENCY

The incidence for congenital limb deficiencies ranges from 2 to 7 per 10,000 live births. This rate has been relatively unchanged over time but varies slightly across geographic areas (Ephraim et al., 2003). The clinical presentation of a child with a congenital limb deficiency depends on the type, level, and number of deficiencies. Almost any combination or variety of limb deficiency is possible, but some are more common, and these are discussed in this chapter in detail. Between 20% and 30% of children have limb deficiencies affecting more than one limb (Krebs & Fishman, 1984) (Fig. 16-3).

Most transverse deficiencies are unilateral, with the transverse below-elbow limb deficiency being the most common (Wright & Jobe, 1991) (Fig. 16-4). Rudimentary finger vestiges called nubbins may be present. This type of deficiency occurs more frequently in females, with a left-sided predominance of almost 2:1 (Shurr & Cook, 1990).

A complex lower extremity congenital limb deficiency has been termed *proximal femoral focal deficiency* (PFFD). Aitken (1969) first described this deficiency, which includes absence or hypoplasia of the proximal femur with varying degrees of involvement of the acetabulum, femoral head, patella, tibia, and fibula. The deficiency may be unilateral or bilateral. Aitken described four classes of severity, A through D, with class A exhibiting the least involvement based on radiographic findings (Fig. 16-5). Gillespie (1998) has developed a classification system for PFFD based on the complexity of medical intervention. Children classified into group A may only require limb lengthening, while those in groups B and C will require some level of amputation or revision and prosthetic fitting.

The clinical manifestations of a child with PFFD are relatively consistent among children. They include a short-

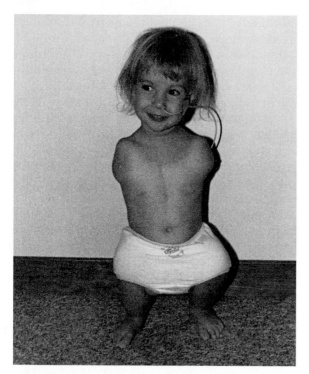

⬧ **Figure 16-3** Child with multiple congenital limb deficiencies including bilateral transverse upper arm deficiency and bilateral proximal femoral focal deficiency.

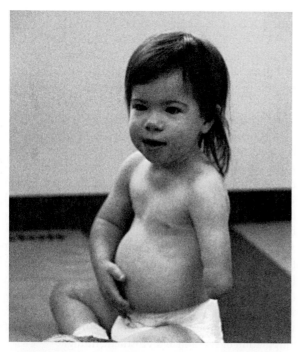

⬧ **Figure 16-4** Child with congenital transverse forearm or below elbow limb deficiency.

ened thigh that is held in flexion, abduction, and external rotation; hip and knee flexion contracture; and severe leg length discrepancy, with the foot often at the level of the opposite knee. These children also have instability of the knee joint secondary to absent or deficient cruciate ligaments and a 70% to 80% incidence of total longitudinal deficiency of the fibula. Fifteen percent of children with PFFD have bilateral involvement (Morrissy et al., 2001). The incidence of PFFD is reported to be 1 per 50,000 live births, and it is usually of unknown etiology (Morrissy et al., 2001).

ACQUIRED AMPUTATIONS

Acquired amputations account for approximately 40% of childhood amputations. Of these, 70% to 85% can be attributed to trauma (Bryant & Pandian, 2001). The remainder of acquired amputations in children are the result of disease (most frequently tumors but also infection and vascular malformations). Ninety percent of acquired amputations involve only one limb, and the lower extremity is involved in 60% of cases (Tooms, 1992).

TRAUMATIC AMPUTATIONS

Accidents involving farm machinery and household power tools are the leading causes of acquired amputations in the pediatric population, followed closely by vehicular accidents, gunshot wounds, and railroad accidents (Tooms, 1992; Trautwein et al., 1996). Incidences vary according to age and geographic location. Lawn mowers and household accidents account for most amputations in the 1- to 4-year-old population. Vehicular accidents, power tools and machinery, and gunshot wounds are common causes of traumatic amputations in the older child (Tooms, 1992; Trautwein et al., 1996).

DISEASE-RELATED AMPUTATIONS

Sarcoma of Bone

Primary bone tumors are rare in children, accounting for only 5% of cancers in children younger than 15 years of age (Miller et al., 1995). Osteosarcoma and Ewing's sarcoma are the most common of the primary bone tumors, with annual incidences in the United States of 3.3 per million for osteosarcoma and 2.8 per million for Ewing's sarcoma (Gurney et al., 1995). There is a slightly higher incidence of both osteosarcoma and Ewing's sarcoma in males than females. Ewing's sarcoma is very rare among the black population (Gurney et al., 1995; Miller et al., 1995).

TYPE		FEMORAL HEAD	ACETABULUM	FEMORAL SEGMENT	RELATIONSHIP AMONG COMPONENTS OF FEMUR AND ACETABULUM AT SKELETAL MATURITY
A	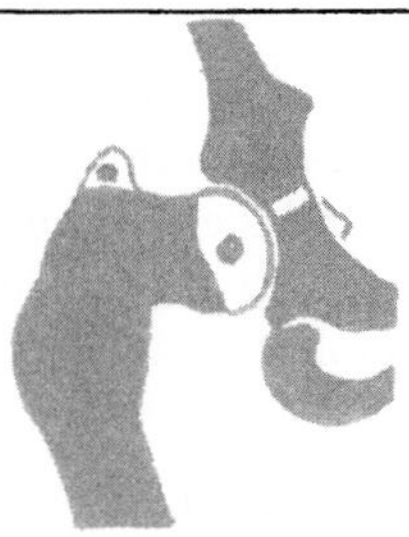	Present	Normal	Short	Bony connection between components of femur Femoral head in acetabulum Subtrochanteric varus angulation, often with pseudarthrosis
B	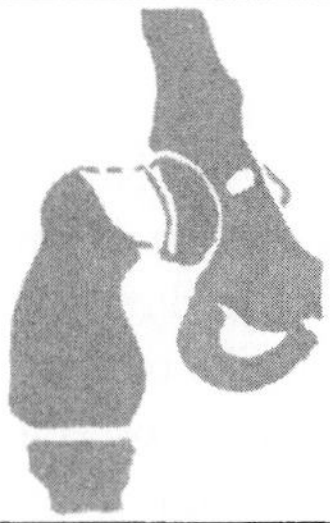	Present	Adequate or moderately dysplastic	Short, usually proximal bony tuft	No osseous connection between head and shaft Femoral head in acetabulum
C	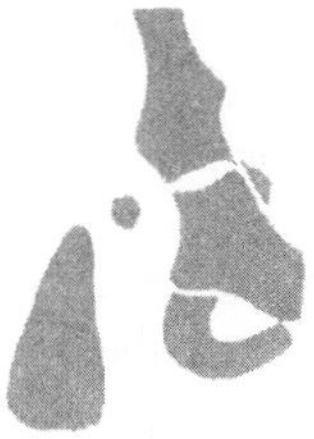	Absent or represented by ossicle	Severely dysplastic	Short, usually proximally tapered	May be osseous connection between shaft and proximal ossicle No articular relation between femur and acetabulum
D	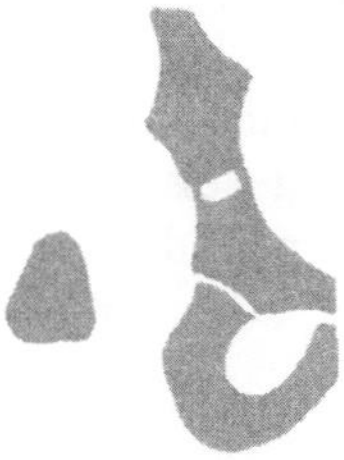	Absent	Absent Obturator foramen enlarged Pelvis squared in bilateral cases	Short, deformed	(none)

• **Figure 16-5**   Aitken classification of proximal femoral focal deficiency. *(From Herring, JA [Ed.]. Tachdjian's Pediatric Orthopedics, 3rd ed. Philadelphia: WB Saunders, 2002, p. 1756.)*

Childhood cancer statistics are based on children younger than 15 years of age; however, both osteosarcoma and Ewing's sarcoma continue to be seen in the late teenage years and beginning of the third decade of life with incidence rates slightly higher for 15- to 19-year-olds than the younger adolescent population (Bleyer, 2002).

Osteosarcoma

Osteosarcoma is a primary malignant tumor of bone derived from bone-forming mesenchyme in which the malignant proliferating spindle cell stroma produces osteoid tissue or immature bone. The cause of osteosarcoma is unknown, but osteosarcoma has been linked with exposure to ionizing radiation. A viral cause has also been suggested based on evidence that bone sarcomas can be induced through viruses in animals, but this has not been replicated in humans (Link et al., 2002). Osteosarcoma is the most common primary malignant bone tumor in children and adolescents (Bleyer, 2002; Dorfman & Czerniak, 1995). The overall annual incidence rate is bidmodal with the primary peak occurring during the second decade of life and the smaller secondary peak occurring near age 70 years (Dorfman & Czerniak, 1995). There is a slightly higher incidence among females in the early adolescent years and a slightly higher incidence among males in the mid to late adolescent years (Bleyer, 2002; Dorfman & Czerniak, 1995). The peak incidence of osteosarcoma coincides with the pubertal growth spurt, and it occurs most frequently at the metaphyseal portion of the most rapidly growing bones in adolescence. As a result, the distal femur, proximal tibia, and proximal humerus are the most common sites for osteosarcoma. This finding supports the theory that these rapidly growing cells are susceptible to oncogenic agents or mitotic errors and that osteosarcoma is the result of an aberration of the normal process of bone growth and remodeling (Link et al., 2002).

Ewing's Sarcoma Family of Tumors

The Ewing's sarcoma family of tumors (ESFT) include a spectrum of neuroepithelial tumors ranging from the undifferentiated round cell tumor of Ewing's sarcoma of bone (ES) to the neural differentiated peripheral primitive neuroectodermal tumors (PNET). Ewing's tumors often involve both bone and soft tissue by the time of diagnosis, including infiltration into the medullary cavity and bone marrow. Ewing's tumors can occur in both flat and long bones with primary sites almost equally distributed between extremity (53%) and central axis (47%) (Ginsberg et al., 2002). The most common primary sites are the pelvis, femur, ribs, humerus, and tibia (Granowetter & West, 1997; Grier, 1997).

Ewing's sarcoma is less common than osteosarcoma and represents 40% of bone tumors in children (Miller et al., 1995). Ewing's sarcoma is seen during times of peak growth rates with 50% of new patients diagnosed between 10 and 20 years of age (Ginsberg et al., 2002).

Diagnosis

The initial complaint for both osteosarcoma and Ewing's sarcoma is pain at the site of the tumor with or without a palpable mass. Localized swelling is present in 63% of children with Ewing's sarcoma. Systemic symptoms are rare in osteosarcoma unless widespread metastatic disease is present. On the other hand, systemic symptoms, most commonly fever and weight loss, are present in 25% of children with Ewing's sarcoma at the time of diagnosis (Link et al., 1991). Because the initial complaint for both osteosarcoma and Ewing's sarcoma is pain at the site of the tumor, diagnosis is often delayed. Duration of symptoms before diagnosis averages 3 months for osteosarcoma and up to 6 months for Ewing's sarcoma (Link et al., 1991). Children presenting to a physical therapist with a complaint of pain, which is often chronic, a negative history of injury, and no evidence of musculoskeletal abnormalities should be referred for further medical workup to rule out a malignant bone tumor.

The key to diagnosis of a bone tumor is radiologic evaluation. Plain-view x-ray films will reveal evidence of a mass and bony destruction; however, a definitive diagnosis is made through biopsy and histologic examination. The extent of the tumor is more precisely defined through magnetic resonance imaging. To complete the workup, a radionuclide bone scan and chest computed tomography are performed to determine the extent of metastases (Ginsberg et al., 2002; Link et al., 2002).

MEDICAL MANAGEMENT OF MALIGNANCIES

Medical management of bony tumors and neoplasms is based upon the following goals: (1) complete and permanent control of the primary tumor, (2) control and prevention of microstatic and metastatic disease, and (3) preservation of as much function as possible. Local control of the primary tumor is most often achieved through surgery and radiation therapy. Surgical options include amputation and limb-sparing procedures. The choice of surgical procedure depends on location and size of the tumor, extramedullary extent, presence or absence of metastatic disease, and the child's age, skeletal development, and lifestyle. Control of microstatic and metastatic disease is achieved through radiation therapy and chemotherapy.

Radiation Therapy

Radiation therapy directs high-energy emissions at the tumor. The energy from the radiation disrupts the structure of atoms and damages essential molecules, including the chromosomes. Cell reproductive capacity is therefore compromised, leading to tumor cell death (Tarbell & Kooy, 2002). Damage can occur to surrounding normal tissue as well.

Osteosarcoma is generally unresponsive to radiation therapy. Osteosarcoma cells seem to repair themselves after radiation injury, whereas Ewing's sarcoma is highly responsive to radiation therapy (Link et al., 2002). Local control of Ewing's sarcoma may be achieved with moderately high doses of radiation directed at the local tumor; however, whole bone radiation is often recommended for tumors larger than 8 cm (Granowetter & West, 1997).

The side effects of radiation therapy are related to the primary site of the tumor, volume, duration, dose rate, age of the patient, and use of chemotherapy. Acute side effects are seen in rapidly dividing tissues such as the skin, bone marrow, and gut. Common side effects are red and tender skin, mouth sores from irradiation to mucous membranes, and nausea and vomiting from irradiation to the abdomen (Tarbell & Kooy, 2002). Children receiving radiation therapy may exhibit a decreased activity level secondary to nausea and vomiting, poor appetite secondary to mouth sores, and generalized malaise. Their physical therapy sessions may need to be altered on a daily basis to accommodate their changing energy levels. Children wearing a prosthesis must be monitored closely for skin irritation and breakdown.

Late side effects of radiation include fibrosis of soft tissues, bony changes ranging from osteoporosis to fractures, and growth disturbances, including damage to the epiphyseal plate and bowing of the metaphysis. Greater growth disturbances are found in younger children (Goldwein, 1991). Butler and colleagues (1990) reported that 77% of patients with Ewing's sarcoma who received radiation therapy developed a leg length discrepancy; in 58% of these patients the leg length discrepancy was significant enough to require treatment. If possible, attempts are made to shield the epiphyseal plate at the opposite end of the involved bone to minimize the radiation-linked growth retardation and still allow for some growth of the extremity. For some young children, an amputation may produce a more functional extremity than an extremity that is significantly shortened as a result of radiation therapy.

Secondary malignant neoplasms of bone and soft tissue resulting from radiation therapy of the primary tumor are well documented, as data from long-term studies suggest that 3% to 12% of survivors of childhood cancer develop these secondary neoplasms (Friedman & Meadows, 2002).

Chemotherapy

Chemotherapy is administered according to several principles including the use of multiple drug combinations, administration of chemotherapy agents at maximally tolerated doses, and administration prior to the development of detectable micrometastatic disease (adjuvant chemotherapy). Most chemotherapy agents interfere with the function of DNA and RNA. However, these agents are nonselective and cause damage to both malignant and normal cells resulting in undesirable and at times toxic side effects. The side effects can be classified as acute and chronic and range from mucositis, vomiting, and neutropenia to cardiotoxicities and growth disturbances (Velaz-Yanguas & Warrier, 1996). Physical therapists working with children receiving chemotherapy should know the specific agents being used with the child and the side effects. The physical therapy interventions may need to be altered or limited depending upon the child's status and development of potentially serious side effects.

The use of adjuvant chemotherapy has increased the survival rates for both osteosarcoma and Ewing's sarcoma. Survival rates are dependent upon age, location of the tumor, and the presence and location of metastatic disease at the time of diagnosis. Five-year event-free survival (EFS) rates for children with Ewing's sarcoma treated with a combination of radiation therapy, chemotherapy, and surgery have improved to 64% to 69% for patients with nonmetastatic disease. For patients with metastatic bone disease the 5-year EFS rate is less than 20% (Wexler et al., 1996; Aparicio et al., 1998). Patients younger than 10 years of age with Ewing's sarcoma have a survival rate of 86% compared to 55% for older adolescents and young adults (Craft et al., 1998). Survival rates are also better for children whose tumors are more distal, rather than located on the axial skeleton. Overall survival rates for children with osteosarcoma treated with a combination of surgery and chemotherapy have also drastically improved from 20% in the 1970s to 60% to 65% more recently. Children with nonmetastatic osteosarcoma of the extremity are more likely to have a favorable outcome than children with more proximal tumors and the presence of metastatic disease (Meyers & Gorlick, 1997; Goorin et al., 2003).

SURGICAL OPTIONS IN THE MANAGEMENT OF ACQUIRED AND CONGENITAL LIMB DEFICIENCIES

AMPUTATION IN THE MANAGEMENT OF TRAUMATIC INJURIES AND MALIGNANT TUMORS

Although most of the basic premises related to management of adults with amputations apply to children, there are important differences. First, skeletal immaturity and future growth are important factors when considering surgical alternatives. Physes should be preserved whenever possible to ensure continued growth of the limb. For the upper extremity the majority of growth occurs in physes around the shoulder and wrist, whereas in the lower extremity the physes around the knee account for most of the growth (Herring, 2002a).

Second, the fact that amputation through long bones may result in terminal overgrowth is an important point that should not be overlooked. Terminal or bony overgrowth is a painful, spike-like prominence of new growth on the transected end of the residual limb. Significant pain can interfere with weight bearing and wearing of the prosthesis. The spike-like growth is not the result of growth from the proximal epiphysis but rather represents osteogenic activity of the periosteum (Gillespie, 1990).

Terminal overgrowth occurs most frequently in the humerus and fibula but is also seen in the tibia and femur (Morrissy et al., 2001). Surgical options include revisions and bone capping. The possibility of terminal overgrowth should not be a reason to elect higher-level amputation, such as a knee disarticulation rather than a below-knee amputation. As in adults, length of the lever arm, function of the extremity, and prosthetic fit remain important considerations when deciding on the level of amputation. Saving the child's life is, of course, the most important consideration, whether the amputation is the result of a malignancy or trauma.

Finally, wound healing in children is rarely a concern as it may be in adults with peripheral vascular disease. Skin grafts therefore may be used to close the amputation site in preference to performing a higher-level amputation for a child with a traumatic injury.

Acquired amputations secondary to trauma may result in a short residual limb. This is especially true of an above-knee amputation in which the distal physes have been resected. It may be possible to increase the length of a residual limb in older children by using one of the limb-lengthening techniques (see Chapter 17). Lengthening of a short residual limb may increase the efficiency of gait and promote a better prosthetic fit (Eldridge et al., 1990).

The traditional approach for malignant bone tumors has been amputation of the limb in which the tumor is found. The surgical margin for an amputation is usually 6 to 7 cm above the most proximal medullary extent of tumor as defined by magnetic resonance imaging. This level of surgical margin allows for removal of microscopic tumor and skip lesions while allowing for the greatest amount of residual limb length for the individual. Local recurrence rates using this level of surgical margin are less than 5% (Link et al., 2002).

For those tumor sites that are in the proximal humerus or femur, amputation results in severe loss of function. For example, a tumor of the proximal humerus treated by amputation would leave the patient with severely diminished function as a result of loss of the hand. Therefore most surgeons elect not to perform an amputation, if possible, for tumors of the upper extremity. Amputation for tumors of the pelvis or proximal femur also results in complete loss of the limb or a very short residual limb, which makes functional ambulation with a prosthesis difficult. Limb-sparing procedures may result in a more functional extremity than a proximal amputation without decreasing the expected rate of survival for the child. The decision regarding an amputation is based on expectations regarding control of the primary tumor and survival of the child and the functional use of the extremity.

AMPUTATION TO REVISE CONGENITAL LIMB DEFICIENCIES TO IMPROVE FUNCTION

Rarely is an amputation necessary with upper extremity limb deficiencies, but it may be indicated for some children with lower extremity limb deficiencies. A child with bilateral PFFD, however, may be more functional without any surgery. They will be of short stature but will walk quite well (Morrissy et al., 2001). For cosmesis, extension prostheses may be an option.

The surgical treatment of a child with unilateral PFFD is case-specific. If the child has a stable hip and foot and a significant portion of normal femur is present, one of the limb-lengthening procedures may be appropriate. Most surgeons agree that 60% of predicted femoral length must be present for a lengthening procedure to be a viable alternative (Gillespie, 1990; Herring, 2002b). If limb lengthening is not an option, one of the surgical options for PFFD is a knee arthrodesis and foot amputation. Usually the Syme or Boyd amputation of the foot is recommended. A Syme amputation involves complete removal of the foot, including the calcaneus, but the Boyd amputation preserves the calcaneus. The Boyd procedure requires an arthrodesis of the calcaneus and the tibia, which adds length to the limb (Morrissy et al., 2001). The knee is usually fused to form one long bone for fitting of an above-knee prosthesis (Herring, 2002b; Morrissy et al., 2001) (Figure 16-6).

Amputation may also be an option for a child with a longitudinal tibial or fibular total deficiency in which a significant limb length difference exists along with deformity of the foot. Frequently the foot is positioned in equinovarus or equinovalgus with absent rays. If the tibia is completely absent, a knee disarticulation and fitting with a prosthesis will provide a very functional lower extremity for the child. If the leg length difference is too significant for limb-lengthening techniques or epiphysiodesis of the uninvolved leg, or if the ankle is significantly unstable, a Syme or Boyd amputation may lead to a more functional lower extremity with the addition of a prosthesis for a child with partial absence of the fibula. When considering an amputation for a child, it is important that alternatives are discussed with the family and child and that the ultimate lifestyle goals are known.

ROTATIONPLASTY

Rotationplasty, or a turnabout procedure, is a typical option for children with congenital limb deficiencies, specifically PFFD, as well as for those with bony tumors of the proximal tibia or distal femur. This procedure involves

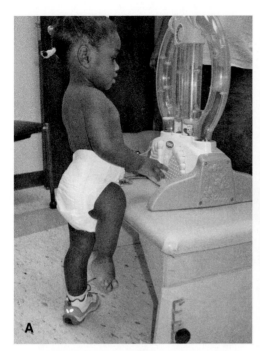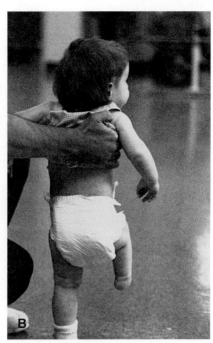

• **Figure 16-6**   **A**, Child with unilateral proximal femoral focal deficiency (PFFD) without any surgical modifications to her leg. **B**, Child with unilateral PFFD following a Boyd amputation of his foot. Note popliteal crease near the diaper line indicating where his knee is located.

excision of the distal femur and proximal tibia; 180° rotation of the residual lower limb, including the distal femur and proximal tibia, ankle joint, foot, and neurovascular supply; and reattachment to the proximal femur (Fig. 16-7). The ankle then functions as a knee joint, with ankle plantar flexion used to extend the "knee" and ankle dorsiflexion to flex the "knee" (Krajbich, 1998) (Fig. 16-8). Rotationplasty requires a functioning hip joint and ankle joint. In the case of malignant tumors, the tumor cannot have invaded the surrounding soft tissue, especially the neurovascular supply. For children with PFFD, the residual foot must be normal with minimal alignment problems for a rotationplasty to be a functional surgical option. If the fibula is absent, alignment of the foot may not be adequate for a successful rotationplasty.

The advantages of a rotationplasty are the increased limb length, improved prosthetic function with the ankle serving as a knee joint, improved weight-bearing capacity, and elimination of the problems of terminal overgrowth and pain from neuromas or phantom limb sensations (Krajbich & Bochman, 1992). Weight is borne through the heel, which is more suitable for weight bearing than the end of a residual limb. Rotationplasty also allows for some growth of the leg. With an appropriate prosthesis, children who have had a rotationplasty procedure can run, jump, and play with their peers.

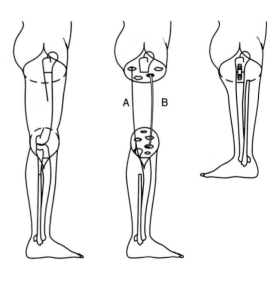

1   2   3

• **Figure 16-7**   A schematic illustration of a rotationplasty procedure. Neurovascular structures (**A** and **B**) are left intact and wrapped into the existing space when the tibia is reattached to the femur.

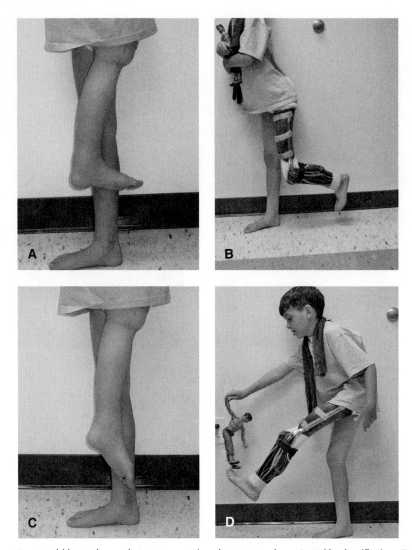

◆ **Figure 16-8**   An 11-year-old boy who underwent a rotationplasty procedure. **A**, Ankle dorsiflexion. **B**, Ankle dorsiflexion produces prosthetic knee flexion. **C**, Ankle plantar flexion. **D**, Ankle plantar flexion produces prosthetic knee extension.

Disadvantages are cosmesis and derotation of the foot. Critics of rotationplasty cite poor cosmesis and psychologic issues as a deterrent to the procedure. In my experience with children who underwent a rotationplasty for either a tumor or congenital PFFD, cosmesis was not a complaint from the child or the child's parents. Krajbich and Bochmann (1992) cite their experience of 27 children with osteosarcoma who underwent a rotationplasty. Twenty-two of these children are alive with no evidence of metastatic disease. No long-term complications related to cosmesis and psychologic decompensation were reported; in fact, virtually all of the children with a rotationplasty now actively participate in sports and other activities with their peers. When a rotationplasty is being considered as a

surgical option, it may be helpful for parents and the child to meet another child who has had the rotationplasty performed. Certainly, the cosmetic disadvantages must be discussed. Additional studies have shown that children with PFFD who underwent a rotationplasty demonstrated a higher walking speed with less oxygen consumption and less compensatory gait deviations than children who underwent an amputation of their foot and knee arthrodesis (Fowler et al., 1996; Oppenheim et al., 1998).

When the procedure is performed on young children, derotation of the foot may occur requiring rerotation of the limb. The limb may derotate secondary to the spiral pull of the muscles proximal and distal to the osteotomy (Herring, 2002b). Both Krajbich (1998) and Gillespie

(1990) discussed surgical options to limit derotation of the limb after a rotationplasty. Derotation is more common in children younger than 10 years of age and is most frequently seen in children when a rotationplasty is performed at 3 or 4 years of age (Gillespie, 1990).

LIMB-SPARING PROCEDURES

With the use of chemotherapy, improvements in diagnostic imaging to determine tumor margins, and new techniques of reconstruction, amputation is not always the treatment of choice for children with bony malignancies. Limb-sparing or limb-salvage procedures may be an alternative to amputation for some children with malignant bone tumors. Limb-sparing procedures involve resection of the tumor and reconstruction of the limb to preserve function without amputation of the limb. Reconstruction of the limb may include excision of bone without replacement of the excised area or replacement with an allograft or endoprosthetic implant.

Appropriate selection of children for limb-sparing surgery is critical. The goal of saving the limb should never compromise the goal of removing all gross and microscopic tumor (Link et al., 2002). Limb-sparing surgery is contraindicated if the tumor has invaded the surrounding soft tissue to a large extent, if it involves the neurovascular supply, or if the tumor has invaded the intramedullary cavity (Link et al., 2002). In addition, limb-sparing surgery for the lower extremity of a young child may not be beneficial when the child is skeletally immature and may be left with a severe leg length discrepancy and nonfunctional lower extremity. In these cases amputation may be a better choice than limb-sparing surgery.

Autologous grafts are rarely appropriate because long segments of bone usually must be excised. Replacement of the excised bone with a near-equal length of noninvolved bone from another portion of the body is often not possible. Cadaver osteoarticular allografts are another option. They involve resection of the tumor and surrounding bone and implantation of a section of cadaver bone. Osteoarticular allografts can preserve some growth plates, especially those of the distal femur and proximal tibia if the tumor resection involves the proximal femur. The grafts are stabilized with plates or intramedullary rods until osteosynthesis has occurred. Once osteosynthesis has occurred and the child's bone has formed a latticework within the implanted bone, the graft is very stable and does not loosen over time (Link et al., 2002). In addition, osteoarticular allografts have fewer complications (infections, nonunion and fractures) over time than metallic endoprosthetic implants. Infections and nonunions are early onset complications and are seen with a greater frequency with children receiving chemotherapy. When fractures occur, they are typically seen later, occurring 3 to 8 years after the procedure. Nonunions or significant infections are serious complications that can ultimately lead to an amputation. Allografts are a viable surgical alternative for children nearing skeletal maturity or those children requiring only excision of a portion of the shaft of the bone. For a child who is skeletally immature, the implanted bone can be cut 1 to 2 cm longer than the portion removed to accommodate some growth. As is true with most limb-sparing procedures, high-intensity activities such as athletic participation are limited for the child with an osteoarticular allograft.

At times a tumor may be excised without replacing the excised bone. The proximal fibula may be resected if the soft tissue involvement is minimal and the peroneal nerve is not included in the soft tissue involvement. The biceps femoris tendon and fibular collateral ligament are reattached to the lateral condyle of the tibia (Herring, 2002a). After healing, full knee motion and a normal gait pattern can be expected. The Tikhoff-Linberg procedure has been successfully used for tumors involving the proximal humerus when the brachial plexus is not included in the soft tissue involvement. With this procedure the proximal humerus is excised and not replaced. The remaining muscles of the upper arm are reattached to the trapezius and pectoralis muscles to suspend the remaining portion of the humerus (Springfield, 1991). The shoulder is unstable, but the elbow and hand are functional. Endoprosthetic devices may be implanted to provide stability and function to the shoulder. In either case the functional outcome is superior to that following amputation of the entire upper extremity.

Endoprosthetic devices are ultimately an extension of joint arthroplasty procedures. These manufactured devices are implanted in the area of the excised bone and can be custom-designed for the proximal humerus, elbow, proximal and distal femur, and proximal tibia. Modular components are also available, sometimes eliminating the need for custom-designed implants. Problems include loosening of the prosthesis, infection, and mechanical failure of the device (Kenan & Lewis, 1991; Unwin & Walker, 1996). Children and adolescents may be very active and create vigorous stresses on prosthetic implants that lead to failures and the need for replacement of the devices over time. They may also not be appropriate for the young, skeletally immature child because these devices are limited in the amount of growth that can be accommodated.

Some endoprosthetic designs incorporate a telescoping unit that can be expanded to accommodate growth. Expansion of the prosthesis involves a surgical procedure at periodic intervals. The expandable prosthesis may function as the permanent prosthesis after skeletal maturity has been achieved or may need to be replaced by a conventional endoprosthesis if the device provides for poor function of the limb (Schindler et al., 1997; Unwin & Walker, 1996). Early clinical experience demonstrated complications with all telescoping endoprosthetic implants over time (Kenan & Lewis, 1991; Schindler et al, 1997). Complications included loosening of the prosthesis, infection after lengthening procedures, mechanical failures, and fractures. Some clinics have begun using an endoprosthesis that can be expanded with the use of an external electromagnetic field. Exposure of the limb to the electromagnetic field unlocks an energy-stored spring and allows for controlled lengthening without a surgical procedure (Wilkins & Soubeiran, 2001).

A review by Eckardt and colleagues (2000) of 32 patients with expandable prostheses included patients ranging from 3 to 15 years of age. Fourteen of the 32 patients had no complications. Eighteen patients had 27 complications including infection, loosening of the device, mechanical failure, fracture, knee flexion contracture, and prosthetic shoulder joint subluxation, and one patient died of a pulmonary embolism. The authors stressed the need for strong family participation during rehabilitation to avoid knee flexion contractures in skeletally immature patients (Eckardt et al., 2000). Several reports demonstrated effective growth of the child's limb with the use of an endoprosthetic device with gains of up to 7 or 8 cm in length (Kenan & Lewis, 1991; Schindler et al., 1997) while Eckardt and colleagues (2000) reported gains of up to 9 cm.

Several studies have reported comparable long-term survival rates between groups undergoing amputation versus a limb-sparing procedure (Rougraff et al., 1994; Finn & Simon, 1991). Limb-sparing procedures may also result in improved function, but these procedures are plagued by higher complication rates than amputation surgery (Renard et al., 2000; Link et al., 2002).

Limb-sparing surgery is as effective in controlling the tumor as amputation when adjuvant chemotherapy is used and when particular attention is given to patient selection, surgical margins, and surgical techniques. Life style of the child is also an important presurgical consideration, because many limb-sparing procedures such as osteoarticular allografts and endoprosthetic implants will limit participation in competitive physical activities. Limb-sparing procedures for the upper extremity clearly result in improved function for the patient when compared to amputation and the use of a prosthesis. Limb-sparing procedures such as rotationplasty and limb lengthening are increasingly used with children with congenital limb deficiencies to avoid an amputation and often result in excellent function for the child.

LIMB REPLANTATION

For children with traumatic amputations, limb replantation may be a surgical option. As with other surgical options, the goal of replantation is directed not only at preserving the amputated limb but also at restoring pain-free function to the extremity that is superior to the function obtained with a prosthesis. For an upper extremity replantation to be considered successful, function of the elbow and hand and distal sensation must be restored. Replantation of a lower extremity must provide a painless, sensate extremity capable of bearing weight during normal daily activities (Beris et al., 1994).

Distal replantations of an upper extremity usually result in a more favorable outcome than proximal replantations. Proximal replantations are often associated with a violent mechanism of injury that result in damage to the nerves, blood vessels, and muscles. A proximal replantation also necessitates a longer distance for the nerves to regenerate for functional use of the hand. Children often achieve better functional results with upper extremity limb replantation than adults, making limb replantation a viable surgical option for some children (Beris et al., 1995).

Physical therapy is indicated for these children for wound care, control of edema, joint range of motion (ROM), strengthening, gait training and self-care activities. Rehabilitation will include close communication with the physician regarding precautions and progression of activities and family instruction while the child is in the hospital and as an outpatient.

PHANTOM LIMB SENSATIONS

Phantom limb sensations are an occurrence in many adults with amputations, but fewer reports are available concerning children with phantom limb sensations. Some persons may believe that if young children do not complain of phantom limb pain, they therefore must not have any pain. Simmel (1962) reported that the incidence of phantom limb sensations increases with the age of the child so that all children older than 8 years of age reported some degree of phantom limb sensations. Melzack and colleagues (1997) reported that 20% of individuals with a congenital limb deficiency and 50% of individuals with an acquired amputation before 6 years of age experienced phantom limb sensations. However, the majority of individuals reporting phantom limb sensations did not report pain but rather the perceived ability to voluntarily move their phantom limb (Melzack et al., 1997).

The phantom limb sensations and pain of adolescents can become intense. If left untreated, phantom limb sensations can become debilitating and interfere with prosthetic wear and daily activities. Some teenagers are able to control the sensations through rubbing or massaging the uninvolved limb at similar points to those in which they are experiencing the phantom limb sensations of the amputated limb. Others feel more in control by keeping a daily log of their sensations and reporting the pain intensities on one of a variety of pain scales. For some adolescents the use of analgesics may be beneficial. If available, a referral to a pain management team should be instituted for children undergoing amputations.

OVERVIEW OF PROSTHETICS

UPPER EXTREMITY PROSTHETICS

Upper extremity prosthetic systems may be body-powered or externally powered. Externally powered prosthetic devices are typically referred to as myoelectric devices. Body-powered components include a terminal device, a wrist unit, possibly an elbow unit, a socket, and are operated by a harness and cable system. With a myoelectric system, a muscle contraction by the child activates an electrode inside the shaft of the device, which generates electrically controlled movement of the terminal device, wrist or elbow. Children may also utilize a prosthesis that is a combination of body- and externally powered components. For example, the child may operate the elbow using a body-powered cable system and operate the hand with a myoelectric system (Farnsworth, 2003).

Terminal devices range from the passive hand or fist to a myoelectric hand. Terminal devices often used in pediatrics include the passive fist or hand, CAPP (Child Amputee Prosthetics Project, Hosmer Dorrance, Campbell, CA), various hooks, including the Dorrance and ADEPT (Anatomically Designed-Engineered Polymer Technology, Therapeutic Recreation Systems, Boulder, CO) models and myoelectric hands such as the Otto Bock Electrohand (Otto Bock) and the New York Mechanical Hand (Hosmer Dorrance) (Fig. 16-9). The child's age and size, as well as the parents' and child's desires and functional goals, determine the appropriate terminal device. The wrist unit allows forearm pronation and supination and accommodates the terminal device.

As a child's activities change, different terminal devices may be needed. Various recreational terminal devices are available to allow participation in a variety of sports activities (Cummings, 2000; Farnsworth, 2003). Teenagers may desire a cosmetic hand for social activities and a functional terminal device for daily activities.

Most upper limb prostheses are suspended with a harness system. Two basic systems are used: the chest strap and the figure-eight. The chest strap or harness fits over the shoulder of the involved limb and around the chest to secure the prosthesis without limiting movement of the shoulders. The figure-eight harness securely anchors the prosthesis so that the child may activate the cable system of an above-elbow prosthesis (Setoguchi & Rosenfelder, 1982). Suction sockets are available for young children. A simple suction socket may be all that is necessary to suspend a below-elbow prosthesis of an infant or toddler. When the cable for the terminal device is added to the prosthesis, an above-elbow pad or cuff to secure the cable can be incorporated. A shoulder disarticulation prosthesis is secured with a chest strap and often with a thigh strap for the young child. A thigh strap can provide added power to operate the control system of a shoulder disarticulation prosthesis and may provide more excursion than the chest strap (Setoguchi & Rosenfelder, 1982).

LOWER EXTREMITY PROSTHETICS

The fact that children are growing and that they may be facing several surgical interventions makes fitting a child with a prosthesis very different than fitting an adult with a prosthesis. Consequently, many prosthetists will fit a child with a prosthesis that accommodates some growth, stage the introduction of components, and utilize components that can be replaced as the child grows. The variety of components available to the pediatric population continues to expand but does not yet compare to the wide variety available for the adolescent or adult population.

The SACH (Otto Bock Orthopedic, Plymouth, MN) foot has long been the mainstay for pediatric prosthetic feet and continues to be used for young toddlers. However, young children can now be fitted with dynamic response or energy storing feet (Fig. 16-10). In two separate retrospective analyses, Anderson found that parents and children preferred the cosmetic appearance of dynamic response feet and stated that these feet improved their child's endurance and possibly stability (Anderson, 1998).

The shank of a lower extremity prosthesis is either an exoskeletal or an endoskeletal design. Exoskeletal shanks are fabricated of wood or a rigid polyurethane foam and laminated to form a hard outer covering. Endoskeletal shanks consist of a pylon made of ultralight material, such as graphite or titanium, and covered with foam. Teenagers often prefer endoskeletal shanks because of their cosmesis and decreased weight. The durability of exoskeletal shanks is often more appropriate for the younger child.

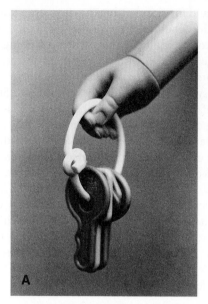

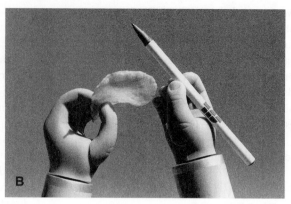

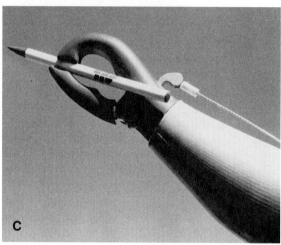

♦ **Figure 16-9** Terminal device options: **A**, Passive Infant Alpha Hand (TRS, Boulder, CO). **B**, L'il E-Z Hand promotes grasping when thumb is moved (TRS, Boulder, CO). **C**, ADEPT voluntary closing hand (TRS, Boulder, CO).

A wider variety of prosthetic knees are now available for the pediatric population, including toddlers just beginning to pull to standing. A single axis constant-friction knee is set to function at a certain walking speed. If the speed of walking increases, the prosthesis lags behind because the shank cannot swing through as quickly as the uninvolved limb. In addition, this type of knee is not very stable and buckles quickly if the ground reaction force is not anterior to the knee joint (Michael, 1999). Another type of knee joint available for the pediatric population is a polycentric knee with a four-bar linkage mechanism (Fig. 16-11). A polycentric knee mimics the anatomic knee joint to increase stability. The axis of motion is posterior during stance to provide added stability and anterior during swing to shorten the shank and assist with clearance. A lower extremity prosthesis with a polycentric knee is shown in Figure 16-12. Polycentric knees are now available for use with toddlers, leading some centers to incorporate a prosthetic knee into a child's first prosthesis.

A larger variety of knee units are available for teenagers, including hydraulic and pneumatic knees. Hydraulic and pneumatic knee units are variable-friction units that allow variable walking and running speeds. Variable-friction units are equipped with a swing control mechanism that sets the drag of the shank through swing phase and a stance control unit that permits knee flexion during stance without collapse of the leg. Swing and stance control mechanisms are excellent options for active teenagers, especially those engaged in physical activities. Drawbacks of hydraulic and pneumatic knees are the added weight to the prosthesis, cost, and intricacy of adjustments.

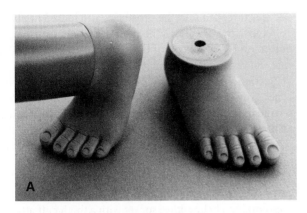

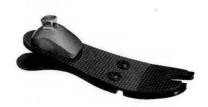

B

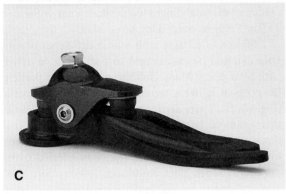

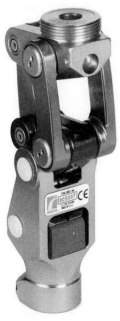

C

• **Figure 16-10**   Prosthetic feet options: **A**, Little Feet (TRS, Boulder, CO). **B**, Flex-Foot Junior. **C**, TruPer Foot (College Park Industries, Fraser, MI). (**B**, *photo courtesy of Ossur of North America.*)

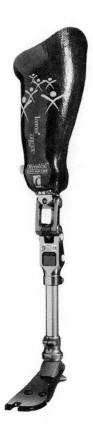

• **Figure 16-11**   Total Knee Junior is a polycentric knee that provides stability and aids in the initiation of a smooth gait pattern. *(Photo courtesy of Ossur of North America.)*

• **Figure 16-12**   Pediatric lower extremity prosthetic system including socket, Total Knee Junior, and Flex-Foot Junior. *(Photo courtesy of Ossur of North America.)*

Like adult sockets, pediatric socket design has changed over the past 15 years. Children with a transfemoral amputation can be fitted with a narrowed medial-lateral ischial containment socket or an ischial weight-bearing quadrilateral socket. The narrowed medial-lateral socket with ischial containment more evenly distributes weight-bearing pressures and allows less lateral movement of the distal femur, thereby providing more stability during stance. Quadrilateral sockets may be indicated for children with a long residual limb while the ischial containment sockets provide greater stability for children with short residual limbs or bilateral transfemoral amputations (Schuch & Pritham, 1999). Adolescents with a below-knee or transtibial amputation may be fitted with the standard patellar-tendon-bearing socket. However, younger children may require a supracondylar socket that offers greater suspension.

Infants and toddlers will require some type of suspension to secure their prosthesis. A Silesian belt or total elastic suspension (TES) belt works well for younger children with an above-knee amputation or PFFD and preschoolers can become independent in their use (Fig. 16-13). Neoprene sleeves and silicone liners with a locking mechanism are additional suspension methods commonly used with young children. The silicone liner is rolled on the residual limb and the pin on the end of the

sleeve is threaded into the prosthesis and locked in place. To remove the prosthesis the pin is released by pushing a button on the distal end of the socket (Cummings, 2000) (Fig. 16-14).

Suction sockets are appropriate for the older child who is not growing rapidly or undergoing weight fluctuations secondary to chemotherapy treatment. Suction sockets utilize negative pressure as air is expelled through a distal valve and surface tension between the skin and socket to maintain the suspension (Cummings, 2000).

Children with a rotationplasty use a prosthesis that incorporates the plantar-flexed foot in the socket. The socket is essentially a below-knee socket with a thigh cuff attachment and external hinges for the knee joint. A Silesian or TES belt may be needed for suspension.

Children of all ages with a limb deficiency or amputation should be encouraged to participate in activities with their peers. Many children may want to participate in sports at either a recreational or a competitive level (Fig. 16-15). There are many prosthetic options available that promote participation in various sports. Recreational prosthetics options are too numerous to mention for this discussion, and the reader is referred to other resources (Kegel, 1992; Anderson, 1998). Information is also available on various upper extremity terminal devices for recreational and sports activities (Radocy, 1992).

Ultimately, any prosthesis for a child must have some cosmetic appeal and be more functional than the limb without a prosthesis (Fig. 16-16). Decision making for infants' and toddlers' prosthetic needs should include the

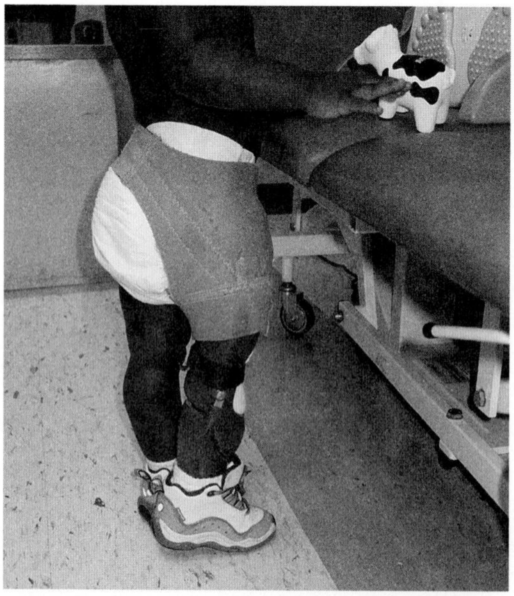

◆ **Figure 16-13** Toddler with a right proximal femoral focal deficiency fitted with a prosthesis prior to any surgical procedures to modify her leg. A neoprene total elastic suspension belt is used as the suspension method to secure the prosthesis.

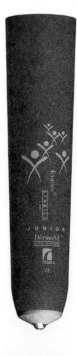

◆ **Figure 16-14** Suspension systems may utilize a silicone liner that is rolled onto the residual limb and attached to the distal end of the socket with a pin locking mechanism.

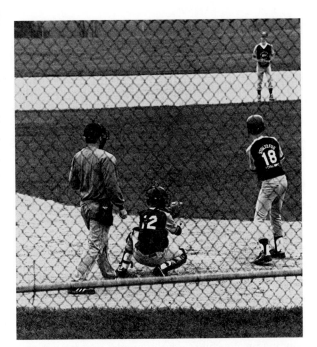

• **Figure 16-15**   Catcher is an adolescent with a left below-knee amputation.

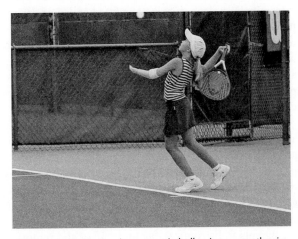

• **Figure 16-16**   Tossing a tennis ball using a prosthesis with a passive hand.

parents, orthopedist, prosthetist, and physical therapist. The older child should be included in the decision-making process.

Appropriate prosthetic components are costly, and a full prosthesis must be replaced at least every 12 to 18 months for growing children and adolescents. If an adolescent chooses to participate in sports or swimming activities, an additional prosthesis or components may be required. Third-party payers are reluctant to pay for multiple prostheses or myoelectric devices. Currently, some health maintenance organizations will pay for only one prosthesis in a lifetime.

Studies are beginning to examine the cost-effectiveness of surgical procedures and various prosthetic options. Grimer and colleagues (1997) compared long-term costs of limb-sparing procedures to amputation with a prosthesis. Limb-sparing procedures are more costly initially, but amputations for children or adolescents are very costly over time because of the need for multiple and sophisticated prostheses.

PHYSICAL THERAPY INTERVENTION FOR THE CHILD WITH A LIMB DEFICIENCY OR AN ACQUIRED AMPUTATION

The parents are an integral part of the rehabilitation team for a child with an amputation or a limb deficiency. The rehabilitation team should also include an orthopedist, a prosthetist, and a physical therapist who are experienced in the management of children with amputations. This may often mean traveling to a major medical center for periodic assessments and prosthetic adjustments. Physical therapy can be delivered in the local community if available, but the therapist must be in communication with the managing rehabilitation team.

The overall goals of physical therapy are to facilitate as normal a sequence of development as possible for the child and prevent or minimize the development of impairments, activity limitations, and participation restrictions. Impairments can include joint contractures and weakness with resultant activity limitations of reduced mobility and a lack of independence in self-care skills. Physical therapy goals are directed toward preventing joint contractures, minimizing muscle strength imbalances, preventing skin breakdown, and developing independence with mobility and self-care skills. Ideally these goals are accomplished through physical therapy intervention for the child, child or parent instruction, and follow-up of a child's progress and functional outcomes. The child's age, type of limb deficiency or level of amputation, and other medical factors will all influence the intensity of physical therapy needed.

Functional outcomes can be assessed using current assessment tools. However, these assessment tools may not be able to determine the functional effectiveness of various prosthetic options. Third-party payers and state-funded programs will opt for the prosthetic options that are less costly if outcomes are not present to justify the more expensive options. Pruitt and colleagues (1996) developed and tested an outcome measure for children with limb deficiencies. The Child Amputee Prosthetics Project—Functional Status Inventory (CAPP-FSI) assesses 40 activities on two scales to determine whether the child performs the activity with or without a prosthesis. The child is also rated for the severity of his or her limb loss. Internal reliability for the two scales that compose the CAPP-FSI was 0.96 (Pruitt et al., 1996). The CAPP-FSIP and the CAPP-FSIT were developed to assess the functional outcome of preschoolers age 4 to 7 years and toddlers age 1 to 4 years respectively (Pruitt et al., 1998; Pruitt et al., 1999).

INFANCY AND TODDLER PERIOD

An infant with a limb deficiency should be referred for an initial examination by a pediatric orthopedist and a physical therapist shortly after birth. Monitoring by the physical therapist with suggestions to parents regarding positioning and ROM exercises may be all that is needed initially. The motor development of children with multiple limb deficiencies or upper extremity deficiencies may become delayed or impaired owing to their inability to use their arms for such activities as pushing up to sit, crawling, and pulling to stand. Physical therapy is necessary to monitor the infant's developmental progress, ROM, and strength needed for later prosthetic use. The physical therapist should also teach the parent or caregiver how to incorporate physical therapy goals into the child's daily activities. This can be accomplished through periodic physical therapy examinations and evaluations, optimally at 1-month intervals, with updated parent instruction provided.

Generally, infants with limb deficiencies do not develop contractures after birth, but ROM should be carefully monitored according to individual needs. The parents of a child with a PFFD may benefit from instruction to decrease the hip flexion and abduction contractures that are typically noted at birth and will later interfere with prosthetic fit. Most children with upper extremity limb deficiencies will maintain ROM and strength through their developmental activities.

Careful monitoring of the developing infant is necessary to evaluate ROM, functional strength, weight-bearing capabilities, and posture while prone, sitting, and standing. Often a child with a limb deficiency will tend to bear weight asymmetrically in prone and during sitting activities. Some children will take increased weight on their limb-deficient side to free their uninvolved side for reaching and movement. Other children may take more weight through their uninvolved side because of weight-shifting and balance difficulties. Suggestions may be given to the

parents and therapy provided to encourage weight-shifting activities to improve symmetry. For the child with an upper limb deficiency this will encourage the co-contraction of shoulder musculature needed later for prosthetic use. For the child with a lower limb deficiency this encourages assumption of an erect trunk with normal balance reactions. Shifting weight to the limb-deficient side is also important for preprosthetic training needed for standing and ambulation activities.

If an infant is not progressing developmentally, physical therapy intervention may be warranted to provide alternative methods of achieving the normal developmental sequence. For example, a child with bilateral upper extremity limb deficiencies may need assistance to learn to stand from sitting or to safely learn to balance in standing.

A child is usually fitted with a prosthesis at a developmentally appropriate age. A child with a lower extremity deficiency will therefore be fitted for a prosthesis when weight bearing is appropriate and the child is beginning to pull to stand (between 8 and 10 months of age depending on the child's developmental progress). A child with a unilateral PFFD may have a Syme or Boyd amputation and be fitted with a prosthesis either before or after the surgery (Morrissy et al., 2001). A child with an upper extremity limb deficiency may be fitted with a prosthesis to assist with early playing skills in sitting or even earlier to assist with weight-bearing skills while prone. A child is best fitted with an upper extremity prosthesis between 3 and 6 months of age or when the child can push to and prop with his or her upper extremities in sitting (Krebs et al., 1991; Hubbard et al., 1998).

When a child first receives a prosthesis, the fit and alignment as well as the overall function of the prosthesis are assessed. The initial session is spent on instructing the parents in proper donning of the prosthesis, in checking the skin, and in developing a wear schedule. The initial goal is to have the infant or toddler wear the prosthesis comfortably for as many hours a day as possible and for the parents to be comfortable in donning and removing the prosthesis. The prosthesis may be removed for naps and should be removed when the child sleeps at night.

A child with an upper extremity prosthesis may initially ignore it. The focus of therapy should be on having the child wear the prosthesis while playing and to begin to use it for bimanual play such as manipulating and holding large toys and during gross motor activities such as pushing up to sitting or quadruped, protective reactions, and propping in sitting.

The child's first upper extremity prosthesis may have one of several terminal device options (see Fig. 16-9). A young infant may have a passive hand that is cosmetically appealing but with limited function (Fig. 16-17). As the

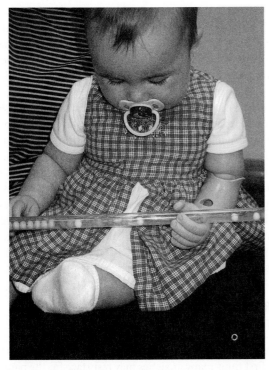

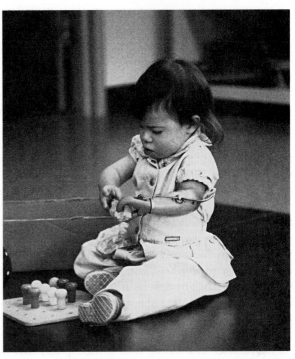

• **Figure 16-17**   Toddler holding a toy with in the passive hand of her prosthesis.

• **Figure 16-18**   Child engaging in bimaual play wearing a forearm prosthesis with an ADEPT voluntary closing hook.

child begins to engage in bimanual play and reaching activities, the decision to use either a body-powered or externally powered myoelectric device is made. Body-powered devices may be a simple split hook terminal device or a CAPP voluntary opening device. The split hook is similar to that used with adult prosthetics except smaller. The CAPP was designed specifically for children, is cosmetically more appealing than a hook terminal device, is safer than a hook for a young child, and provides an efficient grip without requiring great operating force (Gover & McIvor, 1992). The goal for the young child at this time is to adjust to the weight of a prosthesis, to begin to use it to manipulate larger toys, and to shake or remove toys placed in the terminal device by an adult (Setoguchi & Rosenfelder, 1982).

A child is not expected to begin to operate the terminal device until 18 months of age or later (Gover & McIvor, 1992; Patton, 1989). An active terminal device and cable as needed should be added to the child's prosthesis by 18 months of age. Training to operate the terminal device is dependent on the child's developmental level. Children can be taught to release objects placed in their terminal device at 15 months of age (Patton, 1989). Generally, children are taught to open the terminal device, place objects in it, and then release them, in that order

(Gover & McIvor, 1992; Setoguchi & Rosenfelder, 1982). This corresponds with the normal developmental sequence of learning to grasp before learning to release objects. The therapist must be familiar with the mechanism that controls the terminal device because it can differ from child to child, depending on the design of the device. The CAPP and Hosmer Dorrance hook are voluntary-opening terminal devices; forward reaching of the arm pulls the cable tight and activates opening of the terminal device. Children with a transverse deficiency of the upper arm will need to use scapular abduction to activate opening of the terminal device with the elbow locked; control of the prosthetic elbow comes at a later age. The ADEPT hook is a voluntary-closing terminal device designed to mimic forward reaching to grasp or close on an object (Fig. 16-18). Enhanced motor development has been reported with the early fitting of a voluntary-closing terminal device (DiCowden et al., 1987).

If the decision is made to fit the child with an externally powered prosthesis, the New York hand (Hosmer Dorrance, Campbell, CA) or the Otto Bock Electrohand are commonly used with young children. Children typically are initially fitted with a myoelectric hand with only one electrode. When this electrode is activated through muscle contraction, the hand opens. When the child relaxes the muscle, the hand closes. Typically by 3 to 4 years of age the child's myoelectric device can be converted to two electrodes so that both opening and closing the hand is controlled by the child (Hubbard et al., 1998; Cummings, 2000) (Fig. 16-19).

Children younger than 2 years of age with a lower limb deficiency or above-knee amputation may be fitted with a prosthesis without a knee. The goal is to begin weight-bearing and ambulation activities and to progress to learning control of a prosthetic knee when they are closer to 3 years of age. The rationale for this decision is that the articulated knee components are often too large to fit into the small prosthetic shaft required with a small child and that the fixed knee extension of the prosthesis provides stability for early gait training and confidence in the use of a prosthesis. More recently, several clinics have begun using articulated prosthetic knees in the initial prosthesis with toddlers. The principle for fitting a young child with a knee component is that knee flexion during gait simulates a more normal gait pattern and may therefore eliminate some of the gait deviations that develop and become ingrained after ambulating with a fixed prosthesis. In addition, the prosthetic knee allows other typical movements seen in young children such as crawling, squatting, and kneeling (Fig. 16-20) (Wilk et al., 1999; Coulter-O'Berry, 2003). Continued advances in prosthetic design have enabled prosthetists to fit the articulating knee in the small shank of a young child's prosthesis.

When fitting toddlers with a lower extremity prosthesis, normal stance and gait patterns for their developmental age should be kept in mind. Children 1 year of age stand and walk with a wide base of support and exhibit increased hip external rotation during swing phase (Sutherland, 1984). For this reason, a toddler's prosthesis may need to be aligned with more hip abduction than that provided to an older child.

Because a goal of physical therapy is symmetry of posture and movements during developmental activities, proper alignment and controlled weight-shifting and balance activities are emphasized for children with a lower limb prosthesis. Many children with lower limb prostheses do not require an assistive device for ambulation; however, initial gait training with an assistive device promotes a reciprocal gait pattern and an erect trunk. As the child develops balance and is able to control weight shifting, he or she will naturally discard the assistive device when he or she is comfortable with independent ambulation.

PRESCHOOL- AND SCHOOL-AGE PERIOD

When a child attends a preschool or kindergarten class for the first time, many anxieties may resurface for the parents of a child with a limb deficiency. Parents will worry that their child may not fit in or will look different from his or her peers. This is also an age by which typical children

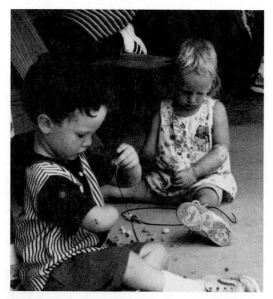

◆ **Figure 16-19**   Young girl using her myoelectric single-site prosthesis to complete a bimanual activity.

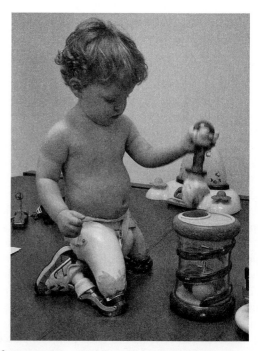

◆ **Figure 16-20**   Toddler with his first bilateral transfemoral prostheses with knee joint to promote age-appropriate ambulation skills and play activities on the floor.

have achieved independence with activities of daily living skills such as eating and dressing and their social relationships with peers increase. The preschool years should emphasize development of independence in self-care skills, mobility, and acquisition of school skills such as coloring, cutting, and writing. If these skills are achieved during the preschool years, the child will enter school with minimal or no activity limitations or participation restrictions.

The child with an upper limb deficiency should be able to activate the terminal device of the prosthesis by this age. Children using an above-elbow prosthesis can begin learning to control the elbow by 3 or 4 years of age. Most above-elbow prostheses have a dual cable system that allows the child to control both elbow flexion and extension and forearm pronation and supination. With control of the elbow and forearm the terminal device of the prosthesis becomes more functional in a variety of positions.

Emphasis should always be on assisting the child to learn skills that are appropriate for his or her age. Play skills involving manipulation of smaller objects, using the prosthesis to hold and turn paper for coloring and cutting activities, holding the handlebars of a tricycle, and self-dressing and feeding skills are important. A child with a unilateral upper limb prosthesis will always use it as a helper hand and not as the dominant hand.

For those children with bilateral upper limb deficiencies the use of a prosthesis should be carefully monitored. These children should always be allowed to use their feet or mouth for play and self-care activities. A prosthesis may aid these children for only some periods of the day and may actually limit their function during some activities. Children with a lower limb deficiency, including those children with unilateral PFFD, should be functional ambulators at this age. A child with a below-knee limb deficiency should be wearing a prosthesis for most of the day and engaging in normal activities with peers. The child with an above-knee limb deficiency should be ready to begin ambulation with a prosthesis with a knee joint by around age 3 years. Initially, children are usually given a constant-friction knee joint. They may need a short period of physical therapy to learn control of the knee joint and weight-shifting activities without falling.

During the preschool years some surgery is usually necessary for the child with a unilateral PFFD. Arthrodesis of the knee joint, usually performed between 2.5 and 4 years of age, increases the lever arm of the thigh and decreases the hip and knee flexion contractures (Gillespie, 1990; Morrissy et al., 2001). Femoral or tibial epiphysiodesis may be performed at the time of knee arthrodesis. The ultimate goal is for limb length on the prosthetic side to be 5 cm shorter than that of the contralateral femur. This enables the prosthetic knee joint to be at approximately the same level as the contralateral knee joint at maturity. Placement of the prosthetic knee joint at the same level as the contralateral knee joint allows for improved cosmesis and improved gait.

For the child with an acquired lower extremity amputation an immediate-fit prosthesis is usually used. This may not be the case if significant trauma was present to the surrounding tissue or if skin grafting was necessary after the injury. The physical therapy examination and evaluation focuses on sensitivity of the residual limb, active movement, strength, bed mobility, transfers for toileting and getting out of bed, and ambulation. The goals of postoperative physical therapy are similar to those developed for an adult with an amputation.

Children are more likely to move about after an amputation than an adult, so contractures are less likely to occur. However, some children undergoing chemotherapy are extremely ill and weak and may tend to lie in bed with their residual limb propped on pillows. They must be monitored for developing contractures, and parents and nursing staff must be instructed in ROM exercises and positioning of the residual limb.

Gait training should begin as soon as cleared by the physician. Young children can safely learn to ambulate with an immediate-fit prosthesis using a walker or crutches. If a child has been hospitalized for a period of time, strengthening exercises of the uninvolved leg and the residual limb may be necessary.

After the removal of the immediate-fit prosthesis the child is fitted with a permanent prosthesis. The exception to this would be a child who is undergoing chemotherapy. These children tend to have weight fluctuations secondary to side effects of the medications. They are better fitted with a socket that allows for weight fluctuations, such as one with Velcro closures or any inner socket that can be removed or added to accommodate changes in size of the residual limb. Children with above-knee amputations should be fitted with a prosthesis with a knee joint. Most children with an above-knee amputation will require a suspension method to help hold the prosthesis in place. Instruction must be given to both the parents and the child in donning and removing the prosthesis, care of the prosthesis, skin checks, and wear schedule.

For the child who undergoes a rotationplasty, the surgical leg is usually casted to allow for healing of the bone. The cast may incorporate a pylon to permit the shortened leg to contact the ground for safe ambulation using a walker or crutches. After the cast is removed and the bone is healed the child with a rotationplasty must work on increasing ROM at the ankle joint, which functions as the child's knee. For ambulation and sitting, 0° to 20° of ankle dorsiflexion is more than adequate. Some children will be able to achieve 30° of ankle dorsiflexion, which will allow for some squatting activities and facilitate bike riding. Maximal plantar flexion will allow for greater extension of the leg in stance. Optimal plantar flexion ROM is at least 45° to 50°; the prosthetist can align the prosthesis to achieve an additional few degrees of plantar flexion for stance. Exercises should begin gently and progress to active and resistive exercises.

The child who undergoes a rotationplasty is fitted with a custom-made prosthesis that incorporates the foot in a position of maximum plantar flexion and allows it to act as a knee joint. An external knee hinge joint must be used with an attached thigh cuff. The prosthesis is usually held in place with a pelvic strap.

A child who has had a limb-sparing procedure will also require physical therapy after surgery. Lower extremity procedures usually require a period of non–weight bearing. Rehabilitation for children with a limb-sparing procedure to either the upper or lower extremity includes exercise through active movement with a progression to strengthening exercises. The progression of the intervention is dictated by the procedure that was performed, the surgeon's protocols, and the amount of bone replaced. Children who have had a limb-sparing procedure involving the femur will also frequently require physical therapy after a lengthening procedure of the endoprosthetic implant. ROM of the knee often becomes restricted, similar to that seen with children who undergo limb-lengthening techniques (see Chapter 17).

Gait training for all children at this age will focus on symmetry and the normal characteristics of gait, such as stride length, step length, and velocity, and all skills that the child needs to participate in play and games with other children. When initially learning to ambulate or after a surgical procedure, most children will use an assistive device. As balance and ambulation speed improve and postsurgical limitations are lifted, many children will begin to discard the assistive device. The assistive device should only be discarded, however, if the child's ambulation is safe and speed is functional to keep pace with the child's peers.

During the school-age years the physical therapist should instruct the child in running techniques so that the child may participate in play and games with her or his peers. This is the age at which the child may also show an interest in participating in various sports or recreational programs designed for persons with amputations.

When attending school for the first time, the child will be questioned about the prosthesis and assistive devices. This is especially true of a child with an upper limb deficiency. A meeting before the beginning of school with the child and his or her parents, the child's teacher, and perhaps the child's physical therapist may be helpful to allay any concerns and to answer or develop a way to answer the questions of the child's peers. The child with a unilateral limb deficiency or amputation should succeed in school with minimal adaptations.

The child with bilateral upper limb deficiencies may need to use a tape recorder or computer to assist with writing skills. In school, a child with bilateral upper limb deficiencies may be able to carry papers or books in the classroom between the chin and shoulder. The child also may use the mouth for manipulation and holding objects such as pencils. Whether the child uses his or her feet in school for manipulation or grasping is something that should be clearly discussed with the child, parents, and teacher before school entrance. Many children opt not to use their feet for grasping objects in public as they get older; however, this can limit their independence, especially with toileting and feeding. If a child is adept with the use of his or her feet and is independent and chooses to use the feet, this should not be discouraged. If the teacher displays a supportive attitude toward the child's use of the feet, the child's classroom peers will soon view this as usual procedure in their classroom. The ultimate outcome is for the child to be functional in our society as an adult; this may mean use of the feet or a combination of use of the feet and prostheses.

ADOLESCENCE AND TRANSITION TO ADULTHOOD

Adolescence, with its hallmark concerns of appearance and acceptance by peers, relationships with the opposite sex, career decisions, and the struggle for independence, can be a trying time for anyone. Restrictions in participation for the child with a limb deficiency may become more apparent during adolescence. The majority of teenagers with a congenital limb deficiency have been adjusting both functionally and emotionally from birth. At this point in their lives they are part of a social network of friends, realize the support of their families, and have attempted and succeeded at various activities in school and the community. They will be dealing with these adolescent issues right alongside their peers, although increased fears concerning dating and social acceptance can be typical at this time and participation in school athletic activities may be limited. A higher percentage of children and adolescents with congenital limb deficiencies exhibit greater behavioral and emotional problems and lower social competence than their peers without a disability (Varni & Setoguchi, 1992).

An amputation of a limb during the adolescent years adds quite an emotional burden to a teenager, who must deal with the loss of a body part and the grieving process and may be facing the possibility of death. Added to the physical appearance difficulties are the possible side effects such as hair loss from chemotherapy. A teenager who is facing a possible amputation as the result of cancer should be included, if he or she desires, in discussions of treatment options, including surgical options. Obviously, this is not possible if the amputation is the result of sudden trauma.

Health care professionals have reasoned that limb-sparing procedures offer cosmetic advantages and an increased quality of life compared with an amputation. Prevailing thought also assumed that limb-sparing surgery offers a more functional outcome than an amputation. However, studies have shown that no significant difference exists in quality of life between adolescents and young adults with amputations compared with those who underwent a limb-sparing procedure (Postma et al., 1992; Weddington et al., 1985). These studies did report that adolescents with an amputation exhibited a lower self-esteem but those who underwent a limb-sparing procedure reported more physical complaints.

The immediate postoperative concerns and physical therapy intervention for adolescents undergoing an amputation or a limb-sparing procedure are similar to those described for school-age children. If an immediate-fit prosthesis is not used, teenagers are more likely to develop edema of their residual limb following surgery. In that case, wrapping of the residual limb or fitting with a shrinker sock should be instituted.

Teenagers who sustain a lower extremity amputation are fitted with a prosthesis when the residual limb has stabilized. They should be involved in the fitting of the prosthesis and in deciding on the design of the socket and type of knee joint and foot to be used. For most teenagers a large variety of prosthetic options are available. These should be fully discussed with the teenager and parents, and the choice should complement the lifestyle of the user. Both the teenager and his or her family should be cautioned that the prosthesis will not function or look exactly like the contralateral limb.

Many teenagers with a high above-knee amputation will attempt to ambulate with a prosthesis but will ultimately opt for no prosthesis and crutches, as ambulation with crutches is faster and more energy efficient. The decision to use or not to use a prosthesis should be the child's and not be based on society's idea of the most appropriate physical appearance. Some teenagers use a prosthesis for certain activities and not for others. The ultimate outcome is for them to be comfortable with their peers and interact socially with their peers at school and in the community.

The use of prosthetics varies for teenagers with upper limb deficiencies. For those who have become adept with a prosthesis since early childhood, they probably will continue to use their prosthesis. The teenager who has an upper limb amputation may learn to operate a body-powered above- or below-elbow prosthesis. To become functional with the prosthesis requires much practice, and the teenager may opt not to use one.

One major milestone for teenagers is the acquisition of a driver's license. Nearly all teenagers with a limb deficiency or amputation can learn to drive. Hand controls can be used for the teenager with bilateral PFFD or with bilateral lower extremity amputation as the result of trauma. For the teenager with a unilateral upper limb deficiency or amputation, minimal adjustments will be necessary. Driving can be done by using the sound hand, or a driving ring can be attached to the steering wheel. The prosthetic terminal device, preferably a hook, slips into the ring to assist with controlling the steering wheel and easily slips out of the ring in emergencies. Driving becomes more difficult for the teenager with bilateral upper limb deficiencies or amputations. A driving ring may be used by the dominant limb. Controls such as light switches or turn signals may need to be moved to the dominant side and within reach of the limb or can be operated by the driver's knee. Unless specifically trained in the area of driver education, physical therapists should assist the teenager and his or her parents to seek information and driver training from a local rehabilitation center.

Career and college decisions are also made during adolescence. Some teenagers may work at a part-time job during high school. All teenagers with limb deficiencies or amputations eventually seek employment. At times, adjustments must be made to a prosthesis, such as a specific terminal device, to assist the young adult in his or her particular career area. Going to college is a true test of independence with self-care skills. Some individuals with bilateral upper limb deficiencies or multiple limb deficiencies will always require some degree of assistance with self-care activities. Toileting, especially wiping after defecation, and dressing, specifically managing underpants and bras, are self-care activities for which it is difficult for anyone with bilateral upper limb deficiencies or short above-elbow amputations to achieve total independence. This does not preclude attending college or independent living, but an aide or other arrangements may be needed. Creativity, experimentation, and talking with other teenagers or adults with limb deficiencies can often produce strategies for accomplishing difficult tasks. High employment rates, active lifestyles, and marriage are reported for adults who underwent an amputation as a child or adolescent (Tebbi, 1993; Nagarajan et al., 2003).

■ SUMMARY

The etiology and classification of congenital limb deficiencies and the causes of acquired amputations were reviewed in this chapter. An overview of the medical and surgical management of congenital limb deficiencies and amputations was presented. Treatment of a child with a congenital limb deficiency or amputation is complex and must involve a team of professionals who recognize the impact of various treatment options on the child's function in both the home and school environment and ultimately as an independent adult. Careful planning and thoughtful discussions with the family are necessary regarding surgical options, the use of chemotherapy and radiation therapy for children with malignant tumors, and prosthetic options. Each child must be assessed as an individual, with consideration given to the child's age and musculoskeletal development, immediate and long-term functional abilities, family and child's activity level and lifestyle choices, and prosthetic and physical therapy intervention needed to meet the child's goals.

The continued proliferation of prosthetic designs and materials available to the pediatric population has opened up many options for recreation and sports, vocation, and self-care, as well as early fitting of infants and toddlers with prostheses. Research is needed in the pediatric population to determine which surgical options, prosthetic designs, terminal devices, and materials best improve function, increase comfort, or decrease energy consumption. Physical therapists can easily contribute their expertise to the literature, as well as initiate clinical research to investigate the effectiveness of various treatment options and prosthetic designs.

CASE STUDIES

SCOTT

Scott is a 7-year-old boy with a congenital right PFFD, Aitken type B. Aitken type B classification signifies presence of an acetabulum and femoral head, although the acetabulum may be dysplastic; ossification of the capital femoral epiphysis is delayed; the proximal portion of the femur is displaced laterally and upward; the femoral neck contains defective cartilage that fails to ossify; and the shaft of the femur is short and deformed (Herring, 2002b). A radiologic assessment shortly after birth revealed an absence of the right distal femoral epiphysis, absence of right proximal tibial and fibular epiphyses, and a fibrous connection between the femoral head and proximal femur.

A Boyd amputation of the right foot was performed at 8 months to allow for fitting of a lower extremity prosthesis and weight bearing. He was followed every 3 to 4 months in an amputee clinic and seen by an orthopedist, a prosthetist, and a physical therapist. Physical therapy focused on assessment of age-appropriate developmental skills and instruction of the family in ROM activities to decrease the hip flexion and abduction contractures typically seen with infants with PFFD.

Scott's first prosthesis was essentially a socket and a pylon without a prosthetic knee to promote standing and weight shifting skills. At 12 months Scott was fitted with a prosthesis with a knee joint and began receiving physical therapy services. Physical therapy focused on weight shifting activities and transitions in and out of sitting, up and down from the floor, and sit to stand utilizing the knee flexion now available with the prosthesis. Initial gait training utilized his own push toys and progressed to a walker.

A knee fusion was performed at 3 years of age to improve the lever arm length needed for an efficient gait. A metaphyseal-epiphyseal synostosis with bone grafting was also performed at that time to achieve stability in the region of the proximal femur. After surgical healing, Scott was fitted with a new prosthesis with a four-bar linkage knee and suspension with a silicone liner and pin mechanism. Scott attended physical therapy to regain the strength in his right leg with emphasis on increasing hip extensor and hip abductor strength, weight shifting activities, and gait training with his new prosthesis. His parents also began to work with instructing Scott in donning the prosthesis as he was already independent with removal of his prosthesis.

At the end of 6 weeks of therapy, Scott was ambulating independently without an assistive device, was able to kick a ball with his noninvolved leg, and was able to run. Scott's running was equal to the speed of his 4-year-old sibling, but asymmetric step lengths necessitated a hop-run pattern. He was pleased with his running speed, and his mother was happy that he was not falling.

Scott presently attends the first grade in his local school. He wears his prosthesis throughout the day. He continues to ambulate independently, runs and climbs with his peers at recess, and is learning to ride a bicycle. He has been independent with donning and removing the prosthesis for several years. Before the start of his first year in school, Scott, his mother, and his physical therapist met with his teacher to discuss Scott's PFFD, use of a prosthesis, and his ability levels. Scott readily answers any questions his peers may ask about his prosthesis. At this time Scott requires no extra help in class or at school.

Scott will probably need to undergo a left distal femoral epiphysiodesis and right proximal tibial epiphysiodesis at age 9 or 10 years to ensure that knee joints are at equivalent height at maturity. Anticipated activity limitations include decreased running speed compared to his peers as he gets older. This may limit his ability to participate in sports at a competitive level. He may benefit from running instruction from a physical therapist with expertise in development of higher level gross motor skills for individuals with an amputation. Scott continues to be followed at 6-month intervals in an amputee clinic by an orthopedist, a prosthetist, and a physical therapist.

ANDREW

Andrew is a 6-year-old boy who was diagnosed with Ewing's sarcoma of the right distal femur at 3 years of age. He had no metastases at the time of diagnosis. Andrew underwent a course of preoperative chemotherapy to destroy any micrometastatic disease. Surgical options were discussed with the family, including amputation and rotationplasty. At his young age an amputation would result in a very short above-knee residual limb. Limb-sparing procedures were not possible because of his young age and significant skeletal immaturity. For these reasons, radiation therapy was not used for local tumor control. A rotationplasty was chosen because it afforded a longer residual limb with more function than an above-knee amputation.

Postoperatively, Andrew was placed in a hip spica cast with his right ankle incorporated in approximately 45° of plantar flexion. A pylon was attached to the cast on the right. He received daily physical therapy while an inpatient with the goals of ambulation with a walker and maintenance of upper body strength. He continued on chemotherapy postoperatively. Andrew was discharged home able to walk with a walker in the hip spica cast; the pylon attachment allowed for earlier and safer postoperative ambulation.

Impairments assessed immediately after cast removal included a 15° right ankle plantar flexion contracture, hip flexion, abduction and extensor muscles strength of 2+/5 bilaterally, right ankle plantar flexor strength of 3/5 and right ankle dorsiflexor strength of 2/5. Andrew attended outpatient physical therapy with goals of achieving increasing right ankle dorsiflexion to 20° and improving strength of the hip and ankle musculature to 5/5 bilaterally with progression to gait training with a prosthesis. His parents were instructed in a home program of ROM and strengthening exercises. Three weeks after cast removal right ankle motion was as follows: dorsiflexion 0° to 15° and plantar flexion 0° to 50°. Andrew could actively move his foot through available ranges, and resistive exercises were added. Cosmetically, Andrew exhibited no

problems looking at or manipulating his foot. Both of his parents had met and spoken with a child who had had a rotationplasty before Andrew's surgery. His mother often expressed the feeling that dealing with the appearance of a "backward foot" was nothing compared with dealing with Andrew's cancer and unknown fate.

Following cast removal Andrew had been fitted with a prosthesis with a socket that holds the foot in maximum plantar flexion. The prosthesis had single-axis external knee hinges attached to a thigh cuff and a waist belt. Family goals related to physical therapy were for Andrew to walk independently and engage in play activities with his older siblings. Andrew's parents were instructed in donning the prosthesis, increasing wearing time, skin checks, and gait training for Andrew using a walker. The parents were able to incorporate wearing of the prosthesis into Andrew's daily routine and readily encouraged ambulation for functional activities within their home. Andrew discarded the walker on his own for independent ambulation.

Presently, Andrew attends fourth grade in his neighborhood school. He runs, climbs on playground equipment, and rides a skateboard. Andrew is monitored for recurrence of his cancer and is followed in an amputee clinic at 6-month intervals. During the summer he goes to the community pool with his family and swims without the prosthesis. He has also participated in Little League within his community. He performs well academically in school and is becoming skilled on the computer. So far Andrew's mother states that he has not expressed any anger at the cosmesis of his leg. She has noticed stares from persons at the pool, but they quickly accept Andrew once they are aware of his medical history.

ANTHONY

Anthony is a 14-year-old boy who sustained a mutilating injury to his left leg when he was hit by a train. He was attempting to jump onto a moving freight train with his friends but he slipped and his leg was crushed by the train. Replantation or limb-sparing procedures were not viable options owing to the extent of the crush injuries and the warm ischemia time. A left transfemoral amputation was performed and a soft dressing was applied for the first week. A rigid cast dressing with pylon and prosthetic foot was applied after the first week. As an inpatient, Anthony received physical therapy on a daily basis for gentle ROM exercises and education for positioning of his residual limb. Physical therapy included gait training after week 1 and progressed to weight bearing as tolerated. After 6 weeks, Anthony was fitted for a permanent prosthesis. Outpatient physical therapy goals included increasing hip extension ROM, increasing strength of residual muscles with an emphasis on hip extensors and hip abductors, and improving strength of upper extremities and the right lower extremity.

Prosthetic components of the permanent prosthesis included a narrowed medial-lateral containment socket, silicone liner with locking pin, four-bar linkage knee, and an energy-storing prosthetic foot. Physical therapy continued on an outpatient basis with goals of independent ambulation with or without an assistive device, independence with transitions including up and down from the floor, and ascending and descending stairs and curbs. Physical therapy intervention included weight shifting and balance activities, gait training, endurance activities and education for skin care and donning and doffing the prosthesis.

Anthony was able to develop the skills to ambulate independently during school using his prosthesis but often did not use his prosthesis when at home. Participation restrictions included difficulty running to participate in activities with his friends and long distance walking with his prosthesis to keep up with his friends. Therefore, Anthony will often ambulate using crutches and no prosthesis when hanging out with his friends.

ACKNOWLEDGMENTS

Thank you to Colleen Coulter-O'Berry, MS, PT, PCS, and Brian Giavedoni, CP, for their assistance in obtaining many of the new photos used in this chapter and for their clinical expertise with the development of the accompanying video.

REFERENCES

Aitken, GT. Surgical amputation in children. Journal of Bone and Joint Surgery (American), 45:1735–1741, 1963.

Aitken, GT. Proximal femoral focal deficiency: Definition, classification, and management. In Proximal Femoral Focal Deficiency: A Congenital Anomaly. Washington, DC: National Academy of Sciences, 1969.

Anderson, TF. Aspects of sports and recreation for the child with a limb deficiency. In Herring, JA & Birch, JG (Eds.). The Child with a Limb Deficiency. Rosemont, IL: American Academy of Orthopedic Surgeons, 1998.

Aparicio, J, Munarriz, B, Pastor, M, Vera, FJ, Aparisi, F, Montalar J, Badal, MD, Gomez-Codina, J, & Herranz, C. Long-term follow-up and prognostic factors in Ewing's sarcoma. Oncology, 55:20–26, 1998.

Beris, AE, Soucacos, PN, Malizos, KN, Mitsionis, GJ, & Soucacos, PR. Major limb replantation in children. Microsurgery, 15:474–478, 1994.

Beris, AE, Soucacos, PN, & Malizos, KN. Micorsurgery in children. Clinical Orthopedics and Related Research, 314:112–121, 1995.

Bleyer, A. Older adolescents with cancer in North America; deficits in outcome and research. Pediatric Clinics of North America, 49:1027–1042, 2002.

Bryant, PR, & Pandian, G. Acquired limb deficiencies in children and young adults. Archives of Physical Medicine and Rehabilitation, 82(Suppl 1):S3–S8, 2001.

Butler, MS, Robertson, WW, Rate, W, D'Angio, GJ, & Drummond, DS. Skeletal sequelae of radiation therapy for malignant tumors. Clinical Orthopedics and Related Research, 251:235–239, 1990.

Coulter-O'Berry, C. Personal communication, 2003.

Craft, A, Cotterill, S, Malcolm, A, Spooner, D, Grimer, R, Souhami, R, Imeson, J, & Lewis, I. Ifosfamide-containing chemotherapy in Ewing's sarcoma: the second United Kingdom children's cancer study group and the medical research council Ewing's tumor study. Journal Clinical Oncology, 16:3628–3633, 1998.

Cummings, DR. Pediatric prosthetics, current trends and future possibilities. Physical Medicine and Rehabilitation Clinics of North America, 11:653–679, 2000.

Day, HJB. The ISO/ISPO classification of congenital limb deficiency. Prosthetics and Orthotics International, 15:67–69, 1991.

DiCowden, M, Ballard, A, Robinette, H, & Ortiz, O. Benefit of early fitting and behavior modification training with a voluntary closing terminal device. Journal of the Association of Children's Prosthetic Orthotic Clinics, 22:47–50, 1987.

Dorfman, HD, & Czerniak, B. Bone cancers. Cancer, 75(S1):203–210, 1995.

Eckhardt, JJ, Kabo, JM, Kelley, CM, Ward, WG, Asavamongkolkul, A, Wirganowics, PZ, Yang, RS, & Eilber, FR. Expandable endoprostheses reconstruction in skeletally immature patients with tumors. Clinical Orthopedics and Related Research, 373:51–61, 2000.

Eldridge, JC, Armstrong, PF, & Krajbich, JI. Amputation stump lengthening with the Ilizarov technique. Clinical Orthopedics and Related Research, 256:76–79, 1990.

Ephraim, PL, Dillingham, TR, Sector, M, Pezzin, LE, & MacKenzie, EJ. Epidemiology of limb loss and congenital limb deficiency: A review of the literature. Archives of Physical Medicine and Rehabilitation, 84:747–761, 2003.

Farnsworth, T. The call to arms, overview of upper limb prosthetic options. Active Living, Health and Activity for the O & P Community, 12:43–45, 2003.

Finn, HA, & Simon, MA. Limb-salvage surgery in the treatment of osteosarcoma in skeletally immature individuals. Clinical Orthopedics and Related Research, 262:108–118, 1991.

Fowler, E, Zernicke, R, & Setoguchi, Y. Energy expenditure during walking by children who have proximal femoral focal deficiency. Journal Bone & Joint Surgery (American), 78:1857–1862, 1996.

Frantz, CH, & O'Rahilly, R. Congenital skeletal limb deficiencies. Journal of Bone and Joint Surgery (American), 43:1202–1204, 1961.

Friedman, DL, & Meadows, AT. Late effects of childhood cancer therapy. Pediatric Clinics of North America, 49:1083–1106, 2002.

Gillespie, R. Principles of amputation surgery in children with longitudinal deficiencies of the femur. Clinical Orthopedics and Related Research, 256:29–38, 1990.

Gillespie, R. Classification of congenital abnormalities of the femur. In Herring, JA, & Birch, JG (Eds.). The Child with a Limb Deficiency. Rosemont, IL: American Academy of Orthopedic Surgeons, 1998, pp. 63–72.

Ginsberg, JP, Woo, SY, Johnson, ME, Hicks, MJ, & Horowitz, ME. Ewing's sarcoma family of tumors: Ewing's sarcoma of bone and soft tissue and the peripheral primitive neuroectodermal tumors. In Pizzo, PA, & Poplack, DG (Eds.). Principles and Practice of Pediatric Oncology, 4th ed. Philadelphia: Lippincott, Williams & Wilkins, 2002, pp. 973–1016.

Goldwein, JW. Effects of radiation therapy on skeletal growth in childhood. Clinical Orthopedics and Related Research, 262:101–107, 1991.

Goorin, AM, Schwartzentruber, DJ, Devidas, M, Gebhardt, MC, Ayala, AC, Harris MB, Helman, LJ, Greier, HE & Link, MP. Presurgical chemotherapy compared with immediate surgery and adjuvant chemotherapy for nonmetastatic osteosarcoma: Pediatric oncology group study pog-8651. Journal Clinical Oncology, 21:1574–1580, 2003.

Gover, AM, & McIvor, J. Upper limb deficiencies in infants and young children. Infants and Young Children, 5:58–72, 1992.

Granowetter, L, & West, DC. The Ewing's sarcoma family of tumors: Ewing's sarcoma and peripheral primitive neuroectodermal tumor of bone and soft tissue. In Walterhourse, DO, & Cohn, SL (Eds.). Diagnostic and Therapeutic Advances in Pediatric Oncology. Boston: Kluwer Academic Publishers, 1997, pp. 253–308.

Grier, HE. The Ewing family of tumors; Ewing's sarcoma and primitive neuroectodermal tumors. Pediatric Clinics of North America, 44:991–1004, 1997.

Grimer, RJ, Carter, SR, & Pynsent, PB. Cost-effectiveness of limb salvage for bone tumors. Journal of Bone and Joint Surgery (British), 79:558–561, 1997.

Gurney, J, Severson, RK, Davis, S, & Robison, LL. Incidence of cancer in children in the United States. Cancer 75:2186–2195, 1995.

Herring, JA (Ed). Growth and development. In Tachdjian's Pediatric Orthopedics, 3rd ed. Philadelphia: WB Saunders, 2002a, pp. 3–21.

Herring JA (Ed). Limb deficiencies. In Tachdjian's Pediatric Orthopedics, 3rd ed. Philadelphia: WB Saunders, 2002b, pp. 1745–1810.

Hubbard, SA, Kurtz, I, Heim, W, & Montgomery, G. Powered prosthetic intervention in upper extremity deficiency. In Herring, JA, & Birch, JG (Eds.). The Child With a Limb Deficiency. Rosemont, IL: American Academy of Orthopedic Surgeons, 1998, pp. 405–416.

Kegel, B. Adaptations for sports and recreation. In Bowker, JH, & Michael, JW (Eds.). Atlas of Limb Prosthetics: Surgical, Prosthetic, and Rehabilitation Principles, 2nd ed. St. Louis: Mosby, 1992, pp. 623–654.

Kenan, S, & Lewis, MM. Limb salvage in pediatric surgery: The use of the expandable prosthesis. Orthopedic Clinics of North America, 22:121–131, 1991.

Krajbich, JI, & Bochmann, D. Van Nes rotation-plasty in tumor surgery. In Bowker, JH, & Michael, JW (Eds.). Atlas of Limb Prosthetics: Surgical, Prosthetic, and Rehabilitation Principles, 2nd ed. St. Louis: Mosby, 1992, pp. 885–899.

Krajbich, JL. Rotationplasty in the management of proximal femoral focal deficiency. In Herring, JA, & Birch, JG (Eds.). The Child with a Limb Deficiency. Rosemont, IL: American Academy of Orthopedic Surgeons, 1998, p. 87.

Krebs, DE, Edelstein, JE, & Thornby, MA. Prosthetic management of children with limb deficiencies. Physical Therapy, 71:920–934, 1991.

Krebs, DE, & Fishman, S. Characteristics of the child amputee population. Journal of Pediatric Orthopedics, 4:89-95, 1984.

Link, MP, Grier, HE, & Donaldson, SS. Sarcomas of bone. In Fernbach, DJ, & Vietti, TJ (Eds.). Clinical Pediatric Oncology, 4th ed. St. Louis: Mosby, 1991, pp. 545–575.

Link, MP, Gebhardt, MC, & Meyers, PA. Osteosarcoma. In Pizzo, PA, & Poplack, DG (Eds.). Principles and Practice of Pediatric Oncology, 4th ed. Philadelphia: Lippincott Williams & Wilkins, 2002, pp. 1051–1089.

Melzack, R, Israel, R, Lacroix, R, & Schultz, G. Phantom limbs in people with congenital deficiency or amputation in early childhood. Brain, 120:1603–1620, 1997.

Meyers, PA, & Gorlick, R. Osteosarcoma. Pediatric Clinics of North America, 44:973–989, 1997.

Michael, JW. Modern prosthetic knee mechanisms. Clinical Orthopedics and Related Research, 361:39–47, 1999.

Miller, RW, Young, JL, & Novakovic, B. Childhood cancer. Cancer, 75:395–405, 1995.

Morrissy, RT, Giavedoni, BJ, & Coulter-O'Berry, C. The limb-deficient child. In Lovell & Winter (Eds.). Pediatric Orthopedics, 5th ed. Philadelphia: Lippincott Williams & Wilkins, 2001, pp. 1217–1272.

Nagarajan, R, Neglia, JP, Clohisy, DR, Yasui, Y, Greenberg, M, Hudson, M, Zevon, MA, Tersak, JM, Ablin, A, & Robison, LL. Education, employment, insurance, and marital status among 694 survivors of pediatric lower extremity bone tumors. Cancer, 97:2554–2564, 2003.

Oppenheim, WL, Setoguchi, Y, & Fowler, E. Overview and comparison of Syme amputation and knee fusion with the Van Nes rotationplasty in proximal femoral focal deficiency. In Herring, JA, & Birch, JG (Eds.). The Child With a Limb Deficiency. Rosemont, IL: American Academy of Orthopedic Surgeons, 1998, pp. 73–86.

Patton, JG. Developmental approach to pediatric prosthetic evaluation and training. In Atkins, DJ, & Meier, RH (Eds.). Comprehensive Management of the Upper-Limb Amputee. New York: Springer-Verlag, 1989, pp. 137–149.

Postma, A, Kingma, A, De Ruiter, JH, Koops, HS, Veth, RPH, Goeken, LNH, & Kamps, WA. Quality of life in bone tumor patients comparing limb salvage and amputation of the lower extremity. Journal of Surgical Oncology, 51:47–51, 1992.

Pruitt, SD, Varni, JW, & Setoguchi, Y. Functional status in children with limb deficiency: development and initial validation of an outcome measure. Archives of Physical Medicine and Rehabilitation, 77:1233–1238, 1996.

Pruitt, SD, Varni, JW, Seid, M, & Setoguchi, Y. Functional status in limb deficiency: Development of an outcome measure for preschool children. Archives of Physical Medicine and Rehabilitation, 79:405–411, 1998.

Pruitt, SD, Seid, M, Varni, JW, & Setoguchi, Y. Toddlers with limb deficiency: Conceptual basis and initial application of a functional status outcome measure. Archives of Physical Medicine and Rehabilitation, 80:819–824, 1999.

Radocy, B. Upper-limb prosthetic adaptations for sports and recreation. In Bowker, JH, & Michael, JW (Eds.). Atlas of Limb Prosthetics: Surgical, Prosthetic, and Rehabilitation Principles, 2nd ed. St. Louis: Mosby, 1992, pp. 325–344.

Renard, AJ, Veth, RP, Schreuder, HW, van Loon, CJ, Koops, HS, & van Horn, JR. Function and complications after ablative and limb-salvage therapy in lower extremity sarcoma of bone. Journal of Surgical Oncology, 73:198–205, 2000.

Rougraff, BT, Simon, MA, & Kneisel, JS. Limb salvage compared with amputation for osteosarcoma of the distal end of the femur. A long-term oncological, functional and quality of life study. Journal of Bone & Joint Surgery (American), 163:1171–1175, 1994.

Sadler, TW (Ed.). Langman's Medical Embryology, 8th ed. Philadelphia: Lippincott Williams & Wilkins, 2000, pp. 172–181.

Schindler, OS, Cannon, SR, Briggs, TWR, & Blunn, GW. Stanmore custom-made extendible distal femoral replacements. Journal of Bone and Joint Surgery (British), 79:927–937, 1997.

Schuch, CM & Pritham, CH. Current transfemoral sockets. Clinical Orthopedics and Related Research, 361:48–54, 1999.

Setoguchi, Y, & Rosenfelder, R (Eds.). The Limb Deficient Child. Springfield, IL: Charles C Thomas, 1982.

Shurr, DG, & Cook, TM. Prosthetics and Orthotics. East Norwalk, CT: Appleton & Lange, 1990, pp. 183–193.

Simmel, ML. Phantom experiences following amputation in childhood. Journal of Neurology, Neurosurgery, and Psychiatry, 25:69–78, 1962.

Springfield, DS. Musculoskeletal tumors. In Canale, ST, & Beatty, JH (Eds.). Operative Pediatric Orthopedics. St. Louis: Mosby, 1991, pp. 1073–1113.

Sutherland, DH. Gait Disorders in Childhood and Adolescence. Baltimore: Williams & Wilkins, 1984, pp. 14–27.

Swanson, AB, Barsky, AJ, & Entin, MA. Classification of limb malformations on the basis of embryological failures. Surgical Clinics of North America, *48*:1169–1179, 1968.

Tarbell, NJ, & Kooy, HM.General Principles of Radiation Oncology. In Pizzo, PA, & Poplack, DG (Eds.). Principles and Practice of Pediatric Oncology, 4th ed. Philadelphia: Lippincott Williams & Wilkins, 2002, pp. 369–380.

Tebbi, CK. Psychological effects of amputation in sarcoma. In Humphrey, GB, Koops, HS, Molenaar, WM, & Postma, A (Eds.). Osteosarcoma in Adolescents and Young Adults. Boston: Kluwer Academic, 1993, pp. 39–44.

Tooms, RE. Acquired amputations in children. In Bowker, JH, & Michael, JW (Eds.). Atlas of Limb Prosthetics: Surgical, Prosthetic, and Rehabilitation principles, 2nd ed. St. Louis: Mosby, 1992, pp. 735–741.

Trautwein, LC, Smith, DG, & Rivara, FP. Pediatric amputation injuries: Etiology, cost and outcome. The Journal of Trauma: Injury, Infection and Critical Care, *41*:831–838, 1996.

Unwin, PS, & Walker, PS. Extendible endoprosthesis for the skeletally immature. Clinical Orthopedics and Related Research, *322*:179–193, 1996.

Varni, JW, & Setoguchi, Y. Screening for behavioral and emotional problems in children and adolescents with congenital or acquired limb deficiencies. American Journal of Diseases in Childhood, *146*:103–107, 1992.

Velez-Yanguas, MC, & Warrier, RP. The evolution of chemotherapeutic agents for the treatment of pediatric musculoskeletal malignancies. Orthopedic Clinics of North America, *27*:545–557, 1996.

Weaver, DD. Vascular etiology of limb defects: The subclavian artery supply disruption sequence. In Herring, JA & Birch, JG (Eds.). The Child with a Limb Deficiency. Rosemont, IL: American Academy of Orthopedic Surgeons, 1998, pp. 25–38.

Weddington, WW, Segraves, KB, & Simon, MA. Psychological outcome of extremity sarcoma survivors undergoing amputation or limb salvage. Journal of Clinical Oncology, *3*:1393–1399, 1985.

Wexler, LH, DeLaney, TF, Tsokos, M, Avila, N, Steinberg, SM, Weaver-McClure, L, Jacobson, J, Jarosinski, P, Hijazi, YM, Balis, FM, & Horowitz, ME. Ifosfamide and etoposide plus vincristine, doxorubicin, and cyclophosphamide for newly diagnosed Ewing's sarcoma of family tumors. Cancer, *78*:901–911, 1996.

Wilk, B, Karol, L, Halliday, S, Cummings, D, Haideri, N, & Stephenson, J. Transition to an articulating knee prosthesis in pediatric amputees. Journal of Prosthetics and Orthotics, *11*:69–74, 1999.

Wilkins, RM, & Soubeiran, A. The Phoenix expandable prosthesis: Early American experience. Clinical Orthopedics and Related Research, *382*:51–58, 2001.

Wright, PE, & Jobe, MT. Congenital anomalies of the hand. In Canale, ST, & Beatty, JH (Eds.). Operative Pediatric Orthopedics. St. Louis: Mosby, 1991, pp. 253–330.

Chapter 17

ORTHOPEDIC CONDITIONS

JUDY LEACH
PT

In the course of their careers, physical therapists may treat patients with a wide variety of diagnoses or they may tend to specialize in one particular area. Almost without exception, however, a strong grounding in orthopedics is a necessary part of a therapist's academic and clinical experience. For therapists specializing in the assessment and treatment of children, this orthopedic knowledge is especially necessary. It is also quite challenging because of one immutable fact—children grow. The human skeleton undergoes an incredible amount of growth and change in the years between birth and skeletal maturity. What may be considered "normal" at one age can be decidedly abnormal at another. For example, most infants have bowlegs (genu varum), but significant genu varum in an 8-year-old child would be cause for concern.

The rotational alignment of the lower extremity provides another example of the need for physical therapists to be familiar with the growth and development of the musculoskeletal system. Internal tibial torsion in the infant is commonly seen and is considered normal for that age. However, a high degree of internal tibial torsion in a 5-year-old child is an impairment that may produce a significant functional deficit, such as difficulty running and frequent falls, and may even require surgical correction.

In addition, as physical therapy practice becomes more autonomous, we are challenged by timely identification of problems outside our scope of practice. These problems require referral to other specialists, and therapists should view this responsibility as a necessary service to our patients. As in so many other areas of life, the Internet is changing the way we do business. Traditionally, parents have relied on the diagnostic information and treatment advice provided by the medical professionals who see their child. Now they can easily obtain additional specific information about a disease or injury from a wide range of sources on the Internet. Obtaining this information can be a blessing or a curse. There is no control over what is posted on the Web, and there is certainly some very inaccurate, overly optimistic, and even downright fraudulent treatment advice given. Physical therapists can provide guidance to parents in determining the quality of the information; for example, is the information coming from a double-blind placebo controlled study from an established research center, or an anecdotal report of a successful treatment for one child? Internet access can also change referral patterns, as parents obtain information on different treatment options and self-refer to a wider geographic range of treatment centers (Morcuende et al., 2003).

In this chapter space will not allow an exhaustive review of all the orthopedic conditions that affect children; however, a number of excellent texts are available for more detailed information on the topics covered in this chapter (Scoles, 1988; Tachdjian, 1990; Wenger & Rang, 1993). Instead, commonly seen conditions and specific areas of concern to physical therapists will be highlighted in the hope that this will provide a basic framework for further independent study.

TORSIONAL CONDITIONS

A chief complaint of either in-toeing or out-toeing is probably the most common reason for elective referral of a child to an orthopedist. Even though these rotational conditions in the lower extremities usually do not require any treatment, they are often a source of significant concern to parents and other family members. This concern often escalates with comments by neighbors, teachers, and strangers on the street: "Why does your child walk funny?" This group of children has been described by Dr. Mercer Rang as "the worried well," an apt phrase that indicates the strong concern of the family and others involved with the child over alignment conditions that are often part of the spectrum of normal musculoskeletal development.

Numerous differences of opinion exist on how to define torsional conditions, how to measure them, and especially on how to treat them, or if they should be treated at all. Most treatment with special shoes, casts, or braces has no proven efficacy, and many orthopedists believe that persistent deformity beyond skeletal maturity is unusual and significant functional disability is rare (Bruce, 1996). Unfortunately the term torsional *deformities* is used in the literature, at national meetings, and in verbal discussions. Patients and parents hear the term *deformity,* and their worst fears are validated. The terms *condition* or *variation* produce less anxiety and are usually more anatomically correct. The Subcommittee on Torsional Deformity of the Pediatric Orthopaedic Society of North America has recommended a classification system in which normal limb alignment and joint range of motion (ROM) are defined as those occurring within

two standard deviations of the mean. These are termed *rotational variations.* Those falling outside the two standard deviations are termed *torsional deformities* (Scoles, 1988).

Once neuromuscular dysfunction or other serious conditions have been ruled out, it is important to spend sufficient time educating the parents about the current reason for their child's condition and why it may not need treatment. Anticipatory guidance about future possibilities should be provided. For example, a 2-year-old child's in-toeing may resolve as his internal tibial torsion (ITT) resolves, but in-toeing may reappear at age 4 to 6 years due to femoral anteversion.

OBTAINING A HISTORY

A specific history provides a wealth of information regarding possible causative factors and indications for possible treatment. Specific information obtained may also direct the examiner to expand the examination to rule out other, more severe conditions that may initially produce a chief complaint of in-toeing or out-toeing. Relevant information to be elicited from the parents includes the following:

1. *Birth history.* Was the infant full term or premature? Was it a vaginal or cesarean delivery? Was oligohydramnios (deficiency of amniotic fluid) present? How many times has the mother been pregnant? What is the birth order of the patient? Many of the torsional problems seen in infants are "packaging" defects (i.e., caused by a restricted intrauterine environment). It is easy to imagine that an infant's lower limbs may "grow" into a particular position if one visualizes a full-term 9-pound fetus in the womb of a gravida 1, para 1 mother.

2. *Age when in-toeing or out-toeing was noted.* Has it improved or worsened since first noted? Has there been any prior treatment? For the walking child, at what age did the child start to walk independently? In the differential diagnosis, there should be an increased index of suspicion when a child has a history of prematurity, difficult birth, or delayed motor milestones or has significant in-toeing or out-toeing that is worsening with time or is very asymmetric. Children with mild spastic diplegia may have in-toeing, and children with Duchenne muscular dystrophy may have out-toeing and flat feet. Conditions such as these must be ruled out.

3. *Family history.* In many cases there is a positive family history for in-toeing or out-toeing, and this should be noted, especially if treatment was

undertaken for the other family member(s).

4. *Sleeping and sitting positions.* Sleeping prone with the legs internally rotated encourages persistent internal tibial torsion and metatarsus adductus (Staheli, 1977). Sitting in a W-sit position encourages the persistence of femoral anteversion.

CLINICAL EXAMINATION AND INTERVENTIONS

Clinical examination of the child with in-toeing or out-toeing should include documentation of the foot progression angle in standing or walking, hip rotation ROM, thigh-foot axis, and alignment of the foot. These four components form the torsional profile described by Staheli (1977). In a later study, Staheli and colleagues (1985) described means and ranges for these parameters in 1000 normal children and adults.

Foot Progression Angle

Foot progression angle (FPA), or "the angle of gait," is defined as the angle between the longitudinal axis of the foot and a straight line of progression of the body in walking (Staheli, 1977). The child is observed while walking, and a value is assigned to the angle of both the right and the left foot. This is a subjective determination and represents an average of the angles noted on multiple steps. There are various footprint techniques to measure FPA, but these are time consuming and usually not practical in a clinical situation. In-toeing is expressed as a negative value (e.g., –30°), and out-toeing is expressed as a positive value (e.g., +20°). This angle gives an overall view of the degree of in-toeing or out-toeing in the walking child. The FPA can also be assessed in supported stance for the child who is not yet walking independently. FPA is variable during infancy. During childhood and adult life, it shows little change, with a mean of +10° and a normal range of –3 to +20° (Staheli et al., 1985).

Hip Rotation, Femoral Anteversion, and Retroversion

Clinical Examination. Hip rotation ROM is measured most accurately in the prone position, with the hip in a position of neutral flexion/extension. (An extremely frightened, crying young child can be examined more easily by having the parent stand up and hold the child against the chest, facing the parent. This allows the child's hips to hang into neutral flexion/extension, and the examiner can then bend the child's knees and evaluate the hip rotation range.) This hip rotation measurement will be a reflection of the flexibility of the soft tissues and the version of the femur.

Version is the normal angular difference between the transverse axis of each end of a long bone. The terms *femoral anteversion* (FA) and *retroversion* refer to this relationship between the neck of the femur and the femoral shaft, ending in the femoral condyles, that dictates the position of the femoral head when the knee is pointing straight ahead (Fig. 17-1). If the femoral head is directed anteriorly, the hip is in anteversion (or "anteverted") and the patient will usually have more hip internal rotation (IR) than external rotation (ER) ROM, assuming no soft tissue tightness. If hip IR is measured at 70° and ER at 25°, for example, the child is said to have FA and may in-toe when walking. In retroversion, the femoral head is directed posteriorly when the knee is aligned straight ahead and the patient will have greater ER range.

Femoral and tibial torsion, or version, can be measured by computed tomography (CT). However, clinical measurements of hip IR and ER have been found to be adequate for diagnosing rotational abnormalities. Cahuzac and co-workers (1992) found that relationships between FA and hip IR were significant, as were relationships between the clinical and CT values of femoral and tibial torsion. Stuberg and associates (1989) found a discrepancy of 10° to 15° between clinical goniometric assessment and CT analysis of femoral torsion, with goniometric measurements less than the femoral anteversion measured by CT. In adulthood, development of pain and osteoarthritis may warrant CT to more precisely measure version of both the femur and acetabulum (Tonnis & Skamel, 2003). Clinical measurements, however, are sufficient for documentation in the majority of children with benign rotational problems.

The sum of hip IR and ER is usually 120° up to age 2 years; over age 2 it is 95° to 110° (Engel & Staheli, 1974). Most infants have FA and also have contractures of the hip external rotator muscles at birth (from the intrauterine position) that mask the anteversion; they tend to hold their legs in an abducted/externally rotated position. True femoral retroversion in an infant is rare; it is usually tightness in the hip lateral rotator muscles and capsular ligaments that is producing the externally rotated position, masking the femoral anteversion (Pitkow, 1975). The tightness of the hip soft tissues gradually stretches out, and the true anteversion of the femur becomes more apparent. This process is often described incorrectly as "femoral anteversion increases"; the amount of femoral version is in fact decreasing, but it is more easily visualized because the muscle tightness of the lateral rotators is decreasing. The FA becomes increasingly more apparent clinically as the child approaches 5 to 6 years of age, as the soft tissue tightness

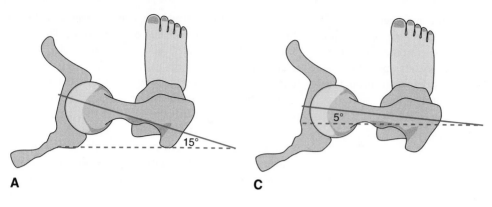

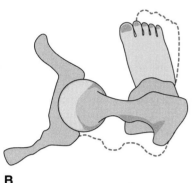

◆ **Figure 17-1**   In the femur, version is the angular difference between the transcondylar axis of the knee (the horizontal line in this drawing) and the axis of the femoral neck. These two lines form an angle and document whether the femur is in anteversion or retroversion. **A**, Normal anteversion: With this small amount of anteversion, the individual can walk comfortably with the foot pointed straight ahead (i.e., a neutral angle of foot progression). **B**, Excessive anteversion with in-toeing: When a large amount of anteversion is present, the individual must internally rotate the femur in order to seat the femoral head in the acetabulum and achieve improved joint congruity. This results in a negative foot progression angle, and the foot is pointed in during gait (in-toeing). **C**, Retroversion: In this drawing, there is a significant reduction in the angle formed between the two axes, depicting retroversion. If this were excessive, the individual would need to externally rotate the femur to seat the femoral head in the acetabulum and would have a positive angle of foot progression (out-toeing). *(Adapted with permission from Neumann, DA. Kinesiology of the Musculoskeletal System. St. Louis: Mosby, 2002, p.395)*

resolves. FA has been measured by radiographs and CT in typically developing children, and the average shows a gradual decrease with age: 35° at age 1 year, to 21° at age 9 years, to 15.5° in adults (Crane, 1959; De Alba et al., 1998; Fabry et al., 1973; Shands & Steele, 1958). By mid-childhood, the femoral head and neck have usually assumed a relatively more neutral position in relationship to the femoral shaft and children typically have approximately equal amounts of hip IR and ER (Fig. 17-2).

Femoral Anteversion: Intervention. Many types of interventions have been tried to correct FA, including braces, twister cables, and special shoes. None of these has been proved effective in clinical trials. Anecdotal evidence of their efficacy abounds, with a tendency to ignore the natural history of the condition (i.e., that spontaneous improvement will occur). One reasonable recommendation is to have the child avoid W-sitting (reverse tailor sitting) and to encourage tailor sitting in maximum external rotation. If significant FA is still present at age 10 to 14 years and is resulting in cosmetically unappealing in-toeing, surgical correction in the form of femoral derotation osteotomies may be considered, although the possible operative risks may outweigh the benefits of

realignment. Surgical intervention may be warranted and has proved successful in children with severe symptomatic torsional malalignment with excessive FA or external tibial torsion (ETT) associated with patellofemoral pathology, when conservative treatment has failed (Cameron and Saha, 1996; Delgado et al., 1996; Meister & James, 1995; Turner, 1994).

Thigh-Foot Axis, Tibial Torsion

Clinical Examination. The alignment of the lower leg can be measured by documenting the thigh-foot axis, which is a reflection of the version of the tibia. Tibial torsion is assessed using the thigh-foot angle, the angular difference between the longitudinal axes of the thigh and foot, as measured in the prone position with the knee flexed. Some examiners measure tibial torsion with the child sitting and the knee flexed to 90°. Tibial torsion can also be described as the angle formed by a straight-line axis through the knee and the axis through the medial and lateral malleoli. By convention, internal tibial torsion (ITT) is expressed as a negative value, such as "tibial torsion of −30." ETT is expressed as a positive value.

The tibia is usually medially rotated in infants (ITT) as a result of intrauterine positioning (Hensinger & Jones,

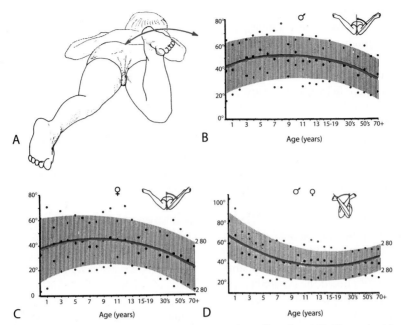

• **Figure 17-2**   **A**, Hip rotation is measured with the patient prone, knee flexed to 90°. Means for hip rotation in mid-childhood and in older subjects. **B**, Medial rotation in males: 50° (range 25°–65°). **C**, Medial rotation in females: 40° (range 15°–60°). **D**, Lateral rotation: 45° (range 25°–65°), with no gender difference. *(From Staheli LT, Corbett, M, Wyss, C, & King, H. Lower extremity rotational problems in children. Journal of Bone and Joint Surgery [American], 67:39–47, 1985.)*

1981). Spontaneous derotation on the long axis takes place during growth. The tibia gradually rotates out into ETT, especially during the first 6 months of independent walking, or by approximately 18 months of age. The normal range of thigh-foot angle is between 0° and 30° of ETT, with a mean of approximately 10° during most of childhood (Staheli & Engel, 1972). Scoles (1988) described the following approximate thigh-foot normative angles:

> Birth: –15° (normal range –30° to +20°)
> Age 3: +5° (normal range –10° to +20°)
> Mid-childhood to skeletal maturity: +10° (normal range –5° to +30°)

ITT in infancy is often not apparent to the parents or the casual examiner because the hips have external rotation muscle contractures and the infant's legs tend to assume an abducted and externally rotated position. The ITT may become noticeable only as the hip contractures stretch out, resulting in a more neutral position of the hip, and especially when the child begins to walk independently.

Internal Tibial Torsion: Intervention. Controversy exists regarding appropriate treatment of ITT, as it does in FA. Many orthopedists believe that it should not be treated at all because the natural history of the condition is gradual improvement. The very small percentage of

children who do not improve and who have a significant functional deficit as a result of ITT can be treated surgically at a later date with external rotational osteotomy of the tibia and fibula. A different school of thought relies on natural improvement up to about 18 months of age, and at that age advocates treating persistent ITT with a Friedman counter splint (a flexible leather strap) or a Denis Browne bar (a metal bar) for night wear, usually for about 6 months. These devices attach to shoes and hold the feet in an externally rotated position.

There may be an association of increased incidence of knee osteoarthritis in adults with decreased ETT or true ITT (Turner, 1994; Yagi, 1994). Turner (1994) observed that patients with patellofemoral instability had greater than normal ETT, patients with panarticular osteoarthritis had decreased ETT, and he noted that abnormal torsion causes gait adaptations that affect external loading on the knee joint. Increased ETT may be a predisposing factor in the onset of Osgood-Schlatter syndrome in male athletes, especially on the side preferentially used for jumping and sprinting (Gigante et al., 2003). However, there may also be a benefit to in-toeing in certain sports. Fuchs and Staheli (1996) studied high school students (50 sprinters and 50 control subjects) and found that the sprinters tended to have low normal thigh-foot angles and in-toed when sprinting.

Surgical correction may be required in severe idiopathic tibial torsion, or in children with cerebral palsy, myelomeningocele, and clubfoot. Dodgin and colleagues (1998) reviewed 63 limbs with same level distal tibial and fibular osteotomies with crossed Kirschner wires and found the procedure to be safe, efficient, and effective.

Metatarsus Adductus

The infant foot is malleable, making it susceptible to deformation and compression from intrauterine positioning. Alterations in alignment of the foot can be divided into two categories: positional or "packaging" problems caused by a restricted intrauterine environment and "manufacturing" defects or true congenital abnormalities such as talipes equinovarus. Metatarsus varus, also called metatarsus adductus (MTA), is one of the most commonly seen positional conditions in infants. Morcuende and Ponseti (1996) noted the possibility of a developmental abnormality of the medial cuneiform as a pathogenic factor. In MTA the forefoot is curved medially, the hindfoot is in the normal slight valgus position, and there is full dorsiflexion ROM. The degree of MTA can be graded as I—mild, II—moderate, and III—severe. Having the child stand on the glass plate of a photocopying machine and xeroxing the feet is an easy, quick way to document the amount of metatarsus adductus. Some clinicians use grade 1/2 to describe dynamic MTA: the foot looks straight at rest, but when the child walks there is a dynamic forefoot varus due to muscle action, with medial motion of the great toe, described as a "searching great toe" (Staheli, 1977). Treatment is rarely required for mild cases (grade I), which usually resolve on their own, generally by about age 4 to 6 months. Moderate cases (grade II) may be treated with stretching exercises and corrective shoes (straight-last or reverse-last shoes or both). Severe cases may be treated with manipulation and serial casting, followed by corrective shoes. Another school of thought advocates no conservative treatment, recommending surgical correction at a later age for those feet that do not improve with time. Thirty-one patients (45 feet) followed an average of 32 years, 6 months, by Farsetti and colleagues (1994) demonstrated good results without intervention in all feet with passively correctable MTA. Twenty-six (90%) of the 29 feet with moderate or severe MTA treated with serial manipulation and casting had good results.

Residual MTA may be a risk factor for stress fractures in adulthood (Theodorou et al., 1999). These authors studied 11 patients ages 25 to 61 years with MTA and stress fractures and noted that 17 of the 22 fractures occurred in the lateral (fourth and fifth) metatarsal bones.

Calcaneovalgus

Calcaneovalgus is a common positional foot problem in newborns, and more than 30% of neonates have bilateral calcaneovalgus (Sullivan, 1999). In this condition, the result of a large infant in a small space, the forefoot is curved out laterally, the hindfoot is in valgus, and there is full or excessive dorsiflexion. The dorsum of the foot may actually be touching the anterior surface of the leg at birth. The positional calcaneovalgus foot corrects spontaneously and does not require treatment. It must be distinguished from more severe conditions, such as a calcaneovalgus foot caused by a vertical talus. In this condition, the talus is vertically oriented and the navicular is displaced onto the dorsal surface of the talus. The forefoot is dorsiflexed but the hindfoot is plantar flexed, and the foot bends at the instep. This characteristic position is described as a rocker-bottom deformity of the foot, and the foot is much more rigid than the typical calcaneovalgus foot. Kodros and Dias (1999) studied 41 patients with 55 feet with congenital vertical talus and found that only 10 were idiopathic. The remaining 45 were associated with neural tube defects, neuromuscular disorders, or congenital malformation syndromes.

Foot Alignment Problems: Summary

Table 17-1 is a decision matrix that provides a quick and easy way to categorize foot conditions (Wenger & Leach, 1986).

TABLE 17-1	**Decision Matrix for Foot Deformity**		
	METATARSUS VARUS	**CLUBFOOT**	**CALCANEOVALGUS**
Side view (Can foot dorsiflex?)	Yes	No	Yes
Foot shape (viewed from bottom)	Kidney shaped (deviated medially)	Kidney shaped	Banana shaped (deviated laterally)
Heel position	Valgus	Varus	Valgus

Torsional Profile

The components that may contribute to in-toeing are femoral anteversion, internal tibial torsion, and metatarsus adductus. Those that may contribute to out-toeing are ER contractures of the hip (and, rarely, femoral retroversion), ETT, and calcaneovalgus. The foot progression angle can be viewed as the "summation" of the rotational alignment of the three segments of the lower limb: the hip and femur, the lower leg, and the foot. For example, significant FA at the hip may be balanced by ETT, with a straight foot (no MTA or calcaneovalgus). The foot progression angle would be 0°/0° (right/left) with the feet pointing straight ahead. When a child toes in or toes out, the condition is usually bilateral, but occasionally one sees "windswept" lower extremities, with one limb toeing in and the other limb toeing out.

A typically developing 8-month-old infant supported in upright might have a torsional profile as follows:

	Right	Left
Foot progression angle	—	— (not yet standing)
Internal rotation of hip	20°	20°
External rotation of hip	90°	90°
Thigh-foot angle	0°	0°
Foot	Neutral	Neutral

In this example, the legs are positioned in external rotation, the usual position for the lower extremities in infancy.

The torsional profile of a 5-year-old child with in-toeing might look like this:

	Right	Left
Foot progression angle	−40°	−30°
Internal rotation of hip	70°	70°
External rotation of hip	20°	20°
Thigh-foot angle	−10°	+15°
Foot	Grade I MTA	Neutral

From this discussion, it is clear that one must determine which component(s) of the lower extremity is causing the torsional condition and then treat that level, if treatment is indicated. For example, using heavy, high-topped orthopedic shoes will not correct femoral anteversion. In fact, the child will probably be more clumsy and stumble more frequently. The concept of a natural history of improvement with time is also pivotal. It is important not to extol the virtues of various treatments too vigorously, because it is difficult to differentiate benefits obtained from the treatment versus benefits that occurred simply with the passage of time as a result of skeletal maturation. In summary, in-toeing is usually attributable to MTA in the infant, ITT in the toddler, and femoral anteversion in older children up to 10 years old (Lincoln & Suen, 2003).

In children with neuromuscular diseases such as cerebral palsy, the basic examination format described previously is useful in helping to delineate the child's problems with gait. This assessment mainly addresses bony alignment. One must also document muscle tone, muscle strength, and motor control. Abnormalities in any of these areas can cause in-toeing or out-toeing, either alone or in conjunction with skeletal malalignment. An example would be a child with cerebral palsy (CP) who ambulates with a foot progression angle of −40°/−30°. This may be due to a combination of FA, ITT, MTA, and spasticity in the hip adductors, medial hamstrings, and posterior tibialis muscles. Bobroff and colleagues (2000) studied 147 patients (267 hips) with CP, comparing femoral anteversion and neck shaft angle (NSA) to those in children without CP. As age increased, those with CP showed little change in FA (FA decreased in the control group) and an increase in NSA compared to the control group. By contrast, a child with Duchenne muscular dystrophy may ambulate with an in-toeing gait at age 6 because of FA and then gradually develop an out-toeing gait by age 10, resulting from resolution of the FA and increasing weakness of the gluteus maximus and quadriceps muscles, plus tightness in the iliotibial band and plantar flexors.

Another area of assessment and treatment in which this multilevel concept is useful is in measurement of other gross motor activities, such as sitting. Many children with increased tone, as well as children with hypotonia, will W-sit. This postural preference is frequently ascribed to problems with spasticity, or it is thought of as a compensatory mechanism to achieve better sitting balance. However, a more detailed examination might reveal that the child has, in addition to spasticity or poor balance, significant FA that simply does not allow comfortable sitting with the hips in external rotation.

ANGULAR CONDITIONS

Genu varum (bowlegs) and genu valgum (knock-knees) are similar to torsional conditions in that they are commonly seen in typically developing children and a specific natural history has been described that results in normal skeletal alignment at maturity.

Moderate genu varum, often referred to as physiologic bowing (apex laterally), is normal for newborns and for infants before they begin walking. This physiologic genu varum generally resolves, and the child gradually develops genu valgum between 2 and 4 years of age. By age 3 years, 80% of children have mild knock-knees. This valgus angulation generally corrects by 5 to 7 years of age, and the child is left with a "normally" straight leg. The normal tibiofemoral angulation in adults is 7° to 9° of valgus in females and 4° to 6° in males (Scoles, 1988). Cahuzac and colleagues (1995) measured the tibio-femoral angle clinically in 427 children ages 10 to 16 years and found that girls had a constant valgus (5.5°), whereas the boys showed a varus evolution (4.4°) during the last 2 years of growth. Bowlegs and knock-knees tend to run in families, however, and some children will inherit this genetic predisposition to one or the other in adulthood.

GENU VARUM

Clinical Examination

The child must be undressed with diaper removed for accurate documentation of genu varum. The child is placed supine with the medial malleoli approximated. The distance between the femoral condyles is measured. Some clinicians use the distance between the knees at the knee joint line. A plastic triangle with centimeters marked on both sides is useful, allowing the examiner to easily obtain accurate measurements, especially of a wiggling child. Infants usually have ITT and genu varum, and this combination tends to make the child look "bowlegged and pigeon-toed," causing many parents and others great concern. Even when the genu varum has resolved and the child may actually have developed genu valgum, the presence of ITT may make the child look bowlegged.

Differential Diagnosis

When a child develops severe genu varum, especially after 4 years of age or worsening over time, systemic disorders such as vitamin D–resistant rickets, achondroplasia, renal osteodystrophy, and osteogenesis imperfecta must be ruled out, along with a variety of skeletal dysplasias and other conditions that cause genu varum (Brooks and Gross, 1995). Radiographs are used to rule out idiopathic tibia vara, also known as Blount's disease.

Physiologic (normal) genu varum in the infant must also be distinguished from pathologic anterolateral bow of the tibia, usually noted at birth (Hensinger & Jones, 1981). In this extremely serious condition, radiographs demonstrate a tibia with a narrowed, sclerotic intra-medullary canal which puts the tibia at severe risk of fracture in the first year of life. In these cases, both tibia and fibula may fail to unite; hence the term "pseudarth-rosis of the tibia" is used to describe this condition. Protective bracing and surgical treatment may be helpful, but many eventually require amputation because of persistent pseudarthrosis.

Treatment

"Physiologic" genu varum does not usually require treatment unless it persists after age 2 years and either shows no tendency to correct or is actually worsening. This latter condition may require bracing in hip-knee-ankle-foot orthoses (HKAFOs) or knee-ankle-foot orthoses (KAFOs) with no knee joint or a hinged knee joint that can be locked. Surgical correction is sometimes required, although this is rare.

GENU VALGUM

Like genu varum, genu valgum can occasionally persist beyond the age range when one expects the legs to become generally straight. Many of the children with persistent genu valgum are overweight, have an out-toeing foot progression angle, an awkward gait, and flat feet. Genu valgum can be measured by documenting the intermalleolar distance in supine or standing, with the medial aspect of the knees lightly touching each other.

Children with significant femoral anteversion may often appear knock-kneed. Once again, a clear under-standing of the three-level concept of torsional condi-tions and the angular conditions of genu varum and genu valgum is necessary to define the specific problem(s). Krivickas (1997) noted that athletes are predisposed to developing overuse injuries from both extrinsic factors (e.g., training errors) and intrinsic or anatomic factors, such as malalignment of the lower extremities. Genu varum or valgum, along with torsional malalignment, may predispose athletes to knee extensor mechanism injuries, iliotibial band syndrome, stress fractures, and plantar fasciitis. Some adolescents with genu valgum present with anterior knee pain, patellofemoral instabil-ity, circumduction gait, and difficulty running (Stevens et al., 1999a). Genu valgum can also be seen in multiple epiphyseal dysplasia (Miura et al., 2000). Asymmetric genu valgum may result from trauma or fracture of the lateral distal femoral epiphysis.

If severe, physiologic genu valgum can be safely and effectively corrected in the teenage years by stapling of the medial femoral growth plate, and genu varum by stapling of the lateral growth plate (Mielke & Stevens, 1996). This allows the unstapled side of the femoral growth plate to continue growing, and the leg gradually grows into better alignment. A second option for surgical treatment is femoral osteotomy.

▌ FLAT FOOT

The subject of flexible flat feet is a controversial one, with a variety of players: unconcerned children, usually with no foot pain and no disability; concerned parents who frequently were treated in childhood for flat feet and now demand treatment for their child; physical therapists concerned about the abnormal appearance of the foot and ankle and the possible secondary negative effects on the more proximal joints; and various other medical practitioners, some well intended, who provide arch supports that are of dubious benefit and need frequent replacement in a growing child.

CLINICAL EXAMINATION

Children with flexible flat feet have a normal-appearing arch in sitting and when asked to walk "on their toes" in maximum plantar flexion. In standing, however, the longitudinal arch decreases or disappears. This is usually due to greater than normal ligamentous laxity in the foot, and the child will typically demonstrate increased laxity throughout the upper and lower extremities, as evidenced by hyperextension at the elbows and knees and ability to approximate the thumb to the forearm. The fat pad noted in the medial part of the foot in many infants and toddlers contributes to the flat-footed appearance. A wide variation of rate and onset of arch development was noted in 160 children studied by Engel and Staheli (1974). Volpon (1994) documented static footprints on 672 children and found rapid spontaneous plantar arch development between 2 and 6 years of age. An interesting study by Sachithanandam and Joseph (1995) of 1846 skeletally mature individuals in India found a significantly higher prevalence of flatfoot in those who began to wear shoes before 6 years of age. They also noted a higher prevalence of flat foot in obese individuals and those with ligamentous laxity. Another study of 1851 Congolese children noted that at age 3 to 4 years, most feet were flat, but the proportion decreased with age in both sexes, reinforcing the concept of gradual improvement with age (Echarri & Forriol, 2003).

TREATMENT

A great deal of anecdotal evidence but little scientific data are available to support the use of special shoes or arch supports for the treatment of flexible flat feet in children. In a prospective study Wenger and colleagues (1989) concluded that wearing corrective shoes or inserts for 3 years does not alter the natural history of flat foot. They studied 129 children randomly assigned to three groups treated with (1) corrective orthopedic shoes, (2) Helfet heel-cups (Apex Foot Health, South Hackensack, NJ), or (3) custom-molded plastic inserts, with a fourth group as a control. A minimum of 3 years of treatment was completed by 98 patients with documented compliance. All groups showed significant improvement, including

the control group, and there was no significant difference between the control group and the treated patients.

It has been widely documented that a low arch is usually less of a problem in adulthood than high-arched (cavus) feet. Michelson and colleagues (2002) studied 196 college athletes with flat feet, who had 227 episodes of lower extremity (LE) injury. Pes planus was not a risk factor for any LE injury, and they therefore discouraged the use of orthotics to prevent future injury. Hogan and Staheli (2002) studied 99 adult grocery store employees and found no relationship between arch configuration and pain scores.

Most pediatric orthopedists who now counsel parents regarding the natural history of improvement in flat feet through childhood advise the use of a lightweight running shoe as the only recommendation. Using shoes with a good arch support and a strong counter will not correct the flat foot but can help decrease wear on the medial border of shoes, thereby decreasing the expense of frequent shoe purchases.

DIFFERENTIAL DIAGNOSIS

A tendo Achillis contracture can produce a secondary flat foot. Examples of conditions in which this may occur are cerebral palsy, congenital or familial tight heel cords, and muscular dystrophy. A fixed valgus of the hindfoot causing symptoms such as pain, callus, ulceration, poor brace tolerance, and excessive shoe wear can be relieved by tendo Achillis lengthenings and other soft tissue and osseus procedures (Mosca, 1995).

Children occasionally have an extra ossicle located at the medial border of the navicular, called an accessory navicular, frequently associated with flat feet. This condition may become symptomatic in late childhood or early adolescence, resulting in pain over the ossicle and along the medial arch, and can be corrected surgically.

Some children with flat foot have a rigid, painful foot with limited subtalar motion. Some of these children carry the diagnosis of peroneal spastic flat foot because of clonus in the peroneal muscles, and may be referred for physical therapy (Kelo & Riddle, 1998). These children deserve further diagnostic scrutiny and a workup for tarsal coalition, a congenital fibrous, cartilaginous or osseous union of two or more tarsal bones. (See section on causes of limping later in this chapter for more information on this condition.)

■ CLUBFOOT

A condition that may be confused with MTA is the congenital deformity of clubfoot, or talipes equinovarus

(TEV). First described by Hippocrates, idiopathic club-foot is characterized by a complex three-dimensional deformity of the foot. The forefoot in this condition is curved in medially (adducted), the calcaneus is small, the hindfoot is in varus, and there is equinus of the ankle. Ankle valgus may evolve with growth and may be mistaken for "overcorrected clubfoot," or hindfoot valgus (Stevens, 1999b). The talar head is small and slightly flattened, the talocalcaneal angle is decreased, subtalar joint facets are misshapened, and the navicular is medially displaced (Ponseti et al., 1981). The calf and the foot are generally smaller on the involved side. In some children, TEV is just one manifestation of more serious malformations such as myelomeningocele or arthrogryposis.

Cuevas de Alba and colleagues (1998) studied 47 children with 70 clubfeet to determine the degree of femoral, tibial, and total limb torsion in both lower extremities. They found no significant difference in torsion of either the femur or tibia, and noted that external tibial torsion increased with age and femoral anteversion decreased with age, consistent with other studies of children without clubfoot.

Although clubfoot clusters in families, suggesting a strong genetic component, it does not fit typical mendelian inheritance patterns. It may be etiologically or genetically heterogeneous, or it may require a pre-disposing gene active with specific polygenes or environmental influences (Dietz, 2002). Congenital clubfoot occurs in 1 per 1000 live births, with a 2:1 male-to-female ratio (Scoles, 1988; Wynne-Davies, 1964). Loren and colleagues (1998) found congenital muscle fiber type disproportion or fiber size variation in 50% of peroneus brevis muscle biopsies performed at the time of postero-medial release, and those feet with such muscle variation had a significantly greater incidence of recurrent equinovarus deformity.

Treatment consists of manipulation and serial casting, which is most effective if started immediately after birth. This used to be routinely followed by surgical posterior medial release (PMR) performed from 3 months to 1 year of age, depending on the surgeon's preference. Extensive surgical procedures have demonstrated complications, including recurrence, overcorrection, stiffness, and pain. Over the last several years, there has been a resurgence of interest in nonsurgical treatment techniques involving serial manipulation and cast treatment as proposed years ago by Ponseti, followed in some cases by minimally invasive surgery (Cummings et al., 2002). The components of the Ponseti method include manipulation – reducing the talonavicular joint by moving the navicular laterally and the head of the talus medially (Kuhns et al.,

2003). Pirani and associates (2001) used MRI (magnetic resonance imaging) studies to document correction of the relationships of the tarsal bones and also the abnormal shapes of the bones involved.

In a report of their first 27 patients with 34 feet undergoing casting with the Ponseti technique, Herzenberg and colleagues (2002) found only 1 of 34 feet (3%) required PMR compared to their control group, in which 32 (94%) of 34 feet required PMR. These authors now believe that PMR is not required for most cases of idiopathic clubfoot.

Heilig and colleagues (2003) surveyed members of the Pediatric Orthopedic Society of North America (POSNA) regarding treatment options for clubfoot. A total of 416 responses were received (totaling 6125 years in practice), providing information on 8595 clubfeet treated in the past year. Great variability was found but the survey reflected renewed interest in the Ponseti technique. Ippolito and colleagues (2003) reviewed 96 clubfeet in 64 patients followed for 19 to 26 years and found that the group treated with Ponseti's method had better long-term results than the group treated with casting and extensive posteromedial release. Colburn and Williams (2003) used the Ponseti method in treating 57 clubfeet in 34 infants. Fifty-four of 57 clubfeet were successfully corrected *without* posteromedial release, and only 3 feet required extensive surgical correction. They had 6 recurrent cases, believed to be related to lack of compliance with the straight last shoes and foot abduction bar regimen.

BLOUNT'S DISEASE

The first case of infantile tibia vara was reported in 1922, and Blount presented a complete description of the condition in 1937 (Wenger & Rang, 1993). In Blount's disease, increased compressive forces across the medial aspect of the knee cause growth suppression of the proximal tibia physis, resulting in a bowleg deformity (Thompson & Carter, 1990). It can be difficult to differentiate physiologic genu varum from early Blount's disease. Radiographic films of children with Blount's disease show varus angulation centered at the knee, mild metaphyseal beaking (appearance similar to a bird's beak), thickening of the medial tibial cortices, and tilted ankle joints.

In Blount's disease, the characteristic beaking of the medial metaphysis is noted on radiographs, especially in younger children, with depression of the proximal tibia medially (Cheems et al., 2003). In 1952 Langenskiold described six stages of infantile tibia vara based on their radiographic appearance (Langenskiold, 1989). Tibia vara is usually seen in children under 3 years of age, although it may be found in older children. Children with Blount's disease may clinically resemble those with physiologic genu varum, except that they are often obese and also have a lateral thrust of the knee during stance phase of gait. Risk factors for Blount's include ligamentous instability, obesity, or postural asymmetry. Females and children of African-American or Hispanic descent are also at increased risk for Blount's disease (Raney et al., 1998). With obesity now the most prevalent nutritional disease of children and adolescents in the United States, the obese child with Blount's disease faces significant morbidity because the excess weight puts extra stress on long bones and joints (Dietz, 1998).

Blount's disease requires aggressive treatment, with bracing in full HKAFOs worn 23 hours per day recommended for patients under 3 years of age (Johnson, 1990). Surgery may be needed to correct the varus deformity, correct the internal tibial torsion, restore normal joint congruity, and prevent or correct limb length discrepancy (Accadbled, 2003). To ensure the best outcome, surgery should be done before permanent physeal damage has occurred, as shown by Hofmann and colleagues (1982) in their series of 19 knees (12 patients) evaluated at a mean of 12 years after osteotomy. Twelve knees were symptomatic, and 8 of those had early degenerative changes. Poor results were directly correlated to the amount of physeal damage that was present prior to surgery.

DEVELOPMENTAL DYSPLASIA OF THE HIP

The term *developmental dysplasia of the hip* (DDH) is replacing the term *congenital dysplasia of the hip*. The term *DDH* is also used as an abbreviation for developmental dislocation of the hip. The term *developmental dysplasia* includes hips that may have been normal, or were believed to be normal, at birth but subsequently were documented to have dysplasia. Ilfeld and co-workers (1986) noted that delayed diagnosis of dislocation is not evidence that these hips were "missed" by inadequate examinations. They describe a separate entity of the delayed subluxed or dislocated hip, possibly the result of a dynamic process due to an increased acetabular index.

The term *dysplasia* describes abnormal development or growth. Normal muscle balance and a femoral head that is concentric, congruent with, and seated deep within the acetabulum are necessary prerequisites for normal hip development. The concave acetabulum develops in response to a spherical femoral head, and the depth normally increases with growth.

The incidence of hip dysplasia in the United States is 1 per 100 persons for dysplasia or subluxation and 1 per 1000 persons for dislocation (Mubarak et al., 1987). Prompt recognition and treatment of DDH, preferably in the newborn period, provides the best chance for subsequent optimal hip development and a normal hip at skeletal maturity.

The etiology of DDH is thought to be multifactorial. In the early fetal period, measurements of femoral head coverage and acetabular anteversion do not show significant variation through the embryonic and early fetal stages (6 to 20 weeks), and the hip stays well covered (Lee et al., 1992). Dislocated fetal hips tend to appear only in the last trimester.

Factors that predispose an infant to DDH include mechanical, physiologic, and environmental factors. Mechanical factors are a small intrauterine space and tight abdominal wall of a primipara mother, breech presentation, and positioning of the fetal hip against the mother's sacrum in utero (Hensinger & Jones, 1981). Physiologic factors include maternal hormonal influence of estrogen and relaxin and the resulting ligamentous laxity of the female infant (Wynne-Davies, 1970). This is thought to account for the 6:1 female-to-male incidence of DDH. Environmental or cultural factors include strapping the child's lower extremities in extension, such as on a cradle board, noted in the Eskimo and some other Native American cultures. Cultures in which infants are routinely carried with their hips in flexion and wide abduction in cloth slings on the mother's back or astride her hip have a decreased incidence of DDH.

Mechanical factors can act to restrict the position of the head, neck, and feet of the developing fetus, as well as the hips. Problems associated with DDH include a 20% incidence of congenital muscular torticollis (Hummer & MacEwen, 1972), although Walsh and Morrissy (1998) reported that the rate of hip disease in those with torticollis is approximately 8%. A 10% incidence of metatarsus adductus or calcaneovalgus is reported in patients with DDH (Dunn, 1976).

CLINICAL EXAMINATION

Based on a careful clinical examination, newborn hips can be classified as follows (Mubarak et al., 1987):

1. Normal—no instability noted.
2. Subluxatable (9.8/1000) (Tredwell & Bell, 1981)—the femoral head is in the socket but can be partially displaced out to the acetabular rim.
3. Dislocatable (1.3/1000)—the femoral head is

reduced but can be dislocated with a Barlow maneuver.

4. Dislocated but reducible (1.2/1000)—the femoral head is out of the acetabulum at rest but can be reduced with an Ortolani maneuver.

5. Dislocated but not reducible—seldom encountered in the newborn to 2-month-old age group. When seen, this type of dislocation is usually teratologic, occurring before birth, typically from a neuromuscular or musculoskeletal abnormality such as myelomeningocele or arthrogryposis.

Clinical examination includes documentation of the ROM of hip abduction in flexion. Most infants have 75° to 90° of abduction. Significant limitation or an asymmetry of even 5° to 10° may indicate hip dysplasia and warrants further workup. Other clinical findings may include asymmetric thigh folds, pistoning, apparent (not true) femoral shortening with uneven knee heights (positive Galeazzi sign), and positive Barlow or Ortolani signs (Fig. 17-3). Hip "clicks" are usually not clinically significant. The experienced examiner can distinguish between hip clicks and the characteristic "clunk" felt during the Barlow maneuver as a hip dislocates. Kane and associates (2003) studied 171 infants with 193 clicking hips and found that those with hip clicks and a normal hip ultrasound examination on initial assessment had a normal radiograph at 6 months of age.

The infant must be completely relaxed for the Barlow and Ortolani maneuvers to have reliable diagnostic value. Even slight muscular contraction around the hip can obscure the instability and negate the examination. These two signs of hip instability usually will disappear by 2 to 3 months of age, because the hip either improves in stability and stays in the socket or becomes fixed in a dislocated position. Often, limited hip abduction is the only clinical sign of hip dysplasia in the infant older than 1 month. It continues to be the most reliable clinical finding in older infants and toddlers with dysplasia. Further diagnostic studies are warranted if there are positive findings on clinical examination and even with a normal clinical examination but a high index of suspicion because of multiple risk factors, such as a female first-born child with breech presentation and a family history of DDH.

The use of ultrasonography to examine infant hips is routine in Europe (Graf, 1992) and is now fairly standard practice in the United States. It is more accurate and helpful than radiographs in diagnosing DDH in infants. Ultrasonography is most useful in the newborn and in infants up to 3 to 6 months of age, before the femoral head starts to ossify and obscure the structures deep to it. It may have some usefulness in detecting DDH in children up to 1 year of age (Harcke, 1992). The secondary ossification center is present in 80% of children at age 6 months (Scoles et al., 1987). Ultrasonography allows assessment of the cartilaginous structures not visualized on plain radiographs and allows stress testing (to document instability), with the additional advantage of no

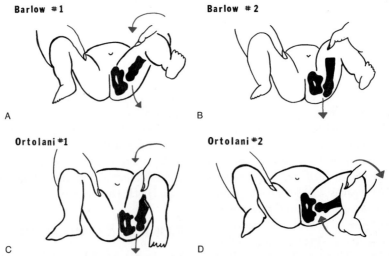

Barlow #1

A

Barlow #2

B

Ortolani #1

C

Ortolani #2

D

◆ **Figure 17-3   A** and **B**, Barlow maneuver: the hip is first flexed and abducted, then gradually adducted with pressure exerted in a posterior direction. Dislocation of the femoral head over the posterior acetabular rim indicates an unstable hip. The head may slide to the edge of the socket (subluxatable) or may dislocate out of the acetabulum (dislocatable). **C** and **D**, Ortolani test: In the Ortolani positive hip, the hip is dislocated in a position of flexion and adduction. Gentle flexion, abduction, and slight traction (the Ortolani maneuver) reduce the hip. A positive Ortolani sign indicates a more unstable hip than a positive Barlow sign. *(From Mubarak, SJ, Leach, J, & Wenger, DR. Management of congenital dislocation of the hip in the infant. Contemporary Orthopaedics, 15:29–44, 1987.)*

radiation exposure. It is a useful tool not only in the diagnosis, but also in the management of DDH, documenting reduction of the dislocated hip in the Pavlik harness (Taylor & Clarke, 1997) and providing information on the status of the hip to aid decisions on altering or stopping treatment. Ultrasonography is superior to radiography for assessing hip position in the harness. Song and Lapinsky (2000) found that hip ultrasound findings agreed with clinical examination in 100% of hips in their study. Provision of ultrasound in pediatric orthopedic offices is has been shown to be efficient, cost effective, and convenient for parents and the treating physician (Davids et al., 1995).

The use of ultrasound screening for DDH in newborns has been studied, especially in Europe. Rosendahl and colleagues (1994) completed a randomized, controlled trial of 11,925 newborns and found no significant reduction in the prevalence of late DDH in the screened group compared with the unscreened group. Donaldson and Feinstein (1997) support targeting high-risk infants for supplemental ultrasound screening as being effective and less expensive than generalized screening.

Radiographs, rather than ultrasound, are used for older infants. Because of the need for a radiograph of the uninvolved side for comparison, and because of the frequency of bilateral involvement, the standard radiograph is an anterior-posterior view of the pelvis. Many parameters of hip development can be measured on hip radiographs (Hensinger & Jones, 1981). Scoles and colleagues (1987) studied 50 boys and 50 girls at each of six age levels: 3, 6, 9, 12, 18, and 24 months. They documented a decrease in acetabular index with age and concluded that this was a helpful parameter in following hip development (Fig. 17-4). J. T. Smith and colleagues (1997) proposed that appearance of the teardrop is the earliest radiographic sign that a stable, concentric reduction of the hip has been achieved. Hips can be classified radiographically as acetabular dysplasia (without subluxation or dislocation); subluxated, with associated acetabular dysplasia; and dislocated.

Between 18 and 24 months of age children with hip dislocation usually have an abnormal gait. With unilateral dislocation the child will limp, demonstrating a positive Trendelenburg sign on the involved side in the stance phase of gait. With bilateral dislocation the child will have a waddling gait.

TREATMENT

Birth to 9 Months

The Pavlik harness was first described by Dr. Arnold Pavlik, who originally called his treatment device

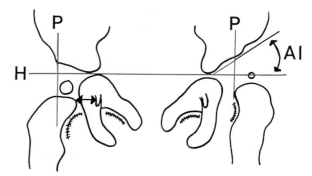

Figure 17-4 Radiographic parameters of hip development involve use of the Hilgenreiner line (*H*) and Perkin's line (*P*) to document proximal and lateral migration of the femoral head, with disruption of Shenton's line (*crosshatched line*). The acetabular index (AI) is the most helpful documentation of acetabular development. In the drawing above, the AI of the left hip is increased, documenting acetabular dysplasia, and Shenton's line is broken, indicating subluxation of the left hip. *(From Mubarak, SJ, Leach, J, & Wenger, DR. Management of congenital dislocation of the hip in the infant. Contemporary Orthopaedics, 15:29–44, 1987.)*

"stirrups." Modifications have been made in the design of the device, but the principles of treatment and the requirements of the harness remain essentially the same as described by him over 50 years ago (Pavlik, 1950). He stressed that one of the main advantages of the harness over casts was that it allowed active motion, thereby decreasing the incidence of avascular necrosis (AVN) of the femoral head (Pavlik, 1957).

The Pavlik harness restricts hip extension and adduction and allows the hips to be maintained in flexion and abduction, the "protective position" (Fig. 17-5). Studies with newborn pigs found that maintaining the hips in extension precipitated hip dislocation (Salter, 1968). The position of flexion and abduction enhances normal acetabular development, and the kicking motion allowed in this "human" position (not as radical as the "frog" position) stretches the contracted hip adductors and promotes spontaneous reduction of the dislocated hip. Because of the biologic plasticity of growing bone, positioning the hip in flexion/abduction can promote acetabular development.

Complications of use of the Pavlik harness include AVN of the femoral head, femoral nerve palsy, inferior dislocation, and erosion of the posterior rim of the acetabulum. Essentially all these complications can be avoided by using a Pavlik harness of proper design, educating the caregiver to apply it correctly, and monitoring the status of the hip carefully over the entire treatment period (Mubarak et al., 1981). The prognosis with Pavlik harness

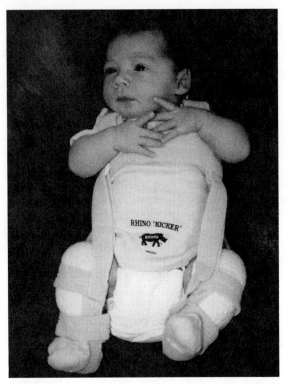

• **Figure 17-5** The Pavlik harness can be used to reduce a dislocated hip, to stabilize a lax hip, and to treat acetabular dysplasia.

treatment is excellent with 90% to 95% success in cases of subluxation and dysplasia and approximately 85% success in cases of dislocation (Fig. 17-6). Cashman and colleagues (2002) studied 332 babies with 546 dysplastic hips treated with a Pavlik harness. The harness failed to reduce 18 hips in 16 patients; (15.2% of the dislocated hips and 3.3% of those with acetabular dysplasia).

If a brief trial (up to 3 weeks) with the Pavlik harness is not successful in reducing a dislocated hip, surgical treatment is indicated. This may include a period of 2 to 3 weeks of traction to reduce the incidence of AVN of the femoral head. Home traction is a safe, effective, and much less expensive alternative to the 2- to 3-week admission required for hospital traction (Mubarak et al., 1986). Surgery includes an arthrogram to define the anatomic landmarks of the femoral head and acetabulum and to detect the presence of soft tissue (pulvinar) interposition between the head and acetabulum; adductor tenotomy; closed or (if necessary) open reduction of the hip; and application of a spica cast. Luhmann and colleagues (2003) reported that delaying reduction of a dislocated hip until the appearance of the ossific nucleus more than doubled the need for future reconstructive procedures.

Age 9 Months and Older

In infants older than 9 months of age who are beginning to walk independently, an abduction orthosis should be considered as an alternative to the Pavlik harness for treatment of acetabular dysplasia with or without subluxation. This orthosis should be designed so the child can walk while in the orthosis. For dislocatable or dislocated hips diagnosed in the 6- to 18-month age group, surgical treatment in the form of closed reduction is usually required. Treatment falls into a gray zone in the 18- to 24-month age group, when either open or closed reduction may be used. Olney and colleagues (1998) used a one-stage procedure combining open reduction and pelvic and femoral osteotomies with success in patients ranging in age from 15 to 117 months.

The diagnosis of hip dislocation in the child age 2 years or older is generally considered to mandate open reduction, because the results of closed reduction are not predictable in these older children. Instead of prior traction, femoral shortening (in which a segment of the femoral shaft is removed) is often used (Galpin et al., 1989) to reduce the compressive forces on the femoral head once it is reduced back into the acetabulum. Wenger and colleagues (1995) described special circumstances in which femoral shortening may also be used in the child younger than 2 years. Older children with continuing acetabular dysplasia will benefit from a pelvic osteotomy, as the remodeling potential of the acetabulum decreases with age. Children 3 to 8 years of age can be treated with an acetabular reshaping osteotomy (e.g., a Pemberton or San Diego osteotomy). In the 8- to 10-year-old group, a triple innominate osteotomy is usually indicated. After age 14 to 15 years, when the triradiate cartilage is closed, the Ganz periacetabular osteotomy is effective (Wenger & Bomar, 2003). Three-dimensional computed tomographic analysis (3-D CT) helps define the nature and degree of acetabular and femoral deformity and can be used to evaluate the results of the surgery (Kim & Wenger, 1997a; BG Smith et al., 1997).

A number of children with acetabular dysplasia are never diagnosed as infants or toddlers. With mild dysplasia, they will walk without a limp, have essentially normal hip ROM, and can actively participate in all childhood activities, including sports. However, the hip is like a tire that is out of alignment—you can drive on it for quite a few miles, but uneven wear will occur. The dysplastic hip, especially the one with subluxation, also develops uneven wear with subsequent articular cartilage damage. The person may develop degenerative arthritis, hip pain, and limp as early as the late teens. Very mild dysplasia may go undetected for many decades and be diagnosed later in life when the patient develops degene-

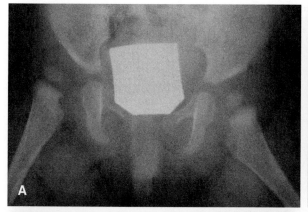

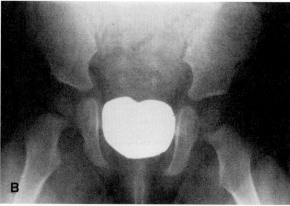

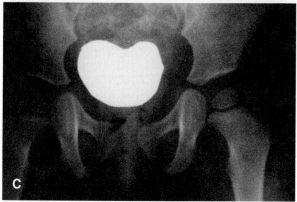

✦ **Figure 17-6**   **A**, Age 4 months: right hip dislocated, severe acetabular dysplasia. **B**, Age 7 months: treated with a Pavlik harness for 3 months full time. Right hip is reduced; continued acetabular dysplasia. Patient continued Pavlik harness treatment for 3 more months, part time (night and naps only). **C**, Age 15 months: both hips centered in the acetabulae with good acetabular development bilaterally.

rative hip joint disease. The age at symptom onset in untreated patients with subluxation is variable, with the mean in the mid-30s for women and the mid-50s for men (Weinstein, 1992). Many middle-aged adults requiring total hip replacement had DDH that was never diagnosed and treated or was treated in childhood without full resolution. A number of studies have documented the association of osteoarthritis (OA) in adults who have residual hip dysplasia (Michaeli et al., 1997) and the increased technical difficulties of total hip arthroplasty with high acetabular component failure rates (Jasty et al., 1995). However, the results of Lane and colleagues (1997) did not support the hypothesis that mild acetabular dysplasia accounts for a substantial proportion of hip OA in adult women.

CAUSES OF LIMPING IN CHILDREN

The acute onset of limp in a child can present a diagnostic dilemma. In this section chronic causes of limp, such as those due to muscle weakness, are not discussed. A review of conditions that cause acute limping will provide an overview of a wide range of orthopedic conditions affect-

ing children. Some are transitory and benign, whereas others can result in lifelong disability, especially if not treated promptly and effectively. A clinical decision tree, as shown in Figure 17-7, is useful in identifying those problems that need immediate medical or surgical attention.

HISTORY AND PHYSICAL EXAMINATION

A careful workup is required when a child has a limp. A detailed history must be taken, including a description of any recent illness or injury that may be related. The examiner should be aware, however, that children do fall frequently and that parents may relate the onset of the limp to a fall or other injury that often turns out to be unrelated. Physical examination includes observational gait analysis, which usually will indicate which leg is involved and perhaps even the location within the leg. An example of an antalgic gait deviation is the Trendelenburg sign, a lean toward the involved side in the stance phase, usually caused by a hip problem. A "sore foot gait" describes a decreased stance time on the involved side and decreased roll-off. This usually results from a problem in the foot, ankle, or lower leg, for example, a toddler's fracture of the tibia.

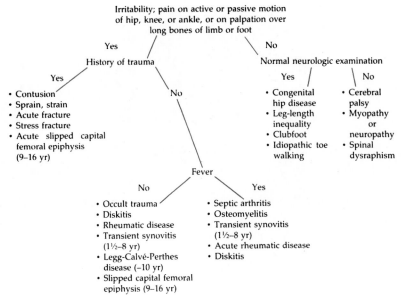

Figure 17-7 A clinical decision tree for children with a limp. *(From Scoles, PV. Pediatric Orthopedics in Clinical Practice, 2nd ed. St. Louis: Mosby, 1988, p. 21.)*

The physical examination should include a complete assessment of the spine, hips, thighs, knees, lower legs, ankles, and feet, including the uninvolved side for comparison. ROM, strength, presence of muscle atrophy, swelling, redness, increased warmth, and pain to palpation must all be assessed. The way in which a child performs functional activities, such as moving from the floor to standing, crawling, and achieving a comfortable sitting position, can provide important information. For example, a child may refuse to walk because of pain but may crawl easily, indicating that the problem is probably in the lower part of the leg rather than the hip or knee. A child may be able to walk short distances with no significant gait deviations but be reluctant to walk because of pain and may move into the seated position with difficulty and sit with a rigidly fixed spine, indicating a problem in the back, such as diskitis.

OTHER DIAGNOSTIC TESTS

In addition to a careful clinical examination, additional tests are often indicated. Radiographs can document fractures or other bony abnormalities, although some occult fractures are not identifiable on radiography until 10 to 14 days after onset, when a repeat radiograph may document callus formation. Laboratory examination of blood samples provides information regarding the presence of infection or other acute processes. The erythrocyte sedimentation rate (ESR) and C-reactive protein (CRP) can indicate the presence of acute inflammation,

as well as response to treatment. More complex diagnostic studies may also be needed to define the problem or evaluate treatment efficacy. These studies include bone scans, MRI (for soft tissue), and CT (for bony structures).

Many causes of limp in children are easily treated on a routine basis, and some require no treatment beyond observation. Many are age dependent in part, and certain common diagnoses are seen most frequently within one of three age groups: birth to 5 years, 5 to 10 years, and 10 to 15 years. Two common causes of limp can occur in any age group: soft tissue injuries (e.g., contusions, ligament and tendon injuries) and fractures. Spine injury or disease may also cause a limp, at any age, with diskitis being the most common pediatric spinal infection (Glazer & Hu, 1996).

COMMON DIAGNOSES BY AGE GROUP

Birth to Age 5 Years

Osteomyelitis. Osteomyelitis is an infection of a bone by bacterial organisms, including *Staphylococcus aureus* and *Haemophilus influenzae* type b (Brook, 2002). In children, osteomyelitis is usually seen in the metaphyseal area. In some cases, the infection starts in the bony metaphysis and spreads to the adjacent joint, creating a septic arthritis. Perlman and colleagues (2000) found 42% of patients with osteomyelitis had evidence of adjacent joint involvement, either septic or nonseptic. Osteomyelitis can be extremely and rapidly destructive, causing permanent damage that can have lifelong consequences for the child. The most common sites of infection are the distal femur and proximal tibia. The origin of the infection is usually hematogenous (blood-borne) and the portal of entry is usually through the skin, secondary to infected scratches, boils, or sore throat (Salter, 1970). Osteomyelitis may occasionally result from an open fracture, a penetrating injury, or something as benign as a stubbed toe (Kensinger et al., 2001). For example, lawn mower injuries can result in multiple complications, including osteomyelitis (Loder et al., 1997) and these injuries are estimated to be 85% preventable by the Research Committee of POSNA.

The child with osteomyelitis can present with a high fever, chills, severe pain, swelling, and tenderness over the metaphysis of the involved bone. In this age group, the child may refuse to walk. Newborns and children with osteomyelitis of the smaller bones tend to be less sick, with fewer symptoms. The leukocyte count and ESR are usually elevated but occasionally are normal. A bone scan is positive early, but needle aspiration may be diagnostic in only about 60% of children (Hughes & Aronson, 1994). Sonography can be useful in early diagnosis with findings of intra-articular fluid collection or subperiosteal abscess formation preceding radiographic changes (Riebel et al., 1996). Radiographs are usually normal initially, with early bone destruction not demonstrated until 7 to 14 days after onset. Subperiosteal new bone formation indicates periosteal stripping with formation of subperiosteal pus; at this stage, the cortex is already dead. Cross-sectional imaging, particularly MRI, provides better characterization of the extent of the disease (Kleinman, 2002). MRI and a heightened awareness of this condition have led to earlier detection and resultant marked decreases in morbidity and mortality rates (Song & Sloboda, 2001). Sequential intravenous and high-dose oral antibiotic therapy are accepted interventions.

Acute hematogenous osteomyelitis can be fatal as a result of overwhelming septicemia, and treatment must be instituted on an emergency basis. It consists of aspiration, antibiotics, and immobilization of the affected part, and possibly surgical decompression if gross purulence is identified. Surgical drainage is usually required when the diagnosis is delayed. Delayed treatment may be lifesaving by controlling the septicemia but may be ineffective in controlling progression of the pathologic process within the bone.

Chronic recurrent multifocal osteomyelitis (CRMO) is a particularly difficult problem, and may cause bone pain, swelling, malaise, fever, and permanent deformity (Duffy et al., 2002). In a review by Huber and colleagues (2002) of 23 patients with a median of 13 years since diagnosis, 78% had no or minimal physical disability.

However, 26% still had active disease and 26% continued to have pain as a result of CRMO.

Septic Arthritis. Septic arthritis (pyogenic arthritis) is defined as an infection of a joint caused by bacterial organisms. This is an extremely threatening condition, because a joint may be destroyed within 48 hours of onset of symptoms. Septic arthritis causes destruction of articular cartilage and long-term growth arrest. The resulting deformities may be permanent and have a wide-ranging, lifelong impact affecting the person's gait, participation in sports, and choice of occupation and leisure activities.

Staphylococcus aureus is the most common organism (Bennett & Namnyak, 1992), and *Haemophilus influenzae* may also be seen in children younger than 3 years of age. Gonococcal arthritis can occur in sexually active adolescents. The organism enters the joint by hematogenous spread (e.g., from an ear infection), direct spread (from adjacent osteomyelitis), or direct inoculation (from a foreign body, needle, or surgical penetration of a joint). An increased incidence of septic arthritis in children with human immunodeficiency virus (HIV) infection has been noted (Hughes & Aronson, 1994). The hip joint is the most commonly involved in this age group, followed by the knee. Septic arthritis of the hip is particularly devastating in the newborn, because the cartilaginous femoral head can be completely destroyed, requiring salvage procedures later in life (Dobbs et al., 2003). Even milder cases have potentially lifelong effects because the increased intra-articular pressure can occlude the blood supply to the femoral head, causing AVN.

The child usually has acute onset of irritability, fever to 104°F (40°C), refusal to move the affected limb, and a warm, swollen joint held in flexion. Laboratory data show an elevated leukocyte count and ESR, although CRP has been shown to be a better independent predictor of disease (Levine et al., 2003). Radiographs and ultrasound examination may show a distended joint capsule. In older children and adolescents there tends to be a more subtle clinical presentation. These patients often do walk and will allow motion. Subjective discomfort and febrile episodes can be prolonged. The incidence of AVN is higher in the older age group (Dales & Hoffinger, 1993). Interestingly, newborns may also have few clinical symptoms, and severe systemic symptoms are rarely seen. Local signs of warmth, swelling, and tenderness may be present. Usually the newborn is unwilling to use an extremity, described as "pseudoparalysis of infancy" (Hensinger & Jones, 1981). Treatment of septic arthritis consists of immediate aspiration and drainage and intravenous administration of antibiotics. Kocher and associates (2003) noted that clinical practice guidelines are a central precept of evidence-based medicine. They developed guidelines for treating septic arthritis of the hip, and then compared a historical control group of 30 children with a prospective cohort group of 30 treated under the practice guidelines. They found less variation in the process of care, improved efficiency of care, but no significant differences in outcome for the two groups.

Transient Synovitis. Transient synovitis (also known as toxic synovitis) is probably the most common cause of a painful hip in children younger than 10 years of age. In the early stages it can be difficult to distinguish from septic arthritis. This condition affects males more than females, in a 4:1 ratio. The child has gradual or acute onset of limp. There may be occasional periods when the child refuses to walk. The child usually complains of mild to moderate hip pain but may complain of knee pain, because hip pain is often referred to the knee. Mild fever may be present, with normal leukocyte count and ESR. The cause is unclear, but often a history can be elicited of a recent upper respiratory tract infection or other illness. The treatment is symptomatic, consisting of limitation of activity, bed rest, and use of crutches if the child is old enough to manage them. Symptoms usually resolve in about 7 days. Occasionally a child will have recurrent hip synovitis, and a small percentage of these patients later develop Legg-Calvé-Perthes disease.

Occult Fractures. Occult fracture is usually a benign condition causing a limp in children. A commonly seen example is a hairline fracture of the tibia called a toddler's fracture. The child usually refuses to walk or walks with a limp, has no history of significant trauma, and has no fever or signs of infection. Laboratory data are normal, and radiographs of the painful area are usually normal initially. The child can be treated with a splint or cast for comfort and observed closely for signs of incipient infection. If an occult fracture is present, radiographs in 10 to 14 days often show evidence of callus (new bone formation) and the diagnosis can be confirmed in retrospect.

Kohler Syndrome. Kohler syndrome is an osteochondrosis affecting the navicular bone, usually occurring in children between ages 2 and 9 years. It was first described by Alban Kohler, a German radiologist (Wenger & Rang, 1993). The child usually has localized pain in the area of the navicular bone and a limp. Radiographic changes are characteristic, with the navicular being sclerotic and small compared with the opposite side. All these cases resolve with time. Children with limited ambulation as a result of severe pain may be best managed with a brief period of casting.

Other orthopedic conditions that can cause an acute limp in children from birth to age 5 years include juvenile rheumatoid arthritis (see Chapter 9), nonaccidental trauma (fractures or soft tissue injuries), hemophilia (see Chapter 10), diskitis, discoid meniscus, popliteal cysts, foreign bodies, and bone tumors.

Ages 5 to 10 Years

Various types of osteochondroses are common causes of limp in the 5- to 10-year-old age group and in the 10- to 15-year-old age group. These are idiopathic conditions (of unknown cause) characterized by a disorder of endochondral ossification. Many may be microtrauma fractures or growth plate injuries not appreciated on plain radiographs. They may be due to repetitive trauma with weight bearing (Lovell & Winter, 1978).

Legg-Calvé-Perthes Disease. Legg-Calvé-Perthes disease (LCPD) is a condition in children who may be referred to physical therapy for treatment of the resulting muscle weakness, ROM limitations, and gait deviations. It was initially described in the early 1900s by three separate authors, Arthur T. Legg in the United States, Georg Perthes in Germany, and Jacques Calvé in France, and is defined as AVN of the ossific nucleus of the femoral head caused by loss of blood supply. The medial femoral circumflex artery is the principal vessel in the complex vascular distribution in the neck and head of the femur.

LCPD usually occurs in children between ages 3 and 12 and most commonly in boys ages 5 to 7 years (Wenger et al., 1991). The male-to-female ratio is 4:1 (Catteral, 1971). These children are frequently small for their age, with retarded bone age (Loder et al., 1995a), are very active, and have a high incidence of learning disabilities (Lahdes-Vasama et al., 1997). The disease is bilateral in 20% of cases. The exact cause is unknown, but it occasionally follows repeated episodes of transient synovitis of the hip. There may be a number of pathologic processes that cause an interruption of the blood flow in vessels ascending the femoral neck, including increased joint pressure secondary to synovitis. There is a relationship of LCPD to parental cigarette smoking during pregnancy, hypofibrinolysis, and thrombophilia (Glueck et al., 1997, 1998). The risk of LCPD in children exposed to second-hand smoke is more than five times higher than in children not exposed (Mata et al., 2000). Gaughan and colleagues (2002) found that similar to adults with HIV who have an increased risk of osteonecrosis of the hip, children with perinatal HIV infections also have an increased risk for LCPD. They recommended that clinicians be alert to this diagnosis when children with HIV present with a limp or hip pain.

The disease is self-limiting and always heals spontaneously in 1 to 3 years' time, as the femoral head revascularizes (Catterall, 1971). Many but not all patients have good clinical outcomes, with good hip ROM and no pain with activity. Prognostic factors include age at onset (younger children tend to do better), extent of the disease, the amount of femoral head deformity, and the amount of incongruity between the femoral head and acetabulum, because hip joint growth and development depends on a well-located, centered, and spherical femoral head (Weinstein, 1997).

Patients tend to have a limp and frequently have a positive Trendelenburg sign resulting from pain or hip abduction weakness. Limited hip ROM is noted, especially in hip abduction and internal rotation. The child complains of pain in the groin, hip, or knee (referred pain). Children who have knee pain may have multiple radiographs of both knees and may be referred to physical therapy for treatment of their "knee pain" (Tippett, 1994). A careful clinical examination and observational gait analysis usually provide the information needed to avoid this situation, with clear indication that the problem is in the hip, not the knee. The radiographic findings reflect the temporary interruption of blood flow, with necrosis, possible subchondral fracture, collapse of the femoral head, and then regeneration of bone in the secondary ossification center. The radiographic "sagging rope" sign results from a portion of the femoral head (false head) protruding anterolaterally and inferiorly (Kim et al., 1995). Two commonly used methods of grading the femoral head changes radiographically are the Catterall grouping (Catterall, 1971) and the Herring lateral pillar classification (Herring et al., 1992), which has been found to be a better predictor of final outcome (Farsetti et al., 1995; Ismail & Macnicol, 1998).

Controversy exists regarding the appropriate treatment for LCPD, or whether treatment is even necessary. The goal of treatment is to maintain the spherical shape of the femoral head (because it may tend to flatten if left untreated) and to prevent extrusion of the enlarged femoral head (coxa magna) from the joint. Treatment is based on the principle of "containment," preserving the contour of the femoral head and keeping it centered in the acetabulum during the active phase of the disease to prevent premature degenerative arthritis. If the entire femoral head cannot be contained, it is still important to obtain and maintain hip motion, especially hip abduction, and to relieve the commonly seen hinge abduction (Reinker, 1996).

Treatment methods include observation only, ROM exercises, bracing, Petrie casts (two long leg casts with a bar between, holding the hips abducted and internally rotated), and surgery (Wang et al., 1995). Proximal femoral varus derotation osteotomy (VDRO) decompresses the femoral head, centers it more deeply in the acetabulum when the limb is in the weight-bearing position, and allows long-term remodeling (Eckerwall et al., 1997; Wenger et al., 1991). A pelvic osteotomy may be used alone or combined with VDRO for certain patients (e.g., with a femoral head so large or subluxated that femoral osteotomy alone will not contain the head). A prophylactic trochanteric arrest is often performed to prevent trochanteric overgrowth and the resulting hip abductor muscle weakness (Matan et al., 1996). Kim and Wenger (1997b, 1997c) described the concept of "functional retroversion" and "functional coxa vara" of the deformed femoral head in severe LCPD and discussed the use of valgus-flexion-internal rotation femoral osteotomy and acetabuloplasty for correction. Bankes and colleagues (2000) described the use of valgus extension osteotomy as a salvage procedure for "hinge abduction" to relieve pain and correct deformity.

Discoid Lateral Meniscus. The lateral meniscus can develop an abnormal discoid shape, possibly a congenital deviation or possibly caused by hypermobility, because the more firmly attached medial meniscus rarely develops this discoid shape. A discoid lateral meniscus may become symptomatic, usually between ages 4 and 12 years (Scoles, 1988). It can cause pain, locking, or clicking of the knee, "giving way," and limp. Twenty-five percent of patients have unilateral symptoms but bilateral discoid menisci, and many symptomatic knees also have a meniscal tear (Connolly et al., 1996). In an MRI study of 1250 knees, Rohren and colleagues (2001) found 56 patients with a discoid lateral meniscus, 71% of whom had one or more meniscal tears compared with 54% of the comparison group. In severe cases, meniscectomy generally resulted in good outcomes (Washington et al., 1995).

Sever Disease. Sever disease, or calcaneal apophysitis, is an osteochondrosis caused by trauma (e.g., traction of the tendo Achillis). This results in the fragmentation or avulsion of cartilage at the point of attachment, disruption of chondrogenesis, reparative callus, fibrosis, and ossification (Siffert, 1981). The child usually has pain in the heel area, exacerbated by sports and especially by running. The condition is usually self-limiting. It may be treated symptomatically with rest, ice, heel cups, heel lifts, reduced activity, and tendo Achillis stretching exercises. A short leg walking cast may be used to relieve severe pain.

Growing Pains. "Growing pains" is a diagnosis frequently made by parents and probably represents pain from a musculoskeletal origin that is manifested in children when increased stresses occur in the musculo-skeletal system, often during periods of rapid growth. Growing pains is a diagnosis of exclusion; that is, all other more serious conditions must be ruled out. The child usually has aching in the legs (typically bilateral and generalized), usually at night and after high levels of activity during the day. Reassurance, symptomatic treatment such as massage and acetaminophen, and time usually resolve the symptoms. The child should be evaluated further if the pain increases or becomes local-ized or if other symptoms such as chronic fatigue appear.

Transient hip synovitis, described in the birth to age 5 years section, can also be seen in this older age group.

Ages 10 to 15 Years

Slipped Capital Femoral Epiphysis. Ambroise Pare first described slipped capital femoral epiphysis (SCFE) in 1572. SCFE (also called epiphysiolysis) occurs when the growth plate of the proximal femoral physis is weak and becomes displaced ("slips") from its normal position. This disorder is classified into three subtypes:

1. Acute: occurs with significant trauma and causes immediate, severe pain and restricted hip abduction and internal rotation.
2. Acute-on-chronic: the patient has already expe-rienced some aching in the hip, thigh, or knee for weeks or even months as a result of a chronic slip. Then, with a significant trauma, the epiphysis suddenly slips farther and acute symptoms are noted.
3. Chronic: in this most common form the child has a history of limp and pain, often for weeks or months, and loss of hip motion, especially internal rotation and abduction.

The cause of SCFE is unclear, although many consider it to be part of a generalized metabolic disorder of puberty. It is thought to involve a mechanical failure of the growth plate to resist displacement (Weiner, 1996). It is probably due to alterations in hormonal balance, with or without the stress imposed by acute trauma or the chronic shearing stresses of weight bearing. The incidence of SCFE is 0.71 to 3.41 per 100,000 (Scoles, 1988). African-Americans are more frequently affected than Caucasians. Loder (1995a, 1995b) reported on an international multicenter study of 1630 children with 1993 slips. Frequency of slips in various populations worldwide was reviewed, and Loder even noted seasonal variations—in children living north of 40°N latitude, slips occurred more often in the summer months. Males were more often affected than females, with a 2:1 to 3:1 male-to-female ratio (Scoles, 1988). Onset of SCFE is closely related to the onset of puberty in males. Slips are bilateral in one quarter to one third of cases (Hurley et al., 1996) and may be more common in younger (11 years, 7 months or less) than older boys (Stasikelis et al., 1996). Obesity is reported in as many as 75% of patients. There is also an association of SCFE in patients with endocrine disorders (Loder et al., 1995), renal failure, and secondary hyperparathyroidism; these slips are usually stable and bilateral (Loder & Hensinger, 1997). Oppenheim and associates (2003), noted slip stabilization in 14 of 16 operated hips in patients with renal disease, but one patient with inadequate disease control had slip progression.

The patient usually has an antalgic limp and pain in the groin, often referred to the anteromedial aspect of the thigh and knee. As with other hip disorders, patients may have only thigh or knee pain (15% according to Matava et al., 1999) and may be referred to a physical therapist for treatment. Knowledge of SCFE and a high index of suspicion will facilitate prompt referral by the physical therapist to an orthopedic surgeon (Pellecchia et al., 1996). The leg is usually held in ER, both when supine and when standing. Decreased hip motion is noted in flexion, abduction, and IR. With attempts to flex the hip, the leg moves into ER.

Radiographs demonstrate that the initial displacement is usually posterior and inferior and therefore may be missed on an anterior-posterior view. A "frog" view of both hips is needed for diagnosis. Slips are classified as grade I (displacement of the femoral head up to one third of the width of the femoral neck), grade II (more than one third but less than one half), and grade III (more than one half) (Fig. 17-8). MRI has been found to delineate physeal changes preslip, as well as SCFE, sometimes earlier than radiographs and CT (Umans et al., 1998).

The goals of treatment are to keep the displacement to a minimum, maintain motion, and delay or prevent premature degenerative arthritis. Treatment is by surgical fixation, using one or two pins or screws, usually in situ (Crawford, 1996) (Fig. 17-9). Percutaneous pin fixation of chronic slips is safe and effective (Rostoucher et al., 1996; Samuelson & Olney, 1996). With higher degrees of slip, the procedure becomes more technically difficult and the incidence of pin penetration into the joint increases, leading to an increased incidence of chondrolysis (Aronson et al., 1992). Chondrolysis (acute cartilage necrosis of the femoral capital epiphysis) is a severe complication of treated and untreated SCFE with no completely successful treatment (Lubicky, 1996; Warner

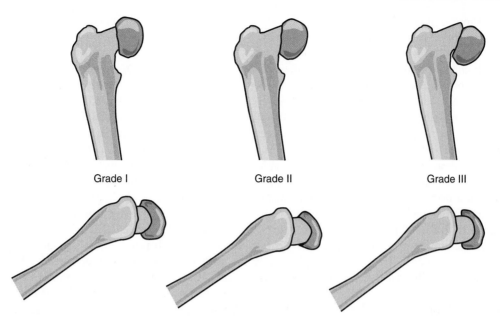

Grade I   Grade II   Grade III

♦ **Figure 17-8**   Three grades of slipped capital femoral epiphysis. Slips are classified as grade I (displacement of the femoral head up to one third of the width of the femoral neck), grade II (more than one third but less than one half), and grade III (more than one half).

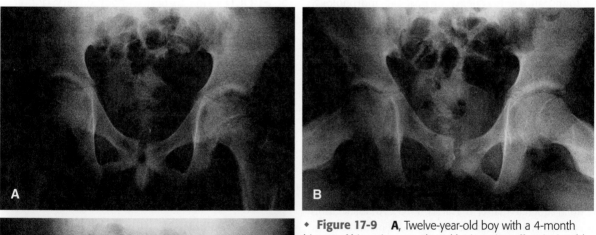

♦ **Figure 17-9**   **A**, Twelve-year-old boy with a 4-month history of hip pain, exacerbated by jumping off a picnic table 2 days previously. The slipped capital femoral epiphysis is not clearly identified on the anterior-posterior view. **B**, Frog view demonstrates a slipped capital femoral epiphysis on the left, thought to be an acute-on-chronic slip by history. **C**, Treatment with percutaneous pin fixation was successful.

et al., 1996). There is also a significant danger of AVN with severe and acute slips (Rattey et al., 1996), especially if a forceful reduction is attempted, if reduction is attempted with chronic slips, or if treatment is delayed past 24 hours (Gordon et al., 2002). However, Peterson and colleagues (1997) found no increased risk of AVN with manipulative reduction in acute slips, with a 7% incidence in hips reduced less than 24 hours after presentation to a care provider. In a series of 240 patients, Tokmakova and colleagues (2003) found the only cases of osteonecrosis (21) had presented with an unstable slip. They found a decreased risk of osteonecrosis with pinning in situ with a single cannulated screw. In unilateral cases, the contralateral hip may be stabilized prophylactically (Hagglund, 1996; Kumm et al., 1996; Seller et al., 2001).

Even though surgically stabilized, most hips with SCFE develop some degenerative changes in later life, especially those with higher-grade slips, along with the complications of chondrolysis and AVN. These changes can affect the person's choice of occupation and recreational activities as an adult and cause secondary impairments, including hip pain. Goodman and colleagues (1997) examined hip joints in 2665 adult human skeletons and found an 8% prevalence of post-slip morphology. They determined that it was a major risk factor for development of OA, unrelated to age. The most severely involved patients may require hip arthrodesis as a salvage procedure (Schoenecker et al., 1997). This provides a good example (along with DDH and LCPD) of how a developmental condition in childhood can cause disability later in life.

Osgood-Schlatter Syndrome. Osgood-Schlatter disease, or syndrome, is characterized by activity-related pain and swelling at the insertion of the patellar tendon on the tibial tubercle caused by minor degrees of separation of the tibial tubercle (Salter & Harris, 1963). An association with patella alta has been demonstrated. This increase in patellar height requires an increase in force needed from the quadriceps for full extension and could be responsible for this apophyseal lesion (Aparicio et al., 1997). Unlike SCFE, it is not felt to be an abnormality of physeal development or structure (Yashar, 1995). It may manifest as acute, severe pain, causing a child to limp, or be noted by the child over a period of months as low-grade discomfort, usually brought on by running or participating in sports. Treatment consists of application of ice and rest, decreasing activity, and avoidance of all squatting and jumping activities. Use of a neoprene knee brace may prove helpful. Severe cases may require cast immobilization initially. The condition is usually self-limiting

and resolves when the tubercle fuses to the main body of the tibia, usually around 15 years of age.

Osteochondritis Dissecans. The term osteochondritis dissecans (OD or OCD) describes the separation of an articular cartilage subchondral bone segment from the articular surface. The mechanism producing this disorder is believed to be ischemic necrosis as a result of repetitive microtrauma, but the cause is not entirely clear. Frequently asymptomatic, OCD is more common in athletically active children, with a male-to-female ratio of 2:1 (Robertson et al., 2003). OCD is most commonly noted in the distal femur, usually on the lateral surface of the medial femoral condyle, although it may occur in other areas such as the femoral capital epiphysis (Wood et al., 1995) or the talus (Higuera et al., 1998). The child with OCD of the distal femur presents with pain, swelling around the knee, and an antalgic gait. If the fragment separates, the loose body may cause locking of the joint. The lesion is identified as a radiolucent area, usually on the posteromedial aspect of the distal femur, and thus often cannot be visualized on a straight anterior-posterior radiograph; a notch, or tunnel, view is needed (Fig. 17-10). MRI can help in determining the potential of an OCD lesion to heal without surgery (Pill et al., 2003). In mild to moderate cases the treatment may consist of cast immobilization and then graduated activity with quadriceps strengthening exercises. Most cases of OCD of the distal femur are self-limiting and heal without surgical intervention. If the defect has separated and an intra-articular loose fragment is present and causing symptoms, surgical treatment is effective in skeletally immature patients. Surgery can include removal or fixation of the loose body, bone grafting, and drilling through the cartilage into the bone in the base of the defect to stimulate healing by growth of new bone (Anderson & Pagnani, 1997; Anderson et al., 1997).

Tarsal Coalition. Tarsal coalition is a failure of segmentation of the hindfoot bones. The connecting tissue may be fibrous, cartilaginous, or osseous. Calcaneonavicular and talocalcaneal coalitions are the most common, and there may be multiple coalitions in the same foot (Clarke, 1997). They are often bilateral and may be asymptomatic (Blakemore et al., 2000). Tarsal coalition usually produces symptoms between ages 8 and 12 years when the abnormal cartilaginous bar begins to ossify. The child usually has foot pain, limp, and a rigid flat foot with decreased subtalar motion and peroneal spasm; there may be a history of frequent sprains. The coalition may be seen on plain radiographs of the foot (oblique views), however CT or MRI provides the most

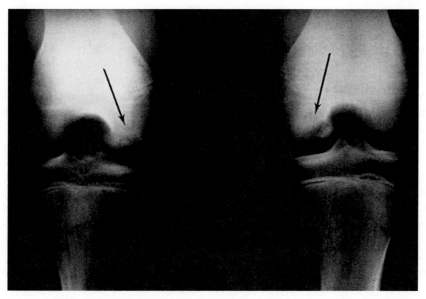

◆ **Figure 17-10**   A notch, or tunnel, view of the distal femurs demonstrates the osteochondritis dissecans lesions, noted by arrows.

definitive information about the site of the bridging, allowing differentiation of osseous from nonosseous coalitions and defining the extent of joint involvement as well as secondary degenerative changes (Newman & Newberg, 2000). Surgical excision of the coalition is frequently necessary and is usually successful in relieving symptoms (Comfort & Johnson, 1998).

Additional Causes of Limp. Patellofemoral pain and recurrent patellar subluxation or dislocation are two common causes of limp in this age group (see Chapter 18 for a detailed discussion). Monoarticular inflammatory arthritis and gonococcal arthritis also can cause acute onset of limp in a child.

Many types of neoplasms and related bone lesions can cause a child to limp. Commonly seen conditions include osteoid osteoma, unicameral bone cyst, osteochondroma (single or multiple), enchondroma, aneurysmal bone cyst, eosinophilic granuloma, and nonossifying fibroma. Symptoms may include limp, pain, and pathologic fracture through the lesion.

MISCELLANEOUS CONDITIONS

BACK PAIN

Back pain in adults is frequently mechanical, but back pain in children (especially preadolescents) is often the result of organic causes (Thompson, 1993). Examples of etiology include spondylolysis and spondylolisthesis, infection (e.g., diskitis or vertebral osteomyelitis), and either benign or malignant tumors. Complaints of back pain in children persisting for more than 1 to 2 weeks should be taken very seriously. The child should be referred to a physician for an appropriate workup, especially if the back pain is accompanied by fever, neurologic signs, or night pain, or the child refuses to walk or walks with a limp (Fernandez et al., 2000).

IDIOPATHIC TOE-WALKING

A number of children tend to toe-walk some of the time when first walking independently. A smaller subset persist in toe-walking, yet have no history of prematurity or difficult delivery and no evidence of hypertonicity or abnormal developmental reflexes that might lead to a diagnosis of cerebral palsy. This "idiopathic toe-walking" (ITW) usually responds well to a conservative treatment program of therapeutic exercise to stretch the gastrocnemius and soleus muscles and strengthen the ankle dorsiflexors. With significant tendo Achillis contractures, patients may require serial casting, perhaps with short leg cutout casts to encourage active dorsiflexion. Operative treatment is rarely required and carries the risk of overlengthening, which can cause a serious functional deficit. Stricker and Angulo (1998) compared outcomes in 85 children with ITW and found that patients in the observation-only group and the cast or brace group showed little change in passive dorsiflexion and poor parental satisfaction. They surgically treated 15 of 85 children with more severe equinus contractures, resulting in improved dorsiflexion and parental satisfaction.

Differences in knee and ankle kinematics between patients with ITW and spastic diplegia can be documented on gait analysis (Kelly et al., 1997). Children with ITW may have "soft" neurologic signs, such as a mild residual asymmetric tonic neck reflex in the quadruped position. Shulman and colleagues (1997) prospectively studied 13 children with persistent toe-walking and found that 10 of 13 had speech or language deficits, with fine motor (4 patients) and gross motor (3 patients) delays as well. There is also a group of idiopathic toe-walkers in which a family history of toe-walking can be documented. This is an autosomal dominant pattern described by Katz and Mubarak (1984).

ACHONDROPLASIA

Achondroplasia (dwarfism) is the most common of a large group of conditions known as the osteochondrodysplasias, a heterogeneous group of disorders characterized by abnormal growth and remodeling of cartilage and bone, affecting from 2 to 4.7 per 10,000 individuals (Baitner et al., 2000). It is an autosomal dominant condition with about 90% of cases representing a new mutation (Smith & Jones, 1982). Orthopedic manifestations of this condition include frontal bossing, cuboid-shaped vertebral bodies that may cause narrowing of the spinal canal and cord compression, with short pedicles, lumbar lordosis, short tubular bones, and short trident-shaped hands. Tibia vara is usually present with the fibula longer than the tibia (Stanley et al., 2002). The incidence of neurologic complications secondary to spinal abnormalities ranges from 20% to 47%, although frequently the symptoms are subtle (Ruiz-Garcia et al., 1997). Persons with achondroplastic dwarfism have abnormal length ratios of limbs to trunk, with more shortening of the proximal limb segments, in contrast to persons classified as midgets, who have proportionate limb and trunk ratios. Some centers advocate surgical lengthening of the lower extremities for children with dwarfism (Yasui et al., 1997).

Many infants with achondroplasia demonstrate hypotonia with transient kyphotic deformity. In 10% to 15% of children this may result in fixed angular kyphosis with serious neurologic sequelae later in life. Discouraging early unsupported sitting is effective, and bracing can also be used (Pauli et al., 1997).

LEG LENGTH INEQUALITY

Leg length inequality (LLI) may also be called leg length discrepancy (LLD) and is often defined as a 2.5 cm or greater difference in leg length. Differences smaller than this tend not to cause clinical problems. The difference in leg lengths may be due to relative overgrowth or shortening.

ETIOLOGY

The etiology of leg length inequality is divided into a number of categories: trauma, congenital, neuromuscular, acquired diseases, infections causing physeal growth arrest, tumors, and vascular disorders. Types of trauma include epiphyseal and diaphyseal injuries. Epiphyseal injuries with growth plate closure may be asymmetric, such as a fracture involving the medial epiphysis of the distal femur. This type of injury can result in an angular deformity (varus) as well as shortening of the femur.

Congenital disorders include hemihypertrophy, in which one half of the body (the arm and leg) is larger than the other. Conversely, in hemiatrophy one half of the body is smaller than the other. These can sometimes be difficult to distinguish, necessitating a decision on which arm and leg best "match" the rest of the body. Proximal focal femoral deficiency, congenital coxa vara, fibular and tibial hemimelia, and other focal dysplasias are additional causes of leg length inequality (see Chapter 16). DDH can also cause a leg length discrepancy, due either to an apparent femoral shortening noted when the hip is dislocated or actual shortening caused by femoral head AVN. Surgical treatment of DDH can change the leg length, including VDRO (shortens the femur) and pelvic osteotomies that may add up to 1 inch to the height of the pelvis.

Neuromuscular disorders can cause asymmetric growth of lower extremity bones. Decreased growth in the affected leg may be due to decreased muscle forces in weak or paralyzed muscles. Examples include myelodysplasia, poliomyelitis, and hemiplegia caused by congenital or acquired cerebral palsy. However, not all cases of LLI should be corrected. A child with hemiplegia will have a short lower limb on the affected side. With weakness and spasticity in that leg, foot clearance may be difficult as a result of decreased hip and knee flexion and equinus. The shortness of the leg makes foot clearance in swing easier.

Acquired conditions such as LCPD and SCFE can also result in a shortened lower extremity, usually as a result of AVN of the femoral head or occasionally as the result of surgical treatment. Fibrous dysplasia and tumors, including benign bone cysts and malignant neoplasms, can change leg length by interference with growth centers or secondarily as a result of fracture or surgical treatment.

IMPAIRMENTS

The effects of LLI vary widely among patients because of the actual amount of difference and how well the patient physically compensates for it, the possibility of progression of the inequality, the patient's perception of the problem, and the overall picture of muscle strength, motor control, and ROM. If the discrepancy is marked or compensation is limited, poor cosmesis may be evident, and a significant increase in energy expenditure may be required to walk. Musculoskeletal adaptations and compensations may result. These secondary impairments include pelvic obliquity with changes in spinal alignment that can cause a functional scoliosis and rotation of the pelvis (Young et al., 2000), or low back pain (Bhave et al., 1996). In 1999 Bhave and colleagues reported that gait characteristics were improved in 18 patients after limb lengthening. Other musculoskeletal adaptations may be observed at the hip, knee, and ankle, including pelvic tilt, contralateral knee flexion, and ipsilateral equinus. These problems may be significant but easily accommodated because of the inherent energy and motivation usually present in children. In adulthood, however, the factors of increased size and weight, increased energy expenditure to walk, increased sensitivity regarding the poor cosmesis of a lurching gait, or long-term effects of asymmetric lumbosacral spinal alignment may combine to significantly reduce the person's ability to walk and even render him or her nonambulatory.

CLINICAL EXAMINATION

The physical therapy examination for patients with LLI starts with obtaining a complete history, including any previous treatment. The physical examination incorporates the following elements:

- Measurement of ROM, joint stability and muscle strength of the trunk, hips, knees, ankles, and feet
- Sensation of the lower extremities
- Anthropometric measurements: sitting and standing height, weight, and arm span; girth of thighs and calves; leg lengths
- Functional activities, such as rising from a chair to standing and moving down to the floor and back up
- Clinical analysis of posture and gait, including observation of the spine and lower extremity alignment and substitution patterns; observation of the patient with and without assistive devices and shoe lift during gait on level ground, ramps, and stairs

Two options are available for clinical measurement of leg lengths. One is to level the pelvis in standing, using blocks under the short leg and then measuring the height of the blocks. The other is to measure the legs using various landmarks with the patient in the supine position: anterior-superior iliac spine to medial malleolus, anterior-superior iliac spine to lateral malleolus, anterior-superior iliac spine to heel pad, and umbilicus to heel pad. In a patient without significant lower extremity contractures, leveling the pelvis in standing with blocks may be the most accurate and reproducible. Radiographic measurement of leg lengths is usually done with scanograms. The patient is positioned on the x-ray table with a ruler alongside the legs, and three radiographs are taken on the same cassette, at the level of the hips, knees, and ankles, with the patient held motionless. These three views with the ruler markings next to them allow the examiner to measure the length of the femur and the tibia and combine them for the total leg length. Landmarks commonly used are the top of the femoral head, the bottom of the medial femoral condyle, and the tibial plafond. A film of the left wrist and hand should be performed in conjunction with the scanogram. This allows determination of the skeletal age of the patient, using a reference such as Greulich and Pyle (1950).

Measurement error is present in any of these techniques, making both clinical and radiographic leg length determinations an inexact science. Validity of the measurement is affected by hip and knee flexion contractures that "shorten" the leg. Determination of bone age is somewhat subjective. Determining the percentage of growth inhibition assists in estimating the eventual discrepancy at skeletal maturity. For example, a 10% inhibition of growth in the short leg may result in a minor discrepancy when the child is quite young. When the leg is 20 cm long, a 10% shortening is only 2 cm. However, as the child matures, when the unaffected leg is 70 cm long a 10% inhibition of growth on the involved side will result in a shortening of 7 cm, which is significant.

If the patient can be followed with serial measurements over time, scanogram measurements of total length of both the long and the short leg and the skeletal age at the time of each scanogram can be plotted on the Moseley graph, which depicts past growth and predicts future growth (Moseley, 1977) (Fig. 17-11). Timing of surgery is based on the predicted LLD at skeletal maturity. The effects of surgery can also be plotted on the

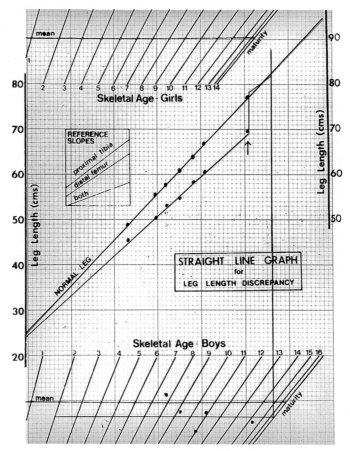

⬩ Figure 17-11   An example of the use of the Moseley graph to plot a patient's serial scanogram measurements and bone ages to determine the discrepancy at maturity and the possibilities for surgical intervention. Growth of the short leg is depicted by the line below the normal leg line. The increase in the length of the short leg (arrow) shows the effects of a leg-lengthening procedure. The two legs are approximately equal at skeletal maturity.

graph to predict the alteration in leg lengths and the eventual impact on discrepancy at skeletal maturity. Paley and colleagues (2000) have developed a mathematical formula that allows these predictions based on as few as one or two measurements.

TREATMENT

Treatment of LLI can be conservative or surgical. Conservative treatment consists of observation only or use of a shoe lift. Surgical treatment is directed at either shortening the long leg or lengthening the short leg. Some patients need both to achieve equality at maturity. Shortening the long leg in the growing child is achieved by epiphysiodesis, the surgical physeal arrest of one or more growth centers in the long leg, which allows the short leg to "catch up" in length. This can be done as an open procedure or percutaneously (Horton & Olney,

1996; Metaizeau et al., 1998). The contribution to growth varies with each growth center, as illustrated in Table 17-2.

Timing of the epiphysiodesis is obviously crucial. Future growth of each leg must be predicted and the surgery performed at a time when the amount of growth denied the long leg will match the amount of growth still available in the short leg, allowing them to be approximately equal in length at skeletal maturity. If epiphysiodesis is performed too early, the long leg may actually become the short leg, with an obviously less than optimal surgical result. One other option for shortening the long leg is a shortening osteotomy, usually considered in a skeletally mature patient who is not a candidate for epiphysiodesis.

Epiphysiodesis can also be performed on only the medial or lateral part of the growth plate to correct angular deformities. For example, a fracture of the distal

TABLE 17-2	Percentage of Growth for Each Growth Center in the Femur and Tibia			

GROWTH CENTER	FOR ENTIRE LEG	TOTAL LENGTH OF FEMUR	TOTAL LENGTH OF TIBIA
Proximal femur	15%	30%	–
Distal femur	35%	70%	–
Proximal tibia	30%	–	60%
Distal tibia	20%	–	40%

femur may cause damage to the medial aspect of the distal femoral growth plate. The lateral part of the growth plate continues to function normally and the leg grows into varus, which also produces a functional shortening. If the medial portion of the growth plate is still open, stapling of the lateral portion can allow the femur to gradually grow out of varus. This type of surgery may also include resection of a bony bar on the involved side of the growth plate.

Limb Lengthening

Surgical lengthening of the short leg has appeal because the surgery is performed on the affected leg, not the "normal" leg, and the opportunity exists for correction of discrepancies of much greater magnitude. Criteria for leg lengthening include a discrepancy of greater than 4 to 6 cm, adequate soft tissue mobility available to allow correction, and a stable joint above and below, although unstable joints can be protected with an external frame. A decision must be made whether to lengthen the femur or the tibia or both. Ideally the final result at maturity will be fairly equal leg lengths and equal knee heights in standing. If the discrepancy is too large to be amenable to these procedures, as in some cases of proximal focal femoral deficiency, amputation of the distal segment to allow the use of a prosthesis would be considered to be the most practical alternative (see Chapter 16). Another option is a rotationplasty of the affected limb (Torode & Gillespie, 1983).

Limb lengthening was first reported in the literature by Codivilla in Italy in 1905 (Coleman & Scott, 1991). Two biologic approaches to lengthening exist: (1) lengthening through bone and (2) lengthening by physeal distraction. Physeal distraction includes the option of subacute epiphysiolysis, initially described by Monticelli and Spinelli and called chondrodiastasis (Coleman & Scott, 1991). It consists of gradual distraction of the growth plate using a circular fixator, leading to a sudden rupture of the growth plate 3 to 4 days after the procedure begins. This is rarely used except for adolescent limb lengthening near the end of the patient's growth, because it may lead to premature closure of the growth plate.

A number of devices have been developed for lengthening bone, including diaphyseal lengthening devices (Wagner, unilateral frame) and metaphyseal lengthening devices, such as the Ilizarov (circular frame). The Wagner technique for lengthening through bone involved an osteotomy of the bone followed by rapid distraction, with cancellous bone grafting and plating of the distraction gap (Wagner, 1978).

Dr. Gavriil Abramovich Ilizarov first developed his technique and device in Russia to treat World War II veterans and later widened the applications (Ilizarov & Ledyaev, 1969). The Ilizarov method of slow distraction does not use bone grafting of the distraction gap. The circular design and the custom fitting of the external fixator allow simultaneous correction of rotational and angular deformities, as well as achieving the lengthening (Stanitski et al., 1996). The standard rate of distraction is usually about 1 mm per day. The frequency of distraction is usually four times per day (0.25 mm each time). After the desired correction has been achieved, the fixator is left in place to allow consolidation of new bone. The Ilizarov technique is used for both adult and pediatric disorders, including limb length discrepancy, angular deformities such as adolescent Blount's disease, congenital tibial pseudarthrosis, resistant or recurrent clubfeet, correction of forearm or humeral shortening and deformity due to trauma or infection, and others (Rajacich et al., 1992). Another, more controversial, indication for leg lengthening is its bilateral use in patients with achondroplasia to achieve a more normal height (Paley, 1988).

Paley and colleagues (1997) have described femoral lengthening over an intramedullary (IM) nail. The IM nail is inserted concomitantly with the external fixator. Once the distraction phase is completed the nail is locked with two screws and the external fixator is removed. The IM nail then protects the bone from fracture during the consolidation phase, and the decreased time with external fixation allows earlier rehabilitation.

As defined by Paley (1990), "problems" following lengthening procedures represent difficulties that do not require operative intervention, "obstacles" require operative intervention, and true "complications" include all problems that do not resolve by the end of treatment. Difficulties encountered during lengthening procedures include the following:

- Bone: angulation, delayed union or nonunion, fractures, pin tract infections, osteomyelitis
- Joint: cartilage degeneration, stiffness, subluxation, dislocation
- Nerves: transient or permanent stretch paralysis
- Muscle: weakness, contracture, ischemia
- Vascular: transient hypertension, probably due to stretching of the sciatic nerve, although this has not been well documented

Barker and colleagues (2001) studied 35 patients undergoing femoral lengthening by the Ilizarov method. They found 92% of patients regained their knee flexion by 12 months and 97% by 18 months. Significant loss of knee flexion occurred in the period prior to lengthening, in response to the application of the fixation device, and they stressed the need for active physical therapy intervention when the fixation device is first applied. Historical guidelines recommend limiting the amount of lengthening to 10% to 20% of the length of the segment prior to surgery. However, Yun and colleagues (2000) undertook 35 lengthenings in 31 patients and achieved a mean gain of 33% with only a 0.9% complication rate by Paley's classification.

Children undergoing leg lengthening must adjust to the pain of the procedure, which can be significant and extended (Young et al., 1994). The child may experience frustration, anger, and fear because of the temporary loss of independence inherent in the procedure. Difficult behavior may require intervention by a psychologist to assist the child and family in developing appropriate coping strategies. Candidates for surgical lengthening must be extremely motivated, with a supportive and committed family. Successful limb lengthening also mandates a comprehensive medical care system, with knowledgeable, experienced physicians, nurses, and therapists to guide the patient and family through the process.

Role of Physical Therapy in Limb Lengthening

An excellent description of the preoperative and postoperative physical therapy goals and interventions for patients undergoing limb lengthening has been provided by Simard and colleagues (1992). The preoperative phase includes the following:

- Comprehensive physical therapy examination
- Crutch fitting and instruction in restricted weight bearing on the involved leg
- Instruction in home exercise and postoperative positioning and splinting in conjunction with the patient, parents, and other caregivers
- Stretching and strengthening exercises to use in preparation for surgery

The greatest challenges for the physical therapist treating children in the postoperative phase include promoting weight bearing in the presence of significant pain, maintaining the child's ROM, and motivating the child to continue with the program both in the hospital and at home over the long period of treatment. There can also be significant difficulty in obtaining funding for physical therapy, an example of environmental factors that can affect the success of the surgery. Insurance carriers require documentation of improved function during the treatment period. For the patient undergoing leg lengthening by the Ilizarov technique, the goal is to maintain ambulation, joint ROM, and strength while undergoing the lengthening, with a long-term goal of improved function after the device is removed.

The postoperative phase includes instruction in functional activities, active assistive and isometric exercise, proper positioning of the extremity, gait training with progressive weight bearing as tolerated, and pin care. Modalities such as ice or transcutaneous electrical nerve stimulation may be useful for pain management. Dynamic splinting may be used in the limb-lengthening stage to provide low-intensity, prolonged stretch to joints with significantly limited ROM. Exercise techniques useful throughout the Ilizarov lengthening include both closed- and open-chain exercise for strengthening and active-assistive or passive exercise for ROM. A stationary bicycle and treadmill may be used. After removal of the fixator, the patient may require additional gait training, monitoring, and adjusting of the exercise program, and possibly refitting and retraining with orthotic or prosthetic devices worn preoperatively. Throughout the course of treatment, children are encouraged to participate in their usual school and leisure activities to the fullest extent possible.

SUMMARY

The pediatric orthopedic conditions presented in this chapter represent a wide range of problems that may be encountered by physical therapists in children referred to them for a specific problem (e.g., clumsy gait), or perhaps a quite specific complaint that turns out to be a "red herring" (e.g. a child referred to physical therapy for intervention of knee pain, who in fact has a slipped capital femoral epiphysis). Alternatively, a child might be referred from a primary care physician or neurologist to physical therapist with one diagnosis (e.g., gross motor developmental delay), but also be under treatment by an orthopedist for developmental dysplasia of the hip. In all these various scenarios, it is essential that the physical therapist be knowledgeable about various pediatric orthopedic conditions, including their signs, symptoms, differential diagnoses, and treatment. As physical therapists, we often have the advantage of following a child intensively over a period of time, as opposed to a physician's visit once every 6 months, and thereby have unique insights into the child's condition and the family dynamics surrounding it. The well-informed physical therapist can often serve to bridge the gap that sometimes occurs between various specialists following a child, including primary care physicians, orthopedists, neurologists, and physiatrists.

CASE STUDY

AMY

Amy was referred for orthopedic consultation at 1 day of age. The following clinical findings were documented: positive Galeazzi sign on the left with the femur approximately 2 cm short, hip abduction right/left 70°/40°, 2 cm shortening of the left tibia measured clinically, a band in the area of the left fibula, and calcaneovalgus of the left foot. Radiographs showed both hips located, with coxa vara and decreased femoral neck length, a slight bow of the left femur, shortening of the left femur by 2 cm and the left tibia 1 cm compared with the right, and complete absence of the left fibula. The diagnosis was made of left proximal focal femoral deficiency and absent left fibula.

The following summary documents the progression of Amy's limb length discrepancy as she grew older, the resulting impairments, her potential activity limitations, and her impressive determination to overcome them. Her extensive treatment is summarized.

Age 1 month: Physical therapy—home exercise program

10 months: Excision of fibular anlage, peroneus longus muscle lengthening; scanogram showed 5.6 cm of shortening of the left leg

13 months: Fitted with a step-in prosthesis, follow-up physical therapy. Options for treatment: (1) knee

fusion and Syme amputation, followed by fitting with a below-knee prosthesis; (2) maintain use of her step-in prosthesis; (3) modified rotationplasty. Her parents opted for a prosthesis

2 years: Using step-in prosthesis, able to run and jump; left leg 7.3 cm short by scanogram

3 years: Left leg 9.2 cm short, continuing with the 20% inhibition of growth noted earlier

8 years: Left leg 12.7 cm short; able to ski with step-in prosthesis

9.75 years: Left Salter pelvic osteotomy to correct mild acetabular dysplasia

At age 10 years, through use of the Canadian Occupational Performance Measure, it was determined that the most important concerns of Amy and her parents included her awkward gait and poor cosmesis. The poor cosmesis had only recently become a concern for Amy, due to her increasing awareness of how she was viewed by her peers. In addition, Amy felt that she was limited in her athletic abilities because of her leg length discrepancy and she wanted very much to participate more actively in competitive sports.

Examination of Amy's left leg showed significant impairments, including shortening of the femur and tibia, external rotational deformity of the femur, genu valgum secondary to a hypoplastic lateral femoral condyle, an apex medial bow in the tibia, and equinus of the ankle. Her projected leg length inequality at skeletal maturity was 18 cm.

Working in concert, Amy's physical therapist and orthopedic surgeon recommended a limb-lengthening procedure. This was agreed to by the child and family, who were very much against the only other surgical alternative, which was amputation. Long-term goals of the surgery included independent ambulation without bracing or assistive devices, a smoother gait with decreased energy expenditure, increased agility in sports, improved cosmesis, and decreased potential for future disability resulting from greatly disparate leg lengths.

Surgery consisted of application of Ilizarov frames to the left femur, tibia, and foot to accomplish femoral lengthening, rotational and angular correction, and tibial lengthening and angular correction. A tendo Achillis lengthening was also performed. Amy's initial lengthening was 0.25 mm four times a day, in both the femur and tibia. This rate provided 1 mm of lengthening in each bone every 24 hours.

The following summary documents her progress during the course of postoperative treatment:

3 weeks: Attending school part time; knee extension (−15°); physical therapy program of active and active-assistive ROM and strengthening exercises

4 weeks: Left tibia subluxating posteriorly on femur; rate of lengthening decreased temporarily

3 months: Foot frame removed; weight bearing as tolerated; ongoing exercise program of ROM exercises of left knee and ankle, strengthening exercises for quadriceps, hip abductor, and hip extensor muscles; able to exercise in a pool

7 months: Tibial frame removed with 3 cm of tibial lengthening achieved; knee passively taken through ROM at the time of surgery, to aid in ROM exercises postoperatively

8 months: Resumed an aggressive knee ROM exercise program; care was taken to support the tibia just distal to the knee during exercise, avoiding a long lever arm across the regenerate bone site

9 months: Losing knee ROM; continuous passive motion machine instituted 4 hours per day; dynamic splint also used

10 months: Femoral frame removed with 13 cm of femoral lengthening achieved

10.5 months: 5-day history of deformity of the proximal femur and increased pain; diagnosis of femoral fracture through one of the half-pin sites; closed reduction, insertion of distal femoral traction pin, and application of Neufeld traction

11 months: Further closed reduction, removal of traction pin, and application of a spica cast

12 months: Total contact HKAFO, with free hip, knee, and ankle joints; worn full time, with time out for bathing; ROM exercise (active only)

13 months: Radiographs showed evidence of an additional, healing pathologic stress fracture of the femur

14.5 months: Able to walk well with HKAFO and one crutch, no pain; extensive stretching and strengthening program through physical therapy, physical education at school, and home exercise program

Even with the added complication of femoral fractures, Amy achieved good results from her surgery. Of the original projected discrepancy of 18 cm, a total of 16 cm was gained through the femoral and tibial lengthenings, and her knees were essentially level. This abbreviated documentation of the process can only hint at the incredible amount of work, time, and commitment required by this type of treatment on the part of everyone involved.

REFERENCES

Accadbled, F, Laville, JM, & Harper, L. One-step treatment for evolved Blount's disease: Four cases and review of the literature. Journal of Pediatric Orthopaedics, 23:747–752, 2003.

Anderson, AF, & Pagnani, MJ. Osteochondritis dissecans of the femoral condyles. Long-term results of excision of the fragment. American Journal of Sports Medicine, 25:830–834, 1997.

Anderson, AF, Richards, DB, Pagnani, MJ, & Hovis, WD. Antegrade drilling for osteochondritis dissecans of the knee. Arthroscopy, 13:319–324, 1997.

Aparicio, G, Abril, JC, Calvo, E, & Alvarez, L. Radiologic study of patellar height in Osgood-Schlatter disease. Journal of Pediatric Orthopaedics, 17:63–66, 1997.

Aronson, DD, Peterson, DA, & Miller, DV. Slipped capital femoral epiphysis: The case for internal fixation in situ. Clinical Orthopaedics and Related Research, 281:115–122, 1992.

Baitner, AC, Maurer, SG, Gruen, MB, & DiCesare, PE. The genetic basis of the osteochondrodysplasias. Journal of Pediatric Orthopaedics, 20:594–605, 2000.

Bankes, MJ, Catterall, A, & Hashemi-Nejad, A. Valgus extension osteotomy for 'hing abduction' in Perthes' disease. Results at maturity and factors influencing the radiological outcome. Journal of Bone and Joint Surgery (British), 82:548–554, 2000.

Barker, KL, Simpson, AH, & Lamb, SE. Loss of knee range of motion in leg lengthening. Journal of Orthopedic Sports Physical Therapy, 31:238–244, 2001.

Bennett, OM, & Namnyak, SS. Acute septic arthritis of the hip joint in infancy and childhood. Clinical Orthopaedics and Related Research, 281:123–132, 1992.

Bhave, A, Herzenberg, JE, & Paley, D. Gait asymmetries with leg length discrepancy (LLD): Symmetry after leg lengthening. Pediatric Orthopaedic Society of North America Annual Meeting, scientific poster, 1996.

Bhave, A, Paley, D, & Herzenberg, JE. Improvement in gait parameters after lengthening for the treatment of limb-length discrepancy. Journal of Bone and Joint Surgery (American), 81:529–534, 1999.

Blakemore, LC, Cooperman, DR, & Thompson, GH. The rigid flatfoot. Tarsal coalitions. Clinics in Podiatric Medicine and Surgery, 17:531–555, 2000.

Bobroff, ED, Chambers, HG, Sartoris, DJ, Wyatt, MP, & Sutherland, DH. Femoral anteversion and neck-shaft angle in children with cerebral palsy. Clinical Orthopedics and Related Research, 364:194–204, 2000.

Brook, I. Joint and bone infections due to anaerobic bacteria in children. Pediatric Rehabilitation, 5:11–19, 2002.

Brooks, WC, & Gross, RH. Genu varum in children: Diagnosis and treatment. Journal of the American Academy of Orthopaedic Surgeons, 3:326–335, 1995.

Bruce, RW, Jr. Torsional and angular deformities. Pediatric Clinics of North America, 43:867–881, 1996.

Cahuzac, JP, Hobatho, MC, Baunin, C, Boulot, J, Darmana, R, & Autefage, A. Classification of 125 children with rotational abnormalities. Journal of Pediatric Orthopaedics, Part B, 1:59–66, 1992.

Cahuzac, JP, Vardon, D, & Sales de Gauzy, J. Development of the clinical tibiofemoral angle in normal adolescents. A study of 427 normal subjects from 10 to 16 years of age. Journal of Bone and Joint Surgery (British), 77:729–732, 1995.

Cameron, JC, & Saha, S. External tibial torsion: An underrecognized cause of recurrent patellar dislocation. Clinical Orthopaedics and Related Research, 328:177–184, 1996.

Cashman, JP, Round, J, Taylor, G, & Clarke, NM. The natural history of developmental dysplasia of the hip after early supervised treatment in the Pavlik harness. A prospective, longitudinal follow-up. Journal of Bone and Joint Surgery (British), 84:418–425, 2002.

Catterall, A. The natural history of Perthes' disease. Journal of Bone and Joint Surgery (British), 53:37–53, 1971.

Cheema, JI, Grisson, LE, & Harcke, HT. Radiographic characteristics of lower-extremity bowing in children. Radiographics, 23:871–880, 2003.

Clarke, DM. Multiple tarsal coalitions in the same foot. Journal of Pediatric Orthopaedics, 17:777–780, 1997.

Colburn, M, & Williams, M. Evaluation of the treatment of idiopathic clubfoot by using the Ponseti method. Journal of Foot and Ankle Surgery, 42:259–267, 2003.

Coleman, SS, & Scott, SM. The present attitude toward the biology and technology of limb lengthening. Clinical Orthopaedics and Related Research, 264:76–83, 1991.

Comfort, TK, & Johnson, LO. Resection for symptomatic talocalcaneal coalition. Journal of Pediatric Orthopaedics, 18:283–288, 1998.

Connolly, B, Babyn, PS, Wright, JG, & Thorner, PS. Discoid meniscus in children: Magnetic resonance imaging characteristics. Canadian Association of Radiology Journal, 47:347–354, 1996.

Crane, L. Femoral torsion and its relation to toeing-in and toeing out. Journal of Bone and Joint Surgery (American), 41:421–428, 1959.

Crawford, AH. Role of osteotomy in the treatment of slipped capital femoral epiphysis. Journal of Pediatric Orthopaedics (British), 5:102–109, 1996.

Cuevas de Alba, C, Guille, JT, Bowen, JR, & Harcke, HT. Computed tomography for femoral and tibial torsion in children with clubfoot. Clinical Orthopaedics and Related Research, 353:203–209, 1998.

Cummings, RJ, Davidson, RS, Armstrong, PF, & Lehman, WB. Congenital clubfoot. Instructional Course Lecture, 51:385–400, 2002.

Dales, MC, & Hoffinger, SA. Septic hip in older children and adolescents (Abstract). Proceedings of the American Academy of Orthopaedic Surgeons Annual Meeting, San Francisco. American Academy of Orthopaedic Surgeons, 1993.

Davids, JR, Benson, LJ, Mubarak, SJ, & McNeil, N. Ultrasonography and developmental dysplasia of the hip: A cost-benefit analysis of three delivery systems. Journal of Pediatric Orthopaedics, 15:325–329, 1995.

De Alba, CC, Guille, JT, Bowen, JR, & Harcke, HT. Computed tomography for femoral and tibial torsion in children with clubfoot. Clinical Orthopaedics and Related Research, 353:203–209, 1998.

Delgado, ED, Schoenecker, PL, Rich, MM, & Capelli, AM. Treatment of severe torsional malalignment syndrome. Journal of Pediatric Orthopaedics, 16:484–488, 1996.

Dietz, F. The genetics of idiopathic clubfoot. Clinical Orthopaedics and Related Research, 401:39–48, 2002.

Dietz, WH. Health consequences of obesity in youth: Childhood predictors of adult disease. Pediatrics, 101:518–525, 1998.

Dobbs, MB, Sheridan, JJ, Gordon, JE, Corley, CL, Szymanski, DA, & Schoenecker, PL. Septic arthritis of the hip in infancy: Long-term follow-up. Journal of Pediatric Orthopaedics, 23:162–168, 2003.

Dodgin, DA, De Swart, RJ, Stefko, RM, Wenger, DR, & Ko, JY. Distal tibial/fibular derotation osteotomy for correction of tibial torsion: Review of technique and results in 63 cases. Journal of Pediatric Orthopaedics, 18:95–101, 1998.

Donaldson, JS, & Feinstein, KA. Imaging of developmental dysplasia of the hip. Pediatric Clinics of North America, 44:591–614, 1997.

Duffy, CM, Lam, PY, Ditchfield, M, Allen, R, & Graham, HK. Chronic recurrent multifocal osteomyelitis: Review of orthopaedic complications at maturity. Journal of Pediatric Orthopaedics, 22:501–505, 2002.

Dunn, PM. Perinatal observations of the etiology of congenital dislocation of the hip. Clinical Orthopaedics and Related Research, 119:11–22, 1976.

Echarri, JJ, & Forriol, F. The development in footprint morphology in 1851 Congolese children from urban and rural areas, and the relationship between this and wearing shoes. Journal of Pediatric Orthopaedics (British), 12:141–146, 2003.

Eckerwall, G, Hochbergs, P, Wingstrand, H, & Egund, N. Magnetic resonance imaging and early remodeling of the femoral head after femoral varus osteotomy in Legg-Calvé-Perthes disease. Journal of Pediatric Orthopaedics (British), 6:239–244, 1997.

Engel, GM, & Staheli, LT. The natural history of torsion and other factors influencing gait in childhood. Clinical Orthopaedics and Related Research, 99:12–17, 1974.

Fabry, G, MacEwen, D, & Shands, AR. Torsion of the femur: A follow-up study in normal and abnormal conditions. Journal of Bone and Joint Surgery (American), 55:1726–1738, 1973.

Farsetti, P, Tudisco, C, Caterini, R, Potenza, V, & Ippolito, E. The Herring lateral pillar classification for prognosis in Perthes disease. Late results in 49 patients treated conservatively. Journal of Bone and Joint Surgery (British), 77:739–742, 1995.

Farsetti, P, Weinstein, SL, & Ponseti, IV. The long-term functional and radiographic outcomes of untreated and non-operatively treated metatarsus adductus. Journal of Bone and Joint Surgery (American), 76:257–265, 1994.

Fernandez, M, Carrol, CL, & Baker, CJ. Discitis and vertebral osteomyelitis in children: An 18-year review. Pediatrics, 105:1299–1304, 2000.

Fuchs, R, & Staheli, LT. Sprinting and intoeing. Journal of Pediatric Orthopaedics, 16:489–491, 1996.

Galpin, RD, Roach, JW, Wenger, DR, Herring, JA, & Birch, JG. One-stage treatment of congenital dislocation of the hip in older children, including femoral shortening. Journal of Bone and Joint Surgery (American), 71:734–741, 1989.

Gaughan, DM, Mofeson, LM, Hughes, MD, Seage, GR, 3rd, Ciupak, GL, & Oleske, JM; AIDS Clinical Trials Group Protocol 219 Team. Osteonecrosis of the hip (Legg-Calve-Perthes disease) in human immunodeficiency virus-infected children. Pediatrics, 109:E74–4, 2002.

Gigante, A, Bevilacqua, C, Bonetti, MG, & Greco, F. Increased external tibial torsion in Osgood-Schlatter disease. Acta Orthopaedica Scandinavia, 74:431–436, 2003.

Glazer, PA, & Hu, SS. Pediatric spinal infections. Orthopaedic Clinics of North America, 27:111–123, 1996.

Glueck, CJ, Brandt, G, Gruppo, R, Crawford, A, Roy, D, Tracy, T, Stroop, D, Wang, P, & Becker, A. Resistance to activated protein C and Legg-Perthes disease. Clinical Orthopaedics and Related Research, 338:139–152, 1997.

Glueck, CJ, Freiberg, RA, Crawford, A, Gruppo, R, Roy, D, Tracy, T, Sieve-Smith, L, & Wang, P. Secondhand smoke, hypofibrinolysis, and Legg-Perthes disease. Clinical Orthopaedics and Related Research, 352:159–167, 1998.

Goodman, DA, Feighan, JE, Smith, AD, Latimer, B, Buly, RL, & Cooperman, DR. Subclinical slipped capital femoral epiphysis: Relationship to osteoarthrosis of the hip. Journal of Bone and Joint Surgery (American), 79:1489–1497, 1997.

Gordon, JE, Abrahams, MS, Dobbs, MB, Luhmann, SJ, & Schoenecker, PL. Early reduction, arthrotomy, and cannulated screw fixation in unstable slipped capital femoral epiphysis treatment. Journal of Pediatric Orthopaedics, 22:352–358, 2002.

Graf, R. Hip sonography—How reliable? Sector scanning versus linear scanning? Dynamic versus static examination? Clinical Orthopaedics and Related Research, 281:18–21, 1992.

Greulich, WW, & Pyle, SI. Radiographic Atlas of Skeletal Development of the Hand and Wrist. Stanford, CA: Stanford University Press, 1950.

Hagglund, G. The contralateral hip in slipped capital femoral epiphysis. Journal of Pediatric Orthopaedics (British), 5:158–161, 1996.

Harcke, HT. Imaging in congenital dislocation and dysplasia of the hip. Clinical Orthopaedics and Related Research, 281:22–28, 1992.

Heilig, MR, Matern, RV, Rosenzweig, SD, & Bennett, JT. Current management of idiopathic clubfoot questionnaire: A multicentric study. Journal of Pediatric Orthopaedics, 23:780–787, 2003.

Hensinger, RH, & Jones, ET. Neonatal orthopaedics. In Oliver, TK (Ed.). Monographs in Neonatalogy. New York: Grune & Stratton, 1981.

Herring, JA, Neustadt, JB, Williams, JJ, Early, JS, & Browne, RH. The lateral pillar classification of Legg-Calvé-Perthes disease. Journal of Pediatric Orthopaedics, 12:143–150, 1992.

Herzenberg, JE, Radler, C, & Bor, N. Ponseti versus traditional methods of casting for idiopathic clubfoot. Journal of Pediatric Orthopaedics, 22:517–521, 2002.

Higuera, J, Laguna, R, Peral, M, Aranda, E, & Soleto, J. Osteochondritis dissecans of the talus during childhood and adolescence. Journal of Pediatric Orthopaedics, 18:328–332, 1998.

Hofmann, A, Jones, RE, & Herring, JA. Blount's disease after skeletal maturity. Journal of Bone and Joint Surgery (American), 64:1004–1009, 1982.

Hogan, MT, & Staheli, LT. Arch height and lower limb pain: an adult civilian study. Foot and Ankle International, 23:43–47, 2002.

Horton, GA, & Olney, BW. Epiphysiodesis of the lower extremity: Results of the percutaneous technique. Journal of Pediatric Orthopaedics, 16:180–182, 1996.

Huber, AM, Lam, PY, Duffy, CM, Yeung, RS, Ditchfield, M, Laxer, D, Cole, WG, Kerr Graham, H, Allen, RC, & Laxer, RM. Chronic recurrent multifocal osteomyelitis: Clinical outcomes after more than five years of follow-up. Journal of Pediatrics, 141:198–203, 2002.

Hughes, LO, & Aronson, J. Skeletal infections in children. Current Opinions in Pediatrics, 6:90–93, 1994.

Hummer, CD, & MacEwen, GD. The coexistence of torticollis and congenital dysplasia of the hip. Journal of Bone and Joint Surgery (American), 54:1255–1256, 1972.

Hurley, JM, Betz, RR, Loder, RT, Davidson, RS, Alburger, PD, & Steel, HH. Slipped capital femoral epiphysis. The prevalence of late contralateral slip. Journal of Bone and Joint Surgery (American), 78:226–230, 1996.

Ilfeld, FW, Westin, GW, & Makin, M. Missed or developmental dislocation of the hip. Clinical Orthopaedics and Related Research, 203:276–281, 1986.

Ilizarov, GA, & Ledyaev, VI. The replacement of long tubular bone defects by lengthening distraction osteotomy of one of the fragments. Vestnik Khirurgii, 6:78, 1969. (Translated by Schwartzman, V. Clinical Orthopaedics and Related Research, 280:7–10, 1992.)

Ippolito, E, Farsetti, P, Caterini, R, & Tudisco, C. Long-term comparative results in patients with congenital clubfoot treated with two different protocols. Journal of Bone and Joint Surgery (American), 85-A:1286–1294, 2003.

Ismail, AM, & Macnicol, MF. Prognosis in Perthes' disease: A comparison of radiological predictors. Journal of Bone and Joint Surgery (British), 80:310–314, 1998.

Jasty, M, Anderson, MJ, & Harris, WH. Total hip replacement for developmental dysplasia of the hip. Clinical Orthopaedics and Related Research, 311:40–45, 1995.

Johnson, CE. Infantile tibia vara. Clinical Orthopaedics and Related Research, 255:13–23, 1990.

Kane, TP, Harvey, JR, Richards, RH, Burby, NG, & Clarke, NM. Radiological outcome of innocent infant hip clicks. Journal of Pediatric Orthopaedics (British), 12:259–263, 2003.

Katz, MM, & Mubarak, SJ. Hereditary tendo Achillis contractures. Journal of Pediatric Orthopaedics, 4:711–714, 1984.

Kelly, IP, Jenkinson, A, Stephens, M, & O'Brien, T. The kinematic patterns of toe-walkers. Journal of Pediatric Orthopaedics, 17:478–480, 1997.

Kelo, MJ, & Riddle, DL. Examination and management of a patient with tarsal coalition. Physical Therapy, 78:518–525, 1998.

Kensinger, DR, Guille, JT, Horn, BD, & Herman, MJ. The stubbed great toe: Importance of early recognition and treatment of open fractures of the distal phalanx. Journal of Pediatric Orthopaedics, 21:31–34, 2001.

Kim, HT, Eisenhauer, E, & Wenger, DR. The "sagging rope sign" in avascular necrosis in children's hip diseases—Confirmation by 3D CT studies. Iowa Orthopaedic Journal, 15:101–111, 1995.

Kim, HT, & Wenger, DR. "Functional retroversion" of the femoral head in Legg-Calvé-Perthes disease and epiphyseal dysplasia: Analysis of head-neck deformity and its effect on limb position using three-dimensional computed tomography. Journal of Pediatric Orthopaedics, 17:240–246, 1997a.

Kim, HT, & Wenger, DR. Surgical correction of "functional retroversion" and "functional coxa vara" in late Legg-Calvé-Perthes disease and epiphyseal dysplasia: Correction of deformity defined by new imaging modalities. Journal of Pediatric Orthopaedics, 17:247–254, 1997b.

Kim, HT, & Wenger, DR. The morphology of residual acetabular deficiency in childhood hip dysplasia: Three dimensional computed tomographic analysis. Journal of Pediatric Orthopaedics, 17:637–647, 1997c.

Kleinman, PK. A regional approach to osteomyelitis of the lower extremities in children. Radiology Clinics of North America, 40:1033–1059, 2002.

Kocher, MS, Mandiga, R, Murphy JM, Goldmann, D, Harper, M, Sundel, R, Ecklund, K, & Kasser, JR. A clinical practice guideline for treatment of septic arthritis in children: Efficacy in improving process of care and effect on outcome of septic arthritis of the hip. Journal of Bone and Joint Surgery (American), 85:994–999, 2003.

Kodros, SA, & Dias, LS. Single-stage surgical correction of congenital vertical talus. Journal of Pediatric Orthopaedics, 19:42–48, 1999.

Krivickas, LS. Anatomical factors associated with overuse sports injuries. Sports Medicine, 24:132–146, 1997.

Kuhns, LR, Koujok, K, Hall, JM, & Craig, C. Ultrasound of the navicular during the simulated Ponseti maneuver. Journal of Pediatric Orthopaedics, 23:243–245, 2003.

Kumm, DA, Schmidt, J, Eisenburger, SH, Rutt, J, & Hackenbroch, MH. Prophylactic dynamic screw fixation of the asymptomatic hip in slipped capital femoral epiphysis. Journal of Pediatric Orthopaedics, 16:249–253, 1996.

Lahdes-Vasama, TT, Sipila, IS, Lamminranta, S, Pihko, SH, Merikanto, EO, & Marttinen, EJ. Psychosocial development and premorbid skeletal growth in Legg-Calvé-Perthes disease: A study of nineteen patients. Journal of Pediatric Orthopaedics (British), 6:133–137, 1997.

Lane, NE, Nevitt, MC, Cooper, C, Pressman, A, Gore, R, & Hochberg, M. Acetabular dysplasia and osteoarthritis of the hip in elderly white women. Annals of Rheumatic Disorders, 56:627–630, 1997.

Langenskiold, A. Tibia vara: A critical review. Clinical Orthopaedics and Related Research, 246:195–206, 1989.

Lee, J, Jarvis, J, Uhthoff, HK, & Avruch, L. The fetal acetabulum. Clinical Orthopaedics and Related Research, 281:48–55, 1992.

Levine, MJ, McGuire, KJ, McGowan, KL, & Flynn, JM. Assessment of the test characteristics of C-reactive protein for septic arthritis in children. Journal of Pediatric Orthopaedics, 23:373–377, 2003.

Lincoln, TL, & Suen, PW. Common rotational variations in children. Journal of the American Academy of Orthopaedic Surgeons, 11:312–320, 2003.

Loder, RT. The demographics of slipped capital femoral epiphysis. An international multicenter study. Clinical Orthopaedics and Related Research, 322:8–27, 1996a.

Loder, RT. A worldwide study on the seasonal variation of slipped capital femoral epiphysis. Clinical Orthopaedics and Related Research, 322:28–36, 1996b.

Loder, RT, Brown, KL, Zaleske, DJ, & Jones, ET. Extremity lawn-mower injuries in children: Report by the Research Committee of the Pediatric Orthopaedic Society of North America. Journal of Pediatric Orthopaedics, 17:360–369, 1997.

Loder, RT, Farley, FA, Herring, JA, Schork, MA, & Shyr, Y. Bone age determination in children with Legg-Calvé-Perthes disease: A comparison of two methods. Journal of Pediatric Orthopaedics, 15:90–94, 1995a.

Loder, RT, Wittenberg, B, & DeSilva, G. Slipped capital femoral epiphysis associated with endocrine disorders. Journal of Pediatric Orthopaedics, 15:349–356, 1995a.

Loder, RT, & Hensinger, RN. Slipped capital femoral epiphysis associated with renal failure osteodystrophy. Journal of Pediatric Orthopaedics, 17:205–211, 1997.

Loren, GJ, Karpinski, NC, & Mubarak, SJ. Clinical implications of clubfoot histopathology. Journal of Pediatric Orthopaedics, 18:765–769, 1998.

Lovell, WW, & Winter, RB. Pediatric Orthopedics, Vols. I and II. Philadelphia: JB Lippincott, 1978.

Lubicky, JP. Chondrolysis and avascular necrosis: Complications of slipped capital femoral epiphysis. Journal of Pediatric Orthopaedics (British), 5:162–167, 1996.

Luhmann, SJ, Bassett, GS, Gordon, JE, Schootman, M, & Schoenecker, PL. Reduction of a dislocation of the hip due to developmental dysplasia. Implications for the need for future surgery. Journal of Bone and Joint Surgery (American), 85-A:239–243, 2003.

Mata, SG, Aicua, EA, Ovejero, AH, & Grande, MM. Legg-Calve-Perthes disease and passive smoking. Journal of Pediatric Orthopaedics, 20:326–330, 2000.

Matan, AJ, Stevens, PM, Smith, JT, & Santora, SD. Combination trochanteric arrest and intertrochanteric osteotomy for Perthes' disease. Journal of Pediatric Orthopaedics, 16:10–14, 1996.

Matava, MJ, Patton, CM, Luhmann, S, Gordon, JE, & Schoenecker, PL. Knee pain as the initial symptom of slipped capital femoral epiphysis: An analysis of initial presentation and treatment. Journal of Pediatric Orthopaedics, 19:455–460, 1999.

Meister, K, & James, SL. Proximal tibial derotation osteotomy for anterior knee pain in the miserably malaligned extremity. American Journal of Orthopaedics, 24:149–155, 1995.

Metaizeau, JP, Wong-Chung, J, Bertrand, H, & Pasquier, P. Percutaneous epiphysiodesis using transphyseal screws (PETS). Journal of Pediatric Orthopaedics, 18:363–369, 1998.

Michaeli, DA, Murphy, SB, & Hipp, JA. Comparison of predicted and measured contact pressures in normal and dysplastic hips. Medical Engineering & Physics, 19:180–186, 1997.

Michelson, JD, Durant, DM, & McFarland, E. The injury risk associated with pes planus in athletes. Foot and Ankle International, 23:629–633, 2002.

Mielke, CH, & Stevens, PM. Hemiepiphyseal stapling for knee deformities in children younger than 10 years: A preliminary report. Journal of Pediatric Orthopaedics, 16:423–429, 1996.

Miura, H, Noguchi, Y, Mitsuyasu, H, Nagamine, R, Urabe, K, Matsuda, S, & Iwamoto, Y. Clinical features of multiple epiphyseal dysplasia expressed in the knee. Clinical Orthopedics and Related Research, 380:184–190, 2000.

Morcuende, JA, Egbert, M, & Ponseti, IV. The effect of the internet in the treatment of congenital idiopathic clubfoot. Iowa Orthopedic Journal, 23:83–86, 2003.

Morcuende, JA, & Ponseti, IV. Congenital metatarsus adductus in early human fetal development: A histologic study. Clinical Orthopaedics and Related Research, 333:261–266, 1996.

Mosca, VS. Calcaneal lengthening for valgus deformity of the hindfoot. Results in children who had severe, symptomatic flatfoot and skewfoot. Journal of Bone and Joint Surgery (American), 77:500–512, 1995.

Moseley, CF. A straight-line graph for leg-length discrepancies. Journal of Bone and Joint Surgery (American), 59:174–179, 1977.

Mubarak, SJ, Beck, L, & Sutherland, D. Home traction in the management of congenital dislocation of the hips. Journal of Pediatric Orthopaedics, 6:721–723, 1986.

Mubarak, SJ, Garfin, SR, Vance, R, McKinnon, B, & Sutherland, D. Pitfalls in the use of the Pavlik harness for treatment of congenital dysplasia, subluxation, and dislocation of the hip. Journal of Bone and Joint Surgery (American), 63:1239–1248, 1981.

Mubarak, SJ, Leach, JL, & Wenger, DR. Management of congenital dislocation of the hip in the infant. Contemporary Orthopaedics, 15:29–44, 1987.

Newman, JS, & Newberg, AH. Congenital tarsal coalition: Multimodality evaluation with emphasis on CT and MR imaging. Radiographics, 20:321–332, 2000.

Olney, B, Latz, K, & Asher, M. Treatment of hip dysplasia in older children with a combined one-stage procedure. Clinical Orthopaedics and Related Research, 347:215–223, 1998.

Oppenheim, WL, Bowen, RE, McDonough, PW, Funahashi, TT, & Salusky, IB. Outcome of slipped capital femoral epiphysis in renal osteodystrophy. Journal of Pediatric Orthopaedics, 23:169–174, 2003.

Paley, D, Bhave, A, Herzenberg, JE, & Bowen, JR. Multiplier method for predicting limb-length discrepancy. Journal of Bone and Joint Surgery (American), 82-A:1432–1446, 2000.

Paley, D. Current techniques of limb lengthening. Journal of Pediatric Orthopaedics, 8:73–92, 1988.

Paley, D. Problems, obstacles, and complications of limb lengthening by the Ilizarov technique. Clinical Orthopaedics and Related Research, 250:81–104, 1990.

Paley, D, Herzenberg, JE, Paremain, G, & Bhave, A. Femoral lengthening over an intramedullary nail. Journal of Bone and Joint Surgery (American), 79:1464–1480, 1997.

Pauli, RM, Breed, A, Horton, VK, Glinski, LP, & Reiser, CA. Prevention of fixed, angular kyphosis in achondroplasia. Journal of Pediatric Orthopaedics, 17:726–733, 1997.

Pavlik, A. Stirrups as an aid in the treatment of congenital dysplasias of the hip in children. LeKarskeListy, 5(3–4):81–85, 1950. (Translated by Bialik, V, & Reis, ND. Journal of Pediatric Orthopaedics, 9:157–159, 1989.)

Pavlik, A. The functional method of treatment using a harness with stirrups as the primary method of conservative therapy for infants with congenital dislocation of the hip. Zeitschrift fur Orthopadie und Ihre Grenzgebiet 89:341, 1957. (Translated by Peltier, LF. Clinical Orthopaedics and Related Research, 281:4–10, 1992.)

Pellecchia, GL, Lugo-Larcheveque, N, & Deluca, PA. Differential diagnosis in physical therapy evaluation of thigh pain in an adolescent boy. Journal of Orthopedic and Sports Physical Therapy, 23:51–55, 1996.

Perlman, MH, Patzakis, MJ, Kumar, PJ, & Holtom, P. The incidence of joint involvement with adjacent osteomyelitis in pediatric patients. Journal of Pediatric Orthopaedics, 20:40–43, 2000.

Peterson, MD, Weiner, DS, Green, NE, & Terry, CL. Acute slipped capital femoral epiphysis: The value and safety of urgent manipulative reduction. Journal of Pediatric Orthopaedics, 17:648–654, 1997.

Pill, SG, Ganley, TJ, Milam, RA, Lou, JE, Meyer, JS, & Flynn, JM. Role of magnetic resonance imaging and clinical criteria in predicting successful nonoperative treatment of osteochondritis dissecans in children. Journal of Pediatric Orthopaedics, 23:102–108, 2003.

Pineda, C, Resnick, D, & Greenway, G. Diagnosis of tarsal coalition with computed tomography. Clinical Orthopaedics and Related Research, 208:282–288, 1986.

Pirani, S, Zeznik, L, & Hodges, D. Magnetic resonance imaging study of the congenital clubfoot treated with the Ponseti method. Journal of Pediatric Orthopaedics, 21:719–726, 2001.

Pitkow, RB. External rotation contracture of the extended hip. Clinical Orthopaedics and Related Research, 110:139–144, 1975.

Ponseti, IV, El-Khoury, GY, Ippolito, E, & Weinstein, SL. A radiographic study of skeletal deformities in treated clubfeet. Clinical Orthopedics and Related Research, 160:30–42, 1981.

Rajacich, N, Bell, DF, & Armstrong, PF. Pediatric applications of the Ilizarov method. Clinical Orthopaedics and Related Research, 280:72–80, 1992.

Raney, EM, Topoleski, TA, Yaghoubian, R, Guidera, KJ, & Marshall, JG. Orthotic treatment of infantile tibia vara. Journal of Pediatric Orthopaedics, 18:670–674, 1998.

Rattey, T, Piehl, F, & Wright, JG. Acute slipped capital femoral epiphysis. Review of outcomes and rates of avascular necrosis. Journal of Bone and Joint Surgery (American), 78:398–402, 1996.

Reikeras, O, Pal Kristiansen, L, Gunderson, R, & Steen, H. Reduced tibial torsion in congenital clubfoot: CT measurements in 24 patients. Acta Orthopaedica Scandinavia, 72:53–56, 2001.

Reinker, KA. Early diagnosis and treatment of hinge abduction in Legg-Perthes disease. Journal of Pediatric Orthopaedics, 16:3–9, 1996.

Riebel, TW, Nasir, R, & Nazarenko, O. The value of sonography in the detection of osteomyelitis. Pediatric Radiology, 26:291–297, 1996.

Robertson, W, Kelly, BT, & Green, DW. Osteochondritis dissecans of the knee in children. Current Opinion in Pediatrics, 15:38–44, 2003.

Rohren, EM, Kosarek, FJ, & Helms, CA. Discoid lateral meniscus and the frequency of meniscal tears. Skeletal Radiology, 30:316–320, 2001.

Rosendahl, K, Markestad, T, & Lie, RT. Ultrasound screening for developmental dysplasia of the hip in the neonate: The effect on treatment rate and prevalence of late cases. Pediatrics, 94:47–52, 1994.

Rostoucher, P, Bensahel, H, Pennecot, GF, Kaewpornsawan, K, & Mazda, K. Slipped capital femoral epiphysis: Evaluation of different modes of treatment. Journal of Pediatric Orthopaedics (British), 5:96–101, 1996.

Ruiz-Garcia, M, Tovar-Baudin, A, Del Castillo-Ruiz, V, Rodriguez, HP, Collado, MA, Mora, TM, Rueda-Franco, F, & Gonzalez-Astiazaran, A. Early detection of neurological manifestations in achondroplasia. Child's Nervous System, 13:208–213, 1997.

Sachithanandam, V, & Joseph, B. The influence of footwear on the prevalence of flat foot. A survey of 1846 skeletally mature persons. Journal of Bone and Joint Surgery (British), 77:254–257, 1995.

Salter, RB. Etiology, pathogenesis and possible prevention of congenital dislocation of the hip. Canadian Medical Association Journal, 98:933–945, 1968.

Salter, RB. Textbook of Disorders and Injuries of the Musculoskeletal System. Baltimore: Williams & Wilkins, 1970.

Salter, RB, & Harris, WR. Injuries involving the epiphyseal plate. Journal of Bone and Joint Surgery (American), 45:587–622, 1963.

Samuelson, T, & Olney, B. Percutaneous pin fixation of chronic slipped capital femoral epiphysis. Clinical Orthopaedics and Related Research, 326:225–228, 1996.

Schoenecker, PL, Johnson, LO, Martin, RA, Doyle, P, & Capelli, AM. Intra-articular hip arthrodesis without subtrochanteric osteotomy in adolescents: Technique and short-term follow-up. American Journal of Orthopaedics, 26:257–264, 1997.

Scoles, PV. Pediatric Orthopaedics in Clinical Practice, 2nd ed. Chicago: Year Book, 1988.

Scoles, PV, Boyd, A, & Jones, PK. Roentgenographic parameters of the normal infant hip. Journal of Pediatric Orthopaedics, 7:656–663, 1987.

Seller, K, Raab, P, Wild, A, & Krauspe R. Risk-benefit analysis of prophylactic pinning in slipped capital femoral epiphysis. Journal of Pediatric Orthopaedics (British), 10:192–196, 2001.

Shands, AR, & Steele, MK. Torsion of the femur: A follow-up report on the use of the Dunlap method for its determination. Journal of Bone and Joint Surgery (American), 40:803–816, 1958.

Shulman, LH, Sala, DA, Chu, ML, McCaul, PR, & Sandler, BJ. Developmental implications of idiopathic toe walking. Journal of Pediatrics, 130:541–546, 1997.

Siffert, RS. Classification of the osteochondroses. Clinical Orthopaedics and Related Research, 158:10–18, 1981.

Simard, S, Marchant, M, & Mencio, G. The Ilizarov procedure: Limb lengthening and its implications. Physical Therapy, 72:25–34, 1992.

Smith, BG, Millis, MB, Hey, LA, Jaramillo, D, & Kasser, JR. Post-reduction computed tomography in developmental dislocation of the hip. Part II: Predictive value for outcome. Journal of Pediatric Orthopaedics, 17:631–636, 1997.

Smith, DW, & Jones, KL. Recognizable Patterns of Human Malformation, Vol. VII. Major Problems in Clinical Pediatrics. Philadelphia: WB Saunders, 1982.

Smith, JT, Matan, A, Coleman, SS, Stevens, PM, & Scott, SM. The predictive value of the development of the acetabular teardrop figure in developmental dysplasia of the hip. Journal of Pediatric Orthopaedics, 17:165–169, 1997.

Song, KM, & Sloboda, JF. Acute hematogenous osteomyelitis in children. Journal of the American Academy of Orthopaedic Surgeons, 9:166–175, 2001.

Song, KM, & Lapinsky, A. Determination of hip position in the Pavlik harness. Journal of Pediatric Orthopaedics, 20:317–319, 2000.

Staheli, LT. Torsional deformity. Pediatric Clinics of North America, 24:799–811, 1977.

Staheli, LT, Corbett, M, Wyss, C, & King, H. Lower extremity rotational problems in children. Journal of Bone and Joint Surgery (American), 67:39–47, 1985.

Staheli, LT, & Engel, GM. Tibial torsion: A method of assessment and a study of normal children. Clinical Orthopaedics and Related Research, 86:183–186, 1972.

Stanitski, DF, Shaheheraghi, H, Nicker, DA, & Armstrong, PF. Results of tibial lengthening with the Ilizarov technique. Journal of Pediatric Orthopaedics, 16:168–172, 1996.

Stanley, G, McLoughlin, S, & Beals, RK. Observations on the cause of bowlegs in achondroplasia. Journal of Pediatric Orthopaedics, 22:112–116, 2002.

Stasikelis, PJ, Sullivan, CM, Phillips, WA, & Polard, JA. Slipped capital femoral epiphysis. Prediction of contralateral involvement. Journal of Bone and Joint Surgery (American), 78:1149–1155, 1996.

Stevens, PM, Maguire, M, Dales, MD, & Robins, AJ. Physeal stapling for idiopathic genu valgum. Journal of Pediatric Orthopaedics, 19:645–649, 1999a.

Stevens, PM, & Otis, S. Ankle valgus and clubfeet. Journal of Pediatric Orthopaedics, 19:515–517, 1999b.

Stricker, SJ, & Angulo, JC. Idiopathic toe walking: A comparison of treatment methods. Journal of Pediatric Orthopaedics, 18:289–293, 1998.

Stuberg, WA, Koehler, A, Wichita, M, Temme, J, & Kaplan, P. A comparison of femoral torsion assessment using goniometry and computerized tomography. Pediatric Physical Therapy, 1:115–118, 1989.

Sullivan, JA. Pediatric flatfoot: Evaluation and management. Journal of the American Academy of Orthopaedic Surgeons, 7:44–53, 1999.

Tachdjian, MO. Pediatric Orthopaedics, Vols. 1–4, 2nd ed. Philadelphia: WB Saunders, 1990.

Taylor, GR, & Clarke, NM. Monitoring the treatment of developmental dysplasia of the hip with the Pavlik harness. The role of ultrasound. Journal of Bone and Joint Surgery (British), 79:719–723, 1997.

Theodorou, DJ, Theodorou, SJ, Boutin, RD, Chung, C, Fliszar, E, Kakitsubata, Y, & Resnick, D. Stress fractures of the lateral metatarsal bones in metatarsus adductus foot deformity: A previously unrecognized association. Skeletal Radiology, 28:679–684, 1999.

Thompson, GH. Back pain in children: An instructional course lecture. Journal of Bone and Joint Surgery (American), 75:928–938, 1993.

Thompson, GH, & Carter, JR. Late onset tibia vara (Blount's disease). Clinical Orthopaedics and Related Research, 255:24–35, 1990.

Tippett, SR. Referred knee pain in a young athlete: A case study. Journal of Orthopedic and Sports Physical Therapy, 19:117–120, 1994.

Tokmakova, KP, Stanton, RP, & Mason, DE. Factors influencing the development of osteonecrosis in patients treated for slipped capital femoral epiphysis. Journal of Bone and Joint Surgery (American), 85-A:798–801, 2003.

Tonnis, D, & Skamel, HJ. Computerized tomography in evaluation of decreased acetabular and femoral anteversion. Radiologe, 43:735–739, 2003.

Torode, IP, & Gillespie, R. Rotationplasty of the lower limb for congenital defects of the femur. Journal of Bone and Joint Surgery (British), 65:569–573, 1983.

Tredwell, SJ, & Bell, HM. Efficacy of neonatal hip examination. Journal of Pediatric Orthopaedics, 1:61–65, 1981.

Turner, MS. The association between tibial torsion and knee joint pathology. Clinical Orthopaedics and Related Research, 302:47–51, 1994.

Umans, H, Liebling, MS, Moy, L, Haramati, N, Macy, NJ, & Pritzker, HA. Slipped capital femoral epiphysis: A physeal lesion diagnosed by MRI, with radiographic and CT correlation. Skeletal Radiology, 27:139–144, 1998.

Volpon, JB. Footprint analysis during the growth period. Journal of Pediatric Orthopaedics, 14:83–85, 1994.

Wagner, H. Operative lengthening of the femur. Clinical Orthopaedics and Related Research, 136:125–142, 1978.

Walsh, JJ, & Morrissy, RT. Torticollis and hip dislocation. Journal of Pediatric Orthopaedics, 18:219–221, 1998.

Wang, L, Bowen, JR, Puniak, MA, Guille, JT, & Glutting J. An evaluation of various methods of treatment for Legg-Calvé-Perthes disease. Clinical Orthopaedics and Related Research, 314:225–233, 1995.

Warner, WC, Jr, Beaty, JH, & Canale, ST. Chondrolysis after slipped capital femoral epiphysis. Journal of Pediatric Orthopaedics (British), 5:168–172, 1996.

Washington, ER, III, Root, L, & Liener, UC. Discoid lateral meniscus in children. Long-term follow-up after excision. Journal of Bone and Joint Surgery (American), 77:1357–1361, 1995.

Weiner, D. Pathogenesis of slipped capital femoral epiphysis: Current concepts. Journal of Pediatric Orthopaedics (British), 5:67–73, 1996.

Weinstein, SL. Congenital hip dislocation: Long range problems, residual signs and symptoms after successful treatment. Clinical Orthopaedics and Related Research, 281:69–74, 1992.

Weinstein, SL. Natural history and treatment outcomes of childhood hip disorders. Clinical Orthopaedics and Related Research, 344:227–242, 1997.

Wenger, DR, & Bomar, JD. Human hip dysplasia: evolution of current treatment concepts. Journal of Orthopaedic Science, 8:264–271, 2003.

Wenger, DR, & Leach, J. Foot deformities in infants and children. Pediatric Clinics of North America, 33:1411–1427, 1986.

Wenger, DR, Lee, CS, & Kolman, B. Derotational femoral shortening for developmental dislocation of the hip: Special indications and results in the child younger than 2 years. Journal of Pediatric Orthopaedics, 15:768–779, 1995.

Wenger, DR, Mauldin, D, Speck, G, Morgan, D, & Lieber, RL. Corrective shoes and inserts as treatment for flexible flatfoot in infants and children. Journal of Bone and Joint Surgery (American), 71:800–810, 1989.

Wenger, DR, & Rang, M. The Art of Pediatric Orthopaedics. New York: Raven Press, 1993.

Wenger, DR, Ward, WT, & Herring, JA. Current concepts review: Legg-Calvé-Perthes disease. Journal of Bone and Joint Surgery (American), 73:778–788, 1991.

Wood, JB, Klassen, RA, & Peterson, HA. Osteochondritis dissecans of the femoral head in children and adolescents: A report of 17 cases. Journal of Pediatric Orthopaedics, 15:313–316, 1995.

Wynne-Davies, R. Family studies and the cause of congenital clubfoot: Talipes equinovarus, talipes calcaneovalgus and metatarsus varus. Journal of Bone and Joint Surgery (British), 46:445–463, 1964.

Wynne-Davies, R. Acetabular dysplasia and familial joint laxity: Two etiological factors in congenital dislocation of the hip. Journal of Bone and Joint Surgery (British), 52:704–716, 1970.

Yagi, T. Tibial torsion in patients with medial-type osteoarthrotic knees. Clinical Orthopaedics and Related Research, 302:52–56, 1994.

Yashar, A, Loder, RT, & Hensinger, RN. Determination of skeletal age in children with Osgood-Schlatter disease by using radiographs of the knee. Journal of Pediatric Orthopaedics, 15:298–301, 1995.

Yasui, N, Kawabata, H, Kojimoto, H, Ohno, H, Matsuda, S, Araki, N, Shimomura, Y, & Ochi, T. Lengthening of the lower limbs in patients with achondroplasia and hypochondroplasia. Clinical Orthopaedics and Related Research, 344:298–306, 1997.

Young, N, Bell, DF, & Anthony, A. Pediatric pain patterns during Ilizarov treatment of limb length discrepancy and angular deformity. Journal of Pediatric Orthopaedics, 14:352–357, 1994.

Young, RS, Andrew, PD, & Cummings, GS. Effect of simulating leg length inequality on pelvic torsion and trunk mobility. Gait and Posture, 11:217–223, 2000.

Yun, AG, Severino, R, Reinker, K. Attempted limb lengthenings beyond twenty percent of the initial bone length: results and complications. Journal of Pediatric Orthopaedics, 20:151–159, 2000.

Chapter 18

Sports Injuries in Children

Donna Bernhardt Bainbridge
PT, EdD, ATC

On playgrounds, fields, and courts, and in gyms and pools, more children than ever before are playing or competing in sports. Current estimates suggest that 20 million to 30 million youths between the ages of 5 and 17 years of age participate in community-sponsored athletic programs (Adirim & Cheng, 2003; Patel & Nelson, 2000). Over 6.5 million teenagers regularly participate in competitive high school team sports (Birrer et al., 2003). Half of all males and one fourth of all females aged 8 to 16 years (approximately 7 million) were reported to be engaged in competitive, organized school sports (Stanitski, 1989). Heath and colleagues (1994) reported that approximately 37% of all students in grades 9 to 12 engaged in vigorous physical activity for at least 20 minutes three or more times per week according to the 1990 Youth Risk Behavior Survey. By 1997 the percentage of participation had increased to 63.8% (Pratt et al., 1999). Participation remained higher for males than for females (72.3% versus 53.5%).

Increase in participation increases the risk of sports-related injury in children. Lack of fitness has also been associated with injury in both children and adults (Caspersen et al., 2000; Centers for Disease Control and Prevention, 2003; Epstein et al., 2001). Fitness levels have declined for boys older than age 14 and for girls older than age 12. One third of American children younger than age 8 are overweight. Fifty percent of children in grades 5 through 12 do not get the vigorous activity necessary to maintain or improve cardiovascular status. Forty percent of children between 5 and 8 years of age show at least one risk factor for heart disease (Thomas et al., 2003).

The child cannot be considered simply a small adult. Children have different structural and physiologic components that must be specifically addressed (Stanitski, 1997). This chapter will provide an extensive overview of sports medicine in children and youth for the pediatric physical therapist. The purposes of the chapter are to review the elements of injury prevention/risk reduction, and to discuss those factors that increase risk for sports-related injury in children with and without disabilities. The types and sites of sports injuries, including those injuries unique to the child, will be addressed with provision of guidelines for rehabilitation.

INCIDENCE OF INJURY

The incidence of injury has escalated as participation has increased. Although varying methodologies and definitions of injury have hindered development of broad epidemiologic data, many studies have documented risk in sports participation. A 1988 National Center for Health Statistics report estimated that 4,379,000 injuries from sports and recreation occur in children aged 5 to 17 years, accounting for 36% of all injuries in children (Bijur et al., 1995). Beachy and colleagues (1997) reported similar rates of injury (35%). The European Home-and Leisure-Accident Surveillance System reported an annual incidence of 73.3 injuries per 1000 children aged 6 to 17 years (Sorensen et al., 1996). Types of injuries included contusions (37%), fractures (22%), sprains (25%), and strains (5%).

Backx and colleagues (1991a) reported 399 sports injuries from a population of 1818 school children aged 8 to 17 years (22%). The most common injuries were contusions (43%) and sprains (21%). Physical contact, a high rate of jumping, and indoor play were the factors that contributed most to injuries. Watkins and Peabody (1996) reported that 62% of injuries were a result of sprains, strains, or contusions, and that high or explosive speed and physical contact were responsible for the majority of injuries. Whieldon and Cerny (1990) reported that collision sports, such as football and wrestling, generated the highest injury rates, followed by contact sports such as baseball and basketball. Boys had higher injury rates than girls only in contact sports. The popularity of football, coupled with the fact that it is the most common participant sport among high school males, make its elevated injury rate a significant economic issue (Dvorak & Junge, 2000; Metzl, 1999).

Taylor and Attia (2000) reviewed all sports-related injuries in children aged between 5 and 18 years seen in an emergency room over a 2-year period. They reported 677 injuries, 71% in males. Sports most commonly implicated were basketball (19.5%), football (17.1%), baseball/softball (14.9%), soccer (14.2%), in-line skating (5.7%), and hockey (4.6%). Sprains and strains were the most frequent types of injuries, followed by fracture, contusions, and lacerations; these accounted for 90% of all injuries. The National Health Interview Survey estimated that the sports-related injury rate for 5- to 24-year-olds was 42% higher than the estimates based on emergency room visits. The highest rate (59.3%) was for 5- to 14-year-olds

(Conn et al., 2003). Lenaway and colleagues (1992) noted that middle school/junior high students had the highest injury rate, followed by elementary school students and then high school students. Sports, which accounted for 53% of all injuries, were an increasing cause of injury as grade level increased. Location of injury was the playground for elementary ages, the athletic field for middle school students, and the gym for high school students.

A recent study by Radelet and colleagues (2002) followed 1659 children aged 7 to 13 years during two seasons of community baseball, softball, indoor and outdoor soccer, and football. Their definition of injury included any injury that was examined on the field by a coach, required first aid, or prevented participation. They reported injury rates of 1.7 for baseball, 1.0 for softball, 2.1 for soccer, and 1.5 for football for 100 athlete exposures. Rates were significantly higher for game versus practice for all sports except softball. However, the frequency of injury per team per season was four to seven times higher in football with more severe injuries. The types of injuries were consistent with findings in other studies. However, contact was a leading cause of severe injury in baseball (contact with ball) and football (contact with player). Interestingly, children between the ages of 8 and 10 years were more frequently injured than younger or older children, related perhaps to their transition to more advanced levels of play.

Children and adolescents are becoming more involved in extreme variations of sports as well as increased risk-taking with everyday sports. Various authors have noted significant injury rates with cycling (Gerstenbluth et al., 2002; Winston et al., 2002); exer-cycling (Benson et al., 2000), riding in all-terrain vehicles (Brogger-Jensen et al., 1990; Brown at al., 2002); diving (Blanksby et al., 1997); snowboarding and skiing (Drkulec & Letts, 2001; Shorter et al., 1999; Skokan et al., 2003); in-line skate, skateboard, or scooter use (Kubiak & Slongo, 2003; Mankovsky et al., 2002; Nguyen & Letts, 2001; Osberg et al., 1998; Powell and Tanz, 2000a; Powell & Tanz, 2000b). Although many of these injuries are contusions, fractures, and sprains/strains, these authors noted significant numbers of abdominal trauma with damage to the kidney, pancreas, or liver; head and neck injury; and hand trauma. Schmitt & Gerner (2001) noted that sports and diving caused 6.8% and 7.7% of 1016 cases of spinal cord injury, respectively, in persons aged 9 to 52 years. The sports implicated were alpine skiing, horse-back riding, airsports (hang gliding and paragliding), gymnastics, and trampoline in decreasing order of incidence. Smith and Shields (1998), who documented 214 trampoline injuries in 1995 through 1997, noted that these children were supervised in 55.6% of the injury occasions.

The incidence of catastrophic injuries and fatalities in high school has been documented for the years 1977 through 1998 (Cantu & Mueller, 2000). Of 384 reported incidents, there were 118 fatalities, 200 nonfatal but permanent cervical injuries with severe neurologic disability, and 66 permanent cerebral injuries. Most cervical injuries occurred with tackling. Attention to the causes of severe injuries or deaths (i.e. proper education about game fundamentals, close monitoring of fair play, higher equipment standards, and improved medical care) have led to a 27% reduction in permanent spinal cord injury in the past 25 years (Cantu & Mueller, 2003a). Brown and Brunn (2001) noted that 27% of cervical injuries seen in a trauma center were related to sports, and football accounted for 29% of those cervical injuries. Head and neck injuries accounted for 23% of all injuries in youth ice hockey players (9–15 years) with 86% caused by body checking (Brust et al., 1992). Baseball also has significant injury potential; the U.S. Consumer Product Safety Commission reported 88 deaths related to baseball between 1973 and 1995. These deaths resulted from impact from the bat, or direct ball contact to chest, head, neck, or throat (Kyle, 1996).

Significant attention has been directed to differences in types and rates of injuries in males and females. Some researchers (Aagaard & Jorgensen, 1996; Backx et al., 1991b; Brynhildsen et al., 1990; Lodge et al., 1990; McLain & Reynolds, 1989) compared boys and girls in similar sports and reported no difference in overall injury rates. Other researchers have noted differences in specific injury type, or in injury rates for targeted joints. A study by de Loes and colleagues (2000) reported that the risk of knee injury was significantly higher for women ages 14 to 20 years than men of the same age in cross country and downhill skiing, gymnastics, volleyball, basketball, and handball. Hosea and colleagues (2000) reported increased risk for grade 1 ankle sprains in women basketball players.

Several studies have noted an increased incidence of anterior cruciate ligament (ACL) injuries in females (Baker, 1998; Smith & Wilder, 1999). The relative risk ranged from 2.44 in collegiate midshipmen (Gwinn et al., 2000), to 3.79 for high school basketball players (Messina et al., 1999). Gomez and colleagues (1996) reported that ACL injuries accounted for 69% of severe knee injuries in basketball. Soderman and colleagues (2002) reported that 38% of soccer players with ACL injuries had sustained the injury before the age of 16 years. Levy and associates (1997) reported higher rates of ACL injury in women playing rugby than soccer or basketball. Although research has yet to define the reasons for this increased risk, several causes including differences in landing angle (Fagenbaum, 2003) or strength (Hewett et al., 1999), hormonal status, or

lower extremity posture such as recurvatum, navicular drop and excessive pronation (Loudon et al., 1996) have been implicated.

PREVENTION OF INJURIES

The key to management of sports injuries in children is prevention. As discussed in Chapter 8, children need proper physiologic conditioning, strength, and flexibility to participate safely in an organized or recreational athletic endeavor. Although lack of fitness, strength, and flexibility does not preclude participation, remediation must be built into conditioning and training programs to decrease the risk of injury. The major elements in the process of injury risk management are preparticipation examination, conditioning and training, proper supervision, protection of the body, and environmental control (Smith & Wilder, 1999).

PREPARTICIPATION EXAMINATION

The preparticipation examination is the initial step in the process of injury prevention. The American Medical Association Committee on Medical Aspects of Sports constructed a Bill of Rights for the Athlete, one part of which is a thorough preseason history and medical examination. The purposes are fivefold: (1) to determine the general health of the athlete and detect conditions that place the participant at additional risk; (2) to identify relative or absolute medical contraindications to participation; (3) to identify sports that may be played safely; (4) to assess maturity and overall fitness; and (5) to educate the athlete. These examinations are also necessary to meet legal and insurance requirements in many states (Bar-Or et al., 1995). The usefulness of these screenings has been demonstrated in several studies (Bratton, 1997; Drezner, 2000; Fuller et al., 1997; Glover & Maron, 1998; Grafe et al., 1997; Kurowski & Chandran, 2000; Linder et al., 1981; Lyznicki et al., 2000; Maron, 2002; Rifat et al., 1995).

Most states require either an individual examination or a multistation screening. The merits and disadvantages of these methods have been evaluated. The primary physician performing an individual examination knows or has access to the athlete's health records, can discuss sensitive health or personal issues, and may be most qualified to oversee any necessary follow-up care. The time and cost are a disadvantage of the individual examination. Additionally, disparate knowledge and interest among physicians regarding sports and the requirements to participate may hinder effective evaluation for all participants. The

TABLE 18-1	Multistation Preparticipation Examination

STATION	PERSONNEL
Sign-in/instructions	Ancillary personnel/coach
Height/weight/vital signs	Nurse, exercise physiologist, athletic trainer, or physical therapist
Visual examination	Nurse or coach
Medical examination	Internist or family practitioner
Orthopedic evaluation	Physician or physical therapist
Flexibility assessment	Physical therapist or athletic trainer
Strength evaluation	Physical therapist, athletic trainer, or exercise physiologist
Body composition	Exercise physiologist, physical therapist, or athletic trainer
Speed, agility, power, balance, endurance	Exercise physiologist, coach, or athletic trainer
Assessment/clearance	Physician

multistation examination is more cost and time efficient, and provides a thorough and appropriate screening for all potential participants. Professional experts assess each athlete in the area of her or his specialization (Table 18-1), increasing the probability of detection of abnormalities (Garrick, 1990; Smith & Laskowski, 1998). North Carolina has adopted a preparticipation examination for their specific needs based on questions that have shown significant yield (Fields, 1994). The use of a Web-based examination has also been reported (Peltz et al., 1999).

The frequency of the preparticipation examination is being debated. Although annual evaluations are most traditional (Powell, 1987), many clinicians advocate evaluation before each season (Grafe et al., 1997). A complete entry-level examination and evaluation, followed by annual reevaluation that includes a brief physical examination, a physical maturity assessment, and an examination/evaluation of all new problems is one current recommendation (Bratton, 1997). The American Academy of Pediatrics (1989) recommends a biannual complete evaluation followed by an interim history before each season. The schedule that meets the primary objectives of the academy, however, is a complete entry-level evaluation followed by a limited annual reevaluation that includes a brief physical examination (to evaluate height, weight, blood pressure, and pulse; perform auscultation; examine the skin; and test visual acuity), a physical maturity

assessment if previous level was less than Tanner stage IV, and an evaluation of all new problems (Powell, 1997).

The components of the preparticipation examination are the medical history; the physical examination, including cardiovascular and eye examinations; musculoskeletal assessment; body composition and height and weight determination; specific field testing; and readiness, both physical and psychologic. The examination should be completed 6 weeks before the practice season to allow adequate time for further evaluation or for correction of any problems (Garrick, 1990; Lombardo, 1991). The components of the examination should be tailored to the specific demands of the sport.

History

The medical history is the cornerstone of the medical evaluation (Lombardo, 1991) and will identify the majority of problems affecting athletes (Grafe et al., 1997; Rifat et al., 1995). Short forms that are easy to complete and written in lay terms are preferable. Forms should be completed and signed by the athlete and parent or legal guardian. Content areas that should be particularly noted include exercise-induced syncope or asthma; family history of heart disease or sudden death; history of loss of consciousness, concussion, or neurologic conditions; history of heat stroke; medications; allergies; history of musculoskeletal dysfunction; dates of hospitalizations or surgery; absence or loss of a paired organ; and immunizations. A Preparticipation Physical Evaluation Form is available at the American Academy of Pediatrics website (http://www.aap.org/sections/sportsmedicine/pubed.htm).

Physical Examination

The physical examination is used to evaluate areas of concern identified in the history (Anderson, 2002). The minimally sufficient examination includes cardiovascular and eye examinations, a maturity assessment, and a review of all body systems. Blood pressure should be measured using appropriately sized sphygmomanometer cuffs (Lombardo, 1991). Blood pressure is most accurately predicted by gender and percentile of height in those under the age of 18 years (NIH, 1996). The 95th percentile upper limit values for normal blood pressure are 110/75 mm Hg below age 6, 120/80 mm Hg for 6- to 10-year-olds, 125/85 mm Hg for 11- to 14-year-olds, and 135/90 mm Hg for 15- to 18-year-olds (Cooper, 1991). A diagnosis of hypertension requires three abnormal readings. If blood pressure is elevated, repeat measures should be taken later in the examination or the next day (Feld et al., 1998). High blood pressure requires further evaluation for clearance to participate in sports (Lombardo, 1991). The remainder of the cardiovascular screening evaluation assesses peripheral pulses and heartbeat for symmetry and rate. Auscultation of the heart should be performed with the young person both seated and supine (Lombardo, 1991). Because as many as 85% of youths have benign heart murmurs, various maneuvers such as squat to stand, Valsalva, and deep inspiration can differentiate functional from pathologic murmurs. Arrhythmias are not abnormal in children, but increases in premature ventricular contractions with exercise require further assessment (Fuller et al., 1997; Glover & Maron, 1998). Paroxysmal supraventricular tachycardia needs to be evaluated, but is not a reason for disqualification (Lyznicki et al., 2000; Maron, 2002; Rifat et al., 1995).

Visual acuity is tested using a Snelling chart and should be correctable to 20/200. Any inequality of pupil diameter or reactivity should be noted so responses after potential injury can be compared with this baseline value. Uncorrectable legal blindness (acuity less than 20/200 or absence of an eye) requires counseling regarding participation in collision or contact sports. The importance of protective eyewear for athletes who wear glasses or have unilateral vision should be stressed (Bar-Or et al., 1995).

Pulmonary status is determined by symmetry of diaphragmatic excursion and breath sounds. Children with asthma, including exercise-induced asthma, should be allowed to participate in activities if the condition is properly controlled with medication (Lombardo, 1991; Wiens et al., 1992). Abdominal assessment determines rigidity, tenderness, organomegaly, or the presence of masses. Par-

ticipation by any athlete with organomegaly is restricted until further tests determine the cause of the enlarged organ (Bar-Or et al., 1995).

Careful examination of the skin is vital in examination of all persons, but it is particularly important for those who will participate in contact sports. Participation in these sports should be deferred for children with evidence of any communicable skin disease, such as impetigo, carbuncles, herpes, scabies, and louse or fungal infections (Bar-Or et al., 1995; Lombardo, 1991).

Genitourinary examination of males is used to assess the child for testicular presence, descended testicles, and possible inguinal hernia. The genital examination is deferred in girls unless a history of amenorrhea or menstrual irregularity warrants referral. A maturational index should be determined for all athletes so that appropriate matching of age and sport can occur (Bar-Or et al, 1995). Guidelines for staging of secondary sexual characteristics are reliable, proven, and practical (Table 18-2).

The musculoskeletal screening examination should include assessment of posture with particular attention to atrophy, spinal asymmetry, pelvic level, discrepancy of leg lengths, and lower extremity deformities such as genu valgus or varus, patellar deformities, and pes planus. Gait should be examined with the child walking and running, as well as walking on toes and heels. Passive range of motion and two-joint musculotendinous flexibility should be screened. Muscle strength can be assessed using a manual muscle test, handheld dynamometer, or isokinetic

| TABLE 18-2 | Maturity Staging Guidelines |

MALE		
PUBIC HAIR	**PENIS**	**TESTIS**
None	Preadolescent	
Slight, long, slight pigmentation	Slight enlargement	Enlarged scrotum, pink slight ruga
Darker, starts to curl, small amount	Longer	Larger
Coarse, curly, adult type, but less quantity	Increase in glans size and breadth of penis	Larger, scrotum darker
Adult—spread to inner thighs	Adult	Adult

FEMALE	
PUBIC HAIR	**BREASTS**
Preadolescent (none)	Preadolescent (no germinal button)
Sparse, lightly pigmented, straight medial border of labia	Breast and papilla elevated as small mound; areolar diameter increased
Darker, beginning to curl, increased	Breast and areola enlarged; no contour separation
Coarse, curly, abundant, but less than adult	Areola and papilla form secondary mound
Adult female triangle and spread to medial surface	Mature, nipple projects, areola part of general breast contour

From McKeag, D. Preseason physical examination for the prevention of sports injuries. Sports Medicine, 2:425, 1985.

device. Special stability testing of the shoulders, knees, and ankles should be conducted if the child has had a previous injury or if the current assessment indicates that instability may be present (Garrick, 1990; Powell, 1987).

Body Composition

Height and weight should be assessed and results compared with standard growth charts. A body mass index (BMI) should also be calculated. Children are considered underweight if calculated BMI-for-age is below the 5th percentile; in the normal range if between the 5th and 85th percentile; at risk for overweight if between the 85th and 95th percentile and overweight if BMI-for-age is over the 95th percentile (CDC, 2004). Because weight alone gives no specific assessment of the percentage of lean mass and fat tissue, assessment of subcutaneous body fat provides a more specific evaluation of body composition, although fat thickness varies from birth to adolescence (see Chapter 8). The most practical method for screening is skinfold measurement. This method has demonstrated correlations of 0.70 to 0.85 with hydrostatic weighing if performed by an experienced examiner (Going, 1988). Although the criterion ranges for body fatness related to optimal health are 15% to 25% for girls and 10% to 25% for boys (Lohman, 1992), 20% for girls and 12% for boys are ideal for most activities. Elevated body fat levels may indicate the need for weight reduction. Low weight or low body fat warrants a thorough evaluation of eating habits, weight loss, and body image to rule out the possibility of an eating disorder. High weight and very low body fat could signal use of anabolic steroids, growth hormone, or other performance-enhancing drugs (Lombardo, 1991; McArdle et al., 2001). Because of unorthodox weight loss methods, nutritional content and patterns should also be evaluated, especially in those athletes who must "make weight" (Perriello et al., 1995).

The preparticipation examination can be utilized to screen for involvement in risky health behaviors such as tobacco and alcohol use, use of recreational drugs or ergogenic aids (Iven, 1998), and unsafe sexual practices (American Medical Association, 1993; Nsuami et al., 2003). In addition to questions, the examiner should be alert for loss of attention, irritability, reported changes in behavior, poor grades, and change in weight (American Medical Association, 1993).

A meta-analysis of the literature in which athletes reported drug use documented an overall doping prevalence of 3% to 5 % among athletes 18 years or younger (Laure, 1997). Risk factors for substance abuse include poor or single parent family situation, poor health perception, other drug consumption, antisocial behavior, depression, and clumsiness, and good communication with a parent, academic achievement, regular sports participation, serious and organized personality, and mother at home were cited as protective (Challier et al., 2000; Green et al., 2001; Peretti-Watel et al., 2003; Stronski et al., 2000).

From 3% to 12% of adolescent males, and 1% to 2% of females report having used steroids (Bahrke et al., 1998; Yesalis & Bahrke, 2000). In addition to the risk factors noted for general use of drugs, attempts to increase strength added another risk for use of steroids (DuRant et al., 1995; Forman et al., 1995). The most compelling reasons for taking steroids are to increase body weight and muscle mass, decrease fatigue, and increase aggressive behavior. The adverse effects, including hypertension, hepatitis, testicular atrophy, loss of libido, hepatic carcinoma, and premature epiphyseal closure, far outweigh the benefits of these drugs (Birrer et al., 2002; Laseter & Russell, 1991; Sachtelben et al., 1993; Stanitski et al., 1994). Warning signs of steroid abuse include irritability; sudden mood swings; puffiness in face, upper arms, and chest; sudden increases in blood pressure and weight; yellowish coloration around the fingernails and eyes; hirsutism; and deepening of voice and acne in girls (Bar-Or et al., 1995; McArdle et al., 2001; Stanitski et al., 1994).

Other substances that have been utilized to increase muscle performance include DHEA, branched chain and essential amino acids, creatine, growth hormone, and dietary supplements containing nandrolone and testosterone (Armsey & Green, 1997; Balsom et al., 1994; Davis, 1995; Kreider et al., 1998; Kreider et al., 1995; van Hall et al., 1995). Most recently, designer steroids have been introduced to provide the effects of steroid use, but avoid detection. Other dietary substances including ephedra and carnitine have been utilized to increase energy and endurance, suppress appetite, and promote weight loss (Bell et al., 2002; Haller & Benowitz, 2000; Heinonen, 1996). These natural elements have been touted in popular literature as aids for growth, performance, immunity, and healing and are used by both high school and college athletes, as well as professional athletes (Naylor et al., 2001; Williams, 1994). Research has not supported the efficacy of these substances for performance enhancement with the exception of creatine (Selsby et al., 2003) and carnitine (Kraemer et al., 2003). The research that exists has examined these substances in young adults; no research has been done in the pediatric population under the age of 18 years. Research has reported potential risk and harm with ingestion of substantial amounts of several substances including steroids and nandrolone, ephedra, and branched chain amino acids. The use of ephedrine-containing compounds has been banned by most professional and collegiate sports organizations, as well as the National Federation of State High School Associations.

Diuretics are frequently used to "make weight" for an event or to mask drug usage (Grana & Kalenak, 1991). Performance may, however, be decreased as a result of dehydration or electrolyte losses (Birrer et al., 2002; Grana & Kalenak, 1991; McArdle et al., 2001). Likewise, stimulants, such as caffeine and amphetamines, are commonly abused in an effort to increase performance in sports. They serve only to mask normal fatigue and to increase aggression, hostility, and uncooperativeness and can lead to addiction and death (Wagner, 1991).

The use of barbiturates, antidepressants, and beta blockers has been noted in sports in which fine control is required, such as shooting and archery. Although they do calm the nervous system and lower heart rate, even therapeutic doses may cause bronchospasm, hypotension, and bradycardia (Millar, 1990).

The use of recreational drugs, including nicotine, smokeless tobacco, alcohol, marijuana, cocaine, and even heroin, is increasing among youth (Sobal & Marquart, 1994). Symptoms including agitation, restlessness, insomnia, difficulty with short-term memory or concentration, and decline in performance might signal behavior indicative of substance abuse (Clarkson, 1996; Green, 1990).

Dietary supplements are not approved by the Food and Drug Administration (FDA), so actual ingredients are not listed on the label, nor are safety and effectiveness validated. The few protections offered to the consumer include a USP label, a nationally known manufacturer, and appropriate and accurate claims supported by research. Overdosage of both fat- and water-soluble vitamins can cause damage to the liver and kidneys (Millar, 1990).

Specific Field Tests

Field testing is done to assess specific athletic potential in a specific sport. The components assessed are muscle strength, muscle power, endurance, speed, agility and flexibility, and cardiovascular performance (Bar-Or et al., 1995). Field test performance has been shown to identify deficits from previous injury that standard physical examination may not define (Nadler et al., 2002).

General muscle strength can be assessed with a maximal activity pertinent to the sport, such as bench presses, pull-ups, or push-ups for the upper extremities and leg presses or sit-ups for the lower extremities. Endurance can be assessed by performing as many repetitions of the task as possible. Muscle power can be evaluated with vertical jumping, performing a standing long jump, or throwing a medicine ball, as appropriate.

Speed is evaluated using a 40- or 50-yard dash, and agility can be assessed with the Vodak agility test (Gaillard et al., 1978) or a similar battery of tests. The most com-mon, standardized methods of assessing flexibility are the sit and reach test, which has norms for children, and active knee extension performed in a supine position with the hips flexed to 90° (Hunter et al., 1985). Cardiovascular performance is most easily assessed using a submaximal test on an appropriate device, such as a cycle ergometer, treadmill, or upper-body ergometer. A field test for cardiovascular performance is the 12-minute run or the timed 1.5-mile run (Bar-Or et al., 1995; Bunc, 1994; Larsen et al., 2002). Field tests that involve jumping and sprinting have been correlated to laboratory results (Baker & Davies, 2002).

The outcome of the preparticipation examination determines the level of clearance to participate in sports. Clearance can be unrestricted for any sport or restricted to specific types of sports in the following manner: (1) no collision (violent, direct impact) or contact (physical touching); (2) limited contact or impact; or (3) noncontact only. The American Academy of Pediatrics has developed a classification system for sports activities and recommendations for restriction of participation that are excellent guides in making decisions for individual athletes (American Academy of Pediatrics, 2001). All decisions or recommendations for further evaluation should be thoroughly discussed with the athletes and their parents (Bar-Or et al., 1995; Powell, 1987).

TRAINING PROGRAM

The preseason examination provides a clear definition of the individual athlete's areas of strength and limitations (Fig. 18-1). The next appropriate step in prevention is the development of an individualized training plan designed to address the particular problems of the athlete as they relate to the requirements of the sport(s). This program could be developed by a sports physical therapist, athletic trainer, or exercise physiologist involved in the preseason screening. Once developed, it should be taught to the athlete, the parent, and the coach.

The training program should be a systematic, progressive plan to address the athlete's weaknesses and to maximally condition the athlete for participation. Training consists of off-season, preseason, in-season, and postseason programs for year-round conditioning and for development of appropriate peak performance. Components should include energy training (aerobic foundation and anaerobic training), muscle training (strength, endurance, flexibility, and power), speed, and proper nutrition. A well-developed, variable, and well-paced program will avoid boredom and potential overuse injury. The psychologic effects of year-round training, or exercise in general, are controversial and not well documented. The risk-benefit

Athletic fitness scorecard for boys

	0	1	2	3	4
Test	Below average	Above average	Good	Very good	Excellent
Strength Pull-ups (no)	Fewer than 7	7 to 9	10 to 12	13 to 14	15 or more
Power Long jump (in)	Fewer than 85	85 to 88	89 to 91	92 to 94	95 or more
Speed 50-yd dash (sec)	Slower than 6.7	6.7 to 6.4	6.3 to 6.0	5.9 to 5.6	5.5 or less
Agility 6-c agility (c)	Fewer than 5-5	5-5 to 6-3	6-4 to 7-2	7-3 to 8-1	8-2 or more
Flexibility Forward flexion (in)	Not reach ruler	1 to 2	3 to 5	6 to 8	9 or more
Muscular endurance Sit-ups (no)	Fewer than 38	38 to 45	46 to 52	53 to 59	60 or more
Cardiorespiratory endurance 12-min run (mi)	Fewer than 1½	1½	1¾	2	2¼ or more

YOUR SCORE

	Strength	Power	Speed	Agility	Flexibility	Muscular endurance	Cardiorespiratory endurance
Your Score							
Rating (0–4)							

Athletic fitness scorecard for girls

	0	1	2	3	4
Test	Below average	Above average	Good	Very good	Excellent
Strength Pull-ups (no)	Fewer than 2	2 to 3	4 to 5	6 to 7	8 or more
Power Long jump (in)	Fewer than 63	63 to 65	66 to 68	69 to 71	72 or more
Speed 50-yd dash (sec)	Slower than 8.2	8.2 to 7.9	7.8 to 7.1	6.9 to 6.0	5.9 or less
Agility 6-c agility (c)	Fewer than 3-5	3-5 to 4-3	4-4 to 5-2	5-3 to 6-2	6-3 or more
Flexibility Forward flexion (in)	Fewer than 3	3 to 5	6 to 8	9 to 11	12 or more
Muscular endurance Sit-ups (no)	Fewer than 26	26 to 31	32 to 38	39 to 45	46 or more
Cardiorespiratory endurance 12-min run (mi)	Fewer than 1¼	1¼	1½	1¾	2 or more

YOUR SCORE

	Strength	Power	Speed	Agility	Flexibility	Muscular endurance	Cardiorespiratory endurance
Your Score							
Rating (0–4)							

◆ **Figure 18-1** Athletic Fitness Scorecards for Boys and Girls. *(Reproduced with permission from Gaillard, B, Haskell, W, Smith, N, & Ogilvie, B. Handbook for the Young Athlete. Boulder, CO: Bull Publishing, 1988.)*

ratio, however, tends to favor exercise for improvement of mood, self-concept, and work behavior when competition is sensibly controlled (Micheli & Jenkins, 2001).

Energy Training

The basis of energy training, a strong aerobic base, should be developed during the off-season. Good training consists of low-intensity, long-duration activity with natural intervals of low- and moderate-intensity work that is sport-specific. Swimming would be a good choice for the field athlete, and cycling or running is appropriate for those in track, soccer, and football. Training on hills or performance of similar resistance efforts should be done once weekly. Children exhibit less efficient movement patterns and a lower maximal acidosis level. Their greater surface area to body mass ratio facilitates greater heat gain on hot days and greater heat loss on colder days. Children produce less sweat, and less total evaporative heat loss. Children produce more metabolic heat per pound of body weight during exercises, such as walking and running. Finally, although children can acclimatize, they do so at a slower rate than adults (Armstrong & Maresh, 1995; Bar-Or, 1995; Falk, 1998). Consequently, intense training in the extreme heat and hard training involving long durations should be minimized until puberty. This avoidance of excessive exercise also helps avert early burnout (Sharkey, 1991).

Anaerobic training programs consist of exertion at 85% to 90% of maximal heart rate for short periods. Anaerobic drills develop a person's ability to tolerate the production of excess lactic acid. Twice-weekly anaerobic training should be performed for maximal benefit. Methods including interval training, fartlek (speed play, or alternate fast and slow running in natural terrain), and pace training are variations of the anaerobic method. Sport-specific anaerobic skills should be developed during preseason and early-season activities (Sharkey, 1991). Young children are less able to use muscle glycogen and produce lactic acid, so this training is difficult for young

athletes and has only minor fitness benefits until they mature. Some training should be used, however, to achieve relaxation and mechanical efficiency at these levels.

Strength Training

Weight training in children has been controversial because of concerns regarding injury to growing bones and the questionable efficacy of this type of training to increase strength. Several research studies have demonstrated that strength can be improved by systematic overload of muscle in postpubescent athletes with results similar to training in adults (Bernhardt et al., 2001; Micheli & Jenkins, 2001).

The area of greatest debate in strength training is how it affects the prepubescent athlete. Because the levels of circulating androgens are low, questions of efficacy have been raised. Strength training for pre- and pubescent athletes has been demonstrated to increase strength without alteration of muscle mass (Faigenbaum et al., 2002; Guy & Micheli, 2001). The trends documenting increased twitch torque and motor unit activation suggest neuromuscular changes, including motor learning and reduction of inhibition (Ramsey et al., 1990; Sharkey, 1991). All authors firmly state, however, that weight lifting in the prepubescent athlete should follow a thorough preparticipation screening for constitutional or anatomic abnormalities (Micheli & Jenkins, 2002; Sharkey, 1991). The program should be closely monitored by an adult with emphasis on form and technique and with careful spotting. Movements should be nonballistic with avoidance of extremely heavy weights. The training apparatus should be scaled to fit the athlete (Kraemer & Fleck, 1993).

Guidelines for strength training are provided in Table 18-3. Athletes will increase strength at a rate of 1% to 3% per week with strength training routines (Sharkey, 1991). Most strength training occurs during the late off-season and preseason periods. Programs should be sport-specific both for the muscles used and the rests between sets. For example, a wrestler, gymnast, or sprinter may

TABLE 18-3	Guidelines for Pediatric Weight Training			
AGES	9–11	12–14	15–16	17+
Exercises per body part	1	1	2	>2
Sets	2	3	3–4	4–6
Repetitions	12–15	10–12	7–11	6–10
Maximum weight (resistance)	Very light	Light	Moderate	Heavy

From Rooks, D, & Micheli, L. Musculoskeletal assessment and training: The young athlete. Clinics in Sports Medicine, 7(3):663, 1988.

TABLE 18-4	Sequence of Muscular Development			
PHASE	**ENDURANCE**	**INTERMEDIATE**	**STRENGTH**	**POWER**
Sets	3–4	3–4	2–3	1–2
Repetitions	10–20	10–15	6–10	4–6
Intensity	Low load	Moderate load	Heavy load	Heaviest load
Training sessions per week	3–5	3–4	2–3	1–2
Rest	Active	Active	Active	Active
Stretching	Before and after session	Before and after session	Before and after session	Before each set, and after last set

take 60- to 90-second rests between exercise bursts whereas a distance runner may move slowly and continuously through all exercises with little rest (Rooks & Micheli, 1988). When athletes have achieved the adequate level for their sport, they should work on the appropriate type of muscle endurance (Table 18-4) with one set of higher-resistance training per week to maintain strength. Endurance work begins in late preseason and continues during the early in-season period.

Power is the ability to do work over a given period of time. As such, it involves both strength and speed in a sport-specific movement. Power is usually developed by performing 15 to 25 repetitions of three sets at 30% to 60% of maximal effort as fast as possible. Although power develops slowly in children, some training can help a child develop the neuromuscular skill of quick movement against low resistance (Sharkey, 1991). Because of the requirements of power training, variable-resistance devices that allow control of speed or resistance are the best approach. Plyometrics, or muscle stretch followed by a burst of contraction, is another available form of power training. Because body weight is approximately 33% of maximal leg strength, these exercises fit the power prescription. An example of a plyometric exercise is step jumping (Voight & Draovitch, 1991).

Power training can cause muscle soreness and potential injury if conducted improperly. Proper technique includes adequate warm-up; slowly increased intensity; performance of jumping activities on dirt, grass, or soft surfaces; and thorough stretching after each session.

Achieving joint and musculotendinous flexibility is an essential part of any training program. Although the effects of flexibility on injury prevention are unclear, enhanced joint mobility, improved comfort of the muscle crossing the joint, and increased blood supply have been documented (Pope et al., 2000; Weimann & Hahn, 1997). Stretching is most effective if nonballistic. Effective methods include static or proprioceptive neuromuscular stretching. The young athlete should be placed on a daily program that stretches all areas of the extremities and trunk with emphasis on the body parts to be used in the sport. Stretches should be easy and simple and demand appropriate levels of neuromuscular control for the age of the child.

Speed

Because the proportion of fast twitch fibers in muscle is inherited, speed is "born" in the child (Sharkey, 1991). All athletes, however, can train the intermediate fibers and improve the components of reaction and movement time. Faster reactions are taught in sport-specific practice drills such as starts, acceleration drills, or play drills that gradually narrow choice. Movement time is enhanced from a base of flexibility and strength with ballistic motions, sprint loading (explosive jump or throw), overspeed, or resisted sprinting (Sharkey, 1991).

Nutrition

Many general articles have been written on nutritional requirements for athletes (Bauman, 1986; Clark, 1991) with recent revisions for pediatric and adolescent athletes (Cooper, 1991; Maughan, 2002; Peterson & Peterson, 1988; Sanders, 1990). The preparticipation screening includes components of a nutritional assessment: skinfold measurements, height, and weight. Skinfold standards for the triceps and calf in children allow one to determine whether the child is overfat (Cooper, 1991). The body fat percentage can be matched to the approximated body fat values developed for various sports, although percentages are not well standarized for younger athletes (Klish, 1995).

Caloric requirements for children are age dependent and vary directly with body weight and surface area. Generally, a young child requires more calories than an adolescent or adult—36 to 40 calories (kcal) per pound per day (Cooper, 1991; Peterson & Peterson, 1988). An additional caloric load is necessary depending on the level of energy output. An approximation for energy expenditure, based on a child weighing 100 lb, is 4 kcal/minute for low-intensity activities, 4 to 7 kcal/minute for moderate-intensity activities, and greater than 7 kcal/minute for high-intensity activities (Peterson & Peterson, 1988). A more complex, but also more accurate, method is to multiply ideal weight in pounds times 10 for basal calories. Basal activity calories are then calculated by multiplying weight in pounds times 3 for sedentary activity, times 5 for moderate activity, and times 10 for vigorous activity. The additional requirements of the sports activity are determined by adding 10 to 14 kcal/minute for boys and 9 to 12 kcal/minute for girls.

Protein requirements of the preadolescent and adolescent athlete approximate those of the adult, but younger athletes have increased protein needs for growth. Small children have special iron needs, as do females after menarche (Peterson & Peterson, 1988; Sanders, 1990). Recommended dietary allowances for children are available online (USDA/ARS Children's Nutrition Research Center at Baylor College of Medicine).

The training diet of the young athlete should routinely consist of 50% to 55% carbohydrate, 15% protein, and 30% to 35% fat, of which only 10% is saturated. Smaller, growing muscles cannot store glycogen as efficiently as larger, strong muscles, so more complex carbohydrates may be necessary if the child complains of fatigue (Peterson & Peterson, 1988). The basic food groups should be included in these plans with attention to total caloric intake (Food Guide Pyramid, 2001). Additional supplements are not necessary if the diet is adequate and may even be dangerous in the growing child (Clarkson, 1996). Glycogen loading, or increased amounts of glycogen to increase muscle stores above their normal levels, is not recommended in young children or in early adolescence because of the side effects of muscle stiffness and water retention, but can be used with caution by teenagers (Birrer et al., 2002; Stanitski et al., 1994).

Dietary recommendations differ during the four phases of training and competition. In the postseason and off-season periods, the athlete should receive all nutritional and caloric needs for optimal weight; during the preseason and in-season periods, optimal weight and performance should guide the nutritional balance and caloric load. The pregame meal should be eaten 2 to 3 hours before competition to guarantee digestion in the stomach and upper intestine. The meal should be easy to digest; be low in fat, protein, salt, and bulk; and have abundant liquid content and complex carbohydrates for adequate energy and hydration. Examples are waffles, pasta, sandwiches, or liquid meals. The goal during competition is maintenance of adequate hydration (and glycogen for endurance events). Postcompetition meals should immediately replenish glycogen stores and restore fluid balance. Two 8-oz cups of water should be consumed for each pound of body weight lost (Clark, 1991; Grana & Kalenak, 1991; Peterson & Peterson, 1988).

Alterations in weight can and should be made carefully. If a special nutrition program and counseling for weight loss or gain is indicated, it should be supervised by a nutritionist or nurse. Difficulties with excess leanness and eating disorders are being identified more frequently in the preadolescent population. Weight gain diets should have a similar composition to the training diet but include additional calories. An added 1000 kcal a day will result in a gain of 2 lb weekly. This gain will occur in lean body tissue if the child is moderately active. Determination of whether an athlete is overfat or overweight must be made before recommendation of a diet for weight loss. If the athlete is excessively fat or has too great a percentage of body fat in relation to total body composition, careful structure of a training plan can decrease fat mass and increase lean muscle mass. If an athlete is also overweight, a weight loss diet of composition similar to that of the normal athlete but with 1000 fewer kcal per day should be constructed. This will result in a safe loss of 2 lb weekly. Additional exercise will hasten weight loss and maintain firmness of body tissue (Peterson & Peterson, 1988).

PROPER SUPERVISION

The first in the series of supervisors is the coach, the key to a successful sports program. Approximately 20 million children, however, are coached by 2.5 million adult volunteers with varying levels of expertise. The American Academy of Pediatrics has stated that coaches should encourage preparticipation screenings every 1 to 2 years, enforce use of warm-up procedures, require suitable protective equipment, and enforce rules concerning safety. In addition, it recommends completion of a certification program that covers teaching techniques, basic sports skills, fitness, first aid, sportsmanship, enhancement of self-image, and motivational skills (American Academy of Pediatrics, 1989).

Qualified officials and professional medical personnel at games and practices are the second level of supervision. These individuals provide game control and immediate injury containment on site. Medical personnel could include physicians, physical therapists, or athletic trainers who have certification in basic first aid and cardiopulmonary resuscitation techniques in addition to their medical skills (American Academy of Pediatrics, 1989; Puffer, 1991).

PROTECTION

Outfitting the child athlete with proper equipment should be mandated and enforced for the protection of the participants. Equipment must be appropriate for the sport. High quality and proper fit are essential to correct function (Stanitski, 1989). Proper footwear with adequate cushioning, rearfoot control, and sole flexibility for the sport should be required (Micheli & Jenkins, 2001; Segesser & Pforringer, 1989). Protective padding in contact or kicking sports, such as shoulder and shin pads, should be required.

Protective headgear for contact and collision in football, baseball, and hockey is necessary to limit the number of head and neck injuries. Schuller and colleagues (1989) have demonstrated a lower risk of auricular damage in wrestlers wearing headgear (26% incidence) versus those with no headgear (52% incidence). Helmets should be approved by the National Operating Committee on Standards for Athletic Equipment and the American National Safety Institute (Grana & Kalenak, 1991; Objective testing group certifies head protection, 1988).

Eye injuries have been on the increase in recent years, particularly in racquet sports, baseball, and basketball (Napier, 1996; Stock & Cornell, 1991; Strahlman et al., 1990). An estimated 100,000 sports-related eye injuries occur yearly and are the most common cause of eye trauma in children younger than age 15 years (Stock & Cornell, 1991) (Box 18-1). Eye protectors that dissipate injury to a wider area without reducing visual field should be required in racquet sports, ice hockey, baseball, basketball, and football and during use of air-powered weapons. They should be cosmetically and functionally acceptable and made of impact-resistant material. Polycarbonate is the most impact- and scratch-resistant material. A list of high-risk sports and recommended protection is given in Table 18-5. All eye protectors should be approved by either the Canadian Standards Association or the American Society for Testing and Materials.

Studies have highlighted the incidence of oral and facial injuries in many sports, particularly football, hockey, baseball, basketball, wrestling, and boxing (Gassner et al., 2003; Maestrello-deMoya & Primosch, 1989). Youth baseball generated the greatest number of head and face injuries in 1980 (Castaldi, 1986; Perkins et al; 2000; Delibasi et al., 2004; Bak & Doerr, 2004). Before mandatory use of mouthguards, oral trauma constituted 50% of all football injuries (McNutt et al., 1989). The mandatory use of mouthguards has cut the injury rate of oral trauma in football to less than 1% of all injuries (Kerr, 1986). The mouth protector serves to prevent injury to the teeth and lacerations of the mouth. Because it absorbs blows to the

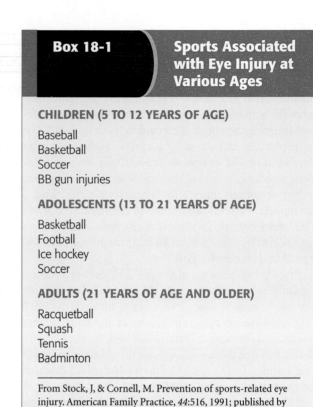

Box 18-1 | **Sports Associated with Eye Injury at Various Ages**

CHILDREN (5 TO 12 YEARS OF AGE)

Baseball
Basketball
Soccer
BB gun injuries

ADOLESCENTS (13 TO 21 YEARS OF AGE)

Basketball
Football
Ice hockey
Soccer

ADULTS (21 YEARS OF AGE AND OLDER)

Racquetball
Squash
Tennis
Badminton

From Stock, J, & Cornell, M. Prevention of sports-related eye injury. American Family Practice, 44:516, 1991; published by the American Academy of Family Physicians.

oral and facial structures, it also prevents fractures, dislocations, and concussions. It should position the bite so the condyles of the mandible do not contact the fossae of the joints. These mouthguards should be inexpensive, strong, and easy to clean and should not interfere with speech or breathing. They should be used alone in field hockey, rugby, wrestling, basketball, and other field events and used in conjunction with face protectors in football, ice hockey, baseball, and lacrosse (Grana & Kalenak, 1991).

ENVIRONMENTAL CONTROL

Assessment and control of the environment is also vital to the safety of the child athlete. The playing area should be well lighted and maintained for safety. Surfaces should be free from obstacles and smooth and even, with good shock-absorbing qualities (wood as opposed to concrete). Modifications of equipment that have been shown to decrease injury (e.g., breakaway bases) should be installed. Sports equipment and playing environments should be scaled down to the size of the athlete (Micheli & Jenkins, 2001; Napier et al., 1996; Stanitski et al., 1994).

Ambient temperature and humidity should be carefully monitored. During exercise, children require more fluid replacement per kilogram of body weight than adults to

TABLE 18-5	Risk Level for Eye Injury with Recommendations for Protective Eyewear

RISK	SPORT	PROTECTIVE WEAR
Unacceptable	Boxing	Not applicable
Very high	Ice hockey	Helmet with full visor
	Squash	Polycarbonate sports protector
	Badminton	Polycarbonate sports protector
	Basketball	Polycarbonate sports protector
	Men's lacrosse	Helmet with full visor
High	Racquetball	Polycarbonate sports protector
	Baseball	Polycarbonate sports protector
	Cricket	Helmet with full visor
	Field hockey	Helmet with full visor
	Rugby football	Debatable
	Soccer	Debatable
	Water polo	Polycarbonate goggles
	Shooting	Polycarbonate sports protector
	Women's lacrosse	Helmet with full visor
Moderate	Tennis	Plastic lens spectacles
	American football	Helmet with polycarbonate visor
Low	Golf	Sports protector if one-eyed
	Volleyball	Sports protector if one-eyed
	Skiing	UV filter goggles ± helmet
	Cycling	Sports protector ± helmet
	Fishing	Polycarbonate protector if one-eyed
	Swimming	Goggles if in water for long periods
	High diving	Not feasible
	Track & field	None required

From Jones, N. Eye injury in sport. Sports Medicine, 7 :178, 1989

avoid dehydration. Children have a greater surface area per body weight, so their rate of heat exchange is greater with lower ability to endure exercise in climatic extremes. They also have a distinctly deficient ability to perspire, so they carry a larger heat load. They acclimatize less efficiently and require more "exposures" for acclimatization to occur (Bar-Or, 1995; Squire, 1990). Exercise should be modified if the wet bulb temperature (an index of climatic heat stress) is above 75°F. (American Academy of Pediatrics, 2000).

Dehydration can be avoided by drinking plenty of liquid before, during, and after play. Thirst is not a valid indicator of the amount of water needed, so every pound (16 oz) lost should be replaced with two cups (16 oz) of water (Peterson & Peterson, 1988). The American College of Sports Medicine recommends that 400 to 500 mL of water be ingested before distance running. They further recommend water intake every 35 to 45 minutes of football practice and nude weighing before and after practice. If residual weight loss from day to day exceeds 2 to 3 lb, practice is restricted until water is replenished. Recommendations for hydration include prehydration of 3 to 12 oz (3–6 oz for <90 lb; 6–12 oz for >90 lb weight) 1 hour before activity, and 3 to 6 oz just prior to activity. During activity 3 to 9 oz (3–5 oz for <90 lb; 6–9 oz for >90 lb) should be ingested every 10 to 20 minutes relative to the temperature and humidity. Eight to 12 oz should be consumed for each pound of weight lost in 2 to 4 hours following activity (Casa et al., 2000) (Table 18-6).

Children will not ingest enough plain water to remain hydrated or to rehydrate following activity. However, if flavor is added to the water, volume of intake is improved substantially (Iuliano et al., 1998; Passe et al., 2000). Sports drinks have been shown to improve energy both in intensive as well as endurance exercise (Bellow et al., 1995; Davis et al., 2001; Galloway & Maughan, 2000; Wilk & Bar-Or, 1996; Utter et al., 1997). In addition to flavor, well-constituted sports drinks have a simple low-carbohydrate content that provides energy, speeds fluid absorption, and provides sodium to stimulate the thirst mechanism (Riviera-Brown, 1999; Shi et al., 1995; Passe et al., 1999).

Successful hydration programs involve not only fluid intake, but also fluid availability. Cool fluids infuse into the system more readily, so accessible liquids should be chilled, or ice provided. Education of everyone involved with the activity, including parents and participants, is of paramount importance to ensure continued compliance. Knowledge of the common signs of dehydration—irritability, headache, nausea, dizziness, weakness, cramps, abdominal distress, and decreased performance—assist those involved with early recognition and intervention (Casa, 2000).

| TABLE 18-6 | Recommended Fluid Intake and Availability for a 90-Minute Practice | | | | |

| WEIGHT LOSS | | MINUTES BETWEEN WATER BREAK | FLUID PER BREAK | | |
LB	KG		OZ	ML	
8	3.6	*			
7.5	3.4	*			
7	3.2	10	8–10	266	
6.5	3.0	10	8–9	251	
6	2.7	10	8–9	251	
5.5	2.5	15	10–12	325	
5	2.3	15	10–11	311	
4.5	2.1	15	9–10	281	
4	1.8	15	8–9	251	
3.5	1.6	20	10–11	311	
3	1.4	20	9–10	281	
2.5	1.1	20	7–8	222	
2	0.9	30	8	237	
1.5	0.7	30	6	177	
1	0.5	45	6	177	
0.5	0.2	60	6	177	

From Peterson, M, & Peterson, K. Eat to Compete: A Guide to Sports Nutrition. Chicago: Year Book Medical, 1988, p. 182.
*No practice recommended.

RISK FACTORS FOR INJURY

Injury can be the result of a single macrotrauma or of repetitive microtrauma (Micheli, 1995). Seven risk factors for repetitive trauma, or "overuse," have been identified: (1) training errors; (2) musculotendinous imbalances of strength, flexibility, or bulk; (3) anatomic malalignment of the lower extremity; (4) improper footwear; (5) faulty playing surface; (6) associated disease states of the lower extremity such as old injury or arthritis; and (7) growth factors (Maffulli, 1990; Micheli, 1995; Taimela et al., 1990).

TRAINING ERROR

Training error is frequently the cause of overuse injuries in children, as it is in adults. The evolution of sport-specific camps from the generalized summer camp experience has dramatically increased the daily level of participation. The sudden transition from casual play to 6 or 8 hours of intense participation has contributed to the increased incidence of overuse injury in children.

MUSCLE-TENDON IMBALANCE

Muscle-tendon imbalance can occur in strength, flexibility, or bulk training. Until recently, little attention was paid to conditioning in children. This attitude may have been appropriate for free play activities but not for organized sport. The repetitive, often predictable, demands of a sport may result in imbalances of muscle and tendon unless the child is on a well-designed training plan. For example, a baseball pitcher or swimmer who does breast stroke might develop a loose anterior capsule and a tight posterior capsule, a situation that could lead to impingement or anterior shoulder subluxation. Repetitive running creates strength and tightness in the quadriceps femoris and triceps surae muscles with relatively weaker hamstrings. This could be problematic if pace and hence stride length are increased.

ANATOMIC MALALIGNMENT

Anatomic malalignment can be a factor in the occurrence of injury because the body may not be able to compensate for the malalignment under the demands of a sport. Femoral anteversion in a young dancer can cause excessive tibial external rotation and ankle pronation as substitutes for natural hip external rotation. Hyperlordosis of the spine or hyperextension of the knee creates abnormal loading on portions of the joint, leading to pain. Pes planus can increase the valgus moment at the knee, as well as allowing the weight of the body to land on a flexible foot. This malalignment can cause pain and abnormal wear on the medial knee joint and foot.

IMPROPER FOOTWEAR AND PLAYING SURFACE

Well-fitting shoes with a firm heel counter, slight heel lift, and flexible toe box are essential for the young athlete. Inadequate footwear that does not support the structures of the foot while playing can lead to a number of foot and lower extremity problems. The shoe should compensate for changes in alignment and shock absorption. Likewise, improper playing surfaces can predispose the child to knee pain, shin splints, or stress fractures. These symptoms have been associated with playing on hard, banked surfaces or synthetic courts, as opposed to clay and hardwood surfaces (Micheli & Jenkins, 2001).

ASSOCIATED DISEASE STATES

Associated disease is occasionally an issue, as in the child with previous Legg-Calvé-Perthes disease who has limited hip rotation. Likewise, a child with juvenile rheumatoid arthritis or hemophilia may have exacerbations of joint pain or synovitis with participation in sports.

GROWTH FACTORS

The first aspect of growth that is a factor in overuse injuries is the articular cartilage (Fig. 18-2). Clinical and biomechanical evidence suggests that growing cartilage has low resistance to repetitive loading, resulting in microtrauma to either the cartilage or the underlying growth plate. Damage may result in osteoarthritis or growth asymmetry (Gerrard, 1993; Micheli, 1995).

Growing articular cartilage is also less resistant to shear, particularly at the elbow, knee, and ankle. Repetitive shear has been implicated in osteochondritis dissecans of the capitellum in Little League pitchers, and of the proximal and distal femur and talus in runners. Studies postulate that a segment of subchondral bone becomes avascular and separates with its articular cartilage from the surrounding bone to become a loose body (Maffulli, 1990; Omey & Micheli, 1999). Shear stress has further been implicated in epiphyseal displacement (Gill & Micheli, 1996).

The final site of growth cartilage weakness is the apophysis. Increasing evidence suggests that traction apophysitis, such as Osgood-Schlatter disease, Sever disease, and irritation of the rectus femoris or sartorius muscle origins, is the result of degeneration of the growth center with tiny avulsion fractures and associated healing (Dalton, 1992; Maffulli, 1990; Micheli & Fehlandt, 1992; Outerbridge & Micheli, 1995; Patel & Nelson, 2000).

The second element of growth involved in overuse injury is the process itself. Longitudinal growth occurs in the bones, with secondary elongation of the soft tissues. During periods of rapid bone growth ("growth spurts") the musculotendinous structures tighten and cause loss of flexibility. A coincidence of overuse injury and growth spurt has been noted (Dalton, 1992; Micheli, 1995).

The biomechanical properties of bone also change with growth and maturation. As bone becomes less cartilaginous and stiffer, the resistance to impact decreases. Sudden overload may cause the bone to bow or buckle. The epiphysis, the area of growth in the long bones, is more susceptible, and may shear or fracture. Examples of this process include avulsion fracture of the anterior cruciate ligament, avulsion fracture of the ankle ligament, and growth plate fractures. Because fractures through the epiphysis can be difficult to visualize on radiographs, any injury to the epiphyseal area is considered a fracture and is treated as such in order to avoid potential growth disturbance (Coady & Micheli, 1997; Maffulli & Bruns, 2000; Micheli & Wood, 1995).

TYPES OF INJURIES

Although injuries in children have some similarity to those in adults, several are peculiar to the growing child. These specific injuries fall into three categories: (1) fractures, (2) joint injuries, and (3) muscle-tendon unit injuries (Micheli, 1995; Gill & Micheli, 1996).

FRACTURES

A relatively new injury in children is the stress fracture, which usually results from repetitive microtrauma or poor training. Repetition causes cancellous bone fractures as opposed to cortical bone fatigue in adults (Coady & Micheli, 1997; Maffulli, 1990). These cancellous bone fractures are often imperceptible on radiographs until 6 to 8 weeks after the onset of pain. Stress fractures cause persistent, activity-related pain that can be reproduced by indirect force to the bone. Suspicion based on clinical signs and symptoms can be reinforced by bone scans if diagnostic uncertainty exists.

Growth plate or epiphyseal fractures are peculiar to the child. The cartilaginous growth plate is less resistant to shear or tensile-deforming force than either the ligament or bony cortex, so mechanical disruption frequently

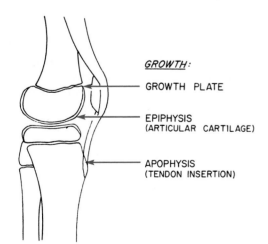

Figure 18-2 Sites of susceptibility of the growth cartilage. *(From Micheli, L. Overuse injuries in children's sports: The growth factor. Orthopedic Clinics of North America, 14:341, 1983.)*

occurs through the plate itself, usually in the zone of hypertrophy (Maffulli, 1990). This disruption can be caused by a single macrotrauma, such as jumping, or by repetitive microtrauma as in distance running. The potential for problems from epiphyseal fracture depends on the specific plate involved and on the extent of the injury. Decreased limb length, angular deformity, joint incongruity, and premature closure are frequent sequelae (Maffulli, 1990; Micheli, 1995). Shaft fractures are more common in the older child who is approaching adult status (Flynn et al., 2003).

JOINT INJURIES

Joint injuries in the young athlete include ligamentous sprains, internal derangement, and musculotendinous insertional injuries. These can result from a single discrete injury or from repetitive trauma. The diagnosis of sprain must be made carefully in the child. During a growth spurt, ligaments may be stronger than the growth plate, so excessive bending or twisting forces cause the plate rather than the ligament to yield. Severe ligamentous injuries can occur, however, so careful examination is necessary to differentiate among these injuries (Micheli, 1995; Gill & Micheli, 1996).

Repetitive microtrauma of the joint articular cartilage often results in softening, followed by frank shredding and thinning of the surface. Compression to the joint causes exacerbation of the symptoms, such as pain, edema, and decreased functional use of the joint (Adirim & Cheng, 2001).

MUSCLE-TENDON UNIT INJURIES

Another area at particular risk of injury in the growing child is the insertion of the musculotendinous unit into the bone through the apophyseal cartilage. Growth occurs at the apophyseal growth plate, where tendons and ligaments are attached. During growth spurts the increased tension on the attachments often leads to detachment of the structure at the apophysis (avulsion fracture). Tendonitis occurs much less frequently in the child than in the adult because the insertion becomes symptomatic before the tendon (Adirim & Cheng, 2001; Micheli, 1995).

Irritation of the insertional area of the musculotendinous unit, the enthesis, can cause pain and inflammation. This area is highly vascular and metabolically active. During exercise, when blood is diverted to the active muscle, these areas may suffer periods of ischemia (Maffulli, 1990). The symptoms cause inhibition of muscle activity with resultant weakness and loss of flexibility. The weakness and tightness then lead to greater irritation and pain (O'Neill & Micheli, 1988).

Children can overuse muscles, resulting in strain, just like adults. The increase in muscle volume during exercise may cause exertional compartment syndromes. Muscle hernias, however, occur in children secondary to tight fascial or musculotendinous structures (Trepman & Micheli, 1988).

SITES OF INJURY

The anatomy and the factor of growth combine to make certain injuries more likely and more serious in the various segments of the child's body.

BRAIN AND CERVICAL INJURIES

The incidence of central nervous system injury in children is low, varying from 1% to 5% of sports-related injuries, but these cases constitute 50% to 100% of the deaths from injury. Cervical spine injuries result in 30% to 50% of cases of childhood quadriplegia (Bruce et al., 1982). The rate of spinal cord injuries in children younger than age 11 years is low, but it escalates dramatically in the 15- to 18-year-old age bracket. Because the brain and spinal cord are largely incapable of regeneration, these injuries take on a singular importance (Cantu, 2000).

Participation in several sports carries a particularly high risk for head and neck injuries. Football accounts for 40% of all concussion injuries in school sports. Although 69% of deaths between 1945 and 1999 were from brain injuries, the incidence of serious head injuries has decreased over the past 20 years (Cantu & Mueller, 2003b). Fatalities in children younger than age 12 have not been reported, but the mortality rate is 0.44 per 100,000 participants in tackle football. The incidence of serious head injury is still 0.75 to 1.5 per 100,000 participants per season, with a mortality rate of 0.5 to 1.09 per season (Bruce et al., 1982). Sosin and colleagues (1996) documented 247 deaths from traumatic brain injury of the 140,000 head injuries in those younger than 18 years between 1989 and 1992.

Severe spinal injuries often result in paralysis and total disability. A population-based study over 7 years identified 32 children younger than 15 years of age who sustained spinal fracture, dislocation, or severe ligamentous injury; sports were the cause of all injuries in children over the age of 10 years (Finch & Barnes, 1998). Rugby, a popular collision sport outside the United States, has head and neck injury rates similar to those of American football. Wrestling has the second highest injury rate of all high school sports, although the central nervous system injury rate is low. The rate of catastrophic wrestling injuries (cervical ligament injury, spinal cord contusion, severe head injury, or herniated disk) is 2.11 per year (1 per 100,000 participants) as a result of direct blows or falls (Boden et al., 2002). Baseball accounts for a large number of concussions secondary to collision with the bat, other players, or the ball, although exact incidence figures have not been reported. Diving accounts for 3% to 21% of all cervical spine injuries in young people (Blanksby et al., 1997). Noguchi (1994) noted that swimming and gymnastics accounted for 51% and 22.8%, respectively, of all spinal injuries in persons younger than 30 years of age.

Concussion, or temporary disturbance of brain function, resulting from a traumatic blow to the head, is considered an important public health problem; approximately 300,000 injuries occur yearly, usually in the young (Thurman et al., 1998). Symptoms are caused by biomechanical or physiologic aberrations, but no permanent pathologic process occurs (Birrer et al., 2003). Concussions are graded according to duration of unconsciousness (Table 18-7). Because of the occurrence of second impact syndrome, in which a series of insults can lead to cerebral damage when one impact would not, decisions regarding return to play are critical (Cantu, 2003; Collins et al., 2002). No universally accepted criteria for return to play exist, but Table 18-8 contains recommendations based on the severity and incidence of prior concussion (Aubry et al., 2002; Cantu, 1998; Echemendie & Cantu, 2003). Postconcussion syndrome, which is characterized by headache, irritability, labyrinthine disturbance, and impaired memory and concentration, is rare but suggests altered neurotransmitter function (Erlanger et al., 2003). Further eva-

luation and good instruction for follow-up is warranted before clearance to play is granted (Cantu, 1998; Genuardi & King, 1995; Kelly et al., 1991).

The leading cause of death from head injury is intracranial hemorrhage. Cantu & Mueller (2003) reported that 86% of brain-injury deaths resulted from subdural hematoma. The most rapidly progressing and universally fatal disorder if missed is the epidural hematoma. Symptoms include initial preservation of consciousness with increasingly severe headache, lethargy, and focal neurologic signs. It is frequently associated with temporal bone fracture. An acute subdural hematoma is the most common fatal head injury and should always be considered as a possible diagnosis in the athlete who loses and does not

TABLE 18-7	**Grading of Severity of Concussion**

GRADE	SEVERITY
1 (mild)	No loss of consciousness; posttraumatic amnesia 30 minutes
2 (moderate)	Loss of consciousness <5 minutes or posttraumatic amnesia >30 minutes
3 (severe)	Loss of consciousness 5 minutes or posttraumatic amnesia 24 hours

Adapted from Cantu, R. Guidelines to return to contact sports after a cerebral concussion. Physician and Sportsmedicine, *14* :76, 1986. Reproduced with permission of McGraw-Hill, Inc.

TABLE 18-8   Guidelines for Return to Play after Concussion

GRADE	FIRST CONCUSSION	SECOND CONCUSSION	THIRD CONCUSSION
1 (mild)	May return to play if asymptomatic* for 1 week	Return to play in 2 weeks if asymptomatic at that time for 1 week	Terminate season; may return to play next season if asymptomatic
2 (moderate)	Return to play after asymptomatic for 1 week	Minimum of 1 month; may return to play then if asymptomatic for 1 week; consider terminating season	Terminate season; may return to play next season if asymptomatic
3 (severe)	Minimum of 1 month; may then return to play if asymptomatic for 1 week	Terminate season; may return to play next season if asymptomatic	

Adapted from Cantu, R. Return to play guidelines after a head injury. Clinics in Sports Medicine, *17*:45–60, 1998. Reproduced with permission from Elsevier Inc.

*No headache, dizziness, or impaired orientation, concentration, or memory during rest.

regain consciousness. A chronic subdural hematoma should be suspected in the athlete who is not quite the same for days or weeks after a head injury. Signs may include headache or mild mental, motor, or sensory signs and symptoms (Bailes & Cantu, 2001).

The intracerebral hemorrhage is also rapidly progressive because the bleeding is into the brain itself. No lucid interval is noted, and death often occurs before arrival at a hospital. The subarachnoid hemorrhage is a brain contusion that causes headache and associated neurologic deficits that are dependent on the area of the brain involved. All injured athletes with potential intracranial hemorrhages should be transported to a hospital for further evaluation and medical or surgical management (Bruce et al., 1982).

Most neck injuries are caused by hyperflexion or hyperextension. Hyperflexion injuries, the most common, result from spearing or butt blocking (Fig. 18-3). Because of the poorly developed musculature in youngsters and the commonly associated fracture, hyperflexion injury can be serious. Hyperextension injuries often occur even in the absence of severe force because the anterior neck musculature is weaker than the posterior musculature. Common causes are face or head tackling (Fig. 18-4). Hyperextension injury with a rotatory component is the most common cause of nerve root damage (Birrer et al., 2002; Stanitski et al., 1994). Evaluation of these injuries should always include radiographs of the cervical spine. In the adolescent, the second cervical vertebra is normally displaced posteriorly over the third secondary to hypermobility. This pseudosubluxation is normal and not the result of injury (Cantu, 2000) but should be referred for assessment.

Another common injury is a "burner," which is a traction injury to the brachial plexus. It is caused by a forceful blow to the head from the side or from depression of the shoulder while the head and neck are fixed. Repeated injuries may cause weakness of the deltoid, biceps, and teres major muscles, which should be resolved with strengthening exercises. If the use of a collar or a change in technique or neck strength does not solve the problem, cessation of participation is warranted (Cantu, 1997). Return to play in a collision or contact sport following any type of cervical injury should be closely monitored (Cantu et al., 1998).

THORACIC AND LUMBAR SPINAL INJURIES

Back injuries in children are very different from those in adults, and require careful evaluation (Gerbino & Micheli, 1995; Kraft, 2002; Waicus & Smith, 2002). Spinal injuries can occur in both the thoracic and the lumbar areas, although thoracic injuries are rare. Costovertebral injury secondary to compression of the rib cage in a pileup in football or from a forceful takedown in wrestling can injure the costovertebral articulations. Complaints include pain and muscle spasm along the associated rib. Axial compression forces on a preflexed spine, as in sledding or tobogganing, can fracture the vertebrae, particularly at the vulnerable T12-L1 level. These injuries can cause pain but are frequently asymptomatic (Birrer et al., 2002; Stanitski et al., 1994).

The most common injuries in the lumbar spine are spondylolysis and spondylolisthesis. One study of 3132 competitive athletes ages 15 to 27 years noted an incidence of spondylolysis of 12.5% (Rossi & Dragoni, 1990). Repeated hyperflexion and hyperextension in football blocking, clean and jerk lift, diving, pole vaulting, wrestling, high jump, or gymnastic maneuvers can place excessive forces on the pars interarticularis and cause a

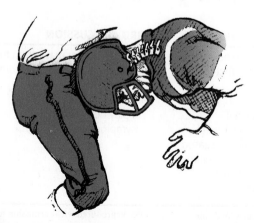

• **Figure 18-3** Hyperflexion damage from head butting. *(From Birrer, R, & Brecher, D. Common Sports Injuries in Youngsters. Oradell, NJ: Medical Economics, 1987, p. 36.)*

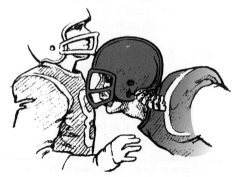

• **Figure 18-4** Hyperextension injury from face blocking. *(From Birrer, R, & Brecher, D. Common Sports Injuries in Youngsters. Oradell, NJ: Medical Economics, 1987, p. 38.)*

stress fracture. Spondylolisthesis, or fracture and slippage of one vertebra on another, usually L5 over S1, is most common at ages 9 to 14 years. Loading of a bilateral spondylolysis, in which there is a defect in the bony connection of the posterior arch with the vertebral body, can cause a spondylolisthesis, as can traumatic or repetitive bilateral loading of a normal spine. The slippage is graded from 1 to 4, depending on the degree of slippage. Athletes with grade 2 or greater slippage should be counseled against participation in weight lifting, baseball, diving, gymnastics, or wrestling. Participation in basketball or football is permissible with use of a brace (Debnath et al., 2003; d'Hemecourt et al., 2000; Kraft, 2002; McTimoney & Micheli, 2003). The growth spurt in the spine causes lumbar lordosis secondary to the enhanced anterior growth with posterior tethering by the heavy lumbodorsal fascia. This biomechanical situation increases the tendency of posterior element failure at the pars and perhaps at the disk (Micheli, 1995). Athletes with spondylolysis are managed in a brace until healing occurs. Physical therapy is indicated to maintain flexibility in the lumbosacral spine and the spinal and hip musculature and to improve trunk and abdominal muscle strength while braced. Surgery is indicated only in cases of unstable lesions or nerve root compression (Birrer et al., 2002; Ogden, 2000; Fu & Stone, 2001).

The incidence of disk lesions in young athletes is unknown, but several studies have demonstrated that disk herniation can occur. Although acute trauma may cause this condition, degenerative changes of the vertebral bodies and intervertebral joints may be the contributing factors, with trauma being the acute precipitating incident (Maffulli, 1990).

SHOULDER INJURIES

Specific shoulder injuries can be predicted based on the biomechanics of the sport and the age of the athlete (Hutchinson & Ireland, 2003; Kocher et al., 2000). Football, wrestling, and ice hockey cause upper extremity fractures and dislocations, and sports with repeated overhead activities, such as volleyball, contribute to overuse injuries (Aagaard & Jorgenson, 1996). The hyperelasticity of juvenile joints, particularly the shoulder, makes them vulnerable to passive and dynamic instability patterns that can predispose the shoulder to injury (Hutchinson & Ireland, 2003; Paterson & Waters, 2000).

Acromioclavicular sprains may occur in the immature athlete without clavicular fracture. The most common mechanism is direct force from a fall or blow to the lateral aspect of the shoulder or a fall on an outstretched arm (Birrer et al., 2002; Kocher et al., 2000; Micheli, 1995; Fu & Stone, 2001). Grade I and II sprains are more common in the athlete whose skeleton is immature. Grade III sprains commonly rupture the dorsal clavicular periosteum, but the acromioclavicular and coracoclavicular ligaments remain intact (Kocher et al., 2000; Paterson & Waters, 2000). These lesions are treated symptomatically with rest, ice, compression, and elevation (RICE) in a sling. Exercises are often necessary to increase scapulothoracic and glenohumeral mobility and strength after the sprain is healed.

Fractures are most common in the middle third of the clavicle from a direct blow. These can be actual fractures in the older child or greenstick fractures in the youngster. They are managed with a figure-of-eight strap until healed.

Because the proximal humerus is an area of bone growth, fractures are more common in children than in adults, who are more prone to dislocation. Epiphyseal displacements occur in the younger child, and metaphyseal fractures are more common in the older child or adolescent (Micheli, 1995). After healing, therapeutic intervention to normalize mobility and strength of the scapular, shoulder, and elbow muscles is frequently indicated (Paterson & Waters, 2000).

Little League shoulder, a relatively common injury in young pitchers and catchers, involves a fracture of the proximal humeral growth plate secondary to rotatory torque. Any athlete who complains of proximal shoulder pain in the absence of trauma should be suspected of having an epiphyseal fracture until proved otherwise. The athlete should not do any throwing until the pain subsides (Hutchinson & Ireland, 2003; Kocher et al., 2000; Paterson & Waters, 2000).

Frank anterior subluxation and dislocation of the glenohumeral joint is rare in children but common in adolescents. Because of the laxity of juvenile joints, a blow or forceful maneuver in abduction, external rotation, or extension can dislodge the head of the humerus (Birrer et al., 2002; Paterson & Waters, 2000; Fu & Stone, 2001; Stanitski et al., 1994). This condition is common in throwing or racquet sports, gymnastics, and swimming. Patients with posterior glenohumeral instability respond better to conservative strengthening of appropriate musculature than those with anterior instability, although a program of scapular and shoulder muscle strengthening in a biomechanically correct range of motion should be attempted. Motion should be limited to ranges that prevent chronic subluxation. Surgery is more often an option with anterior or multidirectional instability than in posterior instability (Kocher et al., 2000; Paterson & Waters, 2000).

Rotator cuff tears are not as common in the skeletally immature athlete as in the older athlete. They occur in throwing and racquet sports, as well as from direct contact blows in collision sports. These tears can be treated successfully with arthroscopic surgery and rehabilitation that includes strength and endurance training for all scapular and shoulder muscles, as well as training with correct biomechanical movements of the shoulder complex (Kocher et al., 2000).

Rotator cuff impingement syndrome (Fig. 18-5) is a frequent injury in athletes younger than 25 years of age. More than 50% of swimmers aged 12 to 18 years complain of shoulder pain (Birrer et al., 2002; Fu & Stone, 2001; Stanitski et al., 1994). One hypothesis is that these athletes develop a characteristic contracture around the shoulder with loss of internal rotation at 90° of abduction and with increased external rotation in all positions of abduction. This might reflect a tightened posterior and a loosened anterior capsule, suggesting a tendency to subluxate anteriorly. Conservative physical therapy with normalization of mobility and strength has been successful in resolving the primary instability (Kocher et al., 2000; Paterson & Waters, 2000; Micheli, 1995). All positions of impingement (anterior, lateral, or overhead) should be avoided until the athlete is pain-free.

ELBOW INJURIES

Supracondylar fracture of the humerus is the second most common fracture in the skeletally immature client. Most of these fractures occur in the age group of 5 to 10 years. They are the result of significant forces into extension. Avulsion fractures of the medial epicondyle are not uncommon and are associated with elbow dislocations or throwing injuries. Anatomic reduction usually requires internal fixation with early protected range of motion to avoid loss of extension (Gill & Micheli, 1996; Kocher et al., 2000). Subsequent to healing, normalization of mobility and strength of the elbow and forearm are necessary for full function.

Repetitive microtrauma from pitching may result in epiphyseal fracture of the radial head. Loss of extension and supination with a history of repetitive loading of the radiocapitellar joint indicates fracture. A radial head fracture is treated with rest (DaSilva et al., 1998; Hutchinson & Ireland, 2003). Forcefully pulling the arm of a child younger than 7 years old can subluxate the radial head because of the poor development of the annular ligament. The child positions the injured arm in flexion and pronation, dangling it at the side of the body (Birrer et al., 2002; Fu & Stone, 2001; Kocher et al., 2000; Stanitski et al., 1994).

Elbow dislocation is seen in contact sports secondary to a fall on an abducted, extended arm. Early reduction will avoid neurovascular damage, and further evaluation and radiographs are necessary to assess the presence of associated fracture. Early protected mobility is necessary to preserve normal elbow motion (Birrer et al., 2002; Fu & Stone, 2001; Kocher et al., 2000). Physical therapy to normalize elbow and forearm mobility and to improve strength at the elbow, forearm, and hand is appropriate.

Little League elbow commonly results from the extreme valgus stress placed on the epicondyles during the acceleration phase of pitching (Fig. 18-6). If this is not recognized and regular throwing continues, mild separation of the medial epicondyle with hypertrophy, irregularity, fragmentation, and avulsion can occur. The most serious damage is the jamming of the radial head against the capitellum on the lateral side, a finding that occurs in 8% to 10% of young pitchers. This jamming can result in osteochondritis of the capitellum, avascular necrosis of the radial head, and loose bodies within the joint. Treatment is RICE and rest from throwing (Birrer et al., 2002; Fu & Stone, 2001; Gill & Micheli, 1996; Ogden, 2000). Eventual alteration of throwing technique may be necessary.

Tennis elbow is seen in a variety of racquet sports as a result of repeated injury to the lateral epicondyle. A faulty stroke initiates the process. The resulting friction between the extensor muscles, the lateral epicondyle, and the radial head causes irritation, microtears in the extensor muscle origin, and adhesions between the annular ligament and the joint capsule. Using tightly strung racquets, racquets with small handles, and old tennis balls will aggravate the situation. Rehabilitation to decrease irritation, reduce adhesions, and strengthen the forearm and hand musculature is required. Alteration of technique and equipment,

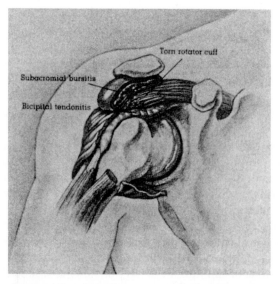

Torn rotator cuff

Subacromial bursitis

Bicipital tendonitis

♦ **Figure 18-5** Common causes of impingement. *(From Birrer, R, & Brecher, D. Common Sports Injuries in Youngsters. Oradell, NJ: Medical Economics, 1987, p. 61.)*

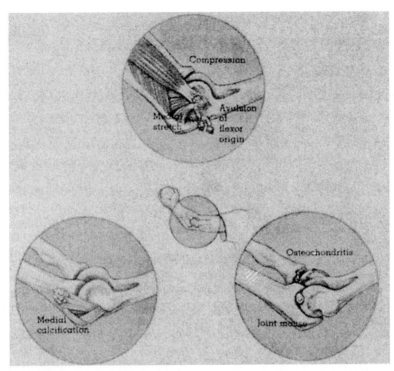

◆ **Figure 18-6**   Little League elbow. *(From Birrer, R, & Brecher, D. Common Sports Injuries in Youngsters. Oradell, NJ: Medical Economics, 1987, p. 74.)*

such as enlargement of the racquet grip area or reduction of string tension, is helpful (Fu & Stone, 2001; Gill & Micheli, 1996; Hutchinson & Ireland, 2003).

WRIST AND HAND INJURIES

Because of the inherent complexity of the anatomy of the wrist joint, potentially serious injuries may be missed or underdiagnosed. Careful diagnosis using knowledge of biomechanics of the wrist and hand is crucial (Birrer et al., 2002; Gill & Micheli, 1996; Kocher et al., 2000; Stanitski et al., 1994).

Fractures about the wrist follow an age-related pattern. In the young child a torus, or buckle fracture, of the distal radial epiphysis is common after a fall. Clinical signs are minimal pain and tenderness, so careful radiologic examination is necessary. Simple splinting is adequate for healing (Birrer et al., 2002; Campbell, 1990; Ogden, 2000; Kocher et al., 2000). Metaphyseal fractures of the distal radius and ulna are more common in the child. Often displaced, they require reduction with the use of anesthesia. In the younger adolescent, fractures through the growth plate are common, again from falls, and require operative reduction to minimize trauma to the growth plate (Kocher et al., 2000). Rehabilitation to regain normal

forearm and wrist mobility as well as wrist and grip strength is desirable. Stress injuries to the distal radial epiphysis have been noted in athletes such as gymnasts who bear weight on their hands. Complaints of pain with wrist dorsiflexion and of wrist stiffness are common. Radiographs demonstrate a widened epiphysis, cystic changes, and breaking of the distal metaphysis. Management consists of cessation of gymnastics with or without casting (Kocher et al., 2000).

Although fracture of most carpal bones is rare, fracture of the navicular or scaphoid bone is common in children from 12 to 15 years of age. This fracture results from a fall on the dorsiflexed hand of an outstretched arm. Although the fracture is not readily visible on a radiograph, early diagnosis is important because of the high incidence of avascular necrosis and nonunion. If tenderness in the anatomic snuffbox occurs with a high degree of suspicion of fracture, use of a short-arm spica cast will be adequate management (Birrer et al., 2002; Fu & Stone, 2001; Gillon, 2001; Stanitski et al., 1994).

Because the hand and fingers are so essential in most sports, the small structures absorb tremendous forces of initial contact, and therefore injuries to the hand and fingers are common (Birrer et al., 2002; Ogden, 2000; Stanitski et al., 1994). Dislocations are uncommon in the child's hand because the forces necessary to produce these injuries are usually dissipated by production of a fracture. If dislocations do occur, it is usually in the adolescent and in patterns similar to those in an adult. Thus, the most common dislocation occurs at the carpometacarpal joint of the thumb, usually secondary to axial compression forces on the thumb tip in contact sports. Although reduction is easy, maintenance is not, and chronic instability can result. The thumb is put in a short-arm thumb spica, and participation in sports should be avoided for 6 weeks. A short opponens splint is advisable for the initial 6 weeks of reentry to play (Beatty et al., 1990; Campbell, 1990; Kocher et al., 2000).

Dorsal dislocation of the thumb metacarpophalangeal joint is the most common dislocation in the hand of a child. A fall or forceful contact hyperextends the metacarpophalangeal joint. If the proximal phalanx is parallel to the metacarpal, the volar plate has been avulsed and surgical reduction is necessary. Cast immobilization for 3 weeks with sports participation permitted is adequate for healing. Physical therapy may be indicated to normalize thumb mobility and strength following casting. Metacarpophalangeal dislocations in the fingers are rare except for those that affect the index finger. After this injury is reduced, splinting in flexion for 3 weeks with immediate mobilization after splint removal is the treatment of choice (Beatty et al., 1990; Birrer et al., 2002; Fu & Stone, 1994; Stanitski et al., 1994).

Joint injuries are common in ball sports and skiing. The metacarpophalangeal joint of the thumb is the most commonly injured joint in skiers. The majority of these injuries in youth are bony gamekeeper's thumb in which the ulnar collateral ligament avulses a segment of bone, as compared with the purely ligamentous injury in adults. If the bony fragment lies close to its origin, good results are obtained with use of a short-arm thumb spica cast for 6 weeks, followed by exercises to normalize mobility and strength. Athletic participation, even molding the cast to fit the ski pole, can be allowed. If the radiograph is negative, integrity of the ulnar collateral ligament must be established by assessing radial deviation in extension and 30° of flexion. Deviation of greater than 30° indicates at least a partial tear. No firm end point in full extension or greater than 45° of deviation in flexion indicates full ligamentous tear with volar plate injury, which will require surgical repair (Beatty et al., 1990; Birrer et al., 2002; Kocher et al., 2000; Stanitski et al., 1994). Hand therapy is necessary to regain normal mobility, strength, and pinch.

Jammed fingers are common injuries in all age groups. Axial compression force to the fingertips causes distal interphalangeal flexion with proximal interphalangeal hyperextension. Reduction is easily accomplished by distal traction. Buddy taping will allow the athlete to return to play (Beatty et al., 1990; Birrer et al., 2002; Stanitski et al., 1994). Caution should be exhibited, however, because fractures through the growth plate of the phalanx are common. These intra-articular, or neck, fractures have a great tendency to displace and then require open reduction with internal fixation (Campbell, 1990; Micheli, 1995). In the absence of a fracture or dislocation, damage to the collateral ligaments can occur and is managed in similar fashion. Jamming at the distal interphalangeal joint can result in "mallet finger," or tearing of the terminal extensor tendon with or without a bony fragment. This injury is easily managed with use of a dorsal extension splint for 6 to 8 weeks. If active and passive extension ranges are equal at 6 weeks, active flexion can be initiated. If not, splinting is continued for another month. Participation is allowed with the splint in place (Birrer et al., 2002; Fu & Stone, 2001; Kocher et al., 2000; Stanitski et al., 1994).

Post-traumatic arthritis of the wrist and hand has been documented in active children. Management requires careful monitoring with nonoperative techniques to permit extensive remodeling, although occasionally surgery is necessary (Peljovich & Simmons, 2000).

PELVIS AND HIP INJURIES

Because the hip and pelvis have complex ossification patterns and fuse late in childhood, the potential for injury is high. The acetabulum has three sections joined by triradiate cartilage. Likewise, three ossification centers exist on the femoral head: the capital femoral epiphysis, the greater trochanter, and the lesser trochanter. The circular vascularity of the femoral head and neck also creates risk for injury in the growing child (Paletta & Andrish, 1995; Waters & Millis, 1988).

Fractures are uncommon but can occur in the epiphyseal plate, the femoral neck, or the subtrochanteric area. Slipped capital femoral epiphysis (SCFE) is not caused by sports but must be suspected in any athlete with persistent hip or knee pain and a limp. SCFE typically occurs during the period of rapid growth in adolescence in either obese or very thin males, but can occur in females as well. Surgical reduction with internal fixation is necessary (see Chapter 17). Hip dislocations, usually posterior, are uncommon but serious; these can be resolved with few long-term consequences if managed carefully (Hamilton & Broughton, 1998).

Fractures of the neck or subtrochanteric area are rare but can be the result of severe trauma, usually incurred during contact sports such as football and rugby. Surgical reduction is necessary to maintain position (Waters & Millis, 1988). More common are avulsion fractures from a sudden violent muscular contraction or excessive muscle stretch. The most common sites are the anterior-superior iliac spine (origin of the sartorius), the ischium (hamstring origin) (Fig. 18-7), the lesser trochanter (insertion of the iliopsoas), the anterior-inferior iliac spine (rectus femoris origin), and iliac crest (abdominal insertion) (Moeller, 2003). These injuries are classic in sprinting, jumping, soccer, football, and weight lifting. Rest with gradual increase of excursion to full mobility followed by progressive resistance exercise and reintegration to play is the treatment sequence (Birrer et al., 2002; Micheli & Smith, 1982; Waters & Millis, 1988; Stanitski et al., 1994). One less traumatic overuse parallel of avulsion is iliac apophysitis, which usually affects adolescent track, field, or cross-country athletes or dancers. Repeated contraction of the tensor fasciae latae, rectus femoris, sartorius, gluteus medius, and oblique abdominal muscles causes nonspecific pain and tenderness over the iliac crest. Rest helps this problem (Birrer et al., 2002; Fu & Stone, 2001), but often exercises to increase strength and normalize two-joint muscle flexibility are required.

Stress fractures and osteitis pubis are being diagnosed more frequently as a result of repetitive microtrauma in runners or athletes who have suddenly increased their involvement in jumping or kicking activities. Persistent pain and tenderness in the groin with limited mobility and activity-related increases in pain could signal either of these conditions. Radiographs showing inflammation, demineralization, and sclerosis confirm the diagnosis of osteitis pubis, but a bone scan is necessary to diagnose a stress fracture. Stress fractures have been seen in the pelvis at the junction of the ischium and pubic ramus and in the femoral neck and shaft (Fu & Stone, 2001; Stanitski et al., 1994; Waters & Millis, 1988). Relative rest, use of crutches, and restriction from percussive activities (running and jumping) are required for resolution of these disorders.

Snapping hip syndrome is an overuse problem noted in gymnasts, dancers, and sprinters. The term *snapping hip syndrome* can refer either to irritation of the iliotibial band over the greater trochanter with hip motion or to tenosynovitis of the iliopsoas tendon near its femoral insertion. Usually, relative rest, use of appropriate modalities, stretching, and improved muscle strength overcome these symptoms (Micheli, 1995; Waters & Millis, 1988).

A serious condition seen in the young athlete age 5 to 12 years is avascular necrosis of the femoral head. Activity can irritate the synovium, leading to joint effusion and reduction of the blood supply to the femoral head. The initial complaint is nonspecific hip pain, but radiographs demonstrate periosteal rarefaction followed by sclerosis and irregular collapse of the femoral head. Bracing or surgery may be required, depending on the degree of progression of the problem (Fu & Stone, 2001; Micheli, 1995; Stanitski et al., 1994) (see Chapter 17).

Contusions are common, but the most frequent is the hip pointer. This iliac crest contusion, occurring typically in football or hockey, is caused by a driving blow by a helmet. The overlying muscle is damaged with a resultant subperiosteal hematoma. RICE and padding will resolve this problem with time (Fu & Stone, 2001; Stanitski et al., 1994). Occasionally, use of ultrasound and soft tissue mobilization with stretching may be necessary.

KNEE INJURIES

As the largest joint in the body and one with minimal anatomic protection, the knee is the focal point of stress forces applied along the tibia and femur. Consequently, it is not only the site of macrotrauma but also the most frequent site of overuse injury (Iobst & Stanitski, 2000; Kujala et al., 1995; Stanitski, 1997).

Fractures about the knee, although not frequent, are significant for their possible influences on growth (Tepper & Ireland, 2003; Zionts, 2002). Distal femoral epiphyseal fractures occur in the young athlete as a consequence of twisting injuries. Careful open anatomic reduction with internal fixation is necessary to avoid subsequent growth disturbances (Steiner & Grana, 1988). Physical therapy is usually necessary for children who sustain distal femoral or proximal tibial epiphyseal fractures. Either open reduction with internal fixation or casting causes loss of knee and ankle mobility and decreased thigh and calf muscle strength. Rehabilitation to reverse these effects and retrain the youngster in balance and agility skills is necessary.

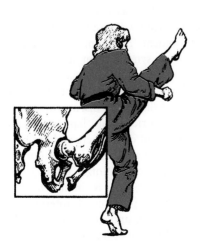

• **Figure 18-7**   Avulsion of the ischial tuberosity. *(From Birrer, R, & Brecher, D. Common Sports Injuries in Youngsters. Oradell, NJ: Medical Economics, 1987, p. 101.)*

Fractures of the proximal tibial epiphysis are rare but treacherous because of associated popliteal artery damage and compartment syndrome. More common is fracture of the tibial tuberosity alone or in association with the proximal tibia. These are most common at the end of adolescence in jumping sports such as basketball and track. These fractures can be managed with extension casting if minimal displacement has occurred or with internal fixation if displaced. Growth disturbances are rare because of the late occurrence of the fracture (Fu & Stone, 2001; Micheli & Jenkins, 2001). Stress fractures were rare but are being reported more commonly in the tibias of runners and swimmers. Reduction of the loading stress of running or of turns in swimming is suggested until healing occurs (Steiner & Grana, 1988). Ligament injuries are becoming more common in the young athlete, with one study reporting medial collateral ligament injury in children as young as 4 years of age (Micheli & Jenkins, 2001). All ligament injuries should be assessed for coincident physis fractures. Medial collateral ligament tears in youth can include both the superficial and the capsular components of the ligament. Nonoperative treatment with splinting and avoidance of valgus stress has been successful in adolescents, so it may be possible to obtain equally good results in younger children (Fu & Stone, 2001). Physical therapy to improve lower extremity strength and retrain coordination is often needed.

Most anterior cruciate ligament tears in the preteen group are in fact avulsion fractures at the tibial insertion (Andrish, 2001; Aichroth et al., 2002). The fracture of the tibial spine usually occurs through the cancellous bone, demonstrating avulsion of the tibial spine on a radiograph. The mechanism of injury is typically a bicycle accident or a fall in preteens and a contact sport in adolescents. Casting in 30° of knee flexion is accepted practice for minimally displaced fractures, but internal fixation is needed for full displacement of the fragment. Midsubstance tears of the anterior cruciate ligament are most common in the adolescent, but are occurring more frequently in children under 15 years of age (Williams et al., 1996). Traditional reconstructive procedures are avoided in the adolescent under the age of 15 years because of fear of injury to the growth plate with the proximal tibial drill hole (Beasley & Chudik, 2001; Guzzanti, 2003; Kouyoumjien & Barber, 2001. Classic management is functional bracing and development of muscular strength and balance for knee stability (Kochy et al., 2002).

Internal derangement of the knee joint can be either juvenile osteochondritis dissecans or meniscal injury. The etiology of juvenile osteochondritis dissecans is still an enigma. Compression of the tibial spine against the medial femoral condyle, interruption of the vascularity, anatomic variations in the knee, and abnormal subchondral bone are all possible causes. Athletic children do not seem to be at greater risk for this injury than more sedentary children. The most common sites of involvement are the lateral side of the medial femoral condyle and the lateral femoral condyle in the weight-bearing region or posteriorly. The condition usually causes pain, recurrent swelling, or catching in the knee. Pain is usually evident as the tibia rotates internally and the knee extends from a flexed position (Fu & Stone, 2001; Micheli & Jenkins, 2001; Stanitski et al., 1994). Because these lesions have a poor prognosis after skeletal maturity, every attempt should be made to gain healing before growth plate closure. In the child younger than 15 years of age, diminished activity to the point of not bearing weight is suggested. Drilling of the condyles with removal of fragments is recommended in children older than 15 years of age (Cain & Clancy, 2001). This procedure usually necessitates restriction of running and jumping for at least 6 weeks with concomitant intensive rehabilitation to regain strength, balance, and agility in the lower extremity (Grana & Kalenak, 1991; Fu & Stone, 2001).

The challenge of meniscal injuries in the young athlete is accurate diagnosis (Moti & Micheli, 2003). Often the initial incident is forgotten and clinical testing is less diagnostic than in the adult. Arthroscopic excision or repair is the treatment of choice if conservative management fails. Excision necessitates physical therapy to regain mobility and strength deficits. Meniscal repair requires further limitations of knee mobility and weight bearing while healing occurs (Boyd & Myers, 2003). Discoid lateral meniscus, which is particularly common in the Japanese, can create joint line tenderness, decreased joint mobility, effusion, and, most notably, a prominent snap in the lateral compartment as the knee is extended (Steiner & Grana, 1988). Normal menisci do not go through a discoid stage during development. The complete type of discoid meniscus, producing symptoms in late adolescence, is distinguished by intact peripheral attachments. Good results are obtained with saucerization of the meniscus. The Wrisberg type of discoid meniscus, which is more common in the pediatric group, has an attachment only through the ligament of Wrisberg and can be resolved by cutting the ligament and removing the portions with no peripheral attachments (Mintzer et al., 1998; Noyes & Barber-Westin, 2002; Steiner & Grana, 1988). As in adults, meniscal tear in the presence of anterior cruciate ligament injury can occur and should be carefully evaluated and managed (Williams et al., 1996).

The majority of problems at the knee in children are disorders of the patellar mechanism (Bergstrom et al., 2001; Steiner & Grana, 1988; van Mechelen, 1992).

Macrotrauma, repetitive microtrauma, and growth all can contribute to the disorders of the patellofemoral joint. Patellofemoral pain is the most frequent problem in the young athlete. Malalignment of the patellofemoral joint is the major cause of this pain. Several factors can cause or contribute to this malalignment. Anatomic factors such as patella alta, large Q angle, hip anteversion, flattened lateral femoral condyle, shallow femoral groove, or pes planus and hyperpronation can cause abnormal tracking of the patella during knee motion (Thomee et al., 1995). Acquired factors such as weakness of the medial quadriceps, tension in the lateral retinaculum and lateral soft tissues, or ligamentous laxity can affect patellar alignment and tracking (Fig. 18-8). The malalignment can assume one of three different patterns: (1) lateral subluxation and tilting, (2) lateral subluxation alone, or (3) isolated tilting. The source of pain has been postulated to be the increased stress on the subchondral bone from abnormal patellar stresses, increased tension in the lateral retinaculum, or formation of synovitis from articular cartilage degeneration (Thomee et al., 1995). Management of patellofemoral pain can be conservative or surgical. Conservative management consists of early relative rest, balancing of muscle strength and length, and correction of abnormal biomechanics with patellar taping or orthotics (Witvrouw et al., 2002). Surgical options include arthroscopic shaving, lateral retinacular release, and patellar realignment (Micheli, 1995; Stanitski et al., 2001).

Apophysitis, or degeneration of the ossification centers where tendons attach with chronic inflammation and

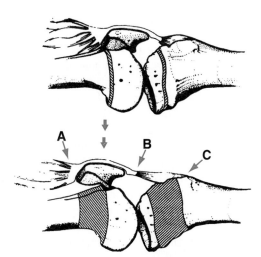

• **Figure 18-8**   Tension resulting from growth. Pain may occur at the patella (**A**), lower pole of the patella (**B**), or patellar tendon insertion on the tibia (**C**). *(From Micheli, L. Overuse injuries in children's sports: The growth factor. Orthopedic Clinics of North America, 14:353, 1983.)*

microavulsion, is common in the knee in girls between ages 8 and 13 years and in boys between 10 and 15 years. These can result from longitudinal traction with bone growth or from repetitive activity of sports participation. The most common apophysitides are Osgood-Schlatter disease of the tibial tubercle and Sinding-Larsen-Johansson disease at the inferior pole of the patella. Careful differential diagnosis is necessary to correctly identify these disorders (see Chapter 17). Relative rest, maintenance of quadriceps muscle strength with pain-free exercise, and possible extension splinting are treatment options (Birrer et al., 2002; Maffulli, 1990; Micheli, 1995; Smith, 2003; Stanitski et al., 1994).

Infrapatellar tendinitis or traction irritation at the inferior pole, otherwise known as jumper's knee, is noted most frequently in the older adolescent. The etiology includes involvement in sports that require running, jumping, climbing, or kicking (Bergstrom et al., 2001). RICE with subsequent strengthening of the knee musculature is important in treatment. Assessment of two-joint muscle length is vital because tightness of the hamstring muscles or iliotibial band may increase the flexion moment at the knee (Birrer et al., 2003; Bergstrom et al., 2001).

Patellar subluxation or dislocation can be seen in young athletes secondary to the stresses of sports requiring cutting and twisting such as soccer, dancing, cheerleading, gymnastics, and track jumping events or as a result of a direct blow to the knee. Imbalance of the length or strength of the extensor muscles, the hamstrings, the retinaculum, or the iliotibial band, as well as anatomic malalignments such as genu valgus, patella alta, or shallow condylar cup, can be etiologic factors. Management of patellar instability may include bracing in conjunction with physical therapy to normalize length-strength relationships. Failure of conservative management, although the exception, may necessitate surgical intervention to realign the patella by release of the tight structures or by alteration of the line of pull of the infrapatellar tendon (Grana & Kalenak, 1991; Micheli, 1995).

ANKLE AND FOOT INJURIES

Because of the peculiarities of their growing skeleton and their penchant for ingenious physical activity, children suffer from foot and ankle problems that may not have counterparts in the adult (Marsh & Daigneault, 2000; Santopietro, 1988). Injuries to the distal tibial and fibular growth plates are common in the young athlete. Gregg and Das (1982) have classified growth plate injuries into a clinically useful system (Fig. 18-9). The most common fractures to the ankle in the skeletally immature athlete are the Salter-Harris type 1 and 2 injuries to the distal

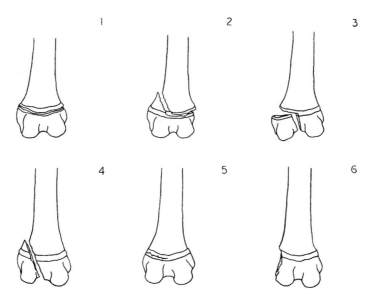

♦ **Figure 18-9** Modified Salter-Harris classification of growth plate injuries: **1**, Disruption entirely confined to the growth plate; distraction or slip injury. **2**, Fracture line runs partially through the growth plate, then extends through the metaphysis. **3**, Fracture line runs partially through the growth plate, then extends through the epiphysis. **4**, Combined disruption of metaphysis, growth plate, and epiphysis. **5**, Crush or compression injury of growth plate. **6**, Abrasion, avulsion, or burn of the perichondrial ring of the growth plate. *(From Gregg, J, & Das, M. Foot and ankle problems in the preadolescent and adolescent athlete. Clinics in Sports Medicine, 1:133, 1982.)*

fibula. Although these fractures can occur with adduction and abduction injury to the distal tibia, they frequently occur alone as a result of inversion injury. The Ottawa Rules for prediction of need for radiograph to rule out fracture has been validated in children (Libetta et al., 1999). The Ottawa Rules state that an ankle series is indicated only for patients with pain in the malleolar zone *and* bone tenderness at the posterior edge of either the medial or lateral malleolus *or* inability to bear weight immediately after injury and take four steps in the emergency room. The Rules further state that a foot series is only required with midfoot pain *and* bone tenderness at the base of the fifth metatarsal *or* bone tenderness at the navicular *or* inability to bear weight immediately and in the emergency room. Treatment with immobilization in a short leg cast for 4 to 6 weeks is suggested, although the fracture will usually heal even if untreated (Kay & Mathys, 2001). Physical therapy after casting to increase ankle and foot mobility and strength and to improve balance may be indicated. Increasing incidence of osteochondral defects of the talar dome has necessitated a review of surgical options for treatment (Toi et al., 2000).

Type 2 injury of the distal tibia is a result of ankle pronation and eversion. Common in football and soccer players, this injury is frequently associated with greenstick fracture of the distal fibula. Care must be taken to

reduce these fractures and immobilize them in a long leg cast with knee flexion to prevent impaction of the tibial metaphysis into the growth plate. The results of this type of fracture are unpredictable; occasionally angulation or premature closure of the plate occurs (Fu & Stone, 2001; Santopietro, 1988). The most common mechanism of injury in type 3 and 4 fractures of the medial malleolus is ankle supination or inversion. Adduction injuries appear in approximately 15% of these injuries and are characterized by medial displacement of part or all of the distal tibial epiphysis. The affected children are usually young, so the incidence of growth disturbance is higher. Internal fixation with restoration of ankle joint congruity is critical (Letts et al., 2001).

Because of the porosity of the bones of the foot in a child, stress fractures are common in the metatarsals in all jumping and distance running activities. If suspected by local tenderness that is aggravated with activity, these injuries should be casted for 3 weeks. After casting, one can progressively and slowly increase activities to former levels over 3 more weeks (Fu & Stone, 2001; Santopietro, 1988).

Several types of ischemia can occur in the bones of the child's foot. Freiberg infarction, or avascular necrosis of the metatarsal epiphysis, occurs in those who walk or perform on their toes. Initial synovitis is followed by sclerosis, resorption, plate fracture and collapse, and bone re-formation. It does not affect children younger than 12 years of age. Most commonly affected is the second metatarsal head. Treatment consists of cessation of toe-walking, wearing high-heeled shoes, and jumping. A negative-heel shoe is fitted. Kohler disease is seen in active boys age 3 to 7 years who have a tendency to cavus feet. Focal tenderness and swelling around the navicular bone are noted clinically. The radiograph reveals sclerosis and irregular rarefaction indicative of ischemia. Conservative treatment calls for use of a walking cast for 6 to 8 weeks followed by use of an arch support and limitation of activity for another 6 weeks (Micheli & Jenkins, 2001).

Although ankle sprains can occur in the young athlete, epiphyseal fractures are more common. Sprains occur in the older adolescent near the end of growth. The common cause of injury is landing on the lateral border of a plantar-flexed foot (Fig. 18-10). Management is similar to that in adults. Quinn and colleagues (2000) have noted a decrease in ankle sprains with external support. Surgery is indicated only in multiple sprains with gross instability.

Sever disease, or apophysitis of the calcaneus, is an Osgood-Schlatter syndrome of the foot (Fig. 18-11). It is seen most frequently in basketball and soccer players with complaint of heel pain on running. The usual age of occurrence is 8 to 13 years. Frequently, tight heel cords, a tendency toward in-toeing, and forefoot varus are noted. Treatment consists of heel cord stretching and initial use of a heel lift in well-constructed shoes (Fu & Stone, 2001).

REHABILITATION AND RETURN TO PLAY

Contrary to some opinions, the young athlete will not return to normal function spontaneously. Children and adolescents require supervised rehabilitation programs that begin with first aid on the field of play (Stanitski, 1989). The goal of first aid is to contain the extent of injury and reduce any possibility of further harm. The long-term goal of rehabilitation is return to play in a safe manner. Short-term goals should include the accomplishment of the component skills needed to reach the long-term goal. The general process of rehabilitation should emphasize maintenance of cardiovascular skills while normalizing mobility and flexibility. Emphasis then shifts to normalization of muscular endurance and strength, of both the injured area and the entire extremity. Eventually attention is directed toward resumption of purposeful, controlled movements at the appropriate speed (Davis, 1986). Utilization of the "10% rule"—no weekly increase greater than 10% of the previous level—is a safe progression for training (Trepman & Micheli, 1988).

Complete rehabilitation is synonymous with return to play. Premature return to activity courts reinjury and the development of chronic problems (Stanitski, 1989). The criteria for return include no edema; full, pain-free, biomechanically normal mobility; normal strength by objective testing; and normal completion of appropriate

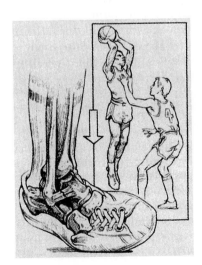

• **Figure 18-10** Plantar flexion-inversion injury. *(From Birrer, R, & Brecher, D. Common Sports Injuries in Youngsters. Oradell, NJ: Medical Economics, 1987, p. 120.)*

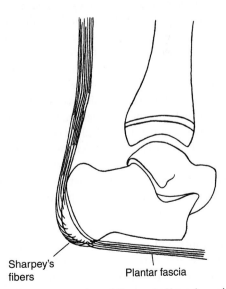

Sharpey's fibers   Plantar fascia

• **Figure 18-11** Insertion of Sharpey's fibers from the Achilles tendon into the calcaneal apophysis. *(From Gregg, J, & Das, M. Foot and ankle problems in the preadolescent and adolescent athlete. Clinics in Sports Medicine, 1:140, 1982.)*

functional tests such as vertical leap, hopping, running, or cutting activities. Supportive or protective devices such as orthoses or braces may be used to supplement rehabilitation and to provide stability and anatomic alignment (Micheli & Jenkins, 2001).

THE YOUNG ATHLETE WITH A PHYSICAL DISABILITY

Children with a disability have the same basic needs as their able-bodied peers (Lai et al., 2000). With the approval in the United States of Public Law 94-142, the Rehabilitation Act of 1973, and the Americans with Disabilities Act in 1991, a variety of physical activity and sports programs are now available to those with impairments (Bernhardt, 1985b; Carek et al., 2002; McCormick, 1985; Webster et al., 2001). Several studies have demonstrated that those with physical disabilities do indeed participate in sports. In a survey of 100 persons with lower extremity amputations, 60% were active in sports. Persons with disabilities of both genders were most active when they are younger (Kegel et al., 1980). Of a group of 67 individuals with spinal cord injury, 72% participated in sports at least once weekly. These sports included basketball, swimming, weight lifting, road racing, and boating. The group included 19 athletes currently involved in competition (Curtis et al., 1986).

Both psychologic and physiologic benefits of sports participation have been demonstrated in individuals with disabilities. Self-concept and self-acceptance were shown to be equal or greater in athletes of various ages with disabilities when compared with control subjects who were able-bodied (Davis et al., 1981; Hanson et al., 2001; Patrick, 1984; Sherrill et al., 1990). Wheelchair basketball players had significantly better mental profiles than players who were able-bodied and nonathletes (Paulsen et al., 1991). When novice and veteran wheelchair athletes were compared, the novice group had lower perceived social adequacy and lower self-perception, suggesting that sports participation might change these perceptions in a positive way (Patrick, 1984). Among children with limb deficiencies, athletic competence was one predictor of higher perceived physical appearance and, in turn, lower levels of depression and higher self-esteem (Varni & Setoguchi, 1991).

Disability often causes some reduction of fitness relative to the general population (Field & Oates, 2001; Patel & Greydanus, 2002; Pitetti et al., 1993; Regan et al., 1993; Rimmer, 2001). Several research studies have demonstrated, however, that fitness training in those with disabilities can reverse this reduction of physiologic status.

In classic studies by Zwiren and Bar-Or (1975) and others, the physiologic capabilities of athletes who participated in wheelchair sports were shown to be only 9% lower than those of athletes without disabilities and fully 50% greater than those of sedentary individuals who used wheelchairs. Other studies have confirmed these findings (Bernhardt, 1985a; Davis et al., 1981). Decreases in body fat and increases in muscle strength and endurance, often beyond that of individuals without disabilities, have also been documented (Davis et al., 1981). In a comparison of the health and functional status of athletes and nonathletes with spinal cord injuries, the athletes had an average of only 2.4 physician visits per year compared with 6.7 physician visits for the nonathletes. Although they were involved in sports significantly more hours per week (10.2 ± 9.6 hours for athletes; 4.9 ± 4.1 hours for nonathletes), the athletes on average had fewer hospitalizations, decubitus ulcers, medical complications, and hours of required attendant care. The researchers concluded that the medical risks associated with intense sports activity for those with spinal cord injuries were minimal (Curtis et al., 1986).

RISK OF INJURY

Little information has been gathered on the incidence and type of sports injuries that occur in persons who are disabled. Although several studies have appeared in the literature, they have had small sample sizes and select groups of individuals with specific disabilities. An exception was a survey distributed to 1200 athletes in regional wheelchair competition during 1981. One hundred two male and 27 female athletes responded. Thirty-two different sports were represented by the group. Seventy-two percent of all athletes had sustained at least 1 injury, with some reporting as many as 14 injuries. The most prevalent injuries were soft tissue trauma (33%), blisters (18%), and lacerations or abrasions (17%). The majority of the injuries occurred in the upper extremity. Most of the injuries were associated with track (26%), basketball (24%), and road racing (22%) (Curtis, 1982). A survey of the 1990 Junior National Wheelchair Games demonstrated injury rates of 97% in track, 22% in field events, and 91% in swimming among 83 athletes (Wilson & Washington, 1993). A 1995 study by Taylor and Williams in the United Kingdom reported a similar overall rate of injury.

The largest study, a retrospective survey of 426 athletes participating in the 1989 competitions of the National Wheelchair Athletic Association (NWAA), the United States Association for Blind Athletes (USABA), and the United States Cerebral Palsy Association (USCPA), demonstrated that 32% of the respondents had at least one time-loss injury. Twenty-six percent of all injuries were from the NWAA, with 57% of this total at the shoulder and elbow. Fifty-three percent of all USABA athletes' injuries were in the lower extremity. The injuries in the USCPA athletes were noted in all areas. Injury rates were the same for athletes with or without disabilities (Ferrara et al., 1992).

Data from the International Flower Marathon showed that 19 athletes experienced 20 medical problems, many caused by climate and spills. Problems were more frequent in groups with disabilities caused by paraplegia and poliomyelitis. Thirteen medical problems were classified as injuries: five were ulcers and abrasions and eight were soft tissue injuries (Hoeberigs et al., 1990).

A study of the injuries at the Special Olympic games demonstrated that 3.5% of the athletes required care for an injury or illness. Track and field events consumed the least time but had the greatest injury rate (McCormick et al., 1990). The Connecticut State Special Olympics Games in 1994 through 1996 noted that the most frequent injuries were sprains/strains to the lower extremities, followed by fractures and dislocations. They also noted a sixfold increase in heat-related dehydration in 1996 (Galena et al., 1998). Data from the 2001 Special Olympics World Winter Games documented 1081 total incidents (58% mild to moderate and 41% moderate to severe). These injuries were 49.5% orthopedic and 49.8% medical with 6% requiring a hospital visit and 2% requiring admission. (Special Olympics inquiry data, 2001).

Because very limited data are available that document the occurrence or management of injuries in the athlete with a disability, more research is needed.

PREPARTICIPATION EXAMINATION

Preparticipation assessment of a young person with a disability is similar to that of someone who is able-bodied, and can be conducted in a multistation fashion. Several areas, however, must be more thoroughly addressed. The personnel performing the assessment must understand not only the physical, physiologic, and psychologic requirements of the sport but also the potential medical risks of participation. The physically challenged athlete may be prone to additional injury or illness secondary to the disability (Smith & Wilder, 1999). In addition, the physician may be involved in classification of the athlete depending on the type and severity of the disability and must be aware of international and national classification systems (Bernhardt, 1991; Davis et al., 1981).

The history should include the date of the onset of disability. Description and dates of all medical problems, hospitalizations, and operations before and after the onset

of disability should be included. Releases for participation from all attending physicians are required. Thorough documentation of medications for comparison with lists of permissible drugs is necessary (Bernhardt, 1991).

Physical examination must include documentation of level of understanding, vocalization, communication abilities, and hearing. Flexibility should be evaluated because greater than normal muscle length may be required for certain activities (e.g., flexible hips for positioning in sports wheelchair). Special consideration should be given to instability in specific disability groups, such as the propensity for cervical instability and subluxation in Down syndrome (Brockmeyer, 1999; Pueschel, 1998). Complete assessment of all sensory systems is required for classification and safety. Documentation of the presence of abnormal muscle tone and primitive, protective, or pathologic reflexes is critical for participation in sports such as archery, horseback riding, and swimming. Assessment of integrity and toughness of the skin and documentation of any history of skin problems are vital in any athlete with sensory impairment (Bernhardt, 1991).

The level of sitting and standing posture and balance as it pertains to the sport is critical for effective and safe participation. The athlete who skis while seated or rides horseback must have adequate balance to perform. The athlete can be placed in a mock-up situation for assessment if necessary. Assessment of gait is mandatory in all clients who are ambulatory. The pattern and efficiency, as well as assistive devices needed, must be reviewed. Estimation of locomotor endurance is helpful.

The assessment of gross and fine motor skills should be performed in tasks similar to those required by the sport. Bilateral comparisons and timing and quality should be noted (Bernhardt, 1991). Muscle strength and endurance should be assessed, if possible, with either manual or mechanical methods. Although this area has received little attention, dominant hand grip force can be used as a partial predictor of upper body strength (Davis et al., 1981; Jackson & Davis, 1983). Davis (1981) has also shown that a good relationship exists between upper body isokinetic strength and habitual activity.

Physiologic assessment should include nutritional analysis, body composition measurement, and exercise testing. Exercise testing may be advisable for assessment of cardiopulmonary functional capacity or the efficacy of medications. Testing must often be adjusted for the disability, such as arm crank, wheelchair, or single leg ergometry (Bernhardt, 1985a, 1991; Bhambhani et al., 1993; Draheim et al., 1999; Pare et al., 1993). Field testing can be completed as long as standard testing principles are followed (Fletcher et al., 1988; Leger et al., 1988). Although maximal oxygen consumption is the best single indicator of cardiovascular fitness, submaximal testing can be performed as an estimation of maximal capacity.

For many athletes with a disability, equipment is part of their participation. Specially designed wheelchairs, skiing outriggers, ergonomic racquet handles, rotation platforms for field events, and custom prostheses are but a few of the technologic advances that have made sports more accessible. The examiner should check the equipment for function, fit, safety, and conformity to rules of competition or participation (Bernhardt, 1991).

TRAINING PROGRAMS

Persons with disabilities should be placed on training programs in a manner similar to those who are able-bodied (Bernhardt, 1985a, 1985b; Curtis, 1981a, 1981b) (Fig. 18-12). Several studies have evaluated the efficacy of these training programs in various disability groups. Research on wheelchair training demonstrated increases in maximal oxygen uptake, decreases in exercise and resting heart rate, and increases in maximal work capacity. Documented increases in muscle force and endurance and peak force have been noted after strength training (Hutzler et al., 1998; Lintunen et al., 1995; Veeger et al., 1991).

▋ SUMMARY

Young athletes, whether able-bodied or disabled, are not small adults. They have unique issues in sports participation that must be specifically addressed. Recognition of these unusual qualities is necessary for effective prevention and management of sports-related injuries.

Physical therapists should play a significant role in the total management of the child athlete. The broad-based and eclectic medical background of physical therapists makes them ideal professionals for the assessment and rehabilitation of sports injuries in athletes with full or altered physical capabilities. Depending on advanced experience or certification in sports physical therapy, athletic training, or exercise physiology, they may be the primary medical professional to administer total management from prevention to return to participation after injury.

If lacking in expertise or time, a physical therapist may alternatively work with a certified athletic trainer and an exercise physiologist to provide comprehensive sports safety management. The certified trainer is appropriately skilled to assist with preparticipation screenings and to provide on-site coverage of practices and games with immediate triage and injury management. The exercise physiologist plays an integral part in the preseason screening and in conditioning and training programs.

The physical therapist can provide assessment and total rehabilitation of sports injuries and aid in phasing the athlete back to play with appropriate progression, supportive devices, or medical limitations. The certified trainer or the exercise physiologist often works with the physical therapist in the return-to-play planning and follow-up.

The goal of these programs is to promote the health and safety of the young athlete. All those involved should work in a manner appropriate to their education, skills, and practice statutes as members of a team, including coaches and parents, toward the goal of safe, rewarding, and successful participation in sport and recreation.

CASE STUDIES

BB

BB is a 14-year-old boy who decided to go out for eighth grade football as a lineman. Two weeks into fall practice he noted left knee pain, especially when in a crouching position, running or cutting, or on stairs. He further experienced left upper back pain. He reported a history of a back injury when loading hay several months ago, but stated that it had improved until football. When questioned, he reported no off-season preparation for football.

His examination revealed tenderness at the inferior patellar pole and over the length of the patellar tendon. He had no tenderness at the tendon insertion on the tibial tuberosity. Knee flexion was limited by 20° when compared with the right, although knee extension was full. Girth measurements of his midthigh and calf were 1 inch smaller on the left. He had a slight antalgic gait with decreased flexion in swing and increased stance time. Active knee extension (popliteal angle) was −50°, indicating hamstring inflexibility.

Examination of his upper back area demonstrated tenderness (6/10) with palpation and use of the rhomboid and lower trapezius muscles on the left. He had a 30° decrease in shoulder flexion and abduction. Strength in the rhomboids was 4/5, lower trapezius 3+/5. His posture was guarded on the left with rounding and depression of his shoulder complex.

A diagnosis of left patellar tendinitis, inferior pole irritation, and strain of the left rhomboid and lower trapezius was made. He received two treatments in the clinic consisting of warmth and inferential stimulation followed by myofascial stretching. He was instructed in stretching for the muscles that elevate the shoulder and adduct the scapula. He was shown shoulder and scapular isolation

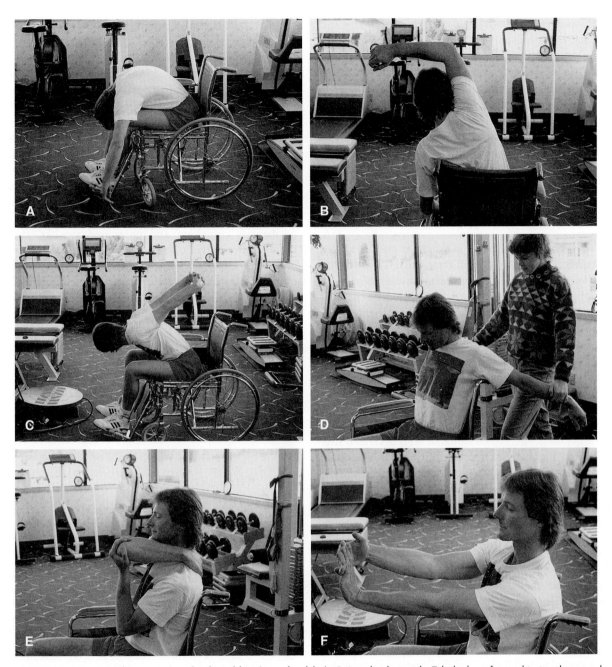

◆ **Figure 18-12** Stretching exercises for the athlete in a wheelchair. **A**, Low back stretch. Exhale; lean forward to touch ground. **B**, Shoulder and lateral trunk muscles stretch. Lift one arm over head and lean to side. Repeat on opposite side. **C**, Anterior chest and wrist stretch. Exhale, clasp hands, lean forward, and lift arms high in back. **D**, Partner anterior chest muscle stretch. Pull arms to side with palms facing forward. Pull back with elbows straight. **E**, Scapular and posterior shoulder muscle stretch. Bend arm across chest. Reach for opposite shoulder blade. Push on elbow. Repeat on opposite side. **F**, Wrist and finger flexor muscle stretch. Straighten elbow. Push wrist and fingers back. Repeat for opposite side.

exercises and correct postural alignment. Additionally, he was given a short home program to increase hamstring flexibility and quadriceps strength. His program consisted of squats, lunges with weights, and 4-inch lateral step-ups to be done on nongame days.

By his second visit, his knee pain was minimal and occasional. Hamstring flexibility had increased 5°. Scapular soreness was decreased (4/10) but still present with play. Postural alignment was now good. He had been compliant with his home program.

His program was advanced to include shoulder and scapular endurance and strength exercises with the green Theraband. He was advanced to 6-inch step-ups and single-leg squats and toe raises. He was instructed to continue his home program and report in 2 weeks.

When he called, his knee pain had resolved, and he could perform functional tests equally well on both legs. His scapular pain was only slight, and he could play without soreness. He was instructed to increase to the blue Theraband and continue his lower extremity exercises. He will come in after football for an off-season program.

N E

NE was a star basketball player in her senior year. She landed off balance during a midseason game and fell, twisting her right knee. Immediate field examination revealed tenderness over the medial joint line. She demonstrated +2 laxity on a Lachman test and could not bear weight on her leg.

Follow-up 2 days later by her orthopedist confirmed the probability of anterior cruciate ligament (ACL) injury. An MRI (magnetic resonance imaging) scan demonstrated both an ACL tear and medial meniscal damage. She was referred for preoperative rehabilitation and scheduled for surgery in 2 weeks.

Initial examination revealed an edematous knee with some bruising. Her gait was antalgic with decreased heel strike and push-off, limited knee motion, and minimal comfortable weight bearing. Although her thigh and calf girth measurements were unchanged, the tone of her right quadriceps was decreased. She performed only a 3+/5 quadriceps isometrically. Knee mobility was −12° extension, 80° flexion. Her pain level was 5 on a scale of 10, and she had difficulty sleeping.

Before surgery, she began a program to reduce edema, increase knee mobility, normalize gait, and maintain leg strength. Her treatment included cooling, inferential stimulation, and gait training. She was instructed in wall slides and heel slides, as well as straight-leg raising (SLR) and short arc knee extension. The final goals for this 2-week period were full knee mobility, normal gait without device, no edema, and strength 80% of normal knee.

Her final preoperative visit consisted of reevaluation and teaching. The surgical procedure, use of crutches, and postsurgical rehabilitation were explained. She was fit for and instructed in the use of a continuous passive motion (CPM) machine and a cooling unit.

Postsurgical rehabilitation after her patellar tendon graft began on postoperative day 1. She was placed in a CPM machine and gradually increased in flexion to 60°. She was instructed in quadriceps setting and assisted SLR. Her CPM mobility was reinforced by supine knee flexion against a wall. Her postoperative brace was unlocked, and she was instructed in correct gait pattern with weight bearing to tolerance with crutches.

Her program progressed from edema and pain reduction, knee mobility, and gait training to endurance and then strength exercises. The CPM was discontinued when she could actively achieve 110° of knee flexion. The majority of her strength exercises were closed-chain exercises with emphasis on correct technique through full available range of motion. She progressed to one crutch, then to no device when her gait was normal without assistance. She was seen three times weekly in the clinic with a full home program.

She was compliant and progressed steadily. Three months after surgery, she was fitted with a functional brace and instructed in a home training program. At this time, mobility and gait were normal. Knee stability was excellent. Thigh and calf strength were still only 50%.

She was monitored every 2 weeks until 5 months, then monthly for 1 year. She was tested on an isokinetic dynamometer at 6 months and 12 months. At the end of 1 year, her strength was 95% of her uninjured leg, so her brace was discontinued and she was released to full function.

◼ REFERENCES

Aagaard, H, & Jorgensen, U. Injuries in elite volleyball. Scandinavian Journal of Medicine & Science in Sports, 6:228–232, 1996.

Adirim, TA, & Cheng, TL. Overview of injuries in the young athlete. Sports Medicine 33:75–81, 2003.

Aichroth, PM, Patel, DV, & Zorrilla, P. The natural history and treatment of rupture of the anterior cruciate ligament in children and adolescents. A prospective review. The Journal of Bone and Joint Surgery (British), 84:38–41, 2002.

American Academy of Pediatrics. Organized athletics for preadolescent children. Pediatrics, 84:583–584, 1989.

American Academy of Pediatrics Committee on Sports Medicine and Fitness. Clinical heat stress and the exercising child and adolescent. Pediatrics, 106:158–159, 2000. Available at http://aappolicy.aappublications.org/cgi/reprint/pediatrics;106/1/158. Accessed September 26, 2005.

American Academy of Pediatrics Committee on Sports Medicine and Fitness. Medical conditions affecting sports participation. Pediatrics, 107:1205–1209, 2001. Available at http://aappolicy.aappublications.org/cgi/reprint/pediatrics;107/5/1205. Accessed September 26, 2005.

American College of Sports Medicine. Inter-Association Task Force on exertional heat illnesses consensus statement, 2003.

American Medical Association: Ensuring the health of the adolescent athlete. Archives of Family Medicine, 2:446–448. 1993.

Anderson, SJ. Lower extremity injuries in youth sports. Pediatric Clinics of North America, 49:627–641, 2002.

Andrish, JT. Anterior cruciate ligament injuries in the skeletally immature patient. The American Journal of Orthopedics, 30:103–110, 2001.

Armsey, TD, Jr, & Green, GA. Nutrition supplements: Science vs. hype. The Physician and Sports Medicine, 25:77–92, 1997.

Armstrong, LE, Maresh, CM, Riebe, D, Riebe, D, Kenefick, RW, Castellani, JW, Sen, JW, Echegaray, M, & Foley, MF. Local cooling in wheelchair athletes during exercise-heat stress. Medicine & Science in Sports & Exercise, 27:211–216, 1995.

Armstrong, N, Kirby, BJ, McManus, AM, & Welsman, JR. Aerobic fitness of prepubescent children. Annuals of Human Biology, 22(5):427–441, 1995.

Aubry, M, Cantu, R, Dvorak, J, Graf-Baumann, T, Johnston, K, Kelly, J, Lovell, M, McCrory, P, Meeuwisse, W, & Schamasch, P. Summary and agreement statement of the First International Conferences on Concussion in Sport, Vienna, 2001. Recommendations for the improvement of safety and health of athletes who may suffer concussive injuries. British Journal of Sports Medicine, 36:6–10, 2002.

Backx, FJ, Beijer, HJ, Bol, E, & Erich, WB. Injuries in high-risk persons and high-risk sports: A longitudinal study of 1818 school children. American Journal of Sports Medicine, 19:124–130, 1991a.

Backx, FJ, Erich, WB, Kemper, AB, & Verbeek AL. Sports injuries in school-aged children: An epidemiological study. American Journal of Sports Medicine, 17:234–240, 1991b.

Bahrke, MS, Yesalis, CE, & Brower, KJ. Anabolic-androgenic steroid abuse and performance-enhancing drugs among adolescents. Child and Adolescent Psychiatric Clinics of North America, 7:821–838, 1998.

Bailes, JE, & Cantu, RC. Head injury in athletes. Neurosurgery, 48:26–45, 2001.

Bak, MJ, & Doerr, TD. Craniomaxillofacial fractures during recreational baseball and softball. Journal of Oral and Maxillofacial Surgery, 62:1209–1212, 2004.

Baker, JS, & Davies, B. High intensity exercise assessment: Relationships between laboratory and field measures of performance. Journal of Science in Medicine and Sport, 5:341–347, 2002.

Baker, MM. Anterior cruciate ligament injuries in female athletes. Journal of Women's Health, 7:343–349, 1998.

Balsom, PD, Soderlund, K, & Ekblom, B. Creatine in humans with special reference to creatine supplementation. Sports Medicine, 18:268–280, 1994.

Bar-Or, O. Child and Adolescent Athlete, Vol. 6. Malden, MA: Blackwell Publishers, 1995.

Bar-Or, O. The young athlete: Some physiological considerations. Journal of Sports Science, 13:S31–S33, 1995.

Bauman, M. Nutritional requirements for athletes. In Bernhardt, DB (Ed.). Sports Physical Therapy. New York: Churchill Livingstone, 1986, pp. 89–105.

Beachy, GKAC, Martinson, M, & Olderr, TF. High school sports injuries: A longitudinal study at Punahou School 1988 to 1996. American Journal of Sports Medicine, 25:675–681, 1997.

Beasley, LS, & Chudik, SC. Anterior cruciate ligament injuries in children: Update of current treatment options. Current Opinions in Pediatrics, 15:45–52, 2003.

Beatty, E, Light, TR, Belsole, RJ, & Ogden, JA. Wrist and hand skeletal injuries in children. Hand Clinics, 6:723–738, 1990.

Bell, DG, McLellan, TM, & Sabiston, CM: Effect of ingesting caffeine and ephedrine on performance. Medicine & Science in Sports & Exercise, 34:1399–1403, 2002.

Below, PR, Mora-Rodriguez, R, Gonzalez-Alonso, J, & Coyle, EF. Fluid and carbohydrate ingestion independently improve performance during 1 h of intense exercise. Medicine & Science in Sports & Exercise, 27:200–210, 1995.

Benson, LS, Waters, PM, Meier, SW, Visotsky, JL, & Williams, CS. Pediatric hand injuries due to home exercycles. Journal of Pediatric Orthopedics, 20:34–39, 2000.

Bergstrom, KA, Brandseth, K, Fretheim, S, Tvilde, K, & Ekeland, A. Activity-related knee injuries and pain in athletic adolescents. Knee Surgery, Sports Traumatology, and Arthroscopy, 9:146–150, 2001.

Bernhardt, DB. Exercise testing and training for disabled populations: The state of the art. In Bernhardt, DB (Ed.). Recreation for the Disabled Child. New York: Haworth Press, 1985a, pp. 3–25.

Bernhardt, DB: The competitive spirit. In Bernhardt, DB (Ed.). Recreation for the Disabled Child. New York, Haworth Press, 1985b, pp. 77–86.

Bernhardt, DB. The physically challenged athlete. In Cantu, RC, & Micheli, LJ (Eds.). ACSM's Guidelines for the Team Physician. Philadelphia: Lea & Febiger, 1991, pp. 242–251.

Bernhardt, DT, Gomez, J, Johnson, MD, Martin, TJ, Rowland, TW, Small, E, LeBlanc, C, Malina, R, Krein, D, Young, JC, Reed FE, Anderson, SJ, Griesemer, BA, Bar-Or, O, & Committee on Sports Medicine and Fitness. Strength training by children and adolescents. Pediatrics, 107:1470–1472, 2001.

Bhambhani, YN, Holland, LJ, & Steadward, RD. Anaerobic threshold in wheelchair athletes with cerebral palsy: Validity and reliability. Archives of Physical Medicine and Rehabilitation, 74:305–311, 1993.

Bijur, PEAT, Harel Y, Overpeck MD, Jones, D, & Scheidt, PC. Sports and recreation injuries in US children and adolescents. Archives of Pediatrics & Adolescent Medicine, 1499:1009–1101, 1995.

Birrer, RB, & Levine, R. Performance parameters in children and adolescent athletes. Sports Medicine, 4:221–237, 1987.

Birrer, RB, Griesemer, BA, & Cataletto, MB. Pediatric Sports Medicine for Primary Care. Philadelphia: Lippincott Williams & Wilkins, 2002.

Blanksby, BA, Wearne, FK, Elliott, BC, & Blitvich, JD. Aetiology and occurrence of diving injuries. A review of diving safety. Sports Medicine, 23(4):228–246, 1997.

Blimke, CJR. Resistance training during preadolescence: Issues and controversies. Sports Medicine, 15:389–407, 1993.

Boden, BP, Lin, W, Young, M, & Mueller, FO. Catastrophic injuries in wrestlers. American Journal of Sports Medicine, 30:791–795, 2002.

Boyd, KT, & Myers, PT. Meniscus preservation: Rationale, repair techniques and results. Knee, 10:1–11, 2003.

Bratton, RL. Preparticipation screening of children for sports. Current recommendations. Sports Medicine, 24:300–307, 1997.

Brockmeyer, D. Down syndrome and craniovertebral instability: Topic review and treatment recommendations. Pediatric Neurosurgery, 31:71–77, 1999.

Brogger-Jensen, T, Hvass, I, & Bugge, S. Injuries at the BMX Cycling European Championship, 1989. British Journal of Sports Medicine, 24:269–270, 1990.

Brown, RL, Brunn, MA, & Garcia, VF. Cervical spine injuries in children: A review of 103 patients treated consecutively at a level 1 pediatric trauma center. Journal of Pediatric Surgery, 36:1107–1114, 2001.

Brown, RL, Koepplinger, ME, Mehlman, CT, Gittelman, M, & Garcia, VF. All-terrain vehicle and bicycle crashes in children: Epidemiology and comparison of injury severity. Journal of Pediatric Surgery, 37:375–380, 2002.

Bruce, DA, Schut, L, & Sutton, LN. Brain and cervical spine injuries occurring during organized sports activities in children and adolescents. Clinical Sports Medicine, 1:495–514, 1982.

Brust, JD, Leonard, BJ, Pheley, A, & Roberts, WO. Children's ice hockey injuries. American Journal of Diseases of Childhood, 146:741–747, 1992.

Brynhildsen, J, Ekstrand, J, Jeppsson, A, & Tropp, H. Previous injuries and persisting symptoms in female soccer players. International Journal of Sports Medicine, 11:489–492, 1990.

Bunc, V. A simple method for estimating aerobic fitness. Ergonomics, 37:159–165, 1994.

Campbell, RM, Jr. Operative treatment of factures and dislocations of the hand and wrist region in children. Orthopedic Clinics of North America, 21:217–243, 1990.

Cantu, RC. Stingers, transient quadriplegia, and cervical spine stenosis: Return to play criteria. Medicine & Science in Sports & Exercise, 29:S233–S235, 1997.

Cantu, RC. Second-impact syndrome. Clinics in Sports Medicine, 17:37–44, 1998.

Cantu, RC. Return to play guidelines after a head injury. Clinics in Sports Medicine, 17:45–60, 1998.

Cantu, RC. Cervical spine injuries in the athlete. Seminars in Neurology, 20:173–178, 2000.

Cantu, RC. Recurrent athletic head injury: risks and when to retire. Clinics in Sports Medicine, 22:593–603, 2003.

Cantu, RC, Bailes, JE, & Wilberger, JE, Jr. Guidelines for return to contact or collision sport after a cervical spine injury. Clinics in Sports Medicine, 17:137–146, 1998.

Cantu, RC, & Mueller, FO. Catastrophic football injuries: 1977–1998. Neurosurgery 47:673–675, 2000.

Cantu, RC, & Mueller, FO. Catastrophic spine injuries in American football, 1977–2001. Neurosurgery, 53:358–362, 2003a.

Cantu, RC, & Mueller, FO. Brain injury-related fatalities in American football, 1945-1999. Neurosurgery, 52:846–852, 2003b.

Carek, PJ, Dickerson, LM, & Hawkins, A. Special Olympics, special athletes, special needs? Journal of Southern Connecticut Medical Association, 98:183–186, 2002.

Casa, DJ, Armstrong, LE, Hillman, SK, Montain, SJ, Reiff, RV, Rich, BSE, Roberts, WO, & Stone, JA. National Athletic Trainers' Association position statement: Fluid replacement for athletes. Journal of Athletic Training, 35:212–224, 2000.

Caspersen, CJ, Pereira, MA, & Curran, KM. Changes in physical activity patterns in the United States by sex and cross-sectional age. Medicine & Science in Sports & Exercise, 32:1601–1609, 2000.

Castaldi, CR. Sports related oral and facial injuries in the young athlete: A new challenge for the pediatric dentist. Pediatric Dentistry, 8:311–316, 1986.

Centers for Disease Control and Prevention: Physical activity levels among children ages 9–13 years—United States, 2002. MMWR Morbity & Mortality Weekly Report, 52:785–788, 2003.

CDC. BMI for Children and Teens. Available at http://www.cdc.gov/nccdphp/dnpa/bmi/bmi-for-age.htm. Accessed September 26, 2005.

Challier, B, Chau, N, Predine, R, Choquet, M, & Legras, B. Associations of family environment and individual factors with tobacco, alcohol, and illicit drug use in adolescents. European Journal of Epidemiology, 16:33–42, 2000.

Clark, N. Nutrition: Pre-, intra-, and post-competition. In Cantu, RC, & Micheli, LJ (Eds.). ACSM's Guidelines for the Team Physician. Philadelphia: Lea & Febiger, 1991, pp. 58–65.

Clarkson, PM. Nutrition for improved sports performance. Current issues on ergogenic aids. Sports Medicine, 21:393–401, 1996.

Coady, CM, & Micheli, LJ. Stress fractures in the pediatric athlete. Clinics in Sports Medicine, 16:225–238, 1997.

Collins, MW, Lovell, MR, Iverson, GL, Cantu, RC, Maroon, JC. & Field, M. Cumulative effects of concussion in high school athletes. Neurosurgery, 51:1175–1179, 2002.

Conn, JM, Annest, JL, & Gilchrist, J. Sports and recreation related injury episodes in the US population, 1997–1999. Injury Prevention, 9:117–123, 2003.

Cooper, K. Kid Fitness. New York: Bantam Books, 1991.

Creath, CJ, Shelton, WO, Wright, JT, Bradley, DH, Feinstein, RA, & Wisniewski, JF. The prevalence of smokeless tobacco use among adolescent male athletes. Journal of American Dental Association, 116:43–48, 1998.

Crews, D. Field testing the wheelchair athlete. Sports n' Spokes, March/April 1982, p. 37.

Curtis, KA. Wheelchair sportsmedicine: II. Training. Sports n' Spokes, July/August 1981a, pp. 16-19.

Curtis, KA. Wheelchair sportsmedicine: III. Stretching. Sports n' Spokes, September/October 1981b, pp. 16–18.

Curtis, KA. Wheelchair sportsmedicine: IV. Athletic injuries. Sports n' Spokes, January/February 1982, pp. 20–24.

Curtis, KA, McClanahan, S, & Hail, KM. Vocational and functional status in spinal cord injured athletes and nonathletes. Archives of Physical Medicine and Rehabilitation, 67:862–865, 1986.

Dalton, SE. Overuse injuries in adolescent athletes. Sports Medicine, 13:58–70, 1992.

DaSilva, MF, Williams, JS, Fadale, PD, Hulstyn, MJ. & Ehrlich, MG. Pediatric throwing injuries about the elbow. American Journal of Orthopedics, 27:90–96, 1998.

Davis, GM. Cardiorespiratory fitness and muscle strength in lower-limb disability. Canadian Journal of Applied Sports Science, 6:159–165, 1981.

Davis, JM, Kuppermann, N, & Fleisher, G. Serious sports injuries requiring hospitalization seen in a pediatric emergency department. American Journal of Diseases in Children, 147:1001–1004, 1993.

Davis, JM. Carbohydrates, branched-chain amino acids, and endurance: The central fatigue hypothesis. International Journal of Sports Nutrition, 5:S29–S38, 1995.

Davis, GM, Kofsky, PR, Kelsey, JC, & Shepard, RJ. Cardiorespiratory fitness and muscular strength of wheelchair athletes. Canadian Medical Association Journal, 125:1317–1323, 1981.

Davis, JM, Welsh, RS, & Alerson, NA. Effects of carbohydrate and chromium ingestion during intermittent high-intensity exercise to fatigue. International Journal of Sport Nutrition and Exercise Metabolism, 10:476–485, 2000.

Debnath, UK, Freeman, BJ, Gregory, P, de la Harpe, D, Kerslake, RW, & Webb. JK. Clinical outcome and return to sport after the surgical treatment of spondylolysis in young athletes. The Journal of Bone and Joint Surgery (British), 85:244–249, 2003.

Delibasi, C, Yamazawa, M, Nomura, K, Iida S, & Kogo, M. Maxillofacial fractures sustained during sports played with a ball. Oral Surgery Oral Medicine Oral Pathology Oral Radiology and Endodontics, 97:23–27, 2004.

deLoes, M, Dahlstedt, LJ, & Thomee, R. A 7-year study on risks and costs of knee injuries in male and female youth participants in 12 sports. Scandinavian Journal of Medicine & Science in Sports, 10:90–97, 2000.

d'Hemecourt, PA, Gerbino, PG, 2nd, & Micheli, LJ. Back injuries in the young athlete. Clinics in Sports Medicine, 19:663–679, 2000.

DiScala, C, Gallagher, SS, & Schneps, SE. Causes and outcomes of pediatric injuries occurring at school. Journal of School Health, 67:384–389, 1997.

Draheim, CC, Laurie, NE, McCubbin, JA, & Perkins, JL. Validity of a modified aerobic fitness test for adults with mental retardation. Medicine & Science in Sports & Exercise, 31:1849–1854, 1999.

Drezner, JA. Sudden cardiac death in young athletes: Causes, athlete's heart and screening guidelines. Postgraduate Medicine, 108:37–44, 47–50, 2000.

Drkulec, JA, & Letts, M. Snowboarding injuries in children. Canadian Journal of Surgery, 44:435–439, 2001.

DuRant, RH, Escobedo, LG, & Heath, GW. Anabolic-steroid use, strength training, and multiple drug use among adolescents in the United States. Pediatrics, 96:23–28, 1995.

Dvorak, J,& Junge, A. Football injuries and physical symptoms: A review of literature. American Journal of Sports Medicine, 28:S3–S9, 2000.

Echemendia, RJ, & Cantu, RC. Return to play following sports-related mild traumatic brain injury: The role for neuropsychology. Applied Neuropsychology, 10:48–55, 2003.

Epstein, LH, Paluch, RA, Kalakanis, LE, Goldfiled, GS, Cerny, FJ, & Roemmich, JN. How much activity do youth get? A quantitative review of heart-rate measured activity. Pediatrics, 108:E44, 2001.

Erlanger, D, Kaushik, T, Cantu, R, Barth, JT, Broshek, DK, Freeman, JR, & Webbe, FM. Symptom-based assessment of the severity of a concussion. Journal of Neurosurgery, 98:477–484, 2003.

Fagenbaum, R, & Darling, WG. Jump landing strategies in male and female college athletes and the implications of such strategies for anterior cruciate ligament injury. American Journal of Sports Medicine, 31:233–240, 2003.

Faigenbaum, AD, Milliken, LA, Loud, RL, Burak, BT, Doherty, CL, & Westcott, WL. Comparison of 1 and 2 days per week of strength training in children. Research Quarterly of Exercise & Sports, 73:416–424, 2002.

Falk, B, & Tenenbaum, G. The effectiveness of resistance training in children: A meta-analysis. Sports Medicine, 3:176–186, 1996.

Feld, LG, Springate, JE, & Waz, WR. Special topics in pediatric hypertension. Seminars in Nephrology, 18:295–303, 1998.

Ferrara, MS, Buckley, WE, McCann, BC, Limbird, TJ. Powell, JW, & Robl, R. The injury experience of a competitive athlete with a disability: Prevention implications. Medicine & Science in Sports & Exercise, 24:184–188, 1992.

Field, SJ, & Oates, RK. Sports and recreation activities and opportunities for children with spina bifida and cystic fibrosis. Journal of Science & Medicine in Sport, 4(1):71–76, 2001.

Fields, KB. Clearing athletes for participation in sports: The North Carolina Medical Society Sports Medicine Committee's recommended examination. North Carolina Medical Journal, 55:116–121, 1994.

Finch, GD, & Barnes, MJ. Major cervical spine injuries in children and adolescents. Journal of Pediatric Orthopedics, 18:811–814, 1998.

Fletcher, GF, Lloyd, A, Waling, JF, & Fletcher, B. Exercise testing in patients with musculoskeletal handicaps. Archives of Physical Medicine and Rehabilitation, 69:123–127, 1988.

Food Guide Pyramid. Washington, DC: U.S. Department of Agriculture, 1992.

Forman, ES, Dekker, AH, Javors, JR, & Davison, DT. High-risk behaviors in teenage male athletes. Clinical Journal of Sports Medicine, 5:36–42, 1995.

Fu, FH. Sports Injuries: Mechanisms, Prevention, and Treatment, 2nd ed. Philadelphia: Lippincott Williams & Wilkins, 2001.

Fuller, CM, McNulty, CM, Spring, DA, Arger, KM, Bruce, SS, Chrysson, B, Drummer, EM, Kelley, FP, Newmark, MJ, & Whipple, GH. Prospective screening of 5,615 high school athletes for risk of sudden cardiac death. Medicine & Science in Sports & Exercise, 29:1131–1138, 1997.

Fullerton, HD, Borckardt, JJ, & Alfano, AP: Shoulder Pain: A comparison of wheelchair athletes and nonathletic wheelchair users. Medicine & Science in Sports & Exercise, 35:1958–1957, 2003.

Gaillard, B. Handbook for the Young Athlete. Palo Alto, CA: Bull Publishing, 1978.

Galena, HJ, Epstein, CR, & Lourie, RJ. Connecticut State Special Olympics: Observations and recommendations. Connecticut Medicine, 62:33–37, 1998.

Galloway, SD, & Maughan, RJ. The effects of substrate and fluid provision on thermoregulatory and metabolic responses to prolonged exercise in a hot environment. Journal of Sports Science, 18:339–351, 2000.

Garrick, JG. Epidemiological perspective. Clinics in Sports Medicine, 1:13–18, 1982.

Garrick, JG: Orthopedic preparticipation screening examination. Pediatric Clinics of North America, 37:1047–1056, 1990.

Gassner, R, Tuli, T, Hachl, O, Rudisch, A, & Ulmer, H. Craniomaxillofacial trauma: A 10 year review of 9,543 cases with 21,067 injuries. Journal of Craniomaxillofacial Surgery, 31:51–61, 2003.

Genuardi, FJ, & King, WD. Inappropriate discharge instructions for youth athletes hospitalized for concussion. Pediatrics, 95:216–218, 1995.

Gerbino, PG, 2nd, & Micheli, LJ. Back injuries in the young athlete. Clinics in Sports Medicine, 14:571–590, 1995.

Gerrard, DF. Overuse injury and growing bones: the young athlete at risk. British Journal of Sports Medicine, 27:14–18, 1993.

Gerstenbluth, RE, Spirnak, JP, & Elder, JS. Sports participation and high grade renal injuries in children. Journal of Urology, 168:2575–2578, 2002.

Gill, TJ, 4th, & Micheli, LJ. The immature athlete: Common injuries and overuse syndromes of the elbow and wrist. Clinics in Sports Medicine, 15:401–423, 1996.

Gillon, H. Scaphoid injuries in children. Accident and Emergency Nursing, 9:249–256, 2001.

Glover, DW, & Maron, BJ. Profile of preparticipation cardiovascular screening for high school athletes. Journal of the American Medical Association, 279:1817–1819, 1998.

Going, S. Physical best: Body composition in the assessment of youth fitness. Journal of Physical Education, Recreation, and Dance, 59:32–36, 1998.

Gomez, E, DeLee, JC, & Farney, WC. Incidence of injury in Texas girls' high school basketball. American Journal of Sports Medicine, 24(5):684–687, 1998.

Grafe, MW, Paul, GR, & Foster, TE. The preparticipation sports examination for high school and college athletes. Clinics in Sports Medicine, 16:569–591, 1997.

Grana, WA, & Kalenak, A. Clinical Sports Medicine. Philadelphia: WB Saunders, 1991.

Green, GA. Drugs, athletes, and drug testing. In Sanders, B (Ed.). Sports Physical Therapy. Norwalk, CT: Appleton & Lange, 1990, pp. 95–111.

Green, GA, Uryasz, FD, Petr, TA, & Bray, CD. NCAA study of substance use and abuse habits of college student-athletes. Clinical Journal of Sport Medicine, 11:51–56, 2001.

Gregg, JR, & Das, M. Foot and ankle problems in the preadolescent and adolescent athlete. Clinics in Sports Medicine, 1:131-147, 1982.

Greydanus, DE, & Patel, DR. Sports doping in the adolescent athlete: The hope, hype and hyperbole. Pediatric Clinics of North America, 49:829–855, 2002.

Guy, JA, & Micheli, LJ. Strength training for children and adolescents. Journal of American Academy of Orthopedic Surgery, 9:29–36, 2001.

Guzzanti, V. The natural history and treatment of rupture of the anterior cruciate ligament in children and adolescents. The Journal of Bone and Joint Surgery (British), 85:618–619, 2003.

Gwinn, DE, Wilckens, JH, McDevitt, ER, Ross, G, & Kao, TC. The relative incidence of anterior cruciate ligament injury in men and women at the United States Naval Academy. American Journal of Sports Medicine, 28:98–102, 2000.

Hamilton, PR, & Broughton, NS. Traumatic hip dislocation in childhood. Journal of Pediatric Orthopedics, 18:691–694, 1998.

Hanson, CS, Nabavi, D, & Yuen, HK. The effect of sports on level of community integration as reported by persons with spinal cord injury. American Journal of Occupational Therapy, 55:332–338, 2001.

Harvey, J. The preparticipation examination of the child athlete. Clinics in Sports Medicine, 1:353–369, 2001.

Haupt, HA. Anabolic steroids and growth hormone. American Journal of Sports Medicine, 21:468–474, 1993.

Heath, GW, Pratt, M, Warren, CW, & Kann, L. Physical activity patterns in American high school students. Results from the 1990 Youth Risk Behavior Survey. Archives of Pediatric & Adolescent Medicine, 148:1131–1136, 1994.

Heinonen, OJ. Carnitine and physical exercise. Sports Medicine, 22:109–132, 1996.

Hergenroeder, AC. The preparticipation sports examination. Pediatric Clinics of North America, 44:1525–1540, 1997.

Hewett, TE, Lindenfeld, TN, Riccobene, JV, & Noyes, FR. The effect of neuromuscular training on the incidence of knee injury in female athletes. A prospective study. American Journal of Sports Medicine, 27:699–706, 1999.

Hoeberigs, JH, Deberts-Eggen, HB, & Debets, PM. Sports medical experience from the International Flower Marathon for disabled wheelers. American Journal of Sports Medicine, 18:418–421, 1999.

Hosea, TM, Carey, OC, & Harrer, MF. The gender issue: Epidemiology of ankle injuries in athletes who participate in basketball. Clinical Orthopedics, 372:45–49, 2000.

Hunter, SC, Etchison, WC, & Halpern, B. Standards and norms of fitness and flexibility in the high school athlete. Journal of Athletic Training, Fall:210–212, 1985.

Hutchinson, MR, & Ireland, ML. Overuse and throwing injuries in the skeletally immature athlete. Instructional Course Lectures, 52:25–36, 2003.

Hutzler, Y, Ochana, S, Bolotin, R, & Kalina, A. Aerobic and non-aerobic arm-cranking outputs of males with lower limb impairments: Relationship with sport participation intensity, age, impairment with functional classification. Spinal Cord, 36:205–212, 1998.

Iobst, CA, & Stanitski, CL. Acute knee injuries. Clinics in Sports Medicine, 19:621–635, 2000.

Iuliano, S, Naughton, G, Collier, G, & Carlson, J. Examination for the self-selected fluid intake practices by junior athletes during a simulated diathlon event. International Journal of Sport Nutrition, 8:10–23, 1998.

Iven, VG. Recreational drugs. Clinics in Sports Medicine, 17:245–259, 1998.

Jackson, RW, & Davis, GM. The value of sports and recreation for the physically disabled. Orthopedic Clinics of North America, 14:301–315, 1983.

Kay, RM, & Matthys, GA. Pediatric ankle fractures: Evaluation and treatment. Journal of American Academy of Orthopedic Surgery, 9:268–278, 2001.

Kegel, B, & Webster, JC, & Burgess, E. Recreational activities of lower extremity amputees. Archives of Physical Medicine and Rehabilitation, 61:258–264, 1980.

Keller, CS, Noyes, FR, & Buncher, CR. The medical aspects of soccer injury epidemiology. American Journal of Sports Medicine, 15:230–236, 1987.

Kelly, JP, Nichols, JS, Filley, CM, Lilleheik, KO, Rubinstein, D, & Kleinschmidt-DeMasters, BK. Concussion in sports: Guidelines for the prevention of catastrophic outcome. Journal of the American Medical Association, 266:2867–2869, 1991.

Kerr, IL. Mouth guards for the prevention of injuries in contact sports. Sports Medicine, 5:415–427, 1986.

Klish, WJ. Childhood obesity: Pathophysiology and treatment. Acta Pediatrica Japan, 37:1–6, 1995.

Knowles, KG, Yakavonis, VJ, & George, F. Overuse syndromes about the elbow. Postgraduate Advances in Sports Medicine, 2:3–17, 1987.

Kocher, MS, Waters, PM, & Micheli, LJ. Upper extremity injuries in the paediatric athlete. Sports Medicine, 30:117–135, 2000.

Kocher, MS, Micheli, LJ, Zurakowski, D, & Luke, A. Partial tears of the anterior cruciate ligament in children and adolescents. American Journal of Sports Medicine, 30:697–703, 2002.

Kouyoumjian, A, & Barber, FA. Management of anterior cruciate ligament disruptions in skeletally immature patients. American Journal of Orthopedics, 30:771–774, 2001.

Kraemer, WJ, & Fleck, S. Strength Training for Young Athletes. Champaign, IL: Human Kinetics, 1993.

Kraemer, WJ, Voleck, JS, French, DN, Rubin, MR, Sharman, MJ, Gomez, A, Ratamess, NA, Newton, R, Jemiolo, B, Craig, BW, & Hakkinen, K. The effects of L-Carnitine tartrate supplementation on hormonal responses to resistance exercise and recovery. Journal of Strength and Conditioning Research, 17:455–462, 2003.

Kraft, DE. Low back pain in the adolescent athlete. Pediatric Clinics of North America, 49:643–653, 2002.

Kreider, RB, Ferriera, M, Wilson, M, Grindstaff, P, Plisk, S, Reinardy, J, Cantler, E, & Almada, AL. Effects of creatine supplementation on body composition, strength, and sprint performance. Medicine & Science in Sports & Exercise, 30:73–82, 1998.

Kreider, RB, Miriel, V, & Bertun, E. Amino acid supplementation and exercise performance: Analylsis of the proposed ergogenic value. Sports Medicine, 16:190–209, 1993.

Kubiak, R, & Slongo, T. Unpowered scooter injuries in children. Acta Paediatrica, 92:50–54, 2003.

Kujala, UM, Taimela, S, Antti-Poika, I, Orava, S, Tuominen, R, & Myllynen, P. Acute injuries in soccer, ice hockey, volleyball, basketball, judo and karate: Analysis of national registry data. British Medical Journal, 311:1465–1468, 1995.

Kurowski, K, & Chandran, S. The preparticipation athletic evaluation. American Family Physician, 61:2696–2698, 2000.

Kyle, SB. Youth baseball protective equipment project: Final report. Washington, DC: US Consumer Product Safety Commission, 1996.

Kyle, SB, Nance, ML, Rutherford, GW, Jr, & Winston, FK. Skateboard-associated injuries: Participation-based estimates and injury characteristics. Journal of Trauma, 53:686–690, 2002.

Lai, AM, Stanish, WD, & Stanish, HI. The young athlete with physical challenges. Clinics in Sports Medicine, 19:793–819, 2000.

Larsen, GE, George, JD, Alexander, JL, Fellington, GW, Aldana, SG, & Parcell, AC. Prediction of maximum oxygen consumption from walking, jogging, or running. Research Quarterly in Exercise & Sport, 71:66–72, 2002.

Laseter, JT, & Russell, JA: Anabolic steroid-induced tendon pathology: A review of the literature. Medicine & Science in Sports & Exercise, 23:1–3, 1991.

Laure, P. Epidemiologic approach of doping in sport: a review. Journal of Sports Medicine and Physical Fitness, 37:218–224, 1997.

Leger, LA, Mercier, D, Gadoury, C, & Lambert, J. The multistage 20 meter shuttle run for aerobic fitness. Journal of Sports Science, 6:93–101, 1988.

Lenaway, DD, Ambler, AG, & Beaudoin, DE. The epidemiology of school-related injuries: New perspectives. American Journal of Preventive Medicine, 8:193–198, 1992.

Letts, M, Davidson, D, & McCaffrey, M. The adolescent pilon fracture: Management and outcome. Journal of Pediatric Orthopedics, 21:20–26, 2001.

Levy, AS, Wetzler, MJ, Lewars, M, & Laughlin, W. Knee injuries in women collegiate rugby players. American Journal of Sports Medicine, 25:360–362, 1997.

Libetta, C, Burke, D, Brennan, P, & Yassa, J. Validation of the Ottawa ankle rules in children. Journal of Accidental and Emergency Medicine, 16:342–344, 1999.

Linder, CW, DuRant, RH, Seklecki, RM, & Strong, WB. Preparticipation health screening of young athletes. American Journal of Sports Medicine, 9:187–193, 1981.

Lintunen, T, Heikinaro-Johansson, P, & Sherrill, C. Use of Perceptual Physical Competence Scale with adolescents with disabilities. Perceptual Motor Skills, 80:571–577, 1995.

Lodge, JF, Langley, JD, & Begg, DJ. Injuries in the 14th and 15th years of life. Journal of Paediatrics and Child Health, 26:316–322, 1990.

Lohman, TG. Advances in Body Composition Assessment. Champaign, IL: Human Kinetics Publishers, 1992.

Lombardo, JA. Preparticipation examination. In Cantu, RC, & Micheli, LJ (Eds.). ACSM's Guidelines for the Team Physician. Philadelphia: Lea & Febiger, 1991, pp. 71–94.

Louden, JK, Jenkins, W, & Louden, KL. The relationship between static posture and ACL injury in female athletes. Journal of Orthopedic & Sports Physical Therapy, 24:91–97, 1996.

Lyznicki, JM, Nielsen, NH, & Schneider, JF. Cardiovascular screening of student athletes. American Family Physician, 62:765–774, 2000.

Macera, CA, Jackson, KL, Hagenmaier, GW, Kronenfeld, JJ, Kohl, HW, & Blair, SN. Age, physical activity, physical fitness, body composition, and incidence of orthopedic problems. Research Quarterly in Exercise & Sport, 60:225–233, 1989.

Maestrello-deMoya, MG, & Primosch, RE. Orofacial trauma and mouth-protector wear among high school varsity basketball players. ASDC Journal of Dentistry in Children, 56:36–39, 1989.

Maffulli, N. Intensive training in young athletes. Sports Medicine, 9:229–243, 1990.

Maffulli, N, & Bruns, W. Injuries in young athletes. European Journal of Pediatrics, 159:59–63, 2000.

Mankovsky, AB, Mendoza-Sagaon, M, Cardinaux, C, Hohlfeld, J, & Reinberg, O. Evaluation of scooter-related injuries in children. Journal of Pediatric Surgery, 37:755–759, 2002.

Maron, BJ. The young competitive athlete with cardiovascular abnormalities: Causes of sudden death, detection by preparticipation screening, and standards for disqualification. Cardiology and Electrophysiological Review, 6:100–103, 2002.

Marsh, JS, & Daigneault, JP. Ankle injuries in the pediatric population. Current Opinions in Pediatrics, 12:52–60, 2000.

Martin, TJ. Technical report: Knee brace use in the young athlete. Pediatrics, 108:503–507, 2001.

Maughan, R. The athlete's diet: Nutritional goals and dietary strategies. Proceedings of the Nutrition Society, 61:87–96, 2002.

McArdle, WD, Katch, FI, & Katch, VL. Exercise Physiology: Energy, Nutrition, and Human Performance. Philadelphia: Lippincott, Williams & Wilkins, 2001.

McCormick, D. Handicapped skiing. In Bernhardt, DB (Ed.). Recreation for the Disabled Child. New York: Haworth Press, 1985, pp. 27–44.

McCormick, DP, Niebiehr, VN, & Risser, WL. Injury and illness surveillance at local Special Olympic Games. British Journal of Sports Medicine, 24:221–224, 1990.

McKeag, D. Preseason physical examination for prevention of sports injuries. Sports Medicine, 2:413–431, 1985.

McLain, LG, & Reynolds, S. Sports injuries in a high school. Pediatrics, 84:446–450, 1989.

McManama, GB. Ankle injuries in the young athlete. Clinics in Sports Medicine, 7:547–562, 1988.

McNutt, T, Shannon, SW, Wright, JT, & Feinstein, RA. Oral trauma in adolescent athletes: A study of mouth protectors. Pediatric Dentistry, 11:209–213, 1989.

McTimoney, CA, & Micheli, LJ. Current evaluation and management of spondylolysis and spondylolisthesis. Current Sports Medicine Reports, 2:41–46, 2003.

Messina, DF, Farney, WC, & DeLee, JC. The incidence of injury in Texas high school basketball. A prospective study among male and female athletes. American Journal of Sports Medicine, 27:294–299, 2003.

Metzl, JD. Strength training and nutritional supplement use in adolescents. Current Opinions in Pediatrics, 11:292–296, 1999.

Metzl, JD. Sports-specific concerns in the young athlete: football. Pediatric Emergency Care, 15:363–367, 1999.

Micheli, L. Musculoskeletal trauma in children. In Green, M, & Haggerty, RJ (Eds.). Ambulatory Pediatrics III. Philadelphia: WB Saunders, 1984, pp. 95–208.

Micheli, LJ. The child athlete. In Cantu, RC, & Micheli, LJ (Eds.). ACSM's Guidelines for the Team Physician. Philadelphia: Lea & Febiger, 1991, pp. 228–241.

Micheli, LJ, Santore, R, & Stanitski, CL. Epiphyseal fractures of the elbow in children. American Family Physician, November:107–116, 1980.

Micheli, LJ, & Smith, AD. Sports injuries in children. Current Problems in Pediatrics, 12:1–54, 1982.

Micheli, LJ. Sports injuries in children and adolescents. Questions and controversies. Clinics in Sports Medicine, 14:727–745, 1995.

Micheli, LJ, & Fehlandt, AF, Jr. Overuse injuries to tendons and apophyses in children and adolescents. Clinics in Sports Medicine, 11:713–726, 1992.

Micheli, LJ, & Wood, R. Back pain in young athletes. Significant differences from adults in causes and patterns. Archives of Pediatric and Adolescent Medicine, 149:15–18, 1995.

Millar, AL. Ergogenic aids. In Sanders B. (Ed.). Sports Physical Therapy. Norwalk, CT: Appleton & Lange, 1990, pp. 79–93.

Mintzer, CM, Richmond, JC, & Taylor, J. Meniscal repair in the young athlete. American Journal of Sports Medicine, 26:630–633, 1998.

Mitchell, LJ, & Jenkins, M. Sports Medicine Bible for Young Athletes. Naperville, IL: Sourcebooks, Inc, 2001.

Moeller, JL. Pelvic and hip apophyseal avulsion injuries in young athletes. Current Sports Medicine Reports, 2:110–115, 2003.

Moti, AW, & Micheli, LJ. Meniscal and articular cartilage injury in the skeletally immature knee. Instructional Course Lectures, 52:683–690, 2003.

Mueller, FD, & Cantu, RC. Catastrophic injuries and fatalities in high school and college sports, Fall 1982–Spring 1988. Medicine & Science in Sports & Exercise, 22:737–741, 1990.

Nadler, SF, Malanga, GA, Feinberg, JH, Rubanni, M, Moley, R, & Foye, P. Functional performance deficits in athletes with previous lower extremity injury. Clinical Journal of Sports Medicine, 12:73–78, 2002.

Napier, SM, Baker, RS, & Sanford, DG. Eye injuries in athletics and recreation. Survey Ophthalmologia, 41:229–244, 1996.

National Federation of State High School Associations. Sport health: Heat stress and athletic participation. March 1, 2005. http://www.nfhs.org/ScriptContent/VA_Custom/vimdisplays/conentpagedisplay.cfm?conent_ID=211&SearchWord=heat%20stress. Accessed September 26, 2005.

National Institutes of Health: Update on the Task Force report on high blood pressure in children and adolescents. National Institutes of Health Publication 96-3790, 1996.

Naylor, AH, Gardner, D, & Zaichkowsky, L. Drug use patterns among high school athletes and nonathletes. Adolescence, 36(144):627–639, 1996.

Nevaiser, RJ. Injuries to and developmental deformities of the shoulder. In Bora FW (Ed.). The Pediatric Upper Extremity. Philadelphia: WB Saunders, 1986, pp. 235–246.

Nevole, GJ, & Prentice, WJ. The effect of anabolic steroids on female athletes. Athletic Trainer 22:297–299, 1987.

Nguyen, D, & Letts, M. In-line skating injuries in children: A ten year review. Journal of Pediatric Orthopedics, 21:613–618, 2001.

Noguchi, T. A survey of spinal cord injuries resulting from sport. Paraplegia, 32:170–173, 2001.

Noyes, FR, & Barber-Westin, SD. Arthroscopic repair of meniscal tears extending into the avascular zone in patients younger than twenty years of age. American Journal of Sports Medicine, 30:589–600, 2002.

Nsuami, M, Elie, M, Brooks, BN, Sanders, LS, Nash, TD, Makonnen, F, Taylor, SN, & Cohen, DA. Screening for sexually transmitted diseases during preparticipation sports examination of high school adolescents. Journal of Adolescent Health, 32:336–339, 2003.

Objective testing group certifies head protection. Occupational Health and Safety, March 1988, pp. 18–20.

Ogden, JA. Skeletal Injury in the Child. New York: Springer-Verlag, 2000.

O'Neill, DB, & Micheli, LJ. Overuse injuries in the young athlete. Clinics in Sports Medicine, 7:591–610, 1988.

Osberg, JS, Schneps, SE, DiScala, C, & Li, G. Skateboarding: More dangerous than roller skating or in-line skating. Archives of Pediatrics and Adolescent Medicine, 52:985–991, 1998.

Outerbridge, AR, & Micheli, LJ. Overuse injuries in young athletes. Clinics in Sports Medicine, 14:503–516, 1995.

Paletta, GA, Jr, & Andrish, JT. Injuries about the hip and pelvis in the young athlete. Clinics in Sports Medicine, 14:591–628, 1995.

Pare, F, Noreau, L, & Simard, C. Prediction of maximal aerobic power from a submaximal exercise test performed by paraplegics on a wheelchair ergometer. Paraplegia, 31:584–592, 1995.

Passe, DH, Horn, M, & Murray, R. Impact of beverage acceptability on fluid intake during exercise. Appetite, 35(3):219–229, 1995.

Patel, DR, & Greydanus, DE. The pediatric athlete with disabilities. Pediatric Clinics of North America, 49:803–827, 2002.

Patel, DR, & Nelson, TL. Sports injuries in adolescents. Medical Clinics of North America, 84:983–1007, 2000.

Paterson, PD, & Waters, PM. Shoulder injuries in the childhood athlete. Clinics in Sports Medicine, 19:681–692, 2000.

Patrick, GD. Comparison of novice and veteran wheelchair athletes' self-concept and acceptance of disability. Rehabilitation Counseling Bulletin, 27:186–188, 1984.

Paulsen, P, French, R, & Sherrill, C. Comparison of mood states of college able-bodied and wheelchair basketball players. Perceptual Motor Skills, 73:396–398, 1991.

Peljovich, AE, & Simmons, BP. Traumatic arthritis of the hand and wrist in children. Hand Clinics, 16:673–684, 2000.

Peltz, JE, Haskell, WL, & Matheson, GO. A comprehensive and cost-effective preparticipation exam implemented on the World Wide Web. Medicine & Science in Sports & Exercise, 31(12):1727–1740, 1999.

Peretti-Watel, P, Guagliardo, V, Verger, P, Pruvost, J, Mignon, P, & Obadia, Y. Sporting activity and drug use: Alcohol, cigarette and cannabis use among elite student athletes. Addiction, 98:1249–1256, 1995.

Perkins, SW, Dayan SH, Sklarew, ED, Hamilton, M, & Bussell, GS. The incidence of sports-related facial trauma in children. Ear Nose Throat Journal, 79:632–638, 2000.

Perriello, VA, Jr, Almquist, J, Conkwright, D, Jr, Cutter, D, Gregory, D, Pitrezzi, MJ, Roemmich, J, & Snyders, J. Health and weight control management among wrestlers. A proposed program for high school athletes. Virginia Medical Quarterly, 122:179–183, 1995.

Peterson, M, & Peterson, K. Eat to Compete: A Guide to Sports Nutrition. Chicago: Year Book Medical, 1988.

Pitetti, KH, Rimmer, JH, & Fernhall, B. Physical fitness and adults with mental retardation: An overview of current research and future directions. Sports Medicine, 16:23–56, 1993.

Pope, RP, Herbert, RD, Kirwan, JD, & Graham, BJ. A randomized trial of pre-exercise stretching for prevention of lower-limb injury. Medicine & Science in Sports & Exercise, 32:271–277, 2000.

Powell, C. Protecting children in the accident and emergency department. Accidents and Emergency Nursing, 5:76–80, 1997.

Powell EC, & Tanz RR. In-line skate and roller skate injuries in children. Pediatric and Emergency Care, 12:259–262, 2000.

Powell, EC, Tanz, RR, & DiScala, C. Bicycle-related injuries among preschool children. Annuals of Emergency Medicine, 30:260–265, 2000.

Powell, EC, & Tanz, RR. Tykes and bikes: injuries associated with bicycle-towed child trailers and bicycle-mounted child seats. Archives of Pediatric & Adolescent Medicine, 154:351–353, 2000.

Powell, EC, & Tanz, RR. Cycling injuries treated in emergency departments: Need for bicycle helmets among preschoolers. Archives of Pediatric & Adolescent Medicine, 154:1096–1100, 2000.

Powell, J. 636,000 injuries annually in high school football. Athletic Trainer, 22:19–22, 1987.

Pratt, M, Macera, CA, & Blanton, C. Levels of physical activity and inactivity in children and adults in the United States: Current evidence and research issues. Medicine & Science in Sports & Exercise, 31:S526–S533, 1999.

Pueschel, SM. Should children with Down syndrome be screened for atlantoaxial instability? Archives of Pediatric & Adolescent Medicine, 152:123–125, pp. 95–100.

Puffer, JC: Organizational aspects. In Cantu, RC, & Micheli, LJ (Eds.). ACSM's Guidelines for the Team Physician. Philadelphia: Lea & Febiger, 1991, pp. 95–100.

Queen, RM, Weinhold, PS, Kirkendall, DT, & Yu, B. Theoretical study of the effect of ball properties on impact force in soccer heading. Medicine & Science in Sports & Exercise, 35(12):2069–2076, 2003.

Quinn, K, Parker, P, de Bie, R, Rowe, B, & Handoll, H. Interventions for preventing ankle ligament injuries. Cochrane Database Systems Review, 2:CD000018, 1990.

Radelet, MA, Lephart, SM, Rubinstein, EN, & Myers, J. Survey of the injury rate for children in community sports. Pediatrics, 110:e28, 1990.

Ramsey, JA, Blunkie, C, & Smith, K. Strength training effects in pre-pubescent boys. Medicine & Science in Sports & Exercise, 22:605–614, 1990.

Regan, KJ, Banks, GK, & Beran, RG. Therapeutic recreation programmes for children with epilepsy. Seizure, 2:195–200, 1995.

Retsky, J, Jaffe, D, & Christoffel, K. Skateboarding injuries in children: A second wave. American Journal of Diseases in Children, 145:188–192, 1995.

Rifat, SF, Ruffin, MT, 4th, & Gorenflo, DW. Disqualifying criteria in a preparticipation sports evaluation. Journal of Family Practice, 41:42–50, 1995.

Rimmer, JH. Physical fitness levels of persons with cerebral palsy. Developmental Medicine and Child Neurology, 43(3):208–212, 2001.

Rivera-Brown, AM, Gutierrez, R, Gutierrez, JC, Frontera, WR, & Bar-Or, O. Drink composition, voluntary drinking, and fluid balance in exercising, training, heat-acclimatized boys. Journal of Applied Physiology, 86:78–84, 1997.

Rooks, DS, & Micheli, LJ. Musculoskeletal assessment and training: The young athlete. Clinics in Sports Medicine, 7:641–677, 1990.

Rossi, F, & Dragoni, S. Lumbar spondylolisthesis: Occurrence in competitive athletes. Journal of Sports Medicine and Physical Fitness, 30:450–452, 1990.

Sachtelben, TR, Berg, KE, Elias, BA, Cheatham, JP, Felix, GL, & Hofschire, PJ. The effects of anabolic steroids on myocardial structure and cardiovascular fitness. Medicine & Science in Sports & Exercise, 25:1240–1245, 1993.

Sanders, B (Ed.). Sports Physical Therapy. Norwalk, CT: Appleton & Lange, 1990.

Santopietro, FJ. Foot and foot-related injuries in the young athlete. Clinics in Sports Medicine, 7:563–589, 1993.

Schmitt, H, & Gerner, HJ. Paralysis from sport and diving accidents. Clinical Journal of Sports Medicine, 11:17–22, 1993.

Schuller, DE, Dankle, SK, Martin, M, & Strauss, RH. Auricular injury and the use of headgear in wrestlers. Archives of Otolaryngological Head Neck Surgery, 115:714–717, 1993.

Segesser, B, & Pforringer, W (Eds.). The Shoe in Sport. Chicago: Year Book Medical, 1989.

Selsby, JT, Beckett KD, Kern, M, & Devor, S. Swim performance following creatine supplementation in division III athletes. Journal of Strength & Conditioning, 17(3):421–424, 2003.

Servedio, FJ, Bartels, RL, Hamlin, D, Teske, T, Schaffer, T, & Servedio, A. The effect of weight training using Olympic style lifts on various physiological variables in prepubescent boys. Medicine & Science in Sports & Exercise, 17:228, 1985.

Sewall, L, & Micheli, LJ. Strength training for children. Journal of Pediatric Orthopedics, 6:143–146, 2003.

Sharkey, B. Training for sports. In Cantu, RC, & Micheli, LJ (Eds.). ACSM's Guidelines for the Team Physician. Philadelphia: Lea & Febiger, 1991, pp. 34–47.

Sherrill, C, Hinson, M, Gench, B, Kennedy, SO, & Low, L. Self-concepts of disabled youth athletes. Perceptual Motor Skills, 70:1093–1098, 1990.

Shi, X, Summers, RW, Schedl, HP, Flanagan, SW, Chang, R, & Gisolfi, CV. Effects of carbohydrate type and concentration and solution osmolarity on water absorption. Medicine & Science in Sports & Exercise, 27:1607–1615, 1995.

Shorter, NA, Mooney, DP, & Harmon, BJ. Snowboarding injuries in children and adolescents. American Journal of Emergency Medicine, 17:261–263, 1999.

Skokan, EG, Junkins, EP, Jr, & Kadish, H: Serious winter sports injuries in children and adolescents requiring hospitalization. American Journal of Emergency Medicine, 21:95–99, 2003.

Smith, AD. The skeletally immature knee: What's new in overuse injuries. Instructional Course Lectures, 52:691–697, 2003.

Smith, GA, & Shields, BJ. Trampoline-related injuries to children. Archives of Pediatric & Adolescent Medicine, 152:694–699, 1998.

Smith, J, & Laskowski, ER. The preparticipation physical examination: Mayo Clinic experience with 2,739 examinations. Mayo Clinic Proceedings, 73:419–429, 1998.

Smith, J, & Wilder, EP. Musculoskeletal rehabilitation and sports medicine. Archives of Physical Medicine and Rehabilitation, 80:S68–S89, 1999.

Soderman K, Pietila T, Alfredson H, & Werner, S. Anterior cruciate ligament injuries in young females playing soccer at senior levels. Scandinavian Journal of Medicine and Science in Sports, 12:65–68, 2002.

Sorenson, L, Larsen, SE, & Rock, ND. The epidemiology of sports injuries in school-aged children. Scandinavian Journal of Medicine and Science in Sports, 6:281–286, 1996.

Sosin, DM, Sacks, JJ, & Webb, KW. Pediatric head injuries and deaths from bicycling in the United States. Pediatrics, 98(5):868–870, 1996.

Special Olympics inquiry data., Washington, D.C: World Winter Games, 2001.

Squire, DL. Heat illness. Fluid and electrolyte issues for pediatric and adolescent athletes. Pediatric Clinics of North America, 37:1085–1109, 1990.

Stanitski, C: Common injuries in preadolescent athletes. Sports Medicine, 7:32–41, 1989.

Stanitski, CL. Pediatric and adolescent sports injuries. Clinics in Sports Medicine, 16:613–633, 1997.

Stanitski, CL, Delee, JC, & Drez, D. Pediatric and Adolescent Sports Medicine. Philadelphia: WB Saunders, 1994.

Steiner, ME, & Grana, WA. The young athlete's knee: Recent advances. Clinics in Sports Medicine, 7:527–546, 1988.

Stock, JG, & Cornell, FM. Prevention of sports-related eye injury. American Family Practice, 44:515–520, 1991.

Strahlman, E, Elman, M, Daub, E, & Baker, S. Causes of pediatric eye injuries. A population-based study. Archives of Ophthalmology, 108:603–606, 1990.

Stronski, SM, Ireland, M, Michaud, P, Narring, F, & Resnick, MD. Protective correlates of stages in adolescent substance use: A Swiss National Study. Journal of Adolescent Health, 26(6):420–427, 2000.

Surgeon General: Call to action to prevent and decrease overweight and obesity. Washington, DC, 2001. http://www.surgerongeneral.gov/topics/obesity. Accessed September 26, 2005.

Taimela, S, Kujala, UM, & Osterman, K. Intrinsic risk factors and athletic injuries. Sports Medicine, 9:205–215, 1990.

Taylor, BL, & Attia, MW. Sports-related injuries in children. Academy of Emergency Medicine, 7:1376–1382, 2000.

Taylor, D, & Williams, T. Sports injuries in athletes with disabilities: Wheelchair racing. Paraplegia, 33:296–269, 1995.

Tepper, KB, & Ireland, ML. Fracture patterns and treatment in the skeletally immature knee. Instructional Course Lectures, 52:667–676, 2003.

Thomas, NE, Baker, JS, & Davies, B. Established and recently identified coronary heart disease risk factors in young people: The influence of physical activity and physical fitness. Sports Medicine, 33:633–650, 2003.

Thomee, R, Renstrom, P, Karlsson, J, & Grimby, G. Patellofemoral pain syndrome in young women: A clinical analysis of alignment, pain parameters, common symptoms, and functional activity level. Scandinavian Journal of Medicine & Science in Sports, 5:237–244, 1995.

Thurman, DJ, Branche, CM, & Sniezek, JE. The epidemiology of sports-related traumatic brain injuries in the United States: recent developments. Journal of Head Trauma Rehabilitation, 13:1–8, 1998.

Tol, JL, Struijs, PA, Bossuyt, PM, Verhagen, RA, & van Dijk, CN. Treatment strategies in osteochondral defects of the talar dome: A systematic review. Foot Ankle International, 21:119–126, 2000.

Trepman, E, & Micheli LJ. Overuse injuries in sports. Seminars in Orthopedics, 3:217–222, 1998.

USDA/ARS Children's Nutrition Research Center at Baylor College of Medicine. Available at http://www.bcm.tmc.edu/cnrc/consumer/archives/percentDV.htm. Accessed September 26, 2005.

Utter, A, Kang, J, Nieman, D, & Warren, B. Effect of carbohydrate substrate availability on ratings of perceived exertion during prolonged running. International Journal of Sport Nutrition, 7:274–285, 1997.

Van Hall, G, Raaymakers, JSH, Saris, WHM, & Wagenmakers, AJM. Ingestion of branched-chain amino acids and tryptophan during sustained exercise in man: Failure to affect performance. Journal of Physiology, 486:789–794, 1995.

Van Mechelen, W: Running injuries: A review of the epidemiological literature. Sports Medicine, 14:320–335, 1992.

Varni, JW, & Setoguchi, Y: Correlates of perceived physical appearance in children with congenital/acquired limb deficiencies. Journal of Developmental and Behavioral Pediatrics, 12:171–176, 1991.

Veeger, HE, Hadj Yahmed, M, van der Woude, LH, & Charpentier, P. Peak oxygen uptake and maximal power output of Olympic wheelchair-dependent athletes. Medicine & Science in Sports & Exercise, 23:1201–1209, 1991.

Voight, M, & Draovitch, P. Plyometrics. In Albert, M (Ed.). Eccentric Muscle Training in Sports and Orthopaedics. New York: Churchill Livingstone, 1991, pp. 45–73.

Wagner, JC. Enhancement of athletic performance with drugs. An overview. Sports Medicine, *12*:250–265, 1991.

Waicus, KM, & Smith, BW. Back injuries in the pediatric athlete. Current Sports Medicine Reports, *1*:52–58, 2002.

Waters, PM, & Millis, MB. Hip and pelvic injuries in the young athlete. Clinics in Sports Medicine, *7*:513–526, 1988.

Watkins, J, & Peabody, P. Sports injuries in children and adolescents treated at a sports injury clinic. Journal of Sports Medicine and Physical Fitness, *36*:43–48, 1996.

Webster, JB, Levy, CE, Bryant, PR, & Prusakowski, PE. Sports and recreation for persons with limb deficiency. Archives of Physical Medicine and Rehabilitation, *82*(3):S38–S44, 2001.

Weiner, HR. Brain injuries in sports: guidelines for managing concussions. Comprehensive Therapy, *27*:330–332, 2001.

Whieldon, TJ, & Cerny, FJ. Incidence and severity of high school athletic injuries. Athletic Trainer, *25*:344–350, 1990.

Wiemann, K, & Hahn, K. Influences of strength, stretching, and circulatory exercise on flexibility parameters of the human hamstrings. International Journal of Sports Medicine, *18*:340–346, 1997.

Wiens, L, Sabath, R, Ewing, L, Gowdamarajan, R, Portnoy, J, & Scagliotti, D. Chest pain in otherwise healthy children and adolescents is frequently caused by exercise-induced asthma. Pediatrics, *90*:350–353, 1992.

Wilk, B, & Bar-Or, O. Effect of drink flavor and NaCl on voluntary drinking and hydration in boys exercising in the heat. Journal of Applied Physiology, *80*:1112–1117, 1996.

Williams, JS, Jr, Abate, JA, Fadale, PD, & Tung, GA. Meniscal and nonosseous ACL injuries in children and adolescents. American Journal of Knee Surgery, *9*:22–26, 1996.

Williams, MH. The use of ergogenic aids in sports: Is it an ethical issue? International Journal of Sports Nutrition, *4*:120–131, 1994.

Wilson PE, & Washington RL: Pediatric wheelchair athletics: Sports injuries and prevention. Paraplegia *31*:330–337, 1993.

Wilson, PE. Exercise and sports for children who have disabilities. Physical Medicine and Rehabilitation Clinics of North America, *13*:907–923, 2002.

Winston, FK, Weiss, HB, Nance, ML, Vivarelli, O, Neill, C, Strotmeyer, S, Lawrence, BA, & Miller, TR. Estimates of the incidence and costs associated with handlebar-related injuries in children. Archives of Pediatric & Adolescent Medicine, *156*:922–928, 2002.

Witvrouw, E, Lysens, R, Bellemans, J, Cambier, D, Cools, A, Danneels, I, & Bourgois, J. Which factors predict outcome in the treatment program of anterior knee pain? Scandinavian Journal of Medicine & Science in Sports, *12*:40–46, 2002.

Yesalis, CE, Wright, JE, & Bahrke, MS. Epidemiological and policy issues in the measurement of long term health effects and anabolic-androgenic steroids. Sports Medicine, *8*:129–138, 1989.

Yesalis, CE, & Bahrke, MS. Doping among adolescent athletes. Baillieres Best Practices Research in Clinical Endocrinology Metabolism, *14*:25–35, 2000.

Zoints, LE. Fractures around the knee in children. Journal of American Academy of Orthopedic Surgery, *10*:345–355, 2002.

Zwiren, L, & Bar-Or, O. Response to exercise of paraplegics who differ in conditioning level. Medicine and Science in Sports, *7*:94–98, 1975.

MANAGEMENT OF NEUROLOGIC IMPAIRMENT

Section Editor
Darl W. Vander Linden
PT, PhD

Chapter 19

❧

DEVELOPMENTAL COORDINATION DISORDERS

KATHRYN STEYER DAVID
PT, MS, PCS

Why are some children considered to be born athletes or graceful dancers? Why do other children always seem to be falling over their feet or bumping into walls?

Forgetting which way to stand when preparing to hit a baseball and how to hold your hands on the bat can result in the appearance of clumsiness. When is clumsiness considered a normal part of growing up and when is it atypical? Is clumsiness simply a delay in normal maturation or does it result from some central nervous system insult? What can physical therapists do to help children with a developmental coordination disorder (DCD)?

Physical therapists have a unique service to offer individuals with DCD. Their background in normal as well as abnormal motor control, motor learning, and motor development can be used to individually assess, plan programs for, treat, and educate children with DCD as well as consult with their families. As members of a collaborative team, physical therapists can improve motor performance and therefore increase participation in home, school, and community life for a group of individuals with very real problems that are often overlooked by members of the medical and educational community.

This chapter describes the process of differential examination that will allow a physical therapist to make evaluation and diagnostic decisions regarding goals, outcomes, and interventions for a child or adolescent with DCD. Evidence is presented to support the need for a multidisciplinary, environmentally referenced, age-appropriate examination followed by an emphasis on selective intervention for collaborative family and school consultation and training at key points during a child's developmental years. A case study will illustrate the decision-making process for a child with DCD from the age of 19 months through high school. The amount of information available on DCD has increased greatly over the past several years. Recommended resources on DCD are listed at the end of the chapter and in the Appendix (p. 589).

559

DEFINITIONS AND INCIDENCE

Developmental coordination disorder is described in the fourth revised edition of the *Diagnostic and Statistical Manual of Mental Disorders* (DSM-IV) (American Psychiatric Association, 1994) as motor coordination markedly below expected levels for the child's chronologic age and intelligence, which significantly interferes with academic achievement or activities of daily living, is not due to a general medical condition, does not meet criteria for a pervasive developmental disorder, and if mental retardation is present, the motor difficulties are in excess of those usually associated with mental retardation. DCD would be included under the *Guide to Physical Therapist Practice* (American Physical Therapy Association, 2001) diagnostic group 5C, Impaired Motor Function and Sensory Integrity Associated With Congenital or Acquired Disorders of the Central Nervous System—Congenital Origin or Acquired in Infancy or Childhood (pp. 347–364). In this chapter, DCD is meant to be closely synonymous with the terms *developmental clumsiness*, *clumsy child*, and *developmental apraxia* (Gubbay, 1975). *Incoordination* has also been associated with a variety of other terms such as *visuomotor problems*, *dyspraxia*, and *somatodyspraxia* (Missiuna & Polatajko, 1994).

By definition, motor incoordination caused by or closely associated with mental retardation, genetic disorders (e.g., Down syndrome), neurologic disorders (e.g., cerebral palsy, traumatic brain damage, Friedreich's ataxia), brain tumors, or loss of sensory function (e.g., visual, auditory) is not discussed in this chapter. One should always consider the possibility, however, that DCD can occur along with any of these other diagnoses. Some children with DCD also are identified as having attention-deficit/hyperactivity disorder (ADHD) (Blondis, 1999). Gillberg (1998) identified the comorbid conditions of DCD and ADHD as deficits in attention, motor control, and perception (DAMP). Kadesjo (1998) found that the rate of ADHD, DCD, and DAMP in a group of Swedish children was 6.1% with an overlap between ADHD and DCD. Others have found evidence for a link between DCD and low birth weight children at age 9 (Holsti et al., 2002; Jongmans et al., 1993). Miller and colleagues (2001) found that within a group of 556 children with potential DCD, 38% had a learning disorder and 41% had a diagnosis of ADD or ADHD. After reviewing the literature, Cermak & Larkin (2002) concluded that there is a significant comorbidity among learning disability (LD), ADHD, and DCD.

It has long been recognized that children with cerebral palsy often exhibit agnosic and apraxic defects that compound the problem of integration of movement (Gubbay, 1975). Deciding when motor incoordination is caused by or closely associated with another disorder such as cerebral palsy rather than occurring along with, but not caused by, that disorder is an important clinical decision. The specific combination of DCD, learning disability, prematurity, and spastic diplegia is further explored in this chapter because it is a combination of which physical therapists need to be especially aware.

Gubbay (1975) proposed that at least 5% of the school-aged population displayed clumsiness or DCD. The DSM-IV estimates that as high as 6% of children between 5 and 11 years of age have DCD. Other estimates project that 5% to 10% of the school-aged population display minimal brain dysfunction (MBD) with soft neurologic signs (Gaddes, 1985; Gillberg et al., 1982) and that 98% of children with MBD have motor problems, as evidenced by poor, slow, labored handwriting (Clements et al., 1971). Reports have indicated that children with educationally identified learning disability compose 4.5% of the school-aged population (U.S. Department of Education, 2001), and it is estimated that 90% of children with learning disability have motor coordination or visuomotor problems (Tarnopol & Tarnopol, 1977). Gillberg (1998) suggested that 1.7% of the children with learning disabilities have severe DAMP, 49% have moderate DAMP, and only 2.2% have severe DCD without ADHD; about half of the population with ADHD also have DCD.

PATHOPHYSIOLOGY

No specific pathologic process or single neuroanatomic site has been definitively associated with DCD (Box 19-1). By definition, DCD is not related to muscle pathology, peripheral sensory abnormality, or central nervous system (CNS) damage that causes spasticity, athetosis, or ataxia. From a systems perspective, smooth motor functioning depends not only on an intact CNS but also on use of appropriate, environmentally referenced inputs.

Gubbay (1978) found that 50% of children identified as clumsy had prenatal, perinatal, or neonatal risk factors. DCD is often associated with prematurity, although the pathophysiology of DCD is unclear. Pinto-Martin and colleagues (1999) found that some low birth weight (LBW) premature children, without major disability including cerebral palsy (CP), had abnormalities indicative of ischemic white-matter injury. These children had poor perceptual motor performance at ages 2, 6, and 9 years. In addition to this group of premature infants, he found that some had small lesions at birth but the lesions resolved without later motor problems. However, Cook and

| Box 19-1 | Relationships among Body Structures and Function, Activity, and Participation for a Child with DCD |

HEALTH CONDITION	BODY STRUCTURE AND FUNCTION	ACTIVITY LIMITATIONS	PARTICIPATION RESTRICTIONS— ENVIRONMENTAL FACTORS	PARTICIPATION RESTRICTIONS— PERSONAL FACTORS
Heterogeneous central nervous system lesions of frontal and parietal areas	Soft signs: Poor strength Poor coordination Jerky movements	Awkward, slow gait	Doors too heavy to open	Depression
Prenatal, perinatal, and neonatal insults	Poor visual perception	Delayed and poor quality of fine and gross motor skills, such as hopping, jumping, ball skills, and writing	Physical education is competitive and skill oriented	Quit trying to participate, unmotivated
	Joint laxity		Late to class because passing time is too short	Low self-esteem
	Poor spatial organization	Delayed oral-motor skills		Poor fitness
	Inadequate information processing		Time to dress and undress reduces participation in recess and readiness for home and community activities	Activities performed without concern for time restrictions
	Poor sequencing			Vocational anxiety
	Poor feedback and feedforward motor control		Slow and messy written communication in class limits academic performance	
	Poor short-and long-term memory		Peers don't wait to try to understand conversations	

Abernethy (1999) did not find an association of cranial lesions in very low birth weight infants with their motor performance as 15- to 17-year-olds. Knuckey and colleagues (1983) used computed tomography (CT) to compare children identified as having perceptual disabilities or defects of motor organization with control subjects. Thirty-nine percent of the children with motor problems had abnormal or variant CT scans compared to 9% of the children with normal motor development. The abnormalities found included ventricular dilatation, peripheral atrophy, and parenchymal lesions.

Recent research by Maruff and colleagues (1999) and Wilson and colleagues (2001) concluded that in some children, DCD occurs because of a deficit of efference copy signals. Control-based learning theory (COBALT)

hypothesizes that an environmental goal triggers activity in the dorsolateral frontal areas of the brain. The frontal areas send signals to the posterior parietal lobes so that intentions can be integrated with previous visual and kinesthetic perceptions. The parietal lobe's specialized circuits connect to the motor areas of the brain. The sequencing of the actions and control parameters take place in the supplemental motor area and the basal ganglia. The primary motor cortex receives these inputs and sends efferent signals to the spinal cord. Immediately prior to execution of the motor action, an efference copy of the motor action is sent via a corollary pathway to the parietal lobe and is stored there. The next time the motor action is attempted, the efference copy serves as an internal representation of the action and can be used as a feedforward "guide" for the action (Willingham, 1998; Rizzolatti et al., 1998). Research with individuals who have had a focal lesion in the parietal lobe has led to the conclusion that the parietal lobe monitors the efference copy signals (Katschmarsky et al., 2001). Once the learner performs the new motor act, feedback is used to begin the creation of a CNS image called an efference copy. Each additional time the novel motor action is performed, past experience, contained in the efference copy, can be used to anticipate which motor control variables should be utilized. After prolonged practice, the learner becomes proficient because a feedforward bias characteristic of skilled actions has been created (Gentile, 1998).

COBALT suggests that if no internal representation of a movement exists in the parietal lobe, either because the motor action is being performed for the first time or because of a deficit in CNS processing, the specific motor control factors such as force, timing, and distance have to be selected without reference to past actions. The learner has no stored previous experience of the intended action and therefore cannot use a feedforward mechanism to generate the intended movement. Without an efference copy, the movement is slow (relying heavily on feedback) and uncoordinated (because of a lack of an internal copy to help smooth out the forces used to generate the movement). An impairment in the ability to generate an internal representation of the motor action (efferent copy) may be responsible for the slow, uncoordinated movement that is so often observed in children with DCD (Wilson et al., 2001).

Blondis (1999) used regional cerebral blood flow (rCBF) and magnetic resonance imaging (MRI) to demonstrate that the supplementary motor area (SMA) and sensory areas are activated during learned sequential movements. As difficulty performing sequential movements is an impairment of body function associated with DCD in some children, the SMA may be implicated in the pathophysiology of DCD. Others, however, have suggested that it is the cerebellum that contributes to DCD, especially in children demonstrating timing or rhythmic coordination deficits (Williams et al., 1992).

Theories related to the pathophysiology of praxis in adults have proposed that multiple mechanisms are involved and that lesions in any of the multiple pathways can result in one of the many forms of apraxia (Kertesz, 1985) (Fig. 19-1). Kertesz suggested that the anterior half of the periventricular white matter and the frontal lobe are the most frequent location of lesions resulting in apraxia. Interestingly, spastic diplegia is the most common form of cerebral palsy likely to result from damage to the periventricular white matter in premature infants (Soltesz & Brockway, 1989). This may be the link between the ob-

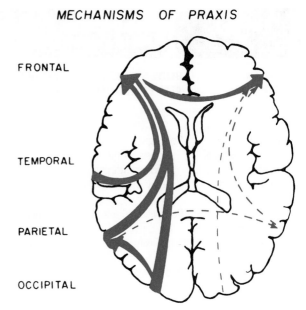

MECHANISMS OF PRAXIS

FRONTAL

TEMPORAL

PARIETAL

OCCIPITAL

♦ **Figure 19-1**   Diagrammatic representation of the neural mechanisms of praxis. Interruption of this network at any point may result in apraxia. Small lesions may affect the system most consistently where convergence of pathways occurs. Dotted lines represent alternate routes that may become active with recovery. *(From Roy, EA [Ed.]. Neuropsychological Studies of Apraxia and Related Disorders. Amsterdam: North-Holland, 1985, p. 175.)*

served comorbidity of prematurity, spastic diplegia, and DCD in some children.

PRIMARY PREVENTION

At the present time, there are no theorized models that would suggest a way to prevent the pathology believed to underlie DCD. Prevention of the impairments related to DCD has not been well addressed, either. General early intervention programs for infants at risk are becoming more common in the United States, especially as a result of the legislative mandates associated with Part C of the Individuals with Disabilities Education Act Amendments of 1997. Interestingly, some of the characteristics described by parents of children with DCD are similar to those used by Als and colleagues (1986, 1988) to describe preterm infants who display state disorganization. Als (1986) has suggested the use of specific positioning and handling techniques to improve state regulation and diminish disorganized behavior to encourage more normal development in infants, toddlers, and preschoolers. Better prenatal care, perinatal monitoring, and newborn care may decrease the occurrence of developmental motor incoordination problems.

This is supported by the research of van Der Fits and colleagues (1999) who used electromyography and video analysis of hyperextended postures during the development of preterm infants' reaching. When compared to term infants, the muscle activity of preterm infants was characterized by increased levels of tonic background activity in neck and lumbar extensors and temporal disorganization. Preterm infants also lacked the ability to modulate their postural output with respect to varying task-specific demands. The authors concluded that preterm infants have a reduced capacity to learn from prior experiences and are unable to integrate prior information for feedforward processing. They suggested this may be related to clumsiness in later motor development. This is similar to the theory that children with DCD have a body function impairment in the processing of an efference copy (Wilson et al., 2001).

ASSOCIATED BODY FUNCTIONS

The number of studies identifying specific characteristics of groups of children with incoordination problems is extensive. Some have even attempted to identify subcategories of DCD (Dewey & Kaplan, 1994; Hoare, 1994; Wright & Sugden, 1996), but most authors agree that children with DCD are a heterogeneous group. The utilization of a variety of assessment instruments to identify the group of children at different ages assumed to have DCD accounts for some of the discrepancy. Unfortunately, as Sugden & Wright (1998) concluded, no meta-analysis has been performed to help establish common characteristics of a DCD syndrome.

A neurologic examination might reveal problems with body functions such as soft neurologic signs including muscle weakness, especially of the hands; poor coordination, especially in finger-to-nose movement and finger-thumb opposition; and possible choreiform movements seen as small jerky twitches of the upper extremities. But not all children with DCD have detectable soft signs. Numerous deviations of typical body functions have been identified in many, but not all, children with DCD (Box 19-2).

This long list of characteristics can be misleading, as no individual child demonstrates all the characteristics. This heterogeneity makes the identification and decisions regarding treatment for an individual child with DCD

Box 19-2	Impairments of Body Functions Identified in Children with DCD
BODY FUNCTION	**REFERENCE**
Visuoperceptual, visual-spatial, and visuomotor impairment	Mon-Williams et al., 1999
	O'Brien et al., 1988
	Wilson & McKenzie, 1998
Inefficient use of visual feedback in fast, goal-directed arm movement	van der Meulen et al., 1991
Impaired visual memory	Dwyer & McKenzie, 1994
More dependent on visuospatial rehearsal to memorize	Skorji & McKenzie, 1997
Difficulty with visual and motor sequencing tasks requiring short-and long-term recall	Murphy & Gliner, 1988
Impairments of size-constancy judgments, spatial position, and visual discrimination	Lord & Hulme, 1987
Slow performance related to reliance on information feedback rather than feedforward programming	Missiuana et al., 2003
	Rösblad & van Hofsten, 1994
	Smyth, 1991
Slow reaction time and movement time related to impaired response selection	Raynor, 1998
	Van Dellan & Geuze, 1988
Prolonged response latency related to the process of searching for and retrieval of the correct responses with reliable timing	Henderson et al., 1992
Poor timing, rhythm, and force control	Lundy-Ekman et al., 1991
	Volman & Geuze, 1998
	Williams et al., 1992
	Hoare & Larkin, 1991
Impaired performance on kinesthetic acuity, linear positioning, and weight discrimination	
Prolonged burst of agonist activity and delayed onset of antagonist activity	Huh et al., 1998
Reduced power and strength	Rayner, 2001
Reduced ability to successfully inhibit an action	Mandich et al., 2002

difficult. More information about the development and the long-term outcomes of children of children with DCD is needed (Geuze et al., 2001).

In summary, children with DCD may have slower response times and have difficulty (1) identifying the important details of the task, (2) analyzing the task to understand its component parts, (3) using past experience to plan a new strategy (feedforward planning), (4) executing the task as planned, and (5) using feedback to make changes for the next attempt. In addition, after a task is performed, retention may be limited owing to difficulty retrieving information from memory processes to perform it again.

Although recent research related to CNS function has increased the knowledge base about children with DCD, physical therapists should remember that most of these studies have used motor learning tasks that were specific to an experimental paradigm and were performed inside a laboratory environment. Whether the performance on these types of tasks is related to functional motor tasks in natural environments requires further study. Future research should focus on functional tasks in natural environments such as measurements of movement times when completing a writing sample, reaction times when asked to stand up from a classroom desk, or sequencing errors when tying shoes after physical education class.

ACTIVITY LIMITATIONS

When children have body function impairments, they often display difficulty in tasks typically measured on norm-referenced or criterion-referenced tests. Parents often report that their children were overly messy when eating and dressing, started walking later than other children and are still awkward, were late talkers, had excessive levels of frustration and crying, and demanded continual adult attention. Gubbay (1975) believed so strongly that clumsiness should be studied by the medical community as an entity separate from MBD or learning disability that he created the Gubbay Tests of Motor Proficiency (Gubbay, 1975), which is reproduced in Appendix I at the end of this chapter. The test items Gubbay found to discriminate between children with and without clumsiness included whistling, skipping, rolling a ball with their foot, clapping while throwing a ball in the air, shoe-tying, threading beads, piercing holes in paper, and placing shapes in a form board. In a later study of 39 children with clumsiness, Gubbay (1978) found that the battery could be shortened to four items: throwing a ball in the air and clapping before it is caught, using a foot to roll a ball along a path, threading beads, and inserting shapes in slots.

In addition to his Tests of Motor Proficiency, Gubbay believed that a full examination for DCD should include eight items related to the general history of the child; six items related to a physical examination; a supplementary neurologic examination; academic testing in the areas of reading, writing, and drawing; an electroencephalogram; a skull radiograph; and psychologic testing.

One of the more recently published examinations for DCD is the Movement Assessment Battery for Children (M-ABC) (Henderson & Sugden, 1992)(see accompanying video). The M-ABC has been normed for children 4 to 10 years old and it includes a screening checklist to be used by teachers and parents and a norm-referenced examination. The checklist has four sections with 12 questions in each section and a fifth section with questions about the child's behaviors related to motor activities. Each of the first four sections has questions regarding the child's performance in one of the following environments: child stationary, environment stable (e.g., cutting); child moving, environment stable (e.g., walking); child stationary, environment changing (e.g., catching); and child moving, environment changing (e.g., running and kicking a ball). A total score is calculated and used to determine if the child is at risk for movement problems (below 15% but above 5% cut-off score) or has movement problems (below the 5% cut-off score).

The norm-referenced examination has three sections, each section containing items for each of three age bands: 4 to 6 years, 7 to 8 years, and 9 to 10 years. Items are divided into manual dexterity, ball skills, and static and dynamic balance sections including activities such as threading beads, putting pegs in a peg board, catching and throwing a bean bag, balancing on one leg, jumping, hopping, and heel-to-toe walking. A total score is used to determine if performance is within normal ranges, if a motor impairment is present, or if the impairment is serious.

The body of evidence examining the use of the M-ABC is growing. Leemrijse and colleagues (1999) concluded that the total score of the M-ABC is sufficiently sensitive to monitor individual child change, and that the cluster scores have moderate sensitivity. They cautioned, however, that using the individual items to measure individual child change is inappropriate.

Others have cautioned that the sensitivity of the M-ABC checklist is so low that many of the children at risk for motor problems were not identified (Junaid et al., 2000). Caution needs to be used when relying only on the judgment of classroom or physical education teachers when using checklists to identify children with DCD. Piek and Edwards (1997) compared the M-ABC checklist results with actual performance on the M-ABC examination. They found that classroom teachers were able to identify only 25% of the children with DCD and physical education teachers identified only 49%. This discrepancy is partially explained by the different environments in which the two types of teachers based their observations. Miyahara and colleagues (2000) cautioned that there may be a cross-cultural issue because typical children in the United States performed at a different level than typical children in Japan. After a literature review of 176 publications, Geuze and colleagues (2001) concluded that the M-ABC is still the best assessment tool for DCD in spite of the fact that it omits tasks related to handwriting.

One of the DSM-IV discriminating criteria for DCD is that the motor coordination is markedly below expected levels for the child's chronologic age. To distinguish DCD from a developmental motor delay, standardized tests of developmentally sequenced gross and fine motor items can be used. The Peabody Developmental Motor Scales, Second Edition (Folio & Fewell, 2000), Battelle Developmental Inventory (Newborg et al., 1984), and Miller Assessment for Preschoolers (Miller, 1988) are examples of developmental motor examinations used to identify motor delay in preschool children. The Test of Gross Motor Development (Ulich, 2000) and The Bruininks-Oseretsky Test of Motor Proficiency (BOTMP) (Bruininks, 1978) are designed to identify motor delay in older children. These are examples of tests to determine developmental motor delay, and they are not designed to be used for the identification of DCD. Developmental motor tests and tests for DCD identify different groups of children (Dugas et al., 1999; Dewey & Wilson, 2001).

PARTICIPATION RESTRICTIONS

Parents know their child's developmental history and have observed his or her functioning in multiple environments. They have the best composite of diagnostic information. When parents of children with DCD were asked what their concerns were, the main concern identified was restricted participation in society, especially in middle school (Segal et al., 2002). Parents identified ongoing problems with everyday participation during dressing, eating, and grooming (see Box 19-1). When their children were preschoolers, these limitations were excused as "slow development" or temperamental differences. Poor performance on everyday activities is tolerated less and less as children with DCD reach school age.

Tying one's shoes is an example of a skilled activity not expected of 3- and 4-year-olds but required at school by the time a student is in first grade. Children with impairments in sequencing skills cannot correctly sequence the

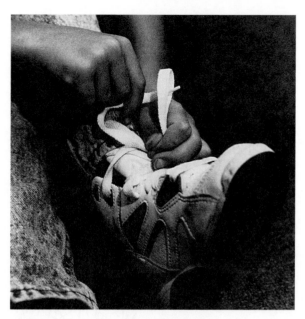

◆ **Figure 19-2** This 8-year-old boy still cannot independently tie his shoes. His verbal cues were "loop around and go through." He forgot to "loop around" and forgot to make a second loop.

steps in shoe-tying even though they have practiced it many times before. When children with DCD make a mistake in one step of the sequence, they have to start over again rather than simply redo the last step. Or they will omit a different step in the sequence each time they try to tie their shoes (Fig. 19-2). Untied shoes can restrict a student's participation in recess and physical education.

Teachers are the next most likely individuals to identify restricted participation related to DCD. Often, the structured demands of the classroom with expectations of increasingly precise motor skills and shorter time frames for performance stress a child with DCD to his or her limit. Teachers are able to compare the performance of children with incoordination to their peers, something parents do not have as many opportunities to do.

Poor written communication is frequently the first activity limitation educators identify (Fig. 19-3). There are many reasons for poor written communication, and poor handwriting associated with DCD is only one of them. Treating handwriting as a motor production problem when the real issue is poor visual form recognition will only frustrate the child and the teacher. The decision to focus interventions toward the underlying processing problem or toward the motor activity limitation is one that the family and the entire educational team should address.

Another common participation restriction identified in early elementary school is poor performance in physical education class. Simple delayed maturation, limited

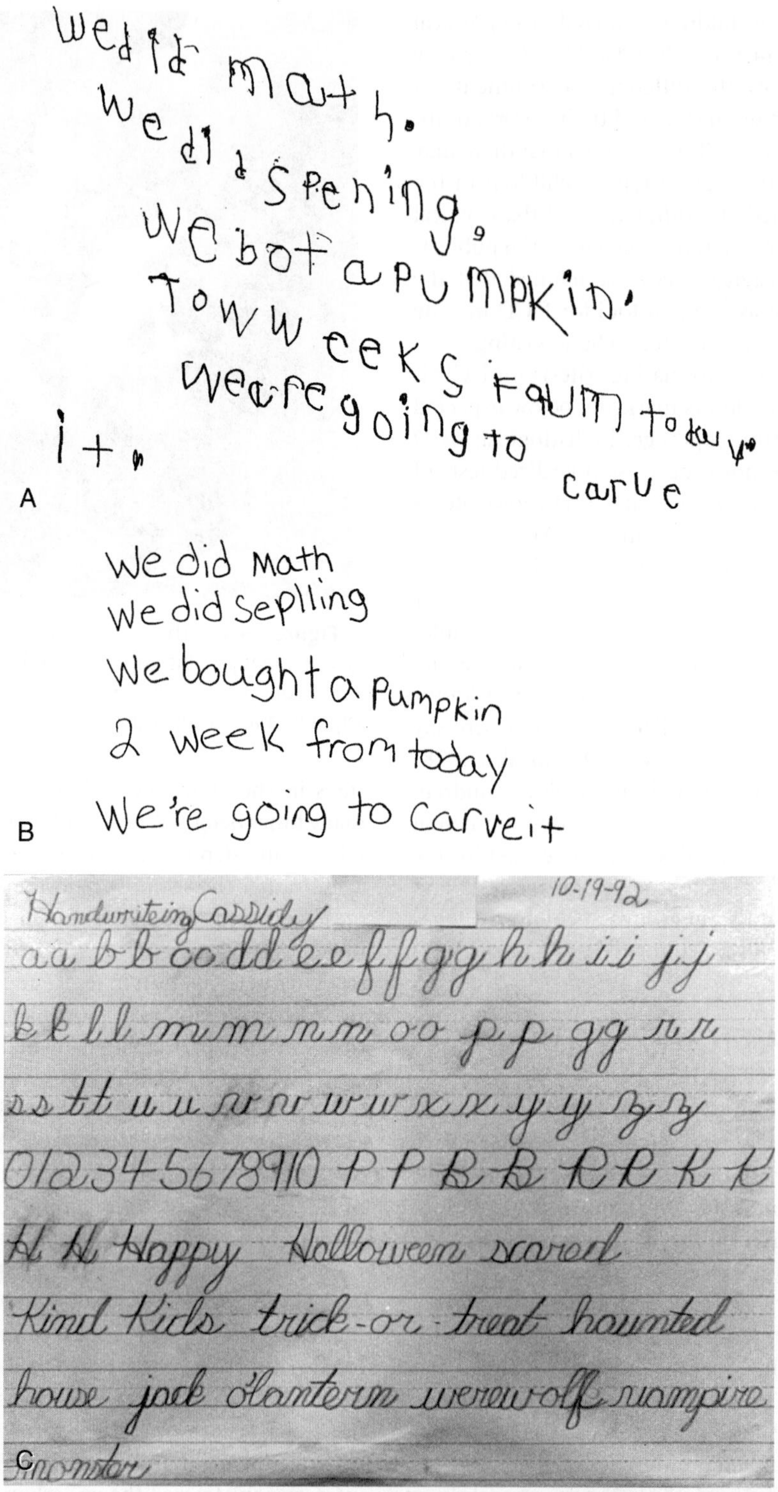

We did math.
we did spening,
we bot a pumpkin,
Tow weeks faum totay
weare going to carve
it.

A

We did Math
We did seplling

We bought a Pumpkin

2 week from today

B   We're going to carve it

Handwriting Cassidy   10-19-92

a a b b o o d d e e f f g g h h i i j j

k k l l m m n n o o p p q g r r

s s t t u u r r w w x x y y z z

0123456789 10 P P B B R R K K

H H Happy Halloween scared

Kind Kids trick-or-treat haunted

house jack o'lantern werewolf vampire

C monster

* **Figure 19-3**   **A**, Handwriting sample of a third-grade child with a developmental coordination disorder and a learning disability. **B**, Handwriting sample obtained for comparison from a randomly selected third-grade peer without motor dysfunction. **C**, Sample of cursive writing from another peer without motor dysfunction demonstrates an even more advanced expectation of third graders.

gross motor play experience, poor motivation, or significant health or medical disorders, as well as DCD, need to be considered as possible reasons for problems in physical education class. Children with DCD have been observed to engage in less vigorous play and spend significantly more time away from the playground area than their peers (Bouffard et al., 1996). Smyth and Anderson (2000) found that children with DCD spend more time alone on the playground and spend less time in formal and informal team play.

CONTEXTUAL FACTORS: ENVIRONMENT

Gubbay (1975) reported that in the younger age groups the environment tends to be less reactive and generally kinder because of the wider range of normal variation. The early signs of clumsiness are often viewed as part of normal developmental awkwardness or normal delay for premature infants.

Peers, parents, teachers, or communities may create unwarranted restrictions, artificial barriers, or rigid expectations as preschoolers become elementary school children. If a physical education class or community recreation program strictly adheres to performance criteria for group activities such as baseball, basketball, or dance class, then a child with DCD has been artificially prevented from participating with peers. If parents prevent their child from going down the street to play at a neighborhood park because they are unduly afraid the child will be hurt or will get lost, then a barrier has been established and peer relationships have been limited.

If a community police department refuses to recognize that an adolescent or adult cannot pass a field sobriety test owing to inherent coordination problems, the individual with DCD may be mistakenly arrested for drunken driving. In this case, society may unnecessarily limit the person's freedom to drive and restrict community mobility and vocational options.

If a restaurant makes a family feel uncomfortable or asks them to leave because their child spills drinks or drops food on the floor, then eating out will occur less often or may be limited to certain environments. Indoor manipulative play can pose just as much of a problem. When limitations exist in fine motor skills of coloring, cutting, and stacking objects, imaginative play with paper, small toy people, or building blocks is very difficult. By not allowing children to play with modified toys or when individualized expectations are not permitted, a child's experiences are artificially limited.

CONTEXTUAL FACTORS: PERSONAL

Children with DCD often self-impose restrictions on their participation. Skinner & Piek (2001) found that children with DCD perceive themselves as less competent than their peers. They had lower self-worth and more anxiety. When poor gross motor skills of running, skipping, hopping, or jumping lead to inactivity and avoidance of physically challenging games, then the child with DCD becomes weak, resulting in increasingly poor fitness and even more avoidance of physical activity. Avoidance of games requiring fine motor skill leads to a decreased amount of practice preventing ongoing skill development. When manipulative games are avoided, random, nonconstructive activities may take their place (Fig. 19-4). Parents have reported that the more difficulty their child had with motor skills, the less willing they were to engage in physical activity (Pless et al., 2002). Self-imposed isolation becomes a self-perpetuating cycle of poor skill development, limited skill practice, poor performance, and further isolation.

Helping families and individuals with DCD to know their rights and identify compensatory means for full participation in meaningful activities is one of the physical therapist's most important roles.

ADOLESCENTS AND YOUNG ADULTS WITH DCD

Although Gubbay (1975) believed that clumsiness was usually not a problem after the age of 12 years because intellectually the older child usually has matured sufficiently to compensate for these problems either by avoidance or concealment, many parents report that adolescence is especially difficult for children with DCD. Teenagers can be verbally and emotionally unaccepting of differences. Even though general motor clumsiness is a developmental characteristic for many adolescents as their body proportions change, motor proficiency is valued because competitive sports play an important role in peer interactions and expectations of some families. Academic demands increase in middle school and high school, and poor written communication skills can seriously interfere with academic achievement.

Increasing numbers of longitudinal studies now exist to support the existence of ongoing motor disability in adolescents with DCD (Cantell et al., 1994; Geuze & Borger, 1993; Gillberg, 2001; Losse et al., 1991). A follow-up study of adolescents who had been identified as having

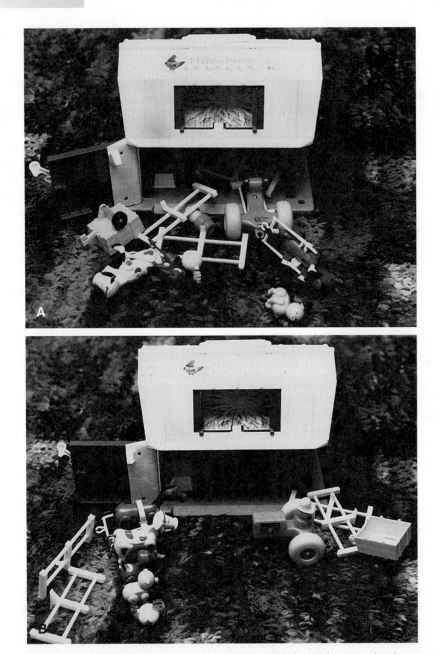

• **Figure 19-4** **A**, Arrangement of toys by a 4-year-old, who was later identified as having a developmental coordination disorder and a learning disability, after he was told to "show me what you can do with these toys." **B**, A 4-year-old with normal development and given the same instructions arranged the toys like this.

DCD when they were in elementary school documented associated problems of lower academic attainment, fewer social contacts, and poorer classroom concentration and behavior than other children (Geuze & Borger, 1993). Losse and colleagues (1991) conducted a 10-year follow-up study of 32 children, including 16 who had been identified as clumsy when they were around 6 years old. Although the 6-year-olds who had been identified as clumsy participated in 1 year of intervention (the specific type and amount of intervention were not identified) to promote learning of motor skills, the gains that were made were not maintained. After extensive retesting, Losse and colleagues concluded that the children with DCD continued to have significant motor difficulties at 16 years of age, with qualitative differences greater than quantitative measures. These children also demonstrated significantly lower academic scores and handwriting problems and had difficulty organizing materials. The teenagers with

DCD had more behavior problems, including being bullied, having poor school attendance, and being easily distractible. Emotional problems such as low self-esteem, depression, and being shy or timid were also found. Losse and colleagues concluded that other studies reporting that some children apparently "outgrew" their clumsiness had used clinical or laboratory-based tests that underestimated qualitative problems and did not reflect competence in natural environments. Not all of the children identified as clumsy at age 6 were having problems at age 16, however. Losse and colleagues found that some bright and well-adjusted children seemed to have come to terms with their ineptitude and appeared to cope well with their school experiences, were able to talk freely about their problems, and evidently enjoyed other aspects of life.

An interesting but not yet understood observation has been made when testing adolescents with and without DCD. While examining the relationship among physical growth, level of activity, and development of motor skills, Visser and colleagues (1998) confirmed that typical adolescents have decreased coordination during periods of rapid growth, but adolescents with DCD did not seem to be affected. In fact, some continued to gain motor skills and even performed at a level similar to their peers. A longitudinal study by Hadders-Algra (2002) found that some adolescents who were identified as typical at a younger age demonstrated minor neurologic dysfunction at puberty. Hadders-Algra hypothesized that this "hidden" dysfunction was present prior to puberty but was not expressed until changes in hormones or body structure created coordination demands that these "typical" children could not accomplish.

Gillberg (2001) summarized data from a long-term study he and colleagues began in 1977 on children with motor coordination problems. An original group of 141 7-year-old children, identified by a questionnaire completed by their teachers, were followed and retested at ages 10, 13, 16, and 22 years. After comprehensive neurologic assessment at the age of 7, the children were assigned to one of the following groups: (1) DAMP ($n = 42$), (2) DCD only ($n = 7$), (3) ADHD only ($n = 12$), and (4) a control group of children ($n = 51$). Over the years some children were lost due to attrition, making the original small sample size even smaller. In addition, comparisons at different ages was affected by changing terminology and availability of specific tests and measurements. In spite of these limitations, Gillberg (2001) concluded that motor control problems that were present in the 7-year-olds are less evident over time, diminishing in this study from 100% at age 7 to 55% in the DAMP group and from 100% to 33% in the DCD only group at age 10. Those children with motor control problems stabilized at about 30% to 35% at ages 13, 16, and 22 years for both groups. Individuals with DAMP (both DCD and ADHD) have the most significant long-term problems affecting their mental health, academic success, and employment. It should be noted that this study originally identified "motor perception dysfunction" and later used the DSM-III and DSM-IV definitions of DCD. No consistent assessment of motor control, such as the M-ABC, was available and utilized over the 15-year span of the study. In summary, adolescents and young adults identified with DCD at a younger age continue to demonstrate a mixed picture of motor, cognitive, and behavioral characteristics. A few had successful graduation from high school and pursued additional education or training. For some, their motor incoordination continued and significantly affected their academic and vocational decisions. For many others, even if their motor incoordination diminished, psychologic problems led to personal factors limiting participation in roles of student or worker. The combination of DCD and ADHD appeared to result in the least positive outcome, as many had significant personality or academic problems that prevented successful vocational endeavors and interpersonal development.

TEAM EVALUATION AND MANAGEMENT OF PARTICIPATION RESTRICTIONS

Unless a young child is receiving physical therapy for some other problem or being closely followed by a high-risk infant program, referral due to processing impairments related to body function such as diminished visual perception, limited motor memory, poor motor sequencing, excessive use of feedback, or poor spatial organization is often not made before kindergarten or early elementary school. Even when referred, standardized evaluations that assess information processing impairments are not currently available, except as part of some neuropsychologic examinations (Kaufman & Kaufman, 1983; Rourke et al., 1986) or as a very specific, nonfunctional and nonenvironmentally referenced kinesthetic task (Laszlo & Bairstow, 1985).

PHYSICAL THERAPY REFERRAL, EXAMINATION, AND EVALUATION

With the passage of the Education of the Handicapped Act in 1975 (amended in 1990 and 1997 and now titled Individuals with Disabilities Education Act), physical therapists working in educational environments in the United

States are often asked to examine children demonstrating problems with motor skills at school. Parents, preschool teachers, and early elementary school teachers are usually the first to raise a concern related to activity limitations or participation restrictions associated with DCD.

Some of these children display the body function and activity limitations associated with DCD such as falling at recess or difficulty putting on a jacket with a zipper. The physical therapist in educational environments has the advantage of screening children in their natural environments while the children participate in everyday, functional activities. Immediate collaborative consultation can occur with the classroom or physical education teacher to problem solve some of the concerns. Often, an initial collection of specific data can solve the problem without a complete physical therapy examination. Data collected during recess may reveal that the child in question really does not fall more frequently than two randomly chosen peers. The child may just come to the teacher more often for help. In this case the problem is not motoric, but behavioral, and an examination by a physical therapist is not needed. When data reveal that the child does indeed fall three times more often than other children during recess, an appropriate physical therapy examination can begin with already collected baseline data related to function. When children with possible DCD are referred and examined in a clinic setting, in-depth interviewing of the parents and teachers and simulation of functional activities are needed to accurately identify true limitations of body function and activities.

When a child's specific motor problem has been defined and it has been determined than an examination is indicated, the physical therapist should avoid repeating examinations already performed by other disciplines. Given the heterogeneous nature of DCD, it is important for a physical therapy examination to utilize multiple sources of information and multiple types of examinations. The *Guide to Physical Therapist Practice* (American Physical Therapy Association, 2001) outlines the following examination and evaluation framework. Initial determination of what practice pattern best describes a child's motor problems begins with the collection of historical information. The following types of information would be pertinent for a child suspected of have a DCD: a medical history including pregnancy, delivery, and past and current health status; developmental history; previous musculoskeletal and neuromuscular examinations; and history of the current functional status from the family and school personnel. Referral to Preferred Practice Pattern 5C would prompt a physical therapist to choose tests of neuromotor development and sensory integration to obtain a current level of motor and sensory functioning.

Physical therapists must make evaluation hypotheses regarding the origin of a child's coordination problems. A typical initial referral in a school-based service environment might be from a physical education teacher regarding a 5-year-old kindergarten student who is falling a lot. Initial hypotheses concerning why Sam is falling more often than his peers might be because (1) he has mild cerebral palsy, spastic diplegia, or hemiplegia, (2) he has early symptoms of muscular dystrophy, (3) he is clumsy and has DCD, (4) he has symptoms of ADHD, and as a result, he is impulsive and distracted to the extent that he bumps into people and objects, (5) his shoes are too big and he trips over the laces, or (6) he has a perceptual or visual impairment.

Direct observation of Sam on the playground and during physical education class could rule out falling related to improper fitting shoes (hypothesis 5) or significant impulsivity and distractibility possibly related to ADHD (hypothesis 4). An observation could identify a positive Gowers sign and large calf muscles suggesting further medical referral for possible muscular dystrophy (hypothesis 2). Observation of movement patterns during play may suggest typical symmetric synergies of hip adduction and internal rotation with knee flexion and ankle plantar flexion (cerebral palsy, spastic diplegia; hypothesis 1), or unilateral shoulder retraction, internal rotation and adduction, elbow supination and flexion, wrist and finger flexion, hip adduction and internal rotation with knee flexion and plantar flexion (cerebral palsy, hemiplegia; hypothesis 1).

Direct observation of activities of daily living (ADLs) in naturally occurring situations is the most valid way to evaluate a concern. If observations and examinations must be performed in a hospital or clinic setting, then behavior might need to be observed in a noisy, distracting, fast-paced environment such as a busy waiting room or children's play area. Putting a coat on surrounded by 25 other 7-year-old children, all struggling in a small space to get dressed and get outside for recess first, is much different from putting on a coat in a quiet room with one adult giving positive encouragement.

Additional information from parent and teacher interviews is vital. A parent may describe her son as having a pattern of general incoordination with delayed speech, messy eating, and general clumsiness present from a young age but without a medical diagnosis related to a neurologic impairment (hypothesis 3). The parent interview combined with information from a teacher can confirm the presence of a significant problem with academic achievement or ADLs, key criteria of the DSM-IV description of DCD (hypothesis 3). However, if the parent describes a pattern of typical motor development followed by a recent decrease in strength and loss of the ability to climb stairs independently, the hypothesis of muscular dystrophy (2) is supported.

A direct examination by the physical therapist might identify muscle hypertonicity that increases with faster movements (possible cerebral palsy; hypothesis 1). On the other hand, if direct examination suggests low muscle tone with shoulder, elbow, and knee hyperextension, DCD again becomes a valid hypothesis (3). If muscle testing reveals a weak gastrocnemius and pseudohypertrophy, the hypothesis of muscular dystrophy (2) is supported. During direct examination the therapist may be able to relate the most striking activity limitations to difficulties in following directions when asked to perform a motor task or to poor attention-to-task. Children with DCD often cannot imitate body postures or follow two- or three-step motor commands. Frequent demonstration and actual physical assistance may be needed to accomplish items on standardized tests.

To rule out problems primarily related to developmental delay consistent with mental retardation, the Peabody Developmental Motor Scales (Folio & Fewell, 1983) or the Bruininks-Oseretsky Test of Motor Proficiency (Bruininks, 1978) are possible choices depending on the age of the child. This developmental motor age needs to be compared to the findings of other team members, especially a psychologist's evaluation of cognitive skills. The DSM-IV definition of DCD states that the child with DCD must have motor incoordination greater than what would be expected secondary to overall developmental delay and a diagnosis of mental retardation. To confirm the diagnosis of DCD with or without developmental delay, the Movement Assessment Battery For Children (Henderson & Sugden, 1992) should be administered as a direct examination of dexterity, agility, and coordination.

There is another group of young children seen by physical therapists who should be considered at risk for DCD. These are the children who were premature and were subsequently diagnosed with spastic diplegic cerebral palsy. Some of these children enter school and have increasing academic difficulties that eventually lead to an educational diagnosis of learning disability. When evaluating and treating a preschool child with spastic diplegia and a birth history of prematurity and perinatal complications, physical therapists need to be aware of early signs of motor incoordination.

REFERRAL TO OTHER DISCIPLINES AND TEAM PLANNING WITH FAMILY AND CHILD OR ADOLESCENT

An evaluation (analysis and synthesis of examination results), diagnosis, and prognosis by the physical thera-

pist will then determine whether intervention and further examinations by other professionals are warranted. It should not be assumed that DCD is an isolated motor problem. Research has found an increased incidence of DCD in combination with ocular motor and oral motor apraxia (Dewey et al., 1988; Rappaport et al., 1987). An examination may be needed by any of the following individuals: (1) a family physician or neurologist when neuromuscular or musculoskeletal concerns are identified; (2) an occupational therapist when fine motor, self-help, or motor planning areas need further examination; (3) a speech and language pathologist when speech, oral-motor dysfunction, or possible cognitive-linguistic problems are observed; (4) a psychologist when intellectual or behavioral issues have surfaced; or (5) an adapted physical education teacher when more thorough gross motor skill training is needed.

In an educational setting, joint planning takes place with the parents, child or adolescent if appropriate, and other educational team members at an individualized education program (IEP) meeting for a student in special education. If the child or adolescent is not in special education but has a disability, a 504 team may be convened. When an examination is performed in a clinic, the clinical judgments and proposed therapy needs are discussed with the family and appropriate medical staff. Team decisions include those related to the child's or adolescent's specific needs, and short- and long-term goals. Decisions related to the need for physical therapy interventions must then be made. This discussion should include an anticipated frequency and duration of therapy sessions needed for this episode of care. Specific and measurable goals and outcomes should be identified because very little research evidence exists that substantiates the successful remediation of DCD. At least one, if not all, of the goals should be environmentally referenced to a problem related to participation in real life situations. Finally, the need to share information with other service agencies is considered. If indicated, parental permission to release reports is obtained, as interagency service coordination is extremely important.

PHYSICAL THERAPY INTERVENTION

Literature reviews of intervention outcomes for children with DCD started to appear in 1998. In their book, *Motor Coordination Disorders in Children,* Sugden and Wright (1998) concluded that there are many skilled therapists using interventions based upon principles from motor learning theory, but there is little evidence to support the effectiveness of any one intervention. Mandich and colleagues (2001a) reviewed intervention literature published over the past 15 years and found that physical therapists have used eclectic treatment approaches to improve motor activities for individual children with DCD. They found that individual therapists used on average five different approaches and concluded that no one intervention approach has been shown to be more effective than another approach. This is also consistent with the review of DCD by Barnhart and colleagues (2003). After comparing five studies related to interventions for children with DCD, they concluded that interventions using principles from systems theory and motor learning theory offer the best opportunity for positive intervention results.

PROCEDURAL INTERVENTIONS

A study by Schoemaker and colleagues (1994) involving physical therapy intervention is often cited as an example of a short-term intervention that was effective. The physical therapist performed eclectic physical therapy for 3 months on 17 children (6–9 years old) who tested clumsy on the Test of Motor Impairment (TOMI) (Stott et al., 1972). Physical therapy intervention consisted of 45-minute visits, twice a week. The physical therapist performed an evaluation and devised individual intervention plans for the children with DCD. The intervention was described as a combination of sensorimotor training and Bobath neurodevelopmental techniques. The TOMI and Movement ABC were used to compare preintervention status with postintervention and 3 months postintervention status. Three TOMI items revealed a significant improvement: moving both hands rapidly during a fine motor skill, catching a ball, and static balance. Improvements were maintained for 3 months. However, the authors acknowledged that improvement was measured in a stable, restricted laboratory setting and that motor activity in natural environments is more complex.

Sigmundsson and colleagues (1998) reviewed intervention procedures used for DCD over a 30-year period. Interventions included perceptual-motor training, sensory integration therapy, and kinesthetic training. They concluded that any given intervention is effective primarily because the therapist is skilled and is able to motivate the child to practice new motor activities. Success is ensured by manipulating the task and environment which improves the child's confidence and willingness to try harder tasks. Sugden and Chambers (1998) came to a similar conclusion. They hypothesized that it is the accurate assessment and decision making related to choosing the appropriate activities for a given child that make the difference.

Three intervention approaches for children with DCD are currently receiving recognition and support: (1) guided imagery based on the efference-copy-deficit hypothesis (Wilson et al., 2002), (2) cognitive approaches based on the hypothesis that children with DCD have poor problem-solving skills (Miller et al., 2001), and (3) task-specific interventions based on motor learning principles (Gentile, 1998).

Brain imaging technology has greatly expanded the knowledge of motor function and dysfunction including dysfunction associated with DCD (Rowe & Frackowiak, 1999). It is possible to identify the changes in brain function that occur before a motor action is performed (effect of feedforward) and compare these changes with the patterns that occur after a motor action has been performed (effect of feedback). Maruff and colleagues (1999) used a motor learning paradigm consisting of a visually guided pointing task to compare strategies used for real tasks with strategies for imagined tasks. They were able to show that children with DCD have an impairment in the ability to generate internal representations of volitional movements suggesting that DCD is related to a deficit of efference copy signals due to an error in processing or generation of the corollary discharge from the efferent motoneuron. Maruff and colleagues (1999) hypothesized that interventions using guided imagery training should improve the performance of children with DCD. Guided imagery training is a cognitive exercise used to imagine a motor action that is not actually being performed. Practice creating a conscious replication of a motor act should help create the missing efference copy that is needed to provide feedforward information for a future actual attempt to achieve the motor goal (Wilson et al., 2001). Training would consist of asking a child to imagine a certain movement with simultaneous attention to the internal signals that are associated with the imagined movement. For example: "Imagine you are bouncing and catching this ball. Which moves first, your wrist or your feet?" Or, "When you practice standing on one foot, what should your other leg be doing?"

As a follow-up to this hypothesis Wilson and colleagues (2002) used an imagery intervention designed to specifically train the forward modeling of purposive actions using an interactive CD-ROM. They randomly assigned 54 children with coordination problems to one of three groups: imagery training, traditional perceptual-motor training, or no treatment. The M-ABC was used as a pretest and posttest measure. Both intervention groups received 5 hours of total training distributed in 60-minute sessions once a week for 5 weeks. Sixteen of the 17 children in the imagery group (significant at $p < 0.001$) and 15 of the 17 children in the perceptual-motor group (significant at $p < 0.001$) improved on the M-ABC. Eleven of the 17 children in the control group demonstrated some change (not significant at $p = 0.190$) and 5 of the control children actually had lower scores on the posttest. The authors concluded that motor imagery training alone with no actual skill practice can improve performance in children with DCD, thus supporting the efference copy deficit hypothesis. They suggested that future research explore the effectiveness of adding motor imagery training to conventional forms of intervention.

Recent emphasis has also been placed on using a cognitive approach to improve activity skills and participation (Cermak & Larkin, 2002). A cognitive approach uses questions to guide the child to identify, analyze, and create solutions to a motor problem that could then be attempted. Both global and task-specific cognitive strategies are discovered by structuring the environment and asking the child to verbalize the strategy they are using. The cognitive approach uses the problem-solving strategy of goal-plan-do-check (Fox, 1998).

The effective use of memory strategies is an important component of a cognitive approach. In a 1985 study, David found that even though 76% of normal 8-year-old children used verbal rehearsal to remember a cognitive sequencing task, only 33% used the same strategy to help them remember a motor sequencing task. Murphy and Gliner (1988) found that 6- to 9-year-old children designated as clumsy have even more trouble than their peers with visual and motor sequencing tasks requiring short- and long-term recall. In addition, some children with DCD have impaired visual memory when compared to their peers (Dwyer & McKenzie, 1994). Verbal self-guidance has been shown to be an effective intervention for children with DCD (Martini & Polatajko, 1998). I successfully used verbal self-guidance to assist a kindergarten student with cerebral palsy and DCD to remember how to sit on the floor with legs crossed during circle time (Fig. 19-5).

Mandich and colleagues (2001b, p. 132) analyzed the videotape of therapists using cognitive strategies and iden-

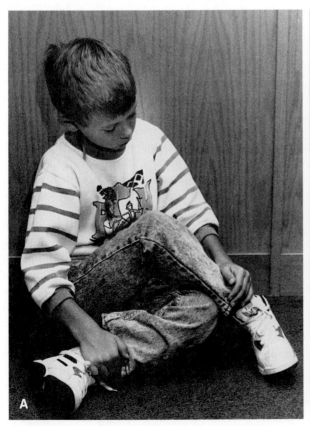 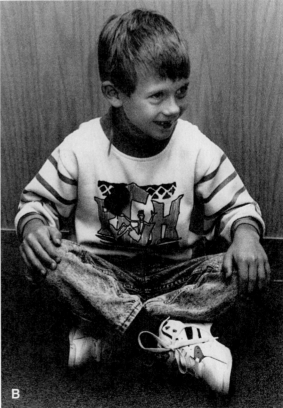

• **Figure 19-5**   **A,** After many therapy sessions with verbal and physical prompts, this child is still unable to sit on the floor and cross his legs independently. **B,** After being reminded of the verbal cues he needs to say to himself, he now successfully crosses his legs.

tified the following specific cognitive strategies that children who have DCD need: task specification/modification, motor mnemonic leading to mental image, body position verbalization, verbalization of the feeling of the movement, verbal cueing of attention to the task, therapist verbal guidance, child self-verbal guidance, and the use of a rote pattern of words to guide the motor sequence.

Polatajko and colleagues (2001) developed a global problem-solving intervention they called Cognitive Orientation to Daily Occupational Performance (CO-OP). CO-OP is a cognitively-based, child-centered approach that focuses on increasing functional performance through the use of specific strategies. CO-OP emphasizes a problem-solving approach and uses adult-guided discovery of child and task-specific strategies. Goals are ecologically valid and performed in a realistic setting. Practice focuses on the child's ability to select, apply, evaluate, and monitor task-specific cognitive strategies. Emphasis is placed on facilitating transfer and generalization of the newly learned strategies.

Miller and colleagues (2001) compared the effectiveness of using CO-OP with a Contemporary Treatment Approach (CTA). The CTA included a variety of approaches such as neuromuscular, multisensory, and biomechanical, focusing on motor aspects of skill acquisition. Both interventions resulted in significant improvement as measured on the Canadian Occupational Performance Measure, with children receiving CO-OP making greater gains than the CTA group. Follow-up data measured by parent perception indicated that children who received CO-OP tended to experience greater long-term maintenance of their motor goals (8 of 8 compared to 2 of 7). Using a scale of 1 to 10, parents reported their perception of how useful the treatment was. They rated the CO-OP intervention as more useful (mean of 8.69 for the CO-OP parent group and mean of 7.71 for the CTA parent group). A complete explanation of the CO-OP approach is found in volume 20 (special issue), number 2/3 of *Physical and Occupational Therapy in Pediatrics*, 2001.

A motor learning approach is the third intervention recommended for children with DCD and includes task-specific interventions. These interventions emphasize focused practice of activity limitations or participation in life situations identified by the child. Motor learning research would suggest that to decrease the problems with body function associated with DCD, procedural interventions must include the specific functional task or motor skill training practiced in its appropriate functional environment (Gentile, 1992; Gentile, 1998).

The physical therapist's role within a motor learning context is to ecologically analyze the task that the child with DCD cannot perform (Burton & Davis, 1996), estab-

lish a hypothesis of why the task is difficult for the child, plan the procedural interventions related to the hypothesis, and use repeated practice in environments where the task occurs. Feedback is provided consistent with the child's current stage of learning, using targeted verbal instructions, demonstration, and modeling strategies. Gentile (1998) stressed that direct handling techniques by the therapist should not be used because handling becomes a variable of the environment which is not present during independent performance of the task. Intervention strategies are changed when the expected outcome is not being achieved. Retention of the task with generalization of the skill to multiple environments is the primary outcome goal.

When underlying problems with body function are hypothesized to be part of the reason a child cannot learn a specific task, procedural interventions should include activities such as the following: (1) improving static balance by standing on one foot to put on a boot, kicking a stationary ball, or standing in line without touching the people or objects in close proximity; (2) increasing muscle strength in hand muscles needed for handwriting; (3) improving memory by verbally identifying and then repeating the sequences for a task such as shoe-tying; (4) improving visual perception used for cutting skills; and (5) practicing attending to visual, auditory, or kinesthetic performance feedback information, such as watching in a mirror or trying to listen to the sounds generated when skipping and using this information to make a different response next time.

If, for example, participation in school is restricted because of the student's inability to quickly and safely climb stairs between classes, isolated time with the physical therapist can initially be used to improve strength and endurance of hip and knee extensor muscles by repeatedly practicing going up and down the school stairs. The therapist can assist the student to verbally identify and rehearse the motor sequence needed to reciprocally climb a flight of stairs and then practice the timing and order of the sequence in isolation until stair climbing can be performed faster and safely (Fig. 19-6**A**). Then, the physical therapist would instruct others so that the task can be repeated during the school day, but with extra time allowances, modified disturbances from other students, and prompted feedback by an educational associate or teacher (Fig. 19-6**B**). This can be combined with additional practice at home in a quieter environment and with prompting from a parent. Finally, reciprocal stair climbing would be performed during normal transition times between classes with typical numbers of other students, without prompts, and without adult guidance (Fig. 19-6**C**).

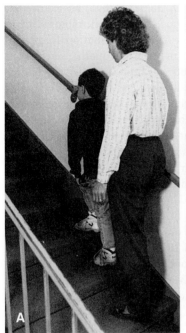
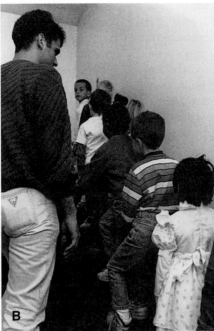
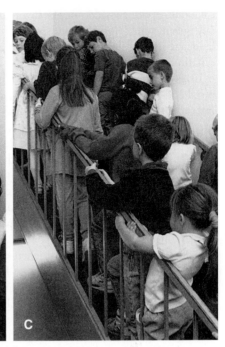

◆ **Figure 19-6**   **A**, During the first stages of learning, natural environments are used with direct instruction from the physical therapist. **B**, During later stages of learning, natural environments and modified distractions are used with faded feedback from the classroom associate. **C**, Stair climbing is now performed in its natural environment with typical environmental distractions. The child is expected to monitor his own performance and make corrections as needed.

INTERVENTION RELATED TO TEACHING, COLLABORATIVE CONSULTATION, AND COMMUNICATION

The *Guide to Physical Therapist Practice* (2001) lists three components of intervention: (1) coordination, communication, and documentation; (2) client-related instruction; and (3) procedural interventions. The previous section focused on procedural interventions directed at changes in body function or activity limitations and in some cases participation restrictions. Some believe that an important (Dewey & Wilson, 2001) or even the primary (Gubbay, 1978) benefit of an evaluation for DCD is the follow-up consultation that allows the physical therapist the opportunity to discuss restrictions in activity and participation with the child, the parents, and school personnel. Interventions related to teaching, coordination, and communication among the family, school personnel, and the community lessen the impact of environmental and personal-contextual factors that may restrict participation. Family members and school personnel are key players in improving outcomes for children with DCD. The physical therapist should always provide parents and school personnel a written activity plan to be imple-

mented at home and at school. Meaningful learning takes place over time and in multiple environments. Daily environmental modifications and task adaptations are critical for improved performance and motor learning for the child with DCD (Gubbay, 1975; Gillberg, 1998; Dewey & Wilson, 2001).

Helping parents to understand their child's motor limitations is an important component of secondary prevention and risk management (Missiuna et al., 2003). Family and cultural expectations can be inconsistent with a child's motor abilities. Expecting proficiency in competitive sports or dance or valuing perfect penmanship can lead to frustration and unhappiness for everyone. Therapists can help families and children match interests and skills with expectations that lead to success. When parents can analyze a play situation in their neighborhood or community recreation program to determine which motor skills are interfering with their child's ability to participate, the play situation can be adapted to maximize their child's participation and help prevent the imposition of societal limitations on full participation in community activities.

Coordination and communication with other disciplines are also important components of physical therapy intervention. DCD is a multifaceted disability and more than one service provider may be involved with a child at any given time. If delays in speech and poor social language skills are associated with developmental incoordination, intervention by a speech and language pathologist is appropriate. Goals related to improved word recall and retrieval or verbal sequencing of multiple-step instructions may be appropriate. If oral-motor impairments are related to motor production, goals should be directed at improving articulation and fluency of speech.

Occupational therapists (OTs) in school settings are often best suited to assist teachers and to provide interventions related to handwriting. OTs can also address classroom and home modifications that can remediate problems related to organization and spatial orientation in changing environments.

Adapted physical education teachers can consult with regular physical education teachers to help modify the curriculum so that the child with DCD can participate and be successful. Children with DCD have a lower activity level than their peers (Bouffard et al., 1996), have decreased anaerobic power, and have decreased muscle strength (O'Beirne et al., 1994). If a child cannot run fast enough or safely without falling, then games such as baseball can be modified so that a designated runner is used or players are grouped in teams for all activities with one person hitting and one person running or one person catching and one person throwing. In addition, peer helpers can be identified to help the child with DCD practice basic motor skills such as hopping, jumping, or skipping. Wilson and Sugden (1998) used a 5-week school-based program carried out by teachers with guidance from a physical educator. All 19 children with DCD demonstrated improvement although they still had significant motor problems.

If distractibility and attending-to-task are identified problems, a school psychologist might consult with the classroom teacher to identify ways that classroom materials can be modified to minimize the number of separate pieces of paper, books, and pencils needed to complete a project. Or a behavior modification program might be started to reinforce class work that is turned in on time and completed consistent with the instructions given. The psychologist can also assist the physical therapist in managing disruptive or otherwise negative behaviors that interfere with learning motor skills.

When concerns regarding distractibility and hyperactivity arise, a referral to a physician should be considered for evaluation of possible attention deficit disorder or ADHD. Many children with ADHD but not DCD will appear clumsy. If they attend poorly, they will bump into and trip over objects in their environment. When ADHD is associated with DCD, Gillberg (2001) has coined the term DAMP (dysfunction of attention, motor control, and perception). If behavioral and emotional problems become apparent, they may warrant another referral to a physician. Distractibility has been identified in children with DCD (Hulme & Lord, 1986). Gubbay (1975) cited temper tantrums, frustration, poor self-esteem, depression, and rejection as possible problems. Shaw and colleagues (1982) concluded that children with learning disability and clumsiness had significantly lower self-esteem and were less happy than other children. If depression is serious, psychiatric intervention, medication, or counseling might be needed. Additional physical symptoms of abdominal pain, loss of bowel or bladder control unrelated to any physical problems, and headaches are often seen as children with DCD grow older (Levine, 1987). These complaints should be taken seriously, and previously unidentified medical conditions should be ruled out before other approaches to deal with the symptoms are implemented.

IS THE INTERVENTION WORKING?

Whatever intervention approach is used, it is imperative that the child benefit from the service. Ongoing reexamination including careful monitoring of outcomes related to the remediation of the identified activity limitation or participation restriction must occur frequently. Very few standardized examinations are useful to monitor and document change in performance of functional activities in children in naturally occurring environments. The School Function Assessment (Coster et al., 1998) was designed to meet this need for elementary school children. It contains three parts: a rating scale for participation in school activities in multiple environments, a rating of the physical and behavioral assistance and supports the student needs, and examination of performance on typical school activities.

IEPs, with measurable annual goals written in behavioral terms with specific performance criteria and evaluation schedules, are designed to be used to monitor individual intervention effectiveness within a school setting. Frequent data collection related to the progress of a specific IEP goal can be used to evaluate the pattern of change as opposed to a one-time posttest. This should lead to intervention changes when progress is not occurring as expected (David, 1996). Another alternative is the use of goal attainment scaling (Palisano et al., 1992). Five possible levels of specific functional attainment are individualized for a child to create a criterion-referenced measurement.

TRANSITION TO ADULTHOOD AND LIFELONG MANAGEMENT OF DCD

High school classes, learning to drive a car, and vocational exploration present new challenges for the adolescent with DCD. High schools have to provide individualized evaluation and modifications in driver education instruction for students with DCD when driver's education is offered as part of the general high school curriculum. If a student is in special education, the 1997 Amendments of IDEA (PL 105-17) state that a student's future needs, as they transition out of high school, must be assessed by age 14 and that a transition plan must be created that includes the identification of needed vocational services by the time the student is 16 years old. Referral to the state vocational rehabilitation agency for evaluation and future service provision can also be pursued before graduation from high school.

It is now apparent that issues related to DCD are lifelong for many, if not all, individuals with DCD. The following quote from a 26-year-old woman with a learning disability supports this conclusion (Cermak & Henderson, 1985, p. 235):

> Motor activities are also a problem; my muscles don't seem to remember past motions. Despite the many times I've walked down steps and through doors, I still have to think about how high to lift my foot and about planning my movements . . . I'm physically inept; I can bump into the same table ten times running. I'm always bruised and as a child people constantly labeled me as clumsy. Physical education courses were hell as a child, especially gymnastics . . . I cannot begin to explain the terror or disorientation.

Physical therapy reexamination needs to include the discussion of the prevention of secondary problems in adolescents with DCD. The identification of strategies to prevent impairments in body function from limiting activity or restricting participation can be one of the most important outcomes of physical therapy intervention. Musculoskeletal or neuromuscular problems that would signal the need for a future episodes of physical therapy care should be discussed, as the changing environment and variables related to growth may place new demands on these systems. Preventive initiatives are needed as adults with DCD often have decreased strength, experience pain, have poor aerobic capacity, and poor endurance. Weight training, treadmill walking, and proper posture and joint protections should be encouraged. The physical therapist can assist the individual with DCD to identify and participate in appropriate community fitness programs.

Goals for lifelong leisure and recreational activity should be discussed with young adults. Activities should minimize competition and the need for quick motor responses. Swimming is likely to be more fun and more successful than playing tennis. Singing in a community choir may be a better choice than playing in a community basketball league. Riding a bike for exercise and enjoyment would be more appropriate than participating in a volleyball competition.

Vocational choices are important decisions for the individual with DCD. Jobs that minimize the need for changing motoric and environmental expectations should be emphasized. Based on Henderson and Sugden's (1992) four level categorization of motor skill difficulty, vocations that have skills in which neither the individual nor the environment is moving or changing would be top choices. Vocations in which the individual is moving and the environment is changing would be difficult (Box 19-3).

◼ SUMMARY

DCD represents a cluster of characteristics affecting approximately 5% of the regular school-aged population. The exact etiology is unknown, but DCD appears to have both motor production and cognitive-linguistic components. Physical therapists play a role both in identifying the impairments of body function and activity limitations associated with DCD and in providing intervention to prevent or minimize the participation restrictions related to the person and environment that might otherwise occur. DCD is a lifelong disability that presents challenges for adults as well as children. Physical therapists function as members of the comprehensive team needed to manage the multiple ramifications of DCD and its many associated learning and medical problems.

CASE STUDY

EVAN

Evan is currently 19 years old. At the adjusted age of 19 months, Evan's pediatrician referred him to a developmental disabilities clinic at a university-affiliated facility. As a part of this evaluation, Evan was seen by a physical therapist. This initial point in the decision making process would correspond to Step 1, the collection of initial data, of the hypothesis-oriented algorithm for

Box 19-3	Examples of Occupations Categorized by Motor Skill Difficulty	
	ENVIRONMENT	
INDIVIDUAL	**STABLE**	**CHANGING**
Stationary	Secondary school and college teaching Managerial occupations Psychologist Data processing Budget analyst	Air traffic controller Preschool and early elementary teaching
Moving	Custodian Mail carrier Gardener Nurse Restaurant waiter	Fire fighter Physical education teacher Athlete in competitive sports Driving a car in urban areas

clinicians (HOAC) by Rothstein and Echternach (1986). The physical therapist reviewed Evan's medical history and interviewed his parents to gather the following information. Evan was born at 32 weeks' gestation and was treated at a neonatal intensive care unit for respiratory distress syndrome and cardiac enlargement. At the adjusted age of 16 months, eye surgery was performed to correct a persistent strabismus on the left. Evan lives with his parents and was enrolled in a community day care program. Evan sat alone at 7 months, creeped on hands and knees at 10 months, and started walking at 16 months (all ages adjusted for prematurity).

The second step in HOAC is to generate a problem statement. The initial problem statements by Evan's family, with the physical therapy–related problem stated in parentheses, were: Does Evan have significant motor delays (impairments or functional limitations)? If so, can he catch up to his age expectations and continue to develop normally (can they be remediated by physical therapy intervention)? What can we, his parents, do to help him (can future motor disabilities and societal limitations be prevented by training and education)? Although Evan's goals were not identified until his first IEP meeting, the HOAC suggests establishing initial goals before the examination. A possible initial goal for Evan could have been: Evan will demonstrate the motor skills of a 2-year-old by the time his adjusted age is 24 months.

The physical therapy examination results when Evan was 19 months old (adjusted age) included the following: joint range of motion within normal limits, posture normal except for a slightly rounded back in sitting, and low muscle tone in Evan's trunk, but slightly increased muscle tone in the lower extremities on physical exertion, especially when Evan tried to move from back-lying to

sitting. Backward protective extension response in sitting could not be elicited, and asymmetric weight bearing was present in standing with the right leg internally rotated and the pelvis retracted on the right. Gross motor skills on the Motor Scale of the Bayley Scales of Infant Development (Bayley, 1969) were around the 13-month level (a raw score of 48 and a Psychomotor Developmen-tal Index of 66). Evan could throw a ball but could not walk sideways or backward. Speech and language and cognitive scores were also around the 13- to 15-month level. Step 3 of HOAC is the examination as just described. A working hypothesis about the feasibility of the pre-established goal can now be made. At this point in time, owing to Evan's young age, the examination resulted in an evaluation diagnosis of developmental delay, not DCD. Referrals to other disciplines included a referral to the local early childhood special education program.

This evaluation represented a crucial point in decision making for the physical therapist. Are Evan's slightly abnormal physical findings and motor delay significant enough to warrant (1) outpatient physical therapy, (2) physical therapy consultation with the family and day care personnel, or (3) recommendations for regular gross motor experiences through the day care? In this case, this decision was left up to the local physical therapist employed by the early childhood special education program.* A follow-up evaluation appointment at the clinic (including physical therapy) was made for 1 year later.

---

* In the state that Evan lived, special education programs were available to all eligible children beginning at birth. With the passage of IDEA Amendments of 1997, Part C, Evan's early intervention needs would now be evaluated and served through the development of an Individualized Family Service Plan (IFSP).

The local physical therapist evaluated Evan at his day care setting and interviewed the day care personnel and Evan's parents. Procedures performed at the developmental disabilities clinic 2 months previously were not repeated. Some gains in gross motor skills were noted. Evan could now walk sideways and backward and up and down stairs with help but still could not stand on one foot alone or jump. Gross motor scores were scattered from 19 to 21 months (chronologic age = 23 months, adjusted to 21 months) on the Early Learning Accomplishment Profile for Young Children (Glover et al., 1978), which was administered by the early intervention preschool teacher.*

Movement quality remained a concern, however. During play, Evan was observed to prefer to "W-sit" and would "bunny-hop" at times rather than creeping reciprocally. Movements lacked trunk rotation, and his gait still had awkward characteristics that included a wide base, low arm guard, and slightly bent hips and knees. No asymmetries were noted during the observation, but day care staff confirmed that asymmetries were sometimes present. Working hypotheses by the local physical therapist were as follows:

1. Delays can be remediated by normal preschool motor experiences.
2. Abnormal movement patterns are a concern and could interfere with future motor development.

Therefore, intervention consisting of consultative physical therapy services is warranted to train family members and day care providers to provide specific motor experiences for Evan so that future problems are prevented. Evan's IEP objectives included the following:

1. When playing spontaneously at day care, Evan will use three different sitting positions during a 20-minute free-play session on three consecutive observations. Day care staff will observe play and record the number and type of sitting positions used during three randomly chosen times per week.
2. When participating in structured gross motor play experiences, Evan will use a walking pattern that includes reciprocal arm swing when observed on three of four occasions per play session. Day care staff will observe and record data once a week.

3. Evan will be able to walk up and down his stairs at home without assistance. His parents will observe this once a week and record Evan's stair climbing pattern on data sheets provided by the physical therapist.*

A home and day care program stressing positioning during play, games to promote trunk rotation, smooth transitions between postures, and general gross motor skills for 2-year-old children was written. Progress monitoring procedures were initiated; a sample is illustrated in Figure 19-7. The preschool teachers collected periodic data, and the early childhood special education teacher monitored the program every week during her visits. Physical therapy reevaluation took place every 3 months (steps 5 and 6 of HOAC). Program modifications were made periodically and the initial episode of intervention consisted of seven visits over 19 months. The return visit to the developmental disabilities clinic was eventually canceled because Evan's parents did not believe that another evaluation was necessary and did not want to take the extra time off work.

After 9 months of service (when Evan was 32 months old) the physical therapist employed by the early childhood education program noted that backward protective extension was observed spontaneously during play and movements with trunk rotation were seen more frequently.

"W-sitting" was still occasionally observed, but so were other types of sitting postures. Evan's gross motor skills as measured on the Brigance Diagnostic Inventory of Early Development (Brigance, 1978) were scattered from a 2-year (jumping off floor) to a 3-year age-level (alternated feet going up stairs with railing).†

Evan's gait pattern still reflected some internal rotation on the right and some toe dragging. Asymmetries inconsistently appeared and then disappeared but were never significant enough to warrant consideration of other diagnoses, such as hemiplegia from cerebral palsy. Day care staff reported that Evan disliked walking outside in the sand and strongly disliked having his socks removed.

The day care and home programs were modified to reflect Evan's new skills and to include activities that

---

* It is not uncommon to see a significant change in gross motor scores in a short time, especially when different examinations are used or when only a few items per age level appear on a test. The achievement of only a few new skills can move a motor score to a higher developmental-age level. For example, within a short time span of a few weeks, a 24-month-old child successfully passes items 56 and 57 on the Motor Scale of the Bayley Scales of Infant Development, "Walks with one foot on walking board" and "Stands up: II" (Bayley, 1969). The Psychomotor Developmental Index then changes from 77 to 87 with age placement changing from 17.8 months to 21.9 months.

* These objectives would now appear as outcomes in Evan's Individualized Family Service Plan, but, when written, Part C of the Individuals with Disabilities Education Act Amendments of 1997 was not in effect.
†This may seem like a large range in developmental levels, but it is very common, especially between 2 and 3 years of age when there are, again, very few items on most motor scales. In addition to wide ranges in motor levels due to test characteristics, clinical experience would support the finding that children with developmental clumsiness often display scattered motor skill profiles.

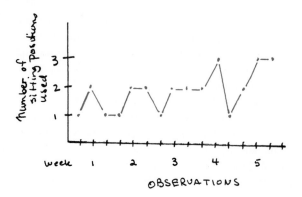

Week	Date	Type of sitting	Total positions used
1	9-10	w-sit	1
	9-12	w-sit, ring sit	2
	9-13	w-sit	1
2	9-17	w-sit	1
	9-18	w-sit, long sit	2
	9-21	w-sit, ring sit	2
3	9-25	w-sit	1
	9-27	w-sit, ring sit	2
	9-28	w-sit, modified ring	2
4	10-1	w-sit, modified ring	2
	10-4	w-sit, long sit, ring	3
	10-5	w-sit	1
5	10-9	w-sit, cross-leg	2
	10-10	w-sit, long, ring	3
	10-12	w-sit, cross-leg, long	3

◆ **Figure 19-7** Progress monitoring chart and graph for Evan.

encouraged sensory experiences, especially involving Evan's hands and feet.

When Evan was 3 years, 6 months old, an educational staffing was held. Reassessment, step 9 of HOAC, revealed that Evan had met his IEP objectives and that no new functional motor goals requiring physical therapy services were identified. Therefore, physical therapy was discontinued.

This is a critical point in the decision-making process for the physical therapist and the IEP team. The primary criteria for discharge, as described in the *Guide to Physical Therapist Practice* (American Physical Therapy Association, 2001), is achievement of anticipated goals and desired outcomes. Continuing physical therapy services beyond a

beneficial level would be an overutilization of service and a violation of some state licensure laws and the American Physical Therapy Association Standards of Practice for Physical Therapy (American Physical Therapy Association, 2000). Physical therapy should continue only when the skilled expertise of a physical therapist is needed. In this case, the IEP team including the physical therapist determined that the early childhood special education teacher had the skills needed to monitor Evan's motor behaviors.

Some concerns still existed because Evan would occasionally bump into objects and at times seemed oblivious to his surroundings. He was starting to avoid some gross motor play experiences, but day care staff believed that this was not yet a significant problem and were aware that the physical therapist could always be asked to consult again, if needed. Other areas of development continued to be slightly delayed and inconsistencies in performance were increasing. For example, with a chronologic age of 3 years, 6 months, Evan's intelligence quotient (IQ) score on the Stanford-Binet Intelligence Scale—Form L-M (Terman & Merrill, 1973) was 91 ± 3. Four subtests from the Illinois Test of Psycholinguistic Abilities (Kirk et al., 1968) indicated that Evan's auditory reception and association were at or slightly above age level, but his scores for visual reception and association were delayed 1 to 1.5 years. The occupational therapist reported that Evan could not imitate block designs but when given verbal guidance, he repeated the directions to himself and successfully completed the design. The team decided that Evan would benefit from a half-day preschool special education program. He returned to the day care program in the afternoon.

Evan's educational program was reviewed when he was 4 years old and referrals for an occupational therapy and adapted physical education evaluation were made. The occupational therapy evaluation revealed joint laxity, especially in Evan's fingers and hands. His fine motor scores were around the 3-year level on the Peabody Developmental Motor Scales (Folio & Fewell, 1983). Dressing skills, as measured by a few items on the Peabody Fine Motor Scales, were also delayed. He was able to remove socks and a cap and lace a shoe through three holes but could not unbutton buttons. Functionally, Evan could not put on his jacket or a pullover shirt. A 6-month trial period of occupational therapy service was recommended. Individual weekly sessions with the physical education teacher were offered in addition to the group gross motor experience he was already receiving.

Evan's parents and preschool teacher were especially concerned about his poor visual skills. An evaluation was requested at the vision clinic at the university-affiliated facility where he was initially evaluated. A computed tomographic scan and electroretinogram were performed with normal results. Slightly decreased visual acuity was identified as well as persistent "lazy eye" syndrome. Eye patching was recommended. Problems with visual perception were noted, and the ophthalmologist anticipated that Evan would have difficulty with depth perception.

After 6 months of occupational therapy, Evan's IEP objectives related to dressing and fine motor skills were implemented by the teacher of the preschool special education class. Occupational therapy was discontinued because the IEP team decided that the early childhood special education teacher could appropriately meet Evan's short-term objectives without the additional expertise of the occupational therapist. The logic behind this decision was similar to the decision to discontinue physical therapy when Evan was 3.5 years old.

This cycle of hypothesis-oriented problem solving was repeated when Evan was 6 years old. A reevaluation by special education personnel identified him as learning disabled and a special class with integration into first grade was recommended for the next school year. Adapted physical education services were continued, and new occupational and physical therapy evaluations were recommended for the following fall.

Shortly after beginning first grade (at age 6.5), Evan was reevaluated by the physical therapist employed by the educational system. Evan's mother, his kindergarten teacher, and his special education consulting teacher were interviewed, and past medical and educational evaluations were read. Evan's teacher was especially concerned about his walking pattern. When walking down the hall, he often "bounced" from step-to-step, landing on his toes. He could walk appropriately on command but soon returned to this atypical pattern. A screening of gross motor skills using the Brigance Diagnostic Inventory of Early Development (Brigance, 1978) was performed by the adapted physical education teacher and revealed that Evan's skills were generally around the 5-year level, but some skills were scattered up to his age level. Evan's mother was pleased with the progress he had made over the years and had no concerns related to his walking or outdoor play.

The physical therapist observed Evan in the classroom, walking down the school hallway, at recess, and in physical education class. Playground skills were observed to be safe and generally consistent with Evan's peer group. Evan's mother was asked to send summer shorts and a tank top to school, and an individual evaluation was performed in the school gymnasium. A postural examination revealed scapular winging (right greater than left), a functional kyphosis, and diminished lordosis when standing. Subjectively, muscle tone appeared to be slightly low with elbow and knee hyperextension bilaterally. The Hughes Basic Gross Motor Assessment (Hughes, 1979) was administered and Evan's overall score was 12 of an expected score of 33 for 6-year-olds (The Hughes Basic Gross Motor Assessment is now out of print and the Movement Assessment Battery for Children [Henderson & Sugden, 1992] would be an appropriate substitution.) Considerable difficulties were noted with any skill requiring motor planning. Movement quality was questionable with awkward, slow, and sometimes jerky responses in attempts at new skills and skills requiring dynamic balance (especially heel-to-toe walking, skipping, hopping, or ball-handling skills). The physical therapist noticed that

Evan had difficulty imitating postures and following verbal directions.*

This time the cycle of hypothesis-oriented problem solving generated a problem statement related to Evan's walking pattern and performance in physical education. Although the term *developmental coordination disorder* had not yet appeared in the Diagnostic and Statistical Manual of Mental Disorders, the description of motor problems by Evan's teacher met the criteria for *clumsy child syndrome*. The problem statement in essence was: Can physical therapy improve Evan's coordination and make his walking look normal? The results of the physical therapy examination were consistent with the current definition of DCD and the physical therapist's working hypothesis was that Evan does have a motor disability that cannot be easily remediated but can be lessened by modifying the environment in the classroom and by removing societal limitations so that Evan can participate in a modified physical education class with peers. Physical therapy intervention beyond an initial consultation was not provided because Evan had safe and functional mobility skills at school. Family and education personnel were made aware of factors that may require a new episode of care.

The collaboration between the physical therapist and the adapted physical education teacher led to the identification of appropriate activities to promote static balance, improve erect postures, and increase shoulder girdle stability and general upper extremity and hand strength. The physical education class was already participating in a unit on general fitness, so the physical education teacher added wheelbarrow walking, crab-walking, and modified push-ups to the other activities the entire class performed. During their next unit on ball skills, the physical education teacher planned to use a variety of different sizes and weights of balls to increase grip strength and two-handed throwing. Students in a fifth-grade peer-helper program helped Evan practice balance skills such as one-foot standing, "Simon-says" games, and "stop-and-go" movements to music to encourage static

posture imitation. Strategies to improve motor planning such as verbal labeling and rehearsing of motor sequences before skill performance were also implemented.

The classroom teacher was asked to monitor Evan's walking pattern and to notify the physical therapist if there was an increase in the number of times Evan fell or tripped. Evan's teacher, with the assistance of the school psychologist, also decided to try a behavior modification system of verbal or visual prompts to change Evan's walking pattern if it did not improve with the added emphasis on motor skills in physical education class. Suggestions were also given to the classroom teacher to modify Evan's desk and chair height to improve his sitting posture in class, especially for written work. A straight, wooden chair was found that allowed Evan's feet to rest flat on the floor. Nonslip material was added to his chair to prevent him from slipping forward. (Evan's previous chair was molded plastic and was very slippery.) These changes also helped to promote an anterior pelvic tilt and back extension (Fig. 19-8).

Evan's fine motor skills in the classroom were becoming more of a concern and, following a reevaluation by occupational therapy, an IEP meeting was held to add occupational therapy consultation. IEP objectives were identified for Evan to promote the use of new learning strategies when writing and when using scissors, and to improve Evan's ability to button, snap, and zip clothing. The entire IEP team including Evan's parents identified strategies to improve visual and motor sequencing during classroom activities and agreed to use the same strategies when Evan dressed at school or home.

At the end of first grade, the occupational therapist reported that Evan could button and unbutton medium-sized buttons on a "dressing vest" he used for practice. He was able to unbutton his own shirt that had small buttons, but he still needed assistance with the two upper buttons. Evan now understood the placement of each of his hands for buttoning and how the button must be manipulated. The occupational therapist reported that much of Evan's improvement was related to his increased attention span and concentration skills. Evan's mother was asked if she could come to school to observe these new dressing skills so that they could be practiced over the summer.

When Evan was in second grade, occupational therapy was discontinued because Evan's dressing skills were functional. Consultation to the classroom teacher was offered to assist with ongoing visuoperceptual problems during academic tasks such as writing. Evan continued to receive instruction in a special class with other students also identified as learning disabled, but he spent 2 hours a day in regular second grade and attended music, art, physical education, lunch, and recess with his second-grade peers.

---

* The apparent discrepancy between Evan's score of approximately 5 years on the Brigance Inventory (Brigance, 1978) and the lower score on the Hughes Basic Gross Motor Assessment (Hughes, 1979) is not surprising. These two tests are designed for different purposes. The Brigance Inventory (Brigance, 1978) is a criterion-referenced, developmental inventory sequenced for task analysis of motor behaviors without rigid administration procedures. The Hughes Gross Motor Assessment (Hughes, 1979) is a test designed specifically to identify minor motor dysfunction in children who appear to perform motor skills reasonably well. Children with DCD would be expected to perform better on a general inventory of skills than on a test with items specifically designed to identify the qualitative factors of performance.

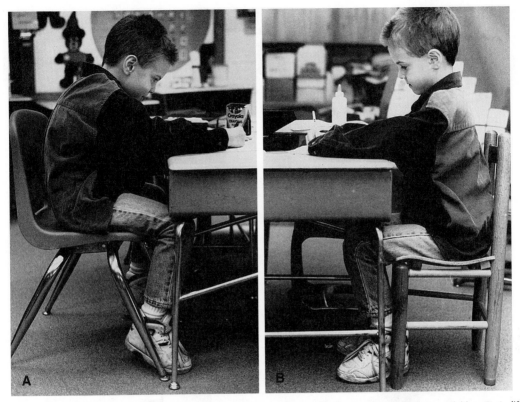

◆ **Figure 19-8** **A**, This child demonstrates poor posture that interferes with fine motor classroom activities. **B**, A different desk and chair improve this child's posture and improve the precision of his fine motor activities.

Adapted physical education collaborative consultation with the regular physical education teacher was continued.

Throughout elementary school Evan's parents and his educational team knew that a physical therapist was available to answer questions, but no new concerns arose. Evan's ongoing problems related to DCD (difficulty planning and sequencing new motor activities, poor balance in environments with changing surfaces and many obstacles, and occasional falls) were managed by other members of his educational team.

In seventh grade at a middle school Evan continues to receive resource instructional assistance and consultative adapted physical education. Evan still stands with his knees slightly bent (right more than left) and demonstrates a "bouncy" gait without a heel-strike. However, he has no difficulty moving around the larger school building. He attends physical education class with other seventh graders (Fig. 19-9). His physical education teacher reports that Evan is weak and small compared with his peers. He participates in all the activities but performs them at his own rate and performance level. Evan is on task 80% to 90% of the time during warm-up activities. The only difficulties

so far are frequent conflicts with the other boys. The physical education teacher believes that sometimes Evan solicits the conflict but that other times Evan is "picked on" by the other boys.

The adapted physical education teacher repeated an examination using the Bruininks-Oseretsky Test of Motor Proficiency (Bruininks, 1978) (Fig. 19-10). Evan's composite gross motor score yielded an age equivalency of 5 years, 9 months (standard score of 16), and his composite fine motor score age equivalency was 5 years, 8 months (standard score of 7). Although this test identifies Evan's developmental motor level, it is inappropriate for Evan to engage in 5- to 6-year-old gross motor activities when he is 12 years old. This information is used, instead, to modify regular middle school physical education activities.

No new motor concerns were expected to arise while Evan is attending middle school. Before the beginning of high school when Evan will move to an even larger building, the physical therapist, the special education consultant, and the adapted physical education teacher will discuss the transition issues that are related to Evan's DCD.

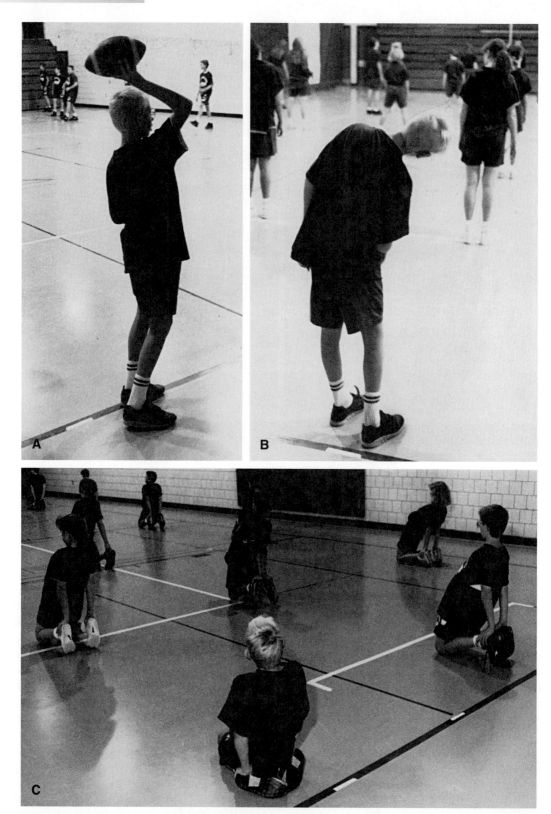

 • **Figure 19-9** Evan participates in regular physical education classes, but his motor performance is still qualitatively and quantitatively below his peers. **A**, Evan and his peers are throwing footballs. His poor form contributes to decreased distance and accuracy. **B**, During warm-up exercises, Evan moves his entire body instead of isolating "neck circles." **C**, Evan has difficulty following instructions for a stretching exercise.

BRUININKS-OSERETSKY TEST OF MOTOR PROFICIENCY / Robert H. Bruininks, Ph.D.

INDIVIDUAL RECORD FORM
COMPLETE BATTERY AND SHORT FORM

NAME _Evan_ _____ SEX: Boy ☒ Girl ☐ GRADE _7_

SCHOOL/AGENCY _Middle School_ CITY _____ STATE _____

EXAMINER _____ REFERRED BY _____

PURPOSE OF TESTING _re-evaluation_

Arm Preference: (circle one)
(RIGHT)   LEFT   MIXED

Leg Preference: (circle one)
RIGHT   (LEFT)   MIXED

	Year	Month	Day
Date Tested	___	___	___
Date of Birth	___	___	___
Chronological Age	12	9	9

Complete Battery:

SUBTEST	POINT SCORE Maximum	Subject's	STANDARD SCORE Test (Table 23)	Composite (Table 24)	PERCENTILE RANK (Table 25)	STANINE (Table 26)	OTHER Age equiv.
GROSS MOTOR SUBTESTS:							
1. Running Speed and Agility	15	6	2				5-11
2. Balance	32	19	3				5-8
3. Bilateral Coordination	20	9	6				7-11
4. Strength	42	16	5				4-11
GROSS MOTOR COMPOSITE			*16 SUM	20-	1-	1	5 9
5. Upper-Limb Coordination	21	7	*1				5-2
FINE MOTOR SUBTESTS:							
6. Response Speed	17	6	5				6-11
7. Visual-Motor Control	24	11	1				5-8
8. Upper-Limb Speed and Dexterity	72	21	1				5-8
FINE MOTOR COMPOSITE			*7 SUM	20-	1-	1	5 8
BATTERY COMPOSITE			*24 SUM	20-	1-	1	5 8

*To obtain Battery Composite: Add Gross Motor Composite, Subtest 5 Standard Score, and Fine Motor Composite. Check result by adding Standard Scores on Subtests 1-8.

Short Form:

	POINT SCORE Maximum	Subject's	STANDARD SCORE (Table 27)	PERCENTILE RANK (Table 27)	STANINE (Table 27)
SHORT FORM	98	___			

DIRECTIONS

Complete Battery:
1. During test administration, record subject's response for each trial.

2. After test administration, convert performance on each item (item raw score) to a point score, using scale provided. For an item with more than one trial, choose best performance. Record item point score in *circle* to right of scale.

3. For each subtest, add item point scores; record total in circle provided at end of each subtest and in Test Score Summary section. Consult *Examiner's Manual* for norms tables.

Short Form:
1. Follow Steps 1 and 2 for Complete Battery, except record each point score in *box* to right of scale.

2. Add point scores for all 14 Short Form items and record total in Test Score Summary section. Consult *Examiner's Manual* for norms tables.

AGS Published by American Guidance Service, Inc., Circle Pines, MN 55014

• **Figure 19-10**   Cover page from Evan's current Bruininks-Oseretsky Test of Motor Proficiency. *(From Bruininks-Oseretsky Test of Motor Proficiency: Individual Record Form by Robert H. Bruininks © 1978 American Guidance Service, Inc., 4201 Woodland Road, Circle Pines, Minnesota 55014-1796. All rights reserved.)*

EPILOGUE

Evan graduated from high school with his peers. He considered his high school experience to be very positive and enjoyed participating in the choir. He was especially excited to have the opportunity to sing the national anthem at the Special Olympics and at the State Fair. Evan's parents are very proud of his 3.2 grade point average. He was integrated into all classes except math. Evan attended a community college with hopes to eventually enter a recording engineering program at a state university.

REFERENCES

Als, H. A synactive model of neonatal behavioral organization: Framework for the assessment of neurobehavioral development in the premature infant and for support of infants and parents in the neonatal intensive care environment. In Sweeney, J (Ed.). The High-Risk Neonate: Developmental Therapy Perspectives. New York: Haworth Press, 1986, pp. 3–55.

Als, H, Duffy, FH, & McAnulty, G. Behavioral differences between preterm and full-term newborns as measured with the APIB system scores: I. Infant Behavior and Development, 11:305–319, 1988.

American Physical Therapy Association. Standards of Practice for Physical Therapy (Amended). Alexandria, VA: American Physical Therapy Association, 2000.

American Physical Therapy Association. Guide to physical therapist practice. Physical Therapy, 81:1–768, 2001.

American Psychiatric Association. Diagnostic and Statistical Manual of Mental Disorders—DSM-IV. Washington, DC: American Psychiatric Association, 1994.

Barnhart, RC, Davenport MJ, Epps SB, & Nordquist VM. Developmental coordination disorder. Physical Therapy, 83:722–731, 2003.

Bayley, N. Bayley Scales of Infant Development. San Antonio, TX: Psychological Corporation, 1969.

Blondis, TA. Motor disorders and attention-deficit/hyperactivity disorder. Pediatric Clinics of North America, 46:899–913, 1999.

Bouffard, M, Watkinson, EJ, Thompson, LP, Dunn, JLC, & Romanow, SKE. A test of the activity deficit hypothesis with children with movement difficulties. Adapted Physical Activity Quarterly, 13:61–73, 1996.

Brigance, AH. Inventory of Early Development. North Billerica, MA: Curriculum Associates, 1978.

Bruininks, R. Bruininks-Oseretsky Test of Motor Proficiency. Circle Pines, MN: American Guidance Services, 1978.

Burton, AW, & Davis, WE. Ecological task analysis: utilizing intrinsic measures in research and practice. Human Movement Science, 15:285–314, 1996.

Cantell, MH, Smyth, MM, & Ahonen, TP. Clumsiness in Adolescence: Educational, motor, and social outcomes of motor delay detected at 5 years. Adapted Physical Activity Quarterly, 11:115–129, 1994.

Cermak, S, & Henderson, A. Learning disabilities. In Umphred, D (Ed.). Neurological Rehabilitation. St. Louis: CV Mosby, 1985, pp. 207–249.

Cermak, SA, & Larkin, D. Developmental Coordination Disorder. Albany, NY: Delmar, 2002.

Clements, SD, David, JS, Edgington, R, Goolsby, CM, & Peters, JE. Two cases of learning disabilities. In Tarnopol, L (Ed.). Learning Disorders in Children: Diagnosis, Medication, Education. Boston: Little, Brown, 1971.

Cooke, RWI, & Abernethy, LJ. Cranial magnetic resonance imaging and school performance in very low birth weight infants in adolescence. Archives of Disease in Childhood Fetal Neonatal Edition 81:F11–F121, 1999.

Coster, W, Deeney, T, Haltiwanger, J, & Haley, S. School Function Assessment. San Antonio: The Psychological Corporation, 1998.

David, KS. Motor sequencing strategies in school-aged children. Physical Therapy, 65:883–889, 1985.

David, KS. Monitoring Progress for Improved Outcomes. Physical and Occupational Therapy in Children, 16:47–76:, 1996.

Dewey, D, & Kaplan, BJ. Subtyping of developmental motor deficits. Developmental Neuropsychology, 10:256–284, 1994.

Dewey, D, & Wilson, BN. Developmental coordination disorder: what is it? Physical & Occupational Therapy in Pediatrics, 20:5–27, 2001.

Dewey, D, Roy, E, Square-Storer, PA, & Hayden, D. Limb and oral praxic abilities of children with verbal sequencing deficits. Developmental Medicine and Child Neurology, 30:743–751, 1988.

Dugas, C, Gervais, C, & Girouard, Y. Clumsiness and developmental coordination disorder (DCD) are two separate motor problems. Actes du 11e Symposium international sur l'activite adaptee (SIAPA) Quebec: Institut de readaptation en deficience physique du Quebec, pp. 142–152, 1999.

Dwyer, C, & McKenzie, BE. Impairment of visual memory in children who are clumsy. Adapted Physical Activity Quarterly, 11:179–199, 1994.

Folio, MR, & Fewell, RR. Peabody Developmental Motor Scales, 2nd ed. San Antonio, TX: The Psychological Corporation/Therapy Skill Builders, 2000.

Fox, MA. Clumsiness in children: Developmental coordination disorder. Learning Disabilities: A Multidisciplinary Journal, 9:57–63, 1998.

Gaddes, W. Learning Disabilities and Brain Function: A Neuropsychological Approach. New York: Springer-Verlag, 1985.

Gentile, AM. The nature of skill acquisition: Therapeutic implications for children with movement disorders. Medical Sport Science, 36:31–40, 1992.

Gentile, AM. Implicit and explicit processes during acquisition of functional skills. Scandinavian Journal of Occupational Therapy, 5:7–16, 1998.

Geuze, R, & Borger, H. Children who are clumsy: Five years later. Adapted Physical Activity Quarterly, 10:10–21, 1993.

Geuze, RH, Jongman M, Schoemaker, M, & Smits-Engelsman, B. Editorial – developmental coordination disorder. Human Movement Science, 20:1–5, 2001.

Gillberg, C. Hyperactivity, inattention and motor control problems: Prevalence, comorbidity and background factors. Folia Phoniatrica et Logopaedica, 50:107–117, 1998.

Gillberg, C. ADHD with comorbid developmental coordination disorder: Long-term outcome in a community sample. The ADHD Report, 9:5–9, 2001.

Gillberg, C, Rasmussen, P, Carlstrom, G, Svenson, B, & Waldenstrom, E. Perceptual, motor and attentional deficits in six-year-old children: Epidemiological aspects. Journal of Child Psychology and Psychiatry, 23:131–144, 1982.

Glover, ME, Preminger, JL, & Sanford, AR. The Early Learning Accomplishment Profile for Young Children: Birth to 36 Months. Chapel Hill, NC, Chapel Hill Training-Outreach Project, 1978.

Gubbay, SS. The Clumsy Child: A Study of Developmental Apraxic and Agnosic Ataxia. London: WB Saunders, 1975.

Gubbay, SS. The management of developmental apraxia. Developmental Medicine and Child Neurology, 20:643–646, 1978.

Hadders-Algra, M. Two distinct forms of minor neurological dysfunction: Perspectives emerging from a review of data on the Groningen

Perinatal Project. Developmental Medicine & Child Neurology, 44:561–571, 2002.

Henderson, SE, & Sugden, D. Movement Assessment Battery For Children. London: The Psychological Corporation, 1992.

Henderson, L, Rose, P, & Henderson, S. Reaction time and movement time in children with a developmental coordination disorder. Journal of Child Psychology and Psychiatry, 33:895–905, 1992.

Hoare, D. Subtypes of developmental coordination disorder. Adapted Physical Activity Quarterly, 11:158–169, 1994.

Hoare, D, & Larkin, D. Kinaesthetic abilities of clumsy children. Developmental Medicine and Child Neurology, 33:671–678, 1991.

Holsti, L, Grunau, RV, & Whitfield, MF. Developmental coordination disorder in extremely low birth weight children at nine years. Journal of Developmental Behavior Pediatrics, 23:9–15, 2002.

Hughes, J. Hughes Basic Gross Motor Assessment. Yonkers, NY: GE Miller, 1979.

Huh, J, Williams, H, & Burke, J. Development of bilateral motor control in children with developmental coordination disorders. Developmental Medicine & Child Neurology, 40:474–484, 1998.

Hulme, C, & Lord, R. Clumsy children: A review of recent research. Child: Care, Health & Development, 12:257–269, 1986.

Jongman, M, Henderson, S, de Vries, L, & Dubowitz, L. Duration of periventricular densities in preterm infants and neurological outcome at 6 years of age. Archives of Disease in Childhood, 69:9–13, 1993.

Junaid, K, Harris, SR, Fulmer, A, & Carswell, A. Teachers' use of the MABC checklist to identify children with motor coordination difficulties. Pediatric Physical Therapy, 12:158–163, 2000.

Kadesjö, B. Attention deficits and clumsiness in Swedish 7-year-old children. Developmental Medicine & Child Neurology, 40:796–804, 1998.

Katschmarcky, S, Cairney, S, Maruff, P, Wilson, PH, & Currie, J. The ability to execute saccades on the basis of efference copy: impairments in double-step saccade performance in children with developmental coordination disorder. Experimental Brain Research, 136:73–78, 2001.

Kaufman, AS, & Kaufman, NL. Kaufman Assessment Battery for Children: Interpretive Manual. Circle Pines, MN: American Guidance Service, 1983.

Kertesz, A. Apraxia and aphasia: Anatomical and clinical relationship. In Roy, EA (Ed.). Neuropsychological Studies of Apraxia and Related Disorders. Amsterdam: North-Holland, 1985, pp. 163–178.

Kirk, SA, McCarthy, JJ, & Kirk, WD. Illinois Test of Psycholinguistic Abilities (rev. ed.). Urbana, IL: University of Illinois Press, 1968.

Knuckey, N, & Gubbay, S. Clumsy children: A prognostic study. Australian Pediatric Journal, 19:9–13, 1983.

Leemrijse, C, Meijer, OG, Vermeer, A, Lambregts, B, & Ader, HJ. Detecting individual change in children with mild to moderate motor impairment: The standard error of measurement of the Movement ABC. Clinical Rehabilitation, 13:420–429, 1999.

Levine, M. Developmental pediatrics: developmental dysfunction in the school-age child. In Behrman, R, & Vaughan, V (Eds.). Nelson Textbook of Pediatrics, 13th ed. Philadelphia: WB Saunders, 1987, pp. 84–95.

Lord, R, & Hulme, C. Kinesthetic sensitivity of normal and clumsy children. Developmental Medicine and Child Neurology, 29:720–725, 1987.

Losse, A, Henderson, SE, Ellimna, D, Hall, D, Knight, E, & Jongmans, M. Clumsiness in children—Do they grow out of it? A 10-year follow-up study. Developmental Medicine and Child Neurology, 33:55–68, 1991.

Lundy-Ekman, L, Ivry, R, Keele, S, & Woollacott, M. Timing and force control deficits in clumsy children. Journal of Cognitive Neuroscience, 3:367–376, 1991.

Mandich, A, Buckolz, E, & Polatajko, H. On the ability of children with developmental coordination disorder (DCD) to inhibit response initiation: the simon effect. Brain Cognition, 50:150–162, 2002.

Mandich, AD, Polatajko, HJ, Macnab, JJ, & Miller, LT. Treatment of children with developmental coordination disorder: What is the evidence? Physical and Occupational Therapy in Pediatrics, 20:51–68, 2001a.

Mandich, AD, Polatajko, HJ, Missiuna, C, & Miller, LT. Cognitive strategies and motor performance in children with developmental coordination disorder. Physical and Occupational Therapy in Pediatrics, 20:125–143, 2001b.

Martini, R, & Polatajko, HJ. Verbal self-guidance as a treatment approach for children with developmental coordination disorder: A systematic replication study. Occupational Therapy Journal of Research, 19:157–181, 1998.

Maruff, P, Wilson, P, Trebilcock, M, & Currie, J. Abnormalities of imaged motor sequences in children with developmental coordination disorder. Neuropsychologia, 37:1317–1324, 1999.

Miller, LT, Missiuna, CA, Macnab, JJ, Malloy-Miller, T, & Polatajko, HJ. Clinical description of children with developmental coordination disorder. Canadian Journal of Occupational Therapy, 68:5–15, 2001.

Missiuana, C, Rivard, L, & Bartlett, D. Early identification and risk management of children with developmental coordination disorder. Pediatric Physical Therapy, 15:32–38, 2003.

Missiuna, C, & Polatajko, H. Developmental dyspraxia by any other name: Are they all just clumsy children? The American Journal of Occupational Therapy, 49:619–627, 1994.

Miyahara, M, & Register, C. Perceptions of three terms to describe physical awkwardness in children. Research in Developmental Disabilities, 21:367–376, 2000.

Mon-Williams, MA, Wann, JJP, & Pascal, E. Visual-proprioceptive mapping in children with developmental coordination disorder. Developmental Medicine & Child Neurology, 41:247–254, 1999.

Murphy, J, & Gliner, J. Visual and motor sequencing in normal and clumsy children. Occupational Therapy Journal, 8:89–103, 1988.

Newborg, J, Stock, JR, Wnek, L, Guidubaldi, J, Svinicki, J, Dickson, J, & Markley, A. Battelle Developmental Inventory Examiner's Manual. Allen, TX: DLM Teaching Resources, 1984.

O'Beirne, C, Larkin, D, & Cable, T. Coordination problems and anaerobic performance in children. Adapted Physical Activity Quarterly, 11:141–149, 1994.

O'Brien, V, Cermak, S, & Murray, E. The relationship between visual-perceptual motor abilities and clumsiness in children with and without learning disabilities. American Journal of Occupational Therapy, 42:359–363, 1988.

Palisano, RJ, Haley, SM, & Brown, DA. Goal attainment scaling as a measure of change in infants with motor delays. Physical Therapy, 72:432–448, 1992.

Piek, JP, & Edwards, K. The identification of children with developmental coordination disorder by class and physical education teachers. British Journal of Educational Psychology, 67:55–67, 1997.

Pinto-Martin, JA, Whitaker, AH, Feldman, JF, Van Rossem, R, & Paneth, N. Relation of cranial ultrasound abnormalities in low-birthweight infants to motor or cognitive performance at ages 2, 6, and 9 years. Developmental Medicine and Child Neurology, 41:826–833, 1999.

Pless, M, Carlsson, M, Sundelin, C, & Persswon, K. Preschool children with developmental coordination disorder: A short-term follow-up of motor status at seven to eight years of age. Acta Paediatrica, 91:521–528, 2002.

Polatajko, HJ, Mandich, AD, Miller, LT, & Macnab, JJ. Cognitive Orientation to Daily Occupational Performance (CO-OP): Part II – The evidence. Physical and Occupational Therapy in Pediatrics, 20:83–106, 2001.

Rappaport, L, Urion, D, Strand, K, & Fulton, A. Concurrence of congenital ocular motor apraxia and motor problems: An expanded syndrome. Developmental Medicine and Child Neurology, 29:85–90, 1987.

Raynor, AJ. Fractional reflex and reaction time in children with developmental coordination disorder. Motor Control, 2:114–124, 1998.

Raynor, AJ. Strength, power, and coactivation in children with developmental coordination disorder. Developmental Medicine and Child Neurology, 43:676–684, 2001.

Rizzolatti, G, Luppino, G, & Matelli, M. Invited review: The organization of the cortical motor system: New concepts. Electroencephalography and Clinical Neurophysiology, 106:283–296, 1998.

Rösblad, B, & von Hofsten, C. Perceptual control of manual pointing in children with motor impairments. Physiotherapy Theory and Practice, 8:223–233, 1992.

Rothstein, JM, & Echternach, JL. Hypothesis-oriented algorithm for clinicians: A method for evaluation and treatment planning. Physical Therapy, 66:1388, 1986.

Rourke, BP, Bakker, D, Fisk, JL, & Strang, JD. The Neuropsychological Assessment of Children: A Treatment-Oriented Approach. New York: Guilford Press, 1986.

Rowe, JB, & Frackowiak, RSJ. The impact of brain imaging technology on our understanding of motor function and dysfunction. Current Opinions in Neurology, 9:728–734, 1999.

Schoemaker, MM, Hijlkema, MGJ, & Kalverboer, AF. Physiotherapy for clumsy children: An evaluation study. Developmental Medicine and Child Neurology, 36:143–155, 1994.

Segal, R, Mandich, A, Polatajko, H, & Cook, JV. Stigma and its management: A pilot study of parental perceptions of the experiences of children with developmental coordination disorder. American Journal of Occupational Therapy, 56:422–428, 2002.

Shaw, L, Levine, MD, & Belfer, M. Developmental double jeopardy: A study of clumsiness and self-esteem in children with learning problems. Developmental and Behavioral Pediatrics, 3:191–196, 1982.

Sigmundsson, H, Pedersen, AV, Whiting, HT, & Ingvaldsen, RP. We can cure your child's clumsiness! A review of intervention methods. Scandinavian Journal of Rehabilitation Medicine, 30:1001–1006, 1998.

Skinner, RA, & Piek, JP. Psychosocial implications of poor motor coordination in children and adolescents. Human Movement Science, 20:73–94, 2001.

Skorji, V, & McKenzie, B. How do children who are clumsy remember modeled movements? Developmental Medicine and Child Neurology, 39:404–408, 1997.

Smyth, TR. Abnormal clumsiness in children: A defect of motor programming? Child: Care, Health & Development, 17:283–294, 1991.

Smyth, MM, & Anderson, HI. Coping with clumsiness in the school playground: Social and physical play in children with coordination impairments. British Journal of Developmental Psychology, 19:389–413, 2000.

Soltesz, M, & Brockway, N. The high-risk infant. In Tecklin, J (Ed.). Pediatric Physical Therapy. Philadelphia: JB Lippincott, 1989, pp. 40–67.

Stott, DH, Moyes, FA, & Henderson, SE. Test of Motor Impairment. Guelph, Ontario: Brook Educational Publishing Limited, 1972.

Sugden, DA, & Chambers, ME. Intervention approaches and children with developmental coordination disorder. Pediatric Rehabilitation, 2:139–147, 1998.

Sugden, DA, & Wright, HC. Motor Coordination Disorders in Children. Developmental Clinical Psychology and Psychiatry, Vol. 39. Thousand Oaks, London: SAGE Publications, 1998.

Tarnopol, L, & Tarnopol, M. Brain Function and Reading Disabilities. Baltimore: University Park Press, 1977.

Terman, LM, & Merrill, MA. Stanford-Binet Intelligence Scale: Form L-M. Chicago: Riverside Publishing, 1973.

Ulrich, DA. Test of Gross Motor Development, 2nd ed. Austin, TX: Pro-Ed, 2000.

U.S. Department of Education. Twenty-third Annual Report to Congress on the Implementation of The Individuals with Disabilities Education Act, Washington, DC, U.S. Government Printing Office, 2001.

Van Dellen, T, & Geuze, R. Motor response processing in clumsy children. Journal of Child Psychology and Psychiatry and Allied Disciplines, 29:489–500, 1988.

van Der Fits, IBM, Flikweert, ER, Stremmelaar, EF, Martijn, A, & Hadders-Algra, M. Development of postural adjustments during reaching in preterm infants. Pediatric Research, 46:1–7, 1999.

van der Meulen, JHP, Denier van der Gon, JJ, Gielen, CCAM, Gooskens, RHJM, & Willemse, J. Visuomotor performance of normal and clumsy children: I. Fast goal-directed arm movements with and without visual feedback. Developmental Medicine and Child Neurology, 33:40–54, 1991a.

van der Meulen, JHP, Denier van der Gon, JJ, Gielen, CCAM, Gooskens, RHJM, & Willemse, J. Visuomotor performance of normal and clumsy children: II. Arm-tracking with and without visual feedback. Developmental Medicine and Child Neurology, 33:119–129, 1991b.

Visser, J, Geuze, RH, & Kalverboer, AF. The relationship between physical growth, level of activity and the development of motor skills in adolescence: Differences between children with DCD and controls. Human Movement Science, 17:573–608, 1998.

Volman, MJ, & Geuze, RH. Stability of rhythmic finger movement in children with a developmental coordination disorder. Motor Control, 2:34–60, 1998.

Williams, HG, Woollacott, MH, & Ivry, R. Timing and motor control in clumsy children. Journal of Motor Behavior, 24:165–172, 1992.

Willingham, DB. A neuropsychological theory of motor skill learning. Psychological Review, 105:558–584, 1998.

Wilson, PH, Maruff, P, Ives, S, & Currie, J. Abnormalities of motor and praxis imagery in children with DCD. Human Movement Science, 20:135–159, 2001.

Wilson, PH, & McKenzie, BE. Information processing deficits associated with developmental coordination disorder: A meta-analysis of research findings. Journal of Child Psychology & Psychiatry, 39:829–840, 1998.

Wilson, PH, Thomas, PR, & Maruff, P. Motor imagery training ameliorates motor clumsiness in children. Journal of Child Neurology, 17:491–498, 2002.

Wright, HC, & Sugden, DA. A school based intervention programme for children with Developmental Coordination Disorder. European Journal of Physical Education, 3:35–50, 1998.

Wright, HC, & Sugden, DA. Two step procedure for the identification of children with developmental coordination disorder in Singapore. Developmental Medicine and Child Neurology, 38:1099–1106, 1996.

Gubbay Tests of Motor Proficiency (Standardized for Children between the Ages of 8 and 12 Years)

THE ASSESSMENT OF THE CLUMSY CHILD

Test 1
Whistle through pouted lips.
The child is required to make a musical note of any pitch and
  intensity by blowing air through pouted lips.
Score: Pass or fail.

Test 2
Skip forward five steps.
Three attempts are allowed after demonstration of the test
  by the examiner (i.e., single hop on left leg, step, single
  hop on right leg, etc—without skipping rope).
Score: Pass or fail.

Test 3
Roll ball with foot.
The child is required to roll a tennis ball under the sole of the
  preferred foot (with or without footwear) in spiral fashion
  around 6 matchboxes placed 30 cm apart. The ball is
  permitted to touch a maximum of 3 matchboxes before
  disqualification. Three attempts are allowed before failure.
Score: Expressed in seconds' time or as failure.

Test 4
Throw, clap hands, then catch tennis ball.
The child is required to clap his or her hands to a maximum
  of 4 times after throwing a tennis ball upward and
  catching the ball with both hands. If able to catch the ball
  after 4 claps, the child is then required to catch the ball
  with one (either) hand after 4 claps. Three attempts are
  allowed before failure at any point.
Score: Expressed in one of the following seven categories:
  1. Cannot catch the ball with both hands.
  2. Can catch the ball with both hands after 0 claps.

3. Can catch the ball with both hands after 1 clap.
4. Can catch the ball with both hands after 2 claps.
5. Can catch the ball with both hands after 3 claps.
6. Can catch the ball with both hands after 4 claps.
7. Can catch the ball with preferred hand after 4 claps.

Test 5
Tie one shoelace with double bow (single knot).
The examiner's right shoelace with approximately 20-cm
  lengths protruding from the shoe is offered.
Score: Expressed in seconds' time or failure if greater than
60 seconds.

Test 6
Thread 10 beads.
The wooden beads are 3 cm in diameter with a bore of 0.8
  cm and the terminal 6 cm of the string is stiffened. (The
  beads are patented Kiddicraft toys that can be readily
  purchased.)
Score: Expressed in seconds' time.

Test 7
Pierce 20 pinholes.
The child is supplied with a stylus (long hatpin) and asked to
  pierce two successive rows of 0.1 inch × 0.1 inch
  (2.5 mm × 2.5 mm) squares on graph paper.
Score: Expressed in seconds' time.

Test 8
Posting box.
The child is required to fit six different plastic shapes in
  appropriate slots. (The posting box is a patented Kiddicraft
  toy that can be readily purchased.)
Score: Expressed in seconds' time or failure if greater than
60 seconds.

Gubbay, SS. The Clumsy Child: A Study of Developmental Apraxic and Agnosic Ataxia. London: WB Saunders, 1975, pp. 155–156.

Chapter 20

CHILDREN WITH MOTOR AND COGNITIVE IMPAIRMENTS

IRENE R. McEwen
PT, PhD

LAURA H. HANSEN
PT, MS

Children with cognitive impairments often have secondary or associated delays in motor development and may have problems with motor learning and motor control. This is especially true of children whose cognitive functioning is moderately or severely limited. Some children's motor problems are minimal, requiring little, if any, physical therapy. Other children have cerebral palsy and other neurologic, musculoskeletal, and cardiopulmonary impairments that require considerable attention by physical therapists and other members of service delivery teams.

Many of the physical therapy examination and intervention strategies used with children who have cognitive impairments differ little from approaches used with any child who has similar motor characteristics, as described in other chapters of this volume. The learning characteristics of children with cognitive impairments, however, can make it necessary to modify or supplement these approaches. These aspects of examination and intervention, along with current evidence-based and "best" practices in educational programs for children with cognitive impairments, are the foci of this chapter. This chapter will cover the definition, incidence, prevalence, etiology, pathophysiology, and prevention of cognitive impairments in children; team assessment; determining goals; intervention to limit impairments and activity limitations, prevent secondary impairments, and promote participation; and considerations for transition to adulthood. The chapter ends with three case studies that illustrate the chapter content. One case also illustrates application of the Guide to Physical Therapist Practice (2001).

DEFINITION OF COGNITIVE IMPAIRMENTS

The definition of cognitive impairments and the means by which children are identified as having cognitive impairments are, and have been, highly controversial (Evans, 1991; American Association on Mental Retardation [AAMR], 2002). Much of the controversy surrounds the risk of inappropriately classifying children of cultural and linguistic minorities as having cognitive impairments. The validity of this concern is supported by overrepresentation of children from cultural and linguistic minorities among children who have been labeled as having cognitive impairments and children placed in special education (Oswald et al., 2001; United States Department of Education [USDE], 2000; Zhang & Katsiyannis, 2002).

Children with motor and sensory impairments also are at risk for being labeled as having cognitive limitations when they do not or for being classified as having a greater degree of cognitive impairment than actually exists (Chinitz & Feder, 1992). This is especially true if the examiner has neither experience nor skill in examining children who require alternative input modes, such as manual signs, or alternative response modes, such as a communication board.

In the United States, the term *mental retardation* is often used by organizations and education and social service agencies to refer to the condition of people whose cognitive impairments were acquired before age 18 (AAMR, 2002). The definition of the term has evolved over the years from primary emphasis on intelligence test scores to an emphasis on individual functioning within natural environments. AAMR has proposed the most widely accepted definitions of mental retardation, which have served as a basis for many other definitions, including those used by school districts for placement of students in special education (AAMR, 2002).

In 2002, the AAMR board of directors adopted a new definition of mental retardation, which was intended to help change the way people with cognitive impairments are viewed. The definition is based on the supports people need within their own environments, rather than on an intelligence quotient (IQ)-derived level of cognitive functioning and incorporates the dimension of participation:

> Mental retardation is a disability characterized by significant limitations both in intellectual functioning and in adaptive behavior as expressed in conceptual, social, and practical adaptive skills. This disability originates before age 18. The following five assumptions are essential to the application of this definition: (1) limitations in present functioning must be considered within the context of community environments typical of the individual's age peers, and culture; (2) valid assessment considers cultural and linguistic diversity as well as differences in communication, sensory, motor, and behavioral factors; (3) within an individual, limitations often coexist with strengths; (4) an important purpose of describing limitations is to develop a profile of needed supports; (5) with appropriate personalized supports over a sustained period, the life functioning of the person with mental retardation generally will improve (AAMR, 2002, p. 1).

Although an IQ of 70 to 75 or below still is required for a diagnosis of mental retardation, the 2002 definition also includes adaptive behavior, participation, interactions and social roles, health, and context consistent with the *International Classification of Function, Disability and Health* (ICF) (World Health Organization [WHO], 2001). The 2002 definition emphasizes identification of the changing supports one needs over a lifetime to live successfully in the community, rather than simply on classification of the individual. Children labeled as having mental retardation who require supports to learn in school settings, for example, may not be labeled in adulthood when participating independently in home, work, and social roles (AAMR, 2002).

Other definitions of cognitive impairment or mental retardation have coexisted with the AAMR definition, including those used in the United States to qualify students for special education and for services for individuals with developmental disabilities. In the United States, Public Law 98-527, the Developmental Disabilities Act of 1984, authorized states to provide habilitation, medical, and social services for children and adults with cognitive impairments and, in some states, for people with other disabilities. The term "developmental disabilities" was defined in the most recent version of the Developmental Disabilities Assistance and Bill of Rights Act of 2000 (Public Law 106-402) as, "a severe, chronic disability that is attributable to a physical or mental impairment that is likely to continue throughout the person's life and results in functional limitations in three or more areas of life activities" (Sec. 102(8)(A)). The only important difference between this definition and the AAMR definition of mental retardation is that the definition of developmental disability has no IQ requirement and the age of onset can be as high as 22 years (AAMR, 2002). Because of the varying definitions of cognitive impairment and eligibility criteria, confusion can exist both within and between states as to who is considered to have cognitive impairment and who qualifies for which services. For this reason, physical therapists often need to seek information about programs in their own areas, the criteria for eligibility, and who is qualified to classify a child as having a cognitive impairment. Some programs provide wheelchairs, splints, and other equipment for children with cognitive impairments; other programs pay for services, such as physical therapy, respite care, and recreational activities.

For any child, a label of cognitive impairment primarily is useful as a "passport" to early intervention, special education, and other educational, social, and medical programs. Such a label provides little, if any, insight into the strengths of the individual or the services that are needed (AAMR, 2002; Evans, 1991) and may limit a child's opportunities if the label causes others to have inappropriate or inadequate expectations of the child's capabilities.

INCIDENCE AND PREVALENCE OF COGNITIVE IMPAIRMENTS

Reported estimates of incidence and prevalence of cognitive impairments vary widely. The differences are thought to be due to a number of factors, including variations in the definition; the methodologies employed; the sex, age, and communities of the samples; and the sociopolitical factors affecting the design and interpretation of the studies (Larson et al., 2001). Larson and colleagues (2001) used data from the 1994 and 1995 Disability Supplement of the National Health Interview Survey to estimate the prevalence of mental retardation and developmental disabilities among community-dwelling people in the United States. They estimated the prevalence of mental retardation to be 7.8 per 1000 people and the prevalence of developmental disability to be 11.3 per 1000 people. The combined prevalence of mental retardation and/or developmental disability was 14.9 per 1000 people. Others have criticized the study because data were collected using a telephone survey and respondents may have underreported disability (USDE, 2000). School districts reported approximately twice as many school-age children with mental retardation as were identified by the telephone survey (USDE, 2000). The U.S. Department of Education report theorized that cultural differences in the concept of disability might be the reason for some of the discrepancies. People with mental retardation may also function independently in home settings, where they are familiar with routines and expectations, yet require supports for more challenging environments such as school and work. A study of the incidence of mental retardation among a birth cohort of children in Minnesota found a rate of children with mental retardation similar to that reported by the U.S. Department of Education Report (Katusic et al., 1996). Using IQ scores from school records as the only criteria for mental retardation, these authors found the cumulative incidence of mental retardation (IQ < 70) by age 8 to be 9.1 per 1000 children. The prevalence of children with severe mental retardation, defined as an IQ score of 50 or below, was 4.9 per 1000 children in this study, and the prevalence of children with mild mental retardation, defined as an IQ of 51 to 70, was 4.3 per 1000 children. Of the 5.5 million school-aged children served by special education, 11% have been identified for reporting purposes as having mental retardation and 1.9% as having multiple disabilities (USDE, 2000).

ETIOLOGY AND PATHOPHYSIOLOGY OF COGNITIVE IMPAIRMENTS

Multiple causes of cognitive impairments exist, many of which have been identified and many of which have not. McLaren and Bryson (1987) reviewed 13 epidemiologic studies of cognitive impairments and concluded that causes could be identified for approximately 70% of those with severe impairments and 50% of those with mild impairments. Understanding the etiology of a child's cognitive impairment may assist physical therapists and others to better predict current or future needs for supports and life planning, and to identify other health-related problems that might be associated with a given diagnosis (AAMR, 2002).

Over 350 etiologies for cognitive impairments have been identified that can be broadly categorized into prenatal, perinatal, and postnatal causes. Prenatal etiologies have been further classified as chromosomal disorders, syndromes, inborn errors of metabolism, developmental disorders of brain formation, and environmental influences. Perinatal causes include intrauterine disorders and neonatal disorders. One meta-analysis of 15 studies that examined cognitive outcomes of children born prematurely provides evidence that prematurity alone may be associated with reduced scores on cognitive tests (Bhutta et al., 2002). The pooled data demonstrated that scores of children born at full gestation were significantly higher than scores of children born prematurely. Classifications of postnatal causes of cognitive impairment include head injuries, infections, demyelinating disorders, degenerative disorders, seizure disorders, toxic-metabolic disorders, malnutrition, environmental deprivation, and hypoconnection syndrome (AAMR, 2002).

Movement dysfunction is more often associated with some etiologies than with others, and in general, children with more severe cognitive impairments are likely to have more severe motor delays and impairments (Anwar, 1986; Chinitz & Feder, 1992). Ellis (1963) proposed that the relatively poor motor performance of people with cognitive impairments is the result of their limited capacity to process information and the rapid decay of that information over time. Such cognitive deficits impede motor learning (Anwar, 1986), leading to the slow and clumsy movements that children with cognitive impairments often have, even when they do not have cerebral palsy or another movement-related diagnosis. Many children also have associated problems, such as vision and hearing impairments, cerebral palsy, low levels of arousal, seizure disorders, cardiopulmonary dysfunction, and various other medical problems that can further negatively influence motor development, motor learning, and motor performance (Anwar, 1986).

PREVENTION

Some forms of cognitive impairment and associated disorders can now be prevented, such as those resulting from phenylketonuria, rubella, and lead poisoning. In addition, amniocentesis, ultrasound, and other techniques have enabled prenatal diagnosis of many conditions, which may help decrease morbidity, such as delivery of a child with myelodysplasia by cesarean section. Genetic counseling also can be offered.

Although the etiologic factors known to cause cognitive impairments may be present in a given child, complex and powerful interactions between those factors and later environmental events can alter the actuality or the severity of cognitive limitations and associated impairments. In a review of current research and theories on the development of intelligences, DiLalla (2000) suggested that about half of a person's IQ may be influenced by environmental factors.

Some infants, for example, who have severe medical problems during the postnatal course, with documented neuroanatomic pathology during this period, have few if any sequelae. On the other hand, children with no known pathology but who experience one or more environmental risk factors may eventually be classified as having cognitive impairment, although the impairment usually is mild (Campbell & Ramey, 1985).

Campbell and Ramey (1985) identified four important environmental factors that contribute to cognitive impairment: (1) malnutrition, (2) teratogens, (3) accidents and injuries, and (4) a poor psychologic environment. These environmental factors are likely to be related to socioeconomic status, which has been found to be one of the most powerful predictors of childhood intellectual functioning (Gibbs, 1990). Kochanek and colleagues (1990) found that, in children from birth to age 3 years, characteristics of their parents, such as the mother's education, more accurately predict whether a child will have a disability as an adolescent than the child's own characteristics.

In the United States, the family-centered services directed by Part C of the Individuals with Disabilities Education Act (IDEA), described in Chapters 30 and 31 of this volume, reflect a belief in the power of early social and physical environments to influence a child's development. It also implies confidence in the capability of physical therapists and other service providers to assist families in providing environments that both prevent unnecessary disability and promote the achievement of a child's potential. Ramey and Ramey (1992) found six components of early intervention programs to be the most critical for children's intellectual development and learning: (1) encouragement to explore and learn from the environment; (2) mentoring by trusted adults in basic cognitive skills; (3) celebration of the child's developmental accomplishments by others; (4) guided rehearsal and elaboration of new skills; (5) protection from inappropriate disapproval, teasing, and punishment; and (6) provision of a rich and responsive language environment.

▌ PRIMARY IMPAIRMENT

The time at which impairments in intellectual functioning and movement become recognized varies widely, both within and between medical diagnoses. In some cases, prenatal or neonatal diagnosis can predict impairments that may not yet be apparent, such as with children with Down syndrome or myelodysplasia. In other cases, a medical diagnosis will not be made until after impaired functioning is noted, perhaps not until months or years after birth.

DIAGNOSIS/PROBLEM IDENTIFICATION

Delay in achievement of developmental motor milestones is often the first indication of cognitive impairment that was present prenatally or perinatally (Chinitz & Feder, 1992). This is particularly true for children with greater than mild cognitive impairments. Some children will develop normally for a period of time and then regress, such as those with Rett syndrome or Tay-Sachs disease. In these cases, too, motor manifestations of the condition often are the first indication of a more global developmental problem (Nomura & Segawa, 1990).

Neuromotor Impairments of Children with Cognitive Impairments

The movement impairments of children with limited cognitive functioning are as diverse as the causes of their primary and associated conditions. Most of the movement problems, however, have their bases in central nervous system pathology that most often leads to impairments in flexibility, force production, coordination, postural control, balance, endurance, and efficiency (Campbell SK, 1991). Cardiopulmonary and musculoskeletal impairments also may contribute to the movement problems.

Although the type and degree of movement and related problems vary greatly, certain medical diagnoses are likely to be associated with specific constellations of neuromuscular, musculoskeletal, and cardiopulmonary impairments. Table 20-1 summarizes impairments that are common among children with selected diagnoses who often receive physical therapy.

Physical therapy examination of the movement impairments of children who have cognitive impairments is similar to that of other children who have problems addressed by physical therapists. Observation, criterion-referenced instruments, norm-referenced tests, and other formats are used, depending on the age of the child, the problem being assessed, and the purpose of the assessment (see other chapters of this volume).

Although the same examination methods and tools may be used for children with and without cognitive impairments, recognizing that a child's intellectual impairment may affect performance of motor activities is important. This is especially the case when a child has to follow directions or perform motor tasks that have major cognitive components. Examination of infants and young children may be less affected by intellectual abilities than that of older children and adolescents, and cognitive function probably will affect examination of impairments less than examination of activity or participation.

Learning in Children with Cognitive Impairments

By definition, impaired learning is what distinguishes children with cognitive impairments from other children. Although their motor problems often are similar to those of children without cognitive impairments and they respond to intervention based on the same physical therapy principles, the application of those principles must be sensitive to the children's learning characteristics. Research demonstrating that physical therapy is less effective with children who have cognitive impairments (Parette & Hourcade, 1984) may at least partially relate to inadequate modification of therapeutic approaches to enhance their learning.

The degree and types of learning impairments of children with cognitive limitations vary considerably, but several common learning characteristics have been identified. Compared with typically developing children, children with cognitive impairments have been found (1) to be capable of learning a fewer number of things; (2) to need a greater number of repetitions to learn; (3) to have greater difficulty generalizing skills; (4) to have greater difficulty maintaining skills that are not practiced regularly; (5) to have slower response times; and (6) to have a more limited repertoire of responses (Brown et al., 1979; Falvey, 1989; Orelove & Sobsey, 1996). Implications of these learning characteristics for physical therapy are described in later sections of this chapter.

TEAM ASSESSMENT

The complex problems of children with both cognitive and motor impairments usually require a team approach for assessment and for planning, implementation, and evaluation of intervention (Foley, 1990; Orelove & Sobsey, 1996; Rainforth & York-Barr, 1997). The team always will include the child's family or another caregiver, with other team members as required by the nature and severity of the child's problems, the child's age, and the service delivery setting. Many children need the services of two or more teams at the same time, such as a clinically based health care team and an early intervention or public school team. Usually, the health care team is primarily responsible for assessment of the child's body functions and structures, with the early intervention or school-based team responsible for addressing activity limitations and ongoing efforts to promote the highest possible level of community participation. When the teams have mutual responsibilities and concerns, overlapping or conflicting services can result, with confusion for the family and unnecessary expenditure of limited resources. To avoid such problems, it is essential that the teams communicate well and that the roles and responsibilities of the members of each team be clear to all (Rainforth & York-Barr, 1997).

MODELS OF TEAM FUNCTIONING

Each team must decide on a model of service delivery that will enable comprehensive evaluation of a child's disabilities and provide the most effective intervention. The transdisciplinary model of service delivery, developed in the mid-1970s by the United Cerebral Palsy National Collaborative Infant Project (1976), is often recommended as best practice in early intervention programs and in special education programs for children with severe and

| TABLE 20-1 | Common Neuromuscular, Musculoskeletal, and Cardiopulmonary Impairments of Children with Mental Retardation Caused by Selected Conditions* | | |

CONDITION	NEUROMUSCULAR	MUSCULOSKELETAL	CARDIOPULMONARY
Cri du chat syndrome Cornish & Bramble, 2002	Hypotonia in early childhood, sometimes hypertonia later	Facial and minor upper extremity anomalies, scoliosis	Congenital heart disease is common
Cytomegalovirus (prenatal) Leung et al., 2003	Cerebral palsy, seizure disorder, microcephaly (hearing problems)	Secondary to neuromuscular problems	Pulmonary valvular stenosis, mitral stenosis, atrial septal defect
de Lange syndrome Berg et al., 1970; Jones, 1997	Spasticity, intention tremor, seizure disorder (10%–20%), microcephaly	Decreased bone age, small stature, small hands and feet, short digits, proximal thumb placement, clinodactyly of fifth fingers, other arm and hand defects, limited elbow extension	Neonatal respiratory problems, cardiac malformations, recurrent upper respiratory infections
Down syndrome Roizen & Patterson, 2003	Low muscle force production, slow postural reactions, slow reaction time (hearing loss)	Joint hyperflexibility, ligamentous laxity, foot deformities, scoliosis, atlantoaxial instability, arthritis	Congenital heart disease (50%)
Fetal alchohol syndrome Prenatal Exposure to Alcohol, 2000	Fine motor and visual motor deficits, balance deficits	Minor facial abnormalities, joint anomalies with abnormal position or function, maxillary hypoplasia	Heart defects
Fragile X syndrome de Vries et al., 1998	Poor coordination and motor planning, seizures	Connective tissue abnormalities, which may lead to congenital hip dislocation in infancy and later to scoliosis and pes planus	Mitral valve prolapse
Hurler's syndrome Carter, 1970; Jones, 1997	Hydrocephalus	Joint contractures, clawlike deformities of hands, short fingers, thoracolumbar kyphosis, shallow acetabular and glenoid fossae, irregularly shaped bones	Cardiac deformities, cardiac enlargement because right ventricular hypertension is common, death frequently due to cardiac failure
Lesch-Nyhan syndrome Jankovic et al., 1988	Hypotonia followed by spasticity and chorea, athetosis, or dystonia; compulsive self-injurious behavior	Secondary to neuromuscular problems	

(continued)

TABLE 20-1	Common Neuromuscular, Musculoskeletal, and Cardiopulmonary Impairments of Children with Mental Retardation Caused by Selected Conditions*—cont'd		
CONDITION	**NEUROMUSCULAR**	**MUSCULOSKELETAL**	**CARDIOPULMONARY**
Prader-Willi syndrome Aughton et al., 1981	Severe hypotonia and feeding problems in infancy, excessive eating and obesity in childhood, poor fine and gross motor coordination	Short stature, small hands and feet	May be associated with cor pulmonale (most common cause of death)
Rett syndrome Percy, 2002	Deceleration in rate of head growth in infancy, gradual loss of acquired skills after 6 to 18 months of age, loss of purposeful hand skills, stereotypic hand movements (clapping, wringing, clenching), apraxia, teeth grinding, seizure disorder	Scoliosis/kyphosis, growth failure, bone demineralization	Breathing irregularities, such as hyperventilation and breath holding
Williams (elfin facies) syndrome Morris & Mervis, 2000	Mild neurologic dysfunction, hypotonia, hyperreflexia, cerebellar dysfunction	Facial abnormalities, slow and abnormal growth, connective tissue abnormalities, radioulnar stenosis, spinal deformities, joint hyperextension when young, contractures when older	Cardiovascular abnormalities

*Not all children with each condition exhibit all impairments.

multiple disabilities (Foley, 1990; Orelove & Sobsey, 1996; Rainforth & York-Barr, 1997).

The transdisciplinary model permits greater coordination of comprehensive services for individuals with complex health, educational, and social needs than most other approaches. Two of the distinguishing features of the model are that assessments are conducted collaboratively by team members and a single, discipline-free service plan is developed to meet the highest-priority needs of the child and family. This mode of operation contrasts with other service delivery models in which service providers conduct separate assessments and develop separate, discipline-referenced intervention plans (McGonigel et al., 1994).

Another distinguishing feature of the transdisciplinary model is that one team member is designated as the primary service provider, usually the person who spends the greatest amount of time with the child or the person who has the skills necessary to address the child's greatest areas of need (McGonigel et al., 1994; Orelove & Sobsey, 1996). The primary service provider will change over time as the child's needs and environments change. A parent or physical therapist may be the primary service provider for an infant or young child, a teacher the primary service provider for an older child, and a personal care assistant the primary service provider for a young adult.

When using a transdisciplinary approach, team members are responsible for determining which of their own disciplinary knowledge and skills are needed by the child, for consulting with and teaching the necessary knowledge and skills to the primary service provider, and for monitoring outcomes. The primary service provider incorporates the knowledge and strategies of other disciplines into ongoing intervention with the child. In effect, team members "release" part of their roles to the primary service provider (McGonigel et al., 1994; Orelove & Sobsey, 1996).

ASSESSMENT OF ACTIVITY AND PARTICIPATION

Assessment of a child's activities and participation is best conducted in the environments in which the child actually participates or environments in which children of similar age and social background participate. Assessment in natural environments is increasingly advocated for all children who have disabilities, but especially for children with cognitive impairments who have difficulty generalizing skills from one setting to another. Such environmentally based assessment also is far more likely to lead to intervention that results in improved abilities to participate in everyday activities and in age-appropriate life roles than assessment that takes place in isolated or clinical settings, is based on a normal developmental sequence, or focuses primarily on identification of impairments, such as range of motion, postural responses, or retention of primitive reflexes (Brown et al., 1979; McEwen & Shelden, 1995; Rainforth & York-Barr, 1997).

ASSESSMENT OF INTELLECTUAL FUNCTIONING

Determining if a child has a cognitive impairment requires a standardized, norm-referenced measure of intelligence, which usually is administered by a psychologist or psychometrist. Even though most physical therapists do not administer intelligence tests, they are often able to promote an environment in which children with motor impairments can perform optimally, such as by providing positioning to enhance a child's communication and eye and hand use (Sents & Marks, 1989) or by assisting the examiner to determine alternative response modes for use by children who have motor impairments.

Assessment of Infants

Physical therapists may be involved in the administration of tests designed to assess the cognitive abilities of infants, because many of these tests focus on an infant's sensorimotor development, such as accomplishment of motor developmental milestones or coordination of vision and hearing with body movement (Chinitz & Feder, 1992; Gibbs, 1990). These tests include instruments described by Campbell in Chapter 2 of this volume.

Unfortunately, sensorimotor-based infant evaluations are poor predictors of cognitive ability at later ages, with little, if any, relationship found between scores on infant tests and children's subsequent scores on intelligence tests for preschool or school-age children (Gibbs, 1990; Zelazo & Weiss, 1990). The most common error is identification of infants as having cognitive delays who later demon-

strate normal intelligence (McCall, 1982). Better predictability has been found with children who have severe cognitive delays and multiple disabilities (Kopp & McCall, 1982), with most children who have severe cognitive delays being identified before they are 2 years old (Katusic et al., 1996). Gibbs (1990) proposed that this is a result of the limited capacity of infants with severe impairments to be influenced by positive environmental circumstances; thus, their range of possible outcomes is more restricted and their test scores are more stable over time.

Some tests of infant cognitive abilities attempt to measure infants' intellectual functioning through evaluation of their information processing capacity rather than their sensorimotor skills. These tests use infants' behavioral responses to novel and previously presented stimuli to assess their visual or auditory memory and their ability to discriminate among stimuli (Chinitz & Feder, 1992; Zelazo & Weiss, 1990). These tests are based on the tendency of infants, almost from birth, to respond for shorter periods of time to stimuli to which they have been previously exposed. Thus, if an infant has a longer response to a new stimulus than to one presented previously, memory for the familiar stimulus and discrimination of the two stimuli are demonstrated. Visual attention to stimuli is often assessed, as with the Fagan Test of Infant Intelligence (FTII) (Fagan & Shepherd, 1987), but changes in heart rate, smiling, and other responses can also indicate an infant's processing of information (Zelazo & Weiss, 1990).

One advantage of information processing tests for infants is that they are essentially motor- and language-free, making them more appropriate for infants with motor and hearing impairments than many other tests (Drotar et al., 1989). Another advantage is that their predictive validity is much better than that of the tests that focus on sensorimotor behaviors (Zelazo & Weiss, 1990). This probably is because they tap information processing capacities that are more similar to requirements of intelligence tests for older children than are the qualities assessed by sensorimotor-based tests (Chinitz & Feder, 1992; Gibbs, 1990).

Assessment of Children

According to the AAMR (2002), the most widely used IQ tests for children are the Stanford-Binet Intelligence Scale-IV (Thorndike et al., 1986) and the Wechsler Intelligence Scale for Children-III (WISC-III) (Wechsler, 1991). Standardized administration of these and most other intelligence tests requires spoken and motor responses that seriously limit their usefulness with children who have communication and motor impairments.

A few intelligence tests have been developed that require children only to indicate a choice from among an array of alternatives. The Columbia Mental Maturity Scale (Burgemeister et al., 1972) is one such test, which was developed specifically to assess the intelligence of children with cerebral palsy and requires only that a child be capable of indicating which pictures are unrelated to others.

Raven's Progressive Matrices (Raven, 1995), requiring selection of missing elements of abstract designs, and the Leiter International Performance Scale – Revised (Rold & Miller, 1998) are other non-language-based tests with minimal motor requirements. They may, however, suggest spuriously low cognitive abilities in children who have visuoperceptual deficits or visual impairments. It is also important to be aware that all of the tests with limited motor and language requirements sample only a narrow range of abilities compared with more traditional tests of intelligence, so they may either overestimate or underestimate more global aspects of a child's intelligence (Chinitz & Feder, 1992). For children with profound multiple disabilities, whose cognitive abilities are the most difficult to assess, tests of visual memory, similar to those developed for evaluation of infants, could provide some of the elusive information about their capacities to store and process information (Switzky et al., 1979).

ASSESSMENT OF ADAPTIVE BEHAVIORS

Although examiners often emphasize intelligence test scores in the diagnosis of cognitive impairment (Evans, 1991), adaptive behaviors are also central in the assessment of cognitive impairment. Nihira (1999) defined adaptive behavior as a person's effectiveness in coping with environmental demands. Assessment of adaptive behavior relies heavily on professional judgment, in both the selection of means to assess adaptive behaviors and in their interpretation. Physical therapists often can provide information about a child's adaptive behaviors, such as self-help and mobility skills, and may also be instrumental in provision of assistive devices that can help improve a child's adaptive skills.

Instruments to measure adaptive behaviors have been developed, but they are of more recent vintage than many of the intelligence tests and there are fewer of them. The Pediatric Evaluation of Disability Inventory (PEDI) (Haley et al., 1992), described in Chapter 2, was developed to measure self-care, mobility, and social function in children age 6 months to 7.5 years with physical or combined physical and cognitive disabilities. This tool is divided into two parts: functional skills and caregiver assistance. Tests that are commonly used for older children include the AAMR Adaptive Behavior Scale-School (ABS-S:2) (Lambert et al., 1993) and the Vineland Adaptive Behavior Scales (VABS) (Sparrow et al., 1984). The ABS-

S:2 was designed for assessment of adaptive behaviors and to help in program planning (Lambert et al., 1993). This tool is divided into two parts: personal independence and social behavior. The tool yields scores in five areas, including personal self-sufficiency, community self-sufficiency, personal-social responsibility, social adjustment, and personal adjustment. The results of a validity study of the ABS-S:2 indicated that the personal independence and social behavior scales of the tool demonstrated the largest difference between typical children and children with mental retardation (Watkins et al., 2002). The results of this study suggested that these two sections of the tool, rather than the scores in all five areas, should be used when assessing children for mental retardation. The VABS is administered as a questionnaire that asks about activities of daily living, cognition, language, play, and social competency. The authors reported that content validity was established through factor analytic techniques (Sparrow et al., 1984). Inter-rater reliability was estimated to be 0.96, with test-retest reliability ranging from 0.77 to 0.98 (Middleton et al., 1990).

ASSESSMENT OF CONTEXTUAL FACTORS

The AAMR definition of mental retardation requires consideration of function within context. Similarly, the ICF views outcomes as resulting from interactions between health conditions and contextual factors. Contextual factors include both personal and environmental factors (WHO, 2001). Environmental factors include "the physical, social, and attitudinal environment in which people live and conduct their lives" (WHO, 2001, p. 10). Factors outside the child can profoundly affect child development, test scores, and intervention planning (Meisels & Atkins-Burnett, 2000). Brook-Gunn and colleagues (1996) found, for example, that differences between IQ test scores of African-American and Caucasian children at age 5 years were nearly eliminated when adjusted for poverty and home environment. Physical therapists may not be able to change the effect of environmental factors on test scores, but should consider the effect of the physical, social, and attitudinal environments on test performance. Participation in everyday activities is considered important for typical child development, and children with combined physical and cognitive impairments are at increased risk for less participation in all settings (King et al., 2003). Some evidence exists to suggest that intervention focused on expanding existing natural learning opportunities in everyday settings can have a positive effect on children's participation (Dunst, 2000). Assessment of environmental factors related to activity and participation is essential for developing interventions that can promote improved participation.

Ecologic Assessments

Physical therapists are often involved in assessing the physical environment and a child's interaction with it. Brown and associates (1979) described an ecologic approach to assessment that others have subsequently promoted as a means to determine functional outcomes and plan programs for people who have cognitive impairments and for children in early intervention programs (Falvey, 1989; Orelove & Sobsey, 1996; Rainforth & York-Barr, 1997; Thurman & Widerstrom, 1990). An ecologic assessment is an approach or format, rather than a specific assessment instrument. Orelove and Sobsey (1996) described four major steps in an ecologic assessment:

1. *Determine the domains to be included in the child's program.* Four domains are considered to be primary: home, community (e.g., school, stores, and church), vocational, and recreation-leisure. Certain critical skills, such as mobility, communication, and hand use, are required for functioning in all domains.

2. *Determine the environments and subenvironments within each domain in which the child currently functions or could function in the future.* A child's team might identify the home, school, and restaurant as especially important. Subenvironments could be the bedroom at home, the cafeteria at school, and the restroom in a restaurant.

3. *Determine the activities the child needs to function in each of the subenvironments.* Activities could include getting out of bed at home, obtaining and eating lunch at school, and using the toilet in a restaurant.

4. *Determine the skills the child needs for each activity.* Skills are determined through task analysis of the activities and identifying the components the child needs to be able to do to accomplish each of them. To get out of bed, for example, one child may need to respond to the alarm, remove the covers, assume a sitting position, and transfer to a wheelchair. A child with less ability could learn to do other components of the task, such as rolling over to sit up after the covers have been removed and assisting with the transfer.

An example of an ecologic assessment is included in the case study of Jeff at the end of the chapter.

Physical therapists often have less experience examining the social and attitudinal aspects of the environment than physical aspects. Children rarely function alone in their environments, however, so social and attitudinal factors need to be considered. Young children are a part of their families, and older children spend their time in classrooms, in after-school activities, and in the community with their peers, family, and other community members. Successful physical therapy services depend on more than developing intervention focused on the physical aspects of a task. Rather, successful intervention often depends on opportunities to practice and a supportive social and attitudinal environment. Standardized tools that measure these aspects of environment do not exist, however, so good understanding of potential environmental facilitators and barriers and good observational skills are important. Informally asking families and children, when they are old enough, about how they spend their time and their social supports can also assist in determining how to design interventions needed to improve social and attitudinal environments.

Personal Factors

In the ICF model, personal factors include those aspects of a person that are not part of the health condition, such as gender, race, coping styles, and those things that are intrinsically motivating (WHO, 2001). Physical therapists need to consider such personal factors to effectively promote children's chosen activities and participation within the context of family, school, and community. A tool that is helpful for identifying the level of supports that adolescents and adults with intellectual disabilities and other developmental disabilities need for quality participation in society is the Supports Intensity Scale (SIS) (AAMR, 2003). The tool was normed with people aged 16 to over 70 years, and measures the supports needed in daily life activities and exceptional medical and behavioral support needs. A supplemental protection and advocacy scale also is included.

COGNITIVE REFERENCING

Cognitive referencing is an assessment approach that has been used to determine whether children are eligible for services, especially for physical therapy, occupational therapy, and speech pathology in public schools (Carr, 1989). The approach is based on an assumption that children's potentials for gains in motor and communication development are related to their cognitive abilities and that children whose cognitive abilities are lower than or equal to their motor or communication abilities would not benefit from services, so they are not eligible for them. Obviously, many children with cognitive impairments could be declared ineligible for physical therapy services under such an assumption, so the use of cognitive referencing has been highly controversial (Giangreco, 1990). Critics have been supported by at least one study that examined the association between IQ scores and progress in occupational therapy or physical therapy over the course of one school year (Baker et al., 1998). Children were divided into two groups based on their IQ scores, and their motor skills were tested before and after 1 year's intervention. Children received approximately 40 minutes of occupational therapy or physical therapy per week. Both groups showed significant change in their age-equivalence scores, but the researchers found no significant correlation between IQ and change in motor test scores. The U.S. Department of Education, Office of Special Education Programs (OSEP) declared cognitive referencing to be an unlawful means to determine whether a child should receive related services in public schools (Rainforth, 1991). The OSEP statement reiterated the authority of each child's educational team to decide on the services necessary for that child to meet individualized educational goals. When goals of children with cognitive and neuromotor impairments focus on reducing activity limitations and improving participation, some type of physical therapy often is needed, as determined through coordination and communication with other team members.

DETERMINING INTERVENTION GOALS AND OUTCOMES

Functional goals have been emphasized in special education for many years and have more recently been supported by pediatric physical therapists and therapists in other areas of practice (Harris, 1991; McEwen & Shelden, 1995; Rainforth & York-Barr, 1997; Randall & McEwen, 2000). Functional skills have been defined as those activities or tasks that someone else will have to do if the child does not (Brown et al., 1979), that are age-appropriate (Falvey, 1989), and that reflect the needs and interests of the child and family (Orelove & Sobsey, 1996). Some children can learn to complete a task or activity, whereas others will be capable of learning to carry out only a part of it. Partial participation, or completion of only part of a task, is a legitimate outcome for some children who have severe disabilities (Ferguson & Baumgart, 1991). A child may, for example, be unable to transfer independently but can learn to unbuckle a seat belt and support weight in standing. Another child may be unable to put a tape into a tape recorder but can learn to turn it on using a switch.

Outcomes of intervention to improve a child's abilities to participate in life must represent specific functional skills that the child will acquire. Team members cannot assume that interventions directed toward remediation of impairments, such as improving postural responses, range of motion, or strength, or toward reducing the degree of activity limitations indicated by failed items on a developmental test, will necessarily lead to meaningful outcomes (Harris, 1991; McEwen & Shelden, 1995; Rainforth

& York-Barr, 1997; Randall & McEwen, 2000). This is especially true of children with cognitive impairments who need many repetitions to learn, forget easily, and generalize poorly. These characteristics make it unlikely that a child with cognitive impairments will be able to synthesize isolated activities or components of movement into meaningful skills.

P.H. Campbell (1991) proposed a "top-down" approach to determining outcomes, in which the desired functional outcomes are determined first, then obstacles to their accomplishment are identified, and then intervention to overcome the obstacles is planned and implemented (Fig. 20-1). This process in similar to the decision-making process of the hypothesis-oriented algorithm for clinicians (HOAC II) (Rothstein et al., 2003), in which a person's goals for intervention are identified first, then the person is examined to generate a hypothesis about why they can or cannot be met at the present time.

As described earlier as a component of an ecologic assessment, functional outcomes can be anything that are a high priority and meaningful to the child and family, are age-appropriate, and are, or could be, a home, community, recreation-leisure, or vocational activity. Giangreco and colleagues (1998, p. 13) proposed five valued life outcomes for all children, including those with severe disabilities:

1. Having a safe, stable home in which to live now or in the future
2. Having access to a variety of places and engaging in meaningful activities
3. Having a social network of personally meaningful relationships
4. Having a level of personal choice and control that matches one's age
5. Being safe and healthy

Teams usually have the most difficulty determining meaningful outcomes for children with profound multiple disabilities who often have extremely limited repertoires of behavior. Evans and Scotti (1989) maintained that even these children can accomplish outcomes that require active behavioral changes, such as indicating a choice of food or activity or increasing body movements used to activate switches. Such active outcomes lead to acquisition of skills that increase participation and are in contrast to passive activities that are done to the child, such as sensory stimulation, range-of-motion exercises, and positioning (often stated as something the child will "tolerate"). Passive activities may be part of the intervention to help a child accomplish a skill, but only the child's active behavior can increase true participation.

One helpful tool for assisting families to identify meaningful outcomes and to measure whether they have been

TOP-DOWN APPROACH

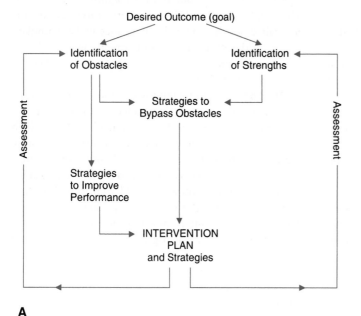

BOTTOM-UP APPROACH

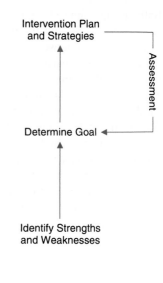

A

B

♦ **Figure 20-1** Comparison of a top-down approach (**A**), in which assessments identify means to achieve desired outcomes, and a bottom-up approach (**B**), in which assessment results determine outcomes. *(From Campbell, PH. Evaluation and assessment in early intervention for infants and toddlers. Journal of Early Intervention, 15:42, 1991. Copyright ©1991 by Division for Early Childhood, the Council for Exceptional Children.)*

accomplished is the Canadian Occupational Performance Measure (COPM) (Law et al., 1994). The COPM was designed as an individualized measure of performance and satisfaction in self-care, productivity (work, household management, play/school), and leisure. Although the COPM was intended for occupational therapists, it is an equally useful tool for physical therapists. This chapter's section on Evaluation of Outcomes gives more information about the COPM.

When desired outcomes are determined first, as with Campbell's (1991) top-down approach, they are discipline-free; that is, they describe the skills the child will accomplish without regard for discipline-related concerns. Only after team members identify the highest-priority outcomes do they decide which disciplines will be needed to help the child accomplish each one (Rainforth & York-Barr, 1997). This team-oriented process for determining outcomes is not necessarily inconsistent with the processes described in the HOAC II (Rothstein et al., 2003) or the *Guide to Physical Therapist Practice (Guide)* (2001), although both the HOAC II and the *Guide* describe primarily a unidisciplinary approach in which the physical therapist makes decisions in collaboration with the patient and perhaps the patient's family. When working

with children whose complex problems require teams of professionals, the process must include other professionals as well. Amy's case history at the end of this chapter provides an example of application of the *Guide* to the decision-making process of a school-based team.

INTERVENTION

During planning and implementation of intervention for children with cognitive impairments, it is important to keep in mind what are widely regarded as best practices for working with children who have cognitive impairments and other developmental disabilities. Some of these practices have been discussed previously and include families and children as full and equal team members, assessment in natural environments, and an emphasis on functional outcomes with active participation by children (McEwen & Shelden, 1995).

Other considerations that influence intervention for children with cognitive impairments include interventions to limit impairments and promote activity and participation, use of teaching methods that are most likely to result in acquisition of skills by children with cognitive impairments, and the role of physical therapists in promoting development in nonmotor domains. Each of these considerations, which are discussed in the following sections, involve one or more of the three components of intervention included in the *Guide to Physical Therapist Practice* (2001): coordination, communication, and documentation; patient/client-related instruction; and procedural interventions.

LIMITING IMPAIRMENTS, MINIMIZING ACTIVITY LIMITATIONS, AND PREVENTING SECONDARY IMPAIRMENTS

Early identification of neuromuscular, musculoskeletal, and cardiopulmonary problems, at whatever age they occur, allows for intervention designed to limit the impairments, thus restricting the development of secondary impairments and activity limitations. Specific intervention will depend on the identified problems and on consequences that can be predicted to follow from the natural history of the condition. Children with Down syndrome and other relatively mild movement impairments, for example, often benefit from activities designed to enhance postural control and force production and accomplishment of motor milestones (Harris & Shea, 1991). Other children with more severe impairments may benefit from positioning and other activities designed to maintain flexibility, prevent musculoskeletal malalignments and deformities, and enhance motor development and control. Such intervention is described in other chapters of this volume.

Limiting Cognitive, Communication, and Psychosocial Impairments and Functional Limitations

Children who have motor impairments that restrict or prevent exploration of their environments may be at risk for secondary delays in domains that are not primarily affected (Campbell SK, 1991), especially cognition, communication, and psychosocial development (Kermoian & Campos, 1988; Telzrow et al., 1987). Campos and Bertenthal (1987) suggested that independent mobility is an organizer of psychologic changes in typically developing infants, especially developmental changes in social understanding, spatial cognition, and emotions. They also proposed theoretic links between independent mobility and the growth of brain structures, self-awareness, attachment to others, and the ability to cope with the environment.

Most of the theoretic links have not been examined empirically, but relations between mobility and spatial cognition have received considerable research attention. Several studies have demonstrated that locomotion, not age per se, is related to changes in such spatial cognitive tasks as recognition of heights (Bertenthal et al., 1984), retrieving hidden toys (Benson & Uzgiris, 1985), and performance on Piagetian spatial search tasks by typical infants and infants with meningomyelocele (Kermoian & Campos, 1988; Telzrow et al., 1987). Self-produced locomotion also has been shown to influence social-communicative behaviors of infants (Gustafson, 1984), and the proposed theoretic link between mobility and development of brain structures has been supported by studies demonstrating that experience shapes the brains of animals (for a review see Kolb et al., 1998). New imaging techniques have shown similar effects of experience on the structure of infants' brains (Chugani, 1998).

Although much of the research has demonstrated an association between motor and cognitive development, other research suggests that the links are indirect, with motor and cognitive abilities facilitating each other but capable of relatively independent development. One study, for example, found that the object permanence task performance of children with cerebral palsy was more closely related to their mental age than to the severity of their motor impairments (Eagle, 1985). This finding is consistent with the well-known capacity for some people to develop average or superior mental abilities in spite of severe motor impairments.

Further research is needed to determine the relative contributions of innate mental capability and sensorimotor experiences on various aspects of cognitive development. It may be that the inborn intelligence of some children enables them to compensate for their motor limitations, thus making them less vulnerable to effects of sensorimotor deprivation than children whose intellectual capacities are more limited.

Assuming that exploration and manipulation of the environment do influence cognitive, communication, and social-emotional development, physical therapy has an obvious role in the development of these nonmotor domains of children who have motor impairments. One means is through intervention strategies designed to improve motor performance, as described in other chapters of this volume. Another potentially important strategy is to provide alternative means of mobility when children's motor impairments prevent exploration of the environment at an age when other children are crawling and walking. In addition, the use of postural support systems to promote interaction with the environment is important when using adaptive equipment and powered mobility.

Use of Power Mobility to Prevent Activity Limitations

Butler (1991) asserted that self-produced locomotion can have such a powerful impact on development that functional means of mobility should be provided for all young children who have mobility restrictions, regardless of whether or not the child is expected to walk eventually. Aided mobility is not seen as "giving up" on walking for young children, but as providing critical assistance at a time when it is needed to promote activity and participation.

Several reports have demonstrated that very young children can learn to use power mobility devices. Zazula and Foulds (1983) reported that an 11-month-old child with congenital limb deformities learned to activate the controls of a motorized cart within 4 hours and controlled all aspects of the cart by 17 months of age. In another study, 12 of 13 children between ages 20 and 37 months, with various disabilities, became competent motorized wheelchair users within their homes after an average of 16.4 days of practice (Butler et al., 1983). More recently, a case report described the development of independent power mobility in a 20-month-old child with spinal muscular atrophy within 6 weeks of the time she received a power wheelchair (Jones et al., 2003).

Although these young children were believed to have normal intelligence, other studies have demonstrated that children with cognitive impairments also can become independent users of power mobility devices (Verburg et al., 1990). Certain cognitive abilities may be necessary to achieve independent power-aided mobility, but the specific abilities that are necessary and the means to assess them have not been determined. Because typically developing children learn to crawl and become independently mobile well before their first birthday, and because children have become independently mobile using power mobility devices before age 2, children with cognitive impairments who have adequate vision and the cognitive skills typical of an 18-month-old (or perhaps younger) are likely to be capable of learning to use powered means of mobility, given appropriate equipment, instruction, and opportunities. Tefft and colleagues (1999) investigated cognitive predictors associated with young children who learn to use power mobility independently after six training sessions in a clinical setting. They found spatial relations and problem-solving abilities were better among children who learned to maneuver a chair than those who did not. Children with poorer spatial relations and problem-solving abilities may be able to learn to use power mobility, however, if practice occurs in their everyday settings and if they have adequate opportunities for practice.

Use of Assistive Positioning to Promote Environmental Interaction

Seating and other assistive positioning devices, as described in Chapter 33, also can influence children's interactions with their physical and social environments through their effects on such variables as hand function (Nwaobi, 1987), switch activation (McEwen & Karlan, 1989), and respiration (Nwaobi & Smith, 1986). One of the most important environmental interactions is communication with others, because it affects not only a child's communication development but also the cognitive and social-emotional development (Campbell, 1989).

To learn to communicate, children must have opportunities to communicate. One study found that teachers initiated interactions at higher rates when children were positioned in wheelchairs than when they were in sidelyers or supine on a mat (McEwen, 1992). Observations suggested that wheelchairs promoted interaction by placing students nearer the normal interaction level of adults than positioning them on the floor. The adults who participated in the study rarely sat on the floor to interact with children unless they were involved in structured programming, a finding that is consistent with other investigations (Houghton et al., 1987).

In addition to providing opportunities for interaction with other persons in the environment, research suggests that positioning can also influence children's own communicative behaviors. Typically developing 3- to 6-month-old infants looked at their mothers for longer periods of time when they were supine than when reclined 45° or seated upright (Fogel et al., 1992). Similarly, children with profound cognitive impairments and physical disabilities interacted with attentive teachers and classroom assistants for longer periods of time when they were in the supine position than when they were seated in their wheelchairs or in a sidelyer (McEwen, 1992).

Positioning also may influence children's interactions with their environments through the effect of position on their behavioral state or arousal. Low levels of arousal and behavioral states that interfere with attention to environmental stimuli are common among children with the most severe cognitive and motor impairments (Guess et al., 1988). Guess and colleagues found that when children with multiple disabilities were positioned upright their behavioral states were more compatible with learning than when they were placed in recumbent positions. Similarly, Landesman-Dwyer and Sackett (1978) found that children's activity levels and receptivity to environmental stimuli were improved when intervention included an upright position. Other studies suggested that oxygenation is improved in the upright position (Navajas et al., 1988), and inadequate oxygenation has been proposed as a factor contributing to the lethargy of children with profound multiple disabilities (Guess et al., 1988).

Although research concerning effects of positioning with children who have multiple disabilities is limited, it does suggest that positioning may influence children's interactions with their environments through a variety of mechanisms. The upright position is more likely to enhance children's receptivity to and opportunities for interaction with the environment than recumbent positions (Campbell, 1989; McEwen, 1992) and thus may help limit or prevent secondary cognitive, emotional, and communication impairments and activity limitations. There are some children, however, especially those functioning at very low levels of communication development, whose own communication may be facilitated by the supine position. Because supine may be socially isolating and physically detrimental, it should be monitored carefully and used only while the child is actively engaged in social interaction.

ENHANCING PARTICIPATION OF CHILDREN WITH COGNITIVE AND MOTOR IMPAIRMENTS

A major way to enhance the participation of children with cognitive and motor impairments is to provide them with the supports necessary to be fully involved with family, friends, and peers in least restrictive environments. The concept of least restrictive environments has its roots in the U. S. Constitution, which affirms that the government shall intrude into peoples' lives in the least restrictive manner possible (Witkin & Fox, 1992). Since the 1960s, this concept has been incorporated into state and federal laws affecting services for people with cognitive impairments, mandating that, to the extent possible, people with disabilities will go to school, live, and work in environments with people who do not have disabilities.

The definition of the least restrictive environment for people with cognitive impairments has been moving steadily away from segregated services and toward full inclusion in community-based settings, as evidenced by closure of many institutions for people with cognitive impairments and court-ordered inclusion of children with cognitive impairments in general education classrooms. In 1992, for example, a judge of the U.S. Court for the District of New Jersey ordered a New Jersey school district to develop a plan to include an 8-year-old boy with Down syndrome in his neighborhood elementary school, with any needed supplementary aids and services. One of the court's findings was that "school districts…must consider placing children with disabilities in regular classroom settings, with the use of supplementary aids and services… before exploring other, more restrictive, alternatives" (TASH Force Strikes Again, 1992, p. 2). The IDEA amendments of 1997 placed additional emphasis on the need for individualized education program (IEP) teams to consider whether a child's needs can be addressed in the general education classroom with supplementary

aids and services. Physical therapists often are involved in coordination and communication with other team members to decide on a child's educational placement.

Physical therapy is one of the services that must follow children with disabilities as they move into their communities and neighborhood schools. Physical therapists must provide all three components of intervention in these settings to promote children's accomplishment of outcomes that will enable them to participate as successfully as possible in inclusive environments (Rainforth & York-Barr, 1997). Giangreco and colleagues (1998) have written a helpful "how-to" manual for inclusion of children with severe disabilities in general education classrooms that addresses provision of physical therapy and other related services. In their book, Downing and associates (2002) also have given practical and creative suggestions including children with severe disabilities in typical classrooms.

TEACHING AND LEARNING CONSIDERATIONS

Much of what physical therapists do is teach children to move more effectively and efficiently. Educational researchers have identified a number of teaching strategies that optimize the learning of students with cognitive impairments, which may be helpful to physical therapists when designing and implementing intervention plans. Although most of the strategies were designed for educational programming of students with cognitive impairments, they can be applied to motor learning as well as academic learning. Many of the strategies are closely related to current motor learning principles (see Chapter 4). Physical therapists should coordinate and communicate with other team members to identify opportunities for students to practice motor skills as well as show parents and teachers how to promote learning during those opportunities. Physical therapists also may apply the principles during direct intervention with children.

Instruction in Natural Environments

One strategy that has received considerable attention over the past two decades and is intended to address several of the learning problems of students with cognitive impairments, especially severe cognitive impairments, is a focus on teaching functional skills in natural environments (Brown et al., 1979; Falvey, 1989). Because students with cognitive impairments may take a long time to learn a few things, and because they have difficulty generalizing and maintaining skills, traditional curricula that build sequentially on fundamental, nonfunctional skills have not generally led to meaningful gains (Downing et al., 2002). Children are often unable to generalize such nonfunctional activities as putting pegs in pegboards, for example, to functional activities such as putting coins in a machine to get a soft drink. Practicing "prerequisite" skills, such as writing the letters of the alphabet, also often fails to result in such functional outcomes as the ability to sign one's name or select the correct restroom in a public place.

Children with severe motor impairments encounter similar difficulties when nonfunctional or presumed prerequisite skills are the focus of physical therapy. Research has largely failed to support children's generalization (carryover) of skills demonstrated during physical therapy sessions to other settings or synthesis of presumed components and prerequisites of movement into measurable functional motor activities (Horn, 1991).

When the emphasis is on acquisition of specific functional skills in natural environments, generalization is unnecessary or less difficult and skills are likely to be maintained by natural reinforcers and ongoing occasions for practice (Orelove & Sobsey, 1996). If several people work with the child on the same skills, learning may be enhanced by providing more opportunities to learn (repetitions) and by varying the stimulus conditions under which the skill is practiced, thus promoting generalization. These principles serve as a basis for integrated models of service delivery that have been advocated for physical therapists and occupational therapists working in early intervention and public school programs (Orelove & Sobsey, 1996; Rainforth & York-Barr, 1997). Although limited research has been conducted to support the effectiveness of teaching motor skills in natural environments, research in other areas, such as life skills, language, and social interaction, has suggested that such an approach would be valuable (Shelden & Rush, 2001).

Behavioral Programming Intervention

Behavioral programming is based on the assumption that behaviors are learned through interactions with the social, physical, and biologic environments; by manipulating such environments, behaviors can then be taught (Bijou, 1966). Following a review of research on the effectiveness of motor skills instruction for children with neuromotor impairments, Horn (1991) concluded that physical therapists and occupational therapists should develop procedures to incorporate behavioral techniques into their intervention programs. This recommendation was made based on the relative success of interventions using behavioral techniques compared with the neuromotor and sensory stimulation techniques commonly used by occupational therapists and physical therapists. By incorporating behavioral techniques into other intervention strategies, physical therapists may not only be able to increase the rate at which children with cognitive

impairments acquire motor skills and the number of skills they acquire but may also promote generalization and maintenance of motor behaviors.

Positive Reinforcement

A child is positively reinforced by a stimulus if a behavior that preceded the stimulus increases (Lutzker et al., 1983). Possible reinforcing stimuli are unlimited, ranging from tangible items, such as food and stickers, to social reinforcers, such as attention or praise, and abstract reinforcers, such as self-approval (Snell & Zirpoli, 1987). With children who have cognitive impairments, especially severe or profound cognitive impairments, common reinforcers such as praise, access to activities, and food often fail to lead to increases in behaviors, and identification of reinforcers can be a challenge (Orelove & Sobsey, 1996). To identify potential reinforcers, Haney and Falvey (1989) suggested (1) identifying natural consequences of the behavior, such as playing in water as a consequence of walking to the sink; (2) surveying the child's likes and dislikes by observing the child, or asking the child, parents, or teachers; and (3) offering paired choices to determine which of several potential reinforcers the child considers to be the most desirable. It is important that reinforcers not be overused, because children can become satiated and the stimuli will no longer have reinforcement value (Snell & Zirpoli, 1987).

Reinforcers have been effective in increasing motor behaviors, such as use of music as biofeedback to increase an erect head position (Maloney & Kurtz, 1982), and a combination of music and food to increase the distance that a child walked independently (Chandler & Adams, 1972). A common limitation of such studies, however, is that few have examined generalization to nonexperimental settings or maintenance of the behaviors beyond the period of intervention. Also, reinforcement has not been shown to result in acquisition of behaviors not previously in the child's repertoire. A combination of reinforcement with antecedent techniques and modification of consequences has, however, resulted in new behavioral responses (Horn, 1991; Reid et al., 1991).

Antecedent Techniques

The first step in shaping a new behavior is to prompt the desired behavior or an approximation by providing instructions, models, cues, or physical prompts (Snell & Zirpoli, 1987). Instructions can take a variety of forms, such as verbal or gestural instructions (e.g., "Reach for the toy") or verbal instructions paired with models, cues, or physical prompts (e.g., "Reach for the toy," paired with facilitation of movement at the shoulder). Modeling provides a demonstration of a behavior that the child attempts to imitate. Cues direct a child's attention to a task that can result in the desired behavior, without a physical prompt. To cue the child to reach for the toy, the toy could be tapped on the table or held above the child to encourage an erect posture, reaching, or assuming a standing position. Many of the handling techniques used by physical therapists provide physical prompts for motor behaviors.

For optimal learning to occur, the type and amount of prompting must be matched to the skills of the child, with the least amount of help necessary being the most conducive to the child's learning (Snell & Zirpoli, 1987). Prompting should be faded as the child responds, so that natural cues eventually provide the stimulus for response. A natural cue is the least intrusive prompt (e.g., the presence of a friend serving as a cue for a child to lift the head) and is the level of prompt required for independent behaviors. Physical prompts, often used by physical therapists, are the most intrusive.

Providing Consequences

Once a behavior has been prompted, it can be improved or expanded through shaping or chaining techniques. Shaping and chaining can also be used to build new behaviors (Snell & Zirpoli, 1987) through reinforcement of behaviors that successively approximate the desired behavior.

New behaviors can be shaped by reinforcing behaviors that are increasingly similar to the target behavior, such as reinforcing components of standing up from a chair, or chaining to link standing, walking, opening doors, and other behaviors necessary to accomplish a goal of walking to lunch. Backward chaining, in which the last step in the sequence is learned first, is often a useful technique because children receive the reward of task completion, often a natural reinforcer, throughout the process of learning the skill (Lutzker et al., 1983; Snell & Zirpoli, 1987).

Behavioral intervention is one of the areas in which physical therapists should take advantage of the expertise of other members of service delivery teams, such as teachers and psychologists. Physical therapy educational prerequisites and curricula rarely provide more than superficial information about behavioral strategies, which limits the extent to which many physical therapists can use them effectively to promote the development of motor skills by children with cognitive impairments.

Positive Behavior Support

Positive behavior support is another approach to intervention for children with developmental disabilities, including cognitive impairments, who may lack knowledge, communication, or social skills necessary to function effectively in their everyday environments. Lucyshyn and colleagues (2002) hypothesized that children with these limitations may develop unwanted behaviors as a means for getting their needs and wants met and for limiting events they find aversive. Positive behavior support interventions involve the use of multiple methods to redesign children's social and attitudinal environments, and sometimes their physical environments, to enhance their ability to enjoy life with behaviors that are more acceptable to others. Intervention is aimed at replacing problem behaviors with more socially acceptable behaviors and rendering problem behaviors ineffective and undesirable (Carr et al., 2002). Positive behavior support shows promise as an intervention that encourages participation in everyday routines without limiting children's personal preferences. The interventionist begins by observing the child in the child's everyday environments to look for antecedents that may be triggering a problem behavior, and identifying any environmental influences on the behavior (Carr et al., 2002). The interventionist must work closely with family members or other primary care providers to develop hypotheses about causes of problem behaviors, learn what motivates the child, and develop a plan that is acceptable for the people in the environments in which the child spends time (Lucyshyn et al., 2002). An effective plan redirects the child before the problem behavior occurs through adapting the task, the environment, or the demands.

Case studies have described use of positive behavior support in a variety of everyday environments (Cole & Levinson, 2002; Vaughn et al., 2002). Vaughn and colleagues (2002), for example, examined positive behavior support intervention to decrease problem behaviors that a 7-year-old with cognitive impairment exhibited while eating out with his family. The authors videotaped and used task analysis of the family's routines while eating out to determine any recurring antecedents and consequences of the child's behavior. With the child's mother, they developed hypotheses about the causes and functions of the behaviors, and determined activities the child most enjoyed doing that could be used as positive reinforcers while eating out. The mother, for example, theorized that the child engaged in disruptive behaviors while standing in line to order because he did not want to wait for a soda, which is what he wanted most when they ate out. As an intervention to reduce disruptive behavior while standing in line, the mother took a cup from home and filled it with soda so he could drink it while they waited to order. With the assistance of the authors, the mother also identified and used reinforcers to decrease the child's disruptive behaviors associated with other aspects of eating out, such as staying at the table to finish eating and leaving the playground equipment when it was time to go home. As measured by direct observation, the interventions were associated with both a decrease in disruptive behavior and an increase in the child's engagement. Using a similar approach, Cole & Levinson (2002) found that providing choice in aspects of unpleasant tasks (such as where to stand in line) reduced occurrence of problem behavior in two school-aged students with developmental disabilities.

Although no randomized controlled studies have examined positive behavior support, the case studies suggest that positive behavior support has promise to assist families, teachers, and other care providers in helping children with cognitive impairments to participate more successfully in everyday routines. As members of teams, physical therapists may participate in task analysis, developing an intervention plan, and using the intervention while working with children. One important aspect of positive behavioral support is promoting children's communication abilities so they can express desires and needs in behaviorally acceptable ways.

PROMOTING CHILDREN'S COMMUNICATION DEVELOPMENT

When working with children who have cognitive impairments, all team members are responsible for promoting development in areas often not considered part of their disciplinary domains. One of the most effective ways physical therapists can contribute to the overall development of children with cognitive impairments is to assist efforts to improve their communication abilities. At its most basic level, communication enables children to influence their social and physical environments to control what happens to them. All children, even those with the most profound multiple disabilities, can communicate. Some communicate in many of the same ways as infants, such as looking at a person, crying, or smiling; others can learn to communicate using signs, communication boards, or electronic voice-output communication aids (Cress, 2002; see also Chapter 33). Ability to control what happens to themselves is often said to be the key to prevention or reduction of these children's pervasive passivity or "learned helplessness," a condition that can effectively block educational efforts and be extremely resistant to change (Campbell PH, 1989).

The critical importance of communication and the need for all team members to participate in communication development was recognized by creation in the United States of the National Joint Committee for the Communicative Needs of Persons with Severe Disabilities in 1986. Representatives of seven organizations, including the American Physical Therapy Association, served on the joint committee and developed guidelines that crossed traditional disciplinary boundaries and reflect a "shared

commitment to promoting effective communication by persons with severe disabilities thus providing a common ground on which the disciplines of the member organizations can unite their efforts to improve the quality of life of such persons" (National Joint Committee for the Communicative Needs of Persons with Severe Disabilities, 1992, pp. 1–2). This means that physical therapists are responsible for promoting effective communication, not only through such traditional means as positioning and improving motor skills to enable access to communication aids but also through provision of environments that acknowledge and address the Communication Bill of Rights (Fig. 20-2) of children who have communication impairments (National Joint Committee for the Communicative Needs of Persons with Severe Disabilities, 1992).

EVALUATION OF OUTCOMES

Because children and young adults with cognitive impairments often progress slowly, particularly those with severe disabilities, it is important to use evaluation methods that are responsive to small changes. This is necessary not only to determine if progress is being made but also to prevent expenditure of time and effort on intervention strategies that are not leading to meaningful outcomes. Three related methods that are especially useful for assessing outcomes of physical therapy intervention for children with cognitive impairments are (1) accomplishment of behavioral objectives, (2) use of the Canadian Occupational Performance Measure (Law et al., 1994), and (3) single-case research methodologies.

Use of Behavioral Objectives

Assessment of outcomes can be relatively straightforward if functional goals and behavioral objectives leading to them are identified before intervention. As described by Randall and McEwen (2000), the components of behavioral objectives should enable therapists to monitor a child's progress toward accomplishment of a goal, determine if it is necessary to modify an intervention, and determine when and if goals have been met. Once a goal has been identified, such as "David will go to the kitchen and make himself a peanut butter sandwich," behavioral objectives leading to achievement of the goal can be developed by comparing David's abilities with the goal's requirements.

Behavioral objectives have five components: *Who* will do *what*, under what *conditions*, *how well*, by *when*. These components permit a measurable evaluation of whether the goal is being met within the projected time frame. One of David's behavioral objectives, leading to the sandwich-making goal, may be to move himself from the living room

All persons, regardless of the extent or severity of their disabilities, have a basic right to affect, through communication, the conditions of their own existence. Beyond this general right, a number of specific communication rights should be ensured in all daily interactions and interventions involving persons who have severe disabilities. These basic communication rights are as follows:

1. The right to request desired objects, actions, events, and persons and to express personal preferences or feelings.

2. The right to be offered choices and alternatives.

3. The right to reject or refuse undesired objects, events, or actions, including the right to decline or reject all proffered choices.

4. The right to request, and be given, attention from and interaction with another person.

5. The right to request feedback or information about a state, an object, a person, or an event of interest.

6. The right to active treatment and intervention efforts to enable people with severe disabilities to communicate messages in whatever modes and as effectively and efficiently as their specific abilities will allow.

7. The right to have communication acts acknowledged and responded to, even when the intent of these acts cannot be fulfilled by the responder.

8. The right to have access at all times to any needed augmentative and alternative communication devices and other assistive devices and to have those devices in good working order.

9. The right to environmental contexts, interactions, and opportunities that expect and encourage persons with disabilities to participate as full communicative partners with other people, including peers.

10. The right to be informed about the people, things, and events in one's immediate environment.

11. The right to be communicated with in a manner that recognizes and acknowledges the inherent dignity of the person being addressed, including the right to be part of communication exchanges about individuals that are conducted in his or her presence.

12. The right to be communicated with in ways that are meaningful, understandable, and culturally and linguistically appropriate.

◆ **Figure 20-2**   Communication bill of rights. *(From Guidelines for Meeting the Communication Needs of Persons with Severe Disabilities by the National Joint Committee for the Communication Needs of Persons with Severe Disabilities, 1992.)*

to the kitchen, which could be written, "David will walk using his reverse walker from the living room to the kitchen in less than 2 minutes on four of five consecutive days after school by December 14, 20__." Assessing whether this objective, or part of it, is accomplished, regardless of the intervention methods used, should not be difficult.

Canadian Occupational Performance Measure

The COPM (Law et al., 1994) was designed to help identify and measure individually meaningful goals for people in the areas of self-care, productivity (work, household management, and play/school), and leisure. An interviewer asks patients or caregivers to think about a typical day to identify activities in these areas that they want to do, need to do, or are expected to do. The interviewer then asks which of the activities the person is able to do

satisfactorily and to rate the importance of these activities on a 10-point scale. Using the importance ratings, the interviewer asks the patient or caregiver to select the five problems that seem to be the most important and asks if the activities should be the focus of intervention. After the patient or caregiver selects activities for intervention, the person rates the current performance of each on a 10-point scale, from "not able to do it at all" to "able to do it extremely well," and rates satisfaction on a 10-point scale, from "not satisfied at all" to "extremely satisfied." Performance, satisfaction, and total scores are then calculated for each activity. Following a period of intervention, outcomes can be measured by asking the patient or caregiver to again rate performance and satisfaction of each activity, and change scores can be calculated. Change scores are a useful measure of change across all goals for one child or as a measure of change across children.

Single-Subject Research Methods

Single-subject research methods are another useful means to assess intervention outcomes in clinical, educational, and other service settings. These methods can be used to assess the outcomes for a single child or can assess effects of intervention across several children (Harris, 1991). Unlike case reports, single-subject research designs have controls that allow identification of cause-and-effect relationships among interventions and outcomes (McEwen, 2001). Several types of single-subject designs exist, including A-B, withdrawal, alternating treatment, and multiple baseline (Portney & Watkins, 2000). Although the designs differ, they all have certain characteristics, such as repeatedly measuring and graphing the outcome variable over time and comparing data in adjacent phases, such as baseline and intervention phases or phases when two or more treatments are alternated (Portney & Watkins, 2000). Graphed data usually are first analyzed visually, by comparing stability, levels, and trends in adjacent phases. Statistical analyses specific to single-subject designs also can be used, such as the two standard deviation bandwidth method and testing the significance of trends in adjacent phases using the split-middle line (Portney & Watkins, 2000).

Many examples of single-subject research exist in rehabilitation literature. McEwen and Karlan (1989), for example, used an alternating treatment single-subject design to compare the effect of positioning in a chair, stander, prone wedge, and sidelyer on the ability of two preschool children to access a switch placed in several locations on a communication board–like grid. As shown in Figure 20-3, the data revealed that it took longer for both of the children to press the switch when they were in the sidelyer than when in the other three positions. Thorpe and Valvano (2002) used a single-subject multiple baseline design across 13 children with cerebral palsy to examine effects of application of motor learning principles on the children's performance of a novel task. Fragala and colleagues (2002) used an A-B design across seven children to determine the effect of botulinum toxin A injections on children's passive range of motion, Modified Ashworth Scale scores, and the COPM. Reid and colleagues (1999) used an A-B-A (withdrawal) design with six children to identify the effect of a wheelchair mounted rigid pelvic stabilizer (RPS) compared with a traditional wheelchair lap belt on task performance and satisfaction with performance as measured by the COPM. Textbooks and research articles are good resources for anyone interested in using single-subject research methods to measure outcomes of intervention. The classic text by Barlow and Hersen (1984) and the chapter on single-subject methods in the text by Portney and Watkins (2000) are excellent.

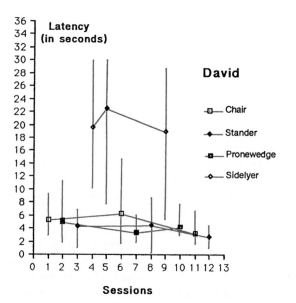
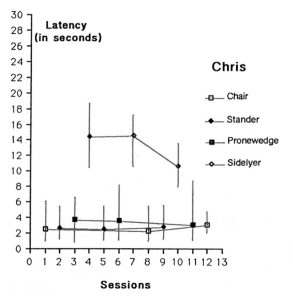

◆ **Figure 20-3**   A single-subject alternating treatment design assessing means and ranges of switch-activation latency when two children were positioned in a chair, stander, prone wedge, and sidelyer. *(From McEwen, IR, & Karlan, GR. Assessment of the effects of position on communication board access by individuals with cerebral palsy. Augmentative and Alternative Communication, 5:238–239, 1989. Copyright ©1989 by the International Society for Augmentative and Alternative Communication.)*

TRANSITION TO ADULTHOOD

Some people with cognitive impairments, especially those with severe and profound multiple disabilities, may receive physical therapy throughout their childhood years and during their transition to adulthood. Others will receive short episodes of physical therapy services as their abilities and needs change over time. The type of services provided, the intensity of services, and the model of service delivery should be individualized to the needs of the person. Therapists working in public schools are especially likely to be involved in the transition to adulthood because Part B of IDEA requires that transition planning begin by at least age 14 for all students with disabilities. The role of physical therapists, along with other IEP and interagency team members, should be to enable students to function meaningfully and as independently as possible in their current and possible future environments (McEwen et al., 2000).

The transition to adulthood is difficult for many young people, regardless of their abilities or disabilities. Until recently, most young adults with cognitive and neuromotor impairments had few options available to them, and the greater their cognitive impairments, the fewer options they had. Employment options either did not exist or were limited to sheltered workshops or activity centers. Residential options usually included staying at home with aging parents or moving into a large residential facility. They also had few choices about how they spent their time, with whom they spent time, or where they could go.

In recent years, more employment and community life options have become available for people with severe cognitive impairments, including those with the most severe multiple disabilities. To be able to take full advantage of these options, young people need to prepare for transition to adult life throughout their years in school and then continue to receive support as the transition takes place and the new life begins. Physical therapy often can make a difference in the options available to young people with both cognitive and neuromotor impairments as they make the transition to adult life and in the success of their transitions. Self-determination and employment are particularly important for most young people.

SELF-DETERMINATION

Youth with disabilities often have difficulty achieving goals, such as independent living, higher education, and employment that their peers without disabilities achieve relatively easily. Teaching and supporting self-determination have been proposed to be important for improving outcomes for youth with disabilities, including youth with cognitive impairments. Wehmeyer and Bolding (2001) defined self-determination at the personal level as "having control over one's life and destiny" (p. 372). Self-determination has four parts: freedom, control over one's own life, support, and responsibility. Each of these parts is defined in Box 20-1.

People exhibit self-determination by making everyday decisions and life decisions for themselves (Wehmeyer & Bolding, 1999). In a review of the self-determination literature, Malian and Nevin (2002) found six curricula for teaching self-determination skills that have been field-tested. Overall, the studies suggested that direct instruction in self-determination skills can lead to positive changes in the knowledge, attitudes, and behaviors associated with self-determination. Wehmeyer and Schwartz (1997) examined the relationship between scores on a self-determination rating scale and outcomes 1 year after leaving school. In their sample of 80 participants, students with higher scores on a self-determination rating scale were more likely to be employed and earn more per hour than students who achieved lower scores on the self-determination rating scale.

Wehmeyer and Bolding (1999, 2001) also studied the relationship between environment and self-determination. In one study, they matched adults by intelligence, age, and gender to examine the relationship between living and working environments and self-determination. They found that those living or working in general community-based settings reported greater self-determination and autonomous function than matched peers living or working in either segregated community-based settings or non-community-based segregated settings. This study suggested that environments and, in particular, inclusive community environments were important for greater self-determination and autonomy for people with cognitive impairments. Wehmeyer and Bolding (2001) also studied change in self-determination with changes in work or living environments. When 31 people moved from a restrictive environment (such as a nursing home or sheltered workshop) to a less restrictive environment, self-determination increased when compared with pre-move test scores.

Physical therapists can help children with cognitive impairments to develop self-determination. This is best accomplished through a team approach that identifies priorities for the child and family and considers the environments in which the child does or will spend time. Self-determination is something that does not start in adolescence. It needs to begin early, with young children being offered opportunities to make choices in any way

---

Box 20-1 **Self-Determination**

Self-determination is the ability for people to control their lives, reach goals they have set, and take part fully in the world around them. Self-determination has four basic rights and responsibilities:

Freedom. Freedom for Americans with disabilities is like freedom for any American. It means deciding for oneself about how to work, live and love; direct one's life; give to the community; and decide what kind of services and supports to use (if any).

People who experience disability do not have to accept segregated schooling, institutional placement, service slots, or forced treatment of any kind.

Authority or control of own life. Americans with disabilities have the right to direct their lives. This includes having control over how to spend their money, having the right to vote, being able to sign legal contracts, and being able to decide how funds available for support services will be spent.

Support agreements must be developed together by individuals and funders. Funds must be assigned to individuals rather than slots. People with disabilities must be allowed to use those funds to purchase the supports they require. They also must be able to personally select (hire) and direct people who provide support or assistance.

Support. People with disabilities may desire support/assistance to care for themselves and be an active part of their communities.

Each person who experiences disability can determine the supports that work for him or her. People with disabilities (together with those they trust, if they want) have the right to figure out their life goals, what kind of supports might work, and how to make and keep track of plans and budgets.

Those who assist people with disabilities will work towards bringing support and access to life opportunities at the highest potential.

Independent brokers must also be available to assist people in designing, setting up, and managing their supports. Fiscal intermediaries must be available to assist with employment paperwork and bill paying. Both must work at the direction of the person with a disability and be free from conflicts of interest.

Responsibility. People with disabilities have the responsibility to fulfill the ordinary obligations of citizenship like voting, obeying laws, directing their own lives, and participating in community life.

Policy barriers must be removed when they prevent people who earn money from receiving health insurance, personal assistance or other needed supports.

From The Oregon Health & Science University Center on Self-Determination. Accessed at http://www.selfdeterminationohsu.org/about/index.html.

---

they are able to indicate preferences. Older children should be expected to be responsible for their choices, and young adults should be expected to thoughtfully decide what is best for them and then be supported in their choices by others.

EMPLOYMENT

Employment options in the United States for people with cognitive impairments and multiple disabilities have expanded greatly over the past several years, particularly in some parts of the country. Many places still offer primarily sheltered workshop and activity center alternatives, but progress is being made nationwide as federal, state, and other public and private initiatives support

development and expansion of employment opportunities for people with disabilities (Cimera, 1998).

Supported employment, one model of employment services, has been responsible for increasing the employment options for many people who have severe disabilities. Rather than working on prerequisite or prevocational skills in sheltered settings until they are "ready" for a job, people in supported employment learn real jobs while they are doing them, with ongoing supports from team members to learn and maintain the job (Flexer et al., 2001).

Since the early 1980s, supported employment has been gaining credibility as a viable employment option and has received significant support from the Vocational Rehabilitation Act Amendments of 1986 (PL 99-506), which authorized new funds for states to provide supported employment services to people with severe disabilities. As yet, however, few communities offer a supported employment alternative to sheltered workshops and day activity centers for those with the most severe disabilities. The economic value of supported employment was documented by Cimera (1998), who studied the cost-efficiency of supported employment programs and found that (1) supported employment is a cost-efficient way to serve people with severe mental retardation and multiple disabilities; (2) supported employment is cost-efficient from the cost-accounting perspective of the client, the taxpayer, and society; and (3) projections of lifelong benefits suggested that all individuals, regardless of the severity or number of disabilities, can be served cost-effectively in supported employment.

Physical therapists can often have a pivotal role in the successful employment of individuals who have both cognitive impairments and limited motor skills. Physical therapists can assist employment specialists to assess an individual's abilities to perform job-related motor skills and to identify jobs that are compatible with those skills. They can also identify assistive technology and environmental modifications that may enable the person to perform a job that might not be possible otherwise. Physical therapists can also help develop training for job-related motor skills and for self-care and mobility during working hours.

SUMMARY

Regardless of their medical diagnoses, children with cognitive impairments have learning characteristics that physical therapists need to consider for effective physical therapy management. Compared with typically developing children, children with cognitive impairments have been shown, for example, to be able to learn a fewer number of things, to need a greater number of repetitions for learning to occur, to have greater difficulty generalizing skills from one environment to another, to have greater difficulty maintaining skills that are not practiced regularly, to have slower response times, and to have a more limited repertoire of responses. Physical therapy intervention strategies that address these learning characteristics and that promote communication, inclusion, and self-determination can have an important role in the meaningful participation of people with cognitive and motor impairments in the lives of their families and communities. Whatever the future of children with cognitive and neuromotor impairments, physical therapy services can often help expand the options, ease the transition,

and promote independence within the community-based environments in which people choose to live and work.

CASE STUDIES

ALISE

Alise is 32 months old and has received home-based early intervention services since age 8 months. She has lissencephaly (also known as smooth brain syndrome), which was identified when she was 5 months old and had a seizure. Alise lives with her parents and 12-year-old brother in a suburb of a large city.

When Alise was 8 months old she did very little. She had great difficulty moving against the force of gravity, did not have head control, and could not roll over, sit, reach for objects, or grasp objects placed in her hands. She did not appear to make eye contact with people or objects and had difficulty sucking from a bottle and swallowing. The evaluation team conducted an arena assessment to document Alise's eligibility for early intervention services, including administration of the Battelle Developmental Inventory (BDI) (Newborg et al., 1984). At age 8 months, Alise's age-equivalent scores were in the birth to 2-month range in all developmental areas.

During the meeting to develop the Individualized Family Service Plan (IFSP), a top-down approach was used to first identify outcomes of intervention and then the strategies to achieve them. Alise's parents said that what they wanted most for Alise was for her to be able to roll over and sit by herself. They were also concerned about her vision and the difficulty she had swallowing without choking while drinking from her bottle.

The early intervention program used a transdisciplinary model of service delivery, and the team selected the physical therapist to be the primary service provider because Alise's parents were primarily concerned about her motor problems. The occupational therapist and a vision specialist would consult with the physical therapist to address the feeding and vision concerns, and other team members would be available for consultation as other needs were identified.

The physical therapist made weekly visits to Alise's home, working with Alise, her parents, and her brother to promote Alise's ability to move in opposition to the force of gravity, to eat more effectively, and to attend visually to people and objects in her environment (Figs. 20-4 and 20-5). A plastic booster chair with a tray, which is widely available for typical infants, was modified to enable Alise

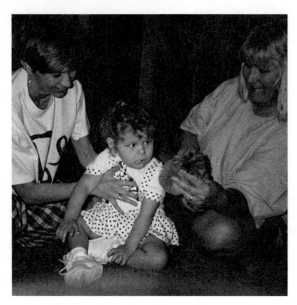

◆ **Figure 20-4** Physical therapist showing Alise's mother how to help her learn to move from a sitting position.

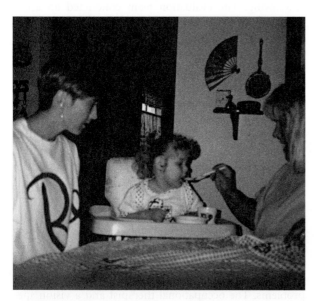

◆ **Figure 20-5** Physical therapist doing an ecologic assessment of Alise's mealtime in her home.

to maintain a seated position while on the floor or at the table. A stroller was also adapted for her.

Two years later, at 2 years 8 months, Alise can now maintain a sitting position when placed on the floor, drink liquids and eat ground foods without difficulty, and easily focus on and track objects and people. She is still

unable to assume a sitting position, roll, or move about on the floor. She has particular difficulty using her hands and holds only her bottle, if it is placed in her hands, and will occasionally reach for her favorite fuzzy rubber ball. She sometimes uses her mouth to get things that she wants and will raise her legs when she is on her back in bed and wants to be picked up. She says approximately 10 words, including "no," "ahm" (mom), "da" (dad), and an approximation of her brother's name. Assistive equipment she now uses includes an adapted high chair, booster chair, and stroller; a prone stander; a walker with a tray; and a bath seat.

Two months ago, when Alise was 30 months old, her IFSP was updated. The desired outcomes identified by her parents were (1) that Alise would learn to get into and out of sitting by herself, (2) that she would learn to move around on the floor, and (3) that she would be able to play with toys with her hands. Because Alise's family continued to be primarily concerned about her motor development, the physical therapist remained the primary service provider. The IFSP also included a plan to prepare for Alise's transition from the early intervention program when she turns 3. Her mother wants Alise to stay at home until she is 5, so the early intervention team must identify the services that Alise and her family will need and determine how they can be obtained through other community agencies, such as the local education agency or developmental disabilities services.

AMY

Amy's case illustrates an application of the *Guide to Physical Therapist Practice* (2001) for a child with cognitive impairment in a public school setting. The process for "patient/client management" described in the *Guide* is not always consistent with the team-oriented process used for making decisions about physical therapy services in schools. The terms "patient" and "client" also are inappropriate for school-based practice, where physical therapists usually refer to children as "students" or "children." Notes throughout the case example indicate other variations in the process described in the *Guide* that are necessary to provide appropriate school-based services.

Based on prior knowledge of Amy, the physical therapist identified the preferred practice pattern as Neuromuscular Pattern 5C: Impaired Motor Function and Sensory Integrity Associated with Nonprogressive Disorders of the Central Nervous System—Congenital Origin or Acquired in Infancy or Childhood. Information about Amy and the process that her school team used to develop her IEP are summarized as follows, according to the *Guide's* five elements of patient/client (student) management.

Examination

History

General demographics. Amy is an 8-year-old girl. English is her family's native language.

Social history. Amy lives with her mother, father, and 12-year-old brother. Her mother is a nurse and her father owns a heating and air-conditioning company. Amy participates in many family activities, such as church, camping, and car trips during the summer.

Employment/work (job/school/play). Amy is in a general third-grade class in her neighborhood elementary school, where she, her teacher, and a classroom assistant receive supports and services from a special education teacher, physical therapist, occupational therapist, and speech-language pathologist. For special education eligibility purposes, Amy is classified as having multiple disabilities.

Growth and development. When Amy was about 6 months old her mother became concerned because she did not seem to look at people and objects, did not reach for objects, and could not roll over. When she was 8 months old she was diagnosed with spastic quadriplegic cerebral palsy. The most recent norm-referenced developmental test was administered when she was 6 years old. At that time her age-equivalent scores on the Battelle Developmental Inventory (Newborg et al., 1984) were personal-social, 7 months; adaptive, 5 months; motor, 4 months; communication, 6 months; and cognitive, 5 months. Her school team believes that further norm-referenced testing would not be helpful.

Living environment. Amy lives with her parents and brother in a one-story house. The family has a van with a lift for Amy's wheelchair.

General health status. Amy's health generally is good, although she usually gets pneumonia at least once a year. Her seizure disorder is well controlled with medication. She usually sleeps through the night if someone turns her once.

Social/health habits. Amy moves very little, leading to a low level of physical fitness, which puts her at risk for cardiopulmonary disease as she grows older.

Family history. Not known.

Medical/surgical history. When Amy was 5 years old she had bilateral Achilles tendon and adductor lengthening. Two years later, she had a right varus derotation osteotomy for a subluxed hip.

Current condition(s)/chief complaints. Amy received home-based early intervention services, including physical therapy, from age 9 months to 3 years. From age 3 to 5 years she was in a half-day neighborhood preschool program, where she received physical therapy, occupational therapy, special education, and speech-language pathology services provided by her school district. When she was 5 years old she entered her neighborhood kindergarten, and since that time she has been included in general education classes.

Note: The *Guide* says that the "current condition/chief complaint" should include "patient/client, family, significant other, and caregiver expectation and goals for the therapeutic intervention." Although families may have expectations for physical therapy at this step in the process, a more appropriate process is for the child's team, including the family, to identify overall educational goals for the child, then later determine if physical therapy is necessary to achieve the goals (Giangreco et al., 1998).

Amy's parents said that they were concerned because Amy is so passive, does so little, and seems interested in so few things. They have three priorities for her education (1) that she learn to choose things, people, and activities that she wants; (2) that she become someone that other people like to be with because one of the things she seems to enjoy is being with other children; and (3) that she learn to help more during caregiving activities because she is becoming heavier and more difficult to handle and move.

Functional status and activity level. Amy will look when her name is called, smiles when people she likes talk with her, and enjoys being around other children. She often will close her eyes and drop her head when she does not have the attention of other people. Amy cannot grasp objects, but occasionally will reach toward objects. She eats ground foods fed from a spoon and drinks liquids from a cup. She is dependent on others for all self-care and mobility.

Medications. She takes Dilantin twice a day for seizures.

Other clinical tests. Amy is below the 99th percentile for weight and height. A report of a nutrition evaluation 6 months ago indicated that Amy was adequately nourished but recommended increasing the amount of calcium and protein in her diet.

Systems Review

Anatomic and physiologic status. Amy's severe neuromuscular impairments are likely to influence her cardiopulmonary, integumentary, and musculoskeletal status, which must be kept in mind when identifying goals and interventions. Her anatomic and physiologic status also may require consultation with or referral to a physician.

Communication, affect, cognition, language, and learning style. Amy is a passive child whose communication and cognitive development are far below those of typical 8-year-olds.

Tests and measures. Note: In a school environment, members of students' educational teams other than the physical therapist often administer tests and measures to examine some of the areas listed in the *Guide*. All team members then share results when developing the IEP. Some information was gathered formally using standardized methods or tools; other information was based on observation or prior knowledge. Other students' teams might have different expertise and be responsible for different areas. An occupational therapist on another team, for example, may know more about swallowing than a speech-language pathologist, or a physical therapist may know more about sensory integration than an occupational therapist.

Evaluation. The team met to discuss the information that each contributed to the development of Amy's IEP. Amy has many impairments, activity limitations, and participation restrictions, most of which the team agreed will not improve with intervention. The team also agreed that Amy's parents' concerns should be priorities in determining Amy's IEP goals. The physical therapist expressed concern that range-of-motion examination indicated that Amy's hip and knee range of motion had decreased since the last measurements 3 months previously.

Diagnosis. The physical therapist decided to use the Gross Motor Function Classification System (Palisano et al., 1997) to identify a diagnosis. Amy was functioning at the most limited level, Level V: Self-Mobility Is Severely Limited Even with the Use of Assistive Technology. This diagnosis is not used for special education and related services purposes.

Prognosis. The physical therapist and the rest of the team agreed that the prognosis for improving Amy's primary neuromuscular impairments was poor, but the prognosis for preventing secondary musculoskeletal impairments was more hopeful. The prognosis for improving activities also was poor, but the team agreed that with consistent and appropriate instruction, Amy probably could learn to help herself more, as her parents wished. Because participation does not necessarily require performance (WHO, 2001), Amy's participation in many activities was limited only by the creativity of others who could support her involvement in various life situations.

Plan of care. Note: The *Guide* states that as the next step in the prognostic process, the physical therapist should develop the plan of care, which includes "specific interventions, proposed frequency and duration of the interventions, anticipated goals, expected outcomes, and discharge plans. In the educational environment, physical therapists do not make these decisions unilaterally. With the physical therapist's input, the team, including the student when appropriate, determines all of these elements when developing a student's IEP. In schools, the term *plan of care* is not used, but the IEP serves a similar purpose.

Amy's team wrote the following goals for her IEP:

Amy will indicate her choice of a person, activity, or object at least 10 times each day at school and 10 times at home for 5 consecutive days by May 20.

When engaged in an activity with her classmates, Amy will interact with them by such means as looking at them, smiling, reaching, or vocalizing for at least 3 of 10 minutes during two activities on 5 consecutive school days by May 20.

Amy will assist in transferring from her wheelchair by leaning forward when touched on the shoulder and asked to stand up and then bear her full weight after being assisted to a standing position during 10 consecutive transfers from her wheelchair by May 20.

The team then wrote a sequence of benchmarks or short-term instructional objectives leading to each goal (not mentioned in the *Guide*, but required by IDEA). After writing the objectives, the team decided who would be necessary to help Amy achieve each objective and what each would contribute. The team also identified the general supports that Amy needs to attend school and to achieve her goals. Giangreco and associates (1998) described five categories of general supports, including supports needed to meet personal, physical, and sensory needs; to teach others about the student; and to provide the student with access and opportunities. The supports identified for Amy were as follows:

Personal: feeding, diaper changing, and other self-care

Physical: positioning and mobility

Sensory: avoiding intense stimuli, which cause Amy to withdraw

Teaching: teaching other children about Amy, her means of communication, and how to help her participate in activities

Access: promoting hand use during classroom activities

The team decided that her educational goals could best be met in a general education classroom, with supplemental aids and services. They agreed that a segregated special education setting was not only unnecessarily restrictive but that a general education classroom was more likely to provide the social and educational environment necessary to help Amy accomplish her goals. Supplemental aids and services in the general education classroom include a half-time assistant assigned to the classroom and ongoing consultation between Amy's classroom teacher and her special education team (a resource teacher, an occupational therapist, a physical therapist, and a speech-language pathologist).

The team decided that Amy's physical therapist was needed to help her achieve the third goal, involving transfers, and with the physical supports of positioning and mobility. The therapist also would help with motor aspects of other goals and consult with the physical education teacher about how to include Amy in activities that are meaningful for her. The physical therapist proposed and the team agreed that the physical therapist would see Amy and her classroom staff (teachers and classroom assistant) for 1 hour three times a week for the first 2 weeks of school, twice a week for the next 2 weeks, then once a week for 3 months, and then twice a month until the end of the school year. Over the school year, the physical therapist would provide 32 hours of service, or 32 "visits" (a term not used on an IEP).

Intervention

Physical therapists working in schools provide (1) coordination, communication, and documentation; (2) student-related instruction; and (3) procedural interventions, as delineated in the *Guide*. To provide the necessary positioning and mobility supports, the physical therapist first determined that Amy's wheelchair was adequate for her needs (procedural intervention). She also consulted with Amy's classroom teacher to determine which alternatives to wheelchair positioning would be used during which activities and who would be responsible for position changes. Positions and activities were matched to enable Amy to function as well as possible throughout the day. She uses a supine stander, for example, during a morning science class, which usually involves groups of students standing around tables as they work on a project together. She also stands in the afternoon during art class because her hand use seems to be better when she is standing.

The therapist taught the teacher and assistant how to place Amy in her wheelchair and other positioning devices (student-related instruction), about some of the basic mechanics of the wheelchair, and how to push the chair safely. She also taught Amy's classmates how to push Amy safely and issued wheelchair pushing licenses to those who demonstrated safe pushing techniques (student-related instruction). Other supports provided by the physical therapist were to teach Amy's teacher, the assistant, and her classmates some ways to encourage Amy to raise her head and use her hands during classroom activities, and to teach the assistant methods to use during caregiving activities, especially diaper changing, to help maintain Amy's joint flexibility (student-related instruction). The assistant also used diaper changing, when Amy was supine, as an opportunity to teach basic social interaction skills.

To help Amy achieve the goal of assisting with transfers, the physical therapist first worked with Amy to identify how best to help her to learn (direct intervention). She found that, although Amy could perform some aspects of a transfer, such as lean forward to prepare to stand, she usually would not, either spontaneously or when asked. She also did not place her feet on the floor as she was moved toward a standing position and did not bear her weight when placed on her feet. To teach Amy to assist with these components of the transfer, the physical therapist consulted with the special education resource teacher to develop a behavioral program. The program included (1) providing verbal and natural cues for a transfer (such as the presence of the supine stander), physical prompts, and reinforcement for leaning forward in her wheelchair, a motor behavior that was already within Amy's repertoire; (2) providing cues, physical prompts, and reinforcement during practice to learn to place her feet on the floor and bear increasing amounts of weight, during transfers and other activities, to shape these skills, which were not yet within Amy's repertoire; (3) chaining the various components of the transfer, as Amy began to learn each one; and (4) eventually fading the verbal cues and physical prompts to permit the natural cues surrounding transfers to prompt Amy's participation.

After she was reasonably sure that the program developed to teach Amy to lean forward was effective, the physical therapist taught Amy's teacher, the classroom assistant, and her parents to implement the techniques whenever Amy transferred (student-related instruction). Because Amy had not demonstrated the ability to place her feet on the floor and bear her weight in standing, the physical therapist worked with Amy during transfers and other classroom activities to determine how best to provide physical prompts and other cues and to teach Amy to begin to learn to stand (direct intervention). She then taught Amy's teacher, the assistant, and her parents how to help Amy continue to develop this skill (student-related instruction).

Reexamination. Part B of IDEA requires that each short-term objective have an evaluation procedure and a schedule for evaluation to determine progress toward the goals and objectives. This is consistent with the "reexamination" step of the *Guide*. The physical therapist and the rest of Amy's team continuously observed her performance to evaluate her progress, and they modified or redirected the intervention, as necessary. Her progress toward meeting each of the IEP objectives was evaluated according to the timelines specified on the IEP.

Criteria for termination of physical therapy services. Note: The *Guide* says that discharge (a term not used in schools) "occurs based on the physical therapist's analysis of the achievement of anticipated goals and expected outcomes." Reasons for discharge or discontinuing services in schools are consistent with the reasons outlined in the *Guide*, except that the physical therapist does not independently make the decision. The physical therapist may give the rest of the team rationale, but the team makes the decision, based on the student's need for physical therapy to achieve goals and provide necessary supports.

JEFF

Jeff is a 20-year-old who recently moved from Sunnyvale, a state residential facility for people with developmental disabilities, to a boarding house in the small town where his parents live. Three other young adults with disabilities live at the boarding house, and they invited Jeff to live with them after he visited with them several months ago.

Jeff has spastic quadriplegic cerebral palsy and moderate cognitive impairments and had lived at Sunnyvale since he was 7 years old. For the first 9 years he spent most of his time in bed, receiving basic care but little education or habilitative services other than passive range-of-motion exercises.

When Jeff was 18, physical therapy and other services were expanded as a result of a court order. Since then, Jeff acquired and learned to use an electronic communication aid and an electric wheelchair. The chair has a custom-contoured seat and back to accommodate his moderate scoliosis, pelvic asymmetry with windswept hips, and lower extremity flexion contractures, which developed in spite of the passive range-of-motion exercises. He also learned to assume a standing position and bear much of his weight during assisted transfers. Bilateral ankle-foot orthoses, improved positioning in bed and wheelchair, active participation during all transfers, and use of good alternative positioning appear to have helped limit progression of his musculoskeletal deformities.

In preparation for Jeff's transition to the boarding house, his physical therapist, occupational therapist, and mother took him there for an ecologic assessment to determine what skills Jeff needed to live there successfully. He can get help with dressing, bathing, and laundry, if necessary, but he has to be able to use the toilet independently and transfer to and from his bed without assistance. He also has to be able to use the telephone, make his own breakfast and lunch, and go shopping in a nearby grocery-variety store (see ecologic assessment in Table 20-2, format from Baumgart et al., 1982).

To prepare for his move, Jeff's physical therapist worked with him on the aspects of toilet transfers and shopping identified by the ecologic assessment, simulating what he will encounter in the community. Before Jeff moved, he, his therapists, and his mother spent several days at the boarding house going through a typical day to help Jeff generalize skills he learned at Sunnyvale to the boarding house and to identify problems and the means to overcome them.

When he moved to the community, Jeff enrolled in the local high school and a new IEP was written. Two of Jeff's educational goals relate to improving his independence at home and obtaining, learning, and keeping a job. His school physical therapist works with Jeff and his personal care assistant to increase his independence in his home and is working with his job coach to identify a job that Jeff can learn. Once a job is found, his physical therapist will also help Jeff learn to use public transportation and to use the toilet at work and will provide ongoing consultation with the job coach to solve problems as they arise.

The physical therapist's involvement to help Jeff become more independent in his home and work environments is directed toward reducing his disabilities. Positioning and orthoses are used to reduce functional limitations and prevent the development of additional musculoskeletal impairments. For Jeff, it is also important that he maintain or increase his flexibility and endurance. For this reason, the physical therapist helped Jeff find a YMCA in his community that has an accessible swimming pool and a gym in which he can work out. In collaboration with YMCA staff, the therapist and Jeff developed an exercise program that is appropriate for Jeff's needs and that he can carry out with the assistance of YMCA personnel. The physical therapist is available to serve as a consultant as needed.

TABLE 20-2   Example of an Ecological Assessment

Name: Jeff
Activity: Shopping
Environment: Dan's One-Stop

STEPS REQUIRED	JEFF'S CURRENT PERFORMANCE	STEPS CAN ACQUIRE	STEPS MAY NOT ACQUIRE	COMPENSATORY STRATEGIES	INTERVENTION*
1. Go from home to Dan's and back using electric wheelchair.	Can open front door (outward), go down ramp and drive to the corner. Cannot go down curb (no curb cut), cross street safely, or go up curb. Once on the sidewalk, can drive to Dan's. Cannot open door from outside. Can maneuver inside store and open door when leaving (outward). Cannot open door of home when returning.	1. Open doors of home and store when the door opens toward him; 2. go down curb; 3. ask for assistance and tell someone how to help him up a curb; and 4. cross the street safely.	Go up a curb without assistance.	Curb cuts.	1. Teach Jeff to open doors, go down curbs, and cross streets safely (PT, PCA). 2. Talk with city about making curb cuts and with store and house manager about modifying doors (Jeff, CM). 3. Program communication aid to request help with curbs and give instructions (mother, PT).
2. Select items in the store.	Does not always remember what he needs to get and cannot make or read a shopping list. Can get items that are at hand level, cannot shift weight or extend arm to reach low or high items.	1. Make and use shopping list; 2. improve ability to reach high and low items; and 3. ask for assistance to get out-of-reach items.	Reach items that are very high or very low.	A reacher?	Teach Jeff 1. to make and use a shopping list (OT, PCA); 2. to use a reacher, if it seems feasible (OT, PCA); and 3. to reach to higher and lower shelves (PT, PCA).
3. Carry items to checkout stand.	Cannot maneuver shopping cart. Items slide off lap, does not want to use tray.	Carry items in a bag or other container on lap or chair.	Push a grocery cart without endangering store and other people	Bag or other container that is accessible to Jeff.	Find container and teach Jeff to use it (OT and PCA).

(continued)

TABLE 20-2 **Example of an Ecological Assessment—cont'd**

STEPS REQUIRED	JEFF'S CURRENT PERFORMANCE	STEPS CAN ACQUIRE	STEPS MAY NOT ACQUIRE	COMPENSATORY STRATEGIES	INTERVENTION*
4. Put items on counter.	Can put items on counter, but is very slow, which annoys people in line behind him.	1. Put container on counter so clerk can remove items; or 2. ask for assistance	1. Increase speed sufficiently; or 2. lift full container to counter	None.	1. Try to improve speed and lifting of container (PT, PCA); and 2. program communication aid and teach Jeff to ask for assistance (mother and PCA).
5. Pay for purchases.	Cannot get wallet out of pocket, cannot get money out of wallet. Does not recognize denominations of bills or coins, cannot pay correct amount or check change.	1. Get money out of suitable container; 2. recognize bills and coins; and 3. give sufficient money to cover the purchase.	1. Get wallet or money out of wallet; and 2. determine if change is accurate.	1. Use an accessible container for money; and 2. ask personal care assistant to compare bill and change occasionally.	1. Find accessible container for money and teach Jeff to use it (OT, PCA); and 2. teach Jeff to use money (OT, mother, PCA).
6. Carry purchases home.	Can carry small bag on lap, cannot carry large bag(s).	Carry purchases in container attached to chair.	Carry large or multiple bags on lap.	Alternate container (probably the same as in 3, above).	Find appropriate container for purchases (OT, PCA).
7. Put purchases away.	Can open cupboards with flat surfaces or knobs, drawers with knobs, and the refrigerator. Cannot open high or low cupboards or drawers with flat surfaces. Can put purchases away in places he can open and reach.	1. Open all drawers he can reach; and 2. put items away in higher and lower places.	Put items in very high or low places.	1. Make adaptations to allow Jeff to open kitchen drawers he can reach. 2. Rearrange cupboards and drawers so items Jeff uses are accessible.	1. Discuss adaptations and rearrangement with house manager (OT); and 2. improve Jeff's reach (also in 2, above) (PT, PCA).

*Note: Those involved with each intervention are determined after the intervention is identified. At this time, Jeff has the assistance of his personal care assistant (PCA), case manager (CM), mother, occupational therapist (OT), and physical therapist (PT).

REFERENCES

AAMR. See American Association on Mental Retardation.

American Association on Mental Retardation. Mental Retardation: Definition, Classification, and Systems of Supports, 10th ed. Washington, DC: American Association on Mental Retardation, 2002.

American Association on Mental Retardation. Supports Intensity Scale. Washington, DC: American Association on Mental Retardation, 2003.

Anwar, F. Cognitive deficit and motor skill. In Ellis, D (Ed.). Sensory Impairments in Mentally Handicapped People. San Diego: College-Hill Press, 1986, pp. 169–183.

Aughton, DJ, & Cassidy, SB. Physical features of Prader-Willi syndrome in neonates. American Journal of Diseases of Children, 144:1251–1254, 1990.

Baker, BJ, Cole, KN, & Harris, SR. Cognitive referencing as a method of OT/PT triage for young children. Pediatric Physical Therapy, 10:2–6, 1998.

Barlow, DH, & Hersen, M. Single Case Experimental Designs: Strategies for Studying Behavioral Change, 2nd ed. New York: Pergamon Press, 1984.

Baumgart, D, Brown, L, Pumpian, I, Nisbet, J, Ford, A, Sweet, M, Messina, R, & Schroeder, J. Principle of partial participation and individualized adaptations in educational programs for severely handicapped students. The Journal of the Association for the Severely Handicapped, 7:17–27, 1982.

Benson, JB, & Uzgiris, IC. Effect of self-initiated locomotion on infant search activity. Developmental Psychology, 21:923–931, 1985.

Berg, JM, McCreary, BD, Ridler, MAC, & Smith, GF. The de Lange Syndrome. New York: Pergamon Press, 1970.

Bertenthal, BI, Campos, JJ, & Barrett, KC. Self-produced locomotion: An organizer of emotional, cognitive, and social development in infancy. In Emde, RN, & Harmon, RJ (Eds.). Continuities and Discontinuities in Development. New York: Plenum, 1984.

Bijou, SW. A functional analysis of retarded development. In Ellis, NR (Ed.). International Review of Research in Mental Retardation, Vol. 1. New York: Academic Press, 1966, pp. 1–19.

Bhutta, AT, Cleves, MA, Casey, PH, Cradock, MM, & Anand, KJS. Cognitive and behavioral outcomes of school-aged children who were born preterm. JAMA, 288:728–737, 2002.

Brookes-Gunn, J, Kelbanov, PK, & Duncan, GJ. Ethnic differences in children's intelligence test scores: Role of economic deprivation, home environment, and maternal characteristics. Child Development, 67:396–408, 1996.

Brown, L, Branston, MB, Hamre-Nietupski, S, Pumpian, I, Certo, N, & Gruenewald, L. A strategy for developing chronological age appropriate and functional curricular content for severely handicapped adolescents and young adults. Journal of Special Education, 12:81–90, 1979.

Burgemeister, BB, Blum, LH, & Lorge, I. Manual: Columbia Mental Maturity Scale, 3rd ed. New York: Psychological Corporation, 1972.

Butler, C. Augmentative mobility: Why do it? Physical Medicine and Rehabilitation Clinics of North America, 2:801–815, 1991.

Butler, C, Okamoto, GA, & McKay, TM. Powered mobility for very young disabled children. Developmental Medicine & Child Neurology, 25:472–474, 1983.

Campbell, FA, & Ramey, CT. High risk infants: Environmental risk factors. In Berg, JM (Ed.). Science and Service in Mental Retardation: Proceedings of the Seventh Congress of the International Association for the Scientific Study of Mental Deficiency (IASSMD). New York: Methuen, 1985, pp. 23–33.

Campbell, PH. Dysfunction in posture and movement with individuals with profound disabilities. In Brown, F, & Lehr, DH (Eds.). Persons with Profound Disabilities: Issues and Practices. Baltimore: Paul H. Brookes, 1989, pp. 163–189.

Campbell, PH. Evaluation and assessment in early intervention for infants and toddlers. Journal of Early Intervention, 15:36–45, 1991.

Campbell, SK. Central nervous system dysfunction in children. In Campbell, SK (Ed.). Pediatric Neurologic Physical Therapy, 2nd ed. New York: Churchill Livingstone, 1991, pp. 1–17.

Campos, JJ, & Bertenthal, BI. Locomotion and psychological development in infancy. In Jaffe, KM (Ed.). Childhood Powered Mobility: Developmental, Technical and Clinical Perspectives: Proceedings of the RESNA First Northwest Regional Conference. Washington, DC: RESNA, 1987, pp. 11–42.

Carr EG, Dunlap G, Horner, RH, et al. Positive behavior support: Evolution of an applied science. Journal of Positive Behavior Interventions, 4:4–16, 2002.

Carr, SH. Louisiana's criteria of eligibility for occupational therapy services in the public school system. American Journal of Occupational Therapy, 43:503–506, 1989.

Carter, CH. Handbook of Mental Retardation Syndromes, 2nd ed. Springfield, IL: Charles C. Thomas, 1970.

Chandler, LS, & Adams, MA. Multiply handicapped child motivated for ambulation through behavior modification. Physical Therapy, 52:339–401, 1972.

Chinitz, SP, & Feder, CZ. Psychological assessment. In Molnar, GE (Ed.). Pediatric Rehabilitation, 2nd ed. Baltimore: Williams & Wilkins, 1992, pp. 48–87.

Chugani, HT. A critical period of brain development: Studies of cerebral glucose utilization with PET. Preventive Medicine, 27:184–188, 1998.

Cimera, RE. Are individuals with severe mental retardation and multiple disabilities cost-efficient to serve via supported employment programs? Mental Retardation, 36:280–292, 1998.

Cole, CL, & Levinson, TR. Effects of within activity choices on the challenging behavior of children with severe developmental disabilities. Journal of Positive Behavior Interventions, 4:29–37, 2002.

Cornish, K, & Bramble, D. Cri du chat syndrome: Genotype-phenotype correlations and recommendations for clinical management. Developmental Medicine & Child Neurology, 44:494–497, 2002.

Cress, CJ. Expanding children's early augmented behaviors to support symbolic development. In Reichle, J, Beukelman, D, & Light, J (Eds.). Exemplary Practices for Beginning Communicators. Baltimore: Paul H. Brookes, 2002, pp. 219–272.

de Vries, BB, Halley, DJJ, Oostra, BA, & Niermeijer, MF. The fragile X syndrome. Journal of Medical Genetics, 35:579–589, 1998.

Developmental Disabilities Assistance and Bill of Rights Act of 2000, P.L. 106–402, 114 Stat. 1678, 2000.

DiLalla, LF. Development of intelligence: Current research and theories. Journal of School Psychology, 38:3–7, 2000.

Downing, J, Eichinger, J, & Demchak, M. Including Students with Severe Disabilities in Typical Classrooms. Baltimore: Paul H. Brookes, 2002.

Drotar, D, Mortimer, J, Shepherd, PA, & Fagan, JF. Recognition memory as a method of assessing intelligence of an infant with quadriplegia. Developmental Medicine & Child Neurology, 31:391–394, 1989.

Dunst, C. Everyday children's learning opportunities: Characteristics and consequences. Children's Learning Opportunities Report, 2:1–2, 2000.

Eagle, RS. Deprivation of early sensorimotor experience and cognition in the severely involved cerebral-palsied child. Journal of Autism and Developmental Disabilities, 15:269–283, 1985.

Ellis, NR. Handbook of Mental Deficiency: Psychological Theory and Research. London: McGraw-Hill, 1963.

Evans, IM. Testing and diagnosis: A review and evaluation. In Meyer, LH, Peck, CA, & Brown, L (Eds.). Critical Issues in the Lives of People with Severe Disabilities. Baltimore: Paul H. Brookes, 1991, pp. 25–43.

Evans, IM, & Scotti, JR. Defining meaningful outcomes for persons with profound disabilities. In Brown, F, & Lehr, DH (Eds.). Persons with Profound Disabilities: Issues and Practices. Baltimore: Paul H. Brookes, 1989, pp. 83–107.

Fagan, JF, & Shepherd, PA. The Fagan Test of Infant Intelligence Training Manual. Cleveland: Infatest Corporation, 1987.

Falvey, MA. Introduction. In Falvey, MA (Ed.). Community-Based Curriculum: Instructional Strategies for Students with Severe Handicaps. Baltimore: Paul H. Brookes, 1989, pp. 1–13.

Ferguson, DL, & Baumgart, D. Partial participation revisited. Journal of the Association for Persons with Severe Handicaps, 16:218–227, 1991.

Flexer, RW, Simmons, TJ, Luft, P, & Baer, RM. Transition Planning for Secondary Students with Disabilities. Upper Saddle, River, NJ: Merrill Prentice-Hall, 2001.

Fogel, A, Dedo, JY, & McEwen, IR. Effect of postural position and reaching on gaze during mother-infant face-to-face interaction. Infant Behavior and Development, 15:231–244, 1992.

Foley, GM. Arena evaluation: Assessment in the transdisciplinary approach. In Gibbs, ED, & Teti, DM (Eds.). Interdisciplinary Assessment of Infants: A Guide for Early Intervention Professionals. Baltimore: Paul H. Brookes, 1990, pp. 271–286.

Fragala, MA, O'Neil, ME, Russo, KJ, & Dumas, HM. Impairment, disability, and satisfaction outcomes after lower-extremity botulinum toxin A injections for children with cerebral palsy. Pediatric Physical Therapy, 14:132–144, 2002.

Giangreco, MF. Letter to the editor. American Journal of Occupational Therapy, 44:470, 1990.

Giangreco, MF, Cloninger, CH, & Iverson, VS. Choosing Options and Accommodations for Children: A Guide to Educational Planning for Students with Disabilities, 2nd ed. Baltimore: Paul H. Brookes, 1998.

Gibbs, ED. Assessment of infant mental ability: Conventional tests and issues of prediction. In Gibbs, ED, & Teti, DM (Eds.). Interdisciplinary Assessment of Infants: A Guide for Early Intervention Professionals. Baltimore: Paul H. Brookes, 1990, pp. 77–89.

Guess, D, Mulligan-Ault, M, Roberts, S, Struth, J, Siegel-Causey, E, Thompson, B, Bronicki, GJB, & Guy, B. Implications of biobehavioral states for the education and treatment of students with the most profoundly handicapping conditions. Journal of the Association for Persons with Severe Handicaps, 13:163–174, 1988.

Guide to Physical Therapist Practice, 2nd ed. Physical Therapy, 81:9–744, 2001.

Gustafson, GE. Effects of the ability to locomote on infants' social and exploratory behaviors: An experimental study. Developmental Psychology, 20:397–405, 1984.

Haley, SM, Coster, WJ, Ludlow, LH, Haltiwanger, JT, & Andrellos, PJ. Pediatric Evaluation of Disability Inventory. Boston, MA: Department of Rehabilitation Medicine, New England Medical Center, 1992.

Haney, M, & Falvey, MA. Instructional strategies. In Falvey, MA (Ed.). Community-Based Curriculum: Instructional Strategies for Students with Severe Handicaps. Baltimore: Paul H. Brookes, 1989, pp. 63–90.

Harris, SR. Functional abilities in context. In Lister, MJ (Ed.). Contemporary Management of Motor Control Problems: Proceedings of the II Step Conference. Alexandria, VA: Foundation for Physical Therapy, 1991, pp. 253–259.

Harris, SR, & Shea, AM. Down syndrome. In Campbell, SK (Ed.). Pediatric Neurologic Physical Therapy, 2nd ed. New York: Churchill Livingstone, 1991, pp. 131–168.

Horn, EM. Basic motor skills instruction for children with neuromotor delays: A critical review. Journal of Special Education, 25:168–197, 1991.

Houghton, J, Bronicki, GJB, & Guess, D. Opportunities to express preferences and make choices among students with severe disabilities in classroom settings. Journal of the Association for Persons with Severe Handicaps, 12:18–27, 1987.

Jankovic, J, Caskey, TC, Stout, JT, & Butler, IJ. Lesch-Nyhan syndrome: A study of motor behavior and cerebrospinal fluid neurotransmitters. Annals of Neurology, 23:466–469, 1988.

Jones, KL. Smith's Recognizable Patterns of Human Malformation, 5th ed. Philadelphia: WB Saunders, 1997.

Jones, MA, McEwen, IR, & Hansen, L. Use of power mobility for a young child with spinal muscular atrophy: A case report. Physical Therapy, 83:253–262, 2003.

Katusic, SK, Colligan, RC, Beard, CM, O'Fallon, WM, Bergstralh, EJ, Jacobsen, SJ, & Kurland, LT. Mental retardation in a birth cohort, 1976–1980, Rochester, Minnesota. American Journal on Mental Retardation, 100:335–344, 1996.

Kermoian, R, & Campos, JJ. Locomotor experience: A facilitator of spatial cognitive development. Child Development, 59:908–917, 1988.

King, G, Law, M, King, S, Rosenbaum, P, Kertoy, MK, & Young, NL. A conceptual model of the factors affecting recreation and leisure participation of children with disabilities. Physical & Occupational Therapy in Pediatrics, 23:63–90, 2003.

Kochanek, TT, Kabacoff, RI, & Lipsitt, LP. Early identification of developmentally disabled and at-risk preschool children. Exceptional Children, 56:528–538, 1990.

Kolb, B, Forgie, M, Gibb, R, Gorny, G, & Rowntree, S. Age, experience and the changing brain. Neuroscience and Biobehavioral Reviews, 22:143–159, 1998.

Kopp, CB, & McCall, RB. Predicting later mental performance for normal, at-risk, and handicapped infants. In Baltes, PB, & Brim, OG (Eds.). Life-Span Development and Behavior. New York: Academic Press, 1982, pp. 33-61.

Landesman-Dwyer, S, & Sackett, GP. Behavioral changes in nonambulatory, profoundly mentally retarded individuals. In Meyers, CE (Ed.). Quality of Life in Severely and Profoundly Mentally Retarded People: Research Foundations for Improvement. Washington, DC: American Association on Mental Deficiency, 1978, pp. 55–144.

Lambert, N, Nihira, K, & Leland, H. AAMR Adaptive Behavior Scale-School, 2nd ed. Austin, TX: Pro-Ed.

Larson, SA, Lakin, KC, Anderson, L, Kwak, N, Lee, JH, & Anderson, D. Prevalence of mental retardation and developmental disabilities: Estimates from the 1994/1995 national health interview survey disability supplements. American Journal on Mental Retardation, 106:231–252, 2001.

Laurance, BM, Brito, A, & Wilkinson, J. Prader-Willi syndrome after age 15 years. Archives of Disease in Childhood, 56:181–186, 1981.

Law, M, Baptiste, S, Carswell, A, McColl, MA, Polatajko, H, & Pollock, N. Canadian Occupational Performance Measure, 2nd ed. Toronto: Canadian Association of Occupational Therapists, 1994.

Leung, AKC, Sauve, RS, & Davies, HD. Congenital cytomegalovirus infection. Journal of the National Medical Association, 95:213–218, 2003.

Lucyshyn, JM, Horner, RH, Dunlap, G, Albin, RW, & Ben, KR. Positive behavior support with families. In Lucyshyn, JM, Dunlap G, & Albin, RW (Eds.). Families and Positive Behavior Support: Addressing Problem Behavior in Family Contexts. Baltimore: Paul H. Brookes, 2002, pp. 3–43.

Lutzker, JR, McGimsey-McRae, S, & McGimsey, JF. General description of behavioral approaches. In Hersen, M, Van Hasselt, VB, & Matson, JL (Eds.). Behavior Therapy for the Developmentally and Physically Disabled. New York: Academic Press, 1983, pp. 25–56.

Malian, I, & Nevin, A. A review of self-determination literature: Implications for practitioners. RASE: Remedial and Special Education, 23:68–74, 2002.

Maloney, FP, & Kurtz, PA. The use of a mercury switch head control device in profoundly retarded, multiply handicapped children. Physical & Occupational Therapy in Pediatrics, 2:11–17, 1982.

McCall, RB. Issues in the early development of intelligence and its assessment. In Lewis, M, & Taft, L (Eds.). Developmental Disabilities: Theory, Assessment and Intervention. New York: SP Medical and Scientific Books, 1982, pp. 177–184.

McEwen, IR (Ed.). Writing case reports: A how-to manual for clinicians. Alexandria, VA: American Physical Therapy Association, 2001.

McEwen, IR. Assistive positioning as a control parameter of social-communicative interactions between students with profound multiple disabilities and classroom staff. Physical Therapy, 72:634–647, 1992.

McEwen, IR, Arnold, S, Jones, M, & Shelden, M. Providing Physical Therapy Services Under Parts B & C of the Individuals with Disabilities Education Act (IDEA). Alexandria, VA: Section on Pediatrics, American Physical Therapy Association, 2000.

McEwen, IR, & Karlan, GR. Assessment of effects of position on communication board access by individuals with cerebral palsy. Augmentative and Alternative Communication, 5:235–242, 1989.

McEwen, IR, & Shelden, ML. Pediatric physical therapy in the 1990s: The demise of the educational versus medical dichotomy. Physical & Occupational Therapy in Pediatrics, 15:33–45, 1995.

McGonigel, MJ, Woodruff, G, & Roszmann-Millican, M. The transdisciplinary team: A model for family-centered early intervention. In Johnson, LJ, Gallagher, RJ, LaMontagne, MJ, Jordan, JB, Gallagher, JJ, Huntinger, PL, & Karnes, MB (Eds.). Meeting Early Intervention Challenges: Issues from Birth to Three, 2nd ed. Baltimore: Paul H. Brookes, 1994, pp. 95–131.

McLaren, J, & Bryson, SE. Review of recent epidemiological studies of mental retardation: Prevalence, associated disorders, and etiology. American Journal on Mental Retardation, 92:243–254, 1987.

Meisels, SJ, & Atkins-Burnett, S. The elements of early childhood assessment. In Shonkoff, JP, & Meisels, SJ (Eds.). Handbook of Early Childhood Intervention, 2nd ed. Cambridge, MA: Cambridge University Press, 2000, pp. 231–257.

Middelton, HA, Keene, RG, & Brown, GW. Convergent and discriminant validities of the Scales of Independent Behavior and the Revised Vineland Adaptive Behavior Scales. American Journal on Mental Retardation, 94:669–673.

Morris, CA, & Mervis, CB. Williams syndrome and related disorders. Annual Review of Genomics & Human Genetics, 1:261–284, 2000.

National Joint Committee for the Communicative Needs of Persons with Severe Disabilities. Guidelines for meeting the communication needs of persons with severe disabilities. ASHA, 34(suppl 7):1–8, 1992.

Navajas, D, Farre, R, Mar Rotger, M, Milic-Emili, J, & Sanchis, J. Effect of body posture on respiratory impedance. Journal of Applied Physiology, 64:194–199, 1988.

Newborg, J, Stock, JR, Wnek, L, Guidubaldi, J, & Svinicki, J. Battelle Developmental Inventory. Chicago: Riverside Publishing, 1984.

Nihira, K. Adaptive behavior: A historical overview. In Shalock, RL (Ed.). Adaptive Behavior and Its Measurement: Implications for the Field of Mental Retardation. Washington, DC: AAMR, 1999, pp. 7–14.

Nomura, Y, & Segawa, Y. Characteristics of motor disturbance in Rett syndrome. Brain Development, 12:27–30, 1990.

Nwaobi, OM. Seating orientations and upper extremity function in children with cerebral palsy. Physical Therapy, 67:1209–1212, 1987.

Nwaobi, OM, & Smith, PD. Effect of adaptive seating on pulmonary function of children with cerebral palsy. Developmental Medicine & Child Neurology, 28:351–354, 1986.

Orelove, FP, & Sobsey, D. Designing transdisciplinary services. In Orelove, FP, & Sobsey, D (Eds.). Educating Children with Multiple Disabilities: A Transdisciplinary Approach, 3rd ed. Baltimore: Paul H. Brookes, 1996, pp. 1–33.

Oswald, DP, Coutinho, MJ, & Nguyen N. Impact of sociodemographic characteristics on identification rates of minority students as having mental retardation. Mental Retardation, 39:351–367, 2001.

Palisano, R, Rosenbaum, P, Walter, S, Russell, D, Wood, E, & Galuppi, B. Gross Motor Function Classification System for Cerebral Palsy. Developmental Medicine & Child Neurology, 39:214–223, 1997.

Parette, HP, Jr, & Hourcade, JJ. How effective are physiotherapeutic programmes with young mentally retarded children who have cerebral palsy? Journal of Mental Deficiency Research, 28:167–175, 1984.

Percy, AK. Rett syndrome: Current status and new vistas. Neurologic Clinics, 20:1125–1141, 2002.

Prenatal Exposure to Alcohol. Alcohol Research & Health, 24:32–41, 2000.

Portney, LG, & Watkins, MP. Foundations of Clinical Research: Applications to Practice, 2nd ed. Upper Saddle River, NJ: Prentice Hall Health, 2000.

Rainforth, B. OSERS clarifies legality of related services eligibility criteria. TASH Newsletter, April 1991, p. 8.

Rainforth, B, & York-Barr, J. Collaborative Teams for Students with Severe Disabilities: Integrating Therapy and Educational Services, 2nd ed. Baltimore: Paul H. Brookes, 1997.

Randall, KE, & McEwen, IR. Writing patient-centered functional goals. Physical Therapy, 80:1197–1203, 2000.

Ramey, CT, & Ramey, SL. Effective early intervention. Mental Retardation, 30:337–345, 1992.

Raven, JC. Raven's Progressive Matrices. San Antonio, TX: The Psychological Corporation, 1995.

Reid, D, Rigby, P, & Ryan S. Functional impact of a rigid pelvic stabilizer on children with cerebral palsy who use wheelchairs: Users' and caregivers' perceptions. Pediatric Rehabilitation, 3:101–118, 1999.

Reid, DH, Phillips, JF, & Green, CW. Teaching persons with profound multiple handicaps: A review of the effects of behavioral research. Journal of Applied Behavior Analysis, 24:319–336, 1991.

Rold, G, & Miller, L. Leiter International Performance Scale – Revised. Wood Dale, IL: Stoelting, 1998.

Rothstein, JM, Echternach, JL, & Riddle, DL. The hypothesis-oriented algorithm for clinicians II (HOAC II): A guide for patient management. Physical Therapy, 83:455–470, 2003.

Rozien, NJ, & Patterson, D. Down's syndrome. The Lancet, 361:1281–1289, 2003.

Sents, B, & Marks, H. Changes in preschool children's IQ scores as a function of positioning. American Journal of Occupational Therapy, 43:685–687, 1989.

Shelden, ML, & Rush, DD. The ten myths about providing early intervention services in natural environments. Infants & Young Children, 14:1–13, 2001.

Snell, ME, & Zirpoli, TJ. Intervention strategies. In Snell, ME (Ed.). Systematic Instruction of Persons with Severe Handicaps, 3rd ed. Columbus, OH: Charles E. Merrill, 1987, pp. 110–149.

Sparrow, SS, Balla, DA, & Cichetti, CV. Vineland Adaptive Behavior Scales. Circle Pines, MN: American Guidance Service, 1984.

Switzky, HN, Woolsey-Hill, J, & Quoss, T. Habituation of visual fixation responses: An assessment tool to measure visual sensory-perceptual cognitive processes in nonverbal profoundly handicapped children in the classroom. AAESPH Review, 4:136–147, 1979.

TASH force strikes again: Laski and Boyd win Oberti case in New Jersey. TASH Newsletter, November 1992, pp. 1–2.

Tefft, D, Guerette, P, & Furumasu, J. Cognitive predictors of young children's readiness for powered mobility. Developmental Medicine & Child Neurology, 41:665–670, 1999.

Telzrow, RW, Campos, JJ, Shepherd, A, Bertenthal, BI, & Atwater, S. Spatial understanding in infants with motor handicaps. In Jaffe, KM (Ed.). Childhood Powered Mobility: Developmental, Technical and Clinical Perspectives: Proceedings of the RESNA first Northwest Regional Conference. Washington, DC: RESNA, 1987, pp. 62–69.

Thorndike, R, Hagen, E, & Sattler, J. Technical Manual for Standford-Binet Intelligence Scale, 4th ed. Chicago, IL: Riverside Publishing, 1986.

Thorpe, DE, & Valvano, J. The effects of knowledge of performance and cognitive strategies on motor skill learning in children with cerebral palsy. Pediatric Physical Therapy, 14:2–15, 2002.

Thurman, SK, & Widerstrom, AH. Infants and Young Children with Special Needs: A Developmental and Ecological Approach. Baltimore: Paul H. Brookes, 1990.

United Cerebral Palsy National Infant Collaborative Project. Staff Development Handbook: A Resource for the Transdisciplinary Process. New York: United Cerebral Palsy Association, 1976.

United States Department of Education. To Assure the Free Appropriate Public Education of All Children with Disabilities: Twenty-second Annual Report to Congress on the Implementation of the Individuals with Disabilities Education Act, 2000.

USDE. See United States Department of Education.

Vaughn, BJ, Wilson, D, & Dunlap, G. Family-centered intervention to resolve problem behavior in a fast-food restaurant. Journal of Positive Behavior Interventions, 4:38–45, 2002.

Verburg, G, Naumann, S, Balfour, L, & Snell, E. Remote training of mobility skills in persons who are physically and developmentally disabled. Proceedings of the RESNA 13th Annual Conference. Washington, DC: RESNA, 1990, pp. 195–196.

Watkins, MW, Ravert, CM, & Crosby, EG. Normative factor structure of the AAMR Adaptive Behavior Scale-School, 2nd ed. Journal of Psychoeducational Assessment, 20:337–345, 2002.

Wechsler, D. Wechsler Intelligence Scale for Children, 3rd ed. San Antonio, TX: Harcourt Assessment, 1991.

Wehmeyer, ML, & Bolding, N. Self-determination across living and working environments: A matched samples study of adults with mental retardation. Mental Retardation, 37:353–363, 1999.

Wehmeyer, ML, & Bolding, N. Enhanced self-determination of adults with intellectual disability as an outcome of moving to community-based work or living environments. Journal of Intellectual Disability Research, 45:371–383, 2001.

Wehmeyer, ML, & Schwartz, M. Self-determination and positive adult outcomes: A follow-up study of youth with mental retardation or learning disabilities. Exceptional Children, 63:245–255, 1997.

WHO. See World Health Organization.

Witkin, SL, & Fox, L. Beyond the least restrictive environment. In Villa, RA, Thousand, JS, Stainback, W, & Stainback, S (Eds.). Restructuring for Caring and Effective Education. Baltimore: Paul H. Brookes, 1992, pp. 325–334.

World Health Organization. International Classification of Functioning, Disability, and Health (ICF). 2001. Accessed July 7, 2003, from: http://www.int/classification/icf/intros/ICF-Eng-Intro.pdf.

Zazula, JL, & Foulds, RA. Mobility device for a child with phocomelia. Archives of Physical Medicine and Rehabilitation, 64:137–139, 1983.

Zelazo, PR, & Weiss, MJ. Infant information processing: An alternative approach. In Gibbs, ED, & Teti, DM (Eds.). Interdisciplinary Assessment of Infants: A Guide for Early Intervention Professionals. Baltimore: Paul H. Brookes, 1990, pp. 129–143.

Zhang, D, & Katsiyannis, A. Minority representation in special education: A persistent challenge. RASE: Remedial & Special Education, 23:180–187, 2002.

Chapter 21

∽

CEREBRAL PALSY

SANDRA J. OLNEY
BSc (P&OT), MEd, PhD

MARILYN J. WRIGHT
BScPT, MEd

Cerebral palsy (CP) is the neurologic condition most frequently encountered by pediatric physical therapists. It is a permanent but not unchanging neurodevelopmental disorder caused by a nonprogressive defect or lesion in single or multiple locations in the immature brain. The defect or lesion can occur in utero or during or shortly after birth and produces motor impairment and possible sensory deficits that are usually evident in early infancy (Scherzer & Tscharnuter, 1990). Progressive musculoskeletal impairment is seen in most children (Graham & Selber, 2003). CP involves one or more limbs and frequently the trunk. It causes disturbances of voluntary motor function and produces a variety of symptoms. Nevertheless, CP is itself an artificial concept, comprising several causes and clinical syndromes that have been grouped together because of a commonality of management. The impaired control and coordination of voluntary muscles is accompanied by cognitive delays or learning disabilities in 50% to 75% of children and by disorders of speech (25%), auditory impairments (25%), seizure disorders (25%–35%), or abnormalities of vision (40%–50%) (Batshaw & Perret, 1992; Schanzenbacher, 1989). Social and family problems may occur secondary to the presence of primary deficits and include seizures, sleep problems, pain, and difficulties with self-care.

In few conditions do physical therapists play such a central role or have as much potential to influence the outcome of children's lives. Their interventions have not only immediate but also lifelong effects, and can be efficient and cost-effective. Treatment of children is specialized: physical therapists provide services that will help them reach their full potential in their homes and communities. Furthermore, decisions about many medical interventions such as orthopedic surgery and spasticity management usually rely on input from physical therapists. The therapist's influence is not restricted to the medical center and treatment gymnasium, but frequently includes consultation regarding the child's functioning in settings within the home, school, recreation, and community environments. Good therapy not only helps the child with CP but also can have a positive influence on the child's family and caregivers. In summary, parents of children with disabilities want services that provide general and specific information about their child as well as coordinated and comprehensive care, and they want these services provided by respectful and supportive professionals (King et al., 1998). The pediatric physical therapist is ideally suited to fill these roles.

NATURE AND CHARACTERISTICS OF CEREBRAL PALSY

CLASSIFICATION, ETIOLOGY, AND PATHOPHYSIOLOGY

CP has been classified in a number of ways. A classification based on the area of the body exhibiting motor impairment yields the designations of monoplegia (one limb), diplegia (lower limbs), hemiplegia (upper and lower limbs on one side of the body), and quadriplegia (all limbs). Another classification, based on the most obvious movement abnormality resulting from common brain lesions, yields spastic, dyskinetic, and ataxic types. The spastic type, in which the muscles are perceived as excessively stiff and taut, especially during attempted movement, results from involvement of the motor cortex or white matter projections to and from cortical sensorimotor areas of the brain. Involvement of the basal ganglia is reflected in dyskinesia or athetosis and sometimes in intermittent muscular tension of the extremities or trunk and involuntary movement patterns. A cerebellar lesion produces ataxia, or general instability of movement. A hypotonic classification, not known to be related to a particular lesion, is characterized by diminished resting muscle tone and decreased ability to generate voluntary muscle force. Symptoms of spasticity and dyskinesia may both be present in a child, with the type of CP referred to as mixed. The degree of severity of CP varies greatly, and the designations mild, moderate, and severe are often applied within types. The Gross Motor Function Classification System (GMFCS) is a five-level, age-categorized system that places children with CP into categories of severity that represent clinically meaningful distinctions in motor function (Palisano et al., 1997; Rosenbaum et al., 2002). Although the proportions of the various subtypes of CP vary with the reporting source, a study from Sweden reported that hemiplegia accounted for 36.4%; diplegia, 41.5%; quadriplegia, 7.3%; dyskinesia or athetosis, 10%; and ataxic forms, 5% (Hagberg et al., 1989a).

CP is a condition with multiple causes leading to damage within the central nervous system. Although the causes are not completely understood, certain prenatal, perinatal, and postnatal factors have been associated with CP (Torfs et al., 1990). Recently an international task force reviewed the literature on the causation of CP and defined an objective template, based upon the evidence, to more accurately identify causes of CP (MacLennan, 1999). About half of the cases of CP are diagnosed in full-term infants. Potentially asphyxiating birth complications, however, are responsible for only a small percentage of CP in these full-term infants. Recent studies have suggested that disorders of coagulation and intrauterine exposure to infection or inflammation are associated with an increased risk of CP. Both may be associated with neonatal encephalopathy, which is associated with CP in term neonates (Nelson, 2002). Epidemiologic research has suggested different mechanisms that may be responsible for brain damage in children diagnosed with CP. One proposed mechanism is insufficient cerebral perfusion. Another is cytokine-mediated damage, triggered by maternal infection, neonatal infection, and neonatal oxygen-induced or ventilator-induced lung injury. In addition, there may also be insufficient levels of developmentally regulated protective substances such as thyroid hormone and glucocorticoids in children diagnosed with CP (O'Shea, 2002).

Of preterm infants diagnosed with CP, about 50% have brain damage that can be detected using cranial ultrasonography through the anterior fontanel (O'Shea, 2002). Preterm birth is associated with up to 33% of all cases of CP, including more than 50% of diplegia (Pharoah et al., 1990), 25% of hemiplegia (Uvebrandt, 1988), and 5% of quadriplegia (Edebol-Tysk, 1989). Prenatal malnutrition, intrinsic developmental problems of the fetus, and poor maternal prenatal condition are also associated with CP (Menkes, 1990). Intracranial hemorrhage, especially among premature infants, is a well-established causal factor. The effects of hyperbilirubinemia and other blood incompatibilities frequently resulting in athetoid CP are a concern, particularly in developing countries. Epidemiologic statistics from developing countries are in sharp contrast to those of developed countries. Studies have suggested that up to 63% of cases of CP in developing countries have preventable causes associated with shortage of care personnel and inadequate financing for effective prenatal services (Karumuna & Mgone, 1990; Nottidge & Okogbo, 1991).

The incidence of CP was reported to be about 2.5 per 1000 live births until about the mid-1950s (Little, 1958), when it decreased to about 1.5 per 1000 and remained at that level for about 15 years. The incidence then increased to near mid-1950s levels (Hagberg et al., 1989b) though numbers from developed countries varied. The current overall prevalence of CP was reported to be 2.0 per 1000 in a five-county U.S. study (Winter et al., 2002), although the United Kingdom reported lower values at 1.7 per 1000 (Surman et al., 2003). The increase in recent years may reflect changes in the live birth rate of preterm infants, although a study of a cohort of 2076 consecutively born infants with birth weights of 500 to 1500 g conducted between 1982 and 1994 does not support this explanation (O'Shea et al., 1998). The risk of CP does, however, increase sharply with decreasing birth weight (Atkinson & Stanley, 1983; Hagberg et al., 1989a; Pharoah et al., 1987) and has been reported to be as much as 40 times higher in infants weighing less than 1000 g compared to infants weighing 3500 g (Hagberg et al., 1989b). Some more recent studies have reported a trend toward improvement in these figures. Evidence from over 400,000 live births in the United Kingdom between 1984 and 1995 showed a decrease in overall CP incidence from 2.5 per 1000 to 1.7 per 1000 live births and a decrease in the rate of severe motor disability among infants weighing less than 1500 g from 24.6% to 12.5% (Surman et al., 2003). The increased risk of CP in preterm infants must be put in perspective. Reports of long-term outcome of extremely premature infants, that is, infants born between 24 and 28 weeks of gestational age, suggest about 75% survive, with more than 50% of those who survive free of major neurodevelopmental impairments, while about 25% have major impairments and about 11% have CP (Msall et al., 1991).

Autopsies of infants have revealed three types of neuropathic lesions (Weinstein & Tharp, 1989): neuropathy resulting from hemorrhage below the lining of the ventricles (subependymal), encephalopathy caused by anoxia or hypoxia, and neuropathy resulting from malformations of the central nervous system. Most subependymal hemorrhages occur in infants of less than 28 weeks of gestational age and those with low birth weight. Intraventricular hemorrhages, present in up to 46% of infants weighing less than 1500 g (Papile et al., 1978), are thought to develop secondary to lesions of ischemic origin. In most cases, blood ruptures into the lateral ventricle and the ensuing connective tissue blocks the cerebrospinal fluid flow, frequently resulting in hydrocephalus. Anoxic or hypoxic encephalopathy results in gray matter and white matter lesions. Gray matter lesions are diffusely present throughout the cortex, basal ganglia and thalamus, brainstem, and spinal cord, whereas lesions in the white matter are frequently in the periventricular zone. Periventricular atrophy has been identified as the most common abnormality found in preterm infants who developed hemiplegic CP, occurring in 50% of cases (Wiklund et al., 1991b). It is unclear, however, whether the lesions occur before, during, or after birth. Although periventricular atrophy is a bilateral lesion thought to be responsible for most cases of preterm spastic diplegia, it has also been reported as an asymmetric or unilateral lesion or one with bilateral lesions expressing only unilateral clinical symptoms (Wiklund et al., 1991b). Malformations of the central nervous system may cause hemorrhagic and anoxic lesions. Many factors may be responsible, including drug ingestion, radiation, and infection by viruses such as herpes simplex and rubella.

Attempts to relate cerebral lesions to the extent of disability have had only limited success. With respect to the side of expression, in the small percentage of children with hemiplegia with bilateral morphologic findings, subtle physical abnormalities were sometimes seen on the non-hemiplegic side, suggesting the existence of a continuum between hemiplegia and diplegia resulting from periventricular lesions (Wiklund & Uvebrant, 1991a). Magnetic resonance imaging demonstrated that, of several measures, only the amount of white matter damage correlated with the severity of disability (Yokochi et al., 1991). In children with hemiplegia, no significant correlations between size of lesion and severity of impairment have been found, although trends toward the association of less impairment with smaller lesions have been reported (Molteni et al., 1987; Wiklund & Uvebrant, 1991a). Quadriplegia has been associated with brainstem and basal nuclei damage in addition to cortical and subcortical lesions (Wilson et al., 1982). Further discussion of the causes of the various types of CP can be found in works by Menkes (1990) and Weinstein and Tharp (1989).

PROGRESS IN PRIMARY PREVENTION

The primary way to reduce the incidence of CP is through improving the prenatal health of at-risk mothers, coupled with maternal education. The role of poverty and low socioeconomic status in the incidence of CP (Dowding & Barry, 1990) and in determining the need for special educational resources (Msall et al., 1991) has frequently been overlooked, yet there is empirical evidence of its importance.

Certain maternal prepregnancy and pregnancy-related risk factors are associated with delivery of a child with a disability (Holst et al., 1989). Studies have suggested that improved intrapartum diagnosis of risk factors, prevention of asphyxia, and medical treatment of children with low Apgar scores would reduce the incidence of disabilities, as would intervention to prevent premature rupture of membranes. However reasonable these hypotheses may seem, no studies are known to have tested them. With the increased awareness of intrauterine factors that may cause CP, more attention is being paid to possible neuroprotective treatments that may prevent CP when these factors are present (Gaudet & Smith, 2001).

The role of the obstetrician in preventing CP before birth occurs is limited (Weinstein & Tharp, 1989). Attention is directed toward developing effective prevention of and intervention for premature delivery, fetal distress, neonatal asphyxia, and mechanical birth trauma. Methods of inhibiting labor have met with much success, although the effects on incidence of CP remain unclear. Methods of antepartum fetal evaluation, including sonographic measurement, electronic fetal monitoring, fetal pH monitoring, and intrauterine pressure monitoring, have provided the obstetrician with powerful tools for assessing the need for active intervention in the labor process. Delivery procedures using high forceps and certain presentations of breech deliveries that were found to be associated with increased perinatal morbidity have dramatically decreased in favor of cesarean section. This is partly due to the increased safety of cesarean birth for both the mother and the fetus.

DIAGNOSIS

CP is diagnosed when a child does not reach motor milestones and exhibits abnormal muscle tone or qualitative differences in movement patterns such as asymmetry (Rosenbaum, 2003). No consensus exists, however, on how early CP can be identified reliably (Campbell & Barbosa, 2003). Complicating the picture is the instability of diagnosis, since CP has been reported to resolve over time in many low birth weight infants (Kitchen et al., 1987). In a study designed to determine the accuracy of diagnosis of CP at 2 years of age (Kitchen et al., 1987), only 55% of those so diagnosed at age 2 were deemed to have CP at age 5, but the diagnosis of those with moderate or severe involvement did not change. Only 1% of children not diagnosed at age 2 were identified at age 5 to have CP. Of those children in whom the diagnosis was no longer accurate at age 5, most had minor neurologic abnormalities and left-hand preference, but their psychologic test scores were no different from those of children who had never been diagnosed as having CP.

Tests of neurologic status, motor function, primitive reflexes, and posture have been assessed for their ability to identify CP (Burns et al., 1989). The sensitivity of the Movement Assessment of Infants (MAI) has been calculated to be 73.5% in a high-risk population (Harris, 1987) identifying considerably more CP children at 4 months of age than the Bayley motor scale (Bayley, 1993). The Bayley scale, however, demonstrated sensitivities of 100% for both spastic diplegia and quadriplegia and 75% for spastic hemiplegia at 1 year corrected age (Bayley, 1993). The MAI has a lower rate of specificity than does the Bayley motor scale; that is, a greater percentage of children with normal outcomes are identified as being at risk. The Alberta Infant Motor Scale (AIMS) identified all children followed longitudinally from birth to 5 years of age as severely delayed in motor development at 6 months of age, though it did not do so at 3 months (Campbell & Barbosa, 2003). Longitudinal assessment using the General Movement Assessment appears more sensitive and shows few false positives (Cioni et al., 1997), but users found it unhelpful in planning interventions (Campbell & Barbosa,

2003). The Test of Infant Motor Performance (TIMP) shows promise of very early detection of CP and in differentiating between the two types of children with delayed motor development (Campbell & Hedeker, 2001): infants with brain insults and those born at less than 30 weeks' gestational age, with birth weight less than 1500 g (high risk) or with chronic lung disease. In summary, given the availability of the tests described here, an experienced physical therapist or pediatrician should be able to accurately diagnose CP in all but the mildest cases by 6 months of age (Samson et al., 2002).

IMPAIRMENTS

Impairments in CP are problems of the neuromuscular and skeletal systems that are either an immediate result of the existing pathophysiologic process or an indirect consequence that has developed over time. Impairments can be classified, somewhat artificially, into single-system impairments and multisystem impairments.

Single-System Impairments

Single-system impairments are expressed in the muscular system and the skeletal system, even though the original pathophysiologic damage occurred in the central nervous system. Primary impairments such as insufficient force generation, spasticity, abnormal extensibility, and exaggerated or hyperactive reflexes are evident in the muscular system; malalignments such as torsion or hip deformities are secondary impairments evident in the skeletal system (Metaxiotis et al., 2000).

CP is characterized by insufficient force generation by affected muscle groups, which is consistent with low levels of electromyographic (EMG) activity and decreased moment of force output (Berger et al., 1982; Engsberg et al., 2000, Ross & Engsberg, 2002). When an activity leads to an active contraction, this impairment may be expressed as a deficiency in power (Olney et al., 1990) or, when considered over time, in work. The term *strength* may refer to any of these measurable factors. Strength measurement in neurologic conditions is problematic, but when measured, strength has frequently been intimately linked with activity capabilities such as speed of walking (Bohannon, 1989).

The clinical term *tone* is used to describe the impairments of spasticity and abnormal extensibility. A sensation of abnormally high tone may be caused by spasticity, a velocity-dependent overactivity that is proportional to the imposed velocity of limb movement. Spasticity is especially evident in children with clonus but is frequently mistaken for problems of extensibility. Supraspinal and interneuronal mechanisms appear to be responsible for spasticity, with increased "gain" in the muscle spindles and increased excitation of Ia afferents having been ruled out as a cause of spasticity (Young, 1994). There is experimental evidence for three pathophysiologic mechanisms: reduced reciprocal inhibition of antagonist motoneuron pools by Ia afferents, decreased presynaptic inhibition of Ia afferents, and decreased nonreciprocal inhibition by Ib afferents. There is considerable evidence indicating that reciprocal inhibition is reduced in CP (Hallett & Alvarez, 1983; Leonard et al., 1991). In addition, studies using transcranial magnetic cerebral stimulation have provided evidence of simultaneous activation of antagonistic muscle groups through abnormal alpha motoneuron innervation (Brouwer & Ashby, 1991). The role of decreased presynaptic inhibition of Ia afferents in spasticity has been deduced from experiments showing that vibration-induced inhibition of the H-reflex is much less in spastic than in normal muscles, a phenomenon that has been shown to be mediated by a presynaptic mechanism in animal models. Finally, nonreciprocal inhibition has been reported to be reduced and even replaced by facilitation in persons exhibiting spasticity with sustained hypertonia (Young, 1994), which suggests that there may be a further mechanism responsible for abnormal alpha motoneuron excitability.

The sense of abnormally high tone can also result from hypoextensibility of the muscle because of abnormal mechanical characteristics. Comparing healthy children with children with CP, Berger and colleagues (1982) found that the EMG activity of leg muscles in nearly all children with CP was reduced in affected limbs and that there were no indications of pathologic reflex effects on muscle activity. A force transducer on the tendo Achillis measured tension that was disproportionate to muscle activity and could best be attributed to mechanical changes in the muscle rather than to increased stretch reflexes from spasticity. These muscles were also seen to be abnormally stiff; that is, they produced more force for a given length change than did muscles in nondisabled children (Tardieu et al., 1982). The most accurate term for this impairment is *hypoextensibility*. The muscle offers resistance to passive stretching at a shorter length than that expected in a normal muscle. In addition, if greater than normal amounts of force are required to produce a change in length, the muscle is said to have increased stiffness. This is represented as the passive tension curve for CP (p,CP) in Figure 21-1, *A*, in contrast to the normal passive tension curve (p,N) in Figure 21-1, *D*, when one moves the ankle from a position of plantar flexion to one of dorsiflexion. When a clinician finds that it is not possible to manually stretch the muscle through a normal range using reasonable amounts of manual force, the muscle group is deemed to have a contracture, represented in Figure 21-2 as "contracture," the difference between the joint angle at

which this extreme resistance is encountered in the CP muscle and that of the normal muscle.

Figure 21-1 shows hypothetical active force-length characteristics of spastic plantar flexors (a,CP; see Fig. 21-1, *B*) and normal plantar flexors (a,N; see Fig. 21-1, *E*), that is, the force generated by the contractile elements of the muscle over the range of muscle lengths from a shortened position (plantar flexed) to a longer position (dorsiflexed). Note that the maximal force is lower for the CP muscle and also that the peak force occurs at a more plantar flexed position in the CP muscle than in the normal muscle. The sum of the combined effects of active force output and passive stiffness for the CP muscle is shown as total tension curve CP, and the corresponding curve for the normal muscle is shown as total tension curve N (see Fig. 21-2). The complexity of the representation in Figure 21-2 underlines the difficulty faced by a physical therapist or physician in correctly determining the cause of increased tone through clinical methods such as passive manipulation of the limb and clinical assessment of muscle strength. Hypoextensibility can result in limitations in mobility, stability, and efficiency.

Muscle normally grows in response to full excursion of the muscle and joint. The conditions for normal growth appear to be regular stretching of relaxed muscle under normal physiologic loading, but in CP the skeletal muscle may not relax during normal stretching activity and, furthermore, greatly reduced forces are generated during movement (Graham & Selber, 2003). In children with CP muscle growth may not keep up with bone growth resulting in *hypoextensibility* (Rang, 1990). If a muscle has become overlengthened, which is usually a secondary impairment resulting from repeated mechanical stretch, it is termed *hyperextensible*. The term does not imply that stiffness is less, nor does it give any information about the force generating capability of the muscle.

The causes of the mechanical behavior of spastic muscle are not yet clear, but a fascinating picture is emerging that is likely to lead to a complex theoretical model that will assist in guiding treatment (Delp, 2003). All studies of the histology and morphology of spastic muscle have shown that differences are present when spastic muscle is compared with normal muscle (Romanini et al., 1989). Spastic muscle has generally been found to have fibers that are shorter than normal because the fibers have fewer sarcomeres in series. When muscle fibers with fewer sarcomeres in series are stretched during movement, excessive passive tension is generated as a result. Muscle fiber segments from subjects with spasticity have been shown to develop passive tension at significantly shorter sarcomere lengths than fibers from normal subjects (Friden & Lieber, 2003). In addition, the stress (force per unit of

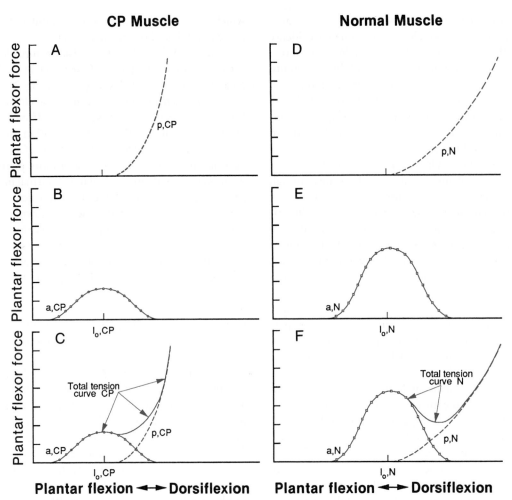

◆ Figure 21-1   Representation of force capabilities of ankle plantar flexor muscle at different joint angles in normal muscle (N) and spastic muscle (CP). **A**, Resistance to passive stretch of spastic muscle (p,CP) increasing with more dorsiflexion. **B**, The force of active contraction (a,CP) varying with the joint angle l_0 denoting resting length. **C**, The sum of the passive and active effects in spastic muscle. **D**, Resistance to passive stretch in normal muscle (p,N). **E**, Force of active contraction in normal muscle (a,N). **F**, The total tension curve comprising the sum of the passive and active effects in normal muscle. Note that (1) the slope (i.e., the stiffness) of p,CP in **A** is greater for the spastic muscle than for the normal muscles (p,N) in **D**; (2) the maximal active force achieved by the spastic muscle (a,CP) in **B** is less than the maximal active force of normal muscle (a,N) in **E**; and (3) the maximal active force for spastic muscle (a,CP) shown in **B** occurs at a more plantar-flexed position than that of the normal muscle (a,N) shown in **E**.

cross-sectional area) borne by spastic fibers was similar to that of normal fibers, but the cross-sectional area of the spastic fibers was less than one third that of the normal fibers. This resulted in greater stress when the spastic fibers were passively stretched. Furthermore, the fiberelastic modulus (change in fiber stress/change in fiber strain) was nearly double that of fibers from normal subjects.

The proposed source of these changes is the giant intramuscular titin (connectin) molecule that connects the myosin filament to the Z-disc, although extracellular matrix protein or collagen could also be implicated. The latter is consistent with the recent finding that the collagen

content of quadriceps biopsy specimens obtained from children with spastic quadriceps muscle was highly correlated with clinical measures of severity of spasticity (Booth et al., 2001). Further research should lead to a better understanding of the structure, behavior, and mechanisms involved, which should in turn lead to improved methods of intervention to address the mechanical changes that are found in spastic muscle.

The presence of impairments, such as low levels of force generation, spasticity, abnormal extensibility, and disturbed reflexes, can result in abnormal weight bearing and malalignment, which can, in turn, affect the orthopedic

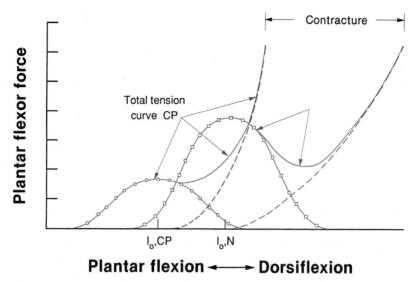

• **Figure 21-2**   Complete representation of force capabilities of ankle plantar flexor muscle at different joint angles in normal muscle (N) and spastic muscle (CP) shown in Figure 20-1. a,CP = force of active contraction of spastic muscle; l_0,CP = resting length of spastic muscle; l_0,N = resting length of normal muscle; a,N = force of active contraction of normal muscle; p,CP = resistance to passive stretch of spastic muscle; p,N = resistance to passive stretch of normal muscle.

development of the spine and the extremities. The application of correct forces is required for optimal skeletal modeling before the skeleton ossifies (LeVeau & Bernhardt, 1984), although the research reported to date has offered little specific guidance. Of particular concern is the effect of increased hip flexion and adduction on acetabular development and hip joint stability. Neck and trunk asymmetry can result in torticollis or spinal deformities. At all ages, children with hypoextensibility and spasticity are prone to developing contractures. Although patterns of tightness vary, commonly at risk for contractures are the shoulder adductors; the elbow, wrist, and finger flexors; the hip flexors and adductors; the knee flexors; and the ankle plantar flexors (Massagli, 1991).

There are no universally accepted methods of measuring spasticity (Katz & Rymer, 1989), and techniques used depend on the purposes of taking the measurement. Methods include measurement of forces in response to standard passive stretches (tonic) or standard hammer stimuli (phasic), Hoffmann's reflex recording (Jones & Mulley, 1982), measurement of responses to sinusoidal cycling or ramp stretches including isokinetic measuring instruments (Lin et al., 1994; Price et al., 1991; Damiano et al., 2002), and use of the pendulum test (Fowler et al., 2000). It is important to consider both the velocity-dependent component and the passive mechanical component of spasticity and measure accordingly. The modified Ashworth scale, though commonly used in clinical situations, is really an undifferentiated measure of spasticity

and extensibility. It has been shown to be reliable in adults with neurologic conditions, although reliability has not been established for children (Bohannon & Smith, 1987). The modified Tardieu scale measures the point of resistance to a rapid velocity stretch to give an indication of the dynamic neural component of tone or the overactive stretch reflex. Moving the limb slowly into a lengthened position indicates the mechanical component of tone or muscle length at rest (Boyd & Graham, 1999). A large difference between the point of the overactive stretch reflex or "dynamic" range and the point of mechanical resistance indicates a large reflexive component to motion limitation and a small difference suggests a more fixed muscle contracture (Boyd & Graham, 1999). There are, however, wide intersessional variations in measures of these differences that limit their use as an outcome measure. Kilgour and colleagues (2003) have suggested that a difference of more than 20° for the popliteal angle and 30° for dorsiflexion is necessary to indicate that a significant change has occurred in range of motion as a result of intervention.

Multisystem Impairments

In the second group of impairments are three multisystem impairments expressed in the neuromuscular system: poor selective control of muscle activity, poor regulation of activity in muscle groups in anticipation of postural changes and body movement (referred to as anticipatory regulation), and decreased ability to learn unique movements.

In CP there is poor selective control of muscle activity. Normal movement is characterized by orderly phasing in and out of muscle activation, coactivation of muscles with similar biomechanical functions, and limited coactivation of antagonists during phasic or free movement. In CP there is abundant evidence of inappropriate sequencing (Nashner et al., 1983) and coactivation of synergists and antagonists (Knutsson & Martensson, 1980).

The reasons for poor selective control of muscle activity are unknown. Failure of the normal reciprocal relationship of activity between agonist and antagonist muscles during voluntary movements has been observed (Berger et al., 1982; Hallett & Alvarez, 1983; Leonard et al., 1990), but whether segmental or supraspinal mechanisms or both are involved is unclear. Although Berbrayer and Ashby (1990) clearly demonstrated the presence of reciprocal inhibition in CP, it is not possible to exclude the possibility that other spinal mechanisms may be impaired (Harrison, 1988). Direct evidence for a supraspinal origin is scant; however, researchers have concluded that in CP, the corticospinal projections are directed equally to the motoneurons of agonist and antagonist muscles of the ankle (Brouwer & Ashby, 1991). Reflex overflow to antagonist muscles in children with CP (Leonard et al., 1991) has been attributed either to exuberant motoneuronal projections or to exuberant projections that extend to motoneurons innervating muscles other than the one being stimulated. From these studies, it appears certain that the neuronal "wiring" in CP is not normal. There is evidence that basic motor programs, including those providing grasp stability, never develop properly in CP (Forssberg et al., 1999).

Poor anticipatory regulation of muscle sequencing when postural correction is attempted has been reported by Nashner and colleagues (1983). In healthy individuals, changes in posture are preceded by preparatory muscle contractions that stabilize the body. In people with CP, the contraction that is needed to produce stability is frequently interrupted by destabilizing synergistic or antagonistic muscle activity.

There is some evidence that motor memory in children with CP is frequently impaired (Lesny et al., 1990; Ehrsson et al., 2001). Functional brain imaging studies in adults have led to identification of the bilateral cortical network involved in primary and secondary parietal and frontal areas involved in the neural control of manipulation (Ehrsson et al., 2002). These findings are important when considering strategies for teaching movement, and further research can be expected to provide guidance in the development of new intervention strategies.

Assessment of multisystem impairments usually involves measurement of a closely associated variable or number of variables and frequently involves different dimensions of functioning. Examination of the impairments of poor selective control of muscle activity, poor anticipatory regulation of muscle groups, and decreased ability to learn unique movements may be specific, such as quantifying active ankle dorsiflexion using the selective motor control test (Boyd & Graham, 1999), or broader with the use of measures of balance, coordination, and motor control. Responses to perturbations can be assessed by disturbing the supporting surface in a variety of ways (Nashner et al., 1983), or by perturbing the subject or environment (Patla et al., 1989). In each case, kinematic, kinetic, and EMG responses are measured. Analysis of EMG during these perturbations makes it possible to detect differences from normal responses in timing of muscle activity onset and duration, in sequencing of agonists, and in co-contraction of antagonists. Gait has been the most commonly observed activity used to examine specific impairments of CP (Perry et al., 1976), and the potential for its wide clinical application has increased with the advent of fast and efficient computer systems.

DETERMINANTS OF PROGNOSIS OR OUTCOME

About 90% of children with CP in developed countries survive to adulthood (Evans et al., 1990). Strauss & Shavelle (1998) found that the key predictors of a reduced life expectancy were lack of mobility and feeding difficulties. Based on a California population of over 45,000 persons with CP, the same authors subsequently reported breast cancer mortality rate in persons with CP to be three times that of the general population, which suggested poorer detection or treatment (Strauss et al., 2000). There was a dramatic increase in death due to brain cancer, especially in children; modest increases due to respiratory diseases and diseases of the circulatory and digestive systems; and a marked increase attributable to external causes such as drowning and being struck by motor vehicles. Survival rate of high-functioning adults was found to be close to that of the general population, but accurate predictions of lifetime functional outcomes in CP are limited.

Using the Gross Motor Function Classification System (GMFCS), Rosenbaum and colleagues (2002) have reported motor development curves of children with CP that offer some prediction of motor outcomes. The rates of attainment and limits of gross motor function for the various levels of severity can be accessed at the CanChild website. Rosenbaum and colleagues (2002) reported that in children with CP 90% of motor potential is reached before the age of 3 years for the most severely affected children (GMFCS Level V) and by the age of 5 years for the least affected children (GMFCS Level I).

Certain observable factors assist in predicting the ambulation potential and general change in motor ability of children with CP. Children with the hemiplegic type of CP usually have a good prognosis for ambulation, whereas the prognosis is less favorable for those with rigid or hypotonic types of CP (Crothers & Paine, 1988). Persistent tonic neck reflexes are associated with decreased likelihood of walking (Crothers & Paine, 1988). Some studies have reported that a remarkably large percentage of children who are able to sit independently by age 24 months eventually walk (Crothers & Paine, 1988) and that nearly all children with CP who eventually walk do so before 8 years of age (Bleck, 1975). Watt and colleagues (1989), examining all survivors of neonatal intensive care, have reported that nearly all who sat by 24 months of age walked 15 meters or more with or without assistive devices or orthoses by age 8 years. Independent sitting by 24 months remains the best predictor of ambulation, despite inclusion of neonatal variables, clinical types, primitive reflexes, and reactions (Watt et al., 1989). A number of factors, expressed as variables and rated by pediatric physical therapists, have been identified as influential in bringing about change in the motor ability of children with CP (Bartlett & Palisano, 2002). These 12 factors are grouped in four constructs: (1) primary impairments (e.g., muscle tone/movement patterns, (2) secondary impairments (e.g., force production, endurance), (3) personality characteristics (motivation), and (4) family factors.

Prediction of future employment has received scant attention. Murphy and colleagues (2000) reported employment rates of 52% for competitive employment in adults with CP. Another 7% had semicompetitive employment, and 18% worked in a noncompetitive environment. Increasing success rates in education and employment over the years have been attributed to advances in and access to technology such as power wheelchairs and computers, environmental access, and supportive legislation. Positive prognostic factors for employment included mild physical involvement, good home support, education, vocational training, and good cognitive skills. Senft and colleagues (1990) reported that more than 60% of registrants in a neuromuscular disability program were dependent on aging parents.

EXAMINATION, EVALUATION, AND INTERVENTION

At all ages, the physical therapy examination of the child with CP involves the identification of abilities as well as participation restrictions, activity limitations, and impair-

ments of body structure and function. Physical therapists integrate information from the many aspects of their examination and evaluation with prognostic knowledge to predict the optimal level of improvement that can be expected, formulate short-term and long-term goals, determine intervention strategies, measure change resulting from intervention, and provide feedback to families.

Children with CP have variable but significant disruptions in the accomplishment of life habits, particularly in the categories of recreation, community roles, personal care, education, mobility, housing, and nutrition, and most are associated with locomotion capabilities (Lepage et al., 1998). From infancy to adulthood, physical therapy goals for clients with CP should focus on the promotion of participation by maximizing the gross motor activity allowed by the organic deficits and helping the child compensate for activity limitations when necessary. Achieving these goals requires the promotion and maintenance of musculoskeletal integrity, the prevention of secondary impairment and deformity, the enhancement of optimal postures and movement to promote functional independence, and maintenance of optimal levels of fitness. Goals are individualized for the particular child and family. They should be determined in collaboration with the family and based on the needs, expectations, and values of the whole family (Rosenbaum et al., 1998). Goal and outcome attainment should be regularly reassessed so that the therapy plan is adapted to reflect changes in the child's progress and the family's needs and wishes. Programs should take into account the child's age, motivation, level of cognition, general health, and periods of transition in the life of the family and child. An important component of therapy programs is education of and sharing of appropriate information with the child and family about CP to enable them to become capable of advocating and taking responsibility for their future. Furthermore, the physical therapist must be cognizant of environmental and personal factors that could enhance activity or participation or, conversely, that could increase existing activity limitations and participation restrictions. The therapist attempts to provide support, guidance, and education for the child, the family, and the community.

The involvement of other health care professionals in the treatment of the child with CP depends on the child's needs and the practices of the institution where the program occurs. Some facilities may have professionals from several disciplines working with the family, whereas at others it may be thought better to have a primary therapist initially, bringing in others for assessment or treatment as necessary. Regardless of practice approach, parents value coordination of care and consistency of service providers.

Increasing emphasis on the costs of provision of services and managed care have led some institutions to develop critical paths. This is a difficult task for CP because of the diversity of presentation and the chronic nature of the condition; however, tools such as clinical practice guidelines that are sensitive to these factors can be beneficial in providing optimal care.

INFANCY

Infants grow and develop in response to being loved and nurtured by parents and caregivers in a home environment. Despite being dependent in most aspects of life, infants interact with and develop an understanding of the people in their lives, their surroundings, and themselves. From the time of birth, a child with CP may not experience the usual activities associated with infancy. As a result, some parents of infants with CP may not receive all aspects of the positive feedback of a typical nurturing experience and the satisfaction of observing the development of motor and social skills. The parents must cope with the impact of the diagnosis and the grieving process that accompanies the awareness that some of the hopes and expectations for their child may not be realized. They may be overwhelmed with the uncertainty that the future holds for them, their child, and their family. Many parents are also concerned with the immediate issues of providing basic infant care and are apprehensive about incorporating the specialized care necessary for their child's optimal development.

Movement is an important component in the learning and interactive processes of infancy. In infants who have CP, the nature and extent of their impairments affect their potential to develop and learn through movement. This may result in activity limitations related to the development of gross motor skills and may affect their ability to interact with their parents and their environment.

Physical Therapy Examination and Evaluation

Infant examination provides information on which to base a prognosis and a baseline for the monitoring of improvement or deterioration, growth, maturation, and treatment effects. Therapists must determine the history and environment of an infant and the capabilities and concerns of the family. At all ages examination of impairment involves qualitative and, when possible, quantitative assessment of single-system and multisystem impairments. Observation of active range of motion (ROM) provides indirect assessment of the force-generating ability of muscle groups and some information about muscle ex-

tensibility. Determination of the passive ROM, using a slow, maintained stretch in a position that promotes relaxation, assesses muscle group extensibility and provides information about joints, such as the presence of subluxation or dislocation. Normal maturational changes in joint range and alignment must be considered in evaluating the significance of measures.

Passive movement performed with greater velocity is used to assess spasticity and the sensitivity of the stretch reflex. Spasticity can be documented descriptively on the basis of resistance to movement and observations of spontaneous active movement and posturing. The severity of spasticity (mild, moderate, or severe), its distribution over the body and limbs, and its variations under different conditions should be noted. Frequently, there are variations in spasticity associated with positioning and the infant's effort and behavior. The modified Ashworth scale (Bohannon & Smith, 1987) or the muscle tone section of the MAI can be used (Chandler et al., 1980).

The presence or persistence of primitive reflexes and the development of the postural reactions of equilibrium, righting, and protective extension are assessed to determine their influence on selective control and anticipatory regulation of muscle group activity. The effects these reflexes and postural reactions have on positioning, handling, and the facilitation or inhibition of functional movement also need to be evaluated (Bly, 1991). The primitive reflex and the automatic reaction sections of the MAI (Chandler et al., 1980) are appropriate to use when evaluating infants with CP.

Selective control and anticipatory regulation of muscle groups are assessed in the context of functional evaluation: for the infant, this is indicated by the assessment of gross motor skills. Standardized tests used by physical therapists when assessing infant movement include the MAI (Chandler et al., 1980), the Test of Infant Motor Performance (Murney & Campbell, 1998), and the Alberta Infant Motor Scale (Piper & Darrah, 1994). The Peabody Developmental Motor Scales (Palisano et al., 1995) and the Gross Motor Function Measure (GMFM), a validated evaluative instrument designed to detect change in children with CP (Russell et al., 1989), can also be used for infant assessment. The GMFM-66 is an interval-level version of the original GMFM that demonstrates improved scoring, interpretation, and overall clinical and research utility (Avery et al., 2003). Various elements of movement and posture combine to produce gross motor skills. These skills include the ability to align one part of the body on another; to bear weight through different parts of the body; to shift weight; to move against gravity; to assume, maintain, and move into and out of different positions;

and to perform graded, isolated, and variable movements with an appropriate degree of effort. When functional motor skills are examined, proficiency in incorporating these elements into purposeful and efficient movement must be evaluated.

Assessments of seating, feeding, or respiratory problems may be necessary for infants with problems in these areas. Growth is often affected in children with CP; therefore, anthropometric measures, including head circumference, weight, and length, should be documented. Growth may influence, or be influenced by, feeding, exercise, and energy efficiency (Campbell et al., 1989). Other factors to be considered during assessment include the reciprocal influences of an infant's temperament and behavior on performance and sensory, social, communication, and cognitive abilities.

Physical Therapy Goals, Outcomes, and Intervention

Physical therapy in infancy is focused on educating the family, facilitating caregiving, and promoting optimal sensorimotor experiences and skills. Intervention must address current and potential problems. Early intervention for children with CP has been advocated to help infants organize potential abilities in the most normal way for them, although there is no definitive support for its efficacy (Barry, 1996; Campbell, 1990).

Family Education

The foremost set of goals at all ages is to educate families about CP, to provide support in their acceptance of their child's problems, and to be of assistance when parents make decisions about managing both their own and their child's lives. Infancy is an important time to foster collaborative goal-setting and programming strategies with the parents and promote ongoing communication between families and service providers. These skills empower them to make decisions, solve problems, and set priorities, as well as to become effective advocates for their children and themselves. Although it is recognized that parents know their children best, at this stage, the parents' goals may be overly optimistic and hopeful. Therapists must be realistic about the prognosis and the efficacy of physical therapy while remaining hopeful and providing options for intervention. They can break down overall goals into objectives that are meaningful, obtainable, sequential, observable, and measurable (Kolobe, 1992). Families value a therapist's honesty, commitment toward their child, and a belief that what they are doing is making a difference for their child. This can be promoted by drawing attention to the gains the child is making,

listening to the parental concerns, and recognizing the personal values and strengths of the child (Piggot et al., 2002).

Handling and Care

Abnormal postures and movements resulting from impairments can make an infant difficult to handle and position. These difficulties can affect an infant's interaction with the environment, reaction to caregiving activities, and development of gross motor skills. Therefore, a second physical therapy goal is to promote the parents' skill, ease, and confidence in handling and caring for their infant. These skills alleviate unnecessary stress for parents and child and also help reduce the influence of the impairments, thereby preventing unnecessary secondary impairments and activity limitations. Parents are taught positioning, carrying, feeding, and dressing techniques that promote symmetry, limit abnormal posturing and movement, and facilitate functional motor activity. The principles guiding these methods are (1) to use a variety of movements and postures to promote sensory variety, (2) to frequently include positions that promote the full lengthening of spastic or hypoextensible muscles, and (3) to use positions that promote functional voluntary movement of limbs.

Facilitating Optimal Sensorimotor Development

A third physical therapy goal in infancy is to facilitate optimal sensorimotor experiences and skills, thereby promoting activity and participation. Therapy should focus on the development of well-aligned postural stability coupled with smooth mobility to allow the emergence of motor skills such as reaching, rolling, sitting, crawling, transitional movements, standing, and prewalking skills. These skills promote the development of spatial perception, body awareness, and mobility to facilitate play, social interaction, and exploration of the environment. Movements that include trunk rotation, dissociation of body segments, weight shifting, weight bearing, and isolated movements should be incorporated into gross motor exercises and activities. These movement components, if experienced with proper alignment, can give the sensory feedback of normal movement patterns and activities. Good sources for the handling and treatment of infants and children of other ages include the works of Finnie (1997), Jaeger (1987, 1989), and Scherzer and Tscharnuter (1990). A practical reference for parents is *Children with Cerebral Palsy* (Geralis, 1991). Careful instruction of the family in specific techniques and activities, ongoing reinforcement, encouragement, and support are essential. Clearly written, illustrated, and updated home programs can be beneficial. Computer-generated programs or videotaping can be used to produce personalized, effective, and efficient information regarding activities, positioning, and exercises.

The normal motor developmental sequence may assist in guiding the progression of motor activities, although research indicates that motor milestones and their components develop in overlapping sequences, with spurts of development interspersed with some plateaus and even regressions (Atwater, 1991). The child with CP does not always proceed along the normal developmental sequence, and therapy becomes more functionally oriented within stage at which this happens depends on the severity of the impairments; in some children, it may occur early in life.

Equipment may facilitate activities when impairments otherwise prevent their development. For example, the sitting position promotes visual attending, upper extremity use, and social interaction. Infants with CP may be unable to sit independently, may sit statically only with precarious balance, or may not even be able to be seated in commercially available infant equipment. Customized seating or adaptations to regular infant seats may be necessary to allow function in other areas of development to progress. Infants with limited upper extremity movement may be unable to bring their hands or toys to their mouths to provide normal oral-motor sensory input. In these cases, mouthing activities should be incorporated into therapy. Toys may need to be adapted to facilitate age-appropriate activities.

The care of an infant exhibiting asymmetry, extensor posturing, and shoulder retraction illustrates these approaches. Such an infant should be carried, seated, and fed in a symmetric position that does not allow axial hyperextension and keeps the hips and knees flexed. A variety of postures is necessary to allow elongation of all muscle groups. Positioning of or playing with the upper extremities to allow the infant to see his or her hands, practice midline play, reach for his or her feet, or suck on fingers can promote sensorimotor awareness. For infants, handling techniques should encourage active movement, and so they experience normal movement sensations.

Active movements, such as the handling of toys that require two hands and that encourage the infant to develop flexor control and symmetry, are incorporated into daily activities. These activities facilitate the use of the neck and trunk muscles, promoting anterior and posterior control. The introduction of lateral control is the next step in achieving functional head and trunk control. In some severely affected children, slight gains in head control may be a goal, whereas in minimally affected children a fairly normal progression of motor development is expected, even without intervention. These therapeutic interventions should not limit infants' spontaneous desires to move and play and explore their environments because even very young children need to be able to assert themselves and manipulate their world (Campbell, 1997).

Role of Other Disciplines

Occupational therapists may be involved in upper extremity function, particularly as it relates to play. In addition, speech and language pathologists may be needed if there are oral-motor problems interfering with feeding or early language development. Community infant development workers may be involved in home-based programs. Social workers may help the parents through the grieving process, explain programs, and direct them to appropriate resources. Parent support groups or meetings with parents who have been through similar experiences may be helpful.

PRESCHOOL PERIOD

During the preschool years, locomotor, cognitive, communication, fine motor, self-care, and social abilities develop to promote functional independence in children. The process is a dynamic one in which all these areas constantly interact with one another. The child's environment remains oriented toward the parents, family, and home during this period, but he or she begins to interact with the outside world. Child care centers, babysitters, nursery schools, and playmates become part of a preschooler's world.

For children with CP, the limitations in motor activities may restrict participation in learning and socialization, as well as reduce independence (Butler, 1991). Concerns of the parents include the impact of impaired performance on all areas of development: for example, their child's ability to participate in and become integrated into normal preschool activities, the development of cognition and language, and the long-term effect of disabilities on future life and independence.

During these years, the child's attainable level of motor skills can be predicted with a greater degree of accuracy as the influences of impairments and activity limitations on each other become apparent. A major area of concern for physical therapists is the child's ability to achieve independent mobility. In addition, skills in gross motor development continue to be a focus of physical therapy to promote play, communication, self-care activities, social skills, and problem-solving skills.

Physical Therapy Examination and Evaluation

Assessment of activity assumes a primary focus, but it is important to determine the interaction of impairment and activity in relation to participation. Tests should be administered at regular intervals to document change that is due to treatment, maturation, or growth and to ensure that goals are appropriate and therapy intervention is being appropriately directed.

Within the dimension of body structure and function, direct testing of the force-generating ability of muscle groups may be difficult because of young age, spasticity, abnormal extensibility, hyperactive reflexes, or poor selective control. Considerable evidence suggests that strength is reduced in muscles affected by CP and that strength is not inversely related to spasticity (Ross & Engsberg, 2002). Although muscle strength can be measured quantitatively using dynamometry, strength should also continue to be assessed in a functional context. Observing activities such as moving between sitting and standing positions or ascending and descending stairs helps to assess both concentric and eccentric power. Endurance should be evaluated by observing the ability to walk age-appropriate distances or propel a wheelchair a comparable span.

During these years, quantitative measures of joint ROM and skeletal alignment, including the rotational and torsional alignment of the pelvis and lower extremities (see Chapter 6), should be documented using consistent and standardized procedures. Measurement errors of 10° to 14° occur in same-day goniometric measurement in children with CP and are even greater for those recorded on different days (McDowell et al., 2000). Some authors have suggested a change of more than 15° to 20° between sessions is required to be 95% confident that a true change in range of motion has occurred in many joints of children with CP (Kilgour et al., 2003). Caution must therefore be used when relying on goniometric measurements to make clinical decisions and measure outcomes. Dynamic tone is noted at the point at which initial resistance is met with high-velocity passive ROM and can be compared to the point of fixed muscle shortening to assist in decision making about spasticity and contracture management. However, it is difficult to accurately and reliably measure dynamic tone from session to session (Kilgour et al., 2003). A major source of error is the difficulty in determining consistent and proper positioning for biarticular muscles.

The Gross Motor Function Measure (Russell et al., 1989) and the Peabody Developmental Motor Scales (Palisano et al., 1995) can continue to be used to monitor the child's progress in attaining motor skills. When motor skills are assessed, the use of equipment to achieve an activity should be taken into consideration. For example, the use of orthoses in ambulation may substantially affect walking abilities.

Assessment should also include mobility and transfers, communication, social function, sleep, self-care and the degree of reliance on caregivers, adaptive equipment, and environmental modifications in the performance of activities of daily living (ADL). The Pediatric Evaluation of Disability Inventory (Feldman et al., 1990) uses parent report through a structured interview to assess many of these functional skills in young children. The Functional Independence Measure for Children (WeeFIM), a pediatric version of the Functional Independence Measure (Msall et al., 1990), measures function as quantified by burden of care. The Canadian Occupational Performance Measure (Law et al., 1990) can be used to measure outcomes and ensure that goals are relevant to the family. Goal Attainment Scaling can be used to evaluate whether specific individualized treatment goals or outcomes have been met, but this form of assessment cannot replace standardized measures, particularly for research (Palisano, 1993). Measures of health-related quality of life take into account various factors and values believed to be important by health care professionals, parents, and children themselves (McCarthy et al., 2002). It is also important to assess and manage pain, particularly in children who have significant movement and communication limitations (Hadden & von Baeyer, 2002).

When assessing children in this age group, environmental and personal factors such as attention, cooperation, the location of the assessment, and the child's reaction to being assessed may affect the evaluation process. Parents or other caregivers can provide information on whether a child's performance is characteristic of his or her abilities.

Physical Therapy Goals, Outcomes, and Intervention

The impact and extent of the child's impairments become more established during the preschool years. Proactive treatment focused specifically on limiting impairments and preventing secondary effects of impairment provides the foundation for interventions aimed at promoting participation in age-appropriate activities of early childhood and family life. Optimal postural alignment and movements of the body that are conducive to musculoskeletal development, neurophysiologic control, fitness, and function, through exercise, positioning, and equipment, are the aims of many interventions. In many cases, physical therapy goals may serve as the building blocks for global interdisciplinary goals in communication, play, social interaction, and self-care activities. Therapists must be willing to respect the priorities of families and other professionals when determining goals, because it may not be possible to work on all areas at once. They must also be sure that treatment is conducive to the goals chosen and is motivating and fun for the child.

Reducing Primary Impairment and Preventing Secondary Impairment

Increasing force generation. Physical therapy interventions to improve force generation of muscles and prevent atrophy in this age group use activities that create increased demands for production of both concentric and eccentric muscle force. Such activities include transitional movements against gravity, ball gymnastics, treadmill use, games, and practice of functional skills such as ascending and descending stairs (Stern & Steidle, 1994).

Spasticity. Several options are available for the management of spasticity. Interventions have been directed toward decreasing the impairment of spasticity with the goals of preventing secondary impairment, ensuring comfort and ease of positioning, and improving functional movement. Decreasing spasticity during the preschool years allows muscle lengthening and growth (Boyd & Graham, 1999; Rang, 1990) and may delay or eliminate the need for orthopedic surgery. These interventions are used if spasticity is interfering with function and conversely are not used if a child appears to be dependent on spasticity for function. Reducing spasticity will not automatically improve motor activity. Therapy that focuses on functional outcomes, but also emphasizes muscle strengthening and lengthening as well as motor learning, is necessary after the spasticity intervention for optimal effectiveness.

Selective dorsal rhizotomy (SDR) is a surgical procedure in which the sensory nerve rootlets from the lower extremities are selectively cut. Intensive physical therapy typically follows such surgical intervention (Fig. 21-3). Although a systematic review of SDR has not yet been completed, one is expected from the Cochrane Library in the near future. A meta-analysis of three randomized clinical trials of SDR demonstrated a small but statistically significant improvement for children who had SDR and physical therapy compared to those who received physical therapy only, as measured by the GMFM (McLaughlin et al., 2002).

The most consistent positive finding across studies of SDR is that the impairment of spasticity is markedly reduced. Gait analysis in children who have had SDR has shown improved sagittal ROM at the hip, knee, and ankle, but there is some concern that children develop a "crouch gait" as a function of muscle weakness that is often unmasked immediately postoperatively (Vaughan et al., 1998). Although postoperative weakness is commonly reported, at least one study has not shown significant deterioration after surgery (Engsberg, 1999).

Improvements in temporal gait measures vary, with stride length generally increased 3 years postoperatively,

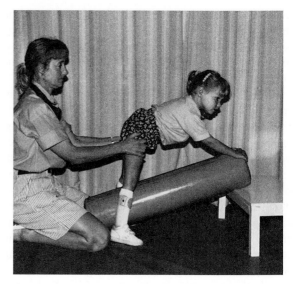

♦ **Figure 21-3** Exercises after rhizotomy are frequently directed toward increasing force generation of extensor muscles.

while changes in gait velocity are inconsistent (Vaughan et al., 1998). Abnormalities in patterns of muscle activation have persisted after SDR and are attributed to continuing problems with motor control, which prohibit the proper sequencing of muscle action (Giuliani, 1991). Some gait improvements have been found to remain 10 years after SDR (Subramanian et al., 1998). Other positive effects that have been noted include improved oral-motor control, increased voice volume and endurance, improved temperament and concentration, improved bowel and bladder control, and improvement in growth parameters (McDonald, 1991). McLaughlin and colleagues (2002) have suggested SDR may be most effective for children aged 3 to 8 years, with GMFCS levels III and IV who have access to and are receptive to physical therapy. Good selective control of muscles, lack of contracture or deformity, good cognitive abilities, and motivation, as well as good parental support, are factors that have been reported to result in the best outcomes after SDR (McDonald, 1991).

A currently popular method of spasticity intervention is the injection of small quantities of botulinum toxin A (BtA) into muscles to prevent the release of acetylcholine at the neuromuscular junction. Neuromuscular junctions near the injection site are inactivated for up to 4 months with peak effects observed 2 weeks after injection. The drug is expensive but this intervention is often covered by insurance. Targeted muscles are those that have good ROM but exhibit spasticity that interferes with function and those that are most prone to developing contractures. These muscles include the gastrocnemius, hamstrings, hip flexors, and hip adductors (Graham et al., 2000). Upper extremity muscles have also been successfully injected (Fehlings et al., 2000). BtA injections can also be used as a diagnostic measure prior to orthopedic surgery or SDR or as an analgesic agent to reduce pain and spasm postoperatively (Barwood et al., 2000). A recent systematic review (Ade-Hall & Moore, 2003) concluded that no strong evidence exists to support or refute the use of BtA for the treatment of leg spasticity in CP, but that ongoing randomized controlled trials are likely to provide useful data on the short-term effects of BtA. The authors of this review recommended that future research examine the longer term use of BtA on impairments and also report effects on outcomes that measure activity and participation.

If interventions directed at spasticity can delay surgery such as tendo Achillis lengthening, recurrence of muscle shortening necessitating repeated surgery may be avoided (Tardieu et al., 1982). Early screening, however, may indicate the need for soft tissue lengthening of hypoextensible or spastic hip adductors to prevent the secondary impairment of subluxation or dislocation of the hip joint for some children (Graham & Selber, 2003). Effectiveness of surgical or pharmacologic interventions for spasticity may be enhanced with concurrent therapeutic interventions such as muscle strengthening, application of motor learning principles, and management of residual contracture through exercise, casting, or positioning.

Hypoextensibility. Various approaches are used to maintain muscle extensibility and joint mobility. Ideally this would be a result of active movement, particularly with muscle activity in a lengthened position. As this is unlikely to happen spontaneously in children with CP, physical therapists may use manual passive stretching programs to maintain muscle length. The usefulness of these passive exercises has been difficult to assess because active exercises, positioning programs, and equipment are usually used simultaneously. Research on the effectiveness of manual stretching on extensibility is inconclusive (Miedaner & Renander, 1987) and ROM exercises have also been reported by some parents to cause pain (Hadden & vonBaeyer, 2002). Tremblay and colleagues (1990) found that a prolonged stretch of 30 minutes to the plantar flexors of children with CP reduced the impairment of spasticity and improved the voluntary activation of the plantar flexors but not the dorsiflexors. The effect lasted for as long as 35 minutes. In a parallel study, the stretching session did not produce a functional improvement in gait (Richards et al., 1991).

The effects of prolonged stretching programs in children with CP have been studied (Tardieu et al., 1988), and

it was found that contractures were prevented if the plantar flexor muscles were stretched beyond a minimum threshold length for at least 6 hours during daily activity. The threshold length was the length at which the muscle began to resist a stretch. The data prompting this statement are suggestive rather than conclusive, however. Lespargot and colleagues (1994) found that physiotherapy and a moderate stretch imposed for 6 hours daily prevented muscle-body contracture but did not prevent shortening of the tendon.

Casting and orthoses. Serial casting with plaster or fiberglass materials has been used as a method of providing prolonged stretch to lengthen hypoextensible calf muscles (Brouwer et al., 2000) and is often used in conjunction with spasticity intervention such as BtA injections (Desloovere et al., 2001). Casting for a 3-week period has been shown to be effective if the hypoextensibility was due to imbalance between the triceps surae and dorsiflexor muscles but not if the primary impairment was lack of appropriate muscle growth in response to bone growth (Tardieu et al., 1982). Serial casting has also been used for other muscle groups, such as the hamstrings and upper extremity musculature. After serial casting of the foot and lower leg from 3 to 6 weeks, eight children with CP demonstrated decreased resistance to passive stretch and increased dorsiflexion end range (Brouwer et al., 2000). Peak strength remained unchanged but occurred at longer muscle lengths. Follow-up 6 weeks after cast removal showed substantial reduction in gains. Although it is clear that at least temporary mechanical changes result from casting, the precise nature of the changes and whether they involve an increase in the number of sarcomeres is unknown.

Lower extremity orthoses may be used to reduce impairment, prevent secondary impairment, and to facilitate activity. The specific goals are to limit inappropriate joint movements and alignment; prevent contracture, hyperextensibility, and deformity; enhance postural control and balance; and provide postoperative protection of tissues (Morris, 2002). Ricks and Eilert (1993) found that although casts and orthoses improved ambulation and preambulation skills, x-rays did not show significant changes in the bony alignment of the foot and ankle during weight bearing.

Many variations of ankle-foot orthoses (AFOs) are available, depending on the biomechanical and functional needs of the individual child (Knutsson & Clark, 1991). In most studies, improvement in gait when compared with the barefoot condition has been reported (Morris, 2002). Solid AFOs are used if maximum restriction of ankle movement is desired. Children who would benefit from freedom of movement at the joint can use hinged AFOs with stops to prevent movement into plantar flexion. Hinged AFOs permit dorsiflexion, which allows stretching of the plantar flexor muscle group during walking and have been found to promote a more normal and efficient gait pattern than do rigid orthotics (Carmick, 1995). Posterior leaf spring orthoses, which are intended to prevent excessive equinus while mechanically augmenting push-off, have been found to reduce equinus in swing, permit ankle dorsiflexion in stance, absorb more energy during midstance, but actually reduced desirable power-generation at push-off (Oonpuu et al., 1996). Foot orthoses, or supramalleolar orthoses, may be used for children with pronation who do not require the ankle stabilization of an AFO (Knutsson & Clark, 1991). Supramalleolar orthoses may not improve ankle motion in the sagittal plane (Carlson et al., 1997), nor is there evidence that they reduce muscle tone (Crenshaw et al., 2000),

In an extensive review of the literature to date Morris (2002) concluded that only orthoses that extend to the knee and have either a rigid ankle, leaf spring, or hinged design with plantar flexion stop can prevent equinus deformities. There is little more than anecdotal observational evidence that using orthoses to control movement into plantar flexion prevents muscle shortening and therefore joint contractures. Controlled trials are difficult to carry out as contractures develop over many years (Morris, 2002).

Orthoses have also been used during sleep to prevent the secondary impairment of hypoextensibility, or contracture. Baumann and Zumstein (1985) found that the use of double-shell foot orthoses as night splints from age 3 years to the end of the skeletal growth period prevented calf muscle contractures from developing and made the need for surgery rare, but these results have not been compared to daytime wearing of orthoses. Other materials such as Lycra (Nichoson et al., 1995, Rennie et al., 2000), neoprene, and tape have been used for splints or actual garments to assist children biomechanically and facilitate function. Caution must be taken concerning the skin tolerance of these materials. Families often find the inconvenience of these garments outweigh the functional gains.

Positioning and alignment. Alignment of the body as a whole 24 hours a day is important. Children should have a variety of positions in which they can optimally function, travel, and sleep. Varying the positions of children who are limited in movement also helps prevent the secondary impairments of positional contractures and deformity, as well as skin breakdown (Healy et al., 1997). At all ages, decreased ability to change body position during sleep can cause discomfort, pain, and respiratory problems, which can result in disrupted sleep for children with CP and their families (Wright et al., 2003). Physical therapists may be involved in promoting safe, comfortable, and biomechanically optimal sleep positions

Positioning can also contribute to pulmonary health. Children with limited movement are at risk for chest complications because of chest wall biomechanics, feeding difficulties, immobility, and poor coughing abilities. Adaptive seating has also been shown to improve pulmonary functioning (Nwaobi & Smith, 1986). For the preschooler, sitting, standing, lying, and a position suitable for playing on the floor are important. When prescribing seating systems, it is necessary to be aware of not only the child's comfort and functional abilities but also the caregivers' concerns and needs and the child's environment. Seating inserts can be used in a variety of situations and with equipment such as strollers and wheelchairs, which are often needed to enable parents to transport their child easily. Specific suggestions are included in Chapter 33. Approved car seats and restraints are necessary for safe and comfortable vehicular transportation (American Academy of Pediatrics, 1999).

Positioning in standing is thought to reduce or prevent secondary impairments by maintaining lower extremity muscle extensibility, maintaining or increasing bone mineral density, and promoting optimal musculoskeletal development (Stuberg, 1992), including acetabular development. A study of bone mineralization in children with hemiplegic CP concluded that bone size and density decrease with increasing neurologic involvement, and weight bearing may slightly lessen the effect (Lin & Henderson, 1996). Optimally, standing involves movement and activity to provide intermittent loading and muscle strain; however, standing programs are often started at 1 year of age if children are not able to bear their weight effectively on their own. Stuberg (1992) recommended positioning in standing for 45 minutes two or three times a day to control lower extremity flexor contractures, and for 60 minutes four or five times per week to facilitate bone development, but notes that there is no definite evidence to support these guidelines. Maintenance of lower extremity weight bearing may allow continued use of standing transfers and reduce the need for older children to be lifted by caregivers.

Interventions of Activity Limitations

Physical therapy to promote activity is often intensive during the preschool years. The frequency of intervention varies, depending on the resources available, complementary programming, client goals, parental needs and desires, and the child's response to treatment. Optimal treatment frequency is unknown, but periods of more intensive intervention have resulted in attainment of specific treatment goals at levels that were maintained when frequency was decreased, provided the skills were incorporated into daily functional activities. Bower and colleagues (1992, 1996, 2001) have conducted a number of studies investigating the intensity of treatment. An initial study found that bursts of intensive physiotherapy directed at achievable specific measurable goals accelerated the acquisition of motor skills compared with conventional physical therapy (Bower et al., 1992). In a more recent study, there was no difference in gross motor outcomes for children treated five times a week for 6 months than those treated twice a week for the same time period (Bower et al., 2001). In addition families had low compliance and were stressed and tired from the intense therapy (Bower et al., 2001). Families and therapists must consider costs, accessibility, time, and the effect of the intervention on family dynamics. A treatment regimen of short periods of intensive therapy (four times a week for 4 weeks) separated by 8 weeks without therapy may allow for optimal motor gain and be less demanding for the children and their families (Trahan & Malouin, 2002). The research on intervention frequencies provides some guidance for developing service delivery models, however, the lower frequency of treatment in the control groups in these studies was often higher than that available at many treatment centers.

Therapy should be challenging and meaningful to the child and involve the integration of the skills learned into functional and cognitively directed skills for carryover. Movement tasks should be goal oriented and interesting to maintain motivation. For example, kicking a soccer ball is a more functional and motivating method of developing balance skills than practicing standing on one foot. Children with CP are able to perform concrete perceptuomotor tasks much more readily than abstract ones, even if the same movements are involved (van der Weel et al., 1991), because more information is available from the environment to direct the task.

Motor control and motor-learning principles (see Chapters 3 and 4) can be used to develop treatment strategies for reducing activity limitations. Feedback is important in the process of learning skilled movement. Information received through the child's sensory receptors provides intrinsic information, whereas extrinsic feedback through various forms of biofeedback provides information from external sources. Knowledge of results contributes information about movement outcome, and knowledge of performance supplies feedback about the nature of the movement (Poole, 1991). The motor learning principles support encouraging movement exploration and self-initiated solutions to new task demands, adapting to changes in the environment, and repetitive practicing of goal-related functional tasks that are meaningful to the child. Ketelaar and colleagues (2001) found that children receiving interventions based upon the foregoing principles demonstrated more improvement in both capability and performance of self-care and mobility activities in daily situations when compared to children receiving intervention designed to normalize movement quality.

Feedforward mechanisms must also be considered, because there is a cognitive component to movement skills. In some instances, cognitive strategies may be able to compensate for some of the inherent motor limitations. Many children with CP do not have normal cognition and behavior, and activities must be adapted accordingly. If a child is limited in the ability to learn, training using memorization of solutions may be necessary, although limited transfer to novel situations will occur (Higgins, 1991). If behavioral factors are negatively affecting treatment, a behavioral approach using appropriate motivators may encourage children to work on certain skills (Horton & Taylor, 1989).

Improvements in functional movement of the preschool-age child are made by reducing the effects of the multisystem impairments of selective control, anticipatory regulation, and learning of unique movements. Although there is a growing body of literature on motor learning, motor control in skill acquisition, and the biomechanics of movement, the profession is still far from being able to provide optimal strategies for interventions that are known to be effective (Fetters, 1991). The therapist who treats children with CP should modify approaches as research produces new insights in the areas of motor learning and motor control. For example, constraint-induced therapy, restraining the unaffected limb of children with hemiplegia while intensely training the involved extremity, has been shown to be effective in improving function (Willis et al., 2002, Bates & Willson, 2003).

Physical therapists may be involved in a variety of roles in addressing a variety of health and well-being issues. Impairments in oral-motor control and swallowing, impaired self-feeding, and difficulties in expressing hunger or food preference can result in eating difficulties. Feeding problems can result in inadequate nutritional intake and poor growth (Reilly & Skuse, 1992). Gastroesophageal reflux and aspiration can also occur. Oral-motor programs, proper positioning, and parent education and support are important issues to address. Malnutrition is common in children with moderate to severe CP; lower energy stores have been associated with poorer health status and restricted social participation as measured by number of hospitalizations, missed school days, and limitations in the child and family's ability to take part in usual activities (Samson-Fung et al., 2002). In extreme cases, gastrostomy and antireflux procedures may be necessary to improve growth and enhance the quality of life for the child and the family (Samson-Fung et al., 2003). Children with this level of involvement may also have chronic pulmonary problems including poor clearance of secretions and susceptibility to pneumonia. Chest physical therapy, suctioning, and other techniques to maintain optimal respiratory function may be necessary (Plioplys et al., 2002).

Drooling, a significant problem in about 10% of children with CP, can cause social embarrassment and affect the quality of social integration (Blasco et al., 2002). It can result from dysfunctional oral-motor activity, oral sensory problems, or inefficient and infrequent swallowing. Management may include waiting for further neurologic maturation, positioning, feeding and oral-motor programs, behavior modification programs to stimulate swallowing, medications, or surgery.

Failure to develop an appropriate toileting routine during the preschool years can result in participation restrictions and negative reactions from peers. Development of bladder control in children with CP may be delayed in comparison to typically developing children, but most become continent. Cognitive abilities and a diagnosis of quadriplegia can influence the development of control (Roijen et al., 2001). Therapists may need to recommend appropriate adaptive equipment as necessary.

Mobility

Ambulation is a major concern of physical therapists during the preschool years. Emphasis in treatment is initially on early ambulation skills, such as attaining effective and well-aligned weight bearing, promoting dissociation and weight shifting, and improving balance. Ambulatory aids, such as walkers and crutches, may be used, either temporarily while the child is progressing to more advanced gait skills or as long-term aids for independent mobility. The use of posterior walkers has been found to encourage a more upright posture during gait and to promote better gait characteristics than does the use of anterior walkers (Fig. 21-4) (Logan et al., 1990). Body weight support harnesses with treadmill training may provide a learning opportunity for the task of walking.

Children in this age group are becoming aware of the concept of achievement, and although ambulation is a coveted skill, it should not become an all-consuming goal, particularly if it may not be attainable. When interviewing adults with significant impairment, Kibele (1989) found that they remembered walking as the most important goal set for them by their parents and therapists. This resulted in feelings of failure from an early age and also in a loss of faith in rehabilitation professionals.

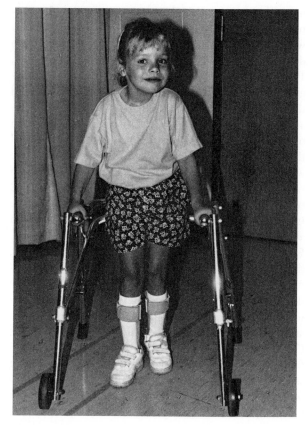

◆ **Figure 21-4** Child using a posterior walker, reported to promote upright posture and higher walking speeds than an anterior walker.

The provision of alternative means to allow children functional, independent mobility when ambulation is impossible or inefficient is recommended. Sometimes this need is met with an adapted tricycle (Fig. 21-5) or manual wheelchair; other children require a power mobility device and may need special controls. These enable children with CP to explore their environment and achieve a sense of independence and competence and increased social participation. Power mobility may also promote the development of initiative (Butler, 1991) and the acquisition of spatial concepts. The lack of self-propelled locomotion can result in apathy, withdrawal, passivity, and dependent behavior that can persist into later life (Butler, 1991).

If power mobility is being considered, fine motor control, cognitive abilities, behavior, environment, visual and auditory abilities, and financial resources must all be taken into account. Children with motor limitations can be safe and effectively mobile in power wheelchairs as young as 17 months of age (Butler, 1991). Parents may initially be hesitant about introducing power mobility to

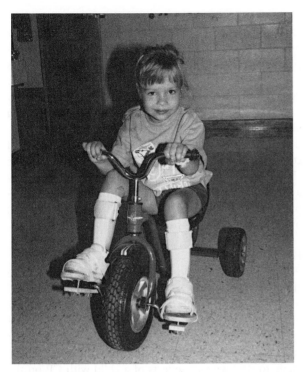

◆ **Figure 21-5**   An adapted tricycle may meet a child's needs for mobility.

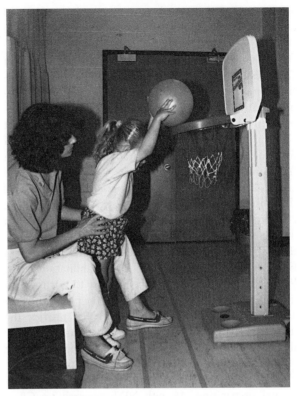

◆ **Figure 21-6**   Therapeutic exercise programs can include highly motivating play activities. Throwing a basketball may be more motivating than trunk extension exercises.

young children, fearing that it signifies giving up on walking. Power mobility does not preclude ambulation-oriented therapy but provides the child with a method of moving about independently in the meantime. For children who will continue to be wholly dependent on power mobility for independence, it provides mobility at an appropriate age and gives the families an indication of the implications of power mobility on housing, schooling, and transportation needs. For more information, see Chapter 33.

Play

Play, the primary productive activity for children, should be intrinsically motivating and pleasurable. The benefits of play include the children's discovering the effects they can have on objects and people in their environment; developing social skills; and promoting the development of perceptual, conceptual, intellectual, and language skills. Limitations in the play of children with physical disabilities may affect their experiential learning derived from play and result in decreased independence, motivation, imagination, creativity, assertiveness, social skills, and self-esteem (Blanche, 1997; Missiuna & Pollock, 1991). Therapy should provide and demonstrate play opportunities (Fig. 21-6). Appropriate toys and play methods

should be suggested to parents and caregivers. If children are physically unable to play with regular toys, a variety of adaptations, such as switch accessing, can make their toys usable (Langley, 1990). Environmental control equipment also can be introduced to preschoolers.

It is important that children not be overprotected in their attempts to play. Parents should be encouraged to let their children enjoy typical play activities, such as rolling down hills and getting dirty in the mud. Therapists must ensure that therapy and home programs promote, rather than interfere with, the normal play experiences parents have with their children.

Intervention Approaches

Some physical therapists may adhere to specific treatment philosophies, although differing treatment approaches often have underlying similarities. An example is neuro-developmental treatment (NDT). Traditionally, NDT was based on the theory that inhibiting or modifying impairments of spasticity and abnormal reflex patterns could improve movement and prevent contracture and deformity. The ultimate aim of the treatment was the acquisition of functional movements that permitted children the greatest degree of independence possible (Bobath & Bobath, 1984).

As an intervention approach, NDT has evolved with advances in the field (Bly, 1991). The theoretical perspective assimilated models of motor control, motor development, and motor learning and recognized the interactions between impairment and motor functioning. Current NDT principles include the encouragement of normal movement patterns through therapeutic handling during functional motor activities. Active participation of the child is encouraged to allow for the gradual withdrawal of therapist feedback. Randomized controlled studies on the effectiveness of NDT for children with CP have been inconclusive (Butler & Darrah, 2001). Conductive education (CE), an approach originated by Andras Peto in Hungary, integrates education and rehabilitation goals. Participants are selected for their ability to learn, which may make some children ineligible for the program. They are usually treated in group settings that provide the incentive of competition and allow more time in therapy than does individual treatment. Functional goals are broken down into small steps. Children initiate the activities on their own, with direct conscious action aided by mental preparation. As with NDT, research on CE is inconclusive, with reviews of the strongest studies in design and conduct revealing no difference in outcomes between conductive education and control groups using conventional approaches (Darrah et al., 2003).

Knowledge of a variety of theoretic models, not necessarily pediatric in origin, can help form a therapist's approach to treating children with cerebral palsy. Carr and Shepherd's task-related movement science-based approach (Shepherd, 1995), the motor control theories of Shumway-Cook and Woollacott (2001), and the dynamic systems theory (Darrah & Bartlett, 1995) can be integrated into physical therapy interventions for children with CP. The family-centered service philosophy of service provision can be applied to all treatment approaches.

It is difficult to compare the effectiveness of different approaches because there are also discrepancies in parameters such as frequency, skill level of individual therapists, compliance of families, and age and abilities of the patients. In a study comparing four treatment approaches, Bower and colleagues (1996) found that parents were most pleased with therapy when they requested the services, when they were present during treatment, and when targeted goals were met. They concluded that the most appropriate approach for a child would be one that would meet the needs of the particular child.

Parents often consider complementary or alternative therapies for their young children with CP with hopes of improving quality of life, augmenting traditional medicine, and relieving symptoms (Hurvitz et al., 2003). For example, some families may have their children participate in hyperbaric oxygen programs, even when studies have shown this treatment not to be effective (Essex, 2003). Alternative therapies are usually expensive and may not be accepted by some professionals. Reasons for seeking alternatives include a desire for more therapy, dissatisfaction with present therapy, and belief that their child could do better (Milo-Manson et al., 1997). If families choose to take an approach other than the one offered by a therapist, it is necessary to respect their choice. Therapists should not react defensively but provide impartial, objective information about the therapies in question.

Family Involvement

Planning of interventions should take into account the child within the context of the family. Therapists should be sensitive to the family's stresses, dynamics, child-rearing practices, coping mechanisms, privacy, values, and cultural variations. Therapists should be flexible in their approach and programming (Kolobe, 1992). Special efforts must be made to deal with the effects of a child with CP on the siblings (Powell & Ogle, 1985).

Family involvement is crucial for integrating treatment into everyday life. Home programs are important for optimal results from therapy programs because strengthening, extensibility, and motor learning often require more input than can be provided by limited treatment resources. It is also important to integrate therapy activities into daily life and for parents to gain insight into the impairments and abilities of their children. It is necessary to be aware of the well-being of the parents and find a balance between providing them with home programs that make them an integral part of their child's therapy and burdening them with activities they cannot realistically be expected to carry out. Obstacles may include constraints on time, energy, skills, or resources or negative effects on the parent-child relationship. Factors that have a positive influence on the participation of parents in home programs include collaborative decision making regarding the content and intensity of programs, sensitivity to the needs of individual families, and use of activities that are integrated easily into daily routines and are not stressful for the child or the caregiver (Jansen et al., 2003).

Siblings can also be included in home programs. Craft and colleagues (1990) studied a group of children with CP whose siblings had been educated about the condition and ways in which they could encourage their brother or sister to be more independent. As a result of this, the children with CP showed increases in ROM and in functional independence.

Role of Other Disciplines

Occupational therapists work closely with the children at this age to develop independence in activities such as dressing, feeding, toileting, and playing. Speech and language pathologists continue to develop efficient methods of communication in children with CP. Psychologists assess cognitive skills and consult with other professionals on the interaction of intellectual abilities with the other areas of development. Social workers and behavior therapists continue to provide ongoing support to the families because the stresses involved in parenting a child with a disability persist (Sternisha et al., 1992). Team assessment and intervention are imperative for addressing issues such as feeding problems, augmentative communication, and transition to school.

SCHOOL-AGE AND ADOLESCENT PERIOD

During the school-age and adolescent years, children typically participate in school and community life while remaining dependent on their families and living in their parental homes. They refine and augment the basic functional skills they have learned and develop life skills activities that will enable them to cope effectively with the demands of daily living and participate in independent adult life.

These years, particularly those spent in high school, can be difficult years for children with CP (Murphy, 2000). They become more aware of the reality, extent, and impact of their disabilities on themselves and their families. As they strive to contend with the normal stresses of growing up, particularly those of adolescence, they must also cope with being different, acknowledge the potential obstacles to attaining independence, and work to overcome them.

Parents remain anxious about how their child's disabilities will affect their participation in educational environments and in social situations. They may worry about their child's future as an adult (Hallum, 1995). While continuing to be naturally attentive, they have to avoid being overprotective and begin to allow their child to take risks and become independent in the outside world (Murphy, 2000). In some cases, there may be financial concerns regarding the need for special equipment, transportation, and home renovations. Parents of children who are dependent in ADL and transfers may suffer from physical stresses, such as back problems.

Typical disabilities encountered during these years include a lack of independent mobility, poor endurance in performing routine activities, and continued difficulty and slowness with self-care and hygiene skills at a time when privacy is becoming increasingly important. Adolescents may also not have the opportunity to develop socially and

sexually and may lack the ability to acquire age-appropriate levels of independence from the family. Environmental factors may reduce access to community and school facilities, thus limiting opportunities for participation in social, cultural, recreational, and athletic activities.

Physical Therapy Examination and Evaluation

Assessment of impairments that could interfere with function, or lead to further secondary impairment, such as scoliosis, continues to be important. Children in this age group may be able to participate in measurement of force production using dynamometry (Damiano et al., 2002). Assessment of gross motor function is appropriate, because children are often making gross motor progress during their school years. They may also change as a result of interventions such as surgery, the use of orthoses, and periods of intensive therapy. Further development of the Gross Motor Performance Measure (Boyce et al., 1995; Thomas, 2001) may help in detecting the fine increments of motor skill gains that are characteristic of children who are severely affected. For children with mild degrees of involvement, the Bruininks-Oseretsky Test of Motor Proficiency (Bruininks, 1978) may be useful in measuring specific components of higher levels of motor function. Tools such as the School Function Assessment may be used to assess participation and environmental factors in educational settings (Coster et al., 1994). Participation in activities of daily living and social roles has been evaluated in children with CP using the Life Habits Assessment (Lepage et al., 1998).

Assessments specific to certain activities or equipment may include evaluations of postural stability (Westcott et al., 1997) and gait (Ounpuu et al., 1996; Olney et al., 1990). Instrumented gait analysis (Gage and Novacheck, 2001; Ounpuu et al., 1996) can provide measurement details that assist in understanding gait, diagnosing specific problems and evaluating outcomes of interventions (Fig. 21-7). Some authors stress the importance of gait analysis in surgical decision making and in providing evidence of its effectiveness (Gage, 1994; Lee et al., 1992), and the development of sophisticated muscle-actuated models offers hope of greater precision in predicting outcomes (Thelen et al., 2003). An understanding of power generation and absorption of muscle groups is of particular importance in assessing outcomes (Zwick et al., 2001). Visual gait assessment using tools such as the Observational Gait Scale have been found to be reliable and valid for many gait parameters and are useful for clinical evaluation and research (Boyd & Hays, 2001; Mackey et al., 2003).

Endurance and efficiency of movement become increasingly important during these years as the children

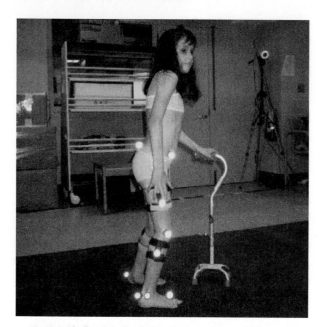

◆ **Figure 21-7** Child taking part in gait analysis. Electromyography shows patterns of muscle activities and aids identification of the presence of co-contraction of muscle groups. Markers at joints allow computer calculation of joint movements; force platforms embedded in floor permit measurement of individual muscle group contributions to the work of walking. *(Courtesy of Human Motion Laboratory at School of Rehabilitation Therapy at Queen's University, Kingston, Ontario.)*

venture into the community on their own or with their peers. The 10-minute walk has been found to be reliable in children with neuromuscular disease. Compared with ambulation measured over short distances, the 10-minute walk more closely simulates community ambulation and may therefore more closely represent the ability to participate in the community (Pirpiris et al., 2003). Physiologic measures such as the physiologic cost index can provide energy cost information (Butler, 1991; Mossberg et al., 1990; Fernhall & Unnithan, 2002) but may be most useful when comparing two or more mobility options for the same person (Rose et al., 1985). A review of methodologies related to physical activity and metabolic issues has been provided by Fernhall and Unnithan (2002). An important consideration in maximizing endurance for daily activities is the effect of excessive weight gain, because it can compromise optimal function and efficiency.

Privacy of individuals at all ages should be respected, but it is particularly important during these years when children are becoming more aware of their bodies and their sexuality. Children should be appropriately dressed when attending therapy sessions and clinics, particularly

if they are being seen by unfamiliar people or are being photographed or videotaped. If it is necessary for children to remove their clothing, their permission should be asked and a reason given for doing so. It is important to include the clients in conversations that involve them and not to converse only with caregivers or other professional staff.

Physical Therapy Goals, Outcomes, and Interventions

As goals change to reflect the adolescent's lifestyle, emphasis is on maintaining or improving the level of activity and participation while considering the stresses of growth, maturation, and increasing demands in life skills and participation in community activities. Although the pathophysiologic impairment of CP is nonprogressive, there are changes related to the stresses of increasing size, accumulative physical overuse, and a more competitive lifestyle. For example, as children advance to higher grades in school, there may be longer distances to walk between classes. Contractures may rapidly develop during periods when bones are growing faster than muscles (Tardieu et al., 1982). Secondary orthopedic impairments must be anticipated and avoided. The maintenance of muscle extensibility and force generation, joint integrity, and fitness is important in preventing secondary impairments that can result from the stresses of aging. This age group also needs to develop problem-solving strategies to overcome environmental and societal barriers to become as independent and active as possible in home, school, recreational, social, and community life.

In many cases, adolescents can and should be involved in setting goals and determining programming. It is important during these years to encourage them to take responsibility for their own health, nutrition, fitness, personal care, and decision making so that they are prepared to assume these responsibilities in adulthood. It is also important to look ahead and set goals that are appropriate for their later life situations and independence. Therapists should strive to foster self-esteem and assertiveness in children and adolescents by emphasizing their abilities, finding areas and activities in which they can excel, and helping them to acknowledge their difficulties with a view toward identifying appropriate compensations and use of attendant care. In the case of children with more severe involvement, goals are oriented toward minimizing impairments to facilitate caregiving and comfort.

Reducing Primary Impairment and Preventing Secondary Impairment

The impairment of deficient muscle force generation that may result in activity limitations and participation restrictions is important to address in this age group, as children with CP are often weak. For example, hip weakness has been proposed as a possible cause of hip deformities in ambulatory children and young adults (Metaxiotis, 2000). Muscle weakness can also contribute to bony deformity, and lower extremity strength has been shown to be related to walking velocity and gross motor function (Damiano et al., 2002). Research has supported the effectiveness of strength training programs in significantly increasing force production in children with CP (Dodd et al., 2003). Some studies have reported concurrent improvements in activity as measured by gross motor function, gait parameters such as stride length and kinematics, and wheelchair propulsion. The improvements have taken place without negative effects such as increased spasticity, increased pain, or decreased range of motion. Programs have typically been at least 4 weeks in duration, with a frequency of three times a week, at 80% to 90% of maximal load with low repetitions arranged in short sets to allow time for the muscle to rest and recover. Free weights and isokinetic equipment have been used. Programs have taken place in the home, clinic, or community. Endurance programs require lower intensities with more repetitions. Children should exercise in positions that are comfortable and allow optimal selective control of selected muscle groups.

Various methods of electrical stimulation have been used as an adjunct to the treatment of CP to attempt to reduce spasticity, increase force production and muscle extensibility, promote the initial learning of selective control, and improve functional activities such as gait (Stanger & Bertoti, 1997). Administration of electrical stimulation at intensities that do not produce a muscle contraction over extended periods has not been shown to have a clinical effect (Dali et al., 2002). Stimulation for short durations at high intensities has been shown to result in an increase in maximum voluntary contraction (Dubowits, 1998; Hazelwood et al., 1994; Wright & Granat, 2000), though a recent well-controlled study did not find an increase in voluntary contraction (van der Linden at al., 2003). Placebo effects may be high (van der Linden et al., 2003). Protocols should be individualized for patients following careful analysis of movement, and application should be closely monitored.

It was once thought that individuals had no control of their spasticity. Subjects with CP, however, have been able to reduce their responsiveness to a stretch reflex stimulus imposed during a lower limb activity (O'Dwyer et al., 1994). These findings encourage further exploration of the possibilities of reducing spastic responses.

Spasticity management is still important in this age group. Botulinum toxin may be effective, but serial casting following the injection may provide more marked and long-lasting effects (Bottos et al., 2003) and address the risk of contracture development (Desloovere et al., 2001). Pharmacologic intervention can be used to control the impairment of spasticity. The use of oral medications has been poorly studied, but medication may be appropriate for some children (Edgar, 2003). Children must be carefully assessed for appropriateness and monitored closely for side effects. Baclofen, a synthetic agonist of aminobutyric acid, has an inhibitory effect on the presynaptic excitatory neurotransmitter release. It has been shown to reduce spasticity in individuals with CP. However, oral doses high enough to give the proper concentration in the cerebrospinal fluid can cause side effects such as drowsiness. If this is a problem, baclofen can be given intrathecally by a continuous infusion pump implanted in the abdomen that releases the drug at a slow, constant rate into the subarachnoid space. The use of intrathecal baclofen reduces spasticity most noticeably in the lower extremities. Improvements in function and ease of care and a reduced need for orthopedic surgery have been documented in studies (Butler & Campbell, 2000). Complications are common but are manageable in most cases. Intrathecal baclofen has also been beneficial in treating patients with generalized dystonia, a difficult problem to manage. In addition to improving the dystonia, subjective improvements have been reported in quality of life, ease of care, speech, swallowing, and upper and lower extremity functioning (Albright et al., 2001).

The secondary impairment of joint or muscle contracture may occur in this age group, particularly in the more severely affected patients. This can be a result of chronic muscle imbalance, abnormal posturing, or static positioning. Casting may be used to increase the range of joint movement by lengthening muscles or tendons or both with no associated loss in strength (Brouwer et al., 1998; O'Dwyer et al., 1989; Tardieu et al., 1982). Anderson and colleagues (1988) found that soft splints made of polyurethane foam were effective in reducing severe knee flexor contractures; this may be a less expensive alternative.

The secondary impairment of joint hypomobility resulting from capsular or ligamentous tightness can be treated with manual therapy techniques (Brooks-Scott, 1995). Joint mobilizations may be used to regain joint mobility, particularly after immobilization. Therapists must ascertain whether joint structures are causing movement restriction and must also be aware of the contraindications and precautions relevant to using mobilizations in growing and neurologically involved patients (Harris & Lundgren, 1991).

Biofeedback providing information about, for example, limb or head position or muscle activation may be used to address single-system and multisystem impairments during these years because by this time children have usually developed abstract thinking and sufficient cognitive ability to use it optimally. Positive results have been reported but carryover is often limited, generalization to real-life situations is not readily demonstrated, and treatment is time consuming (James, 1992). Toner and colleagues (1998) found that a program of biofeedback improved active ROM, strength, and motor control of dorsiflexion in a group of children with CP. Using a crossover design of biofeedback or physical therapy treatment Colborne and colleagues (1994) reported increases in gait symmetry, greater peak ankle power for push-off, and increases in positive work done by the hip and ankle during gait after biofeedback but not after physical therapy. Uses in controlling posture have also met with some success (Bolek et al., 2001; Kramer et al., 1992).

Osteopenia with an increased rate of fracture in moderately to severely involved children with CP has been associated with the use of anticonvulsants, feeding problems, and low muscle mass (Henderson et al., 2002a). Physical activity that involves weight bearing and bisphosphonate therapy have been shown to have a positive effect on bone mineral density in children and adolescents with CP (Chad, 1999; Henderson et al., 2002b).

Orthopedic surgery. Despite new and effective methods of spasticity, many children will still develop progressive musculoskeletal deformities as they grow. Surgical intervention may be used to correct contracture or bony deformity, or to restore biomechanical alignment to improve function, posture, cosmesis, and hygiene and prevent pain in adulthood. Possible surgical procedures include muscle/tendon lengthenings and transfers, tenotomies, neurectomies, osteotomies, and fusions. Although some types of orthopedic surgery have been evaluated, there are few comparative studies or well-controlled studies on the long-term effects of orthopedic surgery in this population (Boyd & Hays, 2001). Single-event multilevel surgery (hip, knee, and ankle) performed after the initial growth period when gross motor function has plateaued and before further deterioration takes place (between 7 and 10 years of age) is one approach used to correct gait problems (Graham & Selber, 2003; DeLuca, 1996). Biomechanical alignment can take place at all joints simultaneously and the children and families will only have to deal with one hospital admission and one period of rehabilitation. As children get older, they should be active participants in surgical decision making. Their interests, priorities, and concerns about interruptions in their lives as a result of hospitalizations, immobilizations, and recovery periods should be respected.

Massagli (1991) has emphasized that patterns of muscle activity are not altered with lengthening, releasing, or transferring muscles. Decreased force production is often a complication of lengthening procedures. Physical therapists play important roles in surgical decision making and the management of pre- and postoperative care. Positioning during the immediate postoperative period is important for comfort and muscle extensibility. Surgery may improve posture and gait, but outcomes can be unpredictable as osteotomies, such as femoral derotations, alter the biomechanics of bones, and decreased force production is a common and significant complication of surgery (Harryman, 1992). The physical therapist must train control of lengthened and transferred muscle in the context of functional motor tasks such as sit to stand, ascent of stairs, and ambulation.

Spasticity, abnormal extensibility of muscles, muscular imbalance, and decreased force generation can result in scoliosis, which, in turn, can affect positioning and respiratory status. Spinal deformity can be a particularly difficult problem in the severely affected patient. Rigid orthoses can result in skin breakdown and patient intolerance; by contrast, the use of a soft orthosis has been found to be beneficial in the management of scoliosis in patients with CP without compromising pulmonary function (Letts et al., 1992; Leopando et al., 1999). Correction of spinal deformities may also be necessary in children with CP; usually those with spastic quadriplegia (see Chapter 11).

Activity, Mobility, and Endurance

In some situations physical therapy services may be reduced as the child reaches adolescence; however, school-aged children can still make gains in gross motor skills (Bower et al., 2001; Woolcott & Shumway-Cook, 2003). Improvements are even possible in children with severe physical and cognitive limitations if goals are realistic, all levels of disability are considered, and appropriate behavioral, communication, and motor learning techniques are incorporated into the treatment programs (Brown et al., 1998).

Gait training can continue throughout the school years, often in conjunction with other interventions such as spasticity interventions or surgery. Treadmill training with partial body weight support harnesses has resulted in clinically relevant improvement in walking as well as improvement in standing transfers in nonambulatory children (Schindl et al., 2000). Treadmills are also a useful method to increase endurance and strength and can be used without harnesses in higher functioning children.

Children and youth with CP are less active than their peers (van den Berg-Emons et al., 1995; Fernhall & Unnithan, 2002). Compensatory strategies can be implemented to promote participation and circumvent disability during the school years. The continued use of power mobility devices is important for independence. Even children who are able to walk independently may need an alternative form of mobility, such as a manual wheelchair or a power scooter, as they become larger and need to travel greater distances to meet their social and educational objectives. Availability of power mobility should not preclude activity to the point of decreased musculoskeletal integrity or physical fitness. Mobility devices may require modifications, such as ramps to buildings or washroom renovations, for accessibility. Driver training offers the freedom to travel independently. For those unable to drive, instruction in the use of public or special transportation should be provided.

It is unclear whether the low level of physical activity in children with CP is related to the physical disability or results from restricted movement and a subsequent relatively sedentary lifestyle. Children with CP have poor cardiorespiratory fitness, lower physical work capacity, and higher oxygen costs. Causes may include inefficiency of breathing, high muscle tone, increased involuntary movements, and a high level of muscle coactivation. Rose and colleagues (1990) found that energy expenditure indices based on oxygen uptake and heart rate measured at a given walking speed were three times higher in children with CP than in nondisabled children. Findings that were similar, but based on mechanical energy analyses, were reported for children with hemiplegia (Olney et al., 1987). Rose and colleagues (1985) also found that children who were ambulatory with wheeled walkers or quadruped canes had high physiologic workloads when walking for 5 minutes, suggesting that it is impractical for such children to walk long distances. Orthoses may also influence energy expenditure, as Mossberg and colleagues (1990) found that the use of AFOs significantly reduced the energy demands of walking in children with spastic diplegia. Increased energy demands as described earlier can result in fatigue and, as a result, have a significant effect on a child's ability to perform everyday activities as well as participate in regular exercise and recreational activities.

School and Community

Because many children with CP have problems with school integration (Lepage et al., 1998), physical therapists should be involved in school-based therapy programs to support participation. Facilities and resources such as support personnel, equipment for accessibility, and computer-based systems may be necessary to meet the physical needs of children in the school system. Therapists working with school personnel may instruct assistants and teachers in positioning, lifting, and transferring the children; carrying out exercise programs; and adapting and developing physical education programs. Therapists may also be involved in accessibility, transportation, evacuation, and other safety issues. Therapists working in school settings must be sensitive to the physical and scheduling constraints of the educational environment and be willing to compromise to meet the educational priorities of the students. Therapy may range from consultation and monitoring for students who are thought to have reached their maximal level of functioning, to active therapy for children who have specific treatment goals. When children are primarily seen through the educational system, effort must be made to keep the family involved in all aspects of care and treatment. See Chapter 32 for further information on this subject based on experiences in the United States.

In addition to educating school staff about the problems associated with CP, therapists can help educate the other children in the classroom and reduce teasing and bullying. In a study by Yude and colleagues (1998), children with hemiplegia who were integrated into regular schools were twice as likely to be rejected and lack friends, and three times more likely to be victimized compared to their nondisabled peers. Knowledge about, and positive interactions with, people with disabilities can create positive attitudes, particularly when children are between 7 and 9 years of age, because their attitudes about people with disabilities are flexible at this age (Morrison & Ursprung, 1987).

It is important for children with disabilities to be involved in community and recreational activities that provide social as well as therapeutic opportunities (Fig. 21-8). This can be particularly important during these years if adolescents are receiving less direct physiotherapy intervention. Many adapted or integrated sports activities are suitable for people with CP, including horseback riding (MacKinnon et al., 1995), swimming, skiing, sailing, canoeing, camping, kayaking, fishing, bungee jumping, yoga, and tai chi. Adapted games can provide athletic competition and participation in team experiences and can facilitate the social aspects of sports. Community fitness programs for adolescents with CP have been shown to improve muscle strength and perception of physical appearance and to result in participants feeling confident and motivated enough to take responsibility for continuing in fitness programs (Darrah et al., 1999). Therapists need to be aware of and address factors that may have a negative impact on participation in recreation and leisure pursuits. These factors include lack of community level supports and barriers such as transportation and accessibility; family factors such as finances, time, preferences, and involvement; as well as the adolescent's

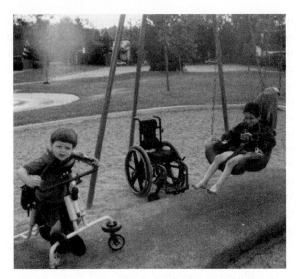

⬧ **Figure 21-8** Environmental adaptations to playgrounds can facilitate participation in normal childhood activities.

physical abilities, interests, and self-perceived competence (King et al., 2003).

All athletes are at risk for sports-related injuries, but relatively minor injuries can incapacitate people with CP. They should be encouraged to be responsible for their bodies during sports activities by following appropriate conditioning, warm-up, and cool-down routines; following comprehensive injury prevention programs, which include strengthening, flexibility, and aerobic and anaerobic training activities and prevention of long-term joint integrity; and using appropriate protective and orthotic equipment. Injuries should be treated promptly. The knee is the most frequently injured body part in athletes with CP. Shoulders, hands, and ankles are also vulnerable (Ferrara et al., 1992). For more information, see Chapter 18.

During these years, children learn about their bodies, their sexuality, and appropriate interactions with other people. Children and adults with disabilities have an increased risk of suffering abuse, including sexual abuse, which can result in physical, social, emotional, and behavioral consequences (Hallum, 1995; Sobsey & Doe, 1991). Some abusers have relationships specifically related to the victim's disability. These people can be personal care attendants, transportation providers, residential care staff, and other disabled individuals. Physical therapists must know how to detect the signs of abuse, be sensitive and receptive to clients who may choose to confide in them, and know the proper procedures to follow if they suspect abuse. They must work with other professionals to promote assertiveness and positive self-esteem in their clients.

All professionals involved with patients who have CP must educate them in being streetwise. Their physical and sometimes cognitive limitations can make them particularly vulnerable to crime. Children and adolescents with disabilities should be taught to avoid threatening situations. They should be warned about carrying valuables (large sums of money or important medications) with them, particularly in a purse that attracts attention and is easy to grab, such as one slung over a wheelchair handle. Self-defense courses specifically designed for people with disabilities may be available.

Health care professionals must realize that although parents have been coping with their child's needs for a number of years, parent education is still important because their child and their needs are constantly changing. Continued attention to education in lifting and transferring is necessary to prevent injury to caregivers as their children grow larger and heavier and parents themselves are aging.

Role of Other Disciplines

Occupational therapists may be involved in promoting independence in ADL. Interdisciplinary life skills training may be offered to focus on self-care, community living, and interpersonal relationships. Prevocational training and related activities, such as money management and employment searching, may be necessary. Psychologists or social workers may be involved in various aspects of adolescent life such as social and sexuality issues.

TRANSITION TO ADULTHOOD

Adults strive to be independently functioning and self-sufficient individuals who have satisfying social and emotional lives and contribute to society. The natural environment for adults is living independently in the community, alone or with others, with employment to support them. The extent to which people with CP can realize these goals depends on factors such as level of cognition, available resources and support, and independence in self-care activities and mobility. Many adults with CP continue to live with their families, in group homes, or in institutions, and only a small proportion of them are employed. For example, one study from the Netherlands found that 30% of adults with CP lived with their parents, 12% with a partner, and 32% alone; 53% had completed some secondary education, and 36% had paid employment (van der Dussen et al., 2001). At a time when most parents are experiencing freedom from caregiving responsibilities, many parents of children with CP continue to have these obligations and have to cope with many anxieties (Hallum, 1995). Their concerns focus on how their child can function as an independent adult, how they can continue to care for their child as they themselves age, and who will care for the child when they are unable to do so. They, and their child, may also be coping with a decrease in the number of relatively organized and available programs and equipment resources that were available for the younger child.

Physical Therapy Examination and Evaluation

Although there is a continuing need to assess body function and structure as well as activity, in adults with CP the focus should be on participation, particularly on living independently. Physical therapy involvement continues to address all levels of function with an emphasis on working together with the individual, the family, and the health care team to provide comprehensive planning to facilitate the transition to adulthood. A variety of functional disability scales, such as the Barthel Index, have been developed for adults in general rather than for adults with a particular disability (Mahoney & Barthel, 1965). These scales measure performance in various self-care, independence, and mobility functions. There are also various health-related quality of life measures such as the SF-36 that have been used to study adults with CP (Jahnsen et al., 2003).

Physical Therapy Goals, Outcomes, and Interventions

The major goal during this period of transition is to maximize the client's capabilities to achieve optimal independence and happiness as an adult. Ideally, the medical, therapeutic, and educational goals of childhood have had this as a long-term goal in earlier intervention. Adults with CP have musculoskeletal problems and urinary complaints (Gajdosik & Cicirello, 2001). In addition, recent studies of higher mortality rates in lower functioning adults with CP from breast cancer, brain cancer, and conditions of the respiratory, circulatory and digestive systems indicate a need for vigilance in detection and treatment (Strauss et al., 2000). In many situations, professionals, the client, and the family are dealing with external environmental forces that make it difficult for a person to overcome disabilities.

Reducing Primary Impairment and Preventing Secondary Impairment

Although there is a focus on participation, therapists must still be cognizant of the impact of impairment on activity. Adults with CP must deal with the normal effects of aging in addition to their existing impairments (Overeynder & Turk, 1998). Insufficient force generation can still respond to therapy, since strength training can result in improve-

ments in walking ability (Andersson et al., 2003). Although secondary impairments such as contracture may appear to be static, there can still be deterioration, so monitoring and treatment, if necessary, should be available.

Poor endurance is the major factor in ambulatory decline in adults with CP, even in young adults (Bottos et al., 2001). Fatigue is a problem in adults with CP, particularly those with moderate motor involvement. It is associated with pain, lack of physical activity, general health problems, deterioration of physical skills, limitation in emotional and physical role function, and low life satisfaction (Jahnsen et al., 2003).

Of particular importance is the prevention of overuse syndromes, early joint degeneration, progression of contractures, osteoporosis, poor endurance, and pathologic fractures. Cervical and back pain, nerve entrapment syndromes, or tendinitis can occur as a result of excessive and repetitive physical stresses (Gajdosik & Cicirello, 2001). A survey of adults found 67% reported one or more areas of pain with lower extremity and back pain most common; 53% had pain of moderate to severe intensity (Engel et al., 1999). Such injuries should be treated with orthopedic therapy techniques, as they would be in the general population. Preventive treatment to minimize the long-term effects of the neuromuscular dysfunction may be beneficial. This may include exercises that minimize excessive joint stress, use of additional mobility aids or devices, orthoses, or surgery. Changes to the adult's environment may be necessary to maintain optimal independence (Overeynder & Turk, 1998). Adults with CP need to find a balance between alleviating unnecessary energy costs in ADL and taking part in programs that stress the body systems to achieve optimal health and fitness (Damiano, 2003).

Adherence to exercise programs of stretching, strengthening, and aerobics may be poor, so encouragement and opportunities should be provided. Poor exercise habits may start during adolescence, if not earlier, and can result in a cycle of poor fitness and endurance (Gajdosik & Cicirello, 2001). Because access to therapy programs may decrease in the adult years, therapists should encourage the use of community and recreational programs that provide the necessary opportunities to promote fitness and activity.

Life Skills

Ongoing involvement in fitness and recreational activities should be planned. This will provide social opportunities, as well as maintain or improve cardiovascular fitness, weight control, and integrity of joints and muscles; help prevent osteoporosis; and generally promote the optimal health that contributes to independent functioning. Fitness clubs, swimming, wheelchair aerobics, and adapted sports are options. Fernandez and Pitetti (1993) found that the values for physical work capacity of ambulatory adults with CP were significantly lower than normal values and concluded that adults with CP would possibly experience fatigue before completing a normal workday. However, physical work capacity and work-related activities improved with training.

Technology is providing adults with CP many options that were not previously available. These include computers for communication, artificial speech devices, environmental control devices, and mobility devices. For more information, see Chapter 33.

Society is becoming more conscious of the rights and needs of the individuals with limitations. This recognition has a positive effect on environmental factors that influence participation. Human rights legislation now exists to accommodate people with disabilities and to prevent discrimination in areas such as employment, accessibility, the legal system, and education. Government programs and services are available to people with disabilities. Theaters, restaurants, libraries, museums, government buildings, educational facilities, shopping areas, parks, campground facilities, and parking lots are becoming accessible, where possible, through the provision of ramps, appropriate washroom facilities, and other modifications. Air and rail travel is also becoming more accessible to people with special mobility needs, and there are now travel organizations that cater to people with disabilities. In some situations, funding for assistive devices, living allowances, and housing and tax exemptions help prevent undue hardship. Therapists should be aware of the facilities available to the disabled and the political policies and issues concerning the disabled and should advocate their advancement.

Transition Planning

Ideally, the planning for the transition to adult services and lifestyle takes place before the actual major life changes. Areas to be addressed when planning for the transition include the following: vocational training or postsecondary educational placement, which may range from higher education to supported work models; living arrangements (independent, with family, institutional, or other supportive care); leisure and recreation (religious groups, community programs, and recreational centers); personal management, including birth control; social skills; and household management. The continuation of professional health services must also be dealt with. This includes the provision of therapy when needed, medical consultation, primary care, and equipment needs and maintenance. Financial planning and education about budgeting, taxes, other governmental benefits, advocacy and legal services, guardianship, conservatorship, wills, and trusts must be addressed (Hallum, 1995).

RESEARCH NEEDS

Research in CP is needed continually. The selection of treatment for an individual with CP requires predictive information about the effects of interventions, if any, on the body function and structure, activity, and participation throughout the life span, yet even descriptive information is limited. To take a simple example, to decide whether orthoses are appropriate for a particular child, we should know whether the impairment of hypoextensibility is preventable by orthoses, as some studies suggest (Tardieu et al., 1988) and, if so, under what conditions. Furthermore, we should know if force generation capability is changed with orthotic wear, how force output changes with growth, and what conditions favor successful long-term outcomes. The multisystem impairments of poor selective control of muscles, poor anticipatory regulation of movement, and decreased ability to learn unique movements have received little attention.

We need better information about the relationships between the domains of activity and participation and their relation to overall health and well-being/quality of life. There is also a need for research that predicts long-term outcomes, and finally, there is a need for specific and sensitive measurements of activity and participation for persons with CP.

GLOBAL ISSUES

The treatment of children with CP varies throughout the world. Physical therapists use many different approaches and combinations of approaches, depending on the facilities available, the child's and the family's needs, the therapist's training and background, and the diversity of client values, beliefs, and priorities. Many of the treatments and technologies discussed are practiced in developed countries, where services, although variable in their extent, quality, and funding, are available and accessible. However, much of the world's population lives in underserved areas, particularly in developing nations or in remote areas of developed nations. Often, many of the principles and equipment ideas developed elsewhere can be adapted to the various situations (Werner, 1987). Using indigenous materials to fabricate effective and affordable equipment, recycling used equipment, and training local personnel or fostering exchange programs can help provide resources to underserviced areas.

It is important to be sensitive to local customs, cultures, and environmental situations when adapting programs for different settings. Often, the direct application of a certain method is impractical or inappropriate because of economic, geographic, or cultural differences. There is an increasing emphasis on community-based rehabilitation, which promotes interventions that are practical and functional for the particular settings, lifestyles, and cultures.

▌PROFESSIONAL ISSUES

Therapists who care for children with CP must realize that the work can be physically demanding. They must practice appropriate lifting and handling precautions and should maintain a suitable level of fitness if they are actively treating patients. Working with children and their families can also be emotionally stressful. Therapists may often be challenged with ethical issues, unrealistic expectations and demands, limited resources, and the pressures of dealing with families during the grieving period and other times of crisis. Therapists need to concentrate on what is positive and realize that they cannot control all the variables in their patients' conditions and lives. Professionals must acknowledge their own needs and reactions and feel comfortable in seeking assistance and support from others.

This chapter concludes with two case studies that illustrate some of the management principles discussed in this chapter.

CASE STUDIES

NOELLE

Noelle was born at 32 weeks of gestation. She weighed 1600 g and had an Apgar score of 8 at 5 minutes. She was admitted to the neonatal intensive care unit and was discharged home to live with her parents and 10 siblings approximately 6 weeks later. She was a healthy, happy baby who was very sociable and interested in play, but her parents felt that she was always behind in her gross motor skills. A developmental pediatrician assessed her at 17 months of age (15 months corrected). At that time, Noelle could roll in both directions and sit unsupported briefly but was not attempting to crawl. She had increased tone in her lower extremities. A diagnosis was made of asymmetric quadriplegic CP with more lower extremity involvement than upper extremity involvement. She was referred to the local children's treatment center for physiotherapy. She was not seen for a few months because

of a waiting list, so her parents enlisted help privately. When seen at the children's center at 23 months of age, a physical therapist, occupational therapist, and speech language pathologist assessed her development. Nicole began attending therapy sessions every 2 to 3 weeks and had a home program. She also attended a gross motor group. Physiotherapy goals included improving postural control through activities that encouraged righting reactions and weight bearing through the extremities, maintenance of ROM, and accomplishment of gross motor skills such as moving in and out of sitting, and reaching activities that would facilitate play. AFOs and supportive equipment for standing were prescribed. By 3 years of age Noelle progressed to walking with a walker using small, adducted steps for short distances and was able to ride an adapted tricycle.

When Noelle was 5 years of age, she had decreased ROM and spasticity in her lower extremities. These impairments were impacting on her gross motor skills and other ADL, such as dressing. She had "scissoring" of her legs and leaned forward when walking. Her parents investigated the possibility of dorsal rhizotomy surgery through research reports and discussions with professionals but decided not to pursue this option. Serial casting to improve ankle ROM resulted in minimal improvements. She proceeded to have orthopedic surgery consisting of bilateral hip flexor (psoas) and adductor releases and medial hamstring and heelcord lengthenings. She had problems with pain management postoperatively and required intensive therapy to maintain ROM and to strengthen muscles after the surgery.

Throughout her school years Noelle received physical therapy services at the children's center, through a school health program, and privately. Communication among therapists was important to provide optimal care. Therapy programs continued to address the impairments of muscle extensibility, strength, and spasticity and focus on activities such as self-care and mobility. She rode an adapted bicycle at home and at her family's summer cottage. This activity provided recreational and fitness opportunities. Treatment strategies included treadmill use, exercises such as step-ups, electrical stimulation to tibialis anterior and quadriceps muscles, and functional activities. She received BtA injections and serial casting for her gastrocnemius muscles and also received injections in her hamstrings. She continued to use hinged AFOs and a posterior walker for ambulating but also had a manual wheelchair for long distances. Noelle also received occupational and speech and language therapy. A computer was used for written communication.

At 12 years of age Noelle functions at Level III on the Gross Motor Function Classification System. She is in grade 7, and her therapist has addressed issues such as participation in physical education, safe and functional mobility, and use of adaptive equipment. She continues to ambulate with a posterior walker but uses a wheelchair for long distances. Noelle's goal is to not use her wheelchair too much so she can maintain her walking abilities. She had a gait assessment to document the characteristics of her walking and to gather information that could contribute to treatment decision making. Specific concerns were difficulty with foot clearance during swing phase and the risk of left hip subluxation over time. Step length was reduced compared to normative data, as were single-limb stance time, cadence, and velocity in barefoot trials. She had inappropriate swing phase activity of her rectus femoris bilaterally and delayed and reduced activity of the tibialis anterior muscle (midswing activity only). When her AFOs were worn, gait symmetry, step length, and velocity were improved but were still different from normative values. With the AFOs, a heel strike was observed, her foot remained plantigrade during stance, and heel rise occurred appropriately at terminal swing with AFOs. Inadequate knee flexion remained a problem with a toe drag in swing bilaterally. Spasticity of the rectus femoris muscle with inappropriate swing phase activity coupled with reduced hip flexor strength could account for the loss of appropriate knee flexion. It was decided that Noelle would receive BtA injections to the rectus femoris muscles and commence a program of strengthening exercises at an afterschool clinic so that therapy would not interfere with school.

A subsequent gait analysis was performed 1 month later to assess changes in gait. She had slight improvement in peak knee flexion bilaterally after Bta injections. There was still a consistent toe drag during initial swing phase on the left but moderate improvement on the right. In order to maintain strength and extensibility to allow participation in gross motor activities, an ongoing program of gym exercises and biking was begun. Prolonged low load stretch through positioning at home or through her positioning during sleep was also implemented. As strengthening of her hip abductors and spinal extensors and knee musculature continues to be important, appropriate exercises have been incorporated into her school gym program.

Noelle participates in many family, school, and community activities such as weddings, horseback riding, swimming programs, and gymnastics. She attends her local school and travels there with her friends on the school bus. She is able to ambulate at school with her walker but may have to consider power mobility when she enters secondary school. She has a service dog, Whisper, who can open doors, pick up objects, bark for help, move things out of the way, pull her coat off, and act as a support to help Noelle stand up.

NICOLE

Nicole was born at 29.5 weeks of gestation after placental separation. She weighed 1300 g and had an Apgar score of 8 at 5 minutes. She remained in the neonatal intensive care unit for 6 weeks and then went home to live with her parents and 3-year-old sister. Nicole was followed up at the screening clinic for high-risk infants where her parents were given suggestions for handling and positioning due to extensor positioning of her neck and trunk and hypertonicity in her legs. At 5 months of age corrected for prematurity, the diagnosis of CP was made on the basis of hypertonicity in her extremities, affecting lower extremities more than upper; strong, persisting primitive reflex activity; and delayed development of head and trunk control. An ultrasound scan at this time showed the left lateral ventricle to be slightly enlarged and the right lateral ventricle to be at the upper limits of normal in size. The periventricular brain parenchyma appeared normal.

Services from a developmental pediatrician, a social worker, an orthopedic surgeon, a physical therapist, and later an occupational therapist were coordinated at the local children's treatment center. Nicole attended physical therapy sessions weekly. Positions that reduced the influence of her extensor posturing were used to encourage active control of movements and functional skills such as play. Bivalved casts were introduced early to maintain muscle extensibility and provide optimal alignment of her feet when she was working on standing activities. The casts also reduced some of the extensor posturing in her lower extremities, resulting in improvements in her alignment in sitting and standing and improvements in the quality of functional activities in these positions. These casts were later replaced with solid AFOs when growth slowed down, and Nicole was eager to wear regular shoes. Customized seating and a standing frame gave her a variety of positions in which she could interact with others, use her hands, and experience weight bearing with her body optimally aligned.

At 2 years of age, the impairments of adductor hypoextensibility and spasticity were treated surgically with bilateral adductor muscle releases and anterior obturator neurectomies. This gave her more functional motion at her hips and put her hip joints in an optimal position for acetabular development to hopefully avoid the potential secondary impairment of hip subluxation or dislocation.

During her preschool years, Nicole attended an integrated child care program. Her therapists visited the center regularly to discuss Nicole's abilities, programs, handling, and equipment. When Nicole was 5 years old, she was progressing slowly in her gross and fine motor skills. Spasticity in her lower extremities resulted in activity limitations in sitting, standing, transitional movements, fine motor activities, and ADL and limited her potential for independence. Ambulation was not functional, but she could move about independently in a power chair and had some limited mobility in a manual wheelchair. The prominence of spasticity and the generally good force-generating capabilities of her musculature prompted the decision to have a selective dorsal rhizotomy. After the rhizotomy, her lower extremity spasticity was greatly reduced and she was weak. Nicole participated in an intensive physical therapy and occupational therapy program for the next year (Figs. 21-9 and 21-10).

A Gross Motor Function Measure evaluation was done preoperatively and 1 year after the surgery. Her scores improved from 88% to 96% in lying and rolling; from 78% to 87% in sitting; from 19% to 57% in crawling and kneeling; from 13% to 32% in standing (with AFOs); and from 7% to 10% in walking, running, and jumping (with AFOs). She had been able to walk 10 m at 0.04 m/s preoperatively but could walk 30 m at 0.15 m/s at her 1-year follow-up. Although these findings indicated that there had been improvements in her gait, the distance and velocity of her walking were still much below age norms and did not result in functional ambulation. She had improved isolated muscle control, which was demonstrated by improved active ROM. Her passive ROM improved, particularly in motions involving the hamstring muscles. Nicole continued to have decreased muscle force production, particularly in her hip and knee extensor muscles (Fig. 21-11).

Nicole improved her self-care skills such as dressing her lower extremities, because she was able to move one leg independently of the other. She was able to function better in activities such as opening jars, printing, and propelling her manual wheelchair. The improvements were believed to be the result of better trunk control and co-contraction in the shoulder musculature rather than of changes in the intrinsic muscles of her hands, motor planning, or visuoperceptual skills—areas that continued to be problems for Nicole.

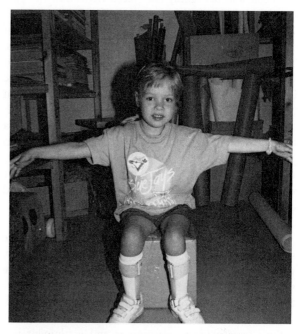

◆ **Figure 21-10**   Nicole, wearing ankle-foot orthoses, doing exercises at school.

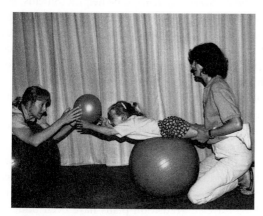

◆ **Figure 21-9**   Mother and therapist with Nicole, encouraging force generation of trunk and hip extensors.

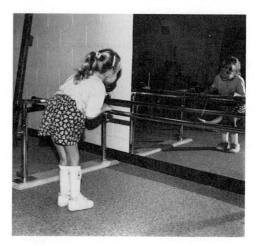

◆ **Figure 21-11**   Despite many improvements after posterior rhizotomy, Nicole still shows diminished force-generating ability in hip and knee muscles.

During her adolescence Nicole has used a power wheelchair in school and community settings but used a manual wheelchair at home. Her inability to support her own weight as she grew taller and heavier has been problematic. She is unable to assist any more than minimally with transfers, although the support of her AFOs does assist in her ability to bear weight. Nicole is able to direct her own care with regard to morning showering and dressing routines with help from personal care workers or her mother.

Nicole and her family have faced environmental barriers. Their home is in the country and had a gravel driveway. The house was not wheelchair accessible because of stairs into the house, stairs inside, and narrow doorways. Thick carpeting made manual wheelchair pushing and walker maneuvering difficult. As a result of prognostic information from all health care professionals involved in her care, Nicole's family built an addition to their home, which made the downstairs fully accessible. There is a large deck that allows Nicole to go outdoors on her own and provides a second entrance to the house. The driveway was paved to enable her to reach her taxi or bus. She needs one-person assistance with transfers, toileting, and dressing, but showers and washes her own hair independently using a commode chair in a wheel-in shower.

Nicole has attended her neighborhood public grade schools and high schools. Her parents worked closely with teachers and administrators of the schools. In grade school a bus with a wheelchair lift provided transportation so she could travel to school with her peers. In high school she used a taxi adapted for wheelchair use. Renovations were made to washrooms and equipment was provided, but obstacles such as inaccessible playground equipment limited participation in some activities. Educational assistants were available to help Nicole with self-care and schoolwork. Her above average knowledge of computer functions allowed her to develop efficient ways of completing her school assignments and communicating with others.

Nicole's therapists provided services at school. Active treatment was provided initially, but during her secondary school years input consisted of consultation and monitoring of her progress. The responsibility for therapeutic exercises has been gradually transferred to Nicole and her family with an emphasis on stretching to maintain ROM. Both have found the motivation to continue difficult, though the assistance of her morning personal support worker was helpful for a short period. She has also attended groups focusing on life skills at the local children's treatment center. These programs provided opportunities for the teens to discuss items of mutual interest.

Nicole has been involved with horseback riding, swimming programs, boating, weddings, camps, birthday parties, and adapted games. Recently she was involved in the Able Sail program, which uses boats designed for sailors with disabilities. Like many teenagers, she uses a chat line on the Internet, and she speaks with her friends on the telephone. Outings with friends, however, are few and far between because of accessibility factors, such as the lack of public wheelchair transportation in their township community. Although obstacles are becoming less common as society becomes more aware of accommodations necessary for people with disabilities, barriers such as buildings without ramps, inadequate parking, and inaccessible washrooms still exist. Impromptu activities, which are so much a part of the teenage lifestyle, are much more difficult when a wheelchair is used for mobility. Her family has found that this can contribute to social isolation and make her friendships harder, though not impossible, to establish and maintain.

Nicole's family has worked with medical, educational, governmental, and community organizations to gain access to services and programs that provide her with normal childhood experiences and minimize disabilities. Nicole's parents are very active advocates for changes that will provide people with disabilities with a full range of life's opportunities. They believe parents must be prepared to play central, responsible leadership roles within groups and agencies that can assist in these endeavors. Nicole's parents have found regular family conferences to discuss short- and long-term goals invaluable in helping to facilitate effective family and school involvement in therapy programs. Such conferences help empower parents and allow them to become effective advocates for their children. They also reinforce the philosophy of teamwork and partnership with the therapists and the treatment center.

Nicole's parents have found Craig Shield's book *Strategies: A Practical Guide for Dealing with Professionals and Human Service Systems* to be helpful (Shields, 1987). They believe that home visits designed to deal with issues of daily routines, integrate treatment goals into home life, and involve all family members are important. Nicole's parents believe that it is particularly important not to withhold any information from the family. They also emphasize the need for feedback and encouragement to the family, especially to the primary caregiver.

Nicole has now graduated from high school (Fig. 21-12) and is preparing to enter college. She has maintained an A average throughout the past 4 years and plans to work in the travel industry as an agent specializing in wheelchair travel and as an organizer of attendant support for the disabled traveler. Transition plans have been under way for the past 18 months and have involved school, college, and treatment center personnel and her physiotherapist. These meetings, held every 4 to 6 months, have proved

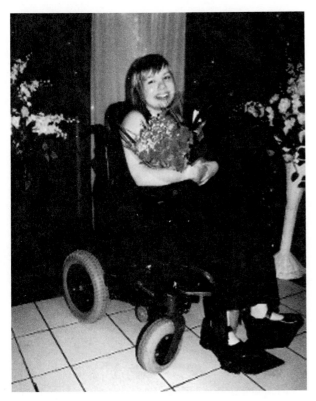

◆ **Figure 21-12**   Nicole's high school graduation!

very helpful in identifying the challenges, in bringing the immediate and long-term goals into focus, and in keeping everyone on Nicole's "team" involved and informed.

ACKNOWLEDGMENTS

Acknowledgments are extended to the Child Development Centre of the Hotel Dieu Hospital, Kingston, Ontario, and to the families of Noelle and Nicole for their support of and contributions to the case studies.

REFERENCES

Ade-Hall, RA, & Moore, AP. Botulinum toxin type A in the treatment of lower limb spasticity in cerebral palsy (Cochrane Review). In The Cochrane Library, Issue 3. Oxford: Update Software, 2003.

Albright, AL, Barry MJ, Shafron, DH, & Ferson, SS. Intrathecal baclofen for generalized dystonia. Developmental Medicine and Child Neurology, 43:652–657, 2001.

American Academy of Pediatrics. Transporting children with special health care needs (RE9852). Pediatrics, 104:998–992, 1999.

Anderson, JP, Snow, B, Dorey, FJ, & Kabo, JM. Efficacy of soft splints in reducing severe knee-flexion contractures. Developmental Medicine and Child Neurology, 30:502–508, 1988.

Andersson, C, Grooten W, Hellsten, M, Kaping, K, & Mattsson, E. Adults with cerebral palsy: Walking ability after progressive strength training. Developmental Medicine and Child Neurology, 45:220–228, 2003.

Atkinson, S, & Stanley, FJ. Spastic diplegia among children of low and normal birthweight. Developmental Medicine and Child Neurology, 25:693–708, 1983.

Atwater, SW. Should the normal motor developmental sequence be used as a theoretical model in pediatric physical therapy? In Lister, MJ (Ed.). Contemporary Management of Motor Control Problems: Proceedings of the II STEP Conference. Alexandria, VA: Foundation for Physical Therapy, 1991, pp. 89–93.

Avery, LM, Russell, DJ, Raina, PS, Walter, SD, & Rosenbaum, PL. Rasch analysis of the Gross Motor Function Measure: Validating the assumptions of the Rasch model to create an interval-level measure. Archives of Physical Medicine and Rehabilitation, 84:697–705, 2003.

Barry, MJ. Physical therapy interventions for patients with movement disorders due to cerebral palsy. Journal of Child Neurology, 11(suppl 1):S51–S60, 1996.

Bates, G, & Willson, SW. Clinical experience of constraint induced movement therapy in adolescents with hemiplegic cerebral palsy—A day camp model. Developmental Medicine and Child Neurology, 45:357–360, 2003.

Bartlett, DJ, & Palisano, RJ. Physical therapist's perceptions of factors influencing the acquisition of motor abilities of children with cerebral palsy: Implications for clinical reasoning. Physical Therapy, 82:237–248, 2002.

Barwood, S, Baillieu, CE, Boyd, RN, Brereton, K, Nattrass, GR, & Graham HK. Analgesic effects of botulinum toxin A: A randomised palcebo trial. Developmental Medicine and Child Neurology, 42:116–121, 2000.

Batshaw, MI, & Perret, YM. Children with Disabilities: A Medical Primer, 3rd ed. Toronto: Paul H. Brookes, 1992.

Baumann, JU, & Zumstein, M. Experience with a plastic ankle-foot orthosis for prevention of muscle contracture. Developmental Medicine and Child Neurology, 27:83, 1985.

Berbrayer, D, & Ashby, P. Reciprocal inhibition in cerebral palsy. Neurology, 40:653–656, 1990.

Berger, W, Quintern, J, & Deitz, V. Pathophysiology of gait in children with cerebral palsy. Electroencephalography and Clinical Neurophysiology, 53:538–548, 1982.

Blanche, EI. Doing with—not doing to: Play and the child with cerebral palsy. In Parham, LD, & Fazio, LS (Eds.). Play in Occupational Therapy for Children. St. Louis: Mosby, 1997, pp. 202–218.

Blasco, PA, Management of drooling: 10 years after the Consortium on Drooling. Developmental Medicine and Child Neurology, 44:778–781, 2002.

Bleck, EE. Locomotor prognosis in cerebral palsy. Developmental Medicine and Child Neurology, 17:18–25, 1975.

Bleck, EE. Orthopedic Management in Cerebral Palsy. Philadelphia: JB Lippincott, 1987.

Bly, L. A historical and current view of the basis of NDT. Pediatric Physical Therapy, 3:131–135, 1991.

Bobath, K, & Bobath, B. The neuro-developmental treatment. In Scrutton, D (Ed.). Management of the Motor Disorders of Children with Cerebral Palsy. Clinics in Developmental Medicine (No. 90). Philadelphia: JB Lippincott, 1984, pp. 6–18.

Bohannon, RW. Is the measurement of muscle strength appropriate in patients with brain lesions? Physical Therapy, 69:225–236, 1989.

Bohannon, RW, & Smith, MB. Interrater reliability of a modified Ashworth scale of muscle spasticity. Physical Therapy, 67:206–207, 1987.

Bolek, J, Moeller-Mansour, L, & Sabet, A. Enhancing proper sitting position using a new sEMG protocol, the "minimax" procedure, with

Boolean logic. Applied Psychophysiology and Biofeedback, 26:9–16, 2001.

Booth, CM, Cortina-Borja, MJF & Theologis, TN. Collagen accumulation in muscles of children with cerebral palsy and correlation with severity of spasticity. Developmental Medicine and Child Neurology 43:314–320, 2001.

Bottos, M, Benedetti, MG, Salucci P, Gasparroni V, & Giannini, S. Botulinum toxin with and without casting in ambulant children with spastic diplegia: A clinical and functional assessment. Developmental Medicine and Child Neurology, 45:758–762, 2003.

Bower, E, & McLellan, DL. Effect of increased exposure to physiotherapy on skill acquisition of children with cerebral palsy. Developmental Medicine and Child Neurology, 34:25–39, 1992.

Bower, E, McLellan, DL, Arney, J, & Campbell, MJ. A randomised controlled trial of different intensities of physiotherapy and different goal-setting procedures in 44 children with cerebral palsy. Developmental Medicine and Child Neurology, 38:226–237, 1996.

Bower, E, Mitchell D, Burnett, M, Campbell, MJ, & McLellan, DL. Randomised controlled trial of physiotherapy in 56 children with cerebral palsy followed for 18 months. Developmental Medicine and Child Neurology, 43:4–15, 2001.

Boyce, W, Gowland, C, Rosenbaum, P, Lane, M, Plews, N, Goldsmith, C, Russell, D, Wright, V, Zdrobov, S, & Harding, D. The Gross Motor Performance Measure: Validity and responsiveness of a measure of quality of movement. Physical Therapy, 75:603–613, 1995.

Boyd, R, & Graham, HK. Objective clinical measures in the use of Botulinum toxin A in the management of cerebral palsy. European Journal of Neurology, 6(suppl 4):23–36, 1999.

Boyd, R, & Hays RM. Current evidence for the use of botulinum toxin A in the management of children with cerebral palsy: A systematic review. European Journal of Neurology, 8(suppl 5):S1–S20, 2001.

Brooks-Scott, S. Mobilization for the Neurologically Involved Child. Tucson, AZ: Therapy Skill Builders, 1995.

Brouwer, B, & Ashby, P. Altered corticospinal projections to lower limb motoneurons in subjects with cerebral palsy. Brain, 114:1395–1407, 1991.

Brouwer, B, Wheeldon, RK, Stradiotto-Parker, N, & Allum, J. Reflex excitability and isometric force production in cerebral palsy: The effect of serial casting. Developmental Medicine and Child Neurology, 40:168–175, 1998.

Brouwer B, Davidson LK & Olney SJ. Serial casting in idiopathic toe-walkers and children with spastic cerebral palsy. Journal of Pediatric Orthopedics, 20:221–225, 2000.

Brown, DA, Effgen, SK & Palisano, RJ. Performance following ability-focused physical therapy intervention in individuals with severely limited physical and cognitive abilities. Physical Therapy, 78:934–950, 1998.

Bruininks, RH. Bruininks-Oseretsky Test of Motor Proficiency: Examiner's Manual. Circle Pines, MN: American Guidance Service, 1978.

Burns, YR, O'Callaghan, M, & Tudehope, DI. Early identification of cerebral palsy in high risk infants. Australian Paediatric Journal, 25:215–219, 1989.

Butler, C. Augmentative mobility: Why do it? Physical Medicine and Rehabilitation Clinics of North America, 2(4):801–815, 1991.

Butler, C & Campbell S. Evidence of the effects of intrathecal baclofen for spastic and dystonic cerebral palsy. AACPCM treatment outcomes committee review panel. Developmental Medicine and Child Neurology, 42:634–645, 2000.

Butler, C, & Darrah, J. Effects of neurodevelopmental treatment (NDT) for cerebral palsy. Developmental Medicine and Child Neurology, 43:772–784, 2001.

Campbell, SK. Introduction to the special issue. Pediatric Physical Therapy, 2:123–125, 1990.

Campbell, SK. Therapy programs for children that last a lifetime. Physical and Occupational Therapy in Pediatrics, 17(1):1–15, 1997.

Campbell, SK, & Barbosa, V. The challenge of early diagnosis. Developmental Medicine and Child Neurology, 45(suppl 94):5–6, 2003.

Campbell, SK, & Hedeker, D. Validity of the Test of Infant Motor Performance for discriminating among infants with varying risk for poor motor outcome. Journal of Pediatrics 139:546–551, 2001

Campbell, SK, Wilhelm, IJ, & Slaton, DS. Anthropometric characteristics of young children with cerebral palsy. Pediatric Physical Therapy, 1:105–108, 1989.

Carlson, WE, Vaughan, CL, Damiano, DL, & Abel, MF. Orthotic management of gait in spastic diplegia. American Journal of Physical Medicine and Rehabilitation, 76:219–224, 1997.

Carmick, J. Managing equinus in a child with cerebral palsy: Merits of hinged ankle-foot orthosis. Developmental Medicine and Child Neurology, 37:1006–1019, 1995a.

Carmick, J. Managing equinus in children with cerebral palsy: Electrical stimulation to strengthen the triceps surae muscle. Developmental Medicine and Child Neurology, 37:965–975, 1995b.

Chad, KE, Bailey, DA, McKay, HA, Zello, GA, & Snyder, RE. The effect of a weight-bearing physical activity program on bone mineral content and estimated volumetric density in children with spastic cerebral palsy. Journal of Pediatrics, 135:115–117, 1999.

Chandler, LS, Andrew, MS, & Swanson, MW. Movement Assessment of Infants: A Manual. Rolling Bay, WA: Infant Movement Research, 1980.

Cioni, G, Ferrari, F, Einspieler, C, Paolicelli, PB, Barbani, T & Prechtl, HFR. Comparison between observation of spontaneous movements and neurologic examination in preterm infants. Journal of Pediatirics, 130:704–711, 1997.

Colborne, GR, Wright FV, & Naumann, S. Feedback of triceps surae EMG in gait of children with cerebral palsy: A controlled study. Archives of Physical Medicine and Rehabilitation, 75:40–45, 1994.

Corry, IS, Cosgrove, AP, Duffy, CM, McNeill, S, Taylor, TC, & Graham, HK. Botulinum toxin A compared with stretching casts in the treatment of spastic equinus: A randomised prospective trial. Journal of Pediatric Orthopedics, 18:304–311, 1998.

Coster, WJ, Deeney, TA, Haltiwanger, JT, & Haley, SM. School Function Assessment. Boston University, 1994.

Craft, MJ, Lakin, JA, Oppliger, RA, Clancy, GM, & Vanderlinden, DW. Siblings as change agents for promoting the functional status of children with cerebral palsy. Developmental Medicine and Child Neurology, 32:1049–1057, 1990.

Crenshaw, S, Herzog, R, Castagno, P, Richards, J, Millar, F, Michaloski, G, & Moran, E. The efficacy of tone-reducing features in orthotics on the gait of children with spastic diplegic cerebral palsy. Journal of Pediatric Orthopedics, 20:210–216, 2000.

Crothers, B, & Paine, RS. The Natural History of Cerebral Palsy, 2nd ed. Philadelphia: JB Lippincott, 1988.

Dali, C, Hansen, FJ, Pedersen, SA, Skov, L, Hilden, J, Bjornskov, I, Strandberg, C, Jette, C, Ulla, H, Herbst, G, & Ulla, L. Threshold electrical stimulation (TES) in ambulant children with CP: A randomized double-blind placebo-controlled clinical trial. Developmental Medicine and Child Neurology, 44:364–369, 2002.

Damiano, DL. Strength, endurance, and fitness in cerebral palsy. Developmental Medicine and Child Neurology, 45(suppl 94):8–10, 2003.

Damiano, DL, Dodd, K, & Taylor, NF. Should we be testing and training muscle strength in cerebral palsy. Developmental Medicine and Child Neurology, 44:68–72, 2002.

Damiano, DL, Quinlivan, ME, Owens, BF, Payne, P, Nelson, KC, & Abel, MF. What does the Ashworth scale really measure and are instrumented measures more valid and precise? Developmental Medicine and Child Neurology, 44:112–118, 2002.

Darrah, J, & Bartlett, D. Dynamic systems theory and management of children with cerebral palsy: Unresolved issues. Infants and Young Children, 8:52–59, 1995.

Darrah, J, Watkins, B, Chen, L, Bonin, C. Effects of conductive education intervention for children with a diagnosis of cerebral palsy: An AACPDM evidence report. Available at http://www.aacpdm.org./ index Accessed July 26, 2005.

Darrah, J, Wessel, J, Nearingburg, P, & O'Connor, M. Evaluation of a community fitness program for adolescents with cerebral palsy. Pediatric Physical Therapy, 11:18–23, 1999.

Delp, SL. What causes increased muscle stiffness in cerebral palsy? Muscle & Nerve, 27:131–132, 2003.

DeLuca, PA. The musculoskeletal management of children with cerebral palsy. Pediatric Clinics of North America, 43:1135–1150, 1996.

Desloovere, K, Molenaers, G, Jonkers, I, De Cat, J, De Borre, L, Nijs, J, Eyssen, M, Pawels, P, & DeCock, P. A randomized study of combined botulinum toxin type A and casting in the ambulant child with cerebral palsy using objective outcome measures. European Journal of Neurology, 8:75–87, 2001.

Dodd, K, Taylor, N, & Damiano, DL. Systemic review of strengthening for individuals with cerebral palsy. Archives of Physical Medicine and Rehabilitation, 83:1157–1164, 2002.

Dowding, VM, & Barry, C. Cerebral palsy: Social class differences in prevalence in relation to birthweight and severity of disability. Journal of Epidemiology and Community Health, 44:191–195, 1990.

Dubowitz, L, Finnie, N, Hyde, SA, Scott, OM, & Vrbova, G. Improvement of muscle performance by chronic stimulation in children with cerebral palsy. Lancet, 1(8585):587–588, 1988.

Edebol-Tysk, K. Epidemiology of spastic tetraplegic cerebral palsy in Sweden. I: Impairments and disabilities. Neuropediatrics, 20:41–45, 1989.

Edgar, TS. Oral pharmocotherapy of childhood movement disorders. Journal of Child Neurology. 18(Suppl 1):S40–S49, 2003.

Ehrsson, HH, Fagergren, E, & Forssberg, H. Differential fronto-parietal activation depending on force used in a precision grip task: An fMRI study. Journal of Neurophysiology, 85:2613–2623, 2001.

Ehrsson, HH, Kuhtz-Buschbeck, JP, & Forssberg, H. Brain regions controlling nonsynergistic versus synergistic movement of the digits: A functional magnetic resonance imaging study. Journal of Neuroscience, 22:5074–5080, 2002.

Engsberg, JR, Ross, SA, Olree, KS, & Park, TS. Ankle spasticity ad strength in children with spastic diplegia cerebral palsy. Developmental Medicine and Child Neurology, 42:42–47, 2000.

Engsberg, JR, Ross, SA, & Park, TS. Changes in ankle spasticity and strength following selective dorsal rhizotomy and physical therapy for spastic cerebral palsy. Journal of Neurosurgery, 91:727–732, 1999.

Essex, C. Hyperbaric oxygen and cerebral palsy: No proven benefit and potentially harmful. Developmental Medicine and Child Neurology, 45:213–215, 2003.

Evans, PM, Evans, SJW, & Alberman, E. Cerebral palsy: Why we must plan for survival. Archives of Disease in Childhood, 65:1329–1333, 1990.

Fehlings, D, Rang, M, Glazier, J, & Steele, C. An evaluation of Botulinum-A toxin injections to improve upper extremity in children with hemiplegia cerebral palsy. Journal of Pediatrics, 137:331–337, 2000.

Feldman, AB, Haley, SM, & Coryell, J. Concurrent and construct validity of the Pediatric Evaluation of Disability Inventory. Physical Therapy, 70:602–610, 1990.

Fernandez, JE, & Pitetti, KH. Training of ambulatory individuals with cerebral palsy. Archives of Physical Medicine and Rehabilitation, 74:468–472, 1993.

Fernhall, B, & Unnithan, VB. Physical activity, metabolic issues and assessment. Physical Medicine and Rehabilitation Clinics of North America, 13:925–947, 2002.

Ferrara, MS, Buckley, WE, McCann, BC, Limbird, TJ, Powell, JW, & Robl, R. The injury experience of a competitive athlete with a disability: Prevention implications. Medicine and Science in Sports and Exercise, 24:184–188, 1992.

Fetters, L. Measurement and treatment in cerebral palsy: An argument for a new approach. Physical Therapy, 71:244–247, 1991.

Flett, PJ, Stern, LM, Waddy, H, Connell, TM, Seeger, JD, & Gobson, SK. Botulinum toxin A versus fixed cast stretching for dynamic calf tightness in cerebral palsy. Journal of Paediatrics and Child Health, 35:71–77, 1999.

Finnie, NR. Handling the Young Cerebral Palsied Child at Home, 3rd ed. Oxford: Butterworth-Heinemann, 1997.

Friden, J, & Lieber, RL. Spastic muscle cells are shorter and stiffer than normal cells. Muscle & Nerve, 26:157–164, 2003.

Fossberg, H, Eliasson, AC, Redon-Zouitenn, C, Mercuri, E, & Dubowitz, L. Impaired grip-lift synergy in children with unilateral brain lesions. Brain, 122:1157–1168, 1999.

Fowler, EG, Nwigwe, AI, & Ho, TW. Sensitivity of the pendulum test for assessing spasticity in persons with cerebral palsy. Developmental Medicine and Child Neurology, 42:182–189, 2000.

Gage, JR, & Novacheck, TF. An update on the treatment of gait problems in cerebral palsy. Journal of Pediatric Orthopaedics, Part B, 10:265–274, 2001.

Gajdosik, CG, & Cicirello, N. Secondary conditions of the musculoskeletal system in adolescents and adults with cerebral palsy. Physical and Occupational Therapy in Pediatrics, 21:4967, 2001.

Gaudet, LM, & Smith, GN. Cerebral palsy and chorioamnionitis: The inflammatory cytokine link. Obstetrics and Gynecology Survey, 56:433–436, 2001

Geralis, E (Ed.). Children with Cerebral Palsy. Rockville, MD: Woodbine House, 1991.

Giuliani, CA. Dorsal rhizotomy for children with cerebral palsy: Support for concepts of motor control. Physical Therapy, 71:248–259, 1991.

Graham, HK, Aoki, KR, Autti-Ramo, IA, Boyd, RN, Delgado, MR, Gaebler-Spira, DJ, Gormley, ME, Guyer, BM, Heinen, F, Holton, AF, Matthews, D, Molenaers, G, Motta, F, Garcia, PJ, & Wissel, J. Recommendations for the use of botulinum toxin type A in the management of cerebral palsy. Gait and Posture, 11:67–79, 2000.

Graham, HK, & Selber, P. Musculoskeletal aspects of cerebral palsy. Journal of Bone and Joint Surgery, 85-B:157–166, 2003.

Hadden, KL, & vonBaeyer, CL. Pain in children with cerebral palsy: Common triggers and expressive behaviors. Pain, 99:281–288, 2002.

Hagberg, B, Hagberg, G, Olow, I, & vonWendt, L. The changing panorama of cerebral palsy in Sweden. V. The birth year period 1979–82. Acta Paediatrica Scandinavica, 78:283–290, 1989a.

Hagberg, B, Hagberg, G, & Zetterstrom, R. Decreasing perinatal mortality—Increase in cerebral palsy morbidity? Acta Paediatrica Scandinavica, 78:664–670, 1989b.

Hainsworth, F, Harrison, MJ, Sheldon, TA, & Roussunis, SHP. Preliminary evaluation of ankle orthoses in the management of children with cerebral palsy. Developmental Medicine and Child Neurology, 39:243–247, 1997.

Hallett, M, & Alvarez, N. Attempted rapid elbow flexion movements in patients with athetosis. Journal of Neurology, Neurosurgery and Psychiatry, 46:745–750, 1983.

Hallum, A. Disability and the transition to adulthood: Issues for the disabled child, the family, and the pediatrician. Current Problems in Pediatrics, 25:12–50, 1995.

Harris, SR. Early detection of cerebral palsy: Sensitivity and specificity of two motor assessment tools. Journal of Perinatology, 7:11–15, 1987.

Harris, SR. Early diagnosis of spastic diplegia, spastic hemiplegia, and quadriplegia. American Journal of Diseases of Children, 143:1356–1360, 1989.

Harris, SR, & Lundgren, BD. Joint mobilization for children with central nervous system disorders: Indications and precautions. Physical Therapy, 71:890–896, 1991.

Harrison, A. Spastic cerebral palsy: Possible spinal interneuronal contributions. Developmental Medicine and Child Neurology, 30:769–780, 1988.

Harryman, SE. Lower-extremity surgery for children with cerebral palsy: Physical therapy management. Physical Therapy, 72:16–24, 1992.

Healy, A, Ramsey, C, & Sexsmith, E. Postural support systems: Their fabrication and functional use. Developmental Medicine and Child Neurology, 39:706-710, 1997.

Henderson, RC, Lark, RK, Gurka, MJ, Worley, G, Fung, EB, Conaway, M, Stallings, VA, & Stevenson, RD. Bone density and metabolism in children and adolescents with moderate to severe cerebral palsy. Pediatrics, 110(1Pt 1):e5, 2002a.

Henderson, RC, Lark, RK, Kecskemethy, HH, Miller, F, Harcke, HT, & Bachrach, SJ. Bisphosponates to treat osteopenia in children with quadriplegic cerebral palsy: A randomized, placebo-controlled clinical trial. The Journal of Pediatrics, 141:644–651, 2002b.

Higgins, S. Motor skill acquisition. Physical Therapy, 71:123–139, 1991.

Holst, K, Andersen, E, Philip, J, & Henningsen, I. Antenatal and perinatal conditions correlated to handicap among 4-year-old children. American Journal of Perinatology, 6:258–267, 1989.

Horton, SV, & Taylor, DC. The use of behavior therapy and physical therapy to promote independent ambulation in a preschooler with mental retardation and cerebral palsy. Research in Developmental Disabilities, 10:363–375, 1989.

Hurvitz, EA, Leonard, C, Ayyangar, R, & Simon Nelson, V. Complementary and alternative medicine use in families of children with cerebral palsy. Developmental Medicine and Child Neurology, 45:364–370, 2003.

Jaeger, DL. Transferring and Lifting Children and Adolescents: Home Instruction Sheets. San Antonio, TX: Therapy Skill Builders, 1989.

Jaeger, L. Home Program Instruction Sheets for Infants and Young Children. San Antonio, TX: Therapy Skill Builders, 1987.

James, R. Biofeedback treatment for cerebral palsy in children and adolescents: A review. Pediatric Exercise Science, 24:198–212, 1992.

Jahnsen, R, Villien, L, Stanghelle, JK, & Holm, I. Fatigue in adults with cerebral palsy in Norway compared with the general population. Developmental Medicine and Child Neurology, 45:296–303, 2003.

Jansen, LMC, Ketalaar, M, & Vermeer, A. Parental experience of participation in physical therapy for children with physical disabilities. Developmental Medicine and Child Neurology, 45:58–69, 2003.

Jones, EW, & Mulley, GP. The measurement of spasticity. In Rose, FC (Ed.). Advances in Stroke Therapy. New York: Raven Press, 1982.

Jonsdottir, J, Fetters, L, & Kluzik, J. Effects of physical therapy on postural control in children with cerebral palsy. Pediatric Physical Therapy, 9:68–75, 1997.

Karumuna, JMS, & Mgone, CS. Cerebral palsy in Dar es Salaam. Central African Journal of Medicine, 36(1):8–10, 1990.

Katz, RT, & Rymer, WZ. Spastic hypertonia: Mechanisms and measurement. Archives of Physical Medicine and Rehabilitation, 70:144–155, 1989.

Ketelaar, M, Vermeer, A, Hart, H, van Petegem-van Beek, E, & Helders, PJM. Effects of a functional therapy program on motor abilities of children with cerebral palsy. Physical Therapy, 81:1534–1545, 2001.

Kibele, A. Occupational therapy's role in improving the quality of life for persons with cerebral palsy. American Journal of Occupational Therapy, 43:371–377, 1989.

Kilgour, G, McNair, P, & Stott, S. Intrarater reliability of lower limb sagittal range-of-motion measures in children with spastic cerebral diplegia. Developmental Medicine and Child Neurology, 45:391–399, 2003.

King, G, Law, M, King, S, & Rosenbaum, P. Parents' and service providers' perceptions of the family-centredness of children's rehabilitation services. Physical and Occupational Therapy in Pediatrics, 18:21–40, 1998.

King, G, Law, M, King, S, Rosenbaum, P, Kertoy, MK, & Young, N. A conceptual model of the factors affecting the recreation and leisure participation of children with disabilities. Physical and Occupational Therapy in Pediatrics, 23:63–90, 2003.

Kitchen, WH, Ford, GW, Rickards, AL, Lissenden, JV, & Ryan, MM. Children of birth weight <1000 g: Changing outcome between ages 2 and 5 years. Journal of Pediatrics, 110:283–288, 1987.

Kluzik, J, Fetters, L, & Coryell, J. Quantification of control: A preliminary study of effects of neurodevelopmental treatment on reaching in children with spastic cerebral palsy. Physical Therapy, 70:65–78, 1990.

Knox, V, & Evans AL. Evaluation of the functional effects of a course of Bobath therapy in children with cerebral palsy: A preliminary study. Developmental Medicine and Child Neurology, 44:447–460, 2002.

Knutsson, LM, & Clark, DE. Orthotic devices for ambulation in children with cerebral palsy and myelomeningocele. Physical Therapy, 71:947–960, 1991.

Knutsson, LM, & Martensson, A. Dynamic motor capacity in spastic paresis and its relation to prime mover dysfunction, spastic reflexes and antagonist co-activation. Scandinavian Journal of Rehabilitation Medicine, 12:93–106, 1980.

Kolobe, THA. Working with families of children with disabilities. Pediatric Physical Therapy, 4:57–63, 1992.

Koman, LA, Mooney, JF, Smith, BP, Goodman, A, & Mulvaney, T. Management of spasticity in cerebral palsy with botulinum-A toxin: A report of a preliminary randomized, double-blind trial. Journal of Pediatric Orthopaedics, 14:299–303, 1994.

Kotagal, S, Gibbons, VP, & Stith, JA. Sleep abnormalities in patients with severe cerebral palsy. Developmental Medicine and Child Neurology, 36:304–311, 1994.

Kramer, JF, Ashton, B, & Brander R. Training of head control in the sitting and semi-prone positions. Child Care and Health Development, 18:365–376, 1992.

Langley, MB. A developmental approach to the use of toys for facilitation of environmental control. Physical and Occupational Therapy in Pediatrics, 10:69–91, 1990.

Law, M, Baptiste, S, McColl, MA, Opzoomer, A, Polatajko, H, & Pollock, N. The Canadian Occupational Performance Measure: An outcome measure for occupational therapy. Canadian Journal of Occupational Therapy, 57:82–87, 1990.

Lee, EH, Goh, JCH, & Bose, K. Value of gait analysis in the assessment of surgery in cerebral palsy. Archives of Physical Medicine and Rehabilitation, 73:642–646, 1992.

Leonard, CT, Hirschfeld, H, Moritani, T, & Forssberg, H. Myotatic reflex development in normal children and children with cerebral palsy. Experimental Neurology, 111:379–382, 1991.

Leonard, CT, Moritani, T, Hirschfeld, H, & Forssberg, H. Deficits in reciprocal inhibition of children with cerebral palsy as revealed by H reflex testing. Developmental Medicine and Child Neurology, 32:974–984, 1990.

Leopando, MT, Moussavi, Z, Holbrow, J, Chernick, V, Pasterkamp, H, & Rempel, G. Effect of a Soft Boston Orthosis on pulmonary mechanics in severe cerebral palsy. Pediatric Pulmonology, 28:53–58, 1999.

Lepage, C, Noreau, L, & Bernard, P. Association between characteristics of locomotion and accomplishment of life habits in children with cerebral palsy. Physical Therapy, 78:458–469, 1998.

Lesny, I, Nachtmann, M, Stehlik, A, Tomankova, A, & Zajidkova, J. Disorders of memory of motor sequences in cerebral palsied children. Brain and Development, 12:339–341, 1990.

Lespargot, A, Renaudin, E, Khouri, N, & Robert, M. Extensibility of hip adductors in children with cerebral palsy. Developmental Medicine and Child Neurology, 36:980–988, 1994.

LeVeau, BF, & Bernhardt, DB. Developmental biomechanics: Effects of forces on the growth, development and maintenance of the human body. Physical Therapy, 64:1874–1882, 1984.

Lin, JP, Brown, JK, & Brotherstone, R. Assessment of spasticity in hemiplegic cerebral palsy. II. Distal lower-limb reflex excitability and function. Developmental Medicine and Child Neurology, 36:290–303, 1994.

Lin, PP, & Henderson, RC. Bone mineralization in the affected extremities of children with spastic hemiplegia. Developmental Medicine and Child Neurology, 38:782–786, 1996.

Little, WJ. On the influence of abnormal parturition, difficult labours, premature births and asphyxia neonatorum on the mental and physical condition of the child, especially in relation to deformities. Transactions of the Obstetrical Society of London 1862. Cerebral Palsy Bulletin, 1:5–34, 1958.

Logan, L, Byers-Hinkley, K, & Ciccone, CD. Anterior versus posterior walkers: A gait analysis study. Developmental Medicine and Child Neurology, 32:1044–1048, 1990.

Mackey AH, Lobb GL, Walt, SE, & Stott, NS. Reliability and validity of the Observational Gait Scale in children with spastic diplegia. Developmental Medicine and Child Neurology, 45:4–11, 2003.

MacKinnon, JR, Noh, S, Lariviere, J, MacPhail, A, Allan, DE, & Laliberte, D. A study of therapeutic effects of horseback riding for children with cerebral palsy. Physical and Occupational Therapy in Pediatrics, 15:17–34, 1995.

MacLennan, A. A template for defining a causal relation between acute intrapartum events and cerebral palsy: International consensus statement. British Medical Journal, 319:1054–1059, 1999.

Mahoney, FI, & Barthel, DW. Functional evaluation: The Barthel Index. Maryland Medical Journal, 14:61–65, 1965.

Massagli, TL. Spasticity and its management in children. Physical Medicine and Rehabilitation Clinics of North America, 2:867–889, 1991.

McCarthy, ML, Silberstein, CE, Atkins, EA, Harryman, SE, Sponseller, PD, & Hadley-Miller, NA. Comparing reliability and validity of pediatric instruments for measuring health and well-being of children with spastic cerebral palsy. Developmental Medicine and Child Neurology, 44:468–476, 2002.

McDonald, CM. Selective dorsal rhizotomy: A critical review. Physical Medicine and Rehabilitation Clinics of North America, 2:891–915, 1991.

McDowell, BC, Hewitt, V, Nurse, A, Weston, T, & Baker, R. The variability of goniometric measurements in ambulatory children with spastic cerebral palsy. Gait and Posture, 12:114–121, 2000.

McLaughlin, JF, Bjornson, KF, Temkin, N, Steinbeck P, Wright, V, Reiner, A, Roberts, T, Drake, J, O'Donnell, M, Rosenbaum, P, Barber, J, & Ferrel, A. Selective dorsal rhizotomy: Meta-analysis of three randomized controlled trial. Developmental Medicine and Child Neurology, 44:17–25, 2002.

Menkes, JH. Textbook of Child Neurology, 4th ed. Philadelphia: Lea & Febiger, 1990.

Metaxiotis, D, Accles, W, Siebel, A, & Doederlein, L. Hip deformities in walking patients with cerebral palsy. Gait and Posture, 11:86–91, 2000.

Miedaner, JA, & Renander, J. The effectiveness of classroom passive stretching programs for increasing or maintaining passive range of motion in non-ambulatory children: An evaluation of frequency. Physical and Occupational Therapy in Pediatrics, 7:35–43, 1987.

Milo-Manson, G, Rosenbaum, P, & Steele, C. Alternative therapies: Prevalence and pattern of use in pediatric rehabilitation. Developmental Medicine and Child Neurology, 39(suppl 75):19, 1997.

Missiuna, C, & Pollock, N. Play deprivation in children with physical disabilities: The roles of the occupational therapist in preventing secondary disability. American Journal of Occupational Therapy, 45:882–888, 1991.

Molteni, B, Oleari, G, Fedrizzi, E, & Bracchi, M. Relation between CT patterns, clinical findings and etiology in children born at term, affected by congenital hemiparesis. Neuropediatrics, 18:75–80, 1987.

Morris, C. A review of the efficacy of lower-limb orthoses used for cerebral palsy. Developmental Medicine and Child Neurology, 44:205–211, 2002.

Morrison, JM, & Ursprung, AW. Children's attitudes toward people with disabilities: A review of the literature. Journal of Rehabilitation, 53:45–49, 1987.

Mossberg, KA, Linton, KA, & Friske, K. Ankle-foot orthoses: Effect on energy expenditure of gait in spastic diplegic children. Archives of Physical Medicine and Rehabilitation, 71:490–494, 1990.

Msall, ME, Buck, GM, Rogers, BT, Merke, D, Catanzaro, NL, & Zorn, WA. Risk factors for major neurodevelopmental impairments and need for special education resources in extremely premature infants. Journal of Pediatrics, 119:606–614, 1991.

Msall, ME, Roseberg, S, DiGuadio, KM, Braun, SL, Duffy, L, & Granger, CV. Pilot test for the WeeFIM for children with motor impairments (Abstract). Developmental Medicine and Child Neurology, 32(9, suppl 62):41, 1990.

Murney, ME, & Campbell, SK. The ecological relevance of the Test of Motor Performance elicited scale items. Physical Therapy, 78:479–489, 1998.

Murphy, KP, Molnar, GE, & Lankansky, BA. Employment and social issues in adults with cerebral palsy. Archives of Physical Medicine and Rehabilitation, 81:807–811, 2000.

Nashner, L, Shumway-Cooke, A, & Marin, O. Stance posture control in select groups of children with cerebral palsy: Deficits in sensory organization and muscular coordination. Experimental Brain Research, 49:393–409, 1983.

Nelson, KB. The epidemiology of cerebral palsy in term infants. Mental retardation and Developmental Disabilities Research Reviews, 8:146–150, 2002.

Nelson, KB, & Ellenberg, J. Antecedents of cerebral palsy: multivariate analysis of risk. New England Journal of Medicine, 315:81–86, 1986.

Nicholson, JH, Morton, RE, & Attfield, S. Assessment of upper-limb function and movement in children with cerebral palsy wearing Lycra garments. Developmental Medicine and Child Neurology, 43:384–391, 2001.

Nottidge, VD, & Okogbo, ME. Cerebral palsy in Ibadan, Nigeria. Developmental Medicine and Child Neurology, 33:241–245, 1991.

Nwaobi, OM, & Smith, PD. Effect of adaptive seating on pulmonary function of children with cerebral palsy. Developmental Medicine and Child Neurology, 28:351–354, 1986.

O'Dwyer, NJ, Neilson, PD, & Nash, J. Mechanisms of muscle growth related to muscle contracture in cerebral palsy. Developmental Medicine and Child Neurology, 31:543–552, 1989.

O'Dwyer, N, Neilson, P, & Nash, J. Reduction of spasticity in cerebral palsy using feedback of the tonic stretch reflex: A controlled study. Developmental Medicine and Child Neurology, 36:770–786, 1994.

Olney, SJ, Costigan, PA, & Hedden, DM. Mechanical energy patterns in gait of cerebral palsied children. Physical Therapy, 67:1348–1354, 1987.

Olney, SJ, MacPhail, HEA, Hedden, DM, & Boyce, WF. Work and power in hemiplegic cerebral palsy gait. Physical Therapy, 70:431–438, 1990.

Ounpuu, S, Bell, KJ, Davis, RB, & DeLuca, PA. An evaluation of the posterior leaf spring orthosis using joint kinematics and kinetics. Journal of Pediatric Orthopedics, 16:378–384, 1996.

Ounpuu, S, Davis, RB, & De Luca, PA. Joint kinetics: Methods, interpretation and treatment decision-making in children with cerebral palsy and myelomeningocele. Gait and Posture, 4:62–78, 1996.

O'Shea, TM. Cerebral palsy in very preterm infants: new epidemiological insights. Mental Retardation and Developmental Disabilities Research Review, 8:135–145, 2002.

O'Shea, TM, Preisser, JS, Klinepeter, KL, & Dillard, RG. Trends in mortality and cerebral palsy in a geographically based cohort of very low birthweight neonates born between 1982 to 1994. Pediatrics, 101:642–647, 1998.

Overeynder, JC, & Turk, MA. Cerebral palsy and aging: A framework for promoting the health of older persons with cerebral palsy. Topics in Geriatric Rehabilitation, 13:19–24, 1998.

Palisano, R. Research on the effectiveness of neurodevelopmental treatment. Pediatric Physical Therapy, 3:143–148, 1991.

Palisano, R. Validity of goal attainment scaling in infants with motor delays. Physical Therapy, 73:651–660, 1993.

Palisano, R, Kolobe, T, & Haley, S. Validity of the Peabody Developmental Gross Motor Scale as an evaluative measure of infants receiving physical therapy. Physical Therapy, 75:939–951, 1995.

Palisano, R, Rosenbaum, P, Walter, S, Russell, D, Wood, E, & Galuppi, B. Development and reliability of a system to classify gross motor function in children with cerebral palsy. Developmental Medicine and Child Neurology, 39:214–223, 1997.

Papile, L, Burstein, J, Burstein, R, & Koffler, H. Incidence and evolution of subependymal and intraventricular hemorrhage: A study of infants with birthweight of less than 1500 gms. Journal of Pediatrics, 92:529–534, 1978.

Parker, DF, Carriere, L, Hebestreit, H, & Bar-Or, O. Anaerobic endurance and peak muscle power in children with spastic cerebral palsy. American Journal of Diseases of Children, 146:1069–1073, 1992.

Patla, AE, Winter, DA, Frank, JS, Walt, JS, & Prasad, S. Identification of age-related changes in the balance control system. Proceedings of the APTA Forum on Balance. Nashville, TN: American Physical Therapy Association, 1989.

Perry, J, Hoffer, M, Antonelli, D, Plut, J, Lewis, G, & Greenberg, R. Electromyography before and after surgery for hip deformity in children with cerebral palsy. Journal of Bone and Joint Surgery (American), 58:201–208, 1976.

Pharoah, POD, Cooke, T, Cooke, RWI, & Rosenbloom, L. Birthweight specific trends in cerebral palsy. Archives of Disease in Childhood, 65:602–606, 1990.

Pharoah, POD, Cooke, T, Rosenbloom, L, & Cooke, RWI. Trends in birth prevalence of cerebral palsy. Archives of Disease in Childhood, 62:379–384, 1987.

Piggot, J, Paterson, J & Hocking, C. Participation in home therapy programs for children with cerebral palsy: A compelling challenge. Qualitative Health Research, 12:1112–1129, 2002.

Pirpiris, M, Wilkinson, AJ, Rodda, J, Hguyen, TC, Baker, RJ, Nattrass, GR, & Graham, HK. Walking speed in children and young adults with neuromuscular disease: Comparison between two assessment methods. Journal of Pediatric Orthopedics, 23:302–307, 2003.

Piper, MC, & Darrah, J. Motor Assessment of the Developing Infant. Philadelphia: WB Saunders, 1994.

Plioplys, AV, Lewis, S, & Kasnicka, I. Pulmonary vest therapy in pediatric long-term care. Journal of the American Medical Directors Association, 3:318–321, 2002.

Poole, JL. Application of motor learning principles in occupational therapy. American Journal of Occupational Therapy, 45:531–537, 1991.

Powell, TH, & Ogle, PA. Brothers and Sisters—A Special Part of Exceptional Families. Baltimore: Paul H. Brookes, 1985.

Price, R, Bjornson, KF, Lehmann, JF, McLaughlin, JF, & Hays, RM. Quantitative measurement of spasticity in children with cerebral palsy. Developmental Medicine and Child Neurology, 33:585–595, 1991.

Rang, M. Cerebral palsy. In Morrissy, RT (Ed.). Lovell and Winter's Paediatric Orthopedics, 3rd ed. Philadelphia: JB Lippincott, 1990, pp. 465–506.

Reilly, S, & Skuse, D. Characteristics and management of feeding problems of young children with cerebral palsy. Developmental Medicine and Child Neurology, 34:379–388, 1992.

Richards, CL, Malouin, F, & Dumas, F. Effects of a single session of prolonged stretch on muscle activations during gait in spastic cerebral palsy. Scandinavian Journal of Rehabilitation Medicine, 23:103–111, 1991.

Ricks, NR, & Eilert, RE. Effects of inhibitory casts and orthoses on bony alignment of foot and ankle during weight-bearing in children with spasticity. Developmental Medicine and Child Neurology, 35:11–16, 1993.

Roijen, LE, Postema, K, & Kuppevelt, VH. Development of bladder control in children and adolescents with cerebral palsy. Developmental Medicine and Child Neurology, 43:103–107, 2001.

Romanini, L, Villani, C, Meloni, C, & Calvisi, V. Histological and morphological aspects of muscle in infantile cerebral palsy. Italian Journal of Orthopaedics and Traumatology, 15:87–93, 1989.

Rose, J, Gamble, JG, Burgos, A, Medeiros, J, & Haskell, WL. Energy expenditure index of walking for normal children and for children with cerebral palsy. Developmental Medicine and Child Neurology, 32:333–340, 1990.

Rose, J, Medeiros, JM, & Parker, R. Energy cost index as an estimate of energy expenditure of cerebral-palsied children during assisted ambulation. Developmental Medicine and Child Neurology, 27:485–490, 1985.

Rosenbaum, P, King, S, Law, M, King, G, & Evans, J. Family-centred service: A conceptual framework and research review. Physical Therapy and Occupational Therapy in Pediatrics, 18:1–20, 1998.

Rosenbaum, PL, Walter, SD, Hanna, SE, Palisano, RJ, Russell, DJ, Raina, P, Wood, E, Bartlett, DJ, & Galuppi, BE. Development and reliabiltity of a system to classify gross motor function in children with cerebral palsy. Journal of the American Medical Association, 288:1357–1363, 2002.

Rosenbaum, PL. Cerebral palsy: What parents and doctors want to know. British Medical Journal, 326(7396):970–974, 2003.

Ross, SA, & Engsberg, JR. Relation between spasticity and strength in individuals with spastic diplegic cerebral palsy. Developmental Medicine and Child Neurology, 44:148–157, 2002.

Russell, D, Rosenbaum, P, Cadman, D, Gowland, C, Hardy, S, & Jarvis, S. The Gross Motor Function Measure: A means to evaluate the effects of physical therapy. Developmental Medicine and Child Neurology, 31:341–352, 1989.

Samson, JF, Sie, LTL, de Groot, L. Muscle power development in preterm infants with periventricular flaring or leukomalacia in relation to outcome at 18 months. Developmental Medicine and Child Neurology, 44:734–740, 2002.

Samson-Fang, L, Fung, E, Satlings, VA, Conaway, M, Worley, G, Rosenbaum, P, Calvert, R, O'Donnell, M, Henderson, RC, Chumlea, WC, Liptak, GS, & Stevenson, RD. Relationship of nutritional status to health and societal participation in children with cerebral palsy. Journal of Pediatrics, *141*:637–643, 2002.

Samson-Fang, L, Butler, C, & O'Donnell, M. Effects of gastrostomy feeding in children with cerebral palsy, an AACPDM evidence report. Developmental Medicine and Child Neurology, *45*:415–426, 2003.

Schanzenbacher, KE. Diagnostic problems in pediatrics. In Pratt, PN, & Allen, AS (Eds.). Occupational Therapy for Children. Toronto: Mosby, 1989, p. 97.

Scherzer, AL, & Tscharnuter, I. Early Diagnosis and Therapy in Cerebral Palsy: A Primer on Infant Developmental Problems, 2nd ed. New York: Marcel Dekker, 1990.

Schwartz, L, Engel, JM, & Jensen, MP. Pain in persons with cerebral palsy. Archives of Physical Medicine and Rehabilitation. *80*:1243–1246, 1999.

Schindl MR, Forstner, C, Kern, J, & Hesse S. Treadmill training with partial body weight support in nonambulatory patients with cerebral palsy. Archives of Physical Medicine and Rehabiltation, *81*:301–316, 2000.

Senft, KE, Pueschel, SM, Robison, NA, & Kiessling, LS. Level of function of young adults with cerebral palsy. Physical and Occupational Therapy in Pediatrics, *10*:19–25, 1990.

Shepherd, RB. Training motor control and optimizing motor learning. In Shepherd, RB (Ed.). Physiotherapy in Paediatrics, 3rd ed. Oxford: Butterworth-Heinemann, 1995.

Shields, CV. Strategies: A Practical Guide for Dealing with Professionals and Human Service Systems. Richmond Hill, Ontario: Human Services Press, 1987.

Shumway-Cook, A, & Woollacott, M. Motor Control: Theory and Practical Applications, 2nd ed. Baltimore: Lippincott, Williams & Wilkins, 1995.

Sobsey, D, & Doe, T. Patterns of sexual abuse and assault. Sexuality and Disability, *9*:243–259, 1991.

Sommerfelt, K, Markestad, T, Berg, K, & Saetesda, I. Therapeutic electrical stimulation in cerebral palsy: A randomized, controlled, crossover trial. Developmental Medicine and Child Neurology, *43*:609–613, 2001.

Stanger, M, & Bertoti, D (Eds.). An overview of electrical stimulation for the pediatric population. Pediatric Physical Therapy, *9*:95–143, 1997.

Stern, L, & Steidle, K. Pediatric Strengthening Program Reproducible Exercises. Tucson, AZ: Therapy Skill Builders, 1994.

Sternisha, C, Cays, M, & Campbell, L. Stress responses in families with handicapped children: An annotated bibliography. Physical and Occupational Therapy in Pediatrics, *12*:89–103, 1992.

Strauss, D, Cable, W, & Shavelle, R. Causes of excess mortality in cerebral palsy. Developmental Medicine and Child Neurology, *41*:580–585, 1999.

Strauss, D, & Shavelle, R. Life expectancy of adults with cerebral palsy. Developmental Medicine and Child Neurology, *40*:369–375, 1998.

Stuberg, WA. Considerations related to weight-bearing programs in children with developmental disabilities. Physical Therapy, *72*:35–40, 1992.

Subramanian, J, Vaughan, CL, Peter, JC, & Arens, LJ. Gait before and 10 years after rhizotomy in children with cerebral palsy spasticity. Journal of Neurosurgery, *88*:1014–1019, 1998.

Surman, G, Newdick, H, & Johnson, A. Cerebral palsy rates among low-birthweight infants fell in the 1990s. Developmental Medicine and Child Neurology *45*:456–462, 2003.

Sutherland, DH, Olshen, R, Cooper, L, & Woo, SY. The development of mature gait. Journal of Bone and Joint Surgery (American), *62*:336–353, 1980.

Tardieu, C, Huet de la Tour, E, Bret, MD, & Tardieu, G. Muscle hypo-extensibility in children with cerebral palsy: I. Clinical and experimental observations. Archives of Physical Medicine and Rehabilitation, *63*:97–102, 1982.

Tardieu, C, Lespargot, A, Tabary, C, & Bret, MD. For how long must the soleus muscle be stretched each day to prevent contracture? Developmental Medicine and Child Neurology, *30*:3–10, 1988.

Tardieu, G, Tardieu, C, Colbeau-Justin, P, & Lespargot, A. Muscle hypoextensibility in children with cerebral palsy: II. Therapeutic implications. Archives of Physical Medicine and Rehabilitation, *63*:103–107, 1982.

Thelen, DG, Anderson, FC, & Delp, SL. Generating dynamic simulations of movement using computed muscle control. Journal of Biomechanics, *36*:321–328, 2003.

Thomas, SS, Buckon, CE, Phillips, DS, Aiona, MD, & Sussman, MD. Interobserver reliability for the gross motor performance measure: preliminary results. Developmental Medicine and Child Neurology, *43*:97–102, 2001.

Toner, LV, Cook, K, & Elder, GCB. Improved ankle function in children with cerebral palsy after computer assisted motor learning. Developmental Medicine and Child Neurology, *40*:829–835, 1998.

Torfs, CP, van den Berg, BJ, & Oechsli, FW. Prenatal and perinatal factors in the etiology of cerebral palsy. Journal of Pediatrics, *116*:615–619, 1990.

Trahan, J & Malouin F. Intermittent intensive physiotherapy in children with cerebral palsy: a pilot study. Developmental Medicine and Child Neurology. *44*:233–239, 2002.

Tremblay, F, Malouin, F, Richards, CL, & Dumas, F. Effects of prolonged muscle stretch on reflex and voluntary muscle activations in children with spastic cerebral palsy. Scandinavian Journal of Rehabilitation Medicine, *22*:171–180, 1990.

Unnithan, VB, Dowling, JJ, Frost, G, & Bar-Or, O. Role of mechanical power estimates in the O_2 cost of walking in children with cerebral palsy. Medicine and Science in Sports and Exercise, *31*:1703–1078, 1999.

Uvebrandt, P. Hemiplegic cerebral palsy. Aetiology and outcome. Acta Paediatrica Scandinavica Supplement, *345*:5–100, 1988.

van den Berg-Emons, RJ, Van Baak, MA, Speth, L, & Saris, WH. Physical training of school children with spastic cerebral palsy: Effects on daily activity, fat mass and fitness. International Journal of Rehabilitation Research, *21*:179–194, 1998.

Van der Dussen, L, Nieuwstraten, W, Roebroeck M, & Stam, HJ. Functional level of young adults with cerebral palsy. Clinical Rehabilitation, *15*:84–91, 2001.

van der Linden, ML, Hazlewood, ME, Aitchison, AM, Hillman, SJ, & Robb, JE. Electrical stimulation of gluteus maximus in children with cerebral palsy: Effects on gait characteristics and muscle strength. Developmental Medicine and Child Neurology, *45*:385–390, 2003.

van der Weel, FR, van der Meer, ALH, & Lee, DN. Effect of task on movement control in cerebral palsy: Implications for assessment and therapy. Developmental Medicine and Child Neurology, *33*:419–426, 1991.

Vaughan, CL, Subramanian, N, & Busse, ME. Selective dorsal rhizotomy as a treatment option for children with spastic cerebral palsy. Gait & Posture, *8*:43–59, 1998.

Watt, JM, Robertson, CMT, & Grace, MGA. Early prognosis for ambulation of neonatal intensive care survivors with cerebral palsy. Developmental Medicine and Child Neurology, *31*:766–773, 1989.

Weinstein, SL, & Tharp, BR. Etiology and timing of static encephalopathies of childhood (cerebral palsy). In Stevenson, DK, & Sunshine, P (Eds.). Fetal and Neonatal Brain Injury. Toronto: BC Decker, 1989.

Werner, D. Disabled Village Children: A Guide for Community Health Workers, Rehabilitation Workers, and Families. Palo Alto, CA: Hesperian Foundation, 1987.

Westcott, SL, Paxhowes, L, & Richardson, PK. Evaluation of postural stability in children: Current theories and assessment. Physical Therapy, *77*:629–643, 1997.

Wiklund, LM, & Uvebrant, P. Hemiplegic cerebral palsy: Correlation between CT morphology and clinical findings. Developmental Medicine and Child Neurology, *33*:512–523, 1991a.

Wiklund, LM, Uvebrant, P, & Flodmark, O. Computed tomography as an adjunct in etiological analysis of hemiplegic cerebral palsy. I: Children born preterm. Neuropediatrics, *22*:50–56, 1991b.

Wilcox, C. Hey, What About Me! Activities for Disabled Children. Toronto: Doubleday Canada, 1988.

Willis, JK, Morello, A, Davie, A, Rice, JC, & Bennett, JT. Forced use treatment of childhood hemiparesis. Pediatrics, *110*:94–96, 2002.

Wilson, ER, Mirra, S, & Schwartz, JF. Congenital diencephalic and brain stem damage: Neuropathologic study of three cases. Acta Neuropathologica, *57*:70–74, 1982.

Winter, S, Autry, A, Boyle, C, & Yeargin-Allsopp, M. Trends in the prevalence of cerebral palsy in a population-based study. Pediatrics, *110*:1220–1225, 2002.

Woolcott, M, & Shumway-Cook, A. Effect of reactive balance training on postural control in children with cerebral palsy. Developmental Medicine and Child Neurology, *45*:19–20, 2003.

Wright, MJ, Yundt, B, Tancredi, AM, & Larin, H. Sleep issues in families of children with physical disabilities. Developmental Medicine and Child Neurology, *45*(Suppl 96):39, 2003.

Wright, PA, & Granat, MH. Therapeutic effects of functional electrical stimulation of the upper limb of eight children with cerebral palsy. Developmental Medicine and Child Neurology, *42*:724–727, 2000.

Yokochi, K, Aiba, K, Horie, M, Inukai, K, Fujimoto, S, Kodama, M, & Kodama, K. Magnetic resonance imaging in children with spastic diplegia: Correlation with severity of their motor and mental abnormality. Developmental Medicine and Child Neurology, *33*:18–25, 1991.

Young, RR. Spasticity: a review. Neurology, *44*(11 suppl 9):512–520, 1994.

Yude, C, Goodman, R, & McConachie, H. Peer problems of children with hemiplegia in mainstream primary schools. Journal of Child Psychology and Psychiatry, *39*:533–541, 1998.

Zwick, EB, Saraph, V, Linhart, WE, & Steinwender, G Propulsive function during gait in diplegic children: Evaluation after surgery for gait improvement. Journal of Pediatric Orthopedics (British), *10*:226–233, 2001.

BRACHIAL PLEXUS INJURY

DARL W. VANDER LINDEN
PT, PhD

ELLEN STAMOS NORTON
PT, PCS

Brachial plexus injuries (BPIs) can occur from a wide variety of traumas to the shoulder and spine. The focus of this chapter is on obstetric brachial plexus injuries (OBPIs), yet the concepts presented apply to resultant impairments, activity limitations, and participation restrictions caused by brachial plexus injury in children at any age. Physical therapists may work with infants and children with OBPI in a variety of settings, including early intervention programs, acute care hospitals, and specialty clinics. Physical therapists may also be involved with these children after neurosurgery to repair damage to nerves in the brachial plexus in infants or after orthopedic surgery to address impairments of muscle strength in toddlers and preschool age children. This chapter will discuss etiology and pathophysiology, physical therapy examination, physical therapy interventions, and medical management of children with OBPI. A case study of a child with OBPI will be presented at the end of the chapter.

ETIOLOGY AND INCIDENCE

Injury to the brachial plexus (Fig. 22-1) usually occurs during a difficult vaginal delivery. Traction on the newborn's shoulder during delivery of the head in a breech delivery can injure the cervical roots, fracture the clavicle or humerus, or sublux the shoulder. Forceful traction and rotation of the head during a vertex presentation to deliver the shoulder tends to injure the C5 and C6 roots. Associated damage to the phrenic nerve at C4 is less common, yet will cause ipsilateral hemiparesis of the diaphragm. Congenital anomalies such as cervical rib, abnormal thoracic vertebrae, or shortened scalenus anticus muscle can also cause pressure on the lower plexus (Shepherd, 1991).

Factors that may contribute to OBPI include birth weight greater than 3500 g, shoulder dystocia (difficult delivery of the shoulder), prolonged maternal labor, maternal diabetes, a sedated hypotonic infant during delivery, and breech delivery (Sjoberg et al., 1998; Bager, 1997; Wolf et al., 2000). Bager (1997) reported that the risk of

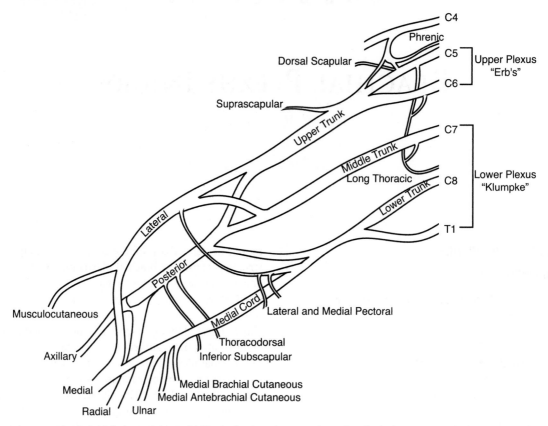

◆ **Figure 22-1** The brachial plexus. The variability in the impairments that a brachial plexus injury can cause is easily understood, because the injury can occur at any point along the nerves as they branch off the spinal cord and weave into the brachial plexus.

OBPI increased as birth weight increased and those infants with a birth weight of over 4500 g had a risk of OBPI 45 times that of infants less than 3500 g. Gilbert and colleagues (2003) found that infants from vaginal breech deliveries of normal weight (2500–3800 g) had a nine times greater risk of OBPI than those from cephalic vaginal deliveries. The risk associated with breech delivery was even five times greater than for macrosomic infants (>4000 g) with cephalic delivery. For infants delivered vaginally with cephalic presentation, high birth weight was found to be the most important risk factor (Wolf et al., 2000). In a prospective study of 62 infants with OBPI of whom 17 had permanent impairment, 16 of the 17 infants had birth weights over 3500 g and only 1 of the 17 had a birth weight less than 3500 g. Twelve of 13 infants (92%) diagnosed with OBPI at birth who weighed less than 3500 g had full recovery, but only 67% of infants (33 of 49) who weighed more than 3500 g had full recovery (Wolf et al., 2000).

In recent prospective studies, the incidence of OBPI has been reported at 1.6 per 1000 (Bager, 1997), 2.9 per 1000 live births (Dawodu et al., 1997), 4.6 per 1000 (Wolf et al., 2000), and 5.1 per 1000 (Hoeksma et al., 2004). These rates are generally higher than the incidence reported earlier by Hardy (1981) of 0.9 per 1000 and by Sjoberg and associates (1988) of 1.9 per 1000. The reasons for the increased incidence is not entirely clear, but may be due in part to more thorough examination of newborns in the recent studies, which identified a higher percentage of children with OBPI. The incidence reported in prospective studies may be greater than that reported in retrospective studies because of the number of children who were identified who exhibited complete recovery within the first 3 weeks (Hoeksma et al., 2004). Bager (1997), however, did find that the incidence increased in Sweden from 1.3 per 1000 in 1980 to 2.2 per 1000 in 1994, which was a statistically significant difference.

PATHOPHYSIOLOGY

Damage can occur at the level of the nerve rootlet attached to the spinal cord, at the anterior or posterior rootlets, or distal to where the rootlets coalesce to form the mixed nerve root that exits the vetebral canal. Roots, trunks, divisions, cords, and peripheral nerves can all suffer neurotmesis (complete rupture), axonotmesis (disruption of axons while neural sheath remains intact), or neurapraxia (temporary nerve conduction block with intact axons). Partial or complete rupture may evolve into a neuroma and a mass of fibrous tissue as disorganized neurons on the proximal end attempt to reach their distal end. Hemorrhage into the subarachnoid space leads to presence of blood in the cerebrospinal fluid, which can be diagnostic of this more serious injury (Shepherd, 1991).

Recovery is usually very limited after ruptures. Prognosis after axonotmesis is better as the neurons reconnect more successfully through the intact neural sheath. As axon regrowth proceeds at approximately 1 mm per day, the majority of recovery usually takes 4 to 6 months in the upper arm and 7 to 9 months in the lower arm. Continued recovery can occur for up to 2 years in the upper arm and 4 years in the lower arm (Gilbert, 1995). Early recovery after neurapraxia occurs as edema resolves is usually quick and complete, sometimes within days or weeks (Hoeksma et al., 2004). In children with OBPI, a combination of these types of lesions is common, which may explain the variability of return of motor function in individual muscles.

CHANGES IN BODY STRUCTURE AND FUNCTION (IMPAIRMENTS)

Injury can occur at any level of the brachial plexus, but the most common injury is to the upper roots (C5 and C6) and results in a condition referred to as Erb's palsy. Strombeck and colleagues (2000) reported that of 247 children followed for OBPI, 52% had C5-C6 involvement and an additional 34% had C5-C7 involvement. As a result of injury to the fibers from the upper roots, the child's shoulder is usually held in extension, internal rotation, and adduction; the elbow is extended; the forearm is pronated; and the wrist and fingers are flexed in the textbook "waiter's tip" position (Fig. 22-2). Paralysis of the rhomboids, levator scapulae, serratus anterior, subscapularis, deltoid, supraspinatus, infraspinatus, teres minor, biceps, brachialis, brachioradialis, supinator, and long extensors of the wrist, fingers, and thumb can be expected. Grasp is left intact, but sensory loss may be present. Elbow and finger extension is compromised if C7 is also involved.

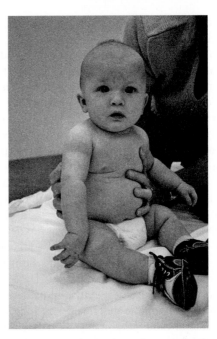

◆ **Figure 22-2**   Infant with Erb's palsy, a C5-C6 brachial plexus injury, resulting in the "waiter's tip" position of the upper extremity, which is typically observed with this type of injury.

Erb-Klumpke palsy is a combination of the injury to the upper and lower roots (C5-T1) resulting in total arm paralysis and loss of sensation. Strombeck and colleagues (2000) reported that 13% of the children with OBPI in their follow-up study had involvement of the C5-T1 roots. Involvement is usually unilateral but has been reported to be bilateral in 4% of cases (Laurent & Lee, 1994). In Erb-Klumpke palsy, the extent of the initial paralysis frequently recedes, with a total paralysis becoming limited to the upper roots. The pattern of motor loss does not always fit the classic definitions, indicating incomplete or mixed upper and lower types. Horner's syndrome, usually a result of avulsion of T1, can cause deficient sweating, recession of the eyeball, abnormal pupillary contraction, myosis, ptosis, and irises of different colors. Considered rare, Eng and colleagues (1978) reported 8 of 135 infants with BPI having Horner's syndrome.

Klumpke's palsy by definition involves only the lower roots of C7-T1. Some authors have reported the incidence of Klumpke's palsy to be 2% of all OBPI cases (Hernandez & Wendle (1990), however in a more recent review, Al-Qattan and colleagues (1995) found Klumpke's palsy in only 20 of 3508 cases of OBPI from papers they reviewed, for an incidence of only 0.6%. When pure Klumpke's palsy is present, the child's shoulder and elbow movements are not impaired, but the resting position of the forearm is typically in supination and there is paralysis of the wrist flexors and extensors and intrinsic muscles of the wrist and hand.

During the period of neural regeneration, children use abnormal muscle substitutions that are the most advantageous given the innervated muscles available (Shepherd, 1991). For example, they may use a medially rotated shoulder with forearm pronation and wrist flexion when grasping an object. They may also neglect the extremity because of sensory loss or the comparative ease with which the opposite arm and hand accomplishes a task. These patterns of neglect or substitution are reinforced with repetition. The problems that arise from these repetitive patterns include soft tissue contracture and abnormal bone growth. The contractures most likely to develop are scapular protraction; shoulder extension, adduction, and internal rotation; elbow flexion or extension; forearm pronation; and wrist and finger flexion. These will obviously vary depending on the individual pattern of paralysis. Common orthopedic abnormalities include flattening of the humeral head, abnormally short clavicle, hypoplasia of the humeral head, or abnormal glenoid fossa (Kon et al., 2004; Hoeksma et al., 2003).

Positional torticollis can develop as a result of the child being positioned away from the involved arm or may be present from the same trauma that caused the OBPI (Clark & Curtis, 1995). See Chapter 12 for more information regarding examination of and interventions for torticollis.

ACTIVITY LIMITATIONS

Activity limitations will vary greatly, depending on the extent of the initial pathology, neurologic regeneration, and residual impairments. The primary activity limitations in children with OBPI relate to an inability to reach, grasp, and perform tasks requiring bilateral manual abilities such as catching a large ball or lifting a large object. Activities of daily living that require bilateral upper extremity use will also be compromised. These activities would include donning and removing shirts and pants, tying shoes, and buttoning. Dressing aids may be necessary to achieve maximum independence. Studies have documented range of motion limitations of these children's affected arms, but no quantitative studies have reported on activity limitations such as dressing and eating, or participating restrictions.

Typical developmental activities may be compromised as a result of OBPI. Movement from prone or supine to sit may always be done from one side, thereby asymmetrically strengthening one side of the trunk or delaying balance reactions. The developmental milestone of creeping on all fours may not occur because the child may not be able to bear weight on the involved arm, and as a result

the child may scoot around in sitting or progress directly to walking at the appropriate age.

Neglect of the involved limb or even self-abusive behavior such as biting can occur because of absent or abnormal sensation. Injuries such as burns, insect bites, and abrasions may go unnoticed if sensation is severely compromised.

Shoulder pain and neuritis in adults is a complication that can interfere not only with the function of the involved arm but also with other aspects of the individual's social or vocational activities.

PHYSICAL THERAPY EXAMINATION

Children may be referred to physical therapy in the days, weeks, months, or years after the initial injury. Physical therapy examination of these children's active and passive range of motion and sensory status is key in establishing a baseline of function and abilities. Screening the developmental status of the infant or child will ensure that other pathologic conditions are not missed. In the neonate, frequent reexamination serves to document motor recovery as neural regeneration occurs. These data aid in program planning whether it be therapeutic exercise, splinting, identification of surgical candidates, or discharge from intervention.

Grossman (1996) recommended that newborns be followed at 2 weeks and at 1, 2, and 3 months of age. Infants not showing evidence of recovery may undergo an MRI (magnetic resonance imaging) scan to define the integrity of the nerve roots. Electromyography (EMG), although of little prognostic value, can determine the extent of involvement and is often recommended as a preoperative baseline. Repeated EMG testing can alert the physical therapist to muscles that are undergoing reinnervation before obvious motor changes occur. Advances in MRI, EMG, computed tomography (CT), and CT with metrizamide (CT-myelogram) have aided in preoperative diagnosis and surgical planning, yet do not replace the careful physical examination of the clinical and functional consequences of neurologic damage and neural regeneration.

RANGE OF MOTION

Physical therapy examination of the neonate with OBPI may be requested before discharge from the hospital. In any age child, range of motion measurements of the involved arm and cervical area are performed. All movements should be performed with great care because the child's joints can be unstable and the limbs may have sensory loss. Baseline range of motion data are essential for future identification of secondary contractures that could be avoided with appropriate intervention and to judge the effectiveness of interventions.

MUSCLE STRENGTH AND MOTOR FUNCTION

In the infant, the physical therapist can observe limb movement or palpate muscle contractions when testing a variety of reactions and reflexes such as visual tracking, neck righting, the Moro reflex, the Galant reflex, or the hand-placing reaction. Arm and head movement can be observed during wakeful play periods as a child tries to bring the hand to the mouth or reach for a toy. Care should be taken to document whether movements are with gravity eliminated or against gravity. Asymmetry of abdominal and thoracic movement may indicate phrenic nerve paralysis. A muscle grading system, called the Active Movement Scale, has been developed specifically for children with OBPI to capture subtle but significant changes in active movement of the arm (Table 22-1) (Clarke & Curtis, 1995). This assessment tool has been shown to have adequate reliability to accurately measure motor function of the upper extremity in infants younger than 1 year of age (Curtis et al., 2002). Curtis and colleagues (2002) also provide a review of other measures of impairment that have been used for children with OBPI including the British Medical Research Council (BMRC) system of manual muscle testing and the modified BMRC that uses a 4-point scale (M0–M3) to measure muscle activity.

Older children can be examined using standard manual muscle tests and dynamometers, which can provide objective measures of muscle and grasp strength. Patterns of movement, abnormal substitutions, and posturing of the arm as a result of muscle imbalance and sensory loss should also be documented. Mallet's classification of upper extremity function (Fig. 22-3) as described by Gilbert (1993) can be used for older children and has been shown to be reliable when used with children with OBPI (Bae et al., 2003).

Any spasticity identified during the examination would suggest an upper motoneuron lesion and therefore warrants further diagnostic evaluation by the child's primary physician or neurologist.

SENSATION

Examination of sensory loss in infants is not sensitive or reliable enough to document the clinical progression of neural regeneration. Attempts should be made, however, to identify areas on the involved extremity that may have compromised sensation. Narakas (1987) has developed the Sensory Grading System for children with BPI. A grade of S0 is no reaction to painful or other stimuli; S1 is reaction to painful stimuli, none to touch; S2 is reaction to touch, not to light touch; and S3 is apparently normal sensation. Sensory loss does not necessarily correspond to the extent of motor involvement (Eng et al., 1978); therefore, care should be taken not to ignore this component of the examination in children with milder involvement.

As neural regeneration proceeds, sensory loss may change to hyperesthesia before achieving normal sensation (Narakas, 1987). Infants or older children may experience pain or discomfort in reaction to sensory stimulation and simple touch. This change should be documented and may indicate progression of regeneration. More definitive sensory testing to a variety of stimuli such as heat, cold, light touch, and two-point discrimination is possible in older children, and specific areas of sensory loss can be mapped. Sensation may take as long as 2 years to recover.

ACTIVITY AND PARTICIPATION

Developmental tests of gross and fine motor performance can be used to establish and track any delays caused by

TABLE 22-1	Hospital for Sick Children Muscle Grading System—Active Movement Scale*

OBSERVATION	MUSCLE GRADE
Gravity Eliminated	
No contraction	0
Contraction, no motion	1
Motion ≤½ range	2
Motion >½ range	3
Full motion	4
Against Gravity	
Motion ≤½ range	5
Motion >½ range	6
Full motion	7

*Full active range of motion with gravity eliminated (muscle grade 4) must be achieved before active range against gravity is scored (muscle grades 5 to 7).
From Clarke, HM, & Curtis, GC. An approach to obstetrical brachial plexus injuries. Hand Clinics, 11(4):567, November 1995.

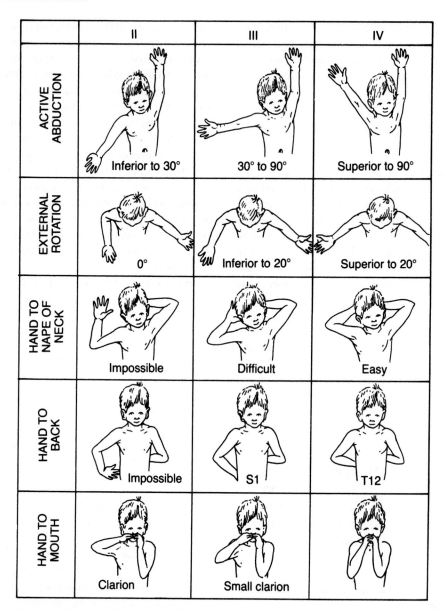

◆ **Figure 22-3** Mallet's classification of function in obstetric brachial plexus palsy. Grade 0 (not shown) is no movement in the desired plane, and grade V (not shown) is full movement. *(From Gilbert, A. Obstetrical brachial plexus palsy. In Tubiana, R [Ed.], The Hand, Vol. 4. Philadelphia: WB Saunders, 1993, p. 579.)*

the upper extremity impairment in infants and toddlers. Older children who can follow verbal commands or copy body positions can be assessed in their abilities to perform functional activities such as bringing the hand to mouth for eating, bringing the hand to the head for brushing hair, and holding a variety of tools (e.g., toothbrush) sufficiently for their intended use. Videotaping of these activities is helpful.

Although several measures have been developed to assess impairments such as muscle strength and sensation as previously described, no specific measure of activity or participation for use with children who have OBPI could be found in the existing literature. Some authors have reported anecdotal information about activity limitations and participation such as difficulty with activities of daily living (ADLs), carrying a tray at school for lunch, or playing a recorder (Sundholm et al., 1998; Sjoberg et al., 1988).

ELECTROMYOGRAPHY

Findings from diagnostic EMG have been used to attempt to assess the extent and severity of the lesion, but may not correlate well with findings upon surgical exploration (Laurent & Lee, 1994; Hearle & Gilbert, 2004). Reinnervation after microsurgery can be identified by EMG immediately following surgery or in the following weeks and months, before clinical signs of motor return are present. This information may change a therapist's goals and intervention, and it may change a patient's prognosis significantly.

NATURAL HISTORY AND PROGNOSIS

The natural history and recovery of OBPI have been difficult to determine because few studies have followed children over a long period of time and authors have primarily used outcome measures of impairment, but not of activity and participation. In addition, many different measures of impairment have been used, but none consistently in a majority of studies, which makes it difficult to determine even the natural history of impairments in children with OBPI. To further complicate matters, neurosurgery as well as secondary orthopedic surgery may be performed on a subset of children studied, and outcomes of these children are often included in data of children who have not had surgical intervention.

A recovery rate of 80% to over 90% has been reported (Hardy, 1981; Michelow et al., 1994; Clark & Curtis, 1995; Gordon et al., 1973), and therefore, the prognosis has been perceived as quite favorable for the majority of infants with OBPI. More recent studies, however, have reported recovery rates of 73% (Hoeksma et al., 2000), 66% (Noetzel et al., 2001), 66% (Hoeksma et al., 2004), and 69% (DiTaranto et al., 2004). In a systematic review designed to better describe the natural history of OBPI, Pondaag and colleagues (2004) reviewed the literature on OBPI outcomes. The inclusion criteria for articles to be used in their systematic review included (1) prospective design, (2) all children with OBPI from a demographic area be followed, (3) minimum of 3-year follow-up with less than 10% lost to follow-up, and (4) outcome well defined with reproducible scoring system and no surgical intervention. Of 103 articles that were identified in the literature, none met all four or even three of the four criteria defined for the systematic review, but 27 of the 103 met two criteria. As a result of their findings, Pondaag and colleagues (2004) concluded that the excellent prognosis often cited for OBPI was not based on sound scientific evidence. It should be noted that the recently published studies by Hoeskma and colleagues (2004) and DiTaranto and colleagues (2004) were not included in the systematic review.

Estimates of spontaneous recovery from OBPI are difficult to establish because many children have neurapraxic lesions that resolve within a few days or weeks, and therefore, these children are not included in many follow-up studies. Hoeksma and colleagues (2004) found, in fact, that 34% of infants (19 of 56) diagnosed with OBPI at birth had full recovery by 3 weeks of age. They also found that 32% (18 of 56) had "late" recovery by 1 year of age, but 19 of 56 (34%) did not have full recovery of muscle strength when assessed at a mean age of 3 years. The authors indicated that if the criteria for a "good" outcome as described by Michelow and colleagues (1994) of "more than 1/2 of normal range of shoulder and elbow motion" had been used with their cohort of 56 children, 93% would have had a "good" outcome (Hoeksma et al., 2004). DiTaranto and colleagues (2004) followed 91 infants in Argentina who did not have access to neurosurgical intervention for at least 2 years. They reported that although 69% had full recovery, 18% of infants had minimal recovery and 13% had global OBPI with flaccid and insensate arms.

In an earlier study, Eng and colleagues (1978) classified 135 children with incomplete recovery from OBPI into three groups based on residual deformities. The mildly affected group (70%) had minimal scapular winging, shoulder abduction of 90° or more, minimal limitation of shoulder rotation and forearm supination, normal hand function, and normal sweat and sensation. These patients were not considered to have functional problems, yet some of their involved limbs were shorter and smaller with some shoulder instability. The moderately affected group (22%) had moderate winging of the scapula, shoulder abduction less than 90° with substitution of the trapezius and serratus anterior in shoulder elevation, flexion contracture of the elbow, no forearm supination, weak wrist and finger extensors, good hand intrinsic muscles, and some loss of sweat and sensation. The third group (8%) was considered to have severe impairment with marked winging of the scapula, total loss of scapulohumeral rhythm, shoulder abduction less than 45°, severe elbow flexion contracture, no forearm supination, poor or no hand function, and severe loss of sweat and sensation resulting in a small atrophic extremity, or agnosia in the arm.

The differences reported in the natural history and outcomes for children with OBPI make it difficult for parents and professionals to predict with any accuracy to what extent children with OBPI will recover. Unfortunately the differences reported may be due primarily to the methodology of the studies as most authors operationally define outcome measures for a specific study, report no information on the reliability or validity of their operationally defined outcome measures, and provide no information on whether the raters were blinded to any interventions that may have taken place. In addition, although more recent reports have specifically defined outcomes based upon strength of specific muscle groups (Hoeksma et al., 2000; Hoeksma et al., 2004), what is still lacking are studies that report outcomes not only of impairments, but also of activity limitations and participation restrictions in children, adolescents, and adults with OBPI.

PHYSICAL THERAPY GOALS

The ideal outcome for the neonate with OBPI is complete return of motor control and sensation with no activity limitations or participation restrictions. The physical therapy goals during the first few months after diagnosis are to support any spontaneous recovery that is occurring and to prevent secondary impairments of muscle contractures and joint injury. If it becomes evident that complete return is not occurring, outcomes and goals must be revised. Depending on the extent of impairment, full range of motion and normal strength may remain a goal in the first 2 years of life, because continued neural regeneration or restored motor control through a variety of orthopedic and neurosurgical procedures may still be possible. The majority of spontaneous recovery occurs by 9 months of age, but continued recovery may occur up to 2 years after the injury (Gilbert, 1995).

At some point between 9 and 24 months of age, it may be apparent that significant neural regeneration is no longer occurring. Goals would need to be revised for children who lose range or plateau in their recovery over several months. Even with the most diligent home program implementation, full range of motion is difficult to maintain when muscle imbalance is present. Children with OBPI continue to need monitoring of their range of motion and functional status. Every attempt should be made to continue encouraging functional bilateral activities. The desired outcomes at this time (2 years of age) would be that the child develop age-appropriate self-care skills such as dressing and grooming using either extremity and participate in age-appropriate movement activities and preschool programs. Goals would include maintaining or increasing range of motion and strength in movements critical to specific activities that the child is currently unable to perform. An example might be increasing elbow flexion motion and strength in order to pick up objects from the ground with both hands and put them on a table.

PHYSICAL THERAPY INTERVENTION

The majority of infants with birth-related BPI require only physical therapy and no surgical intervention (Laurent & Lee, 1994). A consultation before discharge from the hospital may be performed; however, an initial rest period of 7 to 10 days is required to allow for reduction of hemorrhage and edema around the traumatized nerves. During this time, no range of motion or other interventions are initiated as the involved limb is positioned gently across the abdomen. Lying on the involved limb is to be avoided.

After this initial period of immobilization, the physical therapist performs the baseline examinations described earlier in this chapter. A home program is developed for the parents that addresses all range of motion at risk for contractures, including precautions about any joints at risk for subluxation or dislocation. The physical therapist explains precautions regarding any areas of sensory loss and teaches the parents how to use positioning and therapeutic play during everyday activities to maintain range of motion and strengthen weak muscles.

ACTIVE MOVEMENT

The objective of the physical therapy program is to facilitate the highest functional outcome possible for the child, particularly in the areas of reach and grasp as they relate to meaningful, developmentally appropriate activities. As previously mentioned, children will use abnormal muscle substitutions that are the most advantageous given the innervated muscles available. The therapist intervenes in several ways, including facilitation of normal movement patterns while inhibiting substitutions during reaching and weight-bearing activities (Shepherd, 1991). This intervention should be in the context of performing concrete versus abstract tasks. For example, strengthening of the shoulder flexors could be done by asking the child to lift 10 toy people up and into a doll house (a concrete task) instead of performing 10 repetitions of shoulder flexion (an abstract task) (van der Weel et al., 1991).

Careful attention to the scapula is critical during reaching activities, because paralysis of the rhomboids and contracture of the muscles that link the humerus to the scapula interfere with the normal 6:1 humeroscapular rhythm in the first 30° of shoulder movement. The scapula can be manually stabilized as the shoulder is assisted in active flexion as the child reaches for a toy. This activity facilitates correct motor training and stretching at the same time.

A variety of opportunities should be provided for weak muscles to participate in normal movement patterns by eliminating gravity for very weak muscles, preventing substitutions, and manually guiding the extremity through movements to accomplish a task. Examples include hand to mouth; transferring objects; weight shifting on propped upper extremities in the prone position, the quadruped position, and in sitting with hands in front or back; creeping; and reaching for toys placed at a variety of angles and heights from the child. Figure 22-4, *A*, illustrates a nonfunctional position that an infant with a classic C5, C6 injury may assume. Figure 22-4, *B*, demonstrates how manually guiding the shoulder into flexion and external rotation allows the infant to experience a more normal, functional movement pattern and obtain more appropriate sensory information through an open palm. The scapula is stabilized at the same time to allow for stretching of the soft tissues connecting the scapula to the humerus. Because active shoulder external rotation and forearm supination is typically lacking in children with C5-C6 injuries, toys should be presented and the upper extremity facilitated such as to encourage these movements during therapy intervention (Shepherd, 1991).

Infants should be placed in a side-lying position on their uninvolved arm to avoid stresses on the involved arm and to free the weak arm to reach and play with toys placed in front of them. Gravity or toys held in the hand can be used as resistance as muscles gain strength. At times, the uninvolved arm may need to be gently restrained when encouraging the child to use the involved arm. Tactile stimulation or facilitation of the weak muscles with gentle joint compression in weight bearing is also helpful.

Normal posture and developmental activities may be compromised as a result of OBPI. Transitional movement into sitting may always be done from one side, and as a result, posture of the trunk may be asymmetric and balance reactions may be delayed on the involved side. To address reliance on the uninvolved side, movement into sitting and other transitional movements can be practiced from the involved side using manual guidance and facilitation as needed. When sitting is achieved, shoulder abduction can be facilitated by challenging protective reactions to the involved side. Normal bilateral upper extremity use will likely be delayed. Opportunities for the child to experience and practice two-handed activities such as holding balls or swinging can be provided. In the older child who has not experienced full return of motor function, adaptations and products to assist in ADLs and recreational activities should be made available for the child's consideration. Many products are available for performing a variety of daily tasks using only one hand, and families can be encouraged to design their own adaptations. Not every child or family wants to use these devices, and their opinions should be respected.

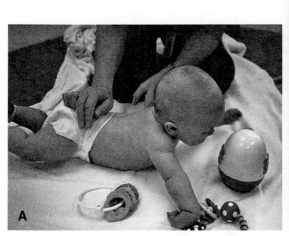
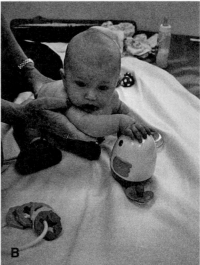

◆ **Figure 22-4**   **A**, Infant with C5-C6 brachial plexus injury trying to prop and reach. **B**, Infant assisted in reaching and grasping with manual guidance.

RANGE OF MOTION

Passive range of motion can be done in the context of normal developmental activities as described previously or during positioning as described later in this chapter. Maintaining range of motion is important as up to 65% of children with incomplete recovery of OBPI have been found to have limited range of motion at the shoulder (Hoeksma et al., 2000). Passive range of motion should never cause pain and should always be gentle. Overstretching can be harmful to joints and joint capsules that are already unstable. For example, forced supination of the elbow may compound the problem of radial head dislocation and ulnar bowing (Eng et al., 1978). Picking the child up under the axilla or by pulling on the arms is discouraged because these actions can damage the unprotected shoulder joint.

Prevention of scapulohumeral adhesions is an important goal of physical therapy intervention. Parents should be educated about the anatomy and kinesiology of the glenohumeral joint. During reach, the scapula can be stabilized or restrained to allow for stretching of the muscles that link the scapula to the humerus during the first 30° of abduction. Beyond 30°, the scapula must rotate along with humeral external rotation to avoid harmful impingement of soft tissues on the acromion process.

The use of botulinum toxin has been shown to improve active motion in muscles antagonist to those injected with the toxin (Disiato & Risina, 2001). The benefits lasted up to 6 weeks and the authors suggested that this intervention is relatively benign when compared to surgical intervention and should be studied further as an intervention to maintain ROM in children with OBPI.

SENSORY AWARENESS

Sensory loss can lead to neglect or even self-mutilation. Parents must be cautioned about the risk of injury to body areas where sensation is compromised and should watch for any signs of self-mutilation such as biting an insensate area. Enlisting the participation of the involved limb in play activities or in holding a bottle allows the child to perceive the extremity as being a purposeful part of the body. Sensory perception can be enhanced by placing objects of different textures and temperatures in the hand, playing games such as finding toys under sudsy water or in rice with the involved hand, or blindfolding the older child and having her name familiar objects placed in her hand. Range of motion can be incorporated into these activities by guiding the hand to different areas of the child's body to experience tactile stimulation. Parents themselves should be encouraged not to neglect the arm,

but to caress and play with it as usual, while holding or guiding it through patterns that must be reinforced.

POSITIONING AND SPLINTING

Placing the child's arm in optimal positions is a time-efficient way to stretch soft tissue restrictions, since this can be done during feeding, carrying, or positioning in a car seat. When sleeping, the arm can be placed toward abduction, external rotation, elbow flexion, and forearm supination on a pillow to the child's side. As the child's arm relaxes during sleep, even more range can be attempted.

Intermittent splinting of the wrist and fingers may sometimes be indicated. Wrist splints may preserve the integrity of the tendons of the fingers and wrist until motor function returns. Resting night splints can help prevent wrist and finger flexion contractures. A wrist cock-up splint maintains a neutral alignment of the wrist yet frees the fingers for play. In an attempt to prevent shoulder adduction and internal rotation contractures, a "statue of liberty" splint or an abduction splint may be used, although some have suggested that these splints may contribute to abduction contractures, hypermobility, and pathology of the glenohumeral and elbow joint (Shepherd, 1991).

Restraining splints such as air splints can be used on the uninvolved extremity to encourage use of the involved arm and hand. For example, if elbow flexion is restrained on the uninvolved side, the child would need to use his involved arm to bring a toy to his mouth or self-feed. These restraints should be used for only brief periods during the day with frustration levels monitored carefully. Some children will not tolerate them at all, particularly if it is unrealistic that the involved arm can perform functional activities with some independence.

ELECTRICAL STIMULATION

Although Eng and colleagues (1978) promoted the use of electrical stimulation for children with OBPI, and electrical stimulation may be used after neurosurgery, no reports were found that described or investigated the use of electrical stimulation for this population. Without such reports, the benefits and risks regarding the use of electrical stimulation for children with OBPI cannot be discussed.

MEDICAL MANAGEMENT

NEUROSURGERY

Neurosurgery to repair the brachial plexus has typically been reserved for the 5% to 10% of children with OBPI who do not exhibit substantial spontaneous recovery. Neurosurgical techniques used in the treatment of OBPI include nerve grafting, neuroma dissection and removal, neurolysis (decompression and removal of scar tissue), and direct end-to-end nerve anastomosis of the nerve ends. These microsurgery techniques have been used to attempt to improve function in those children with OBPI who have significant impairments and activity limitations and who are no longer exhibiting spontaneous improvement. Although some authors have reported improvement in 75% to 95% of children who have had neurosurgery (Laurent et al., 1993; Laurent & Lee, 1994; Sherburn et al., 1997; Clark et al., 1996), Strombeck and colleagues (2000) reported that for children with total arm involvement (C5-T1), children who had surgery had no significant improvements in active motion at the shoulder, elbow, or hand when compared to a group of children who did not have surgery. They did, however, report that children with C5-C6 lesions who had surgery had slightly better shoulder function than children who did not have surgery (Strombeck et al., 2000). In a systematic review of outcomes for children with OBPI who underwent neurosurgery, McNeely and Drake (2003) found no randomized controlled trials that reported the effects of neurosurgery compared to conservative treatment for children with OBPI. Although outcomes from case-series studies without control groups (Level III evidence) were generally favorable, the authors concluded that there was no conclusive evidence demonstrating a benefit of surgery over conservative management in the treatment of children with OBPI (McNeely & Drake, 2003).

A lack of biceps function and elbow flexion has been used in the past to predict which infants would lack complete recovery and therefore be candidates for surgery (Gilbert, 1995), however, Hoeksma and colleagues (2004) found that shoulder external rotation and forearm supination were more accurate predictors of full recovery than elbow flexion. Hence, lack of active external rotation and forearm supination may be better markers to use when determining if an infant should have surgery to repair the brachial plexus.

Neurosurgeons have typically recommended that brachial plexus repair by microsurgery be done between 3 and 8 months of age for optimal results (Laurent & Lee, 1994; Clarke & Curtis, 1995), however, Grossman and colleagues (2004) found that children who underwent late nerve reconstruction (9–21 months of age) demonstrated significant improvement in shoulder function. Because a small number of children (3 of 19) who demonstrated incomplete elbow flexion at 9 months of age went on to have full elbow flexion function at 12 months (Hoeksma et al., 2004), it may be prudent to delay neurosurgery until 12 months of age in those children with only upper nerve root involvement.

Based upon the findings of McNeely and Drake (2003) it would seem essential that randomized, controlled trials of the effects of neurosurgery on outcomes in children with OBPI be started as soon as possible. These trials should use standardized, reliable, and valid outcome measures in each of the three domains of impairment, activity, and participation. Because Grossman and colleagues (2004) have demonstrated that late nerve reconstruction resulted in improvement of shoulder function, it would seem reasonable that a control group for these trials could include a group of children who have late rather than early surgery if the parents so choose after a period of conservative treatment. Only through such randomized controlled trials can it be determined if neurosurgery results in improved outcomes for children with OBPI.

ORTHOPEDIC CONCERNS AND ORTHOPEDIC SURGERY

Despite therapy and neurosurgery, contractures and secondary deformities are likely to occur in children who do not experience complete return and may even occur in children who have been categorized as having full return of muscle strength and activity (Hoeksma et al., 2003). Several authors have reported that glenohumeral deformity is present in up to 67% of children with OBPI (Kon et al., 2004; Ter Steeg et al., 2003; Hoeksma et al., 2003). These osseous deformities were even found to be present in children who had full passive range of motion of the shoulder and full functional recovery. Hoeskma and colleagues (2003) found that even mild contracture is strongly associated with osseous deformity of the shoulder. Ter Steeg and colleagues (2003) suggested that physical therapists may want to consider the use of splints to protect the shoulder during the flaccid period of OBPI, before muscle function returns.

The severity and type of contracture will vary depending on the pattern of return and type of intervention the child has undergone. The most common injury, to C5 and C6, will likely result in absence or weakness of shoulder external rotation and abduction, elbow flexion, and forearm supination. Therefore, the most common contractures are shoulder adduction and internal rotation, elbow flexion or extension (depending on the involvement of the triceps), and forearm pronation.

The main goal of orthopedic surgery is to provide the necessary active and passive range of motion that will enable the patient's hand to reach the head and mouth for meaningful activities of daily living. Price and Grossman (1995) provide a thorough discussion of historical and current orthopedic surgery for patients with OBPI. Common surgeries include soft tissue releases (at muscle insertions or by Z-plasty), reductions of glenohumeral joint dislocations, transfers of muscles, and osteotomies (Waters, 1999; Dodds & Wolfe, 2000; Hearle & Gilbert, 2004). Hoffer and Phipps (1998) achieved an increase in abduction of one grade and external rotation of two grades by releasing the pectoralis major, latissimus dorsi, and teres major and then transferring the latissimus dorsi and teres major to the rotator cuff. Functionally, the patients could then reach above their head for a variety of ADLs. Transferring a muscle can be expected to result in the loss of one muscle strength grade; therefore, the muscle chosen for transfer should be as strong as possible before surgery. Grossman (1996) reported releasing the subscapularis by 2 years of age in children with persistent internal rotation contractures. He recommended delaying hand and wrist reconstruction until 8 years of age when spontaneous recovery has reached a plateau and the child can fully participate in postoperative hand therapy. Any parents pursuing orthopedic surgery for their child should become intimately knowledgeable of the most current research on the technique and outcome of any procedure being considered. Clearly identified functional goals should be established before any surgery.

OUTCOMES

Little information is available on long-term outcomes in adults with a history of OBPI. Discussion in chat rooms on the Internet would suggest that a number of adults are looking for treatment suggestions for persistent residual arm and shoulder pain. Gjorup (1965) published a long-term follow-up study of adults that included clinical examinations and a lengthy questionnaire of their functional and social status, their vocational and avocational activities, and their feelings about how OBPI had affected their lives. Although this study is descriptive in nature, it is unique in its attempt to document how OBPI affects people as adults. Out of 222 respondents, approximately one third thought they had a usable arm, one third thought they had a useless arm, and the remainder reported transitional stages between these extremes (Gjorup, 1965). Slightly more than one third thought they were disabled. Gjorup (1965) concluded that patients with OBPI manage well socially, and no correlation was found between the severity of the arm defect and social status achieved by the patient.

Unfortunately, no other studies could be identified that investigated activity limitations or participation restrictions in school-age young children, adolescents, or young adults. Outcomes research using health-related quality-of-life measures as described by Jette (1993) would be extremely helpful for physical therapists and parents to help in long-term planning for children with OBPI.

PREVENTION

Risk factors for OBPI can be identified before birth. O'Leary (1992) identified maternal birth weight, prior shoulder dystocia, abnormal pelvis, maternal obesity, multiparity, and advanced maternal age as risk factors for delivering a child with shoulder dystocia. Cesarean section should be considered when a mother has multiple risk factors for a child being born with shoulder dystocia.

SUMMARY

Children with OBPI present with impairments of flaccidity or reduced muscle activity that are readily apparent at birth. Shoulder dystocia as a result of macrosomia is the most common cause of OBPI. Physical therapists can provide important early intervention for these children by working with parents to ensure that the joints of the flaccid extremity are protected during the first few weeks. If spontaneous recovery does not occur within a few weeks, physical therapists provide interventions to maintain muscle extensibility and joint range of motion as well as developmental activities to enhance motor recovery of the involved extremity. Neurosurgery may be indicated if substantial spontaneous recovery is not apparent by the age of 6 to 9 months, however, the evidence for the benefits of neurosurgical intervention compared to conservative treatment is not strong.

CASE STUDY

BLAIR K.

Mrs. K. was at 36 weeks of gestation with her third child. She requested an ultrasound to determine the size of her baby because her second child had been born after 38 weeks of gestation at 9.7 pounds with the complication of shoulder dystocia. Her obstetrician reluctantly agreed. The fetus was estimated to be 7 pounds at 36 weeks of gestation. The physician declined Mrs. K.'s request to be induced or to have a cesarean section at 40 weeks. At 42 weeks of gestation, Mrs. K. was induced and delivered an 11-pound baby after a difficult delivery complicated by shoulder dystocia. Blair was in fetal distress with a limp left arm. Radiographs were inconclusive in establishing if there was a clavicular fracture. The intern told the family that Blair had Erb's palsy and that her hand would be in the waiter's tip position for life. On seeing the pediatric neurologist, the family was told that Blair had a "mild stretching" of the nerves, that the condition was not permanent, and that she would recover fully.

The physical therapist saw Blair on her second day of life, before discharge. The family was educated about the disorder, including precautions and prognosis. Instruction in range of motion and positioning was provided, with the parents given the opportunity to practice on a doll. They were told not to begin the exercises until the next week. They were given a packet of information on the diagnosis, exercises, terminology, support groups, and the National Brachial Plexus Association.

Initial examination at 2 days of age: Blair's left arm demonstrated no movement in the shoulder or arm except for palpable contractions in the pectoralis muscle. Her upper trapezius was active, which she used to splint the shoulder area, causing her left shoulder to be held close to her left ear. Range of motion was full in all joints. No reaction to pinching of the skin on the left arm was observed. A screening of her motor development was normal for a newborn.

Physical therapy was begun once a week at 3 weeks of age. Direct therapy was provided in the form of guided movements through developmentally appropriate gross and fine movement patterns as the weeks progressed. Tactile stimulation to individual muscles began to elicit muscle contractions in the triceps and pectoralis muscles after 4 weeks. About the same time, a weak grasp was developing when a finger was placed in Blair's hand. Range of motion in the cervical area and all upper extremity joints remained full.

The Internet and a local OBPI support group provided a great deal of information to Blair's family in the ensuing weeks. The support group informed them about a hospital specializing in the management of OBPI. Their local neurologist was not supportive of their pursuing surgical options for Blair because the neurologist thought the surgery was experimental. They decided to visit this hospital when Blair was 3 months of age.

Age 3 months: Range of motion was full for all joints. Strength was returning to some muscle groups as follows: shoulder flexion (2), shoulder abduction (0), shoulder extension (2), elbow flexion (1), elbow extension (2), supination (0), wrist extension (1), and wrist flexion (3). Finger flexion and extension appeared normal. It was difficult to determine whether elbow flexion was being performed by the brachioradialis or biceps. Sensation was returning yet was not normal because responses to light touch did not elicit a response in the lower left arm.

Blair was taken to a hospital specializing in OBPI at this time. She was evaluated and told to return at 6 to 7 months of age. Therapy continued once a week, and Blair continued to gain more strength in her shoulder, elbow, and hand. Her home program was modified weekly to add resistance in the form of gravity, handheld toys, or bracelet weights to muscle groups gaining strength in the grade 3 to 4 range. Manual guidance techniques to emerging gross motor activities were taught. Careful attention was paid to identifying muscles regaining innervation and facilitating them appropriately. Other aspects of the treatment program were followed as described in the intervention section of this chapter.

Age 6 months: Range of motion continued to be full. Blair no longer elevated her shoulder toward her ear. Strength was as follows: shoulder flexion (2+), shoulder abduction (0), shoulder extension (3), elbow flexion (1+), elbow extension (3), supination (0), wrist extension (1), and wrist flexion (3). Finger flexion and extension appeared normal. Wrist flexion was accompanied by a strong pull into ulnar deviation. A wrist cock-up splint to support weak wrist extension and prevent the ulnar deviation was provided for daytime use.

It was still unclear whether elbow flexion was being performed by the biceps, brachialis, or brachioradialis muscle. Developmentally, Blair progressed normally except for assuming quadruped and creeping, which she could not do. Sitting was asymmetric because she was afraid to shift her weight to the left (there were no functional protective reactions to that side). Weight-shifting activities while seated on balls and the caregiver's lap while Blair was supported at the trunk were done while she was encouraged to reach for toys.

Age 7 months: Blair returned to the hospital specializing in OBPI. The family was instructed to come on a Monday and be prepared for possible exploratory surgery if indicated, on the following day. Exploratory surgery was recommended. Decisions on the surgery to be performed were determined at the time of exploration during which EMG was performed. Nerve conduction to the deltoid was present, but not to the biceps. Surgery included removal of a neuroma and nerve grafting using the sural nerve as a donor. Blair was discharged on postoperative day 4, and her arm was placed in a sling for 10 days because of the nerve graft. Therapy resumed 10 days after surgery, twice a week. At this time, deltoid muscle activity could be palpated, but biceps strength remained at 1+. Two months after surgery, elbow flexion strength increased from 1+ to 2.

Age 1 year: Range of motion continued to be full except for some mild scapulohumeral tightness. The left arm was slightly smaller in girth. Blair continued to prefer to use her right hand for ADLs, yet would use her left hand if encouraged to do so or if bilateral participation was required. Scapular winging was minimal, and based on Mallet's functional classification (see Fig. 22-3), Blair had grade III function. Active range of motion was not full yet was functional for activities such as hand to mouth, using some shoulder abduction to substitute for decreased elbow flexion. She also used substitutions for the lack of wrist supination. Therapy continued once a week, and sensation and muscle strength continued to improve. Substitutions were being replaced with more normal movements, and new strategies for gaining and maintaining shoulder range were needed. Therapy activities included picking up objects from the floor and then placing them up on a table while a caregiver facilitated shoulder flexion with external rotation and forearm supination; use of a vibrator on the biceps during activities requiring elbow flexion, such as self-feeding; and utilization of fine motor skills, such as stacking rings, which require elbow flexion and supination.

Age 18 months: Electrical stimulation was prescribed at this time to stimulate the deltoid and biceps. Shoulder abduction was at 3−, elbow flexion 3−. Use of a stimulator that provided alternating current assisted these two active contractions to achieve close to full-range motions against gravity (3+). After 1 month of experimentation and parent instruction with the stimulator, therapy was reduced to once a week, and the parents used the stimulator 3 to 5 days a week for 30- to 60-minute sessions. At this age, Blair loved being prone on a platform swing doing push and pull activities that encouraged bilateral shoulder and elbow movements, and fast movements while prone over bolsters that elicited protective reactions and shoulder flexion.

Age 2 years: Residual impairments at this time included mild sensory loss, decreased active shoulder and elbow range of motion (grade IV on Mallet's scale), and smaller limb girth. Passive range of motion was full, yet the family had learned that the shoulder would quickly become tight if exercises were neglected. Active ranges, as mentioned, were slightly limited yet functional for toothbrushing and hair brushing, with some substitution of shoulder abduction for lack of full elbow flexion. Some neglect of the involved arm was noticed in situations such as stair climbing because she would only use her uninvolved arm on a railing and in crayon-to-paper activities. No residual disability was apparent at this age; Blair performed all gross and fine motor activities at age-appropriate levels, with some abnormal substitutions. Electrical stimulation was discontinued because strength gains were occurring minimally. The frequency of physical therapy was decreased to once a month to monitor progress or regression and continue working on the acquisition of bilateral upper extremity skills without abnormal substitutions.

ACKNOWLEDGMENT

We would like to thank Barry Chapman, PT, Developmental Services Center, Champaign, Illinois, for completing the video case for a child with obstetrical brachial plexus injury that accompanies this book on the DVD.

REFERENCES

Al-qattan, NM, Clarke, HM, & Curtis, CG. Klumpke's birth palsy: Does it really exist? Journal of Hand Surgery (British), *20B*:19–23, 1995.

Bae, DS, Waters, PM, & Zurakowski, D. Reliability of three classification systems measuring active motion in brachial plexus birth palsy. Journal of Bone and Joint Surgery, *85A*:1733–1738, 2003.

Bager, B. Perinatally acquired brachial plexus palsy—A persisting challenge. Acta Paediatrica, *86*: 1214–1219, 1997.

Clarke, HM, & Curtis, CG. An approach to obstetrical brachial plexus injuries. Hand Clinics, *11*:563–580, 1995.

Curtis, C, Stephens, D, Clarke, HM, & Andrews, D. The active movement scale: An evaluative tool for infants with obstetrical brachial plexus injury. Journal of Hand Surgery (American), *27A*: 470–478, 2002.

Dawodu, A, Sankaran-Kutty, M, & Rajan, TV. Risk factors and prognosis for brachial plexus injury and clavicular fracture in neonates: A prospective analysis from the United Arab Emirates. Annals of Tropical Pediatrics, *17*:195–200, 1997.

Desiato, MT, & Risina, B. The role of botulinum toxin in the neurorehabilitation of young patients with brachial plexus palsy. Pediatric Rehabilitation, *4*:29–36, 2001.

DiTaranto, P, Campagna, L, Price, AE, & Grossman, JA. Outcome following nonoperative treatment of brachial plexus birth injuries. Journal of Child Neurology, *19*:87–90, 2004.

Dodds, SD, & Wolfe, SW. Perinatal brachial plexus palsy. Current Opinion in Pediatrics, *12*:40–47, 2000.

Eng, GD, Koch, B, & Smokvina, MD. Brachial plexus palsy in neonates and children. Archives of Physical Medicine and Rehabilitation, *59*:458–464, 1978.

Gilbert, A. Obstetrical brachial plexus palsy. In Tubiana, R (Ed.). The Hand, Vol. 4. Philadelphia: WB Saunders, 1993, p. 579.

Gilbert, A. Long-term evaluation of brachial plexus surgery in obstetrical palsy. Hand Clinics, *11*:583–593, 1995.

Gilbert, WM, Hicks, SM, Boe, NM, & Danielsen, B. Vaginal versus cesarean delivery for breech presentation in California: A population-based study. Obstetrics & Gynecology, *102*:911–917, 2003.

Gjorup, L. Obstetrical lesion of the brachial plexus. Acta Neurologica Scandinavica Supplementum, *18*:31–58, 1965.

Gordon, M, Rich, H, Deutschberger, J, & Green, M. The immediate and long-term outcome of obstetric birth trauma. I. Brachial plexus paralysis. American Journal of Obstetrics and Gynecology, *117*:51–56, 1973.

Grossman, AL, Ditaranto, P, Yaylali, I, Alfonso, I, Ramos LE, & Price, AE. Shoulder function following late neurolysis and bypass grafting for upper brachial plexus birth injuries. Journal of Hand Surgery (British), *29B*:356–358, 2004.

Grossman, JAI. Multidisciplinary treatment of patients with obstetrical brachial plexus palsy. Acta Neuropediatrica, *2*:151–152, 1996.

Hardy, AF. Birth injuries of the brachial plexus; incidence and prognosis. Journal of Bone and Joint Surgery (British), *63B*:98–101, 1981.

Hearle, M, & Gilbert, A. Management of complete obstetrical brachial plexus lesions. Journal of Pediatric Orthopedics, *24*:194–200, 2004.

Hernandez, C, & Wendel, GD. Shoulder dystocia. Clinical Obstetrics and Gynecology, *33*:526–534, 1990.

Hoeksma, AF, Wolf, H, & Oei, SL. Obstetrical brachial plexus injuries: Incidence, natural course and shoulder contracture. Clinical Rehabilitation, *14*:523–526, 2000.

Hoeksma, AF, ter Steeg, AM, Dijkstra, P, Nelissen, RG, Bellen, A, & de Jong, BA. Shoulder contracture and osseous deformity in obstetrical brachial plexus injuries. Journal of Bone and Joint Surgery (American), *85A*:316–322, 2003.

Hoeksma, AF, ter Steeg, AM, Nelissen, RG, van Ouwerkerk, WJ, Lankhorst, GJ, & de Jong, BA. Neurological recovery in obstetric brachial plexus injuries: An historical cohort study. Developmental Medicine & Child Neurology, *46*:76–83, 2004.

Hoffer, MM, & Phipps, GJ. Closed reduction and tendon transfer for treatment of dislocation of the glenohumeral joint secondary to brachial plexus birth palsy. Journal of Bone and Joint Surgery (American), *7*:997–1001, 1998.

Kon, DS, Darakjian, AB, Pearl, ML, & Kosco, AE. Glenohumeral deformity in children with internal rotation contractures secondary to brachial plexus birth palsy: Intraoperative arthorgraphic classification. Radiology, *231*:791–795, 2004.

Jette, AM. Using health related quality of life measures in physical therapy outcomes research. Physical Therapy, *73*:528–537, 1993.

Laurent, JP, Lee, R, Shenaq, S, Parke, JT, Solis, IS, & Kowalik, L. Neurosurgical correction of upper brachial plexus birth injuries. Journal of Neurosurgery, *79*:197–203, 1993.

Laurent, JP, & Lee, RT. Birth related upper brachial plexus injuries in infants: Operative and nonoperative approaches. Journal of Child Neurology, *9*:111–117, 1994.

McNeely, PD, & Drake, JM. A systematic review of brachial plexus surgery for birth-related brachial plexus injury. Pediatric Neurosurgery, *38*:57–62, 2003.

Michelow, BJ, Clarke, HM, Curtis, CG, Zuker, RM, Seifu, Y, & Andrews, DF. The natural history of brachial plexus palsy. Plastic and Reconstructive Surgery, *93*:675–680, 1994.

Narakas, AO. Obstetrical brachial plexus injuries. In Lamb, DW (Ed.). The Hand and Upper Limb, Vol. 2: The Paralyzed Hand. Edinburgh: Churchill Livingstone, 1987, p. 116.

Noetzel, MJ, Park, TS, Robinson, S, & Kaufman, B. Prospective study of recovery following neonatal brachial plexus injury. Journal of Child Neurology, *16*:488–492, 2001.

Pondaag, W, Malessy, MJ, van Dijk, JG, & Thomeer, RT. Natural history of obstetric brachial plexus palsy: A systematic review. Developmental Medicine & Child Neurology. *46*:138–144, 2004.

Price, AE, & Grossman, JAI. A management approach for secondary shoulder and forearm deformities following obstetrical brachial plexus surgery. Hand Clinics, *11*:607–614, 1995.

Shepherd, RB. Brachial plexus injury. In Campbell, SK (Ed.). Pediatric Neurologic Physical Therapy, 2nd ed. New York: Churchill Livingstone, 1991, pp. 101–130.

Sherburn, EW, Kaplan, SS, Kaufman, BA, Noetzel, MJ, & Park, TS. Outcome of surgically treated birth-related brachial plexus injuries in twenty cases. Pediatric Neurosurgery, *27*:19-27, 1997.

Sjoberg, I, Erichs, K, & Bjerre, I. Cause and effect of obstetric (neonatal) brachial plexus palsy. Acta Paediatrics Scandinavia, *77*:357–564,1988.

Strombeck C, Krumlinde-Sundholm, & Forssberg H. Functional outcome at 5 years in children with obstetrical brachial plexus palsy with and without microsurgical reconstruction. Developmental Medicine & Child Neurology, *42*:148–157, 2000.

Sundholm, LK, Eliasson, AC, & Forssberg, H. Obstetric brachial plexus injuries: Assessment protocol and functional outcome at age 5 years. Developmental Medicine & Child Neurology, *40*:4–11, 1998.

Ter Steeg, AM, Hoeksma, AF, Kijkstra, PF, Nelissen, RGHH, & De Jong, BA. Orthopedic sequelae in neurologically recovered obstetrical brachial plexus injury. Case study and literature review. Disability and Rehabilitation, *25*:1–8, 2003.

van der Weel, FRR, van der Meer, ALH, & Lee, DN. Effect of task on movement control in cerebral palsy: Implications for assessment and therapy. Developmental Medicine and Child Neurology, *33*:419–426, 1991.

Waters, PM. Comparison of the natural history, the outcome of microsurgical repair, and the outcome of operative reconstruction in brachial plexus birth palsy. Journal of Bone and Joint Surgery (American), *81*:649–659, 1999.

Wolf, H, Hoeksma, AF, Oei, SL, & Bleker, OP. Obstetric brachial plexus injury: Risk factors related to recovery. European Journal of Obstetrics & Gynecology and Reproductive Biology, *88*:133–138, 2000.

∾

SPINAL CORD INJURY

KRISTINE A. SHAKHAZIZIAN
PT

TERESA L. MASSAGLI
MD

Acquired lesions of the spinal cord occur far less commonly in children than in adults, but the unique aspects of growth and development can make treatment of the child with spinal cord injury (SCI) a challenge for pediatric physical therapists. The rehabilitation process may take years because the young child requires time to achieve adequate upper body strength, adult body proportions, and cognitive skills for maximal independence. The child who is not skeletally mature may develop orthopedic problems during growth, which may result in altered function. Direct intervention, monitoring skill acquisition, and assessing equipment needs are important roles for the physical therapist.

This chapter describes the pathophysiology and resulting neurologic changes and changes in body functions and structures and their impact on activity and participation of children with SCI. Examination, prognosis, goals and outcomes, and physical therapy intervention for the child with pediatric SCI are then discussed.

EPIDEMIOLOGY

The most common cause of SCI for all ages is trauma. The overall incidence is estimated to be 40 injuries per million persons per year, or around 11,000 new cases each year in the United States. Children younger than 16 years of age account for less than 5% of these cases. Motor vehicle crashes, sports, violence, and falls are the leading causes, and traumatic SCI more frequently occurs in boys, during the summer, and on weekends (Nobunaga et al., 1999). Traumatic SCI is more common in children 10 to 15 years old and from birth to 5 years old than in children who are 5 to 9 years old (Kewalramani et al., 1980). Violence as a cause of SCI is increasing in frequency, particularly in older teenagers of African-American or Hispanic ethnicity (Nobunaga et al., 1999). Child abuse accounts for some cases of SCI, particularly in younger children, but its frequency as a cause of SCI is unknown. Developmental anomalies of the cervical vertebrae can place the spinal cord at increased risk of injury. These anomalies include instability of the atlantoaxial joint, as seen in

Down syndrome, juvenile rheumatoid arthritis, or os odontoideum (a congenital failure of fusion of the odontoid process to the C2 vertebral body) and dysplasia of the base of the skull or upper cervical vertebrae, as seen in achondroplasia.

Nontraumatic myelopathy can be difficult to diagnose because imaging studies may be nonspecific. Nontraumatic causes of SCI in children include tumor, transverse myelitis, epidural abscess, arteriovenous malformation, multiple sclerosis, and spinal cord infarction due to thromboembolic disorders. Treating the child with SCI resulting from the presence of a tumor is especially challenging because the child's overall medical condition and the progression of disease dramatically influence the formulation of goals or attainment of outcomes.

PATHOPHYSIOLOGY

The site or level at which SCI occurs is often related to the cause of injury and the child's age. Most of the nontraumatic causes of SCI occur in the thoracic spinal cord. By contrast, vertebral dysplasias place the upper cervical spinal cord or lower brainstem at risk. Birth trauma due to traction and angulation of the spine at a breech delivery most commonly causes SCI at the cervicothoracic junction. In the child younger than 8 to 10 years old, the cervical spine has greater mobility than it does in adults because of ligamentous laxity, shallow angulation of the facets, incomplete ossification of vertebrae, and relative underdevelopment of the neck muscles for the size of the head (Wilberger, 1986). Young children are therefore more likely to experience injury at the upper cervical spine than are adults (Bohn et al., 1990), and SCI may occur without any signs of bone damage by radiography, a finding referred to as spinal cord injury without radiographic abnormality, or SCIWORA (Bosch et al., 2002). In children, 55% of cases of traumatic SCI result in tetraplegia owing to injury between the first cervical and first thoracic root levels, and 45% result in paraplegia from injury below the first thoracic level (Nobunaga et al., 1999).

Most cases of traumatic SCI are caused by a blunt, nonpenetrating injury to the spinal cord in which the cord is not lacerated or transected, and in the majority of cases, some white matter tracts remain intact across the lesion. The direct effect of the trauma is immediate disruption of neural transmission in the gray and white matter of the spinal cord at and below the injury site, resulting in spinal shock. Reactive physiologic events evolve over a period of hours and induce secondary injury to the spinal cord (Kakulas, 1999). The exact sequence of events between transfer of kinetic energy to the cord and subsequent neuronal death is unknown. Animal models have shown that ischemia, hemorrhage, edema, calcium influx into cells, and generation of free radicals contribute to cell membrane degradation and death of neurons (Hall, 2001). In gray matter, neurons that die are not replaced. In white matter, axonal segments distal to the injury degenerate and synapses no longer function. Although axonal sprouting does occur to a limited degree in the central nervous system, it appears to be functionally insignificant, and most of the recovery observed in patients with incomplete lesions is probably due to resolution of neurapraxic injury. Case reports of neurologic improvement years after SCI are rare, but provide hope that therapies can be developed to enhance function in the remaining spinal cord tissue (McDonald et al., 2002).

The zone of injury within the spinal cord is usually large enough to cause a transition in neurologic function from normal to abnormal or from normal to absent over several spinal root levels. Soon after SCI, the level of injury may appear to move cephalad as the secondary or indirect processes set in. Later, the level of injury may move caudally as these factors resolve, as sprouting develops (either within the spinal cord or peripherally to denervated muscles), or as hypertrophy of weak muscles occurs. Research has shown that the extent of injury may diminish for as long as 1 year (Wu et al., 1992), and it is obvious that until the natural history of SCI and recovery is delineated, experimental treatments may be inappropriately credited with enhancing recovery.

If some function below the zone of the spinal cord injury remains and motor function or sensation is present in the lowest sacral segment, the child has an incomplete SCI. After traumatic SCI, incomplete lesions are found in 40% of children with paraplegia and in 55% of those with tetraplegia (Go et al., 1995). Several distinct patterns of clinical syndromes have been described. Injury to the anterior spinal cord produces variable motor paralysis, with reduced sensation of pain and temperature but with preserved dorsal column function. Hemorrhage in the central part of the cervical spinal cord produces flaccid weakness of the arms and strong but spastic legs, with preservation of bladder and bowel function. Posterior cord lesions are rare and produce selective loss of proprioception. Stab wounds may produce a Brown-Sequard lesion with ipsilateral paralysis and proprioceptive loss and contralateral loss of pain and temperature sensation. Injury to the lumbosacral nerve roots results in cauda equina syndrome, with lower extremity weakness and areflexia of the legs and bladder.

Delayed cavitation (syringomyelia) within the damaged spinal cord can occur in patients with complete or incomplete lesions. The occurrence of a cystic cavitation, or syrinx, appears to be common after SCI, occurring in

51% of children in a study reported by Backe and colleagues (1991). In a small number of such patients the cyst may progressively enlarge, resulting in further loss of neurologic function months to years after SCI. Signs and symptoms that may herald presence of a syrinx include loss of motor function, ascending sensory level, increased spasticity or sweating, and new onset of pain or dysesthesia.

PREVENTION

Proper use of vehicle restraints, water safety instruction, and preparticipation sports physical examinations are important measures in preventing traumatic SCI in children. Lap seat belts must be placed across the pelvis, not across the waist, and shoulder harnesses should cross the clavicle, not the neck, to avoid lumbar or cervical spine injury in the event of a collision. Children should use a booster seat until the lap belt and shoulder harness fit correctly. This typically occurs when the child is about 4 feet 9 inches tall, 8 years old, or 80 pounds. Health care professionals and schools have supported cooperative programs to reduce diving injuries (the most common sports-related cause of SCI) and other high-risk activities (Greene et al., 2002). "Feet first, first time" is a slogan adopted by many public swimming areas to avoid shallow water diving injuries. Because children with Down syndrome have some risk of atlantoaxial instability, the American Academy of Pediatrics (Committee on Genetics, 2001) recommends screening radiographs to assess cervical spine stability for this population of children between the ages of 3 and 5 years. This radiographic screening is most helpful for children who may participate in sports or who are symptomatic. The Committee on Genetics (1995) also recommends that children with achondroplasia be encouraged to participate in activities such as biking or swimming, but to avoid gymnastics and contact sports because of the potential for neck or back injury.

MEDICAL DIAGNOSIS AND MANAGEMENT

The early management of a child with SCI is focused on stabilization of the spine to prevent further damage to the intact but injured spinal cord. The spine is immobilized during transport and throughout all assessments and procedures. At the hospital, a thorough neurologic examination is performed to determine the motor and sensory level of SCI and the completeness of injury. Spinal shock is usually present, although occasionally it has resolved by the time the patient is treated in the emergency department. In spinal shock, the muscles are flaccid below the SCI and all cutaneous and deep tendon reflexes are absent. This state persists for hours to weeks and is said to be over when sacral reflexes, including the bulbocavernous and anal reflexes, are present.

Further evaluation is undertaken with plain radiographs of the whole spine from the first cervical to the sacral vertebrae to identify any fractures, facet subluxations, or dislocations. A small but significant number of patients may have more than one site of injury to the spine and spinal cord. Computed tomography and magnetic resonance imaging are used to diagnose root impingement, presence of bone fragments in the spinal canal, cord compression, and spinal cord hemorrhage.

Whether immediate surgical intervention to correct bone injury and decompress the spinal cord is effective in reducing paralysis is unknown because the numerous surgical procedures have never been subjected to randomized clinical trials. Surgery often allows a patient to be mobilized more quickly, but ultimate levels of independence or recovery do not appear to be altered (Murphy et al., 1990). The main goal of surgery is to prevent later deformity, pain, or loss of neurologic function. Surgery may not be necessary if spinal alignment can be achieved with traction and maintained with an orthosis. Surgery is indicated if there is a penetrating injury, if traction has failed to reduce a dislocation, if nerve root impingement exists, if the spine is highly unstable and at risk of further damaging the cord, or if bone fragments are compressing the cauda equina (Fehlings et al., 2001). Regardless of whether surgery is performed, if bone injury has occurred, patients usually wear an external orthosis until bone fusion is complete, often for 3 or more months. There is, however, regional variation in practice among orthopedic surgeons in the use of spinal orthoses after spinal fusion. For some lower lumbar (L4 or L5) injuries, the surgeon may have the child wear an orthosis with a thigh piece (Fig. 23-1), which permits only limited hip flexion (e.g., to only 60°). This is done to reduce torque on the immature fusion mass, which could occur from pull of the hamstrings on the pelvis in a position of hip flexion.

Researchers have tried pharmacologic interventions to halt the chain of secondary events producing neural damage and to protect compromised but viable cells. Antioxidants, free radical scavengers, opiate antagonists, vitamins, thyrotropin-releasing hormone, and calcium channel blockers are a few of the agents that have been tested (Rhoney et al., 1996). It is a slow process to bring new pharmacotherapies into clinical practice, owing to the necessary steps of animal trials, followed by preliminary and then larger-scale trials in humans. Human trials must be placebo controlled and have a sufficient period of

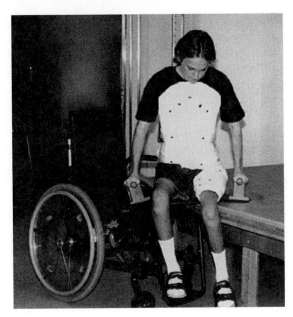

♦ Figure 23-1 Teen wearing a thoracolumbosacral orthosis with a thigh piece that restricts hip flexion uses a sliding board and push-up blocks to begin learning transfers.

follow-up to assess the efficacy of the treatment. Because spinal cord injury is not very common, clinical trials usually require collaboration among many medical centers. High doses of corticosteroids (methylprednisolone) administered within the first 8 hours and continued for 24 to 48 hours have been shown to slightly enhance motor recovery in humans (Hall, 2001). At this time, methylprednisolone is the only medication used in standard clinical practice.

Trauma to the spinal cord provokes the development of scar tissue, which includes both connective tissue elements and glial hyperplasia. Scientists have not yet determined why axons are unable to grow across this scar tissue area. Some researchers have proposed that the glial cells act as a surrogate target for the regrowing axons, whereas others have argued that the glial cells engender a nonpermissive substrate for axonal growth. Strategies to promote spinal cord regeneration have included use of neurotrophic factors, monoclonal antibodies directed against glial cells, and intraspinal transplants of peripheral nerve tissue, fetal spinal cord tissue, or omental tissue from the abdomen. Both in vitro techniques and animal models have been used to demonstrate that injured axons can survive and grow under certain environmental conditions, but the feat of effecting axonal growth across scar tissue and through appropriate myelin sheaths to reach and innervate appropriate muscles remains elusive. Significant progress has occurred in understanding the inhibi-

tory factors, as well as those promoting axonal sprouting. It is difficult to envision a timetable for a cure for SCI, but there are and will be many clinical trials involving human subjects as in vitro or animal work on regeneration progresses. Clinical trials involving human subjects in the next several years will most likely involve neurorestorative agents to stimulate surviving neurons, antibodies against growth-inhibiting substances in the spinal cord, and building cellular bridges across injured spinal cord using fetal spinal cord or fetal glial transplants (Giovanini et al., 1997; Hall, 2001; Schwab, 1996). Researchers have also experimented with nonpharmacologic treatments, including acupuncture and functional electrical stimulation to enhance recovery after SCI (Wong et al., 2003; McDonald et al., 2002), but these therapies have not been subjected to randomized clinical trials. In a highly publicized case, a man with C2 ventilator-dependent tetraplegia participated in an intensive 3-year program of electrical stimulation, aqua therapy, and range of motion and breathing exercises. Improvements in cardiorespiratory endurance, increased muscle mass, decreased spasticity, decreased infections, changes in motor strength of some muscles, and improved light touch sensation were reported, but no changes in bladder, bowel, sexual function, or requirement for a ventilator and power wheelchair were noted (McDonald et al., 2002).

Patients and families have been and will continue to be tempted by unproved therapies, often at considerable personal financial expense. Therapists can help patients and families evaluate the evidence regarding potential therapies. Any purported cure should be subjected to randomized clinical trials before being offered to hopeful but vulnerable patients. It is reasonable for patients and therapists to hold out hope for a cure for SCI. It is often just this hope that motivates patients and caregivers to be meticulous about preventing secondary complications.

With ongoing appropriate medical care, long-term survival after traumatic SCI is not only possible but also likely. Life expectancy is approximately 85% of average for those with paraplegia and incomplete tetraplegia, and about 75% of average for those with tetraplegia (DeVivo & Stover, 1995).

■ IMPAIRMENTS AND ACTIVITY LIMITATIONS

All professionals should use a common terminology when describing the motor or sensory level of SCI in children or adults. The most widely used standards are those published by the American Spinal Injury Association (ASIA) (2000). These standards have been developed by consensus of a multidisciplinary group of clinical experts and have been revised periodically since their initial publication in 1982. The ASIA standards define right and left motor levels, right and left sensory levels, and incomplete and complete injuries.

DEFINING THE LEVEL OF SPINAL CORD INJURY

The ASIA standards accept the widely used system of muscle grading: 0 = absence, total paralysis; 1 = trace, palpable, or visible contraction; 2 = poor, active movement through full range of motion (ROM) with gravity eliminated; 3 = fair, active movement through full ROM against gravity; 4 = good, active movement through full ROM against moderate resistance; and 5 = normal, active movement through full ROM against full resistance. Motor levels may differ for right and left sides of the body. The key muscles for determination of motor level are listed in Table 23-1. Because all muscles have innervation from more than one root level, the presence of innervation by one root level and the absence by the next lower level results in a weakened muscle. The ASIA-defined motor level is the most caudal root level in which muscle strength is grade 3 or more and the next most rostral muscle a grade 5. By convention, if a muscle has grade 3 strength and the next most rostral muscle is grade 5, the grade 3 muscle is considered to have full innervation by the higher root level, for which it is named. For example, for a patient with a grade 2 C8 key muscle, grade 3 C7 key muscle, grade 4 C6 key muscle, and grade 5 C5 key muscle, the motor level as defined by ASIA is C6. One disadvantage to using only the ASIA key muscles to define a level of function is the omission of examination of hip extensors, hip abductors, and knee flexors. These other L5 and S1 muscles play an important role in activities such as transfers, ambulation, and stair climbing. Strength grades of the key muscles can be added together for both sides of the body to create a composite ASIA motor score. This score has been used in research studies assessing efficacy of pharmacologic treatment of SCI. It can also be used to predict function and need for assistance (Saboe et al., 1997). Waters and colleagues (1994) found that if the sum of the key muscles from both lower extremities (L2-S1) is 30 or higher, the patients were community ambulators. Those with scores less than 20 were limited ambulators who required knee-ankle-foot orthoses (KAFOs) and crutches.

The sensory level may not correspond exactly to the motor level. Determining the sensory level is especially helpful in injuries above C5, or to the thoracic spinal cord, where there are no key muscles to define the level of SCI. Rather than relying on dermatome charts, which vary from one text to another, the ASIA standards rely on the presence of normal light touch and pinprick sensation at a key point in each of the 28 dermatomes on the right and left sides of the body (Fig. 23-2 and Table 23-2). Proprioception should also be assessed below the level of injury in patients with incomplete SCI to determine integrity of dorsal column function.

A patient is said to have an incomplete SCI only if motor or sensory function is present in the lowest sacral segment, implying voluntary control of the external anal sphincter or sensation at the mucocutaneous junction or both. To be motor incomplete, the patient must also have motor function preserved more than three levels below the motor level (ASIA, 2000). Incomplete lesions are referred to in two ways: by the ASIA Impairment Scale (Table 23-3) and by neuroanatomic description. Distinct neuroanatomic patterns of incomplete lesions include the central cord syndrome, Brown-Séquard syndrome, anterior cord syndrome, and posterior cord syndrome previously described in the section on pathophysiology. The cauda equina syndrome may be complete or incomplete.

Precise description of the motor and sensory loss after SCI is important for two reasons. First, it helps predict the likelihood of further neurologic recovery in both complete and incomplete syndromes. For instance, in motor complete C5 tetraplegia, most if not all patients gain one full motor level, achieving grade 3 wrist extensor movement (a C6 muscle) during the first 8 months after injury

TABLE 23-1	**Key Muscles for Motor Level Classification**

C5	Elbow flexors (biceps, brachialis)
C6	Wrist extensors (extensor carpi radialis longus and brevis)
C7	Elbow extensors (triceps)
C8	Finger flexors to the middle finger (flexor digitorum profundus)
T1	Small finger abductors (abductor digiti minimi manus)
L2	Hip flexors (iliopsoas)
L3	Knee extensors (quadriceps)
L4	Ankle dorsiflexors (tibialis anterior)
L5	Long toe extensors (extensor hallucis longus)
S1	Ankle plantar flexors (gastrocnemius, soleus)

From American Spinal Injury Association. International Standards for Neurological and Functional Classification of Spinal Cord Injury. Chicago: American Spinal Injury Association, 2000 (revised 2002).

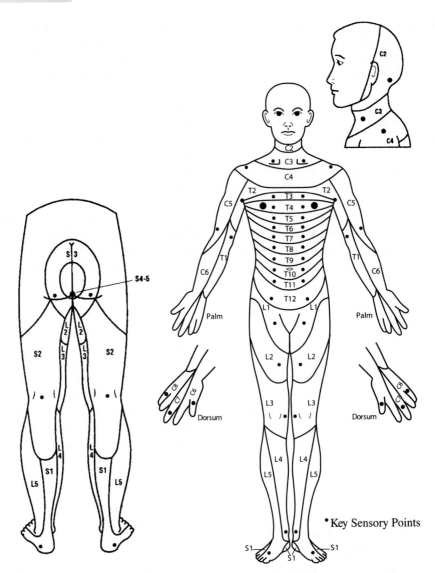

♦ **Figure 23-2** Key sensory areas by dermatome. *(From American Spinal Injury Association. International Standards for Neurological and Functional Classification of Spinal Cord Injury, Chicago: American Spinal Injury Association, 2000.)*

(Ditunno et al., 2000). Researchers have also determined that in SCI above T11, preservation of pinprick sensation has predictive value for return of motor function and independent ambulation, probably because of the proximity of the ascending pain fibers and descending motor fibers in the spinal cord (Poynton et al., 1997).

Some generalizations about recovery can be stated for the neuroanatomic incomplete syndromes. Anterior cord syndrome is usually due to damage to the anterior spinal artery, causing infarction in the spinal cord. Prognosis for return of function is poor. In posterior cord syndrome, motor function is preserved but the loss of proprioception means ambulation is unlikely. In Brown-Séquard and

central cord syndromes, prognosis for ambulation and bladder and bowel control is very good but hand function may be impaired, depending on the level of injury. Lesions of the cauda equina are essentially lesions of the peripheral nerve or lower motoneuron and may show recovery over several years owing to resolution of neurapraxia or to regrowth of damaged axons, as well as to peripheral sprouting.

The second reason for the importance of precise definition of the level of SCI is that it helps predict the ultimate level of independence a patient can expect to achieve in the areas of mobility, self-care, and even communication. Tables 23-4 and 23-5 delineate the optimal functional

TABLE 23-2	Key Sensory Areas

C2	Occipital protuberance
C3	Supraclavicular fossa
C4	Top of the acromioclavicular joint
C5	Lateral side of the antecubital fossa
C6	Thumb, dorsal surface, proximal phalanx
C7	Middle finger, dorsal surface, proximal phalanx
C8	Little finger, dorsal surface, proximal phalanx
T1	Medial (ulnar) side of the antecubital fossa
T2	Apex of the axilla
T3	Third intercostal space
T4	Fourth intercostal space (nipple line)
T5	Fifth intercostal space (midway between T4 and T6)
T6	Sixth intercostal space (level of xiphisternum)
T7	Seventh intercostal space (midway between T6 and T8)
T8	Eighth intercostal space (midway between T6 and T10)
T9	Ninth intercostal space (midway between T8 and T10)
T10	Tenth intercostal space (umbilicus)
T11	Eleventh intercostal space (midway between T10 and T12)
T12	Inguinal ligament at midpoint
L1	Half the distance between T12 and L2
L2	Midanterior thigh
L3	Medial femoral condyle
L4	Medial malleolus
L5	Dorsum of the foot at the third metatarsal phalangeal joint
S1	Lateral heel
S2	Popliteal fossa in the midline
S3	Ischial tuberosity
S4-S5	Perianal area (taken as one level)

From American Spinal Injury Association. International Standards for Neurological and Functional Classification of Spinal Cord Injury. Chicago: American Spinal Injury Association, 2000 (revised 2002).

TABLE 23-3	ASIA Impairment Scale

A **Complete**—No sensory or motor function is preserved in the sacral segments S4-S5.

B **Incomplete**—Sensory but not motor function is preserved below the neurologic level and includes the sacral segments S4-S5.

C **Incomplete**—Motor function is preserved below the neurologic level, and more than half of key muscles below the neurologic level have a muscle grade less than 3.

D **Incomplete**—Motor function is preserved below the neurologic level, and at least half of key muscles below the neurologic level have a muscle grade of 3 or more.

E **Normal**—Sensory and motor function are normal.

From American Spinal Injury Association. International Standards for Neurological and Functional Classification of Spinal Cord Injury. Chicago: American Spinal Injury Association, 2000 (revised 2002).

MEDICAL COMPLICATIONS

A host of medical complications can occur after SCI and may affect a child's ability to participate in physical therapy and rehabilitation (Massagli & Jaffe, 1990). With lesions of the cervical or thoracic spinal cord, altered respiratory function may occur, ranging from total paralysis of the diaphragm to diminished vital capacity or weakened forced expiration during coughing. SCI at a midthoracic level or above can interrupt sympathetic outflow, leading to orthostatic hypotension, impaired ability to sweat or shiver, and autonomic dysreflexia. Autonomic dysreflexia is a massive reflex sympathetic discharge that occurs after SCI above midthoracic levels in response to noxious stimuli. Clinical features include headache, flushing, sweating, pilomotor activity, rapid or reduced heart rate, and hypertension. The hypertensive crisis poses a danger to patients and can cause stroke, seizures, or even death. School-age children and adolescents are capable of reporting headaches, but younger children may have difficulty in verbalizing symptoms, and autonomic dysreflexia is often overlooked in these youngsters. In the first weeks after SCI, gastrointestinal bleeding from stress ulcers may occur, but the frequency (20%) is no greater than that in patients with other acute serious medical conditions (Sugarman, 1985). Paralyzed and dependent lower extremities can develop edema and deep vein thromboses.

abilities for each level of motor complete SCI. Patients with incomplete SCI may exceed the expectations for any given level of injury. Such expectations for independence must also be tempered by consideration of the child's age, which influences developmental expectations. It can take years for a preschooler to reach the expected level of independence, or he or she may fall short if complications, particularly orthopedic problems, arise. Environmental and personal factors also play an important role in determining the child's participation in home life, education, community activities, and social relationships.

TABLE 23-4	Mobility in Complete Tetraplegia: Expected Function and Necessary Equipment

MOBILITY FOR LEVEL OF INJURY

FUNCTIONAL SKILL	C1–C4	C5	C6	C7–T1
Bed mobility	D	A: Even with electric bed	I: May use equipment; electric bed helpful	I: Electric bed helpful
Transfers	D: May need mechanical lift	D: May need mechanical lift	Some I with or without sliding board	I: May need sliding board
Wheelchair	I: PWC, head, chin, mouth, or tongue control	I: PWC, hand control with splint	I: MWC, may use adapted rims; likely to use PWC in community	I: MWC
Pressure relief	D: Bed, MWC I: Power tilt PWC	D: Bed, MWC I: Power tilt PWC	I: Leaning to side	I: Push-up on open hands
Transportation	U: Driving; van with lift needed	I: Upper extremity controls; van with lift needed	I: Hand controls A: Load MWC	I: Hand controls I: Load MWC

Adapted from Massagli, TL, & Jaffe, KM. Pediatric spinal cord injury: Treatment and outcome. Pediatrician, *17*:244–254, 1990. Reprinted with permission of S. Karger, Basel.
A, Assistance required; *D*, dependent; *I*, independent; *MWC*, manual wheelchair; *PWC*, power wheelchair; *U*, unable.

TABLE 23-5	Mobility in Complete Paraplegia: Expected Function and Necessary Equipment

LEVEL OF INJURY

FUNCTIONAL SKILL	T2–T10	T11–L2	L3–S2
Manual wheelchair	I: Indoors and in community	I: Indoors and in community	May not need MWC except long distances, recreation
Ambulation	SBA: Exercise only; need KAFOs or RGOs and forearm crutches or walker; not practical for T2–T6	I: Indoors with KAFOs or RGOs and forearm crutches; some can do stairs with railing	I: Indoors and community with AFOs; may need forearm crutches or cane
Driving	I: Hand controls I: Load MWC	I: Hand controls I: Load MWC	Can drive automatic transmission; may prefer hand controls

Adapted from Massagli, TL, & Jaffe, KM. Pediatric spinal cord injury: Treatment and outcome. Pediatrician, *17*:244–254, 1990. Reprinted with permission of S. Karger, Basel.
AFOs, Ankle-foot orthoses; *I*, independent; *KAFOs*, knee-ankle-foot orthoses; *MWC*, manual wheelchair; *RGOs*, reciprocating gait orthoses; *SBA*, standby assistance.

Deep vein thrombosis occurs less frequently in children with SCI (5%) than in adults (10%) (Chen et al., 1999). Neurogenic pain can occur after SCI at, above, or below the level of injury and is relatively more common with cauda equina lesions. Loss of descending input to the sacral spinal cord or damage to the sacral nerve roots leads to impairment of bladder and bowel emptying, loss of sexual response, and male infertility.

Almost unique to children is the problem of immobilization hypercalcemia. During the first year after SCI, approximately 40% of bone mineral density is lost via calcium excreted in the urine. Children are more likely to have rapid bone turnover, resulting in a larger load of calcium than the kidneys can excrete. This produces elevated serum calcium level, or hypercalcemia. Nonspecific symptoms include lethargy, nausea, altered mood, and anorexia. Remobilization is an important aspect of treatment in persons without SCI (e.g., the child with a femur fracture), but it is not known if this is effective in reducing hypercalcemia after SCI. The mainstays of treatment are primarily medical and are aimed at reducing calcium loss from bones or at enhancing urinary excretion. Pathologic fractures, which occur at an increased rate in persons with bone mineral density below 40% of normal, are a potential complication of osteopenia. Deposition of new bone in periarticular soft tissue can also occur in paralyzed extremities. This heterotopic ossification can be asymptomatic, or it may interfere with ROM around a joint or even cause ankylosis. The most commonly affected joints are hips, knees, shoulders, and elbows.

Spasticity is a frequent occurrence after SCI and usually evolves over a period of 1 to 2 years. Although initially the patient is flaccid, hypertonus gradually appears, and in the first 3 to 6 months after SCI the patient develops hyperreflexia, clonus, and flexor spasms. Later, extensor spasms usually predominate. Evolution of spasticity after central nervous system insult is common and is seen in other conditions such as cerebral palsy and stroke. In SCI, the immediate effects of loss of supraspinal inhibition and the later-developing effects of denervation supersensitivity and sprouting by afferent and collateral neurons probably all contribute to the development of spasticity, but the sequence of events behind the evolution of clinical manifestations of spasticity is not known.

REHABILITATION MANAGEMENT

The acute rehabilitation and long-term treatment of children with SCI require a comprehensive interdisciplinary approach involving both hospital and school-based personnel. Team members typically include physicians, nurses, a dietitian, occupational therapists, therapeutic recreation specialists, a social worker, an orthotist, a clinical psychologist, and teachers, as well as physical therapists, the child, and the family.

A pediatric physiatrist provides medical management of the complications noted earlier and serves as a team leader. In some centers, an orthopedist, a neurologist, or a pediatrician may fill this role. Researchers, however, have shown that timely referral of patients with SCI to comprehensive, multidisciplinary SCI centers is more cost-effective, with improved patient outcomes, reduced hospital and long-term nursing care charges, and improved prospect for long-term patient earnings, compared with unspecialized care for SCI patients (Cardenas et al., 2001). The lead physician may also request consultation by other physicians such as an orthopedic surgeon or neurosurgeon to monitor spine stability and alignment, a urologist to monitor urinary tract function, and a pulmonologist for ventilator management.

Physical therapists develop age-appropriate ROM and strengthening programs. They address functional mobility, including bed mobility, transfers, sitting balance, ambulation, and wheelchair skills. The physical therapist makes recommendations on lower extremity orthoses and plays a primary role in the ordering of a wheelchair.

Rehabilitation nurses manage bladder and bowel care, monitor skin for pressure ulcers, provide emotional support to patients, and train the patient and family to carry out these tasks at home. Children can be taught self-management of bladder and bowel emptying at about age 5, but may need reminders or supervision for many more years. The dietitian educates the child and family in meal selection to avoid protein catabolism or, conversely, obesity and to choose high-fiber foods to facilitate bowel management.

Occupational therapists provide training in self-care management, in use of orthoses to aid hand function in tetraplegia, and in use of adaptive writing equipment. They often assist physical therapists with upper extremity strengthening and wheelchair prescriptions. Goals for self-care management must be set according to usual expectations for age. For the older teenager, the occupational therapist may also provide training in home and money management, prevocational skills, travel within the community, and use of adaptive equipment for driving. An orthotist is needed if either functional hand orthoses or lower extremity orthoses are necessary. Therapeutic recreation specialists find leisure activities, including sports, which allow the child to be more independent and participate in school and community leisure activities.

Social workers or case managers are indispensable for working with funding agencies. Inpatient and outpatient rehabilitation funding may be determined by visit, day, or dollar amount. A child may be eligible for a combination of funding through private insurance, Medicaid, and state developmental disability programs. The social worker or case manager helps determine eligibility and benefits and works with the family, rehabilitation team, and third-party payers in making the best use of available rehabilitation resources. The social worker also assists with discharge planning and provides support to the patient and family.

A team member skilled in mental health should monitor the child's adaptation to disability and be available to help the child verbally process the injury and rehabilitation treatment. This could be a skilled social worker, but if a behavior management program using reinforcers is needed, a clinical psychologist should be consulted. In some rare cases, the child may truly be clinically depressed, and a psychiatrist can be consulted if a medication trial is contemplated. As described by Fordyce (1981), acquisition of SCI accompanied by pain, medical complications, altered cosmesis and body image, and the new and challenging rehabilitation procedures can be expected to have a significant impact on the patient's affect, self-esteem, and behavior. The child's adjustment to SCI does not necessarily follow predictable stages of crisis response such as shock, denial, depression, and adaptation. Adjustment to SCI probably occurs over several years. The verbal or attitudinal expressions of children with new SCI are less predictive of outcome than are their behaviors. Physical therapists can facilitate adjustment by actively engaging the child in acquiring the skills needed to maximize independence. The psychologist or psychiatrist may also need to confront issues of premorbid risk-taking behavior or even substance abuse. Psychologists, nurses, and pediatric physiatrists collaborate in discussing sexuality and changes in sexual functioning with teenagers who have had SCI.

Teachers are particularly important during the acute rehabilitation phase because the length of hospitalization after SCI is often 1 to 3 months and the child must keep up with his or her curriculum. The teacher can be instrumental in assisting the receiving school to prepare for the child's return. Schools and state agencies should be asked to participate in vocational planning and counseling with teenagers.

THE YOUNG CHILD WITH SPINAL CORD INJURY

PHYSICAL THERAPY EXAMINATION

Infants, toddlers, and preschoolers can incur SCI as a result of birth trauma, child abuse, motor vehicle crashes, tumor, or even transverse myelitis. In infants, determination of the motor and sensory levels of SCI can be challenging and may require multiple examinations to determine what movement is voluntary and what is reflexively mediated. Examination of passive ROM should be performed, as for any infant. The therapist can determine activity limitations by comparing the infant's motor skills such as head control, rolling, sitting balance, transitional movements, crawling, and standing with expected developmental milestones. Very young children with SCI require careful follow-up over time to ensure that they meet functional goals and are not infantilized by caregivers.

Examination of the performance of preschool children with a recent SCI is rarely completed in one session. These children are commonly anxious in the presence of health care professionals. Trust must be established in the child and the parents. This means taking extra time to play and talk with the child and to interact with the parents. Some children are initially fearful of movement, whereas others act fearlessly. In the former case, it will take time to build their confidence. In the latter case, the child may attempt to remove the cervical collar or body jacket or may assume body positions that stress the healing spinal fusion. Thus, additional adult supervision may be necessary to make sure the child complies during the healing phase.

Quantification of changes in body structure and function in the young child is often unreliable because young children are unable to cooperate consistently with formal testing. Passive ROM measurement is possibly an exception to this, but its reliability in children with SCI has not been established. In children without SCI and in children with myelodysplasia, manual muscle testing is generally unreliable if the child is younger than 5 years of age (McDonald et al., 1986; Molnar & Alexander, 1999). In young children, strength testing is often estimated by encouraging and observing movement. Ideally, the therapist places the child in various positions and encourages him or her to reach for toys with a single extremity. This allows examination of gravity-eliminated and antigravity movements, as well as comparison of left and right extremities. Resistance can be provided with small wrap weights (0.25 lb) or the weight of handheld toys. In reality, the best choice may be for the physical therapist to observe spontaneous play and record descriptions of available movements. The physical therapist also facilitates the child's basic postural responses, such as positive support of the lower extremities or protective extension of the upper extremities. Ruling out substitutions can be challenging. Muscle strength is recorded as 0 through 5, as with adults (rarely with the finer + or − gradations). Scores of 4 and 5 are subjective measures, particularly in growing children, but with experience, the therapist can become a more accurate evaluator.

Cardiorespiratory endurance is commonly diminished in children with recent SCI but is difficult to quantify because they cannot complete the available standardized tests requiring walking or running (see Chapter 8). Therapists can make clinical estimates of endurance by recording the length of time a child can engage in an activity or the number of repetitions of a movement completed before the child needs to rest. Accurate recording of these data can be used to document changes in endurance over time.

Both the Functional Independence Measure for Children (WeeFIM) (Granger et al., 1988; Ottenbacher et al., 1996) and the Pediatric Evaluation of Disability Inventory (PEDI) (Haley et al., 1992; Nichols et al., 1996) are used as measures of functional skills for children with SCI. Regardless of which assessment tools are used, the physical therapist must establish a complete baseline of the child's abilities and activity and determine whether limitations are due to the child's age, primary neurologic changes in body function, secondary changes in body functions such as contractures, the need to wear a spinal orthosis, or other causes. Any standard physical therapy examination includes testing of the child's ability to reach, roll, position in bed, come to sitting, balance in sitting, scoot, crawl, transfer, come to kneel, stand, and ambulate. Some or all of these may not be possible, so the type and amount of assistance needed are recorded, or the therapist may simply record the movement as "unable."

Physical therapists should include parents as active participants during the examination phase. Parents need to receive accurate, understandable information about their child's condition. Because they are trying to adapt to the sudden change in their child's health, they often are unable to generate therapy outcomes for their child beyond wanting the child "to walk again." The therapist and SCI team must assist the family and child in establishing realistic outcomes. One must consider the child's level of injury (see Tables 23-4 and 23-5), the completeness of injury, the age of the child, and the family's expectations for the child. If the wearing of a spinal orthosis limits some activities, some goals may need to be postponed until it is removed, which may be after discharge from inpatient rehabilitation.

INTERVENTIONS FOR IMPAIRMENTS AND ACTIVITY LIMITATIONS

The child's anxiety with strangers and fear of movement often persist beyond the examination phase and affect treatment. The physical therapist should start with brief sessions that have low demand and high success and then gradually increase the duration and expectations of the therapy sessions. The therapist can provide predictability and promote trust by establishing routines for scheduling, treatment session locations, and safe play space, and whenever possible should give the child choices regarding play activities.

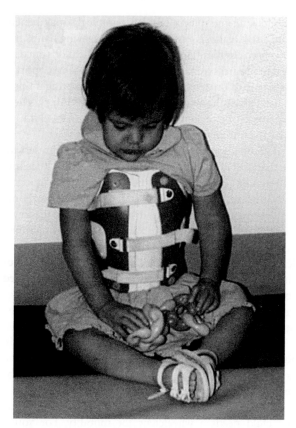

⬩ Figure 23-3   A soft orthosis provides external support, improving sitting balance and allowing this child with a high thoracic spinal cord injury to use both hands in play.

Parents should be included in treatment sessions whenever possible. Although many children work better in therapy sessions in the absence of parents, parents should be regularly included to see the new skills their child can independently accomplish and the emerging skills that require assistance. Parents must become experts in all aspects of their child's mobility and use of adaptive equipment. Parent education and training should be an ongoing process that begins soon after the initial examination and is completed in time for practice on day or overnight outings.

During physical therapy sessions with the child, it is nearly impossible to do isolated treatment of impairments, with the exception of ROM activities. The child's motivation for play gives overall structure for the sessions. Within that, the therapist designs activities that encourage strengthening, balance, reaching, rolling, sitting, transitions, and mobility in various combinations.

Sitting balance is often one of the major goals of therapy. Balance is impaired by altered strength and sensation and often by the presence of a spinal orthosis. Conversely, a child with tetraplegia or high paraplegia may benefit from a soft orthosis to facilitate sitting, leaving hands free for other activities (Fig. 23-3). The seated child is encouraged to progress from therapist support to self-support at a table top or on a mat and to independent sitting if this is realistic given the level and completeness of injury. These goals may be achieved by distracting the child or engaging the child in play activities.

If some lower extremity function has been preserved, the therapist helps children progress to crawling, kneeling, and standing activities when the functioning lower extremity muscles can be appropriately strengthened. Some children require orthoses for distal weakness in the lower extremities. Table 23-5 outlines the expected functional ambulation by level of SCI. Preschool-age children can learn to use reciprocating gait orthoses and KAFOs, but they generally rely on a front-wheeled walker, as opposed to crutches, until age 7 to 8 years. Further discussion of gait training and use of orthoses is presented in the section on school-age and adolescent children.

Orthoses may also be needed by children to maintain ROM in the hands or at the ankles when muscle function is absent. As with any insensate area, the skin must be regularly examined to avoid pressure ulcers.

If community ambulation is not an expected outcome, the child needs a wheelchair for mobility. For young children with SCI at or above C6, a power wheelchair is needed for independent mobility. Some young children with lower levels of cervical SCI, or even high thoracic injuries, may be able to propel a manual wheelchair for only limited distances on smooth, level surfaces owing to lack of upper body strength and endurance. For these children to be exposed to a broader range of environments, such as preschool playgrounds or uneven or steep terrain around the family home, prescription of a power wheelchair is justifiable to promote age-appropriate functional mobility. A child as young as 18 to 24 months may be trained to use a power wheelchair but requires adult supervision for safety. In addition, a manual wheelchair is necessary to provide these children with a substitute when the power chair needs repairs. The manual wheelchair is also useful for transport in places where the larger, heavier power chair is impractical. Many families do not have a home with hallways or doors large enough to accommodate a power wheelchair, so a power wheelchair may be used primarily in community and school settings and the manual wheelchair is used in the home.

The seating components of either a power or manual wheelchair are prescribed with skin protection and spinal alignment in mind (see Chapter 33 for additional information). A level pelvis avoids undue pressure over the ischial tuberosities and facilitates a straight spine (Hobson & Tooms, 1992). A solid seat and back are preferred to sling upholstery in this age group. Several types of wheelchair cushions are available, but none is universally effective for all persons with SCI, and individual assessment is required to prevent pressure ulcers (Garber & Dylerly, 1991). Children who use a wheelchair and their parents must be trained to complete transfers. Children younger than 4 years often lack the upper body strength to transfer independently and typically require a one-person lift transfer. Use of a sliding board or pivot transfer is appropriate for older children (5 to 7 years). Pressure-relief techniques must also be taught. Younger children often rely on caregivers for tilt-back pressure relief. Older children may be able to complete one of the techniques independently, depending on the level and completeness of injury (see Table 23-4).

PREVENTION OF SECONDARY IMPAIRMENTS

As discussed in the section on medical management, a number of secondary impairments can arise after SCI. Many of these can lead to activity limitations and participation restrictions. Physical therapists contribute to prevention, treatment, and monitoring of pressure ulcers, contractures, edema, spasticity, pathologic fractures, and scoliosis. Pressure ulcers occur as a result of improper positioning or inadequate pressure relief and can limit ability to sit. Very young children may not need frequent pressure relief because body weight is not great enough to impair tissue blood flow and they are often held and handled frequently enough that they do not remain in one position too long. As children grow older, however, it is often difficult for them to understand the importance of routine pressure-relief activities.

Contractures can arise as a result of static positioning, spasticity, or heterotopic bone formation and may interfere with positioning or voluntary movement. Hip subluxation and dislocation are common in children who have onset of SCI before age 5, so stretching of hip adductors and hip flexors is important. Dependent edema is more common in children with flaccid lower extremities. When it develops, it predisposes skin to breakdown by increasing fragility and by altering the fit of garments and braces. Spasticity may be present and cause no activity limitations, or it may impair positioning, transfers, or other voluntary movements. Conversely, spasticity may be helpful for those with incomplete SCI who use it to achieve or maintain standing. Pathologic fractures can occur to osteopenic extremities as a result of improper transfers, falls, or forceful ROM exercises. No treatment, including passive standing and electrical stimulation, has yet been found to reverse osteopenia in paralyzed extremities, so the presence of osteopenia and the risk of pathologic fractures should be assumed for all children with SCI, even for those with spasticity. Research using functional electrical stimulation (FES) to prevent osteopenia after acute SCI in adults appears promising, but protocols have yet to be developed for this use, and it is not known if the benefits are lasting (Jacobs & Nash, 2001). Scoliosis occurs in virtually all children with SCI in this age group and can affect comfortable seating and respiratory function. Although it is important to provide proper pelvic alignment and trunk support in wheelchairs, external devices do not prevent the ultimate development of scoliosis, and many children require treatment with bracing and then spinal fusion after they have achieved the majority of their expected height. Both braces and spinal fusion can dramatically reduce trunk mobility, so it becomes imperative to maximize passive hip ROM in children with SCI.

Although family training and positioning needs are initially managed or determined by inpatient physical therapists, outpatient and school physical therapists have an important role in monitoring and maintaining ROM and in using stretching and positioning to minimize spasticity. They monitor and promote the upper body strength that allows the growing child to perform independent pressure relief. They also monitor positioning in seating devices and the fit of adaptive equipment, including wheelchairs and orthoses.

MAXIMIZING ACTIVITY AND PARTICIPATION

While hospitalized, the child must practice mobility skills outside the structured therapy sessions. Thus children must be encouraged to partially or fully self-propel during daily activities. Family and other team members must be familiar with each child's skills and routines to maximize the child's independence across settings and activities. For instance, nurses should be updated on progress in mobility skills so that the child can be encouraged to incorporate these abilities into play activities or getting to meals.

The child must eventually be trained in using these new skills in the community. Community reentry activities are often the combined responsibility of physical therapists, occupational therapists, and therapeutic recreation specialists. Children must become familiar with common architectural barriers such as curbs, heavy doors, and high shelves and learn how to negotiate them or ask for help. Caregivers need to be trained in the type and amount of assistance to provide and cautioned against being overly helpful. Discharge planning and long-term management

should address mobility issues in the child's home, school, and community. Whenever possible, a home evaluation should be conducted early in the child's hospital stay. If home modifications are necessary for wheelchair accessibility or safety, the family needs time to gather financial resources and complete modifications. These modifications can be evaluated during weekend passes. Public schools employ physical and occupational therapists who can provide accessibility information while the child is still hospitalized. Upon school entry, the child can be assisted with accommodations under the provisions of Section 504 of the Vocational Rehabilitation Act of 1973. The therapist plays a major role as a consultant to the faculty, family, and student regarding accessibility issues and needed modifications to architectural barriers or curriculum. For children living great distances from the hospital, physical therapists in the school can provide a local perspective and become a resource to the family. Another area of concern in community reentry is safe transportation. The physical therapist can assist the family with evaluating safe transportation of their child. If a van will be used, wheelchair tie-downs will be necessary. If the child can sit in a vehicle seat, appropriate car seats, booster seats, or restraints are needed, depending on the child's age and amount of trunk and neck control.

ONGOING MONITORING

The key to ensuring maximal participation in young children with SCI is to provide ongoing examination of impairments and activity and to regularly update expected outcomes that are appropriate. At least two mechanisms are available to accomplish this objective. Children who are discharged from rehabilitation centers are routinely seen in follow-up visits two or more times each year. These reevaluations include medical follow-up to reexamine the level and completeness of injury, to evaluate changes in bladder and bowel function and skin integrity, to monitor the spine for development of scoliosis, and to determine the need for medications to treat spasticity or bladder or bowel incontinence.

Reexamination by the physical therapist is an important part of these follow-up visits. For children who have developed sufficient upper extremity strength, a standard push-up for pressure relief in the wheelchair may be taught, and children should learn to check their skin each day. These children are often gaining more independence in self-propelling outdoors and on inclines. They may need instruction and training to participate more in transfers. The child's wheelchair should be reassessed and adapted as needed to accommodate the child's growth and to ensure that any modifications enhance independence.

The physical therapy reexaminations at the rehabilitation facility follow a consultative model. The ongoing progress toward age-appropriate outcomes may occur in a hospital-based outpatient therapy program, but it is more typically accomplished through therapy services offered in early intervention programs or in publicly funded developmental preschools. Therapists in these programs ideally are in contact with the rehabilitation centers on a regular basis to update progress and goals and to identify new concerns and equipment needs.

A small number of children with SCI may actually experience more activity limitations over time. These are usually children with SCI caused by progressive or metastatic tumor. It can be unsettling and challenging for rehabilitation professionals to care for such patients, but it is an important aspect of their work. Often such children need more assistive devices over time, such as more bracing or a wheelchair with more supportive seating. These children can often be very ill from ongoing chemotherapy or radiation treatments, and it may be more practical to rent equipment than to purchase it. Coordination of efforts among oncology and rehabilitation staff, the patient, and the family is crucial.

THE SCHOOL-AGE CHILD AND ADOLESCENT WITH SPINAL CORD INJURY

PHYSICAL THERAPY EXAMINATION

The examination of older children is usually more straightforward than that of preschoolers, toddlers, or infants and can be conducted as for an adult. ROM measurements and manual muscle testing are completed. As previously noted, endurance testing is limited because standardized testing requires lower extremity function. Research is needed in this area, particularly in standardization of upper extremity ergometry. The same basic mobility skills must be assessed as with younger children, that is, rolling, coming to sit, sitting balance, transfers, and locomotion. Functional examination may include the PEDI or Functional Independence Measure (FIM) (Hamilton et al., 1987). The FIM measures activity and the amount of assistance needed by patients older than 7 years. It can be used to assess the same categories of function (using the same seven-level scale) as the WeeFIM. The FIM is widely used in national databases of persons with SCI.

Parents may or may not be present during the actual examination. They should be provided with accurate, understandable information, and as previously noted,

families and children in their early crisis phase often need the rehabilitation team to assist them with realistic outcome setting. The therapist must nevertheless keep in mind that these children may be confronting the potential permanence of their condition. The therapist may notice the adolescent being withdrawn or angry or in denial or even enthusiastic to begin therapy. These behaviors may fluctuate and change rapidly. Children who have returned to school may be better able to identify personal goals. Although age plays a smaller role in outcome development, level and completeness of injury must be considered.

INTERVENTIONS FOR IMPAIRMENTS AND ACTIVITY LIMITATIONS

When planning physical therapy sessions, it is important to be sensitive to the child's current emotional status. Treatment session demands can be modified to most appropriately challenge the child. An issue commonly expressed by teenagers is that of not being able to trust their bodies. The altered motor and sensory processes and potential changes in bowel and bladder function can make their bodies feel foreign to them. In addition, teenagers are accustomed to privacy and independence in their lives. Both their injury and subsequent reliance on a hospital environment and adaptive equipment can disrupt their sense of control. The rehabilitation team should respect their privacy and allow them to participate in scheduling therapy, nursing care, and free time.

Parents need to be included regularly in sessions to observe their child's progress and receive updated training for transfers, wheelchair mobility, pressure relief, use of orthoses, and ambulation. It can be helpful to allow close friends to observe therapy and attend outings. If friends feel comfortable with the injured adolescent, their presence may help lessen social isolation.

Treatment sessions are more structured with older children than with younger children. The first step is to get the child upright and out of bed. If orthostatic hypotension is a problem, this process may require several sessions and use of a wheelchair with a reclinable back to allow the child to gradually assume a fully upright posture. Protocols for remobilizing the newly injured older child or teenager with SCI often use a tilt table to gradually elevate the child's head, although use of this tactic has not yet been proved to hasten resolution of orthostatic hypotension. Other useful measures include support stockings, wrapping the legs with Ace bandages, and using abdominal binders to deter venous pooling. In addition, the therapist should be alert for any complaints of headaches that may signal autonomic dysreflexia, a problem described in the section on medical management. The therapist should monitor heart rate and blood pressure and, when appropriate, alert the medical staff.

Teenagers are familiar with the concept of exercise, so they can participate in progressive resistive exercises beginning with powder board and progressing to weight lifting. All innervated musculature must be strengthened, including muscles that have normal grade 5 strength because they will need to compensate for weakened or paralyzed muscles. Full ROM at the shoulders must be maintained for ease of dressing. Patients with tetraplegia who have wrist extension but no hand function should be allowed to develop mild finger flexor tightness. This provides a tenodesis grasp, which occurs with wrist extension. Stretching the hamstrings to allow 100° to 110° of hip flexion and having adequate hip external rotation is necessary for dressing and self-care. It is important to have excessively flexible hamstrings to prevent overstretching of the low back. Maintaining a tight low back is crucial for transfers and bed mobility to ensure that head and shoulder movements maximally effect lower body mobility. Ankle ROM must be maintained at neutral for proper placement on the wheelchair footrest.

A small number of children with tetraplegia have upper cervical injuries (C1-C3) that necessitate mechanical ventilation (see Chapter 26). Physical therapy intervention for these children and for those with C4 tetraplegia has a more narrowed focus, because the child is dependent with bed mobility, transfers, and sitting balance (see Table 23-4). Spasticity tends to be more problematic with this population, although daily passive ROM can help reduce tone and facilitate positioning. The family must be thoroughly trained in all aspects of the child's mobility and care, and the child must be trained to instruct others in his or her care, including use and maintenance of the wheelchair and any other equipment. Caregivers need to learn pivot transfers and use of a mechanical lift. The child will need a power and a manual wheelchair. The wheelchairs must be ordered as soon as possible, but it is likely that they will not arrive before discharge, so rental wheelchairs may be necessary. Environmental controls and a more complex power wheelchair are needed for independent mobility. The joystick is replaced with head, tongue, or sip-and-puff controls, and the power tilt must allow for ventilator placement. The manual wheelchair should have tilt-in-space capability as well. All wheelchairs and environmental control systems should be chosen by the rehabilitation team, child, and family in consultation with a knowledgeable vendor (see Chapter 33). The therapist should be aware of available funding for wheelchairs and other durable medical equipment. There may be limitations in coverage, and the therapist can assist the family in prioritizing equipment needs.

For children and teenagers with C5 or lower tetraplegia, the focus of physical therapy is on maintaining ROM, upper extremity strengthening, bed mobility, sitting balance, transfer training, and the ordering and training in use of adaptive equipment. Those with tetraplegia at C5 and C6 or above (and even some at C7) need a power wheelchair in addition to a manual wheelchair. Pressure relief may be accomplished by lateral or forward weight shift. Those without adequate trunk control for weight shifting will need the addition of a power tilt-in-space feature on the wheelchair. Ordering the appropriate wheelchair can be challenging because approximately half these children have incomplete injuries and the extent of their recovery may not be clear for months.

For children with paraplegia, transfer training initially includes sliding board transfers. Push-up blocks can also be helpful when first learning transfers (see Fig. 23-1). As upper extremity strength increases, the child may be able to transfer without a sliding board. Older children must also practice car transfers and how to get up from and down to the floor with and without assistance. Wheelchair mobility must be practiced on even and uneven terrain and up and down ramps and curbs. Wheelies can be taught at about age 8 years to facilitate managing curbs and uneven terrain. Pressure-relief techniques must also be taught (see Table 23-4). The child with paraplegia can lift the buttocks off the seat for 20 to 60 seconds two or three times an hour. If the child with paraplegia is not able to ambulate long distances, a manual wheelchair should be prescribed. Lightweight components should be used, and if it is anticipated that the child will be very active or frequently traverse rough terrain, a rigid frame, as opposed to a folding frame, is more appropriate. If the teenager has completed most of his or her growth and has a low thoracic or lumbar level SCI, a low sling back with a taut sling seat may be used in place of the solid seat and back.

For teenagers with incomplete SCI with preserved or recovered lower extremity function, ambulation may be a realistic outcome. Often, an orthosis is needed (see Table 23-5). Donning and removing orthoses must be practiced, as well as controlled sit-to-stand maneuvers and finding the balance point in standing. As with most ambulation training, practice begins in the parallel bars and progresses to use of other assistive devices when the child gains enough control. Body weight supported treadmill training is currently being studied in adults with incomplete SCI. Cases reported in the literature suggest that the technique can result in improvements in ambulation on static surfaces (Behrman & Harkema, 2000). Ambulation is most practical for those who have at least grade 3 strength in one set of quadriceps muscles. At higher injury levels, the child requires KAFOs and some type of upper extremity assistive device. A four-point gait is possible for those with strong hip flexors or with the use of reciprocating gait orthoses. The swing-through gait pattern is, however, much more efficient. Five to 12 times as much energy is expended walking with KAFOs compared with that required for normal gait on even terrain (Jaeger et al., 1989). Numerous follow-up studies of adults have found that more than half of patients who have reciprocating gait orthoses (RGOs) or KAFOs prescribed do not use them at all in the long term, and the majority of the rest of patients use them only for standing or exercise (Jaeger et al., 1989). The most common reasons for discontinuing use of the braces are the excessive energy costs and the need for assistance to don and remove them for ambulation. Given the significant expense of brace manufacture and ambulation training, it is often best to complete initial rehabilitation outcomes and master independent wheelchair mobility before ordering braces. Periodic reexamination of the child's physical abilities and outcomes as an outpatient can then be used to determine whether ambulation with braces is a reasonable goal. Many patients become less interested over time in ambulation requiring extensive bracing as the permanence of the injury becomes more apparent. Those who remain interested may have more specific needs for standing or limited walking that increase the likelihood of long-term use of the orthoses.

FUNCTIONAL ELECTRICAL STIMULATION

Functional electrical stimulation (FES) has been applied in many areas in SCI, including muscle strengthening, cardiovascular conditioning, ambulation, and hand function. In all of these areas, research continues into the effectiveness, efficiency, and long-term outcome of FES. With all uses of FES, it is important that there be realistic expectations by the family and child.

FES for strengthening is useful only in cases of upper motoneuron paralysis in which the intact peripheral nerve is stimulated, causing muscle contraction. In lower motoneuron injuries to the cauda equina, the peripheral nerve, and its muscular branches undergo Wallerian degeneration, so the muscle must be stimulated directly, and larger pulse widths and current amplitudes are necessary to produce contractions. The whole muscle must be flooded with current, and the contraction response is often inadequate. The stimulation parameters can be painful in those who have some preservation of sensation.

FES has been used as a strengthening modality for partially paralyzed muscles. In crossover studies of FES-assisted exercise versus conventional resistive exercise, no significant increases in maximal strength have been found with use of FES (Seeger et al., 1989). However, FES-assisted exercise has been found to be more effective than upper extremity ergometry for strengthening the triceps muscles (Needham-Shropshire et al., 1997). FES does improve strength, muscle mass, and endurance of totally paralyzed muscles and can improve aerobic capacity. Because degenerative joint disease of the shoulder is a significant problem for aging persons with SCI, one advantage of FES over conventional exercise as an aerobic training strategy is that more muscle groups are exercised, placing less stress on the upper extremities (Jacobs & Nash, 2001).

Exercise must be performed regularly to maintain positive effects. Home bicycle ergometer units with FES are now available, but follow-up studies have shown that patients with SCI are often too busy to use this expensive equipment on a regular and long-term basis (Sipski et al., 1993). In patients who do exercise consistently, increase of muscle bulk occurs concomitantly with increase of strength in paralyzed muscles. In addition, blood flow to muscles is increased during stimulation, and the combination of increased bulk and improved circulatory flow may help prevent pressure ulcers. When used after recent SCI, FES may delay bone loss (Rodgers et al., 1991). Researchers and clinicians hoped that FES could help reverse osteopenia after chronic SCI, but to date, none of the protocols used, including those combined with ambulation, has been shown to restore bone mass. FES may actually be dangerous in those with the most severe osteopenia because it may cause pathologic fractures. Complications reported with FES exercise and ambulation include fractures or joint dislocation in persons with severe spasticity, autonomic dysreflexia, postexercise hypotension, and skin burns from electrodes (Jacobs & Nash, 2001).

FES has also been applied to facilitate standing and walking after SCI. Surface, percutaneous, or implanted electrodes are used to deliver current to lower extremity nerves innervating muscles such as the quadriceps and gluteals. The development of sensors to determine leg position, force, acceleration, and muscle fatigue has lagged behind progress in stimulation but is necessary to improve the quality and efficiency of movement. None of the currently available technologic methods permits standing or walking without upper extremity assistive devices. Hybrid systems using FES and orthoses have also been developed, and less expensive garments with surface electrodes sewn into them for easier application are available. The energy costs of walking with FES are comparable to those of using KAFOs but may be slightly reduced when FES is combined with reciprocating gait orthoses (Hirokawa et al., 1990; Yarkony et al., 1992). At present, this technology remains imperfect, expensive, and not widely available. Data on long-term use other than in a limited number of research subjects have not been published.

FES has been used in patients with tetraplegia to improve or restore hand function. For adolescents with C5 and C6 tetraplegia who are skeletally mature and who lack grasp and release, surgical reconstruction at the forearm and hand in conjunction with implanted electrodes can provide palmar and lateral grasp. An external unit is worn and small shoulder movements control hand movements. This may allow the child to perform activities such as basic hygiene, eating, and writing more independently and without the use of an orthosis (Mulcahey et al., 1997). As with other complex technologies, subjects have had variable patterns of long-term use because they need to rely on others to don the stimulator (Mulcahey et al., 1993).

PREVENTION OF SECONDARY IMPAIRMENTS

The secondary impairments facing older children and adolescents with SCI are similar to those for younger children, with a few additions. In this older age group, cardiovascular fitness and overuse syndromes are important to consider. Studies of adults with chronic SCI have shown that physical work capacity inversely correlates with lesion level and that cardiovascular responses to exercise are abnormal because of a deficient sympathetic nervous system (Schmid et al., 1998). Such persons may be at increased risk for cardiovascular compromise and disease. Clinicians should encourage regular aerobic exercise in older children and young adults with SCI to help them develop lifelong habits of health promotion. School therapists can facilitate participation in an adaptive physical education program, community-based recreational programs for people with disabilities, or competitive wheelchair sports. Stotts (1986) found that athletes with paraplegia were less likely to incur avoidable medical complications than nonathletes with paraplegia. Consideration of such participation must be balanced against the recognized propensity for overuse syndromes in these athletes, including such problems as carpal tunnel syndrome, tendonitis, rotator cuff impingement, and degenerative disease of shoulder joints. Patients with tetraplegia and wheelchair athletes at any level have a high incidence of impingement syndrome and rotator cuff tears. An imbalance of strength at the shoulder with relative weakness of humeral head depressors may be contributory, and patients should engage in a program of balanced shoulder exercises (Curtis et al., 1999).

MAXIMIZING ACTIVITY AND PARTICIPATION

Getting into the community as soon as is feasible is important for older children and adolescents with SCI. As is the case with younger children, outings are practice sessions for return to the community. In addition to the usual home and school assessments, the complex issue of transportation must be addressed. The teenager's friends may need to be trained in car transfers so that he or she can stay socially active. The teenager returning to driving needs to be independent with transfers and with loading and unloading the wheelchair. Above all, teenagers should be encouraged to problem solve the management of architectural barriers and ask for assistance if safety is jeopardized. On return to the community, the teenager's primary resource for mobility and seating issues is the school therapist. Some teenagers, especially those with higher levels of injury, may benefit from use of animal aids, such as dogs trained by the program Canine Companions for Independence (P.O. Box 446, Santa Rosa, CA 95402).

ONGOING MONITORING AND TRANSITION TO ADULTHOOD

Unlike younger children, school-age children and adolescents with SCI are usually closer to their predicted function for level of injury by the time of discharge from the rehabilitation unit. As mentioned previously, however, neurologic changes may continue for some months; for example, children with C5 complete tetraplegia may develop antigravity wrist extension during the first 8 months after injury, and outpatient or school therapists may need to formulate new goals. In many children, upper body strength of intact muscles continues to improve, enabling smoother transfers or easier wheelchair propulsion up inclines. In general, however, the majority of physical therapy intervention after discharge eventually becomes a consulting and monitoring role; for example, making sure that mobility skills learned in the hospital environment are generalized to the child's home and community, monitoring ROM or spasticity, and updating equipment. Any deterioration in motor strength should be referred for medical evaluation because it may signify development of a syrinx, which is a fluid-filled collection in the spinal cord that can progressively enlarge and compress the cord.

Older children and adolescents require reexamination similar to that of younger children in a rehabilitation center once or twice a year. The focus of these examinations is on medical issues, equipment needs, and efficacy of home or outpatient stretching or exercise programs. For teenagers, such visits should include discussions related to sexuality and reproduction (Lisenmeyer, 2000). Fertility in women is not impaired by spinal cord injury but sexual response and orgasm may be. Pregnant women with SCI should be managed at high-risk centers to avoid respiratory and urinary tract complications, detect threatened preterm births, and prevent autonomic dysreflexia during delivery. Although the majority of males with SCI can have erections, these are often fleeting and not adequate for vaginal penetration. Few men with SCI have ejaculations, and sperm quality decreases over time for reasons that are not entirely clear. New techniques for retrieval of sperm and for artificial insemination have helped some men with SCI to father children. In addition to this physiologic information, it is important to include issues of intimacy and relationships in discussions of sexuality.

We have found that although the majority of young school-age children with SCI receive direct physical and occupational therapy services in school, few adolescents receive such services. The therapist works from a consultant model, using the faculty and student to carry out programs and recommendations. Issues may include supporting the teen to continue with regular pressure releases, stretching and other home programs, and progressing mobility skills to community distances. The physical and occupational therapist should also consult with the faculty and student regarding an appropriate physical education program; modification of classroom and desk setup; and accessibility to lockers, bathroom, and lunchroom. In reality, many adolescents with SCI have no physical education program, face problems of accessibility at school, and report that breakdown of wheelchairs (both power and manual) contributes to absences at school (Massagli et al., 1996). Although completion of education is supported by accommodations and modifications, such supports are more often implemented to enhance the child's participation in classroom activities and are not geared toward competitive performance and productivity. Therapists should assist adolescents in achieving independence with assistive technology for mobility, communication, and environmental control. Skills development in directing and managing human assistants may also be needed (Dudgeon et al, 1997). We have also found that few adolescents with SCI receive educational or vocational counseling beyond selection of classes each term (Massagli et al., 1996). Such students may qualify for transition planning under the Individuals with Disabilities Education Act, Public Law 105-17. School physical therapists might participate in a transition program by assessing functional mobility skills in the community or work-study setting. When the teenager with SCI becomes 18 years of age, she or he is eligible for state vocational counseling services. Such services are often

important sources of funding for vocationally related education or even equipment. The importance of facilitating education and employment is underscored by research showing that life satisfaction of adults with pediatric onset SCI is associated with education, income, satisfaction with employment and social opportunities, but not with level of, age at, or duration of SCI (Vogel et al., 1998).

Three case studies illustrate the application of the principles discussed in this chapter. The first describes the experiences of a child injured as an infant; the second, those of a young school-age child; and the third, those of a teenager.

SUMMARY

Physical therapy for the child with SCI can, at first glance, appear straightforward. Preserving ROM and promoting strength and endurance are the cornerstones for the functional achievement predicted by the level of injury. Yet predicting realistic long-term outcomes and attaining them require respect for the broader and more complex picture. The physical therapist must consider the cause of the injury (progressive versus stable), the completeness of the injury (preserved motor function, sensory function), and the potential for, or presence of, secondary complications (scoliosis, skin breakdown, contractures). The therapist must also be sensitive to the child's age, personal and environmental factors, and the child's ability to meet age-appropriate expectations in the home, school, and community. Unlike adults with SCI, who may be very close to expected levels of independence at discharge from inpatient rehabilitation, children often require years of outpatient therapy to achieve optimal outcomes. Thus, it becomes imperative to provide the child and the family with a team approach, incorporating multiple disciplines and settings to maximize the child's potential for functional independence and participation in life roles.

CASE STUDIES

STACY

This case study demonstrates the physical therapy management of a very young child with complete tetraplegia and highlights the importance of parent education and training. The need to monitor the acquisition of skills is also discussed.

Stacy was injured at 9 months of age. She was an unrestrained passenger in a motor vehicle crash. Although she did not sustain bone injury to the spine, magnetic resonance imaging revealed a C6 to T1 intracord hemorrhage. Formal manual muscle testing could not be conducted because of her age, so gross estimates of muscle strength were made. Shoulder flexion was estimated at grade 4, elbow flexion at grade 3, and elbow extension at grade 2. Wrist extension was estimated at grade 3, with movements of the fingers graded at trace. Her sensory examination was difficult to interpret, but she did not appear to have reliable pinprick in the lowest sacral dermatome. Pinprick in the lower extremities induced triple flexion involuntary responses. She was diagnosed with C5 tetraplegia, ASIA Impairment Scale level A. Even though the key muscles for C6, wrist extensors, were grade 3, the next higher key muscle was not grade 5. Therefore, a level of C5 was assigned.

At her initial physical therapy examination, Stacy had normal passive ROM with the exception of tightness noted at the end range of shoulder flexion and abduction and elbow extension. Functionally, Stacy was unable to roll, and when placed in prone-on-elbows could sustain the position only very briefly. When placed in sitting with full trunk support, she could raise her head to within about 20° of vertical.

After approximately 2 weeks of acute medical care, Stacy was transferred to an inpatient pediatric rehabilitation facility. Considering her age and level of injury, physical therapy interventions and outcomes were targeted at three major areas (Fig. 23-4).

Within approximately 2 weeks, Stacy's caregivers had learned and demonstrated competence in all aspects of her care, and she was discharged to home. At that time, she continued to show good ROM and some increase in using her upper torso musculature. From an activity standpoint, Stacy was able to reach against gravity when lying supine and to assist minimally in rolling herself to the side. When positioned in prone on her elbows, she was able to maintain her head upright intermittently for 1 to 2 minutes. She was unable to roll out of prone into

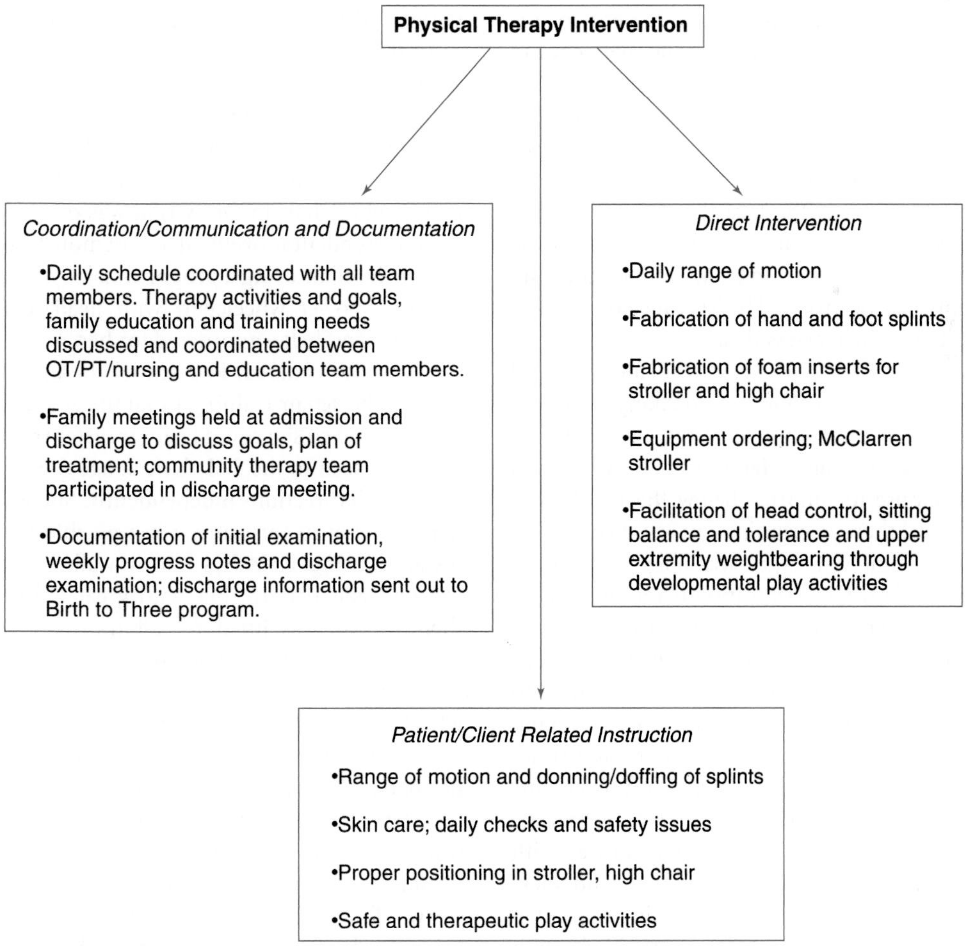

Physical Therapy Intervention

Coordination/Communication and Documentation

•Daily schedule coordinated with all team members. Therapy activities and goals, family education and training needs discussed and coordinated between OT/PT/nursing and education team members.

•Family meetings held at admission and discharge to discuss goals, plan of treatment; community therapy team participated in discharge meeting.

•Documentation of initial examination, weekly progress notes and discharge examination; discharge information sent out to Birth to Three program.

Direct Intervention

•Daily range of motion

•Fabrication of hand and foot splints

•Fabrication of foam inserts for stroller and high chair

•Equipment ordering; McClarren stroller

•Facilitation of head control, sitting balance and tolerance and upper extremity weightbearing through developmental play activities

Patient/Client Related Instruction

•Range of motion and donning/doffing of splints

•Skin care; daily checks and safety issues

•Proper positioning in stroller, high chair

•Safe and therapeutic play activities

◆ **Figure 23-4**   Physical therapy intervention for an infant with C5 tetraplegia.

supine. When in sitting, she was able to prop herself on the upper extremities with some success.

Therapy services were transitioned to a community Birth to Three program, and she began to receive physical therapy and occupational therapy two times per week with a focus on trunk control, upper extremity weight bearing, and the facilitation of developmental milestones.

By 1 year after SCI, her elbow extensor strength had improved to grade 3 and she had a pincer grasp bilaterally but weak finger flexion and no finger extension. She did not show substantial changes in ROM or tone, but demonstrated continued improvement in her functional skills. She was able to move from prone to supine independently. When placed in sitting she could sit but needed to use her hands for support. Stacy was able to move from sitting to prone by moving onto her forearms over her legs. She was able to "commando crawl" 5 to 10 feet by pulling with the upper extremities.

Her family reported two major concerns. The first was whether Stacy would eventually be able to walk with braces. Her prognosis was discussed and the concept of the use of a wheelchair was introduced. Benefits of increasing her strength and increasing her independence in mobility were emphasized. It was also emphasized that the use of the wheelchair would in no way hinder her potential ability to walk someday if she were to have neurologic return of function. The other concern was that of headaches and flushing of the face that the family had noted. This raised the question of autonomic dysreflexia. The family was instructed in taking Stacy's blood pressure when these episodes occurred. The visiting home nurse was also contacted to help assess this.

When Stacy was 2.5 years old, her examination revealed continued gains in finger flexion but no change in finger extension. Formal manual muscle testing was still not possible because of her age. Her sensory examination revealed no response to pinprick below the C7 dermatome. Her physical therapy examination revealed further improvements in function. Stacy was able to independently commando crawl and transition from prone to sit without difficulty. Her sitting balance had improved, and she could reach for and play with toys but needed to keep one hand on the floor for support. She was beginning to scoot backward in sitting and pivot in prone. Her hand strength was notably improved, and overall hand function was better. Owing to her growth and improvements in upper extremity function, a trial use of a manual wheelchair was conducted. Stacy was able to sit well with hip pads and a hip belt on a solid seat with a solid back. She was able to propel only minimally during the initial trial. A wheelchair prescription was provided, with recommendations for a solid seat and back, hip supports

and belt, and a headrest and knee adductors. Over the next months, Stacy learned to self-propel short distances with some difficulty.

By age 3.5, Stacy was receiving physical therapy once a week at school and once a week at a local hospital. Stacy was fitted for a pair of hip-knee-ankle-foot orthoses (HKAFOs) because her parents were very interested in a trial of standing and ambulation. It was explained that with Stacy's level of injury, this would probably only be a therapeutic activity and would not result in independent functional ambulation. Her community therapists provided gait training with the orthoses and a posture control walker. The other issue discussed at the SCI clinic was prescription of a car seat. She had outgrown her car seat but had poor trunk control, necessitating an adapted car seat instead of a standard booster seat.

Stacy returned to the SCI clinic at age 4. Therapy services were unchanged. She was now able to sit briefly without upper extremity support. With moderate to maximal assistance she could walk a short distance with a walker and HKAFOs, employing a swing-through gait pattern. Although Stacy exhibited improving upper extremity function, it was discussed with her family that she would probably not attain enough strength in the upper extremities to keep up with her peers at school or in her rural home setting in a manual wheelchair and that a power wheelchair would be necessary. They agreed, and a power wheelchair mobility trial was done. Stacy enjoyed the independent movement and demonstrated good control of the chair using a proportional joystick with a small knob. A power wheelchair with head, trunk, and hip supports and belt was ordered for her. A wheelchair cushion was also ordered. Her school therapist supervised a power wheelchair training program. A sliding board was also ordered so she could begin transfer training.

When seen in the SCI clinic at age 6, Stacy was able to scoot in all directions independently. She was able to pull herself up onto furniture. She was able to walk a short distance using HKAFOs and a walker using a swing-through gait pattern, but with great effort and only in therapy. She was lifted for all transfers. She used her power wheelchair at school and used her manual wheelchair at home. She was often pushed in her manual wheelchair, as she had difficulty with directionality and endurance when she self-propelled. It was emphasized to her parents that it was important for Stacy to learn to do transfers and to improve her manual wheelchair skills in order to give her more independence.

Stacy was again seen in the clinic at age 7. At this visit, she was finally able to cooperate for formal manual muscle testing and sensory examination. She had grade 5 shoulder flexion and abduction, elbow flexion, and wrist extension and grade 4 elbow extension. Finger flexors were grade 3 and finger abductors grade 2. Grip strength was 1 kg bilaterally. She had intact sensation to C7. Her level of injury was redefined as C7 tetraplegia, ASIA Impairment Scale level A. She was now receiving therapy only at school. She was able to transfer with moderate assistance using the sliding board. She used her HKAFOs infrequently and had become fearful of standing in them. She was able to propel her manual wheelchair only over level indoor surfaces and preferred the power wheelchair for mobility. Adjustments for growth were ordered for her manual wheelchair. It was recommended that therapy continue to focus on transfer training and wheelchair skills. Ambulation training was discussed, and the relative benefits of this for lower extremity ROM and upper extremity exercise were contrasted with the need to develop functional independence in transfers and wheelchair use. It was suggested that Stacy continue to use the orthoses if she was interested and motivated but that the main focus in therapy should be on transfer training and wheelchair skills.

Reflections on practice

Therapists will frequently encounter families who remain hopeful that their child will ambulate. In fact, even limited ambulation may be more practical than using a power wheelchair inside a small home. In helping the family and child set realistic goals and outcomes, the therapist must also keep an eye to the future, to consider the functional environments a child will face in the home, school, community, and ultimately the workplace. The basic skills of transfers, wheelchair mobility, and being able to direct one's own care must be incorporated at appropriate developmental stages. In addition, whereas an adult with C7 tetraplegia would be expected to be independent with transfers and a manual wheelchair, a young child is unlikely to have the upper body strength to perform these tasks and will have greater independence at a young age in a power wheelchair. In the first year after SCI, Stacy would have benefited from the now available soft trunk orthosis (see Fig. 23-3) to facilitate sitting and to free her hands for play.

ALEX

This case study illustrates the acquisition of skills with growth and development in a young school-age child with a spinal cord injury. Medical complications, both in the acute phase and over time, are also discussed because of their impact on function.

Alex was injured in a high-speed motor vehicle crash at age 5. He had an L3-L4 ligamentous tear with right facet dislocation and a right T10 pedicle fracture with cord damage. He was diagnosed with T10 paraplegia, ASIA Impairment Scale level A. He underwent L3-L4 open reduction and internal fixation and fusion, using a right posterior iliac bone graft. He had intestinal injuries and underwent small bowel resection and had a colostomy. A gastrostomy tube was placed several days later to help decompress his stomach. He was fitted with a thoraco-lumbar sacral orthosis with a cutout for his gastrostomy tube and colostomy. Two weeks after injury, Alex was transferred to a pediatric inpatient rehabilitation unit.

It took several sessions to complete tests and measures for the physical therapy examination. The therapist initially scheduled short sessions and spent much of the time playing, developing rapport, and employing strategies that helped decrease Alex's anxiety and improve participation. Upper extremity strength was within normal limits, although endurance for activities was decreased. Straight leg raise was to 50° bilaterally. All other passive ROM was within normal limits. Sensation and movement were absent below the T10 level. There was no lower extremity spasticity. Alex required maximal assistance for all of his mobility, including rolling, getting into and out of sitting, sitting balance, and transfers. He could not self-propel a wheelchair. He frequently complained of stomach pain, and pancreatitis was diagnosed.

Over the next month, Alex adjusted well to the hospital rehabilitation environment. His cooperation and participation improved. Therapy was done in the context of play. Skills were taught starting with small components, and therapy was structured to ensure maximal success. Intervention focused on sitting balance, bed mobility, and transfers. Sliding board, push-up blocks, and leg loops were used to facilitate transfers and bed mobility.

ROM was provided with a focus on hamstring stretching. Alex began learning basic wheelchair skills. Purchase of his own lightweight wheelchair with a pressure-relieving cushion was initiated. Plastic ankle-foot orthoses were fabricated for night wear. After 3.5 months, Alex met the discharge outcomes, which were set based on his age and level of injury, and was discharged home (Box 23-1).

Integration into school was carefully coordinated with his school district. He began half-day kindergarten and received occupational therapy two times per week at school. Physical therapy was initially provided on a consultative basis through the SCI clinic.

Alex was seen 1 year after injury in the clinic. Lower extremity spasticity had developed, and hip flexor tightness was noted. He was referred for outpatient physical therapy for upper extremity strengthening, lower extremity ROM, and more advanced wheelchair skills (Box 23-2).

In the first years after injury, Alex was introduced to adaptive sports, and he became an enthusiastic and

Box 23-1

Box 23-1 **Skills Acquired during Inpatient Rehabilitation at Age 5 in a Patient with T10 Paraplegia**

- Independent bed mobility
- Independent short and long sitting balance
- Independent transfers from wheelchair to bed and back using a sliding board
- Independent push-up pressure releases with reminders
- Self-propel wheelchair over level terrain

Box 23-2 **Skills Acquired from Ages 6 to 9 in a Patient with T10 Paraplegia**

- Independently perform self range of motion
- Perform all transfers without a sliding board independently, including from floor to wheelchair
- Independently assume, maintain, and move in a wheelie position
- Ascend and descend low curbs independently
- Self-propel over mild uneven terrain in a wheelie position
- Ascend and descend mild hills

talented skier, swimmer, and track competitor. Mild hip flexion contractures developed during these years, and scoliosis was diagnosed at age 7.

Three years after injury, Alex expressed interest in a walking trial. This was done over the summer and was an episode of more intense physical therapy at the regional children's hospital. KAFOs were fabricated initially and a pelvic piece was added later. Because of his hip flexion contractures and lower extremity spasticity, he had a difficult time donning the orthotics. He was unable to lock his hips into extension when standing. Thus, while able to walk in the parallel bars, he was unable to independently walk outside of them with a walker. He decided to continue to work on walking with his outpatient physical therapist during the school year. Nine months later, Alex stopped his ambulation attempts because of lack of progress. He asked about the use of FES for ambulation and,

after learning that the current state of technology did not result in functional ambulation, decided to not pursue this. He was discharged from outpatient physical therapy at age 10.

By age 12, wheelchair skills improved to include negotiating steeper inclines and higher curbs. Alex was fully independent in wheelchair mobility with the exception of loading his wheelchair into a vehicle. He competed in sports at the national level. At 12.5 years of age, he developed painful right forearm tendonitis. He used a rental power wheelchair for several months because propelling his manual wheelchair aggravated the tendonitis. Anti-inflammatory drugs were prescribed along with outpatient physical therapy for strengthening. Later that same year at the SCI clinic, he described posterior axillary pain. Examination revealed muscular imbalance with weak external rotators as a likely cause. He was instructed in a home program of strengthening. Hip flexor tightness was worsening despite a program of active stretching and passive stretching using the prone position.

By age 14 his scoliosis had increased to 55°. A posterior spinal fusion was done. Postoperatively, Alex was restricted in his sports activities. At the SCI clinic that year, his hip flexion contractures were found to be increased at –30° on the right and –20° on the left.

Alex was seen again in the SCI clinic at age 15. He was still not very active because of restrictions from his spinal surgery. Hip flexion contractures had increased to –45° on the right and –30° on the left. His right hip was subluxing. The physiatrist discussed hip management options. Alex also complained of upper back pain. Posterior shoulder and scapular strengthening and anterior shoulder stretching to avoid impingement syndrome were reviewed with him by the physical therapist.

Alex was then seen in clinic at age 16 to discuss management of his subluxed hip. Although he was now cleared for sports activities, his lumbar mobility had decreased significantly as a result of the spinal fusion and he could no longer compensate for the limitation in hip extension. Although this did not affect his skiing or track skills, his position in the water changed because his hips were now in a much greater degree of flexion (Fig. 23-5). This caused him to swim more slowly and he sustained a significant loss in his competitive standing.

Reflections on Practice

The need for episodic physical therapy can occur years after initial rehabilitation. The physical therapist must be knowledgeable about typical musculoskeletal problems such as overuse and shoulder impingement syndromes that can occur as a result of a spinal cord injury, paralysis,

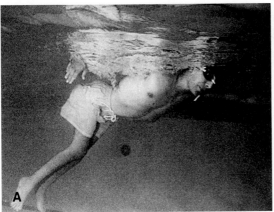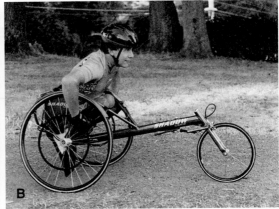

+ **Figure 23-5** Decreased lumbar mobility resulting from back surgery for scoliosis significantly worsens positioning and performance in the water, but has no effect on positioning for track events. **A,** Position in water. **B,** No effect for track.

and resulting wheelchair usage. Wheelchair athletes propel their chairs with shoulders flexed and internally rotated, placing them at increased risk for impingement. They need to actively exercise humeral depressors, especially external rotators. Compared with adults, children who sustain SCI are at risk for unique orthopedic complications that may interfere with achieving maximal function.

ADAM

This case demonstrates the long-term physical therapy management of a teenager with incomplete paraplegia caused by cauda equina injury. This teenager continued to experience long-term functional improvements owing to a combination of neurologic recovery and active strengthening programs. Four years of treatment and follow-up were needed before he reached a plateau of function.

Adam was injured at age 14 when he fell from a tree. He sustained a burst fracture of the L3 vertebra and a complete anterior dislocation of L3 on the L4 vertebra. On the day after his injury, he underwent surgery to reduce the dislocation, and instrumentation was placed across the two vertebrae for stabilization. Postoperatively, Adam was given a thoracolumbosacral orthosis (TLSO) to wear 24 hours a day for the next 3 to 4 months until fusion was complete. Owing to the instability of the initial injury and the short segment of fusion and instrumentation, a thigh piece was added to the TLSO to prevent hip flexion beyond 80° (see Fig. 23-1).

Eight days after his injury, Adam was admitted to a pediatric rehabilitation program. His cauda equina spinal cord injury was classified as L2 paraplegia, ASIA Impairment Scale level B. His impairments included deficits in motor and sensory functioning, loss of voluntary bladder

and bowel control, and orthostatic hypotension. Motor examination, functional skills, and physical therapy intervention are outlined in Table 23-6. Passive range of motion was normal throughout, except straight leg raising was possible to only 30° bilaterally because of posterior thigh pain. His sensory examination to pinprick showed that he had lost normal sensation below the medial femoral condyles and had decreased sensation in the L4 and L5 dermatomes, absent sensation at S1, but preservation of pinprick at S4-S5, perianally. There were no problems with spasticity because cauda equina injuries result in lower motoneuron deficits with flaccid paralysis.

His sitting tolerance was limited by orthostatic hypotension, and he could only sit up with the wheelchair back reclined 45°. From such a position, he could not propel his wheelchair. Support stockings and Ace wraps around his legs were used in conjunction with progressively increasing his upright sitting. His FIM scores were complete independence (7) in communication and social cognition. In self-care, he was completely independent (7) for eating and grooming but needed moderate assistance (3) for bathing, set-up assistance (5) for upper body dressing, maximal assistance (2) for lower body dressing, and total assistance (1) for toileting and bladder and bowel management. For mobility and locomotion, he needed maximal assistance (2) for all transfers and total assistance (1) for locomotion, using a wheelchair. He was unable to ascend stairs.

His activity limitations on admission included lack of independence in bed mobility, transfers, and indoor and community mobility. With his level of injury, realistic long-term outcomes were independence in bed mobility and transfers and ambulation at home and in the community using ankle-foot orthoses (AFOs) and crutches.

TABLE 23-6	Physical Therapy Intervention during Inpatient Rehabilitation for Teen with Cauda Equina Spinal Cord Injury		

DATE	LOWER EXTREMITY STRENGTH		FUNCTIONAL STATUS	PHYSICAL THERAPY INTERVENTION
Admission to rehabilitation unit	Grade 3 hip flexion and knee extension. Grade 0 for all other lower extremity muscles.		Assist needed for bed mobility and transfers. Unable to self-propel wheelchair, stand, or walk.	Direct intervention for bed mobility, transfers, wheelchair skills, and upper/lower extremity strengthening.
One month after SCI	Grade 3+ hip flexion and knee extension. Grade 0 for all other lower extremity muscles.		Independent bed mobility. Transfers with a sliding board. Independent wheelchair mobility. Beginning to stand in parallel bars.	Direct intervention with focus on upper and lower extremity strengthening and gait training. Referred for solid-ankle AFOs.
Four months after SCI: discharge from inpatient rehabilitation program		**Right Left**	Ambulates independently with wheeled walker and AFOs up to 150 ft. Uses wheelchair for long distances.	Direct outpatient intervention for lower extremity strengthening and gait training. School-based consultation for adaptive physical education and mobility in school.
	Hip flexion	4− 4−		
	Hip abduction	0 2		
	Hip extention	1 1		
	Knee extension	4+ 4+		
	Knee flexion	2 2		
	Ankle dorsiflexion	0 1		
	Long toe extensors	0 1		
	Ankle plantar flexion	0 1		

Short-term goals included tolerance to the upright position, improved hamstring ROM to allow long-sitting, improved upper extremity strength and endurance to allow independent transfers and wheelchair propulsion, and lower extremity strengthening of the weakened muscle groups.

After 2 weeks, he had only rare episodes of symptomatic orthostatic hypotension. A lighter-weight wheelchair was substituted for the recliner wheelchair.

One month after admission to rehabilitation, there was minimal change in lower extremity strength, but significant improvement with his functional skills (see Table 23-6). Hamstring ROM continued to be limited owing to complaints of pain with stretching. Upper body strength improved, so that Adam could lift his trunk to do independent pressure relief and could transfer himself without a sliding board to level heights.

Two months after injury, Adam had increased knee extensor strength to grade 4. Solid-ankle AFOs were fabricated, and he began to stand in the parallel bars. Within another month he had adequate standing balance to begin gait training with a walker. He had also begun to get return of hamstring function. Several weeks later he was independently ambulating with a walker and had met all of his inpatient discharge outcomes and so was discharged to home. Functional skills and lower extremity strength at discharge are shown in Table 23-6. He was reclassified as having L2 paraplegia, ASIA Impairment Scale level C. Passive straight leg raising was to 85° bilaterally, and all other passive ROM was normal. Adam's FIM scores had improved to complete independence (7) in all areas of self-care except bathing; to modified independence (6) for bathing and bladder and bowel management; to complete independence (7) in transfers to bed, chair, wheelchair, and toilet; and to modified independence (6) for transfers to the bathtub chair and for locomotion using a wheelchair or ambulating with the walker and AFOs. He needed moderate assistance (4) to ascend stairs.

At reexamination 1 year after SCI, Adam demonstrated improved strength, particularly in knee flexors, hip extensors, and hip abductors. These resulted in improved function, but his classification remained L2 paraplegia, ASIA Impairment Scale level C, because he had weakness in the L4, L5, and S1 key muscles used by the ASIA scale. Adam had discontinued his participation in the outpatient physical therapy program the month before but was continuing to work on stretching and strengthening at home. He demonstrated significant improvements in strength and ambulation skills (Table 23-7). His left AFO was changed to one with a hinged ankle to allow free dorsiflexion but no plantar flexion past neutral to allow motion and the possibility of strengthening these muscle groups while walking. Continued home ROM and strengthening exercises were recommended.

Reexamination 2 years after his SCI demonstrated a grade increase in left hip extension and abduction and a half-grade increase in right hip extension. This additional strength allowed Adam to ambulate without crutches (see Table 23-7). His level of SCI was now L3 paraplegia, ASIA Impairment Scale level C. He needed new AFOs because of wear and tear. He had developed skin breakdown on the lateral border of his left foot and on his right shin from rubbing against the AFO and the Velcro closure. He no longer used his forearm crutches. ROM was well maintained. He was provided with new AFOs and counseled regarding care of insensate skin. Because he was working out in a gym several times a week, specific exercises were recommended for strengthening hip girdle and knee flexor muscles.

At his last examination 4 years after SCI, Adam had shown some improvement in right lower extremity strength of the targeted muscle groups (see Table 23-7). He also demonstrated activity of plantar flexor muscles at the right ankle. Bilateral hinged AFOs with plantar flexion stops were prescribed. Adam was a senior in high school and worked after school in a gas station. He had returned to an outdoor lifestyle, hiking, fishing, and hunting on a regular basis. He planned to enroll in a community college

| **TABLE 23-7** | **Physical Therapy Intervention and Consultation during Outpatient Rehabilitation for Teen with Cauda Equina Spinal Cord Injury** |

DATE	LOWER EXTREMITY STRENGTH			FUNCTIONAL STATUS	PHYSICAL THERAPY INTERVENTION
One year after SCI		**Right**	**Left**	Ambulates with forearm crutches and AFOs using bilateral reciprocal gait pattern. Starting to walk without crutches. Wheelchair . discontinued	Outpatient physical therapy discontinued; instructed in home exercise program. Consultation through rehab clinic. Home exercise program updated at clinic visit. Hinged AFO on left recommended due to increased plantar-flexion strength.
	Hip flexion	4−	4		
	Hip abduction	3−	3		
	Hip extension	2	3		
	Knee extension	5	5		
	Knee flexion	3	4		
	Ankle dorsiflexion	0	2		
	Long toe extensors	0	3		
	Ankle plantar flexion	0	2		
Two years after SCI		**Right**	**Left**	Ambulates without forearm crutches and with AFOs. Works out at a gym several times per week.	Consultation through rehab clinic; instructed in specific exercises for right leg muscles.
	Hip flexion	4	4		
	Hip abduction	3−	4		
	Hip extension	3−	4		
	Knee extension	5	5		
	Knee flexion	3	4		
	Ankle dorsiflexion	0	2		
	Long toe extensors	0	3		
	Ankle plantar flexion	0	3		
Four years after SCI		**Right**	**Left**	Has returned to all preinjury recreational and leisure activities, including hiking, fishing, and hunting.	Consultation through rehab clinic. Recommended hinged AFO on right due to increase in plantar-flexion strength.
	Hip flexion	5	5		
	Hip abduction	4	4		
	Hip extension	3+	4		
	Knee extension	5	5		
	Knee flexion	4	5		
	Ankle dorsiflexion	0	2		
	Long toe extensors	0	3		
	Ankle plantar flexion	2	3		

to study forestry. He was advised of state vocational rehabilitation services available to him and was referred to an adult SCI rehabilitation program for long-term monitoring of renal function and prescription of orthoses.

Reflections on Practice

At various points in his course of recovery, Adam demonstrated functional improvement, sometimes as a result of neurologic improvement and other times as a result of targeted functional skills training, strengthening, and gait training. Comprehensive reexaminations, including precise manual muscle testing, were critical in order to set new goals and implement appropriate interventions to meet these goals.

▌ REFERENCES

American Spinal Injury Association. International Standards for Neurological and Functional Classification of Spinal Cord Injury. Chicago: American Spinal Injury Association, 2000 (reprinted 2002).

Backe, HA, Betz, RR, Mesgarzadeh, M, Beck, T, & Clancy, M. Post-traumatic spinal cord cysts evaluated by magnetic resonance imaging. Paraplegia, 29:607–612, 1991.

Behrman, AL, & Harkema, SJ. Locomotor training after human spinal cord injury: A series of case studies. Physical Therapy, 80:688–700, 2000.

Bohn, D, Armstrong, D, Becker, L, & Humphreys, R. Cervical spine injuries in children. Journal of Trauma, 30:463–469, 1990.

Bosch, PP, Vogt MT, & Ward, WT. Pediatric spinal cord injury without radiographic abnormality (SCIWORA): The absence of occult instability and lack of indication for bracing. Spine, 27:2788–2800, 2002.

Cardenas, DD, Haselkorn, JK, McElliot, JM, & Gnatz, SM. A bibliography of cost-effectiveness practices in physical medicine and rehabilitation: AAPM&R white paper. Archives of Physical Medicine and Rehabilitation, 82:711–719, 2001.

Chen, D, Apple, DF, Hudson, LM, & Bode, R. Medical complications during acute rehabilitation following spinal cord injury—current experiences of the model systems. Archives of Physical Medicine and Rehabilitation, 80:1397–1401, 1999.

Committee on Genetics, American Academy of Pediatrics. Health supervision for children with achondroplasia. Pediatrics, 95:443–451, 1995.

Committee on Genetics, American Academy of Pediatrics. Health supervision for children with Down syndrome. Pediatrics, 107:442–449, 2001.

Curtis, KA, Tyner, TM, Zachary, L, Lentell, G, Brink, D, Didyk, T, Gean, K, Hall, J, Hooper, M, Klos, J, Lesina, S, & Pacillas, B. Effect of a standard exercise protocol on shoulder pain in long-term wheelchair users. Spinal Cord, 37:421–429, 1999.

DeVivo, MJ, Richards, JS, Stover, SL, & Go, BK. Spinal cord injury: rehabilitation adds life to years. Western Journal of Medicine, 154:602–606, 1991.

DeVivo, MJ, & Stover, SL. Long term survival and causes of death. In Stover, SL, DeLisa, JA, & Whiteneck, GG (Eds.). Spinal Cord Injury: Clinical Outcomes from the Model Systems. Gaithersburg, MD: Aspen, 1995, pp. 289–316.

Ditunno, JF, Cohen, ME, Hauck, WW, Jackson, AB, & Sipski, ML. Recovery of upper-extremity strength in complete and incomplete tetraplegia: A multicenter study. Archives of Physical Medicine and Rehabilitation, 81:389–393, 2000.

Dudgeon, BJ, Massagli, TM, & Ross, BW. Educational participation of children with spinal cord injury. American Journal of Occupational Therapy, 51:553–561, 1997.

Fehlings, MG, Sekhon, LHS, & Tator, C. The role and timing of decompression in acute spinal cord injury. Spine, 26:S101–S110, 2001.

Fordyce, WE. Behavioral methods in medical rehabilitation. Neuroscience and Biobehavioral Reviews, 5:391–396, 1981.

Garber, SL, & Dyerly, LR. Wheelchair cushions for persons with spinal cord injury: An update. American Journal of Occupational Therapy, 45:550–554, 1991.

Giovanini, MA, Reier, PJ, Eskin, TA, Wirth, E, & Anderson, DK. Characteristics of human fetal spinal cord grafts in the adult rat spinal cord: Influences of lesion and grafting conditions. Experimental Neurology, 148:523–543, 1997.

Go, BK, DeVivo, MJ, & Richards, JS. The epidemiology of spinal cord injury. In Stover, SL, DeLisa, JA, & Whiteneck, GG (Eds.). Spinal Cord Injury: Clinical Outcomes from the Model Systems. Gaithersburg, MD: Aspen, 1995, pp. 21–25.

Granger, CV, Hamilton, BB, & Kayton, R. Guide for the Use of the Functional Independence Measure for Children (WeeFIM) of the Uniform Data Set for Medical Rehabilitation. Buffalo, NY: State University of New York, Research Foundation, 1988.

Greene, A, Barnett, P, Crossen, J, Sexten, G, Ruzicka, P, & Neuwelt, E. Evaluation of the THINK FIRST For KIDS injury prevention curriculum for primary students. Injury Prevention, 8:257–258, 2002.

Haley, SM, Faas, RM, Coster, WJ, Webster, H, & Gans, BM. Pediatric Evaluation of Disability Inventory. Boston: New England Medical Center, 1992.

Hall, ED. Pharmacological treatment of acute spinal cord injury: How do we build on past success? Journal of Spinal Cord Injury Medicine, 24:142–146, 2001.

Hamilton, BB, Granger, CV, Sherwin, FS, Zielezny, M, & Tashman, JS. A uniform national data system for medical rehabilitation. In Fuhrer, MJ (Ed.). Rehabilitation Outcomes: Analysis and Measurement. Baltimore: Paul H. Brookes, 1987, pp. 137–147.

Hirokawa, S, Grimm, M, Le, T, Solomonow, M, Baratta, RV, Shoji, H, & D'Ambrosia, RD. Energy consumption in paraplegic ambulation using the reciprocating gait orthosis and electric stimulation of the thigh muscles. Archives of Physical Medicine and Rehabilitation, 71:687–694, 1990.

Hobson, DA, & Tooms, RE. Seated lumbar/pelvic alignment. A comparison between spinal cord injured and noninjured groups. Spine, 17:293–298, 1992.

Jacobs, PL, & Nash MS. Modes, benefits, and risks of voluntary and electrically induced exercise in persons with spinal cord injury. Journal of Spinal Cord Injury Medicine, 24:10–18, 2001.

Jaeger, RJ, Yarkony, GM, & Roth, EJ. Rehabilitation technology for standing and walking after spinal cord injury. American Journal of Physical Medicine and Rehabilitation, 68:128–133, 1989.

Kakulas BA. A review of the neuropathology of human spinal cord injury with emphasis on special features. Journal of Spinal Cord Injury Medicine, 22:119–124, 1999.

Kewalramani, LS, Krauss, JF, & Sterling, HM. Acute spinal-cord lesions in a pediatric population: Epidemiological and clinical features. Paraplegia, 18:206–219, 1980.

Lisenmeyer, TA. Sexual function and infertility following spinal cord injury. Physical Medicine and Rehabilitation Clinics of North America, 11:141–156, 2000.

Massagli, TL, Dudgeon, BJ, & Ross, BW. Educational performance and vocational participation after spinal cord injury in childhood. Archives of Physical Medicine and Rehabilitation, 77:995–999, 1996.

Massagli, TL, & Jaffe, KM. Pediatric spinal cord injury: Treatment and outcome. Pediatrician, 17:244–254, 1990.

McDonald, CM, Jaffe, KM, & Shurtleff, DB. Assessment of muscle strength in children with meningomyelocele: Accuracy and stability of measurements over time. Archives of Physical Medicine and Rehabilitation, 67:855–861, 1986.

McDonald JW, Becker D, Sadowsky CL, Jane JA, Conturo TE, Schultz LM. Late recovery following spinal cord injury: Case report and review of the literature. Journal of Neurosurgery (Spine 2), 97:252–265, 2002.

Molnar, GE, & Alexander, MA. History and examination. In Molnar, GE (Ed.). Pediatric Rehabilitation, 3rd ed. Philadelphia: Hanley & Belfus, 1999, pp. 1–12.

Mulcahey, MS, Betz, RR, Smith, BT, Weiss, AA, & Davis, SE. Implanted functional electrical stimulation hand system in adolescents with spinal injuries: An evaluation. Archives of Physical Medicine and Rehabilitation, 78:597–607, 1997.

Mulcahey, MS, Smith, BT, Betz, RR, Triolo, RJ, & Peckham, PH. Functional neuromuscular stimulation: Outcomes in young people with tetraplegia. Journal of the American Paraplegia Society, 17:20–35, 1993.

Murphy, KP, Opitz, JL, Cabanela, ME, & Ebersold, MJ. Cervical fractures and spinal cord injury: Outcome of surgical and nonsurgical management. Mayo Clinic Proceedings, 65:949–959, 1990.

Needham-Shropshire, BM, Broton, JG, Cameron, TL, & Klose, KJ. Improved motor function in tetraplegics following neuromuscular stimulation-assisted arm ergometry. Journal of Spinal Cord Medicine, 20:49–55, 1997.

Nichols, DS, & Case-Smith, J. Reliability and validity of the Pediatric Evaluation of Disability Inventory. Pediatric Physical Therapy, 8:15–24, 1996.

Nobunaga, AI, Go, BK, & Karunas RB. Recent demographic and injury trends in people served by the Model Spinal Cord Injury Care Systems. Archives of Physical Medicine and Rehabilitation, 80:1372–1382, 1999.

Ottenbacher, KJ, Taylor, ET, Msall, ME, Braun, S, Lane, SJ, Granger, CV, Lyons, N, & Duffy, LC. The stability and equivalence reliability of the Functional Independence Measure for children (WeeFIM). Developmental Medicine and Child Neurology, 38:907–916, 1996.

Poynton, AR, O'Farrell, DA, Shannon, F, Murray, P, McManus, F, & Walsh, MG. Sparing of sensation to pin prick predicts recovery of a motor segment after injury to the spinal cord. Journal of Bone and Joint Surgery, 79:952–954, 1997.

Rhoney, DH, Luer, MS, Hughes, M, & Hatton, J. New pharmacological approaches to acute spinal cord injury. Pharmacotherapy, 16:382–392, 1996.

Rodgers, MM, Glaser, RM, Figoni, SF, Hooker SP, Ezenwa, BN, Matthew, T, Suryaprasad AG, & Gupta, SC. Musculoskeletal responses of spinal cord injured individuals to functional neuromuscular stimulation-induced knee extension exercise training. Journal of Rehabilitation Research and Development, 28:19–20, 1991.

Saboe, LA, Darrah, JM, Pain, KS, & Guthrie, J. Early predictors of functional independence 2 years after spinal cord injury. Archives of Physical Medicine and Rehabilitation, 78:644–650, 1997.

Schmid, A, Huonker, M, Barturen, JM, Stahl, F, Schmidt-Truckssass, A, Konig, D, Grathwohl, D, Lehmann, M, & Keul, J. Catecholamines, heart rate, and oxygen uptake during exercise in people with spinal cord injury. Journal of Applied Physiology, 85:635–641, 1998.

Schwab, ME. Molecules inhibiting neurite growth: a minireview. Neurochemical Research, 21:755–761, 1996.

Seeger, BR, Law, D, Creswell, JE, Stern, LM, & Potter, MB. Functional electrical stimulation for upper limb strengthening in traumatic quadriplegia. Archives of Physical Medicine and Rehabilitation, 70:663–667, 1989.

Sipski, ML, Alexander, CJ, & Harris, M. Long term use of computerized bicycle ergometry for spinal cord injured subjects. Archives of Physical Medicine and Rehabilitation, 74:238–241, 1993.

Stotts, KM. Health maintenance: Paraplegia athletes and nonathletes. Archives of Physical Medicine and Rehabilitation, 67:109–114, 1986.

Sugarman, B. Medical complications of spinal cord injury. Quarterly Journal of Medicine, 54:3–18, 1985.

Vogel LC, Klaas SJ, Lubicky JP, & Anderson CJ. Long-term outcomes and life satisfaction of adults who had pediatric spinal cord injuries. Archives of Physical Medicine and Rehabilitation, 79:1496–1503, 1998.

Waters, RL, Adkins, R, Yakura, J, & Vigil, D. Prediction of ambulatory performance based on motor scores derived from standards of the American Spinal Injury Association. Archives of Physical Medicine and Rehabilitation, 75:756–760, 1994.

Wilberger, JE. Spinal Cord Injuries in Children. New York: Futura, 1986.

Wong AMK, Leong C, Su T, Yu S, Tsai W, & Chen CPC. Clinical trial of acupuncture for patients with spinal cord injuries. American Journal of Physical Medicine and Rehabilitation, 82:21–27, 2003.

Wu, L, Marino, R, Herbison, GJ, & Ditunno, JF. Recovery of zero-grade muscles in the zone of partial preservation in motor complete quadriplegia. Archives of Physical Medicine and Rehabilitation, 73:40–43, 1992.

Yarkony, GM, Roth, EJ, Cybulski, G, & Jaeger, RJ. Neuromuscular stimulation in spinal cord injury. I: Restoration of functional movement of the extremities. Archives of Physical Medicine and Rehabilitation, 73:78–86, 1992.

∾

Chapter 24

BRAIN INJURIES:
TRAUMATIC BRAIN INJURIES,
NEAR-DROWNING, AND BRAIN TUMORS

GINETTE A. KERKERING
PT

TRAUMATIC BRAIN INJURY
Incidence
Etiology
Medical and Surgical Management

NEAR-DROWNING
Incidence
Etiology
Medical and Surgical Management

BRAIN TUMORS
Incidence
Types of Pediatric Brain Tumors
Medical and Surgical Management

DIAGNOSTIC TESTS FOR CHILDREN WITH BRAIN INJURIES

COGNITIVE CHANGES IN CHILDREN WITH BRAIN INJURIES
Memory Functioning
Executive Skills
Visuospatial Skills
Language

PHYSICAL THERAPY MANAGEMENT
Examination
Evaluation
Diagnosis and Prognosis
Plan of Care
Intervention
Outcomes
Optimization of Health Status
Prevention

CASE STUDIES

Pediatric physical therapists see a large number of children with central nervous system (CNS) dysfunction. Many of these children have neurologic involvement from birth, but many acquire neurologic insults later in childhood. This chapter will focus on brain injuries acquired by children after birth. Three primary acquired brain injuries are traumatic brain injuries, near-drowning injuries, and brain tumors. Although these three etiologies of brain injury are different and will be discussed as such, physical therapy management of children with acquired brain injury will be discussed as a whole.

It is important to remember that although all three forms of these types of brain injury can occur in the adult population, children will be different in terms of medical management and rehabilitation management. These differences are based on the anatomic and physiologic differences in children as well as developmental milestones achieved before injury.

TRAUMATIC BRAIN INJURY

INCIDENCE

Traumatic brain injury is the leading cause of death and injury-related disability among children and young adults. Among children in the United States ages 0 to 14 years, traumatic brain injury results in an estimated 3000 deaths, 29,000 hospitalizations, and 400,000 emergency department visits (Langlois, 2001). According to the National Pediatric Trauma Registry boys are twice as likely as girls to suffer a traumatic brain injury. Children are especially at risk in the afternoon hours after they have been dismissed from school.

ETIOLOGY

There are numerous mechanisms of traumatic brain injury in the pediatric population. These causes may be differentiated by age. In the infant population, more than two thirds of the injuries sustained are from falls. In the preschool population, the primary injuries sustained are from falls (51%) and motor vehicle accidents (22%). School-age children, from 5 to 9 years, are equally divided among motor vehicle accidents (31%), falls (31%), and sports and recreation-related activities (32%). A greater percentage of sports and recreation injuries (43%) is found among 10- to 14-year-olds (Kraus et al., 1990).

Brain injury that results from closed head injury may be related to both primary and secondary factors. Primary injuries are related to the forces that occur at the time of initial impact. Secondary injuries are related to the systemic response to the primary trauma.

Primary Injuries

Primary injuries, or those injuries related to the forces that occur at the time of initial impact, may be grouped with respect to the role played by acceleration factors. *Acceleration-dependent injuries* are related to the effects that occur when a force is applied to a movable head. These forces may be translational or rotational.

In the case of translational injuries, a vector related to the force applied to the head passes approximately through the head's center of mass. For example, the response to a force applied to the side of the skull is lateral movement of both the skull and the brain. As the skull contacts an immovable object such as the door frame of an automobile, it rapidly decelerates. The brain, however, continues to move laterally until it is stopped by the lateral aspect of the skull. The injury that results from the initial impact of the brain on the skull is translational and is termed a *coup* lesion. The lesion that occurs as the brain reacts secondarily to the initial force against the skull (moving in the opposite direction against the skull on the opposite side) is termed *contrecoup* (Fig. 24-1).

In rotational injuries, the resultant force vector does not pass through the center of mass of the head, and angular acceleration results. *Rotational injury* occurs when the brain remains stationary while the skull rotates. The resultant forces are angular. Rotational injuries have been related to shearing trauma, which may be manifested as brain surface contusions and lacerations (Pang, 1985). Diffuse axonal injuries have also been related to shearing trauma. For most force vectors, the result is not purely translational or rotational but a combination of the two (Fig. 24-2).

Primary injuries can also result from factors not related to acceleration. Brain injury that results from skull depression into brain tissue is one example.

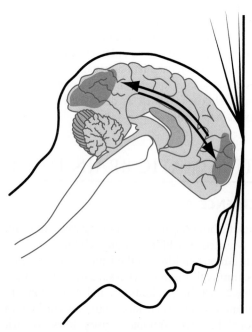

◆ **Figure 24-1**   Mechanism of coup-contrecoup injury.

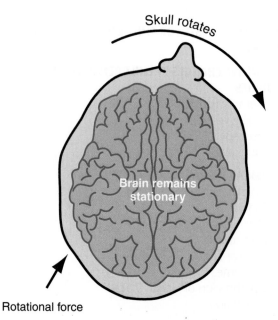

◆ **Figure 24-2**   Mechanism of rotational injury.

Secondary Injuries

Secondary injuries, or those that occur due to processes evoked in response to the initial trauma, account for a significant amount of the overall damage that occurs in traumatic brain injury. Secondary brain injury is a primary determinant of outcome in severe head injury (Wright, 1999).

Epidural hematomas result when the middle meningeal artery, vein, or venous sinus bleeds into the epidural space between the dura and the skull. This usually follows a skull fracture or bending of the skull into the brain. As the skull recoils, the space between the skull and dura may fill with blood, creating the hematoma. The rate of blood collection, and the resultant increase in intracranial pressure, determines the prognosis. The prognosis for rapidly accumulating hematomas is grave. The location of the hematoma also affects outcome, with temporal or posterior fossa hematomas more likely to cause brain shift and brainstem compression than a hematoma in the frontoparietal area (Pang, 1985).

Acute subdural hematomas are related to extensive cortical injury and lacerated cortical vessels. Edema in underlying brain tissue develops rapidly. Acute cerebral hematomas must be removed expediently. Recovery from a subdural hematoma depends on both the time between development and evacuation of the hemorrhage and on the extent of damage to underlying brain tissue.

After traumatic brain injury, cerebral swelling invariably develops from increased cerebral blood volume or cerebral edema (Kochanek et al., 2001). Cerebral edema develops by one of three mechanisms: cellular swelling, blood-brain barrier injury, or osmolar swelling. *Increased intracranial pressure* frequently occurs after brain injury as a result of edema and hematoma. Unchecked cerebral edema and the resultant increase in intracranial pressure can lead to brain herniation, multiple cerebral infarctions, permanent brainstem necrosis, and irreversible coma (Pang, 1985).

Ischemia also plays a role in secondary brain injury. Ischemia may be caused by hypotension, cell sludging, endothelial cell swelling, and compression by edematous tissue (Wright, 1999). These processes decrease the cerebral blood flow, which then results in ischemic brain tissue.

Because of the traumatic nature of these brain injuries, there will frequently be other injuries to assess as well. These other injuries can be fractures, skin abrasions, and internal injuries. At times a child will suffer both a spinal cord injury and a brain injury during a traumatic event.

Shaken Baby Syndrome

A discussion of pediatric traumatic brain injury would not be complete without a description of shaken baby syndrome. Shaken baby syndrome is the most common cause of death or serious neurologic injury resulting from child abuse (Blumenthal, 2002). Shaking is usually in response to prolonged inconsolable crying. The injuries sustained are a result of the combination of the mechanism of the shaking and the unique anatomic features of an infant: a relatively large head with weak neck muscles. In the past, the damage to the infant brain from shaking has been described as diffuse axonal injury or axonal shearing. It has more recently been reported that this diffuse axonal injury is an uncommon sequela of inflicted head injury (Geddes et al., 2001). In cases in which cortical axonal trauma is noted, there is typically an external impact associated with the shaking.

With advances in neuropathology imaging and staining methods, it has been discovered that with violent shaking, the initial brain injury is from hypoxia (Blumenthal, 2002). When an infant is shaken, the pivotal movement of the head on the neck is thought to cause a stretch injury from cervical hyperextension and flexion. This stretch injury occurs at the craniocervical junction and can damage axons in the cortispinal tracts and cervical cord roots. This damage could account for the typically observed period of apnea, which in turn could lead to hypoxic damage and brain swelling (Geddes et al., 2001). Subdural hemorrhages may also be caused by movement of the brain within the subdural space, which stretches and tears the veins that cross the subdural space (Blumenthal, 2002). Other injuries commonly seen in infants with shaken baby syndrome are retinal hemorrhages and skeletal injuries.

MEDICAL AND SURGICAL MANAGEMENT

Children are assessed for level of coma throughout the initial traumatic episode. Level of coma is monitored using criterion-based behavioral scales such as the Glasgow Coma Scale (Teasdale & Jennett, 1974) and the Rancho Los Amigos Scale (Hagen et al., 1979). Both of these scales assess a child's ability to respond to various stimuli ranging from a painful stimulus to a complex verbal command. A child's orientation to time and place is also assessed. An increase in summary score of the Glasgow Coma Scale on successive administrations is an indicator of improvement. The administration of the Rancho Los Amigos Scale results in classification of a child into one of eight cognitive levels. Progression to a numerically higher level is an indicator of progress. The Children's Orientation and Amnesia Test (COAT) (Ewing-Cobbs et al., 1989) is also used to evaluate level of coma in children. Test items of the COAT, particularly those that assess the appropriateness of verbal responses to orientation questions, are based on facts commonly known by children.

Interventions for the child with traumatic brain injury to address the areas of swelling and pressure may include surgery, the use of pharmacologic agents, and the use of mechanical ventilation. All these interventions are aimed at sustaining life and preventing secondary injuries to the brain. Treatment of cerebral swelling and increased intracranial pressure represents the backbone of cerebral resuscitation following traumatic brain injury (Kochanek et al., 2001). Pressure is monitored by an intracranial pressure bolt. Surgical interventions include the evacuation of subdural or intracerebral hematomas. In patients who fail conventional therapy to manage cerebral swelling, decompressive craniectomy has been investigated as a safe method to quickly reduce intracranial hypertension (Guerra et al., 1999).

Several medical complications are commonly found in children who have had a traumatic brain injury. Fever and infection are common responses to trauma. McLean and colleagues (1995) have suggested that children who sustain a traumatic brain injury may have a suppressed immune system as a result of the trauma. Endocrine dysfunctions that can occur after traumatic brain injury in children include diabetes insipidus, syndrome of inappropriate antidiuretic hormone (SIADH), and precocious puberty. Skin and gastrointestinal disorders have also been noted in children who have suffered a traumatic brain injury. Orthopedic complications are generally fractures, including skull fractures, and heterotopic ossification (McLean et al., 1995).

Pediatric patients who sustain a traumatic brain injury are at risk of developing heterotopic ossification (HO), which is pathologic bone formation around a joint in the pericapsular space (Citta-Pietrolungo et al., 1992). It is frequently characterized by pain, decrease in range of motion, and swelling of the joint. The etiology of HO is still unclear, but it has been found to be related to an increase in muscle tone around a joint, immobility, and coma (Citta-Pietrolungo et al., 1992). Research has shown that 3% to 20% of children who sustain a traumatic brain injury may develop HO (Hurvitz et al., 1992; Kluger et al., 2000). A bone scan is the best method of detection of HO. Children who have tremendously increased tone or are in a persistent vegetative state seem to be at the highest risk. (Kluger et al., 2000). As a prophylactic regimen for those children at risk, salicylates are recommended. Baclofen or botulinum toxin may be considered for those children with severe increases in muscle tone (Kluger et al., 2000). Aggressive physical therapy aimed at maintaining range of motion and strength around the joint should be implemented if HO is suspected or diagnosed. Because

some joints with HO may progress to ankyloses, splinting and casting may be necessary in severe cases to maintain the joint in a functional position.

NEAR-DROWNING

INCIDENCE

Drowning is the fourth leading cause of fatal injuries in children between 0 and 19 years of age. The most common age groups affected are children younger than 4 years of age and adolescents (Fields, 1992). In the infant population, 78% of drownings are in bathtubs, and 20% occur in artificial pools or fresh water. Among children 1 to 4 years old, 56% of drownings occur in artificial pools and 26% occur in fresh water. In the older population, 63% of drownings are in bodies of fresh water (Centers for Disease Control, 2003).

Near-drowning has been defined as an episode in which someone survives a period of underwater submersion (Fisher, 1993). Near-drowning may also be referred to as a submersion injury. Survivors may experience cardiac, CNS, or respiratory system complications and may require rehabilitation.

ETIOLOGY

To understand the injuries caused from a near-drowning incident, it is necessary to understand the pathophysiology that occurs with near-drowning. It is hypothesized that in the sequence of drowning, the victim undergoes a period of panic, struggling, and automatic swimming movements. Apnea occurs and water is aspirated. Once the person is unconscious, fluid is passively introduced into the airways (Fields, 1992). Evolving hypoxemia causes neuronal injury and eventually leads to circulatory collapse and myocardial damage and dysfunction of multiple organ systems, with further ischemic brain injury (Ibsen & Koch, 2002).

The most devastating outcome of near-drowning is the sequelae of global hypoxic-ischemic brain injury. During the first few minutes of submersion, the brain is deprived of oxygen, leading to the hypoxic effects. The cardiovascular system subsequently fails, leading to decreased cerebral blood flow and ischemic injury (Ibsen & Koch, 2002).

In general, neuronal cells are not able to tolerate periods of complete ischemia lasting longer than 5 minutes without sustaining permanent injury; irreversible neuronal injury has been demonstrated to increase significantly after 10 minutes (Safar, 1988). The magnitude of the neuronal injury that occurs is also related to both the level of blood flow during the complete ischemic interval and the total duration of the ischemia. Despite numerous studies attempting to predict outcome at initial presentation, no one factor or combination of factors has been identified to reliably predict outcome (Gonzales-Luis et al., 2001; Ibsen & Koch, 2002). Because of this lack of predictability, it has been advocated that resuscitation attempts be made, at least briefly, in all patients who arrive in the emergency department after submersion injury (Ibsen & Koch, 2002).

Traumatic injuries are seldom observed in near-drowning victims. When other injuries are present, they are generally cervical spine injuries and there is typically a clear history of diving (Hwang et al., 2003).

MEDICAL AND SURGICAL MANAGEMENT

Once the patient is in the hospital, medical interventions are focused on supporting respiration and attempting to prevent further neurologic injury. Traditional and high-frequency mechanical ventilation are used to treat acquired respiratory distress syndrome and may indirectly prevent further CNS complications. Extracorporeal membrane oxygenation (ECMO) is a respiratory system intervention in which blood is oxygenated mechanically outside the body, allowing the lungs to "rest." Ventilation is frequently used in conjunction with pharmacologic paralysis of the musculoskeletal system, placing the child at risk for contractures, muscle weakness, and atrophy.

Cardiac function continues to be monitored in the initial phases if persistent myocardial dysfunction occurs after resuscitation. Therapies for the cardiac dysfunction are based on the specific hemodynamics and adequacy of oxygenation found.

Although once advocated, monitoring and treating for changes in intracranial pressure have not been shown to be of benefit for near-drowning victims. Although high intracranial pressures (ICPs) (>20 mm Hg) have been correlated with a poor outcome, low ICPs (<20 mm Hg) have not been correlated with a good outcome (Ibsen & Koch, 2002).

▌ BRAIN TUMORS

INCIDENCE

In the United States, approximately 2200 children and adolescents are diagnosed with malignant CNS tumors each year (Gurney et al., 1999; American Brain Tumor Association, 1998). Over 90% of primary CNS malignan-cies in children are located within the brain (Gurney et al., 1999). Primary CNS tumors are those that originate in the brain rather than tumors that are a result of metastasis to the brain. Young children have a relatively high occurrence of malignancies in the cerebellum and the brainstem. In children younger than 10 years old, brainstem malignancies are nearly as common as cerebral tumors. Cerebellar malignancies are far more common than cerebral malignancies (Gurney et al., 1999).

TYPES OF PEDIATRIC BRAIN TUMORS

Pediatric brain tumors may be generally classified according to their location and their biologic characteristics (Fig. 24-3). The tentorium is a flap of meninges that separates the cerebral hemispheres from the cerebellum in the posterior fossa of the cranium. Pediatric brain tumors are generally classified as being supratentorial or infratentorial (see Fig. 24-3).

Infratentorial Tumors

Infratentorial tumors occur in the posterior fossa, which is below the tentorium cerebelli, and contains the cerebellum, the brainstem, and the fourth ventricle. About half of all pediatric brain tumors occur in this area.

Three of the most common cerebellar tumors that occur in childhood are cerebellar astrocytomas, medulloblastomas, and ependymomas. Astrocytomas are usually well circumscribed and may be cystic. Cerebellar astrocytomas represent about 15% of pediatric brain tumors (American Brain Tumor Association, 1998). Ten-year survival rates range from 29% to 96%, depending on tumor subtypes (Menkes & Till, 1990). Medulloblastomas infiltrate the floor or lateral wall of the fourth ventricle and extend into its cavity. These are fast-growing tumors and they may spread throughout the CNS via cerebrospinal fluid. Medulloblastomas represent 15% to 20% of childhood brain tumors. The prognosis for medulloblastomas is variable according to subtype. Infratentorial ependymomas represent about 7% of childhood brain tumors. Ependymomas are found in the infratentorial region about 65% of the time, and represent 10% of all childhood brain tumors. These tumors arise from ependymal cells in the ventricles and spinal column (American Brain Tumor Association, 1998).

Clinical symptoms of posterior fossa tumors are related to increased intracranial pressure and involvement of cerebellar structures. Headaches that are nonlocalized or frontal are an early symptom. Vomiting is the most common sign of cerebellar tumors and may be related to increased intracranial pressure or to direct pressure on the medullary vagal nuclei.

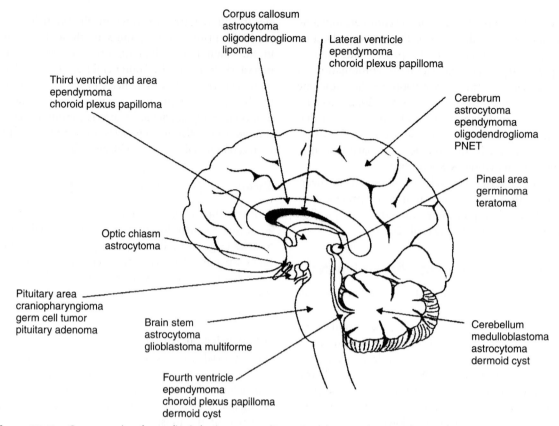

Figure 24-3   Common sites for pediatric brain tumors. *(From American Brain Tumor Association. A Primer of Brain Tumors. Des Plaines, IL: ABTA, 1998, p. 101.)*

Motor signs of cerebellar involvement are ataxia, dysmetria, dysdiadochokinesia, intention tremor, and hypotonia. Hemiplegia and oculomotor signs may be clinical manifestations of cerebellar astrocytoma. When tumors extend into the brainstem, unilateral hearing loss and facial weakness may be found (Epstein & Wisoff, 1987). When the tumor extends rostrally or caudally from the medulla, quadriparesis, neck pain, and torticollis may be present (Epstein & Wisoff, 1987, 1988).

Supratentorial Tumors

These tumors are found in the area above the tentorium cerebelli. The supratentorial region contains the cerebral hemispheres, the lateral ventricles, and the third ventricle.

Craniopharyngiomas, optic tract gliomas, and pineal tumors are examples of tumors that occur in midline brain regions. Clinical signs and symptoms of midline tumors are determined by the tumor's size and location and its relationship to adjacent brain structures. Cranio-pharyngiomas are benign tumors located near the pituitary gland. This tumor causes problems from compression rather than invasion of tissue (American Brain Tumor Association, 1998). Progression of the

tumor is related to symptoms of increasing intracranial pressure, visual complaints, and endocrine disturbances (Epstein & McCleary, 1986; Menkes & Till, 1990). In the case of optic nerve gliomas, visual disturbances are the predominant clinical symptom. Optic nerve gliomas are generally slow-growing astrocytomas. They account for about 4% of childhood brain tumors (American Brain Tumor Association, 1998). Symptoms of pineal tumors are often related to increased intracranial pressure and include headache. The inability to direct eye movement outward bilaterally is sometimes also present.

Examples of cerebral hemisphere tumors are astro-cytomas and ependymomas. Symptoms of increased intracranial pressure are frequently the initial signs and symptoms of cerebral hemisphere tumors. Headache is most typical of these and is often transitory, occurring in the morning or during the night. Vomiting is another common sign of increased intracranial pressure. Although vomiting may occur in conjunction with nausea, it is not usually projectile. It often occurs in the morning and is not related to the child's eating pattern. Seizures are also a common clinical sign of cerebral hemisphere tumors.

MEDICAL AND SURGICAL MANAGEMENT

Medical treatment of pediatric brain tumors includes surgery, radiation therapy, chemotherapy, or a combination of these therapies. The treatment selected depends on the type, location, and characteristics of the tumor and the age of the child. The standard treatment for most pediatric brain tumors is surgery followed by radiation or chemotherapy.

Surgery

Surgical excision of a brain tumor may be performed as a primary treatment or may be performed in conjunction with other treatments such as radiation therapy or chemotherapy. In cases in which full surgical excision of the tumor is not possible, an adjunct therapy such as radiation therapy or chemotherapy is administered in an attempt to eradicate residual tumor cells. When hydrocephalus is present secondary to the obstruction of cerebrospinal fluid by a tumor, surgical intervention may include the placement of a shunt (Cochrane et al., 1994).

Radiation Therapy

Radiation therapy is a common treatment for brain tumors. However, because the brains of young children are so susceptible to radiation damage, generally radiation is not administered to children under the age of 3. Radiation is administered by a radiation beam directed at the tumor as a predetermined dose of energy is administered. This process is repeated on a regular schedule for several days or weeks. Radiation damages the DNA of cells, and as a result radiated tumor cells die while attempting to divide and reproduce. Adjacent cells and physiologic structures are often also affected, which results in various immediate and long-term side effects.

Acute radiation encephalopathy occurs when vascular damage caused by the radiation results in increased vessel wall permeability. Side effects noted in the patient who is undergoing radiation include lethargy, nausea, and vomiting. Neurologic signs that existed before surgical intervention may reappear. Corticosteroids are often administered to treat edema and related symptoms.

Chemotherapy

The aim of chemotherapy is to kill significant numbers of tumor cells in each of the successive administrations of the chemotherapy. Antineoplastic drugs are frequently administered together to act against the tumor cells at different biochemical sites. Chemotherapy is the adjunct treatment of choice if the child is under the age of 3. Frequently chemotherapy will be used in this age group to slow tumor progression until the child is old enough to undergo radiation therapy.

Antineoplastic drugs that affect tumor cells also affect other rapidly growing, normal tissues, such as bone marrow, gastrointestinal epithelium, and hair follicles. The toxic effect of antineoplastic drugs on normal tissues causes the frequently experienced side effects of hair loss, nausea and vomiting, and immune system depression.

Although medical interventions such as surgery, radiation therapy, and chemotherapy are often effective in the treatment of pediatric brain tumors, adjacent brain tissues and structures may be negatively affected.

DIAGNOSTIC TESTS FOR CHILDREN WITH BRAIN INJURIES

Several diagnostic tests are commonly used in children with brain pathology. It is important for the physical therapist to have an understanding of these tests, because this will allow a more complete understanding of the patient's injuries and clinical presentation.

Magnetic resonance imaging (MRI) is a diagnostic tool based on signals emitted by protons when placed in a magnetic field. Different tissues in the body have different proton concentrations, and this difference allows for a clear contrast between tissues. MRI is a frequently used diagnostic tool in the evaluation of pediatric CNS problems. In fact, MRI has been suggested to be superior to other diagnostic tools for this purpose (Gusnard & Zimmerman, 1990). For example, bone artifacts often noted on computed tomography (CT) of the posterior fossa are not a problem with MRI. MRI may also differentiate between benign structures such as a collection of cerebrospinal fluid and malignant masses such as cystic tumors. Additionally, MRI is very sensitive in the detection of blood and is particularly useful in the evaluation of hemorrhage. MRI may also be utilized several days after injury to evaluate hypoxic-ischemic damage from a near-drowning event.

CT is used to show thin slices though the brain on the basis of x-rays. Various planes of sectioning may be chosen by the examiner. CT is most successful in the assessment of areas of calcification, the evaluation of a foreign body in a sensitive location, and the identification of skull and bony abnormalities. CT may also be the evaluative tool of choice at times when a screening must be performed quickly. CT is less costly than MRI, and financial restraints may influence the selection of CT versus MRI diagnostic testing (Fig. 24-4). The role of CT in the early evaluation of a hypoxic-ischemic event is limited (Ibsen & Koch, 2002).

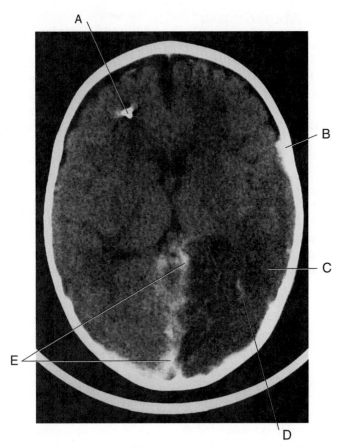

+ **Figure 24-4** Computed tomography scan of a child with a traumatic brain injury sustained in a motor vehicle accident. The left border of the photo is the right hemisphere. Clockwise from the top: **A**, Intracranial pressure bolt placed in the right frontal cortex; **B**, small left subdural hematoma; **C** and **D**, area of ischemia in left parietal, temporal, and occipital lobes; **E**, subarachnoid hemorrhage.

Electroencephalography (EEG) is the recording of brain activity from externally applied electrodes. EEG records waveforms representing brain activity. In a non-stimulated situation, EEG primarily shows slow waves. With an increase in stimulation in the brain, the waveforms become faster with a lower amplitude. The evaluator notes frequency, amplitude, and organization of the waveform. Different neurologic conditions have characteristic encephalographic changes, and EEG plays a primary role in diagnosing seizure disorders.

The visually evoked response (VER) is another electrodiagnostic test used in evaluating brain injuries. This test uses electrical impulses with visual stimuli to detect abnormalities in the visual pathways. A similar test is the brainstem auditory evoked response (BAER). The BAER also uses electrical impulses to determine abnormalities along the auditory pathways and other abnormalities in the brainstem.

COGNITIVE CHANGES IN CHILDREN WITH BRAIN INJURIES

Cognitive processes are essential to motor control, learning, and participation in therapy. Injuries from chemotherapy, radiation, anoxia, and hemorrhage will affect not only a child's motor patterns but also the ability to attend, follow directions, complete complicated motor tasks, and use executive functioning. Although cognitive changes can be functionally screened by a physical therapist, formal testing by a psychologist is critical for a detailed assessment.

MEMORY FUNCTIONING

Memory is evaluated, particularly with respect to the child's ability to learn new material. Although the child may retain and remember material learned before a brain injury, learning new information may be problematic. Difficulties in the area of memory skills pose obvious problems for the child who will be returning to school. Less obvious are the influences of memory deficits on rehabilitative treatment.

The child who demonstrates difficulty learning new material may not progress as quickly as would be expected in learning an exercise program or in achieving independence in functional skills. For example, a child who demonstrates sufficient strength and coordination skills to perform a home exercise program may not be able to achieve the goal of independence in performing the program because of an inability to remember the component parts from one treatment session to the next.

Memory deficits may also be demonstrated by unsafe performance of functional skills. The omission of safety-related behaviors when performing transfers, for example, may limit the functional independence of a child whose balance and coordination skills are sufficient for the performance of the task.

The limiting effect of memory deficits may be particularly frustrating for parents. A change in memory skills may increase the child's level of dependence. Such an apparent developmental regression may be perceived by a parent as the child's unwillingness to "try hard" or as a behavior problem that is within the child's control to change. The results of an evaluation of a child's memory skills and capacity for new learning will be helpful in the development of an appropriate rehabilitation program and establishment of appropriate functional goals. Working with the family, the speech therapist, and the pediatric psychologist, the pediatric physical therapist may help determine the effect of memory and learning deficits on the child's functional abilities and the related need for assistance, environmental modification, or both.

EXECUTIVE SKILLS

The ability to formulate and switch conceptual sets, the ability to use feedback to initiate behavioral change, and the ability to exercise judgment in social and community settings are included under the rubric of "executive skills." Deficits in executive functioning are often associated with frontal lobe injury and may be expressed as impulsive behavior resulting in failure to observe safety precautions or an inability to recognize socially appropriate behaviors.

The inability to change conceptual sets may be demonstrated in perseveration on a task or the inability to change activities without becoming disorganized. Difficulty switching conceptual sets may also influence

the ability to perform reciprocal movements, alternating patterns of movement, or tasks with reciprocal or alternating components.

Arousal level and attentional ability may be impaired by frontal lobe lesions or lesions affecting the brainstem. A child's ability to follow commands or to benefit from feedback while learning motor and functional skills may be affected by level of arousal. A child who is able to maintain a level of arousal at which incoming environmental stimuli are neither overstimulating nor insufficient to elicit the child's attention is likely to benefit more from training or instruction than the child who is hypoaroused or hyperaroused.

When possible, a determination of the time of day at which arousal level is optimal or an alteration of therapeutic goals within a given treatment session in response to current arousal status may increase the effectiveness of intervention. Medications such as antiseizure or pain agents may also affect arousal. A knowledge of pharmacologic agents being used and time administered may assist in optimizing treatment.

VISUOSPATIAL SKILLS

Visuospatial and perceptual deficits can affect a child's perception of the environment. These deficits may influence cognitive tasks and motor performance and functional mobility skills (Fig. 24-5). Such deficits are frequently associated with lesions in the temporal or occipital lobes of the brain. A figure-ground deficit, or the inability to distinguish a given form from the background, may be related to difficulty with functional mobility skills. For example, problems with foot placement or the placement of an assistive device on a complex surface such as a step or a ramp may be related to visuospatial skills. Visuospatial deficits may also limit the

Figure 24-5   Math problem completed by a 12-year-old girl 2 days after removal of a brain tumor. The therapist asked the child to subtract 24 from 76. Note the correct answer, despite the perceptual difficulties with constructing the problem.

level of functional independence achieved. For example, a child who is unable to put on an orthosis because of visuospatial deficits may ultimately be dependent in functional mobility even though he or she is able to ambulate on flat surfaces independently after the orthosis is on. A child with visuospatial deficits related to memory skills may demonstrate difficulty developing a cognitive map of his or her environment. Consequently, this child may have difficulty moving independently from place to place in the home, school, or community.

LANGUAGE

Temporal lobe lesions may result in deficits in expressive or receptive language skills that can affect communication between therapist and patient, and can ultimately affect rehabilitation treatment. Language deficits are addressed in depth by speech and language pathologists. A basic understanding by the physical therapist will assist in communication during treatment sessions.

Receptive language deficits impair a child's ability to comprehend the instructions that are given for the performance of a task or activity. Determination of the extent of a child's receptive language impairment and the most effective means of communication will increase the results from treatment and decrease the therapist's and child's frustration.

Expressive language disorders impair a child's ability to communicate information to others. A child with an expressive disorder may fully comprehend verbally communicated information and successfully formulate a cognitive response. A breakdown occurs, however, between the formulation of the response and the execution or verbal expression of what was intended. In this case, the child may not be able to express a related idea or concern. In this situation, as in the case of the child with a receptive disorder, knowledge of the child's most efficient mode of communication may lessen frustration related to the inability to express an intended response.

▌ PHYSICAL THERAPY MANAGEMENT

Given the complexity of the developing brain, the wide range of injury severity and recoveries, there is no one appropriate set of activities for children with brain injuries. Utilizing the World Health Organization model of International Classification of Functioning, Disability and Health, strengths and concerns can be identified in each domain. This model of classification is discussed

in detail in Chapter 1. The *Guide to Physical Therapist Practice* provides an excellent framework to complete the physical therapy examination, diagnosis, prognosis, and intervention (American Physical Therapy Association, 2001).

Physical therapy management of the child with an insult to the brain will be outlined according to the practice guidelines in the *Guide*. Examination and intervention of children with insults to the brain, regardless of the cause of the insult, will be similar in many respects. Differences specific to traumatic brain injury, near-drowning, and brain tumors will be discussed as appropriate.

EXAMINATION

Many of the children described in this chapter will be transferred from one setting to another during the course of their recovery. These settings may include an acute care hospital, a rehabilitation center, an outpatient therapy center, or a school. A thorough examination should be performed on entry into each new setting.

A detailed history is the first component of the examination. In children with brain injury, it is important to carefully review the medical record. MRI, CT, and EEG reports provide the therapist with critical information regarding the anatomic and physiologic changes that have taken place as a result of the insult. Previous and current medications should be reviewed. In the acute care environment, for those patients on ventilator support, it is important to know if they are receiving paralytics. These drugs reduce the child's ability to move actively in order to maximize the respiratory support. This puts the child at risk for muscle atrophy and loss of range of motion. If a child has demonstrated EEG changes consistent with seizures, the child will probably be administered antiseizure medication. These commonly have side effects of drowsiness and decreased level of alertness. Other medications may be given to the child who is still in an agitated state. These may help the child sleep, participate in therapies, and tolerate changes in stimulation.

The history should also record any other injuries from the event. This could include orthopedic injuries sustained in a traumatic injury or cardiac changes from an anoxic event. Any surgical procedures should be noted in the history as well. If a child has received other therapy services before the examination, that should be noted, and ideally contact should be made with the therapists who provided those services. Any prior medical history that would affect physical therapy intervention should also be noted. An example of this is the child with a brain injury who had a premorbid diagnosis of developmental dyspraxia.

Including the child and family during the history process allows the family to express expectations and desired outcomes. This information will allow the therapist to more fully understand the family's perception of the extent of injuries and deficits present and will be utilized in setting functional goals.

The systems review is a brief screening that will allow the therapist to focus the physical examination. For a child with brain injury, this screening should include information that will allow referral to other disciplines as well. Screenings may include a gross assessment of activities of daily living, feeding, and cognitive issues. For example, consider a child who had a submersion injury. A screening may quickly demonstrate that the child has no independent mobility, is unable to complete age-appropriate activities of daily living, and coughs when she drinks thin liquids. Because of the review of systems, an appropriate referral is made to both occupational therapy and speech therapy.

After completing the history and review of systems, the therapist then selects the appropriate tests and measures to complete the evaluation. If chosen appropriately, the tests and measures should allow the physical therapist to make an accurate evaluation, diagnosis, and prognosis. For children with brain injuries, a variety of tests and measures can be used. These may be broken down into tests for impairments in body structure and function, tests for activity limitations, and tests for participation. See Box 24-1 for common impairments, activity limitations, and participation restrictions seen in children with brain injuries.

Tests and Measures for Body Structures and Function

Loss of functional active or passive range of motion (ROM) may be a risk for the child who is unable to continue with normal levels of activity either because of direct effects of the injury or because of the side effects of medical intervention. A child with a brainstem glioma may demonstrate limited volitional movement of the lower extremities related to spasticity and, without ROM exercises, may develop hypoextensibility or contractures. On the other hand, a child who does not demonstrate motor dysfunction directly related to the brain injury may experience limited mobility related to the general or specific side effects of medical treatment. Those children receiving respiratory support through a ventilator or ECMO may be paralyzed pharmacologically, which may lead to a loss of both ROM and strength. A child whose activity level is limited by nausea and vomiting or fatigue may also be at risk for loss of flexibility and ROM. Specific side effects of chemotherapy have also been related to limited ROM or flexibility. Vincristine, an antineoplastic agent used in the treatment of medulloblastoma and other tumors, has been associated with peripheral neuropathy, especially when levels approach toxicity (Kosmidis et al., 1991).

Passive ROM may be assessed regardless of the cognitive abilities of the child. Changes in passive ROM should be documented and should include information as to why the change has occurred. Active ROM should be assessed frequently, with documentation of changes that are noted. With the child or adolescent who remains cognitively intact, this task is relatively straightforward. For the young infant or child, active ROM information is typically obtained by careful observation of the child's movement during play.

Changes in muscle tone may be noted at the same time as assessment for ROM. Passive movement at different velocities is used to examine muscle tone changes at rest. Active movements must be carefully observed to determine any differences in tone with volitional movement.

Box 24-1	**Common Impairments, Activity Limitations, and Participation Restrictions in Children with Brain Injuries**

IMPAIRMENTS	ACTIVITY LIMITATIONS	PARTICIPATION RESTRICTIONS
Abnormal muscle tone	Decreased age-appropriate mobility	Dependent mobility
Postural asymmetry	Delayed gross motor skills	Dependent self-help skills
Decreased muscle strength	Poor school performances	Social isolation
Loss of range of motion	Poor ability to follow directions	Limited play with peers
Ataxia	Decreased attention to environment	
Poor balance		
Behavior state changes		
Poor motor planning		
Poor visual perceptual skils		
Impaired cognition		

Frequently, a child will be observed to have lower muscle tone at rest but, with activity, appears to have increased tone because of postural fixing in an attempt to stabilize the joint. Symmetry of tone is often disturbed with brain injuries; therefore, tone should be assessed thoroughly bilaterally.

Impairments in strength are also a common finding among children with brain insults. Muscle weakness that results from generally decreased activity may be present in children who are undergoing chemotherapy or radiation therapy. Less frequently administered treatments such as bone marrow transplant will also put children at risk for muscle weakness. After extended periods of bed rest or sedentary behavior, muscle atrophy may be expected. In the case of a child with a peripheral neuropathy related to vincristine chemotherapy, atrophy is also likely to result. Children whose tumors cause alterations in postural tone will also experience weakness. In the case of a child who has spasticity in agonist muscle groups, weakness can be expected in the antagonist groups. The child whose tumor caused hypotonia may also experience weakness related to less frequent functional use of muscle groups, especially antigravity muscles.

In the pediatric brain injury population, standardized manual muscle testing is difficult because of the need for the child to follow specific instructions. Because of age and cognitive deficits, many of these children are unable to accurately follow the instructions. Therefore, it is again necessary to complete a careful observation of the child's active movements. Documentation may report the child's ability to move against gravity, to support weight, to support an object, or to complete a movement requiring strength in a certain muscle group.

With increases in active movement and in positions against gravity, impairments in equilibrium and righting reactions may be observed. These reactions may be tested in a variety of positions and activities. Completion, symmetry, and speed of the reactions are qualitative information that should be noted when testing these reactions. In the young infant or the child who shows significant involvement, deep tendon reflexes and primitive reflexes should be assessed. These primitive reflexes may include the Babinski reflex, which, beyond age 7 months, is pathologic. Other reflexes such as the asymmetric tonic neck reflex and the tonic labyrinthine reflex should also be assessed.

Sensory testing in the pediatric brain injury population is challenging for a variety of reasons. First of all, by virtue of injury, these children may have cognitive deficits that impair their ability to be able to accurately respond to sensory input. Their young age may also lead to inability to accurately respond to sensory input.

Sensory inputs should be introduced selectively with careful observation to determine the response. Responses to input are noted as being either generalized, with a full-body response and physiologic changes with any input, or localized. Localized responses are more appropriate responses with the response specific to the system being stimulated. For example, if a nail bed is squeezed to assess for a pain response, a generalized response would be to see an increase in heart rate with a total body flexion withdrawal. A localized response to this same input is to observe withdrawal of the stimulated extremity, or the child may look toward the pain. As the child begins more active movement, sensory assessment can be completed in more depth, adding proprioception and kinesthesia to the systems assessed.

Coordination deficits may also be demonstrated in children who experience alterations of postural tone or weakness. A child demonstrating poor balance or motor control may be impaired by sensory integration disorders. This is characterized by either inadequate perception of sensory input or an inappropriate motor response to the input. Deficits in balance and coordination abilities may be anticipated in children whose tumors are located in the posterior fossa and affect the cerebellum (Menkes & Till, 1990). Visuoperceptual skills are commonly impaired in children with a brain insult. Deficits such as neglect and poor proprioception are also commonly noted. The classic "foam and dome" test, designed by Shumway-Cook and Horak (1986), is an excellent method of determining sensory integration deficits and their effect on balance in older children. For infants and young children, selective introduction of different sensory input and careful observation of the motor response is necessary to determine sensory integration difficulties.

Ataxia may become apparent as the child begins to initiate purposeful movement characterized by the loss of muscle coordination. Ataxia is a movement disorder that can be caused by damage to several different nervous system structures. Common causes of ataxia are damage to the cerebellum or to the sensory structures. These two types of ataxia are distinguishable because sensory ataxia worsens significantly when the child's eyes are closed (Bastian, 1997). Oscillations during movement will be observed with an increase in the oscillations as the tasks increase in difficulty. Limb ataxia will be observed in tasks such as active reaching and tying shoes. Proximal, or truncal, ataxia is more evident in upright postures with increasing antigravity demands. Assessment and documentation focus on movements and positions that affect ataxia.

Apraxia may also be present in children who have sustained a brain injury. Apraxia is difficulty in the child's ability to plan and execute a motor task. The child will be unable to demonstrate a requested task but may be able to complete the task automatically. For example, the child will be unable to lift his leg on demand, but if a ball were rolled to him, he would be able to kick the ball. Apraxia of speech may also be seen and is demonstrated by the child's inability to coordinate oral, laryngeal, and respiratory muscles for functional speech.

Particularly in the acute care setting, impairments may be noted in the cardiorespiratory system. For all three diagnoses, the cardiorespiratory system may be limited by a variety of factors. Children with brain trauma may also have thoracic trauma. They may also be limited by an overall state of lethargy that can occur with head trauma. Children who experience a submersion injury may have had damage to the myocardium, leaving them with limited endurance. Children with brain tumors may be limited by side effects from chemotherapy. The cardiorespiratory status should be assessed in the physical therapy examination by monitoring heart rate, respiratory rate, blood pressure, and oxygen saturation during activities. This is convenient in the pediatric intensive care setting because of the close nursing supervision and monitors available, but may also be done in other settings with the appropriate monitoring devices.

Assessment of arousal, attention, and cognition is another critical area. Children who have injuries to their brain will most likely show changes in one or all of these areas. Knowledge of a child's behavior states and what assists the child in reaching an optimal behavior state will increase the efficiency of physical therapy intervention. Position changes, motoric demands, and fatigue may affect arousal and attention and should be documented.

Physical therapists may also do a quick scan of cranial nerve integrity when evaluating children with brain injury. It is common to find that children with an insult to the brain often have difficulties with vestibular input. This may be evident from nausea and dizziness observed with movement. The use of swings, visual tracking, and functional reach tests will allow an assessment of the integrity of the vestibular system. If a child has difficulty swallowing and controlling secretions, a referral should be made to a speech pathologist.

Measures of Activity and Participation

Activity is the execution of a task or action by an individual integrating the use of body functions. Activities may vary in complexity, and appropriate activities for a child will depend on the age of the child. For example, a child who has lost ROM into dorsiflexion may be unable to ambulate because of poor ankle strategies. In the participation domain, a child's ability to function and be integrated into the community at large is a concern. Standardized tests are available for the physical therapist's use to determine both activity strengths and participation abilities for children with brain injuries.

Two tests specifically assess functional skills. These tests were designed to be utilized for the pediatric rehabilitation population and work well for those children who have brain insults. The Pediatric Evaluation of Disability Inventory (PEDI) (Haley et al., 1992) and the WeeFIM (Uniform Data System for Medical Rehabilitation, 2000) are both criterion-referenced indicators of change in functional skills such as mobility and self-care. The WeeFIM is the pediatric equivalent of the Functional Independence Measure (FIM) used for adult rehabilitation patients. The WeeFIM measures a child's independence in the areas of self-care, sphincter control, transfers, locomotion, communication, and social cognition. The PEDI is standardized for children ages 6 months to 7.5 years. It measures skills in three content domains: (1) self-care, (2) mobility, and (3) social function. The PEDI focuses on the function of specific tasks and also rates caregiver assistance and modification. This allows a good overall assessment of many skills. The use of standardized measures to monitor motoric and functional change is useful to document progress as required by third-party payers. The PEDI has demonstrated good sensitivity to both global and item-specific changes in acquired brain injury (Tokcan et al., 2003).

Neuromotor development is also important to assess in children with brain injury. Several standardized tests assess motor development. The Bayley Scales of Infant Development II is appropriate to use for children from birth to 42 months of age. This test scores the children on a mental and motor scale and is useful for a full evaluation of all skills. It gives the examiner an index score, as well as an age equivalence score, which may be needed to qualify for funding and state programs. The Peabody Developmental Motor Scales (PDMS) (Folio and Fewell, 2000) is appropriate for children from birth to 83 months of age and assesses both gross and fine motor skills. The Bruininks-Oseretsky (Bruininks, 1978) is standardized for children from ages 4.5 to 14.5 years and also is used to assess fine and gross motor tasks. See Chapter 2 for more detailed information on these standardized tests.

EVALUATION

After a thorough examination is complete, the therapist must then make several judgments based on the results. Included in these judgments is severity of impairment, activity limitation, and participation restrictions. Knowledge of environmental and personal factors are critical when making these determinants.

When making decisions regarding the severity of impairment, there are several factors to address. First, of course, are the specific strengths and challenges noted in the examination. It is critical to determine if the impairment is causing activity limitations and whether the impairment can be modified by physical therapy intervention. Knowledge of the pathophysiology of the various brain insults and other physiologic processes will help predict expected improvements in function. Length of time since the brain injury and any prior interventions should also be taken into account. If the impairment, such as muscle contracture or strength, is not expected to improve spontaneously, the therapist must decide what type, frequency, and duration of intervention is needed to address each identified impairment.

Activity limitations should be assessed relevant to age of the child and severity of the limitation. For instance, if an infant has significant motor deficits as a result of an insult, it may be reasonable to discharge the child home with the family and provide both home and outpatient physical therapy intervention. On the other hand, if the child is an adolescent with significant mobility needs and poor judgment of safety issues, the family may not be able to care for the child at home, and the child may benefit from a rehabilitation stay to address these issues and to train the family in home management. Activity limitations must then be related to participation.

Participation and restrictions in participation not only reflect variance in injury but also perceptions and expectations of the child and family. Participation should be addressed in relation to the age of the child. As children grow and mature, their function in society expands. Their role increases from that of an infant, whose primary role is to play and explore, to a child who interacts on an increasing basis with the world. Again, an infant may not necessarily show severe participation restrictions initially after an insult, but restrictions may appear as the child grows and matures. An adolescent who sustains an insult will generally demonstrate participation restrictions in the motor areas immediately, but it may not be until return to school that some of the cognitive deficits become apparent.

Knowledge of the living environment and social supports should be considered in the evaluation process. A 10-year-old child with significant motor needs may be a perfect candidate for a power wheelchair. However, if that child lives in a single-wide trailer, a power wheelchair may not be a functional means of mobility. An infant with significant motor and feeding needs who is to be placed with a parent who has also sustained an injury may need significantly more intervention and training than the same infant who is cared for by an intact family unit, capable of carrying out some activities at home.

DIAGNOSIS AND PROGNOSIS

From the information gained in the examination, the physical therapist develops a diagnosis and prognosis for children with brain insults. For example, a child with a traumatic brain injury who also has a fractured humerus may fit the diagnostic groups of skeletal deficits, impaired balance, impaired arousal and attention, and impaired motor function. The diagnosis is then used to guide the therapist in determining the most appropriate intervention.

Based on the diagnosis, the physical therapist must consider the likely outcomes of intervention. For children who have a brain injury, the prognosis will depend on the severity of their injury, the rate of recovery, and the social and physical supports available to them at home and at school. Determining prognosis and outcomes in children is more complex than in adults because children are growing and developing while they are recovering. Children who have acquired a brain injury may have achieved only a portion of their developmental milestones prior to injury. A key component when determining the prognosis is to assess the child in relation to what age-appropriate activities the child would normally be participating in at home, at school, and in the community.

PLAN OF CARE

The plan of care should be formulated once the physical therapist has determined the diagnosis and prognosis. The plan of care should include long- and short-term goals and outcomes, specific interventions, duration and frequency of intervention necessary to achieve the desired outcomes, and discharge criteria. Goals should be related to changes in impairments, and outcomes should be related to changes in activity and participation. Goals and outcomes are determined based on the clinical evaluation, resources available, knowledge of pathophysiology, and the child's age. For infants, outcomes are focused on the infant being able to explore the environment with continuing progression in development. Because of dramatic changes in growth that an infant will undergo, goals and outcomes should be addressed for long-term needs as well. For the school-age child or adolescent, outcomes should focus on mobility in terms of interaction with peers and safety. For children with brain insults who are not involved in school at the time of examination, the plan of care should include goals related to integration back into the educational setting.

INTERVENTION

Physical therapy intervention consists of purposeful and skillful interactions of the therapist with the child and family to produce changes that are consistent with the diagnosis and prognosis. The physical therapist provides direct intervention, as well as instruction and coordination, communication, and documentation.

Intervention interactions of coordination, communication, and documentation for the child with a brain insult consist of communication and coordination with all involved with the child's care. For this population, communication may be with the physician, other health care team members, third-party payers, and educational personnel. Participation in care conferences and discharge planning fall under this intervention. Communication and coordination relating to goals of integration or reintegration into the school setting are vital to a child's successful return into the community.

Instruction is a cornerstone of physical therapy intervention. A child with brain insult may have many deficits, some obvious and others subtle. Instruction may be directed to the child, family, educational supports, and other people involved in the care of the child. Proper instruction will lead to an increased carryover of therapeutic activities and a decreased level of frustration and helplessness for both the child and family.

Direct interventions, of course, will take up a major part of the time spent with the patient and should focus on addressing specific impairments, activity limitations, and restrictions in participation. Direct interventions include but are not limited to therapeutic exercise, manual therapy techniques, selection of assistive or adaptive devices, electrotherapeutic modalities, physical agents, mechanical modalities, functional training in self-care, and functional training in community and school settings.

Intervention for Impairments

Traditional medical treatments in brain injury management address intervention at the impairment level. These treatments involve chemotherapy and radiation, respiratory support, surgical management, and cardiopulmonary support. Physical therapy management and intervention at the impairment level focuses on specific component deficits. Examples are ataxia and hypotonia or related weakness, which may be considered manifestations of the brain pathology at the organ systems level.

Weakness is a common impairment in children with brain injury. Strengthening activities will therefore be a large part of the physical therapy intervention. Strength has been shown to be correlated with an increase in motor performance in children with cerebral palsy (Damiano & Abel, 1998). In Damiano and Abel's study, children with spastic cerebral palsy demonstrated strength gains in specific muscle groups, increased velocity of gait, and improvement in the ambulatory subtest of the Gross Motor Function Measure after a 6-week strengthening program.

How strengthening activities are carried out will vary depending on the age of the child and the severity of the brain injury. With an adolescent, the therapist may be able to complete a rote therapeutic exercise program with standard exercises and repetitions. Adolescents may also enjoy strengthening activities in a weight room with their peers. With a younger child, the therapist may need to choose appropriate developmental activities that will facilitate muscle strengthening in a given muscle group or pattern of movement. For example, if a 5-year-old child is demonstrating lower extremity weakness as a result of a traumatic brain injury, therapeutic activities could consist of climbing on equipment, squat to stand to retrieve game pieces, or step-stance activities while drawing on the wall. A pool is an excellent modality for this population. If a child is very weak with minimal active movements, the principles of buoyancy will assist with movement. For the stronger child, the principles of resistance of water will allow for increased strengthening. For the child who demonstrates ataxia, proximal strengthening will assist in the child's stability. For the pediatric physical therapist, therapeutic exercise is limited only by the imagination of the therapist (Fig. 24-6).

Contraindications to strengthening must be noted before initiating an exercise program. Limitations caused by fractures, skin involvement, or myocardial involvement must be noted. In the child who has a brain tumor, a specific set of guidelines should also be followed as side effects of medical treatment may limit the child's performance. For example, the child who is fatigued after radiation therapy or who is nauseated after chemotherapy may be scheduled for physical therapy before radiation or chemotherapy. Because chemotherapy frequently affects blood parameters that are associated with clotting and tolerance of activity, blood cell counts should be considered when an exercise program is developed or modified. According to the hematology-oncology protocol at Egleston Children's Hospital, which was adapted from the work of Dietz (1980), exercise is recommended only for children whose hematocrit is greater than 25%, hemoglobin levels are greater than

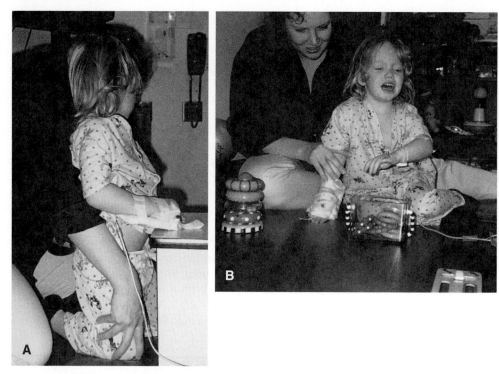

⬩ **Figure 24-6**   Three-year-old child with weakness and right hemiplegia after a traumatic brain injury. **A**, Strengthening for hip extensors in tall kneeling position. **B**, Right upper extremity weight bearing during play activity.

10 mg/dL, platelet counts are greater than 50,000/mm³, and white blood cell counts are greater than 500/mm³.

Neuromuscular electrical stimulation (NMES) may be a useful adjunct to therapy in children with brain injury. NMES was found to increase ankle dorsiflexion at heel strike in children with cerebral palsy (Comeaux et al., 1997). Carmick (1997) published a guideline for clinical application of NMES for children with cerebral palsy that may also be useful for children with brain injury. Care must be taken to introduce electrical stimulus slowly to the child and to let the child initiate the movement during functional activities.

When impairments in ROM are present, the pediatric physical therapist has many options for intervention. For the child who demonstrates an increase in muscle tone and little active movement, passive ROM and positioning are the primary means of preventing contracture. Children who suffer severe submersion injury impairments may demonstrate severe spasticity and abnormal posturing, and as a result, adaptive equipment fabrication may constitute a significant component of intervention. Splinting or serial casting may also be used to maintain optimal ROM over time. For children who demonstrate active movement, ROM activities may be used in conjunction with strengthening and functional activities to maximize function and therapy time.

Joint mobilization or soft tissue massage in children with CNS disorders may help maintain ROM. Although much more research in the area of joint mobilization for children in general is needed, some basic precautions and contraindications should be noted. Absolute contraindications include malignancy involving the spinal cord, cauda equina lesions producing bowel and bladder dysfunction, bone disease of the spine, active inflammatory and infective arthritis, and rheumatoid collagen necrosis of vertebral ligaments (Harris, 1991). Aside from training in manual therapy techniques, the therapist should have knowledge in developmental biomechanics. Caution and care should be exhibited when using this method, particularly if the patient is unable to report pain or discomfort.

Changes in the child's cognitive status will also be an important consideration in the development of an exercise program that focuses on the improvement of balance and coordination skills, as well as other aspects of rehabilitation. Short-term memory deficits may make it difficult for a child to become independent in performing an exercise program. A lack of mastery at this task may be frustrating for both the child and the family. Variable levels of arousal within a session or from session to session will affect a child's ability to attend to instructions and to stay on task. A treatment plan for a given session may then need to be adjusted accordingly.

Intervention for Activity Limitations

The systems theory of motor control as defined by Woollacott and Shumway-Cook (2001) suggests that examination and intervention focus not only on the impairments within individual systems but also on the effect of interacting impairments among multiple systems. Activity limitations can contribute to secondary impairments. In the activity domain, increased independence in mobility skills, including bed mobility, transfer training, gait activities, and wheelchair mobility training, is emphasized.

Once again, the child's cognitive status must be considered. Difficulty learning new tasks and material or short-term memory problems may influence the method selected for instruction in transfer and mobility training. A child who demonstrates perseveration may have difficulty with reciprocal tasks or may become upset when asked to change from one activity to another. A child's short-term memory deficits or variable levels of arousal may necessitate frequent repetition of instructions and additional cueing while learning a task. These factors will also influence safety. For example, a child may be physically capable of performing a transfer but may not be able to attend to the task sufficiently to observe the necessary safety precautions, such as positioning a wheelchair or locking the brakes, to safely complete the task independently.

Children whose injuries are the result of a traumatic event may have other associated complications, such as fractures. This may change the management of mobility-related skills. For example, a child who demonstrates hemiplegia related to a brain injury but also has a fractured femur and humerus will be considerably more limited in mobility skills than the child who experiences neurologic or orthopedic injuries exclusively.

Functional training at home, at school, and in the community is important for children with brain injuries. Because brain injuries can lead to deficits in a broad range of skills, it is not appropriate to simply address impairments such as strengthening. A child with hemiplegia may be able to demonstrate adequate strength for independent ambulation but may be lacking visual-perceptual and cognitive skills that would allow him or her to do this functionally. The physical therapist must treat the whole child and treat the child in settings that will allow the child to practice functional skills. For a 1-year-old child with severe spasticity from a submersion injury, intervention involving functional training may involve work in sitting so that the child may be able to play in a functional sitting position. For an 11-year-old child with hemiplegia, a functional training session may involve work on bicycle riding so that the child can ride to school with friends.

Assessing for and fabricating assistive devices and equipment is an intervention that will lead to increased independence for the child with brain insult. Assessment is difficult in the early stages of recovery because of the difficulty in determining the amount of recovery a child may make. In this case, it may be best to create temporary devices before spending time and money on a permanent device. If a child is unable to ambulate initially after injury, a rental wheelchair may be more appropriate than purchase of a chair. Therapists can fabricate splints for the lower extremities initially to assess for later use of a foot orthosis in a child with poor motor control in the lower extremities. If complete neurologic recovery does not occur, custom orthoses and adaptive equipment may be purchased to facilitate independent functioning in the child's environment. Because of the potential for changes and growth in this population, equipment needs may change frequently.

Intervention for Participation Restrictions

In the participation domain, a child's ability to function and be integrated into the community at large is a concern. Intervention is directed at assisting the child in the achievement of the highest possible levels of independent functioning in his or her home, school, and residential community. Intervention will be focused on the adaptive equipment, orthoses, and environmental modifications to allow the child to function as independently as possible in his or her natural environment.

Traumatic brain injury is a disability category under the Individuals with Disabilities Educational Act (IDEA) (Public Law 105-17). Therefore, any child who has a documented traumatic brain injury must be evaluated by school personnel for special services, including physical therapy, on reentry to schools. Although children who have sustained a submersion injury or a brain tumor do not fit specifically under this category, they should also be evaluated by school personnel on reentry because of the similar nature of their impairments, activity limitations, and participation.

The role of the school physical therapist in intervention with a child who has undergone treatment and rehabilitation for a brain tumor provides an illustration of treatment focused at preventing disability. Goals of treatment may include determination of the mode of mobility and required assistive devices to promote efficient functioning in the classroom and school building. An evaluation of the child's general endurance in relation to the demands of daily activity and the formulation of recommendations for modifications in the child's schedule will also be included.

Education of and support for parents as they adapt to changes in their child's transition to school and community living are appropriate goals to prevent disability and facilitate coping with inevitable societal barriers to full integration in society.

Intervention that focuses on helping the child become reintegrated into the community through the implementation of provisions in federal legislation such as the Americans with Disabilities Act (Public Law 101-336) may also be considered as an illustration of intervention to prevent disability. For example, working on improving the child's mobility in the community by securing public transportation mandated by federal legislation influences the child's ability to fully participate in the life of the community.

Referrals to support groups and community agencies can be valuable to the family, child, and siblings. In the case of the child with a brain tumor who experiences regrowth or for whom further treatment is not possible, physical therapists work with hospice organizations or home health agencies. In such cases, the physical therapist collaborates with the family and the child to help them cope with a progressively debilitating process in the child.

OUTCOMES

Outcomes in the pediatric population who have sustained brain injuries are variable. Cerebral water content, extent of myelination, degree of brain development, stage of development of localization of cortical function, and neurochemical content vary in children of different ages, and each of these factors may affect brain plasticity and potential recovery of function (Michaud et al., 1993).

In children who suffer traumatic brain injuries, the prognosis is also variable with factors such as extent of primary injury, other injuries sustained, and amount of secondary damage. Severity of injury has been found to be related to mobility outcomes. Children who have a traumatic brain injury have been found to have a significant decline in motor performance as injury severity increases (Jaffe et al., 1992). In contrast, children who sustained a mild head injury did not demonstrate clinically detectable deficits in fine or gross motor skills at 3 weeks and 1 year after injury (Fay et al., 1993). It has also been suggested that children who have had inflicted traumatic brain injuries have a poorer motor outcome than those experiencing other mechanisms of injury (Kriel et al., 1989; Ewing-Cobbs et al., 1989). Recovery has been studied over time with findings suggesting that children with moderate injuries showed a large initial deficit in motor skills with improvement at 1 year and performing slightly worse at 3 years. Children with severe

injuries have the largest initial deficit, again showed improvement at 1 year, and then little change was noted thereafter (Jaffe et al., 1995). Another study divided the study group into mild and severe injuries with almost all the subjects with the mild traumatic brain injury demonstrating gross motor functioning within the normal range. Forty percent of the severe group showed impairments at 6-month follow-up with continued impairments in gross motor skills at 2 years (O'Flaherty et al., 2000).

Children who have sustained more severe injuries have also been noted to have long-term cognitive and behavioral consequences. Cognitive outcomes include previously mentioned declines in intelligence, memory, language, nonverbal skills, attention, and executive functioning. Behavioral outcomes include impulsivity, irritability, agitation, confusion, apathy, and emotional lability (Barry et al., 1996). Academic achievements and school performance are also negatively affected (Fay et al., 1994). A recent study found that children with severe traumatic brain injury demonstrated selective, long-term deficits in their social problem-solving skills that may help to account for their poor social and academic outcomes (Janusz et al., 2002). All these factors create struggles for children and their families as they return to home, school, and their community.

In the case of the child with a diagnosis of brain tumor, the amount of function that will be regained depends on whether the limitation is related to the lesion itself, to pressure effects, or to the effects of medical treatment such as surgery or radiation therapy. For example, if a child's hemiparesis is related to direct pressure of a tumor or associated edema, surgical excision of the tumor or treatment that shrinks it will probably be followed by recovery of function. If the hemiparesis is related to an exacerbation of symptoms that has been noted to occur with radiation therapy (Menkes & Till, 1990), recovery of some function may also be expected. If the hemiparesis is related to infiltration of the tumor into healthy tissue, function is less likely to be regained. Similarly, if healthy tissues have been surgically excised or damaged by radiation therapy, recovery is less likely to occur. Future recurrence of the tumor will also, of course, have an effect on the outcome of treatment.

Duration of the hypoxic-ischemic event is the primary determinant of prognosis of victims of submersion incidents. Studies vary, but most recently have suggested that if patients do not die, or are not left in a persistive vegetative state, they are likely to have only minimal neurologic deficits (Fields, 1992).

The therapist should consider outcomes at every level of care. Therapeutic outcomes should include maximization of activity and participation, optimization of health status, and optimization of patient and family satisfaction. To minimize activity limitations and prevent further participation restriction, the therapist must be proactive in all aspects of intervention. Aside from therapy services, the patient and family should be directed to community support groups.

OPTIMIZATION OF HEALTH STATUS

In a recent study, adults who had sustained a traumatic brain injury were surveyed to determine what long-term health issues may be common in the traumatic brain injury population. The most frequently reported health issues were suggestive of ongoing neuroendocrine dysfunction, neurologic difficulties, and arthritic complaints (Hibbard et al., 1998). Children who acquired a brain injury due a tumor have been noted to have long-term health issues related to endocrine dysfunction and cardiovascular dysfunction, particularly if they were treated with radiation and chemotherapy in addition to surgery (Gurney et al., 2003). Endocrine issues were related to obesity, growth disturbances, and osteoporosis (Gurney et al., 2003; Muirhead et al., 2002). Cardiovascular effects were noted to be arrhythmia, stroke, blood clots, and angina-like symptoms (Gurney et al., 2003). It is important to remember that pediatric patients may have health issues that affect them for a lifetime, and therefore, intervention should consider the possible long-term sequelae of brain injury.

Wellness is an area of rehabilitation for the child with a brain insult that is an integral but often overlooked part of the rehabilitation process. One way that a physical therapist can assist with wellness activities is to assist the child in maintaining activities that promote cardiovascular health and strength. A recent study found that adult patients with traumatic brain injury who exercised regularly had improved mood, fewer impairments, less disability, and perceptions of better health than those who did not exercise (Gordon et al., 1998). Early and closely monitored exercise programs will also be critical for those children at risk for obesity and osteoporosis secondary to endocrine dysfunction.

For children with chronic neurologic sequelae, the therapist may need to help the child adapt an exercise program to maintain a level of cardiovascular fitness and strength. For example, a group of children with various mild motor impairments from traumatic head injuries may be seen weekly for a fitness group. Intervention could include strengthening and cardiovascular activities, as well as some general instruction about health and wellness. Children with more significant motor impairments may participate in a swimming program to address strength and cardiovascular endurance in a gravity-limited, buoyancy-assisted environment.

PREVENTION

A large part of the practice of physical therapy is education, and part of our educational efforts should be focused on prevention of brain injuries. Education of our patients should also extend to education of the general public. Brain injury prevention efforts have focused on use of helmets and appropriate motor vehicle restraints in children. There have also been educational efforts regarding safe-proofing houses and eliminating the use of baby walkers. It has been documented that after sustaining one traumatic brain injury, the risk of a further traumatic brain injury increases (Annegers et al., 1980). Some communities have local chapters of the Brain Injury Association that give free helmets and car seats to children who have suffered or are at risk for a traumatic brain injury.

Near-drowning prevention efforts have focused on general water safety. The U.S. Consumer Product Safety Commission has begun to look at regulations regarding pools in residential properties. Owners are being advised to have childproof barriers around their pool and have cardiopulmonary resuscitation training. Parent education about household dangers such as the bathtub, buckets, and other dangerous water sources is also necessary.

Although brain tumors are largely unpreventable, physical therapists must be aware of early signs and symptoms. Children who are examined by a therapist for motor signs and symptoms of unknown etiology may benefit from a further workup by a neurologist to rule out tumor. This may allow for earlier identification and treatment of tumors.

Many local and national organizations have prevention efforts aimed at reducing injury in the pediatric population. The National SAFE Kids Coalition sponsors SAFE Kid Week nationally and other safety-related events throughout the year. Nonaccidental injuries such as shaken baby syndrome are being targeted in national "Babies Are Fragile" campaigns.

CASE STUDIES

K.F.

Examination

History. K.F. is a 14-month-old boy who was admitted to the pediatric intensive care unit in November 2002 with a very large ependymoma in the posterior fossa. K.F. was 7 months old when he was initially diagnosed. He was hospitalized for 6 months and underwent numerous procedures. His first surgery shortly after initial diagnosis was to partially resect the tumor. After this initial surgery, he was noted to have bilateral vocal cord paralysis and was unable to protect his airway, necessitating a tracheostomy placement. After his initial surgery to resect the tumor, he had an externalized ventricular shunt placed. There have been numerous attempts to internalize this shunt. The last surgery to internalize the shunt was successful, and he now has an internal ventricular atrial shunt. He has been unable to eat orally and is fed through a gastrostomy tube. He has been through several rounds of chemotherapy with some calcification noted in the remaining tumor. His hospital course was also complicated by occasional neutropenia following his chemotherapy and one significant episode of sepsis with pneumonia.

K.F. is the third child in a very supportive family. His older sisters are 4 and 6 years of age. His parents alternate being at the hospital so that one of them is present for all sessions. Physical therapy services were initiated shortly after the first surgery to resect the tumor, when K.F. was approximately 8 months old. Family contact was made and the following family goals were expressed:

1. K.F. will be able to tolerate being held and interacting for play.
2. K.F. will sit by himself.
3. K.F. will be able to walk.

Review of systems. On initial examination of this child, the following findings were noted:

1. The child had a tracheostomy and was ventilated.
2. The child had no observable antigravity movement.
3. The child was positioned in supine at all times.
4. The child did not demonstrate active dorsiflexion of his left foot.
5. The child did not tolerate handling by persons other than his mother and father.
6. The child's family was supportive of rehabilitation services.

Speech and occupational therapy services were initiated at the same time as physical therapy services. After individual evaluations were completed, the therapists met as a team to discuss goals and plans of care.

Tests and Measures

Body structure and function. K.F. was noted to have weakness throughout his trunk and extremities as evidenced by very little antigravity movement in supine. He did demonstrate some gravity eliminated hip and knee flexion as well as dorsiflexion of the right foot. He was unable to dorsiflex his left ankle. He did not use his abdominals actively in supine and had made no attempts to roll to his side. His ROM throughout all of his extremities was within age-appropriate limits with the exception of his left ankle, which was lacking 10° of dorsiflexion. He responded to light and firm touch on all extremities. He tolerated very little handling. He became very irritable and had significant changes in his vital signs with movement.

Activity and Participation

Because of K.F.'s very limited tolerance of handling and movement, and his limited endurance, standardized testing was not completed initially. A clinical assessment of his activity level and participation was completed instead. K.F. was observed to need assistance for any exploration of his environment. He was unable to change his own position in bed, or move himself to a new position for play. He was unable to reach out for toys. When a small toy was placed in his hand, he was unable to bring that toy to midline or manipulate it beyond partial wrist rotation. He had a very minimal tolerance for sitting. His up time consisted primarily of sitting in his mother or father's lap in a reclined position. Because of the paralyzed vocal cords and the tracheostomy, K.F. was unable to vocalize his needs.

K.F. was very comfortable with his parents. He would seek his parents out visually and was easily comforted by either his mother or father. K.F. was very animate with his facial expressions and his mother and father quickly became adept at reading his cues. He had a fleece blanket that he liked to hold for comfort. When he was calm and quiet, K.F. would enjoy looking at toys presented by his parents.

Diagnosis

Based on the examination information, the following diagnoses were determined: impaired motor function and sensory integrity associated with progressive disorder of the CNS.

Prognosis

The size, type and location of K.F.'s brain tumor were very significant in terms of long-term outcomes and survival. These factors, as well as the medical complications of shunt malfunctions and mechanical ventilation, led us to a guarded prognosis for long-term outcomes. However, because of his significant weakness, limited endurance, and ROM limitations in his left ankle, physical therapy goals were easily established and felt to be achievable in the duration of his hospital stay. K.F.'s outstanding parental and extended family support were also factors in determining goals.

Plan of Care

Because of K.F.'s significant changes in activities and participation since his diagnosis and subsequent surgeries, it was determined that physical therapy services would work in conjunction with occupational therapy and speech therapy on a 5 day per week schedule toward the following goals and outcomes:

Goals

1. K.F. will move all of his extremities antigravity.
2. K.F. will tolerate supported upright sitting for 5 minutes.
3. K.F. will have full active and passive ROM of his left ankle.
4. K.F. will utilize his upper extremities in prone.
5. K.F. will support some weight through his lower extremities.

Outcomes

1. K.F. will tolerate routine care.
2. K.F. will explore his environment with set-up.
3. K.F. will roll to change his position or reach for a toy.
4. K.F. will be able to actively play in prone, supine, and sitting.
5. K.F. will tolerate a mobility system for routine infant transport.

Intervention

Indirect physical therapy intervention consisted of parent education in the role of physical therapy, ROM activities, and developmental play. Education and communication also took place with the nursing and medical staff. Nursing staff were instructed in how to maximize function and development with positioning in bed, as well as during routine care. Nurses were encouraged to provide care from both sides of his bed to encourage head turning to both sides. They were also given options for positioning to include supine on a "Boppy" pillow, up in a Tumbleform chair, brief periods in a high chair with support, and side lying as an alternative to supine for bedtime. As discharge neared, communication was broadened to discussions with therapists and the Birth-to-Three coordinator in K.F.'s home community.

Direct physical therapy intervention occurred approximately 5 days per week unless physiologic status or medical procedures prohibited therapy intervention for the day. Physical therapy fabricated a splint for K.F.'s left ankle to stretch and support until function returned. When K.F. started showing functional ROM and active dorsiflexion at his left ankle, the splint was discontinued. At that time, more functional activities such as lower extremity weight bearing in bench sitting were utilized to continue to maintain ROM and strengthening around the ankles. Strengthening activities consisted primarily of challenging K.F. to move actively in a variety of positions. Because of the gastrostomy tube, multiple abdominal scars from shunt revisions, and the tracheostomy, prone was an especially difficult position for K.F. A "Boppy" pillow was used to support K.F. under the chest in prone to avoid direct weight bearing on the gastrostomy or tracheostomy. Transitional movements were also addressed with work on rolling and upper extremity weight bearing while reaching in sitting.

Equipment that was obtained for K.F. when discharge from the hospital neared included a hospital crib and a mobility system. The crib allowed more flexibility in terms of changing positions than a standard crib. These position changes were crucial to accommodate variations in shunt function, and the height of the crib allowed easier caregiving for activities such as suctioning the tracheostomy. The mobility system that was ordered for K.F. was the Kid Kart (Fig. 24-7). This system allowed for excellent trunk and extremity support as well as tilt options for pressure release. It had attachments for intravenous lines, oxygen tanks, and a ventilator if that should be needed in the future. It also was an adequate height to allow K.F.

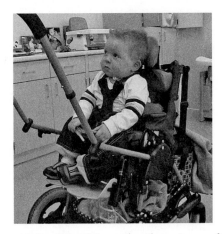

◆ **Figure 24-7**   K.F. at 19 months of age, 1 year after initial diagnosis. Shown sitting in Kid Kart with trunk, head, and pelvic supports. Note that he continues to have tracheostomy in place.

Box 24-2	Bayley Scales of Infant Development II Scores for K.F.	
SCORES	**MOTOR SCALE**	**MENTAL SCALE**
Raw score	36	64
Index score	<50	59
Age-equivalent score	5 months	6 months

to sit at home and socialize with family members at mealtime.

Outcomes

Just prior to discharge, K.F. was assessed utilizing the Bayley Scales of Infant Development II. The scores obtained from this test provided an objective baseline developmental level and assisted in the transition into the Birth to Three Program in K.F.'s home community. Scores for the BSID-II are shown in Box 24-2.

At discharge from the hospital, K.F. was demonstrating a much improved tolerance of handling. His endurance had increased to tolerating 45 minutes of activity. He demonstrated full passive ROM in all extremities, although he still had limited passive or active trunk mobility. He was able to sit independently for 3 to 5 seconds at a time. With support at the pelvis he was able to play and reach from ring sitting and bench sitting. He was able to roll from supine to side lying on either side. He could reach against gravity for objects in supine and supported sitting and would explore anything within his reach. He had briefly, on two occasions, taken some weight on his lower extremities, but this was inconsistent. Prone continued to be a difficult position, and he had yet to utilize his upper extremities in prone for weight bearing on elbows or extended arms, or for reaching. His parents were well educated in therapy activities and performed these activities regularly.

K.F. was discharged home in the care of his local Birth to Three program. He would receive twice weekly visits in the home from physical therapy.

L . L .

Examination

History. L.L. is an 18-month-old girl who was an unrestrained passenger in a motor vehicle accident. She sustained a small subdural hematoma, a subarachnoid hematoma, a skull fracture, an ischemic infarct, and bilateral retinal hemorrhages. She was in the pediatric intensive care unit (PICU) for 2 weeks following her injury and had her intracranial pressure (ICP) monitored while in intensive care. Other medical procedures included a period of assisted ventilation and placement of a nasogastric tube for nutrition. Physical therapy services were initiated immediately after removal of the ICP bolt in the PICU.

L.L. was the daughter of a teenage mother who was living in a converted school bus on her parent's property in the mountains, 30 miles from the nearest town, and 60 miles from the nearest pediatric rehabilitation center. The child had shown some mild delays early in her life and was being followed on a monthly basis by a educational development team prior to injury. At the time of initial evaluation, L.L.'s mother was unable to specifically identify any deficits or goals other than to take her child back home.

Review of Systems

Upon initial examination of this child, the following findings were noted:

1. The child was not responding to any stimuli presented.
2. The child was unable to control her secretions.
3. The child was positioned in a left-facing-only posture.
4. The child occasionally demonstrated random movement of the left side of her body.
5. The child was not vocalizing.

At this point, it was recommended that the child receive speech therapy and occupational therapy in conjunction with physical therapy services to address feeding, cognition, and developmental skills.

Tests and Measures

Body Structures and Function

Initially, L.L. was noted to have flaccid extremities on the right side. Her left extremities were demonstrating some

Box 24-3	Admission PEDI Scores for L.L.		
DOMAIN	**RAW SCORE**	**NORMATIVE STANDARD SCORE**	**SCALED SCORE**
Mobility Functional skills	5	Below 10	20.9
Mobility Caregiver assistance	0	Below 10	0
MODICATION FREQUENCIES (7 ITEMS)			
NONE	**CHILD**	**REHAB**	**EXTENSIVE**
0	3	4	0

movement and some resistance to passive movement. Her muscle tone in the left extremities was felt to be near normal. She demonstrated full passive ROM of all extremities but active ROM was limited due to weakness in the extremities. She was unable to control her head in any upright position. Vital signs were stable during the examination activities. As noted in the review of systems, L.L. was not responding to tactile, visual, or auditory input. She did, however, show an increase in heart rate and respiratory rate with vestibular input.

Activity and Participation

The PEDI was administered to determine activity level. Scores for initial administration are shown in Box 24-3.

L.L. was unable to demonstrate any active exploration of her environment, and her mother was unable to respond to her change in needs.

Diagnosis

Based on the examination information, the following diagnoses were determined: impaired vision, impaired arousal and attention, impaired motor function, and impaired sensory integration.

Prognosis

Because of the severity of both the physiologic changes and the resulting profound impairments and activity limitations, it was thought that L.L.'s prognosis was guarded as to the amount of motor function and skills that she would regain. However, because she was still so young and so recently injured, it was thought that she had potential to regain some motor skills.

Plan of Care

Because of the distance of L.L.'s home from rehabilitation services and her continued medical and nutritional needs, it was determined that a stay in a rehabilitation center would provide the family and child with the best possible outcomes. For the rehabilitation stay, the following physical therapy goals and outcomes were established.

Goals

1. L.L. will tolerate change in positions without significant changes in vital signs.
2. L.L. will hold her head independently in supported sitting.
3. L.L. will support weight through her lower extremities.
4. L.L. will actively use all extremities in play.

Outcomes

1. L.L. will tolerate handling for routine care.
2. L.L.'s mother will recognize deficits and strengths in the child's sensory motor system and respond accordingly.
3. L.L. will explore the environment with caregiver modification.
4. L.L. will sit independently and stand with assistance.
5. L.L. will demonstrate two play skills.

Intervention

L.L. received extensive physical therapy services in the rehabilitation center over 2.5 months. Intervention involved weekly care conferences, staff training in developmental activities for nontherapy times, and extensive family training.

Box 24-4	Admission PEDI Scores for L.L.		
DOMAIN	RAW SCORE	NORMATIVE STANDARD SCORE	SCALED SCORE
Mobility Functional skills	7	Below 10	25.4
Mobility Caregiver assistance	9	54.4	40.9
MODICATION FREQUENCIES (7 ITEMS)			
NONE	CHILD	REHAB	EXTENSIVE
0	4	3	0

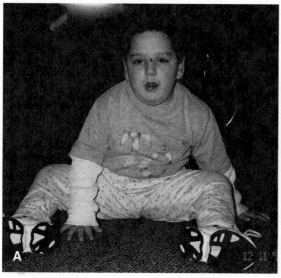

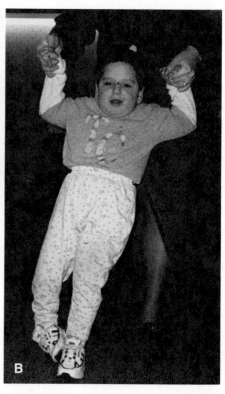

• **Figure 24-8** L.L. 3 years after injury, at age 4.5. **A**, Preferred sitting posture; note continued low muscle tone and stabilizing patterns of upper extremity propping and wide base of support. **B**, Ambulation with caregiver assistance; note the posturing of the right foot with attempts to progress the right lower extremity forward.

Direct physical therapy intervention was done twice daily. Emphasis was on sensorimotor stimulation, strengthening, postural stability, and establishing some forms of independent movement. Physical therapy sessions frequently coincided with speech therapy sessions. Multiple goals were accomplished during these sessions. First, L.L. was more active vocally with more active body postures. She also demonstrated more active oral motor skills in terms of feeding in more dynamic positions. Also, because of the need for extensive handling, co-treatment with the speech therapist facilitated play.

Outcomes

L.L. was discharged from the rehabilitation center 3 months following her initial injury with discharge PEDI scores as shown in Box 24-4. At time of discharge she could roll from supine to prone independently, sit for brief periods of time independently with upper extremity propping, and take weight through her lower extremities. With assistance she was able to pull to sit, although still with a slight head lag. She demonstrated some purposeful movements in her left extremities. Movements of the right extremities were random and less frequent than movements of the left extremities. She responded intermittently to stimuli on the right side of her body. She appeared to track some toys and was able to reach for toys with variable accuracy with her left upper extremity. She continued to have significant deficits, and it was determined that L.L. would benefit from an intensive outpatient therapy program. Because of the rural area where she lived and the family's limited resources for transportation, she would be followed by a home health therapy team. No therapists on the home health team had pediatric experience, so a video demonstrating intervention techniques was made by the pediatric team on the day of discharge. L.L. was also scheduled to be followed every 3 months for reassessment by the pediatric therapy team at the rehabilitation center.

L.L.'s last follow-up visit was 3 years after her injury (Fig. 24-8). She was receiving therapy 4 days weekly in a developmental preschool. She was able to ambulate with a walker, using bilateral fixed ankle-foot orthoses to assist with stability. She demonstrated an improved repertoire of play and had increased her vocabulary to include some two-word sentences. Her family continues to be thrilled with her progress and are very involved in her therapy activities.

■ REFERENCES

American Brain Tumor Association. A primer of brain tumors. Des Plaines, IL: ABTA, 1998, pp. 100–105.

American Physical Therapy Association. Guide to Physical Therapist Practice. Physical Therapy, 81:51–573, 2001.

Annegers, JF, Garbow, JD, Kurland, LT, & Laws, ER, Jr. The incidence, causes and secular trends of head trauma in Olmstead County Minnesota. Neurology, 30:912–919, 1980.

Barry, CT, Taylor, HG, Klein, S, & Yeates, KO. The validity of neurobehavioral symptoms reported in children after traumatic brain injury. Child Neuropsychology, 2:213–226, 1996.

Bastian, AJ. Mechanisms of ataxia. Physical Therapy, 77:672–675, 1997.

Blumenthal, I. Shaken baby syndrome. Postgraduate Medical Journal, 78:732–735, 2002.

Bruininks, RH. Bruininks-Oseretsky Test of Motor Proficiency. Circle Pines, MN: American Guidance Service, 1978.

Carmick, J. Guidelines for the clinical application of neuromuscular electrical stimulation (NMES) for children with cerebral palsy. Pediatric Physical Therapy, 9:128–136, 1997.

Centers for Disease Control, National Center for Injury Prevention and Control: WISQARS. Available at http://www.cdc.gov/ncipc/wisqars/. Accessed June 2003.

Citta-Pietrolungo, TJ, Alexander, MA, & Steg, NL. Early detection of heterotopic ossification in young patients with traumatic brain injury. Archives of Physical Medicine and Rehabilitation, 73:258–262, 1992.

Cochrane, DD, Gustavsson, B, Poskitt, KP, Steinbok, P, & Kestle, JR. The surgical and natural morbidity of aggressive resection for posterior fossa tumors in childhood. Pediatric Neurosurgery, 20:19–29, 1994.

Comeaux, P, Patterson, N, Rubin, M, & Meiner, R. Effect of neuromuscular electrical stimulation during gait in children with cerebral palsy. Pediatric Physical Therapy, 9:103–109, 1997.

Damiano, DL, & Abel, MF. Functional outcomes of strength training in spastic cerebral palsy. Archives of Physical Medicine and Rehabilitation 79:119–125, 1998.

Dietz, JH. Adaptive rehabilitation in cancer: A program to improve quality of survival. Postgraduate Medicine, 68:145–153, 1980.

Epstein, F, & McCleary, EL. Intrinsic brain stem tumors of childhood: surgical indications. Journal of Neurosurgery, 64:11–24, 1986.

Epstein, F, & Wisoff, JH. Intra-axial tumors of the cervico medullary junction. Journal of Neurosurgery, 67:483–487, 1987.

Epstein, F, & Wisoff, JH. Intrinsic brain stem tumors in childhood: Surgical indications. Journal of Neuro-oncology, 6:309–317, 1988.

Ewing-Cobbs, L, Lewin, HS, Fletcher, JM, Miner, ME, & Eisenberg, HM. Post-traumatic amnesia in children: Assessment and outcome. Paper presented at the meeting the International Neuropsychological Society. Vancouver, British Columbia, 1989.

Fay, GC, Jaffe, KM, Polissar, ML, Liao, S, Rivara, JB, & Martin, KM. Outcome of pediatric traumatic brain injury at three years: A cohort study. Archives of Physical Medicine and Rehabilitation, 75:73–741, 1994.

Fields, AI. Near-drowning in the pediatric population. Progress in Pediatric Critical Care, 8:113–129, 1992.

Fisher, DH. Near-drowning. Pediatric Review, 14:148–151, 1993.

Folio, MR, & Fewell, RR. Peabody Developmental Motor Scales, 2nd ed. Austin, TX: Pro-Ed, Inc., 2000.

Geddes, JF, Vowles, GH, Hackshaw, AK, Nichols, CD, Scott, IS, & Whitwell, HL. Neuropathology of inflicted head injury in children. II. Microscopic brain injury in infants. Brain, 124:1299–1306, 2001.

Gonzales-Luis,G, Pons, M, Cambra, FJ, Martin, JM, & Palomeque, A. Use of the Pediatric Risk of Mortality Score as predictor of death and serious neurologic damage in children after submersion. Pediatric Emergency Care, 17:405–409, 2001.

Gordon, WA, Sliwinski, M, Echo, J, McLoughlin, M, Sheerer, M, & Meili, T. The benefits of exercise in individuals with traumatic brain injury: A retrospective study. Journal of Head Trauma Rehabilitation, 13:58–67, 1998.

Guerra, WK, Gaab, MR, Dietz, H, Mueller, JU, Piek, J, & Fritsch, MJ. Surgical decompression for traumatic brain swelling: Indications and results. Journal of Neurosurgery, 90:187–196, 1999.

Gusnard, DA, & Zimmerman, RA. Computed tomography versus magnetic resonance imaging. Clinical Pediatrics, 29:136–157, 1990.

Gurney, JG, Kadan-Lottick, NS, Packer, RJ, Neglia, JP, Sklar, CA, Punyko, JA, Stovall, M, Yasui, Y, Nicholson, HS, Wolden, S, McNeil, DE, Mertens, AC, & Robison, LL. Endocrine and cardiovascular late effects among adult survivors of childhood brain tumors. Cancer, 97:663–673, 2003.

Gurney, JG, Smith, MA, & Bunin, GR. CNS and miscellaneous intracranial and intraspinal neoplasms. Washington, DC: National Cancer Institute SEER Pediatric Monograph, 1999.

Hagen, C, Makmus, D, Durhham, P, & Bowman, K. Levels of cognitive functioning. In Rehabilitation of the Head-Injured Adult: Comprehensive Physical Management. Downey, CA: Professional Staff Association of Rancho Los Amigos Hospital, 1979, pp. 87–90.

Haley, SM, Coster, WJ, Ludlow, LH, Halliwanges, JT, & Andrellos, PJ. Pediatric Evaluation of Disability Inventory (PEDI), version 1.0. Boston: New England Medical Center, 1992.

Harris, SR, & Lundgren, BD. Joint mobilization for children with central nervous system disorders: Indications and precautions. Physical Therapy, 71:890–896, 1991.

Hibbard, MR, Uysal, S, Sliwinski, M, & Gordon, WA. Undiagnosed health issues in individuals with traumatic brain injury living in the community. Journal of Head Trauma Rehabilitation, *13:*47–57, 1998.

Hurvitz, EA, Mandac, BR, Davidoff, G, Johnson, JH, & Nelson, VH. Risk factors for heterotopic ossification in children and adolescents with severe traumatic brain injury. Archives of Physical Medicine and Rehabilitation, *73:*459–462, 1992.

Hwang, V, Shofer, F, Durbin, D, & Baren, J. Prevalence of traumatic injuries in drowning and near drowning in children and adolescents. Archives of Pediatrics and Adolescent Medicine, *157:*50–53, 2003.

Ibsen, LM, & Koch, T. Submersion and asphyxial injury. Critcal Care Medicine, *30:*402–408, 2002.

Jaffe, KM, Polissar NL, Fay, GC, & Liao, S. Recovery trends over three years following pediatric traumatic brain injury. Archives of Physical Medicine and Rehabilitation, *76:*17–26, 1995.

Jaffe, KM, Fay, GC, Polissar, NL, Martin, KM, Shurtleff, H, Rivara, JB, & Winn, HR. Severity of pediatric traumatic brain injury and early neurobehavioral outcomes: A cohort study. Archives of Physical Medicine and Rehabilitation, *73:*540–547, 1992.

Janusz, JA, Kirkwood, MW, Yeates, KO, & Taylor, HG. Social problem solving skills in children with traumatic brain injury: Long term outcomes and prediction of social competence. Child Neuropsychology, *8:*179–194, 2002.

Kluger, G, Kochs, A, & Holthausen, H. Heterotopic ossification in childhood and adolescence. Journal of Child Neurology, *15:*406–413, 2000.

Kochanek, PM, Clark, RS, Ruppel, RA, & Dixon, CE. Cerebral resuscitation after traumatic brain injury and cardiopulmonary arrest in infants and children in the new millennium. Pediatric Clinics of North America, *48:*661–681, 2001.

Kosmidis, HV, Bouhoutsouu, DO, Varroutsi, MC, Papadatos, J, Stefanidis, CG, Vlachos, P, Scardoutsou, A, & Kostakis, A. Vincristine overdose experience with three patients. Pediatric Hematology and Oncology, *8:*171–178, 1991.

Kraus, JF, Rock, A, & Hemyari, P. Brain injuries among infants, children, adolescents and young adults. American Journal of the Disabled Child, *144:*684–691, 1990.

Kriel, RL, Krach, LE, & Panser LA. Closed head injury: Comparison of children younger and older than 6 years of age. Pediatric Neurology, *5:*296–300, 1989.

Langlois, J, & Gotsch, K. Traumatic Brain Injury in the United States: Assessing Outcomes in Children. Atlanta: National Center for Injury Prevention and Control, Centers for Disease Control and Prevention, 2001.

McLean, DE, Kaitz, ES, Keenan, CJ, Dabney, K, Cawley, MF, & Alexander, MA. Medical and surgical complications of pediatric brain injury. Journal of Head Trauma and Rehabilitation, *10:*1–12, 1995.

Menkes, JH, & Till, K. Tumors of the nervous system. In Menkes, JH (Ed.). Textbook of Child Neurology. Philadelphia: Lea & Febiger, 1990, pp. 526–582.

Michaud, LJ, Duhaime, AC, & Batshaw, ML. Traumatic brain injury in children. Pediatric Clinics of North America, *40:*553–565, 1993.

Muirhead, SE, Hsu, E, Grimard, L, & Keene, D. Endocrine complications of pediatric brain tumors: Case series and literature review. Pediatric Neurology, *27:*165–170, 2002.

O'Flaherty, SJ, Chivers, A, Hannan, TJ, Kendrick, LM, McCartney, LC, Wallen, MA, & Dogget C. The Westmead Pediatric TBI Multidisciplinary Outcome study: Use of functional outcomes data to determine resource prioritization. Archives of Physical Medicine and Rehabilitation, *81:*723–729, 2000.

Pang, D. Pathophysiologic correlates of neurobehavioral syndromes following closed head injury. In Ylviasaker, M (Ed.). Head Injury Rehabilitation. Austin, TX: Pro-Ed, 1985, pp. 3–70.

Public Law 101-336, Americans with Disabilities Act (1990), 42 USC Section 12101.

Public Law 105-17, Individuals with Disabilities Education Act Amendments of 1997, 105 USC Section 602.

Safar, P. Resuscitation from clinical death: Pathophysiologic limits and therapeutic potentials. Critical Care Medicine, *16:*923–941, 1988.

Shumway-Cook, A, & Horak, FB. Assessing the influence of sensory interaction on balance: suggestions from the field. Physical Therapy, *66:*1548–1550, 1986.

Shumway-Cook, A, & Woollacott, MH. Motor Control: Theory and Practical Applications. Baltimore: JB Lippincott, 2001, p. 22.

Teasdale, G, & Jennett, B. Assessment of coma and impaired consciousness: A practical scale. Lancet, *2:*81–84, 1974.

Tokcan, G, Haley, S, Gill-Body, KM, & Dumas, HM. Item Specific Functional Recovery in Children and Youth with Acquired Brain Injury. Pediatric Physical Therapy, *15:*16–22, 2003.

Uniform Data System for Medical Rehabilitation. The WeeFIM System Clinical Guide, Version 5.01. Buffalo: UDSMR, 2000.

Wright, MM. Resuscitation of the multitrauma patient with head injury. AACN Clinical Issues, *10:*32–45, 1999.

MYELODYSPLASIA

KATHLEEN A. HINDERER
PT, PhD
STEVEN R. HINDERER
PT, MD
DAVID B. SHURTLEFF
MD

Children and adolescents with myelodysplasia, perhaps more than most diagnostic groups of children with disabilities, challenge pediatric physical therapists to use and integrate many facets of their knowledge and skills. The multiple body systems affected by this congenital malformation make intervention of these patients highly complex, more than the congenital spinal cord defect alone might imply. Awareness of the many possible manifestations of this condition, knowledge of methods to examine and detect their presence, and the ability to evaluate the relative contribution of each manifestation to current activity limitations are important. This knowledge, combined with the ability to anticipate future needs and potential problems, empowers the physical therapist to select interventions that will optimize function and prevent the development of secondary impairments. Conversely, lack of awareness of these issues is not without consequences, as significant secondary permanent impairments can result when clinicians are not aware of or do not recognize early signs and symptoms of preventable complications related to myelodysplasia.

The objectives of this chapter are to familiarize the physical therapist with the numerous manifestations of myelodysplasia; describe its impact on body systems and functional skills; provide developmental expectations and prognosis based on the level of involvement; outline the roles of the various disciplines involved in team management; discuss methods of examination, evaluation, and diagnosis; and highlight intervention strategies for specific problems.

GENERAL OVERVIEW

TYPES OF MYELODYSPLASIA

Dorland's Medical Dictionary defines myelodysplasia as "defective development of any part (especially the lower segments) of the spinal cord." The various types of myelodysplasia are illustrated in Figure 25-1. *Spina bifida* is a commonly used term referring to various forms of myelodysplasia. Spina bifida is classified into *aperta* (visible or open) lesions and *occulta* (hidden or not visible) lesions (Lemire et al., 1975). The degree of motor and sensory loss from these lesions can range from no loss to severe impairment. Regardless of initial level of neurologic impairment, individuals with *any* of these lesions are at risk for further loss of function over time. Paralysis may occur later in life as a complication of abnormal tissue growth (dysplasia) causing pressure on nerves (e.g., lipomatous or dermoid tissue). Lack of proper growth of associated connective tissues around the malformed spinal cord can also cause ischemia and progressive neurologic impairment by tethering of the cord.

Spina bifida aperta is commonly thought of as *myelomeningocele*, which is an open spinal cord defect that usually protrudes dorsally. Myelomeningoceles are not skin covered and are usually associated with spinal nerve paralysis (see Fig. 25-1**A** and **B**). Meninges and nerves can also protrude anteriorly or laterally, making them not visible externally but still associated with nerve paralysis. Some individuals with myelomeningocele do not have associated paralysis.

Meningoceles are also classified as spina bifida aperta. They are skin covered and are initially associated with no paralysis (see Fig. 25-1**C**). Meningoceles contain only membranes or nonfunctional nerves that end in the sac wall (Lemire et al., 1975). Other skin-covered lesions, however, can be associated with paralysis.

The next most common form of myelodysplasia is a *lipoma* of the spinal cord. Lipomas are classified as spina bifida occulta, but most are visible. They may be large or small and manifest as distinct, subcutaneous masses of fat, frequently associated with abnormal pigmentation of the skin, hirsutism, skin appendages, and dimples above the gluteal cleft. A lipomatous or fibrous tract descends ventrally from the subcutaneous lipoma to varying extents into the subdural space adjacent to the spinal cord. Lipomas of the spinal cord are therefore classified based on the location of the tract. They can be (1) lipomyelomeningocele with paralysis, (2) lipomeningoceles with no paralysis, (3) lipomas of the filum terminale usually with no paralysis, and (4) lipomas of the cauda equina or conus medullaris with or without paralysis at birth. If paralysis is absent at birth, it is acquired over time, and if present at birth, it will worsen with time. Some lipomas involving the spinal cord are not associated with an extension to subcutaneous fat. Lipomas of the spinal cord may or may not be associated with bifid vertebrae (true spina bifida occulta).

Diastematomyelia is a fibrous, cartilaginous, or bony band or spicule separating the spinal cord into hemicords, each surrounded by a dural sac. It can occur as an isolated defect along with vertebral anomalies or in conjunction with either myelomeningocele or lipomyelomeningocele. Depending on the associated involvement of the spinal cord and meninges, diastematomyelia may be associated with paralysis initially, or progressive weakness can develop later in occulta lesions as a result of cord tethering.

The least common of the myelodysplasias are separate or septated cysts. These *myelocystoceles* are separate from the central canal of the spinal cord and from the subarachnoid space. They occur in the low lumbar and sacral area and are skin covered. They may or may not be associated with nerve impairment or lipomas of the spinal cord. When a myelocystocele is associated with a primitive gut and an open abdomen, it is classified as an *exstrophy of the cloaca*. When the bony elements of the sacrum are missing or abnormal, such myelocystic lesions are termed *sacral agenesis*.

PATHOEMBRYOLOGY

Embryologically, myelodysplastic lesions can be related to two different processes of nervous system formation: abnormal neurulation or canalization. *Neurulation* is the

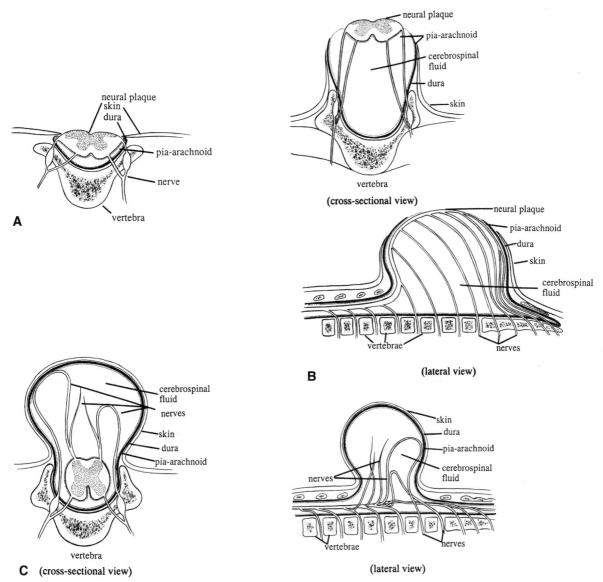

◆ **Figure 25-1**   Types of myelodysplasia. **A**, An illustration of a myelocele with no cystic subarachnoid space anterior to the spinal cord as is observed with myelomeningocele. **B**, A myelomeningocele may barely protrude from the back or may be a large sessile lesion as pictured here. There is a covering membrane with nerves imbedded in the dome of the sac. These spinal nerves occasionally return to their appropriate neural foramina to exit from the spinal canal. **C**, This type of lesion may be incompletely covered or have a full-thickness skin covering as shown here. When such a lesion is completely skin covered and is associated with no paralysis, it is classified as a meningocele. Meningoceles have only a few or no nerves attached to the dome of the sac. *(Adapted from Shurtleff, DB [Ed.]. Myelodysplasias and Exstrophies: Significance, Prevention, and Treatment. Orlando, FL: Grune & Stratton, 1986, pp. 44 and 45.)*

folding of ectoderm (primitive skin and associated structures) on each side of the notochord (primitive spinal cord) to form a tube that extends from the hindbrain to the second sacral vertebra. Meningoceles can therefore occur both over the skull and along the spinal column. Encephaloceles (containing brain if along the midline of the skull) and myelomeningoceles, which can occur along the spinal canal from the C1 to S2 vertebrae, result from a failure of complete entubulation with associated abnormal mesodermal (primitive connective tissue, muscle, and nervous tissue) development. Abnormal mesodermal development produces epidermal sinus tracts, lipomas, and diastematomyelia, as well as unfused posterior vertebral laminae (i.e., true spina bifida occulta) (Lemire et al., 1975). Neurulation occurs early in development, before day 28 of gestation.

The spinal cord distal to the S2 vertebra develops by *canalization*. Groups of cells in the dorsal, central midline of the mesoderm, distal to the S2 vertebra, become nerve cells. These cells clump together into masses, which develop cystic structures that join to form many canals. The canals ultimately fuse into one tubular structure that joins with the distal end of the spinal cord, which was developing from the neurulation process described previously. Failure of proper canalization, with subsequent retrogressive development of this region, embryologically explains the occurrence of skin-covered meningoceles, lipomas of the spinal cord, and myelocystoceles, all of which most frequently develop caudal to the L3 vertebra (Lemire et al., 1975).

The much better formed, essentially normal, central nervous system (CNS) observed in lesions associated with abnormal canalization and the frequency of CNS malformations (e.g., Arnold-Chiari type II, mental impairment, cranial nerve palsies, and hydrocephalus) associated with neurulation can be explained by the way that neurulation takes place. The neural crests first fuse at approximately the C1 vertebra, and closure of the neural tube progresses simultaneously in cephalad and caudal directions. The same embryologic neurulation processes are simultaneously forming the CNS from the tectal plate to the midlumbar area. It is therefore logical that an influence sufficient to interfere with neurulation along the spinal canal would also interfere with development of the cephalad end, producing CNS malformations above the spinal cord level, which are commonly exhibited in this population (Lemire et al., 1975). Because canalization occurs by different embryologic processes at a different time period than neurulation, any factor interfering with canalization will not necessarily affect neurulation, so the CNS usually forms normally above the midlumbar area.

ETIOLOGY

The cause of canalization disorders is unknown. This discussion therefore focuses on disorders of neurulation and, in particular, on myelomeningocele. These causes may also apply to other neural tube defects that can result from defective neurulation (anencephaly, encephalocele, meningocele, and lipomyelomeningocele, all with or without diastematomyelia). For brevity, we refer to all these lesions throughout this chapter as MM for myelomeningocele and its associated malformations (Shurtleff et al., 1986a).

Genetics

MM is often associated with genetic abnormalities, including chromosomal aberrations and other classic "syndromes." Each child born with MM, therefore, warrants a careful physical examination by a pediatrician because the "syndrome" is usually more important than the spinal lesion for defining prognosis. The recurrence risk for siblings in the United States is 2% to 3% (Shurtleff et al., 1986a).

The occurrence of MM varies among races and regions of the world. African blacks have the lowest incidence at 1 in 10,000. Celts (Eastern Irish, Western Scots, and all Welsh) have had a birth incidence recorded as high as 1 in 80. The Spanish also have a high birth incidence; however, these patients have unusually good leg function and minimal CNS abnormalities considering their thoracic and high lumbar level lesions. Sikhs living in Vancouver, British Columbia, have another form of MM, with a higher frequency in birth incidence than many other genetically related groups. One can conclude from these data that either there are many different genetic causes for MM or that there are many different genetically determined responses to one or more teratogens (Shurtleff et al., 1986a).

Teratogens

Teratogens can cause MM. Excess maternal alcohol intake can produce a classic fetal alcohol syndrome with MM. Ingestion of valproic acid (an anticonvulsant medication) during pregnancy is also associated with an increased birth incidence of MM. Many other possible teratogens have been studied, but inadequate descriptions of the pathology of the lesions and the relative infrequency of their occurrence have resulted in inconclusive observations. The rachitic lesion illustrated by Jacobson and Berlin (1972) suggests that the MM they observed among progeny of street-drug abusers is a specific entity that is probably due to nutritional deprivation, teratogens, or a combination of these influences. More studies combining detailed family histories, pathologic anatomy, and detailed physical examinations must be conducted to determine the relative contribution of teratogens to MM formation (Shurtleff et al., 1986a).

Nutritional Deficiencies

Inadequate levels of dietary folic acid have been identified as a cause of MM and anencephaly in some populations. A significant decrease in the incidence of MM births and abortions was observed for MM diagnosed prenatally in the United Kingdom during a placebo-controlled trial of prenatal folic acid administration for women who had given birth to a previous baby with a neural tube defect (CIBA, 1994; MRC Vitamin Study Research Group, 1991). With the introduction of more foods containing folic acid in the Celtic regions of the United Kingdom, particularly during winter and early spring when such foods were unavailable in the past, there has been a decrease in the birth incidence of MM predating the research on folic acid supplementation (Elwood & Elwood, 1980).

The decrease in birth incidence in the United Kingdom reflects a current worldwide trend. Four reports have suggested that the European and United Kingdom studies regarding the benefit of supplementation of folic acid can be applied to the culturally and genetically more diverse populations of Canada, Mexico, and China, where there are different racial and regional differences in the birth incidence of MM (De Villarreal et al., 2002; Gucciardi et al., 2002; Persad et al., 2002; Beery et al., 1999). The data from the United States does not include pregnancies terminated because of in utero diagnosis of neural tube defects and, therefore, has led to controversy (Birth Defects and Genetic Diseases Branch of Birth Defects and Developmental Disabilities Office, 1991; Mills et al., 1989; Milunsky et al., 1989; Seller & Nevin, 1984).

Regardless of the applicability of these studies to the population of the United States, we recommend advising women to take folic acid in an effort to reduce both the recurrence in families (MRC,1991) and the occurrence in families without a member with MM (Berry et al., 1999; Czeizel & Dudas, 1992). Women with a first-degree relative with MM or with history of having an open neural tube defect in a previous child or fetus should be advised to take 4 mg per day, and women without a positive history should be advised to take 0.4 mg per day. Both should begin the folic acid at least 3 months before conception. Folic acid is believed to be harmless in this age group because the only possible concern is the masking of pernicious anemia due to cobalamin deficiency, allowing progression of the subacute combined degeneration of the spinal cord resulting from cobalamin deficiency. Cobalamin deficiency is rare in this age group, and awareness of the possibility of neurologic loss from spinal cord degeneration should lead to early detection before significant harm occurs. The only other precaution is to warn the women that taking folic acid reduces their risk by 70% but does not eliminate the occurrence of open neural tube defects and has no known effect on the occurrence of closed neural tube defects.

INCIDENCE AND PREVALENCE

Superimposed on a general worldwide decrease in the birth incidence of MM are a number of influences to cause both a reduction in birth incidence and increased prevalence due to improved survival. Better nutrition mentioned earlier for the Celtic region of the United Kingdom and Ireland applies to many areas of the industrialized world. Wider availability of maternal serum alpha-

fetoprotein screening and more highly refined resolution of diagnostic ultrasonography for fetal examination have given parents an option to terminate pregnancies because their fetus has MM (Main & Mennuti, 1986; Babcook, 1995). Conversely, prenatal diagnosis has allowed other parents to select cesarean section prior to rupture of the amniotic membranes and onset of labor, avoiding trauma to the neural sac from vaginal delivery. The outcome of cesarean delivery compared to vaginal delivery has been children with less paralysis and with minimal risk for CNS infection, both of which were previously a cause for increased morbidity and early death (Liu et al., 1999; Shurtleff et al., 1994). Improved medical care has resulted in increased survival and, secondarily, an increased prevalence of MM. Incidence at birth in the United States has been reported to range from 0.4 to 0.9 per 1000 births, depending on the reporting source (Shurtleff et al., 1986a).

PERINATAL MANAGEMENT

The past decade has altered the intervention of MM from a postnatal crisis of horrendous magnitude to a prenatal option of either pregnancy termination or improved pregnancy outcome by prelabor cesarean section birth. This advance has been made possible by widespread use of maternal serum alpha-fetoprotein screening and improved resolution of ultrasonography (Main & Mennuti, 1986). Unfortunately, this type of screening will not detect skin-covered neural defects such as meningoceles, lipomyelomeningoceles, or other rare lesions covered by skin.

Technical improvements are being made rapidly in ultrasonography so that minor variations in the frontal bones of the fetus and encapsulation of the midbrain by the cerebellum can be interpreted as the "lemon" and "banana" signs (Babcook, 1995). These ultrasonographic signs are more accurate in defining the cranial malformations associated with MM than in detecting abnormalities of the spine. As discussed in the section on pathoembryology, these ultrasonographic signs are pertinent to neural tube defects cephalad to the S2 vertebra (i.e., neurulation defects) but not to canalization defects, which are usually not associated with cranial malformations responsible for the Arnold-Chiari type II malformation (Shurtleff, 1986e), the cause of the "lemon" and "banana" signs. Some spinal dysraphic states and dorsal lumbosacral masses consistent with canalization defects such as myelocystocele or lipomyelomeningocele can be identified with ultrasonography. Other anomalies consistent with syndromes or organ malformations that are incompatible with survival beyond intrauterine life (e.g., anencephaly) can also be detected.

A third modality for prenatal diagnosis, amniotic fluid analysis, is critical in the evaluation of a fetus with a neural tube defect. Up to 10% of fetuses with a neural tube defect, detected in the first half of the second trimester or before, have an associated chromosome error, usually trisomy 13 or 18 (Luthy et al., 1991). Chromosome analysis of amniotic cells is therefore essential to the parental decision-making process regarding abortion of the pregnancy. From the same amniotic fluid specimen obtained for chromosome analysis, the acetylcholinesterase level can be determined. This test is more accurate than determination of the amniotic fluid level of alphafetoprotein used previously because the former is positive only in a fetus with an open neural tube defect (Main & Mennuti, 1986). The presence of a dorsal spine lesion and a negative result of an acetylcholinesterase test suggest a skin-covered meningocele or other skin-covered MM, which is an indication for normal vaginal delivery. A MM lesion containing nerves protruding dorsal to the plane of the back, in the presence of fetal knee or ankle function observed on ultrasonography, warrants prelabor cesarean section, sterile delivery, and closure of the open-back lesion to preserve nerve function (Luthy et al., 1991).

Prenatal diagnosis has allowed the introduction of repair of the MM sac in utero. Tulipan and associates (2003) report a decreased need for a cerebrospinal fluid shunt when intrauterine repairs are performed. The authors also claim improvement in the Chiari II malformation, as evidenced solely by improved appearance on magnetic resonance imaging (MRI). Bannister (2000) has cautioned that the MRI appearance is not as important as function. Many believe the Chiari II symptoms are due to abnormalities in neurulation causing failure of brainstem nuclei to develop properly. Tulipan and associates' (2003) claims, however, are not substantiated by the results of cases sent for intrauterine repair by several referral centers to the two surgical treatment centers cited by these authors. Twenty-one of the 26 cases have required cerebrospinal fluid shunts. Additional complications for the 26 infants included the following: 3 had severe Chiari II symptoms, 6 had prolonged neonatal intensive care hospitalizations for apnea due to a combination of prematurity (30–31 weeks' gestational age) and Chiari II symptoms, and 4 had dehiscence in utero, with 3 of these 4 developing gramnegative meningitis. In order to resolve the controversial issues surrounding intrauterine MM repair, the U.S. federal government has funded a prospective study, Management of Myelomeningocele (MOMS), in three centers with prior experience with intrauterine surgery. Patients are referred via a fourth center, the Biostatistics Center of George Washington University (1-866-ASK-MOMS). This center assigns cases to one of three treating centers and to either the treatment group (cesarean section delivery with intrauterine repair) or a control group (cesarean section delivery without intrauterine repair). The results of this study will determine the value of intrauterine repair of MM.

IMPAIRMENTS

The discussions of pathoembryology and diagnosis describe the potential involvement of the brain and brainstem in addition to the spinal cord in individuals with MM. The multifocal involvement of the CNS results in several possible complex problems, making the care of these individuals more challenging than and substantially different from that of children with traumatic spinal cord injuries. The broad spectrum of problems encountered with MM requires a multidisciplinary team approach in a comprehensive care outpatient clinic setting. In this section the variety of impairments that can occur with MM are described. In addition, general examination and intervention issues related to each impairment are discussed. *Impairment*, for the purpose of this discussion, is defined as a change in body structure and function, whereas *activity limitation* is the inability to perform tasks as a consequence of impairments. Activity limitations and participation restrictions encountered at specific age levels, along with age-specific examination, evaluation, and intervention issues, are discussed in subsequent sections of this chapter.

MUSCULOSKELETAL DEFORMITIES

Spinal and lower limb deformities and joint contractures occur frequently in children with MM. Orthopedic deformities and joint contractures negatively affect positioning, body image, weight bearing (both in sitting and standing), activities of daily living (ADL), energy expenditure, and mobility from infancy through adulthood. Several factors contribute to abnormal posture, limb deformity, and joint contractures, including muscle imbalance secondary to neurologic dysfunction, progressive neurologic dysfunction, intrauterine positioning, coexisting congenital malformations, arthrogryposis, habitually assumed postures after birth, reduced or absent active joint motion, and deformities after fractures (Mayfield, 1991; Shurtleff, 1986d). The upper limbs can also be involved as a result of spasticity or poor postural habits. The upper limb region most likely to have restricted motion is the shoulder girdle due to overuse of the arms for weight bearing and poor postural habits.

Postural stability is essential to effectively perform functional tasks. Symmetric alignment is important to minimize joint stress and deforming forces and to permit muscles to function at their optimal length. Uncorrected postural deficits can result in joint contractures and deformities, stretch weakness, and musculoskeletal pain. Deficits that may appear insignificant during childhood often become magnified once an individual has adult body proportions, resulting in activity limitations and discomfort (e.g., low back pain resulting from an increased lumbar lordosis and hip flexion contractures). Consequently, limb, neck, and trunk range of motion (ROM), muscle extensibility, and joint alignment should be monitored throughout the life span so that appropriate interventions can be implemented as indicated.

Typical postural problems include forward head, rounded shoulders, kyphosis, scoliosis, excessive lordosis, anterior pelvic tilt, rotational deformities of the hip or tibia (in-toeing, out-toeing, or windswept positions), flexed hips and knees, and pronated feet. It is important to observe posture and postural control after a given position has been maintained for a period of time to determine the effects of fatigue. Static and dynamic balance should be observed in sitting, four-point positioning, kneeling, half-kneeling, and standing, as well as during transitions between these positions. Symmetry and weight distribution should also be noted. In addition, typical sleeping and sitting positions should be identified to determine if habitual positioning is contributing to postural or joint deformities (e.g., "frog-leg" position in prone or supine, W-sitting, ring sitting, heel sitting, cross-legged sitting, and crouch standing). These habitual positions should be avoided because they may produce deforming forces and altered musculotendon length that result in the development of secondary impairments such as the progression of orthopedic deformities, joint contractures, and strength deficits. Photographs or videotapes of sitting and standing postures are often useful to document current status and to provide a visual baseline for future reference.

Postural deviations and contractures that are typical for individual lesion levels are summarized as follows. Individuals with high-level lesions (thoracic to L2) often have hip flexion, abduction, and external rotation contractures; knee flexion contractures; and ankle plantar flexion contractures. The lumbar spine is typically lordotic. Individuals with mid- to low-lumbar (L3-L5) lesion levels often have hip and knee flexion contractures, an increased lumbar lordosis, genu and calcaneal valgus malalignment, and a pronated position of the foot when bearing weight. They often walk with a pronounced crouched gait and bear weight primarily on their calcaneus. Individuals with sacral level lesions often have mild hip and knee flexion contractures and an increased lumbar lordosis, and the ankle and foot can either be in varus or valgus, combined with a pronated or supinated

forefoot. They may walk with a mild crouch gait and may bear weight primarily on their calcaneus unless plantar flexor muscles are at least grade 3/5.

Crouch standing is a typical postural deviation that is observed across lesion levels and is characterized by persistent hip and knee flexion and an increased lumbar lordosis. The crouch posture often occurs because of muscle weakness (e.g., insufficient soleus strength to maintain the tibia vertical) and orthopedic deformities (e.g., calcaneal valgus, which results in obligatory tibial internal rotation and knee flexion). Hip and knee flexion contractures often occur secondarily, in response to adaptive shortening of muscles from prolonged positioning in the crouch-standing posture. Altered postures, such as crouch standing, negatively affect both the task requirements (by increasing the muscle torque required to maintain the position) and the torque-generating capacity of the musculoskeletal system (Hinderer, 2003). Such increased demands placed upon the musculoskeletal system when standing and walking in a crouched posture may negatively impact function and result in secondary impairments (Andersson & Mattsson, 2001; Brown, 2001; Hinderer, 2003; Lollar, 1994; Murphy et at., 1995; Nagankatti et al., 2000; Shurtleff & Dunne, 1986; Turk & Weber, 1998; Winter, 1983). It is important that appropriate intervention be implemented to ameliorate crouch standing so that the excessive physical demands and stress placed on the musculoskeletal system are reduced and the development of secondary impairments is prevented.

Scoliosis occurring with MM can be congenital or acquired; the congenital form is usually related to underlying vertebral anomalies and the curve is often inflexible, whereas the acquired type is usually caused by muscle imbalance and the curve is flexible until skeletal maturity is reached (Mayfield, 1991), at which point little further progression is usually observed (Shurtleff, 1986d). Scoliosis is more frequently observed in higher lesion level groups and becomes more prevalent and increasingly severe with age in all groups (Mayfield, 1991).

Other spinal deformities that can occur in conjunction with or separate from scoliosis are kyphosis and lordosis deformities (Fig. 25-2). Congenital kyphosis occurs in 10% to 15% of infants with MM (Mintz et al., 1991; Torode & Godette, 1995). Paralytic kyphosis is acquired in approximately one third by early adolescence (Brown, 2001), progressing at a rate of 7% to 8% per year (Banta & Hamada, 1976). Kyphosis can occur in the lumbar spine with reversal of the lumbar lordosis, or the kyphosis can be more diffusely distributed over the entire spine. Hyperlordosis of the lumbar spine is another commonly observed deformity. Like scoliosis, both kyphosis and lordosis are more commonly observed in children with

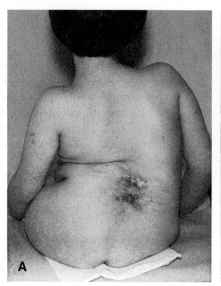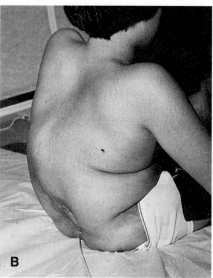

♦ **Figure 25-2** Spinal deformities. **A**, Collapsing type of lordoscoliosis. **B**, Kyphotic spinal deformity.

higher spinal lesions and the curves tend to progress with age (Mayfield, 1991). Severe kyphosis and scoliosis can limit chest wall expansion with consequent restriction of lung ventilation and frequent respiratory infections. The resulting restrictive lung condition can limit exercise tolerance and can be life-threatening in extreme cases (Mayfield, 1991). Poor sitting posture, muscle imbalance, and recurrent skin ulcerations are additional problems encountered (Brown, 2001).

The goal of treatment of spinal deformities is to maintain a balanced trunk and pelvis (Karol, 1995). Orthotic intervention, usually with a bivalved Silastic thoracolumbosacral orthosis (TLSO), is helpful in maintaining improved trunk position for functional activities but does not prevent progression of acquired spinal deformity (Mayfield, 1991). For children with progressive spinal deformities, orthotic intervention is continued until the child reaches a sufficient age to allow surgical fusion of the spine to prevent further progression of these deformities. Long spinal fusions before the skeletal age of 10 result in greater loss of trunk height because of ablation of the growth plates of vertebral bodies included in the fusion mass (Mayfield, 1991). In addition, surgery at too young a skeletal age is associated with an increased frequency of instrumentation failure as a result of fragile bones and skin breakdown over the bulky spinal instrumentation (Mayfield, 1991). The ideal minimum age for spinal fusion is 10 to 11 years old in girls and 12 to 13 years old in boys (Mayfield, 1991). In general, children with spina bifida reach puberty and their growth spurt earlier than their able-bodied peers, so only minimal

truncal shortening occurs as a consequence of long spinal fusion when it is performed at the appropriate age.

Hip joints also are prone to deformity in children with MM. Fixed flexion deformities often require surgical intervention because they interfere with ambulation and orthotic fit. Correction after surgery should be maintained by encouraging standing and walking (Dias, 1999b; Menelaus, 1999). Children with high lumbar lesions (L1, L2) have unopposed flexion and adduction forces that gradually push the femoral head superiorly and posteriorly. The resulting contractures and secondary bony deformities of the proximal femur and acetabulum can lead to subluxation or dislocation (Fig. 25-3, A and B) in nearly one third to one half of children with MM (Dias, 1999b).

In children with hip subluxation or dislocation, long-term follow-up studies have indicated that reduction of the hips is not a prerequisite for ambulation (Sherk et al., 1991). Mayfield (1991) stated that a level pelvis and good ROM are more important for function than hip reduction. Furthermore, he stated that the presence of the femoral head in the acetabulum does not necessarily improve ROM at the hip or the ability to ambulate. In addition, unlike in children with cerebral palsy, it does not appear to affect the amount of orthotic support required, hip pain, or gait deviation (Ryan et al., 1991). The indications for hip surgery in children with MM continue to be controversial; however, a basic principle practiced at many centers is to operate only on children with a lesion level at or below L3, when quadriceps muscle function is present, because these children are

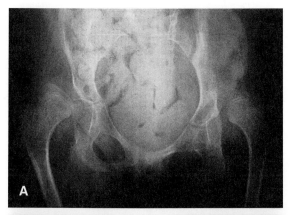

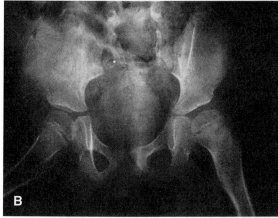

• **Figure 25-3**   Lower limb deformities. **A**, Hip dislocation. **B**, Hip dysplasia and subluxation.

more likely to be functional ambulators into adulthood (Mayfield, 1991; Shurtleff, 1986d). Fixed pelvic obliquity caused by unilateral subluxation or dislocation interferes with sitting or standing posture, contributes to scoliosis, and makes skin care unmanageable. It is another indication for surgical relocation of the hip, regardless of lesion level or ambulatory potential, along with painful hip dysplasia in ambulators (Staheli, 2001).

Shurtleff (1986d) evaluated the frequency of all types of hip contractures in large numbers of children with various spinal lesion levels. He noted that contractures measured in infancy tended to decrease in severity until approximately age 3 to 4 years, then increased to much higher values by adolescence. The initial decrease in severity of hip contractures can potentially be explained as a normal physiologic phenomenon resulting from intrauterine positioning. The increase in severity of contractures by adolescence, however, is of special concern to physical therapists. Mild contractures of minimal functional significance in young children can increase dramatically during later childhood and adolescence,

necessitating persistent intervention and follow-up by the therapist to prevent significant functional loss. Consequently, physical therapists should be proactive in preventing the progression of contractures. Thoracic and high lumbar (L1, L2) groups of children have a higher incidence and greater severity of contractures owing to unopposed iliopsoas function, regardless of whether they were participating in a standing program or not (Liptak et al., 1992). Shurtleff (1986d) reported progressively declining frequency and severity of contractures in groups of children with lesions at L3, L4 to L5, and sacral levels, respectively. An unexpected finding from Shurtleff's study was that only a certain percentage of children in each lesion level group had hip contractures, subluxation, or both. These relative percentages were not altered by surgical procedures on the hip and stayed constant across age groups. No clear reasons were discerned why certain individuals were susceptible to contractures while others with similar neurologic function were not.

The knee joints of children with MM frequently have contractures or deformities. These include both flexion and extension contractures; the former more commonly occur in children who primarily use a wheelchair for mobility (Liptak et al., 1992), and the latter often occur after periods of immobility from fractures, decubitus ulcers, or surgical procedures. Varus and valgus deformities (see Fig. 25-3, C and D) are also observed. Flexion deformities may make walking difficult or impossible, and extension deformities may complicate sitting. If either flexion or extension deformities are significant, they may need to be ameliorated via surgical release (Staheli, 2001). Wright and associates (1991) reported that 60% of individuals with fixed flexion contractures less than 20° and a lesion level higher than L3 were still biped ambulators in late adolescence, as compared to fewer than 5% of individuals with fixed flexion contractures greater than 20°. They also concluded that muscle imbalance and spasticity do not appear to be major causative factors; rather, the lack of normal joint movement may lead to joint stiffness. As described earlier for the hip joints, Shurtleff (1986d) studied the frequency of knee contractures and deformities in children with different lesion levels. An initial decrease from the contractures measured in infants was also noted at the knees, with the lowest prevalence occurring at age 4 to 5 years for patients with L3 or higher lesions, and at age 2 to 3 years for children with lesions below L3. The frequency and severity of contractures increased in all groups from early childhood into adolescence. Knee joint contractures occurred in 65% to 70% of the thoracic and high lumbar groups by age 6 to 8, 20% to 25% of the L4 to L5 group by age 9 to 12, and sporadically among the children with sacral level lesions. Valgus and

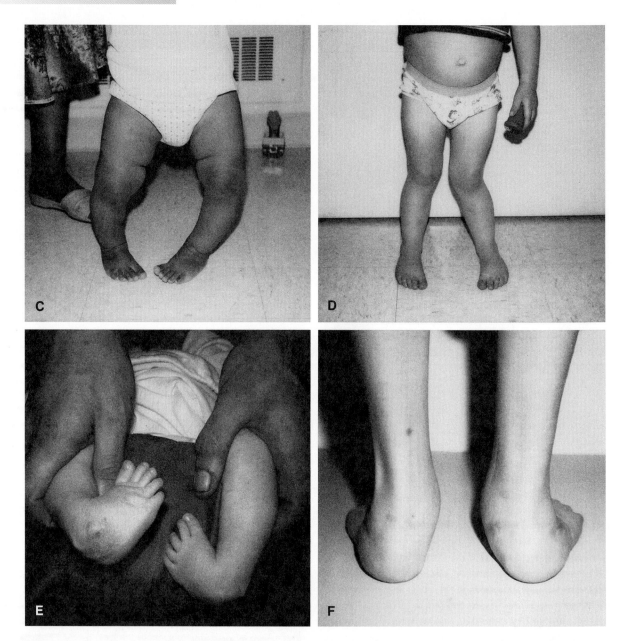

• **Figure 25-3 (*con't*)** Lower limb deformities. **C**, Genu varus. **D**, Genu valgus. **E**, Equinovarus. **F**, Calcaneal valgus.

varus deformities were most frequently observed in the L3 and above groups, with a slight increase during adolescence.

Deformities of the ankles and feet can occur in both ambulatory and nonambulatory children and are most common in children with lesion levels at L5 and above (Shurtleff, 1986d). Partial innervation and consequent muscle imbalance determine the type of deformity that occurs. Even with surgical correction these deformities will recur unless the deforming forces are removed. Progressive ankle and foot deformities can also be observed in conjunction with the development of spasticity and motor strength loss associated with tethering of the spinal cord. Children with "skip" lesions (see section on motor paralysis) are particularly prone to progressive foot deformities (Shurtleff, 1986d).

A variety of foot and ankle deformities can occur (see Fig. 25-3, *E* and *F*), including ankle equinovarus (clubfeet), forefoot varus or valgus, forefoot supination or pronation, calcaneal varus or valgus, pes cavus and planus, and claw-toe deformities. The most frequent contracture observed is of the ankle plantar flexor muscles. The frequency of foot deformities has been reported to vary from 20% to 50% between lesion level groups (Shurtleff, 1986d) and has been reported to be as high as 90% for high level paralysis and 60% to 70% for lower level paralysis (Broughton et al., 1994; Frawley et al., 1998; Staheli, 2001). Although some deformities are more frequently associated with certain neurosegmental levels (e.g., clubfeet in thoracic and high lumbar lesions, claw-toes in sacral lesions), all types of ankle and foot deformities are observed in children at every lesion level. Congenital club feet are common and surgery is indicated once the child is developmentally ready to stand (Brown, 2001). Other foot deformities may develop over time as a result of muscle imbalance. Dias (1999a) noted that ankle valgus occurs in the presence of fibular shortening, the latter being highly correlated with paralysis of the soleus muscle. Surgical treatment of a valgus ankle is indicated when the deformity cannot be functionally alleviated with orthotics. The presence of ankle and foot deformities can greatly affect sitting and standing posture, balance, mobility, foot ulcerations, and shoe fit, regardless of lesion level. Weight-bearing forces often result in ankle and foot deformities. Even partial weight bearing on wheelchair footrests in poor alignment over time can result in deformities and foot ulcerations. Consequently, achieving a plantigrade position of the feet is a priority, regardless of ambulatory status. Surgical procedures are often necessary and are effective (Staheli, 2001). Orthoses and assistive devices should be adjusted properly to maintain neutral subtalar alignment and a plantigrade foot position.

Torsional deformities are common. Excessive foot progression angles and windswept positions of the lower limbs are often present (Fig. 25-4) as a result of hip anteversion, hip retroversion, or tibial torsion. These torsional deformities negatively affect sitting and standing balance, weight distribution, and walking. See Cusick and Stuberg (1992) for factors that contribute to torsional deformities in individuals with developmental disabilities, examination procedures, normative values, and intervention suggestions.

Joint alignment and evidence of abnormal joint stress are often most apparent during dynamic activities, such as walking or wheelchair propulsion. Joint stresses are often magnified when walking on uneven surfaces, stairs, or curbs. Observing wear patterns on shoes and orthoses can provide additional clues to abnormal stress and malalignment. If joint deformities are supple, they may respond to stretching, combined with orthoses or positioning splints to maintain alignment. Fixed deformities may respond to serial casting (e.g., foot deformities) but will often require surgical intervention (e.g., scoliosis, unilateral hip dislocation, or tibial torsion). If muscle imbalance is severe and the deforming forces are not effectively counteracted by stretching, strengthening, or positioning, muscle transfers may be indicated (e.g., partial transfer of the anterior tibialis muscle to the calcaneus to achieve a plantigrade foot position by balancing the unopposed dorsiflexion force in a child with L5 motor function).

There are several reasons for maintaining joint ROM. Limited ROM can interfere with ADL, bed mobility, and transfers. Bed mobility is more efficient and self-care is easier for individuals who have maintained their flexibility (Hinderer & Hinderer, 1988). Restricted ROM, combined with muscle weakness, can result in poor postural habits and gait deviations. Adequate ROM must be maintained to perform ADL, such as bathing and toileting. Restricted joint motion can result in overlengthening of weak muscles, not permitting them to function in the optimal range of the length-tension curve. Limited ROM may result in discomfort, especially when lying down (e.g., tight hip flexors pulling on the lumbar spine). Severe contractures also can negatively affect body image. Contractures that may seem insignificant during childhood may become functionally limiting once the individual has adult-sized body proportions (e.g., knee extension contractures can interfere with the ability to maneuver in a wheelchair). In extreme cases, difficulty in managing paralyzed limbs because of joint contractures can put individuals at risk for skin breakdown and possibly amputations because of the increased incidence of injury (Hinderer et al., 1988). The impact of limited ROM on functional performance should be considered before deciding whether intervention is indicated.

ROM and positioning of paralytic limbs should be done carefully, without excessive force, to avoid fractures (Schneider et al., 2001). Caution should also be exercised when adducting the hips to avoid hip dislocation. The prone hip extension test (Staheli, 1977) for measuring hip extension is the method of choice in this population because of interference of spinal and pelvic deformities and lower limb spasticity with the traditional Thomas test method (Bartlett et al., 1985). Ankle ROM should always be measured with the ankle joint in subtalar neutral so that measurements are comparable.

The long-term effects of surgical interventions and weight bearing on insensate joints are becoming evident as individuals with MM reach adulthood (Brown, 2001). Secondary impairments of knee joint deterioration and arthritis occur with increased frequency in older individuals (Lollar, 1994). Nagarkatti and associates (2000) reported a prevalence of 1 per 100 cases of Charcot arthroplasty in the MM population.

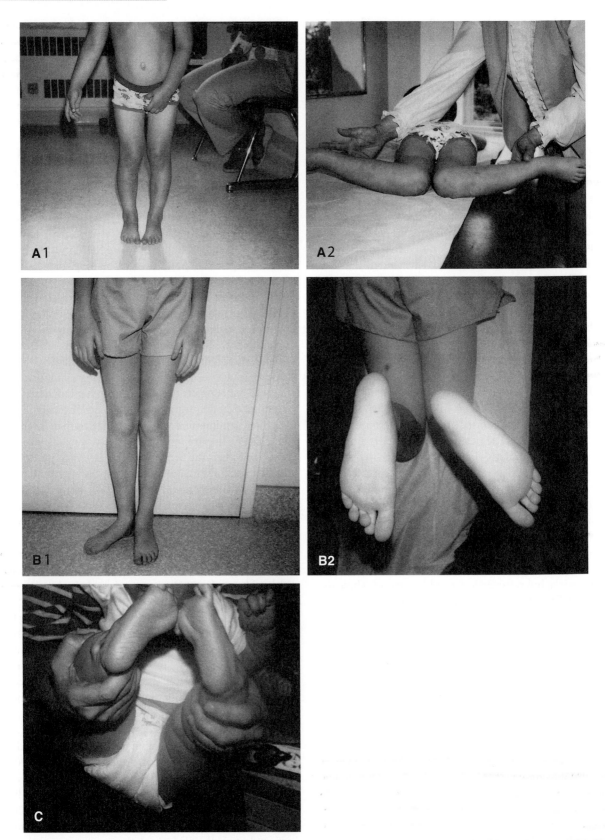

♦ **Figure 25-4**   Torsional deformities. **A**, Femoral neck anteversion. **B**, External tibial torsion. **C**, Internal tibial torsion.

There are several ways to minimize musculoskeletal stress and reduce the incidence of acquired orthopedic deformities. Improving traction of the hands by providing biking gloves for community wheelchair mobility reduces the grip forces required for wheelchair propulsion. Wheelchair seat positions influence propulsion effectiveness and the amount of stress on upper limb joints and muscles (Masse et al., 1992). For ambulators, shoes with nonskid soles improve foot traction. Symmetric neutral joint alignment should be maintained in both sitting and standing via appropriate orthotics or seating devices. It is important to avoid shifting weight to one leg when standing and to avoid crossing the legs when sitting. Extreme ROM should be avoided, especially when bearing weight. Crutch and walker handgrips should be angled to avoid hyperextension of the wrists, and weight should be distributed across a broad, cushioned area. Orthoses should provide total contact to minimize the risk of development of pressure areas. Excessive pressure on tendons and the palms of the hand should be avoided to reduce the risk of developing carpal tunnel syndrome. Overhead reaching and work activities should be minimized by adapting the home, school, and work environments. In addition, long-distance mobility options should be provided to reduce joint stresses. When sitting, weight bearing should be symmetric, pelvic tilt should be neutral with a slight lumbar lordosis, the hips and knees should be at 90°, and the feet should be flat on the floor. Good lumbar support should be provided. Inclining the seat backward 15° minimizes stress on the lumbar spine and helps keep the pelvis seated back in the chair (Chaffin et al., 1999). Tilting the desk or table top upward improves the position of the upper trunk, head, and shoulders.

OSTEOPOROSIS

Decreased bone mineral density, thought to be secondary to hypotonic or flaccid musculature combined with decreased loading of long bones from altered mobility, is frequently observed in children with MM and often results in osteoporotic fractures. Stuberg (1992) suggested that standing programs are beneficial for children with developmental disabilities. He reported that the use of a standing program (60 minutes four or five times per week) appears to increase bone mineral density and enhance acetabular development in children with cerebral palsy. These issues must be studied further in the MM population, however. Bone responses in children with flaccid paralysis may be quite different. Rosenstein and associates (1987) examined this issue in the MM population and reported that bone mineral density was 38% to 44% higher in household or community ambulators compared with

nonfunctional ambulators (exercise-only ambulators or nonambulators). Salvaggio and associates (1999) reported that walking ability was a highly significant determinant of bone density in prepubertal children with MM. Because the effects of lesion level were not controlled in either of these studies, however, the potential contribution of muscle activity versus weight-bearing status to the differences in bone mineral density cannot be determined. In addition, neither study addressed the issue of reduction of the incidence of osteoporotic fractures.

Studying the frequency of fractures is a more direct and clinically significant method of examining the benefits of standing programs. Shurtleff (1986d) asked the question, "Are fractures less common among those patients in standing or ambulatory programs than among similarly paralyzed sedentary peers?" Asher and Olson (1983) showed no correlation between fractures and the use of wheelchairs. DeSouza and Carroll (1976) reported no fractures in 7 nonambulators and 38 fractures in 16 ambulators. Their data implied that exposure to forces that can produce fractures (i.e., upright mobility) is the important risk factor for fractures, rather than the level of flaccid paralysis, as would be expected. Liptak and associates (1992) found no difference in the frequency of fractures between a group of children who were wheelchair users and a comparable group of children who ambulated with orthoses. Clinically, the use of standing frames, parapodiums, or hip-knee-ankle-foot orthoses (HKAFOs) in children with high lumbar and thoracic lesions does not appear warranted for the purpose of fracture prevention. For children with lower lumbar and sacral lesion levels, for whom upright positioning and mobility is an important functional skill, undue restriction of physical activity for fear of a fracture is not indicated. The fact that passive weight bearing does not decrease the risk of fractures in these children makes sense if one considers that bone density is more likely maintained by torque generated from volitional muscle activity. Active muscle contraction generates forces through the long bones that are several times greater than the forces from passive weight bearing.

Fractures often present subacutely due to lack of sensation, with swelling and warmth at the fracture site and a low-grade fever often being the only symptoms. Fractures frequently occur after surgery, immobilization in a cast, or as a sequela to foot arthrodesis. Because of the correlation between the duration of casting and the incidence of fracturing, immobilization in a cast is kept to a minimum and fractures are contained in soft immobilization for alignment (Brown, 2001). Weight bearing is resumed as soon as possible to avoid the risk of additional fractures (Karol, 1995).

MOTOR PARALYSIS

The inherently obvious manifestation of MM is the paraplegia resulting from the spinal cord malformation. Upper limb weakness can also occur in this population, regardless of lesion level, and is often a sign of progressive neurologic dysfunction. Knowledge of the motor lesion level is useful for predicting associated abnormalities and for prognostication of functional outcome. A detailed discussion regarding developmental and functional expectations for each motor lesion level is provided later in the section on outcomes and their determinants. Strategies for assessing strength and planning intervention programs to enhance motor function are provided in the section on age-specific examination and physical therapy intervention strategies.

The motor level is defined as the lowest intact, functional neuromuscular segment. For example, an L4 level indicates that the fourth lumbar nerve and the myotome it innervates are functioning, whereas segments below L4 are not intact. Table 25-1 provides the International Myelodysplasia Study Group (IMSG) criteria for assigning motor levels from manual muscle strength test results (IMSG, 1993). The IMSG criteria have been shown to best reflect the innervation patterns of individuals with MM as opposed to other spinal segment classification systems. MM spinal lesions can be asymmetric when motor or sensory function of the right and left sides of the body are compared. Consequently, motor function should be classified individually for the right and left sides.

Neuromuscular involvement of individuals with MM may manifest in one of three ways: (1) lesions resembling complete cord transection, (2) incomplete lesions, and (3) skip lesions (Shurtleff, 1986d). Lesions resembling complete cord transection manifest as normal function down to a particular level, below which there is flaccid

TABLE 25-1	International Myelodysplasia Study Group Criteria for Assigning Motor Levels

MOTOR LEVEL	CRITERIA FOR ASSIGNING MOTOR LEVELS
T10 or above	Determined by sensory level and/or palpation of abdominal muscles.
T11	
T12	Some pelvic control is present in sitting or supine (this may come from the abdominals or paraspinal muscles). Hip hiking from the quadratus lumborum may also be present.
L1	Weak iliopsoas muscle function is present (grade 2).
L1-L2	Exceeds criteria for L1 but does not meet L2 criteria.*
L2	Iliopsoas, sartorius, and the hip adductors all must be grade 3 or better.
L3	Meets or exceeds the criteria for L2 *plus* the quadriceps are grade 3 or better.
L3-L4	Exceeds criteria for L3 but does not meet L4 criteria.
L4	Meets or exceeds the criteria for L3 and the medial hamstrings *or* the tibialis anterior is grade 3 or better. A weak peroneus tertius may also be seen.
L4-L5	Exceeds criteria for L4 but does not meet L5 criteria.
L5	Meets or exceeds the criteria for L4 and has lateral hamstring strength of grade 3 or better *plus one* of the following: gluteus medius grade 2 or better, peroneus tertius grade 4 or better, or tibialis posterior grade 3 or better.
L5-S1	Exceeds criteria for L5 but does not meet S1 criteria.
S1	Meets or exceeds the criteria for L5 *plus at least two* of the following: gastrocnemius/soleus grade 2 or better, gluteus medius grade 3 or better, or gluteus maximus grade 2 or better (can pucker the buttocks).
S1-2	Exceeds criteria for S1 but does not meet S2 criteria.
S2	Meets or exceeds the criteria for S1, the gastrocnemius/soleus must be grade 3 or better, *and* gluteus medius and maximus are grade 4 or better.
S2-3	All of the lower limb muscle groups are of normal strength (may be grade 4 in one or two groups). Also includes normal-appearing infants who are too young to be bowel and bladder trained (see "no loss").
"No loss"	Meets all of the criteria for S2-S3 *and* has no bowel or bladder dysfunction.

*When description states "meets criteria …," strength of muscles listed for preceding levels should be increasing respectively.

Adapted with permission from Patient Data Management System. Myelodysplasia Study Data Collection Criteria and Instructions, 1994. (Available from D.B. Shurtleff, MD, Professor, Dept. of Pediatrics, Univ. of Washington, Seattle, WA 98195.)

paralysis, loss of sensation, and absent reflexes. Incomplete lesions have a mixed manifestation of spasticity and volitional control. Skip lesions are also observed, where more caudal segments are functioning despite the presence of one or more nonfunctional segments interposed between the intact more cephalad spinal segments. Individual skip motor lesions manifest either with isolated function of muscles noted below the last functional level of the lesion or with inadequate strength of muscle groups that have innervation higher than the lowest functioning group (Patient Data Management System, 1994). Consequently, it is important to evaluate muscles with lower innervation than the last functional level to determine whether a skip lesion exists. The presence of spasticity and reflexes should also be carefully documented.

McDonald and associates (1991b) demonstrated that muscle strength grades for the gluteus medius and medial hamstring muscles correlate more highly with strength grades of the hip adductors, hip flexors, and knee extensors than lower limb anterior compartment muscles that have been previously described as being innervated by the L4, L5, and sacral nerve roots. These data potentially explain the clinical observation that individuals with MM often have functional strength in the gluteus medius and medial hamstrings, despite having weak or nonactive lower limb anterior compartment muscles. It was concluded from this study that it is more useful clinically to group individuals with MM by the strength of specific muscle groups, as outlined in Table 25-1, rather than by traditional neurosegmental levels.

SENSORY DEFICITS

Sensory deficits are not clear-cut in this population, because sensory levels often do not correlate with motor levels and there may be skip areas that lack sensation. Because skip areas can occur within a given dermatome, it is important to test all dermatomes and multiple sites within a given dermatome to have an accurate baseline examination. Deficits should be recorded on a dermatome chart with areas of absent and decreased sensation color coded for the various sensory modalities (e.g., light touch, pinprick, vibration, and thermal). Proprioception and kinesthetic sense should also be evaluated in both the upper and lower extremities.

Based on the results of a study conducted on 30 adults with MM, testing with both light touch and pinprick stimuli is not necessary in this population because there is little discriminating value for detecting insensate areas (Hinderer & Hinderer, 1990). In contrast, vibratory stimuli could be felt one dermatome below light touch and pinprick sensation. Based on these results, vibration sensa-

tion should be evaluated in addition to either light touch or pinprick sensation.

It is important for individuals with MM to be aware of their sensory deficits and to be taught techniques to compensate by substituting other sensory modalities (e.g., vision). The impact of decreased sensation on safety should be emphasized, especially when checking temperature (e.g., bath water or when sitting near a fireplace) and when barefoot. Skin inspection and pressure relief techniques should be taught early so that they are incorporated into the daily routine. The importance of pressure relief cushions and sitting push-ups for pressure relief should be emphasized. Proper intervention of lower limbs and joint protection techniques should be taught when learning how to perform ADL, such as transfers.

The impact of sensory deficits on functional performance should be kept in mind when teaching functional tasks. Individuals with MM may rely heavily on vision to compensate for sensory deficits (Shaffer et al., 1986). They may lack kinesthetic acuity that permits subconscious completion of many repetitive motor tasks. Consequently, visual attention may not be available to be directed at other factors in the environment (Andersen & Plewis, 1977). Adding small amounts of weight to the ankles or a walker may enhance proprioceptive awareness and facilitate gait training. Use of patellar tendon-bearing orthoses (Fig. 25-5) instead of traditional ankle-foot orthoses (AFOs) may also facilitate foot placement for individuals with innervation through L3 because the orthosis contacts the skin in an area of intact sensation.

HYDROCEPHALUS

Hydrocephalus is excessive accumulation of cerebrospinal fluid (CSF) in the ventricles of the brain. Approximately 25% or more of children with MM are born with hydrocephalus. An additional 60% develop it after surgical closure of their back lesion (Reigel, 1992). If left untreated, the continued expansion of the ventricles can cause loss of cerebral cortex with additional cognitive and functional impairment. Cerebellar hypoplasia with caudal displacement of the hindbrain through the foramen magnum, known as the Arnold-Chiari type II malformation, is usually associated with hydrocephalus.

The hydrocephalus will occasionally arrest spontaneously; however, 80% to 90% of children with hydrocephalus will require a CSF shunt (Shurtleff et al., 1986b). A ventriculoperitoneal catheter shunts excess CSF from the lateral ventricles of the brain to the peritoneal space, where the CSF is resorbed. Because a shunt is a foreign body, it can be a nidus for infection or can become obstructed, requiring neurosurgical intervention. Repeated

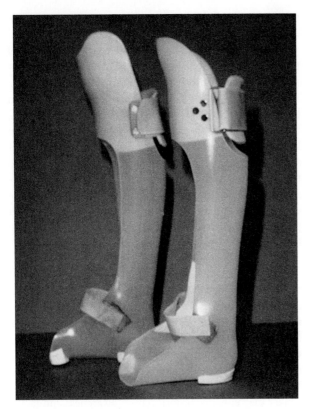

+ **Figure 25-5** Ground-reaction ankle-foot orthosis. Polypropylene patellar tendon-bearing ground-reaction ankle-foot orthoses molded with the foot in a subtalar neutral position. Note the zero heel posts and posts under the first metatarsal heads.

Box 25-1	**Early Warning Signs and Symptoms of Shunt Dysfunction**

Changes in speech
Fever and malaise
Recurring headache
Decreased activity level
Decreased school performance
Onset of or increased strabismus
Changes in appetite and weight
Incontinence begins or worsens
Onset or worsening of scoliosis
Onset of or increased spasticity
Personality change (irritability)
Decreased or static grip strength
Difficult to arouse in the morning
Decreased visuomotor coordination
Decreased visual acuity or diplopia
Decreased visuoperceptual coordination
Onset or increased frequency of seizures

Adapted with permission from Shurtleff, DB, Stuntz, JT, & Hayden, P. Hydrocephalus. In Shurtleff, DB (Ed.), Myelodysplasias and Exstrophies: Significance, Prevention, and Treatment. Orlando, FL: Grune & Stratton, 1986, p. 142.

or prolonged shunt dysfunction and infections often lead to additional functional and cognitive decline of the child. Shunt dysfunction is often gradual, with subtle symptoms. Therapists should be familiar with these symptoms to facilitate early detection and appropriate referral to a physician for further evaluation. Box 25-1 provides a list of early symptoms and signs of shunt obstruction. Of particular interest are the findings of Kilburn and associates (1985), which suggest that static or declining grip strength measurements are potentially an early indicator of neurologic dysfunction such as shunt malfunction or symptomatic Arnold-Chiari malformation. Hydrocephalus persists throughout life with consequent need of ongoing follow-up by a physician who is familiar with the medical complications associated with MM.

COGNITIVE DYSFUNCTION

Early closure of spinal lesions with antibiotic intervention to prevent meningitis and improved CSF shunt intervention have increased the expected cognitive function of chil-

dren born with MM. The majority of children without hydrocephalus or with uncomplicated hydrocephalus (no infections or cerebral hemorrhage) will have intellect falling within the normal range on intelligence testing. The distribution of scores tends to be skewed toward the upper and lower ends of normal, however, with fewer children scoring in the middle of the curve and a greater proportion scoring at the lower end of the range (Shaffer et al., 1986). The intellectual performance of children who have had significant CNS infections is lower than those who have not had infection (Shurtleff et al., 1986b). Intelligence scores tend to be higher in lumbar and sacral lesion level groups than in thoracic lesion level groups (Shaffer et al., 1986). Verbal subtest scores usually exceed performance subtest scores (Shaffer et al., 1986). The poorer scores on performance subtests, however, may not represent true differences in verbal versus nonverbal reasoning skills. Instead, these differences can potentially be explained by upper limb dyscoordination (discussed later) and by memory deficits (Shaffer et al., 1986). Dyscoordination and memory deficits are manifested as distractibility on subtests assessing acquired knowledge (e.g., arithmetic), integrated right-left hemisphere function (e.g., picture arrangement, block design, and coding), speed of motor response (e.g., coding), and memory (e.g., digit span, coding, and arithmetic). Further controlled studies must be conducted to determine the source or sources of discrepant verbal versus performance intelligence scores observed in individuals with MM.

Dise and Lohr (1998) demonstrated the need for individual analysis of "higher order" cognitive functions, including conceptual reasoning, problem solving, mental flexibility, and efficiency of thinking for individuals with MM, regardless of lesion level or general intelligence level. They contend that such neuropsychologic deficits underlie the "motivational" and academic difficulties observed in this population, especially for those with an average IQ.

The "cocktail party personality" is a cognitively associated behavioral disorder that occurs in some individuals with hydrocephalus, regardless of age or intelligence level (Hurley, 1992). These individuals are articulate and verbose, superficially appearing to have high verbal skills. Close examination of the content of their speech, however, shows frequent and inappropriate use of clichés and jargon. Individual words are often misused. Despite the initial appearance of being capable, these individuals are often impaired, their performance in daily life is below what they superficially appear capable of (Hurley, 1992), and they lack social skills (Simeonsson et al., 1999). It is important for the physical therapist to directly observe skills that these children report that they can perform and to confirm regular performance of the task at home with parents and care providers to determine if information provided by the patient is accurate.

LANGUAGE DYSFUNCTION

Children with MM and hydrocephalus have been observed to have deficits in discourse, characterized by a high frequency of irrelevant utterances and poorer performance with abstract rather than concrete language. Culatta and Young (1992) administered the Preschool Language Assessment Instrument (PLAI) at four different levels of abstraction to children with MM and comparable language-age control children. Children with MM performed comparably to control subjects on concrete tasks of the PLAI, but they produced more "no response" and irrelevant responses than control participants on abstract tasks.

LATEX ALLERGY

A range of 18% to 40% of children with MM have been reported to have latex allergies (Shapiro et al, 1992; Zsolt et al, 1999) compared to 1% to 5% of control groups. Unfortunately, 2% of latex is major IgE sensitizing pro-

teins that are ubiquitous in our culture, and some children with MM have life-threatening anaphylaxis. Latex-containing materials are most common in operating rooms but are also present in many products used elsewhere in the hospital and in the general community. Furthermore, these proteins are present in wheelchair seats and tires, foam rubber lining on splints and braces, elastic on diapers and clothes, pacifiers, balls, examination gloves used for bladder and bowel programs, and many other everyday objects. Whereas almost all children's hospitals have latex precaution policies, it is important for therapists in schools and clinics in the community to be aware of the need for children with MM to avoid exposure to latex products.

UPPER LIMB DYSCOORDINATION

Upper limb dyscoordination is frequently observed in children with MM, especially in those with hydrocephalus (Shaffer et al., 1986). The dyscoordination can potentially be explained by three possible causes: (1) cerebellar ataxia most likely related to the Arnold-Chiari type II malformation; (2) motor cortex or pyramidal tract damage secondary to hydrocephalus; or (3) motor learning deficits resulting from the use of upper limbs for balance and support rather than manipulation and exploration. These children perform poorly on timed fine motor skill tasks (Shaffer et al., 1986). Their movements can be described as halting and deliberate, rather than the expected smooth, continuous motion of able-bodied children. It often appears that there is a heavy reliance on visual feedback instead of kinesthetic sense. Consequently, even with extensive training, these children often have difficulty integrating frequently used fine motor movements at a subconscious level (Shaffer et al., 1986). Practicing fine motor tasks has been found to be beneficial, however, and often carries over into functional tasks (Fay et al., 1986). These coordination deficits have been described by some authors as apparent motor apraxias or motor learning deficits (Brunt, 1980; Land, 1977). Given the frequent occurrence of upper limb dyscoordination in these children, true apraxias are probably less common than these studies indicate.

An additional factor that may contribute to upper limb dyscoordination is delayed development of hand dominance (Shaffer et al., 1986). A large number of children with MM have mixed hand dominance or are left-handed, suggestive of possible left hemisphere damage (Shaffer et al., 1986). Brunt (1980) indicated that delayed hand dominance may contribute to deficits in bilateral upper limb function integration, resulting in further difficulty with fine motor tasks.

VISUOPERCEPTUAL DEFICITS

Studies assessing visual perception have not clearly determined whether deficits in children with MM are common, as has been described in the literature (Miller & Sethi, 1971; Sand et al., 1973; Tew & Laurence, 1975). Tests that require good hand-eye coordination, such as the Frostig Developmental Test of Visual Perception, may artificially lower scores of children with MM as a result of the upper limb dyscoordination described earlier. When upper limb motor function has been removed as a factor in testing by using the Motor Free Visual Perception Test, children with MM have performed at age-appropriate levels (Shaffer et al., 1986). Consequently, results of visuoperceptual tests must be interpreted carefully, in conjunction with other examinations, before a diagnosis of a visuoperception deficit is made.

CRANIAL NERVE PALSIES

The Arnold-Chiari malformation, along with hydrocephalus or dysplasia of the brainstem, may result in cranial nerve deficits. Ocular muscle palsies can occur (Shurtleff, 1986e), such as involvement of cranial nerve VI (abducens) with consequent lateral rectus eye muscle weakness and esotropia on the involved side. Correction with patching of the eye, prescription lenses, or minor outpatient surgery is necessary to prevent amblyopia and for cosmesis (Reigel, 1992). Gaston (1991) studied 322 children with MM for 6 years to monitor them for ophthalmic complications. Forty-two percent of these children had a manifest squint, 29% had an oculomotor nerve palsy or musculoparetic nystagmus, 14% had papilledema, and 17% had optic nerve atrophy. Only 27% of those surveyed had definite normal vision. Seventy percent of proven episodes of raised intracranial pressure (ICP) from CSF shunt malfunction had positive ophthalmologic evidence of the ICP. Shunt surgery is the first priority but may not restore normal ocular motility and visual function, requiring further compensatory interventions.

Cranial nerves IX (glossopharyngeal) and X (vagus) can also be affected with pharyngeal and laryngeal dysfunction (croupy, hoarse cry) and swallowing difficulties (Shurtleff, 1986e). Apneic episodes and bradycardia may occur with a severely symptomatic Arnold-Chiari type II malformation and can potentially be life-threatening. These severe symptoms usually appear within the first few weeks of life but can occur at any time (Reigel, 1992). The survival rate is only about 40% in these severe cases (Shurtleff, 1986c). Those infants who do survive, however, have been noted to have gradual improvement in cranial nerve function. Neurosurgical posterior fossa decompression and high cervical laminectomies do not seem to substantially improve the outcome (Griebel et al., 1991; Shurtleff, 1986c). In contrast, surgical decompression of the Arnold-Chiari malformation has been shown to be beneficial for the intervention of progressive upper and lower limb spasticity (Griebel et al., 1991).

SPASTICITY

The muscle tone of infants and children with MM can range from flaccid to normal to spastic. Stack and Baber (1967) found that some upper motoneuron signs were present in approximately two thirds of children with MM whom they examined; however, only about 9% had true spastic paraparesis. The remainder of this group had predominantly a lower motoneuron presentation with scattered upper motoneuron signs (e.g., flexor withdrawal reflex). In the group of children without upper motoneuron signs, most had totally flaccid paralysis below the segmental level of their spinal lesion, but a small percentage had normal tone. In contrast, Mazur and Menelaus (1991) stated that approximately 25% of individuals with MM exhibit lower extremity spasticity because of associated CNS abnormalities. As with other CNS conditions, spasticity and abnormal reflexes can affect function, positioning, or comfort in individuals with MM.

PROGRESSIVE NEUROLOGIC DYSFUNCTION

Minor improvements in strength or development of sensation, although rare, can occur even as late as the fourth decade of life. More important, however, is the deterioration from neurologic changes that are due to treatable complications. These changes that can occur in the upper or lower extremities or trunk include loss of sensation, loss of strength, pain at the site of the sac repair, pain radiating along a dermatome, initial onset or worsening of spasticity, development or rapid progression of scoliosis, development of a lower limb deformity not explained by previously documented muscle imbalance, or change in bowel or bladder sphincter control. Such changes can be due to CSF shunt obstruction, hydromyelia (syringohydromyelia, syrinx), growth of a dermoid or lipoma at the site of repair, subarachnoid cysts of the cord, or spinal cord tethering and can be detected via MRI. Cord tethering occurs from scarring of the neural placode or spinal cord to the overlying dura or skin with resultant traction on neural structures (Shurtleff et al., 1997). The tethered cord syndrome may also result from other congenital anomalies, including thickening of the filum terminale and diastematomyelia (Rekate, 1991). An acquired cause of progressive spinal cord dysfunction that has been reported is severe herniation of intervertebral disks into the spinal canal, causing compression of the cord (Shurtleff & Dunne, 1986). Lais and associates (1993) stated that slow deterioration of neurologic function is not uncommon.

Progressive deterioration of spinal cord function due to any of these causes can be arrested by neurosurgical interventions. Deterioration of the gait pattern is frequently the first complaint by patients or their parents. Because physical therapists see these patients more frequently than physicians or surgeons, the therapist often will be the first to observe these changes and should be alert to the need for immediate referral to a neurosurgeon. Owing to this risk of progressive loss of function, it is *essential* that individuals with MM be closely monitored throughout their life span.

SEIZURES

Seizures have been reported to occur in 10% to 30% of children and adolescents with MM (Shurtleff & Dunne, 1986). The etiologies of seizure activity include associated brain malformation, CSF shunt malfunction or infection, and residual brain damage from shunt infection or malfunction. Anticonvulsant medications, which are necessary for prophylaxis against seizures, unfortunately can also accentuate any cognitive deficits or dyscoordination already present (Gadow, 1986; Reynolds, 1983). Untreated seizures, however, can lead to permanent cognitive or neurologic functional loss, or even death.

NEUROGENIC BOWEL

Fewer than 5% of children with MM develop voluntary control of their urinary or anal sphincter (Reigel, 1992). Abnormal or absent function of spinal segments S2 through S4, which provide the innervation to these organs, is the primary reason for the incontinence. The anal sphincter can be flaccid, hypotonic, or spastic, causing different manifestations of dysfunction during defecation. Anorectal sensation is also often impaired, preventing the individual from receiving sensory input of an imminent bowel movement so that he or she can take appropriate action. In addition to incontinence, constipation and impaction can also occur. Fortunately, conscientious attention to individually designed bowel programs can have effective results, minimizing problems of incontinence and constipation (King et al., 1994; Reigel, 1992; Wicks & Shurtleff, 1986a, 1986b). The presence of a bulbocavernosus or anal cutaneous reflex (indicating that lower motoneuron innervation of the sphincter is present) is highly predictive of success with a bowel training program (King et al., 1994). King and

associates (1994) also reported that instituting bowel training before age 7 years correlates with improved outcomes by means of better compliance. When stool incontinence is interfering with a child's school and social activities, the physical therapist may want to become involved to help address the problem. Incontinence often affects feelings of self-image and competence, which in turn can affect performance in other activities pertinent to the therapist's intervention program.

NEUROGENIC BLADDER

Just as the nerves to control defecation are impaired, so are the nerves that produce bladder control. A variety of different types of dysfunctions can occur, depending on the relative tonicity of the detrusor muscle in the bladder wall and the outlet sphincters of the bladder. Bladder intervention strategies are directed toward the point or points of dysfunction. The goal is infection-free social continence with preservation of renal function. Retrograde flow of urine from the bladder up the ureters to the kidneys, termed *vesicoureteral reflux*, can occur without symptoms or signs being evident until the later stages of irreversible renal failure. Inadequate emptying of the bladder with residual urine retention within the bladder provides an optimal culture medium for bacteria, causing recurrent urinary tract infections and possible generalized sepsis. Adequate bladder intervention is therefore an essential component of health maintenance and normal longevity of people with MM, in addition to being an important social issue.

For most individuals, effective bladder intervention is achieved with clean intermittent catheterization on a regularly timed schedule for voiding. A small catheter is inserted into the bladder through the urethra until urine begins to flow. After the bladder is empty or urine stops flowing, the catheter is withdrawn, cleansed with soap and water, and stored for future use. It has been shown that the clean method of catheterization, as opposed to sterile technique, is sufficient for prevention of urinary tract infections (Reigel, 1992). The risk of injury to the urethra or bladder from clean intermittent catheterization is sufficiently low to allow young children to be taught to catheterize themselves. Mastery of the technique is usually achieved by age 6 to 8 years depending on the severity of the involvement (Shurtleff & Mayo, 1986). Supplementation of clean intermittent catheterization with oral medication for spastic detrusor muscle function (e.g., oxybutynin [Ditropan] or propantheline [Pro-Banthine]), spastic sphincter function (phenoxybenzamine), or hypotonic sphincter function (ephedrine) is required in some children to achieve intervention goals. It is recommended that individuals with MM have regular follow-up with a urologist every 6 months until age 2, and yearly thereafter, throughout the life span (Kimura et al., 1986). The physical therapist must be aware of the method used for urine drainage as it relates to wheelchair positioning, transfer techniques, and orthoses so that assistive devices do not interfere with effective performance of urine drainage techniques. It is important to allow adequate time for patients with MM to attend to bowel and bladder needs before and after examination and therapy sessions so that they are comfortable and continent during physical activities. Discomfort from a distended bladder or rectum may impair performance. Patients are often not assertive in requesting necessary time for personal care, and therapists should encourage them to do so to avoid embarrassing accidents.

SKIN BREAKDOWN

Decubitus ulcers and other types of skin breakdown occur in 85% to 95% of all children with MM by the time they reach young adulthood (Shurtleff, 1986a). Okamoto and associates (1983) performed an extensive study of skin breakdown on 524 patients with MM who were 1 to 20 years old. Perineal decubiti and breakdown over the apex of the spinal kyphotic curve (gibbus) occurred in 82% of children with thoracic level lesions, 62% of those with high lumbar level lesions, and 50% to 53% of those with lower level lesions. Lower limb skin breakdown was approximately equivalent in all lesion level groups (30%–46%). Although the sites and causes of skin breakdown varied among lesion level groups, the overall frequency was the same. The prevalence of skin breakdown at any one time was 20% to 25% for the population sampled. Several etiologies for skin breakdown were ascertained. In 42% of the children, tissue ischemia from excessive pressure was the cause. In 23% a cast or orthotic device produced the breakdown. In another 23% urine and stool soiling produced skin maceration. Friction and shear accounted for another 10%; burns accounted for 1%; and 1% of causes were not recorded or were unknown. Other authors have described additional causes of skin breakdown (Shurtleff, 1986a). These include excessive weight bearing over bony prominences of the pelvis as a result of spinal deformity, obesity, lower limb autonomic dysfunction with vascular insufficiency or venous stasis, and tenuous tissue postoperatively over bony prominences.

Age is an important factor in the etiology of skin breakdown. Shurtleff (1986a) showed that young children who are not toilet trained have the greatest problem with breakdown from skin soiling (ammonia burns). Young active children with MM have the greatest fre-

quency of friction burns on knees and feet from scooting along rugs, hot water scalds, and pressure ulcers from orthoses or casts. Older children, adolescents, and young adults develop skin breakdown over lower limb bony prominences (even if they did not have ulcers when they were younger) from the increased pressure of a larger body habitus, asymmetric weight bearing resulting from deformities, abrasions of the buttocks or lower limbs due to poor transfer skills, improperly fitted orthoses, and lower limb vascular problems. Strategies for prevention taught by the physical therapist therefore should be directed to the likely causes of skin breakdown for the age of the individual. Helping the child develop an awareness of his insensate extremities is important during the early years in order to later develop independence with personal care. Mobley and associates (1996) found that preschoolers with MM exhibited altered self-perception as evidenced by their drawing fewer trunks, legs, and feet on self-portraits than their able-bodied peers.

Pressure sores can result in a delay or loss of ambulation (Diaz Llopis et al., 1993). Skin breakdown of the insensate foot is often a cause of decreased ability to ambulate. Predictors of skin breakdown resulting from excessive pressure during ambulation or while resting feet on wheelchair footrests are foot rigidity, nonplantigrade position, and surgical arthrodesis (Maynard et al., 1992). Clawing of the toes may be another contributing factor that also affects shoe wear. To avoid foot ulcerations, physical therapists should examine and document foot deformity, level of sensation, and pressure areas. The insensate foot can be protected with appropriate footwear, orthotics, or surgery. Total contact casting can be useful in healing ulcers (Brown, 2001).

OBESITY

Obesity is a common and difficult multifactorial problem occurring in children with MM that complicates orthotic and wheelchair fitting and can affect independence and proficiency with transfers, mobility, and self-care activities. For children who are ambulatory, a greater expenditure of energy is required to participate in physical play activities, so it is likely that less time will be spent engaged in physical play and that more sedentary activities (e.g., watching television) will be adopted. Children with mobility limitations, whether they are ambulatory or wheelchair mobile, may not be well accepted by able-bodied peers when they attempt to participate in physically challenging play, or they may feel conspicuous because they have difficulty keeping up. The likelihood of participation under these circumstances is diminished. As obesity develops, this further complicates participation and negatively affects self-image, creating an undesirable cycle perpetuating weight gain. In addition, children with MM probably are at a disadvantage physiologically. Studies evaluating the caloric intake required for children with MM (Shurtleff, 1986b) have shown that the intake should be lower than for able-bodied obese peers. This is probably not just a function of the decreased activity level of children with MM. Decreased muscle mass of large lower limb muscle groups diminishes the ability to burn calories (i.e., the basal metabolic rate of children with MM is probably lower than normal). This is consistent with the observation that children with high lumbar and thoracic lesions have greater problems with obesity. Decreased muscle mass coupled with lower extremity inactivity reduces the daily caloric needs such that a young adult who uses a wheelchair as his primary means of mobility will need less than 1500 calories a day to maintain his current weight (Lutkenhoff & Oppenheimer, 1997). Weight control is not just a function of decreased caloric intake for children with MM, however, and must involve a regular exercise program. The challenge of the physical therapist is to find age-appropriate physical activities for their clients that are fun and at which they can succeed; in this way, physical activity is positively reinforced and a lifelong pattern of engaging in such activities is developed.

The usual mechanism to screen for obesity in the general population is height-weight ratios; however, arm span-weight ratios are more appropriate for monitoring individuals with MM. Shurtleff (1986b) noted that height-weight ratios are not useful in children with MM because of their short stature, decreased linear length secondary to spine or lower limb deformities, and decreased growth of paretic limbs. He recommended monitoring individuals with MM by measuring serial subscapular skinfold thickness, linear length measured along the axis of long bones to take into consideration hip and knee joint contractures, arm span measured with a spanner, and weight measured on a platform scale (subtracting the weight of the wheelchair or adaptive aids). Results should be recorded on National Center for Health Statistics percentile charts (Hamill et al., 1979). Arm span measurements should be adjusted using correction factors to avoid underestimating body fat content: 0.9 arm span for children with no leg muscle mass (thoracic and high-lumbar levels), 0.95 arm span for those with partial loss of muscle mass (mid- and low-lumbar lesions), and 1.0 arm span for children with minimal or no muscle mass loss. Del Gado and associates (1999) reported that in comparison to a control group, 32 children with MM had significantly lower stature, higher weights, and greater subcutaneous fat deposits in their trunks, the latter being associated with cardiovascular disease risk factors.

AGE-SPECIFIC EXAMINATION AND PHYSICAL THERAPY INTERVENTION

There are issues of particular importance for specific age groups with MM. Intervention should be provided to keep pace with the normal timing of development (Bleck & Nagel, 1982; Shurtleff, 1966). Throughout the life span, it is important to keep in mind the overall picture of the needs of the patient and family. The medical problems and the number of health care professionals involved in the care of individuals with MM can be overwhelming. Many members of other disciplines in addition to the physical therapist may also be making requests of the family's time. Each professional should prioritize his or her goals, relative to those of other disciplines, and coordinate planning so that the demands placed on the patient and the family are realistic. It is best to work as a team with the family and other disciplines to integrate appropriate intervention programs into the patient's daily routine. In addition, if conflicting information is provided to parents, they often become confused and may lack appropriate information to set realistic goals for their children and adolescents (e.g., goals for mobility, self-care, employment, and independent living). Consequently, multidisciplinary team collaboration with the family is important to establish appropriate goals and expectations.

The following sections focus on special considerations throughout the life span. Four age groups are discussed: infancy, preschool age, school age, and adolescence. Participation restrictions that are typically present as well as the causes and impact of activity limitations on expected life roles are discussed for each of the four age groups. Examination and evaluation of body structure and function, activity limitations, and participation restrictions, along with recommendations for ongoing monitoring, typical physical therapy goals, intervention, and strategies to prevent secondary impairments and activity limitations, are also discussed. In addition, typical secondary participation restrictions and activity limitations encountered during adolescence and their impact on the transition to adulthood are discussed in the section on adolescence and transition to adulthood. The information presented in this latter section has important implications for preventive intervention during childhood and adolescence to minimize the incidence of acquired impairments and activity limitations that often surface later in life.

It is important to keep in mind that the interaction of a multitude of impairments may affect an individual's functional performance, yet only a few key impairments are discussed for each age group. The reader is referred to the previous section on impairments for a more thorough discussion of other factors. Similarly, only key examination and intervention strategies that are specific to a given age category are discussed in each section. Common goals across the life span are to prevent joint contractures, correct existing deformities, prevent or minimize the effects of sensory and motor deficiency, and optimize mobility (Mazur & Menelaus, 1991).

INFANCY

Typical Participation Restrictions: Causes and Implications

The multiple impairments and overwhelming medical needs of a newborn with MM may interfere with parent-infant interaction. Parents are often afraid to handle their infant with MM, and the opportunities for handling and interacting with their child may be further limited by medical complications. Parents and extended family members may be cautious in handling the infant, resulting in decreased stimulation. Naturally occurring opportunities for early environmental stimulation, observation and exploration, and social interaction also may be limited as a result of somatosensory and motor deficits, hypotonia, and visual deficits. Family and infant interaction may be further impeded by the additional parental duties required (e.g., bowel and bladder intervention), frequent medical visits, and hospitalizations for complications.

The achievement of fine motor and gross motor developmental milestones is usually delayed during infancy because of multiple impairments, including joint contractures and deformities, motor and sensory deficits, hypotonia, upper limb dyscoordination, CNS dysfunction, visual and perceptual disorders, and cognitive deficits. The lack of normal infant movements, combined with impaired sensation, results in decreased kinesthetic awareness and inhibits perceptuomotor development. Independence with early ADL, such as holding a bottle or finger feeding, is also negatively affected by impairments resulting from MM, especially swallowing disorders, upper limb dyscoordination, and visuoperceptual deficits.

Examination of Impairments

As discussed in Chapter 6, therapists must be aware of normal physiologic flexion of the hips and knees when assessing newborns. Limitations of up to 35° are present in normal newborns. These contractures may be more pronounced at birth in the infant with MM after prolonged intrauterine positioning of the relatively inactive fetus. Physiologic flexion spontaneously reduces in able-bodied infants from the effects of gravity and sponta-

neous lower limb movements. Physiologic flexion of infants with MM typically does not spontaneously reduce, because of decreased or absent spontaneous lower limb activity secondary to muscle weakness. Consequently, contractures may develop even in children with sacral level function if they lack full strength of the gluteal muscles.

Two primary orthopedic concerns during this period are to identify and manage dislocated hips and foot deformities. Early orthopedic intervention of these deformities results in improved potential for standing balance and more timely achievement of motor milestones such as sitting and walking (Mayfield, 1991; Menelaus, 1976). Achieving a plantigrade foot position is important, regardless of ambulatory prognosis. Plantigrade alignment is optimal for shoe fit, positioning and weight distribution in sitting, and stability when bearing weight for standing pivot transfers or ambulation.

When assessing muscle tone in infants, the Movement Assessment of Infants (Chandler et al., 1980) is a useful tool. Hypotonia is typical in infants with MM, even if sacral level function is present (Wolf & McLaughlin, 1992). Poor head control, delayed neck and trunk righting, automatic reactions, and low trunk and lower limb muscle tone are typical. A mixture of hypotonia, hypertonia, and spastic movements may be present in the limbs. It is important to distinguish between voluntary and reflexive movements when assessing muscle function.

One of the key physical therapy considerations in managing the newborn with MM is to establish a reliable baseline of muscle function before and after back closure. This baseline is important for predicting future function and for monitoring status. In addition, it is important to identify muscle imbalance around joints and existing joint contractures that are unlikely to reduce spontaneously.

In the newborn, muscle function is assessed before and after surgical closure of the back to determine the extent of motor paralysis. Side lying is usually the position of choice for testing the newborn, to avoid injury to the exposed neural tissue (Schneider et al., 2001). The state of alertness must be considered and documented when testing newborns or infants. Repeated examinations may need to be conducted at different times of the day to observe the infant's muscle activity in various behavioral states. Optimal performance cannot be elicited if the infant is in a sleepy state. Muscle activity is best observed when the infant is alert, hungry, or crying. If the infant is drowsy, several techniques can be used to arouse the infant, including assessing limb ROM, rocking vertically to stimulate the vestibular system, and providing tactile and auditory stimulation (Hinderer & Hinderer, 1993; Schneider et al., 2001). Ideally, the infant's spontaneous activity should be observed in supine, prone, and side-lying positions before the examiner starts handling the infant. Handling the infant may suppress spontaneous activity. Movement can often be elicited through sounds, visual tracking, reaching for toys, tickling, placing limbs in antigravity positions to elicit holding responses, and moving limbs to end-range positions to see if the infant will move out of the position (Hinderer & Hinderer, 1993). For older infants, muscle activity can be observed, palpated, and resisted in developmental positions.

Therapists often do not record specific strength grades for infants and young children. Instead, either a dichotomous scale (present or absent) or a 3-point ordinal scale (apparently normal, weak, or absent) is often advocated (Murdoch, 1980; Pact et al., 1984; Schneider et al., 2001). This 3-point scale, however, lacks sensitivity and predictive validity (Murdoch, 1980). In contrast, specific manual muscle test strength scores (grades 0 to 5) have been found to provide useful information for infants and young children with MM and are predictive of later function (McDonald et al., 1986). Consequently, when strength is assessed manually, we recommend using the full manual muscle testing scale, regardless of age. The estimated quality of the examination should also be recorded, indicating the examiner's degree of confidence in the results, based on the child's level of cooperation. Neck and trunk musculature should be graded as "normal for age" if the child is able to perform developmentally appropriate activities (Kendall et al., 1999).

Testing sensation in infants and young children presents special challenges. Complete testing of multiple sensory modalities is not possible until the child has acquired sufficient cognitive and language abilities to accurately respond to testing (Schneider et al., 2001). Parents can often provide useful information to help focus on probable insensate areas. It is best to test the child in a quiet state. Testing with a pin or other sharp object should begin at the lowest level of sacral innervation and progress to more proximally innervated dermatomes until a noxious response is noted (e.g., crying or facial grimace).

Ongoing Monitoring

During the first year of life, it is important to monitor joint alignment, muscle imbalance, and the development of contractures. Typical lower limb contractures that develop are hip and knee flexion contractures, combined with external rotation at the hips. Children with weak or absent hip musculature often lie in a "frog-legged" position with the hips flexed and externally rotated and the knees flexed. Consequently, these muscle groups are typically in a shortened position. It is important to closely monitor ROM and muscle extensibility during periods of rapid growth. Soft tissue growth typically lags behind

skeletal changes, resulting in decreased extensibility. Stretching exercises should be initiated early on, if indicated, when contractures are relatively flexible and respond well to intervention. If orthoses or night-positioning splints are used to correct orthopedic deformities, the fit of these devices should be monitored to prevent skin breakdown.

Changes in muscle tone and muscle function are observed with progressive neurologic dysfunction. Baseline measurements, therefore, are essential, and these parameters should be closely monitored. Therapists should also watch for behavioral changes, decreases in performance, and other subtle signs of shunt malfunction (see Box 25-1) or seizure disorders. Motor development must also be observed to determine whether an infant is keeping pace with normal developmental expectations. Abnormalities in any of these areas should be reported to the child's primary care physician.

Typical Physical Therapy Goals and Strategies

During the newborn period, physical therapists must be sensitive to the feelings and needs of parents and other extended family members who are learning to cope with the overwhelming problems of a child with MM. Parents go through a period of tremendous adjustment. They are required to meet the demands of a normal infant, plus deal with the extensive medical and surgical needs of their newborn and adjust to the long-term implications of their child's multiple impairments. Not all instructions may be assimilated at any one time given the large amount of information to which parents are asked to attend. Often instructions must be reviewed and reinforced during subsequent visits. Written instructions should be provided to augment verbal explanations.

If ROM is limited, parents should be instructed in positioning techniques. It is optimal to maintain ROM by means of positioning because little additional time is required of the family. If contractures do not resolve with positioning, or if contractures are not supple, parents should also be instructed in stretching exercises and soft tissue mobilization techniques. It is usually most efficient to perform stretching exercises and soft tissue mobilization techniques in conjunction with diaper changes.

For infants who exhibit hypotonia, parents should be instructed in handling techniques to facilitate head and trunk control. Techniques advocated for children with hypotonic cerebral palsy (e.g., Finnie, 1975) are often beneficial. Parents should be encouraged to provide sitting opportunities for the infant to facilitate the development of head and trunk control. Additional head and trunk support is often required in high chairs, strollers, and car seats. If motor development is significantly delayed and requires therapeutic intervention, a combination of neurodevelopmental intervention and proprioceptive neuromuscular facilitation techniques is beneficial. Therapeutic interventions and adaptive equipment should ideally be planned to keep pace with the normal timing of development so that the child is provided with typical developmental experiences. During the latter half of the first year, preparatory activities for mobility are indicated. Emphasis should be placed on balance, trunk control, and facilitating an upright posture as the child progresses through the developmental sequence.

Prevention of Secondary Impairments and Activity Limitations

Parents should be instructed in proper positioning, ROM, and handling techniques with the lower limbs in neutral alignment to prevent the development of contractures. If the hips are dislocated or subluxed, parents should be instructed in proper positioning, double diapering, and the use of a night-positioning orthosis, if indicated (Rowley-Kelly & Kunkle, 1992; Schafer & Dias, 1983). If surgery is indicated to relocate hip dislocations (see previous section on orthopedic deformities), it is generally performed after 6 months of age. Foot deformities are generally treated through serial casting or positioning splints.

Parents should also be instructed to inspect insensate skin areas during diaper changes and dressing for signs of pressure or injury. Parents need to understand the importance of skin inspection and that insensate areas should be inspected on a daily basis throughout the life span.

TODDLER AND PRESCHOOL YEARS

Typical Participation Restrictions: Causes and Implications

The achievement of fine motor and gross motor developmental milestones continues to be delayed. Mobility is typically impaired in this population owing to orthopedic, motor, and sensory deficits. As the child nears the end of the first year of life, it is important to provide opportunities for environmental exploration. If the child does not have an efficient, effective mode of independent mobility by the end of the first year, provision of a mobility device is indicated.

Environmental exploration is essential for the development of initiative and independence. Limited early mobility may result in a lack of curiosity and initiative and may negatively affect other aspects of development (Becker, 1975; Butler et al., 1984; Shurtleff, 1986d). If a toddler does not have an effective means of independently exploring

and interacting with the environment, he or she may learn to be passively dependent. The negative influence of limited early mobility on personality and behavior development can persist throughout life. Passive-dependent behavior is a commonly observed personality trait of adolescents and adults with MM.

Limited mobility also negatively affects socialization, especially interaction with other children. If a stroller is used as the primary mode of community mobility beyond the normal age of weaning a child from a stroller, other children will view the child with MM as a "baby." Play opportunities are also limited if a child does not have an effective means of mobility.

Independence with ADL is often impaired in this population because of fine and gross motor impairments, upper limb dyscoordination, and CNS dysfunction. Children who are not independent with ADL may miss out on normal childhood experiences (e.g., play time) while waiting for others to assist them with basic skills. Their self-esteem may also be negatively affected if other children tease them regarding their dependency.

It is important that parents, child care personnel, and preschool teachers be aware of other motor deficits that are often exhibited in this population, such as poor eye-hand coordination. The potential impact of these deficits on functional performance in handwriting and the acquisition of ADL skills such as feeding and dressing should be realized so that reasonable goals can be established and the use of appropriate adaptive equipment implemented.

Examination and Evaluation of Impairments and Activity Limitations

By the end of the first year, ROM is expected to be within normal limits. If limited ROM persists, it is important to distinguish between fixed and supple contractures, determine muscle extensibility, and evaluate orthopedic deformities to determine whether they are fixed or flexible.

To assess strength, functional muscle testing techniques are advocated for young children 2 to 5 years old because they may not cooperate with traditional test procedures (Hinderer & Hinderer, 1993; Pact et al., 1984). Functional activities that are helpful in determining the strength of key lower limb muscle groups include gait observations, heel- and toe-walking, climbing up and down a step, one-legged stand, toe touching, squat to stand, bridging, bicycling while supine, the Landau position, prone kicking, the wheelbarrow position, sit-ups, pull to sit, and sitting and standing push-ups. It is often possible for young children to cooperate with isolated muscle actions by having them push against a puppet to show how strong they are. To elicit the cooperation of older preschoolers (3- to 4-year-olds), it is often helpful to name the muscle and describe its "job" (the muscle action). The children think that the muscle names are humorous, maintaining their attention. Asking children to have the muscle do its "job" makes strength testing more understandable (Hinderer & Hinderer, 1993). We have found it possible to obtain objective, reliable measures of strength from children as young as 4 years of age using handheld myometry techniques (Hinderer & Hinderer, 1993). The degree of confidence regarding whether the child's optimal performance was elicited should be recorded.

Once the child is 2 years of age, light touch and position sense can usually be assessed by eliciting tickling responses or having the child respond to the touch of a puppet. Other sensory modalities can ordinarily be accurately tested once the child is 5 to 7 years old. The accuracy of responses often must be double-checked because of short attention span and response perseveration. Two sensory testing techniques help minimize perseveration of responses. The first is to randomly alternate between testing light touch and pinprick and have the child identify the type of sensation. The second is to have the child point to the spot that was touched and correctly state when no area was touched.

Fine and gross motor development should be assessed using appropriate standardized tests such as those discussed in Chapter 2. Examination of ADL should focus on what the individual actually does on a daily basis, in addition to what he or she is capable of doing. If independence with ADL is limited, appropriate adaptations and interventions should be implemented to foster independence. The Functional Activities Assessment (Okamoto et al., 1984; Sousa et al., 1976, 1983) is useful for this population (Fig. 25-6). Items may be scored by direct observation or by parent report. Assistive devices required to perform a given task are also documented. The "Can" and "Does" scoring format permits the examiner to record what the child can do versus what the child actually does on a regular basis. In addition, if the child is directly observed performing the task, the degree of independence and the time to complete the task are recorded.

Ongoing Monitoring

Joint alignment, muscle imbalance, contractures, posture, and signs of progressive neurologic dysfunction should continue to be monitored. Contractures that seem insignificant during childhood may become functionally limiting once the individual has adult-sized body proportions. For example, knee extension contractures can interfere with the ability to maneuver in a wheelchair.

Typical Physical Therapy Goals and Strategies

Joint alignment, contractures, muscle strength, and postural alignment should continue to be treated, as necessary. Proper positioning in sleeping and sitting should continue. If stretching or strengthening exercises are indicated, it is often helpful to involve other family members in the exercise program so that the child does not feel singled out. For ambulatory candidates with weak hip and knee musculature, strengthening activities may be beneficial if the child is cooperative. In addition to traditional posture exercises (Kendall et al., 1999), many play activities promote strengthening and the development of good posture (Embrey et al., 1983). The use of therapy ball techniques to strengthen postural muscles is also beneficial. Muscle reeducation techniques, such as functional electrical stimulation and biofeedback, are useful to teach muscles to function in new ROM after stretching exercises. Electrical stimulation has also been found to be beneficial in increasing strength and enhancing functional performance in this population (Karmel-Ross et al., 1992).

During the preschool years, the focus is on improving the independence, efficiency, and effectiveness of ADL and mobility. Development of independence with dressing and feeding should be encouraged. Appropriate guidance should be provided so that parents have age-appropriate expectations. It is important for young children to actively participate in skin inspection, bowel and bladder intervention, donning and removing orthoses, wheelchair intervention, and other ADL tasks. Teaching these skills early on and actively involving the child facilitates independence and incorporation of these activities into the daily routine. As a result, these extra responsibilities required of the child with MM become as natural as other ADL, such as brushing teeth. Waiting to introduce tasks until the child is older often is met with resistance, especially when the child observes that siblings do not have the same requirements.

By kindergarten age, children without disabilities are able to dress and toilet themselves (with the exception of some fasteners), eat independently, and be mobile (Fay et al., 1986). These skills must be emphasized at an early age in children with MM so that independence is achieved by the time the child begins school. A wide range of age of achievement of independence with ADL is evident in this population when examining the normative data provided on the Functional Activities Assessment (see Fig. 25-6). This wide variability in age of achieving skills within a given motor level suggests that a significant percentage of children are delayed in ADL skill acquisition because of attitudes and expectations. Fay and associates (1986)

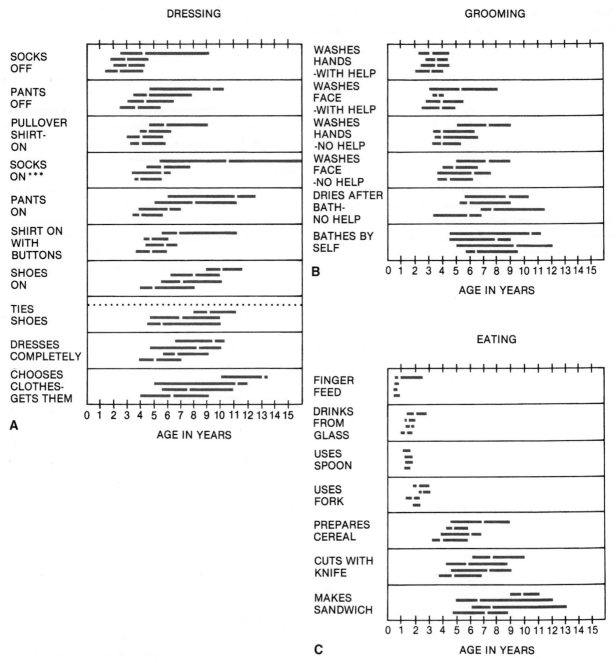

• **Figure 25-6**   Functional activities assessment. The age at which 20%, 50%, and 80% of a group of 173 children learned dressing (**A**), grooming (**B**), and eating (**C**) skills is indicated by the beginning of, space between (white space), and end of the black bars, respectively. Triple asterisks indicate that this group never achieved an 80% learning proportion. Dotted line indicates activity was attempted with this group. The bars in each category represent, from top to bottom: (1) thoracic and L1-L2; (2) L3 and mixed lesions, L2-L4; (3) L4-L5; and (4) sacral-level groups. All data were recorded as the child achieved the skill during the 2.5-year period of the study, within 4 months of entering the study, or when the caretaker entered a specific date of achievement in the child's diary. These charts were created from data published by Okamoto and associates (1984) and Sousa and associates (1983). *(From Shurtleff, DB [Ed.]. Myelodysplasias and Exstrophies: Significance, Prevention, and Treatment. Orlando, FL: Grune & Stratton, 1986, p. 376.)*

suggested that these delays may be partially caused by low parental expectations and protective attitudes, perceptions that it is faster for the parent to perform the task, and parental difficulty accepting the reality of the child's activity limitations. Showing parents the ADL normative data for children with MM and promoting positive parental expectations of independence are beneficial. It is important for parents to positively reinforce the child's attempts to be independent so that he or she is motivated to achieve. It is also important to help the parents understand how incontinence retards their child's normal sexual exploration, learning, and social inhibitions that normal preschool children learn. Alternative opportunities should be offered to children with MM (Brazelton, 1992; Shurtleff et al., 2004).

Skin inspection and pressure relief techniques should be taught early so that they are incorporated into the daily routine. Proper intervention of lower limbs and joint protection techniques should be taught to avoid injury of insensate areas when learning how to perform ADL, such as transfers. The impact of sensory deficits on functional performance should be kept in mind during gait training and when teaching other functional tasks.

Provision of an effective means of independent mobility is *essential* for young children. Consequently, if a child does not begin maneuvering effectively within the environment by 1 year of age, alternative means of mobility must be considered to achieve independent home and short-distance community mobility (Butler et al., 1984; Shurtleff, 1986d). Mobility options should be explored and implemented as frequently as is needed so that the child is able to actively participate in normal childhood activities. Various mobility options are available, from manual devices such as a caster cart to electric wheelchairs. Electric wheelchair use has been found to be feasible and beneficial for children as young as 24 months of age (Butler et al., 1984). If a wheelchair is indicated, it is important to present this option to the parents in a positive way. The use of a wheelchair does not preclude walking. In fact, children who use wheelchairs at an early age generally are more interested in mobility, independence, and environmental exploration. Consequently, they tend to be more independent in all forms of mobility later in life. Ryan and associates (1991) recommended introducing a wheelchair as early as 18 months to enable children to keep up with their peers, boost self-confidence, facilitate independence, and increase activity levels.

Preparatory activities for mobility are indicated for 1- to 2-year-olds. Emphasis should be placed on balance, trunk control, and facilitating an upright posture. For ambulatory candidates, once the child begins to pull to stand, the need for orthoses to improve weight-bearing alignment should be considered. It is important to anticipate future ambulatory needs when recommending orthoses to maximize their utility.

For children with high-level lesions (thoracic to L3), preparatory activities for wheelchair mobility should be emphasized (e.g., sitting balance, arm strengthening, transfer training, wheelchair propulsion, and electrical switch operation if indicated). The focus of wheelchair training for toddlers and preschoolers with high-level lesions should include mobility, environmental exploration, safety, and transfer skills. Household distance ambulation using a parapodium, HKAFO, knee-ankle-foot orthosis (KAFO), or reciprocating gait orthosis (RGO) may be attempted, but energy expenditure is very high. Consequently, wheelchairs are generally used for community mobility of children with thoracic to L3 motor function, particularly once body proportions increase.

Effective biped ambulation is feasible for toddlers and preschoolers with L4 and below motor function. They will require wheelchair skills as older children, however, to participate in sports and prolonged activities. It is essential to maintain adequate ROM and to emphasize an upright posture so that weight-bearing forces are properly distributed and muscles can function at their optimal length. Therapeutic activities that promote trunk control and balance are beneficial. Children with lumbar level lesions will require upper limb support for walking. In general, a reverse-facing walker is best when learning to walk because it allows the child to be upright and minimizes upper limb weight bearing. Reverse-facing walkers have been found to promote better postural alignment than anterior-facing walkers (Logan et al., 1990). Once an upright gait is established, the child can be advanced to forearm crutches.

If children with sacral level motor function require upper limb support to begin walking, a reverse-facing walker is also usually best to minimize upper limb weight bearing. Alternatively, forearm crutches can be used if the child is able to walk upright while manipulating the crutches. Children with L5 and S1 level lesions often abandon their upper limb aids when they are young and their center of mass is low to the ground. Upper limb aids may still be indicated for endurance and to decrease trunk sway when walking long distances, for balance when walking on rough terrain, or to minimize the stress on weight-bearing lower limb joints. The need for upper limb aids should be reevaluated when the child is older and body proportions and environmental demands have changed.

The use of positive reinforcement is often recommended for this population to enhance cooperation with examination procedures and intervention programs. In general, food is not an appropriate form of reinforcement because obesity is often a concern. Verbal reinforcement is preferred at this age.

Prevention of Secondary Impairments and Activity Limitations

Individuals are at risk for joint contractures when there is muscle imbalance around joints, when a substantial portion of the day is spent sitting, when there is a prolonged period of immobilization or bed rest, following surgery, and during periods of rapid growth when soft tissue growth may lag behind skeletal changes. It is important to closely monitor individuals with MM during these periods so that intervention can be initiated early on, if needed, when contractures are still flexible and respond well to intervention. Early detection and intervention of contractures is important to prevent fixed deformities and stretch weakness of overlengthened muscles. Similarly, the importance of skin inspection of insensate areas, use of pressure relief cushions, and sitting push-ups for pressure relief should be emphasized at an early age so that these preventive measures become routine. Daily monitoring of insensate areas can be taught at an early age by jointly inspecting the skin and verbalizing that there are no red areas. Body image can be promoted by playing games that involve touching and finding body parts.

Habitual postural positions that contribute to deforming forces should be discouraged. It is essential to emphasize an upright posture when a child is learning to walk. If children are permitted to stand and walk in a crouched posture, habit patterns become established and it is difficult to teach a more upright posture because of the development of secondary impairments (e.g., joint contractures and stretch weakness of excessively lengthened muscles). Therapists should closely observe joint alignment and posture when a child is standing. Postural deviations that look insignificant when a child is young are often magnified once body proportions increase.

SCHOOL AGE

Typical Participation Restrictions: Causes and Implications

Independence with ADL often continues to be impaired in this age group. Children who are not independent with ADL may miss out on normal childhood experiences (e.g., play time or recess) while waiting for parents or teachers to assist them with basic skills. Their self-esteem may continue to be negatively affected if other children tease them regarding their dependency.

Mobility limitations are magnified once a child begins school because of the increased community mobility distances and skills required. Advanced mobility skills are needed because of environmental barriers such as curbs, ramps, uneven terrain, and steps. Ineffective or inefficient community mobility can further reinforce dependent behaviors if other children carry his or her school books and lunch tray or push the wheelchair.

The negative effects of limited mobility and physical limitations on socialization become more apparent at this age. Play and recreational opportunities are restricted if a child does not have an effective method of mobility. Often children with MM are excluded from recess or physical education class. Consequently, they miss out on opportunities for social interaction. Even if they are included in these activities, often their involvement is peripheral (e.g., score keeper during physical education class). Mobility limitations, dependency with ADL, difficulties with toileting, and the difficulty of managing adaptive equipment often interfere with other aspects of peer interaction, such as going over to friends' houses to play or spending the night with friends.

Finally, it is important that parents and teachers be aware of perceptuomotor, visuoperceptual, and sensory deficits. The potential impact of these deficits on writing speed, legibility, and accuracy; the efficiency and effectiveness of performing ADL skills; problem solving; and cognitive abilities should be realized so that reasonable goals can be established and the use of appropriate adaptive equipment can be implemented. Multiple hospitalizations or medical complications can also negatively affect school performance.

Examination and Evaluation of Impairments and Activity Limitations

As with younger children, joint alignment, strength, muscle imbalance, contractures, muscle extensibility, and posture should continue to be monitored. Other parameters that should be assessed include sensation, coordination, fine motor skills, ADL, mobility, gait, body awareness, and functional skills.

Reliable, sensitive, objective measures of strength can be obtained in school-age children (Hinderer & Hinderer, 1993). We recommend that objective methods of strength examination, such as handheld myometry, be used to serially monitor strength of individuals with MM who are old enough to cooperate (typically age 4 or older). Stationary isokinetic or strain gauge devices can also provide objective measures of strength, but these devices are not available in the typical clinic or school setting.

Independence with ADL should be assessed. In addition to the basic ADL skills evaluated in the Functional Activities Assessment, the school-age child's ability to carry items and assist with basic household chores should be evaluated. The adequacy of clearance, duration, frequency, and reliability of performance of wheelchair push-ups are also assessed by the physical therapist. Bowel and bladder function and the degree of continence are usually evaluated by a nurse. It is important that the physical therapist understand these and degree of independence with bowel and bladder function, however, because positioning, adaptive equipment, and mobility issues can often restrict independence with bowel and bladder intervention programs.

The home, school, and community environments should be accessible so that individuals with MM can participate fully in all activities. The Americans with Disabilities Act of 1990 mandates access to all buildings, programs, and services used by the general public in the United States. Even partial exclusion from a school program can have lasting negative effects on a student's social and emotional development (Baker & Rogosky-Grassi, 1992). Providing accessibility to the entirety of school, home, and community activities lets individuals with MM know that they have the same opportunities and rights of access as everyone else. Limited access broadcasts a message of exclusion and estrangement. Both physical and social barriers to participation must be addressed. For a more thorough discussion of evaluating environmental accessibility in the school setting, see Baker and Rogosky-Grassi (1992). Community accessibility should also be evaluated. Ideally, the patient should have access to the community school, church, grocery and drug stores, post office, bank, cleaners, stores and shopping malls, library, restaurants, theaters, sports arenas, hospital, physician's office, work environment, and public transportation. Streets, sidewalks, crosswalks, and parking lots should also be accessible.

Ongoing Monitoring

Joint alignment, muscle imbalance, contractures, posture, and signs of progressive neurologic dysfunction should continue to be monitored. As school-age children mature, they should become more responsible for daily inspection of insensate skin areas when they are bathing and dressing. Appropriate performance of pressure relief strategies should also be monitored. Areas of skin breakdown should be noted so that appropriate adjustments in equipment and preventive behaviors can be implemented or reviewed.

School-age children should be observed closely during periods of rapid growth because they are at risk for loss of function as a result of cord tethering. Parents and teachers should be made aware of signs of progressive CNS complications so that they know when to refer the child to a primary care physician.

Typical Physical Therapy Goals and Strategies

The stretching and strengthening strategies discussed for the two previous age groups also apply to the school-age child. Improving the flexibility of low back extensor, hip flexor, hamstring, and shoulder girdle musculature should be emphasized. When possible, stretching and strengthening exercises should also be incorporated into the physical education program. It is important that children with MM participate in physical education classes and sports activities in a meaningful way. As noted earlier, if children dependent on braces and crutches learn wheelchair skills and use at an early age, they will not be depressed and perceive wheelchair use as a failure when they arrive at adolescence.

Proper positioning while sleeping and sitting should continue. In the classroom, seating should provide stability and symmetric alignment. Feet should be flat on the floor or on wheelchair footrests. The seat and desk height should be adjusted to fit the child's body proportions. The desk top should be tilted up to improve neck and upper trunk alignment. Appropriate cushioning should be provided. The child's chair should be positioned in the room so that the teacher and blackboard can easily be viewed while maintaining neutral alignment, without having to turn in the chair.

If a child has not achieved independence with a given ADL task by the age at which 50% of the normative group achieved independence on the Functional Activities Assessment, the child's performance should be assessed to determine if adaptive equipment is required or if further interventions are indicated. Goals for ADL performance should include efficiency in addition to independence. If the child is not as efficient as the primary caretaker, the caretaker will most likely perform the task. The target goal, therefore, is for the child to be able to perform the task as efficiently as the primary caretaker. Showing parents the ADL normative data for children with MM and promoting positive parental expectations of independence are beneficial (see Fig. 25-6). It is important for parents to positively reinforce the child's attempts to be independent so that he or she is motivated to achieve. Pressure relief techniques should be incorporated into the daily routine. Joint protection measures should also be implemented early on to prevent the development of future degenerative changes.

Once children with MM begin school, it is important that they have an independent, efficient, and effective means of mobility for home and long community distances. Alternative means of mobility may need to be considered for long distances to ensure that children with MM are able to keep up with their peers and still have energy left to attend to classroom activities. Various mobility options should be evaluated according to the criteria outlined in Box 25-2 to determine the most effective means of mobility for a given environment. Community-level wheelchair and ambulation skills should be taught, emphasizing efficiency and safety. Community, home, and school environments should be assessed to determine if there are architectural barriers that interfere with daily activities. It is essential for normal social development to permit accessibility to all school, home, and community activities, including recess, physical education, and field trips (Baker & Rogosky-Grassi, 1992).

A functional environment should be created at home and school by removing obstacles and adapting the environment to facilitate efficient and independent function.

Adaptive equipment and effective mobility devices should be provided to maximize function. Community mobility skills may need to be practiced to facilitate independent function. Endurance training may also be indicated to ensure that the individual has sufficient endurance and efficiency to function effectively in all activities.

Recreation and physical fitness are important for physical, psychologic, and social reasons. Psychosocial benefits of participation in recreational activities include enhancing confidence and self-esteem, increasing socialization, improving group participation skills, provision of a means of exercising in a more normal way, and increasing interest and motivation in maintaining flexibility, strengthening, and endurance. In contrast, perceived physical restrictions result in a sedentary

---

Box 25-2 Feasibility of Wheelchair and Biped Ambulation: Criteria for Evaluation

HOUSEHOLD DISTANCES

Endurance
Adequate to go between rooms in house?
Adequate to get to yard and car?

Efficiency
Record heart rate and calculate energy expenditure.
Record normal and fast household walking speeds.
Is fast pace adequate for emergency situations?
Is normal pace practical for everyday activities?

Effectiveness
Independent with all transfers?
Able to carry, reach, lift, and climb?
Able to perform activities of daily living?
Able to go forward, backward, sideways, and turn?

Safety
Has good stability and balance?
Observes joint and skin protection?
Able to maneuver around obstacles?
Safe on smooth surfaces and rugs?
Safe when turning?

Accessibility
Maneuvers in and out of house independently?
Necessary household rooms accessible?
Emergency exit routes accessible?

COMMUNITY DISTANCES

Endurance
Sufficient at a functional speed for average community distances (e.g., going to school, store, medical appointments, and social activities)?
Adequate for play and recreational activities (e.g., playground, park, beach, theater, sports arenas, sports participation)?
Adequate for long-distance community distances (e.g., shopping mall, zoo, concert, sporting events, hiking)?

Efficiency
Record heart rate and calculate energy expenditure.
Record normal and fast walking paces.
Adequate speed to cross intersections?
Is typical pace practical for community distances?

Effectiveness
Independent with all transfers?
Able to maneuver in all directions?
Able to climb and step over obstacles?
Able to carry packages and groceries?
Able to reach and lift items from shelves?

Safety
Has good stability and balance?
Observes joint and skin protection?
Safe on wet or slippery surfaces?
Able to maneuver around obstacles?
Able to maneuver in congested areas?
Safe on uneven terrain, curbs, inclines, and steps?

Accessibility
Maneuvers in and out of car and bus independently?
Necessary community buildings accessible?

lifestyle, potentially predisposing these individuals to problems with obesity and degenerative diseases. It is important to stimulate a lifelong interest in fitness and recreation. In addition, community resources, feasibility of transportation, and the family's lifestyle must be taken into account.

Recreation activities must be carefully selected to ensure that they are beneficial and feasible yet enjoyable so they will be continued on a regular basis. Ideally, recreation activities should incorporate forms of aerobic exercise, along with socialization. It is important for individuals with MM to be involved in regular aerobic exercise to maintain their physical fitness and effectively control their weight. Recreational and physical fitness goals include maintaining and improving flexibility, strength, endurance, aerobic capacity, cardiovascular fitness, and coordination and controlling weight. Low-impact aerobics are preferred to minimize stress on joints. Aerobic exercise videotapes have been developed for individuals with disabilities. Swimming is an ideal sport for this population, because they are often able to be competitive with their able-bodied peers and there is minimal stress on joints. Other low-impact activities include cycling, rowing, cross-country skiing, roller and ice skating, and aerobic dance.

Verbal reinforcement or implementation of a token economy system to earn special privileges is preferred at this age to enhance cooperation with examination procedures and intervention programs. As mentioned above, food is not an appropriate form of reinforcement.

Prevention of Secondary Impairments and Activity Limitations

Deficits that may appear insignificant during childhood often become magnified once an individual has adult body proportions, resulting in activity limitations and discomfort (e.g., low back pain resulting from an increased lumbar lordosis and hip flexion contractures). Joint protection is also important, beginning in early childhood. Joint trauma from excessive stress is cumulative over the life span. Children do not typically complain of pain, and children with MM may not be able to reliably detect pain in insensate areas. Consequently, sources of excess joint stress must be identified by carefully observing children while they perform ADL and transfers, walk, and propel their wheelchair. Permitting school-age children to assume responsibility for daily skin inspection checks with supervision helps prepare them for independence in adolescence (Peterson et al., 1994). One method of teaching careful skin inspection involves letting the child locate a small colored adhesive dot that is placed randomly on insensate skin.

Children and their parents should be involved as much as possible in the decision-making process and intervention of their disability. The rationale for assistive devices and therapeutic interventions should be explained so that they are in agreement with intervention plans and become knowledgeable regarding acquisition of medical care and services, rather than being passive recipients.

ADOLESCENCE AND TRANSITION TO ADULTHOOD

Typical Participation Restrictions: Causes and Implications

If normal developmental stages for early childhood development have not been taught, adolescence can present a crisis (Shurtleff et al., 2004). The preparation of individuals with MM for a successful transition into adult life must be based on developmental concerns and timely issues from infancy through all stages of development to young-adult life (Peterson et al., 1994). Adolescence brings expanded domains of travel for individuals with MM. School buildings become larger, with more environmental barriers for people with physical disabilities. To keep up with peers, community mobility must include mobility skills to travel long distances quickly and efficiently between classrooms, out to athletic fields as a participant or spectator, around shopping malls, and into crowded movie theaters, dances, and night clubs. Independent adult living also requires mobility and balance skills that permit completion of advanced ADL tasks such as cooking, cleaning, clothes washing, shopping, yardwork, house and equipment maintenance, driving, riding on public transportation, and going to work. Children who have gotten by with slow, inefficient ambulation skills using cumbersome adaptive equipment or who have had basic wheelchair mobility on level surfaces but suddenly cannot handle ramps, hills, curbs, and uneven ground find themselves lagging behind their peers. Nearly all of the adults in a study of 30 individuals with MM (Hinderer et al., 1988) required referral to a physical therapist to address advanced mobility or equipment issues. It has been the observation of the authors that many adolescents and young adults do not have sufficient mobility skills to succeed independently in the community and must play "catch-up" to achieve their functional potential. The price paid for this delayed development of functional community mobility and lack of independence is social incompetence, dependence for advanced living skills, and unemployability, all of which must subsequently be addressed once mobility skills are improved. It is also important to train for competence and self-reliance. Blum and associates (1991) reported that young people with MM who perceived that they were overprotected had less happiness, lower self-esteem, higher anxiety, lower self-perceived popularity, and greater self-consciousness.

Changes in functional mobility skills often occur concurrently with the rapid changes of adolescence. Individuals who have previously been ambulatory often become more reliant on a wheelchair. Dudgeon and associates (1991) reported that adolescents with MM often exhibit changes in ambulation that are not explained by progressive complications. They suggested that these changes reflect adaptation of mobility to new environmental and social demands that require different speed, accessibility, and energy demands than those encountered in childhood. If orthotic stabilization of the hip, knee, or both is required, it is unlikely that adolescents with MM will maintain community ambulation; instead, most become nonambulators (Dudgeon et al., 1991). Brinker and associates (1994) reported a decline in the ability to walk in 11 of 35 adults with sacral level MM (19 to 51 years old). Of the 34 adults who were initially community ambulators, 5 had become household ambulators, 2 were nonfunctional ambulators, and 4 were nonambulators. The one adult who had been a household ambulator became a nonambulator. The most common reasons for their declining ambulatory status were foot ulcerations, infections, and amputations. Wheelchair transfer skills have also been observed to decline during the transition from adolescence to adulthood. In a study of 30 adults with MM who had thoracic through sacral level motor function, 43% had declined in their mobility status from previous examinations performed during adolescence (Hinderer et al., 1988). Several potential factors can play a role in this decreased function.

Changes in body proportions and body composition occur throughout the growing years, but the rate of these changes is accelerated dramatically during adolescence (Hinderer & Hinderer, 1993). Increases in limb length affect the torque generated by muscles due to altered muscle length and resistance force moment arms. In addition, increases in height raise the location of the center of mass higher off the ground, making upright balance more difficult and energy expenditure greater to perform mobility tasks. Changes in body composition also alter the biomechanics of movement and affect performance. The relative percentage of force-generating muscle to fat and bone tissue changes the ratio of force-producing tissue to the load of the limbs. The development of obesity often occurs during adolescence and can further accentuate these changes. Banta (1999) stated that body mass increases by the cube or volume whereas strength increases only by the square or cross-sectional

area. The inevitable result during the adolescent growth spurt is that walking efficiency declines as the energy demands increase. Furthermore, it is known that during the adolescent growth spurt, the rate of skeletal growth exceeds the increase in muscle mass; the latter catches up after skeletal growth slows in late adolescence. Decreased flexibility of the trunk and two-joint limb muscles is often observed as part of this process. Normal adolescents frequently become clumsy during this period of adjustment while learning how to coordinate their longer limb lengths and increased muscle mass. Adolescents with MM already have a mechanical disadvantage and are consequently more susceptible to dyscoordination and decreased flexibility. It is likely that these developmental changes contribute to the decline in mobility that often occurs in adolescents with MM.

Progression of the neurologic deficit is another potential cause for decline in mobility function, and adolescents are particularly at risk during rapid periods of growth. Forty percent of the participants in our adult follow-up study (Hinderer et al., 1988) had lower limb strength loss compared with previous strength examinations as adolescents. Twenty-seven percent had a reduction in lower limb sensory perception. The greatest motor and sensory losses occurred in the group with lesions at L5 and below—the individuals with the most function to lose. In addition, 10% of study participants demonstrated upper limb strength loss. Progressive neurologic loss, therefore, appears to be an important factor in the changes in mobility status of many individuals during the transition from adolescence to adulthood.

Immobilization for intervention of secondary complications of MM can also contribute to decreased mobility skills. The development of decubiti, fractures, and orthopedic surgeries such as spinal fusions often require extended periods of immobilization with consequent disuse weakness, decreased endurance, and contracture development, all of which can contribute to decreased performance of mobility and transfer tasks.

Prolonged periods of bed rest are often necessary to heal decubitus ulcers to avoid bearing weight on pressure areas. Adolescents often have an increased incidence of decubiti compared with younger children. This is due to their increased body mass causing greater pressure over bony prominences around the buttocks and because of the development of adult sweat patterns in these areas. Fifty-six percent of the adults evaluated in our study (Hinderer et al., 1988) had a history of skin breakdown since their last examination as adolescents; nearly 17% had breakdown present at the time of the examination. An alarming number of these people had little insight into the causes or methods for preventing skin breakdown despite their previous care in a large multidisciplinary pediatric clinic. Even more disturbing was the fact that three individuals (10%) had sustained lower limb amputations since adolescence (two bilateral, one unilateral) as a result of nonhealing ulcers that had progressed to osteomyelitis. Clearly, functional mobility is affected by decubitus ulcers and especially by limb loss.

Musculoskeletal problems can also affect the mobility of adolescents. Progression of spinal deformities often occurs during the growth spurt or in conjunction with one of the neurologic complications previously discussed. Sitting and standing balance can be affected by these spinal changes, leading to decreased mobility and transfer skills. Spinal orthoses prescribed to maintain optimal postural alignment also limit trunk ROM and hip flexion, interfering with wheelchair transfers and moving from sitting to standing. Surgical fusion of the spine to correct deformity and prevent its further progression can lead to immobilization with its consequent effects on mobility described earlier. Lower limb fractures secondary to osteoporosis can also necessitate immobilization with increased risk of functional loss.

Adolescents often begin to develop degenerative changes of weight-bearing joints and overuse syndromes as a result of the excessive loading of these joints necessitated by their neurologic deficit. Joint pain, ligamentous instability, or tendinitis can further limit mobility capabilities. Fifty percent of the adult study participants (Hinderer et al., 1988) complained of joint pain and 100% had joint or spinal deformities noted at the time of their examination.

Several other issues become important for the physical therapist to be cognizant of during adolescence. Independence with self-care and other daily activities is essential for normal socialization and for preparing individuals to lead normal adult lives. Bowel and bladder continence and independent intervention of bowel and bladder emptying are essential for social acceptance by peers and are even more critical at this stage because of the impact on dating, sexuality, higher education, employment, and independent living. Design and fit of wheelchair equipment, mobility aids, and orthoses affect independence with these tasks. Cosmesis is also a consideration with regard to equipment selection because body image and appearance become increasingly important issues during adolescence. Improper design or fit of equipment can significantly limit normal development in these areas.

Examination and Evaluation of Impairments and Activity Limitations

Based on the discussion of participation restrictions and their causes, several impairments should be assessed by the physical therapist. Emphasis of specific impairments should be based on the known or suspected concurrent medical problems.

Joint ROM and muscle extensibility of two-joint muscles (especially hip and knee flexors) and trunk muscles should be assessed. Neck and low back motions are often restricted, particularly in adolescents and adults, because of muscle imbalance and poor postural habits. Joint swelling, ligamentous instability, crepitus, and pain with or without joint motion should be documented. If these conditions are progressive or severe enough to interfere with function, the patient should be referred to a physician for further evaluation and intervention. The distribution of degenerative joint changes should be noted with regard to performance of mobility tasks and obesity to determine the contribution of abnormal joint stresses to joint pain and dysfunction.

Muscle strength should continue to be monitored for all major upper and lower limb muscle groups. When progressive neurologic dysfunction is suspected, coordination testing and serial grip strength measurements can also be helpful. Posture and trunk balance in sitting and standing (for ambulators) should be assessed. Real or apparent leg length discrepancy may be present in individuals with foot and ankle deformities, lower limb contractures, unilateral or bilateral hip dislocation, or pelvic obliquity related to spinal curves.

Thorough examination of bed mobility, floor mobility, wheelchair mobility and transfers, and appropriateness and fit of wheelchair equipment is essential for wheelchair users. Endurance and effectiveness of mobility should be assessed to determine whether the individual's current mode of mobility is practical for community-level function. Box 25-2 provides further detail regarding important areas to assess. When orthoses are needed to maintain proper alignment or to facilitate efficient ambulation, the appropriateness and fit of the orthoses must be assessed by the physical therapist. Boxes 25-3 and 25-4 provide further information regarding lower limb orthoses used in this population (see pp. 778–779).

Ongoing Monitoring

Given the multitude of potential problems that can occur during adolescence and adulthood, comprehensive examinations should continue on at least a yearly basis, and potentially more frequently when problems are suspected or known to be present. Without regular reexamination, these individuals often "fall through the cracks" and endure permanent loss of function that was avoidable. An unfortunate example was one of the adult study participants with a diagnosis of lipomeningocele and a neurosegmental classification of "no loss" as an adolescent. His lesion level was reclassified at an L5 level at the time of our study. His loss of neurologic function was caused by a recurrent lipoma on his spine that went undetected and was not surgically removed until permanent neurologic loss had occurred. This individual thought that because his original lesion was removed as an infant with preservation of his spinal cord function, he had no risk of future problems and therefore did not seek medical care until neurologic loss was irreversible. Early detection of progressive muscle strength loss, scoliosis, progression of spasticity, or contractures by the physical therapist with timely referral to a physician familiar with the potential complications associated with MM, along with aggressive physical therapy to reverse lost function (see section on prevention of secondary impairments and activity limitations), can prevent this scenario. This patient's story underscores the need for all individuals with MM to be followed *throughout life*, even if there are seemingly no current problems or their lesion has been classified as "no loss" after surgical closure.

Typical Physical Therapy Goals and Strategies

Functional goals for adolescents and adults are based on a number of factors that have been discussed in preceding sections of this chapter. The section on outcomes and their determinants provides guidelines for outcome expectations based on neurologic system function. In general, the goal for all but the most severely involved patients is to achieve independent basic and community mobility skills. The physical therapist must, therefore, be aware of all environments, distances, and barriers the individual is required to negotiate to adequately prepare the patient for all eventualities. Instruction in advanced community skills, along with endurance training, is often indicated. Physical and occupational therapists often need to be involved with driver's education programs and with the provision of adaptive equipment required for driving.

Goodwyn (1990) expanded the Functional Activities Assessment format to include adolescent skills required for independent living. The items were selected from existing adult-oriented skill achievement tests, and normative data were studied in this population. The Assessment of Motor and Process Skills (AMPS) was also studied in a group of individuals ranging in age from 6 to 73 years old (mean = 21.3 years) and was found to be a valid assessment of ADL performance (Kottorp et al., 2003). The AMPS assesses motor and process skills in terms of efficiency, effort, safety, and level of independence. The Kohlman Evaluation of Living Skills (McGourty, 1988) is also a useful screening tool for determining independence with adult living skills such as self-care, safety, health maintenance, money management, transporta-

tion, telephone use, and work and leisure activities. For adolescents and adults, the ability to lift and carry items such as a hot dish, grocery bags, a laundry basket, and heavy household items is also important to evaluate. It is particularly important to observe safety issues and the use of proper body mechanics for advanced living skills. In addition, the maximum carrying distance should be determined and contrasted with functional demands. If independence and effectiveness with ADL are limited, appropriate adaptations and interventions should be made to foster independence. Environmental adaptations or assistive devices required to perform functional tasks should be determined and specifically selected for application to social, educational, vocational, and work capacity requirements of the adolescent and adult. Vocational counseling and planning should begin early during the high school years. A social worker may need to be involved with the family to assist with the transition to independent living because a mutually dependent relationship is often fostered by the intense lifelong involvement of parents and siblings in assisting the individual with MM. Recreation therapy may be used to assist with shopping for and purchasing personal items, use of public transportation, and developing appropriate adult leisure activities. Occupational therapy may be useful to address advanced living skills such as cooking, cleaning, laundry, money management, and driver's training for appropriate candidates. A social worker can assist with locating accessible housing and obtaining appropriate support services for physical tasks that are too difficult for the patient. Depending on the practice setting, however, it may be necessary for the physical therapist to manage these areas. The expectation for individuals with MM who have intelligence in the normal range and sufficient motor function to care for themselves is the ability to thrive as an independent adult in our society.

Prevention of Secondary Impairments and Activity Limitations

The physical therapist plays an important role in anticipating the potential for functional loss when one of the medical complications of MM previously described increases the risk of secondary impairments. For example, when an adolescent undergoes a surgical procedure that requires extended bed rest, maintenance of muscle extensibility, joint ROM, and strength at the bedside followed by resumption of physical mobility tasks as soon as possible postoperatively can prevent long-term or permanent decline in mobility skills. Unfortunately, care providers are often not aware of these issues and intervention is not instituted until it is too late to recover lost function. The physical therapist must serve as an advocate for the patient under these circumstances. Regular skin inspection continues to be important to monitor skin integrity. Another mechanism for preventing secondary impairments is education of patients and their parents regarding the fit, specifications, condition, and maintenance of their adaptive equipment. They should know how to monitor skin tolerance and the fit of adaptive equipment. They should also understand the rationale for equipment and design features that are recommended. Knowledgeable consumers can detect and report potential problems before they result in complications such as decubiti. They need to be aware of the potential consequences of poorly fitted equipment so that they can advocate for the provision of quality equipment. The majority of adults in our follow-up study had improperly fitted equipment or lacked equipment that was essential for optimal function. These adults were also unaware of proper equipment maintenance techniques (Hinderer et al., 1988). As a result, many adults were functioning well below their capabilities and had skin breakdown, back pain, or joint pain as a result of poorly fitted orthoses or improper wheelchair design and seating.

OUTCOMES AND THEIR DETERMINANTS

Survival, disability, health, and lifestyles were investigated in a complete cohort of adults with MM in Cambridge, England (Hunt & Oakeshott, 2003). Outcomes were investigated at age 35 for 117 individuals who were born between 1963 and 1971. Sixty-three (54%) had died, primarily the most severely affected. The mean age of the survivors was 35 years (range 32 to 38) and 39 of the 54 survivors had an IQ above 80. Sixteen could walk for community distances (50 meters or more) with or without aids. These 16 individuals all had a sensory lesion level at or below L3. Thirty had pressure sores, 30 were overweight, and only 11 were fully continent. In terms of independent living status, 22 survivors lived independently in the community, 12 lived in sheltered accommodations where help was available if required, and 20 needed daily assistance. Twenty of the survivors drove cars and another nine had given up driving. Thirteen were employed, with five of them being in wheelchairs. Seven females and two males had had a total of 13 children (none with visible MM). Hunt and colleagues (1999) also reported that shunt revisions, particularly after the age of 2, were associated with poor long-term achievement in this same group of adult survivors with MM. Achievement was operationally defined according to their independent living status, employment, and use of a car.

McDonnell and McCann (2000) in a commentary to Hunt and associates' article reported more optimistic outcomes in terms of mobility and employment for shunt-treated survivors of MM in Belfast, Northern Ireland. Hunt (1990) reported that only 50% of adults were capable of living independently based on a sample of 69, of whom 68% had normal intelligence. In a sample of 18 patients 16 to 47 years old in Japan, Oi and associates (1996) reported that patients with spina bifida occulta (spinal lipoma) have a risk of neurologic deterioration, whether or not they have undergone radical preventive surgery in infancy. This deterioration is primarily related to lower spinal functions, such as ambulation and bowel and bladder control, which likely result from tethered cord, re-expansion of the residual lipoma, or syringomyelia. In contrast, these authors reported psychologic problems in patients with spina bifida aperta. Pandua and associates (2002) reported that adolescents with MM who have relatively mild activity limitations (i.e., they are able to walk and run) but who have urologic problems need psychologic support to a greater extent than adolescents with severe activity limitations and limited independence. There are many factors that contribute to the observed outcomes.

The motor function present is an important factor for predicting outcomes. Common characteristics of each lesion level are described in this section. The functional motor level does not always correspond to the anatomic lesion level because of individual variations in nerve root innervation of muscles. The information presented here is intended to serve as general guidelines for expectations at a given level of motor function. Many factors besides muscle strength influence an individual's functional potential and result in variations of performance within a given lesion level group. These factors include age, body proportions, weight, sensation, orthopedic deformities, joint contractures, spasticity, upper limb function, and cognition. The relative contribution of these factors is highly individual, and a thorough examination and follow-up of each child is necessary to maximize potential capabilities.

THORACIC LEVEL

Individuals with thoracic level muscle function have innervation of neck, upper limb, shoulder girdle, and trunk musculature, but no volitional lower limb movements are present. Banta (1999) stated that at the thoracic level the orthopedic goals are to maintain a straight spine, level pelvis, and symmetric lower limbs. Neck, upper limb, and shoulder girdle muscle groups are innervated by the C1 to T4 spinal nerves; back extensors by the C2 to L4 spinal nerves; intercostals by the thoracic nerves; and abdominals by T5 to L1. Consequently, individuals with motor function at or above T10 have strong upper limbs and upper thoracic and neck motions, but their lower trunk musculature is weak. They have difficulty with unsupported sitting balance and may have decreased respiratory function. Sliding boards may be required to perform wheelchair transfers because of the combination of poor trunk control and upper limb dyscoordination.

Individuals with motor function at T12 have strong trunk musculature and good sitting balance and may have weak hip hiking by means of the quadratus lumborum (innervated by T12 to L3). Ambulation may be attempted for exercise at this level using a parapodium; however, it is generally not an effective means of mobility (Liptak et al., 1992). A wheelchair is required for functional household and community mobility.

Children with thoracic level lesions also tend to have greater involvement of other areas of the CNS, with corresponding cognitive deficits. Consequently, even though many of these people achieve independence with basic self-care skills and mobility by late childhood, they often require a supervised living situation throughout life. They are rarely competitively employed but often participate in sheltered workshop settings or perform volunteer work (Hinderer et al., 1988).

HIGH LUMBAR (L1-L2) LEVEL

Individuals with high lumbar motor function have weak hip movements. The iliopsoas muscle is supplied by nerve roots L1 through L4, with its primary innervation at L2 and L3. The sartorius muscle is supplied by L2 and L3 and the adductors by L2 through L4. With L1 motor function, weak hip flexion may be present, and with L2 motor function the hip flexors, adductors, and rotators are grade 3 or better. According to Schafer and Dias (1983), unopposed hip flexion and adduction contractures are often present at the L2 motor level, and this muscle imbalance often results in dislocated hips. Short-distance household ambulation is possible with high lumbar innervation (L1 and L2) when body proportions are small, using KAFOs or RGOs and upper limb support. These children generally use a wheelchair for community distances. By the second decade of life, a wheelchair is typically the sole means of mobility commensurate with increased energy requirements and enlarged body proportions (Hinderer et al., 1988; Shurtleff, 1986d).

The prognosis of children with high lumbar lesions for function and independent living as adults is similar to that of the thoracic group described earlier (Hinderer et al., 1988). More individuals in this group, however, achieve independent living status (approximately 50%), but they are rarely able to maintain competitive employment as adults.

L3 LEVEL

Individuals with L3 muscle function have strong hip flexion and adduction, weak hip rotation, and at least antigravity knee extension. The quadriceps muscle group is innervated by nerve roots L2 through L4. Children with grade 3 quadriceps strength usually require KAFOs and forearm crutches to ambulate for household and short community distances and a wheelchair for long community distances. By adulthood, most individuals with L3 level lesions are primarily wheelchair mobile (Hinderer et al., 1988; Shurtleff & Lamers, 1978; Stillwell & Menelaus, 1983).

Approximately 60% of individuals with lesions at this level achieve independent living status as adults (Hinderer et al., 1988). Despite their higher level of independence, only a small percentage (about 20%) actively participate in full-time competitive employment (Hinderer et al., 1988).

L4 LEVEL

At the L4 motor level, antigravity knee flexion and grade 4 ankle dorsiflexion with inversion may be present. The medial hamstrings are innervated by nerve roots L4 through S2, and the anterior tibialis is innervated primarily by L4 and L5, with some innervation from S1. An individual is considered to have L4 motor function if the medial hamstrings or anterior tibialis is at least grade 3. Calcaneal foot deformities are common at this motor level as a result of the unopposed action of the tibialis anterior muscle (Schafer & Dias, 1983). Knee extension is usually strong, and these individuals are generally functional ambulators with AFOs and forearm crutches. When first learning to walk, however, KAFOs, a walker, or both may be required. A wheelchair is often needed for long distances.

In the adult follow-up study that we conducted, only 20% of individuals with L4 motor function continued to ambulate as adults (Hinderer et al., 1988). Many individuals stopped ambulation after their adolescent growth spurt. Others were unable to maintain ambulation because of ankle and knee valgus joint deformities and elbow and wrist pain resulting from years of weight bearing in poor alignment. To increase the likelihood of maintaining biped ambulation for individuals with L4 motor function throughout adulthood, upright posture should be emphasized when ambulating to minimize the weight-bearing stress on upper limb joints. Orthoses must be aligned properly and posted to support the ankle in a subtalar neutral position. If the ankle joint is malaligned, the knee joint position is adversely affected. It is essential to maintain the knee and ankle in neutral alignment when weight bearing. A flexed and valgus position should not be permitted. Ounpuu and associates (1992) demonstrated that 30% of the mechanical work occurs at the ankle during normal gait, underscoring the importance of controlling the ankle in order to provide proper alignment of the body to the ground reaction force. Often a patellar tendon-bearing, ground-reaction force orthotic design is optimal to protect the knee and increase the knee extension moment. The proximal medial trim line can be extended higher to provide additional medial knee support, if needed, to reduce a genu valgus deformity (see Fig. 25-5). Knee musculature should be strengthened to assist in maintaining the knee in neutral alignment when weight bearing. Every effort should be made to progress ambulation to using AFOs and forearm crutches to allow short-distance ambulation to easily be combined with long-distance wheelchair mobility. Crutches can be transported on the wheelchair, and AFOs are optimal because, unlike KAFOs, they do not interfere with dressing or toileting and do not cause skin breakdown when sitting. The prognosis for independent living and employment is similar to that for the group with L3 lesions.

L5 LEVEL

According to the IMSG criteria, classification of an L5 motor level is based on the presence of lateral hamstring muscles with at least grade 3 strength, and either grade 2 gluteus minimus and medius muscles (L4-S1), grade 3 posterior tibialis muscles (L5-S1), or grade 4 peroneus tertius muscles (L4-S1). Therefore, an individual with an L5 motor level has at least antigravity knee flexion and weak hip extension using the hamstrings and may have weak hip abduction, as well as weak plantar flexion with inversion, strong dorsiflexion with eversion, or both. Weak toe movements may also be present. Hindfoot valgus deformities or calcaneal foot deformities are common as a result of muscle imbalance. Individuals with motor function through L5 are able to ambulate without orthoses, yet require them to correct foot alignment and substitute for lack of push-off. A gluteal lurch is typically evident unless upper limb support is used. Bilateral upper limb support is usually recommended for community distances to decrease energy expenditure, decrease gluteal lurch and trunk sway, maintain symmetric alignment, protect lower limb joints, and improve safety. The need for upper limb support often becomes more apparent

with increased height following growth spurts. Traversing uneven terrain is often difficult. A wheelchair may be required when there is a rapid change in body proportions (e.g., pregnancy) or for long distances on rough terrain. A bike is also useful for long community distances.

Approximately 80% of individuals with lesions at L5 and below achieve independent living status as adults (Hinderer et al., 1988). About 30% are employed full time and an additional 20% part time, well below the average employment rate of the general adult population.

S1 LEVEL

With muscle function present through S1, at least two of the following additional muscle actions are present: gastrocnemius/soleus (grade 2), gluteus medius (grade 3), or gluteus maximus (grade 2). Individuals with S1 motor function have improved hip stability and can walk without orthoses or upper limb support. A weak push-off is evident when running or climbing stairs. A mild to moderate gluteal lurch is often present. Vankoski and associates (1995) documented the benefits of crutch use for this lesion level, which resulted in improved pelvis and hip kinematics during gait. Gait deviations and activity limitations are often more pronounced after the adolescent growth spurt. The toe musculature is generally strong. Foot deformities are less common at this level, but foot orthoses or AFOs may be required to improve lower limb alignment and permit muscle groups to function at a more optimal length. Medial and lateral stability at the ankle is required for adequate function of the plantar flexor muscles during push-off (Lehmann et al., 1986).

S2, S2-S3, AND "NO LOSS" LEVELS

Motor function is classified at the S2 level if the plantar flexor muscles are at least grade 3 and the gluteals grade 4. The only obvious gait abnormality present at this level is generally a decreased push-off and stride length when walking rapidly or running as a result of the decreased strength of the plantar flexor muscles. If all lower limb muscle groups have grade 5 strength except for one or two groups with grade 4 strength, the motor level is classified as S2-S3, according to the IMSG criteria. The term *no loss* is used if the bowel and bladder function normally and lower limb strength is judged to be normal through manual muscle testing. Functional deficits may be present, however, for individuals classified as having no loss. Foot orthoses are often beneficial to maintain the ankle in the subtalar neutral position and optimize ankle muscle function by maintaining optimal muscle length.

EXAMINATION, EVALUATION, AND DIRECT INTERVENTIONS FOR MUSCULOSKELETAL ISSUES, MOBILITY, AND FUNCTIONAL SKILLS

There are three primary reasons for evaluating the individual with MM: (1) to define an individual's current status so that appropriate program planning can occur, (2) to identify the potential for developing secondary impairments so that preventive measures can be implemented, and (3) to monitor changes in status that could indicate progressive neurologic dysfunction. Because of the complexity of problems associated with MM, numerous dimensions of disability must be assessed by various disciplines. The physical therapist provides essential information to other team members for program planning and to monitor status. Careful documentation is important for communication among team members and for serial comparisons over time. General examination and intervention strategies will be discussed in this section. Considerations that are specific to certain age categories are discussed in the section on age-specific examination and physical therapy interventions.

EXAMINATION STRATEGIES

The dimensions typically assessed by physical therapists include ROM, muscle extensibility, joint alignment or orthopedic deformities, muscle tone, muscle strength and endurance, sensation, posture, motor development, ADL, mobility skills, equipment needs, and environmental accessibility. It is important to use standardized protocols, when available, that have good reliability and validity to permit comparison within and between individuals (Hinderer & Hinderer, 1998). If more than one measurement method exists (e.g., hip extension ROM), the specific method employed should be documented and used consistently. Comprehensive examinations should be conducted at regular intervals throughout the life span on all individuals with MM. In addition, it is recommended that therapists remain blind to previous results of the more subjective measures (e.g., manual muscle testing scores or gait deviations) until the examination is complete to avoid potential biases from previous results. Videotapes and photographs are often a useful adjunct to clinical examination of gait, joint deformities, and posture. These visual records provide an excellent baseline for comparison purposes if deterioration in status is suspected. It is

beneficial to conduct examination of activities that are influenced by environmental or endurance factors (e.g., wheelchair mobility, gait, or ADL) in more natural settings.

The IMSG recommends a comprehensive, multidisciplinary evaluation for *all* individuals with MM, regardless of functional level, because they all are at risk for progressive neurologic dysfunction, as discussed earlier. The following examination intervals are recommended: newborn preoperatively, newborn postoperatively, 6 months, 12 months, 18 months, 24 months, and annually thereafter, continuing through adulthood (Shurtleff, 1986c). Annual examinations are suggested to occur around an individual's birth date so that they are not forgotten. ROM, muscle extensibility, strength, endurance, coordination, and functional parameters should be monitored more closely during periods of rapid growth, when individuals with MM are at increased risk for loss of function. Preintervention and postintervention measurements should be obtained for individuals undergoing surgery or other therapeutic procedures. More frequent evaluation of specific goal attainment is indicated for individuals receiving ongoing therapeutic intervention. Mobility and independence with ADL should be reevaluated when body proportions or environmental demands change to determine if the individual has the strength, endurance, coordination, and adaptive equipment required to function effectively.

Shurtleff (1986c, 1991) advocated using the Patient Data Management System (PDMS) standardized protocol and recording format to serially monitor individuals with MM. The PDMS is composed of a comprehensive, interdisciplinary recording format, which consists of the dimensions typically assessed by each discipline. In addition, intervention data (e.g., surgery, medications, and therapy) are also documented. Scoring and recording criteria can be obtained by contacting the IMSG (IMSG, 1993). The PDMS computerized recording format is beneficial for monitoring this population because serial test results from birth to present can be efficiently scanned for each parameter to detect improvements or deterioration in status. In addition, an individual patient's status can be directly compared with that of other individuals with similar characteristics by using the interactive database. The standardized format facilitates communication between and within disciplines and intervention centers and promotes clinical research. Duplication of effort by the various health care professionals involved in the intervention of individuals with MM is minimized because each discipline is assigned specific PDMS areas to assess, yet all disciplines share the information in the combined database. The PDMS format has also been applied to several other pediatric populations, including those with cerebral palsy, cystic fibrosis, hemophilia, and traumatic brain injury (Shurtleff, 1991).

Individuals with MM should be evaluated on at least a yearly basis by multiple disciplines at a comprehensive care center. It is important, however, for comprehensive care centers and local school and intervention settings to coordinate their examinations, goals, and intervention programs to avoid duplication of effort and to ensure appropriate prioritization of intervention goals. The use of the PDMS facilitates communication. The School Needs Identification and Action Forms (Rowley-Kelly & Kunkle, 1992) also provide a useful format for identifying impairments, academic and activity limitations, and the remedial action recommended. The areas assessed by the school needs forms include health-related services required, physical intervention instructions, accessibility, safety and fire drills, preparation for school entry, educational rights and related services, academic difficulties, psychologic evaluation, perceptuomotor deficits, visuo-perceptual deficits, self-help skills, social acceptance, social and emotional issues, parent and school relationships, transitional services, and other needs.

INTERVENTION STRATEGIES

Once primary and secondary impairments, activity limitations, and participation restrictions are identified through a comprehensive evaluation, the functional significance must be determined to plan appropriate intervention strategies. Intervention of an impairment is indicated if it currently interferes with function or if the deficit can progress to a point where it may negatively affect future function. Intervention is also indicated if the efficiency, effectiveness, or safety of performance can be improved. Strength, endurance, and efficiency of performing tasks should be emphasized. Weight-bearing joints must be protected to prevent early onset of osteoarthritis and to prolong mobility. In addition, the most efficient and effective means of mobility for a given environment should be determined. Goal setting for intervention must consider the impact of the multiple impairments discussed earlier on functional performance expectations. The cognitive, social, and behavioral issues discussed in the impairments section should also be considered.

Fay and associates (1986) recommended three specific intervention approaches for developmental delays in this population. The first is developmental programming in which children are encouraged by parents, teachers, and therapists with a "high dose" of normal developmental activities in "at-risk" areas. The philosophy behind this approach is that supplemental early emphasis and practice in potential problem areas will minimize later deficits.

These early intervention programs are often initiated for children with MM before measurable delays are identified. The second approach, remediation, is implemented once problem areas are clearly identified. This approach consists of repetition of a set of graded tasks in the domain of concern. Improved performance through practice theoretically carries over into functional activities. The third approach is teaching compensatory skills. Compensation is often implemented when the other two approaches have not produced sufficient results or when the child is older or more severely impaired. This intervention approach involves identifying and developing strategies to help the child become as independent as possible or providing adaptive equipment to compensate for underlying problems and minimize disability in daily life.

SPECIFIC EXAMINATION AND INTERVENTION STRATEGIES

Specific examination and intervention strategies as they pertain to strength, mobility, gait, and equipment issues are highlighted in this section because of the magnitude of the impact of these factors on function in this population, regardless of age or lesion level. Suggestions for impairment-specific parameters (e.g., ROM, orthopedic deformities, and sensation) were discussed in the section on impairments. Developmental issues were discussed in the section on age-specific examination and physical therapy interventions.

Strength

Upper limb, neck, and trunk musculature should be screened for weakness. If evidence of weakness exists, a more specific examination of strength should be conducted. For individuals with thoracic or high lumbar level involvement, it is important to palpate trunk musculature to determine which portions of muscle groups are functioning. Dynamometer values of grip and pinch strength should also be obtained. Kilburn and associates (1985) suggested that grip strength measurements can be a sensitive measure of progressive neurologic dysfunction. A standardized protocol for obtaining grip strength measurements and normative values for children has been provided by Level (1984).

Specific testing of isolated motions of lower limb muscles is essential to determine if individual muscles are functioning. Standardized test protocols should be used (e.g., Hislop & Montgomery, 2002; Janda, 1983; Kendall et al., 1999). It is *essential* to detect changes in strength in this population as soon as possible, because loss of strength can be a sign of progressive neurologic dysfunction. As a result, we recommend using quantitative strength measurements in conjunction with traditional manual muscle testing techniques. It is also important to distinguish between reflexive and voluntary movements. Reflexive movements should be documented, but they should not be considered when determining motor lesion levels.

Manual muscle testing is the most common method used to assess strength in this population because of its adaptability in a typical clinic setting. Manual muscle testing is the method of choice for screening muscle strength to determine the presence of volitional activity in specific muscles and to determine whether an individual muscle's function varies throughout the ROM. There are several limitations to relying only on manual muscle testing scores for serially monitoring strength, as discussed in Chapter 6.

Manual muscle testing has limited interrater and test-retest reliability (Hinderer & Hinderer, 1993). Manual muscle test scores must change more than one full grade to be confident that a true change in strength has occurred. In addition, manual muscle testing has poor concurrent validity compared with more quantitative measures. Several studies have demonstrated that deficits in strength exceeding 50% are *not* detected by manual muscle testing (Agre et al., 1987; Aitkens et al., 1989; Bohannon, 1986; Griffin et al., 1986; Miller et al., 1988). Agre and colleagues (1987) examined this issue in 33 adolescents with MM. Individuals who had been classified as having "no motor deficits" by means of manual muscle testing actually had strength deficits compared with normative data. These deficits were 40% for the hip extensor and 60% for the knee extensor muscles. The lack of concurrent validity of manual muscle testing compared with quantitative measurements demonstrates that the sensitivity of manual muscle testing in detecting weakness is very limited and is inadequate for detecting early strength loss in individuals with MM.

The *predictive validity* of manual muscle testing has been examined in two studies on children with MM. Murdoch (1980) examined the predictive validity of neonatal manual muscle testing examinations using a truncated 3-point scale. The correlation between muscle power of the newborn and subsequent mobility of the child at age 3 to 8 years was "very poor." In contrast, McDonald and associates (1986) examined the predictive validity of manual muscle testing for individual muscle groups on 825 children with MM using the complete 0- to 5-point grading scale. Predictive validity of manual muscle testing generally increased from birth to age 5. The probability that a given manual muscle test score precisely predicted future scores varied with age and the particular muscle group tested. These probabilities ranged from 23% to 68% for newborns and from 54% to 87% for older children. The

probability that a single test score predicted future strength within ±1 manual muscle test grade, however, was considerably higher, ranging from 70% to 86% for newborns and from 87% to 97% for older children. These results indicate that manual muscle testing is useful for predicting future muscle function within one manual muscle test grade. Strength test results obtained in infancy using the complete manual muscle test scale, therefore, appear to provide useful information for prognosis and for planning the course of intervention.

The limited reliability and concurrent validity of manual muscle testing indicates that it is not the method of choice for monitoring changes in strength over time. In contrast, strength testing using handheld instruments has been found to be a reliable and sensitive method for assessing strength in children and adolescents with MM. Intraclass interrater and test-retest correlation coefficients using this technique ranged from 0.73 to 0.99 (Effgen & Brown, 1992; Hinderer, 1988). Other authors report good to high levels of reliability when testing the strength of other populations of children and adolescents with handheld instrumentation (Florence et al., 1988; Hinderer & Gutierrez, 1988; Hinderer & Hinderer, 1993; Hosking et al., 1976; Hyde et al., 1983; Mendell & Florence, 1990; Stuberg & Metcalf, 1988). Several portable, handheld instruments are available for use in conjunction with manual muscle testing (Hinderer & Hinderer, 1993). The advantages of these instruments over nonportable instruments are that they are easily applied in typical clinic settings and can be used with standard manual muscle testing techniques to obtain objective force readings from most muscle groups.

It is best to obtain three myometry trials and report the average score because the mean is more stable over time and between raters (Hack et al., 1981; Hinderer, 1988). Torque values should be reported (force times lever arm length) to permit comparison over time, regardless of changing body proportions, at least until skeletal maturity has been attained. Torque values also permit direct comparison of force production capabilities between individuals with different body proportions. Standardized testing techniques must be implemented when assessing strength with handheld instruments to ensure the consistency of measurements. Many factors influence test results and must be controlled for when testing, including test positions, instructions and commands provided, use of reinforcement and feedback, application of resistance, the type of contraction, and the examiner's body mechanics. For more information regarding techniques used in testing with handheld instruments, see Hinderer and Hinderer (1993).

Several factors should be considered when testing the muscle strength of children with MM, including age, developmental level, cognitive level, ability to follow directions, attention span, motivation, motor planning skills, sensation, and proprioception. The examiner must carefully watch for muscle substitutions. This is particularly challenging in the MM population because of altered angles of pull from orthopedic deformities. It is often difficult for multijoint muscles such as the hamstrings to initiate motions. Any differences in function between end-range and midrange positions should be noted. Special considerations when testing infants and young children are discussed in the section on age-specific examination and physical therapy interventions.

As discussed in the impairments section, several CNS complications can account for loss of muscle function in this population, necessitating serial strength testing for early detection. There are many factors that can result in normal variations in strength, however, that should also be considered when interpreting test results. These factors include changes in body proportions, hormonal influences, motor learning, illness, injury, surgery, immobilization, physical or psychologic fatigue, the prior state of activity, seasonal variations, temporal factors, motivation, cooperation, and comprehension. Discussion of the specific influences of these factors is beyond the scope of this chapter. For further information regarding the impact of these factors on force production, see Hinderer and Hinderer (1993). Because of the multiple factors that can influence force production, it is important to repeat the testing at more frequent intervals, if strength loss is suspected, to determine whether consistent test results are obtained. Several variables should be considered when interpreting muscle test results, including the reliability and standard error of measurement of the testing method used, the concurrent and predictive validity of test results, and factors that can account for fluctuations in strength (Hinderer & Hinderer, 1993).

Static strength measurements should be correlated with functional measures to observe effects of fatigue and to determine the effect of reduced strength and limited endurance on function. Individuals with neurogenic muscle weakness may have a higher degree of variability in force production as a result of the lower threshold of fatigue and slower rate of recovery of weak musculature. Local muscle endurance appears to be deficient in some neuromuscular diseases (Bar-Or, 1986; Milner-Brown & Miller, 1989). Although this issue has not been specifically tested in the MM population, these results suggest that force production may be more variable in weak muscle groups of individuals with MM.

If function is present but weakness exists in muscle groups that are important for postural stability, ADL, mobility, or balance of muscle forces around joints,

strengthening exercises are indicated. The specific muscle groups to emphasize vary depending on the lesion level and functional requirements. In general, strong upper limb muscle groups are required for performing transfers, for wheelchair propulsion, and when using assistive devices to walk. Increasing the strength of trunk musculature improves sitting balance and postural stability. Increasing the strength of key lower limb muscle groups that are critical for ambulation can improve gait and can possibly minimize the need for orthoses and assistive devices. For example, increasing the quadriceps and hamstrings strength in an individual with L4 motor function may enable progression of ambulation from using KAFOs to using AFOs (see the case study at the end of this chapter).

Muscle groups should be strengthened within functional ROM. In addition to traditional strengthening exercises, many play activities promote strengthening (Embry et al., 1983). Muscle reeducation techniques such as functional electrical stimulation and biofeedback are useful to teach muscles to function in new parts of the ROM. Electrical stimulation has also been found to be beneficial to increase strength and enhance functional performance in this population (Karmel-Ross et al., 1992). Strengthening programs should be implemented during periods when an individual is at risk for loss of muscle strength and endurance (e.g., after recent surgery, immobilization, illness, or bed rest) and during periods of rapid growth when individuals often lose function as a result of changes in body proportions.

Endurance activities are also important for weight control and to enhance aerobic capacity. Individuals with MM must have adequate endurance to meet the challenges of community mobility. Low-impact aerobic activities to minimize joint stress are preferable. In general, jumping activities should be avoided because joint stress is increased as a result of the inadequate deceleration provided by weak lower limb muscles. Indications for endurance training and instruction in energy conservation techniques include decreased aerobic capacity, high energy cost of mobility, and limited endurance.

Mobility

Ineffective mobility is a hallmark of MM. *Effective mobility* is defined as any efficient and effective means of moving about in space that enables the individual to easily traverse and explore the environment, grow and develop, and independently pursue an education, vocation, or avocation (Shurtleff, 1986d). Mobility options provided should meet these criteria for all environments encountered by the individual so that lifestyle is not limited by endurance and difficulty traversing uneven terrain.

Changes in body proportions can significantly affect mobility. Mobility options, orthoses, and assistive device requirements that are ideal at one time may not be effective once body proportions, environmental demands, or both change. Consequently, the appropriateness of adaptive equipment and mobility options must be reevaluated throughout the life span. Emphasis of this point to patients by their health care providers helps prevent the feeling of failure if alternative mobility options are required in the future. Too often, individuals with MM grow up being praised for walking instead of using a wheelchair or for walking without assistive devices, depending on their lesion level. This emphasis gives the impression that normal biped ambulation is the only socially acceptable form of mobility. Several of the adults in our follow-up study reported that it was difficult to accept the use of a wheelchair or other assistive devices as they grew up because they felt that they were a failure or that they would disappoint their parents and health care providers (Hinderer & Hinderer, 1988). It is important to emphasize that wheelchairs and other assistive devices are aids for effective mobility and that their use does not represent a failure of biped ambulation.

Bed mobility, floor mobility, wheelchair mobility, ambulation, and transfers should be assessed and compared with the requirements for independent function. Criteria for assessing mobility parameters are endurance, efficiency, effectiveness, safety, degree of independence, and accessibility. Objective information regarding these parameters is often helpful to convince patients and their parents that alternative methods of mobility should be considered. Efficiency can be estimated by measuring the time required to complete a task. Energy expenditure can be estimated by measuring heart rate (HR). Regression equations have been determined for this population to equate heart rate with the energy expenditure required for a given task (Williams et al., 1983). The regression equations for energy expenditure and efficiency of this population are as follows:

Energy cost (mL O_2/kg min) = 0.073 (HR) + 6.119.
Energy efficiency (mL O_2/kg meter) = 0.006 (HR) – 0.313.

Criteria for determining the most practical and effective mode of mobility for household and community distances are provided in Box 25-2. Standardized tests that are useful for evaluating mobility in this population are discussed in Chapter 2. In addition, the Timed Test of Patient Mobility (Jebsen et al., 1970) is beneficial for assessing the efficiency of mobility because the time required to perform bed mobility, transfers, wheelchair mobility, and gait mobility tasks is documented. Normative data are available for comparison purposes. We suggest augmenting the efficiency time score of the Timed Test of Patient Mobility with a rating scale for the level of independence, safety, practicality, and assistive devices required for each task (Hinderer & Hinderer, 1988). Other evaluations that are specific to function in wheelchairs include the Functional Task Performance Wheelchair Assessment of positioning, reaching, and driving tasks (Deitz et al., 1991) and the Seated Postural Control Measure for sitting posture and functional movements (Fife et al., 1991).

Gait

Delays in achieving ambulation can be expected for all children with MM, including those with sacral level lesions, and children with high level lesions may cease walking after a period of 3 to 4 years of biped ambulation (Williams et al., 1999). Thorough examination and documentation of gait status are essential to monitor functional motor status and to watch for signs of progressive neurologic dysfunction. Patients or their parents typically notice changes in gait patterns and walking endurance before they notice increased muscle weakness. Careful gait observation is also needed to determine the most appropriate orthoses and assistive devices. Examination of orthoses and assistive devices for wear patterns helps determine if they are being used on a regular basis or just to perform in the clinic setting. Gait should be evaluated in a natural environment on a variety of walking surfaces. Patients should be observed walking for typical household and community distances to determine the effects of fatigue.

All too often decisions regarding gait problems and the need for orthoses and assistive devices are made by observing short-distance ambulation on a smooth clinic floor. Performance in the home or community environment may be vastly different than in a clinic situation, especially when walking around a number of obstacles, when in congested areas, when traversing uneven terrain, or with inclement weather. The impact of these factors must be considered when making recommendations.

Requirements for orthoses and ambulatory aids should be documented. Gait deviations should be closely observed and recorded. If possible, gait deviations and efficiency parameters should be observed both with and without orthoses and assistive devices. Typical gait parameters evaluated include arm swing, trunk position and sway, pelvic tilt and rotations, compensated or uncompensated Trendelenburg position, excessive hip flexion and rotation, excessive knee flexion or hyperextension, toe clearance, foot position, push-off effectiveness, and foot progression angle.

Observational gait analysis is the technique used most commonly to assess gait in clinical settings (Krebs et al., 1985). Video analysis augments clinical observations by allowing the evaluator to observe gait multiple times at slow speeds and by providing a permanent record that is invaluable for comparison purposes if deterioration of functional status is suspected. The interrater reliability of observational analysis through videotapes, however, has been reported to be low to moderate (Eastlack et al., 1991; Krebs et al., 1985). Footprint analysis is a low-cost method of obtaining objective information regarding velocity, cadence, foot progression angle, base of support, toe clearance, stride length, and step length (Shores, 1980). More sophisticated methods of objective gait analysis are described in Chapter 5.

Criteria for the effectiveness, efficiency, and safety of household and community ambulation are provided in Box 25-2. Efficiency and practicality of ambulation can be estimated by monitoring heart rate, normal and fast walking velocity, and maximum walking distance. Other time-distance variables (e.g., step and stride length, cadence, and cycle time) provide useful information regarding symmetry, stability, and function. These variables can be used for comparison purposes if they are normalized (adjusted) for stature (Rose et al., 1991).

Time-distance variables provide information about gait symmetry by comparing right-left differences in step lengths and stance-to-swing phase ratios. Examining cadence and the percentage of time spent in the stance phase versus the swing phase provides information regarding the stability of gait. For instance, a high cadence or an imbalance in the stance versus swing phase duration may indicate instability. Parameters such as walking velocity and cadence provide information regarding the functional practicality of gait. If the velocity is too low or step rate is too high, the individual may not be able to meet environmental demands.

It is essential to normalize time-distance variables for stature to compare these parameters serially over time for a given individual or to compare between individuals of different stature (e.g., comparing with normative data). These parameters are normalized by dividing by leg length. An alternative but less precise method of normalizing time-distance parameters is to divide by height because overall height is closely correlated to individual limb lengths. If these parameters are not normalized for stature, conclusions regarding differences in function may be confounded by changes in body proportions over time.

Indications for lower limb orthoses are provided in Box 25-3. Specifications and their effect on gait are outlined in Box 25-4. Indications for gait training include when a child is first learning to walk; when there is potential for progression to a new type of orthosis or upper limb aid; for progression to a more efficient gait pattern (e.g., from a four-point to a two-point alternative gait);

when there is potential for improving gait (e.g., crouched gait pattern, excessive foot progression angle); to improve safety and confidence with advanced walking activities (e.g., walking on inclines, rough terrain, steps; learning to fall safely and stand up independently from floor; carrying and lifting objects); and to improve the efficiency and safety of gait, transfers, and intervention of aids.

Strength of the quadriceps muscles has been suggested by some authors to be the best predictor of ambulatory potential in children with MM (Schopler & Menelaus, 1987; Williams et al., 1983); others indicate that iliopsoas muscle strength is better (McDonald et al., 1991a). McDonald and associates (1991a) examined the relationship between the patterns of strength and mobility in 291 children with MM who had received at least three serial standardized strength examinations after age 5 and who were classified for their mobility status as community ambulators, partial (household) ambulators, and nonambulators. Iliopsoas muscle strength was found to be the best predictor of ambulation. The quadriceps, anterior tibialis, and gluteal muscles also were determined to have significant importance for ambulation in these children. Grade 0 to 3 iliopsoas strength was always associated with partial or complete reliance on a wheelchair. Patients with grade 4 to 5 iliopsoas and quadriceps muscle strength were almost all community ambulators, and no members of this group were completely wheelchair dependent. Children with grade 4 to 5 gluteal and anterior tibialis muscle strength were all classified as community ambulators and did not require the use of an assistive device or orthosis.

Key muscle groups for community ambulation, listed in order of importance, are the iliopsoas, gluteus medius and maximus, quadriceps, anterior tibialis, and hamstring muscles (McDonald et al., 1991a). Specific strength of these muscles accounted for 86% of the variance in mobility status. Gluteus medius muscle strength was found to be the best predictor of requirements for aids or orthoses. In individuals with gluteus medius strength grade 2 to 3, 72.2% required aids, orthoses, or both. If activity in this muscle was absent or trace, 95.7% required aids, orthoses, or both. In contrast, if gluteus medius strength was grade 4 to 5, only 11.2% required aids, orthoses, or both. Mazur and Menelaus (1991) reported that 98% of all individuals with quadriceps strength of grade 4 to 5 were at least household ambulators, with 82% being community ambulators. In contrast, for individuals with quadriceps strength of grade 3 or less, 88% were exclusive wheelchair users.

Agre and associates (1987) reported that maximum walking velocity was correlated with hip and knee extensor muscle strength. They compared the energy expenditure and efficiency of ambulation in children with MM versus able-bodied peers and found that children with

Box 25-3 Indicators for Lower Limb Orthoses

FOOT ORTHOSES AND SUPRAMALLEOLAR ORTHOSES

Advantages
Permits full active dorsiflexion and plantar flexion.
Maintains the subtalar joint in neutral alignment.
Provides medial and lateral ankle stability.

Motor function
S1 to "no loss."
Must have adequate toe clearance and sufficient gastrocnemius/soleus strength to provide adequate push-off and decelerate forward movement of tibia.

Indications
Unequal weight distribution, resulting in skin breakdown, foot deformities, or abnormal shoe wear.
Medial and lateral ankle instability, resulting in balance problems, especially difficulty traversing uneven terrain.
Poor alignment of the subtalar joint, forefoot, or rearfoot.

ANKLE-FOOT ORTHOSES (STANDARD AFOS AND GROUND-REACTION FORCE AFOS)

Advantages
In general, the ground-reaction force (see Fig. 23-5) is advantageous for this population. The proximal trim line can be extended medially to control genu valgus. The ground-reaction force AFO also facilitates push-off and knee extension during the stance phase and improves static standing balance. The ground-reaction force AFO has a patellar tendon-bearing design. This design distributes pressure across a broad area, preventing skin breakdown and lower leg deformities, which are common when traditional AFO anterior straps have been worn for an extended period of time. If traditional AFOs are used in this population, the anterior straps must be well padded.

Motor function
L4 to S1
Weak or absent ankle musculature
Knee extensors at least grade 4

Indications
Medial and lateral instability of knee or ankle
Insufficient knee extension moment (ground-reaction force AFO)
Lack of or ineffective push-off
Inadequate toe clearance
Crouched gait pattern

KNEE-ANKLE-FOOT ORTHOSES

Advantages
If unable to maintain upright posture because of joint contractures or muscle weakness, or if the knee joints are unstable, KAFOs are indicated.

If the knee joint is primarily required for medial and lateral stability so the knee joint is unlocked, or if there is potential to progress to ambulation with the knee joints unlocked, it is best to incorporate the ground-reaction force AFO component into the KAFO design to provide the advantages listed earlier in the AFO section.

Motor function
L3 to L4
Weak knee musculature
Absent ankle musculature

Indications
Medial and lateral instability of knee
Weak quadriceps (grade 4– or less)

RECIPROCATING GAIT ORTHOSES OR HIP-KNEE-ANKLE-FOOT ORTHOSES

Advantages
The reciprocating gait orthosis (RGO) cable system facilitates hip extension during stance phase and hip flexion during swing phase by coupling flexion of one hip with extension of the opposite hip.
Release of both cables permits hip flexion when sitting.
The RGO reduces the energy required for ambulation compared with walking with traditional KAFOs.

Motor function
L1 to L3 (some centers also advocate for thoracic level).
Weak hip flexion is required to effectively operate the cables.

Indications
Unable to maintain an upright posture with the hip joints extended.
RGO is indicated to facilitate hip extension and swing phase.

THORACIC-HIP-KNEE-ANKLE-FOOT ORTHOSES, PARAPODIUMS, OR VERLOS

Advantages
Upright positioning for high-level lesions
Generally for exercise walking only

Motor function
Thoracic to L2. Walking is usually nonfunctional for these high-level lesions because of the high energy expenditure required and the slow, cumbersome walking pace.

Indications
Limited distance mobility
Upright positioning
"Exercise" walking

Box 25-4   Lower Limb Orthotic Specifications, Objectives, and Examination Criteria

ORTHOTIC SPECIFICATIONS

Shoe heel height

A low heel ($1/4$ to $1/2$ inch) may improve balance by shifting the center of gravity forward in a person with a calcaneal weight-bearing position.

A low heel ($1/4$ to $1/2$ inch) may decrease knee hyperextension by shifting the center of gravity forward.

A high heel shifts the center of gravity too far forward and causes balance problems in a person with weak plantar flexors.

A high heel may result in increased hip and knee flexion, combined with an increased lordosis or swayback posture.

Ankle angle

Ideally molded or set in 5° *plantar flexion* with a rigid anterior and posterior stop to reduce energy requirements and to increase the knee extension moment (Lehmann et al., 1985), as long as toe clearance is adequate and the knee does not hyperextend. If foot clearance is a problem, set angle more acutely, no higher than neutral, at the minimum angle required to clear the foot during swing phase. Plastic orthoses must enclose the malleoli to effectively resist dorsiflexion and provide a rigid anterior stop (Lehmann et al., 1983).

Do not set ankle angle more acutely than a neutral angle unless trying to control a knee hyperextension problem, because the energy expenditure will increase.

Keel

Generally, keel should be rigid to the distal aspect of the metatarsal heads (to decrease energy expenditure by providing a longer lever). The plastic should extend to the end of the toes to maintain proper toe alignment, but it must be pulled thin distal to the metatarsal heads to provide a flexible toe break. If a flexible toe break is not provided, the knee extension moment may be excessive, resulting in knee hyperextension. The alternative is to trim the plastic at the metatarsal heads, but the toes are not adequately supported in this latter case.

Extending a rigid keel out to the end of the toes may be indicated to increase the extension moment at the knee. Do not extend the rigid lever arm to the end of the toes if it results in knee hyperextension or difficulty with balance (especially on stairs).

Plantar aspect

Posting may be required to accommodate the hindfoot and rearfoot position so that the subtalar joint is maintained in a neutral position, yet a plantigrade position is achieved (Weber & Agro, 1990).

Posting helps distribute the weight across the plantar aspect and prevents varus or valgus.

Straps

All straps should be well padded.

An instep strap angled at 45° helps hold the heel in place and prevents pistoning and friction.

KAFOs should have a three-point pressure distribution.

A combined suprapatellar and infrapatellar strap distributes the pressure best. A spider knee cap pad can also be used but results in greater shear forces through the knee joint.

An infrapatellar strap often deforms the lower leg when worn for a prolonged period of time because the pressure is not well distributed. The patellar tendon-bearing orthotic trim line is preferred in this population because the pressure is better distributed.

ORTHOTIC FABRICATION OBJECTIVES

Increase medial and lateral stability

Mold in subtalar neutral position (Knutson & Clark, 1991; Weber & Agro, 1990).

Proximal trim line should be sufficiently proximal and anterior to provide adequate leverage to control the ankle and to distribute pressure evenly.

Increase base of support and equalize weight-bearing forces by means of external posting.

Valgus or pronated foot

Post medially under first metatarsal head and medial aspect of calcaneus.

Flare posting medially to increase the base of support and to prevent deviation into valgus.

Varus or supinated foot

Post medially under first metatarsal head to accommodate supinated position of forefoot and equalize pressure distribution.

Zero posting under calcaneus (with lateral flare if needed) to prevent deviation into supination at heel strike.

Orthoses must sit level in shoes, and the shoes should be fastened securely so they do not slide on orthoses.

continued

Box 25-4 **Lower Limb Orthotic Specifications, Objectives, and Examination Criteria—con't**

Decrease energy expenditure

Ankle angle ideally molded or set at 5° plantar flexion with rigid anterior stop (see ankle angle, earlier)

Distal trim line at metatarsal heads to provide a long rigid lever arm

Provide adequate toe clearance and simulate push-off

Plantar flexion stop, ideally set at 5° of plantar flexion if able to adequately clear toe without increasing knee flexion during swing phase (see ankle angle, earlier).

Generally a rigid dorsiflexion stop is required, unless the patient has sufficient plantar flexor strength to control forward movement of tibia during stance phase.

Increase knee extension moment

Ground-reaction force, patellar tendon-bearing orthosis

Solid ankle, cushioned heel, or wedge heel anteriorly to move ground-reaction force forward at heel strike

Rigid dorsiflexion stop set in 5° plantar flexion (see ankle angle, earlier)

Keel rigid to distal aspect of metatarsal heads to provide a long rigid lever and yet still permit a flexible toe break (see keel, earlier). An even greater extension moment can be provided by extending the rigid lever to the end of the toes. This is usually contraindicated, however, because it results in difficulties with balance (especially on stairs).

Prevent knee hyperextension

Prevent knee hyperextension by increasing knee flexion moment.

Flare heel posteriorly to move ground-reaction force behind knee joint axis at heel strike to produce a flexion moment.

Ankle set at neutral angle with rigid dorsiflexion and plantar flexion stop (if this does not adequately prevent knee hyperextension, the angle may need to be set more acutely, into dorsiflexion). The more acute the angle, however, the greater the energy expenditure (Lehmann et al., 1985).

A low heel (1/4 to 1/2 inch) may decrease knee hyperextension by shifting the center of gravity forward.

Keel rigid to the distal aspect of the metatarsal heads to provide a long rigid lever to decrease energy expenditure. Plastic must be pulled thin beyond

this point, however, to provide a flexible toe break (do not extend the rigid keel to the end of the toes because this will increase the knee extension moment at push-off).

If knee hyperextension cannot be adequately controlled with previously described modifications, use KAFOs with knee extension stops.

Improve pressure distribution

Use total contact orthoses.

All straps should be well padded.

Bony prominences should be padded (e.g., malleoli, prominent naviculi, patellar tendon region).

Posting to equalize pressure distribution on foot and minimize pressure on malleoli and naviculi.

Patellar tendon-bearing orthosis distributes pressure better than a proximal strap.

KAFOs: the combination of a suprapatellar and infrapatellar strap distributes pressure most effectively.

Improve balance

Adding a low heel (1/4 to 1/2 inch) may improve balance by shifting the center of gravity forward in a person with a calcaneal weight-bearing position.

A high heel shifts the center of gravity too far forward and causes balance problems, particularly in a person with weak or absent plantar flexors.

ORTHOTIC EXAMINATION CRITERIA

Check for pressure areas.

Heel must seat well in orthosis.

Check for rigid keel and flexible toe break.

Check knee alignment and congruency of knee joint axis.

All straps and bony prominences should be well padded.

Check medial and lateral alignment and make sure the orthosis is posted properly with subtalar joint in neutral.

Check angle at ankle (anterior/posterior and medial/lateral).

Check anterior and posterior stops to make sure they adequately control motion, facilitate push-off, and permit toe clearance during swing phase.

Insert orthosis in shoe to check alignment. If molded properly, the orthosis should be able to balance and stand without support on a flat surface.

MM used almost twice as much energy when walking and had a 41% lower ambulation velocity. They also reported that mobility in a wheelchair was considerably more efficient than walking, approximating normal gait in terms of energy requirements. In addition, individuals classified as having "no loss" by means of manual muscle testing had a decreased walking velocity and increased energy expenditure compared with able-bodied peers.

Equipment

A wide variety of adaptive equipment typically is required for individuals with MM. Equipment needs vary considerably with level of lesion and age. Therapists must be aware of the available options and be able to select the most appropriate type of equipment for a given situation. In addition, it is important to educate parents and patients regarding the fit and appropriateness of adaptive equipment so that they can be knowledgeable consumers. It is beyond the scope of this chapter to discuss specific equipment items. See Baker and Rogosky-Grassi (1992), Knutson and Clark (1991), and Pomatto (1991) for further information regarding adaptive equipment and orthoses for this population. In the following section the focus is on factors to consider when evaluating the appropriateness and fit of adaptive equipment. Indications for lower limb orthotics are provided in Box 25-3. Design specifications, objectives, and considerations when evaluating the components and fit of orthoses are included in Box 25-4.

Examinations of adaptive equipment and orthotics should be conducted on at least a yearly basis. Examinations should occur more often during periods of rapid growth; when environmental demands change (e.g., changing school or work settings); when there are changes in lifestyle, goals, or vocation; or when there is a change in status that may affect motor control or mobility.

▋ SUMMARY

Few populations challenge the skill and knowledge domains of the physical therapist as extensively as individuals with MM. The previous discussion has highlighted the multitude and complexity of problems encountered by children and adolescents with MM. Each lesion level group has general functional expectations that help direct physical therapy goals from an early age. Although MM is a congenital-onset problem requiring intervention by the physical therapist during infancy and childhood, most of the impairments and functional deficits described in this chapter occur throughout the life span. Individuals with MM should be followed on a regular basis, even as adults, in multidisciplinary specialty clinics by care providers familiar with this population. Because the physical therapist has extended contact with these individuals from infancy through adolescence, the therapist plays an important role in screening and triaging for potential problems, in addition to more traditional physical therapy roles. The challenges and rewards of working with this population are therefore extraordinary. The following case studies illustrate the principles of examination and intervention discussed in this chapter.

CASE STUDIES

SALLY

History

Sally is a 6-year-old girl with L4 level paraplegia resulting from a myelomeningocele. She was referred for physical therapy assessment to determine if her ambulation skills could be improved. She had a ventriculoperitoneal CSF shunt placed as an infant with one revision secondary to shunt infection. According to her mother Sally performs fine motor activities slowly. She is social, happy, and self-confident, however, and makes friends easily.

At 7 months Sally rolled from prone to supine position but could not sit independently. At 15 months she commando crawled and was able to get into quadruped position. She pulled to stand and had a modified quadruped crawl with little lower limb reciprocation at 2 years of age. She did not have an effective method of mobility until 3.5 years of age when she was able to walk with AFOs and a wheeled anterior-facing walker. By 4 years of age, her gait with AFOs and the walker was crouched with little reciprocation and a wheelchair was her primary method of mobility. Her walking improved by switching to use of long leg braces (knees locked) at age 4.5 years, and she began to walk with forearm crutches and KAFOs at age 5 years.

Systems Review

Sally has frequent urinary tract infections that often cause her to miss school. Sally's mother performs intermittent catheterization every 4 hours, except when Sally is at school.

Tests and Measures

ROM was within functional limits except for bilateral 15° hip flexion contractures and 20° knee flexion contractures. Her forefeet and hindfeet had a varus inclination when examined in a non-weight-bearing position with her subtalar joint positioned in neutral. This resulted in a valgus, everted position of her feet when bearing weight.

Motor level was L4 with weak quadriceps muscle strength (grade 4–), particularly in the shortened part of the range (from 40° to 20° of active knee extension), and grade 3+ hamstring muscle strength. Weakness in the terminal knee extension range had not been noted previously but was consistent with her history of knee flexion contractures and crouched gait. No volitional activity was present in the gluteal muscles or distal to the knee. Minimal spasticity was present in the hip adductor and hamstring muscles. Sensory level was intact through L3 but absent below this level.

Sally propelled independently in a lightweight wheelchair on level surfaces and on gradual inclines. She was independent for all transfers except to and from the floor because she was unable to independently operate the knee locks on her KAFOs. She walked with locked KAFOs and forearm crutches using a four-point gait pattern and was independent on level surfaces and gradual inclines. She had difficulty traversing uneven terrain and more severe inclines. When she attempted to walk without upper limb support, she had a severe gluteal lurch with lateral trunk sway and lost her balance after a few steps. She was a short-distance community ambulator (primarily walked at home and school and used a wheelchair for long distances). When bearing weight without orthoses or with the knees of her KAFOs unlocked, her hips and knees were severely flexed and her feet were dorsiflexed, everted, and pronated.

Her KAFOs were set in 5° of dorsiflexion and were aligned in valgus at the subtalar joint. The KAFO knee joint axis was not congruent with her anatomic knee joint axis. Only a narrow, infrapatellar anterior knee strap was present, and there was no padding on any of the KAFO straps. She was unable to independently manipulate the knee locks because of her knee flexion contractures. She had pressure marks from the infrapatellar straps and decubiti on her heels.

Evaluation

At the time of her initial assessment, Sally's orthoses did not fit properly and were causing pressure sores. Her parents requested that she progress to AFOs, if possible, so that she could be more independent with transfers. Her hip and knee flexion contractures prevented her from achieving the stable upright stance required for efficient ambulation with AFOs. Her weakness in terminal knee extension, in conjunction with the contractures, presented further difficulties for maintaining upright posture and ambulating with AFOs. Because this weakness had not been noted previously, and she exhibited mild lower limb spasticity, it was important to serially monitor her strength and muscle tone over the next several months to determine if she was experiencing progressive neurologic loss.

Despite the problems, in Sally's favor were the volitional quadriceps and hamstring muscle function present, a supportive family, and her personality with a willingness to try new and difficult tasks. Hip and knee flexion contracture reduction and healing of the heel decubitus ulcers were initial steps that had to be completed before AFOs could be fabricated. The unavailability of physical therapy at school provided an additional challenge. Her father worked full time and her mother had four other children to care for in addition to Sally, so frequent outpatient physical therapy sessions were not a practical alternative. Discontinuance of the improperly fitting KAFOs and good wound care healed the decubitus ulcers. In the meantime, an aggressive program of stretching and strengthening was implemented.

Direct Interventions

An initial physical therapy session consisting of soft tissue mobilization followed by passive stretching resulted in 10° reductions in the hip and knee contractures. Sally's mother was instructed by the therapist in techniques for stretching the hip and knee flexors, which Sally performed daily. Strengthening exercises for the quadriceps and hamstring muscles were also implemented, including short arc quads, straight leg raises, knee flexion, and squat-to-stand exercises. Sally was seen biweekly by the therapist for reexamination and progression of her program. After 2 weeks of therapy, she continued to have difficulty with terminal knee extension and initiation of knee flexion. A home program of functional electrical stimulation was implemented to enhance volitional contractions of the quadriceps and hamstring muscles and to assist with muscle reeducation (Karmel-Ross et al., 1992). Strengthening exercises augmented with functional electrical stimulation resulted in significant increases in strength.

After 2 months of intervention, Sally had only 5° hip flexion contractures and her knees could fully extend. Quadriceps and hamstring muscle strength were grades 4 and 4–, respectively. Her decubiti were fully healed and she was anxious to resume bipedal ambulation. She could stand and walk short distances with her knees and hips extended when she used a reverse-facing walker and concentrated on walking with an upright posture. She fatigued and was distracted easily, however, and still required support at the knees for community distances. The long-term goal remained progression to independent ambulation using AFOs and forearm crutches. Ground-reaction force AFOs (see Fig. 25-5) would most likely be the optimal design for advancing her to ambulation with AFOs, for the reasons outlined in Box 25-3. KAFOs were still currently indicated, however, to maintain an upright posture for community distances. If she regressed to a crouch gait pattern, contractures and stretch weakness could recur. After consultation with the orthotist, new KAFOs were fabricated that incorporated a ground-reaction force AFO component, along with removable metal knee joints, uprights, and thigh cuff sections. These orthoses enabled Sally to practice upright walking using a posture-control walker at home, with the knee joints either locked or unlocked. In therapy sessions, and under her mother's supervision, the thigh and knee components could be removed so that she could practice walking with the ground-reaction force AFOs.

Orthotic specifications included those listed in Box 25-4 for increasing medial and lateral stability, enhancing the knee extension moment, decreasing energy expenditure, providing adequate toe clearance, simulating push-off, distributing pressure evenly, and improving balance. The orthotist molded the feet in subtalar neutral, and the footplates of the AFOs were posted to accommodate forefoot and hindfoot varus and forefoot supination. The posting provided a wider base of plantigrade support to improve balance and prevented her feet from rolling over into pronation when weight bearing, thus maintaining good biomechanical alignment of the ankles and knees. The ankles were set in 5° of plantar flexion, providing an extensor moment at the knees to encourage more upright stance and gait.

Strengthening exercises and functional electrical stimulation were continued. Gait training began at home and in therapy sessions, initially using a posture-control walker and then progressing to forearm crutches. Gait training emphasized an upright posture and terminal knee extension with the KAFO knee joints unlocked and removed. Functional electrical stimulation was used in conjunction with gait training for muscle reeducation (Kieklak & DeVahl, 1986; Packman & Ewaski, 1983). Videotaping of her gait pattern was used throughout the intervention process to provide visual feedback. Sally quickly progressed to ambulation with forearm crutches with the knee joints unlocked. Strength continued to increase; after 3 months of strengthening and gait training, quadriceps and hamstring muscle strength were grades 4+ and 4, respectively, and she was able to walk with ground-reaction force AFOs and forearm crutches for short community distances using a four-point gait pattern. She continued to use a wheelchair for long distances.

Progression to a more efficient two-point gait was then emphasized. She mastered the two-point gait pattern following another month of gait training. Strengthening exercises and stretching have continued prophylactically three times a week. Her mother understood that it was essential to avoid regression to a crouched gait pattern and continued to monitor her ROM and posture closely, especially during periods of rapid growth. Sally continues to ambulate independently for short community distances with ground-reaction force AFOs and forearm crutches and uses a wheelchair for longer distances. She also has mastered wheelchair-to-floor transfers.

Sally was referred by the physical therapist for evaluation by a urologist because of her recurrent urinary tract infections. This physician started her on a daily suppressive dose of antibiotic medication and referred her to a nurse to learn self-catheterization. Owing to Sally's upper limb dyscoordination, it took her several months to master this skill, but the ability to catheterize herself, especially during school hours so that she no longer went 7 hours between catheterizations from before to after school, resulted in resolution of the recurrent infections.

Prognosis

It will be important to continue to teach Sally advanced wheelchair skills, including ramps and curbs, so that she is independent with the chair in the community; like many individuals with L4 level function, Sally will most likely continue to use the chair for long-distance community mobility as an adolescent and adult. Fortunately, neither Sally's lower limb weakness nor her spasticity progressed to suggest the presence of tethered cord syndrome, but monitoring should continue at least annually throughout her life.

MEGAN

History

Megan is a 6-year-old girl with S1-S2 level paraplegia resulting from a myelomeningocele. She receives physical and occupational therapy through the public schools. She has both ventriculoperitoneal and spinal CSF shunts, which have required multiple revisions. She has also had ophthamologic surgery for strabismus and three decompressions for Arnold-Chiari malformation. She is very happy, social, self-confident, and makes friends with peers easily, but she prefers to interact with adults.

Megan rolled from prone to supine at 5 months of age and from supine to prone at 7 months. She sat independently at 12 months and crawled on level surfaces and stairs at 18 months. She pulled to stand at 2 years of age and began cruising and walking with a walker using AFOs at 2.5 years of age. Megan's fine motor skills are delayed, which affects her personal care, dressing, and handwriting activities.

Systems Review

Megan has frequent urinary tract infections that are treated with Ditropan. She is catheterized three times a day and is independent with self-catheterization at school. She has no history of skin breakdown or cardiopulmonary complications.

Tests and Measures

Current examination results for Megan at 6 years of age are summarized here. ROM and muscle extensibility were within functional limits. Her forefeet and hindfeet had a varus inclination when examined in a non-weight-bearing position with her subtalar joint positioned in neutral. This resulted in a valgus, everted position of her feet when bearing weight.

Megan's motor level was determined to be S1 on the left and S2 on the right with hip extensors, adductors, and abductors grade 4– on the left and grade 4 on the right; knee extensors were grade 5 bilaterally, and knee flexors, ankle dorsiflexors, invertors, evertors, toe flexors and extensors were grade 4 on the left and grade 5 on the right; and ankle plantar flexors were grade 2 on the left and grade 3 on the right (on a 5 point MMT scale). Sensation was intact through S2.

Megan walked using supramalleolar AFOs with a crouch gait pattern and bilateral gluteal lurch combined with lateral trunk sway. She was independent on level surfaces and gradual inclines. She had difficulty traversing uneven terrain and steeper inclines. She was a short-distance community ambulator with limited endurance. She walked at home and school for distances up to 300 feet and was carried or pushed in a grocery cart for longer distances. The maximum distance she had ever been able to walk with her supramalleolar AFOs was approximately $\frac{1}{4}$ mile with one hand held, according to her mother. She was beginning to learn to use a tricycle.

Evaluation

Although her supramalleolar AFOs maintained her foot alignment and subtalar joint in neutral in the frontal plane, the strength of her plantar flexors was not sufficient to control advancement of the tibia during the stance phase of gait, resulting in a crouch gait posture.

Direct Interventions

The physical therapist determined that ground-reaction force AFOs (see Fig. 25-5) would improve her crouch gait pattern for the reasons outlined in Box 25-3. Orthotic specifications included those listed in Box 25-4 for increasing medial and lateral stability, enhancing the knee extension moment, decreasing energy expenditure, providing adequate toe clearance, simulating push-off, distributing pressure evenly, and improving balance. The orthotist molded the feet in subtalar neutral, and the footplates of the AFOs were posted to accommodate forefoot and hindfoot varus and forefoot supination. The posting provided a wider base of plantigrade support to improve balance and prevented her feet from rolling over into pronation when weight bearing, thus maintaining good biomechanical alignment of the ankles and knees. The ankles were set in 5° of plantar flexion, providing an extensor moment at the knees to encourage more upright stance and gait. Gait training began at home and in therapy sessions, using a posture-control walker for balance in combination with walking independently. Gait training emphasized an upright posture, symmetric steps, and reciprocal arm swing. The improvement in Megan's posture and endurance was immediately apparent with the ground reaction AFOs. Her posture was significantly more upright with hip and knee extension. The first weekend that Megan had her new orthoses, she hiked 1.5 miles on uneven terrain with one hand held, only requiring three short rest periods. Megan continues to ambulate independently for short distances in the community with ground-reaction force AFOs.

Prognosis

It will be important to continue lower extremity strengthening exercises and to progress Megan to be independent with community ambulation, including inclines, uneven terrain, and curbs. It will also be important to encourage alternative means of long distance mobility such as bike riding. Her parents understand that it is essential to avoid regression to a crouched gait pattern and continue to monitor her ROM and posture closely, especially during periods of rapid growth. Monitoring her strength should continue at least annually throughout her life, ideally using objective methods of strength assessment.

▌ REFERENCES

Agre, JC, Findley, TW, McNally, MC, Habeck, R, Leon, AS, Stradel, L, Birkebak, R, & Schmalz, R. Physical activity capacity in children with myelomeningocele. Archives of Physical Medicine and Rehabilitation, 68:372–377, 1987.

Aitkens, S, Lord, J, Bernauer, E, Fowler, W, Lieberman, J, & Berck, P. Relationship of manual muscle testing to objective strength measurements. Muscle and Nerve, 12:173–177, 1989.

Andersen, EM, & Plewis, I. Impairment of motor skill in children with spina bifida cystica and hydrocephalus: An exploratory study. British Journal of Psychology, 68:61–70, 1977.

Andersson, C, & Mattsson, E. Adults with cerebral palsy: A survey describing problems, needs, and resources, with special emphasis on locomotion. Developmental Medicine & Child Neurology, 43:76–82, 2001.

Asher, M, & Olson, J. Factors affecting the ambulatory status of patients with spina bifida cystica. Journal of Bone and Joint Surgery (American), 65:350–356, 1983.

Babcook, CJ. Ultrasound evaluation of prenatal and neonatal spina bifida. Neurosurgery Clinics of North America, 6:203–218, 1995.

Baker, SB, & Rogosky-Grassi, MA. Access to the school. In Rowley-Kelly, FL, & Reigel, DH (Eds.). Teaching the Student with Spina Bifida. Baltimore: Paul H. Brookes, 1992, pp. 31–70.

Bannister, CM. The case for and against intrauterine surgery for myelomeningocele. European Journal of Obstetrics, Gynecology & Reproductive Biology, 92:109–113, 2000.

Banta, J, & Hamada, J. Natural history of the kyphotic deformity in myelomeningocele. Journal of Bone and Joint Surgery, 58A:279, 1976.

Banta, JV. Bracing for ambulation: Basic principles, brace alternatives by motor level and predictive long-term goals. In Matsumoto, S, & Sato, H (Eds.). Spina Bifida. New York: Springer Verlag, 1999, pp. 307–311.

Bar-Or, O. Pathophysiological factors which limit the exercise capacity of the sick child. Medicine and Science in Sports and Exercise, 18:276–282, 1986.

Bartlett, MD, Wolf, LS, Shurtleff, DB, & Staheli, LT. Hip flexion contractures: A comparison of measurement methods. Archives of Physical Medicine and Rehabilitation, 66:620–625, 1985.

Becker, RD. Recent developments in child psychiatry: I. The restrictive emotional and cognitive environment reconsidered: A redefinition of the concept of therapeutic restraint. Israeli Journal of Psychiatry and Related Sciences, 12:239–258, 1975.

Berry, RJ, Li, Z, Erickson, JD, et al. Prevention of neural-tube defects with folic acid in China. New England Journal of Medicine 341:1485–1491, 1999.

Birth Defects and Genetic Diseases Branch of Birth Defects and Developmental Disabilities Office, National Center for Environmental Disease and Injury. Use of folic acid prevention of spina bifida and other neural tube defects, 1983–1991. Morbidity and Mortality Weekly Report, 40:1–4, 1991.

Bleck, EE, & Nagel, DA. Physically Handicapped Children-A Medical Atlas for Teachers. Orlando, FL: Grune & Stratton, 1982.

Blum, RW, Resnick, MD, Nelson R, & St. Germain, A. Family and peer issues among adolescents with spina bifida and cerebral palsy. Pediatrics, 88:280–285, 1991.

Bohannon, RW. Manual muscle test scores and dynamometer test scores of knee extension strength. Archives of Physical Medicine and Rehabilitation, 67:390–392, 1986.

Brazelton, TB. Touchpoints: Your Child's Emotional and Behavioral Development. Reading, MA: Perseus Book, 1992.

Brinker, M, Rosenfeld, S, Feiwell, E, Granger, S, Mitchell, D, & Rice, J. Myelomeningocele at the sacral level: Long-term outcomes in adults. Journal of Bone and Joint Surgery, 76A:1293–1300, 1994.

Broughton, NS, Graham, G, & Menelaus, MB. The high incidence of foot deformity in patients with high-level spina bifida. Journal of Bone and Joint Surgery, 76B:548–550, 1994.

Brown, JP. Orthopedic care of children with spina bifida: You've come a long way, baby! Orthopaedic Nursing, 20:51–58, 2001.

Brunt, D. Characteristics of upper limb movements in a sample of meningomyelocele children. Perceptual Motor Skills, 51:431–437, 1980.

Butler, C, Okamoto, GA, & McKay, TM. Motorized wheelchair driving by disabled children. Archives of Physical Medicine and Rehabilitation, 65:95–97, 1984.

Chaffin, DB, Andersson, GBJ, & Martin, BJ. Occupational Biomechanics, 3rd ed. New York: John Wiley & Sons, 1999.

Chandler, LS, Andrews, MS, & Swanson, MW. Movement Assessment of Infants: A Manual. Rolling Bay, WA: Authors, 1980.

CIBA. CIBA Symposium No. 191: Neural Tube Defects. London: CIBA Foundation, 1994.

Culatta, B, & Young, C. Linguistic performance as a function of abstract task demands in children with spina bifida. Developmental Medicine and Child Neurology, 34(5):434–440, 1992.

Cusick, BD, & Stuberg, WA. Assessment of lower extremity alignment in the transverse plane: Implications for management of children with neuromotor dysfunction. Physical Therapy, 72:3–15, 1992.

Czeizel, AE, & Dudas, I. Prevention of first occurrence of neural tube defects by periconceptual vitamin supplementation. New England Journal of Medicine, 327:131–137, 1992.

Deitz, JC, Jaffe, KM, Wolf, LS, Massagli, TL, & Anson, DK. Pediatric power wheelchairs: Evaluation of function in the home and school environments. Assistive Technology, 3:24–31, 1991.

Del Gado, R, Del Gaizo, D, Brescia, D, Polidori, G, & Tamburro, A. Obesity and overweight in a group of patients with myelomeningocele. In Matsumoto, S, & Sato, H (Eds.). Spina Bifida. New York: Springer Verlag, 1999, pp. 474–475.

DeSouza, L, & Carroll, N. Ambulation of the braced myelomeningocele patient. Journal of Bone and Joint Surgery (American), 58:1112–1118, 1976.

De Villarreal, LM, Perez, JZ, Vasquez, PA, Herrera, RH, Campos, M del R, Lopez, RA, Ramirez, JM, et al. Decline of neural tube defects after a folic acid campaign in Neuvo Leon, Mexico. Teratology, 66:249–256, 2002.

Dias, L. Management of ankle and hindfoot valgus in spina bifida. In Matsumoto, S, & Sato, H (Eds.). Spina Bifida. New York: Springer Verlag, 1999a, pp. 374–377.

Dias, L. The management of hip pathology in spina bifida. In Matsumoto, S & Sato, H (Eds.). Spina Bifida. New York: Springer Verlag, 1999b, pp. 321–322.

Diaz Llopis, I, Bea Munoz, M, Martinez Agullo, E, Lopez Martinez, A, Garcia Aymerich, V, & Forner Valero, JV. Ambulation in patients with myelomeningocele: A study of 1500 patients. Paraplegia, 31:28–32, 1993.

Dise, JE, Lohr, ME. Examination of deficits in conceptual reasoning abilities associated with spina bifida. American Journal of Physical Medicine and Rehabilitation, 77:247–251, 1998.

Dudgeon, BJ, Jaffe, KM, & Shurtleff, DB. Variations in midlumbar myelomeningocele: Implications for ambulation. Pediatric Physical Therapy, 3:57–62, 1991.

Eastlack, ME, Arvidson, J, Snyder-Mackler, L, Danoff, JV, & McGarvey, CL. Interrater reliability of videotaped observational gait-analysis assessments. Physical Therapy, 71:465–472, 1991.

Effgen, SK, & Brown, DA. Long-term stability of hand-held dynamometric measurements in children who have myelomeningocele. Physical Therapy, 72:458–465, 1992.

Elwood, JM, & Elwood, JH. Epidemiology of Anencephalus and Spina Bifida. Cambridge: Oxford University Press, 1980.

Embrey, D, Endicott, J, Glenn, T, & Jaeger, DL. Developing better postural tone in grade school children. Clinical Management in Physical Therapy, 3:6–10, 1983.

Fay, G, Shurtleff, DB, Shurtleff, H, & Wolf, L. Approaches to facilitate independent self-care and academic success. In Shurtleff, DB (Ed.). Myelodysplasias and Exstrophies: Significance, Prevention, and Treatment. Orlando, FL: Grune & Stratton, 1986, pp. 373–398.

Fife, SE, Roxborough, LA, Armstrong, RW, Harris, SR, Gregson, JL, & Field, D. Development of a clinical measure of postural control for assessment of adaptive seating in children with neuromotor disabilities. Physical Therapy, 71:981–993, 1991.

Finnie, NR. Handling the Young Cerebral Palsied Child at Home, 2nd ed. New York: EP Dutton, 1975.

Florence, JM, Pandya, S, King, W, Schierbecker, J, Robison, JD, Signore, LC, Mandel, S, & Arfken, C. Strength assessment: Comparison of methods in children with Duchenne muscular dystrophy (Abstract). Physical Therapy, 68:866, 1988.

Frawley, PA, Broughton, NS, & Menelaus, MB. Incidence and type of hindfoot deformities in patients with low-level spina bifida. Journal of Pediatric Orthopedics, 18:312–313, 1998

Gadow, K. Children on Medication. San Diego: College Hill Press, 1986.

Gaston, H. Ophthalmic complications of spina bifida and hydrocephalus. Eye, 5:279–290, 1991.

Goodwyn, MA. Biomedical Psychological Factors Predicting Success with Activities of Daily Living and Academic Pursuits. Unpublished doctoral dissertation. Seattle: University of Washington, 1990.

Griebel, ML, Oakes, WJ, & Worley, G. The Chiari malformation associated with myelomeningocele. In Rekate, HL (Ed.). Comprehensive Management of Spina Bifida. Boca Raton, FL: CRC Press, 1991, pp. 67–92.

Griffin, JW, McClure, MH, & Bertorini, TE. Sequential isokinetic and manual muscle testing in patients with neuromuscular disease: Pilot study. Physical Therapy, 66:32–35, 1986.

Gucciardi, E, Pietrusiak, MA, Reynolds, DL, & Rouleau, J. Incidence of neural tube defects in Ontario, 1986-1999. Canadian Medical Association Journal 167:237–240, 2002.

Hack, SN, Norton, BJ, & Zahalak, GI. A quantitative muscle tester for clinical use (Abstract). Physical Therapy, 61:673, 1981.

Hamill, PV, Drizd, TA, Johnson, CL, Reed, RB, Roche, AF, & Moore, WM. Physical growth: National Center for Health Statistics percentiles. American Journal of Clinical Nutrition, 32:607–629, 1979.

Hinderer, KA. Reliability of the Myometer in Muscle Testing Children and Adolescents with Myelodysplasia. Unpublished master's thesis. Seattle: University of Washington, 1988.

Hinderer, KA. The Relationship Between Musculoskeletal System Capacity and Task Requirements in Simulated Crouch Standing. Doctoral dissertation. Ann Arbor, MI: University of Michigan, 2003.

Hinderer, KA, & Gutierrez, T. Myometry measurements of children using isometric and eccentric methods of muscle testing (Abstract). Physical Therapy, 68:817, 1988.

Hinderer, KA, & Hinderer, SR. Mobility and transfer efficiency of adults with myelodysplasia (Abstract). Archives of Physical Medicine and Rehabilitation, 69:712, 1988.

Hinderer, KA, & Hinderer, SR. Muscle strength development and assessment in children and adolescents. In Harms-Ringdahl, K (Ed.). International Perspectives in Physical Therapy. Vol. 8, Muscle Strength. London: Churchill Livingstone, 1993, pp. 93–140.

Hinderer, SR, & Hinderer, KA. Sensory examination of individuals with myelodysplasia (Abstract). Archives of Physical Medicine and Rehabilitation, 71:769–770, 1990.

Hinderer, SR, & Hinderer, KA. Quantitative methods of evaluation. In DeLisa, JA, & Gans, BM (Eds.). Rehabilitation Medicine: Principles and Practices, 3rd ed. Philadelphia: Lippincott-Raven, 1998, pp. 109–136.

Hinderer, SR, Hinderer, KA, Dunne, K, & Shurtleff, DB. Medical and functional status of adults with spina bifida (Abstract). Developmental Medicine and Child Neurology, 30(suppl 57):28, 1988.

Hislop, HJ, & Montgomery, J. Daniels and Worthingham's Muscle Testing, 7th ed. Philadelphia: WB Saunders, 2002.

Hosking, GP, Bhat, US, Dubowitz, V, & Edwards, RHT. Measurements of muscle strength and performance in children with normal and diseased muscle. Archives of Disease in Childhood, 51:957–963, 1976.

Hunt, GM. Open spina bifida: outcome for complete cohort treated unselectively and followed into adulthood. Developmental Medicine and Child Neurology, 32:108–118, 1990.

Hunt G, Oakeshott, P. Outcome in people with open spina bifida at age 35: Prospective community based cohort study. British Medical Journal, 326:1365–1366, 2003.

Hunt, GM, Oakeshott, P, & Kerry S. Link between the CSF shunt and achievement in adults with spina bifida. Journal of Neurology, Neurosurgery, and Psychiatry, 67:591–595, 1999.

Hurley, AD. Conducting psychological assessments. In Rowley-Kelly, FL, & Reigel, DH (Eds.). Teaching the Student with Spina Bifida. Baltimore: Paul H. Brookes, 1992, pp. 107–124.

Hyde, S, Goddard, C, & Scott, O: The myometer: The development of a clinical tool. Physiotherapy, 69:424–427, 1983.

IMSG. International Myelodysplasia Study Group Database Coordination. David B. Shurtleff, MD, Department of Pediatrics, University of Washington. Seattle, WA, 1993.

Jacobson, CB, & Berlin, CM. Possible reproductive deterrent in LSD users. Journal of the American Medical Association, 222:1367–1373, 1972.

Janda, V. Muscle Function Testing. Boston: Butterworths, 1983.

Jebsen, RH, Trieschman, RB, Mikulic, MA, Hartley, RB, McMillan, JA, & Snook, ME. Measurement of time in a standardized test of patient mobility. Archives of Physical Medicine and Rehabilitation, 51:170–175, 1970.

Karmel-Ross, K, Cooperman, DR, & Van Doren, CL. The effect of electrical stimulation on quadriceps femoris muscle torque in children with spina bifida. Physical Therapy, 72:723–731, 1992.

Karol, L, Orthopedic management in myelomeningocele. Neurosurgery Clinics of North America, 6:259–268, 1995.

Kendall, FP, McCreary, EK, & Provance, PG. Muscles: Testing and Function, 4th ed. Baltimore: Williams & Wilkins, 1999.

Kieklak, H, & DeVahl, J. Respond II: Protocol for Pediatric Applications. Minneapolis, MN: Medtronics, Inc., 1986.

Kilburn, J, Saffer, A, Barnes, L, Kling, T, & Venes, J. The Vigorimeter as an early predictor of central neurologic malformation in myelodysplastic children. Paper presented at the meeting of the American Academy for Cerebral Palsy and Developmental Medicine, Seattle, 1985.

Kimura, DK, Mayo, M, & Shurtleff, DB. Urinary tract management. In Shurtleff, DB (Ed.). Myelodysplasias and Exstrophies: Significance, Prevention, and Treatment. Orlando, FL: Grune & Stratton, 1986, pp. 243–266.

King, JC, Currie, DM, & Wright, E. Bowel training in spina bifida: Importance of education, patient compliance, age, and anal reflexes. Archives of Physical Medicine and Rehabilitation, 75:243–247, 1994.

Knutson, LM, & Clark, DE. Orthotic devices for ambulation in children with cerebral palsy and myelomeningocele. Physical Therapy, 71:947–960, 1991.

Kottorp, A, Bernspang, B, & Fisher, AG. Validity of a performance assessment of activities of daily living for people with developmental disabilities. Journal of Intellectual Disability Research, 47(8):597–605, 2003.

Krebs, DE, Edelstein, JE, & Fishman, S. Reliability of observational kinematic gait analysis. Physical Therapy, 65:1027–1033, 1985.

Lais, A, Kasabian, NG, Dryo, FM, Scott, RM, Kelly, MD, & Bauer, SB. The neurosurgical implications of continuous neurological surveillance of children with myelodysplasia. Journal of Urology, *150*:1879–1883, 1993.

Land, LC. Study of the sensory integration of children with myelomeningocele. In McLaurin, RL (Ed.). Myelomeningocele. Orlando, FL: Grune & Stratton, 1977, pp. 115–140.

Lehmann, JF, Condon, SM, de Lateur, BJ, & Price, R. Gait abnormalities in peroneal nerve paralysis and their corrections by orthoses: A biomechanical study. Archives of Physical Medicine and Rehabilitation, *67*:380–386, 1986.

Lehmann, JF, Condon, SM, de Lateur, BJ, & Smith, C. Ankle-foot orthoses: Effect on gait abnormalities in tibial nerve paralysis. Archives of Physical Medicine and Rehabilitation, *66*:212–218, 1985.

Lehmann, JF, Esselman, PC, Ko, MJ, de Lateur, BJ, & Dralle, AJ. Plastic ankle-foot orthoses: Evaluation of function. Archives of Physical Medicine and Rehabilitation, *64*:402–404, 1983.

Lemire, RJ, Loeser, JD, Leech, RW, & Alvord, ED (Eds.). Normal and Abnormal Development of the Human Nervous System. Hagerstown, MD: Harper & Row, 1975.

Level, MB. Spherical Grip Strength of Children. Unpublished master's thesis. Seattle: University of Washington, 1984.

Liptak, GS, Shurtleff, DB, Bloss, JW, Baitus-Hebert, E, & Manitta, P. Mobility aids for children with high-level myelomeningocele: Parapodium versus wheelchair. Developmental Medicine and Child Neurology, *34*:787–796, 1992.

Liu, SL, Shurtleff, DB, Ellenbogen, RG, Loeser, JD, & Kropp, R. 19 year follow up of fetal myelomeningocele brought to term. Proceedings of the 43rd Annual Meeting of the Society for Research into Hydrocephalus and Spina Bifida. European Journal of Pediatric Surgery, *9*(Suppl 1):12–14, 1999.

Logan, L, Byers-Hinkley, K, & Ciccone, CD. Anterior versus posterior walkers: A gait analysis study. Developmental Medicine and Child Neurology, *32*:1044–1048, 1990.

Lollar, D. Preventing Secondary Conditions Associated with Spina Bifida or Cerebral Palsy: Proceedings and Recommendations of a Symposium. Washington, D.C.: Spina Bifida Association of America, 1994, pp. 54–64.

Luthy, DA, Wardinsky, T, Shurtleff, DB, Hollenbach, KA, Hickok, DE, Nyberg, DA, & Benedetti, TJ. Cesarean section before the onset of labor and subsequent motor function in infants with myelomeningocele diagnosed antenatally. New England Journal of Medicine, *324*:662–666, 1991.

Lutkenhoff, M, & Oppenheimer, S. Spinabilities: A Young Person's Guide to Spina Bifida. Bethesda, MD: Woodbine House, 1997.

Main, DM, & Mennuti, MT. Neural tube defects: Issues in prenatal diagnosis and counseling. Journal of the American College of Obstetrics and Gynecology, *67*:1–16, 1986.

Masse, LC, Lamontagne, M, & O'Riain, MD. Biomedical analysis of wheelchair propulsion for various seating positions. Journal of Rehabilitation Research and Development, *29*:12–28, 1992.

Mayfield, JK. Comprehensive orthopedic management in myelomeningocele. In Rekate, HL (Ed.). Comprehensive Management of Spina Bifida. Boca Raton, FL: CRC Press, 1991, pp. 113–164.

Maynard, J, Weiner, J, & Burke, S. Neuropathic foot ulceration in patients with myelodysplastia. Journal of Pediatric Orthopedics, *12*:786–788, 1992.

Mazur, JM, & Menelaus, MB. Neurologic status of spina bifida patients and the orthopedic surgeon. Clinical Orthopaedics and Related Research, *264*:54–63, 1991.

McDonald, CM, Jaffe, KM, Mosca, VS, & Shurtleff, DB. Ambulatory outcome of children with myelomeningocele: Effect of lower-extremity muscle strength. Developmental Medicine and Child Neurology, *33*:482–490, 1991a.

McDonald, CM, Jaffe, K, & Shurtleff, DB. Assessment of muscle strength in children with meningomyelocele: Accuracy and stability of measurements over time. Archives of Physical Medicine and Rehabilitation, *67*:855–861, 1986.

McDonald, CM, Jaffe, KM, Shurtleff, DB, & Menelaus, MB. Modifications to the traditional description of neurosegmental innervation in myelomeningocele. Developmental Medicine and Child Neurology, *33*:473–481, 1991b.

McDonnell, GV, & McCann, JP. Link between the CSF shunt and achievement in adults with spina bifida. Journal of Neurology, Neurosurgery, and Psychiatry, *68*:800, 2000.

McGourty, LK. Kohlman Evaluation of Living Skills (KELS). In Hemphill, BJ (Ed.). Mental Health Assessment in Occupational Therapy. Thorofare, NJ: Black, 1988, pp. 131–146.

Mendell, JR, & Florence, J. Manual muscle testing. Muscle and Nerve, *13*(suppl):16–20, 1990.

Menelaus, MB. Orthopedic management of children with myelomeningocele: A plea for realistic goals. Developmental Medicine and Child Neurology, *18*(suppl 37):3–11, 1976.

Menelaus, MD. The hip—current treatment. In Matsumoto, S, & Sato, H (Eds.). Spina Bifida. New York: Springer Verlag, 1999, pp. 338–340.

Miller, E, & Sethi, L. The effect of hydrocephalus on perception. Developmental Medicine and Child Neurology, *13*(suppl 25):77–81, 1971.

Miller, LC, Michael, AF, Baxter, TL, & Kim, Y. Quantitative muscle testing in childhood dermatomyositis. Archives of Physical Medicine and Rehabilitation, *69*:610–613, 1988.

Mills, JL, Rhoads, GG, Simpson, JL, Cunningham, GC, Conley, MR, Lassman, MR, Walden, ME, Depp, R, & Hoffman, HJ. The absence of a relation between the periconceptual use of vitamins and neural tube defects. New England Journal of Medicine, *321*:430–435, 1989.

Milner-Brown, HS, & Miller, RG. Increased muscular fatigue in patients with neurogenic muscle weakness: Quantification and pathophysiology. Archives of Physical Medicine and Rehabilitation, *70*:361–366, 1989.

Milunsky, A, Jick, H, Jick, SS, Bruell, CL, MacLaughlin, DS, Rothman, KJ, & Willett, W. Multivitamin/folic acid supplementation in early pregnancy reduces the prevalence of neural tube defects. Journal of the American Medical Association, *262*:2847–2852, 1989.

Mintz, L, Sarwark, J, Dias, L, & Schafer, M. The natural history of congenital kyphosis in myelomeningocele. Spine, *16*(Suppl. 5):348–350, 1991.

Mobley, C, Harless, L, & Miller, K. Self perceptions of preschool children with spina bifida. Journal of Pediatric Nursing, *1*:217–224, 1996.

MRC Vitamin Study Research Group. Prevention of neural tube defects: Results of the Medical Research Council vitamin study. Lancet, *338*:131–137, 1991.

Murdoch, A. How valuable is muscle charting? A study of the relationship between neonatal assessment of muscle power and later mobility in children with spina bifida defects. Physiotherapy, *66*:221–223, 1980.

Murphy, KP, Molnar, GE, & Lankasky, K. Medical and functional status of adults with cerebral palsy. Developmental Medicine & Child Neurology. *37*:1075–1084, 1995.

Nagankatti, D, Banta, J, & Thomson, J. Charcot arthropathy in spina bifida. Journal of Pediatric Orthopedics, *20*:82–87, 2000.

Oi, S, Sato, O, & Matsumoto, S. Neurological and medico-social problems of spina bifida patients in adolescence and adulthood. Child's Nervous System, *12*:181–187, 1996.

Okamoto, GA, Lamers, JV, & Shurtleff, DB. Skin breakdown in patients with myelomeningocele. Archives of Physical Medicine and Rehabilitation, *64*:20–23, 1983.

Okamoto, GA, Sousa, J, Telzrow, RW, Holm, RA, McCartin, R, & Shurtleff, DB. Toileting skills in children with myelomeningocele: Rates of learning. Archives of Physical Medicine and Rehabilitation, 65(4):182–185, 1984.

Ounpuu, S, Davis, RB, Banta, JV, & DeLuce, PA. The effects of orthotics on gait in children with low-level myelomeningocele. Proceedings of the North American Congress on Biomechanics, Chicago, IL, 1992, pp. 323–324.

Packman, RA, & Ewaski, B. Respond II: Gait Training Protocol. Minneapolis, MN: Medtronics, 1983.

Pact, V, Sirotkin-Roses, M, & Beatus, J. The Muscle Testing Handbook. Boston: Little, Brown, 1984.

Padua, L, Rendeli, C, Rabini, A, Girardi, E, Tonali, P, & Salvaggio, E. Health-related quality of life and disability in young patients with spina bifida. Archives of Physicial Medicine and Rehabilitation, 83:1384–1388, 2002.

Patient Data Management System. Myelodysplasia Study Data Collection Criteria and Instructions, 1994.

Persad, VL, Van den Hof, MC, Dube, JM, & Zimmer, P. Incidence of open neural tube defects in Nova Scotia after folic acid fortification. Canadian Medical Association Journal, 167:241–245, 2002.

Peterson, P, Rauen, K, Brown, J, & Cole, J. Spina bifida: The transition into adulthood begins in infancy. Rehabilitation Nursing, 19:229–238, 1994.

Pomatto, RC. The use of orthotics in the treatment of myelomeningocele. In Rekate, HL (Ed.). Comprehensive Management of Spina Bifida. Boca Raton, FL: CRC Press, 1991, pp. 165–183.

Reigel, DH. Spina bifida from infancy through the school years. In Rowley-Kelly, FL, & Reigel, DH (Eds.). Teaching the Students with Spina Bifida. Baltimore: Paul H. Brookes, 1992, pp. 3–30.

Rekate, HL. Neurosurgical management of the newborn with spina bifida. In Rekate, HL (Ed.). Comprehensive Management of Spina Bifida. Boca Raton, FL: CRC Press, 1991, pp. 1–28.

Reynolds, EH. Mental effects of antiepileptic medication: A review. Epilepsia, 24(suppl 2):S85–S95, 1983.

Rose, SA, Ounpuu, S, & DeLuca, PA. Strategies for the assessment of pediatric gait in the clinical setting. Physical Therapy, 71:961–980, 1991.

Rosenstein, BD, Greene, WB, Herrington, RT, & Blum, AS. Bone density in myelomeningocele: The effects of ambulatory status and other factors. Developmental Medicine and Child Neurology, 29:486–494, 1987.

Rowley-Kelly, FL, & Kunkle, PM. Developing a school outreach program. In Rowley-Kelly, FL, & Reigel, DH (Eds.). Teaching the Student with Spina Bifida. Baltimore: Paul H. Brookes, 1992, pp. 395–436.

Ryan, KD, Pioski, C, & Emans, JB. Myelodysplasia—The musculoskeletal problem: Habilitation from infancy to adulthood. Physical Therapy, 71:935–946, 1991.

Salvaggio, E, Mauti, G, Ranieri, P, Venuti, L, Pulitano, S, Ferrara, P, & Caradonna, P. Ability in walking is a predictor of bone mineral density and body composition in prepubertal children with myelomeningocele. In Matsumoto, S, & Sato, H (Eds.). Spina Bifida. New York: Springer Verlag, 1999, pp. 298–301.

Sand, PL, Taylor, N, Rawlings, M, & Chitnis, S. Performance of children with spina bifida manifest on the Frostig Developmental Test of Visual Perception. Perceptual Motor Skills, 37:539–546, 1973.

Schafer, MF, & Dias, LS. Myelomeningocele: Orthopaedic Treatment. Baltimore: Williams & Wilkins, 1983.

Schneider, JW, Krosschell, K, & Gabriel, KL. Congenital spinal cord injury. In Umphred, DA (Ed.). Neurological Rehabilitation, 4th ed. St. Louis: Mosby, 2001, pp. 454–483.

Schopler, SA, & Menelaus, MB. Significance of strength of the quadriceps muscles in children with myelomeningocele. Journal of Pediatric Orthopaedics, 7:507–512, 1987.

Seller, MJ, & Nevin, NC. Periconceptual vitamin supplementation and the prevention of neural tube defects in south-east England and northern Ireland. Journal of Medical Genetics, 21:325–330, 1984.

Shaffer, J, Wolfe, L, Friedrich, W, Shurtleff, H, Shurtleff, D, & Fay, G. Developmental expectations: Intelligence and fine motor skills. In Shurtleff, DB (Ed.). Myelodysplasias and Exstrophies: Significance, Prevention, and Treatment. Orlando, FL: Grune & Stratton, 1986, pp. 359–372.

Shapiro, E, Kelly, KJ, Setlock, MA, Suwalski, KL, & Meyers, P. Complications of latex allergy. Dialogues in Pediatric Urology, 15:1–5, 1992.

Sherk, H. Uppal, G, Lane, G, & Melchionni, J. Treatment versus nontreatment of hip dislocations in ambulatory patients with myelomeningocele. Development Medicine & Child Neurology, 33:491–494, 1991.

Shores, M. Footprint analysis in gait documentation. Physical Therapy, 60:1163–1167, 1980.

Shurtleff, DB. Timing of learning in the myelomeningocele patient. Journal of the American Physical Therapy Association, 46(2):136–148, 1966.

Shurtleff, DB. Decubitus formation and skin breakdown. In Shurtleff, DB (Ed.). Myelodysplasias and Exstrophies: Significance, Prevention, and Treatment. Orlando, FL: Grune & Stratton, 1986a, pp. 299–312.

Shurtleff, DB. Dietary management. In Shurtleff, DB (Ed.). Myelodysplasias and Exstrophies: Significance, Prevention, and Treatment. Orlando, FL: Grune & Stratton, 1986b, pp. 285–298.

Shurtleff, DB. Health care delivery. In Shurtleff, DB (Ed.). Myelodysplasias and Exstrophies: Significance, Prevention, and Treatment. Orlando, FL: Grune & Stratton, 1986c, pp. 449–514.

Shurtleff, DB. Mobility. In Shurtleff, DB (Ed.). Myelodysplasias and Exstrophies: Significance, Prevention, and Treatment. Orlando, FL: Grune & Stratton, 1986d, pp. 313–356.

Shurtleff, DB. Selection process for the care of congenitally malformed infants. In Shurtleff, DB (Ed.). Myelodysplasias and Exstrophies: Significance, Prevention, and Treatment. Orlando, FL: Grune & Stratton, 1986e, pp. 89–116.

Shurtleff, DB. Computer data bases for pediatric disability: Clinical and research applications. In Jaffe, KM (Ed.). Physical Medicine and Rehabilitation Clinics of North America: Pediatric Rehabilitation. Philadelphia: WB Saunders, 1991, pp. 665–688.

Shurtleff, DB, Duguay, S, Duguay, G, Moskowitz, D, Weinberger, E, Roberts, T, & Loeser, J. Epidemiology of tethered cord with meningomyelocele. European Journal of Paediatric Surgery, 7(suppl 1): 7–11, 1997.

Shurtleff, DB, & Dunne, K. Adults and adolescents with myelomeningocele. In Shurtleff, DB (Ed.). Myelodysplasias and Exstrophies: Significance, Prevention, and Treatment. Orlando, FL: Grune & Stratton, 1986, pp. 433–448.

Shurtleff, DB, & Lamers, J. Clinical considerations in the treatment of myelodysplasia. In Crandal, DB, & Brazier, MAB (Eds.). Prevention of Neural Tube Defects: The Role of Alpha-Fetoprotein. New York: Academic Press, 1978, pp. 103–122.

Shurtleff, DB, Lemire, RJ, & Warkany, J: Embryology, etiology and epidemiology. In Shurtleff, DB (Ed.). Myelodysplasias and Exstrophies: Significance, Prevention, and Treatment. Orlando, FL: Grune & Stratton, 1986a, pp. 39–64.

Shurtleff, DB, Luthy, DA, Benededetti, TJ, & Mack, LA. Meningomyelocele: Management in utero and post partum. Neural tube defects. CIBA Foundation Symposium 181, 1994, pp. 270–286.

Shurtleff, DB, & Mayo, M. Toilet training: The Seattle experience and conclusions. In Shurtleff, DB (Ed.). Myelodysplasias and Exstrophies: Significance, Prevention, and Treatment. Orlando, FL: Grune & Stratton, 1986, pp. 267–284.

Shurtleff, DB, Sobkowiak, C, & Walker, W. Transition/Separation, Toilet Training and Sexuality. In Wyszynski, DF (Ed.). Neural Tube Defects: From Origin to Treatment. New York: Oxford University Press (in press).

Shurtleff, DB, Stuntz, JT, & Hayden, PW. Hydrocephalus. In Shurtleff, DB (Ed.). Myelodysplasias and Exstrophies: Significance, Prevention, and Treatment. Orlando, FL: Grune & Stratton, 1986b, pp. 139–180.

Simeonsson, RJ, Huntington, GS, McMillen, JS, Halperin, D, & Swann, D. Development factors, health, and psychosocial adjustment of children and youths with spina bifida. In Matsumoto, S, & Sato, H (Eds.). Spina Bifida. New York: Springer Verlag, 1999, pp. 543–551.

Sousa, JC, Gordon, LH, & Shurtleff, DB. Assessing the development of daily living skills in patients with spina bifida. Developmental Medicine and Child Neurology, 18(suppl 37):134–142, 1976.

Sousa, JC, Telzrow, RW, Holm, RA, McCartin, R, & Shurtleff, DB. Developmental guidelines for children with myelodysplasia. Journal of the American Physical Therapy Association, 63:21–29, 1983.

Stack, GD, & Baber, GC. The neurological involvement of the lower limbs in myelomeningocele. Developmental Medicine and Child Neurology, 9:732, 1967.

Staheli, LT. Practice of Pediatric Orthopedics. Philadelphia: Lippincott Williams & Wilkins, 2001.

Staheli, LT. Prone hip extension test: Method of measuring hip flexion deformity. Clinical Orthopedics, 123:12–15, 1977.

Stillwell, A, & Menelaus, MB. Walking ability in mature patients with spina bifida. Journal of Pediatric Orthopedics, 3:184–190, 1983.

Stuberg, WA. Considerations related to weight-bearing program in children with developmental disabilities. Physical Therapy, 72:35–40, 1992.

Stuberg, WA, & Metcalf, WK. Reliability of quantitative muscle testing in healthy children and in children with Duchenne muscular dystrophy using a hand-held dynamometer. Physical Therapy, 68:977–982, 1988.

Tew, B, & Laurence, KM. The effects of hydrocephalus on intelligence, visual perception, and school attainments. Developmental Medicine and Child Neurology, 17(suppl 35):129–134, 1975.

Torode, I, & Godette, G. Surgical correction of congential kyphosis in myelomeningocele. Journal of Pediatric Orthopedics, 15:202–205, 1995.

Tulipan, N, Sutton, LN, & Cohen, BM. The effect of intrauterine myelomeningocele repair on the incidence of shunt-dependent hydrocephalus. Pediatric Neurosurgery, 38:27–33, 2003.

Turk, MA & Weber, RJ. Adults with congenital and childhood onset disability disorders. In DeLisa, JB, & Gans, BM, (Eds.). Rehabilitation Medicine: Principles and Practice. 3rd ed. Philadelphia: Lippincott-Raven; 1998, pp. 953–962.

Vankoski, S, Moore, C, Satler, K, Sarwark, JF, & Dias, L. The influence of forearm crutches on pelvic and hip kinematic parameters in childhood community ambulators with low-level myelomeningocele—Don't throw away the crutches. Developmental Medicine & Child Neurology, 37(Suppl 75):5–6, 1995.

Weber, D, & Agro, M. Clinical Aspects of Lower Extremity Orthotics. Winnipeg, Manitoba: Canadian Association of Prosthetists and Orthotists, 1993.

Wicks, K, & Shurtleff, DB. An introduction to toilet training. In Shurtleff, DB (Ed.). Myelodysplasias and Exstrophies: Significance, Prevention, and Treatment. Orlando, FL: Grune & Stratton, 1986a, pp. 203–219.

Wicks, K, & Shurtleff, DB. Stool management. In Shurtleff, DB (Ed.). Myelodysplasias and Exstrophies: Significance, Prevention, and Treatment. Orlando, FL: Grune & Stratton, 1986b, pp. 221–242.

Williams, EN, Broughton, NS, & Menelaus, MB. Age-related walking in children with spina bifida. Developmental Medicine & Child Neurology, 41:446–449, 1999.

Williams, LV, Anderson, AD, Campbell, J, Thomas, L, Feiwell, E, & Walker, JM. Energy cost of walking and of wheelchair propulsion by children with myelodysplasia: Comparison with normal children. Developmental Medicine and Child Neurology, 25:617–624, 1983.

Winter, DA. Knee flexion during stance as a determinant of inefficient walking. Physical Therapy, 63:331–333, 1983.

Wolf, LS, & McLaughlin, JF. Early motor development in infants with myelomeningocele. Pediatric Physical Therapy, 4:12–17, 1992.

Wright, J, Menelaus, M, Broughton, N, & Shurtleff, D. Natural history of knee contractures in myelomeningocele. Journal of Pediatric Orthopedics, 11:725–730, 1991.

Zsolt, S, Seidl, R, Bernert, G, Dietrich, W, Spitzauer, S, & Urbanek, R. Latex sensitization in spina bifida appears disease-associated. Journal of Pediatrics, 134:344–348, 1999.

MANAGEMENT OF CARDIOPULMONARY CONDITIONS

Section Editor
Suzann K. Campbell
PT, PhD, FAPTA

Chapter 26

CHILDREN REQUIRING LONG-TERM VENTILATOR ASSISTANCE

M. KATHLEEN KELLY
PT, PhD

The U.S. Office of Technology Assessment defined the technology-dependent child as "one who needs both a medical device to compensate for the loss of a vital body function, and substantial and ongoing nursing care to avert death or further disability" (Office of Technology Assessment, 1987). As a result of continuing advances in medical care, use of aggressive respiratory management for critically ill infants and children, and improved technology, the number of children who are dependent on mechanical ventilation continues to increase (Criner et al., 1994; Haffner & Schurman, 2001; Office of Technology Assessment, 1987). By definition, an individual is considered to be a long-term ventilator user if the individual requires ventilator assistance for more than 6 hours per day for at least 3 weeks (Make, 2001). Geographic differences in the prevalence of children with ventilator dependence may also exist largely as a result of differing parental attitudes and differing medical practices with respect to the incidence of ventilator-dependent children (Mallory & Stillwell, 1991; Office of Technology Assessment, 1987). One particular factor that has contributed to the increase in numbers of children requiring long-term ventilatory assistance is parental expectations of long-term survival. Often, in spite of differing physician attitudes, parents and caregivers "force" a change in the treatment plan toward initiation of long-term ventilatory use. Lastly, the ongoing introduction of new respiratory equipment for home care use has also added to the presumptive ease of care for children at home on a ventilator (Teague, 2001). Unfortunately, no central tracking system exists for following these children and the impact of such care (Gracey & Hubmayr, 2001).

INCIDENCE

A distinctive aspect of children requiring long-term ventilator assistance is that they are united by dependence on technology and not by a common diagnosis. Rather, a wide variety of diagnoses exist in which chronic respiratory failure results. Although the degree of care and support varies from child to child, each requires a high cost of care that demands sophisticated equipment and round-the-clock vigilance and monitoring. The child with ventilator dependence represents a unique challenge for all health care professionals as we have moved beyond the goal of increasing their survival; rather, we are now in the era of defining best practices as those that result in optimal quality-of-life outcomes. For the pediatric patient, this goal includes optimizing their developmental potential, reducing the incidence of activity limitations and disabilities, and ultimately maximizing their participation in home, school and community activities. The role of the pediatric physical therapist is an important one in addressing these issues. This chapter attempts to move beyond individual diagnostic categories to which the children belong, and instead suggests a framework for examination, diagnosis and intervention strategies for these children based on their need for ventilatory assistance. The pathophysiologic processes that are commonly seen in pediatric practice are discussed, as well as the common modes of ventilatory support. The reader is referred to several sources for a more in-depth discussion of ventilatory strategies and clinical management.

PATHOPHYSIOLOGY OF CHRONIC RESPIRATORY FAILURE

Adequate respiratory function requires effective pulmonary exchange of oxygen and carbon dioxide. Respiration requires an organ of gas exchange, the lungs, a "pump" mechanism consisting of the rib cage and respiratory muscles, and the neural control centers (Watchko et al., 1991). Under normal conditions, this pump mechanism can adapt to satisfy the changing metabolic needs that may occur during exercise, hyperthermia, or other demands (Bureau & Begin, 1983), but when these systems are unable to deliver oxygen and remove carbon dioxide from the pulmonary circulation, respiratory failure ensues and gas exchange is impaired (Pagtakhan & Chernick, 1983).

Chronic respiratory failure is not a specific disease entity but a pathophysiologic state defined by treatment with mechanical ventilation for more than 28 days, usually as a result of abnormal gas exchange caused by either primary lung failure or failure of the respiratory pump (Roussos, 1985). In essence, chronic respiratory failure "is the result of an uncorrectable imbalance in the respiratory system, in which ventilatory muscle power and central respiratory drive are inadequate to overcome the respiratory load" (Make et al., 1998). Primary lung failure is typically associated with acute respiratory diseases such as respiratory distress syndrome (RDS), in some cases leading to bronchopulmonary dysplasia (BPD). In this case, primary lung or airway disease compromises pulmonary gas exchange. On the other hand, failure of the respiratory pump may be caused by impaired neural control of respiration or by inadequate force generation of the respiratory muscles as the result of primary muscle disease, spinal cord injury, chest wall defects, or muscle fatigue. As a result, respiratory muscles are unable to sustain adequate alveolar ventilation (Amin & Fitton, 2003).

A number of conditions may predispose children to chronic respiratory failure, but the most common pathophysiologic process is respiratory distress leading to respiratory failure (Box 26-1). Some of the more common diagnoses requiring long-term ventilation in the pediatric

---

Box 26-1   **Clinical Signs of Respiratory Failure**

RESPIRATORY

Tachypnea
Altered depth and pattern of respiration (deep, shallow, apnea, irregular)
Chest wall retractions
Nasal flaring
Cyanosis
Decreased or absent breath sounds
Expiratory grunting
Wheezing or prolonged expiration

GENERAL

Fatigue
Excessive sweating

CARDIAC

Tachycardia
Hypertension

Bradycardia
Hypotension
Cardiac arrest

CEREBRAL

Restlessness
Irritability
Headache
Mental confusion
Papilledema
Seizures
Coma

LABORATORY FINDINGS

Hypoxemia (acute or chronic)
Hypercapnia (acute or chronic)
Acidosis (metabolic or respiratory)

From Pagtakhan, RD, & Chernick, V. Intensive care for respiratory disorders. In Kendig, EL, & Chernick, V (Eds.), Disorders of the Respiratory Tract in Children. Philadelphia: WB Saunders, 1983, p. 148.

TABLE 26-1	Common Pathophysiologic Mechanisms Leading to Chronic Respiratory Failure		
CENTRAL NERVOUS SYSTEM	**INTRINSIC MUSCLE DISEASE**	**INTRINSIC PULMONARY DISEASE**	**CONGENITAL AIRWAY ABNORMALITIES**
Congenital hypoventilation syndrome	Congenital abnormalities of thoracic rib cage	Congenital heart disease	Tracheoesophageal fistula
Viral encephalitis	Congenital myopathies	Respiratory distress syndrome or bronchopulmonary dysplasia	Subglottic stenosis
Brain tumors	Duchenne muscular dystrophy	Tumors	Laryngomalacia
Arnold-Chiari malformation	Phrenic nerve trauma	Aspiration syndromes	Choanal atresia
Traumatic spinal cord injuries	Diaphragmatic dysfunction	Pneumothorax	Various syndromes
Anterior horn cell disease	Myasthenia gravis		
Apnea of prematurity	Botulism		
Intracranial hemorrhage			
Hypoxic encephalopathy			

Data from Mallory, GB, & Stillwell, PC. The ventilator-dependent child: Issues in diagnosis and management. Archives of Physical Medicine and Rehabilitation, 72:43–55, 1991; Goldsmith, JP, & Karotkin, EH. Introduction to assisted ventilation. In Goldsmith, JP, & Karotkin, EH (Eds.), Assisted Ventilation of the Neonate, 2nd ed. Philadelphia: WB Saunders, pp. 1–21; 1988; and Pagtakhan, RD, & Chernick, V. Intensive care for respiratory disorders. In Kendig, EL, & Chernick, V (Eds.), Disorders of the Respiratory Tract, 4th ed. Philadelphia: WB Saunders, 1983, pp. 205–224.

population include BPD, progressive and nonprogressive myopathies, traumatic or congenital spinal cord injuries, congenital anomalies such as congenital heart disease and various airway abnormalities, and congenital central hypoventilation syndrome (CCHS, aka "Ondine's curse") (Teague, 2001). The mechanisms that can lead to respiratory failure can be broadly categorized into four major groups: central nervous system (CNS) disease; muscle disease and musculoskeletal abnormalities; intrinsic pulmonary disease; and airway abnormalities (Table 26-1).

CNS disease is characterized by disorders affecting the central respiratory centers (i.e., the brainstem or cervical spinal cord) (Fig. 26-1). Congenital central hypoventilation syndrome (CCHS) is a rare disorder that presents very shortly after birth or early in infancy. Although categorized as a disorder of the CNS, it is thought to be characterized by a failure of the autonomic control of ventilation in the absence of primary pulmonary or neuromuscular disease or the absence of a brainstem lesion. It is typically more severe during sleep versus wakeful periods and is most apparent during non-REM sleep, when breathing is almost entirely under autonomic control (Trang et al., 2003; Teague, 2001). The anatomic and biochemical mechanisms of central dysfunction are not completely known, but are postulated to be due to abnormalities in chemoreceptor input to the central control of breathing (Woo et al., 1992; Cutz et al., 1997),

and more specifically abnormal development of neural crest–derived cells (American Thoracic Society, 1999). This disorder is generally diagnosed in the neonatal period when the infant experiences apneic episodes during sleep or while awake. CCHS is known to be associated with other systemic or oncologic conditions such as Hirschsprung's disease or neuroblastoma (American Thoracic Society, 1999; Woo et al., 1992) and with genetic disorders (for a review, see Silvestri et al., 2002).

Although the incidence of CCHS is low, this group of patients faces a lifelong dependence on mechanical ventilation. The severity of CCHS varies, as does the degree of dependence on a mechanical ventilator. Because these children have absent or negligible ventilatory sensitivity to hypercapnia and variable sensitivity to hypoxemia, they are dependent on a ventilator during the night or during sleep (Weese-Mayer et al., 1992; Woo et al., 1992). In addition, extra caution needs to be taken during physical activity. Even with adequate ventilation, these children do not perceive a sense of hypoxia and hypercarbia that may accompany exertion and thus require constant vigilance during exercise. Artificial ventilation in these patients is done almost exclusively with positive-pressure ventilators or diaphragmatic pacemakers. For children who require 24-hours-a-day ventilation, these options seem to be the most reasonable and the least invasive.

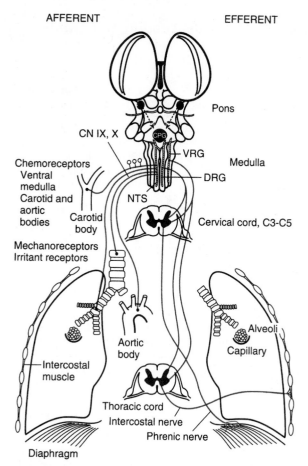

AFFERENT   EFFERENT

Pons

CN IX, X

VRG

Medulla

Chemoreceptors
Ventral
medulla   DRG
Carotid and
aortic   NTS
bodies   Carotid
body   Cervical cord, C3-C5

Mechanoreceptors
Irritant receptors

Alveoli

Aortic   Capillary
body

Intercostal
muscle

Thoracic cord
Intercostal nerve
Phrenic nerve

Diaphragm

- **Figure 26-1** Schema outlining the various contributions to the neural control of respiration. NTS, nucleus tractus solitarius; VRG, ventral respiratory group; DRG, dorsal respiratory group. *(From Brazy, JE, Kinney, HC, & Oakes,WJ. CNS structural lesions causing apnea at birth. Journal of Pediatrics, 111:163–175, 1987.)*

Children with CCHS may have otherwise unremarkable medical histories. The most vulnerable period is before the diagnosis is made when the infant may experience hypoxic episodes resulting in permanent neurologic damage. With early diagnosis and aggressive management of respiratory failure, the adverse sequelae of hypoxia should be minimized and most of these children can enjoy a relatively "normal" and productive life.

Acquired disorders of the brainstem that affect respiration typically result from either infectious disease processes, brainstem tumors, or complications of Arnold-Chiari malformations. In these instances chronic respiratory failure may be transient or long term. Spinal cord injury or disease can also result in chronic respiratory failure, leading to dependence on mechanical ventilation. The rate of recovery of breathing and motor function

after the injury separates those infants and children with satisfactory outcomes from those with poor outcomes (i.e., complete dependence on mechanical ventilation). The level of spinal cord injury dictates the degree of respiratory compromise. Typically, with injuries involving the upper cervical or cervicothoracic area, respiration is compromised because of phrenic and intercostal nerve root damage affecting the function of the diaphragmatic and accessory muscles of respiration. Patients with cervical-level injuries usually require mechanical ventilation either throughout the entire day or only at night. The prognosis for dependence on mechanical ventilation depends on the level of the lesion, the extent of nerve damage, and the nature of the lesion (MacKinnon et al., 1993).

Anterior horn cell disease represents another group of disorders affecting the spinal cord. Spinal muscular atrophy is one of the most common anterior horn cell diseases seen in children since the polio era (Mallory & Stillwell, 1991). There are different types of spinal muscular atrophy, the most common being type I (Werdnig-Hoffmann disease). Werdnig-Hoffmann disease is an hereditary and progressive disease that typically leads to respiratory failure within a few months after birth. The infant with Werdnig-Hoffmann disease typically presents with generalized hypotonia and paralysis of the limb and trunk musculature with facial sparing. The presence of bulbar weakness results in difficulty with swallowing and sucking, putting these infants at great risk of aspiration, which complicates their already compromised respiratory status. If respiratory involvement is present and noted in the early postnatal period, it is usually severe, leading to respirator dependence very early in the child's life (see Chapter 15).

Intrinsic muscle disease is another common cause of chronic respiratory failure in children. Those with congenital myopathies typically manifest symptoms of respiratory failure early in the course of the disease, whereas those with muscular dystrophies typically do not present with respiratory compromise until late childhood or early adolescence. In either case, mechanical ventilation may be warranted to compensate for the significantly reduced respiratory muscle function (Bureau & Begin, 1983; Teague, 2001).

Congenital anomalies of the thorax may also predispose the infant to respiratory failure due to hypoventilation. Thoracic abnormalities are associated with a variety of syndromes (e.g., asphyxiating thoracic dystrophy and dwarfism) as well as scoliosis. In all cases, the rib cage abnormalities may result in pulmonary hypoplasia and significantly decreased lung volumes. Treatment of these various impairments will vary; however, in some cases the child may require mechanical ventilation.

Respiratory failure associated with preterm birth is a common cause of ventilator dependence in infants and is a major cause of neonatal death. Acute respiratory distress syndrome (RDS) in neonates accounts for approximately 30% of all neonatal deaths and 50% to 70% of preterm infant deaths. Because of anatomic and physiologic immaturities, the infant is predisposed to respiratory dysfunction such as atelectasis, airway obstruction, increased pulmonary vascular resistance, and pulmonary edema. As well, they are predisposed to diaphragmatic fatigue and instability in the neural control of breathing (Make, 2001). As smaller and more immature babies survive, they are at risk for the unfortunate sequelae of ventilator-induced lung injury resulting in bronchopulmonary dysplasia (BPD) (Attar & Donn, 2002; Rodriguez, 2003).

BPD, first described by Northway in 1967, is the most common type of chronic lung disease in infants (Bregman & Farrell, 1992). BPD is associated with low birth weight, prematurity, and severe initial lung disease, but it has also been described in full-term infants treated with extracorporeal membranous oxygenation (ECMO) (Gannon et al., 1998; Kornhauser et al., 1998). It is thought that structural changes in the lung parenchyma occur as a result of both increased ventilatory pressures over a period of time and prolonged exposure to high levels of oxygen tension. Only after the acute disease has subsided can BPD be accurately distinguished from complications of other acute lung injury (Northway, 1979). BPD was originally defined as oxygen dependence greater than 30% beyond 28 to 30 days with accompanying radiographic changes in the lungs. In this initial cohort of infants, however, the mean gestational age (GA) at birth was greater than 31 weeks and only one of the infants weighed less than 1500 g. More recently, a newer and milder form of BPD has emerged as a result of surfactant administration and improved critical care practices that are more lung-protective (Coalson, 2003; Robin et al., 2004). Currently, the prevalence of BPD is low in infants greater than 1200 g or 30 weeks GA (Coalson, 2003; Gregoire et al., 1998; Jobe and Bancalari, 2001). The classification of the disease is based on several factors, first defined by the GA being either less than or more than 32 weeks. From that point, disease severity is categorized as mild, moderate, or severe based on the need for supplemental oxygen or positive pressure ventilation at 36 weeks postmenstrual age (for infants <32 weeks GA at birth) or 56 days postnatal age (for infants born at 32 weeks or after). This new phenotype is characterized by impaired/disrupted alveolar development, rather than the airway damage and fibrosis seen in the "old" BPD (Jobe & Bancalari, 2001; Robin et al., 2004). Both structural and functional immaturities predispose the lungs to injury. In addition, there are suggestions that pre- or perinatal exposure to cytokines may contribute to the evolution of chronic lung disease. Proinflammatory cytokines have also been implicated in the development of periventricular leukomalacia (Rezaie & Dean, 2002; Viscardi et al., 2004).

Although there have been no major breakthroughs in the prevention of BPD, the long-term outcomes have improved and the disease severity is reduced as a result of medical and pharmacologic improvements (Bancalari & Sosenko, 1990). Two of the most recent additions to the armamentarium for treatment of neonatal respiratory distress are the use of high-frequency ventilators and surfactant replacement in the early neonatal period. The goal of high-frequency ventilation is to adequately ventilate at lower intrapulmonary pressures and smaller tidal volumes, thereby reducing the degree of barotrauma and volutrauma to the immature airways, and to reduce the risks of pulmonary air leaks. The use of surfactant therapy is now standard practice for the treatment of RDS and its use has contributed substantially to reduced morbidity rates. A wide variety of surfactant types exist, including both artificial surfactant and surfactant derived from animal sources. A recent review of several clinical trials assessing the efficacy of synthetic surfactant replacement concluded that there were improved clinical outcomes (Soll, 2000). The treatment of BPD, as well as of other forms of chronic lung disease, includes nutritional support, respiratory support (often in the form of supplemental oxygen and ventilatory strategies), pharmacologic interventions such as bronchodilators, anti-inflammatory drugs, sedatives and diuretics, and developmental care and follow-up. These infants and children require ongoing monitoring of their physiologic status to ensure physiologic stability.

Postnatal lung tissue development confers an advantage for infants with chronic lung disease. Many "recover" from BPD and eventually function independent of assisted ventilation and supplemental oxygen if conditions for growth are optimized (Farrell & Fost, 1989). Nevertheless, a small proportion of the infants with BPD will go on to require prolonged ventilation.

MECHANICAL VENTILATION

Mechanical ventilators have played an important role in critical care medicine for both adults and children since the modern era of long-term ventilatory assistance began in the 1950s. By the mid 1980s, there were reports of successful long-term ventilator use by children in the home (see review by Teague, 2001). Although the underlying disease processes and severity of respiratory failure differ considerably among individuals, mechanical ventilation is the final common treatment approach for individuals with chronic respiratory failure (Table 26-2) (Amin & Fitton, 2003; Pilmer, 1994). Mechanical ventilation and the artificial airways used to facilitate it are designed to either assist or substitute for a person's respiratory efforts (i.e., moving air into and out of the lungs) (Luce, 1996; Pagtakhan & Chernick, 1983; Tobin, 2001). In addition to the major goal of restoring adequate gas exchange, it is also essential that complications be avoided at best, and minimized at the very least (Cheifetz, 2003; Dick and Sassoon, 1996). The decision to institute long-term mechanical ventilation is increasingly being made electively to preserve physiologic function and to improve quality of life. In many instances, the clinical decision is made to take advantage of the growth and developmental potential of the lungs (Make, 2001) and to maximize the developmental potential of the infant or child. Thus, the desired outcome for many patients is medical stability with adequate growth and healing of the lungs, and eventual withdrawal of the assisted ventilation.

Since the beginning of the modern era of mechanical ventilation in the 1950s, ventilators have undergone, and continue to undergo, significant technologic advances (Goldsmith & Karotkin, 1988; Make, 2001; Perel & Stock, 1992). Since the 1950s, 300 to 400 different types of ventilators have been on the market at one time or another (Perel & Stock, 1992; Tremolieres, 1991). Specifically, pediatric mechanical ventilation has undergone continual changes that reflect an increased knowledge, understanding, and appreciation of the developing cardiorespiratory system. Currently, ventilation approaches utilize protective strategies to avoid atelectotrauma and lung overdistention through the use of maximal alveolar pressures, minimal positive end-expiratory pressure, and permissive hypercapnia (Elixson et al., 1997; Gannon et al., 1998; Make, 2001). Contemporary knowledge of respiratory physiology and a more detailed understanding of the pathophysiologic mechanisms underlying diseases of the respiratory system continue to drive research and development in this area. Although it is beyond the scope and intent of this chapter to detail the technical information that exists on mechanical ventilation, a brief overview of assisted ventilation will be provided.

Assisted ventilatory support may be accomplished noninvasively (e.g. negative pressure ventilation) or with an invasive approach (positive pressure ventilation with a tracheostomy). Positive pressure ventilation (PPV) is the most commonly used assisted ventilation strategy and is the preferred method for children who are at home on

---

TABLE 26-2	**Selection Criteria for Mechanical Ventilation**

PARAMETER	FINDINGS
Clinical	
Respiratory*	Apnea; decreased breath sounds; rigorous chest wall movement; weakening ventilatory effort
Cardiac	Asystole; peripheral collapse; severe bradycardia or tachycardia
Cerebral	Coma; lack of response to physical stimuli; uncontrolled restlessness; anxious facial expression
General	Limpness; loss of ability to cry
Laboratory†	
$Paco_2$	Newborn: >60-65 mm Hg
	Older child: >55-60 mm Hg
	Rapidly rising >5 mm Hg
Pao_2	Newborn: <40-50 mm Hg
	Older child: <50-60 mm Hg

From Pagtakhan, RD, & Chernick, V. Intensive care for respiratory disorders. In Kendig, EL, & Chernick, V (Eds.), Disorders of the Respiratory Tract in Children. Philadelphia: WB Saunders, 1984, p. 160.

*More than one episode of apnea with bradycardia or an episode of cardiac arrest is an adequate indication for initiating mechanical ventilation even in the absence of blood gas data.

†Laboratory values less extreme than those indicated must be supplemented by clinical evidence of severity to warrant initiating mechanical ventilation.

portable ventilators. Most often, PPV is delivered via an endotracheal or tracheostomy tube with pressurized gas being delivered into the airways and ventilator circuit during inspiration. There is, however, increasing support for the use of noninvasive methods of PPV in treating children with acute and chronic respiratory failure (Hess, 2002; Cheifetz, 2003; Simonds, 2003; Gali & Goyal, 2003). In addition to the obvious reason of avoiding a tracheostomy, this form of PPV reduces the risk of acquired infections and allows patients to be more mobile (Cheifetz, 2003). Despite a limited number of studies on this form of PPV in children, rapid technologic and medical advances should lead to an increased utilization of this mode of assisted ventilation in the near future.

The more common strategy for noninvasive ventilation is the use of negative pressure ventilators (NPV). NPV provides a pressure gradient, which is established by creating a negative pressure around the person's entire body (from the neck down) during inspiration, causing air to enter the lungs. The typical interface used with this type of ventilation is a customized chest shell, wrap/poncho, or a tank ventilator. The major advantage of NPV is avoiding or delaying the need for a tracheostomy, thereby reducing the risk of infection. Another advantage of NPV is that ventilation is not interrupted when suctioning (Dougherty, 1990; Make, 2001; Teague, 2001). NPV has been used most successfully for patients with normal lung mechanics and hypoventilation as seen in patients with neuromuscular diseases and pulmonary disease requiring periodic or nocturnal ventilatory support (McPherson, 1995). The limitations of NPV is that it may cause airway occlusion in infants and young children during sleep, and the chest shell or wrap is not effective for children who require high respiratory rates, tidal volumes, or distending pressures; thus NPV are not commonly used in the latter (Make et al., 1998).

Mechanical ventilators using PPV are classified by varying parameters and attributes. Unfortunately there is no uniform system nor standardized nomenclature for classifying ventilators or ventilatory modes. Chatburn (1991) proposed that ventilator classifications be conceptualized according to respiratory mechanics, rather than according to mechanical features. Chatburn suggested that this framework is more useful because the mechanics of respiration will remain constant, despite the constant changes in technology. Using this scheme, ventilators can be classified according to their *control* parameters of pressure, volume, flow, or time; their *phase* parameters of trigger, limit, and cycle (Table 26-3); and the mode of delivery with respect to amount of ventilatory assistance (pattern of spontaneous and mandatory breaths) (Box 26-2).

Because there are so many combinations of ventilatory attributes that can obtain desirable results, practices are far from uniform and often scientific research is lacking (Branson, 2004; Make, 2001; Make et al., 1998). The optimal settings for each patient vary and are determined by their metabolic requirements, respiratory drive, and pulmonary mechanics (Amin & Fitton, 2003; Shneerson, 1996). The type of mechanical ventilation and the various parameters chosen depend on a number of considerations. These include the age of the patient, an understanding of

TABLE 26-3	**Classification of Positive Pressure Ventilators**
CONTROL VARIABLES	**PHASE VARIABLE CATEGORIES**
Variables that the ventilator manipulates to cause inspiration; only *one* variable can be controlled at a time	Control variables *measured and used* by the ventilator to initiate some phase of the breath cycle
Pressure: ventilator has a set pressure, thus mechanical ventilation terminates when a preselected peak inspiratory pressure is achieved.	**Trigger variable:** these variables reach some preset threshold to begin inspiration.
Volume: ventilator maintains a constant volume irrespective of changes in pulmonary mechanics.	**Limit variable:** these variables reach a preset level before inspiration ends.
Flow: ventilator maintains a constant tidal volume.	**Cycle variable:** these control variables are used to end inspiration.
Time: ventilator maintains a constant time between inspiration and expiration.	**Baseline:** these control variables are controlled during expiratory time.

Adapted from Chatburn R. A new system for understanding mechanical ventilators. Respiratory Care, *36*:1123–1155, 1991; and Chatburn, RL, & Primiano, FP. A new system for understanding mechanical ventilation. Respiratory Care, *46*(6):604–621, 2001.

Box 26-2	Modes of Invasive Positive Pressure Ventilation

- Continuous mandatory ventilation (CMV)—all breaths are mandatory; full ventilator support
- Continuous spontaneous ventilation—all breaths are spontaneous
- Intermittent mandatory ventilation (IMV)—intermittent breaths are at a fixed rate and are not synchronized to the patient
- Assist/control (AC) ventilation—mandatory breaths are triggered by patient's inspiratory effort (or within a preset time)

- Synchronized intermittent mandatory ventilation (SIMV)—patient can take unassisted spontaneous breaths, which are synchronized with mandatory breaths at some preset volume and rate
- Proportional assisted ventilation—every ventilator breath is proportional to the patient's respiratory effort

Note: Portable positive pressure ventilation may not be designed to operate within certain limits and may not be able to handle dynamic changes in respiratory physiology.

Adapted from numerous sources, listed in the references at the end of the chapter (Chatburn, 1991; Chatburn & Primiano, 2001; Donn & Sinha, 2002; Gali & Goyal, 2003; Make et al., 1998).

the underlying disease process that precipitated ventilatory failure, available equipment, knowledge of the current literature, previous experience with specific types of machines, and site of care (intensive care unit [ICU] or home environment?) (Perel & Stock, 1992; Teague, 2001). Although mechanical ventilation has had a significant impact on the outcomes of children with respiratory failure, one needs to appreciate the unwanted effects of secondary lung injury that can occur with PPV (Cheifetz, 2003).

There are numerous complications that can occur with invasive PPV (Box 26-3). It is essential that individuals working with children who require long-term ventilatory assistance have a knowledge of normal and pathologic respiratory physiology, the anatomic and physiologic changes of the developing respiratory system, and an intimate knowledge and understanding of how the machine interfaces with the patient's physiology (Branson, 2004; Cheifetz, 2003; Kondili et al., 2003; Make et al., 1998). To avoid the complications related to controlled mechanical ventilation, there is an increasing emphasis on the use of partial ventilatory assistance. Ideally, the desirable mode of ventilation is one with optimal synchrony and patient-ventilator interface, along with the use of lung-protective strategies (Donn & Sinha, 2002; Navalesi & Costa, 2003). With the advent of microprocessor technology, newer models of ventilators are able to offer greater flexibility with respect to their modes of ventilatory delivery (Branson, 2004; Chatburn & Primiano, 2001; Donn & Sinha, 2002). The other major disadvantage of invasive PPV is the need for a tracheostomy. Although the tracheostomy provides instantaneous access to the airway, it also increases the complexities

of care, especially for children who are at home using ventilatory assistance. As well, an artificial airway interferes with speech and nutrition (Make et al., 1998). Despite the tremendous flexibility of the various ventilators on the market, the ultimate decision needs to be based on whether the machine is the right match for the child at a given point in time. For children who are cared for outside of the ICU environment, it is mandatory that they are assessed using the ventilator with which they will ultimately be discharged. Home ventilators do not provide the same ventilation as do hospital ventilators, and thus, the specific settings need to be adjusted to meet the physiologic needs of the child (Make et al., 1998).

For the infant or child who is facing the need for long-term ventilator assistance, the possibilities and options for being cared for at home should weigh heavily in the decision-making process. Technologic advances in design, efficiency, and portability have contributed to an increase in use of mechanical ventilation outside the hospital environment. In the past decade or more, there has been an increasing emphasis on home care and it is now standard practice for medically stable children with ventilator dependence to be cared for outside the hospital (Haffner & Schurman, 2001). A number of studies have demonstrated that appropriately selected infants and children can be safely cared for at home (for review, see Ambrosio et al., 1998; Make, 2001). The transition to home carries with it other circumstances that can contribute to increased stress, financial burden, and significant changes in a family's lifestyle and relationships. The shift in responsibility for medical care from health care professionals to the family has resulted in "a spectrum of issues that demand psychological, social,

> ## Box 26-3   Complications Associated with Mechanical Ventilation
>
> ### RESPIRATORY
>
> Tracheal lesions (erosion, edema, stenosis, granuloma, obstruction, perforation)
> Accidental endotracheal tube displacement or actual extubation
> Air leaks (pneumothorax, pneumomediastinum, interstitial emphysema)
> Infection (tracheitis, pneumonitis)
> Trapping of gas (hyperinflation)
> Excessive secretions (atelectasis)
> Oxygen hazards (depression of ventilation, bronchopulmonary dysplasia)
> Pulmonary hemorrhage
>
> ### CIRCULATORY
>
> Impairment of venous return (decreased cardiac output and systemic hypotension)
> Oxygen hazard (retrolental fibroplasia, cerebral vasoconstriction
> Septicemia
>
> Intracranial hemorrhage
> Hyperventilation (decreased cerebral blood flow)
>
> ### METABOLIC
>
> Increased work of breathing ("fighting the ventilator")
> Alkalosis (potassium depletion, excessive bicarbonate therapy)
>
> ### RENAL AND FLUID BALANCE
>
> Antidiuresis
> Excess water in inspired gas
>
> ### EQUIPMENT MALFUNCTION
>
> Power source failure
> Improper humidification (overheating of inspired gas, inspiratory line condensation)
> Improper tubing connections (kinked line, disconnection)
> Ventilation malfunction (leaks, valve dysfunction)
>
> Adapted from Pagtakhan, RD, & Chernick, V. Intensive care for respiratory disorders. In Kendig, EL, & Chernick, V (Eds.), Disorders of the Respiratory Tract in Chilren. Philadelphia: WB Saunders, 1983, p. 162.

ethical, financial and policy solutions" (Wang & Barnard, 2004). Although these added burdens do not necessarily outweigh the tremendous benefits of children being raised at home and integrated into their communities, they can be overwhelming and impact the quality of life for the child and their family (Haffner & Schurman, 2001; O'Brien & Wegner, 2002). Fortunately, there seem to be increased efforts to formulate social and public policies around their unique needs (Mentro, 2003; Wang & Barnard, 2004). It has been suggested that a social model of disability more appropriately captures the needs of these individuals and their families and highlights the responsibilities of society to meet the needs of individuals with disabilities (Wang & Barnard, 2004).

WEANING

The transition to unassisted breathing is a complex issue. Weaning the patient from the support of a mechanical ventilator is quite individualized, but it should be the ultimate goal for most patients. The primary assessment of weaning capability is to determine at what point the patient is capable of maintaining adequate alveolar ventilation while breathing spontaneously. This requires

that the patient's ventilatory pump be able to support the work required for breathing (Hess, 2001). Prolonged mechanical ventilation has deleterious effects on diaphragmatic function, which would affect weaning potential. Knisely and co-workers (1988) found an association between prolonged ventilatory dependence in infants and diaphragmatic muscle atrophy. These investigators suggested that these changes could certainly affect the weaning process because the diaphragm would be predisposed to fatigue. A similar result was seen in a study by Anzueto and associates (1997), who used a baboon model of ventilator dependence. After 11 days on a ventilator, there were decreases in transdiaphragmatic pressures and a decrease in endurance. Various determinants of physiologic and medical stability such as pulmonary function, gas exchange, neuromuscular function, respiratory muscle strength, and ventilatory pattern are used to determine weaning capabilities.

The process of weaning is often done by trial and error whereby the time off the ventilator is variable, dependent on when hypercapnia and hypoxia develop (Gozal et al., 1993). There are three commonly used approaches that may be used to wean: (1) spontaneous breathing trial with the use of a T-piece (with or without continuous positive airway pressure, or CPAP); (2) pressure-support ventilation (PSV) in which all breaths are patient-triggered and pressure-limited; more patient effort is required as the level of pressure support is decreased; and (3) synchronized intermittent mandatory ventilation (SIMV) in which breaths can be either mandatory ventilator-controlled or spontaneous. The latter is the least favored strategy among the three (Hess, 2001; Gracey & Hubmayr, 2001). Thus far, there are "no widely accepted criteria for weaning and extubation of pediatric patients" (Kercsmar, 2003).

Weaning can be an arduous task both physiologically and psychologically, and it must be done with caution (Gracey & Hubmayr, 2001). During this time, the child's schedule of activities may need to be altered. It is imperative that the physical therapist coordinate and communicate with the medical team as to the amount of physical exertion that can be tolerated safely. At all costs both muscular and respiratory fatigue during this period of time must be avoided.

ACTIVITY LIMITATIONS ASSOCIATED WITH LONG-TERM VENTILATOR ASSISTANCE

Chronic dependence on assisted ventilation has created a new category of developmental disabilities. As elucidated previously, a wide range of pathophysiologic mechanisms underlie dependence on mechanical ventilation, hence this "medical" diagnosis represents a diverse and heterogeneous group of children with varying impairments and capabilities. Despite differences, these children are similar in that they are medically fragile and at risk for physical, mental, and psychosocial disabilities. Although the predictive value of any one risk factor is not well established, it appears that long-term outcome depends on the interaction of biologic and environmental risk factors. In the recent revision of the ICIDH (International Classification of Impairments, Disabilities and Health) disablement model—now termed the International Classification of Function (ICF)—the environment is recognized as a major influence on body structure/function, daily activities, and social participation (World Health Organization, 2001). In fact, the ICF conceptualizes manifestations of disability as being bidirectional. In other words, there is the recognition that the disabling process is not a linear process.

In general, a paucity of literature exists on the long-term developmental outcomes for infants and children with BPD or other diagnoses requiring prolonged ventilatory assistance. One group that has probably been studied most extensively are infants and children with BPD. The morbidity associated with BPD includes not only the associated chronic respiratory problems but other growth and development-related factors (Barbosa, Campbell, et al., 2003). For example, linear and anthropometric growth are often adversely affected by BPD (Bregman & Farrell, 1992; Huysman et al., 2003; Kurzner et al., 1988). Although optimal nutrition is an important goal in the care of infants with respiratory distress, it is often difficult to achieve because of the increased energy expenditure, increased work of breathing, and limited fluid intake (Bregman & Farrell, 1992; Kurzner et al., 1988). Weinstein and Oh (1981) reported a 25% increase in resting oxygen consumption of preterm infants with BPD compared with typical infants. In addition, the caloric requirements of the infants with BPD are 25% to 50% greater than those of typical infants. Kao and colleagues (1998) found that when pulmonary mechanics were improved and work of breathing decreased, oxygen consumption did not decrease. More recent work by deMeer and colleagues (1997) showed that infants with BPD have greater total energy expenditure, which is strongly correlated with their respiratory status. These results suggest that factors such as inflammation, repair processes of the lung, and pulmonary tension might account for the increased metabolic rate, and hence the increased oxygen consumption. Children with BPD may also experience a failure to thrive because of intolerance for feeding secondary to oral motor sensitivity, a poor suck, or decreased physical stamina to sustain the demands of feeding (Bregman & Farrell, 1992; Yu et al., 1983).

Discrepancies exist regarding the impact of chronic lung disease on developmental outcomes beyond infancy. Bozynski and colleagues (1987) assessed the relationship between mechanical ventilation and developmental outcome. They found prolonged ventilator dependence to be the best predictor of poor developmental progress during the first 18 months. Even when the effects of intracranial hemorrhage were controlled, chronic lung disease was associated with lower scores on the Bayley Scales. Bregman and Farrell (1992) suggest that length of mechanical ventilation does not necessarily correlate with developmental outcome. More recently, O'Shea and associates (1996) found that chronic lung disease was associated with long-term effects on cognitive development. In this study, IQ tests were administered to 4- to 5-year-old children who had very low birth weights and had similar medical outcomes, and all were without evidence of major abnormalities on cranial ultrasound. Those children who had recovered from severe chronic lung disease had significantly lower full scale and performance IQ scores. Singer and colleagues (1997) reported poorer performance on developmental indices for infants with BPD followed longitudinally to 3 years of age. Regression analyses revealed that BPD predicted a poor motor outcome. Gregoire and colleagues (1998) discuss these discrepancies in terms of the definitions of BPD being used and whether or not there were associated neurologic lesions that coexisted with the chronic lung disease. In their study, the developmental outcomes of two groups were compared: one with traditionally defined BPD (O_2 dependence at 28 days) and the other with the "revised" definition of O_2 dependence at 36 weeks' postconceptional age. In their cohort, those with O_2 dependence at 36 weeks had a greater incidence of developmental delay, but not greater neurologic impairments, at 18 months. The presence of chronic lung disease (and ventilator dependence) alone puts a child at the same risk of neurodevelopmental impairments as the child with only a neurologic insult such as an intra- or periventricular hemorrhage (I/PVH) or periventricular leukomalacia (PVL). For example, of 10 children with cerebral palsy identified in a longitudinal study of 96 infants with varying risk for poor developmental outcome, 6 came from a group with brain insults and 4 from a group with BPD and no brain insult (except one with Grade II IVH) (Barbosa et al., 2003). Thus, the presence of both, as is commonly seen, would certainly place the child at an even higher risk for chronic developmental disabilities.

Even in the presence of an otherwise unremarkable medical history, the child on a ventilator is at risk for activity limitations related to communication, mobility, and fatigue related to poor cardiorespiratory endurance, to name a few. This is not surprising when one considers the extent of the child's "world" when they are ventilator dependent. The context for motor learning is quite limiting for the child who is hospitalized for prolonged periods or who is constrained by life-saving equipment. The lack of practice and of variable practice opportunities makes skill acquisition difficult, and thus the repertoire of skills in a variety of developmental domains is limited (see Chapter 4 for further details on motor learning concepts). As a point of illustration, the acquisition of independent mobility in typically developing children allows them to acquire information about their world and develop perceptions upon which they can act. Thus, development of cognitive skills such as object permanence is facilitated through motoric competencies (Bai & Bertenthal, 1992). This interleaving of developmental domains and their interdependence is a well-known phenomenon, so the impact of atypical circumstances and a lack of environmental affordances

can be quite substantial. It is easy to see why these children often present with global developmental delays, despite having no history of neurologic insults.

In addition to the aforementioned developmental risks, the additive effects of secondary complications such as recurrent hypoxic episodes, recurrent infections, poor weight gain, and poor physical growth can directly result in any number of impairments (Bos et al., 1998; Singer et al., 1997). For example, because of the often prolonged periods of immobility or restricted activity early in the course of their disease, these children may demonstrate such problems as sensory defensiveness, generalized weakness, and soft tissue or muscular tightness. Likewise, if the child has had some type of hypoxic or ischemic episode, there may be neurologic damage that additionally limits motor skill acquisition and execution. However, if these children have been spared the associated problems (most commonly the frequent hypoxic episodes), then there is a good chance that they can grow and develop normally. For example, children with CCHS have a favorable prognosis and the capacity for normal or near-normal intelligence if they are diagnosed early and managed aggressively (American Thoracic Society, 1999; Weese-Mayer et al., 1992). Similarly, infants with BPD who have not had major neurologic insults also have an excellent chance of being weaned from oxygen dependence and the ventilator, as well as functioning independently in their school years (Mallory & Stillwell, 1991).

Regardless of the reason for being dependent on assisted ventilation, appreciation of the fact that the child is at a disadvantage in terms of developmental risks is a compelling reason to begin early intervention as soon as the infant or child is medically stable. Because of the risks for abnormal neurodevelopmental sequelae in this population and in other children who are ventilator dependent, physical therapists should be involved with providing developmental intervention early in the course of an infant's hospitalization. Delays in the initiation of rehabilitation or habilitation may place the child at risk for developing secondary impairments and activity limitations that could otherwise be prevented.

ELEMENTS OF PATIENT MANAGEMENT

The physical therapy examination and evaluation of the infant or child who is mechanically ventilated needs to encompass a wide range of skills and observations. In addition to an understanding of typical and atypical motor skill development, one needs to have knowledge of

TABLE 26-4	Commonly Encountered Noninvasive Monitoring Devices*

EQUIPMENT	PHYSIOLOGIC PARAMETERS MONITORED
Cardiorespiratory monitors	Heart rate and respiratory rate
Pulse oximeter[†]	Transcutaneous arterial oxygen saturation to monitor hypoxemia
Ventilator alarms	Various modes chosen for the individual case, as well as airway pressures, gas concentrations, and expiratory tidal volumes
Transcutaneous P_{O_2} and P_{CO_2}	Partial pressure of oxygen and carbon dioxide in the arterial blood
Oxygen analyzers on the ventilator	Oxygen supply in the ventilator circuit
Sphygmomanometer	Blood pressure

*These are some noninvasive devices that one may use to monitor response to activity and general status. Before any examination or treatment session the therapist should be familiar with all of the equipment used for the child.
[†]Pulse oximeters are not useful for discriminating hyperoxia because the blood is fully saturated at Pa_{O_2} of 150 mm Hg.

cardiorespiratory physiology and the implications of a compromise to that system in the developing infant or child. The complexity of the technical environment also makes this a challenging population. First, the physical therapist needs to be comfortable with the ventilator equipment in addition to the physiologic monitoring devices (Table 26-4). Although the infant or child may be medically stable, the presence of an artificial airway creates a critical situation because of the potential for its being dislodged or occluded. Because the infant or young child may not yet communicate well, it is up to the therapist to interpret any signs of impending or actual distress. The essence of our intervention is to ensure that no harm be done in the delivery of services and to optimize the child's developmental potential.

Before any examination or treatment session, the therapist should confer with the child's primary nurse or caregiver to determine the child's most recent medical status, in addition to their baseline physiologic parameters. Depending on the nature and severity of the predisposing condition, the cardiorespiratory parameters may vary from what is considered to be typical for the child's age (Table 26-5). It is always prudent to establish the "safe" physiologic parameters within which to work. Typically, heart rate, respiratory rate, and oxygen saturation are monitored while the child is on the ventilator. In the home or outpatient setting, one may choose to monitor these parameters periodically; however, *there is no substitute for the keen visual observation of signs of distress.*

PHYSICAL THERAPY EXAMINATION

Although the most obvious impairment in patients on ventilators is in their cardiopulmonary system, it is

essential that the approach to patient management be multidimensional. It is likely the case that these patients have coexisting impairments, functional and activity limitations, and disabilities in various areas. Thus, once the necessary history and systems review is completed, the appropriate tests and measures are chosen to adequately examine aerobic capacity and endurance, adequacy of respiration, motor function, musculoskeletal performance, and general adaptive behaviors that are age-appropriate.

In terms of the respiratory examination, at a minimum the therapist should be comfortable observing the patient for signs of respiratory distress, skin color changes indicative of hypoxia, changes in respiratory rate, breathing pattern, symmetry of chest expansion, posture, and general comfort (DeCesare & Graybill, 1990). In neonates, visual inspection for hypoxia is not effective because neonates generally do not appear cyanotic until the Pa_{O_2} is dangerously low, below 40 mm Hg (Null et al., 1990). Signs of respiratory distress such as retractions, nasal flaring, expiratory grunting, and stridor may not be evident when a child is on a mechanical ventilator. For more information specific to the assessment of the cardiorespiratory system, the reader is referred elsewhere (DeCesare and Graybill, 1990; Gould, 1991; Waring, 1983).

The neuromuscular examination should provide information about the child's general musculoskeletal status and includes strength, sensation, posture, and general movement competencies. The examination procedures vary depending on the age and cognitive level of the child, and the areas of emphasis may be different depending on the diagnosis. Lastly, an important component is the measurement of neuromotor development and motor control. This is an important aspect of the examination for these children because they are at great

TABLE 26-5	Normal Ranges of Physiologic Values*	
PARAMETER	**NEWBORN**	**OLDER INFANT AND CHILD**
Respiratory rate	40-60	20-30 (≤6 years)
		15-20 (>6 years)
Heart rate	120-200	100-180 (≤3 years)
		70-150 (>3 years)
P_{O_2} (mm Hg)	60-90	80-100
P_{CO_2} (mm Hg)	30-35	30-35 (≤2 years)
		20-24 (>2 years)
Blood pressure (mm Hg)		
Systolic	60-90	75-130 (≤3 years)
		90-140 (>3 years)
Diastolic	30-60	45-90 (≤3 years)
		50-80 (>3 years)
Arterial oxygen saturation (%)	87-89 (low)	95-100
	94-95 (high)	
	90-95 (preterm infant)	

Data from Comer, DM. Pulse oximetry: Implications for practice. Journal of Obstetric, Gynecologic and Neonatal Nursing, 21:35-41, 1992; and Pagtakhan, RD, & Chernick, V. Intensive care for respiratory disorders. In Kendig, EL, & Chernick, V (Eds.), Disorders of the Respiratory Tract in Children, 4th ed. Philadelphia: WB Saunders, 1983, pp. 145-168.

*These values represent "normal" physiologic values; in the case of infants and children with varying pathophysiologic processes, the "normal" values may be different.

risk for global developmental delays that may or may not have a pathophysiologic component.

The physical therapy examination alone does not begin to represent the wide range of competencies that need to be monitored. Ideally, all aspects of the child's development will be assessed periodically by members of the health care team. It cannot be emphasized enough that a multidisciplinary team approach is necessary in the management of these children and should be the standard of practice, regardless of the physical therapist's practice setting.

The child needs to be functional within the context of his or her environment, therefore, an examination of the child's functional level is as important as the respiratory and neuromotor assessments that the physical therapist would typically perform. The functional examination should include age-appropriate basic and instrumental activities of daily living; general mobility skills; communication skills; and an assessment of the child's role within the family and within the relevant environment. At the very least, the functional assessment provides an indication of how well the child is integrated into the family and community lifestyle.

Haley and colleagues (1993) stress the significance of assessing motor skills during spontaneous activity and of obtaining parental impressions of function. Their emphasis on functional considerations is translated into the recommendation that the environment and social context be an essential part of any examination to determine the nature of the child's activity limitations and participation. The child requiring assisted ventilation exemplifies this concept because it would be impossible to isolate the effects of the restrictive environment in an examination of the child's sensorimotor development. This concept is very much congruent with the framework of the ICF in which the importance of the environment is recognized (see Chapter 30 for more on this topic).

The types of formal developmental tests used will vary with the age of the child (see Chapter 2). Although useful to some degree with this population, most developmental tests are inadequate because they fail to take into account the effects of medical and physiologic instability; long-term hospitalization; decreased mobility; and separation from typical social, emotional, and physical life experiences. As a result, the use of any standardized test requires that the therapist be familiar with the purpose of the test, its limitations, and its relevance to the outcome measures of interest. Specifically, the user needs to understand the generalizability of the test results because many assessments are normed on children without disabilities. Judgment-based assessments can provide additional information as a useful adjunct to the information obtained from standardized or criterion-based tests. Judgment-based assessments do not require observation of the *actual* performance of the motor task; however, the respondent is asked to make a judgment about the ability of the child to perform a task based on prior observations and knowledge of how the child would typically perform (Haley et al., 1993). This allows one to distinguish between what the child is capable of and how the child actually performs during day-to-day functional tasks. Parent or caregiver participation should be encouraged in the actual examination, as well as in the formulation of therapy goals (see Chapters 30 and 31).

EVALUATION AND DIAGNOSIS

Considering the complexity of impairments in many children who are ventilator dependent, the evaluation is especially important. Ideally, a multidimensional approach to the use of tests and measures should be employed and the results correlated to the relevant activity limitations and disabilities interfering with the child's quality of life. This important step in the process will be used to define the physical therapy diagnosis and to describe the specific plan of care for the child. For the child with ventilator dependence, the range of diagnoses can be quite broad. For example, the child with chronic lung disease and mechanical ventilator dependence secondary to BPD may have coexisting neurologic impairments, gastrointestinal abnormalities, and growth disturbance. The diagnosis might therefore include developmental delay, aerobic capacity and endurance limitations, and decreased repertoire of movement patterns. On the other hand, a child with the neurologic diagnosis of CCHS may be otherwise medically stable and is at risk for developmental delay only if he or she are hospitalized for a prolonged period of time. With appropriate attention to ensuring adequate and appropriate developmental intervention, these children can lead fairly typical lives. Thus, at this stage of clinical decision making, the diagnostic and prognostic determinations will vary depending on the age of the child, the severity and chronicity of the lung disease, and the coexisting diagnoses.

INTERVENTION CONSIDERATIONS

Regardless of the cause for requiring chronic mechanical ventilation, once a child is diagnosed with chronic respiratory failure and the decision is made to begin artificial ventilation, prevention and treatment of the associated complications need to be primary goals of medical and rehabilitative management. These children require early and aggressive developmental intervention.

Although the degree and intensity may vary, the intervention strategy should maximize the child's developmental and functional potential. After the acute medical condition of any of these patient groups is stabilized, considerable efforts should be aimed at promoting growth and development. In many centers, specialized units exist that exclusively serve the medical and developmental needs of infants and children who are ventilator dependent (Mallory & Stillwell, 1991; O'Brien et al., 2002; Schreiner et al., 1987). These units often attempt to provide individualized care and management while trying to maintain as normal an environment as possible.

No one intervention strategy is unanimously embraced by physical therapists for any diagnostic group. Similarly, in the case of children with ventilator dependence, physical therapy varies widely because of differing philosophies of management and the wide range of problem areas that might be identified. Thus, the intent of this section is not to prescribe specific treatment but to present a conceptual framework from which one can organize an appropriate plan of care and to emphasize considerations unique to this group of children.

Typically developing infants and children are capable of using a variable repertoire of motor skills to explore and learn. This normal acquisition of skills presumes an interaction of the cardiopulmonary and musculoskeletal systems, as well as the presence of the necessary cognitive requirements. Inactivity in children is never normal, and they usually require minimal encouragement to be active and spontaneous. In the case of a child with chronic respiratory insufficiency, however, compromised physiologic stability alone may limit the seemingly endless exploration and practice in which children typically engage. In children with a chronic illness a reduced capacity for activity or exercise can be a direct or indirect result of their underlying pathophysiologic process (Bar-Or, 1986). Regardless of the cause, a vicious circle of inactivity ensues: inactivity→ reluctance to move and explore→ decreased endurance and "fitness"→ inactivity. Another consideration is that these children may associate movement with negative experiences such as fatigue, hypoxia, and pain, which limits their "motivation" to be as active as their peers. It is not always easy to distinguish among the various factors that lead to a paucity of movement, especially in the absence of neurologic deficits.

A major goal of the physical therapist in the management of children who are dependent on ventilators should be secondary prevention, that is, to prevent deprivation of sensory and motor experiences and all the various sequelae that result from that deprivation. Regardless of the child's medical diagnosis, treatment should be aimed at providing a variety of opportunities for movement challenges and for exploration, as well as to increase their capacity for exercise. Depending on whether the child has a specific motor impairment, these goals may be accomplished with or without the use of assistive devices. For example, in the case of a child with BPD who also had an IVH, adaptive equipment may be needed for positioning because of poor antigravity trunk control, or for ambulation because of lower extremity weakness and spasticity. Alternatively, the child with CCHS and no neurologic injuries leading to motor impairments may be completely independent in all motor skills. In the context of functional limitations, exercise intolerance is certainly a problem in this group of children. Any activity in which these infants or children engage should be viewed as "exercise" and seen as a means of improving their tolerance for movement. A paucity of literature exists on the role developmental intervention plays in improving cardiopulmonary status and exercise tolerance, *in addition to* achieving developmental goals.

Simply stated, the "normal" response to exercise is an increase in heart rate, followed by a return to baseline. Ventilation also increases linearly with the metabolic rate until approximately 60% of the oxygen consumption at which time it increases more rapidly. (See Chapter 8 for a summary of the cardiorespiratory and musculoskeletal components of exercise and fitness.) These relationships, as well as the other physiologic processes that support adequate ventilation and perfusion during exercise, are altered in conditions of lung disease. Whereas exercise is normally cardiac-limited, in those with chronic lung disease exercise may be ventilatory-limited as a result of deficient exercise capacity, gas exchange, or poor pulmonary mechanics (Darbee & Cerny, 1990). Each child's specific pathophysiologic process determines the response to exercise and the capacity for improvement.

The beneficial effects of exercise have been well documented in certain populations such as those individuals with cystic fibrosis and asthma (Darbee & Cerny, 1990), but less information exists that objectively documents the effects of any type of structured exercise program on either short- or long-term outcomes of children who need assistance with ventilation. Bader and colleagues (1987) examined the long-term pulmonary sequelae and exercise tolerance of 10 children with BPD at a mean of 10 years of age. All children in the study had required either mechanical ventilation or oxygen therapy for at least 30 days. Half of the group had exercise-induced bronchospasms, but no significant differences from normal values were found in maximal oxygen consumption, suggesting that their aerobic fitness was comparable to the "normal" group. Despite similar cardiovascular function to typical children, those with BPD demon-strated pulmonary limitations to exercise evidenced by a decrease in arterial oxygen saturation and an increased $PaCO_2$. Although some of the children were mechanically ventilated for a very short time during their acute disease course, it would be erroneous to extrapolate the findings to the population of children who remain chronically dependent on mechanical ventilation. Certainly there is a need for more long-term studies to determine the effectiveness of exercise programs in this group.

One of the ultimate goals for pediatric physical therapists should be to promote the concept of lifelong fitness with our patients. Regardless of the underlying medical diagnosis there is usually no reason not to encourage some type of physical activity in children who are dependent on a ventilator. The long-term benefits of physical activity and lifelong fitness go even further than physiologic and health-related ones, but also include mental health benefits such as improved self-esteem and confidence.

In all circumstances the physical therapist needs to recognize the potential for physiologic jeopardy when implementing any intervention program with these infants and children. The amount and type of motor activities must be individualized and graded to the child's level of tolerance so that the risks associated with the physiologically immature or unstable systems are not magnified. Decisions regarding the mode, intensity, and frequency of activity should be made in conjunction with the other members of the child's medical team and modified as the disease process changes.

COMMUNICATION AND COLLABORATION

Although physical therapists play an important role in direct treatment, consultation, parent teaching, and discharge planning, they represent only one aspect of the care that children dependent on ventilators require. The lives of these children are complex, so it is imperative that they be managed by a multidisciplinary team rather than by fragmented individual service providers. Typically, the multidisciplinary team might consist of physician and nurse specialists, therapists, nutritionists, and other professionals who address the psychosocial aspects of the child and family in their community. Communication and collaboration among team members are essential to the child and family's well-being and to an understanding of the disability (Aday & Wegener, 1998). Short-term and long-term goals developed by the team should be formulated in conjunction with the family, keeping in mind the ultimate goal of maximizing function from a physical, cognitive, social-emotional, and family dynamics perspective. It is not uncommon for parents to be naive to the disease process and the implications for future function. As a protective mechanism, many parents are often overprotective of a "sick" child and actually contribute to sustaining the child's fear of movement challenges or lack of activity. Especially in relation to functional mobility and fitness, the physical therapist has an important role to play in educating the family toward maximizing the child's *abilities* rather than imposing limitations because of the child's *disabilities*. In the case of the child who is at home, this role may extend to community therapists and school personnel as well. The most effective outcomes occur when the focus of the team is on the integration of the child into the family and then, at the right time, into the community. In fact, it is the integration of the child into their community – be it their schools, play groups, structured social activities, etc.—that represents optimal outcomes when considering quality-of-life measures. This is a challenge that requires and deserves the attention of numerous professionals and the child's family (Make et al., 1998; Sevick & Bradham, 1997).

Family-centered intervention is mandated by law, in the United States, but for reasons other than legal ones the involvement of the parents and family in the life of the child with a disability is essential for optimal child development and family dynamics. Probably no situation better demonstrates the need for inclusion of the family in the child's entire care plan more than in the case of the child who is dependent on mechanical ventilation. The role of the family in shaping the child's environment to be the most conducive to learning, optimal development, and participation is crucial. More important, from a practical point of view, the child's life depends on the parents' knowledge of the intensive care needed to maintain the child's fragile life.

HOME CARE OF THE CHILD REQUIRING LONG-TERM VENTILATOR ASSISTANCE

Once the decision has been made to mechanically ventilate an infant or child for an extended length of time, immediate thoughts should be toward the long-term impact of a prolonged hospitalization. It is unfortunate that despite the well-known benefits of being in one's natural environment, far too many children with ventilator dependence stay in an ICU setting long past the point of clinical stability and readiness for discharge (Make et al., 1998). Although most would agree that it is

beneficial to have a child who is dependent on a ventilator remain at home, the impact of caring for a child with chronic medical needs and disabilities causes varying degrees of stress on families (American Thoracic Society, 1990; Noyes, 2002; Wilson & Morse, 1998). The dilemma of whether a child with ventilator dependence can be cared for at home is not made solely on the basis of medical stability. Rather, family and social supports, as well as financial resources, are as important as the medical and technical management skills that are required (Teague, 2001). The parents of a child who is dependent on mechanical ventilation also have the added burden of needing highly qualified child care resources, making leisure time or needed respite care difficult to arrange. As the degree and complexity of impairment, activity limitations, and disabilities increase, the quality of life usually decreases—especially if financial, psychosocial, and emotional supports dwindle. Keeping this in mind, one of the most important roles of the various disciplines is to work closely with family members as the child is being considered for discharge. Parents should expect the health care professionals to give them as much information as needed to make an informed decision about their abilities to care for their child at home, as well as the risks and benefits (Hewitt-Taylor, 2004). The family's coping skills and lifestyle needs should always be at the forefront of any parent-professional relationship and a major consideration of any rehabilitation program that might be recommended (Mallory & Stillwell, 1991). It is essential that the child's therapy program be integrated into the family's daily routine and not be the sole focus of the family's daily schedule.

It is imperative that the family or designated caregivers be involved in, and capable of learning, all aspects of the child's care (Edwards et al., 2004; Noyes, 2002; Make et al., 1998; Mallory & Stillwell, 1991). This care includes not only managing the ventilator and other monitoring equipment, but also being able to provide emergency medical procedures if the child experiences distress and, most important, the ability to recognize signs of distress. The high degree of medical and technologic expertise required by parents or caregivers can be a tremendous drain on a family, and it "strains the traditional conceptions of parental responsibilities" (Mallory & Stillwell, 1991). The critical nature of this type of family teaching goes beyond our normal expectations of the family unit, so caregivers need extensive support from the various team members. Parents who decide *not* to have their child cared for at home on a ventilator, or those who do not have a choice, will also need ongoing support as they continue to be parents from a distance and without the luxury of the home environment.

The reality is that home care is only possible and feasible when the financial costs and caregiver needs are adequately met (Campbell & Pierce, 1998). Unfortunately, in many instances the rate-limiting factor for discharge is the excessive amount of time it takes to process the paper trail associated with applying for home care funding (Downes & Parra, 2001). In recent years there has been a rapid growth in high-tech pediatric home care and increasing support for managing children with chronic illnesses at home (Haffner & Schurman, 2001). Changes in health care financing also reflect a greater acceptance of home care as an alternative to hospitalization. Since 1981, U.S. legislative efforts in the area of financial assistance have made it economically more feasible for families to care for children at home. The Omnibus Reconciliation Act of 1981 (OBRA) resulted in an expansion of Medicaid benefits for U.S. children by financing medical and nonmedical support services and allowing the purchase of equipment to be used in the home. It also expanded Medicaid eligibility by considering only the child's income and essentially disregarding parental income when calculating the allotment of funds. Originally, these waivers were individually approved through the Health Care Financing Administration (HCFA), but in 1982 the Medicaid Home and Community Based waiver program (also known as the Katie Beckett waiver) was developed, allowing each state to establish its own program under the waiver (Burr et al., 1983).

Provided the home is safe and nurturing, children with chronic illnesses or disabilities have a much better chance of optimal development when cared for at home. The cost of home care, although thought to be less than that of hospital care, is still high because many of the children are expected to survive well beyond early childhood. In many cases an often overlooked indirect cost is that the primary caregiver has to leave the work force to care for the child (Billeaud et al., 1992; Make et al., 1998; Office of Technology Assessment, 1987). Even in the best of situations, the burden on the family continues to be great not only because they are expected to bear some portion of the financial cost, but also because the psychologic, social, and personal resources necessary to keep a child who is dependent on technology at home are great. As a result, the cost savings often associated with home care can be attributed to the family's willingness to assume the major responsibilities for the day-to-day care of the patient (Sevick & Bradham, 1997). Despite this burden, the majority of caregivers report that caring for their child at home is less stressful than the separation of the child being hospitalized, and that they feel that they provide better care than the hospital personnel (Make et al., 1998).

SUMMARY

Because of improved medical and technologic management, the prevalence of infants and children dependent on mechanical ventilation is increasing. More than likely, the rate of medical and technologic progress will continue to exceed the strides made in the rehabilitation and prevention of disabilities and the policies that support an uncomplicated transition into the home and community.

Although physical therapists can do little to prevent chronic respiratory failure and ventilator dependence, they have an important role to play in fostering the child's development and endurance for physical activity. Uncertainty regarding the prognosis for weaning from the ventilator or a child's prognosis for a productive and independent life may persist for an extended period of time. For the family there is the additional stress relating to the child's fragile medical status and the constant possibility of sudden death if the mechanical equipment should fail. When children go home on mechanical ventilation, normal family routines are replaced with highly structured schedules with little room for spontaneity. It is essential that health care professionals present the parents with a realistic picture of the benefits, cost, and burden of caring for a child at home and help them to realize that advanced technologic capacity does not necessarily ensure or equate to a benefit for the patient or the family.

From early on in the neonatal intensive care unit (NICU) through school age, physical therapists are in a unique position to be involved with these children and families. Some aspects of care may be specific medically related interventions, such as percussion and postural drainage; however, the majority of time is spent addressing various aspects of the child's development. In dealing with any population at risk for disability, one of the major roles of the physical therapist is to integrate treatment goals into everyday activities and help the caregivers or parents appreciate the relevance of their involvement. The ecologic validity of the treatment goals increases if those goals are made a part of functionally relevant tasks.

The care of this group of children will continue to be a challenge to physical therapists and other health care professionals because they possess a wide range of impairments, activity limitations, and disabilities. The conceptual framework offered by the International Classification of Functioning, Disability and Health provides the opportunity for us to re-think how we measure the impact of chronic medical conditions on individuals. The model suggests a bidirectional impact of the environment, in addition to personal factors. Thus, the ICF provides a structure for broadening our thoughts about health and wellness, extending it to factors not only within, but external to the individual. This move away from the medical model of disease and disability will hopefully force us to think about the needs of the child with respect to their roles in their home, school, and community (Simeonsson et al., 2003).

CASE STUDY

HELENE DUMAS, MS, PT, PCS

This case illustrates the physical therapy management of a child with ventilator-dependence and several comorbidities and uses the *Guide to Physical Therapist Practice* (American Physical Therapy Association, 2001) and the ICF (WHO, 2001) as a framework for aligning the intervention strategies and supports with the problem areas.

Manny is a 2-year-old boy with chronic lung disease and history of mechanical ventilator dependence. Manny was born at 28 weeks' gestation to a 29-year-old gravida[3], para[2-3] mother. The pregnancy was remarkable for poor fetal growth for the 2 weeks prior to delivery. Upon delivery, Manny was intubated in the delivery room. Apgar scores were 4 at 1 minute and 6 at 5 minutes as Manny demonstrated increased muscle tone, respiratory rate, and heart rate. An echocardiogram revealed a large patent ductus arteriosus (PDA) that was treated successfully. A left grade III intraventricular hemorrhage and mild stage I retinopathy diagnosed at birth have reportedly resolved. A tracheostomy tube was placed at 3 months of age, as Manny was unable to be weaned from mechanical ventilation. Prior to transfer to an inpatient pediatric pulmonary rehabilitation program, Manny spent the first 4 months of his life in a neonatal intensive care unit (NICU).

The anticipated outcomes of Manny's transfer to an inpatient pediatric pulmonary rehabilitation program were (1) elimination or reduction of primary body function and structure impairments (chronic lung disease) and of secondary body function and structure impairments (altered muscle tone, decreased force production, diminished aerobic capacity and endurance, decreased tolerance to movement and tactile stimulation), (2) elimination or reduction of activity limitations (mobility, self-care, speech-language, behavior, cognition), and (3) promotion of participation in life situations (readiness for home and family life). Manny's team at the rehabilitation hospital includes his family, a pediatrician, nurse practitioner, pediatric pulmonologist, primary nurse, associate nurses, physical therapist, occupational therapist, speech-language pathologist, respiratory therapists, social worker, dietitian, case manager, pastoral care associate, and a child-life specialist.

Manny would be classified into the following physical therapy practice patterns:

Cardiovascular/Pulmonary

Practice Pattern G—Impaired ventilation, respiration/gas exchange, and aerobic capacity/endurance associated with respiratory failure in the neonate

Manny would have been originally placed in this classification of practice patterns because of his chronic lung disease. Because Practice Pattern G only includes infants up to 4 months of age, Manny would need to be reclassified into the following two patterns at his current age of 2 years:

Practice Pattern B—Impaired aerobic capacity/endurance associated with deconditioning

Practice Pattern F— Impaired ventilation, respiration/gas exchange associated with respiratory failure

Neuromuscular

Practice Pattern B—Impaired neuromotor development

Manny's physical therapy problem list and anticipated goals were developed from the projected hospitalization outcomes at admission and the results of his initial physical therapy examination and monthly reexaminations. The initial physical therapy examination at 4 months of age, and subsequent reexaminations, included a review of his current health status, progress toward projected hospitalization outcomes and physical therapy goals, and the application of physical therapy tests and measures. Tests and measures were chosen based on personal contextual factors such as Manny's age, medical diagnosis, medical history/current medical status, and functional capabilities. Tests and measures were also chosen based on environmental factors such as service delivery setting (hospital, hospital crib) and equipment (ventilator or oxygen, physiologic monitoring devices).

The following tests and measures were used:

Arousal, Attention, and Cognition/Sensory Integrity —responses to tactile, auditory and visual stimuli

Aerobic Capacity and Endurance—tolerance to physical activity using clinical signs of shortness of breath and use of pulse oximetry

Range of Motion/Posture—passive and active ROM and postural alignment in age-appropriate developmental positions

Reflex Integrity—present or emerging reflexes and reactions

Muscle Performance—axial and appendicular muscle tone assessed in gravity-eliminated and antigravity positions

Motor Function/Neuromotor Development and Sensory Integration—voluntary postures and movement patterns, a developmental checklist of motor performance

Assistive and Adaptive Devices

The child-related/personal factors influencing Manny's recovery included his neuromuscular and cardiopulmonary impairments. In general, the environmental factors influencing Manny's functioning include his dependence on pulmonary support (mechanical ventilation and oxygen) and his extended hospitalization. Manny was given a physical therapy diagnosis of developmental delay (Practice Pattern 5B).

Manny's history of ventilator assistance includes placement on an LP6 continuous PPV at 3 months of age. Manny was weaned from mechanical ventilation by gradually decreasing the pressure and number of assisted breaths per minute, while gas exchange and other clinical indicators (i.e., respiratory rate, oxygen saturation) were carefully monitored. Manny was dependent on the ventilator 24 hours per day until 18 months of age when he progressed to using oxygen mist via a tracheostomy collar as the length of time off his ventilator each day was increased. Gas exchange and other clinical indicators (i.e., respiratory rate, oxygen saturation) were carefully monitored. Manny progressed to the use of oxygen mist during waking hours and then to using oxygen mist 24 hours per day with oxygen saturation remaining above 95% as measured by pulse oximetry. Presently, at 2 years of age, Manny is progressing to using a heat moisture exchanger (HME) over his tracheostomy when not using his oxygen mist. At 2 years of age, a smaller tracheostomy tube was tried but Manny was unable to tolerate the downsizing (exhibiting an increased respiratory rate, decreased oxygen saturations) and required that the larger tracheostomy tube continue to be used at the present time.

Using the ICF as a framework, Table 26-6 provides an overview of Manny's cardiopulmonary and physical functioning since his admission to the inpatient pulmonary rehabilitation program.

Manny has been receiving physical therapy intervention up to three times per week since admission to the inpatient rehabilitation program. Manny's *current* problem list and goals and objectives are shown in Table 26-7.

The physical therapist interventions utilized as part of Manny's current treatment plan include the following:

a. Coordination, communication, and documentation, with physical therapist participation

b. Patient care rounds; case conferences; family/team meetings; hospital discharge planning; medical record documentation

c. Patient/client-related instruction: instruction and education of family and other rehabilitation team members regarding body functions and structures, activity limitations and participation restrictions; risk factors (i.e., aerobic capacity and endurance); physical therapy plan of care including positions for play and feeding, activities and equipment for promotion of muscle strength and ambulation; and equipment use

d. Therapeutic exercise: developmental activities training; task-specific performance training; flexibility exercises; active, active assistive, active and resisted exercises; balance and coordination training; body-weight-supported treadmill training; gait and locomotion training

e. Functional training in self-care and home management: bed mobility and transfer training (sit ↔ quadruped, sit ↔ stand)

f. Prescription, application, and as appropriate, fabrication of devices and equipment: seating systems (highchair, stroller, walker)

g. Environmental adaptation: maximize positioning and mobility options limited by hospital crib, length of ventilator and oxygen tubing and safety monitoring equipment (pulse oximeter)

h. Airway clearance techniques: chest percussion, vibration, postural drainage, and suctioning are used by physical therapist in conjunction with the nursing and respiratory staff to manage Manny's airway

Manny was admitted to the inpatient pediatric pulmonary rehabilitation program and it was anticipated that Manny would wean from his mechanical ventilation. In this case, Manny's decreased dependence on pulmonary support paralleled his gains in physical functioning. The decrease in pulmonary support from mechanical ventilation to oxygen mist lessened Manny's environmental barriers (short tubing and being restricted to a hospital crib) and minimized his personal barriers (decreased aerobic capacity and endurance) to promote increased mobility.

Physical therapy is projected to continue throughout Manny's hospitalization to continue to promote Manny's physical functioning. Manny's projected discharge

TABLE 26-6	Manny's Cardiopulmonary and Physical Functioning

AGE	FUNCTIONING AND DISABILITY	CONTEXTUAL FACTORS
4 months	Easily stressed (inaudible cry, distress noted by facial expression, oxygen desaturations) with movement; increased truncal arching at rest; actively moving all extremities, lifts head briefly when held at caregiver's shoulder	*Environment*—hospital inpatient with multiple caretakers, excessive noise and lighting, frequent medical interventions, mobility limited by ventilator tubing and cardiac and pulse oximetry wiring, positioning in crib and infant seat
6 months	Easily stressed as described above; actively turning head side to side	*Personal*—age, inaudible cry, tracheostomy and gastrostomy tubes in place limiting prone positioning, frequent family visits
9 months	Rolling side to supine; lifts head if propped in prone with support under chest	*Environment*—as above, now able to be placed in infant swing and high chair outside of crib *Personal*—as above
1 year	No longer exhibiting stress signals, tolerant of handling and movement, maintains sitting when placed (using arms for propping), able to lift one arm off of the supporting surface; maintains quadruped when placed; assists supine to sit transition	*Environment*—continues as hospital inpatient; beginning to participate in physical therapy when on oxygen mist via tracheostomy collar allowing for increased distance with movement (including provision of physical therapy in unit playroom) *Personal*—as above, increasing distractibility
15 months	Rolls side to prone; maintains standing with assist when placed (demonstrates lower extremity hypertonia)	
18 months	Transitioning sit to quadruped; creeping with assist; bouncing in standing (decreased lower extremity hypertonia to maintain upright posture); cruises with assist	*Environment*—continues as hospital inpatient; on oxygen mist via tracheostomy collar allowing for movement around unit with caregivers using stroller *Personal*—as above
21 months	Creeping independently; cruising independently; pulling to stand in crib; beginning to take forward step with hands held	*Environment*—continues as hospital inpatient; continuing improved respiratory status—on oxygen mist via tracheostomy collar allowing for use of body-weight-supported treadmill training off of nursing unit in physical therapy department
2 years current status	Independent ambulation with high guard; wide base of support; creeping up/down stairs (Fig. 26-2)	*Environment*—continues as hospital inpatient but able to be out of room off of hospital unit with trained caregiver *Personal*—continuing improved respiratory status; able to leave oxygen mist on unit when with trained caregiver

disposition is home to the care of his family with medical, educational, and social support services. At the time of hospital discharge, Manny will be referred for physical therapy at home or at school to continue to promote motor function and to address personal and environmental barriers to Manny's current level of physical functioning and health.

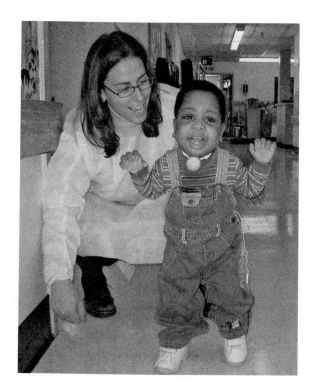

◆ **Figure 26-2** At 2 years of age, Manny is beginning to ambulate independently. Manny displays a high guard position of his upper extremities and a wide base of support. Around his neck are his tracheostomy ties with the heat moisture exchanger (HME) in place over his tracheostomy tube.

TABLE 26-7	Manny's Current Problems and Goals

PROBLEMS	GOALS AND OBJECTIVES
Body functions and structure: Decreased force production of axial and appendicular musculature in antigravity positions with lower extremity extensor muscle hypertonia	Goal: Promote stability and mobility in antigravity positions without use of hypertonia for stability in trunk and extremity extensor musculature Short-term objective: Manny will stand unsupported for up to 10 seconds with the supervision of the physical therapist or a caregiver trained to promote safety and assess respiratory response to physical activity
Body functions and structure: Diminished aerobic capacity and endurance	Goal: Maximize aerobic capacity and endurance for mobility and self-care tasks Short-term objective: Manny will participate in physical therapy activities as outlined in the plan of care without oxygen saturation declining below preset levels of 95% as measured by pulse oximetry
Activity limitation: Delayed motor development and mobility (Figs. 26-3 and 26-4)	Goal: Promote age-appropriate motor and mobility skills Short-term objective: Manny will take 1 or 2 unsupported steps with the guarding of the physical therapist or a caregiver trained to promote safety and assess respiratory response to physical activity Short-term objective: Manny will ambulate up to 50 feet with one hand held once per day with the physical therapist or a caregiver trained to promote safety and assess respiratory response to physical activity
Participation restriction: Limited mobility for participation in hospital environment secondary to ventilator and oxygen equipment, safety monitoring and caregiver supervision needs (Fig. 26-5)	Goal: Instruct caregivers (family and program staff) to promote safety and assess respiratory response to physical activity with ambulation activities Goal: Provide appropriate equipment for mobility (walker) and positioning (highchair) to promote participation with family and program staff

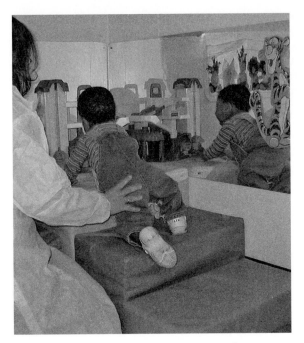

◆ **Figure 26-3**   Uneven surfaces are a new phenomenon for Manny after spending most of his early life in a hospital crib. In this picture, Manny is learning to creep up the stairs with the help of his physical therapist.

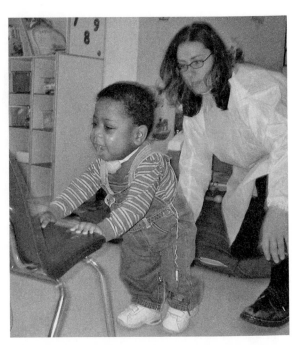

◆ **Figure 26-4**   At approximately 18 months of age, children typically will climb into a chair without assistance. At 2 years of age, when presented with a child-size chair, Manny did not attempt to climb up onto the chair but began to push it as if it were a push toy or an assistive device for ambulation. The only chairs Manny has used are a highchair and a stroller, and he has always been lifted by a caregiver from his crib to one of these two seats.

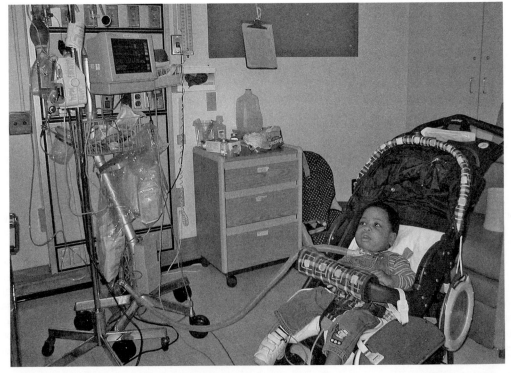

◆ **Figure 26-5**   Manny in his stroller in his hospital room with his oxygen mist, gastrostomy tube feeding, and cardiac and respiratory monitors connected. The oxygen mist tubing is approximately twice as long as his ventilator tubing used to be, thus significantly limiting his mobility within his crib and within his room.

References

Ambrosio, IU, Woo, MS, Jansen, MT, & Keens, TG. Safety of hospitalized ventilator-dependent children outside of the intensive care unit. Pediatrics, 101(2):257–259, 1998.

American Physical Therapy Association. Guide to Physical Therapist Practice, 2nd ed. Physical Therapy 81(1). 2001.

American Thoracic Society. Home mechanical ventilation of pediatric patients. American Review of Respiratory Disease, 141:258–259, 1990.

American Thoracic Society. Idiopathic Congenital Central Hypoventilation Syndrome. American Journal of Respiratory Critical Care Medicine, 160:368–373, 1999.

Amin, R, & Fitton, C. Tracheostomy and home ventilation in children. Seminars in Neonatal Medicine, 8:127–135, 2003.

Anzueto, A, Peters, J, Tobin, M, de los Santos, R, Seidenfeld, J, Moore, G, Cox, W, & Coalson, J. Effects of prolonged controlled mechanical ventilation on diaphragmatic function in healthy adult baboons. Critical Care Medicine, 25:1187–1190, 1997.

Attar, MA, & Donn, SM. Mechanisms of ventilator-induced lung injury in premature infants. Seminars in Neonatal Medicine, 7:353–360, 2002.

Bader, David, Ramos, Angela D, Lew, Cheryl D, Platzker, Arnold CG, Stabile, Michael W, & Keens, Thomas G. Childhood sequelae of infant lung disease: Exercise and pulmonary function abnormalities after bronchopulmonary dysplasia. Journal of Pediatrics, 110(5):693–699, 1987.

Bai, D, & Bertenthal, B. Locomotor status and the development of spatial search skills. Child Development, 63:215–226, 1992.

Bancalari, Eduardo, & Sosenko, Ilene. Pathogenesis and prevention of neonatal chronic lung disease: Recent developments. Pediatric Pulmonology, 8:109–116, 1990.

Bar-Or, O. Pathophysiologic factors which limit the exercise capacity of the sick child. Medicine and Sport Science, 18:276–282, 1986.

Barbosa, V, Campbell, S, Sheftel, D, Singh, J, & Beligere, N. Longitudinal performance of infants with cerebral palsy on the Test of Infant Motor Performance and on the Alberta Infant Motor Scale. Physical & Occupational Therapy in Pediatrics, 23(3):7–29, 2003.

Billeaud, Claude, Piedboeuf, Bruno, & Chessex, Philippe. Clinical and Laboratory Observations: Energy expenditure and severity of respiratory disease in very low birth weight infants receiving long-term ventilatory support. Journal of Pediatrics, 120(3):461–464, 1992.

Bos, AE, Martijn, A, van Asperen, RM, et al. Qualitative assessment of general movements in high-risk preterm infants with chronic lung disease requiring dexamethasone therapy. Journal of Pediatrics, 132(2):300–306, 1998.

Bozynski, Mary Ellen A, Nelson, Michael M, Matalon, Terence AS, O'Donnell, Karen J, et al. Prolonged mechanical ventilation and intracranial hemorrhage: impact on developmental progress through 18 months in infants weighing 1200 grams or less at birth. Pediatrics, 79(5):670–676, 1987.

Branson, R. Understanding and implementing advances in ventilator capabilities. Current Opinion in Critical Care, 10:23–32, 2004.

Bregman, Joanne, & Farrell, Elaine E. Neurodevelopmental outcome in infants with bronchopulmonary dysplasia. Clinics in Perinatology, 19(3):673–694, 1992.

Bureau, M, & Begin, R. Chest wall diseases and dysfunction in children. In Kendig E, & Chernick, V (Eds.). Disorders of the Respiratory Tract in Children. Philadelphia: WB Saunders, 1983, pp. 606–616.

Burr, B, Guyer, B, Todres, I, Abrahams, B, & Chiodo, T. Home care for children on respirators. New England Journal of Medicine, 21:319–1323, 1983.

Campbell, D, & Pierce, R. Long term ventilatory support at home: Any progress? Medical Journal of Australia, 168:7–8, 1998.

Chatburn, R. A new system for understanding mechanical ventilators. Respiratory Care, 36:1123–1155, 1991.

Chatburn, RL, & Primiano FP Jr. A new system for understanding modes of mechanical ventilation. Respiratory Care, 46(6):604–621, 2001.

Cheifetz, Ira M. Invasive and noninvasive pediatric mechanical ventilation. Respiratory Care, 48(4):442–453, 2003.

Coalson, JJ. Pathology of new bronchopulmonary dysplasia. Seminars in Neonatal Medicine, 8:73–81, 2003.

Criner, Gerard J, Tzouanakis, Alexander, & Kreimer, Diane T. Overview of improving tolerance of long-term mechanical ventilation. Critical Care Clinics, 10(4):845–863, 1994.

Cutz, E, Ma, TKF, Perrin, DG, Moore, AM, & Becker, LE. Peripheral chemoreceptors in congenital central hypoventilation syndrome. American Journal of Respiratory and Critical Care Medicine, 155:358–363, 1997.

Darbee, J, & Cerny, F. Exercise testing and exercise conditioning for children with lung dysfunction. In Irwin, S, & Tecklin, J (Eds.). Cardiopulmonary Physical Therapy. St. Louis: Mosby, 1990, pp. 461–476.

DeCesare, J, & Graybill, C. Physical therapy for the child with respiratory dysfunction. In Irwin, S, & Tecklin, J (Eds.). Cardiopulmonary Physical Therapy. St. Louis: Mosby, 1990, pp. 417–460.

deMeer, K, Westerterp, K, Houwen, R, Brouwers, H, Berger, R, & Okken, A. Total energy expenditure in infants with bronchopulmonary dysplasia is associated with respiratory status. European Journal of Pediatrics, 156:299–304, 1997.

Dick, C, & Sassoon, C. Patient-ventilator interactions. Clinics in Chest Medicine, 17:423–438, 1996.

Donn, SM, & Sinha, SK. Newer techniques of mechanical ventilation: An overview. Seminars in Neonatology, 7:401–407, 2002.

Dougherty, J. Negative pressure devices in pediatric practice. Pediatric Nursing, 16:135–138, 1990.

Downes, John J, & Parra, MM. Costs and reimbursement issues in long-term mechanical ventilation of patients at home. In Hill, NS. 1(152), 353–374. 2001. New York, Marcel Dekker.

Edwards, EA, O'Toole, M, & Wallis, C. Sending children home on tracheostomy dependent ventilation: Pitfalls and outcomes. Archives of Disease in Childhood, 89:251–255, 2004.

Elixson, E Marsha, Myrer, Mary L, & Horn, Mary H. Current trends in ventilation of the pediatric patient. Critical Care Nurse, 20(1):1–13, 1997.

Farrell, P, & Fost, N. Long-term mechanical ventilation in pediatric respiratory failure: Medical and ethical considerations. American Review of Respiratory Disease, 140:S36–S40, 1989.

Gali, B, & Goyal, D. Positive pressure mechanical ventilation. Emergency Medicine Clinics of North America, 21:453–473, 2003.

Gannon, Catherine M, Wiswell, Thomas E, & Spitzer, Alan R. Volutrauma, $PaCO_2$ levels, and neurodevelopmental sequelae following assisted ventilation. Clinics in Perinatology, 25(1):159–175, 1998.

Goldsmith, J, & Karotkin, E. Assisted ventilation of the neonate. Philadelphia: WB Saunders, 1988.

Gould, A. cardiopulmonary evaluation of the infant, toddler, child and adolescent. Pediatric Physical Therapy, 3:9–13, 1991.

Gozal, David, Shoseyov, David, & Keens, Thomas G. Inspiratory pressures with CO_2 stimulation and weaning from mechanical ventilation in children. American Review of Respiratory Disease, 147:256–261, 1993.

Gracey, DR, & Hubmayr, RD. Weaning from long-term mechanical ventilation. In Hill, NS. 1(152), 431–448. 2001. New York, Marcel Dekker.

Gregoire, Marie-Claude, Lefebvre, Francine, & Glorieux, Jacqueline. Health and developmental outcomes at 18 months in very preterm infants with bronchopulmonary dysplasia. Pediatrics, *101*(5):856–860, 1998.

Haffner, J, & Schurman, S. The technology-dependent child. Pediatric Clinics of North America, *48*:751–764, 2001.

Haley, S, Baryza, M, & Blanchard, Y. Functional and naturalistic frameworks in assessing physical and motor disablement. In Wilhelm, I (Ed.). Physical Therapy Assessment in Early Infancy. New York: Churchill Livingstone, 1993, pp. 225–256.

Hess, Dean. Ventilator modes used in weaning. Chest, 120:474S–476S, 2001.

Hess, DR. Mechanical ventilation strategies: What's new and what's worth keeping? Respiratory Care, *47*(9):1007–1017, 2002.

Hewitt-Taylor, Jaqui. Children who require long-term ventilation: Staff education and training. Intensive and Critical Care Nursing, *20*:93–102, 2004.

Huysman, WA, Ridder, M de, Bruin, NC, Helmond, G, Terpstra, N, Goudoever, JB, & Sauer, PJJ. Growth and body composition in preterm infants with bronchopulmonary dysplasia. Archives of Disease in Childhood Fetal Neonatal Ed 88:F46–F51, 2003.

Jobe, Alan H, & Bancalari, Eduardo. Bronchopulmonary dysplasia. American Journal of Respiratory Critical Care Medicine, *163*: 1723–1729, 2001.

Kercsmar, CM. Current trends in neonatal and pediatric respiratory care: Conference Summary. Respiratory Care, *48*(4):459–464, 2003.

Knisely, AS, Leal, Susana M, & Singer, DB. Abnormalities of diaphragmatic muscle in neonates with ventilated lungs. Journal of Pediatrics, *113*(6):1074–1077, 1988.

Kondili, E, Prinianakis, G, & Georgopoulos, D. Patient-ventilator interaction. British Journal of Anaesthesia, *91*(1):106–119, 2003.

Kornhauser, MS, Baumgart, S, Desai, SA, Stanley, CW, Culbane, J, Cullen, JA, Wiswell, Thomas E, Graziani, LJ, & Spitzer, Alan R. Adverse neurodevelopmental outcome after extracorporeal membrane oxygenation among neonates with bronchopulmonary dysplasia. Journal of Pediatrics, *132*(2):307–311, 1998.

Kurzner, Sharon I, Garg, Meena, Bautista, Daisy B, Sargent, Charles W, Bowman, Michael, & Keens, Thomas G. Growth failure in bronchopulmonary dysplasia: Elevated metabolic rates and pulmonary mechanics. Journal of Pediatrics, *112*(1):73–80, 1988.

Luce, John M. Reducing the use of mechanical ventilation. The New England Journal of Medicine, *335*(25):1916–1917, 1996.

MacKinnon J, Perlman M, Kirpalani H, Rehan V, Sauve R, & Kovacs L. Spinal cord injury at birth: Diagnostic and prognostic data in twenty-two patients. Journal of Pediatrics, *122*:431–437, 1993.

Make, BJ. Epidemiology of long-term ventilatory assistance. In Hill, NS. Long-term mechanical ventilation. 1(1), 1–18. 2001. New York, Marcel Dekker.

Make, B, Hill, N, Goldberg, AI, Bach, J, Criner, GJ, Dunne, P, Gilmartin, M, Heffner, JE, Kacmarek, R, Keens, T, McInturff, S, O'Donohue, W, Oppenheimer, E, & Dominique, R. Mechanical ventilation beyond the intensive care unit: Report of a consensus conference of the American College of Chest Physicians. Chest, *113*:289–344, 1998.

Mallory, George B Jr, & Stillwell, Paul C. The ventilator-dependent child: Issues in diagnosis and management. Archives of Physical Medicine and Rehabilitation, *72*:43–55, 1991.

McPherson, S. Respiratory Care Equipment. St. Louis: Mosby, 1995.

Mentro, A. Health care policy for medically fragile children. Journal of Pediatric Nursing, *18*:225–232, 1995.

Navalesi, Paolo, & Costa, Roberta. New modes of mechanical ventilation: Proportional assist ventilation, neurally adjusted ventilatory assist, and fractal ventilation. Current Opinion in Critical Care, 9:51–58, 2003.

Northway, William H Jr. Observations on bronchopulmonary dysplasia. Journal of Pediatrics, 95(5, part 2):815–817, 1979.

Noyes, J. Barriers that delay children and young people who are dependent on mechanical ventilators from being discharged from hospital. Journal of Clinical Nursing, 11:2–11, 2002.

Null, D, Berman, L, & Clark, R. Neonatal and pediatric ventilatory support. In Kirby, R, Banner, M, & Downs, JB (Eds.). Clinical Applications of Ventilatory Support. New York: Churchill Livingstone, 1990, pp. 199–238.

O'Brien, JE, Dumas, HM, Haley, SM, O'Neil, ME, Renn, M, Bartolacci, TE, & Kharasch, VS. Clinical findings and resource use of infants and toddlers dependent on oxygen and ventilators. Clinical Pediatrics, *41*(3):155–162, 2002.

O'Brien, ME, & Wegner, CB. Rearing the Child Who Is Technology Dependent: Perceptions of Parents and Home Care Nurses. J Spec Pediatr Nursing, *7*(1):7–15, 2002.

O'Shea, T Michael, Goldstein, Donald J, deReginier, Raye-Ann, Sheaffer, Christopher I, Roberts, Dia D, & Dillard, Robert G. Outcome at 4 to 5 years of age in children recovered from neonatal chronic lung disease. Developmental Medicine and Child Neurology, *38*:830–839, 1996.

Office of Technology Assessment. Technology Dependent Children: Home vs Hospital Care. A Technical Memorandum. Washington, D.C.: U.S. Government Printing Office, 1987.

Pagtakhan, R, & Chernick, V. Intensive care for respiratory disorders. In Kendig, E, & Chernick, V (Eds.). Disorders of the Respiratory Tract in Children. Philadelphia: WB Saunders, 1983, pp. 145–168.

Perel, A, & Stock, M. Introduction to ventilatory support. In Perel, A, & Stock, M (Eds.). Handbook of Mechanical Ventilatory Support. Baltimore: Williams & Wilkins, 1992, pp. 3–6.

Pilmer, Sharon L. Prolonged mechanical ventilation in children. Respiratory Medicine II, *41*(3):473–512, 1994.

Rezaie, P, & Dean, A. Periventricular leukomalacia, inflammation and white matter lesions within the developing nervous system. Neuropathology, *22*:106–132, 2002.

Robin, Beverley, Kim, Young-Jee, Huth, Jaimee, Klocksieben, Jim, Torres, Margaret, & Tepper, Robert. Pulmonary function in bronchopulmonary dysplasia. Pediatric Pulmonology, *37*:236–242, 2004.

Rodriguez, Ricardo J. Management of respiratory distress syndrome: An update. Respiratory Care, *48*(3):279–287, 2003.

Roussos, C. Ventilatory failure and respiratory muscles. Lung Biology in Health and Disease, *29*:1253–1279, 1985.

Schreiner, MS, Downes, John J, Kettrick, Robert G, & Ise, C. Chronic respiratory failure in infants with prolonged ventilator dependency. JAMA, *258*(23):3396–3404, 1987.

Sevick, M, & Bradham, D. Economic cost of home-based care for ventilator-assisted individuals. Heart and Lung, *26*:148–157, 1997.

Shneerson, JM. Techniques in mechanical ventilation: Principles and practice. Thorax, *51*:756–761, 1996.

Silvestri, J, Chen, M, Weese-Mayer, D, McQuitty, J, Carveth, H, Nielson, D, Borowitz, D, & Cerny, F. Idiopathic congenital central hypoventilation syndrome: The next generation. American Journal of Medical Genetics, *112*:46–50, 2002.

Simeonsson, RJ, Leonard, M, Lollar, D, Bjorck-Akesson, E, Hollenweger, J, & Martinuzzi, A. Applying the International Classification of Functioning, Disability and Health (ICF) to measure childhood disability. Disability and Rehabilitation, 25(11):602–610, 2003.

Simonds, A. Home ventilation. European Respiratory Journal Supplement, *47*:38–46, 2003.

Singer, Lynn, Yamashita, Toyoko, Lilien, Lawrence, Collin, Marc, & Baley, Jill. A longitudinal study of development outcome of infants with bronchopulmonary dysplasia and very low birth weight. Pediatrics, *100*(6):987–993, 1997.

Soll, RF. Synthetic surfactant treatment for respiratory distress in preterm infants. Cochrane Database Systematic Review, (2):CD001149, 2000.

Teague, WG. Long term mechanical ventilation in infants and children. In Hill, NS. Long-term mechanical ventilation. 1(8), 177–214. 2001. New York, Marcel Dekker.

Tobin, Martin J. Advances in Mechanical Ventilation. New England Journal of Medicine, *344*(26):1986–1996, 2001.

Trang, H, Boureghda, S, Denjoy, I, & Kabaker, M. 24-hour BP control in children with congenital central hypoventilation syndrome. Chest, *124*:1393–1399, 2003.

Tremolieres, F. Description of a ventilator. In Lemaire, F (Ed.). Mechanical Ventilation. New York: Springer-Verlag, 1991, pp. 3–18.

Viscardi, RM, Muhumuza, CK, Rodriguez, A, Fairchild, KD, Sun, CC, Gross, GW, Campbell, AB, Wilson, PD, Hester, L, & Hasday, JD. Inflammatory markers in intrauterine and fetal blood and cerebrospinal fluid compartments are associated with adverse pulmonary and neurologic outcomes in preterm infants. Pediatric Research, *55*(6):1009–1017, 2004.

Wang, K, & Barnard, A. Technology-dependent children and their families: A review. Journal of Advanced Nursing, *45*:36–46, 2004.

Waring, W. The history and physical examination. In Kendig, E, & Chernick, V (Eds.). Disorders of the Respiratory Tract in Children. Philadelphia: WB Saunders, 1983, pp. 57–78.

Watchko, Jon F, Maycock, Dennis E, Standaert, Thomas A, & Woodrum, David E. The Ventilatory Pump: Neonatal and Developmental Issues. St. Louis: Mosby YearBook, 1991, pp. 109–134.

Weese-Mayer, DE, Silvestri, JM, Menzies, LJ, et al. Congenital central hypoventilation syndrome: Diagnosis, management, and long-term outcome in thirty-two children. Journal of Pediatrics, *120*:381–387, 1992.

Weinstein M, & Oh, W. Oxygen consumption in infants with BPD. Pediatrics, *99*:958–961, 1981.

Wilson, S, & Morse, JM. Absolute involvement: the experience of mothers of ventilator-dependent children. Health and Social Care in the Community, *6*(4):224–233, 1998.

Woo, MS, Woo, MA, Gozal, D, Jansen, MT, Keens, TG, & Harper, RM. Heart rate variability in congenital central hypoventilation syndrome. Pediatric Research, *31*(3):291–296, 1992.

World Health Organization. International Classification of Impairments, Disabilities and Health. Geneva: World Health Organization, 2001.

Yu, VYH, Orgill, AA, Lim, SB, Bajuk, B, & Astbury, J. Growth and development of very low birthweight infants recovering from bronchopulmonary dysplasia. Archives of Disease in Childhood, *58*:791–794, 1983.

Chapter 27

CX

CYSTIC FIBROSIS

JENNIFER L. AGNEW
BScPT

JO A. ASHWELL
BScPT, BHK

SHARI L. RENAUD
BHScPT, BKIN

Cystic fibrosis (CF) was first defined as a clinical entity over 60 years ago when Andersen published a paper describing the clinical course of a number of children who had died of pulmonary and digestive problems. She labeled the disorder "cystic fibrosis of the pancreas" (Andersen, 1938). This disease was thereafter classified as a disorder of exocrine gland function, influencing the respiratory system, pancreas, reproductive organs, and sweat glands. At times the first presenting sign has been the subjective report "my child tastes salty to kiss"; the "sweat test" often confirms the diagnosis. Subsequent study and interest led to clearer understanding of the disease and a coordinated approach to treating the

associated impairments. Over time the disorder that had so intrigued Andersen has come to be known as cystic fibrosis, and research has continued, yielding a vast knowledge base about this chronic illness. In 1989 a major scientific breakthrough occurred with discovery of the precise locus on chromosome 7 of the gene responsible for CF (Riordan et al., 1989). Investigations and research have followed to define the pathologic basis of the physical manifestations of CF.

Although at present the time-honored definition of this disease as the most commonly inherited life-shortening illness in the white population remains appropriate, our present growing understanding of CF may prove to temper its impact. More research must be done before treatment may allow people with CF to lead lives free of the complications currently implicit in this diagnosis. Current management of the manifestations of CF has, however, promoted improved quality of life and a better prognosis for life expectancy for people with CF (MacLusky & Levison, 1998).

Classified as a hereditary disease, CF has long been understood to be inherited in an autosomal recessive pattern (MacLusky & Levison, 1998). Two copies of the gene responsible for CF are inherited by an affected individual. Both parents of a child diagnosed with CF are, therefore, known to be carriers of at least one copy of a mutation at the gene locus responsible for CF. Those persons with one copy of the CF gene are termed *heterozygote carriers* and are not diagnostically positive for CF.

CF is diagnosed in 1 in 2500 children born to white parents, and statistical analysis of this incidence yields a best estimate of the rate of heterozygote carriers as about 5% of the population in areas of the world where significant white populations have settled (Boucher et al., 2000). The incidence of CF in black and Asian peoples is considerably lower than that in whites—approximately 1 in 17,000 births in the black population and an estimated 1 in 90,000 births in Asian societies (Boucher et al., 2000). Recent research and new possibilities for carrier screening are producing more precise statistical estimates of the actual incidence of individuals who are heterozygote CF carriers, suggesting that previous rates were underestimated (Witt et al., 1992). Prenatal diagnosis of CF is now sometimes possible, as is screening for carrier status, which is discussed in detail later in this chapter.

The identification in 1989 of the site of the gene responsible for CF by an international team of researchers, led by Drs. Tsui, Collins, and Riordan, was an extraordinary achievement in molecular genetics (Kerem et al., 1989). Subsequent research advances in numerous laboratories worldwide have yielded an unprecedented quantity of data on the genetic and pathologic components of CF. Over 1000 distinct mutations within the CF gene have been identified (Brennan & Geddes, 2004). A specific trinucleotide deletion (delta-F508, resulting in the loss of phenylalanine from the product protein) is the most common mutation associated with clinical CF, identified in 66% of more than 20,000 patients with CF analyzed worldwide (Boucher et al., 2000). Various degrees of disease expression are associated with the different mutations, and significant variability exists in the incidence of the different mutations in ethnic populations (MacLusky & Levison, 1998).

The nature of the disease, its multisystemic involvement, and the variety of needs of affected individuals and their families dictate that professional intervention in the management of CF is generally concentrated in regional CF clinics. Comprehensive treatment programs for CF were established over 45 years ago (Doershuk et al., 1964) and are now the primary mode of delivery of associated health care needs. CF centers can offer their clients the services of respirologists, gastroenterologists, physical therapists, dietitians, psychologic and genetic counselors, social workers, and specialty care nursing personnel. These multidisciplinary teams are dedicated to the delivery of the most effective and palatable treatments available in promoting the optimal level of well-being for their patients with CF. The team can offer crucial support to affected families. Worldwide, CF centers are also dedicated to the collaborative process, as clinical expertise and the knowledge base expand to suggest new possibilities in the treatment of this disease and new hopes for an ultimate cure.

In this chapter considerations for choosing appropriate intervention for patients with CF are outlined. An increasing number of people with CF are reaching the third and even fourth decades of life (Orenstein, 2003), with a few patients living into their 60s and 70s (Boucher et al., 2000). Surgical advances in lung transplantation offer hope of prolonging life for people with chronic pulmonary disabilities. Physical therapists are serving an expanded role in management programs for people with CF. It is of crucial importance that clinical decisions be directed by careful consideration of the available scientific evidence and that therapists continue to seek out the means to scientifically evaluate empiric experiences. A clear understanding of the pathophysiology, etiology, diagnostic indicators, methods of examination, and medical management is essential for the physical therapist working with the CF population to ensure a comprehensive incorporation of the issues in developing management strategies and goals. A discussion of the evolution of self-management through infancy, for preschool and school-age children, and during adolescence and adulthood is included. Improving adherence to a plan of care through the promotion of self-efficacy may prove to enhance the effectiveness of treatment and help prevent or delay the onset of disability characteristic of this disorder. As a result, well-being and improved quality of life will be promoted.

PATHOPHYSIOLOGY

The primary pathologic feature of CF is obstruction of mucus-secreting exocrine glands by hyperviscous secretions (MacLusky et al., 1987). Blockage of exocrine gland products prevents their delivery to target tissues and organs and creates clinical abnormalities in these body systems. The most impaired organs are the lungs and pancreas, with significant involvement of the reproductive system, sinuses, and sweat glands. An elevated level of sodium chloride in the sweat has been the principal diagnostic indicator for CF for more than 50 years (MacLusky & Levison, 1998).

The pulmonary impairments of CF are characterized by accumulation of hyperviscous secretions leading to progressive airway obstruction, secondary infection by opportunistic bacteria, inflammation, and subsequent bronchiectasis and irreversible airway damage. Airways may be further obstructed by bronchoconstriction. Impaired respiratory muscle function under conditions of malnutrition and weakness or deconditioning also has an impact on progression of the functional limitations of the respiratory system in patients with CF, as does the mechanical disadvantage that results from chronic lung hyperinflation.

The obstruction of the small airways in CF and subsequent air trapping and atelectasis result in ventilation and perfusion mismatching, which leads to hypoxemia. Long-standing hypoxemia may result in pulmonary artery hypertension and cor pulmonale or right ventricular failure. Large airway bronchiectasis combined with small airway obstruction reduces vital capacity and tidal volume and results in decreased volumes of airflow at the alveolar level and a progressively increasing arterial carbon dioxide tension ($PaCO_2$), which may lead to hypercapnic respiratory failure (Yankaskas, 1992). Respiratory failure accounts for 95% of the mortality rate in CF (Orenstein, 2003).

Viscous secretions begin to obstruct the pancreatic duct in utero, and periductal inflammation and fibrosis cause the loss of the pancreatic exocrine function. The resulting maldigestion of fats and protein leaves the pancreatic-insufficient patient with clinical steatorrhea (Durie et al., 1984); the stools are described as bulky, frequent, and "greasy" and, perhaps most noticeably, as having a strongly offensive odor. In infancy, patients with CF can display evidence of protein-calorie malnutrition with a protruding abdomen, muscle wasting, and initial diagnosis of failure to thrive despite the reports from parents of these children's hearty appetites (MacLusky & Levison, 1998). Compensating for loss of pancreatic function remains a critical feature of management throughout these children's lives.

Another pathologic finding that presents in 10% to 15% of diagnosed cases of CF is meconium ileus, which is demonstrated in neonates (Park & Grand, 1981). The combination of abnormal pancreatic function and hyperviscous secretions of the intestinal glands creates an altered viscosity of the meconium causing an obstruction at the distal ileum, thus preventing passage of meconium in the first neonatal days (MacLusky & Levison, 1998). Distal intestinal obstruction is seen in some older patients, associated with abnormal intestinal secretions and increased adherence of mucus in the intestines (Durie, 1988).

Abnormal secretions may cause hepatobiliary involvement, recurrent pancreatitis, and, for about 13% to 28% of patients with CF, diabetes mellitus (MacLusky & Levison, 1998; Solomon et al., 2003). Obstruction of the vas deferens causes infertility in 98% of males with CF (Wilschanski et al., 1996). The fertility rate in females with CF is estimated as 20% of normal (Flume & Yankaskas, 1999).

In the upper respiratory tract, sinusitis may cause persistent headache, and nasal polyps occur in 6% to 36% of patients with CF and often necessitate surgical resection. Within 12 months there is a 60% recurrence rate of nasal polyps once polypectomy is performed (MacLusky & Levison, 1998). Hypertrophic pulmonary osteoarthropathy is often associated with advanced severity of pulmonary disease and is most noticeable in the clinical finding of "clubbing," which is rounded hypertrophic changes in the terminal phalanges of the fingers and toes (MacLusky & Levison, 1990).

ETIOLOGY

The etiology of CF is traced to the abnormal gene product, the cystic fibrosis transmembrane conductance regulator (CFTR) protein, which seems to be most abundantly expressed in the apical membrane surface of epithelial cells of the respiratory, gastrointestinal, reproductive, and sweat glands (Collins, 1992). Normal epithelial cells secrete fluid by allowing chloride (a negatively charged ion) to pass through the luminal membrane of the cell. Because this membrane is permeable to sodium (positively charged), it passively follows; increased levels of sodium chloride then stimulate fluid secretion. Fluid levels in the airways must be maintained at a sufficient level to provide for normal mucociliary transport. Structural defects in the CFTR protein lead to abnormalities in cell membrane function. The resulting electrolyte abnormality (chloride impermeability and sodium hyperpermeability) leads to abnormal amounts of fluid being removed from the airway lumen, resulting in reduced airway surface liquid volume and underhydrated mucus. These impairments in turn lead to impaired mucociliary clearance (Brennan & Geddes, 2004; MacLusky & Levison, 1998). Abnormal expression of the CFTR protein in airway epithelial cells is the primary cause of the respiratory manifestations of CF.

A main focus of current research in CF is aimed at normalizing the defective electrolyte transport of the epithelium. This may be achieved in various ways, either by transferring normally functioning genes into the CFTR gene locus or by mediating the chloride channel by other means (Orenstein, 2003). Recently, researchers have shown that it is possible to correct the CFTR defect (using a compound in the spice turmeric called curcumin) in the most common mutation delta-F508 in the mouse model (Egan et al., 2004). Research on various gene transfer techniques will be further discussed in this chapter.

DIAGNOSIS AND MEDICAL MANAGEMENT

Early diagnosis, including prenatal determination of the presence of CF gene mutation, has enabled researchers to follow the expression and progression of the disease from birth in many patients. Impairment of the respiratory system does not manifest immediately, and at birth the lungs appear normal on radiologic examination. In the most distal small airways, however, dilation and hypertrophy of mucus-secreting goblet cells begins early in life and subsequent impaired mucociliary clearance can cause obstructive mucus plugs and associated air trapping and atelectasis. Signs of hyperinflation may be present on radiography. The presentation of infants with failure to thrive and nutritional losses through steatorrhea accounts for up to 85% of the cases of CF diagnosed in infancy. A history of respiratory illness such as repeated respiratory tract infections, recurrent bronchiolitis, or even pneumonia is often reported, but in 80% of newly diagnosed cases, there is no known family history of CF (MacLusky & Levison, 1998).

A quantitative pilocarpine iontophoresis sweat test, an analysis of chloride levels in the sweat, is the accepted test to confirm the diagnosis of CF. Because of the quantity of sweat required to provide an accurate analysis and the difficulty in inducing adequate amounts when testing infants in the first couple of months of life, positive diagnosis may be delayed until a valid test can be performed. Values greater than 50 mEq/L in children and 60 mEq/L in adults of sweat chloride are considered positive for CF. Approximately 1% to 2% of patients have borderline sweat chloride levels (40 to 60 mEq/L) or even normal range values and with further investigations have been given the diagnosis of CF (Boucher et al., 2000; MacLusky & Levison, 1998).

In the few centers with the capacity (the specialized laboratory and the trained personnel), another diagnostic test, nasal potential difference (PD), is possible. This test measures the electrical charge (potential difference) across the epithelial surface (mucous membrane) of the nose. In normal subjects a small charge of –5 to –30 mV is present, whereas subjects with CF demonstrate values between –40 and –80 mV (Orenstein, 2003).

Screening tests for prospective parents who are known carriers (with prior offspring with CF or with CF themselves) are now possible and raise a number of ethical issues when CF is suggested prenatally. Genetic counseling is therefore available at CF centers. Analysis of the blood of known heterozygote parents and tissue from the fetus obtained through amniocentesis or chorionic villi sampling can determine the presence of the CF gene mutation common to the family history. With identity of the same pattern of inherited genetic material in the fetus as in an affected sibling, there is a 98% probability the fetus is also affected (Dean et al., 1987). Mass carrier screening in prenatal populations of up to 4000 women

has been undertaken in both the United States and England to investigate the value and feasibility of population screening for CF heterozygotes. In California, where 6 to 12 of the most common mutations were sought, this type of screening identified more than 90 female heterozygotes. Screening of their partners revealed five male heterozygotes and therefore five high-risk pregnancies (Witt et al., 1992). Among adults with CF and parents of affected children, attitudes and debate about prenatal diagnosis and heterozygote screening reflect a variety of concerns. Although up to 74% of questioned adults with CF in one study reported supporting carrier testing of their siblings (Lemke et al., 1992) and 93% supported screening for carriers in the general population, only a minority saw prenatal diagnosis as an absolute indication for termination of pregnancy (Conway & Allenby, 1992). The future of carrier screening and any possible effects prenatal diagnosis may have on the incidence rate of CF remain to be seen.

Most diagnoses of CF are made in infancy; however, the diagnosis of CF is being made in adults with increasing frequency. Patients diagnosed as adults usually have milder lung disease and are pancreatic sufficient. There is often a delay in their diagnosis because of the belief it is a pediatric disease and the finding that some adults have normal to borderline sweat test results. The criteria, however, for making a diagnosis are the same for adults and children (Yankaskas, 2004).

Medical management of pulmonary disability in CF generally focuses on attempts to limit the effects of impairments in the disease, namely, the airway obstruction due to chronic bronchorrhea (abnormal mucus secretions) and the progressive inflammation that is secondary to chronic bacterial infection (MacLusky et al., 1987). Nutritional management is also vitally important because most patients with CF will have some pancreatic insufficiency and therefore require enzyme supplementation to compensate for losses of enzymes crucial to fat and protein digestion. Patients are followed periodically, and quantitative sputum cultures are regularly performed. (Clinics vary as to frequency of assessment; generally, appointments are made every 3 months.) Radiologic assessment, pulmonary function testing (PFT), nutritional status, and any pattern of weight loss combined with subjective reports of treatment adherence assist the CF clinical team to gauge the ever-changing therapeutic needs of patients with CF and to initiate treatment regimens with the aim of preventing or slowing development of the functional limitations of CF.

Throughout their lives, most people with CF battle the tendency toward malnutrition that comes from protein and calorie deficits. Special attention to a properly balanced, high-calorie diet with supplementary pancreatic enzymes requires acceptance and compliance in patients of all ages with CF but may aid in slowing the rate of deterioration of lung function. During acute episodes of respiratory exacerbations, the anorexia that accompanies the frequent racking cough, increase in mucus production, and increased work of breathing poses a challenge to provide adequate nutritional intake. Levels of resting energy expenditure have been shown to be in excess of 150% of normal in patients with CF with more progressive pulmonary disease or malnutrition (MacLusky & Levison, 1998), and this has implications for the degree of caloric input necessary for patients with advanced pulmonary dysfunction. Caloric supplementation may be necessary in the form of feedings given nasogastrically or intravenously. Nutritional management for patients with intractable weight loss can be provided by nocturnal feedings through indwelling gastrostomy or jejunostomy tubes (MacLusky & Levison, 1998).

Most of the morbidity seen in CF is associated with deteriorating pulmonary status; medical intervention is, therefore, focused on attempts to influence the rate of progression of the pathogenesis of pulmonary dysfunction in CF. Antibiotic therapy appears to have significantly influenced the effects of the chronic endobronchial infection that typifies CF and has been a mainstay of treatment regimens for 40 years (MacLusky & Levison, 1998). Optimally the choice of antibiotics should be based on the results of sputum culture and sensitivity tests (Boucher et al., 2000). Sputum cultures show infection by a number of organisms in a common pattern that changes with severity of disease and age of the patient. *Staphylococcus aureus, Pseudomonas aeruginosa, Burkholderia cepacia, Haemophilus influenzae,* and *Klebsiella* are the organisms most commonly seen. Combinations of infectious organisms are common, particularly when disease severity and age of the patient advance. Prophylactic antibiotics are advocated by some but remain controversial. There is some evidence that early and vigorous use of antibiotics produces better results than delaying their administration until symptoms are well developed or advanced (Boucher et al., 2000). Inhaled antibiotics, such as the aminoglycosides tobramycin and gentamicin, which have shown some effect on *Pseudomonas* species, have not shown universal therapeutic value (MacLusky et al., 1989). Ceftazidime and aminoglycosides are used intravenously to target *Pseudomonas* infections in the hospitalized patient, but eradication of this organism is rare. *Pseudomonas aeruginosa* is now the most common pathogen in CF, with reported clinic rates as high as 70% of patients affected (Corey et al., 1984a). Pharmacologic therapies are needed

to inhibit the adherence of the initiating bacteria in *P. aeruginosa* infection because this pathogen has demonstrated an extraordinary affinity for the airways of patients with CF (Prince, 1992).

Burkholderia cepacia is an opportunistic pathogen in hospitalized patients and other compromised hosts. Although normally nonpathogenic in healthy immunocompetent individuals, patients with CF are at significant risk of infection (MacLusky & Levison, 1998). *Burkholderia cepacia* is recognized as a particularly virulent pathogen because of its high level of intrinsic antibiotic resistance, its tenacity to persist in the lungs, and its association with more advanced pulmonary disease. Synergy studies combining antibiotics may help identify a more effective antimicrobial therapy for patients with these organisms (Burns, 1997). Evidence that transmission of this organism may occur through interpatient mechanisms (Pegues et al., 1994; Tablan et al., 1985) has initiated segregation practices and attempts to control cross-contamination of equipment in many centers.

Several of the virulent products of bacterial infection cause airway inflammation and progressive epithelial destruction and therefore contribute significantly to the severity of the pulmonary impairment in CF (MacLusky & Levison, 1998). Anti-inflammatory corticosteroids may slow the progressive pulmonary deterioration (Auerbach et al., 1985) but are associated with numerous side effects when used on a long-term basis and require careful consideration before use (MacLusky & Levison, 1998). They may be used in a small percentage of patients for specific indications such as the fungal infection allergic bronchopulmonary aspergillosis (Boucher et al., 2000).

Influenza, rubeola, and pertussis infections are particularly harmful to individuals with CF and could trigger a downward spiral of lung function. Early immunization is highly recommended, and a routine yearly influenza vaccine should be addressed in the regular clinic routine (Boucher et al., 2000).

Although 25% to 50% of patients with CF have evidence of increased airway hyperactivity, the mechanism for bronchoconstriction in CF appears to differ from that of asthma (MacLusky & Levison, 1998). When assessed by methacholine challenge, higher doses are necessary to produce a response, and the bronchodilation achieved through albuterol therapy is both slower and less dramatic than in patients with asthma (Skorecki et al., 1976). Evaluation by exercise challenge, using a bicycle ergometer or treadmill and using the change in peak expiratory flow rate as a measure of lung function, indicates that a majority of children with CF demonstrate bronchial hyperreactivity with the increased respiratory effort of exercise (Day & Mearns, 1973). Inhaled

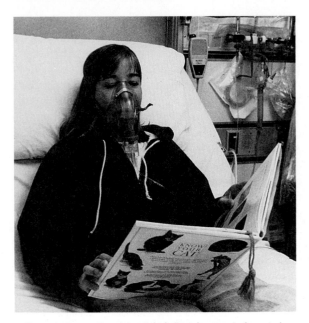

‣ **Figure 27-1** Receiving inhalation therapy in hospital.

sympathomimetic agents do demonstrate the effect of bronchodilation in many patients and may also improve mucociliary function and therefore serve to complement airway clearance techniques (Ormerod et al., 1980) (Fig. 27-1). When used immediately before exercise or pulmonary physical therapy, bronchodilators may help prevent induced bronchospasm and are therefore often prescribed as an important adjunct to physical therapy (MacLusky & Levison, 1998).

Many medications employed in the treatment of CF require nebulization. As a result, the performance characteristics of the nebulizer must be considered when selecting a method of delivery for inhaled medications. Studies comparing the efficiency of different aerosol delivery systems found that there was a significant difference among systems in particle size, total delivery of fluid, and time taken to deliver the medication (Coates et al., 1998; Loffert et al., 1994). Less drug wastage, reduced treatment time, and a more specific match of the delivery system to the breathing pattern of the individual is therefore possible (Coates et al., 1998).

Providing effective pulmonary hygiene by promoting improved clearance of mucus-obstructed airways benefits the pulmonary environment, allowing for improvements in gas exchange and limiting the tissue damage associated with infection. Physical therapy techniques to promote airway clearance include postural drainage and manual or mechanical percussion of segmental lobes, vibratory facilitation of ciliary function, directed breathing techniques such as the active cycle of breathing technique

(ACBT) (formerly known as FET, for forced expiratory technique) and autogenic drainage, use of positive expiratory pressures (PEP) through valve-equipped facial masks and oscillating PEP (Flutter and Acapella), and high-frequency chest wall oscillations (HFCWO), as well as exercise prescription, assisted coughing, and postural realignment exercises.

More research is needed to scientifically support the efficacy of the use of pulmonary physical therapy modalities in CF. In a recent review it was suggested that despite clinical observation and anecdotal association between secretion clearance and improvements in respiratory function there is little high-level evidence to support airway clearance techniques (Hess, 2001). A comparative study of the literature and a meta-analysis demonstrated a need for more adequate controls, randomized design and sampling, larger sample sizes, and use of valid outcome measures (Boyd et al., 1994; Thomas et al., 1995). The studies reviewed by Boyd and colleagues were evaluated and classified according to the level of evidence supported by the research design as proposed by Sackett (1986). The analysis suggested support for exercise, "conventional" physical therapy (postural drainage, percussion, and vibration), and PEP mask therapies in treatment of children with CF in chronic stages of the disease when PFT results were used as an outcome measure. In acute exacerbations of respiratory status, both PEP mask therapy and conventional physical therapy showed some evidence of improving pulmonary function scores. A 2-year study of 66 subjects found that PEP therapy is a valid alternative to conventional physical therapy (Gaskin et al., 1998). In another long-term study, pulmonary function scores improved in subjects using PEP versus conventional physical therapy and indicated that PEP was preferred by subjects, thereby increasing adherence (McIlwaine et al., 1997). A recent study demonstrated the physiologic basis for the efficacy of PEP by confirming that both low PEP and high PEP improve gas mixing in individuals with CF and that these improvements were associated with increased lung function, sputum expectoration, and arterial blood oxyhemoglobin saturation (Darbee et al, 2004). Oscillating PEP (Flutter) has gained popularity as an airway clearance mechanism, and short-term studies indicate its usefulness as an alternative modality to conventional physical therapy (Konstan et al., 1994). A long-term comparison of Flutter versus PEP found that Flutter was not as effective as PEP in maintaining pulmonary function over a 1-year period and was more costly as a result of increased hospitalizations and antibiotic use (McIlwaine et al., 2001). Exercise should be included in the management of CF. In a study at the Hospital for Sick Children in Toronto that evaluated the effects of a 3-year home exercise program, it was found that pulmonary function declined more slowly in the exercise group versus the control group, suggesting a benefit for patients with CF participating in regular aerobic exercise (Schneiderman-Walker et al., 2000).

New strategies for treating CF by pharmacologic means (gene therapy) continue to show promise (Collins, 1996). Research has demonstrated that to successfully treat the respiratory dysfunction of CF, 5% to 10% of the airway epithelial cells must be corrected with normal CFTR expression. To achieve this, a method of delivering the normal gene to the airways is needed. Three different vector delivery systems—modified adenovirus, adeno-associated virus, and liposomes—are being extensively investigated worldwide (Crystal, 1997). An undesirable immune response that targets and destroys corrected epithelial cells remains problematic. A new vector virus that does not carry any of its own viral genes and causes less inflammation than earlier viral vectors has recently been developed. This type of viral vector helps to alleviate the risk of cancer by not inserting itself into the patient's DNA (Koehler et al., 2003).

Studies with high-dose preservative-free aerosolized tobramycin have demonstrated improved pulmonary function, decreased sputum bacterial densities, and decreased risk for hospitalization (Ramsey, 1997). Other drugs under investigation include ibuprofen (to decrease airway inflammation), recombinant human DNAse (to improve mucous surface properties and transportability) (Galabert et al., 1996), azithromycin (to decrease inflammation, reduce sputum viscosity, and prevent bacterial airway adhesion) (Peckham, 2002), and other mucolytic agents such as hypertonic saline.

The unprecedented volume of current research and the emergence of new, successful therapies for CF dictate a need for conscientious practitioners to remain educated and receptive to adjusting their management plans and critical pathways for care of patients with CF.

LUNG TRANSPLANTATION

Organ transplantation is now a treatment option in many different terminal illnesses, including CF. Advances in surgical technique and postoperative care with improved immunosuppressive therapies have given some patients with CF a new lease on life. (See Chapter 29 for a more detailed discussion of the involvement of physical therapy in postsurgical care.)

In North America, both heart-lung and double-lung transplants have been performed on patients with CF with end-stage pulmonary disease. The Toronto Lung Transplant Group were pioneers in this field and performed the world's first successful double-lung transplant in 1987 (Pizer, 1991). Cystic fibrosis has steadily increased as an indication leading to lung transplantation and accounts for 67% of adolescent lung recipients and 16% of adults (Boucek et al., 2003). Survival rates have not significantly improved in the past few years. The current estimate for 3- and 5-year survival is 59% and 49.5%, respectively (Starnes et al., 2004). Living-donor lobar lung transplantation has been performed since 1993, but because it involves recruitment of two donors and the surgical procedure carries inherent risks to the donors, it is not without its problems. This technique's impact on survival statistics appears comparable to that of other approaches, but long-term analysis is needed (Starnes et al., 2004). Most complications arise from infections or development of graft rejection. The development of obliterative bronchiolitis may be evidence of chronic rejection and is a leading cause of death after pediatric lung transplantation (Boucek et al., 2003). The problem with malabsorption that patients with CF have dictates difficulties with the therapeutic regimen for adequate immunosuppression after transplantation. Individual transplant centers should direct and monitor the immunosuppressive regimen because close monitoring of serum levels and adjustment of doses are vital to successful posttransplant management (Yankaskas et al., 1998).

Criteria for acceptance on a waiting list for lung transplantation include severe pulmonary disease with marked hypoxemia, increased frequency and duration of hospitalizations for pulmonary exacerbations, increasing antibiotic resistance of infectious bacteria, no significant dysfunction or disease of other vital organs, a history of compliance with medical treatment, and an acceptable psychosocial profile (Yankaskas et al., 1998). A referral for transplant (and acceptance onto the waiting list) must be made early enough to allow for a substantial wait for a suitable donor and creates a need for the development of a preoperative program of conditioning for these patients, which is a component of the lung transplantation program in many centers. These conditioning programs are designed to optimize the patient's functional ability and exercise tolerance, as well as help maintain emotional well-being during the long wait for a transplant (Craven et al., 1990). Physical therapists play a primary role in development and implementation of both preoperative and postoperative exercise programs, which are described later in this chapter.

Double-lung transplantation is now most often performed by bilateral anterolateral thoracotomies using bilateral submammary incisions as first described in

1990 (Pasque et al., 1990). The lungs are transplanted as sequential single-lung grafts. The lung with the worst pulmonary function is replaced first while oxygenation and ventilation are maintained by the native lung. Replacement of the second lung can then proceed with the newly implanted lung supporting the patient (Winton, 1992). Use of this technique has reduced to 30% to 35% the number of patients requiring anticoagulation and cardiopulmonary bypass during surgery (Winton, 1992). This surgical innovation has also reduced the degree of complication from perioperative bleeding, which can be a significant problem for patients with CF because of the presence of inflammatory adhesions within the pleural space (Winton, 1992).

Single-lung transplants are not performed on patients with CF because the remaining native lung continues to be ventilated after transplantation and its overexpansion will compress the transplanted lung (MacLusky & Levison, 1990). Contamination of the native lung could also spread infection to the transplanted lung (Egan, 1992).

BODY FUNCTIONS AND STRUCTURES

EXAMINATION AND IMPLICATIONS

The primary physiologic abnormalities in CF include (1) a dysfunctional chloride channel in transepithelial electrolyte transport, creating abnormal increases in the concentrations of sodium and chloride in serous gland secretions; (2) blocked exocrine gland function due to obstruction by hyperviscous secretions; and (3) an extraordinary susceptibility to chronic endobronchial infection by specific groups of bacteria, apparently compounded by impaired or deficient ciliary clearance. Although patients with CF show significant differences in levels of clinical impairment, all patients with CF have these three abnormalities (MacLusky & Levison, 1990).

The degree of limitations that the abnormal pathology imposes varies greatly among people with CF. Proper measurement of these limitations is crucial to determining the proper interventions. Examination techniques to quantify the abnormal pathology seen in CF measure the functioning of the respiratory and gastrointestinal systems and the limitations in exercise tolerance. Quality-of-life questionnaires and other subjective reports provide information on the patient's perceived level of functioning.

A number of clinical scoring systems have been proposed in an attempt to standardize measurement of CF severity. The most commonly used is the Shwachman score (Shwachman & Kulczycki, 1958). Points are awarded under four categories: (1) chest radiography, (2) growth and nutrition, (3) pulmonary (physical findings and cough), and (4) case history, which includes subjective reports of activity tolerance. Findings that reflect no limitation ("normal" findings) are awarded 25 points; therefore a "perfect" Shwachman score is 100. The lower the score, the worse the clinical condition of the patient. A patient scoring 40 points may have an increased anterior-posterior diameter on chest radiography with atelectatic patches and noticeable hyperinflation, subnormal weight and height, poor muscle strength, marked reduction of fat on skinfold testing, chronic productive cough, rapid respiration and pulse, moderate to severe overexpansion of the lungs, rattles and wheezes on auscultation, breathlessness on exertion, listlessness or lethargy, poor school attendance, limited exercise tolerance, postural abnormalities of protracted shoulders and extended neck, clubbing of the phalanges, and poor appetite or anorexia (Shwachman & Kulczycki, 1958) (Fig. 27-2). This scoring system has good interobserver reliability and correlates well with PFT scoring systems

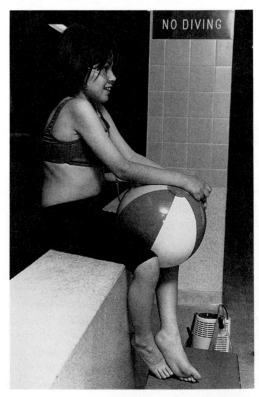

♦ **Figure 27-2** An example of postural changes in one individual: elevation of the shoulders and an increased anterior-posterior diameter of the chest. Note intercostal indrawing.

(Lewiston & Moss, 1987), permitting use in clinical comparisons of disease morbidity.

MEASURING PULMONARY FUNCTION

PFT (pulmonary function test) scores provide incremental knowledge of the extent of bronchial obstruction and a means of tracing the degree of restriction of lung function. PFTs include measurement of static and dynamic lung volumes and airflow. Evidence of reactive airway disease can be quantified. Spirometry can be used to record acute deterioration of pulmonary function and to monitor recovery. Vital capacity (VC), inspiratory reserve volume (IRV), and expiratory reserve volume (ERV) are directly measured by spirometry. Spirometry can measure airflow rates during different phases of expiration, yielding an indication of the amount of bronchial obstruction. The measure of forced expiratory volume in 1 second (FEV_1) chronicles the early portion of expiration and is often reported as a ratio to forced vital capacity (FVC). In a healthy individual, FEV_1/FVC is 0.70 to 0.80, indicating that 70% to 80% of the FVC is expired in the first second of a forced exhalation (Miller, 1987). Changes in this ratio can reflect an obstructed expiratory airflow.

Analysis of spirometric flow-volume curves enables the early detection of abnormalities in the smaller airways (Orenstein, 2003). Convexity of the curve in relation to the volume axis is one of the most sensitive indicators of early obstruction of the peripheral airways (Mellins, 1969). Forced expiratory flow between 25% and 75% ($FEF_{25-75\%}$) is the measurement of flow between 25% and 75% of vital capacity and reflects airflow in the small airways. Miller (1987) suggests that $FEF_{25-75\%}$ is more sensitive than FEV_1 or FEV_1/FVC in detecting changes in small airway obstruction and provides an important indication of early pulmonary disease in individuals with CF because initial abnormalities involve the small airways (Mellins et al., 1968). Timed volumes at high lung volumes (e.g., FEV_1) may remain within typical limits because the contribution of the small airways to overall resistance is low (Kattan, 1987). FEV_1 is therefore not a sensitive test in early lung disease but indicates obstruction of the central bronchi and becomes markedly abnormal as disease progresses (MacLusky & Levison, 1998).

With more severe pulmonary dysfunction, air trapping results in increases in residual volume (RV) and functional reserve capacity (FRC) (both are measured by a more complicated PFT than spirometry) and an increase in RV/TLC (total lung capacity). Restrictive disease can be reflected in decreases in TLC and VC (Altose, 1979). The presence of both restrictive and obstructive components of pulmonary dysfunction may compensate for each other in some measurements (Miller et al., 1987). For example, restrictive disease (in the absence of an obstructive component) results in a normal RV/TLC and obstructive disease (in the absence of a restrictive component) results in an increase in this ratio. When both components coexist, RV/TLC "may not reflect the anatomic changes" (Miller et al., 1987).

Spirometry is the simplest type of PFT performed in the hospital or clinic. Spirometric measurements are all generated by "effort-dependent" means. Children younger than age 6 years cannot perform the standard test of forced expiration in 1 second in a reliable way. Modifications to the classic methods of measuring ventilatory parameters in infants and young children are described in the literature (Buist et al., 1980; Doershuk et al., 1970; England, 1988; Sammut & Morgan, 1987; Taussig, 1977; Tepper et al., 1988). A recent study examining children ages 2 to 5 years found that modifying the FEV_1 test to $FEV_{0.75}$ gave a reliable measure of pulmonary function for young children (Aurora et al., 2004.)

In older children and adults, many other factors, such as sputum retention, poor nutrition, and fatigue, can influence the individual's performance on spirometric PFTs. Notably, many children with CF show performance scores on repeat tests that have a significantly greater range of variability than that of scores of typical test subjects (Cooper et al., 1990). Interpretation of the pulmonary function of an individual with CF therefore also must include other PFTs, such as the closed-circuit helium dilution method, the open-circuit nitrogen washout technique, or a method colloquially known as the "body box"—total-body plethysmography. Ruppel (1991) provides detailed descriptions of these tests. In the plethysmograph, the volume of air is a constant; the test measures the changes in air pressure within the sealed chamber as the patient breathes through a mouthpiece. These measures yield an accurate calculation of the patient's lung volumes, the FRC and RV (Altose, 1979). Some claustrophobia may be experienced by subjects undergoing testing in the "body box," and plethysmography may not be appropriate for all young children.

The U.S. National Institutes of Health's comparative review of 307 cases of CF reported that PFT scores showed a common pattern: progressive declines in flow rates and VC and an increase in the RV/TLC ratio, correlating with clinically gauged worsening of disease (di Sant'Agnese & Davis, 1979). As pulmonary disease becomes progressively more severe, deteriorating PFT scores can be used to help predict life expectancy. In one study patients with poor arterial gases and an FEV_1 of less than 30% of predicted value had 2-year mortality rates of greater than 50% (Kerem et al., 1992). Individuals with CF demonstrate a characteristic decline in midexpiratory flow rate ($FEF_{25-75\%}$); noting the rate of this decline becomes an important prognostic indicator (Gurwitz et al., 1979). Steadily worsening PFT scores reliably correlate with declining clinical condition and are used as an indicator in assessment for lung transplantation (Khaghani et al., 1991).

Progressive hypoxemia is one of the earliest signs of increasing pulmonary disease and can occur before any other detectable abnormality in lung function (Lamarre et al., 1972). Mucous plugging and bronchiolitis in the patient's airways cause ventilation-perfusion abnormalities, and the subsequent hypoxemia worsens as severity of the obstruction increases (MacLusky & Levison, 1990). Further declines in arterial oxygenation can occur during sleep, so blood gases may have to be monitored throughout the night to assess the need for nocturnal supplementation of oxygen (Muller et al., 1980). Increased oxygen demands during exercise can be a contributing factor to hypoxemia in the patient with CF. Although arterial blood gas measures are considered the "gold standard" in blood gas analysis (Zadai, 1992), they are not commonly used in patients with CF because of their invasive nature. Other noninvasive techniques such as pulse oximetry are preferred. Pulse oximetry to gauge the level of oxygen saturation in the blood as the patient performs exercise contributes to assessment of the suitability of supplemental oxygen during exercise.

Other changes in blood gas readings forewarn of serious advanced pathology. Hypercapnia in CF indicates advanced pulmonary disease and carries a poor prognosis. In a study of survival patterns of patients with CF who demonstrated hypercapnia, it was found that death usually occurred within 1 year of the development of chronic hypercapnia (Wagener et al., 1980).

Chest radiographs can provide detailed evidence of the progressive nature of pulmonary disease in CF. In the initial stages of pulmonary involvement, the chest radiograph may reveal signs of hyperinflation and peribronchial thickening. As the disease progresses, bronchiectasis can become apparent, particularly in the upper lobes, and pulmonary infiltrates appear as nodular shadows on radiographs. With severe pulmonary disease the hyperexpanded lungs can precipitate flattening of the diaphragm, thoracic kyphosis, and bowing of the sternum, all detectable on radiography (MacLusky & Levison, 1990) (Fig. 27-3). Confirmation of the development of a pneumothorax can also be provided by examining the chest radiographs. When pulmonary disease is advanced,

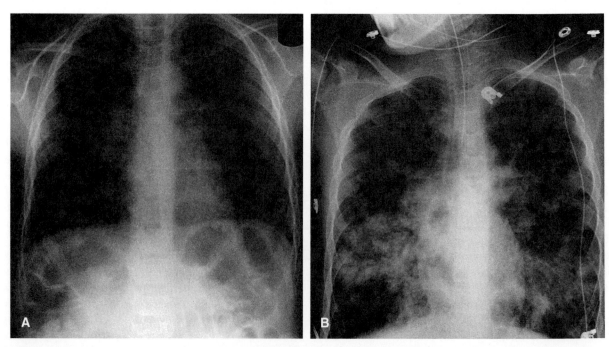

• **Figure 27-3** Two chest radiographs of same individual showing marked deterioration over course of 8 years. **A**, At the time of diagnosis there is evidence of bronchial wall thickening and slight prominence of pulmonary arteries. **B**, At the preterminal stage there is diffuse bilateral bronchiectasis and fibrosis, with severe hyperinflation and bilateral areas of consolidation.

pulmonary artery hypertrophy may be noticed on radiography as a sign of the pulmonary hypertension associated with cor pulmonale (MacLusky & Levison, 1990).

Cultures from sputum of a patient with CF identify the variety of bacteria that has infected the lower respiratory tract (Gilljam et al., 1986). Sensitivity studies can then be performed to identify effective antibiotic therapies (Orenstein, 2003). CF centers perform regular sputum bacteriologic tests to ensure adequate antibiotic coverage for their patients and to help monitor the state of bacterial infection (MacLusky et al., 1987).

Physical examination of the patient also gathers valuable information. Chest assessment includes inspection, palpation, percussion, and auscultation. Inspection can reveal postural abnormalities, modifications of breathing pattern (Fig. 27-4), or signs of respiratory distress. Evidence of a chronic productive cough may be apparent. Examination of the comparative dimensions of the chest in the anterior-posterior and transverse planes may reveal the barrel chest deformity common to obstructive lung diseases (Humberstone, 1990). Palpation and accurate evaluation of the findings of tactile fremitus will reveal atelectasis, pneumothorax, or large airway secretions (Humberstone, 1990). Examination of the resonance pattern of the chest, as demonstrated by audible changes on percussion, can provide an indication of abnormally dense areas of the lungs (Humberstone, 1990).

Age of the patient may highly influence the reliability and clinical usefulness of different components of the physical examination. In an infant, measurement of chest wall expansion may be difficult and percussion may not be appropriate (Crane, 1990).

Careful auscultation of the chest can contribute information on the quality of airflow and evidence of obstruction in different areas of the lungs. Reduced ventilation is suggested by decreased breath sounds or presence of inspiratory crackles (also called rales). If crackles are heard throughout the ventilatory cycle, it suggests impaired secretion clearance. Diffuse airway obstruction may cause polyphonic wheezing (Humberstone, 1990).

The examiner must be aware that chronically hyperinflated lungs tend to mask or make it difficult to hear adventitious sounds on auscultation (Humberstone, 1990). It is also important to note that use of a stethoscope, described as the "most frequently used tool in medicine" (Loudon, 1987), is not consistent or reliable among health care providers (Pasterkamp et al., 1987). Validity and reliability of auscultation may be affected by a disparity in nomenclature, the quality of the stethoscope used, and a lack of correlation between pathologic findings and lung sounds (Aweida & Kelsey, 1989). When various health care workers were compared, significant differences were noted in the terminology used to describe tape-recorded adventitious sounds (Pasterkamp et al., 1987). Despite auscultation's limitations in interobserver reliability, it continues to serve as a valuable element of clinical examination. Familiarization with the usual pattern of a patient's lung sounds can be a critical component of evaluation of examination results because an alteration of the typical pattern may signal a pulmonary change that might otherwise have gone undetected.

The long-term prognosis of CF patients with significant pulmonary disease worsens when there is also evidence of protein-calorie malnutrition (Park & Grand, 1981). Patients who are pancreatic insufficient need oral supplementary enzymes to enable them to absorb adequate nutrients from their diet and prevent the devastating effects of malnutrition. Identifying the need for enzyme supplementation is, therefore, a critical component in the treatment of CF. Pancreatic function may be determined by a number of testing methods, including fecal fat assessment, pancreatic substrate assays, and direct collection of pancreatic secretions by duodenal intubation (MacLusky & Levison, 1998). Individuals with

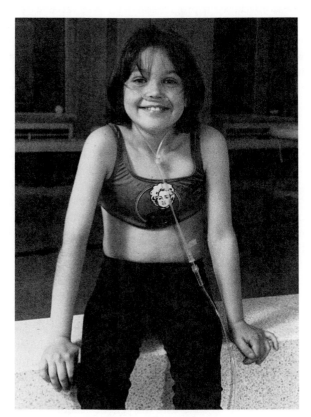

◆ **Figure 27-4**　Use of accessory muscles of respiration is apparent on physical inspection.

CF who have significant preservation of pancreatic function and therefore can maintain normal fat absorption have less pulmonary dysfunction and a better prognosis than those individuals who have pancreatic insufficiency (Corey et al., 1984b).

A number of clinicians and researchers have examined various prognostic indicators in CF. Sustaining adequate nutritional requirements to ensure the maintenance of appropriate growth percentiles is one such indicator (Corey et al., 1984b). Other factors that are associated with a preferred prognosis include single-organ involvement at diagnosis, absent or single-organism sputum colonization, and a normal chest radiograph 1 year after diagnosis. Multiple organ involvement, abnormal chest radiographs at diagnosis, colonization of multiple organisms in the sputum, a falloff from typical growth curves, and recurrent hemoptysis are all factors associated with a poor prognosis. There also appears to be a gender bias in severity of disease expression, with male patients possessing a better prognosis than their female counterparts (MacLusky et al., 1987).

PHYSICAL THERAPY: EXAMINATION AND INTERVENTION

INFANCY

Newborn screening for CF is currently carried out in the United States as well as many other countries. The current method of screening suggests that many but not all newborns can be identified. Studies have suggested that through newborn screening, nutritional deficits are detected and that early intervention may be useful to protect against loss of lung function (Boucher et al., 2000).

A diagnosis of CF for their child can mean many things to parents. At the most basic level, it means they have a child with "special needs," and those needs can be seen to influence the family dynamics (Lloyd-Still & Lloyd-Still, 1983). The child's family members are forced to familiarize themselves with CF and both the psychologic and practical demands implicit with this diagnosis. Education of the family is a crucial goal, and this seems best achieved by regional CF centers because a number of different specialty services can be provided in one place. A physical therapist at a CF center is part of a cohesive team of interested investigators and caregivers. Educating the patients and their families while measuring and treating the myriad complications in this disease is the ongoing goal of a CF center's staff.

Promoting Function: Parental Education

Intervention often must be implemented immediately on diagnosis, and the family needs assistance in making the necessary adjustments and provisions to ensure adherence with any suggested therapeutic regimen. Physical therapists evaluate which essential elements of the child's care must be addressed by them and then provide instruction for the family in the proper administration of the physical therapy modalities that appear appropriate. The therapist should demonstrate sensitivity and equanimity while interacting with these children and their families, remembering that this is a very stressful time for those involved and that what the family may "hear" can differ from what is actually said to them (Bush, 1997).

What families seem to need most is information that acknowledges the seriousness of the disease while still emphasizing the likelihood of a happy and fulfilling family life. Developing the types of strategies that permit some flexibility in intervention regimens promotes a better integration of the child's treatment needs into the family's routines (Maxwell, 1991). Parents may have many concerns and a host of questions and can be especially confused by all the uncertainty that typifies the disease. Because the progression of CF is so variable from case to case, an ongoing examination of the child's status is the only way to ensure meeting the child's individual requirements. This means that the family members must have continued association with the CF center and need to appreciate their role as integral members of the caregiving team.

Children with a chronic condition have been shown to have increased risk of psychosocial dysfunction, particularly when parental anxiety is overwhelming (Cappelli et al., 1989; Green & Solnit, 1964). Because excessive parental overprotection is strongly linked to the existence of psychosocial maladjustment in children, the parents of a child with CF must be alerted to the dangers of unnecessarily shielding their child from aspects of normal life. In infancy, this may take the form of overdressing the child to guard against drafts or neglecting to allow the child to participate in normal exploratory play. Physical therapists should reassure parents that infants with CF have the same requirements as other infants with respect to physical and emotional development. Excellent reference materials are available in most CF centers. Teaching manuals, designed to supplement the information imparted by the CF center staff, are often distributed to families and can be made available to other interested caregivers such as child care workers or school teachers. Orenstein's book *Cystic Fibrosis: A Guide for Patient and Family* (Orenstein, 2003) is highly recommended.

Management of Body Functions and Structures

In the neonate, the most frequently seen symptoms of CF are meconium ileus, malabsorption of nutrients, and failure to thrive, all of which are associated with the gastrointestinal tract (Rosenstein & Langbaum, 1984). Overt pulmonary involvement is not apparent in the neonatal period because the lungs are morphologically normal at birth (Hardy et al., 1989; MacLusky & Levison, 1990). Within a few months, however, some infants with CF develop signs of impaired respiratory function, manifesting symptoms suggesting bronchiolitis. Pronounced wheeze, an indication of hyperactive airways, is sometimes apparent, and chest radiographs can reveal evidence of hyperinflation (Phillips & David, 1987). Obstruction of airflow in these infants may be related to airway inflammation, mucosal edema, copious mucus secretions, and increased airway tone (Tepper, 1992). The bronchioles are considered the main site of airflow obstruction in infancy (Taussig et al., 1984). Studies using bronchoalveolar lavage revealed that every infant with CF—whether symptomatic or not—has evidence of small airway obstruction in the form of bronchial mucous casts (Wood,1993).

Measurements to assess possible limitation of pulmonary function cannot be taken in the conventional way (e.g., spirometry) in infants; therefore, researchers have had to modify standard methods by using the raised-volume rapid thoracoabdominal compression technique (RVRTC). $FEV_{0.5}$ was measured and was found to be significantly lower in infants with CF shortly after diagnosis (median age of 28 weeks) and 6 months later on retest (Ranganathan et al., 2004).

Infants with CF demonstrate low values of pulmonary compliance (Phelan et al., 1969), decreased lung compliance, and a less homogeneous distribution of ventilation when compared with typical control subjects (Tepper et al., 1988). Tepper and colleagues (1987) found these changes in both symptomatic and asymptomatic infants. Abnormalities in flow-volume curves (Godfrey et al., 1983) and low values of maximal expiratory flow (Hiatt et al., 1988) indicate that the limitations to airflow in infancy are associated with bronchoconstriction (Hardy et al., 1989). Infants with CF have indeed displayed altered bronchial tone after the administration of a bronchodilator, as revealed by the fact that airflow rates showed significant increases not seen in a control group (Hiatt et al., 1988). Methacholine challenge testing also revealed heightened airway responsiveness (Ackerman et al., 1991).

These research studies have yielded valuable insight into the early pulmonary manifestations of CF in infancy.

The formal PFTs used in these studies, however, are not feasible or practical for the infant population of most clinics or CF centers. Examination of pulmonary involvement in infancy is usually limited to physical findings, history of respiratory symptoms, and chest radiographs. Carefully observing for signs of respiratory distress, such as nasal flaring, expiratory grunting, retractions of the chest wall, tachypnea, pallor, or cyanosis, produces an indication of respiratory status. Auscultation of an infant or young child is less than ideal owing to the deceptively easy transmission of sounds from the close structures underlying the thin chest wall (Crane, 1990), but careful auscultation is necessary to ascertain if there is any evidence of wheezing. Changes visible on radiography are the most reliable indication of early pulmonary involvement, because it has been demonstrated that airflow obstruction may precede the presence of overt respiratory symptoms and because lack of cooperation in this population diminishes the reliability of the physical examination. Historical accounts of respiratory illness must also be carefully considered.

It has been suggested that the rate of deterioration of pulmonary function in individuals with CF might be slowed by early initiation of treatment (Taussig et al., 1984). Because research has shown changes in respiratory patterns and mechanics in asymptomatic infants newly diagnosed with CF (Tepper et al., 1988) and evidence of small airway obstruction in the form of bronchial mucous casts (Wood, 1993), early therapeutic intervention might actually delay the onset of overt symptoms of respiratory impairment. The value of initiating pulmonary treatment before development of symptoms remains controversial, but various theoretic arguments for initiating therapy as soon as possible can be presented. Adherence to a therapy routine may be improved if it is accepted as a routine part of life, and prevention of respiratory impairment is an easily supported goal (Wood, 1993).

A study was conducted to evaluate the combined effect of a bronchodilator and cardiopulmonary physical therapy on infants newly diagnosed with CF, addressing the controversy surrounding treatment for asymptomatic children (Hardy et al., 1989). Baseline, preintervention measurements of the mechanics and energetics of breathing were obtained for all subjects. Twenty minutes after the inhalation of a bronchodilator, cardiopulmonary physical therapy was given to the subjects, consisting of 20 minutes of chest percussions and vibrations applied in five different postural drainage positions. Immediately after the physical therapy session, repeat pulmonary function measurements were taken. Most of the infants (10 of 13) demonstrated decreases from baseline values in pulmonary resistance, with subsequent decreases in the work of breathing, after the administration of the bronchodilator and physical therapy (Hardy et al., 1989). The researchers postulated that the bronchodilator relieved subclinical bronchospasm and aided the reduction of mucosal edema, and that physical therapy, assisting the immature mucociliary system, was effective in mobilizing secretions, thereby improving the patency of the airways (Hardy et al., 1989). When serial PFTs are possible, objective measures of the progression of impairment and the effects of specific treatments may provide future evidence of the efficacy of early intervention (Hardy et al., 1989).

Prevention of obstructive mucous plugging is the initial goal of pulmonary physical therapy in this population. The primary modalities used for promotion of clearance of secretions for infants with CF are postural drainage, percussion, and vibrations. The physiologic rationale and precise methodology of these modalities are well described in most comprehensive texts on physical therapy (e.g., Frownfelter, 1987; Irwin & Tecklin, 1990; Mackenzie, 1989), but important modifications to the proper use of these modalities for infants will be discussed.

In obstructive airway diseases such as CF, the effectiveness of the antireflux mechanism at the esophagogastric junction is reduced (Orenstein & Orenstein, 1988). The increases in intra-abdominal pressure that can be associated with coughing also promote gastroesophageal reflux (Scott et al., 1985). Of newly diagnosed infants with CF, 35% had symptomatic gastroesophageal reflux in one study (Vinocur et al., 1985), and 24-hour esophageal monitoring revealed abnormalities in 10 successive infants newly diagnosed with CF in another (Dab & Malfroot, 1988). There are suggestions that reflux can worsen lung disease in CF (Malfroot & Dab, 1991) and cause upper respiratory symptoms (Yellon, 1997). A 5-year comparison study by Button and colleagues (2003) compared tipped position versus modified (no tip) in 20 asymptomatic infants. They found that the modified group had significantly fewer days with upper respiratory tract symptoms and shorter courses of antibiotics in the first year of life than those with standard conventional physical therapy. They also had better chest x-ray scores at 2.5 years old and better pulmonary function at 5 years.

Timing the physical therapy around feeding schedules may also be necessary to reduce the risk of gastroesophageal reflux. Postural drainage positions are easily achieved by arranging the infant in the required manner on the caregiver's lap. Holding the small child in this way also seems to offer the child an extra measure of security. Adapting hand position (by "tenting" of the middle

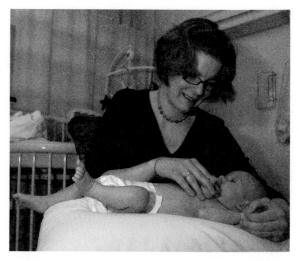

◆ **Figure 27-5**   Infant postural drainage and percussion performed by therapist using an infant palm cup.

finger) or using a rubber finger held cup suits the application of percussion on a tiny chest wall (Fig. 27-5). The applied force of percussion should vary with size and condition of the infant, and conscientious monitoring of the infant's response to treatment should guide the amount of vigor used in percussion. Timing of manual vibrations to coincide with the expirations of an infant is difficult owing to the infant's rapid respiratory rate, and this technique may be very difficult to teach to parents.

Education for the family in the application of prescribed physical therapy modalities should be ongoing. Periodically asking the parent or caregiver to demonstrate treatment positions and manual technique allows the therapist to identify possible problems with proper application. Instructing parents to perform breathing games with their infants and toddlers can eventually lead them to perform diaphragmatic breathing and huffing (Davidson, 2002). Breathing exercises can promote use of collateral ventilation and introduce concepts of techniques that will be used in the future. In some CF centers the physical therapist is also responsible for ordering, demonstrating, and arranging for the maintenance of the equipment necessary for the aerosol delivery of medications. Instruction in the care and use of these nebulizers is vitally important to ensure correct delivery of prescribed medications.

Adherence with any suggested therapeutic regimen requires commitment on the part of the caregiver. The demands of caring for a child with CF can seem extreme when considering the extra attention to nutritional issues, medications, and physical therapy that this diagnosis entails. Signs of excessive stress or evidence that the family is having difficulty in coping with the caregiving requirements may become obvious. Referral to a social worker or a psychologist might help identify the family in crisis and aid the family in developing strategies to enable adjustment to the various challenges that lie ahead of them as they nurture their child with CF.

PRESCHOOL AND SCHOOL-AGE PERIOD

Approximately 75% of children with CF are now diagnosed before their third birthday (Lloyd-Still & Lloyd-Still, 1983). When there is a positive family history of CF, parents are familiar with the disease, but in many cases there is no prior knowledge of the disorder and the diagnosis can be startling. Initial shock may be followed by disbelief, anger, or grief (Lloyd-Still & Lloyd-Still, 1983). The age of the child when diagnosed affects parental reaction to some extent. The longer the pre-diagnostic stage (the older the child), the greater the likelihood of the parents experiencing extreme shock at the time of diagnosis (Burton, 1975). Sensitivity for the anguish experienced by the family must be shown.

The clinical status of children with CF is highly variable. Some toddlers may have already experienced pulmonary complications and been hospitalized repeatedly, whereas others exhibit little or no detrimental impact on their respiratory status. The effects of protein-calorie deficits due to malabsorption may be manifest in stunted development such as small stature or a lower than average weight-to-height ratio; therefore, a difference in appearance from their healthy siblings or friends may already be perceptible.

Participation

Young children need to develop the ability to function socially outside the family circle. Demands of school and new friendships dictate a lessening of parental attachments and a capacity for some measure of independence (Lloyd-Still & Lloyd-Still, 1983). This type of autonomy may be difficult to achieve for the child with CF. If parents perceive that their child is fragile with exceptionally vulnerable health, they may become overprotective. McCollum and Gibson (1970) examined issues of family adaptation to CF and found that 47% of parents in the study admitted granting less independence to their child with CF than to their healthy children. Cappelli and colleagues (1989) found a strong correlation between parental overprotection and psychologic maladjustment in the child. Behavior problems such as restlessness, excessive daydreaming, and inattentiveness are found more often in children with medical conditions such as CF than in their healthy peers (McCollum &

Gibson, 1970). Encouraging children with CF to participate in a variety of social and physical activities could prove beneficial to both their physical and emotional health. The physical therapist should stress the importance of incorporating an active lifestyle into the family dynamic.

Assisting children to gain a sense of self-efficacy is an important goal at this time. A key factor of lifelong adherence to necessary treatment is incorporating a sense of self-efficacy (the confidence that one has the ability to perform a behavior). This results from exposure to a credible role model, the encouragement to perform the tasks of self-management, and developing competency (Bartholomew et al., 1993). Self-management workshops at the Hospital for Sick Children in Toronto, Canada, have been implemented to increase the knowledge and commitment to treatment for children and their families by teaching age-appropriate tasks in a multisensory, multidisciplinary setting. Individual care plans are developed with each child, and a self-care manual is provided to the families to act as a guide. By initiating this education when the child is young, it is hoped that it may influence the negative correlation between adherence and aging identified by Passero and colleagues (1981).

The CF Family Education Project at Baylor College of Medicine and Texas Children's Hospital developed an educational program that emphasized self-management by providing individual learning packages for parents and patients in early childhood, middle childhood, and adolescence. The curriculums were developed based on social cognitive theory and target behavioral capability, self-efficacy, and outcome expectations. The program was designed to be implemented as an integral component of the health care of these families, facilitating learning by the reciprocity between the clients and the health care environment (Bartholomew et al., 1996).

Measurement of Function and Activity

Measurement of impairment and activity limitations in the young child includes history, physical examination, chest radiographs, blood gases, oximetry, and sputum bacteriology. The pulmonary function of children who are able to execute the necessary voluntary maneuver (usually by age 6) can be assessed by spirometry.

Examination by the physical therapist should include thorough history taking, a physical examination including posture, and, when applicable, some type of exercise tolerance testing. Young children with CF may have a chronic cough, hypoxemia, and decreased compliance of the lungs (Tepper et al., 1988), leading to restrictions in maximal oxygen consumption, an increase in work of breathing, and an increase in resting energy expenditure (Shepherd et al., 1988). These factors will all compromise exercise tolerance.

Exercise testing is an objective method in which the physical therapist can quantify the subject's pulmonary deterioration, as well as determine the subject's response to physical therapy. Individuals with CF will often not be aware of the extent of their physical limitations owing to the slow progression of their disease (Cerny & Darbee, 1990). An exercise test can detect mild pulmonary dysfunction, which may go undetected during investigations at rest, and will also help reveal how the individual copes with work despite his or her disability (Godfrey, 1974).

When choosing an exercise test protocol, the purpose for the test and the age and disease severity of the subject should be carefully considered. Choosing the appropriate exercise test depends on the specific question being asked (Orenstein, 1998). For example, to evaluate activity limitations in aerobic performance, the exercise test should be progressive and stress the subject's cardiorespiratory system to a symptom-limited maximum. The test should also be reproducible and capable of providing meaningful results (Singh, 1992).

Cycle ergometers are often used for testing exercise capacity in children with pulmonary disease (Cerny et al., 1982; Nixon et al., 1992). An accurate prediction of oxygen consumption can be obtained because the mechanical efficiency for pedaling a cycle is independent of body weight and therefore is almost identical for all individuals (Cerny & Darbee, 1990). Although the treadmill test generally yields higher oxygen consumption values, the cycle ergometer has the advantages of being relatively inexpensive, portable, and safe. Because cycling is also a familiar exercise for many people, it is less likely to cause apprehension. As with the treadmill test, cycle ergometry is reproducible (Fox & Mathews, 1981). In addition, the subject is relatively stationary and therefore vital signs are more easily monitored. Most ergometers have adjustable seat heights suitable for children, and it is important to be able to adjust handlebars and pedal crank length.

Several progressive exercise protocols are used on the cycle ergometer to determine maximum oxygen consumption or individual peak work capacity (see Chapter 8). Cerny and colleagues (1982) examined subjects with CF matched to a typical control sample to monitor cardiopulmonary response to incrementally increased workloads with cycle ergometry. Workloads were increased every 2 minutes until the subject could not continue. The study demonstrated that control subjects needed an increased workload of 0.32 W/kg on average for an increase in heart rate of 10 beats per minute. Subjects with CF required workload increases ranging from 0.15 to 0.35 W/kg, depending on the severity of their disease, to demonstrate the same change in heart rate. Cerny and colleagues concluded that the limiting factor in exercise tolerance was severity of pulmonary involvement and not cardiovascular limitation (Cerny et al., 1982).

If the child is too small to successfully use a cycle ergometer, a treadmill can be used because only the ability to walk is required (Fig. 27-6). The child should be monitored closely to maintain a sense of confidence during the test. The elevation and speed are adjusted according to the size and skill of the subject and should be selected to allow even the subject with severe dysfunction to exercise at two to three levels of difficulty (Cerny & Darbee, 1990).

For individuals with severe lung disease, field walking tests such as 6- or 12-minute walks (Butland et al., 1982) or the shuttle walking test (Scott et al., 1990) may be

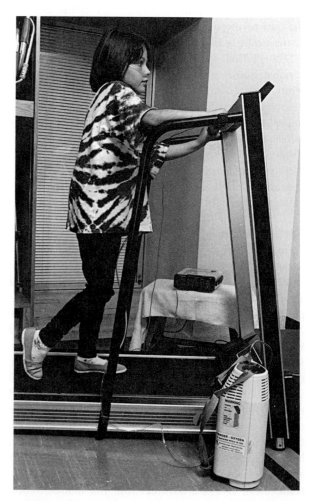

♦ Figure 27-6 Treadmill testing with a young patient on oxygen.

preferred. The reliability and validity of the 6-minute walk test (Gulmans et al., 1996) and the shuttle test (Selvadurai, 2003) with children with CF has been demonstrated. Walking tests are simple, are inexpensive, and can be performed by individuals of all ages and abilities with little risk of injury (Porcari et al., 1989). Because they are highly reproducible, walking tests correspond closely to the demands of everyday activity (Guyatt et al., 1985). Another quick and portable test that may prove useful in a clinical setting is the 3-minute step test, which illustrated similar results as the 6-minute walk test when outcome measures were arterial oxygen saturation, maximum pulse rate, and the Modified Borg Dyspnea Scale (Balfour-Lynn et al., 1998). Narang and colleagues (2003), however, found that when the 3-minute step test was compared to the cycle ergometer, the 3-minute step test provided limited information relating to exercise performance in a group with mild lung disease. They suggest that a more suitable test for this group must be at a higher intensity and equate more to typical levels of physical activity.

Subjects performing an exercise test must be closely monitored and special notice must be given to signs of increased work of breathing, disproportionate to what is expected (Cerny & Darbee, 1990). Subjective measures of the perceived level of respiratory labor with a dyspnea scale such as Borg's Scale of Ratings of Perceived Exertion (Borg, 1982) can be taken before, during, and after the exercise test. Borg's scale is a good indicator of both physiologic and psychologic strain and allows individuals to interpret the intensity of their exercise according to subjective impressions (Paley, 1997). For more information on quantifying increased work of breathing, a 15 count breathlessness scale is an objective measure that can be used with the Borg scale or a visual analogue scale (Prasad, 2000).

Maximal work capacity is limited by ventilation in individuals with pulmonary disease (Cerny & Darbee, 1990). Deficiencies in gas exchange and poor pulmonary mechanics compound the effects of decreased exercise capacity (Cerny et al., 1982; Henke & Orenstein, 1984). That limitation to exercise due to pulmonary restrictions is further evidenced by the failure to reach predicted peak heart rates in exercise test subjects with CF, suggesting that exercise capacity is not limited by cardiovascular factors (Canny & Levison, 1987).

A complete physical examination should assist in revealing the individual's level of fitness, thus aiding the physical therapist in choosing the most appropriate exercise testing protocol. Individual exercise programs can then be designed to improve exercise capacity and fitness level.

Management of Body Functions and Structures

People with CF demonstrate a wide variance in the severity of illness, because the disease progresses in individuals at different rates, but some amount of chronic airflow obstruction is often already present in childhood. The small peripheral airways are the site of most of these early pulmonary changes, and patchy atelectasis and ventilation-perfusion abnormalities lead to increases in functional dead space and discernible hypoxemia (MacLusky & Levison, 1990).

The goals of a physical therapy program for the young child should encompass the improvement of exercise tolerance with continued attention to secretion clearance techniques. Correction and maintenance of proper postural alignment are also stressed. Goals of treatment should be designed with the child and her or his family and account for the developmental stage of the child and the uniqueness of the family's circumstances. The learning environment must accommodate the child's learning style and avoid prescriptive tasks that are beyond the child's capabilities in order to promote self-efficacy and adherence. Education of the caregivers must incorporate similar strategies because their full cooperation and participation is essential.

Postural drainage, percussion, and vibration (conventional physical therapy) are common modalities for secretion mobilization in this population. Once children have grown too large to be positioned in the caregiver's lap for postural drainage, equipment such as a drainage board will have to be introduced. Mechanical percussors may be used to ease the work involved with manual percussion and to provide the child with an aid for self-treatment. Children with a chronic illness should be encouraged to assume a degree of responsibility for their own treatment. Feeling some level of control over one's own health fosters self-esteem and helps subdue anxiety (Kellerman et al., 1980). Children with CF may find it difficult to sustain the performance of manual percussion, even on easily accessible lung segments, and mechanical percussors can therefore help alleviate this problem.

Although conventional physical therapy has long been used in the treatment of CF, it has been criticized as being too time-consuming and difficult to perform independently. Adherence with a daily physical therapy regimen is reported as lower than with all other aspects of treatment (Passero et al., 1981). Proof of efficacy might promote adherence, but research studies to examine the effectiveness of conventional physical therapy are difficult to evaluate because they use a wide variety of outcome measures, including different PFTs, volume of secretions produced, and participants' subjective impressions (Starr,

1992). It is also problematic to compare studies done in different stages of the disease or with differences in study populations. Identifying the independent variable is sometimes troublesome because of the diverse combinations of techniques used; for example, percussion is rarely performed independently of postural drainage and coughing, making it difficult to definitively state which aspect of the treatment investigated has proved effective. Recent reviews suggest the usefulness of designing studies comparing treatment versus no treatment, but the ethical considerations of withholding treatment have prevented researchers from conducting this type of study at the present time (Hess, 2001).

In a study by Lorin and Denning (1971), the short-term effect of conventional physical therapy for patients with CF, compared with cough alone, was production of more sputum. Other studies support the effectiveness of conventional physical therapy in increasing amounts of sputum expectorated by subjects when excess secretion production is already a feature of the patient's condition (Bateman et al., 1979; Mazzacco et al., 1985). The amount of sputum produced may be quantified by volume or weight, but caution must be used when interpreting the findings from this type of measurement. Because many individuals may swallow a portion of their sputum, the output can underestimate the true volume produced. The amount of saliva that contaminates the product is difficult to determine, and this has resulted in the measurement of the dry weight of sputum in some studies. Measurement of dry weight is not practical in most clinical settings. In addition, the amount of sputum produced does not indicate where it originated.

Alternative methods for mobilizing secretions and stimulating cough have been suggested, usually involving directed breathing techniques. These include huffing, PEP, oscillating PEP (Flutter and Acapella), autogenic drainage, and active cycle of breathing (formerly known as FET).

The rationale for use of huffing, a type of forced expiration with a similar mechanism to coughing, was suggested by a study that bronchoscopically demonstrated that maintenance of an open glottis throughout the maneuver stabilized the collapsible airway walls of subjects with chronic airflow obstruction (Hietpas et al., 1979). The glottis normally closes in the compression phase of a cough, translating high compressive pressures on the tracheobronchial tree that may cause bronchiolar collapse (Starr, 1992). Uncontrolled coughing is often nonproductive and exhausting. To perform huffing, the subject is asked to take a deep inspiration and then, without allowing the glottis to close, to render a strong contraction of the abdominal muscles to aid in forceful expiration. Maintaining an open glottis can be compared

to vocalizing "ha" (Starr, 1992). Huffing is an uncomplicated breathing technique that can be easily taught to young children, and performing huffs can introduce the child to the concept of controlled or directed breathing techniques.

Descriptions of the forced expiratory technique vary in the literature. Generally, it employs forceful expirations combined with an open glottis as in huffing, interspersed with controlled breathing at mid to low lung volumes. A 3-year study was conducted by Reisman and associates (1988) to compare the treatment effects of FETs in isolation (without postural drainage) versus conventional physical therapy in subjects with mild to moderate pulmonary involvement. The study assessed the rates of deterioration in PFT scores, exercise challenge tests, and Shwachman clinical scores for all study subjects. The subjects who performed only FETs had significantly greater rates of decline in measures of FEV_1, midexpiratory flow rates ($FEF_{25-75\%}$), and Shwachman score than the group performing conventional physical therapy.

Clarification of the use of FET that always includes finer breathing control techniques and thoracic expansion exercises required that FET be reclassified as active cycle of breathing techniques by Pryor and associates (Pryor, 1991). The three components are combined in a set cycle: relaxation and breathing control and three to four thoracic expansion exercises repeated twice, then relaxation and breathing control followed by one or two forced expirations. When secretions reach the larger, proximal airways they may be cleared by a huff or a cough at high lung volume. Postural drainage positions may augment the effect, but the sitting position may be used if a gravity-assisted position is contraindicated (Webber & Pryor, 1998).

Use of PEP (Fig. 27-7) as a means of secretion mobilization for individuals with CF has been proposed. Introduced for use in this population in the 1980s in Denmark, PEP has been shown to be as effective as traditional cardiopulmonary physical therapy in both chronic (baseline) stages of CF (Gaskin et al., 1998; McIlwaine et al., 1997b; Oberwaldner et al., 1986) and during an acute exacerbation of pulmonary complications (Oberwaldner et al., 1991). The transmural pressure generated by maintaining resistant pressure throughout the expiration phase is thought to allow airflow to reach some obstructed alveoli through use of collateral airway channels. Airways are "splinted open" through the maintenance of PEP, thereby facilitating movement of peripheral secretions toward central airways (Lannefors, 1992). The reader is urged to refer to the studies mentioned earlier to gain a better understanding of PEP as an airway clearance modality for CF.

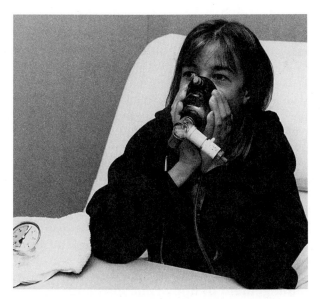

• **Figure 27-7**   Use of a positive expiratory pressure mask.

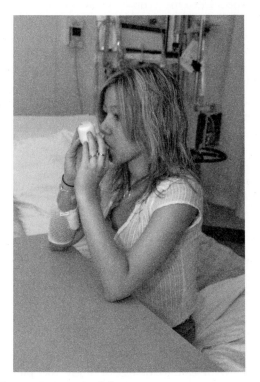

• **Figure 27-8**   Use of Flutter.

Oscillating PEP (Flutter therapy and the Acapella) was developed to generate a controlled oscillating positive pressure and interruptions to the airflow during expiration through a handheld device (Fig. 27-8). The Flutter uses the force of gravity, whereas the Acapella uses the force of magnetic attraction (Volsko et al., 2003). A long-term comparative trial study found that using Flutter in

isolation from other airway clearance techniques did not prove as effective as PEP in maintaining pulmonary function and was more costly due to the increased number of hospitalizations and antibiotic use (McIlwaine et al., 2001). Flutter may be useful as an adjunct to other airway clearance techniques, and short-term studies indicate its usefulness (Konstan et al, 1994). The Acapella is a new device for which little research has been conducted. One study comparing Acapella versus Flutter found that they had similar performance characteristics. They suggested Acapella may have some advantages over Flutter because it is not position-dependent and can be used at very low expiratory flows (Volsko, 2003).

An inflatable fitted vest attached to a pump that generates high-frequency oscillations applied to the external chest wall has been developed and is currently used in some CF centers. The high-frequency chest wall oscillation (HFCWO) helps to mobilize secretions and can be used simultaneously with other airway clearance techniques. The device is costly, however, and long-term studies of efficacy are still necessary (Hardy, 1994). Studies have found that HFCWO and conventional physical therapy are comparable for airway clearance (Grece, 2000; Tecklin et al., 2000; Warwick & Hanson, 1991), but caution must be used when comparing these studies because there are a number of manufacturers producing this device that use different protocols (Phillips et al., 2004).

Exercise has also been shown to be a useful therapeutic modality for secretion clearance, as evidenced by improved expiratory flow rates in subjects with stable CF with mild pulmonary disease (Zach et al., 1981). A 30-month study of the effects of discontinuing other airway clearance modalities in favor of participation in aerobic exercise activities demonstrated no significant declines in clinical status (Shwachman score), radiographic results, or PFT outcomes (Andreasson et al., 1987). In an acute exacerbation, exercise proved as effective as conventional physical therapy for the study subjects when pulmonary function was reviewed. The group assigned to "exercise" continued to receive one bronchial hygiene treatment session by a physical therapist daily, whereas the conventional physical therapy group received three of these sessions per day. Cerny concluded that hospitalized patients could substitute exercise for part of the standard in-hospital care (Cerny, 1989).

Benefits of an exercise program extend beyond increases in peak oxygen consumption, increased maximal work capacity, improved mucus expectoration, and improved expiratory flow rates (Heijerman et al., 1991; Orenstein et al., 1981; Zach et al., 1981). Participation in a prescribed exercise program has also been shown to improve self-concept (Folkins, 1972) and may provide increased social interaction. Fitness level has implications as a prognostic indicator. An improved survival rate is found in individuals with CF who demonstrate higher levels of aerobic fitness. Although this may simply reflect less severe illness, the ability to maintain aerobic fitness appears to have value in improving longevity (Nixon et al., 1992). In a habitual physical activity study of 101 patients age 7 to 18 years, girls in the highest physical activity group were characterized by a positive rate of change in FEV_1 over a 2-year period while the girls in the lowest activity groups had steeper rates of decline in their FEV_1 over the same period (Wilkes et al., 2003). In another habitual physical activity study, Nixon found that children with CF engage in less vigorous physical activities than their non-CF peers despite having good lung function. Therefore, it was concluded that individuals with CF should be encouraged to engage in more vigorous activities to promote aerobic fitness that may ultimately have an impact on survival (Nixon et al., 2001).

Young children with CF should be encouraged to use those treatments that best suit their requirements for adequate secretion clearance and prevention of deterioration of clinical status. Attitudes toward adherence with treatment can greatly influence the effectiveness of any therapeutic regimen, and the challenge for the physical therapist is to design a treatment strategy that is both useful for efficacy and practicality. Factors that must be considered in designing a therapy program include disease presentation and severity; patient's age; motivation and ability to concentrate; physician, caregiver, and patient goals; documented effectiveness; training considerations; work required; need for assistance or equipment; and costs (Hardy, 1994). Children who learn to adopt their physical therapy as an aspect of daily living, as opposed to a burden or punishment, will be more likely to comply with treatment plans.

ADOLESCENCE

Adolescence is a time of rapid transformation in many areas of development. Sexual maturation comes about as a result of the major changes in circulating hormones occurring around the time of maturity of the skeletal system, typically when the child is about 11 or 12 years old. These hormonal secretions cause a "growth spurt" in the adolescent (Green, 1983). "Delay of maturity" occurs when there has been slowed or prolonged skeletal maturation. This is often the cause of delayed puberty in adolescents with CF (di Sant'Agnese & Davis, 1979; Mitchell-Heggs et al., 1976). Arrested sexual development, combined with a smaller than average physical

build, can intensify feelings of isolation from healthy peers (McCollum & Gibson, 1970). Osteopenia (low bone mass) is a possible complication of CF and may be linked to nutritional factors, delayed puberty, reduced exercise or weight bearing activities, treatment with corticosteroids, and chronic infection (Conway, 2001). The prevention of osteoporosis and risk of fractures in patients with signs of osteopenia must be considered when developing a therapy program.

A need for increasing independence can conflict with the demands of daily medical care, making adherence with the routine seem arduous. The adolescent with CF who looks and feels disparate from the perceived "norm" may rebel against the continuation of time-consuming treatments that reinforce his or her sense of being dissimilar or abnormal (Boyle et al., 1976).

Management of Body Functions and Structures

Adherence with the "conventional" physical therapy routine of daily postural drainage and percussion sessions is poor in the adolescent population (McCollum & Gibson, 1970; Passero et al., 1981). One challenge with this population is to promote self-efficacy with alternative methods of treatment. The use of PEP, active cycle of breathing technique, or a program of regular exercise may help promote independence and has already been discussed. Autogenic drainage (AD) is another treatment modality involving self-controlled breathing techniques.

AD requires no equipment or special environment to execute and relies on the user's ability to control both inspiratory and expiratory airflow to generate maximum airflow within the different generations of bronchi (Chevaillier, 1984). Three separate phases of the technique are believed to "unstick" mucus in the peripheral airways, "collect" the mucus in the middle airways, and "evacuate" it from the central airways according to the volume level of the controlled breaths (McIlwaine et al., 1992). Mobilization of airway secretions by AD does not rely on the gravity assistance needed for postural drainage and can be performed in a sitting position.

There is a scarcity of research studies validating the long-term efficacy of AD. A study was published comparing AD with conventional physical therapy and PEP in patients with CF (McIlwaine et al., 1988), and a 2-year comparison trial of AD and conventional physical therapy has also been reported and showed no significant differences between treatment groups when clinical status and PFT scores were used as outcome measures (Davidson et al., 1992).

Learning the technique of AD poses difficulties for both the subject and the trainer. It requires concentration and the ability to use proprioceptive and sensory cues to localize the secretions in the various levels of bronchi. A hands-on approach is essential, with a minimum of environmental distractions. Frequent training sessions and reviews are necessary. This type of concentrated self-directed activity is usually not achievable by children younger than age 12. The mechanism for collateral ventilation through the channels of Lambert and pores of Kahn is not fully developed in young children (DeCesare & Graybill, 1990), providing another limitation to the use of AD.

Maintenance of proper posture is important for individuals with CF to provide efficient breathing mechanics. The changes in the length-tension relationships of the respiratory musculature that may occur with increases in FRC create a mechanical disadvantage and contribute to increased work of breathing and muscle fatigue (Cerny & Darbee, 1990). Several postural changes are found in CF to varying degrees, associated with chronically hyperinflated lungs, including increased anterior-posterior diameter of the chest, shoulder elevation, and forward protraction and abdominal flexion (Rose & Jay, 1986). The incidence of thoracic kyphosis in CF is approximately 15% (Denton et al., 1981), which predisposes affected individuals to chronic back pain. Estimates of the rate of back pain among people with CF are as high as 80% (Rose & Jay, 1986).

The physical therapist must examine the patient for postural deviations and signs of osteoporosis and determine which changes may be reversible or amenable to treatment. Exercises to promote improved posture include a strengthening program for the supporting muscles of the back and spine, stretching of contractured musculature, and training the subject to develop a keener sense of his or her postural alignment. Weight-bearing exercises should be included to promote bone formation. An innovative way to keep the adolescent active that can address the above issues is "ball therapy" (Fig. 27-9). Ball therapy can also be used to promote aerobic fitness, balance, coordination, and relaxation (Spalding et al., 1999). Projecting a good appearance is usually very important to adolescents, and informing the teenager with CF of the benefits of a good postural maintenance and weight-bearing program may provide the incentive necessary to ensure adherence to recommendations for exercises.

Secondary effects of strength training with weights may be an improvement in self-confidence in the adolescent because training has been shown to be beneficial in promoting weight gain (Strauss et al., 1987). As pulmonary impairment worsens, nutritional status is a consideration that requires a great deal of focus. Reduced anaerobic performance in CF is predominately due to poor nutritional status (Klijn et al., 2003). The dietitian serving the population with CF contributes considerable expertise in identifying situations in which intervention is necessary and may be a valuable ally to reinforce the message that exercise can promote weight gain when appropriately managed. A liaison with the dietitian can ensure coordination of dietary and physical therapy recommendations.

TRANSITION TO ADULTHOOD

When CF was first described in 1938, fewer than half of the patients survived their first year (Davis, 1983), but CF is no longer a purely pediatric disease. With contemporary methods of management, almost 80% of patients should reach adulthood (MacLusky & Levison, 1990), with an estimated life expectancy of 32 years (Yankaskas et al., 2004). Although many of the issues physical therapists are concerned with in the pediatric patient are similar for adults, some special differences should be considered.

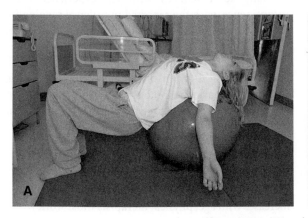
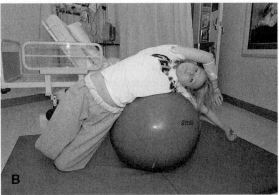

◆ **Figure 27-9** Exercise on the therapy ball.

Standard programs of transition from a pediatric to an adult center should include all team members to ensure the continuity of the patient's care (Flume et al., 2004). Continuity of care enhances the effectiveness of care, as well as minimizing uncertainty and distress for young individuals and their families. Transition from the pediatric to the adult CF team is an important milestone for patients and must be handled sensitively. Transfer is more easily achieved when the pediatric and adult clinics work closely together (Landau, 1995).

The psychosocial issues in adulthood are distinct because the normal progression of psychologic maturation brings new concerns with each developmental stage (Davis, 1983). Greater clinical awareness, early treatment, and more effective management of CF have all contributed to the improvement of prognosis (Pinkerton et al., 1985). Choices regarding education, employment (medical insurance), marriage, and family will have to be made. These choices are more complex than usual for the adult with CF, who not only has to consider present health status but also must attempt to predict future health status.

Consideration should be made concerning medical insurance coverage, flexible work hours, and sick time when choosing employment (Yankaskas et al., 2004). Physically demanding occupations may not be appropriate for the adult with CF with pulmonary limitations; therefore, a careful consideration of the physical demands of any task must be undertaken. Jobs involving constant exposure to dust, chemical fumes, or smoke should be avoided (Davis, 1983; Orenstein, 2003). Adults with CF will face few restrictions on choice of employment; however, infection control issues should be well thought out when choosing a career in health care (Yankaskas et al., 2004). Physical therapists should help to accommodate the adult's busy lifestyle and help to incorporate strategies for fitting treatment into work schedules. Methods that are more convenient and promote independence, such as the PEP mask, Flutter, or AD, may be more agreeable to the adult at work or school.

Because many adults with CF witness death among their peers, deterioration of their own health may have heightened significance for them. The adult who as an adolescent chose to be nonadherent with a physical therapy regimen may decide to initiate one again. Generally, individuals with CF have a strong positive outlook and are able to fully enjoy many of the typical pleasures of adulthood despite having to contend with unusual difficulties (Orenstein, 2003). Patients' attitudes and outlook on life can have a tremendous influence on the medical progression of CF and are considered in prognostic scores (Davis, 1983).

Because of the progressive nature of CF, many adults will have more symptoms and activity limitations than they had as children (Orenstein, 2003). Minor hemoptysis occurs in up to 60% of adults with CF (di Sant'Agnese & Davis, 1979), and in most cases, the cause is an increase in bronchial infection that has irritated a blood vessel (Orenstein, 1997). *Massive hemoptysis*, which is also strongly related to advancing age (Davis, 1983), is defined as a rupture of a bronchial blood vessel into the airways, producing greater than 300 mL of blood in 24 hours (Cohen, 1992). It is reported to occur in 5% to 7% of adults with CF (Porter et al., 1983) and warrants hospitalization and possible blood transfusion (Lloyd-Still, 1983).

Pneumothorax, which is one of the most common respiratory complications in adulthood, occurs in approximately 19% of individuals older than 13 years of age (MacLusky & Levison, 1990). A common cause of pneumothorax is the spontaneous rupture of apical bullae, which develop due to increased air trapping and microabscess formation in the diseased lung (MacLusky & Levison, 1990).

Episodes of hypertrophic pulmonary osteoarthropathy also increase in prevalence with advancing age (Davis, 1983). Digital clubbing can become more noticeable in people whose pulmonary disease is severe (Orenstein, 2003).

In general, cardiac status is related to severity of pulmonary involvement: the more severe the pulmonary adaptation to hypoxemia, the worse the pulmonary hypertension and right-sided heart strain. With comparable degrees of pulmonary disease, adults, especially those with mild lung disease, have more severe echocardiographic abnormalities than children. This may reflect the accumulative effects of episodes of mild hypoxemia and nocturnal oxygen desaturation that occur in even minimally affected individuals (Davis, 1983).

Many adult females with CF experience urinary incontinence, with the reported prevalence ranging from 30% to 68% on anonymous questionnaires. Respondents indicated that this problem was not reported due to embarrassment (Moran et al., 2003; Orr et al., 2001). The repeated physical strain of coughing, physical therapy, and exercise may contribute to its development. Addressing this issue should become part of the routine management and follow-up appointments in CF centers.

Management of Body Functions and Structures

Because the incidence of respiratory complications increases with age, physical therapists must work with the individual to adapt the treatment program accordingly.

For the individual experiencing hemoptysis, physical therapy may have to be altered, although there are conflicting opinions in the literature as to the extent of the modification necessary. Orenstein (2003) believes that if the cause of minor hemoptysis is an increase in bronchial infection irritating a blood vessel, treatment should be the same as for other types of increased infection. He believes that bleeding within the lungs can worsen infection by providing a more hospitable environment for bacteria. He does caution that if a particular treatment position aggravates the bleeding, that position should be avoided. Webber and Pryor (1998) also believe that physical therapy should be continued with blood streaking; however, with frank hemoptysis downward chest tilted and chest percussions should be discontinued. The use of postural drainage, percussion, and shaking, along with huffing or FETs, may be less likely to increase the amount of bleeding than the frequent uncontrolled coughing that may occur with abandonment of the manual techniques (Starr, 1992). In summary, it would seem logical that if a particular technique, such as percussion, makes the individual's situation worse, it should be discontinued. Other modalities using breathing techniques may be beneficial at this time.

Cardiopulmonary physical therapy is contraindicated in the presence of an untreated, progressing, or tension pneumothorax (DeCesare & Graybill, 1990); however, treatment can continue with a small, stable pneumothorax (DeCesare & Graybill, 1990; Mackenzie, 1989) and with a pneumothorax that has resolved through treatment with a thoracotomy and insertion of a chest tube for vacuum drainage of air (DeCesare & Graybill, 1990). Percussion must not be performed directly over the chest tube site owing to the danger of displacement, but percussion may be safely performed elsewhere on the thorax as tolerated. The PEP mask would not be the treatment of choice, because theoretically it could make the pneumothorax worse as a result of increased pressures generated in the airways.

Standard anti-inflammatory agents are used to treat the joint pain associated with hypertrophic pulmonary osteoarthropathy (Phillips & David, 1986). Physical therapists have a role in helping to relieve pain while maintaining joint range of motion. A home treatment program consisting of stretching, muscle strengthening, and range-of-motion exercises for the specific joints involved can be easily added to the individual's existing exercise program.

Management of urinary incontinence can be addressed by physical therapists prescribing pelvic floor muscle strength training. In the general population it was reported that pelvic floor muscle training was effective in 53% of the patients studied, with this group demonstrating a 66% success rate in the management of urinary incontinence for at least 10 years (Cammu et al., 2000).

When pulmonary disease becomes so disabling that the individual is having difficulty performing activities of daily living, physical therapy goals should encompass these needs. The patient may have to be instructed in energy conservation techniques such as diaphragmatic pursed-lip breathing and assuming positions that relieve breathlessness. These positions should promote comfort and relaxation and should encourage mobility of the thorax and support of the spinal column. They should also include hip flexion to relax the abdominal musculature and aid in increasing intra-abdominal pressure for coughing (DeCesare & Graybill, 1990). Examples of energy conservation positions are shown in Figure 27-10. Retraining of the respiratory pattern using pursed-lip breathing in conjunction with diaphragmatic excursion has shown temporary benefits in increased tidal volume, decreased respiratory rate, reduction in $Paco_2$ levels, and improved Pao_2 levels, as well as subjective benefits reported by patients (Ciesla, 1989). It may be that pursed-lip breathing improves confidence and decreases anxiety by providing some temporary control over oxygenation (Ciesla, 1989).

Oxygen needs with exercise may have to be assessed at this time. Continuation of an active lifestyle should be promoted for all individuals with CF to optimize physical condition and maintain an optimistic outlook. If the individual is considering lung transplantation as an option, physical therapists must involve the individual in a formalized exercise program. The Toronto Lung Transplant Program at the Toronto Hospital has a well-established rehabilitation program. Exercise capacity is determined by using a 6-minute walk test and ear oximetry, or the Modified Bruce Protocol on the treadmill (Craven et al., 1990). For a 6-minute walk test, the subject is instructed to walk as quickly and comfortably as possible on a level, measured distance for 6 minutes. If the patient becomes short of breath or too exhausted to continue, he or she is allowed to rest but then must continue the test as soon as symptoms subside. The distance traveled and the rest periods the subject takes are recorded. Subjects' pulse and respiratory rates and oxygen saturation are measured and recorded before, during, and at the conclusion of the test. The purpose of performing a test of exercise capacity is to help determine if severity of disability warrants consideration for transplant. A 6-minute walk test result of less than 400 meters was found to be a significant indicator for a patient to be listed for transplantation (Kadikar et al., 1997).

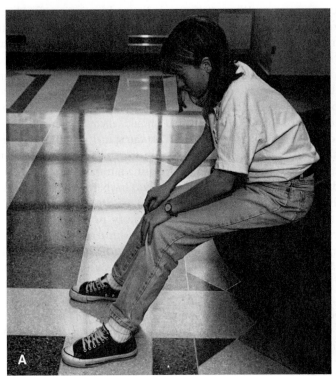
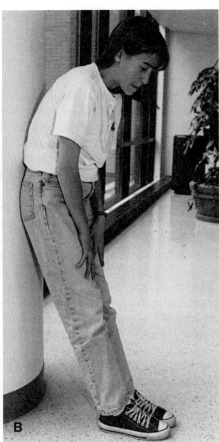

+ **Figure 27-10** **A** and **B**, Positioning for energy conservation, promoting relaxation and ease of breathing.

Individuals can also be monitored at regular intervals with these tests to gauge potential deterioration in their functional status. Once accepted into the lung transplantation program, most centers require attendance at a formal rehabilitation program (Grossman, 1988) featuring aerobics, muscle strengthening, stretching, and light calisthenics.

Expected physical therapy outcomes for the adult with CF include optimizing functional ability, physical exercise tolerance, and emotional well-being. For the individual awaiting a lung transplant, improvement in overall function should enable him or her to handle the actual surgery and immediate postoperative period with less difficulty (Craven et al., 1990). Arnold and associates (1991) found that 13 patients with end-stage CF showed improvement in their functional exercise capacity by participation in pulmonary rehabilitation while awaiting double-lung transplantation. Pulmonary rehabilitation entailed treadmill walking and lower extremity ergometry three to five times per week, initiated at the time of listing for double-lung transplant. Six-minute walks

were performed biweekly to assess changes in functional exercise capacity, and workload on the treadmill and bicycle ergometer was recorded. Six-minute walk distances and treadmill and bicycle workloads all increased significantly. The conclusions from this data confirm the possibility of improving functional exercise capacity in patients with end-stage CF awaiting double-lung transplantation, despite severe limitations in pulmonary function.

Noninvasive ventilation, most commonly biphasic positive airway pressure (BIPAP), may benefit CF patients who are experiencing respiratory failure and awaiting lung transplantation. Although nocturnal oxygen therapy has not been shown to improve long-term prognosis, nighttime BIPAP reduces hypoxia, hypercarbia, and work of breathing and may enhance airway clearance and reduce pulmonary hypertension (Wagener & Headley, 2003).

The physical therapist's contact with those individuals in the terminal stages of their disease should not be discontinued. Intervention at this stage must include the provision of comfort measures and be directed by the patient's wishes. Treatment sessions may have to decrease in duration and be offered with increased frequency throughout the day. Adaptations to postural drainage positions may have to be adopted so treatment can be tolerated. As the work of coughing becomes too tiring or painful, other modalities such as splinting and huffing can be reviewed. Pain control measures and relaxation and anxiety-reducing techniques, such as massage, may be the primary need of the dying patient. Simply listening to the concerns of these patients can be therapeutic. The value of a compassionate ear should not be underestimated. Physical therapists treating terminally ill patients should be careful to incorporate the families' needs, respecting the fact that this is an emotionally volatile time for all involved.

▌ SUMMARY

The management of CF poses many challenges for physical therapists. The multisystemic involvement and chronicity of the disorder compel physical therapists to continually interact with a team of professionals to shape appropriate treatment plans. Collaboration with this type of multidisciplinary health care team is always stimulating and fosters creative and fulfilling practice of physical therapy. New advances suggest exciting possibilities for the future care of people with CF, and physical therapists serving this population are required to continually adapt their management approach in light of new research. The aspiration to discover a cure seems to be approaching fulfillment. Meanwhile, the challenge for all those involved is in finding effective means to slow (or prevent) the disabling effects of this disease.

CASE STUDY

TRISTAN

The following case study documents the diagnosis and symptomology of a male with CF, who we will call Tristan, over the course of a 16-year period.

Tristan's state of health has fluctuated a great deal, especially during times of poor adherence, both to the suggested physical therapy regimen and to the diet and medications prescribed. Tristan's history of poor adherence does not represent all CF patients but is illustrated in this case history to identify the challenges

multidisciplinary team members struggle with. His parents have often reported having difficulty with obtaining cooperation from Tristan, and frequent residential moves have tended to exacerbate the problem of establishing beneficial routines. We can draw inferences from the evidence, which demonstrates correlations between adherence and overall health or frequency of admission to hospital. Perhaps the greatest benefit of examining a case such as this one is to ask ourselves if more could have been done to stimulate or inspire Tristan and his parents to engage in a proactive way with the treatment regimen.

Tristan was diagnosed with CF at the age of 2 months with a sweat chloride reading of 124 mEq/L. As is common among children diagnosed in infancy, Tristan had been admitted to hospital because of his failure to thrive. Tristan's parents underwent the newly diagnosed CF teaching program to learn how to care for Tristan once he was discharged home. They were instructed by all team members including the doctor, nurse, dietitian, social worker, and the physical therapist. Tristan's parents were provided with information and education from the physical therapist regarding anatomy and physiology of the lungs, how CF affects the lungs, the purpose of physical therapy, signs of respiratory distress, and the importance of exercise. His parents obtained a compressor and nebulizer for inhalation treatments and were instructed with a home program consisting of postural drainage and manual percussion. Goals for physical therapy were established and included maintaining good ventilation and promoting secretion clearance.

When Tristan was seen in the clinic at age 2, his mother reported that adherence to the therapy was sporadic, as she was having difficulty keeping Tristan in position on her lap. A postural drainage board was ordered to assist in placing Tristan in proper positions. During the following 2 years, Tristan was seen in clinic with increased cough, elevated sputum quantity, decreased appetite, and poor exercise capacity. His mother reported that he was having difficulty keeping up with his brothers. At age 4, his sputum cultures grew *Staphylococcus aureus* and *Streptococcus pyogenes* and his cough was persistently harsh, often culminating in vomiting. This greatly affected his ability to gain weight and he presented below the third percentile in growth for his age. At this time Tristan was admitted to the hospital. A fecal fat collection, upper gastrointestinal series, and immunologic workups were initiated upon admission. The dietitian felt that the abnormally high fecal fat percentage in his stool and low vitamin levels was due to poor adherence with enzymes at home. This admission provided an opportunity for the social worker to interview and offer aid to the family. The importance of enzyme therapy was reviewed and a need for assistance with the physical therapy regimen was requested by the family. A referral was initiated to obtain physical therapy services through the Home Care Program. This was welcomed by the parents, who had been feeling overwhelmed with all the time demands of Tristan's treatment and raising three other boys. During the admission, Tristan received ceftazidime and tobramycin intravenously, and a physical therapy program of postural drainage, manual percussions, expiratory vibrations, breathing exercises, and an exercise program was performed three times a day. Near the end of the admission he showed marked improvement and was clearing secretions comfortably with little to no vomiting after being taught proper huffing technique. He was discharged home on oral cephalexin owing to his acquisition of *Staphylococcus aureus* infection.

At age 4 years 9 months, Tristan's sputum cultures grew *Pseudomonas aeruginosa* and he was started on inhaled tobramycin. Since the referral to Home Care there were no identified problems with the physical therapy regimen; however, the importance of regular exercise was reviewed. At age 5 years 6 months, Tristan's first PFT revealed a FEV_1 of 69% predicted. His chest x-ray findings demonstrated mild air trapping with increased peribronchial thickening and some small nodular cystic areas. His medications included inhaled tobramycin and salbutamol three times daily. Over the next few years, his FEV_1 fluctuated, from 54% to 64% to 71%. These changes seemed directly related to his adherence to therapy. At the time of his eighth birthday Tristan's mother reported that there was some friction between Tristan and herself; there was an ongoing struggle around adherence to the treatment regimen, in particular, the physical therapy. A chest x-ray revealed bronchiectatic changes, particularly in the left lower lobe. It was suggested that Tristan and his family attend the annual teaching day focusing on self-management skills in the hope that Tristan would take responsibility and have more understanding of his disease. In an attempt to improve his self-efficacy, a log book (Junior Passport) was provided to Tristan to keep track of his treatments and any questions he may have for the clinic team.

Over the next year, Tristan had no admissions to hospital. He reported his spirits improved after meeting other children with CF at the teaching day. Having the chance to discuss how CF affects other kid's lives and how they cope with the heavy treatment regimen gave him new motivation to improve his adherence. Tristan, however, was hesitant to change his physical therapy program from postural drainage and percussion to a more independent treatment (PEP therapy) demonstrating his continued reliance on his parents to assist in his treatment.

Tristan's pulmonary function values continued to decline despite all efforts to improve his adherence. This steady decline was accompanied by noticeable respiratory changes such as tachypnea and indrawing. Tristan also continued to experience frequent emesis with coughing. His chest x-ray showed new markings in the upper lobes and continued deterioration of his lower lobes. His parents resisted having him hospitalized but finally agreed to an admission when his FEV_1 was 57% predicted. He was also feverish with cough and vomiting and had significant weight loss. During this admission, physical therapy of manual percussions and expiratory vibrations in classical positions was supplemented by 20 to 30 minutes of stationary bike riding. Tristan was released home on inhaled tobramycin and oral cephalexin as well as a home exercise program designed to accommodate his interests and routine.

A few months later Tristan required another admission to hospital with a chest exacerbation. By this time Tristan was 11 years old and showing evidence of stubbornness and an urgent need for an independent method of chest therapy. In consultation with the physical therapist, Tristan and his parents decided to pursue PEP therapy. During his time in hospital Tristan was supervised with five to six cycles of PEP therapy including abdominal breathing and huffing. Tristan demonstrated good technique and tolerance and was able to produce large amounts of sputum. At the time of discharge his FEV_1 improved to 77% predicted. At his next clinic appointment, 5 months later, Tristan admitted to using the PEP mask only sporadically, but reported he was enjoying learning to play the saxophone at school, which was encouraged by the CF team. Once again, an attempt was made through counseling to impress on him the importance of adhering with the treatment regimen. Less than a year later, Tristan was again admitted to hospital, with an FEV_1 of 56%. His coughing was extremely harsh and frequently caused vomiting. On auscultation, Tristan had diffuse crackles and decreased air entry to the bilateral bases, with very little airflow audible in the left side. During this stay consistent exercise and PEP mask treatment three times a day after inhalation therapy were maintained. His FEV_1 climbed back up and was measured a month later as 80% predicted.

His next hospital admission occurred just 6 months later, when his FEV_1 dropped again, this time to 61% predicted. His coughing and repeated vomiting continued to haunt his attempts to gain or maintain his weight and there was new evidence on chest x-ray of deteriorating lung status. The dietitian suggested that he eat frequent smaller meals and reviewed high-energy caloric foods.

It was a year later when he was next admitted to hospital with an increased cough and a plummeting FEV_1 of 57% predicted. With his decreasing lung function, his resistance on the PEP mask was adjusted to maintain proper pressures for optimal airway clearance. He showed improvement on pulmonary function testing with a discharge FEV_1 of 74% predicted. The improvement was short-lived, however, as 1 month later he was readmitted with symptoms of mononucleosis: lethargy and poor energy levels, episodes of fever and chills, tonsillitis, and thrush with mouth sores. He had lost another 3 kg (6.7 lb) and was showing evidence of moderate respiratory distress, with tachypnea and severe indrawing. His FEV_1 was only 50% predicted. The team worked to stabilize and improve his overall status. While in hospital, Tristan had extensive interaction with the social worker, dietitian, and physical therapist, who once again reinforced the importance of adherence with the treatment regimens.

Over the next year, admissions to hospital increased in frequency, and Tristan was in hospital every 2 to 3 months. Monitoring adherence with his physical therapy program was facilitated when he was an in-patient, and he did apply himself to the exercises of ball therapy, bicycling, and stair climbing. He continued to lose weight, however, and at age 15, in April, was admitted for a G-tube insertion. Within a month, he had gained 1.4 kg (3.08 lb), but was readmitted with a chest exacerbation, blood streaked sputum, and a racking cough. During this admission, the team discovered that his frequent absences from school had resulted in him failing his year, prompting his mother to request summer admissions in the future so as not to jeopardize his schooling. Counseling was offered to both Tristan and his mother, and again, a social work referral was initiated through his local Home Care Agency. Tristan's FEV_1 was at a new low of 41% and he was complaining of chest tightness. Additional physical therapy techniques, autogenic drainage, and active cycle of breathing were initiated in an attempt to find the most effective airway clearance technique for his current chest status. Tristan demonstrated the technique of AD very effectively and was able to clear secretions even with his feelings of chest tightness. He also enjoyed working on postural chest expansion exercises on a therapy ball and on discharge had resolved to continue with this combination of treatments.

Three months later, at the end of the summer, Tristan was readmitted to hospital with the by now familiar scenario of falling FEV_1 and vomiting with heavy coughing. A 1-month trial of DNase was initiated. Tristan admitted to not being 100% compliant with the suggested physical therapy. Within 1 month he was back in hospital with deteriorating status: an FEV_1 of 36%, daily vomiting and fevers, and significant weight loss. Evidence of his deteriorating respiratory status was also apparent in his chest x-rays: nodular densities in lateral aspects of both right and left upper lobes and worsening lesions that likely represented areas of mucoid impaction. Tristan's ranitidine dosage was adjusted and his gastro-intestinal symptoms decreased. Tristan agreed to follow the same course of physical therapy, and adherence was stressed once again; however, within a month Tristan attended clinic and reported continued difficulty sleeping, night sweats, and fevers. He was not admitted but was prescribed a 21-day course of azithromycin, an anti-inflammatory agent, and a 5-day course of prednisone. Unfortunately, financial difficulties arose and Tristan did not take the suggested 3-week trial of azithromycin. Subsequently, the team's social worker investigated and obtained funding for the drug and Tristan did have good response to the drug.

The next few months were quiet ones. Tristan continued to do well but things deteriorated again when he stopped taking his ranitidine (the excuse for this was that it got misplaced during a residential move). As this situation came to light, Tristan also revealed that he had not been taking the azithromycin during the last few weeks because he had also lost this medication. He was complaining of abdominal pain again and was demonstrating low PFT scores with an FEV_1 of 43% predicted. Tristan was skipping school and lying in front of the television all day. A referral to psychology was made because he was despondent. Tristan was given the opportunity to relate his fears and concerns regarding his future with the psychologist, and life strategies were discussed. The correlation between adhering with the prescribed treatment regimen and his overall health status appeared to be finally accepted by Tristan. Quality of life issues and ideas to boost both his energy levels and his mood were proposed by all members of the team. Once again, Tristan appeared to understand and agreed to try to be more diligent with the treatment program.

As he left the clinic, he was boosted by the support of the team, and we remain hopeful that as he continues to mature he will be able to apply himself with a new resolve.

REFERENCES

Ackerman, V, Montgomery, G, Eigen, H, & Tepper, R. Assessment of airway responsiveness in infants with cystic fibrosis. American Review of Respiratory Disease, 144:344–346, 1991.

Altose, MD. The physiological basis of pulmonary function testing. Clinical Symposia, *31*(2):1–39, 1979.

Andersen, DH. Cystic fibrosis of the pancreas and its relation to celiac disease: A clinical and pathologic study. American Journal of Diseases of Children, *56*:344–395, 1938.

Andreasson, B, Jonson, B, Kornfalt, R, Nordmar, E, & Sandstrom, S. Long-term effects of physical exercise on working capacity and pulmonary function in cystic fibrosis. Acta Paediatrica Scandinavica, *76*:70–75, 1987.

Arnold, CD, Westerman, JH, Downs, AM, & Egan, TM. Benefits of an aerobic exercise program in C.F. patients waiting for double lung transplant. Pediatric Pulmonology Supplement, *6*:287, 1991.

Auerbach, HS, Williams, M, Kirkpatrick, JA, & Colten, HR. Alternate-day prednisone reduces morbidity and improves pulmonary function in cystic fibrosis. Lancet, *2*:686–688, 1985.

Aurora, P, Stocks, J, Oliver, C, Saunders, C, Castle, R, Chaziparasidis, G, & Bush, A. Quality control for spirometry in pre-school children with and without lung disease. American Journal of Respiratory and Critical Care Medicine, *169*:1152–1159, 2004.

Aweida, D, & Kelsey, CJ. Accuracy and reliability of physical therapists in auscultating tape-recorded breath sounds. Physiotherapy in Canada, *42*(6):279–282, 1989.

Balfour-Lynn, IM, Prasad, SA, Laverty, A, Whitehead, BF, & Dinwiddie, R. A step in the right direction: Assessing exercise tolerance in cystic fibrosis. Pediatric Pulmonology, *25*(4):223–225, 1998.

Bartholomew, LK, Czyzewski, DI, & Swank, PR. Short-term outcomes of the CF Family Education Program (CF FEP): What we know and what we don't know. Pediatric Pulmonology Supplement, *13*:154–155, 1996.

Bartholomew, LK, Parcel, GS, Swank, PR, & Czyzewski, DI. Measuring self-efficacy expectations for the self-management of cystic fibrosis. Chest, *103*:1524–1530, 1993.

Bateman, JRM, Newton, SP, Daunt, KM, Pavia, D, & Clarke, SW. Regional lung clearance of excessive bronchial secretions during chest physiotherapy in patients with stable chronic airway obstruction. Lancet, *1*:294–297, 1979.

Borg, GAV. Psychophysical bases of perceived exertion. Medicine and Science in Sports and Exercise, *14*:377–381, 1982.

Boucek, MM, Edwards, LB, Keck, BM, Trulock, EP, Taylor, DO, Mohacsi, PJ, & Hertz, MI. The registry of the international society for heart and lung transplantation: Sixth official pediatric report—2003. The Journal of Heart and Lung Transplantation, *22*:636–652, 2003.

Boucher, RC, Knowles, MR, & Yankaskas, JR. Cystic fibrosis. In Textbook of Respiratory Medicine, 3rd ed. Vol. 2. Toronto: WB Saunders, 2000, pp. 1291–1323.

Boyd, S, Brooks, D, Agnew-Coughlin, J, & Ashwell, J. Evaluation of the literature on the effectiveness of physical therapy modalities in the management of children with cystic fibrosis. Pediatric Physical Therapy, *6*(2):70–74, 1994.

Boyle, IR, di Sant'Agnese, PA, & Sack, S. Emotional adjustment of adolescents and young adults with cystic fibrosis. Journal of Pediatrics, *88*:318–326, 1976.

Brennan, AL & Geddes, DM. Bringing new treatments to the bedside in cystic fibrosis. Pediatric Pulmonology, *37*:87–98, 2004.

Buist, AS, Adams, BE, Sexton, GJ, & Azzam, AH. Reference values for functional residual capacity and maximal expiratory flow in young children. American Review of Respiratory Disease, *122*:938–988, 1980.

Burns, JL. Treatment of cepacia: In search of the magic bullet. Pediatric Pulmonology Supplement, *14*:90–91, 1997.

Burton, L. The Family Life of Sick Children: A Study of Families Coping with Chronic Childhood Disease. London: Routledge & Kegan Paul, 1975.

Bush, A. Giving the bad news—Your child has cystic fibrosis. Pediatric Pulmonology Supplement, *14*:206–208, 1997.

Butland, RJA, Pang, J, Gross, ER, Woodcock, AA, & Geddes, DM. Two, six and 12-minute walking test in respiratory disease. British Medical Journal, *284*:1607–1608, 1982.

Button, BM, Heine, R, Catto-Smith, A, Olinsky, A, Phelan, PD, & Story, I. Chest physiotherapy in infants with cystic fibrosis: To tip or not? A five-year study. Pediatric Pulmonology, *35*(3):208–213, 2003.

Button, BM, Heine, R, Catto-Smith, A, Olinsky, A, Phelan, PD, & Story, I. A 12 month comparison of standard vs. modified chest physiotherapy in 20 infants with cystic fibrosis. Pediatric Pulmonology Supplement, *14*:299a, 1997.

Cammu, H, Van Nylen, M, & Amy, JJ. A 10-year follow-up after Kegel pelvic floor muscle exercises for genuine stress incontinence. British Journal of Urology International, *85*:655–658, 2000.

Canadian Association for Health, Physical Education and Recreation. Fitness Performance: Second Test Manual—Canadian Youths, Ages 6–17. Ottawa: CAHPER, 1980.

Cappelli, M, McGrath, PJ, MacDonald, NE, Katsanis, J, & Lascelles, M. Parental care and overprotection of children with cystic fibrosis. British Journal of Medical Psychology, *62*:281–289, 1989.

Cerny, FJ. Relative effects of bronchial drainage and exercise for in-hospital care of patients with cystic fibrosis. Physical Therapy, *69*:633–639, 1989.

Cerny, FJ, & Darbee, J. Exercise testing and exercise conditioning for children with lung dysfunction. In Irwin, S, & Tecklin, JS (Eds.). Cardiopulmonary Physical Therapy. St. Louis: Mosby, 1990, pp. 461–475.

Cerny, FJ, Pullano, TP, & Cropp, GJA. Cardiorespiratory adaptations to exercise in cystic fibrosis. American Review of Respiratory Disease, *126*:217–220, 1982.

Chevaillier, J. Autogenic drainage. In Lawson, D (Ed.). Cystic Fibrosis: Horizons. New York: Wiley, 1984, p. 235.

Ciesla, N. Postural drainage, positioning and breathing exercises. In Mackenzie, CF (Ed.). Chest Physiotherapy in the Intensive Care Unit. Baltimore: Williams & Wilkins, 1989, pp. 93–133.

Coates, AL, MacNeish, CF, Lands, LC, Meisner, D, Kelemen, S, & Vadas, EB. A comparison of the availability of tobramycin for inhalation from vented vs. unvented nebulizers. Chest, *113*(4):951–956, 1998.

Cohen, AM. Hemoptysis: Role of angiography and embolization. Pediatric Pulmonology Supplement, *8*:85–86, 1992.

Collins, FS. The C.F. gene: Perceptions, puzzles and promises. Pediatric Pulmonology Supplement, *8*:63–64, 1992.

Collins, FS. CF Research: Highlights of 1996. Pediatric Pulmonology Supplement, *13*:74, 1996.

Conway, SP. Impact of lung inflammation on bone metabolism in adolescents with cystic fibrosis. Paediatric Respiratory Review, *2*(4):324–331, 2001.

Conway, SP, & Allenby, K. Parental and patient attitudes in an adult CF clinic to prenatal screening programmes. Pediatric Pulmonology Supplement, *8*:238, 1992.

Cooper, PJ, Robertson, CF, Hudson, IL, & Phelan, PD. Variability of pulmonary function tests in cystic fibrosis. Pediatric Pulmonology, *8*:16–22, 1990.

Corey, M, Allison, L, Prober, C, & Levison, H. Sputum bacteriology in patients with cystic fibrosis in a Toronto hospital during 1970–1981. Journal of Infectious Diseases, *149*:283, 1984a.

Corey, M, Gaskin, K, Durie, P, Levison, H, & Forstner, G. Improved prognosis in C.F. patients with normal fat absorption. Journal of Pediatric Gastroenterology and Nutrition, *3*(suppl 1):99–105, 1984b.

Crane, L. Physical therapy for the neonate with respiratory disease. In Irwin, S, & Tecklin, JS (Eds.). Cardiopulmonary Physical Therapy. St. Louis: Mosby, 1990, pp. 389–416.

Craven, JL, Bright, J, & Dear, CL. Psychiatric, psychosocial, and rehabilitative aspects of lung transplantation. Clinics in Chest Medicine, *11*:247–257, 1990.

Crystal, RG. Gene therapy for cystic fibrosis: Where have we been and where are we going? Pediatric Pulmonology Supplement, *14*:73, 1997.

Dab, I, & Malfroot, A. Gastroesophageal reflux: A primary defect in cystic fibrosis. Scandinavian Journal of Gastroenterology Supplement, *143*:125–131, 1988.

Darbee, JC, Ohtake PJ, Grant BJ, & Cerny FJ. Physiologic evidence for the efficacy of positive expiratory pressure as an airway clearance technique in patients with cystic fibrosis. Physical Therapy, *84*(6):524–537, 2004.

Davidson, AGF, McIlwaine, PM, Wong, LTK, & Pirie, GE. Long-term comparative trial of conventional percussion and drainage physiotherapy versus autogenic drainage in cystic fibrosis. Pediatric Pulmonology Supplement, *8*:a298, 1992.

Davidson, KL. Airway clearance strategies for the pediatric patient. Respiratory Care, *47*:823–828, 2002.

Davis, PB. Cystic fibrosis in adults. In Lloyd-Still, JD (Ed.). Textbook of Cystic Fibrosis. Stoneham, MA: Wright, 1983, pp. 351–370.

Day, G, & Mearns, M. Bronchial lability in cystic fibrosis. Archives of Disease in Childhood, *48*:355–359, 1973.

Dean, M, O'Connell, P, Leppert, M, Park, M, Amos, JA, Phillips, DG, White, R, & Vande Woude, GF. Three additional DNA polymorphisms in the met gene and D7S8 locus: Use in prenatal diagnosis of cystic fibrosis. Journal of Pediatrics, *111*:490–495, 1987.

DeCesare, JA, & Graybill, CA. Physical therapy for the child with respiratory dysfunction. In Irwin, S, & Tecklin, JS (Eds.). Cardiopulmonary Physical Therapy. St. Louis: Mosby, 1990, pp. 417–460.

Denton, JR, Tietjen, R, & Gaerlan, PF. Thoracic kyphosis in cystic fibrosis. Clinical Orthopaedics and Related Research, *155*:71–74, 1981.

di Sant'Agnese, PA, & Davis, PB. Cystic fibrosis in adults: 75 cases and a review of 232 cases in the literature. American Journal of Medicine, *66*:121–132, 1979.

Doershuk, CF, Downs, TD, Matthews, LW, & Lough, MD. A method for ventilatory measurements in subjects one month to five years of age: Normal results and observations in disease. Pediatric Research, *4*:165–174, 1970.

Doershuk, CF, Matthews, LW, & Tucker, AS. A five-year clinical evaluation of a therapeutic program for patients with cystic fibrosis. Journal of Pediatrics, *65*:1112–1113, 1964.

Durie, PR. Gastrointestinal motility disorders in cystic fibrosis. In Willa, JP (Ed.). Disorders of Gastrointestinal Motility in Childhood. New York: Wiley, 1988, pp. 91–99.

Durie, PR, Gaskin, KJ, Corey, M, Kopelman, H, Weizman, Z, & Forstner, GG. Pancreatic function testing in cystic fibrosis. Journal of Pediatric Gastroenterology and Nutrition, *3*:89–98, 1984.

Eakin, EG, Resnikoff, PM, Prewitt, LM, Ries, AL, & Kaplan, RM. Validation of a new dyspnea measure: The UCSD Shortness of Breath Questionnaire. University of California, San Diego. Chest, *113*(3):619–624, 1998.

Egan, ME, Pearson, M, Weiner, SA, Rajendran, V, Rubin, D, Glockner-Pagel, J, Canny, S, Du, K, Lukacs, GL & Caplan, MJ. Curcumin, a major constituent of turmeric, corrects cystic fibrosis defects. Science, *304*:600–602, 2004.

Egan, TM. Overview of lung transplantation for cystic fibrosis. Pediatric Pulmonology Supplement, *8*:204–205, 1992.

England, SJ. Current techniques for assessing pulmonary function in the newborn and infant: Advantages and limitations. Pediatric Pulmonology, *4*:48–53, 1988.

Flume, PA, Taylor LA, Anderson DL, Gray, S, & Turner, D. Transition programs in cystic fibrosis centers: Perceptions of team members. Pediatric Pulmonology, *37*:4–7, 2004.

Flume, PA, & Yankaskas, JR. Reproductive issues. In Yankaskas JR, Knowles, MR (Eds). Cystic Fibrosis in Adults. Philadelphia: Lippincott-Raven, 1999, pp. 449–464.

Folkins, C. The effects of physical training on mood. Journal of Clinical Psychology, *32*:583–588, 1972.

Fox, EL, & Mathews, DK. The Physiological Basis of Physical Education and Athletics, 3rd ed. Philadelphia: Saunders College, 1981.

Fried, MD, Durie, PR, Tsui, LC, Corey, M, Levison, H, & Pencharz, PB. The cystic fibrosis gene and resting energy expenditure. Journal of Pediatrics, *119*:913–916, 1991.

Frownfelter, DL (Ed.). Chest Physical Therapy and Pulmonary Rehabilitation. Chicago: Year Book Medical, 1987.

Galabert, C, Zahm, JM, Chaffin, C, de Bentzmann, S, Grosskopf, C, Chazalette, JP, & Puchelle, E. Improvement by rhDNASE of cystic fibrosis mucus transport capacity is related to the release of surface active molecules. Pediatric Pulmonology Supplement, *13*:283a, 1996.

Gaskin, L, Shin, J, Reisman, JJ, Thomas, J, & Tullis, E. Long term trial of conventional postural drainage and percussion vs. positive expiratory pressure. Pediatric Pulmonology Supplement, *15*:345a, 1998.

Gibson, LE, & Cooke, RE. A test for the concentration of electrolytes in sweat in cystic fibrosis of the pancreas utilizing pilocarpine by iontophoresis. Pediatrics, *23*:545–549, 1959.

Gilljam, H, Malmborg, A, & Strandvik, B. Conformity of bacterial growth in sputum and contamination free endobronchial samples in patients with cystic fibrosis. Thorax, *41*:641–645, 1986.

Godfrey, S. Exercise Testing in Children. Philadelphia: WB Saunders, 1974.

Godfrey, S, Bar-Yishay, E, Arad, I, Landau, LI, & Taussig, LM. Flow-volume curves in infants with lung disease. Pediatrics, *72*:517–522, 1983.

Grece, CA. Effectiveness of high frequency chest compression: A 3-year retrospective study. Pediatric Pulmonology Supplement, *20*:302, 2000.

Green, M, & Solnit, AJ. Reactions to the threatened loss of a child: A vulnerable child syndrome. Pediatrics, *34*:58–66, 1964.

Green, OC. Endocrinological complications associated with cystic fibrosis. In Lloyd-Still, JD (Ed.). Textbook of Cystic Fibrosis. Stoneham, MA: Wright, 1983, pp. 329–349.

Grossman, RF. Lung transplantation. Medical Clinics of North America, *24*:4572–4579, 1988.

Gulmans, VAM, van Veldhoven, NHMJ, de Meer, K, & Helders, PJM. The six-minute walking test in children with cystic fibrosis: Reliability and validity. Pediatric Pulmonology, *22*:85–89, 1996.

Gurwitz, D, Corey, M, Francis, PJ, Crozier, D, & Levison, H. Perspectives in cystic fibrosis. Pediatric Clinics of North America, *26*(3):603–615, 1979.

Guyatt, GH, Sullivan, MJ, Thompson, PJ, Fallen, EL, Pugsley, SO, Taylor, DW, & Berman, LB. The 6-minute walk: A new measure of exercise capacity in patients with chronic heart failure. Canadian Medical Association Journal, *132*:919–923, 1985.

Hardy, KA. A review of airway clearance: New techniques, indications, and recommendations. Respiratory Care, *39*(5):440–452, 1994.

Hardy, KA, Wolfson, MR, Schidlow, DV, & Shaffer, TH. Mechanics and energetics of breathing in newly diagnosed infants with cystic fibrosis: Effect of combined bronchodilator and chest physical therapy. Pediatric Pulmonology, *6*:103–108, 1989.

Heijerman, HGM, Bakker, W, Sterk, P, & Dijkman, JH. Oxygen-assisted exercise training in adult cystic fibrosis patients with pulmonary limitation to exercise. International Journal of Rehabilitation Research, *14*:101–115, 1991.

Henke, KG, & Orenstein, DM. Oxygen saturation during exercise in cystic fibrosis. American Review of Respiratory Disease, *129:*708–711, 1984.

Hess, DR. The evidence for secretion clearance techniques. Respiratory Care, *46*(11):1276–1293, 2001.

Hiatt, P, Eigen, H, Yu, P, & Tepper, RS. Bronchodilator response in infants and young children with cystic fibrosis. American Review of Respiratory Disease, *137:*119–122, 1988.

Hietpas, B, Roth, R, & Jensen, W. Huff coughing and airway patency. Respiratory Care, *24:*710, 1979.

Humberstone, N. Respiratory assessment and treatment. In Irwin, S, & Tecklin, JS (Eds.). Cardiopulmonary Physical Therapy. St. Louis: Mosby, 1990, pp. 283–322.

Kadikar, A, Maurer, J, & Kesten, S. The six-minute walk test: A guide to assessment for lung transplantation. Journal of Heart and Lung Transplantation, *16*(3):313–319, 1997.

Kattan, M. Pediatric pulmonary function testing. In Miller, A (Ed.). Pulmonary Function Tests: A Guide for the Student and House Officer. Philadelphia: WB Saunders, 1987, pp. 199–212.

Kellerman, J, Zeltzer, L, & Ellenberg, L. Psychological effects of illness in adolescence: Anxiety, self-esteem and perception of control. Journal of Pediatrics, *97:*126–131, 1980.

Kerem, BS, Rommens, JR, Buchanan, JA, Markiewicz, D, Cox, TK, Chakravarti, A, Buchwald, M, & Tsui, LC. Identification of the cystic fibrosis gene: Gene analysis. Science, *245:*1073–1080, 1989.

Kerem, E, Reisman, J, Corey, M, Canny, GJ, & Levison, H. Prediction of mortality in patients with cystic fibrosis. New England Journal of Medicine, *326:*1187–1191, 1992.

Khaghani, A, Madden, B, Hodson, M, & Yacoub, M. Heart-lung transplantation for cystic fibrosis. Pediatric Pulmonology Supplement, *6:*128–129, 1991.

Klijn, PH, Terherggen-Largo, SW, van der Ent, CK, van der Net, J, Kimpen, JL, & Helders, PJ. Anaerobic exercise in pediatric cystic fibrosis. Pediatric Pulmonology, *36:*223–229, 2003.

Koehler, DR, Sajjan, U, Martin, B, Kent, G, Tanswell, AK, McKerlie, C, Forstner, JF, & Hu, J. Protection of Cftr knockout mice from acute lung infection by a helper-dependent adenoviral vector expressing Cftr in airway epithelia. Proceedings of the National Academy of Sciences of United States of America, *100:*15364–15369, 2003.

Konstan, MW, Stern, RC, & Doershuk, CF. Efficacy of the Flutter VRP1 in airway mucus clearance in cystic fibrosis. Pediatrics, *124:*689–693, 1994.

Lamarre, A, Reilly, BJ, & Bryan, AC. Early detection of pulmonary function abnormalities in cystic fibrosis. Pediatrics, *50:*291–298, 1972.

Landau, LI. Cystic fibrosis: Transition from paediatric to adult physician's care. Thorax, *50:*1031–1032, 1995.

Lannefors, L. Different ways of using positive expiratory pressure to loosen and mobilize secretions. Pediatric Pulmonology Supplement, *8:*136–137, 1992.

Lemke, A, Lester, L, Lloyd-Still, J, & Powers, C. Attitudes toward genetic testing among adults with cystic fibrosis. Pediatric Pulmonology Supplement, *8:*238, 1992.

Lewiston, N, & Moss, R. Interobserver variance in clinical scoring for cystic fibrosis. Chest, *91:*878–882, 1987.

Lloyd-Still, DM, & Lloyd-Still, JD. The patient, the family and the community. In Lloyd-Still, JD (Ed.). Textbook of Cystic Fibrosis. Stoneham, MA: Wright, 1983, pp. 443–446.

Lloyd-Still, JD. Pulmonary manifestations. In Lloyd-Still, JD (Ed.). Textbook of Cystic Fibrosis. Stoneham, MA: Wright, 1983, pp. 165–198.

Loffert, DT, Ikle, D, & Nelson, HS. A comparison of commercial jet nebulizers. Chest, *106:*1788–1792, 1994.

Lorin, MI, & Denning, CR. Evaluation of postural drainage by measure-ment of sputum volume and consistency. American Journal of Physical Medicine and Rehabilitation, *50:*215–219, 1971.

Loudon, RG. The lung exam. Clinics in Chest Medicine, *8:*265, 1987.

Mackenzie, CF. Undesirable effects, precautions, and contraindications of chest physiotherapy. In Mackenzie, CF (Ed.). Chest Physiotherapy in the Intensive Care Unit. Baltimore: Williams & Wilkins, 1989, pp. 321–344.

MacLusky, IB, Canny, GJ, & Levison, H. Cystic fibrosis: An update. Paediatric Reviews and Communications, *1:*343–384, 1987.

MacLusky, IB, Gold, R, Corey, M, & Levison, H. Long-term effects of inhaled tobramycin in patients with cystic fibrosis colonised with *Pseudomonas aeruginosa.* Pediatric Pulmonology, *7:*42–48, 1989.

MacLusky, IB, & Levison, H. Cystic fibrosis. In Chernick, V (Ed.). Kendig's Disorders of the Respiratory Tract in Children, Vol. 5. Philadelphia: WB Saunders, 1990, pp. 692–730.

MacLusky, IB, & Levison, H. Cystic fibrosis. In Chernick, VI (Ed.). Kendig's Disorders of the Respiratory Tract in Children, Vol. 6. Philadelphia: WB Saunders, 1998, pp. 838–882.

Malfroot, A, & Dab, I. New insights on gastro-oesophageal reflux in cystic fibrosis by longitudinal follow–up. Archives of Disease in Childhood, *66:*1339–1345, 1991.

Maxwell, B. Nursing aspects of C.F. care. Pediatric Pulmonology Supplement, *6:*85–86, 1991.

Mazzacco, MC, Owens, GR, Kirilloff, LH, & Rogers, RM. Chest percussion and postural drainage in patients with chronic bronchiectasis. Chest, *88:*360–363, 1985.

McCollum, AT, & Gibson, LE. Family adaptation to the child with cystic fibrosis. Journal of Pediatrics, *77:*571–578, 1970.

McIlwaine, PM, Davidson, AGF, Wong, LTK, & Pirie, GE. Autogenic drainage. Pediatric Pulmonology Supplement, *8:*134–135, 1992.

McIlwaine, PM, Davidson, AGF, Wong, LTK, Pirie, GE, & Nakielna, EM. Comparison of positive expiratory pressure and autogenic drainage with conventional percussion and drainage therapy in the treatment of cystic fibrosis. Pediatric Pulmonology, *4*(supplement 2):132a, 1988.

McIlwaine, PM, Wong, LT, Peacock, D, Davidson, AG. Long-term comparative trial of positive expiratory pressure versus oscillating positive expiratory pressure (flutter) physiotherapy in the treatment of cystic fibrosis. Journal of Pediatrics, *138:*845–850, 2001.

Mellins, R. The site of airway obstruction in cystic fibrosis. Pediatrics, *44:*315–318, 1969.

Mellins, R, Levine, OR, Ingram, RH, Jr, & Fishman, AP. Obstructive disease of the airways in cystic fibrosis. Pediatrics, *41:*560–573, 1968.

Miller, A. Spirometry and maximum expiratory flow-volume curves. In Miller, A (Ed.). Pulmonary Function Tests: A Guide for the Student and House Officer. Philadelphia: WB Saunders, 1987, pp. 15–32.

Miller, WF, Scacci, R, & Gast, LR. Laboratory Evaluation of Pulmonary Function. Philadelphia: JB Lippincott, 1987, pp. 105–176.

Mitchell-Heggs, P, Mearns, M, & Batten, JC. Cystic fibrosis in adolescents and adults. Quarterly Journal of Medicine, *45:*479–504, 1976.

Moran, F, Bradley, JM, Boyle, L, Elborn, JS. Incontinence in adult females with cystic fibrosis: A Northern Ireland survey. International Journal of Clinical Practice, *57:*182–183, 2003.

Muller, N, Frances, P, Gurwitz, D, Levison, H, & Bryan, AC. Mechanisms of hemoglobin desaturation during rapid-eye movement sleep in normal subjects and in patients with cystic fibrosis. American Review of Respiratory Disease, *119:*338, 1980.

Narang, I, Pike, S, Rosenthal, M, Balfour-Lynn, IM, & Bush, A. Three-minute step test to assess exercise capacity in children with cystic fibrosis with mild lung disease. Pediatric Pulmonology, *35:*108–113, 2003.

Nixon, PA, Orenstein, DM, & Kelsey, SF. Habitual physical activity in children and adolescents with cystic fibrosis. Medicine and Science in Sports and Exercise, *33*(1):30–35, 2001.

Nixon, PA, Orenstein, DM, Kelsey, SF, & Doershuk, CF. The prognostic value of exercise testing in patients with cystic fibrosis. New England Journal of Medicine, *327*:1785–1788, 1992.

Oberwaldner, B, Evans, JC, & Zach, MS. Forced expirations against a variable resistance: A new chest physiotherapy method in cystic fibrosis. Pediatric Pulmonology, *2*:358–367, 1986.

Oberwaldner, B, Theissl, B, Rucker, A, & Zach, MS. Chest physiotherapy in hospitalized patients with cystic fibrosis: A study of lung function effects and sputum production. European Respiratory Journal, *4*:152–158, 1991.

Orenstein, DM. Cystic Fibrosis: A Guide for Patient and Family, 3rd ed. New York: Lippincott-Raven, 2003.

Orenstein, DM, Franklin, BA, Doershuk, CF, Hellerstein, HK, Germann, KJ, Horowitz, JG, & Stern, RC. Exercise conditioning and cardiopulmonary fitness in cystic fibrosis. Chest, *80*:292–298, 1981.

Orenstein, DM, Henke, KG, & Cerny, FJ. Exercise and cystic fibrosis. Physician and Sports Medicine, *2*:57–63, 1983.

Orenstein, SR, & Orenstein, DM. Gastroesophageal reflux and respiratory disease in children. Journal of Pediatrics, *112*:847–858, 1988.

Orenstein, DM. Exercise testing in cystic fibrosis. Pediatric Pulmonology, *25*:223–225, 1998.

Ormerod, LP, Thompson, RA, & Anderson, CM. Reversibility of airways obstruction in cystic fibrosis. Thorax, *35*:768–772, 1980.

Orr, A, McVean, RJ, Webb, AK, & Dodd, ME. Questionnaire survey of urinary incontinence in women with cystic fibrosis. British Medical Journal, *322*:1521, 2001.

Paley, CA. A way forward for determining optimal aerobic exercise intensity? Physiotherapy, *83*(12):620–624, 1997.

Paradowski, LJ. The CF patient post lung transplant: The UNC experience. Pediatric Pulmonology Supplement, *8*:210–212, 1992.

Park, RW, & Grand, RJ. Gastrointestinal manifestations of cystic fibrosis: A review. Gastroenterology, *81*:1143–1161, 1981.

Pasque, MK, Cooper, JD, Kaiser, LR, Haydock, DA, Triantafilloy, A, & Trulock, EP. Improved technique for bilateral lung transplantation: Rationale and initial clinical experience. Annals of Thoracic Surgery, *49*:785–791, 1990.

Passero, MA, Remor, B, & Solomon, J. Patient-reported compliance with cystic fibrosis therapy. Clinical Pediatrics, *20*:264–268, 1981.

Pasterkamp, H, Montgomery, M, & Wiebicke, W. Nomenclature used by health care professionals to describe breath sounds in asthma. Chest, *92*:346–352, 1987.

Peckham, DG. Macrolide antibiotics and cystic fibrosis. Thorax, *57*:189–190, 2002.

Pegues, DA, Carson, LA, Tablan, OC, FitzSimmons, SC, Roman, SB, Miller, JM, Jarvis, WR, and the Summer Camp Group. Acquisition of *Pseudomonas cepacia* at summer camps for patients with cystic fibrosis. Summer camp study group. Pediatrics, *124*:694–702, 1994.

Phelan, PD, Gracey, M, Williams, HE, & Anderson, CM. Ventilatory function in infants with cystic fibrosis. Archives of Disease in Childhood, *44*:393–400, 1969.

Phillips, BM, & David, TJ. Pathogenesis and management of arthropathy in cystic fibrosis. Journal of the Royal Society of Medicine, *79*(suppl 12):44–49, 1986.

Phillips, BM, & David, TJ. Management of the chest in cystic fibrosis. Journal of the Royal Society of Medicine, *80*(Supplement 15):30–37, 1987.

Phillips, GE, Pike, SE, Jaffe, A, & Bush, A. Comparison of active cycle of breathing and high-frequency oscillation jacket in children with cystic fibrosis. Pediatric Pulmonology, *37*:71–75, 2004.

Physiotherapy in the Treatment of Cystic Fibrosis (CF). International Physiotherapy Group for Cystic Fibrosis Mucoviscidosis Association, 2002. (Available by the secretary of IPG/CF, contact www.ipg-cf.fw.hu

Pinkerton, P, Trauer, T, Duncan, F, Hodson, M, & Batten, J. Cystic fibrosis in adult life: A study of coping patterns. Lancet, *2*:761–763, 1985.

Pizer, HF. Organ Transplants: A Patient's Guide. Cambridge, MA: Harvard University Press, 1991.

Porcari, JP, Ebbeling, CB, Ward, A, Freedson, PS, & Rippe, JM. Walking for exercise testing and training. Sports Medicine, *8*:189–200, 1989.

Porter, DK, Van Every, MJ, Anthracite, RF, & Mack, JW, Jr. Massive hemoptysis in cystic fibrosis. Archives of Internal Medicine, *143*:287–290, 1983.

Prasad, SA, Randall, SD, Balfour-Lynn, IM. Fifteen-count breathlessness score: An objective measure for children. Pediatric Pulmonology, *30*:56–62, 2000.

Prince, A. *Pseudomonas aeruginosa* gene products associated with epithelial colonization. Pediatric Pulmonology Supplement, *8*:75–76, 1992.

Pryor, JA, Webber, BA, Hodson, ME, & Batten, JC. Evaluation of the forced expiration technique as an adjunct to postural drainage in treatment of cystic fibrosis. British Medical Journal, *2*:417–418, 1979.

Pryor, JA. The forced expiratory technique. In Pryor J (Ed.). Respiratory Care. London: Churchill Livingstone, 1991, pp. 79–100.

Ramsey, BW. New clinical developments: From the test tube to the bedside. Pediatric Pulmonology Supplement, *14*:137–138, 1997.

Ranganathan, SC, Stocks, J, Dezateux, C, Bush, A, Wade, A, Carr, S, Castle, R, Dinwiddie, R, Hoo, A, Price, J, Stroobant, J, Wallis, C, & The London Collaborative Cystic Fibrosis Group. The evolution of airway function in early childhood following clinical diagnosis of cystic fibrosis. American Journal of Respiratory and Critical Care Medicine, *169*:928–933, 2004.

Reisman, JJ, Rivington-Law, B, Corey, M, Marcotte, J, Wannamaker, E, Harcourt, D, & Levison, H. Role of conventional physiotherapy in cystic fibrosis. Journal of Pediatrics, *113*:632–636, 1988.

Riordan, JR, Rommens, JM, Kerem, BS, Alon, N, Rozmahel, R, Grzelczak, Z, Zielensky, J, Lok, S, Plavsic, N, Drumm, ML, Iannuzzi, MC, Collins, FS, & Tsui, LC. Identification of the cystic fibrosis gene: Cloning and characterization of complementary DNA. Science, *245*:1066–1073, 1989.

Rose, J, & Jay, S. A comprehensive exercise program for persons with cystic fibrosis. Journal of Pediatric Nursing, *1*:323–334, 1986.

Rosenstein, B, & Langbaum, T. Diagnosis. In Taussig, LM (Ed.). Cystic Fibrosis. New York: Thieme-Stratton, 1984, pp. 85–115.

Ruppel, G. Manual of Pulmonary Function Testing. St. Louis: Mosby, 1991.

Sackett, DL. Rules of evidence and clinical recommendations on the use of antithrombotic agents. Chest, *89*(suppl):25–35, 1986.

Sammut, P, & Morgan, WJ. Volume-independent assessment of forced expiratory flow in young children. American Review of Respiratory Disease, *135*:A238, 1987.

Schneiderman-Walker, J, Pollock, S, Corey, M, Wilkes, D, Canny, G, Pedder, L, & Reisman, J. A randomized controlled trial of a 3-year home exercise program in cystic fibrosis. Journal of Pediatrics, *136*:304–310, 2000.

Scott, RB, O'Loughlin, EV, & Gall, DG. Gastroesophageal reflux in patients with cystic fibrosis. Journal of Pediatrics, *106*:223–227, 1985.

Scott, SM, Walters, DA, Singh, SJ, Morgan, MDL, & Hardman, AE. A progressive shuttle walking test of functional capacity in patients with chronic airflow limitation. Thorax, *45*:781a, 1990.

Selvadurai, HC, Cooper, PJ, Meyers, N, Blimkie, CJ, Smith, L, Mellis, CM, & Van Asperen, PP. Validation of shuttle tests in children with cystic fibrosis. Pediatric Pulmonology, *35*:133–138, 2003.

Shepherd, R, Vasques-Velasquez, L, Prentice, A, Holt, TL, Coward, W, & Lucas, A. Increased energy expenditure in young children with cystic fibrosis. Lancet, *2*:1300–1303, 1988.

Shwachman, H, & Kulczycki, LL. Long-term study of 105 patients with cystic fibrosis. American Journal of Diseases of Children, 96:6–15, 1958.

Singh, S. The use of field walking test for assessment of functional capacity in patients with chronic airways obstruction. Physiotherapy, 78:102–104, 1992.

Skorecki, K, Levison, H, & Crozier, DN. Bronchial lability in cystic fibrosis. Acta Paediatrica Scandinavica, 65:39–44, 1976.

Solomon, MP, Wilson, DC, Corey, M, Kalnins, D, Zielenski, J, Tsui, LC, Pencharz, P, Durie, P, & Sweezey, NB, Glucose intolerance in children with cystic fibrosis. Journal of Pediatrics, 142:128–132, 2003.

Spalding, A, Kelly, L, Santopietro, J, & Posner-Mayor, J. Kid on the Ball: Swiss Balls in a Complete Fitness Program. Windsor: Human Kinetics, 1999.

Spicher, V, Roulet, M, & Schultz, Y. Assessment of total energy expenditure in free-living patients with cystic fibrosis. Journal of Pediatrics, 118:865–972, 1991.

Starnes, VA, Bowdish, ME, Woo, MS, Barbers, RG, Schenkel, FA, Horn, MV, Pessotto, R, Sievers EM, Baker, CJ, Cohen, RG, Bremner, RM, Wells, WJ, & Barr, ML. A decade of living lobar lung transplantation: Recipient outcomes. The Journal of Thoracic and Cardiovascular Surgery, 127:114–122, 2004.

Starr, JA. Manual techniques of chest physical therapy and airway clearance techniques. In Zadai, CC (Ed.). Pulmonary Management in Physical Therapy. New York: Churchill Livingstone, 1992, pp. 99–133.

Strauss, GD, Osher, A, Wang, CI, Goodrich, E, Gold, F, Colman, W, Stabile, M, Dobrenchuk, A, & Keens, T. Variable weight training in cystic fibrosis. Chest, 92:273–276, 1987.

Sutton, PP, Lopez-Vidriero, MT, Pavia, D, Newman, SP, & Clay, MM. Assessment of percussion, vibratory-shaking and breathing exercises in chest physiotherapy. American Review of Respiratory Disease, 66:147–152, 1985.

Sutton, PP, Parker, RA, Webber, BA, Newman, SP, & Garland, N. Assessment of the forced expiration technique, postural drainage and directed coughing in chest physiotherapy. European Journal of Respiratory Disease, 64:62–68, 1983.

Tablan, OC, Chorba, TL, Schidlow, DV, White, JW, Hardy, KA, Gilligan, PH, Morgan, WM, Carson, MS, Martone, WJ, Jason, JM, & Jarvis, WR. Pseudomonas cepacia colonization in patients with cystic fibrosis: Risk factors and clinical outcome. Pediatrics, 107:382–387, 1985.

Taussig, LM. Maximal expiratory flows at functional residual capacity: A test of lung function for young children. American Review of Respiratory Disease, 116:1031–1038, 1977.

Taussig, LM, Landau, LI, & Marks, MI. Respiratory system. In Taussig, LM (Ed.). Cystic Fibrosis. New York: Thieme-Stratton, 1984, pp. 115–174.

Taussig, LM, Lobeck, CC, di Sant'Agnese, PA, Ackerman, DR, & Kattwinkel, J. Fertility in males with cystic fibrosis. New England Journal of Medicine, 287:587–589, 1972.

Tecklin, JS, Clayton, RG, & Scanlin, TF. High frequency chest wall oscillation vs. traditional chest physical therapy in CF: A large, 1-year, controlled study. Pediatric Pulmonology Supplement, 20:304, 2000.

Tepper, RS. Assessment of pulmonary function in infants with cystic fibrosis. Pediatric Pulmonology Supplement, 8:165–166, 1992.

Tepper, RS, Hiatt, P, Eigen, H, Scott, P, Grosfeld, J, & Cohen, M. Infants with cystic fibrosis: Pulmonary function at diagnosis. Pediatric Pulmonology, 5:15–18, 1988.

Tepper, RS, Hiatt, PW, Eigen, H, & Smith, J. Total respiratory compliance in asymptomatic infants with cystic fibrosis. American Review of Respiratory Disease, 135:1075–1079, 1987.

Thomas, J, Cook, DJ, & Brooks, D. Chest physical therapy management of patients with cystic fibrosis. A meta-analysis. American Journal of Respiratory Critical Care Medicine, 151(3 Pt 1):846–850.

Van Hengstrum, M, Festen, J, & Beurskens, C. Conventional physiotherapy and forced expiration technique maneuvers have similar effects on tracheobronchial clearance. European Respiratory Journal, 1:758, 1988.

Vinocur, CD, Marmon, L, Schidlow, DV, & Weintraub, WH. Gastroesophageal reflux in the infant with cystic fibrosis. American Journal of Surgery, 149:182–186, 1985.

Volsko, TA, DiFiore, JM, & Chatburn, RL. Performance comparison of two oscillating positive expiratory pressure devices: Acapella versus Flutter. Respiratory Care, 48:124–130, 2003.

Wagener, JS, & Headley, AA. Cystic fibrosis: Current trends in respiratory care. Respiratory Care, 48:234–244, 2003.

Wagener, JS, Taussig, LM, Burrows, B, Hernried, L, & Boat, T. Comparison of lung function survival patterns between cystic fibrosis and emphysema or chronic bronchitis patients. In Sturgess, JM (Ed.). Perspectives in Cystic Fibrosis. Mississauga, Canada: Imperial Press, 1980, pp. 236–245.

Warwick, WJ, & Hansen, LG. The long term effect of high frequency chest compression therapy on pulmonary complications of cystic fibrosis. Pediatric Pulmonology, 11:265–271, 1991.

Webber, BA, & Pryor, JA. Physiotherapy for Respiratory and Cardiac Problems, 2nd ed. New York: Churchill Livingstone, 1998.

Wilkes, D, Schneiderman-Walker, J, Strug, L, Selvadurai, HC, Lands, LC, Corey, M, Coates, AL. Habitual activity and disease progression in boys and girls with cystic fibrosis. Pediatric Pulmonology Supplement, 25:330, 2003.

Wilschanski, M., Corey, M., Durie, P, Tullis, E, Bain, J, Asch, M, Ginzburg, B, Jarvi, K, Buckspan, B, & Hartwick, W. Diversity of reproductive tract abnormalities in men with cystic fibrosis. Journal of the American Medical Association, 276:607–608, 1996.

Wilson, CB. The immune system: The devil within or the good guy. Pediatric Pulmonology Supplement, 13:75, 1996.

Winton, T. Double lung transplantation for cystic fibrosis: Operative technique and early post-operative care. Pediatric Pulmonology Supplement, 8:208–209, 1992.

Witt, DR, Blumberg, B, Schaefer, C, Fitzgerald, P, Fishbach, A, Holtzman, J, Kornfeld, S, Lee, R, Nemzer, L, Palmer, R, Sato, M, & Jenkins, L. Cystic fibrosis carrier screening in a prenatal population. Pediatric Pulmonology Supplement, 8:235, 1992.

Wood, RE. Why commence conventional chest physiotherapy for CF at diagnosis? Pediatric Pulmonology Supplement, 9:89–90, 1993.

Yankaskas, JR. Respiratory failure in CF: Pathophysiology and treatment, including the role of mechanical ventilation. Pediatric Pulmonology Supplement, 8:87–88, 1992.

Yankaskas, JR, Mallory, GB, and the Consensus Committee. Lung transplantation in cystic fibrosis: Consensus conference statement. Chest, 113(1):217–226, 1998.

Yankaskas, JR, Marshall, BC, Sufian, B, Simon, RH, & Rodman, D. Cystic fibrosis adult care: Consensus conference report. Chest, 125(1):1S–39S, 2004.

Yellon, RF. The spectrum of reflux-associated otolaryngologic problems in infants and children. American Journal of Medicine, 103:125–129, 1997.

Zach, MS, Purrer, B, & Oberwaldner, B. Effect of swimming on forced expiration and sputum clearance in cystic fibrosis. Lancet, 2:1201–1203, 1981.

Zadai, CC. Comprehensive physical therapy evaluation: Identifying potential pulmonary limitations. In Zadai, CC (Ed.). Pulmonary Management in Physical Therapy. New York: Churchill Livingstone, 1992, pp. 55–78.

Chapter 28

Asthma: Multisystem Implications

Mary Massery
PT, DPT

Cynthia L. Magee
PT, MS

PATHOPHYSIOLOGY

PRIMARY IMPAIRMENT
  Diagnosis
  Impairment in Infancy and Early Childhood
  Impairment Childhood
  Impairment in Adolescence
  Medical Management

SECONDARY IMPAIRMENTS
  Restrictions in Daily Life and Physical Activity
  Medication Side Effects
  Growth and Development
  Impact on Financial Costs to Family and Society

SUMMARY OF THE MEDICAL ASPECT OF ASTHMA

PHYSICAL THERAPY EXAMINATION, EVALUATION, AND INTERVENTIONS

SUMMARY

CASE STUDY

Nearly one in ten children in the United States has a diagnosis of asthma (CDC, 2004). This frequency has been increasing for decades (Sunyer et al., 1999; Kaiser, 2004) both here and abroad for reasons that are not yet clearly understood (Frischer et al., 1993; Taggart & Fulwood, 1993; von Mutius et al., 1993; Krishnamoorthy et al., 1994; Kussin & Fulkerson, 1995; Schaubel et al., 1996; Meza & Gershwin, 1997; Bruce, 1998; Evans et al., 1998; Strachan & Cook, 1998; Kennedy, 1999; Patterson & Harding 1999; Hartert & Peebles, 2000; Pianosi & Fisk 2000; Doyle et al., 2001; Kaiser, 2004; Malo et al., 2004; Zmirou et al., 2004). According to the Centers for Disease Control and Prevention (CDC) in the United States, from 1979 to 1995, the incidence of asthma increased over 160% for children ages 0 to 4 years and 74% for children ages 5 to 14 years. Similarly, morbidity rate increased 63% for children ages 0 to 4 years and 20% for children ages 5 to 14 years (according to physician office visits for asthma), and mortality rate increased 12% for children ages 0 to 4 years and 146% for children ages 5 to 14 years in that same time interval (CDC, 1998). Follow-up data in a CDC 2002 report indicates that some of these morbidity and mortality figures may have peaked in the mid-1990's (CDC, 2002).

Pragmatically, the incidence figures mean that nearly 10% of all children seen by pediatric physical therapists may have asthma. Does this disease impact a child's motor performance? If so, what kind of impact does it have and what clinical implications does the presence of asthma have for the physical therapist treating pediatric patients?

The purpose of this chapter is to achieve the following:
  1. Define asthma and discuss the medical ramifications of the disease.
  2. Demonstrate the process of a differential physical therapy diagnosis for potential physical and activity limitations secondary to asthma through the illustration of a clinical case.
  3. Identify the types of cardiopulmonary, neuromuscular, musculoskeletal, integumentary, and gastrointestinal impairments that may be associated with this diagnosis.
  4. Present possible treatment strategies and specific interventions.
  5. Present potential long-term outcomes of physical therapy interventions on the maturation and physical performance of a child with asthma.

PATHOPHYSIOLOGY

Asthma is a pulmonary disease with three significant characteristics: (1) airway obstruction that is reversible either spontaneously or with pharmacologic intervention; (2) airway inflammation; and (3) airway hypersensitivity to stimuli that are classified as either extrinsic or intrinsic (Wagner, 2003; Morris & Perkins, 2004). It is a disease of both the large and the small airways. Complex interactions occur between various cells and cellular elements, resulting in recurrent episodes of shortness of breath, chest tightness, and coughing. Bronchial hypersensitivity to a variety of stimuli is increased (National Heart, Lung and Blood Institute, 1997). These stimuli are classified as extrinsic or intrinsic. Extrinsic or allergic stimuli include pollen, mold, animal dander, cigarette smoke, foods, drugs, and dust. Intrinsic or nonallergic stimuli include viral infections, inhalation of irritating substances, exercise, emotional stress, and environmental factors such as the weather or climate changes. An individual may be sensitive to either type of stimuli or to both types (National Heart, Lung and Blood Institute, 1997).

Researchers have found genetic causes for the development of asthma (Apter & Szefler, 2004; Birkisson et al., 2004), but genetics alone does not account for all types and severities of the expression of the disease (Harik-Khan et al., 2004). The physical, environmental, neurogenic, chemical, and pharmacologic factors that are associated with asthma are specific to each individual. They stimulate or trigger the immune system to release chemical mediators, which in turn cause constriction of the bronchial muscles, increased mucus production, and swelling of the mucous membranes. These effects result in increased resistance to airflow, increasing the work of breathing and decreasing pulmonary ventilation. Mucus accumulation, which has been shown to be abnormal in asthma, may cause blockage of the airways, resulting in further air trapping, hyperinflation, and, eventually, atelectasis (Kurashima et al., 1992). In fact, airway obstruction from mucous plugs has been identified as a primary cause of death associated with asthma (Kuyper et al., 2003). In some patients, there is hypertrophy of the smooth muscles of the airways with new vessel formation, an increase in the number of goblet cells, and deposition of interstitial collagen, which may not be reversible and results in fibrosis of the basement membrane (National Heart, Lung and Blood Institute, 1997). In the acute stage, the early recruitment of cells results in inflammation. In the subacute stage, the recruited and activated resident cells result in a more persistent inflammation. Persistent cell damage and ongoing repair result in chronic inflammation.

In addition to the medical manifestation of asthma, numerous studies have shown that a diagnosis of asthma in childhood results in recurring, chronic respiratory problems, frequent hospitalizations, poorer growth and development than peers, and endurance impairments, all of which result in an increased number of missed school/work days and limitations on the child's participation in normal childhood activities. (Chryssanthopoulos et al., 1984; Ramazanoglu & Kraemer, 1985; McKenzie & Gandevia, 1986; Taggart & Fulwood, 1993; Chye & Gray, 1995; Schaubel et al., 1996; Meza & Gershwin, 1997; Berhane et al., 2000; Pianosi & Fisk, 2000; Abrams, 2001; Mellinger-Birdsong et al., 2003; CDC, 2004).

PRIMARY IMPAIRMENT

DIAGNOSIS

The diagnosis of asthma is made on the basis of history, physical examination, auscultation and palpation, and pulmonary function tests (PFTs), especially in response to a methacholine challenge (Joseph-Bowen et al., 2004). Wheezing and rhonchi may be detected and may even be present when the child demonstrates no breathing difficulty. Coughing, wheezing, difficulty breathing, and chest tightness may be reported as being worse at night or early in the morning. Hyperexpansion of the thorax, decreased use of the diaphragm with increased use of accessory muscles, postural changes, increased nasal secretions, mucosal swelling, nasal polyps, "allergic shiners" (darkened areas under the eyes), and evidence of an allergic skin condition may be noted on physical examination. During an acute asthma attack, the child may evidence an increased respiratory rate, expiratory grunting, intercostal muscle retractions and nasal flaring, an alteration in the inspiration-expiration ratio, and coughing. In severe cases, a bluish color of the lips and nails may be noted.

Attempts have been made to produce a national classification system for the severity of the disease based on clinical findings, but follow-up studies found those systems to inconsistently reflect the severity of the disease (Baker et al., 2003; Braganza et al., 2003; Powell et al., 2003). In spite of the shortcomings, one of the most common severity classification systems was published by the U.S. National Institutes of Health (NIH) Heart, Lung and Blood Institute in 1997 and the details are listed in Table 28-1. (NIH, 1997) The NIH classification system lists asthma by clinical symptoms as (1) intermittent, (2) mild persistent, (3) moderate persistent, or (4) severe persistent.

| TABLE 28-1 | Clinical Classification of the Disease Severity of Asthma |

CLASSIFICATION	INDICATIONS AND BEHAVIORS
Step 1 Intermittent	Intermittent symptoms occurring less than once a week Brief exacerbations Nocturnal symptoms occurring less than twice a month Asymptomatic with normal lung function between exacerbations FEV_1 or PEFR rate greater than 80%, with less than 20% variability
Step 2 Mild persistent	Symptoms occurring more than once a week but less than once a day Exacerbations affect activity and sleep Nocturnal symptoms occurring more than twice a month FEV_1 or PEFR rate greater than 80% predicted, with variability of 20-30%
Step 3 Moderate persistent	Daily symptoms Exacerbations affect activity and sleep Nocturnal symptoms occurring more than once a week FEV_1 or PEFR rate 60-80% of predicted, with variability greater than 30%
Step 4 Severe persistent	Continuous symptoms Frequent exacerbations Frequent nocturnal asthma symptoms Physical activities limited by asthma symptoms FEV_1 or PEFR rate less than 60%, with variability greater than 30%

Practical Guide for the Diagnosis and Management of Asthma Based on Expert Panel Report 2. NIH Publication No. 97-4053. Bethesda, MD: National Institute of Health, National Heart, Lung and Blood Institute, 1997, p.10; and Morris, M, & Perkins, P. Asthma. e-Medicine, available at http://www.emedicine.com/med/topic177.htm, last updated 5/9/04.

Pulmonary Function Tests

PFTs are performed to determine the location and degree of the respiratory impairment as well as the reversibility of bronchoconstriction following administration of a bronchodilator (methacholine challenge). Test values are compared with predicted values based on age, sex, and height (Cherniack & Cherniack, 1983). PFT measurements may reveal decreases in (1) forced vital capacity (FVC), (2) forced expiration during the first second of FVC (FEV_1), (3) forced expiratory volume compared with forced vital capacity (FEV/FVC), (4) peak expiratory flow rate (PEFR) due to airway obstruction in large or small airways; (5) decreases in forced expiratory flow (FEF) during 25% to 75% of FVC ($FEF_{25\%-75\%}$) due to airway obstruction specifically in small airways; and (6) increases in residual volume (RV) and functional residual capacity (FRC) due to air trapping. Generally, patients with asthma are instructed to monitor their daily pulmonary fluctuations and adjust their medication levels by testing their PEFR with a peak flowmeter. However, recent studies have shown that FEV_1 and midexpiratory $FEF_{25\%-75\%}$ are better indicators of disease status than PEFR (Hansen et al., 2001). Peak flowmeters are cheaper and more readily available in a home environment, so they

will probably continue as the home equipment of choice until FEV_1 and $FEF_{25\%-75\%}$ can be readily tested at home.

IMPAIRMENT IN INFANCY AND EARLY CHILDHOOD

A diagnosis of asthma is not typically made until the child is 3 to 6 years of age when numerous episodes of pulmonary problems have been demonstrated and are consistent with asthma (Joseph-Bowen et al., 2004). In the meantime, children may be diagnosed with "reactive airway disease." More objective tests such as PFTs are not possible until the child is around 6 years of age and capable of cooperating and performing the tests. The child diagnosed with asthma at 3 to 6 years old will typically present with a history of episodes of wheezy bronchitis, croup, recurrent upper respiratory tract infections, chronic bronchitis, recurrent pneumonia, difficulty sleeping, or respiratory syncytial virus (RSV) infection. Severe RSV infection in infancy is highly associated with a later diagnosis of asthma. Currently, it is not known if children with asthma have a more severe reaction to the virus or if a severe infection with RSV actually causes asthma to develop later in childhood

(Openshaw et al., 2003; Gern, 2004; Silvestri et al., 2004). In addition to normal childhood illness, complications associated with prematurity and very low birth weight also have a high correlation with a later diagnosis of asthma. Like the RSV, it is not known if prematurity causes asthma or simply makes the infants more predisposed to asthma (Koumbourlis et al., 1996; Evans et al., 1998; Kennedy, 1999). Thus, pediatric physical therapists should pay careful attention to a child's medical history to note a history that may indicate a risk for asthma and consider all the ramifications on that child's health, growth, and development when planning treatment interventions.

IMPAIRMENT IN CHILDHOOD

During childhood, PFT measures become an easy and effective diagnostic tool. Overt wheezing is the major presenting sign. Numerous other childhood problems have been associated with a later diagnosis of asthma including an increased prevalence of chronic or recurrent otitis media with effusion (Fireman, 1988) or gastro-intestinal problems such as gastroesophageal reflux disease (GERD) (Eid, 2004; Eid & Morton, 2004). Some children may exhibit respiratory difficulty only after exercise, at night, or in cold air (de Benedictis et al., 1990). Other children may have trouble keeping up with peers or with strenuous exercise. Routine PFT results may be normal; however, the history may indicate that an allergen or exercise challenge test should be performed. The prevalence of exercise-induced bronchospasm (EIB) is 70% to 90% in individuals with documented asthma who have performed an exercise challenge test; however, a positive history of EIB is not always given (Sly, 1986; Voy, 1986).

IMPAIRMENT IN ADOLESCENCE

By adolescence, symptoms often decrease. Even when free of symptoms, however, the adolescent may have significant impairment revealed by PFT measures. Continued decrease in severity and frequency of asthma attacks during adolescence results in the belief that children "outgrow" asthma. Research has not demonstrated this to be true. In a study of 286 subjects at age 28, first studied at age 7 and again at ages 10, 14, and 21, it was found that asthma severity at age 28 was similar to that at age 14 (Kelly et al., 1988).

MEDICAL MANAGEMENT

Episodes of asthma attacks are usually reversible and can be prevented or modified to some degree when the

individual-specific triggers have been identified. The frequency, duration, and severity of attacks are highly variable even for the same individual. Acute treatment is aimed at reversing the bronchoconstriction. Broncho-dilator medications are administered by inhalation or injection. If the asthma attack is severe and does not respond to bronchodilator medications, the diagnosis of status asthmaticus may be made. This is considered a life-threatening medical emergency (Papiris et al., 2002). Hospitalization will be required to administer medications intravenously, to monitor blood gases, and to administer oxygen.

The goals of long-term management are to prevent chronic and troublesome symptoms, to maintain pulmonary function and physical activity level, to prevent recurrent exacerbations, to minimize the need for emergency room visits or hospitalizations, to provide optimal pharmacotherapy, and to meet the patient's and family's expectations of and satisfaction with asthma care (National Heart, Lung and Blood Institute, 1997). This is accomplished through periodic examination, ongoing monitoring, and education. The patient should be taught to self-monitor asthma symptoms and patterns, response to medications, quality of life, and functional status and to perform and record peak flow readings. A written action plan should be developed and reviewed and revised periodically. This action plan should be shared with school and other personnel who are involved with the child. Some allergens such as cigarette smoke, animal dander, and dust can be handled by environmental control. Desensitization ("allergy shots") may be used for triggers such as pollen or mold. Triggers such as emotional stress may be handled by relaxation exercises and education.

The medical management of asthma is primarily through the use of pharmacologic agents that are either intended for short-term relief or long-term management of the condition. (See Table 28-2 for details of current medications.) They can be ingested or inhaled directly to the airways via a variety of metered dose inhalers or nebulizers. Inhaled medications deliver a concentrated dose most effectively with fewer systemic side effects and a shorter onset of action than other means of administration. However, no single delivery system is superior for all patients. The patient's age and compliance, and other factors, such as the type of medication, determine the most effective method (O'Riordan, 2002).

Pharmacologic management is complex and individualized according to the patient's particular needs. Morris and Perkins (2004) of the Brooke Army Medical Center summarized the current intervention strategy as the following:

TABLE 28-2	Current Medications for the Quick Relief and Long-Term Management of Asthma

TYPE OF DRUG	DRUG NAMES AND FUNCTION
Bronchodilators Provide symptomatic relief of bronchospasm due to acute asthma exacerbation (short-acting agents) or long-term control of symptoms (long-acting agents). Also used as the primary medication for prophylaxis of EIA. A metered-dose inhaler can be used for administration.	Albuterol (Ventolin, Proventil) — Beta-agonist for bronchospasm. Relaxes bronchial smooth muscle by action on beta-2 receptors, with little effect on cardiac muscle contractility. Metaproterenol (Alupent, Metaprel) — Beta-2 adrenergic agonist that relaxes bronchial smooth muscle with little effect on heart rate. Salmeterol (Serevent) — Can relieve bronchospasms by relaxing the smooth muscles of the bronchioles in conditions associated with bronchitis, emphysema, asthma, or bronchiectasis. Effect also may facilitate expectoration. Adverse effects are more likely when administered at high doses or more frequent doses than recommended; prevalence of adverse effects is higher. Regular use in patients with EIA associated with smaller decrease in FEV_1 during exercise. Ipratropium (Atrovent) — Decreases vagal tone in the airways through antagonism of muscarinic receptors and inhibition of vagally mediated reflexes. Chemically related to atropine. Has antisecretory properties and, when applied locally, inhibits secretions from serous and seromucous glands lining the nasal mucosa. Only 50% of patients who are asthmatic bronchodilate with ipratropium and, to a lesser degree, with beta-adrenergic agonists. Used primarily in conjunction with beta-agonists for severe exacerbations. No additive or synergistic effects observed with long-term treatment of asthma. Theophylline (Slo-bid, Theo-Dur, Uniphyl) — Mild-to-moderate bronchodilator used as an adjuvant in the treatment of stable asthma and prevention of nocturnal asthma symptoms. Potentiates exogenous catecholamines and stimulates endogenous catecholamine release and diaphragmatic muscular relaxation, which, in turn, stimulates bronchodilation.
Leukotriene receptor antagonists Direct antagonist of mediators responsible for airway inflammation in asthma. Used for prophylaxis of EIA and long-term treatment of asthma as alternative to low doses of inhaled corticosteroids.	Montelukast (Singulair) — Selective and competitive receptor antagonist of leukotriene D4 and E4, components of slow-reacting substance of anaphylaxis. Indicated for treatment of stable, mild, persistent asthma or prophylaxis for EIA. Zafirlukast (Accolate) — Selective and competitive receptor antagonist of leukotriene D4 and E4, components of slow-reacting substance of anaphylaxis. Indicated for treatment of stable, mild, persistent asthma or prophylaxis for EIA.
Corticosteroids Highly potent agents that are the primary drug of choice for treatment of chronic asthma and prevention of acute asthma exacerbations. Numerous inhaled corticosteroids are used for asthma and include beclomethasone (Beclovent, Vanceril), budesonide (Pulmicort Turbuhaler), flunisolide (AeroBid), fluticasone (Flovent), and triamcinolone (Azmacort).	Fluticasone (Flovent) — Alters level of inflammation in airways by inhibiting multiple types of inflammatory cells and decreasing production of cytokines and other mediators involved in the asthmatic response. Triamcinolone (Azmacort) — Alters level of inflammation in airways by inhibiting multiple types of inflammatory cells and decreasing production of cytokines and other mediators involved in the asthmatic response. Beclomethasone (Vanceril, Beclovent, QVAR) — Alters level of inflammation in airways by inhibiting multiple types of inflammatory cells and decreasing production of cytokines and other mediators involved in the asthmatic response.

(continued)

TABLE 28-2	Current Medications for the Quick Relief and Long-Term Management of Asthma—*cont'd*
TYPE OF DRUG	**DRUG NAMES AND FUNCTION**
Mast cell stabilizers Prevent the release of mediators from mast cells that cause airway inflammation and bronchospasm. Indicated for maintenance therapy of mild-to-moderate asthma or prophylaxis for EIA. **5-Lipoxygenase inhibitors** Inhibit the formation of leukotrienes. Leukotrienes activate receptors that may be responsible for events leading to the pathophysiology of asthma, including airway edema, smooth muscle constriction, and altered cellular activity associated with inflammatory reactions.	Prednisone (Deltasone, Orasone, Meticorten) — Systemic steroidal anti-inflammatory medication. Used primarily for moderate-to-severe asthma exacerbations to speed recovery and prevent late-phase response. May be used long term to control severe asthma. Budesonide (Pulmicort Turbuhaler, Rhinocort) — Inhibits bronchoconstriction mechanisms, produces direct smooth muscle relaxation, and may decrease number and activity of inflammatory cells, which, in turn, decreases airway hyperresponsiveness. Cromolyn (Intal) — Inhibits degranulation of sensitized mast cells following exposure to specific antigens. Attenuates bronchospasm caused by exercise, cold air, aspirin, and environmental pollutants. Nedocromil (Tilade) — Inhibits activation and release of mediators of a variety of inflammatory cell types associated with asthma, to include eosinophils, mast cells, neutrophils, and others. Zileuton (Zyflo) — Inhibits leukotriene formation, which, in turn, decreases neutrophil and eosinophil migration, neutrophil and monocyte aggregation, leukocyte adhesion, capillary permeability, and smooth muscle contractions.

Adapted from Morris, M, & Perkins, P. Asthma. e-Medicine, available at http://www.emedicine.com/med/topic177.htm, last updated 5/9/04.

Medications used for asthma are generally divided into 2 categories, quick relief (also called reliever medications) and long-term control (also called controller medications). Quick relief medications are used to relieve acute asthma exacerbations and to prevent EIA [exercise-induced asthma] symptoms. These medications include short-acting beta-agonists, anticholinergics (used for severe exacerbations), and systemic corticosteroids, which speed recovery from acute exacerbations. Long-term control medications include inhaled corticosteroids, cromolyn sodium, nedocromil, long-acting beta-agonists, methylxanthines, and leukotriene antagonists. Other medications that have been used to reduce oral systemic corticosteroid dependence include cyclosporine, methotrexate, gold, intravenous immunoglobulin, dapsone, troleandomycin, and hydroxychloroquine. Their use in patients with asthma is extremely limited because of variable responses, adverse effects, and limited experience. Only an asthma specialist should administer these medications. The newest asthma medication is omalizumab (Xolair), a recombinant DNA-derived humanized immunoglobulin G monoclonal antibody that binds selectively to human immunoglobulin E on the surface of mast cells and basophils. The drug reduces mediator release, which promotes an allergic response.

Indicated for moderate-to-severe persistent asthma in patients who react to perennial allergens, in whom symptoms are not controlled by inhaled corticosteroids.

Newer drugs are constantly being researched and brought on the market; thus, any listing of medications is relevant only within that timeframe. The overall goal of medication research is to find drugs that will stop the inflammatory process at an earlier point or prevent the presentation of asthma altogether. As the understanding of the pathophysiology and genetics of asthma increases, new medications with more specific but fewer side effects will probably be developed. Physical therapists should check with the physician about current medications.

SECONDARY IMPAIRMENTS

RESTRICTIONS IN DAILY LIFE AND PHYSICAL ACTIVITY

Recurrent asthma attacks may result in secondary physical and medical impairments, eventually causing the child and the family to place limitations on normal childhood activities. In a study of 1083 children in first through sixth grades, Hessel and colleagues found that 70.5% of the children with asthma had limited their activities for a health reason compared with 6.6% of the children without asthma (Hessel et al., 1996). Asthma may result in the family focusing on the medical needs of the child rather than normal childhood activities. A study by Braback and Kalvesten (1988) found that 32.7% of the children with asthma had missed 2 or more days of school in the preceding month compared with 14.8% of the children without asthma; this finding is replicated in numerous other studies. As the child then approaches adolescence, self-esteem concerns and emotional items such as frustration, anger, and fear of an asthma attack become problems (Townsend et al., 1991). As adulthood is reached, concerns such as choice of vocation and living location become increasingly more important to consider.

MEDICATION SIDE EFFECTS

Although the medications used in the management of asthma are necessary, the side effects of these medications also may have an impact on daily life. For example, oral corticosteroids may cause an increased appetite and weight gain, fluid retention, increased bruising, and mild elevation of blood pressure. Other side effects reported from a variety of asthma medications are nervousness, headache, trembling, heart palpitations, dizziness or light-headedness, dryness or irritation of the mouth and throat, heartburn, nausea, bad taste in the mouth, restlessness, difficulty concentrating, and insomnia, to mention a few (Morris & Perkins, 2004). To determine if motor, cognitive, or emotional behaviors are related to the medication, consult with the child's physician.

GROWTH AND DEVELOPMENT

Another aspect of asthma that is particularly important for self-esteem in adolescence is growth and development. New data contradict the previous belief that children with asthma eventually catch up to their peers in terms of skeletal maturation (Turktas et al., 2001; Allen, 2002; Baum et al., 2002; Wong et al., 2002). For example, Baum and colleagues (2002) found that children with severe asthma have a significantly shorter stature, skeletal retardation, and delayed puberty. Researchers question whether asthma itself or the prolonged use of steroids is responsible for such findings. Long-term studies are needed before definitive conclusions can be reached.

IMPACT ON FINANCIAL COSTS TO THE FAMILY AND SOCIETY

Asthma is associated with the highest related costs of routine pediatric care, reportedly topping $3 billion a year in the United States (Mellon & Parasuraman, 2004). A study of 71,818 children ages 1 to 17 years who were enrolled in a health maintenance organization (Lozano et al., 1997) was conducted to measure the impact of asthma on the use and cost of health care. The children with asthma incurred 88% more costs than children without asthma. Thus, having a child with asthma not only increases the family's focus on their medical needs but also consumes their financial resources. For some families this cost may be at the expense of other needs, placing a financial burden on the family and the community.

SUMMARY OF THE MEDICAL ASPECT OF ASTHMA

Asthma is a common childhood disease that can result in severe functional limitations and restrictions in childhood activities. The disease itself is complex with multiple system interactions such that each child's presentation of asthma is unique. The physical therapist needs to know how this disease affects that particular child's ability to participate in physical activities and what role the therapist can play in optimizing the child's potential for normal development, participation, and health.

PHYSICAL THERAPY EXAMINATION, EVALUATION, AND INTERVENTIONS

Physical therapists are traditionally involved in exercise programs for children with asthma, and studies have shown the efficacy of such programs in improving endurance and decreasing asthmatic symptoms (Cambach et al., 1999; Emtner, 1999; Bing'ol Karako et al., 2000; Ram et al., 2000; van Veldhoven et al., 2001). The specifics of exercise testing and the development of a fitness program are covered in Chapter 8 and will not be covered here. Endurance programs such as treadmill training, which are also common, will not be covered either, as this author prefers to find ways to improve fitness and endurance through participation in typical childhood activities rather than in contrived activities. If physical fitness is seen as an "exercise duty," it is my experience that the child and family are less likely to follow through, seeing physical exercise as a chore rather than an opportunity for growth. Thus, my intent for the physical therapy section of this chapter is to (1) help the clinician understand the process of a differential diagnosis for the potential physical and activity limitations that may occur in a child secondary to the interaction of asthma with their growing and maturing bodies, and (2) to present strategies and interventions that endeavor to get these children back among their peers, playing and competing in age-appropriate physical activities, rather than participating in adult-supervised exercise programs.

Nevertheless, the child with asthma may need more than a nudge and emotional support to engage in age-appropriate physical activities. Few studies address possible secondary physical impairments, such as adverse musculoskeletal changes/alignments, and neuromuscular recruitment problems that could limit the child's functional potential. (Cserhati et al., 1982, 1984; Fonkalsrud et al., 2000; Holloway & Ram, 2001; Temprado et al., 2002; Roux et al., 2003). In the *Guide to Physical Therapist Practice*, physical therapy is defined as a "profession with ... widespread applications in the restoration, maintenance and promotion of optimal physical function" (American Physical Therapy Association, 2001). Thus, if physical and functional limitations were identified as occurring secondary to asthma, then physical therapy would be the appropriate service to restore, maintain, and promote optimal physical functioning. Physical therapy examinations and evaluation and considerations for physical therapy interventions will be discussed within the context of a single case to illustrate how to perform a differential diagnosis through a multisystem review and how to appropriately plan interventions to address both the medical and physical deficits. Impairment categories listed in the *Guide*, plus an additional category of "internal organs," will be specifically evaluated for their impact on movement potential for the child with asthma (Box 28-1). Long-term outcomes from these interventions will also be presented.

CASE STUDY

MARY MASSERY, PT, DPT

"Jonathan" was referred to physical therapy by his pediatric pulmonologist at 9 years of age. He was in fourth grade and lived with both parents and two older

> ### Box 28-1   Motor Impairment Categories
>
> 1. Neuromuscular system
> 2. Musculoskeletal system
> 3. Integumentary system
> 4. Cardiovascular/pulmonary system
> 5. Internal organs, especially gastrointestinal system*
>
> ---
>
> Adapted from American Physical Therapy Association. Guide to Physical Therapist Practice, 2nd ed. Physical Therapy, *81*(1):29, 2001.
> *The APTA's impairment categories do not have a category for dysfunction of internal organ systems other than the cardiovascular/pulmonary system; thus "internal organs" was added by this author to correct for this deficit.

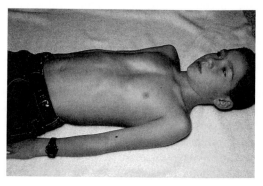

• **Figure 28-1**   Jonathan at age 10 years. Note pectus excavatum (cavus deformity of the lower chest and sternum).

siblings in a large metropolitan area with access to excellent pediatric care. He had two significant diagnoses: exercise-induced asthma (EIA) and a pectus excavatum. Figure 28-1 shows Jonathan at 10 years old.

A pectus excavatum is a skeletal lower chest wall deformity, particularly of the body of the sternum and the surrounding costal cartilage. The cartilage is collapsed inward giving the visual presentation of a hollowing out of the chest, otherwise called a "cavus," "caving-in," or a "funneling" deformity of the lower sternum (Hebra, 2004) (Fig. 28-2). Jonathan's mother reported that his chest "always looked that way" from birth (Fig. 28-3). The thoracic surgeon recommended surgery to correct the deformity, but the family refused any surgical intervention.

Jonathan's mother reported a history of frequent bouts of recurring bronchitis from 3 to 6 years old prior to the eventual diagnosis of asthma at age 6 by a pediatric pulmonologist. He had no history of pneumonia or hospitalizations. Jonathan's asthma has been managed with medications since then, including Flovent twice a

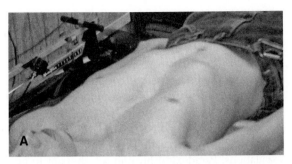
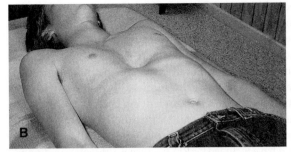

• **Figure 28-2**   **A**, This 16-year-old male has asthma and a more severe congenital pectus excavatum deformity. **B**, Note lower sternal depression (or funnel), bilateral rib flares, and elevated and protracted shoulders.

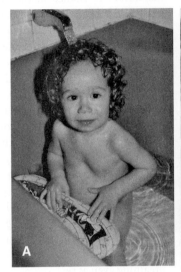
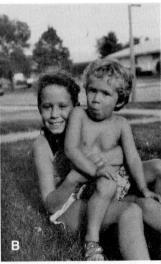

• **Figure 28-3**   Comparison picture of Jonathan at ages 2 and 3 years old. Note the pectus excavatum is more severe at 3 years of age.

day (2 puffs), and Intal and Ventolin as necessary before participation in soccer. In spite of the medications, the patient and his mother reported frequent episodes of extreme EIA symptoms, including chest tightness, wheezing, and shortness of breath after 5 to 10 minutes of soccer, resulting in a termination of the activity. The pulmonary physician reported that Jonathan's PFTs indicated that his pulmonary limitations were minor (i.e., minor peripheral airway resistance). No other significant deficits were found on four different testing dates over a year's time. Cardiac testing was negative. Even on an exercise challenge test by the pulmonologist, Jonathan showed no significant change in lung function, nor a positive response to a bronchodilator challenge. The diagnosis of EIA was made primarily on the basis of the child's clinical presentation rather than PFT results.

If his lung function tests did not show significant impairment from his EIA, and his chest deformity was not causing lung or heart impairments, then what could

explain his level of functional limitations? The pulmonologist believed that the medical status of his EIA alone could not have caused such a severe activity limitation. She knew that the patient and his family were motivated to follow his asthma management program especially because Jonathan wanted to qualify for the travel soccer team. As a result, she referred Jonathan to physical therapy to rule out physical impairments that might account for some of the severity of his disease presentation.

PHYSICAL THERAPY EXAMINATION AND EVALUATION

Medical History and Multisystem Screening of the Neuromuscular, Musculoskeletal, Integumentary, Cardiovascular/Pulmonary, and Gastrointestinal Systems

A multisystem approach to screening medical and physical deficits was performed starting with an extensive medical history, followed by identifying the child's limitations in activities and participation, and then working "backward" with this information to try to uncover the primary impairment(s) that might explain the presenting signs and symptoms. In this case, the pulmonologist had already done an extensive medical history and pertinent tests to rule out other underlying medical pathologies that could account for his participation limitations. Other medical reasons for an increase in asthmatic symptoms could have included GERD, nocturnal asthmatic conditions, pulmonary ciliary dysfunction, or vocal fold dysfunction (Wood et al., 1986; Hayes et al., 1993; Krishnamoorthy et al., 1994; Imam & Halpern, 1995; Elshami & Tino, 1996; Houtmeyers et al., 1999; Patterson & Harding, 1999; Pierce & Worsnop, 1999; Andrianopoulos et al., 2000; Kraft et al., 2001; Roger et al., 2001; Eid, 2004; Malagelada, 2004). Jonathan never had any clinical symptoms of reflux or nocturnal dysfunction, and thus no tests were done. His mother did not recall any testing for ciliary dysfunction (which results in impaired airway secretion motility due to dysfunction of the beating cilia), and the lack of any recurrent respiratory infection, such as repeat pneumonias, made this diagnosis unlikely (Houtmeyers et al., 1999; Cole, 2001). At the time of the physical therapy evaluation, vocal fold dysfunction and supraesophageal manifestations of GERD were not commonly understood to be a possible cause of asthmatic symptoms, and this possibility was thus not explored (Elshami & Tino, 1996; Pierce & Worsnop, 1999; Andrianopoulos et al., 2000; Malagelada, 2004). However, physical therapists currently assessing children with asthma should include gastric and vocal fold disorders as a routine part of the asthma examination.

Screening Assessment of Functional Limitations Related to Asthma

Following a medical history review, the physical therapy examination and evaluation focused on looking at Jonathan's breath support throughout everyday activities to determine if there was a specific area of impairment or a pattern of limitation that could explain his endurance limitations (Table 28-3). Jonathan's functional screening summary is included in Table 28-4. These findings are not unique to Jonathan. In my view, functional breath support screening at age-appropriate levels should be considered a basic examination tool for children with asthma, regardless of the primary reason for the physical therapy referral, in order to identify the contribution that asthma may have to that child's motor performance and health presentation. Functional limitations are identified by behaviors, in this case motor behaviors that require

adequate lung volumes and coordinated breath support for optimal performance; thus, they can be assessed through observations and questions to the family about the child's performance. Thus, infants as well as adolescents can be assessed with similar methods.

Breathing: Increased effort was noted with Jonathan's quiet breathing pattern, including (1) occasional paradoxical breathing (i.e., inward movement of the chest or abdomen during inhalation), and (2) frequent forced exhalations. Paradoxical breathing is thought to be due to the significant negative inspiratory pressures that the child with asthma must exert in order to overcome inspiratory resistance in the airways (Han et al., 1993; Massery, 1996). The paradoxical movements of his chest wall indicated a muscle imbalance between the respiratory muscles, usually associated with weak intercostals and abdominal muscles in relation to the diaphragm (Han et al., 1993; Bach & Bianchi, 2003). This weakness in the chest muscles, combined with the unbalanced descent of the diaphragm, may be the result of the pectus excavatum or it may have contributed to the further development of the pectus (the "chicken and the egg" syndrome). On the other hand, Jonathan's forced exhalations were probably secondary to the obstructive lung component of asthma, which constricts the conducting airways during exhalation. This forces the child to recruit expiratory muscles (primarily the abdominals and internal intercostals) to push the air out of the chest even during quiet exhalation, causing increased work of breathing even at rest.

These patterns indicated that Jonathan's motor planning for ventilation muscle recruitment did not appear to be optimal for activities that required greater oxygen consumption because he was already overusing his diaphragm and recruiting his upper accessory muscles at rest, all the while underutilizing his intercostal muscles. All these observations led me to believe that his respiratory muscle imbalance may be significantly contributing to his decreased endurance, and poor musculoskeletal alignment of his chest and overall postural alignment and could account for the endurance limitations not attributed to asthma itself by the pulmonologist.

Coughing: The patient demonstrated an effective cough. The only reports from the family of ineffective coughing or impaired airway clearance strategies during respiratory episodes came from his mother, noting that sometimes when he is sick, his secretions are so thick that they get "stuck" in his chest. Jonathan reported that he rarely drank water at school. This would indicate a need for increased hydration and a possible screening for ciliary dysfunction to rule out the possibility that the cilia themselves were dysfunctional rather than that the mucus

TABLE 28-3	**Assessing Functional Limitations Associated with Asthma or Other Ventilatory Dysfunction***

FUNCTIONAL ACTIVITY	SECONDARY PROBLEMS†
Breathing	Inadequate breath support and inefficient trunk muscle recruitment at rest or with activities such that breathing or postural control are compromised
	Asthmatic triggers such as rapid airflow caused by sudden increase in physical activity, dry air or extreme air temperatures, or other triggers that trip an asthmatic reaction
Coughing	Ineffective mobilization and expectoration strategies
Sleeping	Breathing difficulties, signs of obstructive or central sleep disorders
	Nocturnal reflux (GERD)
Eating	Swallowing dysfunction
	Reflux (GERD)
	Dehydration
	Poor nutrition
Talking	Inadequate lung volume and/or inadequate motor control for eccentric and concentric expiratory patterns of speech
	Poor coordination between talking (refined breath support) and moving (postural control)
Moving	Inadequate balance between ventilation and postural demands
	Breath holding with more demanding postures: use of the diaphragm as a primary postural muscle for trunk stabilization
	Inadequate lung volume to support movement
	Inadequate and/or inefficient muscle recruitment patterns for trunk/respiratory muscles causing endurance problems or poor motor performance
	Ineffective pairing of breathing with movement, especially with higher level activities

*The following activities require adequate lung volumes and coordination of breathing with movement for optimal performance.

† These typical secondary problems associated with asthma should be screened for to determine their possible contribution to the child's motor impairment or motor dysfunction.

was simply thicker due to dehydration (Mossberg et al., 1978). He did not report vomiting associated with forceful coughing as many children with asthma report. (Gagging or vomiting is a common occurrence following a hard cough in the pediatric patient, most likely due to the close proximity of the esophagus and trachea, as well as a higher sensitivity in children to noxious stimuli in general [Sontag et al., 2003; Eid & Morton, 2004].)

Sleeping: The patient reported that he sleeps on his back with his arms by his side, and occasionally he sleeps on his side. No breathing difficulties (including apnea, snoring, or irregularities), coughing, or drooling at night were reported that could indicate upper airway obstruction or GERD (D'Ambrosio & Mohsenin, 1998). However, a preference for the supine position at night may indicate a recruitment of upper accessory muscles even while sleeping owing to the optimal length-tension relationship of those muscles in supine along with increased posterior stabilization. Jonathan reports that he does not "curl up" to sleep. It is my clinical observation

that children who are primarily upper chest breathers instead of diaphragmatic breathers will often choose to sleep supine with their arms thrown up over their heads rather than prone or curled up on their side, probably because of the improved length-tension relationship of all the anterior and superior chest muscles in supine. They may also report that they start out on their side or stomach, but find themselves on their backs in the morning. Depending on the rest of the findings, one may want to recommend a change in sleep postures for Jonathan, but only if that still allows him to sleep through the night.

Eating: Jonathan did not report problems with chewing or swallowing any foods or textures, nor any difficulties with drinking any type of liquid at any speed. In addition, there was no history of aspiration, choking, or gagging episodes. He did not present with any clinical signs of reflux, which is a common association with asthma and should be ruled out as a contributor to the motor or health restrictions (Sontag et al., 2003).

TABLE 28-4	Synopsis of Jonathan's Initial Physical Therapy Examination and Evaluation

EVALUATION	JONATHAN'S RESULTS
Medical diagnoses (pathology)	Asthma, primarily exercise induced (EIA) Pectus excavatum
Impairment (summary of body functions and structure)	**Cardiopulmonary:** Inflammation and hyperresponsiveness of airways particularly after initiation of exercise with PFTs indicating mild peripheral airway resistance Marked endurance limitations (5–10 minute tolerance) especially with higher level activities (particularly soccer) Occasional dehydration and decreased secretion mobility Increased work of breathing even at rest, RR 20 breaths/min (high end of normal) Auscultation clear in all lung fields No cardiac deficits per cardiologist **Musculoskeletal:** Marked pectus excavatum and elevated sternal angle Rib flares, L > R, with weakness noted in oblique abdominal muscles L > R (patient is right-handed) Functional midthoracic kyphosis of the spine particularly at the level opposite the pectus Decreased lateral side bending, indicating chest wall and quadratus lumborum restrictions Rib cage mobility restrictions greatest in mid chest nearest the pectus Mid trunk "fold" in sitting (rib cage collapsing onto the abdomen in sitting) "Slouched" sitting and standing postures: shoulders protracted and internally rotated Shortened neck musculature, hypertrophy No shoulder range-of-motion limitations **Neuromuscular:** Muscle imbalances in trunk muscles with significantly weaker/underutilized intercostal muscles, oblique abdominal muscles, and scapular adductors Inefficient neuromuscular recruitment patterns for inspiratory and expiratory efforts as well as for postural demands **Integumentary:** No restrictions noted **Internal organs, especially gastrointestinal system:** No reflux, constipation, or other gastrointestinal dysfunction
Functional limitations (breathing, coughing, sleeping, eating, talking, moving)	Breathing pattern was inefficient showing muscle imbalance among the diaphragm, abdominals, intercostals, and upper accessory muscles Movement and participation limitations secondary to medical impairments, endurance impairments, postural impairments, and breath support impairments In addition to movement limitations due to the medical component of asthma, his movements were limited by the simultaneous postural and respiratory demands presented during higher level activities such as soccer and the ventilatory needs to support such tasks No functional breath support limitations noted in sleeping, eating, coughing, or talking activities
Activity and participation limitations	According to mother, Jonathan was beginning to withdraw from participation in physical activities, especially organized athletics, secondary to his "deformed chest" and fear of asthmatic episodes

TABLE 28-4	Synopsis of Jonathan's Initial Physical Therapy Examination and Evaluation—*cont'd*

EVALUATION	JONATHAN'S RESULTS
	EIA caused him to stop playing soccer after typically 5 to 10 minutes
	Patient had already stopped swimming to avoid taking off his shirt among his friends
Diagnosis	9-year-old boy, with history of severe EIA and marked pectus excavatum
	Significant restrictions in chest wall mobility and posture, as well as motor planning deficits, contributed to limitations in adequate breath support, postural control and endurance for desired functional activities and contributed to the continued development of the pectus and other postural deformities
	Dehydration also appeared to play a significant role in triggering a bronchospasm (EIA) during the rapid change in inhalation volume and negative force associated with participation in sports such as soccer
Prognosis	Excellent
	Capable of developing new motor plans
	Musculoskeletal deformities were functional, not fixed; still prepubescent
	Motivated by his desire to "make" the traveling soccer team, and be "normal"
	Supportive family
	Good medical care

Asthma is typically associated with a higher sensitivity or reactivity to dry air in the airway; thus adequate hydration to keep the airway moist (humidity) is necessary to decrease external triggers to asthmatic reactions (Moloney et al., 2002). Hydration is also necessary to keep secretions thin and mobile (Anderson & Holzer, 2000; Moloney et al., 2003). Jonathan did not have a "feeding problem," but he did have a hydration problem, which most likely exacerbated his EIA symptoms.

Talking: Jonathan demonstrated a normal number of syllables per breath (at least 8 to 10) as noted during conversational speech (Hixon, 1991; Deem & Miller, 2000). He was capable of excellent sustained vocalization: 20 seconds (twice the expected length) (Deem & Miller, 2000). He could also talk in all postures at multiple volume levels with good postural control and controlled eccentric breath support. This was clearly the patient's strongest demonstration of breath control within a functional task. I anticipated using this "strength" to reinforce eccentric trunk control and pacing activities with soccer. Speech breathing is primarily eccentric control of the inspiratory muscles; thus I can use his excellent eccentric motor planning for the trunk muscles during speech to recruit the same muscles for eccentric control during other eccentric trunk and postural maneuvers (Deem & Miller, 2000).

Moving: Jonathan reported episodes of extreme shortness of breath (dyspnea) and asthmatic episodes within 5 to 10 minutes of participating in strenuous activities such as soccer. He reported that he "warms up for a minute" before starting to run in soccer. This quick change from rest to running would cause a rapid acceleration in inspiratory volume and flow rates and could possibly trigger his EIA response secondary to upper airway hyperresponsiveness or increased airway resistance (Tecklin, 1994; Milgrom & Taussig, 1999; Anderson & Holzer, 2000; Massie, 2002; Moloney et al., 2002). He also reported that he used his bronchodilator inhaler immediately prior to team practice, which doesn't allow for maximal benefit of the drug; thus incorrect use of medications may also be contributing to his EIA (Physicians' Desk Reference, 2001). It was interesting that Jonathan did not report breathing problems with quiet activities in spite of the fact that his breathing demonstrated inconsistent recruitment patterns and an increased work of breathing at rest. No breath holding was noted with any developmental posture or transitional movement. Discoordination between breathing and movement appear to be contributing to his limitations in higher level activities such as sport participation but not during quiet activities.

Summary of Functional Screening

The functional screening indicated impairment at the level of muscle recruitment for breath support at rest and during strenuous exercise, with resultant endurance impairments. Activities that demanded greater oxygen consumption and faster inspiratory flow rates, such as soccer, immediately used up his pulmonary reserves, causing Jonathan to hit an early "ceiling" effect, forcing him to terminate the activity due to dyspnea and asthmatic symptoms. It also caused a rapid influx of dry air, which most likely triggered the EIA response. No significant problems were noted with functional tasks requiring less oxygen demand and slower inspiratory flow rates such as sleeping, coughing, eating, or talking. In fact, breath support for talking was extremely well developed and was noted as his strongest asset on the functional assessment. Inadequate daily hydration, which would decrease his secretion mobility and produce heightened airway hyperresponsiveness (bronchospasm) was also a significant finding. Jonathan's functional screening results are summarized along with his other examination and evaluation findings in Table 28-4.

ASSESSING THE IMPAIRMENTS RELATED TO FUNCTIONAL LIMITATIONS

When limitations are noted during the functional limitation screening assessment, further impairment testing should be done (age appropriately) to assess the extent of the initial limitations and as a baseline for assessing future progress. A baby or young child would not be capable of performing or cooperating with some tests, such as PFTs, and thus the physical therapist must assess the appropriateness of any impairment test for each specific patient.

According to Jonathan's pulmonologist, his lung pathology alone could not have caused his marked functional limitations noted during athletics such as soccer. Results of our functional screening concur with that opinion, and thus further impairment tests and measures were taken. A summary of the impairment results are found on Table 28-4. A few key findings from his examination will be interpreted here to explain their relevance to his functional limitations.

Jonathan demonstrated a muscle imbalance between his three primary respiratory muscles (diaphragm, abdominals, and intercostals) and his upper accessory muscles of respiration (Primiano, 1982; Cala, 1993; Han et al., 1993). All play a dual role in simultaneously meeting his breathing needs and his postural needs (Hodges & Gandevia, 2000; Gandevia et al., 2002). Because of his

asthma, Jonathan had to overcome increased inspiratory resistance even at rest, which forced him to overrecruit the upper accessory muscles from a very young age, setting up a pattern of overuse, which leads to fatigue (endurance factor). When he needed more oxygen during exercise, he recruited those same accessory muscles even more so, reaching a "ceiling" on his respiratory reserves. He had no "extra" muscles to recruit when he needed more oxygen (again with an impact on endurance). Thus, when his postural demands increased, such as during soccer, and his oxygen demands couldn't support these needs, his oxygen requirements limited the activity (Hodges et al., 2001).

Typical of many patients who have an increased work of breathing, Jonathan used his accessory muscles of respiration at the expense of his diaphragm and external intercostals, seen clinically as occasional paradoxical breathing and forced expiratory maneuvers at rest. I suspect this pattern contributed to the sternal abnormalities that formed early in life. In my clinical observations, children with an early onset of asthma who overuse their sternocleidomastoid, scalene, and trapezius muscles cause a greater force on the anterior-superior pull on the sternal angle, resulting in an elevated sternal angle. The manubrium (the top portion of the sternum) is calcified at birth, while the body of the sternum is primarily cartilaginous. Perhaps that is why the solid manubrium tilts superiorly with the pull of the sternocleidomastoid while the less stable sternal body is less likely to be drawn upward. This in turn causes greater *superior* expansion of the chest at a loss of *anterior* chest excursion (decreased circumferential chest wall excursion) leading to chest wall restrictions. In addition, children like Jonathan tend to initiate inspiration with a greater effort to overcome the increased airway resistance from asthma, creating a larger negative inspiratory force (NIF) and more collapsing forces on the chest wall (Han et al., 1993). Clinically, this is observed as an excessive inferior descent of the diaphragm (low abdominal excursion) with flat or paradoxical intercostal movement (inward movement of the mid or lower chest wall). I believe that, over time, the repeated excessive NIF contributed to a decreased developmental stimulus for the activation of the intercostal muscles, thus setting up a pattern of muscle imbalance along Jonathan's chest wall and contributing to the further development of his pectus and associated rib cage and thoracic spine restrictions.

This is a pattern that I see repeated in numerous other cases in which asthma limits the child's participation in normal activities from infancy through puberty. I believe that the neuromuscular recruitment patterns developed early in life due to the child's ventilatory needs result in musculoskeletal abnormalities and neuromuscular imbalance of the respiratory/postural trunk muscles for movement. This is unique to childhood asthma because of the maturation and development of their systems versus adult-onset asthma where the motor systems have already completed typical development.

Evaluation: Impairments of the Neuromuscular, Musculoskeletal, Integumentary, Cardiovascular/Pulmonary, and Gastrointestinal Systems

1. From a medical perspective, Jonathan's asthma was well managed, but it was still limiting participation in typical childhood activities. Thus, his cardiopulmonary system was not the only system with impairment. Typical secondary medical impairments such as GERD were not present, but daily underhydration was likely a significant contributor to his EIA response (Anderson & Holzer, 2000; Moloney et al., 2002).
2. Jonathan demonstrated muscle imbalance in quiet and strenuous breathing. It appeared that he could benefit from learning new motor strategies to breathe effectively and efficiently (neuromuscular retraining) to attempt to better support ventilatory needs simultaneously with the postural demands of the task.
3. Jonathan demonstrated numerous chest wall and spine restrictions, but no integumentary restrictions. He needed more musculoskeletal mobility in order to support adequate internal lung expansion at low energy cost and decrease the triggers that caused his EIA response, such as rapid inspiratory airflows (Leong et al., 1999; Wilson et al., 1999). This mobility was necessary before neuromuscular retraining could be effectively undertaken, and before adaptive cardiopulmonary strategies could be optimized. Thus, with his asthma well managed from a medical perspective, the *musculoskeletal* system presented the primary obstacles to his optimal physical function and endurance.

Therefore, in spite of the fact that his primary diagnosis was cardiopulmonary, this examination pointed to significant musculoskeletal and neuromuscular impairments associated with Jonathan's medical diagnosis. Yet, the literature rarely mentions this possibility. An extensive search of Medline, Cochrane Reviews, and CINAHL databases showed a plethora of articles identifying endurance impairments, quality of life issues, and poor overall health as consequences of childhood asthma, but only a very few articles identified potential secondary physical impairments such as those observed in Jonathan:

1. Musculoskeletal restrictions and deformities of the chest wall, upper extremity, or spine (Cserhati et al., 1982, 1984; Fonkalsrud et al., 2000).
2. Inefficient neuromuscular recruitment for breathing and postural control (Weiner et al., 2002; Cooper et al., 2003; McConnell & Romer, 2004).
3. Ineffective coordination of breathing with movement (no articles were found on this topic).

Of particular interest, large-scale literature reviews of breathing retraining such as the Cochrane Reviews have been more plentiful in the past few years. Although authors of these reviews continue to conclude that the evidence for strengthening respiratory muscles or neuromuscular retraining of breathing patterns is inconclusive based on a lack of controlled studies or the small number of available controlled studies, they specifically state that that doesn't mean that breathing retraining doesn't work, just that there is not enough hard evidence to make a decision either way (Holloway & Ram, 2001; Steurer-Stey et al., 2002; Ram et al., 2003; Gyorik & Brutsche, 2004; Markham & Wilkinson, 2004).

DIAGNOSIS

Jonathan is a 9-year-old boy with a history of severe EIA and marked pectus excavatum. Significant restrictions in his chest wall mobility and posture, as well as motor planning deficits and underhydration, appear to contribute to limitations in breath support and endurance for his desired functional activities and contribute to the continued development of the pectus excavatum and other postural deformities by perpetuating trunk muscle imbalance and an increased work of breathing.

PROGNOSIS

Jonathan's parents have rejected a surgical option to reduce his pectus and thus his prognosis was related to the potential success of a noninvasive physical therapy program. I believed that Jonathan had an excellent prognosis for the following reasons: (1) he was closely followed from a medical perspective, (2) he was neurologically intact and capable of developing new motor plans, (3) his musculoskeletal deformities were functional, not fixed, and he was still prepubescent, and (4) just as important, Jonathan was extremely *motivated* by his desire to "make" the traveling soccer team and his desire to be able to take his shirt off without embarrassment due to the pectus. His mother was completely committed to helping her son maximize any opportunity to improve his health and well-being, including doing daily exercises at home under her supervision, if necessary. With this high level of support from the patient and his family, I anticipated making maximal progress with about 6 to 12 visits over a 1-year timeframe.

TABLE 28-5	**Goals of Physical Therapy Program**

PHYSICAL THERAPY GOALS	JONATHAN'S GOALS
Long-term goal	**Reduce secondary impairments** that limit Jonathan's ability to achieved his desired level of physical activity performance and participation (soccer, baseball, swimming, etc.) and health (missed days of school, ER visits, sicknesses)
Short-term goals	**Increase joint mobility** of rib cage and thoracic spine to promote full ROM for optimal breath support, full trunk movements to optimize skilled movements of the trunk musculature, decrease forces promoting developing kyphosis, as well as decrease forces promoting developing pectus excavatum.
	Improve muscle strength and muscle balance between diaphragm, intercostals, abdominals, paraspinals, scapular retractors, and neck muscles to normalize forces on the developing spine (decrease kyphosis), ribs (increase individual rib movement potential), sternum (decrease pectus forces), and shoulder (decrease anterior humeral head positioning and potential shoulder ROM losses).
	Improve motor planning of trunk muscle recruitment for respiration and posture by: Changing the sequence of activation of respiratory muscles to promote sooner activation of intercostal muscles, thus preventing paradoxical chest wall movement, which increases pectus forces (greater negative inspiratory forces reinforce development of a pectus if intercostals are weak, paralyzed, or delayed). Refining the respiratory pattern during quiet and stressful breathing to improve endurance by teaching Jonathon to utilize his diaphragm (endurance muscle) for a greater percentage of the ventilatory workload, and to decrease his over-recruitment of accessory muscles (short burst supporters) during quiet breathing. Refining recruitment pattern of postural muscle to: Increase recruitment of intercostals, oblique abdominal and transverse abdominal muscles, scapular retractors, and paraspinals. Decrease over-recruitment of rectus abdominus and sternocleidomastoid (SCM). Improve core trunk movements so that the intercostals, oblique abdominals, and transverse abdominal muscles become the primary stabilizers of the mid trunk, thus avoiding the SCM being overutilized as the primary trunk flexor, which can cause rib elevation, forward head, and eventually rib flares from underuse of oblique abdominals.
	Improve coordination of breathing with movement to improve oxygen transport during an activity (improving endurance) and to optimize the coordination between the respiration and postural demands of any physical task in order to improve overall physical performance from simple tasks such as activities of daily living to demanding tasks such as soccer.
	Improve patient and family's understanding of how they can more effectively manage the adverse effects of asthma on Jonathan's posture and movement patterns in order to reduce external triggers that precipitate his asthma attacks. This includes improving his overall hydration levels especially during athletic activities, decreasing activities that result in rapid changes in inspiratory airflow demands (slower warm-ups), and improving the timing of his asthma medications with strenuous activities.

PHYSICAL THERAPY INTERVENTIONS AND OUTCOMES

The goals of Jonathan's physical therapy program are listed in detail in Table 28-5, and the physical therapy interventions are summarized in Table 28-6. These represent typical goals and intervention strategies for many children with asthma and can be adapted for any other case or age range.

Asthma (Cardiovascular/Pulmonary and Gastrointestinal) Management Interventions

Jonathan was instructed in immediate changes that he could implement at school, home, and on the soccer field to decrease the triggers that set off his EIA response. He was extremely sensitive to a sudden increase in inspiratory volumes and flow rates that occurred secondary to soccer warm-ups, which started with laps around the

TABLE 28-6	Physical Therapy Interventions

IMPAIRMENT CATEGORY	INTERVENTIONS FOR JONATHAN

Asthma (cardiopulmonary) management strategies	Increased hydration to decrease extrinsic EIA triggers
	Improved timing of medications with activity level to get maximal benefit of medication
	Developed and implemented a new warm-up protocol for soccer practices and games that slowly increased his respiratory work load to avoid dramatic changes in inspiratory lung volumes and speed to avoid EIA trigger such as initiating a walk/run warm-up rather than running only, with gradual increase in running time and speed and stretching all trunk musculature prior to soccer
	Coordinated ventilatory strategies with movement and stretching to
	   Decrease respiratory work load and EIA trigger
	   Improve efficiency of movement with resultant improved endurance
	Implement breath control techniques to prevent or minimize EIA attacks
	   Improve awareness of oncoming EIA symptoms
	   Use controlled breathing techniques to ward off EIA attack when possible

Musculoskeletal interventions	Rib cage mobilization to increase chest wall and thoracic spine mobility in order to reduce respiratory workload and increase likelihood of recruiting intercostal muscles for more efficient respiration and support for developing thorax (reducing pectus excavatum forces) Intercostal muscle release to optimize length-tension relationship Quadratus lumborum muscle release to promote activation of oblique and transverse abdominis muscles for lower trunk stabilization instead of quadratus Active assistive anterior and axial glides to thoracic spine Home program to maintain newly gained trunk mobility
Neuromuscular interventions	Specific diaphragmatic training from recumbent to upright positions, and eventually to sporting conditions Emphasis on slow, easy effort during initiation of inhalation to prevent overpowering developing intercostal muscles Increased recruitment and strength of intercostals for all breathing patterns, postural control, and skeletal development (reducing pectus, paradoxical breathing, and thoracic kyphosis) Specific coordination of inhalation/exhalation patterns with all activities (ventilatory strategies) Increased recruitment and strength of scapular adductors, shoulder external rotators, and paraspinals for increased posterior stabilization Lengthening of neck accessory muscles through active stretching Midtrunk stabilization exercises (reducing rib flares and improving midtrunk interfacing between intercostals and abdominals)
Integumentary interventions	None needed at this time
Internal organs (gastrointestinal) interventions	Increase hydration, especially during sporting activities

soccer field. It was likely that the combination of (1) the *dryness* in his airway caused by the change from nose breathing to mouth breathing due to the sudden need for increased inspired air during the running activity and (2) the *large, fast moving volume* of air required to perform this high level of exercise played a significant role in triggering an acute attack (Anderson & Holzer, 2000; Moloney et al., 2002). Within 5 to 10 minutes of soccer, he would typically experience such extreme shortness of breath that he was forced to stop playing. Often he did not recover in time to rejoin his teammates.

Jonathan's management program included several steps:

1. Instruction in increasing his hydration overall, and specifically to use hydration before and throughout the games and practices in order to keep his upper airway moist (Anderson & Holzer, 2000; Moloney et al., 2002).

2. He began to take his medications sooner, at least a full 15 to 30 minutes prior to the start of soccer, in order to receive the maximum benefit from the drugs.

3. He started a new warm-up that slowly increased his activity level so that the oxygen demand slowly increased, allowing him to breathe through his nose for a longer period of time and allowing the necessary inspired air volume to also increase slowly.

4. He stretched his trunk, spine, rib cage and shoulders prior to the game to maximize mobility (compliance) of his chest wall movements, thus decreasing his work of breathing.

5. He coordinated his breathing specifically with the relationship of the trunk movement and rib cage during each stretching exercise and movement in general to reinforce normal pattern combinations of movement and breathing (ventilatory strategies) (Massery & Frownfelter, 1996; Temprado et al., 2002).

6. He was taught two particular breath control techniques to help him regain control of breathing during the early stages of an asthmatic attack: (a) repatterning controlled breathing technique and (b) an enhanced Jacobsen's progressive relaxation exercise. The repatterning technique is described by Frownfelter and Dean (1996) in their cardiopulmonary textbook (p. 393):

> The patient is asked to start with exhalation. "Try to blow out easily with your lips pursed. Don't force it just let it come out." Suggesting that the patient visualize a candle with a flame which their exhalation makes flicker but not go out will help to produce a prolonged, easy exhalation. Doing this allows the respiratory rate to decrease automatically. When the patient feels some control of this step, then ask him or her to "hold your breath at the top of inspiration just for a second or two." Make sure the patient does not hold his or her breath and bear down as in a Valsalva maneuver. Last, ask the patient to take a slow breath in, hold it, and let it go out through pursed lips. Patients learn that when they are short of breath, this technique often helps them to gain control, making them feel less panicky.

Jacobsen's modified technique utilizes ventilatory strategies to help the patient experience the difference between inhaling and contracting the upper trapezius versus exhaling and relaxing the trapezius in order to develop new motor plans to keep the trapezius from being over recruited (Massery & Frownfelter, 1996).

Asthma Management Outcomes

Jonathan rigorously followed the regimen including carrying a water bottle with him everywhere, even in the classroom. He noticed an immediate decrease in chest tightness and dyspnea during soccer practice and games. Of particular note, prior to using the repatterning controlled breathing technique, Jonathan said he had no way to stop the progression of his asthma attack once it started. Now, he said that if the attack was mild, he was able to "work through it" with the repatterning and it did not develop into a full-blown attack. He could now play a whole game of soccer without EIA preventing his participation. In fact, he made the travel soccer team and could play four consecutive games of soccer in 1 day without EIA symptoms. As a consequence of decreasing EIA triggers, Jonathan began having fewer and fewer asthmatic attacks, such that all asthma medications were discontinued 2 months after starting physical therapy. This was not an intended consequence of physical therapy, but a welcome one. Jonathan reported only one incident of bronchitis in the following year, and no asthma attacks after 2 months of physical therapy.

Musculoskeletal Interventions

Jonathan needed increased chest wall and spine mobility before attempting neuromuscular training of muscles along that tight rib cage. Manual rib mobilization was performed to all 10 ribs bilaterally (Johnson, 1989) to increase individual rib movement potentials, to increase rib cage compliance, and to increase the potential for axial rotation of his thoracic spine (a tight rib cage makes lateral or axial movements of the thoracic spine less possible). Jonathan was positioned in side lying with a large towel roll placed under his lower ribs to maximize rib expansion on the uppermost side. From the results of my testing, the intervention was focused more on the left side than the right, and more in the midchest than the upper or lower chest. This was followed by intercostal muscle release techniques to maximize intercostal spacing and optimize their length-tension relationship for neuromuscular retraining. Finally, his quadratus lumborum was released bilaterally to allow for more separation between the rib cage and the pelvis. Posteriorly, the thoracic spine was only mildly restricted in anterior glides (extension of spine) and axial rotation, so active assisted mobilizations were incorporated into his home program. Jonathan worked on maintaining his new-found trunk mobility with a home stretching program.

TABLE 28-7 Lateral Trunk Flexion Mobility Test for Rib Cage and Quadratus Lumborum

TEST	INITIAL DATE	DISCHARGE DATE 11 MONTHS LATER	REEVALUATION 4 YEARS AFTER DISCHARGE
Lateral side bend toward L: mobility of right rib cage	2 1/4"	4 1/2"	3 5/8"
Lateral side bend toward L: mobility of right quadratus lumborum	1"	3"	2 3/8"
Lateral side bend toward R: mobility of left rib cage	1 1/2"	3 3/4"	3"
Lateral side bend toward R: mobility of left quadratus lumborum	1 1/4"	2 1/2"	2 3/8"

Note: From initial evaluation to discharge 11 months later, Jonathan's rib cage mobility doubled on the right, and more than doubled on the left. His quadratus lumborum length tripled on the right and doubled on the left. At the 4-year follow up examination, he had lost some mobility at all levels except the left quadratus lumborum.

TABLE 28-8 Other Tests and Measures

TEST	INITIAL DATE	DISCHARGE DATE 11 MONTHS LATER	REEVALUATION 4 YEARS AFTER DISCHARGE
Pectus volume displacement (typical: zero or minimal volume)	34 mL (taken 4 months after initial evaluation)	18 mL	17 mL
Respiratory rate (typical 10 – 20)	20	11	—
Auscultation	Clear	Clear	Clear
Phonation (typical 10 seconds)	20 sec	25.5 sec	28.6 sec
PFTs (pulmonary function tests)	Normal lung volumes and flow rates	Not taken	Normal lung volumes and flow rates

Note that Jonathan's pectus excavatum, which was 34 mL H_2O when measured 4 months into treatment, was reduced by half to 18 mL H_2O at discharge and was maintained relatively at the same level when remeasured 4 years later.

Musculoskeletal Outcomes

Jonathan made tremendous progress in trunk mobility as measured by range of motion in lateral trunk flexion (Table 28-7). His rib cage mobility doubled on the right, and more than doubled on the left. His quadratus lumborum length tripled on the right and doubled on the left. His anterior glides and axial rotation glides of thoracic spine were now normal. His pectus excavatum, which was 34 mL H_2O when measured 4 months into treatment, was reduced by half to 18 mL H_2O at discharge 7 months later (Table 28-8). Even though his pectus volume was not measured until midway through his physical therapy timeline, he still showed a reduction of approximately 50% within 8 months. There was no

initial photo to compare his pectus, as the patient was uncomfortable having his picture taken at that time.

Postural assessment showed elimination of functional kyphosis in sitting and standing postures. Jonathan no longer showed a midtrunk "fold" in a sitting posture. Mother and son reported that his teachers no longer continually reminded him to "sit up straight" in school. Inferior rib flares were no longer apparent as his abdominal muscles now adequately stabilized the rib cage at the midtrunk and his primary neuromuscular recruitment pattern now utilized his abdominal muscles instead of his sternocleidomastoid muscles as his primary trunk flexor. His sternal angle elevation appeared slightly reduced but was not objectively measured.

Neuromuscular Interventions

The priorities of Jonathan's physical therapy program were to address his medical needs first, then his musculoskeletal restrictions, and finally his neuromuscular impairments. Jonathan needed to balance the strength and recruitment patterns of his respiratory and postural muscles to optimize breath control at a low energy cost while simultaneously providing appropriate muscle force to his trunk that would promote normalizing forces on his developing spine and rib cage (Han et al., 1993; Hodges & Gandevia, 2000).

Respiration can be achieved through numerous combinations of muscles and activation patterns. The literature shows variability in the percentage of work that the diaphragm does during normal quiet breathing, with the range generally noted from about 60% to 85% of the total muscular effort (Cherniack & Cherniack, 1983; Frownfelter & Dean, 1996). The intercostals, paraspinals, upper accessory muscles, and abdominal muscles supplement the diaphragmatic effort (Primiano, 1982; Saumarez, 1986; Dean & Hobson, 1996). Clinicians have observed, and researchers have confirmed, that the body attempts to recruit the most efficient combination of respiratory muscles for a specific respiratory or motor task in different postures (Wolfson et al., 1992; Nava et al., 1993; Estenne et al., 1998; Wilson et al., 1999; Aliverti et al., 2001; Temprado et al., 2002). Thus, the neuromuscular retraining of Jonathan's respiratory muscles started with specific diaphragmatic training in a side-lying posture to facilitate a more optimal length-tension relationship of the diaphragm while simultaneously facilitating a less optimal length-tension relationship of the upper accessory muscles to minimize their recruitment during quiet breathing. Jonathan did not respond with increased diaphragmatic recruitment and excursion with positioning and verbal cues alone, so manual techniques were added.

Several techniques were used, but the one that produced the greatest consistency, reproducibility, and appropriate timing of activity in the diaphragm was the "diaphragm scoop" technique (see Massery & Frownfelter, 1996). This technique provides specific quick stretch input to the central tendon of the diaphragm via the patient's abdominal viscera at the end of the expiratory cycle in an effort to recruit the central tendon as the initiator of the next inspiratory effort. Continued manual cueing was provided throughout the entire inspiratory phase to facilitate greater inferior excursion of the diaphragm. An emphasis was placed on initiating inspiration with an "easy, slow onset" to avoid recruitment of the upper accessory muscles and an overpowering

of his intercostal muscles (paradoxical breathing). Once the patient could consistently succeed in recruiting the diaphragm in side lying, he was challenged by decreasing manual input and increasing postural demands by using positions such as sitting and standing. At this point Jonathan was instructed to practice this technique using "visualization" at home just before sleeping to take advantage of a relaxed state. Eventually, he was trained to use the diaphragm breathing technique in sports as well as static postural holds. Auditory cues for the rate, rhythm, and depth of inspiration were included in all breathing retraining techniques. Objective measures of his success were taken with assessment of chest wall excursion (CWE) (Massery et al., 1997; LaPier et al., 2000).

Jonathan demonstrated poor recruitment of his external intercostal muscles, which are needed to stabilize the chest wall during inspiration to prevent paradoxical breathing and the potential development of a pectus excavatum secondary to this inward movement (Han et al., 1993). Jonathan demonstrated this paradoxical chest wall movement even at rest in his mid rib cage. Thus, weak intercostals could be, in part, responsible for the development of his pectus. I used manual facilitation techniques with (1) upper extremity flexion, abduction, and external rotation activities (D2 diagonals from proprioceptive neuromuscular facilitation [PNF]) (Knott & Voss, 1968); combined with (2) thoracic extension and rotation; intentionally paired with (3) large inspiratory efforts, in order to utilize optimal length-tension relationships and function of the external intercostals; and (4) a maximal inspiratory effort followed by a peak inspiratory hold to increase positive outward pressure on the anterior chest wall (Decramer et al., 1986; Saumarez, 1986; Han et al., 1993; Rimmer et al., 1995; Wilson et al., 2001; Temprado et al., 2002). Jonathan was instructed to visually follow his arm motions to maximize the trunk rotation. Thoracic rotation produces greater intercostal muscle recruitment than straight plane motions (Decramer et al., 1986; Rimmer et al., 1995; Wilson et al., 2001). Jonathan was instructed to continue the exercises at home once he could demonstrate the proper recruitment pattern.

Jonathan's abdominal muscles were often recruited concentrically for exhalation. To retrain the abdominals for quiet breathing, Jonathan was given simple eccentric trunk exercises to be done during his warm-up for soccer. He was told to pair eccentric exhalation (quiet speech) with the eccentric trunk movements to reinforce the natural coupling and avoid the concentric forceful expiratory pattern (Massery, 1994). Jonathan's speech breathing pattern was highly developed, so I incorporated it into his independent neuromuscular retraining program.

A second chest wall stabilizer exercise was added. The patient was positioned supine on top of a vertical thoracic towel roll to maximize thoracic extension and stabilization. Jonathan was then instructed to externally rotate his shoulders while "pinching his shoulder blades" back to the towel roll to maximize anterior chest expansion by recruiting the external intercostals and the pectoralis muscle (using the pectoralis muscles to act as a chest wall expander rather than an upper extremity adductor). The position also stretched his neck flexors. During this activity, he was instructed in take in a deep breath and "hold it" during PNF hold-relax technique to maximize the response from his scapular retractors (Sullivan et al., 1982). This provided maximal positive pressure from within his chest cavity, which provided a greater force to "push out" his chest wall, in order to reduce the pectus forces (Bach & Biandi, 2003; Lissoni, 1998).

Lastly, Jonathan was instructed in specific recruitment of internal intercostals and oblique abdominal muscles as the primary stabilizers of the inferior rib cage to (1) decrease the rib flare deformity, (2) improve midtrunk stabilization to offer the diaphragm better mechanical support, (3) reduce his overdependence on the rectus muscle for stabilization, which again reinforced the development of the pectus, and (4) provide stability of the rib cage during activation of the sternocleidomastoid muscles to prevent the chest from being lifted toward the head when Jonathan's intended movement was to bring his head to the chest. Once again, a PNF D2 upper extremity pattern was used (Knott & Voss, 1968). This time, the patient was positioned supine with his arm positioned in flexion, abduction, and external rotation while lying over a vertical towel roll. The patient's arm was stabilized distally. The patient was asked to "try to lift his arm up in the diagonal pattern" but was not allowed any movement. The result was a strong isometric contraction of the midtrunk muscles (oblique and transverse abdominis and internal intercostals), which are required for stabilization of the trunk before the distal extremity could be moved off the ground. This allowed him to perform small concentric contractions of his internal intercostals and obliques without being over-powered by the rectus. When the patient successfully demonstrated consistency in recruiting these muscles, which was observed by a flattening of the rib flares during the active contractions of the intercostals and obliques, he was instructed to carry over the training independently with higher level postures.

To improve recruitment of thoracic paraspinal muscles, rather than primarily lumbar extensors (to decrease kyphotic forces), Jonathan was instructed in (1) full upper extremity swings in standing during soccer warm-up routine, (2) coordinating slow inhalation with shoulder abduction and scapular adduction, and (3) coordinating eccentric exhalation (counting out loud) when he returned his arms down to his side. He was instructed to focus on recruiting diaphragm and inter-costal muscles during inhalation (which should recruit more thoracic extensors) and to concentrate on controlling the eccentric component of the arm and trunk muscles during exhalation.

Neuromuscular Outcomes

Jonathan now demonstrated an effective balance between the primary respiratory muscles (diaphragm, intercostals, and abdominals) during volitional and spontaneous breathing in both quiet breathing and maximal inspiratory maneuvers in multiple postures and activities. Paradoxical movement of the chest wall was no longer noted (improved functional strength of intercostal muscles). No functional thoracic kyphosis was noted during quiet stance or during active recruitment of trunk extensors. Quiet breathing now demonstrated a normal recruitment pattern: (1) initiation of inhalation with the diaphragm and simultaneous chest wall movement, (2) easy inspiratory onset, no apparent effort (low work of breathing, low negative inspiratory force which reduces pectus forces), and (3) smooth continuous movements throughout the inspiratory cycle. Objectively, this was seen with (1) significant increases in mid chest wall excursion measurements (intercostal recruitment) during quiet breathing (tidal volume) in both supine and standing (Table 28-9), (2) a respiratory rate that decreased from 20 to 11 breaths/minute, and (3) phonation support in syllables/breath that increased by 28% (see Table 28-8). Midtrunk stabilization showed marked improvement in strength of oblique abdominal muscles, right still stronger than left. Posturally, this was noted by the elimination of his rib flares and appropriate timing recruitment of the abdominals during trunk stabilization activities both in therapy and as reported by the patient during sports activities. Functionally, the patient reported that he could now run the mile at school without excessive dyspnea or asthmatic symptoms.

Jonathan needed maximal sensory and motor input to change his motor plans for respiration. Verbal cues alone did not produce satisfactory results. Manual, visual, auditory, and positional input in each activity was specifically applied to assist Jonathan in developing new motor plans to improve breathing efficiency and appropriate skeletal forces that promoted normal development of his rib cage and spine.

TABLE 28-9   Chest Wall Excursion (CWE) in Sitting and Supine Positions

TIDAL VOLUME SITTING (QUIET SPONTANEOUS BREATHING)	INITIAL DATE	DISCHARGE DATE 11 MONTHS LATER	REEXAMINATION 4 YEARS AFTER DISCHARGE
Upper chest (level of 3rd rib) upper accessory muscles	$1/2''$	$1/2''$	—
Mid chest (level of xiphoid) intercostals	$1/4''$	$3/8''$	—
Lower chest (half the distance from xiphoid process to naval) lower intercostals and diaphragm	$1/8''$	$3/8''$	—

TIDAL VOLUME SUPINE (QUIET SPONTANEOUS BREATHING)	INITIAL DATE	DISCHARGE DATE 11 MONTHS LATER	REEXAMINATION 4 YEARS AFTER DISCHARGE
Upper chest (Level of 3rd rib) upper accessory muscles	$1/8''$	$1/2''$	$1/16''$
Mid chest (level of xiphoid) intercostals	$0''$	$1/4''$	$0''$
Lower chest (half the distance from xiphoid process to naval) lower intercostals and diaphragm	$3/8$-$1/2''$	$5/8''$	$3/4''$

Note that, in sitting, improvements were noted in mid and lower chest expansion. No 4-year follow-up measurements.
In supine, all levels increased by discharge, but at the 4-year follow-up examination, the gains in the mid and upper chest had disappeared. Only the lower chest expansion continued to show similar levels to the discharge values.

Integumentary Interventions

No interventions.

FUNCTIONAL OUTCOMES AND QUALITY OF LIFE ISSUES

Following his physical therapy program, Jonathan and his mother noted important functional improvements (Table 28-10). He made the travel soccer team and could play four consecutive games without EIA attacks. His last EIA episode occurred 2 months after starting physical therapy. Prior to physical therapy, he had an EIA episode almost every time he played soccer. At discharge, he could also run the mile in gym class at school without EIA or excessive dyspnea.

He did not miss any days of school for EIA after initiating physical therapy. His mother said that before the physical therapy program, "he would miss 5 to 8 days a year due to sickness related to EIA, but those sick days don't take into account the weekends, holidays, and summer days that Jonathan was incapacitated with asthma-related problems." He had two severe EIA episodes prior to physical therapy that resulted in emergency room (ER) visits. During his physical therapy interval, he did not have any ER visits.

His mother said that in addition to making it possible for him to rejoin his classmates in regular physical activity such as soccer and baseball, following the year of physical therapy, Jonathan began to go swimming again. He had all but given up swimming the year before because of "his deformed chest" and the derogatory comments that were directed at him by other children.

When asked for a general statement about how the physical therapy program affected her son's quality of life, Jonathan's mom said: "It was a miracle. Before we began to see you, Jonathan and I had to focus on his medical condition rather than focusing on being a kid. It completely changed his life." Jonathan and his mother no longer saw him as "disabled" by his pulmonary disease.

DISCUSSION

Jonathan was seen for eight visits over 11 months. The family's motivation to follow through diligently on home programs, and the child's excellent ability to learn new motor strategies, resulted in a minimal number of visits to accomplish the goals of treatment. Under different circumstances, achieving the intervention goals in a similar case may take longer or goals may be less attainable.

TABLE 28-10 Functional Outcomes

FUNCTIONAL OUTCOMES	INITIAL DATE	DISCHARGE DATE 11 MONTHS LATER	REEXAMINATION 4 YEARS AFTER DISCHARGE
EIA attacks or symptoms during sports activities	Frequent	None	None
Length of participation in a sporting activity	5 to 10 minutes before EIA symptoms forced him to stop	Full participation: up to four soccer games per day	Full participation: plays baseball in high school
Complete the "mile test" in gym class	No	Yes	Yes
Average number of days absent from school due to asthma-related complications	5 to 8	0	0
Emergency room visits	2	0	1
Hospitalizations	0	0	0
Daily asthma medications	Yes	No	No

Note that Jonathan's greatest improvements are in activity and health gains.

The results of this particular case were marked, but not unrepeatable. Jonathan's physical therapy program was developed from a multisystem and multidiscipline perspective to develop better "external support" for his "internal" asthma. I believe the keys to his success were threefold:

1. A team approach to his condition: recognition by his pulmonologist that his functional limitations were more severe than his medical condition alone indicated, her belief that physical interventions are an integral part of effective management of pulmonary diseases, and her belief that a surgical intervention for his pectus should be the last, not his first, option.

2. A detailed physical therapy examination that focused on identifying the underlying impairments outside of his "asthma and the pectus diagnoses alone," examining both medical and physical impairments to determine which system(s) could account for the severity of his functional limitations.

3. A specific intervention program targeted to reverse or minimize those impairments with a major emphasis on the patient's responsibility in the program (education), and on applying new strategies directly into his daily life (functional).

Although it is possible that his changes were due to maturation, it is unlikely according to his mother, who noted that all of his improvements came after the initiation of physical therapy compared to the previous school year without physical therapy.

Jonathan had a complete remission of his pulmonary symptoms following physical therapy, which was not anticipated by this author or his pulmonologist. Physical therapy does not "cure" asthma. Could it be that the EIA diagnosis was not completely accurate? Jonathan had all the symptoms of EIA, but his pulmonary function tests did not confirm the diagnosis. Recently, doctors have begun to explore other possible explanations for EIA symptoms that do not fit the classic picture of asthma, such as vocal fold dysfunction or supraesophageal manifestations of GERD, which present with similar symptoms: high sensitivity to fast inspiratory flow rates, a lack of typical asthmatic responses on pulmonary function tests, and a lack of significant improvement with asthma medications (Wood et al., 1986; Elshami & Tino, 1996; Pierce & Worsnop, 1999; Chandra et al., 2004; Malagelada, 2004; Ay et al., 2004). Because of Jonathan's dramatic improvement with physical interventions, his pulmonologist is now reconsidering his original diagnosis.

The tests and measures used in this case have varied levels of reliability and validity. The medical tests, such as pulmonary function tests and respiratory rates, have long-established reliability and validity (Leiner et al., 1963; Cherniack & Cherniack, 1983). Tests for the physical impairments are not as well established. Tests for phonation length were established in the speech therapy field (Deem & Miller, 2000). Tests for CWE were recently shown to have inter- and intratester reliability, but normative standards for quiet breathing and maximal effort are just beginning to be established (Massery et al., 1997; LaPier et al., 2000). Lateral trunk flexion and the pectus volume measurement have not been validated by research.

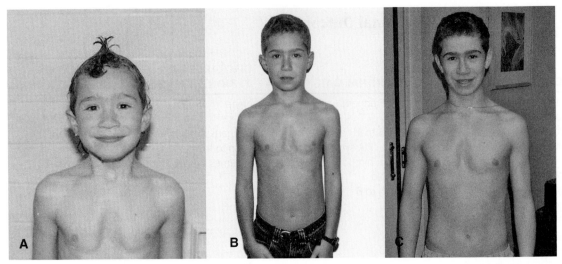

• **Figure 28-4** Comparison of pectus excavatum and postural alignments. **A**, Jonathan at 6 years old. **B**, Jonathan at 10 years old. **C**, Jonathan at 14 years old. By 14, Jonathan's pectus has become narrower and more localized. Shoulders are less protracted, resulting in a more neutral resting position. His trapezius is less elevated, and although there is no rib flare noted in either standing posture, adequate abdominal stability is more apparent at age 14.

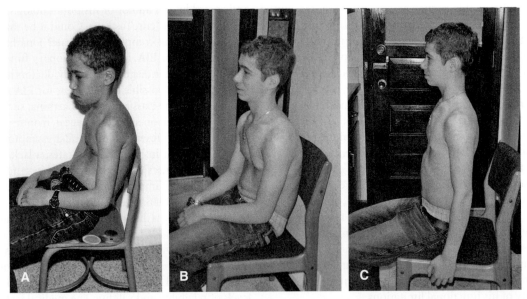

• **Figure 28-5** Comparison of sitting postures. **A**, Typical sitting posture in school per his mother: age 9 and younger. This is a reenactment picture taken at age 10. Jonathan was too embarrassed to have his picture taken of his "deformed chest" when he was initially evaluated at age 9. Note slouched posture (functional kyphosis) with midtrunk fold, pectus, elevated sternal angle. By age 10, patient no longer regularly postured himself like this in sitting. **B**, Jonathan at 14 years old. When asked to slouch in sitting, the midtrunk fold and kyphosis are barely noticeable. Prominent sternal angle is still noticeable. **C**, Straight sitting posture at age 14 years old. Note normal back posture. Mild pectus and mild rib flare still present at base of sternum.

FOUR-YEAR FOLLOW-UP AT AGE 14 YEARS

Jonathan participated in physical therapy for 1 year. Four years after discharge (5 years after initiating physical therapy), Jonathan was contacted, interviewed, and re-examined to assess the long-term effects of this program on his pathology (asthma), his impairments, activity limitations, and participation. Jonathan was 14 years old and a freshman in high school (Figs. 28-4 to 28-6).

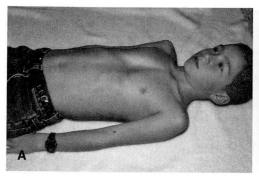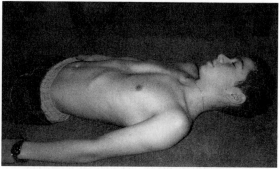

⬩ **Figure 28-6**   Comparison of supine postures. **A,** Discharge picture at age 10. Pectus was reduced almost in half from 34 to 18 mL H_2O displacement measurement during the 11 months of physical therapy. Lower rib flares functionally integrated with abdominal muscles. Neck muscles more elongated. Slight shoulder protraction still noted. **B,** Four years later at age 14. Pectus slightly deeper, but narrower (volume unchanged from discharge at 17 mL). Rib flares more prominent than at discharge. Patient stated that he stopped doing his trunk exercises about 4 months after discharge because he was doing so well. Neck muscles more elongated. Shoulders less protracted.

Medical Update

An examination by his pulmonologist showed no limitations noted in PFT volumes or flow rates. He was also reevaluated by his cardiologist who diagnosed an asymptomatic mitral valve prolapse, which is not uncommon with a pectus excavatum (Fonkalsrud, 2003). No treatment was needed. He had had only one respiratory episode in the last 5 years: a croup-type virus that resulted in a severe bronchitis and his only trip to the ER. He did not have any EIA episode during the 4-year interval. He did not use daily asthma medication. He did, however, report use of his bronchodilator prophylactically when he had a cold "just in case."

Test and Measures

See Tables 28-7 through 28-9 for results of tests.

Functional Outcomes and Quality of Life Update

See Table 28-10 for Jonathan's functional outcomes.

Jonathan received a "perfect attendance award" in eighth grade, which his mother commented was a complete reversal of his school years prior to physical therapy. Endurance is no longer a limitation according to both Jonathan and his mother.

Jonathan's mother reported that he continues to gain confidence both socially and athletically following the physical therapy intervention. She no longer sees any signs of self-consciousness regarding his chest wall deformity. This may be a result of maturation, but she thought it was worth noting because it changed so significantly during and following the intervention period.

Even with 4 to 5 years' reflection since the onset of physical therapy, Jonathan's mother still says that the physical, medical and emotional benefits to her son were incredible. She said that they kept up the home exercises for approximately 4 months after his discharge from physical therapy, but slowly drifted away from them, which may explain some of the minor loss of chest wall mobility upon reevaluation. Jonathan did keep using the strategies that he learned in physical therapy such as maintaining adequate hydration levels and proper warm up before exercise.

Impression

Jonathan has maintained his pulmonary health since discharge 4 years ago with no apparent signs of EIA or its impairments, especially as it affected his endurance and participation in activities and his overall health. At this point, it appears that his asthma or other undiagnosed pulmonary disease is resolved or benign. His spinal alignment is now completely normal, avoiding what appeared to be the likely development of a true thoracic kyphosis. His chest wall deformities are still present but more localized, less noticeable, and do not cause any activity limitations. Recent medical tests also show that his chest wall deformities do not have any measurable impact on his cardiac or pulmonary function. His remarkable gains in individual rib cage mobility from the initial visit to discharge (lateral side bending test) have been nearly retained. Jonathan and his mother stated that they wished they had continued with periodic physical therapy rechecks to maintain all the gains he made during that first year.

I believe Jonathan's physical therapy program worked so well because it was tailored to address his specific EIA pattern and chest wall deformities from a multisystem perspective and included educational, medical, psychologic, and physical perspectives. Interventions by physical therapists can have a tremendous positive impact on the impairments, activity limitations, and resultant disabilities that occur as a result of a primary pulmonary pathology, especially in a maturing system. If the patient cannot breathe efficiently and effectively, then that patient cannot function at his or her highest level. The concepts presented here for Jonathan can certainly be adapted to infants and toddlers as well as older children. The key is to develop a program that keeps the patient, his family, and his resources in mind while developing a targeted intervention strategy.

Following the reevaluation, Jonathan's home program was updated and reinitiated with an emphasis on maintaining his musculoskeletal alignment and trunk control. I recommended quarterly check-ups throughout puberty to modify the program as necessary.

SUMMARY

This chapter presented the pathophysiology and current medical management strategies associated with childhood asthma. In addition, through the use of a single case, ideas for the physical therapy diagnosis and management of physical limitations associated with asthma and its resultant functional limitations were presented through a multisystem and multidiscipline perspective. Impairments in the cardiopulmonary, neuromuscular, musculoskeletal, integumentary, and gastrointestinal systems were assessed for their contribution to the activity and participation limitations that could not be fully explained by asthma alone. An individualized physical therapy program was then presented as a template for other pediatric physical therapy programs. Short-term and long-term results from the physical therapy interventions used with this single case were presented to give the reader an indication of the potential success of such interventions. Obviously, each individual case is unique and must be developed within the context of that particular patient's situation.

REFERENCES

Abrams, SA. Chronic pulmonary insufficiency in children and its effects on growth and development. Journal of Nutrition, *131*(3): 938S–941S, 2001.

Aliverti, A, & Dellaca, R. Compartmental analysis of breathing in the supine and prone positions by optoelectronic plethysmography. Annals of Biomedical Engineering, *29*(1):60–70, 2001.

Allen, DB. Safety of inhaled corticosteroids in children. Pediatric Pulmonology, *33*(3):208–220, 2002.

American Physical Therapy Association. Guide to Physical Therapist Practice, 2nd ed. Physical Therapy, *81*(1):744, 2001.

Anderson, SD, & Holzer, K. Exercise-induced asthma: Is it the right diagnosis in elite athletes? Journal of Allergy & Clinical Immunology, *106*(3):419–428, 2000.

Andrianopoulos, MV, Gallivan, GJ, et al. PVCM, PVCD, EPL, and irritable larynx syndrome: What are we talking about and how do we treat it? Journal of Voice, *14*(4):607–618, 2000.

Apter, AJ, & Szefler, SJ. Advances in adult and pediatric asthma. Journal of Allergy & Clinical Immunology, *113*(3):407–414, 2004.

Ay, M, Sivasli, E et al. Association of asthma with gastroesophageal reflux disease in children. Journal of the Chinese Medical Association, *67*:63–66, 2004.

Bach, JR & Bianchi, C. Prevention of pectus excavatum for children with spinal muscular atrophy type I. American Journal of Physical Medicine & Rehabilitation, *82*:815–819, 2003.

Baker, KM, Brand, DA, et al. Classifying asthma: Disagreement among specialists (see comment). Chest, *124*(6): 2156–2163, 2003.

Baum, WF, Schneyer, U, et al. Delay of growth and development in children with bronchial asthma, atopic dermatitis and allergic rhinitis. Experimental & Clinical Endocrinology & Diabetes, *110*(2):53–59, 2002.

Berhane, K, McConnell, R, et al. Sex-specific effects of asthma on pulmonary function in children. American Journal of Respiratory & Critical Care Medicine, *162*(5):1723–1730, 2000.

Bing'ol Karako, C, Yilmaz, M, et al. The effects of daily pulmonary rehabilitation program at home on childhood asthma. Allergologia et Immunopathologia, *28*(1):12–14, 2000.

Birkisson, IF, Halapi, E, et al. Genetic approaches to assessing evidence for a T helper type 1 cytokine defect in adult asthma. American Journal of Respiratory & Critical Care Medicine, *169*(9):1007–1013, 2004.

Braback, L, & Kalvesten, L. Asthma in schoolchildren. Factors influencing morbidity in a Swedish survey. Acta Paediatrica Scandinavica, *77*(6):826–830, 1988.

Braganza, S, Sharif, I, et al. Documenting asthma severity: Do we get it right? Journal of Asthma, *40*(6):661–665, 2003.

Bruce, J. Review: Parental tobacco smoke increases the risk of asthma and respiratory symptoms in school age children. [Commentary on Cook, DG, & Strachan, DP. Parental smoking and prevalence of respiratory symptoms and asthma in school age children. Thorax, *52*:1081–1094, 1997.] Evidence-Based Nursing, *1*(3):86, 1998.

Cala, SJ. Abdominal compliance, parasternal activation, and chest wall motion. Journal of Applied Physiology, *74*(3):1398–1405, 1993.

Cambach, W, Wagenaar, RC, et al. The long-term effects of pulmonary rehabilitation in patients with asthma and chronic obstructive pulmonary disease: A research synthesis. Archives of Physical Medicine & Rehabilitation, *80*(1):103–111, 1999.

CDC. Surveillance for Asthma — United States, 1960–1995. Atlanta: CDC, 1998.

CDC. Surveillance for Asthma — United States, 1980–1999. Atlanta: CDC, 2002.

CDC. Asthma Fast Facts. Atlanta: Center for Disease Control, National Center for Health Statistics, 2004.

Chandra, A, Moazzez, R, et al. A review of the atypical manifestations of gastroesophageal reflux disease. International Journal of Clinical Practice, *58*(1):41–48, 2004.

Cherniack, RM, & Cherniack, L. Respiration in Health and Disease, 3rd ed. Philadelphia: WB Saunders, 1983.

Chryssanthopoulos, C, Maksud, MG, et al. Cardiopulmonary responses of asthmatic children to strenuous exercise. Effect of theophylline. Clinical Pediatrics, 23(7):384–388, 1984.

Chye, JK, & Gray, PH. Rehospitalization and growth of infants with bronchopulmonary dysplasia: A matched control study. Journal of Paediatrics & Child Health, 31(2):105–111, 1995.

Cole, P. Pathophysiology and treatment of airway mucociliary clearance. A moving tale. Minerva Anestesiologica, 67(4):206–209, 2001.

Cooper, S, Oborne, J, et al. Effect of two breathing exercises (Buteyko and pranayama) in asthma: A randomised controlled trial (see comment). Thorax, 58(8):674–679, 2003.

Cserhati, E, Mezei, G, et al. The prognosis of severe bronchial asthma in childhood on the basis of late reexaminations. Acta Paediatrica Academiae Scientiarum Hungaricae, 23(4):473–482, 1982.

Cserhati, EF, Gregesi, KA, et al. Thorax deformity and asthma bronchial. Allergologia et Immunopathologia, 12(1):7–10, 1984.

D'Ambrosio, CM, & Mohsenin, V. Sleep in asthma. Clinics in Chest Medicine, 19(1):127–137, 1998.

de Benedictis, FM, Canny, GJ, et al. The progressive nature of childhood asthma. Lung, 168(Suppl):278–285, 1990.

Dean, E, & Hobson, L. Cardiopulmonary Anatomy. Principles and Practice of Cardiopulmonary Physical Therapy, 3rd ed. St. Louis: Mosby-YearBook, 1996, pp. 23–51.

Decramer, M, Kelly, S, et al. Respiratory and postural changes in intercostal muscle length in supine dogs. Journal of Applied Physiology, 60(5):1686–1691, 1986.

Deem, JF, & Miller, L. Manual of Voice Therapy, 2nd ed. Austin: PRO-ED, Inc., 2000.

Doyle, LW, Cheung, MM, et al. Birth weight <1501 g and respiratory health at age 14. Archives of Diseases in Childhood, 84(1):40–44, 2001.

Eid, NS. Gastroesophageal reflux is a major cause of lung disease-pro. Pediatric Pulmonology Supplement, 26:194–196, 2004.

Eid, NS, & Morton, RL. Rational approach to the wheezy infant. Paediatric Respiratory Reviews, 5(Suppl A):S77–S79, 2004.

Elshami, AA, & Tino, G. Coexistent asthma and functional upper airway obstruction. Case reports and review of the literature. Chest, 110(5):1358–1361, 1996.

Emtner, M. Physiotherapy and intensive physical training in rehabilitation of adults with asthma. Physical Therapy Reviews, 4(4):229–240, 1999.

Estenne, M, Derom, E, et al. Neck and abdominal muscle activity in patients with severe thoracic scoliosis. American Journal of Respiratory & Critical Care Medicine, 158(2):452–457, 1998.

Evans, M, Palta, M, et al. Associations between family history of asthma, bronchopulmonary dysplasia, and childhood asthma in very low birth weight children. American Journal of Epidemiology, 148(5):460–466, 1998.

Fireman, P. Otitis media and its relationship to allergy. Pediatric Clinics of North America, 35(5):1075–1090, 1988.

Fonkalsrud, EW. Current management of pectus excavatum. World Journal of Surgery, 27(5):502–508, 2003.

Fonkalsrud, EW, Dunn, JC, et al. Repair of pectus excavatum deformities: 30 years of experience with 375 patients. Annals of Surgery, 231(3):443–448, 2000.

Frischer, T, Kuehr, J, et al. Risk factors for childhood asthma and recurrent wheezy bronchitis. European Journal of Pediatrics, 152(9):771–775, 1003.

Frownfelter, D, & Dean, E. Principles and Practice of Cardiopulmonary Physical Therapy. St. Louis: Mosby-YearBook, 1996.

Gandevia, SC, Butler, JE, et al. Balancing acts: Respiratory sensations, motor control and human posture. Clinical & Experimental Pharmacology & Physiology, 29(1–2):118–121, 2002.

Gern, JE. Viral respiratory infection and the link to asthma. Pediatric Infectious Disease Journal, 23(1 Suppl):S78–S86, 2004.

Gyorik, SA, & Brutsche, MH. Complementary and alternative medicine for bronchial asthma: Is there new evidence? Current Opinion in Pulmonary Medicine, 10(1):37–43, 2004.

Han, JN, Gayan-Ramirez, GG, et al.. Respiratory function of the rib cage muscles. European Respiratory Journal, 6:722–728, 1993.

Hansen, EF, Vestbo, J, et al. Peak flow as predictor of overall mortality in asthma and chronic obstructive pulmonary disease. American Journal of Respiratory & Critical Care Medicine, 163(3 Pt 1):690–693, 2001.

Harik-Khan, RI, Muller, DC, et al. Serum vitamin levels and the risk of asthma in children. American Journal of Epidemiology, 159(4):351–357, 2004.

Hartert, TV, & Peebles, RS, Jr. Epidemiology of asthma: The year in review. Current Opinion in Pulmonary Medicine, 6(1):4–9, 2000.

Hayes, JP, Nolan, MT, et al. Three cases of paradoxical vocal cord adduction followed up over a 10-year period. Chest, 104(3):678–680, 1993.

Hebra, A. Pectus excavatum. e-Medicine, accessed at http://www.emedicine.com/ped/topic2558.htm., 2004.

Hessel, PA, Sliwkanich, T, et al. Asthma and limitation of activities in Fort Saskatchewan, Alberta (see comment). Canadian Journal of Public Health (Revue Canadienne de Sante Publique), 87(6):397–400, 1996.

Hixon, TJ. Respiratory Function in Speech and Song. San Diego, CA: Singular Publishing Group, 1991.

Hodges, PW, & Gandevia, SC. Activation of the human diaphragm during a repetitive postural task. Journal of Physiology, 522(Pt 1):165–175, 2000.

Hodges, PW, & Gandevia, SC. Changes in intra-abdominal pressure during postural and respiratory activation of the human diaphragm. Journal of Applied Physiology, 89(3):967–976, 2000.

Hodges, PW, Heijnen, I, et al. Postural activity of the diaphragm is reduced in humans when respiratory demand increases. Journal of Physiology, 537(Pt 3):999–1008, 2001.

Holloway, E, & Ram, FSF. Breathing Exercises for Asthma. Oxford: The Cochrane Library, 2001.

Houtmeyers, E, Gosselink, R, et al. Regulation of mucociliary clearance in health and disease. European Respiratory Journal, 13(5):1177–1188, 1999.

Imam, AP, & Halpern, GM. Pseudoasthma in a case of asthma. Allergologia et Immunopathologia, 23(2):96–100, 1995.

Johnson, G. Functional Orthopedics I. Chicago: The Institute of Physical Art, 1989.

Joseph-Bowen, J, de Klerk, NH, et al. Lung function, bronchial responsiveness, and asthma in a community cohort of 6-year-old children. American Journal of Respiratory & Critical Care Medicine, 169(7):850–854, 2004.

Kaiser, HB. Risk factors in allergy/asthma. Allergy & Asthma Proceedings, 25(1):7–10, 2004.

Kelly, WJ, Hudson, I, et al. Childhood asthma and adult lung function. American Review of Respiratory Disease, 138(1):26–30, 1988.

Kennedy, JD. Lung function outcome in children of premature birth. Journal of Paediatrics & Child Health, 35(6):516–521, 1999.

Knott, M, & Voss, D. Proprioceptive Neuromuscular Facilitation. New York: Harper & Row, 1968.

Koumbourlis, AC, Motoyama, EK, et al. Longitudinal follow-up of lung function from childhood to adolescence in prematurely born patients with neonatal chronic lung disease. Pediatric Pulmonology, *21*(1):28–34, 1996.

Kraft, M, Pak, J, et al. Distal lung dysfunction at night in nocturnal asthma. American Journal of Respiratory Critical Care Medicine, *163*(7):1551–1556, 2001.

Krishnamoorthy, M, Mintz, A, et al. Diagnosis and treatment of respiratory symptoms of initially unsuspected gastroesophageal reflux in infants. American Surgeon, *60*(10):783–785, 1994.

Kurashima, K, Ogawa, H, et al. Thromboxane A2 synthetase inhibitor (OXY-046) improves abnormal mucociliary transport in asthmatic patients. Annals of Allergy, *68*:53–56, 1992.

Kussin, PS, & Fulkerson, WJ. The rising tide of asthma. Trends in the epidemiology of morbidity and mortality from asthma. Respiratory Care Clinics of North America, *1*(2):163–175, 1995.

Kuyper, LM, Pare, PD, et al. Characterization of airway plugging in fatal asthma (see comment). American Journal of Medicine, *115*(1):6–11, 2003.

LaPier, TK. Chest wall expansion values in supine and standing across the adult lifespan. Physical and Occupational Therapy in Geriatrics *21*:65–81, 2002.

LaPier, TK, Cook, A, et al. Intertester and intratester reliability of chest excursion measurement in subjects without impairment. Cardiopulmonary Physical Therapy, *11*(3):94–98, 2000.

Leiner, GC, Abramowitz, S, et al. Expiratory peak flow rate; standard values for normal subjects. American Review of Respiratory Disease, *88*:644–651, 1963.

Leong, JC, Lu, WW, et al. Kinematics of the chest cage and spine during breathing in healthy individuals and in patients with adolescent idiopathic scoliosis. Spine, *24*(13):1310–1315, 1999.

Lissoni, A, Aliverti, A, et al. Kinematic analysis of patients with spinal muscular atrophy during spontaneous breathing and mechanical ventilation. American Journal of Physical Medicine & Rehabilitation *77*:188–192, 1998.

Lozano, P, Fishman, P, et al. Health care utilization and cost among children with asthma who were enrolled in a health maintenance organization. Pediatrics, *99*(6):757–764, 1997.

Malagelada, JR. Review article: supra-oesophageal manifestations of gastro-oesophageal reflux disease. Alimentary Pharmacology & Therapeutics, *19*(Suppl 1):43–48, 2004.

Malo, JL, Lemiere, C, et al. Occupational asthma. Current Opinion in Pulmonary Medicine, *10*(1):57–61, 2004.

Markham, AW, & Wilkinson, JM. Complementary and alternative medicines (CAM) in the management of asthma: An examination of the evidence. Journal of Asthma, *41*(2):131–139, 2004.

Massery, MP. What's positioning got to do with it? Neurology Report, *18*(3):11–14, 1994.

Massery, MP. The patient with neuromuscular or musculoskeletal dysfunction. In Frownfelter, DL, & Dean, E (Eds.). Principles and Practice of Cardiopulmonary Physical Therapy, 3rd ed. St. Louis: Mosby-YearBook, pp. 679–702.

Massery, MP, Dreyer, HE, et al. Chest wall excursion and tidal volume change during passive positioning in cervical spinal cord injury (abstract). Cardiopulmonary Physical Therapy, *8*(4):27, 1997.

Massery, MP, & Frownfelter, DL. Facilitating ventilatory patterns and breathing strategies. In Frownfelter, DL, & Dean, E (Eds.). Principles and Practice of Cardiopulmonary Physical Therapy, 3rd St. Louis: Mosby-YearBook, pp. 383–416.

Massie, J. Exercise-induced asthma in children. Paediatric Drugs, *4*(4):267–278, 2002.

McConnell, AK, & Romer, LM. Dyspnea in health and obstructive pulmonary disease: The role of respiratory muscle function and training. Sports Medicine, *34*(2):117–132, 2004.

McKenzie, DK, & Gandevia, SC. Strength and endurance of inspiratory, expiratory, and limb muscles in asthma. American Review of Respiratory Disease, *134*(5):999–1004, 1986.

Mellinger-Birdsong, AK, Powell, KE, et al. Prevalence and impact of asthma in children, Georgia, 2000. American Journal of Preventive Medicine, *24*(3):242–248, 2003.

Mellon, M, & Parasuraman, B. Pediatric asthma: Improving management to reduce cost of care. Journal of Managed Care Pharmacy, *10*(2):130–141, 2004.

Meza, C, & Gershwin, ME. Why is asthma becoming more of a problem? Current Opinion in Pulmonary Medicine, *3*(1):6–9, 1997.

Milgrom, H, & Taussig, LM. Keeping children with exercise-induced asthma active. Pediatrics, *104*(3):e38, 1999.

Moloney, E, O'Sullivan, S, et al. Airway dehydration: A therapeutic target in asthma? Chest, *121*(6):1806–1811, 2002.

Moloney, ED, Griffin, S, et al. Release of inflammatory mediators from eosinophils following a hyperosmolar stimulus. Respiratory Medicine, *97*(8):928–932, 2003.

Morris, M, & Perkins, P. Asthma. e-Medicine, accessed at http://www.emedicine.com., 2004.

Mossberg, B, Afzelius, BA, et al. On the pathogenesis of obstructive lung disease. A study on the immotile-cilia syndrome. Scandinavian Journal of Respiratory Diseases, *59*(2):55–65, 1978.

National Heart, Lung and Blood Institute. Expert Panel Report 2: Guidelines for the Diagnosis and Management of Asthma. Pub. No. 97-4051. Bethesda, MD: National Institutes of Health, 1997.

Nava, S, Ambrosino, N, et al. Recruitment of some respiratory muscles during three maximal inspiratory manoeuvres. Thorax, *48*(7):702–707, 1993.

NIH. Practical Guide for the Diagnosis and Management of Asthma Based on Expert Panel Report 2. NIH Publication No. 97-4053. Bethesda, MD: National Institutes of Health, National Heart, Lung and Blood Institute, 1997, p. 60.

Openshaw, PJ, Dean, GS, et al. Links between respiratory syncytial virus bronchiolitis and childhood asthma: Clinical and research approaches. Pediatric Infectious Disease Journal, *22*(2 Suppl): S58–S64; discussion S64–S65, 2003.

O'Riordan, TG. Optimizing delivery of inhaled corticosteroids: Matching drugs with devices. Journal of Aerosol Medicine, *15*(3):245–250, 2002.

Papiris, S, Kotanidou, A, et al. Clinical review: Severe asthma. Critical Care (London), *6*(1):30–44, 2002.

Patterson, PE, & Harding, SM. Gastroesophageal reflux disorders and asthma. Current Opinion in Pulmonary Medicine, *5*(1):63–67, 1999.

Physicians' Desk Reference. Montvale, NJ: Medical Economics Company, 2001.

Pianosi, PT, & Fisk, M. High frequency ventilation trial. Nine year follow up of lung function. Early Human Development, *57*(3):225–234, 2000.

Pierce, RJ, & Worsnop, CJ. Upper airway function and dysfunction in respiration. Clinical & Experimental Pharmacology & Physiology, *26*(1):1–10, 1999.

Powell, CV, Kelly, AM, et al. Lack of agreement in classification of the severity of acute asthma between emergency physician assessment and classification using the National Asthma Council Australia guidelines (1998). Emergency Medicine (Fremantle, WA), *15*(1):49–53, 2003.

Primiano, FP, Jr. Theoretical analysis of chest wall mechanics. Journal of Biomechanics, *15*(12):919–931, 1982.

Ram, FS, Robinson, SM, et al. Effects of physical training in asthma: A systematic review. British Journal of Sports Medicine, *34*(3):162–167, 2000.

Ram, FS, Wellington, SR, et al. Inspiratory muscle training for asthma. Cochrane Database of Systematic Reviews, 4:CD003792, 2003.

Ramazanoglu, YM, & Kraemer, R. Cardiorespiratory response to physical conditioning in children with bronchial asthma. Pediatric Pulmonology, 1(5):272–277, 1985.

Rimmer, KP, Ford, GT, et al. Interaction between postural and respiratory control of human intercostal muscles. Journal of Applied Physiology, 79(5):1556–1561, 1995.

Roger, G, Denoyelle, F, et al. Dysfonction laryngee episodique. Archives de Pediatrie, 8(Suppl 3):650–654, 2001.

Roux, C, Kolta, S, et al. Long-term safety of fluticasone propionate and nedocromil sodium on bone in children with asthma. Pediatrics, 111(6 Pt 1):e706–713, 2003.

Saumarez, RC. An analysis of action of intercostal muscles in human upper rib cage. Journal of Applied Physiology, 60(2):690–701, 1986.

Schaubel, D, Johansen, H, et al. Neonatal characteristics as risk factors for preschool asthma. Journal of Asthma, 33(4):255–264, 1996.

Silvestri, M, Sabatini, F, et al. The wheezy infant — Immunological and molecular considerations. Paediatric Respiratory Reviews, 5(Suppl A):S81–S87, 2004.

Sly, RM. History of exercise-induced asthma. Medicine & Science in Sports & Exercise, 18(3):314–317, 1986.

Sontag, SJ, O'Connell, S, et al. Asthmatics with gastroesophageal reflux: Long term results of a randomized trial of medical and surgical antireflux therapies. American Journal of Gastroenterology, 98(5):987–999, 2003.

Steurer-Stey, C, Russi, EW, et al. Complementary and alternative medicine in asthma: Do they work? (see comment). Swiss Medical Weekly, 132(25–26):338–344, 2002.

Strachan, DP, & Cook, DG. Health effects of passive smoking. 6. Parental smoking and childhood asthma: Longitudinal and case-control studies. Thorax, 53(3):204–212, 1998.

Sullivan, PE, Markos, PD, et al. An Integrated Approach to Therapeutic Exercise: Theory and Clinical Application. Reston, VA: Reston Publishing Co., 1982.

Sunyer, J, Anto, JM, et al. Generational increase of self-reported first attack of asthma in fifteen industrialized countries. European Community Respiratory Health Study (ECRHS). European Respiratory Journal, 14(4):885–891, 1999.

Taggart, VS, & Fulwood, R. Youth health report card: Asthma. Preventive Medicine, 22(4):579–584, 1993.

Tecklin, JS. Pediatric Physical Therapy, 2nd ed. Philadelphia: JB Lippincott, 1994.

Temprado, JJ, Milliex, L, et al. A dynamic pattern analysis of coordination between breathing and rhythmic arm movements in humans. Neuroscience Letters, 329(3):314–318, 2002.

Townsend, M, Feeny, DH, et al. Evaluation of the burden of illness for pediatric asthmatic patients and their parents. Annals of Allergy, 67(4):403–408, 1991.

Turktas, I, Ozkaya, O, et al. Safety of inhaled corticosteroid therapy in young children with asthma. Annals of Allergy, Asthma, & Immunology, 86(6):649–654, 2001.

van Veldhoven, NH, Vermeer, A, et al. Children with asthma and physical exercise: Effects of an exercise programme. Clinical Rehabilitation, 15(4):360–370, 2001.

von Mutius, E, Nicolai, T, et al. Prematurity as a risk factor for asthma in preadolescent children. Journal of Pediatrics, 123(2):223–229, 1993.

Voy, RO. The U.S. Olympic Committee experience with exercise-induced bronchospasm, 1984. Medicine & Science in Sports & Exercise, 18(3):328–330, 1986.

Wagner, CW. Pathophysiology and diagnosis of asthma. Nursing Clinics of North America, 38(4):561–570, 2003.

Weiner, P, Magadle, R, et al. The relationship among inspiratory muscle strength, the perception of dyspnea and inhaled beta$_2$-agonist use in patients with asthma. Canadian Respiratory Journal, 9(5):307–312, 2002.

Wilson, TA, Angelillo, M, et al. Muscle kinematics for minimal work of breathing. Journal of Applied Physiology, 87(2):554–560, 1999.

Wilson, TA, Legrand, A, et al. Respiratory effects of the external and internal intercostal muscles in humans. Journal of Physiology, 530 (Pt 2):319–330, 2001.

Wolfson, MR, Greenspan, JS, et al. Effect of position on the mechanical interaction between the rib cage and abdomen in preterm infants. Journal of Applied Physiology, 72(3):1032–1038, 1992.

Wong, CA, Subakumar, G, et al. Effects of asthma and asthma therapies on bone mineral density. Current Opinion in Pulmonary Medicine, 8(1):39–44, 2002.

Wood, RP, 2nd, Jafek, BW, et al. Laryngeal dysfunction and pulmonary disorder. Otolaryngology Head & Neck Surgery, 94(3):374–378, 1986.

Zmirou, D, Gauvin, S, et al. Traffic related air pollution and incidence of childhood asthma: results of the Vesta case-control study. Journal of Epidemiology & Community Health, 58(1):18–23, 2004.

Chapter 29

THORACIC SURGERY

BETSY A. HOWELL
PT, MS

PATRICIA REYNOLDS HILL
PT, MA

Approximately 6 to 10 in 1000 children are born each year with moderate and severe forms of congenital heart defects (Hoffman, 2002). Early detection, often prenatal, and improved medical and surgical management combine with the type of defect and the individual child to determine the impact. For example, two children, each diagnosed with a ventricular septal defect, may have entirely different histories. One child may go undiagnosed for several years, whereas the other child may require surgery in infancy. As technologic advances are incorporated into patient care, the diagnosis of congenital heart defect during fetal development is occurring with increasing regularity. Formerly, most congenital heart defects were repaired when the child was at least 1 year old, often older. More of these surgeries are now being performed during the first days and months of life, which is likely to affect how children with congenital heart defects grow and develop. The likelihood of treating a child who has previously had open-heart surgery is greater now that more children survive open-heart surgery.

Physical therapists examining this population should closely monitor and document the nature and extent of developmental differences that may result from earlier surgical repair, as well as potential neurologic deficits possibly secondary to deep hypothermic circulatory arrest. To prepare therapists for this task, this chapter describes congenital heart defects; surgical repairs, including heart and heart-lung transplantation; acute and chronic physical impairments secondary to heart defects and surgery; profound cyanosis or neurologic complications; and physical therapy intervention for the population of children with cardiac defects.

CONGENITAL HEART DEFECTS

Although embryologists can identify at what point during fetal development certain defects occur, and what risk factors may contribute to their development, the cause of congenital heart defects remains unknown. The presence of more than one child with congenital heart defect in the same family or in the family history suggests a possible genetic component. Approximately 10% of children with congenital heart defects also have other physical malformations (Noonan, 1981). Heart defects may be associated with Down syndrome, Turner syndrome, Williams syndrome, Marfan syndrome, Costello syndrome, DiGeorge syndrome, and the VATER association. Infants of diabetic mothers also have an increased incidence of congenital heart disease (Clarke et al., 1991).

Diagnosis of cardiac problems may occur during prenatal life or at birth. Some congenital heart defects require immediate attention and others may be followed by further evaluation. Even with improved diagnostic techniques, some infants with severe cyanotic disease are not diagnosed before they are discharged to home, but several weeks later they may be diagnosed with a heart defect when they develop symptoms of septic shock. Other cardiac defects may not be diagnosed until much later, even as late as adolescence. For example, coarctation of the aorta is occasionally diagnosed during a sports physical examination when a large difference between upper and lower extremity blood pressure or an abnormally high upper extremity blood pressure is observed.

The infant with a congenital heart defect often has abnormal respiratory signs, including a labored breathing pattern and an increased respiratory rate. The infant may be diaphoretic and tachycardic. Edema around the eyes and decreased urine output (evidenced by dry diapers) may also be observed. Eating problems result from difficulty in coordinating sucking and swallowing with breathing at an increased rate. Irritability that is difficult to assuage may be noted. These symptoms of congestive heart failure can lead to the diagnosis of a cardiac defect or provide evidence of the worsening of a known defect.

Congenital heart defects are usually classified as acyanotic or cyanotic. In acyanotic lesions, the child is pink and has normal oxygen saturation. If there is mixing or shunting of blood within the heart, the blood shunts from the left side of the heart to the right side, so oxygenated blood goes to the lungs as well as to the body.

Common acyanotic lesions include atrial septal defects, ventricular septal defects, patent ductus arteriosus, coarctation of the aorta, pulmonary stenosis, and aortic stenosis.

In cyanotic defects, blood is typically shunted from the right side of the heart to the left side. Unoxygenated blood is then returned to the body, resulting in arterial oxygen saturation levels 15% to 30% below normal values.

Common cyanotic lesions include tetralogy of Fallot, transposition of the great arteries, tricuspid atresia, pulmonary atresia, truncus arteriosus, total anomalous pulmonary venous return, and hypoplastic left-sided heart syndrome.

Type and timing of intervention depend on the defect and the child's age. Some defects are repaired immediately, whereas others require a staged procedure, with the first several surgeries being palliative rather than corrective. Some acyanotic defects are not repaired until the child is several years old. Less impairment of growth and weight gain, however, occurs when surgery is performed in the first 2 years of life (Rosenthal, 1983; Suoninen, 1971). Concerns regarding neurologic complications following surgery and their impact on long-term functional and cognitive development continue to be examined as an increasing number of infants survive earlier and more complex surgeries (duPlessis, 1997; Limperopoulos et al., 2001). Low-flow cardiopulmonary bypass (Zimmerman et al., 1997) and neurophysiologic monitoring during surgery help to minimize the possibility of neurologic complications (Austin et al., 1997). Acyanotic and cyanotic defects are described in the next two sections and may be compared with normal anatomy of the heart (Fig. 29-1).

ACYANOTIC DEFECTS

ATRIAL SEPTAL DEFECT

Atrial septal defect, one of the most common congenital heart defects, is an abnormal communication between the left and right atria (Fig. 29-2). The defect is classified by its location on the septum. Blood is generally shunted from the left atrium to the right atrium. This defect has traditionally been repaired when a child is between 4 and 6 years old because of slow progression of damage to the heart and lungs. If a child has more severe symptoms, the defect is repaired sooner (Mee, 1991). Some adults with

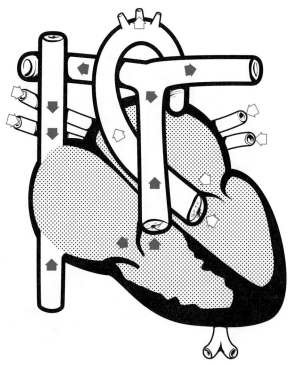

• **Figure 29-1**   Anatomy of the heart.

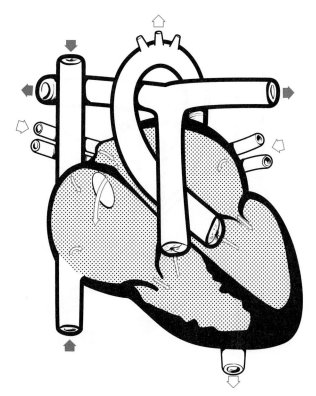

• **Figure 29-2**   Atrial septal defect.

signs of heart failure are found to have a previously undiagnosed atrial septal defect. As medical technology advances, late diagnoses should become rare.

Surgical repair has traditionally been made through a median sternotomy incision; however, a right thoracotomy approach has also been used primarily for cosmetic reasons. Minimal access techniques are being used with increasing frequency and include smaller incisions centered over the xiphoid process. These techniques can also result in shortened length of hospitalization (Ohye & Bove, 2001). The defect is usually sutured together, or a patch closure is used when necessary (Kopf & Laks, 1991). The timing of surgery depends on the age of the child, when the diagnosis is confirmed, and how symptomatic the child is, but it typically occurs during the first 5 years of life. A longitudinal study of patients undergoing closure of an atrial septal defect during childhood showed excellent survival and low morbidity rates (Roos-Hesselink et al., 2003).

VENTRICULAR SEPTAL DEFECT

Ventricular septal defect is the most common congenital heart defect (20%–30% of all children with congenital defects) (Graham et al., 1989). It can be present alone or in association with other defects such as the tetralogy of Fallot and transposition of the great arteries. Ventricular

septal defect alone is discussed here. A ventricular septal defect is a communication between the ventricles that allows blood to be shunted between them, generally from left to right (Fig. 29-3). The increase in blood flow through the right ventricle to the lungs may lead to pulmonary hypertension. In severe cases, in which pulmonary pressures exceed systemic pressures, shunting switches from right to left, which is often termed Eisenmenger syndrome (Graham et al., 1989). A large defect may lead to early left ventricular failure. An infant with a large ventricular septal defect has signs of severe respiratory distress, diaphoresis, and fatigability, especially during feeding, when the infant's endurance is stressed (Giboney, 1983). The infant's weight is dramatically affected in this situation. A child this severely affected has a much earlier surgical repair than a child who is asymptomatic.

Small defects may close spontaneously. Defects that compromise the clinical status of the patient must be surgically closed. The timing of surgery varies, depending on the child's tolerance of the defect. A child with a larger defect undergoes surgery earlier to diminish the negative effects on growth and the pulmonary system.

Surgical intervention is through a mediastinal approach and usually requires a synthetic patch closure (Arciniegas, 1991).

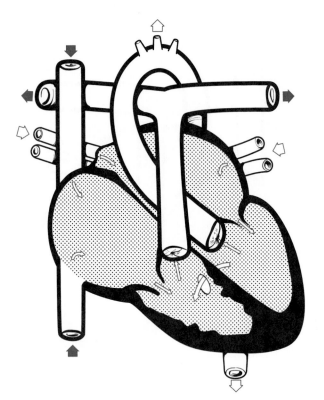

• **Figure 29-3**   Ventricular septal defect.

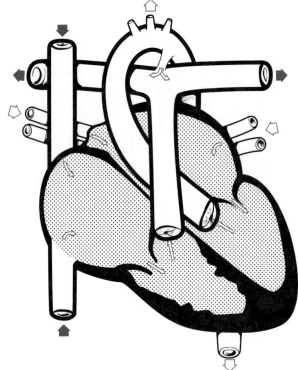

• **Figure 29-4**   Patent ductus arteriosus.

PATENT DUCTUS ARTERIOSUS

The ductus arteriosus is a large vessel that connects the main pulmonary artery to the descending aorta (Fig. 29-4). It usually closes soon after birth but dilates (remains patent) in response to hypoxia or prosta-glandins E_1 and E_2 (Levitsky & del Nido, 1991). The ability to maintain patency of the ductus arteriosus becomes important in certain cyanotic heart defects to be discussed later. The spontaneous closing of the ductus arteriosus can create a critical situation in the infant with an undiagnosed heart defect. A high incidence of patency is found in premature infants because of respiratory distress syndrome and the resulting hypoxia.

Several surgical options are currently available. The traditional left thoracotomy incision is the standard operative approach. Recent advances include video-assisted thoracoscopic surgery, which involves several small thoracostomies and results in no chest wall muscles being cut and no rib retraction (Hines et al., 2003). Another surgical intervention is transcatheter coil occlusion performed by cardiac catheterization, which can be an outpatient procedure. Video-assisted and coil occlusion techniques are less traumatic, can reduce hospital stay (Jacobs et al., 2003), and may also decrease

the risk of scoliosis which is associated with thoracotomy. The ductus is ligated and sutured.

COARCTATION OF THE AORTA

Coarctation of the aorta is defined as a narrowing or closing of a section of the aorta (Fig. 29-5). Patent ductus arteriosus was observed in approximately 23% of diagnosed cases of coarctation of the aorta (Waldhausen et al., 1991). Infants with a severe narrowing may develop left ventricular failure (Girlando et al., 1988). Early repair is necessary when a child is severely symptomatic. The child or adult without symptoms may go undiagnosed until a routine physical examination reveals an abnormally high upper extremity blood pressure.

Surgical intervention is the primary method of treating coarctation of the aorta. Access to the aorta is through a left thoracotomy, after which the aorta is repaired with an end-to-end anastomosis, a subclavian flap, or a patch aortoplasty (Waldhausen et al., 1991).

PULMONARY STENOSIS

Pulmonary stenosis is a narrowing of the right ventri-cular outflow tract and is classified by the location of the narrowing relative to the pulmonary valve. It often occurs

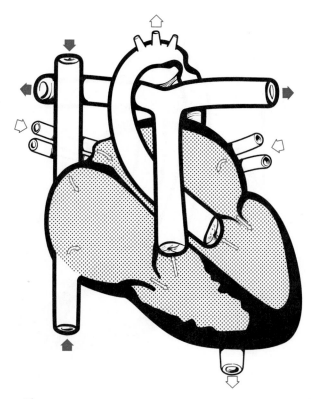

♦ **Figure 29-5**   Coarctation of the aorta.

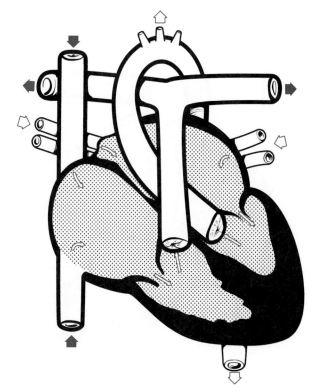

♦ **Figure 29-6**   Aortic stenosis.

in association with other heart defects. Timing of surgery depends on the severity of the narrowing and the degree of functional compromise. Surgery is performed through a median sternotomy; the type of surgical procedure depends on the site of narrowing. A valvotomy may be performed, or in severe cases, the valve may need to be replaced (Moulton & Malm, 1991).

AORTIC STENOSIS

Aortic stenosis is a narrowing of the left ventricular outflow tract and is classified by its relation to the aortic valve (supravalvular, valvular, or subvalvular) (Fig. 29-6). An aortic valvotomy is performed through a median sternotomy in infants and children with severe stenosis. In severe cases, a valve replacement may be necessary if a valvotomy cannot be performed (Weldon et al., 1991).

CYANOTIC DEFECTS

TETRALOGY OF FALLOT

The tetralogy of Fallot is the most common cyanotic cardiac defect, accounting for almost 50% of all cyanotic

lesions. The primary abnormalities that occur in the tetralogy of Fallot are a ventricular septal defect, right ventricular outflow tract obstruction, an aorta that overrides the right ventricle, and hypertrophy of the right ventricle (Laks & Breda, 1991a) (Fig. 29-7). Clinical manifestations of the defect depend on severity of the obstruction of the right ventricular outflow tract. With increasing obstruction, an increase in cyanosis is observed that becomes more marked when the child is overexerted or upset. Clubbing of the nailbeds occurs and becomes more apparent after the first 6 to 8 months. The child's height and weight are often affected. Cyanotic or blue episodes occur, which are thought to be caused by an abrupt decrease in pulmonary blood flow and are characterized by dyspnea, syncope, and deepening cyanosis (Laks & Breda, 1991a; Page, 1986). The cyanotic episodes are typically relieved by squatting or by bringing the knees to the chest. These maneuvers are believed to increase systemic vascular resistance and ultimately to increase pulmonary blood flow. Oxygen or morphine or both may also need to be administered (Laks & Breda, 1991a).

Surgical intervention depends on the patient's symptoms and overall clinical picture. Early palliation may be necessary if an infant is severely involved and would probably not survive corrective surgery. The

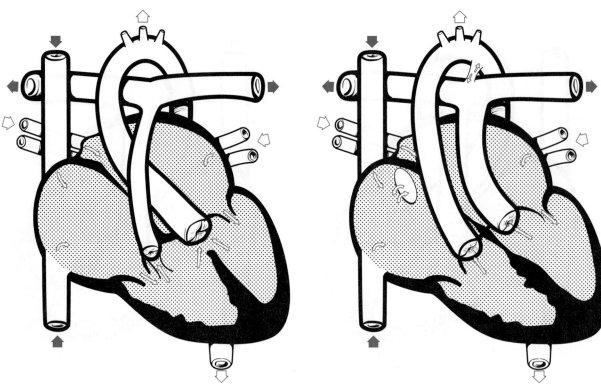

◆ **Figure 29-7**   Tetralogy of Fallot.

◆ **Figure 29-8**   Transposition of the great arteries.

palliative procedure used most often is a Blalock-Taussig (BT) shunt performed through a thoracotomy. The BT shunt involves an anastomosis of the subclavian artery to the pulmonary artery, providing increased pulmonary blood flow while the infant gains more time to grow before undergoing corrective surgery. Mild growth retardation may occur in the upper extremity on the side of the shunt, but it has not been viewed as a major problem (Page, 1986). Another important consequence of early palliation is continued cyanosis until complete repair is performed.

Corrective surgery involves closing the ventricular septal defect and relieving the right outflow tract obstruction. After surgical repair, an exercise stress test is warranted before the initiation of an exercise program because of a 14% incidence of ventricular arrhythmias at rest and a 30% incidence during exercise (Garson et al., 1980). Early and late mortality rate was observed to be 4.5% (Cho et al., 2002).

TRANSPOSITION OF THE GREAT ARTERIES

In transposition of the great arteries, the pulmonary artery arises from the morphologic left ventricle, and the aorta arises from the right ventricle (Callow, 1989)

(Fig. 29-8). In the absence of other defects, the systemic blood returns to the body unoxygenated and pulmonary blood returns to the lungs fully oxygenated. This situation is obviously not compatible with life unless the ductus arteriosus remains patent. Immediate intervention, usually with the infusion of prostaglandin E_1, is necessary to keep the ductus arteriosus open. An atrial septostomy is performed by a cardiac catheterization to keep the child alive until surgical intervention occurs.

The type of surgical intervention used for correction of transposition of the great arteries depends largely on the surgeon's preference. In some institutions, a Mustard or Senning technique is used to redirect the venous return to the atria, either by baffles or flaps of atrial wall, respectively (de Leval, 1991; Trusler, 1991). These techniques leave the right ventricle as the pumping chamber for the systemic system.

The Rastelli procedure is a surgical technique used when a severe left ventricular outflow tract obstruction and a ventricular septal defect coexist. Repair usually occurs when the child is between 4 and 6 years old. A conduit diverts blood from the left ventricle through the ventricular septal defect and right ventricle to the aorta, a right ventricle to pulmonary artery conduit is formed, and any previous shunts are eliminated (Williams, 1991).

Reoperation for conduit enlargement is not un-common. Depression of right ventricular function over time has been reported in some patients whose defects were corrected with these procedures (Jarmakani & Canent, 1974; Nakazawa et al., 1986).

The preferred technique, when anatomically possible, is the arterial switch procedure. Surgery during the first 2 to 4 weeks of life is preferred so that the left ventricle meets the systemic demands. Surgical repair occurs through a median sternotomy and involves transecting the aorta and pulmonary artery. The coronary arteries are excised with a wide button of aortic tissue and reimplanted in the old pulmonary arterial vessel; the great vessels are then switched and anastomosed so that the aorta connects to the left ventricle and the pulmonary artery connects to the right ventricle. The arterial switch procedure produces results that are free of the dysrhythmias and right ventricular failure associated with the techniques described previously (Callow, 1989).

TRICUSPID ATRESIA

Tricuspid atresia is the failure of development of the tricuspid valve, resulting in a lack of communication between the right atrium and right ventricle. Usually, an atrial septal defect or a ventricular septal defect or both exist to allow pulmonary blood flow (Fig. 29-9). The right-to-left shunt allows mixing of unoxygenated and oxygenated blood, causing the child to be cyanotic. The right ventricle is frequently underdeveloped.

Surgical repair is staged, with the initial operation shunting blood from the body to the lungs with a BT shunt through a thoracotomy. However, if the ventricular septal defect is large and too much blood is going to the lungs, a band may be placed around the pulmonary artery to decrease blood flow to the lungs. The child remains cyanotic for several years. The next stage of surgical repair is often the Fontan procedure (or a modification thereof) performed through a median sternotomy in which the right atrium is attached to the pulmonary artery or directly to the right ventricle, using a conduit or baffle. The ventricular septal defect may be surgically closed (Laks & Breda, 1991b). It is not un-common to have significant chest tube drainage for weeks after the Fontan surgery, thereby increasing the length of hospital stay.

In some institutions, a bidirectional Glenn procedure performed before the Fontan procedure leads to an improved outcome. In the Glenn procedure, the superior vena cava is anastomosed to the right pulmonary artery. The child remains cyanotic but gains time for growth before undergoing the Fontan operation.

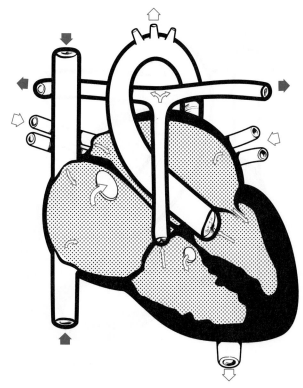

◆ **Figure 29-9**   Tricuspid atresia.

PULMONARY ATRESIA

Pulmonary atresia occurs when the pulmonary valve fails to develop, resulting in obstruction of blood flow from the right side of the heart to the lungs. Blood flow to the lungs is initially maintained by a patent ductus arteriosus. An atrial septal defect or a ventricular septal defect may also be present, allowing shunting of blood from the right to the left side of the heart and ultimately back to the body. The size of the right ventricle may vary, affecting later surgical decisions. Early intervention involves maintaining patency of the ductus arteriosus to increase blood flow to the lungs until surgery can be performed. An atrial septostomy is usually performed during the initial cardiac catheterization. A BT shunt is often performed as soon as possible. Later surgery involves ligating the previous shunt, closing the atrial septal defect, and opening the pulmonary valve by a valvulotomy, an infundibular graft, or a right ventricle-to-pulmonary artery conduit. If the ventricle is poorly developed, the Fontan procedure may be performed to provide communication through a conduit between the right atrium and pulmonary artery (Puga, 1991). Children remain cyanotic during their early developmental years until the Fontan operation is performed.

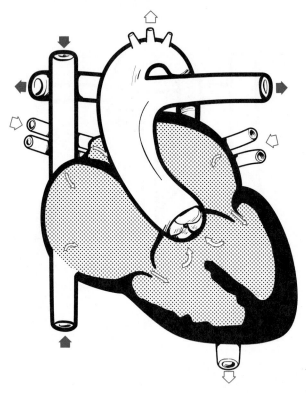

♦ **Figure 29-10** Truncus arteriosus.

TRUNCUS ARTERIOSUS

Truncus arteriosus occurs when the aorta and pulmonary artery fail to separate in utero and form a common trunk arising from both ventricles (Fig. 29-10). Four grades of the condition are differentiated, depending on the location of the pulmonary arteries. Early surgical intervention is necessary. Surgical repair is through a median sternotomy and involves removing the pulmonary arteries from the truncus, closing the ventricular septal defect, and connecting the pulmonary arteries to the right ventricle by an extracardiac baffle. Mortality rates are lower in patients operated on in the first 6 months of life (9% versus 18% for later repair) (Milgalter & Laks, 1991; Peetz et al., 1982).

TOTAL ANOMALOUS PULMONARY VENOUS RETURN

Total anomalous pulmonary venous return occurs when the pulmonary veins fail to communicate with the left atrium and instead connect to the coronary sinus of the right atrium or to one of the systemic veins. The ductus arteriosus often remains patent (Fig. 29-11). The increase in flow through the right side of the heart and into the lungs may lead to congestive heart failure. Anastomosis of

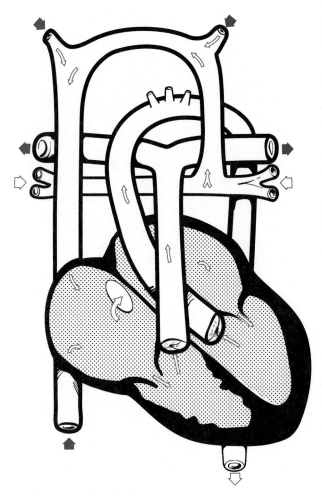

♦ **Figure 29-11** Total anomalous pulmonary venous return.

the pulmonary veins to the left atrium through a median sternotomy is usually performed as soon as possible. Postoperative ventilation may be difficult because of stiffness and wetness of the lungs from the previous excessive blood flow (Byrum et al., 1982; Hammon & Bender, 1991). Mortality rates continue to improve but remain nearly 30% for infants (Hammon & Bender, 1991).

HYPOPLASTIC LEFT-SIDED HEART SYNDROME

Hypoplasia (incomplete development or underdevelopment) or absence of the left ventricle and hypoplasia of the ascending aorta mark hypoplastic left-sided heart syndrome, the most common form of a univentricular heart, often coexisting with severe aortic valve hypoplasia. A patent ductus arteriosus provides systemic circulation until surgical intervention. Without surgical intervention, death is certain; however, the surgical mortality rate at 24% is still higher than the rate for other congenital heart surgeries (Lloyd, 1996). Lloyd (1996) reported that the survival rate after the second-stage palliation is now 97%, and the survival rate is 81% after the Fontan operation. However, Lloyd also reported that some of the survivors of the Fontan operation were observed to have neurologic conditions (6%) and respiratory conditions (11%).

Three options are available to parents of infants diagnosed as having hypoplastic left-sided heart syndrome. One option is no surgical intervention. As a second option, the child's name may be placed on a waiting list for a heart transplant, or as a third, the child may undergo a series of palliative procedures (Chang et al., 2002).

The initial surgical procedure (Norwood I) involves enlarging the atrial septal defect, transecting the main pulmonary artery and anastomosing it to the aorta, and reconstructing the aortic root. A BT or central shunt is placed to allow pulmonary blood flow. The second stage is a bidirectional Glenn procedure anastomosing the superior vena cava to the pulmonary arteries and ligating the BT shunt. The Fontan procedure may be performed several months to a few years later. This procedure provides continuity between the right atrium and pulmonary artery, and the pulmonary venous return is separated from the systemic system. As a result, the right ventricle pumps fully oxygenated blood to the body (Johnson & Davis, 1991; Norwood, 1991a, 1991b). Heart transplantation is also offered as a second-stage possibility. The postoperative stay is usually lengthy, and children often have difficulty in being weaned from the ventilator. Although infants who survive the first stage may die (10%) before reaching the second stage, surgical interventions continue to lower the mortality rate (Bailey & Gundry, 1990).

Table 29-1 summarizes the common types of congenital heart defects, their typical surgical repair, and associated impairments and functional limitations.

TRANSPLANTATION

HEART TRANSPLANTATION

Cardiac transplantation is a viable option for children with end-stage heart failure secondary to congenital malformations or for children with cardiomyopathy. Introduction of immunosuppressive medications to control rejection has increased survival rates to 65% after 5 years, and a 92% survival rate in infants has been reported (Bauer et al., 1998).

The previous indication for transplantation in children was largely cardiomyopathy (62%). Since 1988, however, the number of transplants for congenital heart defects has surpassed that of cardiomyopathy (Kriett & Kaye, 1991; Pennington et al., 1991). The increase is at least partly related to the fact that cardiac transplantation is being offered more frequently as an option for children with hypoplastic left-sided heart syndrome. As a result, a greatly increased number of children under 1 year of age have received a cardiac transplant (Bailey et al., 1988; Bove, 1991; Pennington et al., 1991; Starnes et al., 1992). Razzouk and associates (1996) have observed an 84% 1-year and 72% 7-year survival rates in infants under 1 year of age undergoing cardiac transplantation.

Surgery is performed through a median sternotomy and involves removal of the recipient heart with residual atrial cuffs remaining. The atria are reanastomosed with the donor heart, and then the great arteries are connected (Haas et al., 1991). Severing of the vagus nerve and the cervical and thoracic sympathetic cardiac nerves leaves the heart denervated (Clough, 1990; Kent & Cooper, 1974). An intrinsic control system exists within the heart, so it is not dependent on innervation for function. Cardiac impulse formation occurs because of spontaneous depolarization of the sinoatrial node (Kent & Cooper, 1974). The sinus node firing rate is faster than the usual heart rate in resting humans, so the heart rate of an individual after transplantation is faster than normal (Uretsky, 1990).

Several other influences on myocardial contractility remain, including the Frank-Starling effect, the Anrep effect, and the Bowditch effect. The Frank-Starling effect is the increase in cardiac output by an increase in stroke volume after an increased input or venous return (Kent & Cooper, 1974). This is an important effect that helps the body meet its early oxygen needs for exercise after transplantation. With the Anrep effect retained, the cardiac muscle increases its contractile force when the aortic pressure rises (afterload). The Bowditch effect describes an augmented contractile force of the heart with an increase in heart rate (Clough, 1990; Kent & Cooper, 1974). The transplanted heart has an increased sensitivity to circulating catecholamines (epinephrine and norepinephrine). Epinephrine increases the heart rate and the force of myocardial contraction, and norepinephrine increases the peripheral vascular resistance (Clough, 1990). The hormonal release takes several minutes to have an effect on the heart's rate and contractility, so it is generally advised that patients perform several minutes of warm-up exercises before vigorous exercise. It also takes several minutes for the body to reduce the hormones to normal levels, so a cool-down period at the end of

| **TABLE 29-1** | **Summary of Congenital Heart Defects, Surgical Repair, and Associated Issues** | | |

TYPE OF DEFECT	SURGICAL REPAIR	ASSOCIATED ISSUES	PHYSICAL THERAPY ISSUES
Atrial septal defect (ASD)	Suture or patch closure		Early mobility
Ventricular septal defect (VSD)	Dacron patch closure	Failure to thrive; pulmonary hypertension	Failure to thrive
Atrial ventricular septal defect/endocardial cushion defect	Pericardial patch	Down syndrome; failure to thrive	Developmental delay
Coarctation of the aorta	Subclavian patch/end-to-end anastomosis	Hypertension	Upper extremity range of motion
Pulmonary stenosis	Valvotomy		
Aortic stenosis	Valvotomy; aortic valve replacement; conduit		
Tetralogy of Fallot	VSD closed; right ventricular outflow tract resected	"Tet" spells	
Transposition of the great arteries (dextro)	Arterial switch operation	Edema; poor left ventricle function	
Pulmonary atresia (PA) with a VSD	Blalock-Taussig shunt (BT); VSD closed; right ventricle-to-pulmonary artery conduit	Developmental delay; poor oral intake	Developmental delay; feeding issues
Pulmonary atresia without a VSD	Valvotomy/BT shunt; right ventricular outflow tract patch, ASD closed, Fontan procedure	Very sick postoperatively, low oxygen saturations	Developmental delay
Total anomalous pulmonary venous return	Anomalous veins connected to left atrium; ASD closed	Failure to thrive	Failure to thrive
Tricuspid atresia	1. Atrial septostomy, BT shunt 2. Bidirectional Glenn or hemi-Fontan procedure 3. Fontan procedure	Low oxygen saturations	Failure to thrive
Truncus arteriosus	VSD closure, right ventricle-to-pulmonary artery conduit	Pulmonary hypertensive crisis	Developmental delay; failure to thrive
Hypoplastic left-sided heart syndrome	1. Division of the main pulmonary artery; suture PA to the aorta; BT shunt and patent ductus arteriosus ligation 2. Bidirectional Glenn or hemi-Fontan procedure 3. Fenestrated Fontan procedure	Low oxygen saturations	Poor oral feeders; developmental delay; may not crawl

exercise is also advised. The resting heart rate is higher than usual in transplant recipients, and the peak heart rate is lower; both should be taken into account when transplant patients are exercising (Uretsky, 1990).

Antirejection treatment begins with triple therapy of tacrolimus, CellCept, and prednisone. The use of steroids is discontinued as soon as possible and reinstituted only if rejection occurs (Bailey et al., 1988; Pennington et al., 1991). The use of steroids should be taken into consideration when the weight and height percentiles of transplant recipients are reviewed. The majority of children increase their weight dramatically without a concomitant increase in height (Fricker et al., 1990; Pennington et al., 1991).

Rejection is an ongoing issue in all transplant patients. Signs and symptoms of rejection range from fever, malaise, poor appetite, weight gain, tachycardia, tachypnea, and low urine output to poor perfusion, complete heart block, pulmonary edema, and shock (Haas et al., 1991). Severe rejection has been observed in several adolescent transplant recipients after missing just one dose of immunosuppressive medicine.

Several complications are common in the pediatric heart transplant population. Hypertension and seizures have been observed in a number of patients. Seizures are believed to be caused by high immunosuppressive medication levels; however, they do not generally recur once the patient is on a therapeutic dose of anticonvulsants (Fricker et al., 1990; Pennington et al., 1991). Other central nervous system (CNS) disturbances have been observed in children, ranging from lethargy and confusion to localized neurologic defects and behavioral disturbances. CNS dysfunction occurs more commonly in children than in adults; fortunately, the impairment is usually transient (Haas et al., 1991). As more children survive successful initial cardiac transplant the potential need for retransplantation increases. The availability of donors, long-term survival, and functional outcomes are factors that need to be investigated.

CONDITIONS REQUIRING LUNG AND HEART-LUNG TRANSPLANTATION

More than 200 heart-lung transplantations take place each year, with only 5% of all transplants in children under 18 years of age (Huddleston, 2002). In 1990, 214 single-lung and 60 double-lung transplants were reported (Kriett & Kaye, 1991). Primary pulmonary hypertension and Eisenmenger syndrome are the indications for over 50% of the heart-lung transplants being done, with a small percentage performed for congenital heart disease and about 30% performed for cystic fibrosis. Primary pulmonary disease is the usual diagnosis of lung transplant recipients; however, some transplants are necessary secondary to lung failure caused by congenital heart defects. Lung transplants in these cases are usually associated with cardiac repair. Previous thoracotomy is no longer considered a contraindication for heart-lung or lung transplantation; however, it does increase the risk of perioperative bleeding (Whitehead et al., 1990). The mortality rate for children has been reported at nearly 30% in the first year after transplant and less than 10% later (Wilkinson, 1989).

The surgical procedure for a heart-lung transplantation is performed through a median sternotomy. The recipient heart and then lungs are removed. The donor organs are placed inside the chest cavity with the trachea anastomosed several rings above the carina. The right atrial anastomosis is performed and followed by anastomosis of the aorta (Bonser & Jamieson, 1990). Because of the risk of tracheal dehiscence, an omentum wrap around the suture line is typically used (Griffith et al., 1987).

The surgical procedure for a single-lung transplantation is performed through a thoracotomy incision. The removal of diseased lung is followed by the placement of the donor lung. The bronchial anastomosis is completed with an omentum wrap and followed by anastomosis of the pulmonary artery (Bolman et al., 1991).

When both lungs are transplanted, pulmonary innervation is lost (Jamieson et al., 1984). An early study observed bronchial hyperresponsiveness to inhaled methacholine, which was thought to be caused by denervation hypersensitivity (Glanville et al., 1989). Since that time, however, the postganglionic cholinergic nerve responses have been observed to be intact, as demonstrated by a normal bronchoconstrictor response to a stimulant. Therefore, airway hypersensitivity is most likely a result of intact postganglionic cholinergic nerve response instead of denervation hypersensitivity (Stretton et al., 1990). Hypersensitivity was not observed during exercise (Glanville et al., 1989).

Because secretions below the tracheal anastomosis in the denervated lung do not excite the cough reflex, percussion, postural drainage, and breathing exercises are required to aid expectoration (Bonser & Jamieson, 1990). A certain amount of atelectasis is observed in all patients, especially when the transplanted lungs must be compressed to fit into the thoracic cage (Jamieson et al., 1984). Pulmonary edema is also commonly observed in the early postoperative period. Positive end-expiratory pressure is often used with mechanical ventilation to reduce atelectasis and pulmonary edema (Whitehead et al., 1990).

The diagnosis of rejection is made based on clinical signs and symptoms suggesting a deterioration in function. Chest radiographic findings and pulmonary function test results are noninvasive indicators. If necessary, a transbronchial biopsy is performed when patients are breathless and febrile and have rales and wheezes on auscultation (Hutter et al., 1988).

Pulmonary infection occurs in most transplant recipients, usually repeatedly. Obliterative bronchiolitis is also a common posttransplant complication that has been reported to affect 71% of long-term survivors (Glanville et al., 1990; Starnes et al., 1991). The acute phase of obliterative bronchiolitis is characterized by varying degrees of bronchiolar obstruction by plugs of granulation tissue; in the chronic phase, the bronchioles are partially to completely occluded (Aziz & Jamieson,

1991). Severe damage may necessitate retransplantation. With improvements in immunosuppression, obliterative bronchiolitis is becoming less common in adults; the same progress is anticipated in children. In spite of all of the progress made in immunosuppression, heart and lung transplant recipients still suffer from many adverse effects including infections, malignancies, organ dysfunction, and toxicities, as well as chronic infections (Reddy & Webber, 2003)

The education of parents and children about the implications and ramifications of a heart, heart-lung, or lung transplantation must be thorough and frank, including discussion of the implications of being on a waiting list and the extent of the postoperative care after transplantation. Geographic and social dislocation may occur during assessment and during the wait for a transplant (Warner, 1991). Warner (1991) stresses that families must be aware that, although transplantation is a last resort, it still may not be the answer. Many centers require transplant candidates to participate in a formal exercise rehabilitation program before receiving the transplant to minimize postoperative complications, maximize the success of the transplant, and assess compliance. Compliance before transplantation may be an indicator of posttransplant compliance. Noncompliance is a contraindication for transplantation because rigid adherence to the immunosuppressive regimen is imperative. Missed doses of immunosuppressants can result in death.

TECHNOLOGIC SUPPORT

Mechanical ventilation is common after open-heart surgery in the pediatric patient but should not deter the physical therapist from beginning treatment. Recent improvements in cardiopulmonary bypass, decreased operating time, and improved postoperative fluid management have allowed early extubation, often within 8 hours of surgery (Prakanrattana et al., 1997). This has led to decreased costs, early patient mobility, and fewer respiratory complications. However, some pediatric patients may require the use of high-frequency jet ventilation in the period after open-heart surgery, and this will prevent initiation of early physical therapy.

High-frequency jet ventilation introduces a small tidal volume at a very rapid rate. Its use allows delivery of oxygen and removal of carbon dioxide at reduced mean airway and peak inspiratory pressures, and it is often used in unstable patients for whom physical therapy is contraindicated (Norwood & Civette, 1991). The three main advantages of high-frequency ventilation over conventional approaches to ventilation are improvement in the ventilation/perfusion ratio, less reduction of cardiac output, and minimized barotrauma (McWilliams, 1987).

Nasal intermittent positive pressure ventilation has been used for short periods in the pediatric surgical patient who has had difficulty in remaining extubated. This type of ventilation provides respiratory support through a preset tidal volume or inspiratory time, resulting in improved arterial blood gas tensions, improved alveolar ventilation, and decreased work of breathing (Bott et al., 1992). Nitric oxide is now being used successfully with patients who have pulmonary hypertension postoperatively (Russell et al., 1998).

Extracorporeal membrane oxygenation (ECMO) may be used for cardiovascular support in children after open-heart surgery. Indications for biventricular support by ECMO in the early postoperative period include progressive hypotension, increased ventricular filling pressures, poor peripheral perfusion, decreased urine output, and decreased mixed venous oxygen saturation (Fenton, 2003; Kolovos, 2003). ECMO is especially effective in treating conditions with right-sided heart failure and has also been used as a support while waiting for a heart, heart-lung, or lung transplantation (Weinhaus et al., 1989). The ECMO pump takes over oxygenation and perfusion of the child's body while the heart and lungs are "rested."

MANAGEMENT OF ACUTE IMPAIRMENT

EDUCATION

The majority of acute impairments after thoracic surgical procedures occur in the immediate or early postoperative period. Rockwell and Campbell (1976) described a preoperative program to assist in minimizing postoperative complications and to educate the parents of children 3 to 12 years of age. Education is facilitated through an audiotape and a puppet show, as well as by a coloring book that shows the child what will happen after surgery. Preoperative programs probably benefit the parents as much as the child in alleviating some anxiety about the surgery. Preoperative education for the child younger than 5 years is also described by Page (1986). The program lists concepts that may be helpful in teaching and preparing the child and family for surgery. A doll is used to educate the child about placement of tubes and incisions; pictures are used for parents. Preparing children before the surgery should assist in obtaining their cooperation after surgery, as well as minimize their fears.

PULMONARY MANAGEMENT

The primary area to be addressed after heart repair is the pulmonary status of the patient. Numerous articles describe pulmonary complications and physical therapy in the postoperative pediatric patient (Ali et al., 1974; Bartlett, 1980, 1984; Bartlett et al., 1973a, 1973b; Gamsu et al., 1976; Krastins et al., 1982; Thoren, 1954; Van De Water et al., 1972; Vraciu & Vraciu, 1977). Although intervention varies with the age of the child, the primary goals are to mobilize secretions, increase aeration, and increase general mobility (Fig. 29-12).

Mucus transport is slowed after surgery and can lead to atelectasis (Gamsu et al., 1976). Atelectasis also occurs secondary to an altered breathing pattern, prolonged positioning in supine, and possible diaphragmatic dysfunction in the early postoperative period (Bartlett, 1984). In early studies by Bartlett and co-workers (Bartlett, 1980; Bartlett et al., 1973a) lack of deep breaths was observed as a causative factor in atelectasis. The yawn maneuver or prolonged inspiration with normal or increased inflation prevented atelectasis (Bartlett et al., 1973b). Bartlett (1984) observed that a collapsed lung expands only after the normal lung is fully inflated. This is achieved with prolonged inspiration. The restriction in ventilation has also been attributed to incoordination and reduction of rib expansion after sternotomy (Locke et al., 1990).

Incentive spirometry is an effective tool for reducing the occurrence of atelectasis in the pediatric population (Krastins et al., 1982). The primary emphasis with incentive spirometry or any other respiratory intervention should be on prolonged inspiration. When the inspiration is held for at least 3 seconds, arterial oxygen tension improves (Ward et al., 1966). Huckabay and Daderian (1990) observed an increase in compliance with breathing exercises after surgery when children were given a choice and some control regarding breathing exercises. With young children, tools such as bubble blowing or blowing on a windmill can be used (Rockwell & Campbell, 1976) (Fig. 29-13). Although these are expiratory maneuvers, a child often takes in a large inspiration before exhaling. Other respiratory techniques can also be performed to mobilize secretions and increase aeration, such as percussion and postural drainage, vibration, segmental expansion, and assisted cough techniques (Hussey, 1992) (Fig. 29-14).

Segmental expansion techniques may be performed to reduce postoperative complications and increase segmental aeration (Vraciu & Vraciu, 1977). This technique is

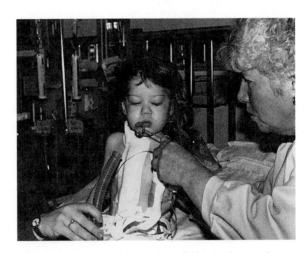

• **Figure 29-13**   Child blowing bubbles 24 hours after open-heart surgery.

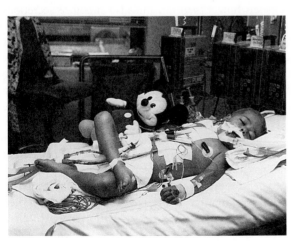

• **Figure 29-12**   Two-year-old boy 24 hours after open-heart surgery.

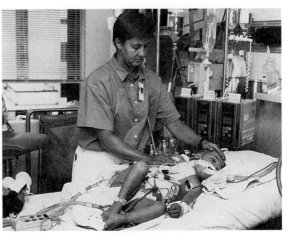

• **Figure 29-14**   Child receiving percussion after open-heart surgery.

performed by placing a hand over a particular segment and allowing it to move with the ventilator or respiratory cycle. Gentle pressure may be applied to the chest wall during exhalation at the end of the expiratory phase just before the inspiratory phase. This facilitates airflow to the specific segment (Massery, 1987). When a specific lobe or segment has decreased aeration, this technique, used in conjunction with gentle sustained pressure on the opposite upper lobe, may increase aeration to the affected area. When the patient is in a side-lying position, gentle rocking may also stimulate segmental expansion and relax the patient (Massery, 1987). This technique is particularly effective when the child is upset or does not tolerate percussion or other treatment techniques. It may also decrease the respiratory rate and is especially useful with infants who cannot respond to verbal relaxation instructions. Segmental expansion techniques are also beneficial when the patient is having excessive bleeding after surgery and use of more vigorous techniques is contraindicated (Johnson, 1991). The authors have used this technique with lung transplant recipients who have been unable to cooperate or follow commands for deep breathing and coughing and found it to work well in decreasing atelectasis and increasing oxygen saturation. Segmental expansion techniques performed before other respiratory techniques may further enhance their benefit. Percussion may need to be performed to assist in removal of excess secretions. Percussion is defined as a rhythmic clapping with cupped hands over the involved lung segment performed throughout the respiratory cycle, with the goal of mechanically dislodging pulmonary secretions (Imle, 1981). Vibration also assists in mobilization of secretions. It is performed by creating a fine oscillating movement of the hand on the chest wall just before expiration and continuing until the beginning of inspiration (Imle, 1981).

Both percussion and vibration techniques can be performed in conjunction with postural drainage. Optimal positions are described by Crane and pictured in Frownfelter's text on chest physical therapy (Crane, 1987). Positioning must be used with caution in the postoperative patient; use of the Trendelenburg position, for example, is often contraindicated after open-heart surgery. It is important to confirm with the nurse or the physician whether it is even suitable for the child to be flat in bed. Despite limitations, percussion and vibration can be performed in the positions available. It has been the authors' experience that children respond well to both percussion and vibration, even on the first postoperative day. Encouraging the child to tell you if the treatment hurts—because it should not be painful—often facilitates cooperation. It may also be helpful to coordinate the treatment with administration of pain medications. Percussion may be contraindicated when platelets are low, pulmonary artery pressures are too high, or the child becomes too agitated with treatment.

Vibration can generally be safely used instead. Blood pressure and intracardiac pressures should be closely monitored throughout the treatment because they are indicators of intolerance to treatment. The physician usually establishes parameters, set on an individual basis.

Massery (1987) described a counterrotation technique for altering respiratory rate in the neurologically impaired patient that has also been safely used in the pediatric patient after open-heart surgery through a median sternotomy only. The technique has been used by the authors to slow the respiratory rate and increase expansion of the lateral segment. It generally relaxes patients and increases their tidal volume. When the technique is used in the postoperative cardiac patient, extreme caution must be exercised to avoid disturbing chest tubes and other intravenous lines. This treatment is recommended only after intracardiac lines have been removed. The sternal incision has not been a problem; because it is stable, it does not undergo any mobilization during application of this technique. The counterrotation technique is performed with the therapist standing behind the side-lying patient near the patient's buttocks. One hand is placed on the anterior iliac spine and the other hand is placed on the patient's posterior shoulder. On inspiration the hand on the buttocks pulls down and posteriorly while the hand on the shoulder gently pushes up and anteriorly. On expiration the therapist's hands and the patient's body return to neutral. This is repeated several times in cycle with the patient's breathing. It should be very relaxing and comfortable for the patient.

The techniques just described not only facilitate increased lung expansion but also mobilize secretions. Once mobilized, secretions act as an irritant in the airway when the child takes a deep breath and a spontaneous cough usually occurs (Bartlett, 1984). The child may need some assistance in removing excess secretions, owing either to lack of cooperation or to inability to cooperate secondary to age. This may be accomplished by coughing or airway suctioning.

If the child is intubated, suctioning is done to clear secretions and maintain patency of the tube. Children who have cyanotic heart defects, such as hypoplastic left-sided heart syndrome, tend to desaturate during suctioning. It is extremely important to hyperventilate these patients with oxygen and a resuscitation bag before and after suctioning and to monitor their oxygen saturation and other hemodynamic parameters (Boutros, 1970; Fox et al., 1978; Hussey, 1992; Rosen & Hillard, 1962). It is also important to monitor how far the suction catheter is inserted so that it only goes approximately 0.5 to 1 cm past the end of the endotracheal tube and does not touch the patient's carina. During suctioning, normal sterile saline may be instilled through the endotracheal tube to thin the thickened secretions. If the child is not intubated and is unwilling to cough, nasal pharyngeal suctioning may be performed to stimulate a cough and clear secretions. If the child is able to drink, a small sip of water or juice may also stimulate a cough. During coughing, a blanket or soft stuffed animal may be used to help splint the incision and minimize discomfort (Johnson, 1991).

PAIN

Postoperative pain can be detrimental to the child's recovery. Pain medications must be given regularly, not only to reduce anxiety (which further increases pain from splinting) but also to encourage deeper breathing. A child in pain does not take deep breaths, even spontaneously. Morphine, a commonly used postoperative narcotic, depresses spontaneous sighing; patients receiving morphine should be encouraged to voluntarily take deep breaths (Egbert & Bendixon, 1964).

Other techniques now being used to manage postoperative pain include epidural morphine administration and patient-controlled analgesia (Asantila et al., 1986; Wilson, 1991). Both have proved effective in management of postoperative pain, especially in thoracotomy patients. Proper pain management is also extremely important in mobilizing the patient.

EARLY MOBILIZATION

Postoperative immobility can lead to a variety of problems, including reduced ventilation and perfusion distribution (Peters, 1979), shallow breathing (Risser, 1980; Scheidegger et al., 1976), fever (Chulay et al., 1982), retention of secretions (Pairolero & Payne, 1991), fluid shifts (Rubin, 1988), and generalized discomfort from immobility. The child should be mobilized as soon as possible to minimize these deleterious effects.

Range-of-motion (ROM) exercises should be initiated as soon as possible. It may not be possible to attain normal ROM immediately because of discomfort or intravenous or arterial lines, but any movement helps to mobilize the patient. ROM exercises are extremely important for the child with a thoracotomy incision because this incision tends to produce more guarding than does a median sternotomy. Passive to active-assisted shoulder ROM to 90° of flexion is usually tolerable. Discomfort often occurs when the arm is returned to a neutral position. The therapist may apply gentle resistance to the arm as the child attempts to return the arm to a neutral position because contraction of the arm muscles tends to minimize discomfort (Johnson, 1991).

The child's position should be changed regularly to avoid retention of secretions in the dependent portion of the lung (Pairolero & Payne, 1991). Regular turning has been observed to decrease postoperative fevers (Chulay et al., 1982). It also assists in decreasing postoperative chest wall immobilization, which is thought to decrease ventilation (Peters, 1979). The supine position alone contributes to airway closure (Dean, 1985; Risser, 1980) and a shift in blood volume to the dependent side (Rubin, 1988).

Arterial oxygen saturation is also affected by body position because of ventilation and perfusion matching (Dean, 1985). The supine position tends to decrease ventilation, which affects ventilation and perfusion matching and may ultimately decrease oxygen saturation. Positioning the patient effectively can reduce the pulmonary dysfunction that occurs most commonly when perfusion is greater than ventilation (Dean, 1985). The prone position has been observed to be associated with a significantly higher arterial oxygen tension than the supine position (Fox & Molesky, 1990), as well as an increased tidal volume and improved lung compliance (Dean, 1985). This position can be especially beneficial in preventing respiratory difficulty in a child who is extubated. The side-lying position has been observed to be a better position than the supine position for improving oxygenation (Banasik et al., 1987; Dean, 1985). In studies, adult patients became better oxygenated when the "good" lung was in the dependent position (Banasik et al., 1987; Todd, 1990). In children, however, the opposite was observed, namely, gas exchange improved with the good lung uppermost (Davies et al., 1985). It has been observed in lung transplant recipients that regional differences in blood flow distribution produced by position changes may lead to significant changes in oxygenation. Positioning the patient in a side-lying position, with the best lung dependent, may improve ventilation and perfusion matching (Todd, 1990). The best lung may or may not be the transplanted lung in the early postoperative period; thus tolerance to having the transplanted lung dependent should be confirmed with the surgeons before placing the patient in this position.

Early ambulation after surgery reduces both pulmonary and circulatory complications (Webber, 1991). It has been observed to be as effective as deep-breathing exercises in minimizing complications in adults (Dull & Dull, 1983). Ambulation was observed to be beneficial in returning respiratory function toward normal by inducing

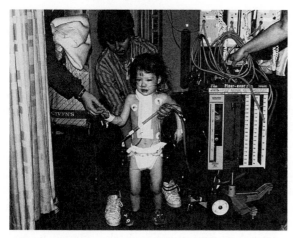

+ **Figure 29-15**   A child walking 1 day after open-heart surgery.

more frequent and deeper sigh respirations (Scheidegger et al., 1976). Activity and mobility have been clinically observed to minimize chest tube output. At our center, children ambulate as soon as atrial lines and groin lines are removed and the child is extubated. Children often ambulate for the first time with any or all of the following: central venous pressure line, peripheral intravenous line, arterial line, chest tubes, temporary pacemakers, and oxygen (Fig. 29-15). The first walk is often only for 5 to 10 feet and may be difficult for the patient. Anxiety often plays as great a role in the perceived difficulty as does the discomfort. It may be beneficial for the patient to receive some pain medication before the first walk. Parents are also anxious, so the benefits of early ambulation should be explained to them ahead of time, with emphasis on the problems that can occur by remaining in bed. This is also a good time to review with parents the importance of picking their child up under the bottom and back as they did when the child was an infant. They should avoid picking up the child under the child's arms for 4 to 6 weeks after surgery to allow the sternum time to heal.

MEDICAL COMPLICATIONS

Several medical complications can affect postoperative function. Secondary to phrenic nerve palsy, some children may have a paralyzed diaphragm after surgery that affects their early postoperative course, as well as their long-term respiratory status and endurance. The paralyzed diaphragm may persist but is seldom permanent (Markland et al., 1985; Morriss & McNamara, 1975). Infants have horizontal ribs and lack the normal bucket handle movement, relying primarily on use of the diaphragm for respiration. Paralysis of the diaphragm by unilateral or bilateral phrenic nerve palsy can cause

further respiratory problems, including difficulty in weaning from the ventilator (Hussey, 1992).

Peroneal nerve palsy is another complication of surgery, usually caused by improper positioning of the lower extremity during surgery. The resultant drastic alteration in the child's gait must be addressed as soon as possible. An ankle-foot orthosis can improve gait and should be necessary for only a short time.

Postoperative neurologic impairments can occur subsequent to prolonged surgical time, usually related to length of hypothermic arrest, low cardiac output, or arrhythmias after surgery (Ferry, 1990; Wells et al., 1983). Hemodynamic instability and coagulation disturbances are risk factors for postoperative neurologic problems in infants (duPlessis, 1997). Thirty-five percent of premature infants weighing less than 2 kg who had open-heart surgery developed neurologic complications (Rossi et al., 1998). Neurologic consequences can also be the result of an air embolus, a prolonged hypotensive period (van Breda, 1985), or complications of long-term cyanosis (Amitia et al., 1984). Choreoathetosis has been observed in some children after they have been on cardiopulmonary bypass. When a basal ganglia lesion is also seen the prognosis is poor (Holden et al., 1998). It is encouraging to note that of almost 700 children who underwent a Fontan operation, less than 3% suffered a stroke (duPlessis et al., 1995). The child who has suffered a neurologic insult requires both early intervention and long-term physical therapy. A child with severe extensor tone may benefit from inhibitive casts on the lower extremities and hand splints to decrease the effects of increased tone and maintain ROM. Parent education concerning the impact of a neurologic insult should begin as soon as the diagnosis is confirmed, including information on handling and positioning the child with increased tone, appropriate stimulation, use of adaptive equipment, and long-term follow-up.

AGE-SPECIFIC DISABILITIES IN THE IMMEDIATE POSTOPERATIVE PERIOD

The infant who undergoes surgery within the first few days of life experiences immediate disruption of all aspects of typical newborn life. The infant is often sedated, restrained, and intubated, all of which interfere with being held, bundled, and fed. Parents need education about the areas of stimulation that are withdrawn from their child during this time and instruction in ways to compensate for this deprivation. The fact that their child is born with a congenital anomaly may further impede the attachment process (Loeffel, 1985). The therapist assists the process by involving the parents in treatment as soon as possible and educating them about engaging and calming their child.

Toddlers who have cardiac surgery often recover very quickly and with few impairments. Anxiety over being left alone during the hospitalization may be the biggest problem interfering with function in this age group (Loeffel, 1985). The child may feel abandoned and react by becoming passive and apathetic or, conversely, by becoming aggressive. These behaviors are more commonly observed in the child who is in the hospital for the first time, such as the child with an atrial septal defect.

Toddlers tend to be limited more by their parents' restrictions than by their own physical limitations (Clare, 1985; Loeffel, 1985). Activity guidelines should be reviewed with parents on an ongoing basis; showing them by example may be even more helpful. Although it is beneficial to explain to the parents ahead of time what their child will experience, it may be helpful to wait to tell the toddler what is happening as it is happening.

Adolescents who have cardiac surgery may need to be encouraged to move and may need to be assisted to become active. The parents are often more reluctant than the child about early mobilization, including ambulation. They should be reassured that it is beneficial for their child to move as soon as possible. Adolescents may choose to assert their independence and try to do everything for themselves, or they may choose to become totally dependent on their parents and hospital staff. Whichever situation occurs, young persons benefit from early education about how to move and what they should be doing. This helps them realize what is expected of them. They should be informed of what they need to do and not given a choice when the task is not optional (van Breda, 1985).

CHRONIC DISABILITIES AND ACTIVITY LIMITATIONS

Various disabilities and activity limitations occur as a result of primary impairments incurred by children with congenital heart defects (see Table 29-1). The disabling process may start very early secondary to poor attachment between parent and infant (Goldberg et al., 1990). Infants who had cardiac surgery showed less positive affect and engagement than typical babies, making it even more stressful for mothers who are already distressed (Gardner et al., 1996). Poor attachment can lead to poor social development. The overprotection and excessive activity restrictions imposed by some parents further compound this disability. Parents have stated that

they were afraid to permit activity in their child with congenital heart disease (Gudermuth, 1975). If this attitude is allowed to persist, the child's developmental and functional level will surely suffer. It has also been observed that maternal perceptions of the child's disease severity were a stronger predictor of emotional adjustment than was disease severity (DeMaso et al., 1991). Emotional maladjustment may contribute to the poor self-esteem that is often noted in children with congenital heart defects. The limitations resulting from decreased activity, delayed development, poor self-esteem, overprotection by parents, and physical illness may all lead to poor peer interactions. This may further limit a child with congenital heart disease from interacting with society. These issues should be addressed with parents and the child as early as possible to try to limit the effect on developmental progression and functional capabilities. Subsequent sections elaborate on various aspects of the disabling process across childhood.

INFANCY

In children with congenital heart disease, several contributing factors can lead to impairment and activity limitations in infancy. Common problems include poor feeding, poor growth, and developmental lag. Parents must constantly watch for signs and symptoms of congestive heart failure in their infant. These signs include the onset of rapid breathing, changes in behavior, edema, excessive sweating, fatigue, vomiting, and poor feeding (Clare, 1985; Zahr & Boisvert, 1990).

Parental frustration and stress can impair early attachment to the infant. It has been observed during the period of 1 year that securely attached infants showed greater improvements in health than did insecurely attached infants (Goldberg et al., 1991). Gardner and associates observed infants with cardiac defects to be consistently less engaging with their mothers when compared to infants without defects (Gardner et al., 1996).

When compared with healthy infants and infants with cystic fibrosis, infants with congenital heart disease were the least attached to their mothers and their parents were the most stressed (Goldberg et al., 1990). Normal attachment may be difficult, particularly with the very sick infant who is frequently hospitalized. The health care team should begin working with the parents as early as possible on how they can interact with their infant to facilitate attachment and avoid overstimulating their infant.

It is not uncommon for infants with congenital heart disease to be poor feeders, which further increases parental stress. An infant expends most of his or her energy during eating. In normal infants decreased ventilation is observed during feeding, creating a decrease in the partial pressure of oxygen and an increase in the partial pressure of carbon dioxide (Mathew, 1988; Mathew et al., 1985). This decrease in ventilation may seriously compromise the child with congenital heart disease compounded by the increase in metabolic rate observed. Not only does the child not eat well, but he or she also requires more calories to thrive (Gingell & Hornung, 1989). Watching their child failing to thrive can be devastating to parents and can further increase their anxiety about feeding their child and trying to encourage adequate caloric intake (Gingell & Hornung, 1989). The prolonged feeding time can be frustrating to parents, as well as make them feel inadequate (Bruning & Schneiderman, 1983; Loeffel, 1985). If alternative feeding methods are used, such as nasogastric or gastrostomy tube feedings, parents should be educated not only in how to administer the feeding but also how to hold and nurture their child during the feeding (Loeffel, 1985). It may be helpful to tell parents that providing time for normal, nonstressful interaction may improve the parent-infant attachment and may ultimately improve the health of their infant. It is also helpful to inform the parents that the overall time that supplemental feedings are necessary varies with each child. Some parents have stated that they were able to remove supplemental feedings within 1 week of leaving the hospital; others have stated that it took months for their child to take enough by mouth to be able to discontinue supplemental feedings. Many parents have stated to these authors that their infant ate better at home, where it was possible to eat on demand and to have a more routine day.

Physical therapy assessment is sometimes needed to observe the infant feeding and parental interaction. There may be other problems unrelated to the poor endurance exhibited by the infant with congenital heart disease. If oral-motor dysfunction exists, it should be addressed with parents as soon as possible. Some parents need assistance in how best to handle and support their child during feeding. It can also be beneficial for the parents to observe that their child does not feed well for anyone.

Poor growth is closely associated with poor feeding. It has been observed that infants with cyanotic heart disease have poor growth in height and weight, whereas infants with acyanotic heart disease, specifically those with a large left-to-right shunt, are severely underweight secondary to the marked increase in metabolism (Gingell & Hornung, 1989). The child's growth improves after surgery but may not achieve typical parameters. This lack of catch-up growth is especially remarkable in children with cyanotic defects with a right-to-left shunt (Gingell & Hornung, 1989; Rosenthal, 1983).

Functional and activity limitations, especially delayed achievement of basic motor skills, can be observed in the infant with cardiac disease. Decreased nutritional status and cardiac function may leave the infant too weak to expend the energy required for typical motor activity (Loeffel, 1985). Some cyanotic children preferentially scoot around on their buttocks and, even after extensive intervention at home, do not crawl. They often go on to walking without ever crawling (Johnson, 1991), probably because of the increased energy expenditure associated with use of both upper and lower extremities in crawling. Cyanotic children also tend to have an internal mechanism that permits them to do only what they are physically capable of doing, given their oxygen saturation (Clare, 1985). They often rest without cueing and can rarely be pushed beyond what they are willing to do. Intervention may or may not improve the child's functional abilities; however, it may do a great deal to relieve parental anxiety. Education should be focused on what the child is doing normally, such as using typical movement patterns, instead of on developmental lag based solely on age. Intervention should include parental education concerning areas the parent can work on with the child throughout the day, rather than in one focused block of time.

The presence of congestive heart failure is significantly associated with mental and motor developmental delay. Infants with congestive heart failure scored less well than expected on the Bayley Scales of Infant Development as early as 2 months of age (Aisenberg et al., 1982). Haneda and associates (1996) observed a significant decrease in Gesell's developmental quotient score in infants and children who had circulatory arrest time greater than 50 minutes. This information is useful when working with parents to help them understand that their child is demonstrating typical developmental skills for a child with congenital heart disease. This does not mean that intervention does not improve the situation. Parents should be encouraged to work with their child on developmental tasks that are challenging. If functional and activity limitations are minimized early, the effect of reparative surgery may be dramatic.

Neurologic impairment and functional limitations may also occur from external forces related to the surgical repair. Discrepancy exists among research study findings regarding the effect of deep hypothermia and circulatory arrest on the psychomotor and intellectual development of infants (Blackwood et al., 1986; duPlessis, 1997; Haka-Ikse et al., 1978; Messmer et al., 1976; Rossi et al., 1998; Settergren et al., 1982). Messmer and associates (1976) observed no delay in psychomotor and intellectual development in infants after deep hypothermia. In another study, the researchers did not observe neurologic impairment after surgery, but they did observe mild developmental delays, most profoundly in cyanotic infants (Haka-Ikse et al., 1978). Bellinger and associates (1997) observed that children who had total circulatory arrest during the arterial switch operation scored lower on the Bayley Scales of Infant Development at 1 year of age than the infants who had low-flow bypass. They were also observed to have expressive language difficulties at 2.5 years of age and exhibited more behavior problems (Bellinger et al., 1997). There is further need to identify those factors that can be consistently utilized to determine risk for neurologic damage in young children after cardiac surgery (Trittenwein et al., 2003). In light of this conflicting information, therapists should realize the potential for problems. Parents should be advised that their child might take longer than usual to accomplish developmental milestones. Long-term developmental review of children after repair or palliation for congenital heart disease observed most children to be functioning within the expected range for most standardized tests (Mahle & Wernovsky, 2001).

PRESCHOOL PERIOD

The preschool child with chronic disabilities caused by congenital heart disease has grown up in the medical environment. This may help alleviate some of the child's and the parents' anxieties. However, parental anxieties can be exacerbated during this period as they begin to realize the impact their child's cardiac disease has on growth and development. The child's symptoms could be worsening, and another surgery may soon be needed. The parents' response and interaction during this period are important; it should be recognized that parents already have the tendency to be overprotective of their child and that this may increase during the preschool period.

The emotional adjustment of the child has been observed to be affected by the mother's perception of the severity of the child's illness more than by its actual severity (DeMaso et al., 1991). If the mother perceives the child's disease to be more severe than it is and limits the child accordingly, the child's physical development and social participation may suffer. In acyanotic children, it has been observed that the intelligence quotient (IQ) was lower when associated with poorer adjustment, greater dependence, and greater maternal pampering and anxiety (Rasof et al., 1967). Activity limitations may be out of proportion compared with what the child is actually capable of doing. Intervention may need to be initiated to instruct parents on what activities the child is capable of performing, as well as how the child self-limits activity without parental intervention.

Children with congenital heart disease have been observed to have some developmental delay—especially those children with cyanotic disease (Bellinger et al., 1997; Feldt et al., 1969; Rasof et al., 1967). Children with cyanosis scored significantly lower than acyanotic and typically developing children in all subscales of the Gesell Developmental Schedules (Haneda et al., 1996) and on Stanford-Binet and Cattell intelligence tests (Rasof et al., 1967). Cyanotic children were observed to sit and walk later than acyanotic and typically developing children and were slower in speaking phrases than were children without disabilities (Feldt et al., 1969; Rasof et al., 1967; Silbert et al., 1969). Curtailment of physical activity in the child with severe cardiac dysfunction interferes with the active manipulation of objects needed for the adequate development of early sensorimotor processes (Rasof et al., 1967; Silbert et al., 1969). This lack of opportunity may affect IQ scores, psychologic development, and participation. Despite these challenges intelligence and behavior are often within typical parameters (Goldberg et al., 2000). In addition to intelligence, other factors to be considered include functional activities and activities of daily living (Limperopoulos et al., 2001).

Educating parents about what they should be allowing their child to do is as important as teaching them precautions pertaining to their child. Children were observed to have significant gross motor advances during the second year of life when parental warmth was combined with a decrease in parental restrictions. It was also observed that children with congenital heart disease performed better on IQ tests when their parents attempted to accelerate their child's development (Rasof et al., 1967). Parents should also be taught that children with cardiac disease, particularly cyanotic disease, limit their own activity and stop and rest when needed (Clare, 1985). Children with Down syndrome were also observed to score higher on developmental tests and achieve feeding milestones earlier if parents followed through appropriately with therapy instructions (Cullen et al., 1981).

SCHOOL-AGE PERIOD

School adjustment and peer interaction have been observed to be altered in children with congenital heart disease. In a study by Youssef (1988), school absenteeism was high in these children and was proportional to the severity of their disease. It has been observed that a child's adjustment to school is affected more by the strain on the family than the child's physical limitations related to the congenital heart disease (Casey et al., 1996). Teachers have noted that children with congenital heart disease had more school problems, and more behavior problems were observed in boys. Children with more behavior problems had a lower self-esteem and more depression (Youssef, 1988). After surgical intervention, some of these problems may be alleviated; the child should miss less school and have an improved physical status and an increased activity level (Linde et al., 1970). Children may need rehabilitation after surgical repair, however, to teach them how much they are capable of doing and to help them deal with any functional limitations or inability to perform a task.

Surgical intervention that corrects a cyanotic defect plays an important role in the child's development. Improvement in IQ has been reported after surgery (Linde et al., 1970; O'Dougharty et al., 1985). The intellectual development was essentially normal in children after the Fontan operation (Uzark et al., 1998). Self-confidence, social confidence, and general adjustment have also improved after surgery (Linde et al., 1970). A significant improvement in self-perception was observed in children after they had their heart defect repaired (Wray & Sensky, 1998). If decreased experiences are a factor in developmental performance, a child who is no longer limited by disease should develop more normally.

Parental overprotectiveness can continue to prove more limiting to a child's development than the defect itself. Parents were found to underestimate their child's exercise tolerance in 80% of the cases studied by Casey and associates (1994). Parental restriction generally begins with the advice of the physician and proceeds from there (Clare, 1985; Kong et al., 1986). Social and emotional maladjustment in children with cardiac disease can be due to maternal maladjustment and guilt (Kong et al., 1986). Psychosocial or therapy intervention by professionals could be beneficial to preserving a more normal parent-child interaction. Some improvement in maternal interaction and attitude has been noted after surgical correction of the child's cardiac defect (O'Dougharty et al., 1985). In contrast to these reports is a study by Laane and associates (1997), which found that children with congenital heart defects reported a higher quality of life than healthy children.

ADOLESCENCE

Adolescents who have congenital heart disease and physical limitations show increased feelings of anxiety and impulsiveness (Kramer et al., 1989). Early professional intervention to assist the parents and child to cope best with the child's physical limitations may be helpful.

A delay in the onset of puberty in adolescents with congenital heart disease may further complicate their social development and participation. The body structure of the adolescent with congenital heart disease was found to be noticeably different from that of typical adolescents. The weight and height were significantly less with the presence of cardiac disease. Adolescents with heart disease had head, neck, and shoulder measurements similar to those of healthy adolescents, but the thorax, trunk, pelvis, and lower extremities were significantly smaller. The anterior-posterior diameter of the pelvis was so reduced that it appeared almost flat (Angelov et al., 1980). Physical differences of this magnitude can only make adolescents with heart disease feel even more different and intensify their low self-esteem.

Intervention that encourages the adolescent to participate in physical activities, including guidelines on how to participate, may improve peer interaction and ultimately self-esteem. Children who participated in an exercise program were observed to have improvement in their self-esteem, as well as in their strength. Parents were found to be less restrictive and had less anxiety about their child after a formal exercise program (Donovan et al., 1983).

Physical activity is important for all children, including children with congenital heart disease. The defect and surgical intervention, as well as possible alterations in response to exercise, must be understood before prescribing an exercise program for a child with congenital heart disease. The American Heart Association has published an extensive review of exercise testing in the pediatric age group, including recommendations for those with various congenital heart defects (James et al., 1982).

Cardiac rehabilitation programs for children with cardiac disease have shown significant and beneficial changes in hemodynamics and improvement in exercise endurance and tolerance (Balfour et al., 1991; Bar-Or, 1985; Goldberg et al., 1981; Koch et al., 1988; Mathews et al., 1983; Perrault & Drblik, 1989; Ruttenberg et al., 1983). Improvement from physical training allowed adolescents to function near typical activity levels (Goldberg et al., 1981). A recent study testing exercise tolerance in children 10 years after arterial switch procedure demonstrated an excellent long-term exercise capacity (Hovels-Gurich et al., 2003). The psychologic improvements were as noticeable and important as the physical improvements (Donovan et al., 1983; Koch et al., 1988; Mathews et al., 1983).

Adolescents who have undergone heart transplantation are able to achieve an increase in cardiac output in response to exercise; however, they do not achieve the same peak workloads or maximal oxygen consumption as do typical adolescents (Christos et al., 1992). During the early phase of rehabilitation, many children with transplanted hearts, lungs, or heart-lungs are so debilitated that they are unable to perform at an intensity that would raise their heart rate. The dyspnea index used as part of the Stanford heart transplant protocol is helpful in monitoring the child's physical tolerance during activity (Sadowsky et al., 1986). The child counts out loud to 15. The goal initially is to attempt to do this on one breath. At first, it may take three breaths to count to 15 while at rest. Exercise should increase the number of breaths to reach the count of 15 by only one or two breaths and should not be resumed until return to resting baseline. Most children progress quickly, usually reaching 15 on one breath within 1 week of beginning exercise. The dyspnea index is an easily used measure for self-monitoring of exercise tolerance at home (Johnson, 1991).

The patient who has had a heart-lung transplant also has an increased ventilatory response to exercise (Banner et al., 1988, 1989; Sciurba et al., 1988). The dyspnea index is again useful with these patients. Heart, heart-lung, and lung transplant recipients have experienced marked rehabilitation after transplantation (Bolman et al., 1991). The authors have found it highly beneficial for adolescents to be enrolled in a formal rehabilitation program after transplant to change their lifestyle, as well as condition them. The quality of life improves, with most children functioning at an age-appropriate level without developmental delays (Dunn et al., 1987; Lawrence & Fricker, 1987; Niset et al., 1988).

SUMMARY

This review of congenital heart defects, surgical and therapeutic intervention, and developmental consequences provides therapists with a foundation for working with this patient population. As surgical intervention occurs earlier and corrective techniques are performed sooner, it will be increasingly important to examine and monitor developmental progression. Children with congenital heart defects cannot be made to perform a developmental task that they do not have the energy to perform. The physical therapist plays an integral role in the habilitation and rehabilitation of children with congenital heart disease. A major part of this role involves parent education concerning typical developmental sequences in children with cardiac conditions and appropriate parent-child interaction.

CASE STUDY

The following case study describes a typical course of surgeries, with complications that resolved, in a child with cyanotic heart disease.

DAVID

David was born with severe cyanotic congenital heart disease. He was diagnosed with total anomalous pulmonary venous return, transposition of the great arteries, hypoplastic left ventricle syndrome, atrioventricular septal defect, and pulmonary atresia. He had two surgeries performed within the first month of life. At 10 days of age, he had ligation of the ductus arteriosus and a modified BT shunt. At 4 weeks of age, he required repair of his right pulmonary artery. Then, at 4 months of age, he underwent surgery to repair his total anomalous pulmonary venous return. After this surgery, it took approximately 4 weeks to wean him from the ventilator, owing to a left phrenic nerve palsy. He was discharged to home on nasogastric feedings, which continued until he was 1 year old. He advanced from nasogastric feedings to baby food and liquid from a "tippy" cup.

David experienced some delay in achieving developmental milestones. He sat independently at 9 months of age. At 16 months of age, David had a bidirectional Glenn procedure and his BT shunt taken down. He did well after this surgery and was discharged to home within 1 week of his surgery date. He developed well over the next 18 months, with marked improvement in his activity level. For instance, David crawled at 17 months of age and then walked at 19 months.

At 3 years of age, David had a Fontan procedure performed, which he tolerated well until seizures occurred on the third postoperative day. A computed tomography scan revealed a right frontal lobe infarct, and increased tone and briskness of reflexes were noted on his left side. He was irritable and difficult to console. Initially, David demonstrated left-sided neglect and a decrease in his protective reactions to the left. Within 1 week, his tone was only minimally increased and he was able to use his left extremities with cueing. Within 2 weeks, his protective reactions were symmetric, and he was shifting his weight and using either extremity readily. His ambulation was typical of a child after surgery, with slight balance problems and the use of a wide base of support. He did have difficulty coming to a standing position from sitting without support, which resolved within 4 weeks.

David's parents are attentive and recognize tasks that are difficult for him. They have continued home exercises to encourage use of his left extremities and have had better cooperation from him than have the therapists. He continued to be followed for reexamination several times a year to monitor his progress and update his home program.

Four years later, David goes to school every day and does well. His overall endurance and risk taking are less than his peers, but generally he gets along well.

REFERENCES

Aisenberg, RB, Rosenthal, A, Nadas, AS, & Wolff, PH. Developmental delay in infants with congenital heart disease. Pediatric Cardiology, 3:133–137, 1982.

Ali, J, Weisel, RD, Layug, AB, Kripke, BJ, & Hechtman, HB. Consequences of postoperative alterations in respiratory mechanics. American Journal of Surgery, 128:376–382, 1974.

Amitia, Y, Blieden, L, Shemtove, A, & Neufeld, H. Cerebrovascular accidents in infants and children with congenital cyanotic heart disease. Israel Journal of Medical Sciences, 20:1143–1145, 1984.

Angelov, G, Tomova, S, & Ninova, P. Physical development and body structure of children with congenital heart disease. Human Biology, 52:413–421, 1980.

Arciniegas, E. Ventricular septal defect. In Baue, AE, Geha, AS, Hammond, GL, Laks, H, & Naunheim, KS (Eds.). Glenn's Thoracic and Cardiovascular Surgery, 5th ed. Norwalk, CT: Appleton & Lange, 1991, pp. 1007–1016.

Asantila, R, Rosenburg, PH, & Scheinin, B. Comparison of different methods of postoperative analgesia after thoracotomy. Acta Anaesthesiologica Scandinavica, 30:421–425, 1986.

Austin, EH, III, Edmonds, HL, Jr, Auden, SM, Seremet, V, Niznik, G, Sehic, A, Sowell, MK, Cheppo, CD, & Corlett, KM. Benefit of neurophysiologic monitoring for pediatric cardiac surgery. Journal of Thoracic and Cardiovascular Surgery, 114(5):707–717, 1997.

Aziz, S, & Jamieson, S. Combined heart and lung transplantation. In Baue, AE, Geha, AS, Hammond, GL, Laks, H, & Naunheim, KS (Eds.). Glenn's Thoracic and Cardiovascular Surgery, 5th ed. Norwalk, CT: Appleton & Lange, 1991, pp. 1623–1638.

Bailey, LL, Assaad, AN, Trimm, RF, Nehlsen-Cannarella, SL, Kanakriyeh, MS, Haas, GS, & Jacobson, JG. Orthotopic transplantation during early infancy as therapy for incurable congenital heart disease. Annals of Surgery, 203:279–285, 1988.

Bailey, LL, & Gundry, SR. Hypoplastic left heart syndrome. In Gillette, PC (Ed.). The Pediatric Clinics of North America. Philadelphia: WB Saunders, 1990, pp. 137–150.

Balfour, IC, Drimmer, AM, Nouri, S, Pennington, DG, Hemkins, CL, & Harvey, LL. Pediatric cardiac rehabilitation. American Journal of Diseases of Children, 145:627–630, 1991.

Banasik, JL, Bruya, MA, Steadman, RE, & Demand, JK. Effect of position on arterial oxygenation in postoperative coronary revascularization patients. Heart and Lung, 16:652–657, 1987.

Banner, N, Guz, A, Heaton, R, Innes, JA, Murphy, K, & Yacoub, M. Ventilatory and circulatory responses at the onset of exercise in man following heart or heart-lung transplantation. Journal of Physiology, 399:437–449, 1988.

Banner, NR, Lloyd, MH, Hamilton, RD, Innes, JA, Guz, A, & Yacoub, MH. Cardiopulmonary response to dynamic exercise after heart

and combined heart-lung transplantation. British Heart Journal, 61:215–223, 1989.

Bar-Or, O. Physical conditioning in children with cardiorespiratory disease. In Terjung, RL (Ed.). Exercise and Sport Science Review. New York: Macmillan, 1985, pp. 305–334.

Bartlett, RH. Pulmonary pathophysiology in surgical patients. Surgical Clinics of North America, 60:1323–1338, 1980.

Bartlett, RH. Respiratory therapy to prevent pulmonary complications of surgery. Respiratory Care, 29:667–677, 1984.

Bartlett, RH, Brennan, ML, Gazzaniga, AB, & Hanson, EL. Studies on the pathogenesis and prevention of postoperative pulmonary complications. Surgery, Gynecology and Obstetrics, 137:925–933, 1973a.

Bartlett, RH, Gazzaniga, AB, & Geraghty, TR. Respiratory maneuvers to prevent postoperative pulmonary complications. Journal of the American Medical Association, 224:1017–1021, 1973b.

Bauer, J, Dapper, F, Kroll, J, Hagel, KJ, Thul, J, & Zickmann, B. Heart transplantation in infants—Experience at the children's heart center in Giessen. Zeitschrift fur Kardiologie, 87:209–217, 1998.

Bellinger, DC, Rappaport, LA, Wypij, D, Wernovsky, G, & Newburger, JW. Patterns of developmental dysfunction after surgery during infancy to correct transposition of the great arteries. Journal of Developmental and Behavioral Pediatrics, 18:75–83, 1997.

Blackwood, MJ, Haka-Ikse, K, & Steward, DJ. Developmental outcome in children undergoing surgery with profound hypothermia. Anesthesiology, 65:437–440, 1986.

Bolman, RM, Shumway, SS, Estrin, JA, & Hertz, MI. Lung and heart-lung transplantation. Annals of Surgery, 214:456–470, 1991.

Bonser, RS, & Jamieson, SW. Heart-lung transplantation. Clinics in Chest Medicine, 11:235–246, 1990.

Bott, J, Keilty, SE, Brown, A, & Ward, EM. Nasal intermittent positive pressure ventilation. Physiotherapy, 78:93–96, 1992.

Boutros, AR. Arterial blood oxygenation during and after endotracheal suctioning in the apneic patient. Anesthesiology, 32:114–118, 1970.

Bove, EL. Transplantation after first-stage reconstruction for hypoplastic left heart syndrome. Annals of Thoracic Surgery, 52:701–707, 1991.

Bruning, MD, & Schneiderman, JU. Heart failure in infants and children. In Michaelson, CR (Ed.). Congestive Heart Failure. St. Louis: Mosby, 1983, pp. 467–484.

Byrum, CJ, Dick, M, Behrendt, DM, & Rosenthal, A. Repair of total anomalous pulmonary venous connection in patients younger than 6 months old. Circulation, 66(suppl I):208–214, 1982.

Callow, LB. A new beginning: Nursing care of the infant undergoing the arterial switch operation for transposition of the great arteries. Heart and Lung, 18:248–257, 1989.

Casey, FA, Craig, BG, & Mulholland, HC. Quality of life in surgically palliated complex congenital heart disease. Archives of Disease in Childhood, 70:382–386, 1994.

Casey, FA, Sykes, DH, Craig, BG, Power, R, & Mulholland, HC. Behavioral adjustment of children with surgically palliated complex congenital heart disease. Journal of Pediatric Psychology, 21:335–352,1996.

Chang, RK, Chen, AY, & Klitzner, TS. Clinical management of infants with hypoplastic left heart syndrome in the United States, 1988–1997. Pediatrics, 110:292–298, 2002.

Cho JM, Puga, FJ, Danielson, GK, Dearani, JA, Mair, DD, Hagler, DJ, Julsrud, PR, & Ilstrup, DM. Early and long-term results of the surgical treatment of tetralogy of Fallot with pulmonary atresia, with or without major aortopulmonary collateral arteries. Journal of Thoracic Cardiovascular Surgery, 124:70–81, 2002.

Christos, SC, Katch, V, Crowley, DC, Eakin, BL, Lindauer, AL, & Beekman, RH. Hemodynamic responses to upright exercise of adolescent cardiac transplant patients. Journal of Pediatrics, *121*:312–316, 1992.

Chulay, M, Brown, J, & Summer, W. Effect of postoperative immobilization after coronary artery bypass surgery. Critical Care Medicine, *10*:176–179, 1982.

Clare, MD. Home care of infants and children with cardiac disease. Heart and Lung, *14*:218–222, 1985.

Clarke, CF, Beall, MH, & Perloff, JK. Genetics, epidemiology, counseling, and prevention. In Perloff, JK, & Child, JS (Eds.). Congenital Heart Disease in Adults. Philadelphia: WB Saunders, 1991, pp. 141–165.

Clough, P. The denervated heart. Clinical Management, *10*:14–17, 1990.

Crane, LD. The neonate and child. In Frownfelter, DL (Ed.). Chest Physical Therapy and Pulmonary Rehabilitation. Chicago: Year Book, 1987, pp. 666–697.

Cullen, SM, Cronk, CE, Pueschel, SM, Schnell, RR, & Reed, RB. Social development and feeding milestones of young Down syndrome children. American Journal of Mental Deficiency, *85*:410–415, 1981.

Davies, H, Kitchman, R, Gordon, I, & Helms, P. Regional ventilation in infancy. New England Journal of Medicine, *313*:1626–1628, 1985.

Dean, E. Effect of body position on pulmonary function. Physical Therapy, *65*:613–618, 1985.

de Leval, MR. Senning operation. In Baue, AE, Geha, AS, Hammond, GL, Laks, H, & Naunheim, KS (Eds.). Glenn's Thoracic and Cardiovascular Surgery, 5th ed. Norwalk, CT: Appleton & Lange, 1991, pp. 1211–1216.

DeMaso, DR, Campis, LK, Wypij, D, Bertram, S, Lipshitz, M, & Freed, M. The impact of maternal perceptions and medical severity on the adjustment of children with congenital heart disease. Journal of Pediatric Psychology, *16*:137–149, 1991.

Donovan, EF, Mathews, RA, Nixon, PA, Stephenson, RJ, Robertson, RJ, Dean, F, Fricker, FJ, Beerman, LB, & Fischer, DR. An exercise program for pediatric patients with congenital heart disease: Psychological aspects. Journal of Cardiac Rehabilitation, *3*:476–480, 1983.

Dull, JL, & Dull, WL. Are maximal inspiratory breathing exercises or incentive spirometry better than early mobilization after cardiopulmonary bypass? Physical Therapy, *63*:655–659, 1983.

Dunn, JM, Cavarocchi, NC, Balsara, RK, Kolff, J, McClurken, J, Badellino, MM, Vieweg, C, & Donner, RM. Pediatric heart transplantation, at St. Christopher's Hospital for Children. Journal of Heart Transplantation, *6*:334–342, 1987.

duPlessis, AJ. Neurologic complications of cardiac disease in the newborn. Clinics in Perinatology, *24*:807–825, 1997.

duPlessis, AJ, Chang, AC, Wessel, DL, Lock, JE, Wernovsky, G, Newburger, JW, & Mayer, JE, Jr. Cerebrovascular accidents following the Fontan operation. Pediatric Neurology, *12*:230–236, 1995.

Egbert, LD, & Bendixon, HH. Effect of morphine on breathing pattern. Journal of the American Medical Association, *188*:485–488, 1964.

Feldt, RH, Ewert, JC, Stickler, GB, & Weidman, WH. Children with congenital heart disease. American Journal of Diseases of Children, *117*:281–287, 1969.

Fenton, KN, Webber, SA, Danford, DA, Ghandi, SK, Periera, J, & Pigula, FA. Long-term survival after pediatric cardiac transplantation and postoperative ECMO support. Annals of Thoracic Surgery, *76*:843–847, 2003.

Ferry, PC. Neurologic sequelae of open-heart surgery in children. American Journal of Diseases of Children, *144*:369–373, 1990.

Fox, MD, & Molesky, MG. The effects of prone and supine positioning on arterial oxygen pressure. Neonatal Network, *8*:25–29, 1990.

Fox, WW, Schwartz, JG, & Shaffer, TH. Pulmonary physiotherapy in neonates: Physiologic changes and respiratory management. Journal of Pediatrics, *92*:977–981, 1978.

Fricker, FJ, Trento, A, & Griffith, BP. Pediatric cardiac transplantation. In Brest, AN (Ed.). Cardiovascular Clinics. Philadelphia: FA Davis, 1990, pp. 223–235.

Gamsu, G, Singer, MM, Vincent, HH, Berry, S, & Nadel, JA. Postoperative impairment of mucous transport in the lung. American Review of Respiratory Disease, *114*:673–679, 1976.

Gardner, FV, Freeman, NH, Black, AM, & Angelini, GD. Disturbed mother-infant interaction in association with congenital heart disease. Heart, *76*:56–59, 1996.

Garson, A, Gillette, PC, Gutgesell, HP, & McNamara, DG. Stress-induced ventricular arrhythmia after repair of tetralogy of Fallot. American Journal of Cardiology, *46*:1006–1012, 1980.

Giboney, GS. Ventricular septal defect. Heart and Lung, *12*:292–299, 1983.

Gingell, RL, & Hornung, MG. Growth problems associated with congenital heart disease in infancy. In Lebenthal, E (Ed.). Textbook of Gastroenterology and Nutrition in Infancy, 2nd ed. New York: Raven Press, 1989, pp. 639–649.

Girlando, RM, Belew, B, & Klara, F. Coarctation of the aorta. Critical Care Nurse, *8*:38–50, 1988.

Glanville, AR, Baldwin, JC, Hunt, SA, & Theodore, J. Long-term cardiopulmonary function after human heart-lung transplantation. Australian and New Zealand Journal of Medicine, *20*:208–214, 1990.

Glanville, AR, Gabb, GM, Theodore, J, & Robin, ED. Bronchial responsiveness to exercise after human cardiopulmonary transplantation. Chest, *96*:281–286, 1989.

Goldberg, B, Fripp, RR, Lister, G, Loke, J, Nicholas, JA, & Talner, NS. Effect of physical training on exercise performance of children following surgical repair of congenital heart disease. Pediatrics, *68*:691–699, 1981.

Goldberg, CS, Schwartz, EM, Brunberg, JA, Mosca, RS, Bove, EL, Schork, MA, Stetz, SP, Cheatham, JP, & Kulik, TJ. Neurodevelopmental outcome of patients after the Fontan operation. A comparison between children with hypoplastic left heart syndrome and other functional single ventricle lesions. Journal of Pediatrics, *137*:646–652, 2000.

Goldberg, S, Simmons, RJ, Newman J, Campbell, K, & Fowler, RS. Congenital heart disease, parental stress, and infant-mother relationships. Journal of Pediatrics, *119*:661–666, 1991.

Goldberg, S, Washington, J, Morris, P, Fischer-Fay, A, & Simmons, RJ. Early diagnosed chronic illness and mother-child relationships in the first two years. Canadian Journal of Psychiatry, *55*:726–733, 1990.

Graham, TP, Bender, HW, & Spach, MS. Ventricular septal defect. In Adams, FH, Emmanouilides, GC, & Riemen Schneider, TA (Eds.). Moss's Heart Disease in Infants, Children, and Adolescents. Baltimore: Williams & Wilkins, 1989, pp. 189–208.

Griffith, BP, Hardesy, RL, Trento, A, Paradis, IL, Duquesnoy, RJ, Zeevi, A, Dauber, JH, Dummer, JS, Thompson, ME, Gryzan, S, & Bahnson, HT. Heart-lung transplantation: Lessons learned and future hopes. Annals of Thoracic Surgery, *43*:6–16, 1987.

Gudermuth, S. Mothers' reports of early experiences of infants with congenital heart disease. Maternal-Child Nursing Journal, *4*:155–164, 1975.

Haas, GS, Bailey, L, & Pennington, DG. Pediatric cardiac transplantation. In Baue, AE, Geha, AS, Hammond, GL, Laks, H, & Naunheim, KS (Eds.). Glenn's Thoracic and Cardiovascular Surgery, 5th ed. Norwalk, CT: Appleton & Lange, 1991, pp. 1297–1317.

Haka-Ikse, K, Blackwood, MA, & Steward, DJ. Psychomotor development of infants and children after profound hypothermia during surgery for congenital heart disease. Developmental Medicine and Child Neurology, *20*:62–70, 1978.

Hammon, JW, & Bender, HW. Anomalous venous connection: Pulmonary and systemic. In Baue, AE, Geha, AS, Hammond, GL, Laks, H, & Naunheim, KS (Eds.). Glenn's Thoracic and Cardiovascular Surgery, 5th ed. Norwalk, CT: Appleton & Lange, 1991, pp. 971–993.

Haneda, K, Itoh, T, Togo, T, Ohmi, M, & Mohri, H. Effects of cardiac surgery on intellectual function in infants and children. Cardiovascular Surgery, 4(3):303–307, 1996.

Hines, MH, Raines, KH, Payne, RM, Covitz, W, Cnota, JF, Smith, TE, O'Brian, JJ, & Ririe, DG. Video-assisted ductal ligation in premature infants. Annals of Thoracic Surgery, 76:1417–1420, 2003.

Hoffman, JI, & Kaplan, S. The incidence of congenital heart disease. Journal of the American College of Cardiology, 39:1890–1900, 2002.

Holden, KR, Sessions, JC, Cure, J, Whitcom, DS, & Sade, RM. Neurologic outcomes in children with post-pump choreoathetosis. Journal of Pediatrics, 132:162–164, 1998.

Hovels-Gurich HH, Kunz D, Seghaye M, Miskova M, Messmer BJ, & von Bermuth G. Acta Paediatrica, 92:190–196, 2003.

Huckabay, L, & Daderian, AD. Effect of choices on breathing exercises post-open heart surgery. Dimensions in Critical Care Nursing, 9:190–201, 1990.

Huddleston, CB, Bloch, JB, Sweet, SC, de la Morena, M, Patterson, GA, & Mendeloff, EN. Lung transplantation in children. Annals of Surgery, 236:270–276, 2002.

Hussey, J. Effects of chest physiotherapy for children in intensive care after surgery. Physiotherapy, 78:109–113, 1992.

Hutter, JA, Despins, P, Higenbottam, T, Stewart, S, & Wallwork, J. Heart-lung transplantation: Better use of resources. American Journal of Medicine, 85:4–11, 1988.

Imle, PC. Percussion and vibration. In MacKenzie, CF, Ciesla, N, Imle, PC, & Klemic, N (Eds.). Chest Physiotherapy in the Intensive Care Unit. Baltimore: Williams & Wilkins, 1981, pp. 81–91.

Jacobs, JP, Giroud, JM, Quintessenza, JA, Morell, VO, Botero, LM, van Gelder, HM, Badhwar, V, & Burke, RP. The modern approach to patent ductus arteriosus treatment: Complementary roles of video-assisted thoracoscopic surgery and interventional cardiology coil occlusion. Annals of Thoracic Surgery, 76:1421–1428, 2003.

James, FW, Blomqvist, CG, Freed, MD, Miller, WW, Moller, JH, Nugent, EW, Riopel, DA, Strong, WB, & Wessel, HU. Standards for exercise testing in the pediatric age group. Circulation, 66:1377A–1397A, 1982.

Jamieson, SW, Stinson, EB, Oyer, PE, Reitz, BA, Baldwin, J, Modry, D, Dawkins, K, Theodore, J, Hunt, S, & Shumway, NE. Heart-lung transplantation for irreversible pulmonary hypertension. Annals of Thoracic Surgery, 38:554–562, 1984.

Jarmakani, JM, & Canent, RV. Preoperative and postoperative right ventricular function in children with transposition of the great vessels. Circulation, 50(suppl II):39–45, 1974.

Johnson, AB, & Davis, JS. Treatment options for the neonate with hypoplastic left heart syndrome. Journal of Perinatal and Neonatal Nursing, 5:84–92, 1991.

Johnson, BA. Postoperative physical therapy in the pediatric cardiac surgery patient. Pediatric Physical Therapy, 2:14–22, 1991.

Kent, KM, & Cooper, T. The denervated heart: A model for studying autonomic control of the heart. New England Journal of Medicine, 291:1017–1021, 1974.

Koch, BM, Galioto, FM, Vaccaro, P, Vaccaro, J, & Buckenmeyer, PJ. Flexibility and strength measures in children participating in a cardiac rehabilitation exercise program. Physician and Sports Medicine, 116:139–147, 1988.

Kolovos, NS, Bratton, SL, Moler, FW, Bove, EL, Ohye, RG, Bartlett, RH, & Kulik, TJ. Outcome of pediatric patients treated with extracorporeal life support after cardiac surgery. Annals of Thoracic Surgery, 76:1435–1442, 2003.

Kong, SG, Tay, JS, Yip, WC, & Chay, SO. Emotional and social effects of congenital heart disease in Singapore. Australian Paediatric Journal, 22:101–106, 1986.

Kopf, GS, & Laks, H. Atrial septal defects and cor triatriatum. In Baue, AE, Geha, AS, Hammond, GL, Laks, H, & Naunheim, KS (Eds.). Glenn's Thoracic and Cardiovascular Surgery, 5th ed. Norwalk, CT: Appleton & Lange, 1991, pp. 995–1005.

Kramer, HH, Aswiszus, D, Sterzel, U, van Halteren, A, & Clafen, R. Development of personality and intelligence in children with congenital heart disease. Journal of Child Psychiatry, 30:299–308, 1989.

Krastins, IR, Corey, ML, McLeod, A, Edmonds, J, Levison, H, & Moles, F. An evaluation of incentive spirometry in the management of pulmonary complications after cardiac surgery in a pediatric population. Critical Care Medicine, 10:525–528, 1982.

Kriett, JM, & Kaye, MP. The registry of the International Society for Heart and Lung Transplantation: Eighth official report, 1991. Journal of Heart and Lung Transplantation, 10:491–498, 1991.

Laane, KM, Meberg, A, Otterstad, JE, Froland, G, & Sorland, S. Quality of life in children with congenital heart defects. Acta Paediatrica, 86:975–980, 1997.

Laks, H, & Breda, MA. Tetralogy of Fallot. In Baue, AE, Geha, AS, Hammond, GL, Laks, H, & Naunheim, KS (Eds.). Glenn's Thoracic and Cardiovascular Surgery, 5th ed. Norwalk, CT: Appleton & Lange, 1991a, pp. 1179–1201.

Laks, H, & Breda, MA. Tricuspid atresia. In Baue, AE, Geha, AS, Hammond, GL, Laks, H, & Naunheim, KS (Eds.). Glenn's Thoracic and Cardiovascular Surgery, 5th ed. Norwalk, CT: Appleton & Lange, 1991b, pp. 1259–1272.

Lawrence, KS, & Fricker, FJ. Pediatric heart transplantation: Quality of life. Journal of Heart Transplantation, 6:329–333, 1987.

Levitsky, S, & del Nido, P. Patent ductus arteriosus and aortopulmonary septal defects. In Baue, AE, Geha, AS, Hammond, GL, Laks, H, & Naunheim, KS (Eds.). Glenn's Thoracic and Cardiovascular Surgery, 5th ed. Norwalk, CT: Appleton & Lange, 1991, pp. 1017–1025.

Limperopoulos, C, Majnemer, A, Shevell, MI, Rosenblatt, B, Rohlicke, C, Tchervenkov, C, & Darwish, HZ. Functional limitations in young children with congenital heart defects after cardiac surgery. Pediatrics, 108:1325–1331, 2001.

Linde, LM, Rasof, B, & Dunn, OJ. Longitudinal studies of intellectual and behavioral development in children with congenital heart disease. Acta Paediatrica, 59:169–176, 1970.

Lloyd, TR. Prognosis of the hypoplastic left heart syndrome. Progress in Pediatric Cardiology, 5:57–64, 1996.

Locke, TJ, Griffiths, TC, Mould, H, & Gibson, GJ. Rib cage mechanics after median sternotomy. Thorax, 45:465–468, 1990.

Loeffel, M. Developmental considerations of infants and children with congenital heart disease. Heart and Lung, 14:214–217, 1985.

Mahle WT, & Wernovsky G. Long-term developmental outcome of children with complex congenital heart disease. Clinics in Perinatology, 28:235–247, 2001.

Markland, ON, Moorthy, SS, Mahomed, Y, King, RD, & Brown, JW. Postoperative phrenic nerve palsy in patients with open-heart surgery. Annals of Thoracic Surgery, 39:68–73, 1985.

Massery, M. Respiratory rehabilitation secondary to neurological deficits: Treatment techniques. In Frownfelter, DL (Ed.). Chest Physical Therapy and Pulmonary Rehabilitation. Chicago: Year Book, 1987, pp. 538–544.

Mathew, OP. Respiratory control during nipple feeding in pre-term infants. Pediatric Pulmonology, 5:220–224, 1988.

Mathew, OP, Clark, ML, Pronske, ML, Luna-Solarzano, HG, & Peterson, MD. Breathing pattern and ventilation during oral feeding in term newborn infants. Journal of Pediatrics, 106:810–813, 1985.

Mathews, RA, Nixon, PA, Stephenson, RJ, Robertson, RJ, Donovan, EF, Dean, F, Fricker, FJ, Beerman, LB, & Fischer, DR. An exercise program for pediatric patients with congenital heart disease: Organizational and physiologic aspects. Journal of Cardiac Rehabilitation, 3:467–475, 1983.

McWilliams, BC. Mechanical ventilation in pediatric patients. Clinics in Chest Medicine, 8:597–607, 1987.

Mee, RB. Current status of cardiac surgery in childhood. Progress in Pediatric Surgery, 27:148–169, 1991.

Messmer, BJ, Schallberger, Y, Gattiker, R, & Senning, A. Psychomotor and intellectual development after deep hypothermia and circulatory arrest in early infancy. Journal of Thoracic and Cardiovascular Surgery, 72:495–501, 1976.

Milgalter, E, & Laks, H. Truncus arteriosus. In Baue, AE, Geha, AS, Hammond, GL, Laks, H, & Naunheim, KS (Eds.). Glenn's Thoracic and Cardiovascular Surgery, 5th ed. Norwalk, CT: Appleton & Lange, 1991, pp. 1079–1987.

Morriss, JH, & McNamara, DG. Residua, sequelae and complications of surgery for congenital heart disease. Progress in Cardiovascular Diseases, 18:1–25, 1975.

Moulton, AL, & Malm, JR. Pulmonary stenosis, pulmonary atresia, single pulmonary artery and aneurysm of the pulmonary artery. In Baue, AE, Geha, AS, Hammond, GL, Laks, H, & Naunheim, KS (Eds.). Glenn's Thoracic and Cardiovascular Surgery, 5th ed. Norwalk, CT: Appleton & Lange, 1991, pp. 1131–1163.

Nakazawa, M, Okuda, H, Imai, Y, Takanashi, Y, & Takao, A. Right and left ventricular volume characteristics after external conduit repair (Rastelli procedure) for cyanotic congenital heart disease. Heart and Vessels, 2:106–110, 1986.

Niset, G, Coustry-Degre, C, & Degre, S. Psychosocial and physical rehabilitation after heart transplantation: 1-year follow-up. Cardiology, 75:311–317, 1988.

Noonan, JA. Syndromes associated with cardiac defects. In Engle, MA (Ed.). Pediatric Cardiovascular Disease. Philadelphia: FA Davis, 1981, pp. 97–115.

Norwood, SH, & Civette, JM. Ventilatory assistance and support. In Baue, AE, Geha, AS, Hammond, GL, Laks, H, & Naunheim, KS (Eds.). Glenn's Thoracic and Cardiovascular Surgery, 5th ed. Norwalk, CT: Appleton & Lange, 1991, pp. 45–66.

Norwood, WI. Hypoplastic left heart syndrome. Annals of Thoracic Surgery, 52:688–695, 1991a.

Norwood, WI. Hypoplastic left heart syndrome. In Baue, AE, Geha, AS, Hammond, GL, Laks, H, & Naunheim, KS (Eds.). Glenn's Thoracic and Cardiovascular Surgery, 5th ed. Norwalk, CT: Appleton & Lange, 1991b, pp. 1123–1130.

O'Dougharty, M, Wright, FS, Loewenson, RB, & Torres, F. Cerebral dysfunction after chronic hypoxia in children. Neurology, 35:42–46, 1985.

Ohye, RG, & Bove, EL. Advances in congenital heart surgery. Current Opinion in Pediatrics, 13:473–481, 2001.

Page, GG. Tetralogy of Fallot. Heart and Lung, 15:390–400, 1986.

Pairolero, PC, & Payne, WS. Postoperative care and complications in the thoracic surgery patient. In Baue, AE, Geha, AS, Hammond, GL, Laks, H, & Naunheim, KS (Eds.). Glenn's Thoracic and Cardiovascular Surgery, 5th ed. Norwalk, CT: Appleton & Lange, 1991, pp. 31–43.

Peetz, DJ, Spicer, RL, Crowley, DC, Sloan, H, & Behrendt, DM. Correction of truncus arteriosus in the neonate using a nonvalved conduit. Journal of Thoracic and Cardiovascular Surgery, 83:743–746, 1982.

Pennington, DG, Noedel, N, McBride, LR, Naunheim, KS, & Ring, WS. Heart transplantation in children: An international survey. Annals of Thoracic Surgery, 52:710–715, 1991.

Perrault, H, & Drblik, SP. Exercise after surgical repair of congenital cardiac lesions. Sports Medicine, 7:18–31, 1989.

Peters, RM. Pulmonary physiologic studies of the perioperative period. Chest, 76:576–585, 1979.

Prakanrattana, U, Valairucha, S, Sriyoschati, S, Pornvilawan, S, & Phanchaipetch, T. Early extubation following open heart surgery in pediatric patients with congenital heart diseases. Journal of the Medical Association of Thailand, 80:87–95, 1997.

Puga, FJ. Surgical treatment of pulmonary atresia with ventricular septal defect. In Baue, AE, Geha, AS, Hammond, GL, Laks, H, & Naunheim, KS (Eds.). Glenn's Thoracic and Cardiovascular Surgery, 5th ed. Norwalk, CT: Appleton & Lange, 1991, pp. 1165–1177.

Rasof, B, Linde, LM, & Dunn, OJ. Intellectual development in children with congenital heart disease. Child Development, 38:1043–1053, 1967.

Razzouk, AJ, Chinnock, RE, Gundry, SR, & Bailey, LL. Cardiac transplantation for infants with hypoplastic left heart syndrome. Progress in Pediatric Cardiology, 5:37–47, 1996.

Reddy, SC, & Webber, SA. Pediatric heart and lung transplantation. Indian Journal of Pediatrics, 70:723–729, 2003.

Risser, NL: Preoperative and postoperative care to prevent pulmonary complications. Heart and Lung, 9:57–67, 1980.

Rockwell, GM, & Campbell, SK. Physical therapy program for the pediatric cardiac surgical patient. Physical Therapy, 56:670–675, 1976.

Roos-Hesselink, JW, Meijboom, FJ, Spitaels, SE, van Domburg, R, van Rijen, EH, Utens, EM, Bogers, AJ, & Simoons, ML. Excellent survival and low incidence of arrhythmias, stroke and heart failure long-term after surgical ASD closure at young age. A prospective follow-up study of 21–33 years. European Heart Journal, 24:190–197, 2003.

Rosen, M, & Hillard, EK. The effects of negative pressure during tracheal suction. Anesthesia and Analgesia, 41:50–57, 1962.

Rosenthal, A. Care of the postoperative child and adolescent with congenital heart disease. In Barness, LA (Ed.). Advances in Pediatrics. Chicago: Year Book, 1983, pp. 131–167.

Rossi, AF, Seiden, HS, Sadeghi, AM, Nguyen, KH, Quintana, CS, Gross, RP, & Griepp, RB. The outcome of cardiac operations in infants weighing two kilograms or less. Journal of Thoracic and Cardiovascular Surgery, 116:29–35, 1998.

Rubin, M. The physiology of bedrest. American Journal of Nursing, 88:50–56, 1988.

Russell, IA, Zwass, MS, Fineman, JR, Balea, M, Rouine-Rapp, K, Brook, M, Hanley, FL, Silverman, NH, & Cahalan, MK. The effects of inhaled nitric oxide on postoperative pulmonary hypertension in infants and children undergoing surgical repair of congenital heart disease. Anesthesia and Analgesia, 87:46–51, 1998.

Ruttenberg, HD, Adams, TD, Orsmond, GS, Conlee, RK, & Fisher, AG. Effects of exercise training on aerobic fitness in children after open heart surgery. Pediatric Cardiology, 4:19–24, 1983.

Sadowsky, HS, Rohrkemper, KF, & Quon, SYM. Rehabilitation of Cardiac and Cardiopulmonary Recipients. An Introduction for Physical and Occupational Therapists. Stanford, CA: Stanford University Hospital, 1986.

Scheidegger, D, Bentz, L, Piolino, G, Pusterla, C, & Gigon, JP. Influence of early mobilisation on pulmonary function in surgical patients. European Journal of Intensive Care Medicine, 2:35–40, 1976.

Sciurba, FC, Owens, GR, Sanders, MH, Bartley, BP, Hardesty, RL, Paradis, IL, & Costantino, JP. Evidence of an altered pattern of breathing during exercise in recipients of heart-lung transplants. New England Journal of Medicine, 319:1186–1192, 1988.

Settergren, G, Ohqvist, G, Lundberg, S, Henze, A, Bjork, VO, & Persson, B. Cerebral blood flow and cerebral metabolism in children following cardiac surgery with deep hypothermia and circulatory arrest. Clinical course and follow-up of psychomotor development. Scandinavian Journal of Thoracic Cardiovascular Surgery, 16:209–215, 1982.

Silbert, A, Wolff, PH, Mayer, B, Rosenthal, A, & Nadas, AS. Cyanotic heart disease and psychological development. Pediatrics, 43:192–200, 1969.

Starnes, VA, Marshall, SE, Lewiston, NJ, Theodore, J, Stinson, EB, & Shumway, NE. Heart-lung transplantation in infants, children, and adolescents. Journal of Pediatric Surgery, 26:434–438, 1991.

Starnes, VA, Oyer, PE, Bernstein, D, Baum, D, Gamberg, P, Miller, J, & Shumway, NE. Heart, heart-lung, and lung transplantation in the first year of life. Annals of Thoracic Surgery, 53:306–310, 1992.

Stretton, CD, Mak, JCW, Belvisi, MG, Yacoub, MH, & Barnes, PJ. Cholinergic control of human airways in vitro following extrinsic denervation of the human respiratory tract by heart-lung transplantation. American Review of Respiratory Disease, 142:1030–1033, 1990.

Suoninen, P. Physical growth of children with congenital heart disease. Acta Paediatrica Supplement, 225:7–50, 1971.

Thoren, L. Post-operative pulmonary complications. Acta Chirurgica Scandinavica, 107:193–205, 1954.

Todd, TR. Early postoperative management following lung transplantation. Clinics in Chest Medicine, 11:259–267, 1990.

Trittenwein, G, Nardi, A, Pansi, H, Golej, J, Burda, G, Hermon, M, Boigner, H, & Wollenek, G. Early postoperative prediction of cerebral damage after pediatric cardiac surgery. Annals of Thoracic Surgery, 76:576–580, 2003.

Trusler, GA. The Mustard procedure. In Baue, AE, Geha, AS, Hammond, GL, Laks, H, & Naunheim, KS (Eds.). Glenn's Thoracic and Cardiovascular Surgery, 5th ed. Norwalk, CT: Appleton & Lange, 1991, pp. 1203–1209.

Uretsky, BF. Physiology of the transplanted heart. In Brest, AN (Ed.). Cardiovascular Clinics. Philadelphia: FA Davis, 1990, pp. 23–55.

Uzark, L, Lincoln, A, Lamberti, JJ, Mainwaring, RD, Spicer, RL, & Moore, JW. Neurodevelopmental outcomes in children with Fontan repair of functional single ventricle. Pediatrics, 101:630–633, 1998.

van Breda, A. Postoperative care of infants and children who require cardiac surgery. Heart and Lung, 14:205–207, 1985.

Van De Water, JM, Watring, WG, Linton, LA, Murphy, M, & Byron, RL. Prevention of postoperative pulmonary complications. Surgery, Gynecology and Obstetrics, 135:229–233, 1972.

Vraciu, JK, & Vraciu, RA. Effectiveness of breathing exercises in preventing pulmonary complications following open heart surgery. Physical Therapy, 57:1367–1371, 1977.

Waldhausen, JA, Myers, JL, & Campbell, DB. Coarctation of the aorta and interrupted aortic arch. In Baue, AE, Geha, AS, Hammond, GL, Laks, H, & Naunheim, KS (Eds.). Glenn's Thoracic and Cardiovascular Surgery, 5th ed. Norwalk, CT: Appleton & Lange, 1991, pp. 1107–1122.

Ward, RJ, Danziger, F, Bonica, JJ, Allen, GD, & Bowes, J. An evaluation of postoperative maneuvers. Surgical Gynecology and Obstetrics, 66:51–54, 1966.

Warner, JO. Heart-lung transplantation: All the facts. Archives of Disease in Childhood, 66:1013–1017, 1991.

Webber, BA. Evaluation and inflation in respiratory care. Physiotherapy, 77:801–804, 1991.

Weinhaus, L, Canter, C, Noetzel, M, McAlister, W, & Spray, TL. Extracorporeal membrane oxygenation for circulatory support after repair of congenital heart defects. Annals of Thoracic Surgery, 48:206–212, 1989.

Weldon, CS, Behrendt, DM, & Haas, GS. Congenital malformations of the aortic valve and left ventricular outflow tract. In Baue, AE, Geha, AS, Hammond, GL, Laks, H, & Naunheim, KS (Eds.). Glenn's Thoracic and Cardiovascular Surgery, 5th ed. Norwalk, CT: Appleton & Lange, 1991, pp. 1089–1106.

Wells, FC, Coghill, S, Caplan, HL, & Lincoln, C. Duration of circulatory arrest does influence the psychological development of children after cardiac operation in early life. Journal of Thoracic and Cardiovascular Surgery, 86:823–831, 1983.

Whitehead, B, James, I, Helms, P, Scott, JP, Smyth, R, Higenbottam, TW, McGoldrick, J, English, TAH, Wallwork, J, Elliott, M, & de Leval, M. Intensive care management of children following heart and heart-lung transplantation. Intensive Care Medicine, 16:426–430, 1990.

Wilkinson, JL. Heart and heart/lung transplantation in children. Australian Paediatric Journal, 25:111–118, 1989.

Williams, WH. Rastelli's operation for "anatomic" repair of transposition of the great arteries with ventricular septal defect and left ventricular outflow tract obstruction. In Baue, AE, Geha, AS, Hammond, GL, Laks, H, & Naunheim, KS (Eds.). Glenn's Thoracic and Cardiovascular Surgery, 5th ed. Norwalk, CT: Appleton & Lange, 1991, pp. 1217–1226.

Wilson, RS. Anesthesia for thoracic surgery. In Baue, AE, Geha, AS, Hammond, GL, Laks, H, & Naunheim, KS (Eds.). Glenn's Thoracic and Cardiovascular Surgery, 5th ed. Norwalk, CT: Appleton & Lange, 1991, pp. 19–29.

Wray, J, & Sensky, T. How does the intervention of cardiac surgery affect the self-perception of children with congenital heart disease? Child: Care, Health and Development, 24:57–72, 1998.

Youssef, NM. School adjustment of children with congenital heart disease. Maternal-Child Nursing Journal, 17:217–302, 1988.

Zahr, LK, & Boisvert, J. Hypoplastic left heart syndrome repair. Dimensions in Critical Care Nursing, 9:88–96, 1990.

Zimmerman, AA, Burrows, FA, Jonas, RA, & Hickey, PR. The limits of detectable cerebral perfusion by transcranial Doppler sonography in neonates undergoing deep hypothermic low-flow cardiopulmonary bypass. Journal of Thoracic and Cardiovascular Surgery, 114:594–600, 1997.

SECTION V

SPECIAL SETTINGS AND SPECIAL CONSIDERATIONS

Section Editor
Robert J. Palisano
PT, ScD

The Environment of Intervention

Thubi H.A. Kolobe
PT, PhD

Ann Taylor

The demand for contextual interventions has expanded the role of pediatric physical therapists in the provision of services for children with disabilities. The expanded role has shifted toward enhancing the capacity of the caregiving environment. To meet this new challenge, therapists must be able to (a) synthesize and apply findings from studies in areas other than child development and motor function; (b) become acquainted with community resources; (c) conduct ecologic assessments; (d) be proficient in providing physical therapy in children's natural environments; (e) engage in collaborative decision making with families; and (f) develop new intervention strategies to enhance the child's participation within the caregiving environment. Providing services in the context of naturally occurring experiences or in the child's natural environments may not be new in physical therapy, but combining both may require advanced knowledge and skills, as well as restructuring many of the service delivery models used by physical therapists.

Simply acknowledging that the caregiving environment is a crucial element in child development is not enough. What is needed is an understanding of (a) how aspects of the environment contribute to optimal or nonoptimal developmental outcomes in children; (b) how families or the environment mediate change in children; (c) intervention programs or approaches that may influence children indirectly through their caregivers; and (d) the types of intervention programs or approaches that influence families and children directly. Studies by pediatric physical therapists that address these aspects of service provision are also needed. Until then, literature from psychology, anthropology, and family therapy, together with theories and theoretical frameworks related to child development, competence, and learning offer a sizable body of knowledge that can be useful to physical therapists.

This chapter will provide an overview of environmental factors as they relate to child development, participation, and physical therapy interventions. We will first discuss the rationale for interventions that focus on the child's caregiving environments and provide an overview of theoretical frameworks that consider the transactional nature of development. The greater part of the chapter will focus on characteristics of the physical and social environments that are relevant to scientific inquiry and service delivery models for children with disabilities. Implications for physical therapy will be integrated throughout the chapter. Finally, we will offer suggestions for how therapists can use this information to build collaborations, enhance information sharing, and plan contextual interventions that are meaningful to families.

Although the chapter focuses on environmental experiences, we acknowledge that biologic factors, discussed in previous chapters, are as important, if not more, in influencing the child's development and the outcome of physical therapy. Physical therapists focus their interventions on motor development and functional mobility, and research on environmental factors has focused on social and cognitive development. Therefore, the focus of the chapter is on environmental factors that (a) may affect or be affected by physical therapy, (b) are important for activity and participation in daily life, and (c) are likely to contribute to the differences in the outcomes of children based on family background. Given the increasing importance placed on family-centered interventions, information that can help physical therapists in their assessments and enhance child and family functioning is crucial. Application for the information presented in this chapter is embedded in other chapters and emphasized in Chapter 31.

RATIONALE FOR FOCUS ON THE ENVIRONMENT

The environment is a term used to describe the physical and social settings in which children develop, grow, and function. The physical environment may be a home, day care center, or school. It includes structural conditions such as space, access, buildings, and equipment (e.g., toys and books), and relates to safety, the quantity of available material that fosters development, learning, and the participation. Although the physical environment includes the presence of toxic agents such as lead or PCBs (Mendola et al., 2002), these issues will not be discussed in this chapter.

The social environment conveys interactions and relationships that nurture development and shape behavior. It encompasses relationships, starting with interactions with parents, siblings, extended families, and extending to peers and other adults in the community. The social environment relates to emotional wellness and the quantity and quality of support. Although physical therapists are often called upon to consult on children's physical environments, to collaborate with families and to develop and implement contextual interventions, they need to understand aspects of the social environment that impact on child functioning. To children and families, these two environments are inextricably intertwined. Two types of environments are described in the literature: proximal (home or child care setting) and distal (neighborhood or community) (Darling & Steinberg, 1993; Kaufman & Rosenbaum, 1992). We will expand on these environments later in the chapter.

DEVELOPMENT, INTERVENTION, AND OUTCOME

A recent report by the National Academy of Sciences (From Neurons to Neighborhoods) (Shonkoff & Phillips, 2001) highlighted 10 core concepts that explain the relationship between biologic and environmental factors in child development (Box 30-1). The report was the result of an extensive analysis of research on early brain

---

Box 30-1	**Core Concepts of Development**

- Human development is shaped by a dynamic and continuous interaction between biology and experience.
- Culture influences every aspect of human development and is reflected in childrearing beliefs and practices designed to promote healthy adaptation.
- The growth of self-regulation is a cornerstone of early childhood development that cuts across all domains of behavior.
- Children are active participants in their own development, reflecting the intrinsic human drive to explore and master one's environment.
- Human relationships, and the effects of relationships on relationships, are the building blocks of healthy development.
- The broad range of individual differences among young children often makes it difficult to distinguish

normal variations and maturational delays from transient disorders and persistent impairments.
- The development of children unfolds along individual pathways whose trajectories are characterized by continuities and discontinuities, as well as by a series of significant transitions.
- Human development is shaped by the ongoing interplay among sources of vulnerability and sources of resilience.
- The timing of early experiences can matter, but, more often than not, the developing child remains vulnerable to risks and open to protective influences throughout the early years of life and into adulthood.
- The course of development can be altered in early childhood by effective interventions that change the balance between risk and protection, thereby shifting the odds in favor of more adaptive outcomes.

From National Research Council and Institute of Medicine. From Neurons to Neighborhoods: The Science of Early Childhood Development. Committee of Integrating the Science of Early Childhood Development, Jack P. Shonkoff and Deborah A. Phillips (Eds.). Washington, D. C.: National Academy Press: Executive Summary, 2000, pp. 3-4.

development and the role of early experiences in shaping development. The findings supported the notion of sensitive periods during which environmental experiences appear to influence development. The sensitive periods were linked to neuroplasticity with motor functioning and memory showing remarkable plasticity throughout the life span. Together with theories such as the neuronal group selection theory proposed by Edelman (1993), the findings from the Neurons to Neighborhoods report provide a compelling argument for the potential for experiential learning to influence brain plasticity and functional activity.

Despite innovations in medical technology and the fact that health and prevention initiatives have reduced diseases and health hazards that contributed to non-optimal development in children, the number of children who are exposed to at-risk environmental and social factors continues to increase (Farran, 2000). For example, childhood poverty, particularly in minority children, has increased in the last 10 years (Roosa et al., 2003). Childhood poverty is associated with multiple physical and social risk factors that further compromise the development and health of children, especially those with developmental disabilities (Farran, 2000).

Children's environments, particularly childrearing practices, are also believed to contribute to differences in the outcomes of a variety of interventions targeted at children with or at risk for developmental delays and disabilities. Two longitudinal interventions studies, one with children with disabilities (Hauser-Cram et al., 2001) and the other with infants who are at risk for developmental delays (Infant Health and Development Program) (McCormick et al., 1998), support the influence of early mother-child interactions on children's functional skills at preschool and school age. The findings from the Infant Health and Development Program (IHDP) also revealed differences that could be associated with cultural childrearing practices. For example, Hispanic-American children made fewer gains in intelligence quotient scores and had more behavior problems compared to Anglo- and African-American children.

A review of studies that investigated the effect of various physical therapy strategies on motor function (Harris, 1997) showed different outcomes based on the target of intervention. Interventions that focused on changing impairments were less effective than those that used assistive technology to adapted specific aspects of the environment. Based on the modest, or insignificant, findings, Harris concluded: "It is hoped that the next generation of early intervention research for children with motor disabilities and their caregivers will include evaluation of the effect of specific, client-centered, functional adaptations and community-based recreational programs on attainment of outcomes that are important to children and to their caregivers" (p. 343).

Harris's observations and the findings from the Neurons to Neighborhoods report are in concert with the service delivery system currently mandated by the Individuals with Disabilities Education Act (IDEA) of 1997 (Public Law 105-17), particularly Part C. At least three provisions target children's environments. These include (a) the development of intervention approaches that focus on enhancing children's participation in their environments, (b) provision of interventions in the context of naturally occurring childrearing experiences, and (c) services that are developed and implemented in collaboration with families. The service delivery system stipulated in IDEA has evolved with each reauthorization and reflect a combination of the current scientific evidence and families' input.

Children's physical environments have always been an important focus of pediatric physical therapy intervention for children with motor disabilities. Concepts of skill acquisition discussed by Gentile (2000), the principles of motor learning (Larin, 2000), and the dynamic system theory (Thelen & Ulrich, 1991; Thelen, 1995) emphasize the significance of the environment for motor development and function. Gentile's taxonomy of tasks (2000) considers the task and the environment to be interrelated, and offers suggestions for using the environment to teach a task or skill. Dynamic system theory considers the interaction of neurologic and psychologic systems and the social environment to be essential for the development of motor function (Thelen, 1995). Recent studies by Palisano and colleagues (2003) and Tieman and colleagues (2004) illustrate how environmental setting can affect the mobility patterns of children with cerebral palsy. Children who were capable of walking with support increasingly needed more assistance ambulating at home, school, and in the neighborhood.

DEVELOPMENTAL THEORIES

Several theories and models view development of children in the context of the environment. The well-known transactional theory, proposed by Sameroff and Chandler (1975), views the child's development as a function of an interaction among the child, family, and the environment. The relationship is considered dynamic in nature, with all three elements having the power to change the nature of the interaction and the outcome of the child's development. The ecologic model of human development, developed by Bronfenbrenner (1986), expands the transactional model to include concentric layers of influence that begin at the level of the family unit (microsystem) and extend to neighborhoods (mesosystem), and policy (macrosystem). The ecologic framework of human development expands the biologic and parent-child views of child development and intervention to include the whole family, its capacities and resources, and the environment (Bronfenbrenner, 1986). This model emphasizes both the multilevel and multifaceted nature of environmental experiences that influence child development and performance. Often terms such as proximal and distal are used to distinguish between the influence that occurs at the family unit level and from neighborhoods and political institutions. The story of Jean, presented in the next section, depicts these interactions very well.

The developmental "niche," developed by Super and Harkness (1986), is another model of child functioning that stipulates three components that encompass the child's sociocultural environment: (1) the physical and social settings of the child's life, (2) culturally regulated customs and practices of child care, and childrearing, and (3) the psychology of the caretakers. These components compose the child's microenvironment and interact together to shape the child through daily life routines.

The few findings on the impact of the physical and social environments, together with the developmental theories reviewed, provide a strong argument for physical therapists to shift their thinking in how to incorporate environmental information in service delivery. The findings underscore the need for interventions that enhance caregiving as well as independent mobility in environmental settings that are important for daily life. Although the developmental theories mentioned above have guided developmental research, it is only recently that attempts have been made to use these models to design intervention programs and to empirically test the models (Sameroff & Fiese, 2000). Each model provides a framework that therapists can use to plan assessments and interventions, and to guide research designs.

CHARACTERISTICS OF THE ENVIRONMENT

PROXIMAL ENVIRONMENT

The distinction between the proximal and distal environments is an important one in terms of the impact each has on children's development and functional skills. Proximal environment refers to home and child care settings, and distal environment refers to the neighborhood and community. The proximal environment represents the microcosm of the child's ecology (Bronfenbrenner, 1986). The greater part of this chapter will focus on the proximal environment, since it is the vehicle through which the family and child's development shape each other (Barnard, 1997; Brooks-Gunn et al., 2000). Within the proximal environment the family, including the child, develops mutual relationships and a sense of cohesion that allows it to function as a unit and to nurture its members.

Figure 30-1 depicts the conceptualization of how factors within the proximal environment interact to influence child functioning and participation. In families with young children, family functioning centers on parenting behaviors and childrearing routines (e.g., caregiver-child interaction, or amount and variety of stimulation). Parenting behaviors and childrearing routines in turn are shaped by several factors such as beliefs and knowledge parents have about child development and competence, cultural expectations, the caregivers' physical and mental health, availability of resources, physical space and play materials, and the neighborhood environment. The parenting behaviors interact with the child's health and developmental abilities/status to influence the child's development, family functioning, and the child's level of participation.

Central to this ecology is the family's home, which provides the child easily accessible opportunities for social and physical interactions that foster development and the child's health. Therefore the framework presented in Figure 30-1 considers the child's developmental status to be a mediator between opportunities and participation, rather than the outcome of interactions. This view of the home and child care environment has several implications for physical therapy. First it expands the concept of how physical therapy may influence child outcome. Second, it requires therapists to look beyond developmental status and to develop measures that assess how the child uses the current levels of development to participate in caregiving and family routines (e.g., daily living skills and levels of independence). It should be noted that despite the dyadic nature of the influences between the child and the environment, there is more evidence that indicates that changing the caregiving environment is more likely to foster change in child outcome than vice versa (Bornstein, 1991; Brooks-Gunn et al., 2000; Maccoby, 1992; Rutter et al., 2001). Third, because the majority of the factors in this environment are interdependent, research that examines the outcomes of physical therapy in children needs to account for the contributions of these factors. The home and child care settings are the natural environments where therapists most often interact with children and their families; we

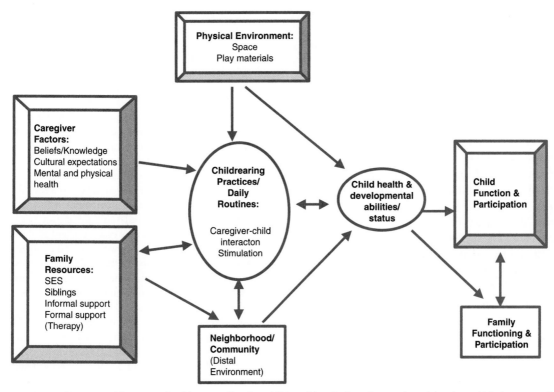

• **Figure 30-1**   Conceptual framework of factors affecting child and family function and participation within home and child care settings (proximal environment).

will expand on the family interactions and functioning within this environment later in the chapter.

DISTAL ENVIRONMENT

In this chapter neighborhood and community are used interchangeably when referring to the distal environment. Neighborhood refers to a specific geographic area, such as a residential area. Community usually refers to a group of people who share not only a geographic area, but also social goals and institutions (Roosa et al., 2003). Neighborhoods may contain social institutions such as schools, churches, and hospitals. The extent to which child development is influenced by proximal and distal environments is related to the time a child spends in each environment. Younger children are influenced more by proximal environments. At school age, the influence of distal environments increases (Darling & Steinberg, 1993; Kaufman & Rosenbaum, 1992). The impact of distal environments on child development may further increase when proximal risk factors are present. For example, children of families with low incomes who live in neighborhoods with limited resources are doubly susceptible to the deleterious effects of poverty than children of families with low incomes who live in relatively affluent neighborhoods (Kaufman & Rosenbaum, 1992). Darling and Steinberg (1993) observed that neighborhood factors explained differences in child outcomes over and above the variance explained by family factors.

The processes by which the factors within the neighborhood and community exert their influence on child development and competence are not clear and are, at best, speculative. Some theorists and researchers propose that frequent contact among parents at common neighborhood places may lead to shared ways of raising children (Klebanov et al., 1997). Parents may use this information to structure family routines and experiences. Others believe that how the family structures and manages resources within their neighborhood determines the types of experiences they will engage in to raise their children (Cook et al., 1997). For example, families who live in neighborhoods with high violence and poor employment opportunities may limit their children's exposure or access to social institutional resources such as the YMCA. Yet another view is that because poor employment opportunities are also associated with long working hours, children may spend a significant amount of time in alternative child care settings (Phillip et al.,

1994). Depending on affordability, child care may be of good or questionable quality.

An emerging role of the physical therapist is consultation with families who express interest in their children's participation in community activities, such as sports, and swimming programs offered by park districts, crafts activities offered by most libraries, and children's theater. The extent to which children and families benefit from community activities will depend on what constitutes an optimal environment, access, and the family's level of participation. Because research indicates that availability of an informal social support network of extended family and friends who live nearby may moderate the impact of the neighborhood on child outcome (Roosa et al., 2003), therapists should consider intervention plans that incorporate informal support networks. Tools such as the Network Survey (NCAST Programs, 1986) offer a quick, easy, and family-centered way of obtaining information on family support systems.

JEAN'S STORY

The story of Jean and her family, narrated by her mother, Annette, illustrates the dynamic interaction among proximal and distal environments and the service delivery system. The story provides an excellent example of how the distal environment shapes and reshapes family functioning, and how the dynamics change over time as the child grows. Such a story, as told by Jean, also illuminates the power of the narrative form of information sharing. There tends to be a good reason for where families choose to begin and end their stories, for making explicit and implicit statements about boundaries and roles, and for what they choose to disclose. A perceptive therapist will hear it all, and reflect on how his/her role will add or detract from the family's experiences. Finally, the story provides a plethora of family experiences that offer opportunities for further discussions, various interpretations, and application to service provision.

In my day no one knew they were having a child with a disability until the birth. I was not allowed to see Jean at first, as there was some possibility that she may not survive. When they wanted me to see her, I didn't want to. I was very concerned about this affecting my other children ages 16, 11, and 8. We had all been so excited about having a new baby in the family. This included my parents, my husband's parents, our friends, and close neighbors. Everyone was stunned. I don't remember who said, "Of course you must find an institution for her; she will need constant care." Well, her heart problem seemed only that it wasn't in the right spot but did work ok. She was alert. She didn't fit any criteria to go to any institution. Besides having quadruple amputation, she couldn't turn her head—we didn't know exactly why.

Two to 3 weeks after Jean's birth, the local Junior League had a conference on birth defects and one of the visiting experts was a doctor from Chicago. He came to see Jean, said she should be fine. He said, "Take her home and love her." He truly was the only positive voice of authority we heard—hope he knows how right he was. He also arranged for her to be on a national program for children with several congenital amputations in Grand Rapids, MI. They wanted her at 1 year. Her grandmother kept her then about 2 weeks more.

Jean had neck surgery when she was 6 weeks old. The problem in her neck was a benign tumor. It was removed. She was casted from head (only the crown was open) down past her buttocks. The cast was changed about 2 to 3 weeks later because she grew and left on another 3 to 4 weeks. When cast came off, she could turn her head for the first time since some time before she was born. She was hysterical—screaming and turning her head from side to side. She only stopped when in a drugged sleep. It took several days before she adjusted. We then had her at home, coping first with the big problem of overheating. We had spent already a lot of time cooling her with cold water and alcohol sponges or she was beet red and very uncomfortable.

Also, all the nerve endings not connected seemed exposed and she overreacted to every sound large or small. She slept only when dosed with liquid Tylenol—a new drug available for babies at that time. This stage lasted forever—4 to 6 months, I guess.

Many times when holding her or feeding her, she seemed to look at me with those big blue eyes as if to say, "It's ok, it's ok!" She did win over her siblings, grandparents, and other family members. When we realized we didn't have to be afraid to handle her, Dan and Katie (siblings) played with her, talked to her, Dan sang to her, her grandfather told her everything—she might have finally known—"It's ok, it's ok!" She grew. Learned all the things babies learn quickly and seemingly easily.

We were advised early on that I should get a job outside the home so I would not become a "slave, martyr, her only caretaker." I didn't agree but went along. It was the *right* thing to do. She learned to trust many people and love them. I became a better parent to her and her siblings as well.

Grandparents are a godsend as they have lots of time and are so nonjudgmental. She and my father became "soul mates." He needed a project—she needed his expertise. Each family member seemed to excel in some particular way for her. Dan and Katie taught her to sit alone, to climb stairs, to read and sing, to play.

Because of her, our family became more dysfunctional—it was inevitable. When Dan was about 14, he developed histoplasmosis. [Histoplasmosis is a very debilitating disease that comes from the pollen put into the air by fungi that grow on bat guano found in caves. It affects respiratory system.] We never knew where he got it. He spent one long summer mostly in bed playing his guitar and playing with Jean. He did recover from that bout. He became very good at playing guitar and singing —he thought he should be in Las Vegas or Hollywood so he kept running away. Surviving all that—it wasn't pretty or easy—at age 16 he was broadsided by a car when on his motorcycle and became a spinal cord victim (actually, midbrain damage). He lived until age 34, in ICU, hospital, at home, in nursing home—a downer for all of us.

It should be noted that from early on Jean's father, who wasn't good at "father knows best behavior," decided his role should be to earn as much money as he could to take care of Jean and Dan. He was good at it—Dan had every opportunity to try experimental treatments and Jean certainly enjoyed traveling and educational opportunities so that she could be self-sufficient in her life. She could attend private school, have tutors, and have attendants and go where she desired to go.

So, then, about the time Jean spent being in a disabled world. When she was 1 year old, we took her to Grand Rapids, Michigan to be enrolled in a federal program for severe amputees.

Available were doctors, nurses, PTs, OTs, and social workers. She went there four times a year, staying from 6 weeks to 3 months in some occasions (being quarantined for measles, chickenpox). She called home once a week and we marveled at her transition to a Michigan accent. She became familiar with the people there, little or no change in personnel.

Each time I went, they reported fully on her actions and gave me instructions and training for what needed to happen at home until the next visit. Looking back I realize each report and instruction was with that individual person but never all together as a team—seems strange now.

She was given an artificial arm—left because she is left-handed. Same arm but powered from two sources, batteries and gas. The arm was mounted on hard plastic caps to hold it in place—eventually there were 2 but not for long—obviously *too* heavy. These were made by a man who made planetarium equipment and broke a lot and had to be sent back. There was also an electric cart, which was about the size of today's wheelchair. They were able to go up and down—about 1 foot, as I recall, but that part of it was finally its demise as it did not work well. Jean stopped going there when it was discovered she had scoliosis. How it got so far advanced before they found it, I don't know. So she went from wearing an arm she disliked to wearing an even more obnoxious brace. After 6 months it was decided surgery was the only answer. Fortunately, a local doctor had been trained by Dr. Harrington to do the rod procedure. The doctor took outstanding pains to assure Jean's surgery would be successful—it was noxious enough but everything went as planned. She was in a cast from shoulder height down

as far as possible to let her be able to still sit. After the cast came off she still spent 6 months back in her brace. She never wore arms again.

The legs. They were mostly my idea all along. I thought she could move about some with them and the appearance definitely was part of it. It was never practical —if she fell she couldn't get up by herself. There were times when transferring her from her chair to the car, etc. was easier. She wore them until she graduated from law school. The federal judge who hired her as a clerk let her know straight away that it would be her decision. That was all for the legs. It should not have been as much my decision—no one questioned me that I recall or asked her if she wanted to wear them. Mothers have great influence over their children and should be challenged, I believe. Perhaps Jean is happier with adaptive aids because she had opportunities to have all the prosthetics.

I do feel good that Jean had so many opportunities to travel, go to private school, to be exposed to many opportunities for a better life than most that are as complicated as hers is. She did, however, add to all that by being very alert, adaptive, open and eager to new situations. I am curious, though, to know if her ability to do complicated procedures in her head and to enjoy many experiences that she did not actively participate in, was present somewhere in her brain. How was she able to learn so many things (cognitively) when she did not have arms? Could other children learn by being exposed to more mind-bending experiences early even if they cannot touch objects with their hands?

Jean's mother concluded her narrative by asking these questions directly to the therapist:

> Can PTs be taught to recognize all these things present in families when they are in the homes of babies or even older children? Can they understand the family dynamics such as guilt or inability to deal with a "different" child? What about the financial strain? How can they be taught? What a challenge!

FAMILY STRUCTURE

First, Jean's story calls attention to the family structure. Who are the family members and what are their roles as they relate to Jean's needs? The family structure and functioning provide an important context for understanding child development (Sameroff & Fiese, 2000). The family as a social system and family units consist of subsystems that represent different levels of interactions. Levels may represent the characteristics of an individual member of the family, a parent-parent, parent-child, and a child-child dyad. In any given situation parents or a child are but one subsystem of the family unit; therefore, interventions directed at a child without regard to other subsystems may be limited.

Family structure and composition influence the type of care the child receives. Families may either be mother-child or father-child households (single parent families), nuclear families (mother, father, and children), extended households (grandparents and aunts and cousins), or foster families. At face value, Jean's family appears to be a nuclear family. The intimate involvement of the grand-parents may be easily overlooked unless the therapists asked, or listened. According to Whiting and Whiting (1975), the nuclear family is common in only a small proportion of all human societies. Given the changing demographics in the United States, definitions of what constitutes a family and family roles are changing, giving way to a more blended or contemporary family. The contemporary family consists of "those significant others who profoundly influence the personal life and health of the individual over an extended period of time" (Sparling & Sekerak, 1992, p. 71).

Family structure has several implications for physical therapy. The structure of the family shapes family resources. Whether or not families are two-parent versus single-parent families not only affects income, but also influences the flexibility parents can have in employment arrangements and child care. The family structure also determines the adult/child ratio and expectations the family may have on the child. In extended households, the infant may be indulged by a large number of adults. As a result, the demand on the child to be independent in areas such as self-help may not be high. In some instances, other family members may influence parent expectations of the child. Research suggests that a high caregiver/child ratio is favorable (Mulligan et al., 1998). Infants are likely to receive a variety of stimulations when the ratio is high.

Findings on the impact of the adult/child ratio on child development, however, are inconclusive (Garrett et al, 1994; Kolobe, 2004; Mulligan et al., 1998). Mulligan and associates (1998) observed that infants with a low caregiver/child ratio had lower motor scores at 9 months but no correlations were found at 6 and 12 months. Garrett and associates (1994) and Kolobe (2004) found no associations between the caregiver/child ratio and infants' scores on motor tests. The advantage of the adult/child ratio is evidenced in situations in which the extended family is closely involved, as in the case of Jean. A high ratio in situations in which the child requires multiple services may be an indication for the need for informal support network. Jean's case also brings to light the importance of considering the siblings' ages in relation to the child with disabilities when determining adult/child ratios. The bigger the age gap, the more likely siblings are to participate in caregiving.

FAMILY FUNCTIONING

The child as a subsystem within a family system influences and is influenced by the interactive nature in which the family performs its functions (family functioning). Family functioning refers to the family's ability to conduct and accomplish everyday activities across various situations (Hayden et al., 1998). Efforts to categorize family behaviors and situations have been depicted in models developed by psychologists and those in related fields. These models assist us in understanding more about family interaction, but most require specialized training for application to a specific family (Ackerman, 1984; Beavers et al., 1985; Morris, 1990; Olson, 1986). Some categorize families according to interaction styles and attitudes that are based on a complexity of assumptions related to demographic variables and stressor conditions.

These models do not always address the continuum of family characteristics and interactions and the unique ways in which individual families interact with their children at different periods in their lives. This point is illustrated by the shifts that take place in the roles played by the individual members of Jean's family not only as she grows, but also as she undergoes the various medical interventions. Her family organizes and reorganizes in their roles in an unpredictable fashion. Because of the innumerable variables involved in family functioning, each family exhibits a different composite of roles and interactions depending on concerns and needs.

Parenting Behaviors and Childrearing Practices

A great deal of family activity or functioning centers on childrearing. Childrearing practices represent goal-directed actions that parents engage in to promote their children's development (Darling & Steinberg, 1993). Other terms used in the literature are family routines (DeGrace, 2003), or parenting behaviors (Goodnow, 1988). That childrearing is the vehicle through which families shape the behavior and development of children is widely accepted (Darling & Steinberg, 1993; Goodnow, 1988; Fox, 1995). The childrearing practices and behaviors that exert the strongest influence on motor development are unclear. Research on childrearing has focused on cognitive, social, emotional, and language development (Barnard, 1997; Kelly & Barnard 2000). The few of the studies that have included the motor domain suggest that teaching motor behaviors within the context of parent-child interactions (Chiarello & Palisano, 1998), and how parents structure the learning and caregiving home environment may promote motor development

(Benasich & Brooks-Gunn, 1996; Garrett et al., 1994; Kolobe et al., 2004).

Parent-Child Interaction. Parent-child interaction is a component of family functioning that represents an intimate transaction between the child and caregivers. Parent-child interaction is considered the basis for subsequent relationships the child forms (Barnard, 1997). The continual and contingent characteristic of parent-child interaction is what is believed to shape relationships and influences skill acquisition. Parent-child interaction is predicated upon the notion that the child and caregiver have a dual responsibility to maintain the interaction (Barnard, 1978). A great deal of parent-child interaction occurs during caregiving and play, which are sensorimotor experiences. Therapists are encouraged to consider how sensorimotor interventions might enhance the quality of parent-child interaction.

Barnard (1978) identified four features of successful parent-child interaction:

a. Sufficient repertoire of behaviors, such as body movements and facial expressions
b. Contingent responses to each other
c. Rich interactive content in terms of play materials, positive affect, and verbal stimulation
d. Adaptive response patterns that accommodate the child's emerging developmental skills

Physical therapists have not fully explored the influence of motor performance on parent-child interaction. Atypical movement patterns of children with motor disabilities may influence the quality of parent-child interaction. If each partner must have a sufficient repertoire of behaviors, then limitations in either the child's movements or the caregiver's facial expressions may result in interactions that are less than satisfying (Kelly & Barnard, 2000). Children with motor disabilities often demonstrate slow responses to external stimulation, which may limit the richness of contingent responses between them and their caregiver. Indeed mothers of children with disabilities were described as initiating play and more directive during play interactions with their children compared to mothers of children with typical development (Marfo, 1992; Shonkoff et al., 1992). Therefore, sharing information with parents about their children's abilities and how it relates to underlying limiting factors, and providing suggestions for encouraging their children's activity and participation may optimize parent-child interactions.

Research suggests that parent-child interactions are amenable to change with interventions and that the quality can improve with time (Barnard, 1997; Chiarello & Palisano, 1998; Hauser-Cram et al., 2001; Spiker et al.,

1993). Using videotaped recordings of parent-child interactions at 30 months of age, Spiker and associates (1993) observed that mothers in the group receiving weekly home visits and center-based program were more supportive and offered more developmentally appropriate stimulation than mothers in the control group. Chiarello and Palisano (1998) reported modest gains in the quality of interaction following physical therapy intervention provided in the context of play and parent-child interaction. Given that children with physical disabilities have limitations in their repertoire of motor skills, it would seem that physical therapy interventions should emphasize adaptive responses and synchronous relationships between children and caregivers. Focusing on motor activities that promote parent-child interaction early in the child's life may provide a foundation for later relationships with adults and peers (Barnard, 1997; Sumner & Spietz, 1994).

The process of caregiver-child interaction is important for providing family-centered interventions in natural environments. Characteristics of positive interactions include flexibility of the caregiver, responsiveness to the child's distress and cues, and contingency in responses by both the child and caregiver. The ability to (a) allow disruption, (b) redirect the child in a supportive manner, and (c) allow the child to initiate an action are reported as distinguishing features of successful and mutually enjoyable interactions (Barnard, 1997; Booth et al., 1989; Marfo, 1992). This information is particularly relevant for families of children with short attention spans who need repeated redirecting, and children with cerebral palsy who may need prompts and extra time to initiate actions. Therapists must capitalize on the essential ingredients of adult interaction that include high levels of maternal responsiveness and moderate to low levels of directiveness.

Therapists may also share and model the "teaching loop" with parents (Sumner & Speitz, 1994, p. 12). The teaching loop has four elements: (a) verbally and nonverbally alerting the child to the task and teaching material, (b) giving clear instructions about how the task it to be performed, (c) allowing the child time to perform the task, and (d) giving the child feedback. Central to the teaching loop is the process of contingency, the immediacy of a response from either the child or the caregiver. The elements of the teaching loop are consistent with the principles of motor learning (Larin, 2000).

Home Environment. For decades the connection between the home environment and children's development and competence has been the subject of research by psychologists, educators, and health professionals (Caldwell & Bradley, 1984). Research during the 1970s and 1980s was largely concerned with understanding the relationship between poverty and child development. As the number of children born prematurely increased, the home environment has again emerged as a topic that merits special attention (Bradley, 1993). Traditionally, motor development was believed to be less sensitive to changes in the home environment. This perspective is supported by studies of children younger than 3 years of age that used the Bayley Scales of Infant Development (McCormick et al., 1998). Recent studies of preschool children, however, suggest there is a positive relationship between the quality of the home environment, measured by the Home Observation Measure of the Environment (HOME), and motor development (Bradley, 1993; Garrett et al., 1994; Kolobe et al., 2004). The findings suggest that the influence of the home environment on motor development may be gradual. There may not be an immediate impact on function, suggesting the need for longitudinal studies to examine the relationship. The HOME assesses various aspects of child participation in family activities and teaching and learning opportunities, including the appropriateness of toys, which are important for therapists and parents to discuss. The HOME also provides a systematic way of gathering information about the caregiving environment at various child ages and can be a valuable asset for service delivery in any setting.

Physical therapists have expertise in modification of the physical environment of the home to increase a child's activities and participation. The focus has been on adapting equipment in the physical space to accommodate the child with disabilities. This can include architectural changes such as ramps or hand rails and special equipment such as special chairs and standers. Because the performance of mobility is needed in many activities of daily living, the child's successful participation will require therapists to consider what Gentile (2000) refers to as regulatory and nonregulatory conditions. Regulatory conditions require individuals to organize their movements around them, for example, the height of the stairs. Nonregulatory conditions are not critical to the performance of a task (e.g., color of the handrail). Tieman and colleagues (2004) have proposed a framework that takes into consideration the context in which a task is performed (regulatory or nonregulatory conditions), and the setting in which the task occurs or is taught. The framework is based on the international classification of functioning (World Health Organization, 2001) and Gentile's taxonomy (Fig. 30-2).

Gibson's social learning theory offers another framework that therapists can apply to promote a child's participation in the home environment. Gibson (1988) uses the term "affordance" to refer to features of the

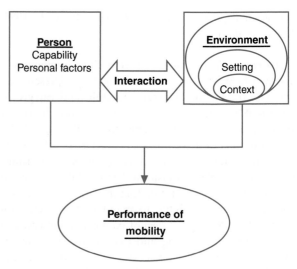

♦ **Figure 30-2**   Person-environment interaction in the performance of mobility. *(Reprinted with permission of The Haworth Press Inc. from Tieman BL, et al. Changes in mobility of children with cerebral palsy over time and across environmental setting. Physical and Occupational Therapy in Pediatrics, 24(1/2):112, 2004.)*

environment that provide the child opportunities for goal-directed actions. Gibson's theory emphasizes the importance of children learning to perceive the opportunities offered and to act on them. A challenge for families and therapists is to structure the environment in ways that encourage the child's self-initiated actions. This requires familiarity not only with the physical organization and types of toys in the home, but also how to create opportunities for play and exploration – the essence of providing therapy in natural environments. For example, depending on age and the social context, a child may perceive a bench as providing the opportunity for pulling up to standing, sitting and playing with a toy, or stepping up and jumping off.

The child's home also offers the therapist an opportunity to put interactions in context. Assessment of the caregiving environment is particularly useful for interventions designed to improve a child's participation in family activities and routines. Examination and evaluation of a child's strengths and needs in the home enables informed decisions on whether intervention should focus on changing the child's abilities, the task, the environment, or some combination to improve activity and participation. The assessment includes, but is not limited to, type of floor surface, space, curbs and steps, door sizes, table heights, and access to toys. Observations can include how the family organizes tasks, environmental demands placed on the child, and opportunities for play and exploration.

Parenting Beliefs

Childrearing practices do not occur in isolation. Childrearing practices that families engage in may reflect the beliefs, ideas, perceptions, expectations, and attitudes families have about parenting and child competence (Kochanska et al., 1989; Mills & Rubin, 1990). Many parents have ideas about how children develop and what they should do to foster specific developmental skills. Parents' beliefs about child development and outcome may also influence decisions about why one approach to childrearing is better than the other (Fox, 1995; Sigel, 1992). The belief-behavior link is believed to have contributed to the many parent education models and programs used by professionals. The underlying assumption is that parents have the power to change the child (change agents) and that educating parents will influence their ideas about parenting and child outcome.

Parenting beliefs of parents of children with disabilities merits special attention for at least two reasons: the source of information and problems with information gaps. A great deal of information about child development and behavior that shape parents' beliefs about childrearing comes from media that are widely endorsed by society (Kochanska, 1990), such as magazines and television. Similar information about children with disabilities, however, is not as readily available, creating information gaps and uncertainty. Parents of children with disabilities have consistently ranked the need for information high (Turnbull et al., 2000). Parents also perceive information sharing as one of the most valuable aspects of therapy (Washington & Schwartz, 1996). These findings have significant implications for therapists. According to Grosec and associates (1997), "parents who have accurate knowledge of their child's ability are better able to match teaching efforts to their child's developmental level" (p. 266), particularly fathers. The findings also underscore the importance of therapists sharing information with families about development, assessment findings, various intervention approaches and their evidence, and resources that are available in their communities, including information on the Internet.

Research is needed to understand how parent beliefs change, and how change in beliefs translates to parent behavior and child motor function. The association between parental beliefs or ideas and parent behavior is lower than expected (Goodnow, 1988; 1992; Kolobe, 2004; Sigel, 1992). A few factors may explain this finding. First, questionnaires used to gather information overlook the fact that parents' beliefs are often dictated by the child's behavior and the conditions under which the behavior occurs (Grosec et al., 1997). Therefore, some beliefs change, while others are stable. Second, self-report measures are subject to distortions (Milner & Crouch, 1997). For example, parents who engage in less than optimal interactions with their children may either exaggerate their responses, or minimize them depending on their perception of how the information will be used. Therapists need to exercise caution when using self-report measures to gather information about families' beliefs and expectations.

Therapists are also interested in parents' beliefs for the purpose of collaborative goal setting. Research findings suggest that beliefs must be understood within the context of the child's characteristics and behavior because of the bidirectional nature of parent-child behavior (Grosec et al., 1997; Hepburn, 2003). Children, as early as infancy. (a) initiate actions that may or may not be acceptable to their caregivers, (b) are capable of evaluating the consequences of such actions, (c) express and negotiate their needs, and (d) make decisions to comply with, or resist, the caregivers' actions or instructions (Hepburn, 2003).

Although parents' beliefs and expectations about child outcome are an important element in collaborative goal setting and intervention, parents' actions or how they structure learning experiences may not be related to their beliefs. Therapists need to consider other sources of information on parental beliefs, such as their cultural expectations, the family's sources of information about child development, and the child's abilities.

Stress and Coping

One rationale for intervening with children with disabilities and their families is to reduce levels of stress and burden of care experienced by families. Stress associated with caregiving is not unique to families of children with disabilities. All families experience unique stressors. The difference between whether or not stress will disrupt family functioning is in how the family perceives the stressful event. Each family reacts to a stressor according to the family's perception, the number of stressful events they are experiencing simultaneously, the family's resources for managing the stressors, and characteristics of the stressor events themselves (McCubbin & Patterson, 1982). Unlike McCubbin and Patterson, who categorized responses to stress in terms of either good or bad adaptation, Boss (1985) has described outcomes more realistically in terms of a continuum.

To study this continuum of adjustment, Petersen and Wikoff (1987) assessed 105 mothers of children with a disability on a combination of home environment and family adjustment variables. The investigators determined that the mere presence of a child with a disability in the family was not sufficient to elicit maladaptation.

The number of child-related stressors and the amount and quality of family resources, such as social support, were the most significant variables in the adjustment of the family. This study suggests that therapists need to be aware of the real and perceived stressors and the unique resources or support available to each family unit, because these factors relate to adaptation and to the potential involvement of the family in the health care of the child. Adaptation appears to be a continuous variable depending on the unique combination of these stressors and resources.

Stress seems to also be related to the number of roles a person assumes (Gottlieb, 2002). Mothers who were the sole responsible provider for their children reported greater stress and poorer psychologic well-being than mothers who were partial providers. Although multiple roles were found to positively influence the mothers' self-esteem, too many roles resulted in depressive symptoms. With more and more single parents working out of the home, the varying and conflicting roles of caregivers should be considered when planning interventions with families. Stress compounds the impact of poverty on children's development. For example, the child outcomes of a parent guidance intervention provided to mothers of low socioeconomic status (SES) were less favorable for mothers experiencing high stress (Brinker, 1994). These findings suggest that therapy interventions, if not well matched with the family's needs, may add to parenting stress.

The findings on stress and coping, and events in Jean's family, provide a compelling reason for physical therapists to assess caregiver stress. A therapist with good communication and observation skills should have little trouble identifying stressors in families. Although type and severity of disability were the only stress factors that applied to Jean's family, several indicators suggested that the family was under a great deal of stress. Not only did this family experience multiple stressors associated with Jean's surgical interventions and Dan's accident, these events were simultaneous. When asked, Annette confirmed that although the support they received from the grandparents and friends helped alleviate the stress, each episode of care that Jean needed (and later Dan) challenged their coping strategies. Because so much has been written about stress as it relates to poverty, professionals tend to overlook other stressors in the lives of families of middle and high SES.

FAMILY RESOURCES

Family resources, or lack thereof, are a major contributing factor to family stress and influence child develop-

ment (Garcia-Coll & Magnusson, 2000; McLoyd, 1998). The family's resources may be internal, such as parents' level of education or knowledge about child development, or external such as income-related resources, or support networks. Part C of the IDEA of 1997 mandates determination of family resources as part of child and family assessment, and as a basis for the development of the individualized family service plan (IFSP). Family resources are numerous, multifaceted, and need-based. Not all the resources that are needed to promote optimal family functioning can be provided through the formal service delivery system. Therefore, the approach recommended is to select family resources that may be related to motor development and participation in the home environment and evaluate how they may be impacted by physical therapy interventions. In this section we will discuss the family's SES and support. SES is an indicator of parental education, occupation, and family structure (Hollingshead, 1975).

Socioeconomic Status

Children of families with low SES are overrepresented among children with disabilities and developmental delays (Shonkoff & Phillips, 2001) and less likely to receive a full complement of services (McLoyd, 1998). The influence of poverty on child development is nonlinear. Younger children are more susceptible to the effects of poverty (Duncan et al., 1994). Children of minority race/ethnicity tend to be the most affected by poverty (Brooks-Gunn & Duncan, 1997; Garcia-Coll & Magnusson, 2000). Two studies reported a positive correlation between SES and motor development of young infants (Garrett et al., 1994; Kolobe, 2004), calling attention to the need for physical therapists to examine the relationship more closely.

How SES influences child development and competence is not well understood. Several mechanisms have been proposed: First, SES organizes family life in terms of determining how much money or time parents allocate to raising their children (Jean's example). Second, factors such as poor maternal and infant malnutrition, stress, and prevalence of toxic environments that are prevalent in low SES environments, affect brain size and growth (Pollitt & Gorman, 1994). Third, maternal and infant malnutrition is linked to small brain size, mental retardation, and birth defects in infants. Finally, other mechanisms are believed to be the types of neighborhoods that parents choose to raise their children (Fig. 30-3), access to community resources that foster child development such as child care, the availability of learning material in the home, and parental stress (Brooks-Gunn & Duncan, 1997; Garret et al., 1994; Halpern, 2000).

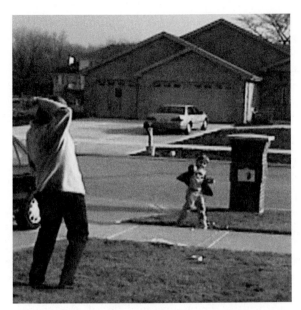

Figure 30-3 Neighborhoods where children grow up influence their development.

Research on resilience and protective factors suggest that infants and young children who live in adverse conditions are most vulnerable when protective factors such as maternal competence are stressed (Werner, 2000). Efforts to ameliorate the negative effects of poverty on children, particularly through parent education, have had mixed results. Halpern (2000) performed an extensive review on the outcomes of early intervention for children and families with low SES and concluded that very little progress has been made over the last decade in improving the lives of families from low SES, including those with children who have special needs.

Of significance to pediatric therapists is the discrepancy that often exists between services provided under research conditions compared with actual practice. Interventions provided under research conditions tend to be more comprehensive and intensive. Depending on program resources, therapists may need to use innovative approaches to service delivery. Frequencies and intensities predetermined by programs may need to be modified to accommodate the families' needs. For example, depending on family needs, therapists may explore with families the feasibility of intensive interventions initially followed by periods of monitoring and consultation. In other words, therapists may need to explore the issue of critical periods for child and family learning. Currently the money allocated to services for children with special needs is far less than the costs associated with providing "best practices" as mandated by the IDEA (Brooks-Gunn et al., 2000). Jean's story

provides a good example of financial resources needed for successful outcomes.

Informal and Formal Support

Support represents the relationship between the need perceived by an individual and the appropriateness of the response. Two forms of support are described in the literature: social and professional, or informal and formal (Dunst & Trivette, 1997). Social support refers to mutually rewarding personal interactions from which an individual derives feelings of being valued and esteemed. The need for social support for children with special needs and their families varies throughout the life span. A shift in support occurs as the child matures, from professional support, to family support, to support from friends. The caretakers of younger children rely on spouse interaction (Flynt et al., 1992) and physician information for support, whereas caretakers of older children rely more on friends and community members (Darling, 1979). Here again Jean's story provides a good example.

An important source of professional support is information sharing. Positive child and family outcomes have been associated with those interventions that focused on providing parents with information pertaining to child development, caregiving for a child with special needs or a chronic disease, and linking families to community resources (Moxley-Haegert & Serbin, 1983; Seitz & Provence, 1990). Therapists are an important source of information for parents in many areas of development, particularly on issues related to mobility and assistive devices.

The impact of social support on parent, child, and family functioning has been studied extensively by Dunst and associates (1997). Overall the findings reveal that social support can buffer the negative effects of stress and impoverished distal and proximal environments. The adequacy of various forms of support enhances positive caregiver interaction styles, positive perception of the child, and family well-being. The authors also discuss various ways of assessing social support. Support may be financial, intellectual, or religious (Heifitz, 1987). Not only is support offered in different ways and perceived to have different meanings by families, but also the concept of support is construed differentially by professionals. Stewart (1989) describes five social support theories that can be applied to clinical practice and, therefore, are germane to our discussion.

1. *Attribution theory* relates to motives for helping, the process of gaining or giving support, and the negative as well as positive aspects of support.
2. *Coping theory* refers to the cognitive aspects of support and its costs to those involved.

3. *Equity theory* describes the reciprocal nature of support.
4. *Loneliness theory* emphasizes the affective aspects of support.
5. *Social-comparison theory* addresses the effects of peer support.

Combining these perspectives, Stewart proposes several recommendations for intervention. Health care professionals and persons providing support need to be in agreement about their intervention approach if the intervention is to be effective. Team members need to understand that support can foster adaptation to stress and prevent health disorders and that therapists have a role in understanding the sources of stress, if not in providing support. Therapists can ascertain whether their clients have a social network that mediates potential loneliness and ultimately helps in modifying their health problems. According to Stewart, recognition of the reciprocal role of social support may encourage the professional to share information and offer support to decrease the family's sense of isolation.

The role of the extended family, particularly grandparents, should not be overlooked. When involved, grandparents provided two types of support—emotional and practical support. As in the case of Jean, grandparents allowed the family to focus on things other than Jean – an important element of coping. Caregiving by older siblings cannot be overlooked. Structured and unstructured teaching through play is largely provided by older siblings in other cultures, even though the siblings may not be expected to take care of the infant's/toddler's other needs (Whiting & Whiting, 1975; Zuniga, 1992). Because infants and toddlers acquire a considerable amount of social and cognitive skills through play, the sibling-child interaction is a valuable resource (Fig. 30-4). Siblings tend to be more adventurous and creative (e.g., Jean's brother); therefore, whenever feasible, therapists should include them in interventions.

Culture

A family's culture is at the heart of parenting and transcends beliefs and expectations about child development and societal roles. The notion that many of the child-rearing practices that parents engage in are embedded in families' ethnic traditions is widely accepted (Garcia-Coll & Magnusson, 1999). Physical therapists are encouraged to consider how a family's culture relates to the child's development and function and plan culturally appropriate interventions. Sensitivity to family culture is particularly imperative in light of the changing population demographics in the United States (US Census Bureau, 2000) and the racial and ethnic disparities in health care reported by the Institute of Medicine (2002). The 2000 Census also indicates that the population of young children in the United States is rapidly becoming racially and ethnically diverse. By 2030, children from racial/ethnic minorities will account for approximately 50% of the country's children (Census, 2000). This shift in demographics gives a new meaning to the task of creating meaningful parent-therapist collaborations and developing mutually agreeable intervention goals.

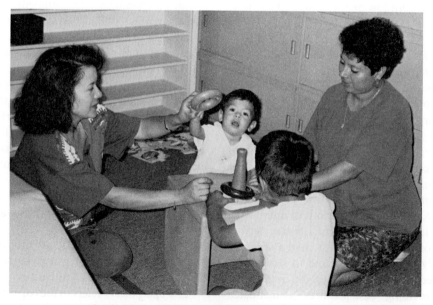

◆ **Figure 30-4** Sibling participation in a therapy session.

Box 30-2	Central Themes to the Definitions of Culture

Blueprint to guide daily behavior
A system of learned patterns of behavior
Shared by other members of a group
Influences peoples' beliefs, values, behaviors and
   perceptions

A way of life
Passed on from one generation to another
Valued by members of the culture and considered to
   be right
Influences not always conscious

A distinction needs to be made between ethnicity and culture, as these terms tend to be used interchangeably. Ethnicity is part of one's identity derived from membership through birth in a racial, national, or linguistic subgroup (Lynch, 1992). Individuals can come from the same ethnic group (e.g., Hispanic), but differ in culture. Therefore, defining culture in terms of ethnicity overlooks the variations within groups and often results in stereotyping of families. Culture is considered to be a shared ideology and valued set of beliefs, norms, customs, and meanings evidenced in a way of life (Super & Harkness, 1997). See Box 30-2 for central themes and other terms that are used to describe culture. Culture influences how families understand life processes, define health and illness, and perceive the causes of illness; it also shapes their attitudes toward wellness and influences their beliefs about the cure. This includes physical therapy. Culture is also believed to play role in the confidence with which childrearing ideas are held by parents, and the flexibility with which they are amenable to change, particularly in light of new information (e.g., parent education) (Garcia-Coll & Magnusson, 1999).

Literature on culture is extensive and a detailed discussion on culture and child development is beyond the scope of this chapter. For more information see Leavitt (1999), Masten (1999), Rogoff and associates (1993), Super and Harkeness (1997), and a special issue on culture in Pediatric Physical Therapy (Knutson, 1995). In this section we will briefly discuss conceptualizations about cultural beliefs and parenting behaviors that we believe will help enhance collaborations between therapists and families from diverse cultures and promote cultural sensitivity—a step toward cultural competence.

Conceptualizations of the cultural environment and how it is linked to the developing child vary. Super and Harkness (1997) describe three core concepts that we believe could be integrated into frameworks and approaches for interventions with families, particularly team-based interventions. These concepts consider the child's cultural environment as (a) representing culturally shared ideas held by parents that inform childrearing, (b) comprising individuals that have assigned roles and responsibilities within a "given frame of routines of daily life" (p. 4), and (c) consisting of shared childrearing practices that integrate the child into the environment. These concepts are distinctive and yet complementary. Cultural beliefs and parent action have implications for collaborative goal setting. Parents who are concerned about the basic survival of their children will organize their caregiving around protection. Parents may hold their infants more and engage in soothing and tactile type of interactions. On the other hand, parents who believe that the lives of their children are not threatened may engage more in talking with the baby than holding it (Richman et al., 1992). Other examples are the practice of passing an infant around from one adult to another in cultures that value interdependence (Zuniga, 1992), and emphasis on structure in cultures that value proper demeanor (Garcia-Coll & Magnusson, 1997). The implicit nature of cultural beliefs suggests that therapists should listen for information that relates to the hierarchical nature of beliefs (e.g., survival/protection before stimulation) when gathering data during assessment and goal development. Skills in interviewing are of utmost importance.

Another view on cultural ideas and child development that provides a good understanding of the link between the cultural beliefs and parenting behaviors comes from Sameroff and Feil's hierarchy of beliefs (1985): *categorical, compensatory,* and *perspectivistic beliefs.* These beliefs influence how parents perceive and respond to their children's behaviors (Gutierrez & Sameroff, 1990) and differ based on acculturation and biculturalism. A categorical belief is associated with attributing a single cause to one outcome. Parents with categorical beliefs are likely to exhibit difficulty in adapting their childrearing practices. A compensatory belief is characterized by a belief that multiple causes lead to multiple outcomes, and parents in this category are likely to pursue several childrearing options. Perspectivistic beliefs are associated with adaptive or flexible parent behaviors. Parents with a perspectivistic view believe that multiple causes may interact with other systems to produce different or alternative outcomes. Take an example of a mother's reaction to her child's inability to crawl at 1 year. A mother who has a categorical belief may suspect heredity and decide to "wait and see." A mother with compensatory beliefs may suspect heredity or illness and consult a professional, while a mother with perspective beliefs may acknowledge the possibility that this is something that runs in the family, but may also investigate other potential causes such as illness, the degree of stimulation or expectations in the home, and may consult both friends and professionals. Guttierez and Sameroff (1990) observed that Mexican-American mothers tended to be categorical, but bicultural Mexican-American mothers were more perspectivistic than Anglo-American mothers. These findings highlight the influence of acculturation on cultural beliefs and parent behavior.

How parents perceive their children's development and behavior has significant implications for assessment, goal setting, and intervention. The flexibility to accept one or a variety of outcomes is also germane to expectations parents may have about the therapists, therapy, and the intervention process as they relate to their children. Perspectivism is associated with ability to accept diversity (of child behavior and outcome). We believe that this would include ideas of outsiders such as health care providers. Although Sameroff & Feil (1985) indicate that neither category is good or bad, they suggest that the explanations given by parents for why things occur be put in the context that applies to each category. In a case of a child with a disability, when the cause of the disability is unknown, or there are multiple causes of functional limitations, or multiple interventions, having a perspectivistic view may be helpful. Parents are more likely to change when new information is in agreement with their views and beliefs (Harwood et al., 1995).

Cultural beliefs that families hold about childrearing and development need to be examined in the context of decisions parents make. One way of understanding the family's perspective is to use scenarios or vignettes. Another is to use questions that focus on both the context and content, particularly circumstantial contexts, and to engage in meta-listening in order to *hear* how parents *explain* their children's behavior and expectations. For example, therapists may ask questions like: "If one were to understand how and why your child moves the way she/he does, what would one need to know or do?" The scenario in which the therapist observes that a young child with Down syndrome prefers to sit and not move around, will eat only certain foods, and enjoy banging objects might generate the following questions. "I notice that Kiesha likes to sit and play by banging objects together. Is this something she likes to do throughout the day? If you or other family members encourage her to move about or play with toys in other ways what does

she do? Are there play activities you would like her to do more often? What about your husband?" What is important is how parents perceive and interpret the child's behavior (Hirsberg, 1996). Hirsberg suggests listening for anxiety and conflict (in terms of decision making). If shifting parent perspective is considered in the best interest of the child (e.g., from categorical to perspectivism), then the therapist should ask parents how their expectations could be realized, the rationale behind the goals they envision for their children, and what they perceive as a consequence if a goal is not attained. This is particularly important for parents from minority cultures who may have a harder time participating in decision making, and for whom barriers to proactive participation and collaboration may exist (Marshak et al., 1999). When working with families from culturally diverse populations, therapists also need to be aware of where the decision making power is within each family. In many families, the father is the decision maker; however, in cultures such as Mexican- or African-American families, extended family members may be the decision maker.

Intervention in a cross-cultural encounter is a reciprocal process between families and therapists, a process in which both parties teach and learn (cultural sensitivity). Cultural sensitivity is only one step toward cultural competence. The term "cultural competent" is used as follows:

> with respect to services, supports, or other assistance that is conducted or provided in a manner that is responsive to the beliefs, interpersonal styles, attitudes, language, and behaviors of individuals who are receiving the services, supports, or other assistance, and in a manner that has the greatest likelihood of ensuring their maximum participation in the program involved.
> Developmental Disabilities Assistance and
> Bill of Rights Act of 2000, Sec 102 (7)

Chan (1990) and Hanley (1999) describe three key factors that contribute to cultural competence: (a) cultural self-awareness, (b) knowledge of information specific to different cultures/experience, and (c) skills in engaging in successful interactions/positive change. Central to the process of cultural self-awareness is the ability to reflect on one's culture and heritage and to examine one's sources of values and beliefs. A similar process should be undertaken at a program or institutional level. Several cultural awareness self-assessments questionnaires are available (e.g., from the Maternal and Child Health website: www.hrsa.gov/OMH/cultural). Knowing about other cultures may be a daunting task. However, activities such as reading about culture, talking and working with individuals from other cultures, participating in celebrations and rituals of families from other cultures are some of the simple ways to learn about other cultures. Because such exposures to culture may be likened to the "tip of the iceberg" (Hanley, 1999), therapists may also consult with professionals from other ethnic and cultural backgrounds who are able to articulate the diverse lifestyles of their communities. Attaining cultural competence (engaging in successful interactions), according to Lynch (1992), requires professionals to do the following: (a) lower their defenses; (b) take risks; (c) practice behaviors that may feel unfamiliar and uncomfortable to them; (d) have a flexible mind and open heart; (e) be willing to accept alternative perspectives; (f) be willing to set aside some beliefs that are cherished to make room for others whose value is unknown; and (g) change what they think, say, and how they behave. Language can be a barrier, but speaking the same language does not guarantee effective cultural communication. For more information on cross-cultural communication, see Lynch (1992).

THE INTERVENTION ENCOUNTER

Interventions with children can only be as successful as what the caregiving environment has to offer. The overarching goal of therapy should be to optimize the child's participation in the home, school, and community (Shelton & Stepanek, 1994). The intervention encounter with children and families should be multifaceted. First, therapists and families should strive to establish a common ground for communication and information sharing. Second, the process of information gathering should involve methods acceptable to both parties. Third, therapists and families should seek to create a good match among the child's functional abilities, the family's resources, the amount of information necessary to level the playing field, and the various environments that are important in the child's daily life. Fourth, intervention should focus on supporting the caregiving environment and the child's participation regardless of the severity of the disability (Fig. 30-5). These facets embrace and expand the provisions of Part B and C of the IDEA of 1997 and are discussed in Chapters 31 and 32.

ESTABLISHING A COMMON GROUND FOR COMMUNICATION

Ordinarily, families begin with little knowledge of the health care and educational systems and are lacking a sense of their own competence in these areas. Similarly, therapists start with very little information about the child and family other than what may be written on referral forms. Traditionally, physical therapists have formally or informally interviewed families to obtain information about the child's birth and developmental history, medical and other interventions, and the family structure and physical home environment. Establishing a common ground for communication, however, requires going beyond asking questions to collaboration on information sharing. That is, therapists need to be aware that the information gaps exists on both sides.

Finding a common ground of understanding is similar to a process parents engage in when teaching their children new skills. It involves collaboration to ensure mutual comprehension (Rogoff et al., 1993), and a stretch on the part of participants—making it a developmental process. From the collaborately constructed common ground, "the participants share in thinking as they extend their understanding together" (Rogoff et al., 1993, p. 8). Parents of children with developmental delays or disabilities constantly try to bridge the gap between what is known and unknown about their child's condition and prognosis. The therapist can either restructure the issue to bring it within the understanding of the parent or can stretch the parents' understanding. This is particularly important when working with families with diverse cultures or beliefs. Either approach requires both parties

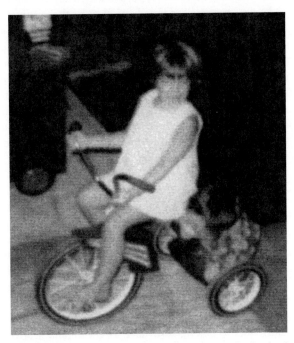

◆ **Figure 30-5** Child with a disability riding at the back of a friend's tricycle.

to understand the rationale behind collaboration and the goals for intervention.

Therapists—Family Collaboration

Collaboration is a shared responsibility whose intent is to capitalize on individual strengths and diversity, and to minimize biases. During the initial encounter families of children with disabilities may rely on physicians, physical and occupational therapists, and case managers for most decisions relating to their child. As can be seen in the case of Jean, at several points the family deferred to the professionals for decisions, particularly when the family encountered a new crisis or transition. Some decisions were good, some not. Yet many families have their own intervention ideas about raising children, including solutions to health-related problems. For some families, professional help may be sought as a last resort. This puts both the family and the therapist in a learner/expert interaction. The therapist needs to explain his or her role to the family, including constraints, and at the same time learn about what the family has to offer, including constraints.

Elements of successful collaborations have been proposed (Turnbull & Turnbull, 2001). Primary skills and attributes are combined in caregiver and therapist competencies in information sharing, mutual trust and respect, conflict resolution, and problem-solving skills (Shelton, 1999; Turnbull & Turnbull, 2001). Initially encounters may be stressful, particularly when roles and needs are not well defined. However, the ultimate goal should be to create a match between the therapist's understanding of the caregiving environment and the parent's understanding of the intervention process. True collaboration occurs when information sharing about the caregiving environment guides the planning of formal assessments. Sharing and exchanging information should also help therapists understand and appreciate the strengths of the child's environment as well as child and family identified needs (Bailey, 2003).

Caregiver Competence

Collaboration elevates and expands the roles of parents. On one hand parents are expected to use their existing parenting skills and resources to meet the needs of their family. On the other hand they must learn new skills that are related to taking care of a child with disabilities, such as advocacy, negotiation, collaboration, and implementing intervention strategies. Some of these roles can be related to Jean's story. Because of the fragmented child health system, parents also have to coordinate services not only within one component, such as developmental services offered within the neighborhood or schools, but also primary health care centers and public health programs such as perinatal outreach programs. Each of these components is independently financed. Therapists must be sensitive to the demands placed on families by building upon the family's readiness and existing resources and when providing suggestions or making recommendations.

Most families of children with disabilities are also families of children who are typically developing. As such, the majority have been successful in caring for and teaching their children without "outside" intervention. Therefore, during the initial encounter, therapists should not only explicitly acknowledge this competence, but also use it as a basis for determining information gaps. For example, finding out about the family's daily routines within their proximal and distal environments prior to or after the diagnosis of the child with disabilities will help determine the extent to which the family has curtailed or enhanced its routines and participation in neighborhood events. Most families may demonstrate the necessary skills and coping in accessing and utilizing services, but some may need more formal support.

Physical Therapist Competencies

Provision of family-centered services in natural environments is mandated by the IDEA of 1997 and competencies are outlined in the Division for Early Childhood (DEC) of the Council for Exceptional Children for best practice (Sandall et al., 2000). The therapist must be resourceful, insightful, have good communication skills, be willing to negotiate, and be eager to learn as well as to educate. A critical component of assessing children within the context of their environments is the sharing of information to enhance the decision-making process. Gathering information about children's environments requires skill in interviewing and observation. Effective communication with the family is characterized by the ability to observe in an unbiased manner and active listening. Observation of movement is a skill of therapists that needs to be extended to include observation of child-family interaction within the context of activities and routines. The long-term benefits that accrue from understanding of the milieu of the child and its environment can be dramatic, albeit time-consuming. Literature on effective interviewing and observation skills is extensive (Adler & Adler, 1998; Fontana & Frey, 1998; Patton, 1990).

Family-Centered Intervention

Collaboration in seeking, gathering, and sharing information is a hallmark of family-centered intervention. The family-centered approach accepts that power resides within the family, but that the family can elect to share the responsibility with the professional. Literature on the family-centered approach to intervention has burgeoned over the last decades (Bailey & Simmeonson, 1990; Dunst, 1996; Kolobe et al., 2000; Rosenbaum et al., 1998; Turnbull et al., 2000) (see also Chapter 31). Studies on the effectiveness of family-centered care have reported that families demonstrate improved decision-making ability (Dunst et al., 1997), coping ability, increasing feelings of empowerment (Brewer et al., 1989; Lewis et al., 1990), and satisfaction with intervention outcomes (Maly et al., 1999). Positive outcomes are partly attributed to sharing of information in ways that allow parents to be equal partners in decision making (Turnbull et al., 2000).

GATHERING INFORMATION ABOUT THE ENVIRONMENT

Families are shaped by so many forces that identifying and assessing them all would be very difficult if not close to impossible for any one given program or professional. The assumption made in this chapter is that the intervention encounter should be team-based. We also assume that parents advance their understanding in many creative ways including becoming active participants in the many child-centered activities within their proximal and distal environments. The method of data gathering may vary but families should be given choices. The open-ended ethnographic interview method (Fontana & Frey, 2001) may provide rich qualitative information in areas such as family structure and functioning, family values, cultural childrearing beliefs, daily family routines, stressors and coping strategies, informal and formal support, and level of family participation. However, some families may prefer the questions and answers method, self-administered questionnaires or assessment scales, or both (Davis & Gettinger, 1995). How the questions are framed holds the key to the quantity, quality, and the flow of information. Methods that have worked well in qualitative research may be valuable to therapists who are inexperienced or having difficulty collaborating with families (Fontana & Frey, 2001).

Several well-known self-report and observational scales can be used to supplement information gathered from interview and to assess other aspects of the caregiving environment. The Home Observation for Measurement of the Environment (HOME) (Caldwell & Bradley, 1984) is particularly useful in gathering information about the quality and quantity of stimulation in a child's proximal environment. The Nursing Child Assessment Satellite Training Feeding (NCAFS) and Teaching scales (NCATS) (Barnard, 1978; Sumner & Spietz, 1994) assess behaviors that the caregiver and child display during interactions with each other. Other family-oriented assessments that can be used to measure aspects of social support and perceptions of family roles and responsibilities are the Inventory of Socially Supportive Behaviors (ISSB) (Berrera, 1981), the Family Needs Survey (Bailey & Simeonsson, 1988), and the Family Routines Inventory (Gallagher et al., 1983). Measures such as the Canadian Occupational Performance Measure (Law et al., 1998) and child health and quality of life measures (Bjornson & McLaughlin, 2001) can be used to gain information about family expectations and their children's quality of life. Efforts have been made to make these assessments unbiased according to ethnicity and other social factors. The scales provide a way of collecting information in a systematic manner.

CHANGING THE CONTEXT

Despite the overwhelming evidence that supports the importance of the ecology in shaping the development and functional independence of children, changing the childrearing environments of children through interventions such as parent education has proved difficult. At the heart of this dilemma is lack of information about the amount of resources or the intensity of interventions that are of sufficient magnitude to bring about change in the child and family. Evidence suggests that families' familiarity with particular teaching strategies, coupled with the importance they place on achievement, plays a major role in the types of activities they will invest in (Goodnow, 1997). Yet seldom do professionals take the time to understand these expectations and strategies. These observations also suggest the need to rethink strategies used in parent education. One such parent education approach that has been found to be effective with mothers of young children is participatory guidance (Rogoff et al., 1993; Stern-Bruschweiler & Stern, 1989).

PARTICIPATORY GUIDANCE

Participatory guidance is a multifaceted approach to learning that emphasizes the child as an active and responsible learner in structured and unstructured activities and in forming diverse relationships with caregivers (Rogoff et al., 1993; Stern-Bruschweiler & Stern, 1989). Participatory guidance focuses simultaneously on individual, interpersonal, and cultural processes of learning. Emphasis is placed on how the caregiver structures and guides the child's learning experiences in novel and routine situations while at the same time adjusting her level of participation according to the child's skill. Mutual understanding of parent and professional roles, learning situations, and strategies to promote the child's development within the context of everyday activities are essential features of participatory guidance. Participatory guidance has been reported to improve mothers' interactional skills, suggesting that parent-child interaction can be improved with instruction (Stern-Bruschweiler & Stern, 1989).

Here is an example of teaching an activity using participatory guidance:

Activity: Teaching Rosa, a 7-year-old girl who has cerebral palsy, how to get in and out of a bathtub independently and safely.

Establishing a Common Ground: First ask Rosa and her mother (individually) why this activity is important, what they think is preventing Rosa from performing the activity, what they have tried to help Rosa perform the activity, how long they think it will take for Rosa to learn the activity, and what would happen if Rosa cannot get in and out of a bathtub independently and safely (cultural beliefs and values, understanding of the disability, and consequences). The key is to understand both the child and the caregiver's perception of the activity. Also ask the mother about her preferred method of learning and teaching. Ask about other skills that require similar ability, that are part of Rosa's daily activities, such as getting in and out of bed or the car, or getting down to the floor. Participatory guidance is believed to be effective when an activity is taught within the context of daily routines (Rogoff et al., 1993).

Observation: Observation of the mother's teaching and Rosa's learning styles is another key element in participatory guidance. Ask the mother and Rosa to demonstrate how they go through the entire routine of taking a bath. During the demonstration, observe her position in relation to Rosa, level and timing of assistance, nonverbal exchanges between her and Rosa. Listen to instructions and verbal interactions. After the demonstration ask her why they do each step the way they do. Within the framework of participatory guidance, the rationale is as important as the manner in which the mother teaches the activity.

Sharing Information: Discuss your analysis of the activity with Rosa and her mother, and relate discussion to Rosa's functional abilities and constraints. Discuss the various options and guide the mother and Rosa (verbally or physically) on how to perform the transfer. The following are three potential methods: (a) first Rosa sits on the outside edge of the tub and then moves her legs into the tub, (b) Rosa holds on to a grab bar and puts one leg in the tub at a time, or (c) Rosa uses a bathtub bench to lower herself into the tub. The key is not only to educate Rosa and the mother about potential options, but to allow them to select their preferred method. This is particularly helpful if any one of the methods can be generalized to other transfer activities. If possible, suggest that the family videotape the practice sessions and analyze the tapes together. Essentially the therapist's role in participatory guidance is that of a coach.

SUMMARY

A challenge to pediatric therapists is to determine strategies for providing evidence-based services that are family-centered, culturally relevant, and environmentally appropriate. The literature on the impact of social and physical environments on child development and function is an important resource for therapists when selecting intervention strategies and providing parents information. Understanding the psychosocial and sociocultural factors that are believed to link family interactions to child outcome will not only enable the therapist to pursue innovative intervention approaches, but will also serve as a resource to families of children with disabilities.

The importance of the environment and Jean's case underscore the need for therapists to rethink several aspects of service provision, particularly parent education, parent-professional collaboration, and cultural competence. First, parent education should focus on information sharing, and should take into consideration the factors such as family stress, socioeconomic status, parent-child interactions, and cultural beliefs about childrearing. Second, central to effective parent-professional collaboration is the willingness by both parties to learn from each other; therefore, therapists must seek to learn from families just as much as they desire to teach them. Third, if professionals are to truly respect families' culture and parenting roles, the process of cultural competence must begin with the examination of one's own culture, proceed to learning about families' cultural beliefs and meanings attached to illness or disabilities, and culminate in mutually rewarding and meaningful interactions.

The importance of the environment does not take precedence over the role of biologic factors in influencing child development and function. On the contrary, best practice requires therapists, together with the child and family, to address impairments in body functions and structures based on an understanding of the child's condition. Effective intervention plans must simultaneously address both biologic and environmental factors that are important for the child's activity and participation. A child's needs change over time. Biologic factors may take precedence over environmental factors at any one time, but at no time can either factor be excluded from consideration. As learned from Jean's case, therapists' must consider a child's needs within the context of family structure and functioning, since recommendations can affect the child and family for years to come.

ACKNOWLEGMENT

The authors would like to thank Irene McEwen for reviewing the chapter.

REFERENCES

Ackerman, NJ. A Theory of Family Systems. New York: Gardner Press, 1984.

Adler, PA, & Adler, P. Observational Techniques. In Denzin, NK, & Lincoln, YS (Eds.). Collecting and Interpreting Qualitative Materials. Thousand Oaks, CA: Sage Publications, 1998, pp 79–109.

Barnard, KE. Nursing Child Assessment Teaching Scale. Seattle: University of Washington, 1978.

Barnard, KE. Influencing parent-child interactions for children at risk. In Guralnick, MJ (Ed.). The Effectiveness of Early Intervention. Baltimore: Brookes Publishing Co., 1997, pp. 249–267.

Bailey, DB. Assessing family resources, priorities, and concerns. In McLean, M, Bailey, DB, & Wolery, M. (Eds.). Assessing Infants and Preschoolers with Special Needs, 3rd ed. Englewood Cliffs: Prentice-Hall, 2003, pp. 173–203.

Bailey, DB, & Simeonsson, RJ. Assessing needs of families with handicapped infants. Journal of Special Education, 22(1):117–127, 1988.

Beavers, R, Hampson, R, & Hulgus, Y. Commentary: The Beavers' system approach to family assessment. Family Process, 24:398–405, 1985.

Benasich, AA, & Brooks-Gunn, J. Maternal attitudes and knowledge of child-rearing: Associations with family and child outcomes. Child Development, 67:1186–1205, 1996.

Bjornson, KF, & McLaughlin, JF. The measurement of health-related quality of life (HRQL) in children with cerebral palsy. European Journal of Neurology, 8(Suppl 5):183–193, 2001.

Booth, CL, Mitchell, SK, Barnard, KE, & Spieker, SJ. Development of maternal social skills in multiproblem families: Effects on the mother-child relationship. Developmental Psychology, 25:403–412, 1989.

Bornstein, MC. Cultural Approaches to Parenting. Hillsdale, NJ: Lawrence Erlbaum Associates, 1991.

Boss, P. Family stress: Perception and context. In Sussman, MB, & Stemmetz, S (Eds.). Handbook on Marriage and the Family. New York: Plenum Press, 1985, p. 704.

Bradley, RH. Children's home environments, health, behavior, and intervention efforts: A review using the HOME inventory as a marker measure. Genetic, Social, and General Psychology Monographs, 119(4):437–490, 1993.

Brewer, EJ, McPherson, M, Magrub, PR, & Hutchins, VL. Family-centered, community-based, coordinated care for children with special health care needs. Pediatrics, 83:1055–1060, 1989.

Bricker, D. Early Intervention for At-risk and Handicapped Infants, Toddlers and Preschool Children, 2nd ed. Palo Alto, CA: Vort Corporation, 1989.

Brinker, RP, Seifer, R, & Sameroff, AJ. Relations among maternal stress, cognitive development, and early intervention in middle- and low-SES infants with developmental disabilities. American Journal of Mental Retardation, 98:463–480, 1994.

Broffenbrenner, U. Ecology of the family as a context for human development research perspectives. Developmental Psychology, 22:723–742, 1986.

Brooks-Gunn, J, Berlin, LJ, & Fuligni, AS. Early childhood intervention programs: What about the family? In Shonkoff, JP & Meisels, SJ (Eds.). Handbook of Early Childhood Intervention. New York: Cambridge University Press, 2000, pp. 549–577.

Brooks-Gunn, J, & Duncan, GJ. The effects of poverty on children and youth. The Future of Children, 7(2):55–71, 1997.

Caldwell, BM, & Bradley, RH. Manual for the Home Observation for Measurement of the Environment, rev. ed. Little Rock: University of Arkansas, 1984.

Chan, SQ. Early intervention with culturally diverse families of infants and toddlers with disabilities. Infants and Young Children, 3:78–87, 1990.

Chen, C, & Stevenson, HW. Homework: A cross-cultural examination. Child Development, 60:551–561, 1989.

Chiarello, LA, & Palisano, RJ. Investigation of the effects of a model of physical therapy on mother-child interactions and the motor behaviors of children with motor delay. Physical Therapy, 78(2):180–194, 1998.

Cook, TD, Kim, JR, Chan, WS, & Setterten, R. How do neighborhoods matter? In Furstenburg, FF, Cook, TD, Eccles, J, Elder, GH, & Sameroff, AJ (Eds.). Managing to Make It: Urban Families in High Risk Neighborhoods. Chicago: University of Chicago Press, 1997.

Cintas, HM. The relationship of motor skill level and risk-taking during exploration in toddlers. Pediatric Physical Therapy, 4(1):165–170, 1992.

Darling, RB. Families against Society: A Study of Reactions to Children with Birth Defects. Beverly Hills, CA: Sage, 1979, p. 78.

Darling, N, & Steinberg, L. Parenting style as context: An integrative model. Psychological Bulletin, 113:487–496, 1993.

Davis, SK, & Gettinger, M. Family-focused assessment for identifying family resources and concerns: Parent preferences, assessment information, and evaluation across three methods. Journal of School Psychology, 33:99–121, 1995.

DeGrace, BW. Occupation-based family-centered care: A challenge for current practice. American Journal of Occupational Therapy, 57:347–350, 2003.

Duncan, GJ, Brooks-Gunn, J, & Klebanov, PK. Economic deprivation and early childhood development. Child Development, 65(2):296–318, 1994.

Dunst, CJ, Trivette, CM, & Jodry, W. Influences of social support on children with disabilities and their families. In Guralnick, M. (Ed.). The Effectiveness of Early Intervention. Baltimore: Paul H. Brookes, 1997, pp. 499–522.

Dunst, CJ, Trivette, CM, Gordon, NJ, & Pletcher, LL. Building and mobilizing informal family support networks. In Singer, GHS, & Irwin, LK (Eds.). Support for Caregiving Families: Enabling Positive Adaptation to Disability. Baltimore: Paul H. Brookes, 1989, pp. 121–141.

Edelman, GM. Neural darwinism: Selection and reentrant signaling in higher brain function. Neuron, 10:115–125, 1993.

Farran, DC. Another decade of intervention for children who are low income or disabled: What do we know? In Shonkoff, JP, & Meisels, SJ (Eds). Handbook of Early Childhood Intervention, 2nd ed. New York: Cambridge University Press, 2000, pp. 510–548.

Flynt, SW, Wood, TA, & Scott, RL. Social support of mothers of children with mental retardation. Mental Retardation, 30:233–236, 1992.

Fontana, A, & Frey, JH. Interviewing: The Art of Science. In Denzin, NK, & Lincoln, YS (Eds.). Collecting and Interpreting Qualitative Materials. Thousand Oaks, CA: Sage Publications, 1988, pp 47–77.

Fox, RA. Maternal factors related to parenting practices, developmental expectations, and perceptions of child behavior problems. Journal of Genetic Psychology, 156:431–441, 1995.

Gallagher, J, Beckman, P, & Cross, A. Families of handicapped children: Sources of stress and its amelioration. Exceptional Children, 50(1):10–19, 1983.

Garcia-Coll, C, & Magnusson, K. Cultural differences as sources of developmental vulnerabilities and resources. In Shonkoff, JP, & Meisels, SJ (Eds.). Handbook of Early Childhood Intervention, 2nd ed. Cambridge: Cambridge University Press, 2000, pp. 94–114.

Garcia-Coll, C, & Magnusson, K. Cultural influences on child development: Are we ready for a paradigm shift? In Masten, AS (Ed.). Cultural Processes in Child Development—The Minnesota Symposia on Child Psychology. Mahwah, NJ: Lawrence Erlbaum, 1999, pp. 1–24.

Garrett, P, Ng'andu, N, & Ferron, J. Poverty experiences of young children and the equality of their home environments. Child Development, 65:331–345, 1994.

Gentile, AM. Skill acquisition: Action, movement, and neuromotor processes. In Carr, JH, & Shepherd, RB (Eds). Movement Science: Foundation for Physical Therapy Rehabilitation. Rockville, MD: Aspen Publishers, 2000, pp. 111–187.

Gibson, EJ. The Ecological Approach to Visual Perception. Boston: Houghton Mifflin, 1988.

Goodnow, JJ. Parents' ideas, children's ideas: Correspondence and divergence. In Sigel, IE, McGillicuddy-DeLisi, AV, & Goodnow, JJ (Eds.). Parental Belief Systems: The Psychological Consequences for Children, 2nd ed. Hillsdale, NJ: Lawrence Erlbaum Associates, 1992, pp. 293–317.

Goodnow, JJ. Parenting and the transmission and internalization of values: From social-cultural perspectives to within-family analysis. In Grusec, JE, & Kuczynski, L (Eds). Parenting Strategies and Children's Internalizations of Values: A Handbook of Contemporary Theory. New York: Wiley, 1997, pp. 331–361.

Goodnow, JJ. Parents ideas, actions, and feelings: Models and methods from developmental and social psychology. Child Development, 59:296–320, 1988.

Gottlieb, AS. Single mothers of children with developmental disabilities: The impact of multiple roles. Family Relations, 46(1):5–13, 2002.

Green, JW. Cultural Awareness in the Human Services: Ethnicity and Social Services. Englewood Cliffs, NJ: Prentice-Hall, 1982.

Grosec, JE, Rudy, D, & Martini, T. Parenting cognitions and child outcomes: An overview and implications for children's internalization of values. In Grusec, JE, & Kuczynski, L (Eds.). Parenting and Children's Internalization of Values: A Handbook of Contemporary Theory. New York: John Wiley & Sons, 1997, pp. 259–282.

Gutierrez, J, & Sameroff, A. Determinant of complexity in Mexican American and Anglo American mothers' conception of child development. Child Development, 61:384–394, 1990.

Haley, SM, & Baryza, MJ. A hierarchy of motor outcome assessment: Self-initiated movements through adaptive motor function. Infants and Young Children, 3(1):1–14, 1990.

Halpern, R. Early intervention for low-income children and families. In Shonkoff, JP, & Meisels, SJ (Eds.). Handbook of Early Childhood Intervention. New York: Cambridge University Press, 2000, pp. 361–386.

Hanley, J. Beyond the tip of the iceberg: Five stages toward cultural competence. Reaching Today's Youth, 3(2):9–12, 1999.

Harris, SR. The effectiveness of early intervention for children with cerebral palsy and related motor disabilities. In Guralnick, MJ (Ed.). The Effectiveness of Early Intervention. Baltimore: Brookes Publishing Co., 1997, pp. 327–347.

Harwood, RL, Miller, JG, & Irizarry, NL. Culture and attachment: Perceptions of the child in context. New York: Guilford, 1995.

Hauser-Cram, P, Warfield, ME, Shonkoff, JP, & Krauss, MW. Children with disabilities: A longitudinal study of child development and parent well-being. Monographs of the Society for Research in Child Development, 66(3, Serial No. 266), 2001.

Hayden, LC, Schiller, M, Dickstein, S, Seifer, R, Sameroff, AJ, et al. Levels of family assessment: I. Family, marital, and parent-child interaction. Journal of Family Psychology, 12:7–22, 1998.

Heifetz, LJ. Integrating religious and secular perspectives in the design of disability services. Mental Retardation, 25:127–131, 1987.

Hepburn, SL. Clinical implications of temperamental characteristics in young children with developmental disabilities. Infant & Young Children, 16:59–76, 2003.

Hirshberg, LM. History-making, not history-taking: Clinical interviews with infants and their families. In Meisels, SJ & Fenichel, E (Eds.). New Visions for the Developmental Assessment of Infants and Young Children. Washington, DC: Zero to Three, 1996, pp. 85–124.

Hollingshead, AB. Four factor index of social status. New Haven: Yale University Press, 1975.

Individuals with Disabilities Act Amendments of 1997. Federal Register, Final Rules, April 1998. 34 CFR Part 303.

Institute of Medicine. Unequal treatment: What healthcare providers need to know about racial and ethnic disparities in health care. National Academy of Sciences, March 2002, pp. 1–7. http://www.iom.edu/Object.File/Master/4/175/0.pdf. Accessed September 27, 2005.

Kaufman, J, & Rosenbaum, J. The education and employment of low-income black youth in white suburbs. Educational Evaluation and Policy Analysis, 14:229–240, 1992.

Kelly, JF, & Barnard, KE. Assessment of parent-child interaction: Implications for early intervention. In Shonkoff, JP, &. Meisels, SJ (Eds.). Handbook of Early Childhood Intervention. New York: Cambridge University Press, 2000, pp. 258–289.

Knutson, LM (Ed.) Cross-cultural and International Health Issues. Pediatric Physical Therapy, vol. 7, 1995.

Kochanska, G, Kuczynski, L, & Radke-Yarrow, M. Correspondence between mother's self-reported and observed child-rearing practices. Child Development, 60:56–63, 1989.

Kochanska, G. Maternal beliefs as long-term predictors of mother-child interaction and report. Child Development, 61(6):1934–1943, 1990.

Kolobe, THA. Childrearing practices and developmental expectations for Mexican-American mothers and the developmental status of their infants. Physical Therapy, 84:439–453, 2004.

Kolobe, THA, Sparling, J, & Daniels, LE. Family-centered intervention. In Campbell, SK, Vander Linden, DW, & Palisano, RJ (Eds.). Physical Therapy for Children, 2nd ed. Philadelphia: WB Saunders, 2000, pp. 881–907.

Kolobe, THA, Bulanda, M, & Susman, L. Predictive validity of the Test of Infant Motor Performance at Pre-school Age. Physical Therapy, 84:1144–1156, 2004.

Larin, HM. Motor learning: Theories and strategies for the practitioner. In Campbell, SK, Vander Linden, DW, & Palisano, RJ (Eds). Physical Therapy for Children, 2nd ed.. Philadelphia: WB Saunders, 2000, pp. 170–197.

Law, M, Baptiste, S, Carswell, A, McCall, M, Polatajko, H, & Pollock, N. Canadian Occupational Performance Measure, 3rd ed. Toronto, Canada: CAOT Publication, 1998.

Leavitt, R. Cross-Cultural Rehabilitation: An International Perspective. Toronto: WB Saunders, 1999.

Levine, RA, Dixon, S, Levin, S, Richman, A, et al. Child Care and Culture: Lessons from Africa. New York: Cambridge University Press, 1994.

Lynch, EW. Developing cross-cultural competence. In Lynch, EW, & Hanson, MJ (Eds.). Developing Cross-Cultural Competence: A Guide for Working with Young Children and Their Families. Baltimore: Paul H. Brookes, 1992.

Maccoby, EE. The role of parents in the socialization of children: An historical overview. Developmental Psychology, 28:1006–1017, 1992.

Mahoney, G, & Filer, J. How responsive is early intervention to the priorities and needs of families? Topics in Early Childhood Special Education, 16(4):437–457, 1996.

Maly, RC, Bourque LB, & Englehardt, RF. A randomized controlled trial of facilitating information giving to patients with chronic medical conditions: Effects on outcomes of care. Journal of Family Practice, 48:356–363, 1999.

Marshak, LE, Seligman, M, & Prezant, F. Disability and the family life cycle: Recognizing and treating challenges. New York: Basic Books, 1999.

Marfo, K. Correlates of maternal directiveness with children who are developmentally delayed. American Journal of Orthopsychiatry, 62:219–233, 1992.

Masten, SA (Ed.). Cultural Processes in Child Development — The Minnesota Symposia on Child Psychology. Mahwah, NJ: Lawrence Erlbaum, 1999, pp. 123–135.

McCormick, MC, McCarton, C, Brooks-Gunn, J, & Gross, RT. The infant health and development program — Interim summary. Journal of Developmental and Behavioral Pediatrics, 19:359–370, 1998.

McCubbin, HI, & Patterson, JM. Systematic Assessment of Family Stress, Resources and Coping. St. Paul: University of Minnesota, 1982, pp. 7–15.

McLoyd, VC. Socioeconomic disadvantage and child development. American Psychologist, 53:185–204, 1998.

Mendola, P, Selevan, SG, Gutter, S, & Rice, D. Environmental factors associated with a spectrum of neurodevelopmental deficits. Mental Retardation and Developmental Disabilities, 8:188–197, 2002.

Mills, RSL, & Rubin, KH. Parental beliefs about problematic social behaviors in early childhood. Child Development, 61:138–151, 1990.

Milner, JS, & Crouch, JL. Impact and detection of response distortions on parenting measures used to assess risk for child physical abuse. Journal of Personality Assessment, 69(3):633–650, 1997.

Morris, TM. Culturally sensitive family assessment: An evaluation of the Family Assessment Device used with Hawaiian-American and Japanese-American families. Family Process, 29:105–116, 1990.

Moxley-Haegert, L, & Serbin, LA. Developmental education for parents of delayed infants: effects on parental motivation and children's development. Child Development, 54L:1324–1331, 1983.

Mulligan, L, Specker, BL, Buckley DD, O'Connor, LS, & Ho, M. Physical and environment factors affecting motor development, activity level, and body composition of infants in child care centers. Pediatric Physical Therapy, 10:156–161, 1998.

NCAST Programs. Network Survey. University of Washington. Seattle, WA: NCAST Publications, 1986.

Olson, DH: Circumplex model VII: Validation studies and FACES III. Family Process, 25(1):337–351, 1986.

Palisano, RJ, Tieman, BL, Walter, SD, et al. Effect of environmental setting on mobility methods of children with cerebral palsy. Developmental Medicine and Child Neurology, 45:113–120, 2003.

Patton, MQ. Qualitative Evaluation and Research Methods, 2nd ed. Newbury Park, CA: Sage, 1990, pp. 277–368.

Petersen, P, & Wikoff, RL. Home environment and adjustment in families with handicapped children: A canonical correlation study. Occupational Therapy Journal of Research, 7(1):67–82, 1987.

Phillip, MJ, Voran, D, Kisker, E, Howes, C, & Whitebook, M. Child care for children in poverty: Opportunity or inequity? Child Development, 65:472–492, 1994.

Pollitt, E, Gorman, KS, Engle, PL, Rivera, JA, & Martorell, R. Nutrition in early life and the fulfillment of intellectual potential, Journal of Nutrition, 125:1111S–1118S, 1995.

Public Law 105-17, Individuals with Disabilities Education Act Amendments of 1997, 111 Stat. 37-157.

Richman, A, Miller, P, & Levine, R. Cultural and educational variations in maternal responsiveness. Developmental Psychology, 28:614–621, 1992.

Rogoff, B, Mistry, J, Concu, A, & Mosier, C. Guided participation in cultural activities by toddlers and caregivers. Monographs of Society for Research in Child Development, 58, Serial No. 236, 1993.

Roosa, MW, Jones, S, Tein, Jenn-Yun, & Cree, W. Prevention science and neighborhood influences on low-income children's development: Theoretical and methodological issues. American Journal of Community Psychology, 31:55–72, 2003.

Rosenbaum, P, King, S, Law, M, et al. Family-centered service: A conceptual framework and research review. Physical & Occupational Therapy in Pediatrics, 18(1):1–20 1998.

Sameroff, AJ, & Chandler, MJ. Reproductive risk and the continuum of caretaking casualty. In Horowitz, FD, Hetherington, M, Scarr-Salapatek, S, & Sigel, G (Eds.). Review of Child Development Research. Chicago: University of Chicago Press, 1975, 4 pp. 187–244.

Sameroff, AJ, & Feil, LA. Parental conception of development. In Sigel IE (Ed.). Parental Belief System: The Psychological Consequences For Children. Hillsdale, NJ: Erlbaum, 1985, pp. 83–105.

Sameroff, AJ, & Fiese, BH. Transactional regulation: The development ecology of early intervention. In Shonkoff, JP, & Meisels, SJ (Eds). Handbook of Early Childhood Intervention, 2nd ed. New York: Cambridge University Press, 2000, pp. 135–159.

Sandall, S, McLean, ME, & Smith, BJ. DEC Recommended Practices in Early Intervention/Early Childhood Special Education. Longmong, CO: Sopris West, 2000.

Seitz, V, & Provence, S. Caregiver-focused models of early intervention. In Meisels, SJ, & Shonkoff, JP (Eds.). Handbook of Early Childhood Intervention. New York: Cambridge University Press, 1990, pp. 400–427.

Shelton, T. Family-centered care in pediatric practice: When and how? Journal of Developmental & Behavioral Pediatrics, 20:117–119, 1999.

Shelton, TL, & Stepanek, JS. Family-Centered Care for Children Needing Specialized Health and Developmental Services, 3rd ed. Bethesda: Association for the Care of Children's Health, 1994.

Shonkoff, JP, Hauser-Cram, P, Krauss, MW, & Upshur, CC. Development of infants with disabilities and their families. Monographs of the Society for Research in Child Development, 57(6, Serial No. 230), 1992.

Shonkoff, JP, & Phillips, DA. From Neurons to Neighborhoods: The Science of Early Childhood Development. Washington, DC: National Academy Press, 2001.

Sigel, IE. The belief-behavior connection: A resolvable dilemma? In Sigel IE, McGillicuddy-Delisi, AV, & Goodnow JJ (Eds.). Parental Belief Systems: The Psychological Consequences for Children, 2nd ed. Hillsdale, NJ: Lawrence Erlbaum Associates, 1992, pp. 433–456.

Sparling, JW, & Sekerak, DK. Embedding the family perspective in an entry level physical therapy curriculum. Pediatric Physical Therapy, 4(1):116–122, 1992.

Spiker, D, Ferguson, J, & Brook-Gunn J. Enhancing maternal interactive behavior and child social competence in low birth-weight, premature infants. Child Development, 64:754–768, 1993.

Stern-Bruscheweiler, N, & Stern, DN. A model for conceptualizing the role of mothers representational work in various mother-infant therapies. Infant Mental Health Journal, 10:142–156, 1989.

Stewart, MJ. Social support: Diverse theoretical perspectives. Social Science and Medicine, 28:1275–1282, 1989.

Sumner, F, & Spietz, A. NCATS/Caregiver/parent-child interaction feeding manual. Seattle, WA: NCATS Publications, 1994.

Super, CM, & Harkness, S. The developmental niche: A concept-ualization at the interface of child and culture. International Journal of Behavioral Development, 9:545–569, 1986.

Super, CM, & Harkness, S. The cultural structuring of child develop-ment. In Berry, JW, Dasen, PR, & Saraswathi, TS (Eds.). Handbook of Cross-Cultural Psychology, 2nd Ed. Boston: Allyn & Bacon, 1997, pp. 1–39.

Thelen, E. Motor Development. A new synthesis. American Psycho-logist, 50:79–95, 1995.

Thelen, E, & Ulrich, BD. Hidden Skills. Monographs of the Society for Research in Child Development, Serial No. 223, 56:1–97, 1991.

Tieman, BL, Palisano, RJ, Gracely, EJ, & Rosenbaum, PL. Gross motor capability and performance of mobility in children with cerebral palsy: A comparison across home, school, and outdoors/community settings. Physical Therapy, 84:419–429, 2004.

Turnbull, A, Turbiville, V, & Turnbull, HR. Evolution of family-professional relationships: Collective empowerment for the early 21st century. In Shonkoff, JP, & Meisels, SJ (Eds). Handbook of Early Childhood Intervention. New York: Cambridge University Press, 2000, pp. 1370–1420.

Turnbull, AP, & Turnbull, HR. Families, Professionals, and Excep-tionality: A Special Partnership, 4th ed. Des Moines: Merrill Prentice-Hall, 2001.

US Census Bureau, Census 2000 Gateway. http://www.census.gov/main/www/cen2000.html.

Vygotsky, L. In Cole, M, John-Steiner, V, Scribner, S, & Souberman, E. (Eds.). Mind in Society: The Development of Higher Psychological Processes. Cambridge, MA: Harvard University Press, 1978.

Washington, K, & Schwartz, I. Maternal perceptions of the effects of physical and occupational therapy services on caregiving compe-tency. Physical and Occupational Therapy in Pediatrics, 16:33–54, 1996.

Werner, E. Protective factors and resilience. In Shonkoff, JP, & Meisels, SJ (Eds). Handbook of Early Childhood Intervention. New York: Cambridge University Press, pp. 115–132, 2000.

Whiting, BB, & Whiting, JWM. Children of Six Cultures: A Psycho-cultural Analysis. Cambridge: Harvard University Press, 1975.

World Health Organization. ICIDH2: International Classification of Functioning, Disability and Health. Geneva: World Health Organ-ization, 2001.

Zuniga, M. Families with Latino roots. In Lynch, EW, & Hanson, MJ (Eds.). Developing cross-cultural competence: A guide for working with young children and their families. Baltimore: Paul H. Brookes, 1992.

Chapter 31

EARLY INTERVENTION SERVICES

LISA A. CHIARELLO
PT, PhD, PCS

THUBI H.A. KOLOBE
PT, PhD

The focus of this chapter is on early intervention services in home and community settings under the Individuals with Disabilities Education Improvement Act (IDEIA) of 2004 (Public Law 108-446). Part C of the IDEIA authorizes federal assistance to states to implement a system of early intervention services for eligible infants and toddlers, birth to 3 years of age, and their families. The law mandates family-centered services in natural environments to promote the child's development and participation in daily activities and routines. Providing services in early intervention can be complex and challenging, but very rewarding. Therapists practicing in early intervention truly have the opportunity to integrate the science and art of physical therapy. In this chapter, theory, policy, and methods of service delivery

are critiqued and research is analyzed. The role of the physical therapist in this unique approach to practice is discussed. Finally, we will present a collaborative model for early intervention service delivery and illustrate application using a case history.

WHAT IS EARLY INTERVENTION?

Early intervention is a multifaceted phenomenon with admirable goals. Early intervention is predicated on the notion that infancy is a sensitive period in development and families assume the primary role of nurturing and providing early learning experiences for their children. The concept of sensitive periods assumes that children are more responsive to experiential learning during the first 3 years of life when there is rapid brain growth and plasticity (Shore, 1997). Shonkoff and Meisels (2000) define early intervention as consisting of "multidisciplinary services provided to children from birth to 5 years of age to promote child health and well-being, enhance emerging competencies, minimize developmental delays, remediate existing or emerging disabilities, prevent functional deterioration, and promote adaptive parenting and overall family functioning. These goals are accomplished by providing individualized developmental, educational, and therapeutic services for children in conjunction with mutually planned support for their families" (pp. xvii–xviii). This definition embraces the concepts of prevention, remediation, experiential learning, individuality, and family-centeredness and is consistent with the definition of early intervention in IDEIA.

IDEIA defines early intervention as "developmental services that are provided under public supervision, are provided at no cost except where Federal or State law provides for a system of payments by families, including a schedule of sliding fees, and are designed to meet the developmental needs of an infant or toddler with disability in any one or more of the following areas: physical development, cognitive development, communication development, social or emotional development, or adaptive development." In addition, IDEIA stipulates that services are selected in collaboration with the parent and "meet the standards of the State including the requirements of the law." This definition emphasizes the service delivery aspect of early intervention; the primary premise is that services must be developmental and involve parent collaboration.

To be effective in early intervention, physical therapists must embrace responsibilities that go beyond technical knowledge and skill. Early intervention providers are required to partner with families and other providers, deliver services in multiple environments, comply with federal and state policy, and provide interventions informed by current evidence and principles of best practice. In addition to expertise in motor development, adaptive function and self-care, physical therapists must have practical knowledge of social, emotional, cognitive, communication, and language development (Shonkoff & Phillips, 2000).

EFFECTIVENESS OF EARLY INTERVENTION

Early intervention services are based primarily on philosophy and knowledge of early childhood development and family function as well as the provisions of federally mandated public laws. Research indicates that the benefits of early intervention are equivocal and vary across children and families (Guralnick, 1997; Ramey & Ramey, 1998; Farran, 2000; Brooks-Gunn et al., 2000). This in part reflects the complex and multifaceted nature of early intervention services and the fact that few states systematically evaluate and report outcomes for children and families. Shonkoff and associates (1992) identified methodologic challenges that have contributed to limited research and ability to generalize findings across children and settings. Research has focused on interventions for infants and toddlers experiencing delays who are at environmental or biologic risk. Interventions tend to be broad in scope with little detail on specific strategies and procedures. The problem of withholding intervention diminishes the potential effect size between the experimental and control group. Consequently, the question of what interventions are most effective based on child and family characteristics remains unclear.

Physical therapists will find it particularly challenging to integrate and apply research findings on early intervention for three reasons: (a) A large proportion of the literature and research comes from the fields of medicine,

psychology, sociology, and early childhood education, and have concentrated on health, cognition, and behavior; (b) the role of physical therapy as part of an early intervention team has seldom been addressed; and (c) well-designed studies with large samples such as the Infant Health Development Program (Ramey et al., 1992) have targeted "at-risk populations" of infants at risk for global developmental delay, speech and language disorders, or social-emotional maladjustment (Ramey et al., 1992; McCormick et al., 1998; Farran, 2000; Brooks-Gunn et al., 2000).

Empirical support for early intervention for children with physical disabilities and their families is inconclusive. A meta-analysis conducted by Shonkoff and associates in 1987 revealed that children with motor disabilities benefited the least from the early intervention services as measured by gains on developmental assessments. More than a decade later, children with motor impairment continue to show less functional gains compared to children with delays in other areas (Harris, 1997; Pakula & Palmer, 1997; Hauser-Cram et al., 2001). Findings for children with disabilities indicate that severity, and not type of physical disability, is a strong predictor of change; children with mild disabilities showed greater gains than children with severe disabilities, regardless of the intensity of services (Shonkoff et al., 1992; Hauser-Cram et al., 2001). Collectively, research indicates that norm-referenced developmental assessments are not responsive to changes that children with severe physical disabilities are capable of achieving. Outcomes for adaptive function, participation in family and community life, and ease of caregiving have not been examined.

Research on the effectiveness of physical therapy for infants has focused on procedural interventions to modify impairments. Outcomes for norm-referenced measures do not support the effectiveness of physical therapy (Piper, 1990; Turnbull, 1993; Harris, 1997; Butler & Darrah, 2001). It is interesting that, despite the small to modest gains in motor function, the findings suggest that physical therapy interventions may enhance parent responsiveness to their children (Palmer et al., 1990). Communication and coordination and patient/client-related instruction are components of physical therapist interventions that are extremely relevant in early intervention. These components of intervention have not been examined.

IMPLICATIONS FOR PHYSICAL THERAPIST PRACTICE

At a program level, research findings underscore the need to consider the interaction among the child's biologic factors and family characteristics when planning physical therapy interventions. Child and family characteristics appear to be more predictive of outcomes than any specific feature of early intervention services (Shonkoff et al., 1992). Family interactions and experiences have had the most direct influence on child developmental outcomes (Guralnick, 1998). Therefore, the environmental context of intervention is as important as the content. Lastly research suggests that services that are comprehensive in nature, that target multiple levels of functioning and outcomes, appear to be more beneficial than a single treatment approach. Consequently, interventions should target all three components of health (body functions and structures, activities, participation) and contextual factors (environmental and personal) of the International Classification of Functioning, Disability, and Health (World Health Organization, 2001).

On an individual level, knowledge and research continue to shape the formulation, refinement, and reexamination of themes for family-centered services such as providing families the opportunity to identify their concerns and needs, sharing information with families, conducting family-friendly culturally sensitive assessments, identifying meaningful outcomes, individualizing services, supporting family efforts, and providing services in natural environments. Because no one discipline can provide services that incorporate all child and family needs, effective interventions will require multiple levels of collaboration (Guralnick, 1998; Jackson, 1998; Filer & Mahoney, 1996). Equally important will be the availability of professionals who are adequately prepared to engage in this expanded scope of practice (Widerstrom & Ableman, 1996).

IDEIA PART C: INFANTS AND TODDLERS WITH DISABILITY

The Education of the Handicapped Act Amendments of 1986 (Public Law 99-457, Part H) provided for family-centered services for infants and toddlers from birth to 3 years of age. This law was subsequently reauthorized and amended as Part C of the Individuals with Disabilities Education Act Amendment (IDEA) of 1997 (Public Law 105-17) and IDEIA of 2004 (Public Law 108-446). Part C mandates early intervention services based on the following declaration:

> [that] Congress finds that there is an urgent and substantial need (1) to enhance the development of infants and toddlers with disabilities and to minimize their potential for developmental delay, and to recognize the significant brain development that occurs during a

child's first 3 years of life; (2) to reduce the educational costs to our society, including our Nation's schools, by minimizing the need for special education and related services after infants and toddlers with disabilities reach school age; (3) to maximize the potential for their independently living in society; (4) to enhance the capacity of families to meet the special needs of their infants and toddlers with disabilities; and (5) to enhance the capacity of State and local agencies and service providers to identify, evaluate, and meet the needs of all children, particularly minority, low-income, inner-city, and rural children and infants and toddlers in foster care

> IDEIA, Part C, Sec. 631

The legislation details the conditions that a state must meet in order to receive federal funding. In addition, Part C clearly articulates particular philosophies of care related to coordination of services, individualized family care, and services in natural environments.

Part C stipulates that early intervention services are designed to meet the developmental needs of an infant or toddler with a developmental delay or disability (or diagnosed physical or mental condition with high probability of resulting in developmental delay) in any one or more of the following areas: physical development, cognitive development, communication development, social or emotional development, and adaptive development. Each state has its own definition of developmental delay and thus eligibility for early intervention varies from state to state (Spiker et al., 2000). In Pennsylvania, children have to demonstrate a developmental delay of 25% in one of five areas; in New Jersey, children have to demonstrate a delay of 33% in one area or 25% in two or more areas; and in Oklahoma, children have to demonstrate a delay of 50% in one area or 25% in two or more areas. The list of early intervention services identified in the legislation is provided in Table 31-1. Services are to be provided by qualified personnel based on state licensing or certification requirements. Physical therapists are included under qualified personnel.

The components of service delivery identified in Part C are included in Box 31-1. The five major components are as follows:

- A public awareness program
- A central directory of information
- A comprehensive child find system
- Comprehensive evaluations and assessments
- Individualized family service plan (IFSP)

To receive funding under Part C, the states must comply with all provisions as detailed in IDEIA. The law also states general guidelines on when, how, and where assessments, IFSPs, and interventions must be planned, conducted, and implemented. For detailed information,

TABLE 31-1	**Early Intervention Services Included in the Individuals with Disabilities Education Improvement Act**

Family training, counseling, home visits
Special instruction
Speech, language pathology, and audiology services
Occupational therapy
Physical therapy
Psychologic services
Service coordination
Medical services only for diagnostic or evaluation purposes

Early identification, screening, and assessment services
Health services necessary to enable the infant or toddler to benefit from the other early intervention services:
Social work services
Vision services
Assistive technology devices and services
Transportation and related costs necessary to receive early intervention services

Box 31-1	**Components of Part C Infant and Toddler Program of the Individuals with Disabilities Education Improvement Act**

- Early intervention services for all infants and toddlers with disabilities from birth to age 3 and their families
- Child Find: a system to identify, locate and evaluate children with disabilities
- Natural environments
- Comprehensive, multidisciplinary evaluation (MDE)
- Individualized family service plan (IFSP)

- Procedural safeguards
- Public awareness program
- Central directory
- Comprehensive system of personnel development
- Administration by a lead agency
- State Interagency Coordinating Council

therapists are advised to read the legislation and regulations which can be accessed through several websites listed in this chapter's resource supplement. The document *Providing Physical Therapy Services Under Parts B & C of the Individuals with Disabilities Education Act* published by the American Physical Therapy Association (McEwen, 2000) elaborates on the federal law and the role of the physical therapist.

FAMILY-CENTERED CARE

Family-centered care is believed to be the key to addressing the multiple levels and facets of care for infants and toddlers with disabilities. The underlying tenet is that optimal family functioning promotes optimal child development (Shonkoff & Phillip, 2000). The emphasis on family-centered care is intended to engender a deeper appreciation of families of children with disabilities, particularly those from minority groups, and the challenges families face in supporting the development of their children.

Several definitions of the concept of family-centered intervention have been presented (Dunst et al., 1991; Shelton & Stepanek, 1994). A common thread is that family-centered care is a philosophical approach with many facets; it is a combination or constellation of beliefs, attitudes, and practices to care and is family-driven. The definition by Dunst and associates is widely used: "a combination of beliefs and practices that define particular ways of working with families that are consumer-driven and competency enhancing" (1991, p. 115). Perhaps the most important difference between family-centered and professional-centered approaches is that the professional's role is partly defined by each child and family's resources and priorities, and not only by the severity of the child's developmental delay or disabilities. Initially, the less defined role may be unsettling to professionals, whose education and expertise is biased toward addressing a child's impairments and functional limitations.

The key elements of family-centered care, proposed by the National Center for Family-Centered Care, influence provision of services to families and children (Shelton & Stepanek, 1994). The elements are listed here:

- Recognition of the family as the constant in a child's life
- Facilitation of family-to-family networking
- Promotion of parent-professional collaboration at all levels of health care
- Incorporating developmental needs of children into health care systems
- Implementation of programs and policies that provide emotional and financial support to meet the needs of the family
- Honoring diversity (racial, cultural, socioeconomic, ethnic)
- Designing health care services that are accessible, flexible, and responsive to families' needs

These elements appear to be common sense, and these simple statements often conceal the complexity of application to practice. Within professions with a history of working with children with disability, service providers may be inclined to regard family-centered care as not being different from what they have always practiced. Implicit in the family-centered approach is that the role of the family extends beyond involvement in the care of the child, to being beneficiaries of interventions (Kolobe et al., 2000; Bailey et al., 1998). The informational, educational, and health needs of the family are addressed in concert with those of the child even though the child is the "ultimate target" of intervention.

A major component of family-centered services is collaboration among providers and the family. Collaboration entails sharing of information to enhance decision making and the intervention process. Service providers recognize and accept the family as the primary decision maker and provide information and support to enable the family to make decisions and to enhance family competency in caring for and nurturing their child (Dunst et al., 1989). Collaboration with families extends beyond parent education, engaging in home-based therapy, obtaining the child's developmental history from parents, or obtaining parental consent for various interventions. It entails "leveling the playing field" by focusing on knowledge gaps on the sides of both parties (Rogoff et al., 1993). Information sharing is reciprocal and acknowledges that families know their children the best (Turnbull et al., 1999). Families share valuable information about the child and family, needs and concerns, and expectations of early intervention. Service providers inquire about the child's health, development, daily activities and routines, and family resources and supports. Service providers are responsive to the family's need for information about their child, community resources, and preparation for the future. As an example, therapists provide family information regarding their

child's diagnosis and prognosis with honesty while embracing hope for the child to participate in life to the fullest potential.

Themes that emerged from a qualitative study in which families described providers that embraced family-centered care were positiveness, responsiveness, orientation to the whole family, friendliness, sensitivity, and demonstration of skills related to child needs and community resources (McWilliam et al., 1998). The importance of the family-service provider relationship in promoting caregiver competency is a theme of a qualitative study by Washington and Schwartz (1996). To provide family-centered care, physical therapists are encouraged to expand their knowledge to include understanding of the multidimensional aspects of family functioning including cultural values, childrearing practices, and the importance of resources and supports. Family functioning is discussed in Chapter 30.

EFFECTIVENESS OF FAMILY-CENTERED CARE

Evidence to support the effectiveness of family-centered care is scarce. In their reviews of studies in this area, Rosenbaum and colleagues (1998) and Brooks-Gunn and colleagues (2000) reported difficulty identifying the literature that has examined family-centered care. Similar to other areas of research in early intervention, a thorough synthesis of findings is challenging because studies vary in how family-centered care is defined, the outcomes measured, and the settings and populations investigated. These reviews suggest that aspects of family-centered care that impact on child skills and adjustment include the following:

- A family's ability to build support networks and to advocate for their children's needs
- Family participation and engagement in intervention programs
- Quality of the home environment for child development
- Maternal mental health
- Quality of parent-child relationships
- Family satisfaction with services

Although long-term maintenance in optimal child behavior has been observed with change in parenting, research is inconclusive in terms of interventions that bring about this change. From the studies reviewed, it appears that (a) programs that targeted parent-child interaction appeared more effective in promoting parent child relationships and children's responsiveness and interactive skills (Barnard, 1997); (b) programs provided within children's everyday experiences were more effective in promoting skill acquisition than those that provided general support; (c) the impact of parent education programs on development is greatest for children from impoverished families (Farran, 2000); and (d) decreased parenting stress was reported in programs that focused on parenting skills and family support (Brooks-Gunn et al., 2000).

FAMILY PARTICIPATION

The family-centered approach, in addition to expanding the role of service providers, expands the role of the family, particularly parents. On one hand, parents are expected to use their skills and resources to meet the needs of their family. On the other hand, they must learn new skills that are related to taking care of a child with special needs, such as advocacy, negotiation, collaboration, and intervention strategies. Because of the fragmented child health system, parents have to coordinate not only developmental services, but also services for primary health care, public health programs such as perinatal outreach programs, and specialized medical services. Some families may not be receiving the services they need and require assistance in accessing and utilizing services and resources (Mahoney & Filer, 1996). Families experiencing difficulty in adapting to caring for a child with special needs may need more formal support from the early intervention team (Barnett et al., 2003).

Family participation in early intervention is encouraged. The extent and type of participation will vary depending on factors unique to each family. The premise is that families have a right and responsibility to select the way in which they will be involved in early intervention services (Simeonsson & Bailey, 1990). Family involvement is viewed as a continuum rather than a hierarchy. Figure 31-1 illustrates the continuum of family involvement. Some parents may elect not to be involved at all, either because of unfamiliarity with the service delivery system, or the difficulty balancing work and family commitments. A family with a demanding work schedule may give permission for professionals to provide early intervention at a child's child care center but not at home

(passive involvement). Another family may actively seek information from the professional team regarding the child's diagnosis, prognosis, and ideias for how the family can enhance the child's development (information seeking). Collaboration and partnership are achieved when a family not only seeks information from professionals, but also offers information and actively participates in the development and implementation of service plans. Service coordination and advocacy represent levels of family participation that involve management of services provided and educating others about children with special needs. Ongoing communication between the family and providers and revisiting family needs and participation are integral to family-centered services.

PROVIDING EARLY INTERVENTION SERVICES

THE ROLE OF THE PHYSICAL THERAPIST

Part C of IDEIA and the American Physical Therapy Association (APTA, 2001; Effgen et al., 1991) support the role of physical therapists in early intervention. Acquisition of motor skills is a major part of early development and young children are sensorimotor learners. Physical therapists as members of the early intervention team provide prevention and intervention strategies for children with impairments in neuromuscular, musculoskeletal, cardiopulmonary, and integumentary systems. Therapists also provide interventions for activity and participation including motor learning, environmental adaptations, assistive technology, family support, and education. Even though physical therapists have a unique role in early intervention, it is recognized that there is overlap of expertise among professional disciplines. Therefore, in early intervention practice, more so than other areas, communication and skills in teamwork are crucial. It is important for providers to openly discuss the overlap in their areas of expertise and respect the contributions of all service providers. Physical therapists may experience overlap in roles and responsibilities with occupational therapy colleagues in the areas of motor and adaptive development as well as assistive technology. Decisions on how each discipline will contribute to the plan of care for a child and family are made based on who can support the identified outcomes.

It is particularly valuable to consider the role of the physical therapist from the consumer perspective. Thirty-six parents of children with disabilities participated in focus groups to explore their perceptions of competent physical, occupational, and speech therapists in early intervention

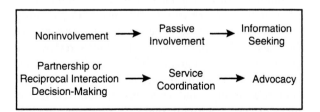

+ **Figure 31-1**   Continuum of caregiver involvement.

Box 31-2   **Families' Perspective of Desired Competencies of Early Intervention Therapists**

1. *Early Intervention Knowledge*: Therapists have previously acquired or have access to general and disability-specific information relevant to family needs or requests related to their child.
2. *Team Coordination*: Therapists actively support the coordination and planning among team members, including the family.
3. *Family as Part of Therapy Visits*: Therapists are able to actively engage and include family members in therapy sessions.
3. *Information Sharing between Therapist and Family*: Therapists share and support the use of therapy techniques throughout child and family daily routines and activities.
5. *Commitment of Therapist*: Therapists view their role as potentially impacting families and children, not simply as a job.

6. *Flexibility of Scheduling*: Therapists are willing to juggle their schedules in order to work with families and children.
7. *Respect for Individual Families*: Therapists have respect for families in that they are sensitive to the family context and changes over time, use parent-friendly language, use active listening, and provide positive feedback to families.
8. *Appreciation for the Child*: Therapists demonstrate appreciation for the child by using a strength-based intervention approach and have the ability to be "in tune" with the child.
9. *Therapist as a Person*: Therapists possess a personality reflective of them as honest, patient, personable, creative, and humorous.

(Milbourne et al., 2003). Parents discussed the skills and attributes of therapists that were important to them. The discussions were audiotaped, transcribed, and analyzed for themes. The nine themes that emerged are described in Box 31-2. The themes reflect interactions among administration issues, expectations for "best practice," and the importance of the family-therapist relationship.

ELEMENTS OF EARLY INTERVENTION

In this section five major elements of intervention included in Part C of IDEIA are presented. The five elements are team collaboration, evaluation and assessment, the IFSP, providing services in natural environments, and transition. These elements are consistent with the recommendations for children from birth to 8 years of age with special needs developed by the Division for Early Childhood (DEC) of the Council for Exceptional Children (Sandall et al., 2000). It is through these elements of service provision that therapists implement family-centered care.

Team Collaboration

Team collaboration is the process of forming partnerships among family members, service providers, and the community with the common goal of enhancing the child's development and supporting the family. Communication and coordination are essential skills for effective collaboration. Communication is the process of passing on knowledge and information to other team members to facilitate coordination of services. Each member must be committed to keeping the team informed of important issues. Communication begins with listening. To avoid miscommunications it is important to restate what was heard and ask for clarification or an example. Prompt follow-through communicates investment in the team. At the same time being patient reflects understanding of group process. When discussing issues it is essential to provide suggestions and options, a solution-focused versus problem-focused approach. A sense of humor helps to bring humanism to day-to-day team struggles.

At the systems level, federal legislation mandates interagency coordination to provide families with efficient and effective mechanisms to access and utilize services from multiple agencies. Service coordination is based on the assumption that integrated and coordinated services will result in improved outcomes for children and families. Within early intervention, the law specifically delineates that service coordinators are responsible for the implementation of the IFSP, coordination with other agencies, and assisting families with access to services. At the service provider level, team collaboration is necessary to address child and family needs. Teams that do not effectively communicate and coordinate care may increase family stress rather than serve as a formal support system.

Characteristics of team collaboration described by Briggs (1997) and supported by the recommendations for early intervention by the Division for Early Childhood (Rapport et al., 2004) are summarized in Box 31-3. Team members demonstrate respect for each other by valuing

---

Box 31-3	**Characteristics of Effective Teams and Collaborative Relationships**

- In developmental phase, team members take time to learn about each other.
- Members demonstrate honesty, trust, and mutual respect for each other.
- Membership is stable.
- All share a common philosophy and goal.
- Group has a structure for interaction, organization.
- All members demonstrate commitment.

- Exchange of information, meaningful discussion, open communication are practiced.
- Equal participation is encouraged.
- Partners contribute specific skills and strengths.
- Plans, priorities, and decisions are made together.
- Action plans are used for implementing team recommendations.

---

cultural differences and acknowledging the expertise and competence each person brings to the team. Parents and service coordinators have reported that a family-centered program philosophy enhances collaboration (Dinnebeil et al., 1999). Opportunities for team members to share information and willingness to release traditional roles were viewed as important for collaboration. The following practices have been reported to enhance collaboration:

- Home visits
- Co-visits by team member
- A teacher/therapist as service coordinator
- Regular communication with the service coordinator
- Appropriate use of individual and group intervention
- Center-based programs for parents
- Service options shared with parents
- Flexibility in scheduling and staffing.

Barriers to collaboration have also been identified. Lack of consistency of staff and problems with contracted employees were cited as interfering with collaboration (Dinnebeil et al., 1999). Issues related to funding, interagency coordination, paperwork requirements, and external policies were reported to negatively influence collaboration (Dinnebeil et al., 1999). Although struggles may exist for "turf," power, or authority more commonly, problems appear to arise from a workplace structure that isolates service providers or one that does not have dedicated time or procedures in place for collaboration (Hinojosa et al., 2001). Providing services in natural environments requires time for travel and reduces direct contact among team members.

Various models of team interaction exist in early intervention. In an interdisciplinary model, team collaboration is necessary because multiple team members with various areas of expertise work together with the family to support one set of outcomes. However, a framework for team collaboration is also essential for a *transdisciplinary* model of service delivery. The transdisciplinary

model involves one primary service provider who implements the IFSP with the family with consultation from other team members. An advantage of the transdisciplinary model is that the family and child interact with a primary service provider. The transdisciplinary model is dependent on role release and crossing of disciplinary boundaries. If services are implemented with poor collaboration and do not include the option for additional team members to provide direct service when needed, then a child may not be receiving the services and strategies necessary to support the IFSP. For a resource on the transdisciplinary model in early intervention the reader is referred to McGonigel et al. (1994).

The need for coordinated care between medial service providers and early intervention for children with special health care needs has long been recognized (Brewer et al., 1989). Families of young children with complex medical conditions expend considerable time and resources to meet their children's health, education, and development needs. Collaboration among health care professionals, early intervention providers, and families is particularly critical to meet the needs of infants and toddlers who are medically fragile. Even though all team members agree that collaboration is needed, problems in communication and coordination among families, service coordinators, early intervention service providers, physicians, and hospital-based therapists have been reported (Ideishi & O'Neil, 2003). Fifty-one family members and professionals participated in focus groups to discuss their perceptions on communication and coordination between medical and early intervention providers. Overall, concerns were expressed about the ability and time to communicate effectively and the challenges in resolving differences in practice philosophies. The focus groups identified strategies to improve coordination and communication. Strategies included providing funding and resources for comprehensive care coordination services; developing interagency communication systems; conducting communication, teamwork, and advocacy training for families and providers; and providing education on the early intervention system for health and medical providers.

Evaluation and Assessment

IDEIA legislation makes a distinction between evaluation and assessment. An evaluation consists of the procedures used to determine initial and continued eligibility for early intervention. No single procedure can be used as the sole criterion for eligibility. The legislation dictates that an evaluation must be comprehensive, multidisciplinary, and timely. The team approach is believed to encourage a holistic view of the child. Assessment refers to the ongoing procedures to identify (1) the child's unique strengths and needs, (2) the services appropriate to meet those needs, (3) the resources, priorities, and concerns of the family, and (4) the supports and services needed to enhance the family's capacity to meet their child's developmental needs.

IDEIA also specifies that evaluations and assessments be nondiscriminatory, performed by qualified and trained personnel, and include informed opinion, review of the child's pertinent medical records, and evaluation of the child's physical, cognitive, communication, social or emotional, and adaptive development. The physical therapist synthesizes findings for motor development and adaptive function within the context of findings for all areas of development, social interactions, activities, and daily routines of the child and family.

Evaluations and assessments are to be provided in a respectful and collaborative manner with families and children. The purpose and process of the evaluation and assessment should be discussed in advance. Family input is requested in deciding *who* should attend, *what* activities and routines will be observed, *where* the evaluation or assessment should take place, and *when* the session will occur (date and time). Family members can take on many different roles during the evaluation or assessment. Some family members may elect to guide the evaluation process, interacting with their child in a variety of activities. Others may prefer to assist the therapist with evaluation activities. Another option for a family member is to be a narrator, reflecting on the child's behaviors and providing commentary and elaboration to the other team members. Some families are comfortable with spontaneous exchange of ideas, and other families prefer to answer specific questions. At times a family member may just want to observe and listen. At the end of the evaluation or assessment, it is important to discuss with the family their perspective on the process (Rocco, 1996).

In order to maximize the value of evaluations and assessments, consideration should be given to the information needed to make decisions on important out-comes, the intervention plan, and how progress will be documented. This process begins with the identification of child and family competencies that serve as a foundation for determining the child's readiness for learning new skills. In addition, an understanding of the family's culture and interests will provide the framework for deciding on meaningful intervention strategies. This information is best gathered and discussed through a family interview and systematic naturalistic observation.

Family Interview. An initial step in the process of evaluation and assessment is a family interview. The purpose of the interview is to obtain information on family perspectives in areas such as resources available or needed to enhance the child's development, child and family daily routines, the child's health and development, perceptions about therapy, and expectations of early intervention. Bernheimer and Keogh (1995) present an approach to family assessment based on gathering information about the family's daily routine. Through open-ended questions, such as "tell me about your child" and "describe for me a typical day in your family," therapists gather information on family members' roles, interests, and daily tasks. The interview process related to early intervention has been described by several authors (Hirshberg, 1996; Chiarello et al., 1992; Patton, 1990). The family interview is considered the first opportunity to establish a trusting relationship and partnership.

Behaviors associated with effective interviewing include maintaining eye contact, eliciting and exploring parental concerns, providing relevant and well-timed information, and attending to the solutions and strategies proposed by parents (Winton & Blow, 1991). An effective interview is characterized by the ability to ask pertinent questions in an unbiased manner and to listen. The manner in which questions are asked also determines the response. Although often unintentional, judgmental questions and comments by service providers not only are a source of parent dissatisfaction, especially with families who represent minority populations, but may contribute to reluctance on the part of these families to offer information (Garcia-Coll & Magnusson, 1999).

Winton and Bailey (1988) described three major types of questions that are used to obtain different information. One type is the linear question that is used to obtain specific information or a "yes" or "no" response. A second type is an open-ended question that is used to facilitate elaboration on an issue. A third type is circular, in which every response facilitates or dictates an additional response. Table 31-2 provides an example of each type of question. For some families the interview process may be a new experience; therefore, therapists must

TABLE 31-2	**Sample Questions for a Family Interview**

QUESTION TYPE	EXAMPLE
Linear	"Is your child taking any medications?"
Open-ended	"What does your family like to do for recreation?"
Circular	"Tell me about your child's personality"

encourage, support, and respect the various levels of involvement and value the information that families provide (Berman & Shaw, 1996).

Active listening is another key to effective interviewing and to establishing partnerships with families and collaboration on the IFSP. Active listening and acknowledging the family's concerns demonstrates respect and value for the family's priorities, and helps the therapist develop a deeper appreciation for the family's daily routines, opportunities for collaboration, how the family frames its resources, and the extent of the family's support network. Another effective interview strategy is the use of silence. There are times when silence is more helpful than questioning. Realini and associates (1992) have developed a scale to assess the use of silence in a medical interview. This tool is extremely helpful in recognizing the importance of silence and the ways in which silence can be used to enhance the interview.

Observation. The second step entails observations of the child and the caregiving environment (natural environment). Natural environment is a broad construct that includes home and community settings such as the park, child care, and recreation centers. This approach is consistent with the Division on Early Childhood recommendation for team interactions and assessment of the child's function in natural contexts (Neisworth & Bagnato, 2000). Observations in the natural environment may focus on family caregiving routines, parent-child interaction, play, and other daily activities such as feeding, bathing and dressing. Within the construct of the International Classification of Functioning, Disability and Health (World Health Organization, 2001), ecologic assessment encompasses the relationships between participation and environmental and personal factors.

The physical therapist's unique role as part of the team is to focus on postural control and mobility during play, exploration of the physical environment, and social interactions. The family and therapist select the settings and activities that are most important for the therapist to observe. While observing, the therapist notes the following:

- What the child enjoys doing
- How the child interacts
- Opportunities for movement and sensorimotor exploration
- How often and under what circumstances the child moves
- Toys and materials that are available
- Areas of the home accessible to the child
- How much adult assistance or guidance is provided
- Skills or resources the child needs to become more successful

Information about the child's activity and participation in settings that are not observed can be gathered during the interview or the therapist may elect to engage the child in an activity that is not the exact context of the daily routine.

The most meaningful observation occurs when watching a child do something enjoyable with someone who is trusted. "The child's relationship and interaction with his or her most trusted caregiver should form the cornerstone of the assessment" (Greenspan & Meisels, 1996, p. 19). Parent-child interactions are sensorimotor experiences. Motor control, sensory integration, and muscle performance are part of parent-child interactions. In addition to looking at the motor components of the interaction, consideration is also given to social patterns of interaction between the child and caregiver. Kelly and Barnard (2000) provide a comprehensive overview of assessment of parent-child interactions. Although not a physical therapist's area of expertise, an appreciation of social interaction helps to focus motor interventions in ways that are holistic and promote a child's self-esteem.

Play is the primary occupational behavior of childhood and is a naturally occurring situation during which children learn and develop new skills. In reference to observing play activities, it is important to look at both independent play as well as play with caregivers, siblings, and peers. Therapists gather information on what toys and play activities the child engages in (sensory/exploratory play, manipulative play, imaginative/dramatic play, or motor/physical play) and the child's likes and dislikes. Therapists consider the interplay between motor abilities

Box 31-4   **Content of the Individualized Family Service Plan**

1. Statement of present levels of development based on objective criteria: cognitive, communication, physical (motor, vision, hearing, health), social or emotional, adaptive
2. Statement of the family's resources, priorities, and concerns related to enhancing the development of the child
3. Statement of measurable outcomes expected with criteria, procedures, and timelines for evaluating the outcomes
4. Specific early intervention services based on peer-reviewed research needed to meet the needs of the child and family, including frequency, intensity and method of delivery
5. Statement of the natural environments in which services to be provided (If services are not going to be provided in natural environments, a justification must be included.)
6. Determination of other services to enhance child's development and plan to secure such services through other public or private resources, such as medical
7. Projected dates for initiation of services and duration of services
8. Identification of the service coordinator
9. Transition plan: steps to be taken to assure smooth transition to preschool services if appropriate (at age 3) or other appropriate services

and play skills. Is the child able to initiate play experiences? What positions can the child play in? Can the child freely move around to reach toys or play activities that interest him? Further analysis considers if the child's movements are goal directed, the variability of movement to meet environmental demands, and the child's reaction to movement (i.e., level of enjoyment, safety, and body awareness). Lastly, a focus on the process of play provides valuable insights into the child's playfulness. Playfulness is concerned with a child's approach to an activity and includes observations related to the child's enjoyment, engagement, responsiveness, motivation, and locus of control (Bundy, 1997).

In addition to the family interview and ecologic observations, therapists use various tests and measures to evaluate motor development, function, and impairments in body functions and structures. These assessment tools are described in Chapter 1 and elsewhere (Long & Toscano, 2002; Tatarka et al., 2000). A caution is noted that measures of child development normed on children without delay are valid for determining present level of development and eligibility but often are not valid for planning intervention and measuring change over time. Based on the top-down approach to evaluation and assessment (Campbell, 1991), measures of body functions and structures are conducted after the team has a clear understanding of the family and child's goals and current abilities and relate to the team's hypothesis for impairments that may be a cause of limitations in activities and social participation.

Individualized Family Service Plan

The culmination of the evaluation and assessment process is the development of the individualized family service plan (IFSP). The principle underlying an IFSP is that families have diverse needs based on their individual structure, values, and coping styles. For intervention to be meaningful for the child, the individuality of each family must be recognized. The team members involved in the development of the IFSP include parents, caregivers, other family members, family advocate, service coordinator, person(s) involved with the evaluation, and as appropriate, persons who will be providing service.

An initial IFSP must be developed in a timely manner at a meeting time and place convenient for the family. Even though family-centered efforts are made, logistics often make it difficult to arrange the meetings at nights or weekends, and thus not all key family members may be able to be involved. If a service provider cannot attend, a representative or written information can be sent. This practice has been an area of concern, for without the team members present it is difficult to truly have a collaborative process.

Although the federal law specifies the content of the IFSP (Box 31-4) it does not specify the format of the document or the process for its development. Typically the service coordinator leads the discussion and records the information. Family members can elect, however, to take the role as a team leader. During the meeting the team discusses the evaluation and assessment findings, exchanges information, and collaborates to develop the IFSP. The team promotes family participation and decisions are made collaboratively. Transferring federal law into practice has been challenging, and research indicates that family involvement during the development of the IFSP is limited (Able-Boone, 1993). The findings from a recent study on quality indicators of IFSP documents were mixed (Jung & Baird, 2003). A high rating was noted for a focus on child strengths and 86% of the outcomes were related to family concerns and priorities. However, the documents contained technical jargon and a low rating was noted for evidence of the family's role.

For families to negotiate for the types of support they need, and to ensure equal partnership and ownership in this process, the family should be provided with information that will enable them to make informed decisions and choices *before* the IFSP meeting. This information may be shared with the family during the information-gathering stages, in the form of a post-evaluation interpretive conference, or in writing in the form of an evaluation report. When feasible, questions the family may have pertaining to the evaluation results should also be addressed before the IFSP meeting, so that questions related to the logistics of service provision can be fully discussed during the meeting. This will also help reduce the prolonged process that sometimes characterizes IFSP meetings. Another benefit to sharing the information at least a few weeks before the IFSP meeting is that the family can decide on whom they want to invite to the meeting, something that families consider to be a valuable form of support.

Identification of child and family outcomes is often challenging. These outcomes must be based on what is important to the family and determined by the family in collaboration with providers, *not* disciplinary goals. It is important for outcomes to focus on activity and participation. Historically therapists have emphasized child outcomes and research indicates that the majority of IFSP outcome statements are child-focused (Boone et al., 1998). Family outcomes on IFSP may be related to resources, supports, and information.

Beckman and Bristol (1991) identified four types of IFSP outcomes or objectives. "Child-related child outcomes" refer to specific child behaviors, such as self-help skills or functional motor tasks. "Family-related child outcomes" are specific child behaviors that will be beneficial to the family's functioning, such as a child's feeding or sleeping schedule. The third type, "child-related family outcomes" refers to needs of the family related to the child, such as accessing respite care. All three types are appropriate IFSP outcomes or objectives. The fourth type, "general family outcomes" is associated with family needs that are not directly related to the child but are beneficial to the family's overall functioning. The fourth type is not specific to early intervention services but is included on the IFSP as an outcome related to interagency coordination.

The outcomes and activities identified by families must be supported; however, problems may arise when the child does not have the readiness or potential to achieve a desired outcome or the family does not have the health insurance or financial resources (American Academy of Pediatrics, 1998; Hughes & Luft, 1998). Further exploration of why specific outcomes are important to the family and detailed explanations and information about the child's condition may be helpful for informed decision making.

All the practical aspects of service provision should be addressed during IFSP process. The IFSP process provides an opportunity for important negotiations and collaborations between the family and professionals about key issues that are likely to affect service provision. These include the prioritization of outcomes, the intervention plan, the appropriate setting and timing for intervention, identification of service providers, interagency coordination, financial issues, and eventually a transition plan for when the child is 3 years old. Issues related to assistive devices such as ankle-foot orthoses or wheelchairs are also best discussed at this time for two reasons: (1) the emotional turmoil that some families experience in making decisions around this issue and (2) the cost involved, particularly in light of financial constraints imposed by most managed care plans. Availability of personnel resources reflecting the current staffing patterns of the program or agency must also be discussed in a candid and open manner so that other options can be explored.

The IFSP is not just a legal document; it is a process of collaboration between the family and providers to design a service plan that is acceptable to the family and addresses the child's needs. The IFSP serves as a means for coordination of services, a guide for intervention, and a standard for evaluating outcomes. The IFSP is reviewed every 6 months and a formal meeting is held annually. The IFSP can be reviewed at another time at the request of a team member. Periodic IFSP reviews allow for renegotiations, or revisions of the service plan, as well as monitoring of goal attainment. During an IFSP review, family satisfaction, effectiveness of the IFSP process, and status of the outcomes should be discussed. If outcomes were not achieved, reflection of the appropriateness of the outcomes, service, and strategies is needed to effectively revise the IFSP.

Therapists practicing in early intervention require effective interpersonal and communication skills to be able to invite and support the family to contribute their insights, recommendations, and priorities. Anecdotal stories indicate that the IFSP process can be overwhelming and intimidating for families, especially when families do not believe that their opinions are valued. It is appropriate for therapists to make recommendations, but they should be consistent with information that was gathered from the family during the interview. Recommendations are framed as questions, thus providing the family the opportunity to agree or disagree. Additional recommendations to make these experiences more positive include a focus on child and family strengths, use of lay language, and flexibility to allow informal conversation and sharing of ideias instead of rigidly following a predetermined format. Therapists may find the book by McGonigel and colleagues (1991) helpful in developing collaborative goals and in addressing some of the challenges of the practical aspects of the IFSP process. Lastly, it is important to acknowledge that variability exists in how states have implemented the IFSP process. Therapists may need to serve as an advocate to ensure that the spirit of family-centered care and individualization are honored.

Natural Environments

In public funded early intervention, services are to be provided in natural environments, defined as "settings that are natural or normal for the child's age peers who have no disabilities." More meaningful is that natural environments are "a variety of settings where children live, learn, and play" (Section on Pediatrics, American Physical Therapy Association, 2001). The natural environment is not limited to the home but rather is defined as any place where children participate in activities and routines that provide learning opportunities that promote a child's behavior, function, and development. This includes child care settings, parks, grocery stores, YMCAs, and libraries.

Providing services in natural environments is a general intervention approach, a process, and a conceptualization. Although natural environment implies a physical location, such as a playground, it goes beyond the physical location. It includes what activities the child and family typically engage in at that location and the learning opportunities afforded by those activities. Dunst and colleagues (2001a) have identified with families a variety of family and community settings and present an approach for discussing with families activities and learning opportunities. These settings include family routines (household chores and errands), caregiving routines (bathing, dressing, eating, grooming, bedtime), family rituals and celebrations (holidays, birthdays, religious events), outdoor activities (gardening, visits to park/zoo), social activities (visiting friends, play groups), play activities (physical play and play with toys), and learning activities (listening to stories, looking at books/pictures). This approach to early intervention has been associated with changes in child competency (Dunst et al., 2001b). The investigators found that learning opportunities that were characterized as being interesting,

engaging, competence-producing, and mastery-oriented predicted positive child outcomes. In a national survey of families and providers, Dunst and Bruder (2002) found child mastery, parent/child interactions, inclusion, and child learning opportunities as important outcomes of natural environments.

The Fact Sheet on Natural Learning Environments (Section on Pediatrics, American Physical Therapy Association, 2001) highlights the rationale for providing interventions in natural environments. First, natural environments match the purpose of early intervention: "to support families in promoting their children's development and participation in community life." This approach embraces family-centered care by recognizing that the family has a primary role in nurturing their child and fostering growth, development, and learning. When providing interventions in natural environments, therapists can easily focus on the children's function, promote socialization with their family and friends, and "strengthen and develop lifelong natural supports for children and families" (Fig. 31-2). For infants and young children, self-regulation, parent-child relationship, and

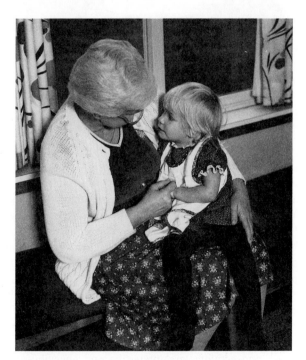

◆ **Figure 31-2**   When providing therapy in the home, family and therapist may consider inviting grandmother to participate in the visit to support her role as a resource for the family in nurturing her grandchild. *(From Wong, DL, Hockenberg-Eaton, M, Winkelstein, ML, Wilson, D, Ahmann, A, & DiVito-Thomas, PA. Whaley & Wong's Nursing Care of Infants and Children, 6th ed. St. Louis: Mosby, 1999, Fig. 4-23, p. 155.)*

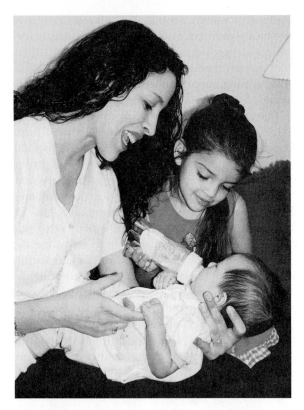

♦ **Figure 31-3** Involvement of siblings in caregiving activities during therapy visits promotes family bonds and supports family routines. *(From Wong, DL, Hockenberg-Eaton, M, Winkelstein, ML, Wilson, D, Ahmann, A, & DiVito-Thomas, PA. Whaley & Wong's Nursing Care of Infants and Children, 6th ed. St. Louis: Mosby, 1999, Fig. 14-6, p. 677.)*

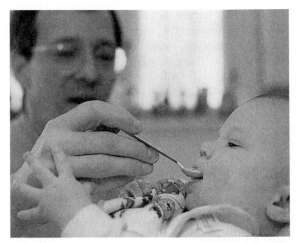

♦ **Figure 31-4** It is important for therapists to partner with fathers and support their role in caregiving activities. *(From Wong, DL, Hockenberg-Eaton, M, Winkelstein, ML, Wilson, D, Ahmann, A, & DiVito-Thomas, PA. Whaley & Wong's Nursing Care of Infants and Children, 6th ed. St. Louis: Mosby, 1999, Fig. 3-7, p. 92.)*

play form the foundation to support the child's role in the family and to prepare the child for interactions with peers and school (Fig. 31-3). Interventions for caregiving and self-care activities such as feeding, bathing, dressing, and moving throughout the environment are essential (Fig. 31-4). "The emphasis in early intervention must not be on creating nearly normal children but on enabling children and their families to have normal life opportunities" (Rocco, 1994).

Second, providing services in natural environments is supported by principles of motor learning. Practice and repetition of activities in natural contexts and settings are more effective for learning and generalization. These places and activities are interesting and engaging and thus naturally motivating to children. This includes the opportunity to learn through modeling by peers and family members. Therapists assist families to provide prompts and cues and, when necessary, physical assistance to enable the child to learn skills in self-care and mobility. Therapists also can provide recommendations to adapt the physical environment, activities, and

materials to enhance the child's access and functional participation. Examples include minor changes to the layout of a room or use of adapted toys or positioning and mobility devices. Assistive technology is an important component of intervention for children with severe physical disabilities (Sullivian & Lewis, 2000). Assistive technology, such as switches to activate toys, needs to become more widespread for children under age 3 (Long et al., 2003). Similarly, power wheelchair mobility may afford children as young as 2 years of age the opportunity for independence (Butler, 1986).

Challenges exist in providing services in natural environments, and therapists are encouraged to seek creative solutions (Hanft & Pilkington, 2000). Challenges include logistic concerns, such as the costs, safety, and time to travel to the child's natural environments as well as philosophical concerns that by mandating a particular approach to service delivery, the system may not be providing options to meet families' individualized needs and circumstances. It is important for agencies to develop and implement policies to ensure staff safety such as use of cell phones, co-visits, and soliciting advocacy efforts from neighborhood child watch organizations. Natural environments include settings other than the home. Visits can occur in a variety of community locations such as the library, town centers, and recreational facilities. When service is provided in a community child care setting, it is important to schedule periodic visits with the family as well as to collaborate with the child care providers. Information on child care regulations, philosophy, and

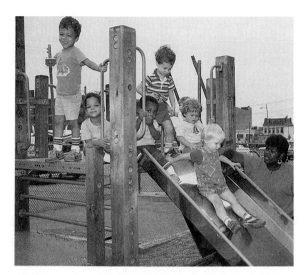

+ **Figure 31-5** Therapy at a child care setting can focus on promoting social interactions with peers and functional mobility to participate in activities on the playground. *(From Wong, DL, Hockenberg-Eaton, M, Winkelstein, ML, Wilson, D, Ahmann, A, & DiVito-Thomas, PA. Whaley & Wong's Nursing Care of Infants and Children, 6th ed. St. Louis: Mosby, 1999, Fig. 2-3.)*

early childhood curriculum will assist the therapist in partnering with child care providers (Fig. 31-5). Lastly, it is important for therapists to advocate for the support and training they need to be able to provide services in natural environments. An annotated bibliography of literature and educational materials provides a useful resource on this topic (Pretti-Frontczak et al., 2003).

The first step in planning an intervention in a natural environment is to consider family-identified outcomes. We believe it is essential to have a match between the information from families regarding their concerns, priorities, and resources and the services provided. The next step is to discuss with the family the activities, routines, and people that are part of their daily life. Box 31-5 provides questions to consider when collaborating with families to identify activities. Therapists are encouraged to identify the functional learning opportunities that occur during each activity. If a family outcome is for their child to be able to play at the park, riding a swing may be an activity that is considered. The therapist may identify a variety of learning opportunities such as grasping with two hands, pumping with your legs, holding head and trunk up, understanding high and low, and making sounds. Therapists integrate their therapeutic intervention strategies within the context of family activities and learning opportunities. Therapeutic techniques are used to improve body functions and structures necessary to achieve a functional ability and to prevent secondary complications related to the cardiopulmonary, musculoskeletal, and neuromuscular systems.

Transition Plan

The transition plan is part of the IFSP process that deserves special attention because of its essential role in assuring the child's progression in the educational system and participation in the community. Similar to the IFSP process as a whole, transition planning has not always been a positive experience for families. Therapists, as early intervention team members, can take an active role in the transition process. The first step is to become knowledgeable about how Part B Preschool Services (IDEIA, 2004) are implemented and about resources and service options in the community. IDEIA provides for increased coordination between Part C and Part B programs. With the permission of the parent a representative from the Part C program is to be invited to the initial Individualized Education Program (IEP) meeting when the child is transitioning to preschool services. In addition IDEIA provides states the flexibility to make Part C services available to children until they enter kindergarten or elementary school. Second, it is important to make the commitment to collaborate with the early intervention and preschool teams. This step includes an open discussion regarding the environmental characteristics that will support the child's learning and development including attention to safety of the child in the new

---

Box 31-5	**Questions to Discuss with Families When Establishing Activities for Services in Natural Environments**

- What activities make up your weekdays and weekends?
- What activities are going well and not going well?
- What activities would you like support for?
- What activities does the child prefer to participate in?
- What activities provide natural learning opportunities?

- What activities provide opportunities for child initiation?
- What activities provide opportunities for peer interaction?
- Are there new activities that you would like to try?

Box 31-6   **Strategies for Collaborating with Families to Support Transition from Early Intervention**

- Listen to the family
- Provide positive, but realistic, support for the preschool program
  - Guide family in gathering information without introducing your bias
  - Provide family with survey and interview guidelines for preschool programs
- Visit a program with the family and help orient the family and child to the new agency
- Discuss separation from the child as a natural process
- Celebrate graduation from early intervention with the family and child
- Consider a follow-up communication with family after transition

---

Box 31-7   **Strategies to Prepare a Child for Preschool**

- Provide the child opportunities to play with other children (i.e., siblings, neighbors, play groups)
- Promote independent play time
- Encourage child participation in a variety of play experiences
- Encourage self-care skills
- Practice following simple directions
- Provide the child responsibility for small tasks like putting away toys
- Have the child make choices and encourage the child to express wants and needs
- Reading stories about school

---

environment and during transportation. Therapists can offer, with family permission, to share information that will assist staff of the preschool program to be prepared to meet the child's needs. Most important, therapists serve as advocates, keeping in mind the family's dreams and vision for their child. Box 31-6 outlines strategies for collaborating with families. Finally, therapists can provide recommendations to prepare the child for preschool. Box 31-7 presents examples of strategies that physical therapists can incorporate during early intervention.

A MODEL FOR EARLY INTERVENTION

A collaborative team model for early intervention service delivery for children with physical disabilities and their families was developed by Palisano, Chiarello, and O'Neil (2004) with input from colleagues and community partners as part of the research activities in the Pediatric Post-Professional Program in Rehabilitation Sciences at Drexel University. The development of the model was supported in part from a Leadership Training Grant of the Maternal and Child Health Bureau. The model provides a framework for implementation of components of early intervention services previously described. Therapists may find intervention strategies from this model useful for their practice as we strive to promote quality service delivery and to support children and family outcomes.

The collaborative model for early intervention service delivery, illustrated in Figure 31-6, integrates the policy embodied in federal law (IDEIA, 2004); the processes of enablement outlined by the World Health Organization (2001); theories on family and child development (Sameroff & Fiese, 2000; Shonkoff & Phillips, 2000); and practice guidelines from physical therapy, occupational therapy, and early childhood education (American Physical Therapy Association, 2001; McEwen, 2000; American Occupational Association, 1999; Sandall et al., 2000). Four broad categories are proposed as outcomes that are meaningful for children with physical disabilities and their families. These outcomes are (1) child achievement of individualized outcomes for activity and participation; (2) meeting family needs; (3) family ease of providing care; and (4) family perception of family-centered behaviors of the service provider team.

The model identifies three components of intervention: *Communication and coordination* among the family, service providers, and community; *information sharing* with the family; and *interventions in natural environments* to meet child and family needs. The double-headed and interconnected arrows in Figure 31-6 indicate that the three components interact in an iterative fashion. Box 31-8 outlines specific intervention strategies for implementation of the model. A case scenario is presented to exemplify how strategies are implemented through a collaborative, family-centered team approach in natural environments.

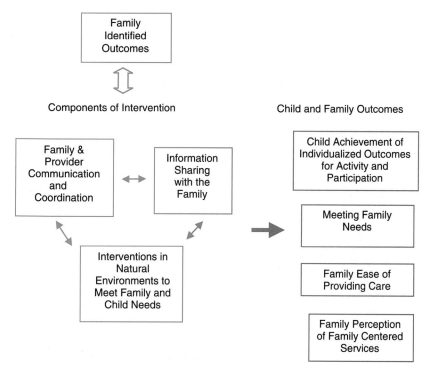

◆ **Figure 31-6**   Collaborative model of early intervention service delivery for children with physical disabilities and their families. *(From Palisano, RJ, Chiarello, LA, & O'Neil, MA. A collaborative model of early intervention service delivery. Presented at Contemporary Therapy Practices in Early Intervention: Second Annual Institute. Malvern, PA, May 14, 2004.)*

Box 31-8   Strategies for Physical Therapist Interventions

COMMUNICATION AND COORDINATION OF SERVICES

- Early intervention team meetings every 3 months
- Co-visits of early intervention team providers every 3 months
- Identification and access of community resources through community mapping
- Visit or phone conference with other health care professionals

INFORMATION SHARING WITH FAMILY

- Provide information on family-identified needs
- Embed intervention strategies into child's and family's daily life (Family Routine and Outcome Matrix, Bricker, 1998)

- Conduct visits when family members who are important in the child's life can participate

THERAPEUTIC INTERVENTION STRATEGIES IN NATURAL ENVIRONMENTS

- Conduct visits at a community location identified by the family
- Provide intervention in different rooms in the home to support a variety of daily activities and routines
- Implement adaptations, functional training, and restorative/preventive techniques to support self-regulation, parent-child interactions, play, self-care, and mobility

---

CASE STUDY

ANDREW

Andrew is a 26-month-old boy with right hemiplegia. His mother, a homemaker, is very involved in his care and

Andrew has two older siblings. The family lives in a two-story row house in an urban environment. Over the past year he has received early intervention services including physical, occupational, and speech therapy. Kate, the physical therapist, has been an integral member of the early intervention team and has established a positive relationship with the family.

The county administrator and provider agency support the need for routine coordination and communication among the early intervention team members. In collaboration with the mother, Kate guides early intervention team meetings every 3 months at the family's home. To gather information necessary to provide family-centered care, at the recent team meeting Kate asked the mother to share with the team information about their family and daily routines as well as people and places in the community that are important to them. The mother indicated that she is planning on returning to work next year and would like information on preschool programs in the neighborhood. The mother explains that the immediate neighborhood including the playground, her older children's schools, and grandmother's house are visited frequently. She also identified key outcomes for Andrew that were important to her for the next year: (1) interacting with children on the playground including riding a tricycle, (2) walking at home and in the neighborhood without falling, and (3) using his right arm more to help with dressing and feeding.

To foster communication and coordination with community programs, the team discusses possible community resources in the neighborhood such as the community recreation center. The team is committed to researching and forming relationships with various family- and child-oriented community programs. As one means of sharing information with the family, the team develops a daily routines and outcomes matrix (Bricker, 1998), shown in Table 31-3. The family identified outcomes are listed across the top row and the family routines are listed down the first column. The team problem solves together to decide on strategies that can be used during the family's day to promote the outcomes, and these are listed in the body of the matrix.

To respond to the family's identified need for information on preschools, Kate compiles a list of neighborhood programs and shares it with Andrew's mother at their next visit. To coordinate care with medical services, Kate accompanies the mother and Andrew to their clinic appointment at the children's hospital to see the orthopedist and orthotist. The group discusses what medical interventions might be needed to support Andrew's goal for safe walking. A plan is established to obtain an orthotic at this time and to keep lines of communication open for the possible need for botulinum toxin injections for management of ankle spasticity.

To support other family members' ability to interact with and care for Andrew, Kate provides one visit at Andrew's grandmother's house and asks the grandmother what is going well and what is not going well when she cares for Andrew. Kate demonstrates strategies to the grandmother on how to provide guidance for Andrew when he goes for walks outside with her. For ongoing communication and coordination among the early intervention team, Kate and the occupational therapist visit Andrew and his mother together to focus on strategies to promote the use of Andrew's right arm during dressing and feeding.

During the summer, Kate and the family have several early intervention visits at the neighborhood playground. Kate adapts Andrew's tricycle with foot pedals, hand rest, and a push handle for the mother. At the playground, Kate and the mother guide Andrew on the climbing gym

---

TABLE 31-3   Sample Activity Matrix for Andrew

	INTERACTING WITH CHILDREN	WALKING AT HOME AND IN THE NEIGHBORHOOD WITHOUT FALLING	USING RIGHT ARM TO ASSIST WITH DRESSING AND FEEDING
Feeding time	Andrew can have a play date over for lunch and build cracker sandwiches together.	Andrew can carry the napkins to the kitchen table at mealtimes.	Andrew can support the bowl with his right hand while scooping food with his left.
Outside play time	With supervision, Andrew can sit on the glider with another child as you sing "Row, row, row your boat."	Support Andrew to walk the block to the playground by having him hold on to your index finger.	Prompt Andrew to push his right arm through his jacket sleeve when getting ready to go outside to play.
Bedtime	Discuss your visit to the playground and ask Andrew to tell you what he liked doing with his friend.	Andrew can walk up the flight of stairs for bath time before bed using the railing.	With Andrew sitting in your lap, have him support a cardboard book with his right hand and turn the pages with his left.

with the neighborhood children and siblings. Andrew's mother asks Kate to visit their home during lunch time so a session in their kitchen can focus on feeding. During other visits Kate provides functional training for independent walking as Andrew goes on a scavenger hunt inside their home and in their yard. She discusses with his mother when it may be appropriate to use verbal and tactile prompts. When the new brace arrives, Kate and Andrew's mother discuss a wearing schedule and the importance of preventing ankle contractures from developing.

At the next team meeting, the therapists and the family discuss Andrew's progress, review the outcomes of the intervention strategies during the past 3 months, and set the stage for working together for the next 3 months to support Andrew and his family.

PROGRAM EVALUATION

Program evaluation determines the extent to which services are provided in an efficient and effective manner. The primary purpose of a program evaluation is to provide feedback to service providers on family satisfaction with how services are provided and the extent child and family outcomes are achieved. A four-tiered approach to program evaluation has been described (Warfield, 2002; Jacobs, 2000, 1988). Through the first tier, a needs assessment, the needs of the population being served are determined, policy or programs to meet the needs are proposed, and a monitoring system is developed to document progress. Through the second tier, monitoring and accountability, services are systematically documented to assist in program planning and decision making. Through the third tier, quality process, the quality of the services is judged to provide information for program improvement. Through the fourth tier, achieving outcomes, the extent in which IFSP outcomes are met and attributed to early intervention services are determined to provide information for program improvement and contribute to the knowledge base.

A need for program evaluations in early intervention is advocated to document how early intervention is actually implemented and to determine its impact on families and children. Bailey (2001) proposed a framework for program evaluation in early intervention to evaluate family involvement and support. He discussed three levels of accountability: (1) providing what is required by legislation, (2) providing services that reflect quality recommended practices, and (3) achieving family outcomes.

Program evaluation includes both consumer satisfaction and effectiveness of achievement of child and family outcomes. An outcomes monitoring system in early intervention is presently being developed to track children's outcomes in the primary developmental domains (Early Childhood Outcomes Center, 2004). To address if early intervention accomplishes family outcomes, Bailey and colleagues (1998) have proposed a framework for evaluating if services have been family-centered. Their first category of family questions relates to the family's belief concerning whether early intervention made a difference in their child's and family's life as well as their perceptions of the professionals and service system. Their second category of questions explores specific outcomes related to the family's ability to assist their child, collaborate with professionals, develop a support system, have hope for the future, and improve quality of life. Program evaluation is challenging secondary to the multidimensional facets of early intervention and the necessary variability to meet the individualized needs of families and children. However, through this process facilitators and barriers to providing quality and effective services are identified and recommendations are provided for program improvements.

SUMMARY

Physical therapists in early intervention support the implementation of IDEIA by establishing collaborative partnerships with children, families, and professionals from multiple disciplines to provide coordinated and comprehensive care. Therapists integrate knowledge and skill from their professional education with knowledge of early childhood development to promote the child's development and participation in family life, as well as support the family. This unique practice setting enables therapists to embrace the art of caring, prepare children for their roles in school, and foster health and well-being.

REFERENCES

Able-Boone, H. Family participation in the IFSP process: Family or professional driven? Infant Toddler Intervention, 3:63–71, 1993.

American Academy of Pediatrics (Committee on Children with Disabilities). Managed care and children with special needs: A subject review. Pediatrics, 102(3):657–660, 1998.

American Physical Therapy Association. Guide to Physical Therapist Practice. Physical Therapy, 81(1):27–50, 2001.

American Occupational Therapy Association. Occupational Therapy Services for Children and Youth Under the Individuals With Disabilities Education Act, 2nd ed. Bethesda: American Occupational Therapy Association, 1999.

Bailey, DB. Evaluating parent involvement and family support in early intervention and preschool programs. Journal of Early Intervention, 24(1):1–14, 2001.

Bailey, DB, McWilliam RA, Darkes LA, Hebbeler K, Simeonsson RJ, Spiker D, & Wagner M. Family outcomes in early intervention: A framework for program evaluation and efficacy research. Exceptional Children, 64(3):313–329, 1998.

Barnard, KE. Influencing parent-child interactions for children at risk. In Guralnick, MJ (Eds.). The Effectiveness of Early Intervention. Baltimore: Brookes Publishing Co., 1997, pp. 249–267.

Barnett, D, Clements, M, Kaplan-Estrin, M, & Fialka, J. Building new dreams: Supporting parents' adaptation to their child with special needs. Infants and Young Children, 16(3):184–200, 2003.

Beckman, PJ, & Bristol, MM. Issues in developing the IFSP: A framework for establishing family outcomes. Topics in Early Childhood Special Education, 11(3):19–31, 1991.

Berman, C, & Shaw, E. 1996. Family-directed child evaluation and assessment under the Individuals with Disabilities Education Act (IDEIA). In Meisels, SJ, & Fenichel, E. New visions for the developmental assessment of infants and young children. Washington, DC: Zero to Three, 1996, pp. 361–390.

Bernheimer, L, & Keogh, B. Weaving interventions into the fabric of everyday life: An approach to family assessment. Topics in Early Childhood Special Education, 15:415–433, 1995.

Boone, HA, McBride, SL, Swann, D, Moore, S, & Drew, BS. IFSP practices in two states: Implications for practice. Infants and Young Children, 10(4):36–45, 1998.

Brewer, EJ, McPherson, M, Magrub, PR, & Hutchins, VL. Family-centered, community-based, coordinated care for children with special health needs. Pediatrics, 83:1055–1060, 1989.

Bricker, D. An Activity-Based Approach to Early Intervention, 2nd ed. Baltimore: Paul H. Brookes Co., 1998.

Briggs, MH. Building Early Intervention Teams: Working Together for Children and Families. Gaithersburg, MD: Aspen Publishers, 1997.

Brooks-Gunn, J, Berlin, LJ, & Fuligni, AS. Early childhood intervention programs: What about the family? In Shonkoff, JP & Meisels, SJ (Eds.). Handbook of Early Childhood Intervention. New York: Cambridge University Press, 2000, pp. 549–577.

Bundy, A. Play and playfulness: What to look for. In Parham, LD, & Fazio, LS (Eds.). Play and Occupational Therapy for Children. Philadelphia: Mosby, 1997, pp. 52–66.

Butler, C. Effects of powered mobility on self-initiated behaviors of very young children with motor disability. Developmental Medicine and Child Neurology, 28:325–332, 1986.

Butler, C, & Darrah, J. Effects of neurodevelopmental treatment (NDT) for cerebral palsy: An AACPDM evidence report. Developmental Medicine and Child Neurology, 43:778–790, 2001.

Campbell, P. Evaluation and assessment in early intervention for infants and toddlers. Journal of Early Intervention, 15:36–45, 1991.

Chiarello, LA, Effgen S, & Levinson, M. Parent-professional partnership in evaluation and development of individualized family service plans. Pediatric Physical Therapy, 4(2):64–69, 1992.

Dinnebeil, LA, Hale, L, & Rule, S. Early intervention program practices that support collaboration. Topics in Early Childhood Special Education, 19(4):225–235, 1999.

Dunst, CJ, Trivette, CM, Gordon, NJ, & Pletcher, LL. Building and mobilizing informal family support networks. In Singer, GHS, & Irwin, LK (Eds.). Support for Caregiving Families: Enabling Positive Adaptation to Disability. Baltimore: Paul H. Brookes Co., 1989, pp. 121–141.

Dunst, C, Johanson, C, Trivetter, C, & Hamby, D. Family oriented early intervention policies: Family centered or not? Exceptional Child, 21(11):115–118, 1991.

Dunst, CJ, & Bruder, MB. Valued outcomes of service coordination, early intervention, and natural environments. Exceptional Children, 68(3):361–375, 2002.

Dunst, CJ, Bruder, MB, Trivette, CM, Hamby, D, Raab, M, & McLean, M. Characteristics and consequences of everyday natural learning opportunities. Topics in Early Childhood Special Education, 21(2):68–92, 2001b.

Dunst, CJ, Bruder, MB, Trivette, CM, Raab, M, & McLean, M. Natural learning opportunities for infants, toddlers, and preschoolers. Young Exceptional Children, 4(3):18–25, 2001a.

Early Childhood Outcomes Center. Considerations related to developing a system for measuring outcomes for young children with disabilities and their families. U.S. Office of Special Education Programs, April 2004. http://www.fpg.unc.edu/~eco/pages/publications.cfm. Accessed September 27, 2005.

Effgen, SK, Bjornson, K, Chiarello, L, Sinzer, L, & Philips, W. Competencies for physical therapists in early intervention. Pediatric Physical Therapy, 3(2):77–80, 1991.

Farran, DC. Another decade of intervention for children who are low income or disabled: What do we know now? In Shonkoff, JP, & Meisels, SJ (Eds.). Handbook of Early Childhood Intervention, 2nd ed. New York: Cambridge University Press, 2000, pp. 510–548.

Filer, JD, & Mahoney, GJ. Collaboration between families and early intervention service providers. Infants and Young Children, 9:22–30, 1996.

Garcia-Coll, G, & Magnusson, K. Cultural influences on child development: Are we ready for a paradigm shift? In Masten, AS (Ed.). Cultural Processes in Child Development—The Minnesota Symposia on Child Psychology. Mahwah, NJ: Lawrence Erlbaum, 1999, pp. 1–24.

Greenspan, SI, & Meisels, SJ. Toward a new vision for the developmental assessment of infants and young children. In Meisels, SJ, & Fenichel, E (Eds.). New Visions for the Developmental Assessment of Infants and Young Children. Washington, DC: Zero to Three, 1996, pp. 11–26.

Guralnick, MJ. The Effectiveness of Early Intervention. Baltimore: Paul H. Brookes Co., 1997.

Guralnick, MJ. Effectiveness of early intervention for vulnerable children: A developmental perspective. American Journal on Mental Retardation, 102(4):319–345, 1998.

Hanft, EH, & Pilkington, KO. Therapy in natural environments: The means or end goal for early intervention? Infants and Young Children, 12(4):1–13, 2000.

Harris, SR. The effectiveness of early intervention for children with cerebral palsy and related motor disabilities. In Guralnick, MJ (Ed.). The Effectiveness of Early Intervention. Baltimore: Paul H. Brookes Co., 1997, pp. 327–347.

Hauser-Cram, P, Warfield, ME, Shonkoff, JP, & Krauss, MW. Children with disabilities: A longitudinal study of child development and parent well-being. Monographs of the Society for Research in Child Development, 66(3, Serial No. 266), 2001.

Hinojosa J, Bedell G, Buchholz ES, Charles J, Shigaki IS, & Bicchieri SM. Team collaboration: A case study. Qualitative Health Research, 11(2):206–220, 2001.

Hirshberg, LM. History-making, not history-taking: Clinical interviews with infants and their families. In Meisels, SJ, & Fenichel, E (Eds.). New Visions for the Developmental Assessment of Infants and Young Children. Washington, DC: Zero to Three, 1996, pp. 85–124.

Hughes, DC, & Luft, HS. Managed Care and Children: An Overview. The Future of Children, 8(2):25–38, 1998.

Ideishi, RI, & O'Neil, M. Facilitating Communication and Coordination Between Medical and Early Intervention Communities to Improve Services for Families and Children with Special Health Care Needs: Final Report to The Division of Early Childhood, Youth and Women's Health. Philadelphia: Department of Public Health, 2003.

Jackson, LL. Who's paying for therapy in early intervention? Infants and Young Children, *11*(2):65–72, 1998.

Jacobs, FH. The five-tiered approach to evaluation: Context and implementation. In Weiss, HB, & Jacobs, FH (Eds.). Evaluating Family Programs. Hawthorne, NY: Aldine de Gruyter, 1988, pp. 37–68.

Jacobs, FH, & Kapuscik, JL. Making it count: Evaluating family preservation services. Medford, MA: Tufts University, 2000.

Jung, LA, & Baird, SM. Effects of service coordinator variables on Individualized Family Service Plans. Journal of Early Intervention, *25*(3):206–218, 2003.

Kelly, JF, & Barnard, KE. Assessment of parent-child interaction: Implications for Early Intervention. In Shonkoff, JP, &. Meisels, SJ (Eds.). Handbook of Early Childhood Intervention. New York: Cambridge University Press, 2000, pp. 258–289.

Kolobe, THA, Sparling, J, & Daniels, LE. Family-Centered Intervention. In Campbell, SK, Vander Linden, DW, & Palisano, RJ (Eds.). Physical Therapy for Children, 2nd ed. Philadelphia: WB Saunders, 2000, pp. 881–907.

Long, T, Huang, L, Woodbridge, M, Woolverton, M, & Minkel, J. Integrating assistive technology into an outcome-driven model of service delivery. Infants and Young Children, *16*(4):272–283, 2003.

Long T, & Toscano K. Handbook of Pediatric Physical Therapy, 2nd ed. Philadelphia: Lippincott Willliams & Wilkins, 2002.

Mahoney, G, & Filer, J. How responsive is early intervention to the priorities and needs of families? Topics in Early Childhood Special Education, *16*(4):437–457, 1996.

McCormick, MC, McCarton, C, Brooks-Gunn, J, & Gross, RT. The infant health and development program—Interim summary. Journal of Developmental and Behavioral Pediatrics, *19*:359–370, 1998.

McEwen, I. Providing Physical Therapy Services Under Parts B & C of the Individuals with Disabilities Education Act (IDEIA), Alexandria, VA, Section on Pediatrics, APTA, 2000.

McGonigel, MJ, Kaufmann, RK, & Johnson, BH (Eds.). Recommended Practices for the Individualized Family Service Plan. Bethesda, MD: Association for the Care of Children's Health, 1991.

McGonigel, MJ, Woodruff, G, & Roszmann-Milican, M. The transdisciplinary team: A model for family-centered early intervention. In Johnson, LJ, Gallagher, RJ, La Montagne, MJ, Jordan, JB, Gallagher, JJ, Hutinger, PL, & Karnes, MB (Eds.). Meeting Early Intervention Challenges: Issues from Birth to Three, 2nd ed. Baltimore: Paul H. Brookes Co., 1994, pp. 95–131.

McWilliam, RA, Tocci, L, & Harbin, GL. Family-Centered Services: Service Providers "Discourse & Behavior." Topics in Early Childhood Special Education, *18*(4):206–221, 1998.

Milbourne, S, Campbell, P, & Chiarello LA. Competent Therapist – Reflective Families: The Crossroads of Quality Early Intervention Services. Division for Early Childhood Conference, Washington, D.C.: October 2003.

Natural Learning Environments Fact Sheet. Alexandria, VA: Section on Pediatrics, APTA, 2001. http://www.pediatricapta.org/graphics/EIFactsheet.pdf.

Neisworth JT, & Bagnato SJ. Recommended practices in assessment. In Sandall, S, McLean, ME, & Smith, BJ (Eds.). DEC Recommended Practices in Early Intervention / Early Childhood Special Education. Longmong, CO: Sopris West, 2000, pp. 17–22.

Pakula, AL, & Palmer, FB. Early intervention for children at risk for neuromotor problems. In Guralnick, MJ (Ed.). The Effectiveness of Early Intervention. Baltimore: Paul H. Brookes Co., 1997, pp. 99–108.

Palisano, RJ, Chiarello, LA, & O'Neil, MA. A collaborative model of early intervention service delivery. Presented at Contemporary Therapy Practices in Early Intervention: Second Annual Institute. Malvern, PA, May 14, 2004.

Palmer, FB, Shapiro, BS, Allen, MC, Mosher, BS, Biler, SA, Harryman, SE, Meinert, CL, & Capute, AJ. Infant stimulation curriculum for infants with cerebral palsy: Effects on infant temperament, parent-infant interaction, and home environment. Pediatrics, *85*(Suppl):411–415, 1990.

Patton, MQ. Qualitative Evaluation and Research Methods, 2nd ed. Newbury Park, CA: Sage, 1990, pp. 277–368.

Piper, M. Efficacy of physical therapy: Rate of motor development in children with cerebral palsy. Pediatric Physical Therapy, *2*:126–130, 1990.

Pretti-Frontczak, KL, Barr, DM, Macy, M, & Carter, A. Research and resources related to activity-based intervention, embedded learning opportunities, and routines-based instruction; An annotated bibliography. Topics in Early Childhood Special Education, *23*(1):29–40, 2003.

Public Law 99-457, Education of the Handicapped Amendments Act of 1986, 100 Stat. 1145-1177.

Public Law 105-17, Individuals with Disabilities Education Act Amendments of 1997, 111 Stat. 37-157.

Public Law 108-446, Individuals with Disabilities Education Improvement Act of 2004, 118 stat. 2647–2808.

Ramey, CT, & Ramey, SL. Early intervention and early experience. American Psychologist, *53*(2):109–120, 1998.

Ramey, CT, Bryant, DM, Wasik, BH, Sparling, JJ, Fendt, KH, & LaVange, LM. Infant health and development program for low birth weight, premature infants: Program elements, family participation, and child intelligence. Pediatrics, *89*(3):454–465, 1992.

Rapport, MJK, McWilliam, RA, & Smith, BJ. Practices across disciplines in early intervention: The research base. Infants and Young Children, *17*(1):32–44, 2004.

Realini, A, Kalet, A, & Sparling, J. Silence in the medical interaction: II. A means of encouraging patient participation in the interaction. Paper presented at the American Academy of Family Physicians 44th Annual Scientific Assembly, San Diego, CA, October 15–18, 1992.

Rocco, S. New visions for the developmental assessment of infants and young children: A parent's perspective. Washington, D.C.: Zero to Three, June/July 1994, pp. 13–15.

Rocco, S. Toward shared commitment and shared responsibility: A parent's vision of developmental assessment. In Meisels, SJ, & Fenichel, E (Eds.). New Visions for the Developmental Assessment of Infants and Young Children. Washington, D.C.: Zero to Three, 1996, pp. 55–57.

Rogoff, B, Mistry, J, Concu, A, & Mosier, C. Guided participation in cultural activities by toddlers and caregivers. Monographs of Society for Research in Child Development, *58*, Serial No. 236, 1993.

Rosenbaum, P, King, S, Law, M, King, G, & Evans, J. Family-centered service: A conceptual framework and research review. Physical & Occupational Therapy in Pediatrics, *18*:1–20, 1998.

Sameroff, AJ, & Fiese, BH. Transactional regulation: The development of ecology in early intervention. In Shonkoff, JP, Meisels, SJ (Eds.). Handbook of Early Intervention, 2nd ed. New York: Cambridge University Press, 2000, pp. 135–159.

Sandall, S, McLean, ME, & Smith, BJ. DEC Recommended Practices in Early Intervention/Early Childhood Special Education. Longmong, CO: Sopris West, 2000.

Shelton, TL, & Stepanek, JS. Family-Centered Care for Children Needing Specialized Health and Developmental Services, 3rd ed. Bethesda, MD: Association for the Care of Children's Health, 1994.

Shonkoff, JP, & Hauser-Cram, P. Early intervention for disabled infants and their families: A quantitative analysis. Pediatrics, *80*:650–658, 1987.

Shonkoff, JP, Hauser-Cram, P, Krauss, MW, & Upshur, CC. Development of infants with disabilities and their families. Monographs of the Society for Research in Child Development, *57*(6, Serial No. 230), 1992.

Shonkoff, JP, & Meisels, SJ. Handbook of Early Childhood Intervention, 2nd ed. New York: Cambridge University Press, 2000.

Shonkoff, JP, & Phillips, DA. From Neurons to Neighborhoods: The Science of Early Childhood Development. Washington, DC: National Academy Press, 2000.

Shore, R. Rethinking the brain: New insights into early development. New York: Families and Work Institute, 1997.

Simeonsson, RJ, & Bailey, DB. Family dimensions in early intervention. In Meisels, SJ, & Shonkoff, JP (Eds.). Handbook of Early Childhood Intervention. New York: Cambridge University Press, 1990, p. 428.

Spiker, D, Hebbeler, K, Wagner, M, Cameto, R, & McKenna, P. A framework for describing variations in state early intervention systems. Topics in Early Childhood Special Education, *20*(4):195–207, 2000.

Sullivan, M, & Lewis, M. Assistive technology for the very young: Creating responsive environments. Infants and Young Children, *12*(4):34–52, 2000.

Tatarka, ME, Swanson, MW, & Washington, KA. The role of pediatric physical therapy in the interdisciplinary assessment process. In Guralnick, MJ (Ed.). Interdisciplinary Clinical Assessment of Young Children with Developmental Disabilities. Baltimore: Paul H. Brookes Co., 2000, pp. 151–182.

Turnbull, AP, Blue-Banning, M, Turbiville, V, & Park, J. From parent education to partnership education: A call for a transformed focus. Topics in Early Childhood Special Education *19*(3):164, 1999.

Turnbull, JD. Early intervention for children with or at risk of cerebral palsy. American Journal of Diseases of Children, *147*:54–59, 1993.

Warfield, ME. Early intervention program evaluation workshop. Philadelphia: MCP Hahnemann University, May 14, 2002.

Washington, K, & Schwartz, IS. Maternal perceptions of the effects of physical and occupational therapy services on caregiving competency. Physical and Occupational Therapy in Pediatrics, *16*(3):33–54, 1996.

Widerstrom, A, & Ableman, D. Team training issues. In Bricker, D, & Widerstrom, A (Eds). Preparing personnel to work with infants and young children and their families: A team approach. Baltimore: Paul H. Brookes Co., 1996, pp. 23–42.

Winton, PJ, & Bailey, DB. The family-focused interview: A collaborative mechanism for family assessment and goal-setting. Journal of the Division of Early Childhood, *12*:195–207, 1988.

Winton, PJ, & Blow, C. Family Interview Performance Rating Scale. Chapel Hill, NC: Frank Porter Graham Child Development Center, 1991.

World Health Organization. ICIDH2: International Classification of Functioning, Disability and Health. Geneva: World Health Organization, 2001.

Chapter 32

THE EDUCATIONAL ENVIRONMENT

SUSAN K. EFFGEN
PT, PhD

Almost from the start of physical therapy in the United States, physical therapists have worked in educational environments. The civil rights movement of the 1960s and federal legislation of the 1970s, however, marked the beginning of major changes in services for all children with special needs in educational environments. In this chapter the history of the delivery of physical therapy in educational environments is reviewed along with a discussion of federal legislation and significant court cases that have changed how children with special needs are educated and receive physical therapy. The focus is on key issues related to physical therapy in educational environments such as inclusive education, models of team interaction, service delivery models, the individualized educational program (IEP), and intervention strategies. Management issues and critical issues facing school-based physical therapists are also discussed.

BACKGROUND

Although the history of physical therapy in the United States is traced to "reconstruction aides" serving the injured of World War I, it can also be traced to the service of "crippled children," especially those with poliomyelitis. These children were served in hospitals and special settings. Special schools and classes began to appear early in the twentieth century in major cities. The children had a variety of diagnoses, including poliomyelitis and spastic paralysis (Cable et al., 1938; Givins, 1938), cardiac disorders, "obstetric arms," bone and joint tuberculosis, clubfeet, and osteomyelitis (Batten, 1933; Cable et al., 1938; Mulcahey, 1936). By the 1930s, numerous articles had been published describing the delivery of physical therapy in these special schools (Batten, 1933; Mulcahey, 1936; Sever, 1938; Vacha, 1933).

The role of physical therapy in schools has continued to expand throughout the century. Epidemics of poliomyelitis increased the need for special schools and physical therapists. After the vaccine for poliomyelitis was developed in the 1950s, the need for special schools was temporarily reduced, until public awareness increased regarding the needs of children with other disabilities.

Historically, most children in special schools had normal or near-normal intelligence. Many schools required children to be toilet trained, and some required children to walk independently. This trend to serve only those with physical disabilities and normal intelligence continued in many areas of the United States until schools were federally mandated in 1975 to serve all children with disabilities by the enactment of Public Law (PL) 94-142, the Education for All Handicapped Children Act.

FEDERAL LEGISLATION AND LITIGATION

A number of social and political events paved the way for the enactment of the Education for All Handicapped Children Act. In 1954, the historic Supreme Court decision regarding segregated schools, *Brown v. Board of Education of Topeka,* was decided. Separate-but-equal schools were found inherently unequal. This Supreme Court decision was to end the segregated education of African-American children. The principles and foundation of this case could apply to segregated schools for those with disabilities. The call for social equality had begun and would eventually include those with disabilities. President Kennedy's personal experience with his sister who had a disability expedited his establishment of a President's Panel on Mental Retardation in 1961.

Television documentaries exposed institutions in New York, and Blatt and Kaplan's book, *Christmas in Purgatory: A Photographic Essay on Mental Retardation* (1966), raised national concern for the care and treatment of individuals with disabilities. Leaders such as Wolfensberger (1971) were influential proponents of deinstitutionalization and normalization. Cruickshank (1980, p. 65) noted that "as is usually the case with major changes in social policy, the normalization trend is not based on empirical data showing greater effectiveness or efficiency of the changes proposed by its advocates." The normalization trend had, rather, an emphasis on the civil rights of individuals, a prevailing anti-institutional attitude—especially governmental institutions—and a commitment "to the democratic, the individualistic, and the humanitarian" (Cruickshank, 1980, pp. 65–66). The federal Developmental Disabilities Assistance and Bill of Rights Act of 1975 (PL 94-103) included a provision that states had to develop and incorporate a "deinstitutionalization and institutional reform plan" (Braddock, 1987, p. 71). Advocacy groups had gained power, and they used the judicial system to win their rights.

The *Pennsylvania Association for Retarded Citizens (PARC) v. Commonwealth of Pennsylvania* (1971) was the historic, decisive court case establishing the uncompromising right to an education for all children with disabilities. This was a class-action suit filed on behalf of 14 specifically named children and all other children who were in a similar "class" to those with trainable mental retardation. In Pennsylvania, these children were excluded from public school if a psychologist or mental health professional certified that a child could no longer profit from attendance at school. The local school board could refuse to accept or retain a child who had not reached the mental age of 5 years. Children who were classified as trainable mentally retarded, therefore, were unable to get a public education in Pennsylvania. The court sided with the children.

In *PARC v. Commonwealth of Pennsylvania,* the court found that all children, between 6 and 21 years of age, regardless of degree of disability, were to be given a "free and appropriate public education (FAPE)." Children with disabilities were to be educated with children without disabilities in the least restrictive environment (LRE). The educational system was ordered to stop applying exclusionary laws; parents were to become involved in the child's program; and reevaluations were to be done. This landmark court case established many important principles that were later incorporated into the Education for All Handicapped Children Act.

Simultaneous with the PARC case, other important court cases were being decided. *Mills v. Board of Educa-*

tion of the District of Columbia (1972) was filed on behalf of all children excluded by public schools for a disability of any kind, including behavioral problems. The major result of this case was that all children, no matter how severe their mental retardation, behavioral problem, or disability, were educable and must be provided for suitably by the public school system. Related services, including physical therapy, were to be part of their educational program.

In *Maryland Association for Retarded Citizens v. Maryland* (1972) it was ruled that children have the right to tuition subsidies, the right to transportation, and the right to be educated with children who are not disabled. These cases and others across the nation began to establish the right of all children to a "free and appropriate public education." It was in this climate that PL 94-142 was enacted.

PL 94-142: EDUCATION FOR ALL HANDICAPPED CHILDREN ACT

PROVISIONS

On November 29, 1975, the U.S. Congress passed PL 94-142, the Education for All Handicapped Children Act. The law included the elements won in individual court cases across the nation and provided for a "free and appropriate public education" for all children with disabilities from ages 6 to 21 years (age 5 years if a state provided public education to children without disabilities at age 5 years). The major provisions of PL 94-142, still in place today, concern the concepts of zero reject, education in the least restrictive environment, right to due process, nondiscriminatory evaluation, individualized educational program, parent participation, and the right to related services, which include physical therapy.

ZERO REJECT

All children are to receive an education, including children with severe or profound disabilities. These children were initially to receive priority for service because they were probably not receiving appropriate service at that time.

LEAST RESTRICTIVE ENVIRONMENT

Public agencies are to ensure the following:

To the maximum extent appropriate, children with disabilities, including children in public or private institutions or other care facilities, are educated with children who are not disabled, and special classes, separate schooling, or other removal of children with disabilities from the regular educational environment occurs only when the nature or severity of the disability of a child is such that education in regular classes with the use of supplementary aids and services cannot be achieved satisfactorily.

PL 108-446, 118 Stat. 2677, § 612 (a)(5)(A)

RIGHT TO DUE PROCESS

The law provides parents with numerous rights. Parents have the right to an impartial hearing, the right to be represented by counsel, and the right to a verbatim transcript of a hearing and written findings. They can appeal and get an independent evaluation. Later, under PL 99-372, the Handicapped Children's Protection Act [1986, 20 USC § 1415(e)(4), (f)], parents would be able to get reimbursed for legal fees if they prevailed in a court case.

NONDISCRIMINATORY EVALUATION

Several court cases had noted the discriminatory nature of the testing and placement procedures used in many school systems. Nondiscriminatory tests were to be used, and no one test could be the sole criterion used for placement. Nondiscriminatory testing is critical in the cognitive and language domain; however, physical therapists should also be careful to determine that their tests are not biased. When possible, standardized tests that have norms for different racial and cultural groups should be used.

INDIVIDUALIZED EDUCATIONAL PROGRAM

Every child receiving special education must have an individualized educational program (IEP). This is the comprehensive program outlining the specific special educational, related services, and supports the child is to receive. It includes measurable annual goals. The IEP is developed annually at an IEP meeting.

PARENT PARTICIPATION

Active participation of parents is encouraged under PL 94-142. Parents are the individuals responsible for the continuity of services for their child and should be the child's best advocates. Parents are major decision makers in the development of the IEP: they must give permission for an evaluation, they can restrict the release of information, they have access to their child's records, and they can request due process hearings.

RELATED SERVICES

Related services, such as transportation, speech pathology, audiology, psychologic services, physical therapy, occupational therapy, recreation, and medical and counseling services, are to be provided "as may be required to assist a child with a disability to benefit from special education" (PL 108-446, 118 Stat. 2657, § 602 (26); PL 94-142, 89 Stat. 775). This quotation from the law has been interpreted in many different ways. Physical therapy "to assist a child with a disability to benefit from special education" in some school systems is limited to only those activities that help the child write or sit properly in class. Other school systems more appropriately interpret the law to mean physical therapy that can help the child explore the environment, perform activities of daily living, improve function in school, prepare for vocational training, and improve physical fitness so as to be better prepared to learn and prepare for life after school.

PL 99-457: EDUCATION OF THE HANDICAPPED ACT AMENDMENTS OF 1986; PL 102-119: INDIVIDUALS WITH DISABILITIES EDUCATION ACT AMENDMENTS OF 1991; PL 105-17: INDIVIDUALS WITH DISABILITIES EDUCATION ACT AMENDMENTS OF 1997; PL 108-446: INDIVIDUALS WITH DISABILITIES EDUCATION IMPROVEMENT ACT OF 2004

Congress must reauthorize PL 94-142 at set intervals. PL 99-457, the Education of the Handicapped Act Amendments of 1986, is critical not only because of the reauthorization of PL 94-142, but because this act extended services to infants, toddlers, and preschoolers with disabilities and their families. Services to infants and toddlers, now covered under Part C of the law, are discussed in Chapter 31. On October 7, 1991, PL 94-142 and PL 99-457 were reauthorized and amended as PL 102-119, the Individuals with Disabilities Education Act Amendments of 1991 (IDEA). PL 105-17 was signed into law in June 1997 and PL 108-446, the Individuals with Disabilities Education Improvement Act of 2004 (IDEIA), was signed on December 3, 2004. PL 108-446 will be in effect until 2010. The key elements of these reauthorizations, really a refinement and reorganization of the previous amendments, consist of four parts.

PART A: GENERAL PROVISIONS

Congress found that "disability is a natural part of the human experience and in no way diminishes the right of individuals to participate in or contribute to society. Improving educational results for children with disabilities is an essential element of our national policy of ensuring equality of opportunity, full participation, independent living, and economic self-sufficiency for individuals with disabilities" [PL 108-446, 118 Stat. 2649, § 601(c)]. The recognition that education is not merely the three "Rs," but that it is intended to prepare children for independent living and self-sufficiency, is critical for therapists. This expands what goals could be considered "educationally relevant." Also, principles of universal design (i.e., design of products that will be usable by all people, to the greatest extent possible, with minimal need for additional adaptations and accommodations) which is part of the Assistive Technology Act of 1998, have been added to IDEIA 2004. This strengthens the physical therapists' role in providing access to the educational environment and learning materials (David, 2005).

PART B: ASSISTANCE FOR EDUCATION OF ALL CHILDREN WITH DISABILITIES

Part B outlines the right to a free appropriate public education to all children ages 3 to 21 years. Children 3 to 5 and 18 to 21 years of age might not be served if inconsistent with state law. States are mandated to identify, locate, and evaluate all children with disabilities. Children eligible for special education and related services are those having one or more of the disabilities listed in Box 32-1.

Children 3 to 5 years of age are to have IEPs, as are school-age children; however, the 1991 reauthorization, PL 102-119, allowed states the option of using the individualized family service plans (IFSP), required for infants and toddlers, for preschool-age children. The 2004 reauthorization also allows states the option to continue to provide early intervention services to children with disabilities until the child enters kindergarten or elementary school [PL 108-446, 118 Stat. 2746, § 632(5)(B)(ii)]. Many professionals believe the problems of preschoolers and their families are better served with the family-centered approach embodied in early intervention.

| Box 32-1 | Federal Definitions of Children with Disabilities |

Autism: A developmental disability significantly affecting verbal and nonverbal communication and social interaction, generally evident before age 3, that adversely affects a child's educational performance. Other characteristics often associated with autism are engagement in repetitive activities and stereotyped movements, resistance to environmental change, change in daily routines, and unusual responses to sensory experiences. The term does not apply if a child's educational performance is adversely affected primarily because the child has a serious emotional disturbance.

Deaf-blindness: Concomitant hearing and visual impairments, the combination of which causes such severe communication and other developmental and educational problems that they cannot be accommodated in special education programs solely for children with deafness or children with blindness.

Deafness: A hearing impairment that is so severe that the child is impaired in processing linguistic information through hearing, with or without amplification, that adversely affects a child's educational performance.

Developmental delay: "The term *child with a disability* for a child aged 3 through 9 may, at the discretion of the State and local educational agency, include a child...experiencing developmental delays, as defined by the State and as measured by appropriate diagnostic instruments and procedures, in one or more of the following areas: physical development, cognitive development, communication development, social or emotional development, or adaptive development, and who, for that reason, need special education and related services" [PL 105-17, 111 Stat. 43, Sec. 602 (3) (B)].

Emotional disturbance: A condition exhibiting one or more of the following characteristics over a long period of time and to a marked degree that adversely affects a child's educational performance: (A) An inability to learn that cannot be explained by intellectual, sensory, or health factors; (B) An inability to build or maintain satisfactory interpersonal relationships with peers and teachers; (C) Inappropriate types of behavior or feelings under normal circumstances; (D) A general pervasive mood of unhappiness or depression; (E) A tendency to develop physical symptoms or fears associated with personal or school problems. (ii) The term includes schizophrenia. The term does not apply to children who are socially maladjusted, unless it is determined that they have an emotional disturbance.

Hearing impairment: An impairment in hearing, whether permanent or fluctuating, that adversely affects a child's educational performance but that is not included under the definition of deafness.

Mental retardation: Significantly subaverage general intellectual functioning, existing concurrently with deficits in adaptive behavior and manifested during the developmental period, that adversely affects a child's educational performance.

Multiple disabilities: Concomitant impairments (such as mental retardation-blindness, mental retardation-orthopedic impairment) the combination of which causes such severe educational problems that they cannot be accommodated in special education programs solely for one of the impairments. The term does not include deaf-blindness.

Orthopedic impairment: A severe orthopedic impairment that adversely affects a child's educational performance. The term includes impairments caused by congenital anomaly (e.g., clubfoot, absence of some member), impairments caused by disease (e.g., poliomyelitis, bone tuberculosis), and impairments from other causes (e.g., cerebral palsy, amputations, and fractures or burns that cause contractures).

Other health impairment: Having limited strength, vitality, or alertness, including a heightened alertness to environmental stimuli, that results in limited alertness with respect to the educational environment, that is due to chronic or acute health problems such as asthma, attention deficit disorder, diabetes, epilepsy, a heart condition, hemophilia, lead poisoning, leukemia, nephritis, rheumatic fever, and sickle cell anemia; and adversely affects a child's educational performance.

Specific learning disability: A disorder in one or more of the basic psychological processes involved in understanding or in using language, spoken or written, that may manifest as an imperfect ability to listen, think, speak, read, write, spell, or do mathematical calculations, including conditions such as perceptual disabilities, brain injury, minimal brain dysfunction, dyslexia, and developmental aphasia. The term does not apply to learning problems that are primarily the result of visual, hearing, or motor disabilities, of mental retardation; of emotional disturbance; or of environmental, cultural, or economic disadvantage.

Speech and language impairment: A communication disorder such as stuttering, impaired articulation, a language impairment, or a

continued

Box 32-1   **Federal Definitions of Children with Disabilities—*cont'd***

voice impairment that adversely affects a child's educational performance.

Traumatic brain injury: An acquired injury to the brain caused by an external physical force, resulting in total or partial functional disability or psychosocial impairment, or both, that adversely affects a child's educational performance. The term applies to open- or closed-head injuries resulting in impairments in one or more areas, such as cognition; language; memory; attention; reasoning; abstract thinking; judgment; problem solving; sensory, perceptual, and

motor abilities; psychosocial behavior; physical functions; information processing; and speech. The term does not apply to brain injuries that are congenital or degenerative or brain injuries induced by birth trauma.

Visual impairment including blindness: An impairment in vision that, even with correction, adversely affects a child's educational performance. The term includes both partial sight and blindness. (34 CFR Subpart A § 300.7)

Least Restrictive Environment

An ongoing area of national effort is the continued emphasis on the education of children with disabilities in the least restrictive environment (LRE). Children should be educated in their local schools to the maximum extent appropriate. The degree of inclusion in the local school and the general education classroom will vary based on what is appropriate for their needs and age. Children are not merely to be "placed" in general education, but they are to fully participate and have goals related to their curricular and social advancement.

Transition

Transition planning was specifically addressed in IDEA 1997 because this important service was often neglected. Transition planning and the needed services must be included in the IFSP and IEP. Consideration must be given to transition from early intervention to preschool, from preschool to school, at critical points during school, and especially from age 16 years to exit from school. Physical therapists and other related service personnel are to be involved in the transition planning for post-school activities, as appropriate.

Assistive Technology

Assistive technology devices and assistive technology services allow the child to fully benefit from her or his educational environment.

The term "assistive technology device" means any item, piece of equipment, or product system whether acquired commercially off the shelf, modified, or customized, that is used to increase, maintain, or improve the functional capabilities of a child with a disability ... "assistive technology service" means any service that directly assists a child with a disability in the selection, acquisition, or use of an assistive technology device.

PL 108-446, 118 Stat. 2652, § 602(1)

Assistive technology services include evaluation, selection, purchasing, and coordination with education and rehabilitation plans and programs. This is an important area, as physical therapists frequently provide assistive devices to improve a child's function and participation at school. Therapists adapt seating so children can function better and safely in the classroom. Therapists also assist other team members in devising the most functional communication systems along with providing access to switching devices and computers. Ambulation devices (e.g., walkers, crutches, and canes) are frequently necessary to allow the child to walk throughout the school. Power mobility devices allow children with severe impairments and limited self-mobility to independently access the school building and grounds and thereby increase participation in all aspects of their education program. The extent of assistive technology services and the purchasing of devices vary among school systems. For additional information, see Chapter 33.

SECTION 504 OF THE REHABILITATION ACT

Section 504 of the Rehabilitation Act of 1973 (PL 93-112) is a broad antidiscrimination statute designed to ensure that federal funding recipients—including schools—provide equal opportunity to people with disabilities (Discipline Under Section 504, 1996). It has been used to broaden a student's eligibility for related services in school. Educational agencies that receive federal funds are not allowed to exclude qualified individuals with disabilities from participation in any program offered by the agency. The definition of "qualified handicapped person" under Section 504 is broader than it is in IDEIA. Under Section 504, handicapped persons means any person who (i) has a physical or mental impairment which substantially limits one or more major life activities (34CFR104.3(j)(1). Major life activities means functions such as caring for one's self, performing manual tasks, walking, seeing, hearing, speaking, breathing, learning, and working. (34CFR104.3(j)(2)(ii).

Thus, it is possible that a child who does not require special education under the accepted definitions of disabilities under IDEA, but who is a "qualified handicapped person," might be able to receive all the aid and services necessary to receive a free and appropriate public education through Section 504 (National Information Center for Children and Youth with Disabilities, 1991).

PL 101-336: AMERICANS WITH DISABILITIES ACT

The Americans with Disabilities Act (ADA) (PL 101-336) was signed into law on July 26, 1990. It "extends to individuals with disabilities comprehensive civil rights protection similar to those provided to persons on the basis of race, sex, national origin, and religion under the Civil Rights Act of 1964" (*Federal Register*, July 26, 1991, p. 3540). The regulations cover employment; public service, including public transportation, public accommodations, and telecommunications; and miscellaneous provisions. Although the law is not specific in reference to issues related to children in school, its provisions assist children with disabilities. The law is especially applicable to day care centers and transition to employment (Pax Lowes & Effgen, 1996). Public buildings, including schools, must be accessible, and children should be able to use public transportation to get to school, work, and social activities. Children with disabilities should expect to use the skills learned at school in an accessible workplace. The ADA is discussed in Chapter 37.

PL 107-110: NO CHILD LEFT BEHIND ACT

Legislation entitled No Child Left Behind Act of 2001 (NCLB) (PL 107-110) was passed as part of title I of the Elementary and Secondary Education Act of 1965 (ESEA). This federal legislation was to ensure that all children, including those with disabilities, receive a quality education. To achieve this goal, all children were to be tested and make adequate yearly progress. There have, however, been significant problems with this legislation and 28% of our nation's schools have failed to make adequate progress (Dillon, 2004). In December 2003, it was recognized that the testing of children with disabilities and meeting yearly goals for closing the achievement gap were not successful, so new federal provisions were announced. Under the new provisions, local school systems will have greater flexibility in meeting the requirements of NCLB (*Federal Register*, 2003). Determination of the definition of significant cognitive disabilities will now be determined by the state. Physical therapists working in school systems should make certain that children are properly positioned and have appropriate writing implements for testing situations to assist with the demands of NCLB.

CASE LAW

A law as comprehensive and complex as IDEA was bound to lead to some controversy. All possible situations could not be anticipated, and some issues were expected to be resolved by the courts. As a result, a number of significant court cases have helped define the scope of the law.

RELATED SERVICES

Tatro v. Texas (1980) was one of the early major cases involving PL 94-142. Amber Tatro had spina bifida and required clean intermittent catheterization several times during the school day. Amber's parents wanted assistance with catheterization at school. The school officials refused, saying catheterization was a medical procedure and Amber could not attend school unless her parents handled the procedure. The parents then initiated what turned out to be a 10-year legal battle. During the legal process, they were told that although catheterization was necessary to sustain Amber's life, it was not necessary to benefit from education; the school system, therefore, was not obligated to provide the service. After a complicated course though the court system, the case was heard by the U.S. Supreme Court. Amber attempted to attend the Supreme Court proceedings, only to discover that the Supreme Court was not readily accessible.

The Supreme Court ruled that clean intermittent catheterization was a related service that enabled the child to benefit from special education:

A service that enables a handicapped child to remain at school during the day is an important means of providing students with the meaningful access to education that Congress envisioned. The Act makes specific provision for services, like transportation, for example, that do no more than enable a child to be physically present in class.

Martin, 1991, p. 45; *Tatro v. Texas*, 1980, at 891

This case led to the "bright-line" physician-non-physician rule that the services of a physician (other than for diagnostic and evaluation purposes) need not be provided by the school system, but that services that can be given by a nurse or qualified layman must be provided by the school. This case is important to physical therapists because the realm of related services was expanded, as was the meaning of "required to benefit from special education."

More recent court cases regarding related services have involved children who are medically fragile and require extensive services of a nurse and others. Some states advocate the use of an extent/nature test. In the extent/nature test, decision making focuses on the individual case and considers the complexity and need for services. The U.S. Supreme Court in *Cedar Rapids Community School District v. Garret F.,* (Supreme Court of the United States, No. 96-1793, March 3 1999), reaffirmed that related services, in this case nursing services, was not an excluded medical service and must be provided in schools, irrespective of the intensity or complicity of the services, under IDEA, thus supporting the right to an education of children with complex health care needs.

Best Possible Education

Rowley v. Board of Education of Hendrick Hudson Central School District (1982) involved Amy Rowley, who was deaf. She had a special tutor, her teachers were trained in basic sign language, and she was provided with a sound amplifier. After experimenting with an interpreter in general education class, the school system decided she did not need the service. Her parents believed she needed the interpreter and went through due process to continue interpreter services. A district court held that Amy was not receiving a free and appropriate public education because she did not have "an opportunity to achieve her full potential commensurate with the opportunity provided to other children." The school system appealed, and the case eventually went to the U.S. Supreme Court. The 1982 Supreme Court decision held that Congress did not intend to give children with disabilities a right to the best possible education (i.e., education that would "maximize their potential"); it rejected the standard used by the lower courts that children with disabilities are entitled to an educational opportunity "commensurate with the education available to nonhandicapped children" and set two standards, namely, that a state is required to provide meaningful access to an education for each child with a disability and that sufficient supportive and related services must be provided to permit the child to benefit educationally from special education instruction.

When the Supreme Court applied these standards in *Rowley* it found that Amy did not need interpreter services because she was making "exemplary progress in the regular education system" with the help of the extensive special services. The Supreme Court was careful to point out that merely passing from grade to grade does not mean a child's education is appropriate.

The *Rowley* decision has had a significant impact on the provision of related services, including physical therapy. Unfortunately, in some school systems the *Rowley* decision has been used to limit the amount of physical therapy provided on the premise that schools are not obligated to provide the "best services." What must be remembered is that Amy was receiving extensive services and was making "exemplary progress in the regular education system." Therapists must recognize that "exemplary progress" may be a reason to terminate services unless significant educational need for physical therapy can be substantiated.

Extended School Year

As children with special needs began to benefit from 9-month educational programs, some parents realized that their children's skills were regressing during the summer and that it took several months to regain those skills when the children returned to class in the fall. Because the U.S. Congress had realized that more than the traditional 12 years of schooling might be necessary for children with disabilities to reach their potential, perhaps it could be inferred that if a child regressed during the summer, extended school year services might be necessary (Martin, 1991).

Several court cases addressed this issue. In both *Battle v. Commonwealth of Pennsylvania* (1981) and *Georgia Association of Retarded Citizens v. McDaniel* (1981), parents sought to extend the school year. In Pennsylvania, it was found that the state's policy of defining a school year as 180 days could not be used to prevent the provision of an extended school year. In Georgia, the court ruled that an extended school year must be based on individual cases. The child must show significant regression, the extended year must be part of the IEP, and an extended year does not mean 5 days a week for 52 weeks but must be based on a program to attain goals.

Eligibility for extended school year services is now based on several criteria. These include "individual need, nature and severity of the disability, educational benefit, regression and recoupment, self-sufficiency and independence, and failing to meet short-term goals and objectives" (Rapport & Thomas, 1993, p. 16). The possibility of receiving services for the entire year has many implications for physical therapy. The children most likely to require extended school year services are usually those with the most severe disabilities, often requiring physical therapy. One criterion used to qualify for extended school year services is documentation of regression during vacation and the length of time it takes to recoup or relearn skills. It is therefore vital for physical therapists to do an examination and evaluation before and after school breaks. Documentation of regression, especially during short breaks, might enable a child to receive physical therapy during the summer. Using the child's status at the end of the summer as the basis for extended school year physical therapy services might be confounded if parents obtain private physical therapy during the summer and regression is prevented.

An ethical dilemma can arise for some physical therapists over the extended school year issue. Some school therapists provide private physical therapy during the summer and might prefer that the school system not provide the service. Others might not want the obligation of having to provide services during the summer, either through the school or privately. Therapists must be careful to recognize this potential conflict of interest.

LEAST RESTRICTIVE ENVIRONMENT

Not only has the issue of LRE, now referred to as inclusion, generated much discussion; it has also generated many due process hearings and lawsuits. The outcomes have been mixed. During the early 1990s, the party seeking inclusion, usually the parent, prevailed in a series of court cases, the most noted being *Oberti* (3d Cir. 1993) and *Daniel R.R.* (5th Cir. 1989) (Zirkel, 1996). Later cases ruled against inclusive, general education placements as the LRE for students who were past elementary school age and had severe disabilities (Special Educator, 1996). A rational approach must prevail in issues regarding inclusion. As discussed later in the chapter, there must be options for the locations and types of services available to the child that can and should change over time.

▌EDUCATIONAL MILIEU

Although physical therapists have served children with disabilities in the general education setting for many years, educational administrators and teachers vary in their perceptions of the role of physical therapy, just as physical therapists have different perspectives of their role in the educational milieu. Hence, there is the need for open communication and collaboration. Physical

therapists must take the time to develop relationships with administrators, teachers, and staff and understand the written and unwritten rules of the educational environment to create an effective working environment.

LEAST RESTRICTIVE ENVIRONMENT

Education of all children in the LRE, no matter how severe their disability, is what the federal laws and "best practices" indicate we must strive to achieve (Meyer et al., 1991; PL 105-17; PL 108-446; Rainforth & York-Barr, 1997; Taylor, 1988). The conceptual framework for education in the least restrictive environment started in the 1960s. Reynolds (1962) advocated a continuum of placement options from most restrictive to least restrictive. Deno (1970) termed this the *cascade* of educational placements. The cascade of environments, from most to least restrictive, includes the residential setting, homebound services, special schools, special classes in neighborhood schools, general classes with resource assistance in neighborhood schools, and general classes in the neighborhood school without resource assistance. Taylor (1988), a long-time advocate for total integration of people with severe disabilities, proposes that the focus of service systems must change from the development of programs in which people must fit to the provision of services and supports necessary for full participation in community life. Terminology used to describe LRE has evolved from *mainstreaming,* to *integrated,* to *inclusive.* The differences in terms are more than merely a change in language.

Inclusive education at its best includes involvement of the whole school where children with disabilities are served in the general education environment with the required "supplementary aids and services" (Lipsky, 2003). Models for meeting a students needs in an inclusive setting include (a) general education and special education teachers co-teaching together during all or part of the curriculum; (b) indirect, consultative support from the special education teacher; (c) material adaptation by the special education teacher; (d) a team model in which the special education teacher is part of a team serving the child, usually in middle and high school; and (e) a schoolwide approach where the entire staff takes responsibility for all students (Lipsky, 2003). Physical therapists who work in systems using any of these models must make certain they interact with all appropriate personnel for maximum communication, team effectiveness, and optimal child outcomes.

Compliance with LRE requirements is occurring to varying degrees across the nation and presents some challenges for physical therapists. Therapists must be prepared to work with administrators, teachers, and staff who may know little about children with disabilities and the role of the physical therapist. Interaction with other physical therapists is often limited. Therapists might also have far to travel to see a single child, and scheduling services and times to meet with teachers is difficult. Physical therapists and teachers must work together so that collaboration and effective service can be achieved in the general education environment. The reader is encouraged to read further for a more in-depth discussion of inclusion (Falvey et al., 1995; Guralnick, 2001; Rainforth & Kugelmass, 2003; Rainforth & York-Barr,1997; Ryndak & Fisher, 2003).

MODELS OF TEAM INTERACTION

There has been an evolution in models of team interaction during the past two decades. The hierarchy of team interaction is presented in Box 32-2. The unidisciplinary model is not a team model and should rarely, if ever, be used in school settings. The multidisciplinary model involves several professionals doing independent evaluations and then meeting to discuss their evaluations and determine goals, objectives, and a plan of action. The meaning of multidisciplinary has changed since 1986 because of its usage in PL 99-457. In the law, the term *multidisciplinary* is used to describe an interdisciplinary model, as noted in Box 32-2; therefore, there is frequently confusion when using this term.

The definition and application of the transdisciplinary model are also ambiguous. For some, the continuous sharing of information across disciplines is sufficient for a transdisciplinary model. For others, there must be complete role release. Role release involves not just the sharing of information but also the sharing of performance competencies. Team members teach each other specific interventions so that all can provide greater consistency and frequency in meeting the child's needs. In a transdisciplinary model occasionally only one individual provides the intervention, thereby increasing consistency and allowing rapport to be established with the child and family.

As the team process has developed, the use of the terms *collaboration* and *collaborative teams* has been used (Rainforth & York-Barr, 1997; Hunt et al., 2003; Snell & Janney, 2000). These are supportive terms and might incorporate a number of models of team interaction based on the needs of educators, therapists, the child, and family. The defining characteristics of collaborative teamwork, as conceptualized by Rainforth and York-Barr (1997), are summarized in Box 32-3. They believe that significant benefits are gained because of the diverse perspectives, skills, and knowledge available from the individuals on the educational team. This combined talent is an enormous resource of problem solving and support. Collaborative teams are of vital importance when working with children having multiple disabilities or with those who are severely or profoundly disabled.

Box 32-2 Models of Team Interaction

UNIDISCIPLINARY

Professional works independently of all others.

INTRADISCIPLINARY

Members of the same profession work together without significant communication with members of other professions.

MULTIDISCIPLINARY

Professionals work independently but recognize and value the contributions of other disciplines. "Little or no interaction or ongoing communication occurs among professionals" (Thurman & Wilderstrom, 1990, p. 225). However, the Rules and Regulations (*Federal Register,* June 22, 1989, p. 26313) for PL 99-457 redefines multidisciplinary to mean "the involvement of two or more disciplines or professions in the provision of integrated and coordinated services, including evaluation and assessment."

INTERDISCIPLINARY

Individuals from different disciplines work together cooperatively to evaluate and develop programs. Emphasis is on teamwork. Role definitions are relaxed.

TRANSDISCIPLINARY

Professionals are committed "to teaching, learning and working with others across traditional disciplinary boundaries" (Rainforth et al., 1992, p. 13). Role release occurs when a team member assumes the responsibilities of other disciplines for service delivery.

COLLABORATIVE

The team interaction of the transdisciplinary model is combined with the integrated service delivery model. Services are provided by professionals across disciplinary boundaries as part of the natural routine of the school and community.

Box 32-3	**Characteristics of Collaborative Teamwork**

- Equal participation in the collaborative teamwork process by family members and service providers
- Consensus decision making in determining priorities for goals and objectives
- Consensus decision making about the type and amount of intervention
- All skills, including motor and communication skills, are embedded throughout the intervention program
- Infusion of knowledge and skills from different disciplines into the design and application of intervention
- Role release to enable team members to develop confidence and competence necessary to facilitate the child's learning

Adapted from Rainforth, B, & York-Barr, J. Collaborative Teams for Students with Severe Disabilities, 2nd ed. Baltimore: Paul H Brookes, 1997.

When joining a team, physical therapists should ask for a clarification and a definition of terms regarding models or expectations of team interaction. All individuals should have the same understanding to avoid miscommunication and conflict.

MODELS OF SERVICE DELIVERY

There is an array of models of physical therapy service delivery. Terms used to describe the various models overlap. To some extent this reflects overlap among models and that more than one model may apply to a practice setting. The models include direct, integrated, consultative, monitoring, and collaborative (Table 32-1).

Direct Model

In the direct model, the therapist is the primary service provider to the child. This is the traditional model used to provide physical therapy across practice settings. Direct intervention is provided when there is emphasis on acquisition of motor skills and when therapeutic techniques cannot be safely delegated. Rarely, if ever, should direct intervention be given without also instructing the child's teachers and parents. Hanft and Place (1996) note that even in a direct service "pullout" model where the child is removed from the natural environment, there should be ongoing consultation with teachers and other team members. It is not unusual for a child to receive direct intervention for a specific goal while other models of service delivery are used to achieve other goals. Rarely should only a direct service model be used. A combination of several models of service delivery is consistent with the integrated and collaborative service delivery models.

Integrated Model

The Iowa State Department of Education (2001) defines the *integrated model* as one in which (a) the therapist

interacts not only with the child but also with the teacher, aide, and family; (b) service delivery is in the learning environment; and (c) many people are involved in implementation of the therapy program. Team collaboration is a feature of the model.

The integrated model of service delivery can, and frequently does, include direct and consultative physical therapy services. The therapist, however, must collaborate with other individuals serving the child. Goals and objectives should be jointly developed, and all individuals serving the child should be instructed in how to incorporate objectives into the child's education program. Direct services, if appropriate, are provided in the LRE. Only when it is in the best interests of the child should the intervention be in a restrictive environment, such as a special room, because generalization of skills learned in one setting do not necessarily generalize to other settings (Brown et al., 1998). Common examples of when therapy might be acceptable in a more restrictive environment are when the child is participating in academic courses, when extensive equipment is required, when the child is highly distractible, or when it is necessary for the child's safety.

Consultative Model

In the consultative model, the therapist interacts with members of the educational team, including the parent and child. The service is provided in the learning environment and the appropriate members of the educational team implement activities. The physical therapist *does not* provide direct intervention. Rather, the therapist meets with, and demonstrates activities to, all appropriate staff. The responsibility for the outcome is with the consultee—the individuals, usually the teachers, receiving the consultation (Dunn, 1991).

Hanft and Place (1996) note that consultation in the school may be included in several service delivery models. Consultation may be child specific, as outlined in Table

TABLE 32-1 Physical Therapy Service Delivery Models in Educational Settings

	DIRECT	INTEGRATED	CONSULTATIVE	MONITORING	COLLABORATIVE
Therapist's primary contact	Pupil	Pupil, teacher, parent, aide	Teacher, parent, aide, pupil	Pupil	Entire team, pupil
Environment for service delivery	Distraction-free environment (may need to be separate from learning environment) Specialized equipment needed	Learning environment and other natural settings Therapy area if necessary for a specific child	Learning environment and other natural settings	Learning environment Therapy area if necessary for a specific child	Learning environment and other natural settings
Methods of intervention	Educationally related functional activities Specific therapeutic techniques that cannot safely be delegated Emphasis on acquisition of new motor skills	Educationally related functional activities Positioning Emphasis on practice of newly acquired motor skills in the daily routine	Educationally related activities Positioning Adaptive materials Emphasis on adapting to learning environment and generalization of acquired skills	Emphasis on making certain that child maintains status to benefit from special education	Educationally related activities
Amount of actual service time	Regularly scheduled sessions, generally at least weekly	Routinely scheduled Flexible amount of time depending on needs of staff or pupil	Intermittent or as needed, depending on needs of staff or pupil	Intermittent, depending on needs of pupil, may be as infrequent as once in 6 months	Ongoing intervention Discipline-referenced knowledge shared among team members so relevant activities occur throughout the day
Implementer of activities	PT, PTA	PT, PTA, teacher, parent, aide, OT, COTA	Teacher, parent, aide	PT	Team
Individualized education plan objectives	Specific to therapy programs as related to educational needs	Specific to educational program	Specific to educational program	Specific to being able to maintain educational program	Organized around life domains in an ecologic curriculum

Adapted from Iowa Guidelines for Educationally Related Physical Services. Des Moines, IA: Department of Education, 1996.
COTA, Certified occupational therapist assistant; *OT*, occupational therapist; *PT*, physical therapist; *PTA*, physical therapist assistant.

32-1, but might also include programmatic consultation involving issues related to safety, transportation, architectural barriers, equipment, documentation, continuing education, and improvement of the program's quality (Lindsey et al., 1980). Programmatic consultation should be the major activity of a therapist at the beginning of each academic year. Issues related to safety, transportation, and positioning are frequently more important than child-specific goals and objectives. Once the environment is safe, the child is properly positioned throughout the day, and a safe means of mobility is determined, the specific intervention program can be initiated.

Monitoring Model

In the monitoring model, the physical therapist shares information and provides instruction to team members, maintains regular contact with the child to check on status, and assumes responsibility for outcome of the intervention. Similar to the consultative model, the therapist *does not* provide direct intervention. Monitoring is important for follow-up of children who have impairments, activity limitations, or participation restrictions that might deteriorate over time. Monitoring allows the therapist to check on the need for modifications in adaptive equipment and assistive devices. Monitoring is also an important way to determine if a child is progressing as necessary for transition to the next level of educational or vocational services. Monitoring is useful for transition from direct or integrated services to no services. Monitoring provides the family, child, and therapist a sense of security that the child is being observed. Also, if the need for direct services is identified, initiation of services is facilitated because physical therapy is already listed on the IEP.

Collaborative Model

Not everyone would consider the collaborative model a model of service delivery; however, because it is defined as a combination of transdisciplinary team interaction and an integrated service delivery model, it is being discussed as part of service delivery (Rainforth & York-Barr, 1997). As noted in Box 32-3 and Table 32-1, services in a collaborative model are provided by all team members, as in an integrated model, but the degree of role release and crossing of disciplinary boundaries is greater. The team assumes responsibility for developing a consensus on the goals and objectives and the implementation of the program activities. The activities are educationally relevant and are implemented in the natural routine of the school and community. In the collaborative model, the amount of time the child practices an

activity should, theoretically, be greater than in other models because implementation involves the entire team. In reality, this might not be the case because of the varied levels of skill of team members, insufficient "natural" opportunities to practice an activity, competition among activities, and difficulty in implementation of some activities (Prieto, 1992; Soccio, 1991). Research by Hunt and associates (2003) suggests that collaborative teaming, with consistent implementation of unified plans of support, results in increased academic skills, engagement in classroom activities, interactions with peers, and student-initiated interactions for students with severe disabilities. The researchers indicated that parents played a critical role in the development and implementation of the programs and flexibility was key to the practicality and applicability of suggestions.

In the past, many believed that state physical therapy practice acts prohibited school personnel from performing procedures used by physical therapists. This generally is not the case as long as the individual does not represent himself or herself as a physical therapist, does not bill for physical therapy, and does not perform a physical therapy evaluation (Rainforth, 1997). In fact, a study by Rainforth (1997) indicates few limitations on the delegation of procedures by others, especially of the nature likely to occur in an educational environment.

PROGRAM DEVELOPMENT

EXAMINATION AND EVALUATION

Throughout this text, language suggested by the *Guide to Physical Therapist Practice* (American Physical Therapy Association, 2001) has been used; however, federal education laws use slightly different terminology. Evaluations (examination and evaluation) are conducted to "assist in determining whether the child is a child with a disability" [PL 108-446, 118 Stat. 27045, § 614(b)(2)] and are used to determine the educational needs of the child.

The evaluation tools used should be technically sound and should be administered by trained and knowledgeable personnel in accordance with instructions and in the child's native language without racial or cultural bias [PL 108-446, 118 Stat. 2705, § 614(b)(3)]. Selection of standardized tests should be based on professional judgment and dictated by the characteristics of the individual child. Therapists should collaborate with school personnel to identify appropriate tests and measures that gather relevant functional and developmental information. The child's abilities should be assessed in the natural environment. This means that the therapist should see the child in the classroom, hallway, and other school settings. If it is not feasible to assess the child in these natural environments, every attempt must be made to make the examination/evaluation setting as close to the natural environment as possible. The School Function Assessment (SFA), developed by Coster and co-workers (1998), is of great assistance in determining the participation of children in all aspects of the education program. The Pediatric Evaluation of Disability Inventory (PEDI) (Haley et al., 1996) provides a useful assessment of the child's functional abilities. Numerous other tests and measures, as discussed throughout this text, may assist in determining the developmental level of a child's physical functioning. Examination should also include a full assessment of all body systems: musculoskeletal, neuromuscular, cardiopulmonary, and integumentary. Impairment of any of these systems can cause limitations in activities and participation affecting school performance. Reduction of impairment of body structures and functions may be necessary before children can improve their activities and participation to assist in meeting their educational needs.

Results of the examination and evaluation are used to determine eligibility for the services; IEP goals; frequency and duration of services; and the need for extended school year programming. As noted previously, for school-age children, a motor delay or disability does not necessarily qualify a child for special education and related services. The children must first have an educational need for special education in one of the categories listed in Box 32-1. Once the child meets the criteria for special education in one of these categories, the related service needs are determined as "required to assist a child with a disability to benefit from special education." If a child is not eligible for special education, he or she may be eligible for related services under Section 504 of the Rehabilitation Act. The need for related services must be based on the individual needs of the child. Several school systems have attempted to develop generalized exclusionary criteria such as performance discrepancy criteria, also called cognitive referencing. Performance discrepancy criteria limit services to children whose cognitive development is below their motor development (Carr, 1989, p. 506). This assumes a positive correlation between the development of cognition and motor skills. Under this interpretation, the child most appropriate for physical therapy has normal intellectual skills but delay in motor skills. Children whose cognitive and motor skills are similar would not be eligible for services. Aside from the legal (Rainforth, 1991) and ethical questions, research

does not support cognitive referencing (Baker et al., 1998; Cole et al., 1991).

Comprehensive, overall reevaluations may be done no more than once a year, unless both the parent and educational agency agree to more frequent evaluations. Reevaluations should be done "at least every 3 years, unless the parent and the local educational agency agree that a reevaluation is unnecessary" [PL 108-446, 118 Stat. 2704, § 614 (a)(2)]. Physical therapy reevaluations might be done more frequently based on the requirements of individual state practice acts and best practice guidelines.

INDIVIDUALIZED EDUCATIONAL PROGRAM

The IEP is the document that guides the program of special education and related services for the school-age child, 5 to 21 years of age. It is also the document used in most states for the educational program of children ages 3 to 5 years attending preschool. The IEP is developed at a meeting involving the child's parents; at least one regular educator (if the child is or will be participating in the regular education environment); not less than one special education teacher; a representative of the local educational agency who is qualified to provide or supervise specially designed instruction and is knowledgeable about the general education curriculum and resources; an individual who can interpret the instructional implications of the evaluation; and "at the discretion of the parent or the agency, other individuals who have knowledge or special expertise regarding the child, including related services personnel as appropriate; and whenever appropriate, the child" [PL 108-446, 118 Stat. 2709, § 614(d)(1)(B)]. The physical therapist has a professional obligation to participate when decisions regarding physical therapy are being made. The physical therapy contribution to the IEP must relate to the educational needs of the child. Individualized measurable annual academic and functional goals are developed at the IEP meeting. Short-term objectives are no longer required under IDEA 2004, except for those children who take alternate assessments; however, they are essential under "best practice" guidelines, and many school systems will continue to require them. If not required locally, therapists should still develop short-term objectives to monitor and report intervention outcomes as required for the plan of care. Table 32-2 describes the different elements of outcomes measures.

IEP attendance may not be mandatory for all members of the team

if the parent of a child with a disability and the local educational agency agree that the attendance of such a

TABLE 32-2	Elements of Outcome Measures				
MEASURE	**PART OF IEP**	**MEASURABLE**	**TIME FRAME**	**DIMENSION**	**DISCIPLINE SPECIFIC**
Annual goal	Yes	Yes	School year	Activity/participation	No
Long-term objective	Yes	Yes	School year	Activity/participation	No
Short-term objective	Not required by federal law except for students who take alternate assessments*	Yes	Months, perhaps a grading period	Body function and structure Activity/participation	Varies, some objectives might clearly be within the domain of one discipline
Benchmark	Yes, but not always included	Yes	School year or months	Activity/participation	No, although some objectives might clearly be within the domain of one discipline

*Might be required by local school system or state physical therapist practice act as part of plan of care.

member is not necessary because the member's area of curriculum or related services is not being modified or discussed. ... A member of the IEP team may be excused ... if the parent and the local educational agency consent to the excusal; and the member submits, in writing to the parent and the IEP team, input into the development of the IEP prior to the meeting.

PL 108-460, 118 Stat. 2710, § 614(d)(1)(C)

Therapists who are presently serving a child would now have to either attend the IEP meeting or receive approval not to attend and then submit in writing their recommendations. This new requirement of written input will hopefully encourage more participation by therapists at IEP meetings.

Under IDEA 2004 the IEP document must include the following:

(I) a statement of the child's present levels of academic achievement and functional performance, including—

(aa) how the child's disability affects the child's involvement and progress in the general curriculum;

(bb) for preschool children, as appropriate, how the disability affects the child's participation in appropriate activities; and

(cc) for children with disabilities who take alternate assessments aligned to alternate achievement standards, a description of benchmarks or short-term objectives;

(II) a statement of measurable annual goals, including academic and functional goals, designed to—

(aa) meet the child's needs that result from the child's disability to enable the child to be involved in and make progress in the general curriculum; and

(bb) meet each of the child's other educational needs that result from the child's disability;

(III) a description of how the child's progress toward meeting the annual goals ... will be measured and when periodic reports on the progress the child is making toward meeting the annual goals (such as through the use of quarterly or other periodic reports, concurrent with the issuance of report cards) will be provided;

(IV) a statement of the special education and related services and supplementary aids and services, based on peer-reviewed research to the extent practicable, to be provided to the child, or on behalf of the child, and a statement of the program modifications or supports for school personnel that will be provided for the child—

(aa) to advance appropriately toward attaining the annual goals;

(bb) to be involved and progress in the general curriculum... and to participate in extracurricular and other nonacademic activities; and

(cc) to be educated and participate with other children with disabilities and nondisabled children;

(V) an explanation of the extent, if any, to which the child will not participate with nondisabled children in the regular class;...

(VI) (aa) a statement of any individual accommodations that are necessary to measure the academic achievement and functional performance of the child on State and districtwide assessments;...

(bb) if the IEP Team determines that the child shall take an alternate assessment ...a statement of why the child cannot participate in the regular assessment...

(VII) the projected date for the beginning of services and modifications...and the anticipated frequency, location, and duration of those services and modifications; and

(VIII) beginning not later than the first IEP to be in effect when the child is 16, and updated annually thereafter—

(aa) appropriate measurable postsecondary goals based upon age appropriate transition assessments related to training, education, employment, and where appropriate, independent living skills;

(bb) transition services (including courses of study) needed to assist the child in reaching these goals; and

(cc) beginning not later than 1 year before the age of majority under State law, a statement that the child has been informed of the child's rights under this title.

PL 108-446, 118 Stat. 2707-2709, § 614(d)(1)(A)

The IEP is a written commitment by the educational agency of the resources necessary to enable a child with a disability to receive needed special education and related services. The IEP also serves as a management, compliance, and monitoring tool and is used to evaluate a child's progress toward achievement of goals and objectives. IDEA does not require that teachers or other school personnel be held accountable if a child with a disability does not achieve the goals set forth in the IEP; however, there are increasing calls for greater accountability.

In the past, the IEP could not be changed without initiating another IEP meeting; however, in IDEA 2004 there are provisions for making changes. The parent "and the local educational agency may agree not to convene an IEP meeting for the purposes of making such changes, and instead may develop a written document to amend or modify the child's current IEP" [PL 108-446, 118 Stat. 2712, § 614(d)(3)(D)]. This change could result in problems for both the child and service providers. For example, therapy services might be added or deleted without input from the therapist. Ongoing team communication and collaboration is essential to ensure that flexibility in modifying the IEP results in positive outcomes.

DEVELOPING GOALS AND OBJECTIVES

The physical therapist, as part of the collaborative team, assists in developing appropriate measurable annual goals, including academic and functional goals. For those children requiring alternate assessment, short-term objectives must also be developed. Short-term objectives are an excellent way of breaking down more global, comprehensive goals into manageable elements. They also assist in clearly identifying when related services might be indicated. For example, instruction by a general or special education teacher might be considered sufficient for an annual goal regarding independently using the cafeteria or the library. But what about a child who is just learning to use a walker around school? General and special education teachers do not have the expertise to teach the child to use a walker and perform the task of opening the library and cafeteria doors, then entering and picking up a book or tray. The expertise required for achievement of the annual goal might require a physical therapist to teach ambulation activities and transfers, an occupational therapist to instruct in feeding activities, and a speech-language pathologist for communication in the food line or library. Without short-term objectives, there is also no guide to assist in determining if the child is progressing in reasonable periods of time and no criteria for the required progress reports.

To determine goals and objectives the desired outcomes must first be identified. Determining a desired outcome might be as simple as merely asking the child, or it might require several team meetings. Outcome statements do not need to be measurable, but they should be functional. Once the desired outcome is identified, the goals that are necessary to achieve the outcome must be expressed. Measurable goals reflect best practice (American Physical Therapy Association, 2001; Lignugaris/Kraft et al., 2001; McEwen & Sheldon, 1992; Randall & McEwen, 2000). Goals are written in an educational setting to be achieved within the school year.

After the desired outcomes and goals are identified, measurable short-term objectives should be developed. "Objectives are developed based on a logical breakdown of the major components of the annual goals, and can serve as milestones for measuring progress towards meeting the goals" (*Federal Register*, 1992, p. 44838). Objectives must relate to the educational program of the child, and *are not* discipline specific (Table 32-2). Short-term objectives are based on a task analysis of the annual goal. The short-term objectives should be functional and educationally relevant and might be written into the IEP. In some situations a short-term objective for reduction of impairment is particularly relevant because that step is limiting the child's achievement of the annual goal. Short-term objectives for reducing impairments are important to document progress toward achievement of the annual goal, but because they are not directly educationally relevant, they are not part of the IEP. To explain the relationships between impairment, activity limitation, and participation restriction, a therapist might use reading as an analogy. Reading is a very important goal of education and few teachers would negate the importance of the child's first knowing the prerequisite alphabet. The alphabet in itself has little value, just as complete knee range of motion has little value as an objective by itself. But knowing the alphabet is critical for reading and writing and knee range of motion is critical for walking and stair climbing. The ability to walk or stair climb expands the child's ability to explore his environment, learn, and most important, achieve the goal of IDEA of " independent living, and economic self-sufficiency for individuals with disabilities" [PL 108-446, 118 Stat. 2649, Part A, § 601(c)(1)]. Eliminating short-term objectives in the IEP is unfortunate because they offer an excellent way of monitoring outcomes and tend to be better indicators of the services required than annual goals.

The physical therapist should participate in the IEP meeting to assist in determining the child's measurable annual goals for the next year. Consensus among experts in pediatric occupational and physical therapy indicated that outcomes should (a) relate to functional skills and activities, (b) enhance the child's performance in school, (c) be easily understood, (d) be free of professional jargon, and (e) be realistic and achievable within the timeframe of the IEP (Dole et al., 2003). These experts suggest that if a skill or activity cannot be observed or measured during the child's normal school day, then it might not be relevant to the child's educational needs. They also note that the therapists surveyed did not reach consensus on whether generalization of skills across settings is important.

An example of a desired outcome and the objectives involving independent stair climbing is given in Box 32-4.

To climb stairs at school independently, a child should have 90° of knee flexion and good strength in the quadriceps muscles. The educationally relevant objectives are included in the child's IEP, and the other short-term objectives, which may or may not be considered educationally relevant, are included in the therapist's plan of care. Documentation of progress toward achievement of each objective is important to share with the child and family. Attainment of short-term objectives should be recognized and rewarded in lieu of waiting, perhaps a long time, for achievement of the long-term goal.

Measurable annual goals and objectives should contain a statement of the behavior to be achieved, under what conditions, and the criteria to be used to determine achievement (Effgen, 1991; Lignugaris/Kraft et al., 2001). When doing a task analysis and developing the short-term objectives, several variables should be considered: (1) changes in the behavior itself, (2) changes in the conditions under which the behavior is performed, and (3) changes in the criteria expected for ultimate performance (Alberto & Troutman, 2003; Effgen, 1991). Changes in the behavior may reflect a progression from basic skills to more complex skills, or increasing levels of functional ability. Changes in conditions may be from simple to complex, such as walking in an empty hallway to walking in a hallway filled with students. Criteria for progression may be qualitative or quantitative. The criterion might include the qualitative measure of hip extension during

---

Box 32-4	**Example of Desired Outcome, Annual Goal, and Short-Term Objectives**

Desired Outcome
Jonathan says: "I want to be able to climb the steps to get into school."

Annual Goal (Long-Term Objective) That Is Measurable and Educationally Relevant
Jonathan will walk up and down the school stairs independently without using the railing.

Short-Term Objectives That Are Measurable and Educationally Relevant
1. Jonathan will climb up 8 stairs at school with standby supervision using a railing.
2. Jonathan will climb up 8 stairs at school with standby supervision without using a railing.
3. Jonathan will climb down 8 stairs at school with standby supervision using a railing.
4. Jonathan will climb down 8 stairs at school with standby supervision without using a railing.
5. Jonathan will climb up 8 stairs at school without supervision or using a railing.
6. Jonathan will climb down 8 stairs at school without supervision or using a railing.

Short-Term Objectives That Are Measurable but Not Directly Educationally Relevant
These objectives, which relate to impairments in body structure and function, are necessary to achieve the educationally relevant short-term and annual goal and would be part of the therapist's intervention plan, but not in the IEP.
1. Jonathan will progress from 30° to 50° of active right-knee flexion.
2. Jonathan will progress from a poor to a fair muscle-strength grade in his left quadriceps.
3. Jonathan will achieve 90° of active right-knee flexion.
4. Jonathan will achieve a good muscle-strength grade in his left quadriceps.

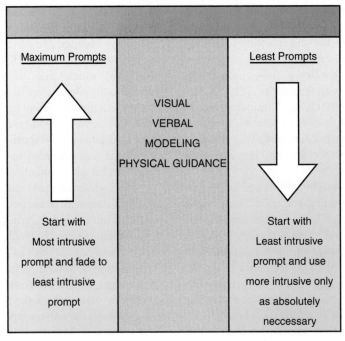

♦ **Figure 32-1**   Hierarchy of prompting assistance.

midstance, which helps make gait more efficient, or a quantitative measure of walking speed. Use of quantitative criteria, such as judgment by three of four trials or 80% of the time, should be considered carefully for their practicability. Successfully crossing the street only 80% of the time can be fatal! Selection of the behavior, conditions, and criteria for judging attainment of each objective for each individual child must be based on sound professional judgment. Books, computer programs, or other materials that provide lists of potential objectives should not replace professional judgment. In addition to the task variables, consideration should be given to the hierarchy of response competence (Alberto & Troutman, 2003). A behavior is first acquired; it is then refined as fluency or proficiency develops. The skill must then be maintained and finally generalized or transferred to multiple environments, individuals, and equipment. *Acquisition, fluency, maintenance,* and *generalization of behaviors* are the terms used by educators. Use of this terminology is important when there is a need to convey the rationale for providing services past the acquisition phase.

Therapists are also encouraged to consider using a prompting system as a strategy to achieve an objective and as a variable in writing the criteria for judging attainment of the objective (Fig. 32-1). A systematic delivery of levels of prompting assistance may be implemented in two ways. One is the "system of maximum prompts," and the other is the "system of least prompts" (Alberto &

Troutman, 2003; Effgen, 1991). The prompts are usually verbal or visual cues, demonstration or modeling, partial assistance or guiding, and maximum assistance. In the system of maximum prompts, the therapist first provides maximum assistance and then gradually, over successive sessions, reduces the amount of assistance as the child achieves more independence. This is also referred to as fading. This is a common technique used by therapists, and it allows for maximal success during learning. This system is best suited for acquisition, when it is important to avoid unsafe movement, and for a complex series of tasks such as some activities of daily living.

In the system of least prompts, the child is initially provided the least amount of assistance, usually a verbal or visual cue, and then progresses to model, guide, or maximal assistance as necessary. This approach allows the child to display his or her best effort before the therapist prematurely provides unnecessary assistance. The system of least prompts is best for tasks in which the child has some ability or is developing fluency or generalization to new settings, individuals, or equipment.

Frequency and Intensity of Intervention

At the IEP meeting the frequency and intensity of all services must be determined by the entire team. The physical therapist must collaborate with other team members to determine the appropriate amount of physical therapy intervention combined with the child's other interventions, educational program, and recreation activities. There must be a careful balance so that other areas of importance are not neglected so the child can receive therapy. The appropriate balance between education, therapy, and leisure (play) is an important topic for discussion with parents, particularly with parents who believe that "more is better."

The frequency and duration of physical therapy services required to achieve a specific goal is not well understood (Iowa Guidelines, 2001). Until there is more research, decisions on how much intervention is required to achieve a goal largely involves professional judgment and consideration of the needs of the individual child. Numerous factors enter into our decision making and include potential for improvement; critical period for skill development; amount of training required to carry out an intervention (if anyone can assist with the intervention, then less therapist time is required); and the significance of the problem to the child's education (Iowa Guidelines, 2001). A matrix of factors to consider when deciding on the amount of physical therapy services are outlined in Table 32-3. Students with several ratings of 4 would probably require more intervention than those with predominant ratings of 1. Note that the availability of physical therapists should never be a factor in determining the frequency and intensity of the intervention.

INTERVENTION

Intervention must be based on the needs of the child, not the system or professionals. The content, goals, frequency, location, and intensity of intervention services are decided at the IEP meeting. As noted in the *Guide to Physical Therapist Practice* (2001) there are three components to intervention: coordination, communication, and documentation; patient/client-related instruction; and procedural interventions. These components are all appropriate and necessary in the educational environment. Coordination, communication, and documentation are particularly important in schools where the therapist might be in the building only occasionally and direct interaction with team members is limited. Lines of frequent communication must be established and maintained. Because practice of motor skills is critical for acquisition, fluency, and generalization, others must be able to assist with the motor program. Therefore, instruction of all staff and parents is a critical component of all intervention plans. Procedural interventions are often not as important as the other two components of intervention. However, as noted in Table 32-3, some factors would indicate a need for direct intervention, such as a child at a critical period of skill acquisition or regression; interventions that should be performed only

by a physical therapist; and when integrating therapy interferes with the educational program. Best practice, research, and federal law indicate that most, if not all, intervention should occur in the natural environment (American Physical Therapy Association, Section on Pediatrics, 1987; TASH, 2000; Effgen & Klepper, 1994; PL 105-17; PL 108-446; Guralnick, 2001; Hanft, Rush, & Shelden, 2004; Noonan & McCormick, 1993; Peck, Odom, & Bricker, 1993; Rainforth & Kugelmass, 2003; Rainforth & York-Barr, 1997). Research suggests that there is little generalization of gross motor skills learned in a physical therapy department to the more natural environments of the home or recreation room (Brown et al., 1998).

Assessment of the school environment and safety considerations take precedent over direct interventions. The physical therapist should first ensure that the child is properly positioned on the bus and in classrooms. The safety of the aisles for ambulation or wheelchair mobility should be assessed. Architectural barriers must be evaluated and appropriate actions taken to eliminate or lessen them. The teachers and family must be consulted regarding their concerns. They should be instructed in proper handling, positioning, and use of body mechanics.

Direct intervention, if indicated, should then start in the natural environment of the classroom. This is accomplished easily with preschoolers and those in special classes for children with severe or profound disabilities (Giangreco et al., 1989; Noonan & McCormick, 1993; Peck et al., 1993). It is more difficult for children whose educational programs consist primarily of academic subjects. Physical therapy in the algebra class or the reading room, after the initial consultation, is generally inappropriate. Common sense must prevail. Perhaps therapy can be given during gross motor time in a preschool or during physical education. This is not always appropriate, however, because this might be the only time the child has to engage in free play and physical activity with her or his peers. Taking this opportunity away from the child might affect motivation, cooperation, and the development of important social skills that occur during these activities.

Merely moving traditional intervention from a special room to a more natural environment is also not in the spirit of best practices. The therapist must adjust intervention to the unique opportunities afforded in the natural environment. Available furniture or classroom items should be used as opposed to bringing in special equipment. Use of these common objects increases the likelihood that the child might use them to practice and develop motor skills when the therapist is not present and allows the therapist to model their use for the parent or teacher.

TABLE 32-3 Factors to Consider When Determining the Intensity and Frequency of Physical Therapy

FACTORS	1*	2	3	4
Potential to benefit from intervention	Student demonstrates minimal potential for change	Student appears to have potential for change but at a slow rate	Student appears to have a significant potential for change	Student appears to have a very high potential to improve skills
Critical period of skill acquisition or regression related to development or disability	Not a critical period	Minimally critical period	Critical period	Extremely critical period
Amount of motor program that can be safely performed by others	Motor program can be carried out safely by others with periodic intervention by therapist	Many activities from the motor program can be safely performed by others in addition to intervention by therapist	Some activities from the motor program can be safely performed by others in addition to intervention by therapist	A few activities can be safely performed by others but most of the motor program requires the expertise of the therapist
Amount of training provided by therapist to others carrying out the program	Teachers, staff, and parents able to meet student's needs and no additional training required	Teacher, staff, and parents require some training and follow-up	Teacher, staff, and parents could be trained to carry out activities	Teacher, staff, and parents might carry out some activities with extensive training and follow-up
Impact of motor problem and environment on educational program	Environment is accommodating and motor difficulties are minimal	Environment is accommodating and motor difficulties moderately interfere with educational program	Environment is accommodating but motor difficulties are significant and interfere with educational program	Environment is not accommodating; or environment is accommodating but problems are severe

Adapted from Iowa Guidelines for Educationally Related Physical Therapy Services. Des Moines, IA: Iowa Department of Education, 2001. Reprinted with permission.
*Numbers are ordered from lowest (1) to highest (4) need for direct services.

In the integrated and collaborative service delivery models the teachers, staff, and parents are usually participants in the delivery of some aspects of the intervention. Their involvement may be as simple as using proper position techniques, or as complicated as handling procedures for transfers and mobility. These individuals must first be instructed in proper positioning, use of adaptive equipment, and then how to encourage selected motor activities. It is generally best to have classroom staff encourage activities at the fluency or generalization stage of motor development. Motor activities at the initial acquisition stage may be too difficult for untrained individuals or may be unsafe without experienced guidance.

Selection of which activities to teach others to assist with is a professional decision that must be based on characteristics of the individual child, the specific activity, and the capabilities and interest of the other individuals. In a series of single-subject design studies, Prieto (1992) found that when teachers are properly instructed in gross motor activities the frequency with which they encourage children to perform those activities generally increases. Soccio (1991) performed a study to examine the frequency of opportunities to practice specific gross motor skills during physical therapy and group early intervention classes. There was no difference in the number of opportunities to practice head control when direct physical therapy was compared with integrated group sessions for a child with severe disabilities. However, two children with cerebral palsy had more opportunities to practice standing and ambulation activities during direct, individual physical therapy sessions than during integrated group sessions in the classroom. The results suggest that the opportunity to practice motor activities in the classroom varies based on the type of movement and the class routines. Therapists must carefully select those activities they expect others to assist with because active gross motor movement is far more limited in classrooms than expected (Ott & Effgen, 2000).

The specific type of intervention provided depends on the needs of the individual child and the education, training, and experience of the therapist. There is no one accepted intervention approach. Information provided throughout this text should assist the therapist in providing state-of-the-art physical therapy. Physical therapy in an educational setting should be based on sound professional judgment and guided by the IEP. If the appropriate intervention cannot be provided for a school-age child because it is not educationally relevant and is not related to the objectives in the IEP, the therapist has a professional obligation to inform the parents. Once the parents are aware of the limitations of school-based physical therapy, they might obtain additional therapy elsewhere.

IDEA 2004 requires that interventions be provided "based on peer-reviewed research to the extent practicable." Although physical therapy intervention has been advancing toward evidence-based practice, many interventions do not have sufficient peer-reviewed research. Throughout this text peer-reviewed research is presented when available. Therapists must learn to search the literature for recent developments in research to support the interventions they use.

Physical therapists in educational settings need not write the daily notes required in other settings. In the United States, however, they must comply with their individual state practice acts. Careful monitoring of progress is critical in determining the effectiveness of and need for continued intervention. David (1996) has outlined a measurement process specifically developed for use by collaborative educational teams. The system involves (a) defining the performance problem; (b) determining operational definitions of the performance expected and outcome criteria; (c) developing a systematic, simple, and time-efficient measure strategy; (d) having a data graphing system; (e) provision of intervention; (f) monitoring progress; and (g) systematic decision making and intervention changes. David (1996, p. 56) stated that "monitoring without decision making is a waste of valuable time and effort." A simple but comprehensive system of data collection using self-graphing data collection sheets is recommended (Effgen, 1991). The availability of laptop computers has also made data collection and its graphic presentation much easier for many therapists. Extensive documentation is necessary to support the need to increase, decrease, or discontinue intervention. Documentation of the child's status before and after short and long school breaks is important in determining the need for extended school year services.

Physical therapy is not a lifelong activity such as learning. Both therapists and parents must recognize that, after a period of time with no documentation of progress, physical therapy should be discontinued or the method of service delivery should be changed to monitoring. A continued desire for walking or similar activity is not sufficient reason for continued therapy after due diligence in trying to achieve an objective. Therapists report that the most important factor in successfully discontinuing therapy services is the child's achievement of functional goals (Effgen, 2000). Determining when to discontinue intervention when goals have not been met continues to be a difficult area of decision making.

TRANSITION PLANNING

Change can be difficult for anyone and the transition from one environment to another environment is particularly stressful for children, especially those with a limited repertoire of response competence. Recognizing that all transitions are important, two critical times were identified in IDEA when specific attention must be paid to transition and the provision of transition services. These times are when a child is to move from the family-centered early intervention services of Part C to provision of educational services under Part B in preschool (Hanson et al., 2000) and transition out of secondary school into the community (Flexor et al., 2001). Under IDEIA 2004, transition services are

a coordinated set of activities for a child with a disability that ... is, designed within an results-oriented process, that is focused on improving academic and functional achievement of the child with a disability to facilitate the child's movement from school to post-school activities, including post-secondary education, vocational education, integrated employment (including supported employment), continuing and adult education, adult services, independent living, or community participation; is based on the individual child's needs, taking into account the child's strengths, preferences, and interests; and includes instruction, related services, community experiences, the development of employment and other post-school adult living objectives, and, when appropriate, acquisition of daily living skills and functional vocational evaluation.

PL 108-446, 118 Stat. 2658, § 602(34)

Transition assessments and services must begin no later that the first IEP to be in effect when the child is age 16 years.

PL 108-446, 118 Stat. 2709, § 614(d)(1)(A)(VIII) or younger if determined appropriate by the IEP team (Federal Registrar, 2005, p. 35865)

Physical therapists as related service providers are not involved in the majority of transition teams serving children with disabilities; however, we should be involved on transition teams for children with physical disabilities and those who have degenerative disabilities involving the neuromuscular system. As a member of the IEP team for an individual student, the physical therapist should become involved in the transition process. The physical therapist should also become involved on the IEP team for a student who had previously received physical therapy, but has not recently received therapy because the educational need for physical therapy might have stabilized. The needs of a young adult in post-school settings will be different from in the protected school environment, and the therapist can assist in evaluating and intervening to facilitate post-school planning and services.

All transition planning should be determined with both the student and the family. There should be an emphasis on self-determination, person-centeredness, and career orientation (Baer, 2001). The role of the physical therapist in transition planning and services for students with physical disabilities might include the following:

- Communication with the family and other transition team members regarding physical expectations and demands of the anticipated new environment;
- Communication with the student's vocational rehabilitation counselor, occupational therapist, and teachers regarding preparation for mobility and functional activities in the new setting;
- Onsite evaluation of the new physical environment to assure the student's ability to physically maneuver throughout the setting;
- Evaluation of the accessibility of the required transportation systems;
- Onsite consultation and education of the student, family, and staff related to the student's physical functioning in that environment;
- Communication with teachers, occupational therapists, and speech-language pathologists regarding augmentative communication access and regarding consultation that might be necessary from the physical therapist;
- With the team determine adaptive equipment and technology needs, assist in securing the equipment and helping the student learn to use the equipment efficiency; and
- Attend IEP and other meetings as appropriate. (McEwen, 2000, pp. 62–63)

A number of issues have been identified that impair collaboration and system linkages for effective transition services. These include a lack of shared information across agencies; lack of follow-up data that could improve services; lack of attention to health insurance and transportation; lack of systematic transition planning with the agencies that will have responsibility for post-school services; difficulties in anticipating the needs of the student post-school; and inefficient and ineffective management practices (Johnson et al., 2002). Although the physical therapist is usually not in a leadership role to make major changes in the transition service system, the therapist can provide assistance in several of the problem areas noted. Specifically the therapist has the ability to provide information on health insurance; evaluation of transportation needs; and anticipation of the physical demands required of the student post-school. A therapist's knowledge of the physical demands of post-school settings, such as college or work environments, would help the team to assist the student in effective transitioning to those environments.

MANAGEMENT OF PHYSICAL THERAPY SERVICES

An important factor in successful management and service delivery in an educational environment is recognition and understanding of the significance of the team process. The physical therapist is part of the educational team. Physical therapists must focus on collaboration with members of all other disciplines and recognize their importance in the total well-being of the child. They cannot work in isolation if they expect maximal effectiveness. The team, including the child and family, must decide on the most appropriate services at each phase in the child's life.

Just as team leaders or case managers are needed in intervention teams, so too a manager or director of physical therapy is needed in school settings. The majority of directors of physical therapy services in school systems across the nation are not physical therapists or, indeed, any type of related service personnel (Effgen & Klepper, 1994). This has serious implications. To understand professional roles and responsibilities and how to nurture a professional, one must understand the profession. Many of the problems encountered in school systems could probably be prevented if an experienced therapist provided supervision. Therapist managers understand the profession and are able to professionally and appropriately address management issues. States such as Iowa, which has therapists working in the state department of education, have become national leaders in related service delivery and policy setting. These therapists help coordinate services throughout the state and educate both therapists and educators regarding the role of physical therapists in educational environments.

Therapists, unlike teachers, are educated to work in a wide variety of settings and therefore have little, if any, opportunity to learn about educational settings. Therapists new to a school system must receive orientation, mentoring, and in-service education. The roles and responsibilities of the therapist and all support staff should be defined clearly in a detailed job description that complies with federal and state laws. Therapists should be introduced to the entire team of professionals with whom they will be working at all sites. They need to know whom to ask for equipment, space, and other items necessary for successful intervention. These introductions should be part of a planned orientation program. Therapists need to know how referrals are received and handled; how workloads and caseloads are determined; how team meetings are planned and when they are scheduled; the written policies and procedures; how peer review or quality improvement is done; the emergency procedures; and the policy for continuing education, to name but a few issues. None of these are unusual requests; they can easily and cost-effectively be addressed in any system.

After the therapist is properly introduced and oriented to the system, administrators and therapists must continue to talk before problems arise. Frequent areas of discontent are the lack of continuing education opportunities, insufficient peer contact, lack of an identified place to work, lack of time allotted for administrative tasks and meetings, and too much travel (Effgen & Klepper, 1994). More time and effort should be spent in retention of physical therapists so that there is not a need for continuous recruitment.

A system for obtaining referrals from physicians, if dictated by state law, must be developed. The referral allows the therapist to examine and evaluate and then determine and provide appropriate intervention for the child. Most physical therapy state practice acts in the United States allow a therapist to examine and evaluate without a referral, and 39 states allow therapists to examine and evaluate and provide intervention without a referral. Depending on the complexity of the child's medical problems and the need for pertinent information, a therapist might still want a referral. Collaboration with physicians and all members of the child's medical and educational team encourages optimal service delivery.

A method must be developed for determination of therapy workloads and caseloads, and guidelines created for determining who should receive intervention and how much intervention should be given. This can be a difficult task. The Florida Department of Exceptional Student Education (1987) developed a matrix that combines clinical judgment factors and a therapy profile to determine the amount of therapy a child should receive. The Iowa Guidelines for Educationally Related Physical Therapy Services (2001) (Table 32-3) relates the potential to benefit from intervention with factors such as critical periods for skill acquisition, the amount of the program that can be performed by others, and the extent that motor problems interfere with the educational program to determine the amount of physical therapy. Children with critical needs for therapy require more intense intervention than do those with lesser needs. A therapist whose caseload includes only children having extensive needs for therapy is able to serve fewer children than a therapist whose caseload includes all children having minimal needs. Having a clear system to determine eligibility for services, amount of services, and termination of services provides needed documentation to support the complex, sensitive decisions regarding allocating services.

ISSUES IN SCHOOL-BASED PRACTICE

SHORTAGE OF PEDIATRIC PHYSICAL THERAPISTS

The shortage of qualified pediatric physical therapists has been an ongoing issue facing school-based physical therapy. The reasons for the shortage are numerous and include the low pay in schools, professional isolation, the benefits of other areas of practice, and difficulty in working with children. Solutions are numerous and sometimes complex, but one of the easiest is often neglected. An effective way to train and then recruit new physical therapists is to have them on clinical affiliations in an educational setting while they are students.

Therapists, especially new graduates and those new to pediatrics, should strive to achieve the competencies for physical therapists in school-based physical therapy (American Physical Therapy Association, 1990; Chiarello et al., 2003). These competencies help therapists to identify minimal standards for practice, as well as encouraging professional growth. The competencies may also be shared with administrators to help define the role of physical therapy and identify the resources necessary for effective service delivery. Therapists should continually read, participate in continuing education, take graduate courses, and engage in dialogue with colleagues. Therapists working in school systems must be aware of the potential for professional isolation and seek opportunities for developing improved competence. Employers must support therapists' efforts at ongoing professional development.

SERVICE DELIVERY SYSTEM

The shortage of qualified therapists has also affected the type of service delivery system used and the roles assumed by personnel. The literature supports integrated or collaborative service delivery models (Dunn, 1991; Rainforth et al., 1992; Rainforth & York-Barr, 1997). The advantages of more frequent practice in the natural setting with the support of all personnel are obvious. An appropriately administrated therapy program in the natural environment might require more and certainly not less personnel. Training all personnel in a truly integrated or collaborative model requires a great deal of time for training and meetings (Giangreco et al., 1989; Rainforth et al., 1992; York et al., 1990). There are those, however, who incorrectly think these models can be used to decrease the time required for physical therapy. It should be noted that TEAMS TAKE TIME (the three Ts). Instead of having a therapist provide the required intervention, unqualified staff might provide activities without adequate supervised instruction, or a teacher might be forced to provide an intervention for which he or she is not properly trained. Instead of providing the intervention in a room with necessary equipment, a classroom or hallway is used in the name of natural environment. Rarely are there sufficient empirical data to support any service delivery system. Educators and therapists alike must step back and ask if they are truly meeting the needs of each individual child.

PROFESSIONAL ROLES

In systems in which there is full staffing, professionals can collaborate to decide on the specific roles of each team member. Overlap of professional roles is acknowledged, and divisions of responsibility are made that are best suited to the needs of the child, system, and professional staff (Commonwealth of Virginia, 2004). In general, the overlap in physical therapy, occupational therapy, and education is greatest when professionals from these disciplines are serving young children. For older children there is less overlap in professional roles. Areas of frequent overlap between occupational therapy and physical therapy include programs for strength and endurance, body awareness, classroom positioning and adaptations, and enhancement of motor experience. Areas of overlap between physical therapists and educators might include advanced gross motor skills, endurance training, and writing. In systems in which there is a critical shortage of physical therapists, the breadth of roles assumed by other staff members increases based on need and not necessarily on professional skill.

EDUCATIONALLY RELEVANT PHYSICAL THERAPY

Educationally relevant versus non–educationally relevant physical therapy is a frequent topic of debate which is nicely summarized by McEwen and Shelden (1995) in

"The demise of the educational versus medical dichotomy." In school systems committed to the comprehensive provision of services to children with disabilities and with adequate therapy staffing, the definition of educationally relevant physical therapy is frequently broad-based and depends on the individual needs of the child addressed at the IEP meeting. IDEIA clearly indicates that education is to prepare students for independent living and economic self-sufficiency, which have broad implications for the provision of physical therapy.

Goals and objectives that are mutually agreed on by the entire educational team help make physical therapy more educationally relevant. The educational system was never meant to provide for all the child's therapy needs. Physical therapy may be provided out of the educational system as appropriate, and all therapists serving the child should collaborate and coordinate services. Therapists and parents must remember that therapy takes time away from other educational and social opportunities that are vital to the total well-being of the child.

LEAST RESTRICTIVE ENVIRONMENT

As more children are educated in the least restrictive environment, therapists must be willing to travel to meet the needs of those students. Unfortunately, travel to many schools is not the most time- and cost-effective method of service delivery. Therapists and administrators must be creative in their approach to serving children in their local schools. Materials such as *Choosing Options and Accommodations for Children: A Guide to Planning Inclusive Education* have been used successfully to encourage inclusive education (Giangreco et al., 1993b).

REIMBURSEMENT FOR SERVICES

The cost of providing related services in educational environments is a serious concern of program administrators. IDEIA provides some federal funding to states, but it has never been sufficient to cover the full spectrum of services needed by children in special education. To cover the costs of physical therapy, some school systems are charging third-party payers. This is a serious concern because of the lifetime cap on many insurance policies, limited therapy coverage, and the possibility of losing insurance if bills are too high. Parents are *not* required to have their insurance company pay for these services, and they should not be intimidated into thinking their child will not receive services without insurance payment. School systems may bill Medicaid directly for physical therapy. A concern regarding using Medicaid is that reimbursement is usually based on direct services and that consultation, team intervention, and group treatment are discouraged. Medicaid rules and regulations are determined by each individual state, and therapists should be active at the state level to make certain that these rules and regulations facilitate and do not hinder appropriate school-based intervention.

THERAPISTS NEW TO SCHOOL SETTINGS

School settings are frequently a place of employment after a physical therapist has worked in adult care or other pediatric care settings. Therapists who are parents like the fact that school system hours coincide with the hours and vacation schedule of their children. Therefore, it is not uncommon to have experienced therapists seek employment in a school setting with little or no background in pediatrics or an understanding of the unique aspects and requirements of working under IDEIA. Therapists new to school settings must first learn the rules and regulations of IDEIA as outlined in this chapter and available from the suggested websites and references. In addition, the therapist must be aware of individual state education laws, special education laws, and the state physical therapy practice act. These all guide practice in school settings. All too often therapists are given inaccurate information regarding the law, and do not seek out the information for themselves. It is the therapist's responsibility to be knowledgeable in the laws that affect practice in a school setting, just as they should know the rules that govern reimbursement and practice in a hospital setting. In this day of limited resources, administrators have been known to say that services are not appropriate for a child with a disability because they do not want to pay for such a service. They might also say that because a therapist is not available, then therapy cannot be recommended in the IEP. That is, of course, incorrect, but most parents and many therapists will not know that unless they are very familiar with the law.

In addition to learning about IDEA, school system therapists must learn about team functioning. Services in school settings require teams and use various team models as discussed in this chapter. Therapists who have worked in other pediatric settings, such as early intervention and pediatric hospitals, will know about team functioning, as will therapists who have worked in rehabilitation settings. Therapists coming from outpatient physical therapy settings are usually not adequately familiar with team functioning and the degree of role release and collaboration required in most school settings. Therapists who gain knowledge of and appreciation of team functioning will be the most successful in a school setting.

Intervention in school settings is also somewhat different from other settings. As already discussed, the goals and objectives must be educationally relevant. Intervention usually focuses on the *Guide's* (2001) intervention aspects of coordination, communication, and documentation, and patient/client-related instruction. For children having many of the factors indicating the need for intervention, as outlined in Table 32-3, then procedural interventions might be provided. This change in focus from direct hands-on intervention can be very difficult for therapists coming from other settings.

Therapists new to school settings would be wise to seek an experienced mentor either within or outside the school system. All too often therapists in schools work in isolation and they do not get the mentoring or support provided in other clinical settings. They work frequently with teachers, but not necessarily with other therapists who can evaluate their knowledge and skills and with whom they can discuss cases. School administrators need to recognize the effect of this professional isolation both for experienced therapists and especially for therapists new to the school environment. They should support the therapist in finding a mentor and providing the time for the therapist to meet with that mentor.

SUMMARY

In the United States, physical therapy is mandated as part of federally sponsored programs to serve infants, toddlers, children, and youth with disabilities. For preschool and school-age children, physical therapy is a related service of the educational program for those children who require special education. The provision of physical therapy in an educational environment is challenging for physical therapists. It is not the high-tech, health-focused environment of the modern hospital setting or the therapy-focused environment of the rehabilitation setting. In the educational environment, the therapist is a member of a team of professionals for whom therapy may or may not carry a high priority in the overall goals and objectives for an individual child. The educational needs of the child have the highest priority.

The therapist must learn to understand the educational milieu to provide the best possible services and be satisfied in the work environment. The federal, state, and local laws and rules and regulations that govern services in the educational environment must be understood and respected. Rules and regulations are meant to help serve the child and family, not hinder service provision.

Therapists who work in the educational environment

have a true picture of the everyday lives of the children they serve. They see first hand the struggles some children with special needs face and are asked daily to solve complex problems to make life better for these children and their families. The education setting is a rewarding and wonderful environment in which to work for those who are willing and able to adjust to its unique demands.

REFERENCES

Alberto, PA, & Troutman, AC. Applied Behavior Analysis for Teachers, 6th ed. Columbus, OH: Merrill, 2003.

American Physical Therapy Association. Physical Therapy Practice in Educational Environments. Alexandria, VA: American Physical Therapy Association, 1990.

American Physical Therapy Association. Guide to Physical Therapist Practice, 2nd ed. Physical Therapy, *81*:1–768, 2001.

American Physical Therapy Association, Section on Pediatrics. TASH Position Statement: On the Provision of Related Services to Persons with Severe Handicaps. Alexandria, VA: American Physical Therapy Association, 1987.

Baer, R. Transition Planning. In Flexer, RW, Simmons, TJ, Luft, P, & Baer, RM. Transition Planning for Secondary Students With Disabilities). Upper Saddle River, NJ: Prentice-Hall, 2001, pp. 333–363.

Baker, BJ, Cole, KN, & Harris, S. Cognitive referencing as a method of OT/PT triage for young children. Pediatric Physical Therapy, *10*:2–6, 1998.

Batten, HE. The industrial school for crippled and deformed children. Physical Therapy Review, *13*:112–113, 1933.

Battle v. Commonwealth of Pennsylvania, 629 F2d 280 (3rd Cir. 1981).

Blatt, B, & Kaplan, F. Christmas in Purgatory: A Photographic Essay on Mental Retardation. Boston: Allyn & Bacon, 1966.

Braddock, D. Federal Policy Toward Mental Retardation and Developmental Disabilities. Baltimore: Paul H. Brookes, 1987, p. 71.

Brown v. Board of Education of Topeka, 347 US 483 (1954).

Brown, DA, Effgen, SK, & Palisano, RJ. Performance following ability-focused physical therapy intervention in individuals with severely limited physical and cognitive abilities. Physical Therapy, *78*:934–949, 1998.

Bruder, MB, & Walker, L. Discharge Planning: Hospital to home transitions for infants. Topics in Early Childhood Special Education, *9*:26–42, 1990.

Cable, OE, Fowler, AF, & Foss, HS. The crippled children's guide of Buffalo, New York. Physical Therapy Review, *16*:85–88, 1938.

Carr, SH. Louisiana's criteria of eligibility for occupational therapy services in the public school system. American Journal of Occupational Therapy, *43*:503–506, 1989.

Chiarello, L, Effgen, S, Milbourne, S, & Campbell, P. Specialty certification program in early intervention and school-based therapy. Pediatric Physical Therapy, *15*:52–53, 2003.

Cole, KN, Mills, PE, & Harris, SR. Retrospective analysis of physical and occupational therapy progress in young children: An examination of cognitive referencing. Pediatric Physical Therapy, *3*:185–189, 1991.

Coster, W, Deeney, T, Haltiwanger, J, & Haley, H. School function assessment. San Antonio: The Psychological Corporation, 1998.

Cruickshank, WM. Psychology of Exceptional Children and Youth, 4th ed. Englewood Cliffs, NJ: Prentice-Hall, 1980, pp. 65–66.

David, KS. Monitoring process for improved outcomes. Physical & Occupational Therapy in Pediatrics, *16*(4):47–76, 1996.

David, K. IDEA 2004, PL 108-446, Impact on physical therapy related services. Feb. 2005. Available at http://www.pediatricapta.org/csm05/9752.pdf.

Deno, E. Special education as developmental capital. Exceptional Children, 37:229–237, 1970.

Dillon, S. Schools resist demands of Bush's law. Lexington Herald-Leader, January 2, 2004, pp. A1, A9.

Discipline Under Section 504. Special Educator, November 22, 1996, p. 7.

Dole, RL, Arvidson, K, Byrne, E, Robbins, J, & Schasberger, B. Consensus among experts in pediatric occupational and physical therapy on elements of Individualized Education Programs. Pediatric Physical Therapy, 15(3):159–166, 2003.

Dunn, W. Integrated related services. In Meyer, LH, Peck, CA, & Brown, L (Eds.). Critical Issues in the Lives of People with Severe Disabilities. Baltimore: Paul H. Brookes, 1991, pp. 353–378.

Effgen, SK. Systematic delivery and recording of intervention assistance. Pediatric Physical Therapy, 3:63–68, 1991.

Effgen, SK. Factors affecting the termination of physical therapy services for children in school settings. Pediatric Physical Therapy, 12(3):121–126, 2000.

Effgen, SK, & Klepper, S. Survey of physical therapy practice in educational settings. Pediatric Physical Therapy, 6:15–21, 1994.

Federal Register, Part II, Department of Education, 34 CFR Parts 300 and 301, Assistance to States for the Education of Children with Disabilities Program and Preschool Grants for Children with Disabilities, Final Rule, Vol. 57, No. 189, September 29, 1992.

Federal Register 34 CFR 111, Part § 300 and § 301, 7-1-02 Edition. Part II, Department of Education, Assistance to States for the Education of Children with Disabilities Program and Preschool Grants for Children with Disabilities. In print and available at: http://www.access.gpo.gov/nara/cfr/waisidx_02/34cfrv2_02.html

Federal Register, Part II, Department of Education, 34 CFR Part 200, Title I—Improving the Academic Achievement of the Disadvantaged; Final Rule, Vol. 68, No. 236, pp. 68697–68708, December 9, 2003. In print and available at: http://www.ed.gov/legislation/FedRegister/finrule/2003-4/120903a.html

Federal Register June 21, 2005. Part II Department of Education. 34 CFR Parts 300, 301, and 304 Assistance to States for the Education of Children with Disabilities; Preschool Grants for Children with Disabilities; and Service Obligations Under Special Education-Personnel Development To Improve Services and Results for Children With Disabilities; Proposed Rule. In print and available at: http://a257.g.akamaitech.net/7/257/2422/01jan20051800/edocket.access.gpo.gov/2005/05-11804.htm

Falvey, MA, Grenot-Scheyer, M, Coots, JJ, & Bishop, KD. Services for students with disabilities: Past and present. In Falvey, MA (Ed.). Inclusive and Heterogeneous Schooling: Assessment, Curriculum, and Instruction. Baltimore: Paul H. Brookes, 1995, pp. 23–40.

Florida Department of Exceptional Student Education. OT/PT Reporting System. Evaluation Protocols for Occupational and Physical Therapists in Public School. Tallahassee, FL: Department of Exceptional Student Education, 1987.

Flexer, RW, McMahan, RK, & Baer, R. Transition models and best practices. In Flexer, RW, Simmons, TJ, Luft, P, & Baer, RM. Transition Planning for Secondary Students with Disabilities. Upper Saddle River, NJ: Prentice-Hall, 2001, pp. 38–68.

Georgia Association of Retarded Citizens v. McDaniel, 511 F. Supp. 1263 (Northern District of Georgia, 1981).

Giangreco, MF, Cloninger, CJ, Dennis, RE, & Edelman, SW. National expert validation of COACH: Congruence with exemplary practice and suggestions for improvement. Journal of the Association for Persons with Severe Handicaps, 18:109–120, 1993a.

Giangreco, MF, Cloninger, CJ, & Iverson, V. Choosing Options and Accommodations for Children: A Guide to Planning Inclusive Education. Baltimore: Paul H. Brookes, 1993b.

Giangreco, MF, York, J, & Rainforth, B. Providing related services to learners with severe handicaps in educational settings: Pursuing the least restrictive option. Pediatric Physical Therapy, 1:55–63, 1989.

Givins, EV. The spastic child in the classroom. Physical Therapy Review, 18:136–137, 1938.

Guralnick, MJ. Early childhood inclusion. Baltimore: Paul H. Brookes, 2001.

Haley, SM, Coster, WJ, Ludlow, LH, Haltiwarger, JT, & Andrellas, PJ. Pediatric Evaluation of Disability Inventory (PEDI). San Antonio, TX: The Psychological Corporation, 1992.

Hanft, BE, & Place, PA. The consulting therapist: A guide for OTs and PTs in schools. San Antonio, TX: Therapy Skill Builders, 1996.

Hanft, BE, Rush DD, & Shelden ML. COACHING families and colleagues in early childhood. Baltimore: Paul H. Brookes, 2004.

Hanson, MJ, Beckman, PJ, Horn, E, Marquart, J, Sandall, SR, Greig, D, & Brennan, E. Entering preschool: Family and professional experiences in this transition process. Journal of Early Intervention, 23:279–293, 2000.

Hunt, P, Soto, G, Maier, J, & Dering, K. Collaborative teaming to support students at risk and students with severe disabilities in general education classrooms. Exceptional Children, 69(3):315–332, 2003.

Iowa Guidelines for Educationally Related Physical Therapy Services. Des Moines, IA: Iowa Department of Education, 2001.

Johnson, DR, Stodden, RA, Emanuel, EJ, Luecking, R, & Mack, M. Current challenges facing secondary education and transition services: What research tells us. Exceptional Children, 68(4):519–531, 2002.

Lignugaris/Kraft, B, Marchand-Martella, N, & Martella, RC. Writing better goals and short-term objectives or benchmarks. Teaching Exceptional Children, 34:52–58, 2001.

Lindsey, D, O'Neal, J, Haas, K, & Tewey, SM. Physical therapy services in North Carolina's schools. Clinical Management in Physical Therapy, 4:40–43, 1980.

Lipsky, DK. The coexistence of high standards and inclusion. School Administrator, 60(3):32–35, 2003.

Martin, EW. Lessons from implementing PL 94-142. In Gallagher, JJ, Trohanis, PL, & Clifford, RM (Eds.). Policy Implementation and PL 99-457: Planning for Young Children with Special Needs. Baltimore: Paul H. Brookes, 1989, pp. 19–32.

Martin, R. Extraordinary Children, Ordinary Lives: Stories Behind Special Education Case Law. Champaign, IL: Research Press, 1991, pp. 45–63.

Maryland Association for Retarded Citizens v. Maryland, Equite No. 100/182/77676 (Cir. Ct. Baltimore County, 1972).

Massey Sekerak, D, Kirkpatrick, DB, Nelson, KC, & Propes, JH. Physical therapy in preschool classrooms: Successful integration of therapy into classroom routines. Pediatric Physical Therapy, 15(2):93–103. 2003.

McEwen, I. (Ed.). Providing physical therapy services under Parts B & C of the Individuals with Disabilities Education Act (IDEA). Alexandria Virginia: Section on Pediatrics, American Physical Therapy Association, 2000.

McEwen, I, & Shelden, M. Writing functional goals: A means to integrate related services in special education. Paper presented at conference of The Association for Persons with Severe Handicaps Annual Convention, San Francisco, November 1992.

McEwen, IR, & Shelden, ML. Pediatric therapy in the 1990s: The demise of the educational versus medical dichotomy. Occupational and Physical Therapy in Pediatrics, 15:33–45, 1995.

Meyer, LH, Peck, CA, & Brown, L (Eds.). Critical Issues in the Lives of People with Severe Disabilities. Baltimore: Paul H. Brookes, 1991.

Mills v. Board of Education of the District of Columbia, 348 F. Supp. 866 (DDC 1972).

Mulcahey, AL. Detroit schools for crippled children. Physical Therapy Review, 16:63–64, 1936.

National Information Center for Children and Youth with Disabilities. Related services for school-aged children with disabilities. News Digest, National Information Center for Children and Youth with Disabilities, 1(2):8, 1991.

Noonan, MJ, & McCormick, L. Early Intervention in Natural Environments. Pacific Grove, CA: Brooks/Cole, 1993.

Ott, DAD, & Effgen, SK. Occurrence of gross motor behaviors in integrated and segregated preschool classrooms. Pediatric Physical Therapy, 12:164–172, 2000.

Parette, HP, & Bartlett, CS. Collaboration and ecological assessment: Bridging the gap between medical and educational environments for students who are medically fragile. Physical Disabilities: Education and Related Services, 15:33–47, 1996.

Pax Lowes, L, & Effgen, SK. The Americans with Disabilities Act of 1990: Implications for pediatric physical therapist. Pediatric Physical Therapy, 8:111–116, 1996.

Peck, CA, Odom, SL, & Bricker, DD. Integrating young children with disabilities into community programs. Baltimore: Paul H. Brookes, 1993.

Pennsylvania Association for Retarded Citizens v. Commonwealth of Pennsylvania, Civil Action No. 71-42, 334 F. Supp. 1257 (ED Pa. 1971), 343 F. Supp. 279 (ED Pa. 1972).

Prieto, GM. Effects of Physical Therapist Instruction on the Frequency and Performance of Teacher Assisted Gross Motor Activities for Students with Motor Disabilities. Unpublished master's thesis, Hahnemann University, Philadelphia, 1992.

Public Law 93-112, Rehabilitation Act (1973), 29 USC § 794.

Public Law 94-103, Developmental Disabilities Assistance and Bill of Rights Act (1975). Stat. 89, pp. 486–507.

Public Law 94-142, Education of All Handicapped Children Act (1975), 89 Stat. 773–796.

Public Law 99-372, Handicapped Children's Protection Act (1986), 20 USC § 1415(e)(4)(f).

Public Law 99-457, Education of the Handicapped Act Amendments of 1986, 100 Stat. 1145–1177.

Public Law 101-336, Americans with Disabilities Act (1990), 42 USC § 12101.

Public Law 102-119, Individuals with Disabilities Education Act Amendments of 1991, 105 Stat. 587–608.

Public Law 105-17, Individuals with Disabilities Education Act Amendments of 1997, 111 Stat. 37–157.

Public Law 107-110, No Child Left Behind Act of 2001, 115 Stat. 1425–2094. Available at http://www.ed.gov/policy/elsec/leg/esea02/107-110.pdf

Public Law 108-446, Individuals with Disabilities Education Improvement Act of 2004, Available at http://www.copyright.gov/legislation/pl108-446.pdf.

Rainforth, B. OSERS clarifies legality of related services eligibility criteria. TASH Newsletter, 17:8, 1991.

Rainforth, B. Analysis of Physical Therapy Practice Acts: Implications for role release in educational environments. Pediatric Physical Therapy, 9:54–61, 1997.

Rainforth, B, & York-Barr, J. Collaborative Teams for Students with Severe Disabilities, 2nd ed. Baltimore: Paul H. Brookes, 1997.

Rainforth, B, & Kugelmass, JW. Curriculum Instruction for All Learners: Blending Systematic and Constructivist Approaches in Inclusive Elementary Schools. Baltimore: Paul H. Brookes, 2003.

Randall, KE, & McEwen, IR. Writing patient-centered functional goals. Physical Therapy, 80:1197–1203, 2000.

Rapport, MJ, & Thomas, SB. Extended school year: Legal issues and implications. Journal of the Association for Persons with Severe Handicaps, 18(1):16–27, 1993.

Reynolds, M. A framework for considering some issues in special education. Exceptional Children, 28:367–370, 1962.

Rowley v. Board of Education of Hendrick Hudson Central School District, 458 US 176 (1982).

Ryndak, DL, & Fisher, D. The Foundations of Inclusive Education: A Compendium of Articles on Effective Strategies to Achieve Inclusive Education, 2nd ed. Baltimore: TASH, 2003.

Savage, RC, Pearson, S, McDonald, H, Potoczany-Gray, A, & Marchese, N. After hospital: Working with schools and families to support the long term needs of children with brain injuries. NeuroRehabilitation, 16:49–58, 2001.

Sever, JW. Physical therapy in schools for crippled children. Physical Therapy Review, 18:298–303, 1938.

Silverstein, R. A user's guide to the 2004 IDEA Reauthorization (PL 108-446 and the Conference Report). Consortium for Citizens with Disabilities, 2004. Available at http://www.c-c-d.org/IdeaUserGuide.pdf.

Snell, ME, & Janney, R. Collaborative Teaming. Baltimore: Paul H. Brookes, 2000.

Soccio, CA. Direct-individual versus integrated-group models of physical therapy service delivery. Unpublished master's thesis, Hahnemann University, Philadelphia, 1991.

Special Educator. Court: Regular class not always LRE. Special Educator 11(21):8, 1996.

Stuart, J, & Goodsitt, JL. From hospital to school: How a transition liaison can help. Teaching Exceptional Children, 4:58–62, 1996.

Supreme Court of the United States, No. 96-1793, March 3, 1999. Cedar Rapids Community School District v. Garret F.

Swinth, Y, & Hanft, B. School-based practice: Moving beyond 1:1 service delivery. OT Practice, Sept. 16, 2002.

TASH. TASH Resolution on Inclusive Quality Education. Baltimore: TASH, March 2000.

Tatro v. Texas, 625 F2d 557 (1980); on rem'd 516 F. Supp. 968 (1981); aff'd 703 F2d 823 (1983); S Ct. No. 83-558 (aff'd July 5, 1984).

Taylor, SJ. Caught in the continuum: A critical analysis of the least restrictive environment. Journal of the Association for Persons with Severe Handicaps, 13(1):41–53, 1988.

Thurman, SK, & Widerstrom, AH. Infants and Young Children with Special Needs, 2nd ed. Baltimore: Paul H. Brookes, 1990.

Vacha, VB. History of the development of special schools and classes for crippled children in Chicago. Physical Therapy Review, 13:21–26, 1933.

Virginia Department of Education. Handbook for Occupational & Physical Therapy Services in the Public Schools of Virginia. Richmond, VA: The Author, April 2004.

Wolfensberger, W. Will there always be an institution? The impact of new service models. Mental Retardation, 9:31–38, 1971.

Wolery, M. Transitions in early childhood special education: Issues and procedures. Focus on Exceptional Children, 22:1–16, 1989.

York, J, Rainforth, B, & Giangreco, MF. Transdisciplinary teamwork and integrated therapy: Clarifying the misconceptions. Pediatric Physical Therapy, 2:73–79, 1990.

Zirkel, P. Inclusion: Return of the pendulum? Special Educator, 12(9):5, 9, 1996.

Chapter 33

∾

ASSISTIVE TECHNOLOGY

ROBERTA KUCHLER O'SHEA
PT, PhD

SHIRLEY J. CARLSON
PT, MS, PCS

CAROLE RAMSEY
OTR/L, ATP

Physical therapists have long been involved in the practice of providing individuals who have physical impairments with technologic equipment designed to help achieve or improve independent function. Attempts to integrate therapy goals in the home and school settings often included homemade adaptive equipment for positioning, mobility, and communication. The application of technologic advances to health care, rehabilitation, and special education settings began slowly several decades ago and has rapidly accelerated. An assistive technology (AT) device is defined by legislation to include any item, piece of equipment, or product system that increases, maintains, or improves an individual's functional status (Parette & McMahon, 2002). In contrast, an assistive technology service is legally defined as any service, such as physical therapy, occupational therapy, or speech therapy, that directly assists someone with a disability in the selection, acquisition, or training of an AT device (Parette & McMahon, 2002). Over recent years, assistive technology has come to encompass a vast range of materials, designs, and applications. It is used to promote the development and acquisition of skills that a client lacks as a result of disease or injury. Assistive technology also enables adaptations in motor function when the attainment of certain skills is unrealistic or impossible

(Dorman, 1998). Also referred to as enabling technology, assistive technology can generate opportunities for social participation for individuals with physical impairments and functional limitations. In the past three decades, a virtual explosion in the number and type of assistive devices has occurred. The creation of federally funded rehabilitation engineering centers in 1972 focused efforts on research and development of new products, as well as on the delivery of services to the consumer (Hedman, 1990). This process brought together professionals from many fields, such as biomedical and rehabilitation engineering, physical therapy, occupational therapy, speech and language pathology, and special education. RESNA, the Rehabilitation Engineering and Assistive Technology Society of North America, an outgrowth of this shared interest, is an interdisciplinary association of professionals interested in applied technology for persons with activity limitations and participation restrictions.

Since 1975, many laws ensure the rights of people with disabilities to be included in natural education and work environments. These laws include Public Law 101-476, Education of All Handicapped Children Act; 1990 Amendment to IDEA); Public Law 101-47, Technology-Related Assistance for Individuals with Disabilities Act of 1988 (TRAIDA/Tech Act); Public Law 93-112, Rehabilitation Act; and Public Law 101-336, Americans with Disabilities Act (ADA). These laws have helped to focus attention on, and create a growing market for, new technologies and products. Consumer demands for increased durability and performance have induced manufacturers to apply technologies created by the aerospace, medical, and information industries. The field of assistive technology is an established cross-disciplinary specialty.

TRAIDA was the first federal legislation to define assistive technology devices and services and to recognize the importance of technology in the lives of individuals with disabilities (Dorman, 1998; Langone et al., 1999). Grants awarded to states and territories provided funds for comprehensive projects to improve access to technology and, subsequently, integration and inclusion of individuals with disabilities within the community and workforce. Services currently offered vary from state to state and may include information and referral services (databases, 800 numbers, and websites), centers for trying out devices and equipment, equipment exchange and recycling programs, funding resource guides, financial loan programs, mobile van outreach services, protection and advocacy services, and training programs on funding and self-advocacy. The Assistive Technology Act of 1998 provides for development of permanent comprehensive technology-related programs. All states and territories are eligible for 10 years of federal funding, and states that

have received 10 years of funding are eligible for an additional 3 years of funding. The 1997 Amendment to the IDEA advocates for consideration of assistive technology devices and services for all individual education plans.

The purpose of this chapter is to discuss five major elements of assistive technology and the role of the physical therapist in selecting and obtaining appropriate equipment for children and their families. The elements include adaptive seating and positioning, wheeled mobility, augmentative and alternative communication (AAC), computers, and electronic aids to daily living (EADLs).

▎ASSISTIVE TECHNOLOGY TEAM

Most technologic devices require modification or customization in design, implementation, or attachment (Hedman, 1990). The complexity and expense of the assistive technology required by individuals with severe physical impairments necessitates a thorough and careful process of selection and construction. All individuals who interact with the child and the equipment on a regular basis need to be considered part of the team. Professionals, the child, family, and caregivers each contribute a particular area of knowledge and expertise. Lahm (Lahm & Sizemore, 2002) argues that, despite laws mandating assistive technology assessment teams, the members of the team often may have individual agendas. Many factors influence the assessment process, including the needs and preferences of the child and family, individual education and experience levels of team members, specialties represented on the team, and the approach advocated by each assessor. Teams need to be cognizant of their strengths and limitations; is the team representative of several disciplines, or just one or two? Are the child and family regarded as integral team members? Lahm's outcomes survey revealed that the professionals with the most experience (therapists) spent the least amount of time with the client, and that the professionals with the least amount of training in disability studies (assistive technology suppliers) spent the most time with the family. Lahm and Sizemore (2002) advocate for more information on assistive technology to be included in professional education programs based on findings that new graduates do not possess sufficient knowledge of services and equipment that are available.

The configuration of the team (Fig. 33-1) will vary depending on child and family needs and on the setting in which the evaluation and prescription are being conducted. Central to the team are the child and family.

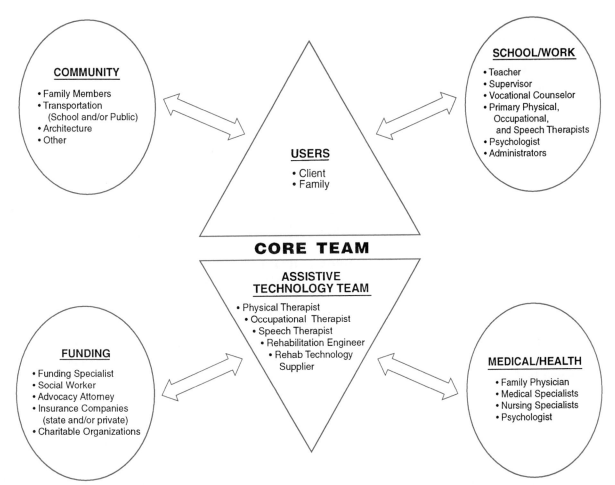

COMMUNITY
- Family Members
- Transportation
  (School and/or Public)
- Architecture
- Other

SCHOOL/WORK
- Teacher
- Supervisor
- Vocational Counselor
- Primary Physical,
  Occupational,
  and Speech Therapists
- Psychologist
- Administrators

USERS
- Client
- Family

CORE TEAM

**ASSISTIVE
TECHNOLOGY TEAM**
- Physical Therapist
- Occupational Therapist
- Speech Therapist
- Rehabilitation Engineer
- Rehab Technology
  Supplier

FUNDING
- Funding Specialist
- Social Worker
- Advocacy Attorney
- Insurance Companies
  (state and/or private)
- Charitable Organizations

MEDICAL/HEALTH
- Family Physician
- Medical Specialists
- Nursing Specialists
- Psychologist

◆ **Figure 33-1**   Core team interactions important in selecting and procuring assistive technology. Members and roles of each component may fluctuate, depending on specific client problems and settings.

Family-centered intervention stresses the need to involve the child and primary caregivers in the goal-setting and decision-making process to ensure realistic and meaningful solutions (Parette & McMahon, 2002). The professional component of the core team should include experts with training and experience in the areas being examined (mobility, seating, augmentative and alternative communication, computers, and activities of daily living). The team usually includes some or all of the following professionals: physical therapist, occupational therapist, speech and language pathologist, rehabilitation engineer, and rehabilitation technology supplier.

Several groups share roles and information that are essential to the core team. In the educational setting, this may include the physical therapist, occupational therapist, speech and language therapist, classroom teachers and aides, administrative personnel, psychologists, vocational counselors, and work supervisors. The development of

goals and strategies must be coordinated with primary service providers. Within the medical setting, the child's family physician, as well as other medical specialists and nurses, may need to be involved. Problems requiring collaboration with medical personnel may include management of deformity and contractures, pressure sores, incontinence, self-injury and safety, and visual and other sensory impairments. The issue of funding establishes a third group of contributors, including third-party payers, state-sponsored medical equipment programs, civic organizations, and other outside funding agencies. Many clinics and centers employ a funding specialist to assist families in identifying and obtaining funding for prescribed technology. A final group within the team includes other community and family members who engage in day-to-day interactions or who provide special support services such as transportation or revision of architectural barriers.

Team makeup and setting are variable. For example, in many hospitals and rehabilitation centers with comprehensive technology service delivery programs, physicians (especially physiatrists and orthopedic surgeons) may be an integral part of the core team. In schools and residential centers, one or more of the client's primary therapists, along with an equipment supplier, may function as the core team. The core team takes responsibility to impart information regarding proper use, training, maintenance, responsibility, and safety relative to the prescribed devices to appropriate individuals.

Effective communication and coordination of care are essential components of intervention to ensure that once obtained, the technology is used. Phillips and Zhao (1993) surveyed 227 adults with various disabilities to identify factors that predict abandonment of assistive technology devices. Nearly 30% of all devices were completely abandoned, with mobility devices abandoned most often. Devices were most frequently abandoned in the first year or after the fifth year. Four factors significantly related to abandonment: lack of consideration, ease of procurement, performance, and priorities. Lack of consideration refers to the child's and family's opinion during the selection process. Ease of procurement was a second factor. Easily obtained items purchased directly from a supplier (without team consultation) were the most likely to be abandoned. A third factor was poor device performance, which reflected the user's perception of the ability of the technology to enhance his or her performance in an easy, reliable, and comfortable manner. The fourth factor was the change in users' needs and priorities over time, including functional changes, as well as changes in lifestyle and activities.

Credentialing of professionals in assistive technology was established in 1995 by RESNA for the purposes of ensuring consumer safeguards and increasing consumer satisfaction. The credential signifies that the professional has specialized training and experience in assistive technology. Two types of credentialing examinations are offered:

- Assistive Technology Practitioner (ATP) Certificate: for service providers involved in analysis of a consumer's needs and training in use of a particular device
- Assistive Technology Supplier (ATS) Certificate: for service providers involved in the sale and service of commercial devices.

Any professional who provides assistive technology services to individuals with disabilities should consider obtaining the credential. This includes, but is not limited to, physical therapists, occupational therapists, speech-language pathologists, rehabilitation engineers, special educators, and rehabilitation technology suppliers. The credential is extremely important for physical therapists working with children and adults with seating, positioning, and mobility needs. There is an increasing need for physical therapists with specialized training and expertise in these areas because many individuals require adaptive equipment to increase functional capabilities.

A rehabilitation technology supplier (RTS) is an individual who provides enabling technology in areas of wheeled mobility, seating and alternative positioning, ambulation assistance, environmental controls, and activities of daily living (note that augmentative and alternative communication and computers are not included). A National Registry of Rehabilitation Technology Suppliers (NRRTS) identifies qualified suppliers by confirming, through a review process, an individual's work experience, references from professional associates, adherence to the Code of Ethics and Standards of Practice and Protocol, and commitment to ongoing continuing education. A Certified Rehabilitation Technology Supplier (CRTS) is a member in good standing of the National Registry of Rehabilitation Technology Suppliers who has successfully completed the RESNA Assistive Technology Supplier examination.

COMPONENTS OF HEALTH AND ASSISTIVE TECHNOLOGY

Throughout the book examples are provided of how assistive technology is used to achieve child and family goals for activity and participation. Assistive technology devices are designed to improve a user's participation in activities that may otherwise be limited by impairments in body structure and function. The benefits of assistive technology can be discussed according to the International Classification of Functioning, Disability, and Health (World Health Organization, 2001). Correctly prescribed and used, assistive technology, especially positioning (adaptive seating), may help prevent secondary impairments such as skin breakdown, cardiopulmonary compromise due to scoliosis or slouched posture, and contractures or deformity due to inadequately supported body segments. Other potential benefits to body function and structure are the reduction of tone or excessive muscle activity and a decrease in nonvolitional movement. By providing a means to compensate for impairments in postural stability and weight shifting, assistive technology can reduce activity limitations in sitting, mobility, use of hands, and speech. Assistive technology also may increase the ability of the child to participate in daily activities and routines. A power wheelchair may allow independent access to school or work. Augmentative and alternative communication may facilitate interactions with peers and promote social skills. An electronic aid to daily living may make the difference between less restricted living in a supervised apartment or living in a nursing home or intermediate care facility.

Social policies and attitudes are important determinants of availability and accessibility of assistive technology. High product and service provider costs require evidence that technology improves the quality of life of users in ways that are associated with cost-efficient care. Documentation of reduction in costs of hospitalizations, surgical procedures, out of home residence, and attendant care would provide evidence of the effectiveness of assistive technology. Technology also has the potential to alter negative attitudes and policies as clients' appearance and visibility improve and their capabilities become recognized.

Documentation of the benefits of assistive technology is often based empirically on clinical experience and observation. The literature is replete with descriptions of creative solutions for individual client problems. More difficult to find are carefully controlled studies of the effectiveness of assistive technology intervention. In this chapter we examine some of the literature in order to provide therapists evidence to assist in decision making.

LIFE-SPAN TECHNOLOGY

The needs of children with physical impairments change with growth and development and, therefore, assistive technology must be applied across the life span. Careful selection, planning, and implementation of assistive technology interventions maximize child and family outcomes and efficient use of health care resources. During infancy, proper positioning helps to promote social interaction and development of early concepts such as cause and effect and object permanence. During the preschool years, switch-activated toys and power-driven mobility toys can help a child learn how to self-initiate movement and control the organization of his or her environment. Children need a reliable way to indicate needs and make choices. The school-age child needs the postural support and comfort to enable learning and adaptive function. The adolescent needs to keep up with peers and be accepted socially. Adolescents should be included in the decision-making process regarding choice

of mobility, seating, or communication options whenever possible. The young adult needs to be able to get to and from a job or day setting and rely as little as possible on others to achieve basic functions, such as position changes, communicating, eating, and toileting. Because individuals with severe limitations in mobility spend many more hours at a time in one position, hygiene and skin care become a priority.

Interestingly, we are experiencing a technology boom in all facets of life. Things only dreamed about just a few years ago are now a readily available reality. Included in this phenomenon are the personal digital assistants (PDAs) used in the classroom by junior high and older students. The PDA is a handheld device that can store digital information. Data is easily inputted via a connected computer, a self-contained minipad, or can be transferred from another PDA via beaming. The PDA offers a flexible learning tool when utilized appropriately. Bauer and Ulrich (2002) investigated academic improvement in children with disabilities who used PDA devices. The students used their PDAs to record homework assignments, socialize with peers by "beaming messages," download information from the Internet, and receive and study vocabulary and spelling lists.

THE SELECTION PROCESS

A person's surroundings or a setting in which he or she spends a great deal of time can be thought of as the environment. Cooke and Hussey (1995) describe the human/activity/assistive technology model (HAAT model). This model dovetails well with the international classification of functioning, disability and health. In the HAAT model, "human" represents someone doing something in some place. "Activity" is the process of doing something, the functional result of human performance. The final component, "assistive technology," is the basis for how the human performance will be enhanced during an activity. Thus, translating the HAAT model into components of health, assistive technology is designed to minimize impairments in body function and structure and maximize activity and social participation. For example, children function in a series of environments throughout the day. Selection of assistive technologies must consider all those environments in which technologies will be used. In addition, the wheelchair itself, with its adaptive seating and communication systems, becomes a primary microenvironment for many children with severe impairments (Bergen, 1992). The ultimate responsibility of the assistive technology team must be to maximize the client's abilities without creating new limitations.

Once a referral has been made, the steps followed by the assistive technology team are similar to the elements of patient/client management in the *Guide to Physical Therapist Practice* (American Physical Therapy Association, 2001):

Step 1. Examination: The process of obtaining a history, performing systems reviews, and selecting and administering specific tests and measures to obtain data. In this step, the team records relevant history and social information. The examination includes assessments and measurements of myotome and dermatome, skin, range of motion, muscle strength, and motor function including sitting, transfer, and mobility. The child/family also report what their goal is when using an AT system.

Step 2. Evaluation: The team makes clinical judgments based on data gathered during the examination. Keeping in mind the information gathered in Step 1, the team begins to determine what devices would benefit the child.

Step 3. Diagnosis: The team organizes findings into categories to determine the most appropriate intervention strategies. The team should mock up several AT device scenarios and test the effectiveness of each demonstration system for the family.

Step 4. Prognosis: Team determines level of optimal improvement that might be attained through AT intervention and the amount of training required.

Step 5. Intervention: Team uses various AT devices and services to implement a system that will provide maximal independence based on findings of the diagnosis and prognosis. The AT device systems are ordered and funding mechanisms are employed. The team may be responsible for gathering prescriptions and writing letters of medical justification based on the data collected from the diagnosis and prognosis stages. The recommended equipment is ordered, delivered, and fit to the user.

Step 6. Outcomes: Results of examination, evaluation, and intervention. Did the child's activity and participation improve with the AT device?

Step 7. Follow-up and reevaluation. For the child using assistive technology, the process described is usually only one of many repetitions of a cycle. Mechanical and electronic equipment wear out and break down, making repairs and fine-tuning necessary. The child's problems and needs change with age, development of new skills, and change of environments. As technologies continue to improve or be introduced, new solutions become available.

SEATING SYSTEMS

The purpose of the seating system is to provide external postural support for the child with functional limitations in sitting as a result of impairments in musculoskeletal alignment, postural control, muscle tone, or strength. Seating is the interface between the child and the mobility device (Galvin & Scherer, 1996). The goal of the seating system is to enable the child to compensate for functional limitations and thereby maximize participation in life activities. In this section, studies that have examined the effectiveness of seating systems are reviewed and considerations in the prescription of seating systems are discussed.

EFFECTS OF ADAPTIVE SEATING

There are several desired outcomes when prescribing seating systems: comfort, neuromuscular management, improved postural control, and maintaining the integumentary system. Comfort is an outcome that spans across all individuals using seating and mobility (Monette et al., 1999; Neilson et al., 2001). Likewise, there are outcomes for specific populations who use assistive technology. Outcomes for individuals with cerebral palsy (CP) or traumatic brain injury may include muscle tone management and improvement of upper body postural control to enhance functional skills of the head and hands. Letts (1991) stated that to achieve stable sitting, biomechanical forces and moments in all planes must be balanced. "Good positioning" usually consists of an upright midline orientation of the entire body with a near-vertical alignment of the trunk and head. In children, the "90-90-90" rule often is used to maintain the hips, knees, and ankles at 90°. As the child grows, it may not be reasonable, due to leg length, to maintain the knees at 90° flexion. In this case, the decision to go with a different angled front rigging must be made. Additionally, if the child has significant contractures of the lower extremities or trunk, it may not be possible to position them in 90° of hip, knee, and ankle flexion. Kangas (1991) has seriously challenged the idea of static positioning, stating that it is unnatural and impedes function. Seating systems can be characterized into three categories: linear/planar; generic contoured/modular; or custom molded. These will all be discussed in more detail later in the chapter.

Much of the research on therapeutic seating for this group has examined the effects of variables such as hip flexion angles (or seat-to-back angles) and orientation of the trunk and head (or angle-in-space). The former is achieved by independently changing the seat back angle; the latter is achieved by tilting/rotating the entire system. There has been considerable interest in the anterior tipped (or forward-inclined) seat, in which the front edge of the seat is tilted downward, thus increasing the seat-to-back angle while maintaining a near-vertical back. Most clients with myelodysplasia or spinal cord injuries tolerate and function well in a typical upright position; however, sitting pressures and the prevention of skin ulcerations are of utmost concern. Various types of sitting surfaces and adjustments to postural alignment have been studied in the attempt to reduce pressure and decrease the incidence of decubiti. In children with muscular dystrophy, prevention of spinal collapse, preservation of upper extremity function, and comfort are desirable outcomes of positioning. Washington and associates (2002) reported that infants with neuromotor impairments demonstrated better postural alignment and engagement with toys when seated on a contoured foam seat as compared to a regular highchair seat or highchair with a thin foam layer. In this study, mothers of the infants reported acceptability for the contoured foam seat within their typical daily routines.

BODY FUNCTION AND STRUCTURE

Neuromuscular Function and Pathologic Movement Patterns

A long-standing principle of therapeutic seating is that increased muscle tone, here defined as muscle activity at rest, can be reduced by altering seating angle. Seats are oriented either horizontally, wedged (front edge raised), or anterior tipped (front edge lowered). Backs are placed vertically, reclined (decreased), or forward inclined (closing the hip angle to more flexion). The seat-back combinations and the degree to which they can be varied are therefore numerous. Several studies have examined the effect of altered seating angles on electromyographic (EMG) activity in children with CP. In a study that varied the hip angle by reclining the back or wedging the seat, lumbar muscle activity was lowest in vertical sitting, with a horizontal seat and a 90° hip angle (Nwaobi et al., 1983). Lumbar muscle activity was higher the more reclined the position regardless of the hip angle. Hip adductor activity was decreased when the back was vertical and the seat was wedged 15° (Nwaobi & Cusick, 1980). When the hip angle was kept constant at 90° and the entire system was tilted 30° posterior, electrical activity of both paraspinal and hip adductor muscle groups was significantly higher (Nwaobi, 1986).

The reclined position also resulted in the highest electrical activity in leg muscles (rectus femoris, adductor longus, biceps femoris, and gastrocnemius) in subjects with CP, as well as in normal control subjects (Myhr & von Wendt, 1993). The addition of an abduction orthosis decreased leg muscle activity in all positions. For subjects with the most severe impairments, EMG responses of back extensors and medial hamstrings to position changes were much more individualized (Fife et al., 1988).

Children with CP who sat on anterior tilted seats without back support showed a decrease in midthoracic muscle activity and an increase in lumbar muscle activity (Bablich et al., 1986) indicating increased firing of low back musculature relative to midback musculature. Myhr and von Wendt (1993) advocate use of anterior tilted seats, but they added an abduction orthosis and a cutout table for upper extremity support of forward leaning. EMG activity of leg muscles was lowest in the forward-leaning position with the abduction orthosis compared with vertical or reclined sitting. The frequency of pathologic movements (a single spastic or tonic reflex pattern defined for each subject) was significantly reduced in the experimental sitting position when compared with the subjects' own systems (Myhr & von Wendt, 1991).

Physiologic Functions

Most studies have measured how pulmonary function is affected by variation of seating parameters. Pulmonary function of children with spastic CP was higher when sitting in a modular seating system with adjustable support components compared to a wheelchair with standard sling seat and back (Nwaobi & Smith, 1986). The differences were attributed to changes in the shape, structure, and capacity of the thorax and abdomen and to improved control of the respiratory muscles in the supported, upright position.

In a group of children with muscle weakness due to neuromuscular disease who were ambulatory and without scoliosis, forced vital capacity (FVC) was slightly decreased in supine position compared with sitting (Noble-Jamieson et al., 1986). In a second group of children with scoliosis who were nonambulators, however, the decrease in FVC while supine compared with sitting was much greater. When tested again in sitting position with their spinal brace on, FVC was further reduced. The more severe the scoliosis, and the greater the reduction of the spinal curve by the brace, the greater the decrease in FVC.

Anterior tilted seats may have some potential to improve respiratory function in children with moderate CP. Tidal volume and minute ventilation in subjects with CP were increased compared with control subjects when seated on a bench tilted 10° anterior without back support (Reid & Sochaniwskyj, 1991).

Skeletal Deformity, Contracture, and Passive Range of Motion

Studies that pertain to musculoskeletal impairments examined the management of scoliosis in patients with

Duchenne muscular dystrophy. Carlson and Payette (1985) used a combination of molded seating systems with soft spinal corsets and found a reduction of curves on radiography. Seeger and associates (1984b), however, found no significant difference in spinal curves when modular seats, custom-molded seats, unmodified wheelchair seats, and spinal jackets were compared.

The assumption that postural support systems prevent contractures and skeletal deformity in children with increased muscle tone has not been examined. In theory, maintenance of balanced forces to the trunk and lower extremities should prevent structural changes such as scoliosis and hip dislocation (Letts, 1991). This theory may apply to young children with asymmetric postures that can be reduced through positioning. Maintenance of balanced forces through a postural control system may not be feasible for children with severely increased tone, strong deforming muscle forces, and asymmetry.

Postural Stability and Control

Research has focused on whether anterior tilted seats improve posture and stability in children with motor impairments. Measurement methods generally include instrumented systems or clinical rating scales. Two typical designs of anterior seats are (1) a flat bench with no trunk support, with feet flat on the floor, and (2) a forward-leaning system with an anterior trunk or upper extremity surface for support. Using the first type of bench seat, Bablich and colleagues (1986) measured postural stability with a three-dimensional tracking system that monitored a point on the top of the head. The anterior tilted seat resulted in a more upright and stable posture compared with a flat seat by increasing trunk extension and decreasing deviation from the midline in subjects with CP.

Reid et al. (1991) reported that when children with neuromuscular impairments were positioned on an anterior tilted seat, trunk posture improved and the effect on sway was variable. The position of the C7 spinous process was tracked to yield a *radius of stability,* with a smaller radius indicating reduced postural sway and thus increased postural stability. During quiet sitting on a flat bench, children with CP and children with head injury showed no significant difference in the amount of postural sway when compared with age-matched control subjects, although they did show more variability. When positioned on a seat with a 10° anterior tilt, half of the children with CP (described as having spasticity with tight hamstrings) had a decrease in sway and a more upright posture (vertical measurement of C7 height). The other half of the children with CP (described as having low trunk tone and tight hamstrings) had an

increase in sway on the anterior seat but also a more upright posture.

McClenaghan and associates (1992) reported that varying seat angle by 10° did not affect postural stability in children with motor impairments. The seating surface was varied between horizontal, 5° anterior tilt, and 5° posterior tilt. Video-digitized displacements of the head, shoulder, hip, knee, and ankle and seat reaction forces were measured as indicators of postural stability. Significant differences were found between children with and without motor impairment, as well as between quiet and active sitting for both groups, but this small degree of seat inclination did not affect postural stability.

Back extension was greatest in children with motor impairments when positioned in an anteriorly tipped seat with a leg support to provide weight bearing through the knees and shins (Miedaner, 1990). Active control of trunk extension was rated using a four-point scale, and trunk extension was measured as the linear distance between defined marks on the spine. Children with motor impairments and delays sat on the floor, a level bench, a bench with an anterior tilt of 20°, a bench with an anterior tilt of 30°, and an TherAdapt Posture Chair (TherAdapt Products, Bensonville, IL) in which the seat is tilted anterior with a leg support to provide weight bearing through the knees and shins rather than the feet. Back extension was greatest in the TherAdapt Posture Chair, perhaps because of the levering action provided by the leg supports.

Myhr and von Wendt (1991) reported that postural control of the head, trunk, and feet improved when children sat in an anterior position. Posture was measured by mean duration of head control during a 5-minute period and rating postural control of the head, trunk, and feet on a four-point scale developed by the authors. Qualitative changes in independent sitting ability, improved or maintained trunk posture in sitting, and power driving ability were observed in 10 children after 3 years of using a seating and mobility system (Pope et al., 1994). The critical features of the seating and mobility system (SAM) are a saddle seat, a solid anterior chest support, and a tray to support forward leaning.

Posture and arm movements of young children with CP was better sitting on a saddle seat with 15° anterior tilt, foot support, and no trunk support compared with sitting on a flat bench (Reid, 1996). Quality of sitting at rest and during upper extremity movements was measured by the Sitting Assessment for Children with Neuromotor Dysfunction (SACND), a standardized, observational rating scale for children over the age of 2 years (Reid, 1996; Reid, 1997). Postural tone and postural alignment items showed the most change, indicating a more upright head and trunk and better alignment between body segments, and correlated with improved spinal extension measured by motion analysis (Reid, 1996).

Seat to back angle and seat pitch should be determined on an individual basis. For most children, a seat to back angle of 90° without any pitch (thus the seat is parallel to the floor) is most practical. If the child assumes a posterior pelvic tilt when sitting, anterior tilt of the seat may facilitate trunk extension. Hence, the seat to back angle is increased or "opened." For a child with increased tone, a seat with a posterior tilt, in which the front edge is relatively higher to the back edge, may reduce extensor spasms and allow the child to maintain a proper seated position. In this case, the seat to back angle is reduced, or "closed."

Pressure and Prevention of Decubiti

Several factors contribute to the development of pressure sores including skin temperature, moisture, and shear and compressive forces (Crenshaw & Vistnes, 1989). Pressure (compressive force) has been the most-studied variable, because it has a clear relationship to the development of decubiti and is relatively easy to measure and manipulate during wheelchair seating. The risk of a pressure sore is directly related to the length of time soft tissue is compressed and inversely related to the area being compressed. Serious pressure sores are a common impairment in children with spinal cord injury and myelodysplasia in which immobility and insensate tissue compound the problem of prolonged sitting. Children with neuromuscular impairments such as CP who use wheeled mobility also need special considerations for

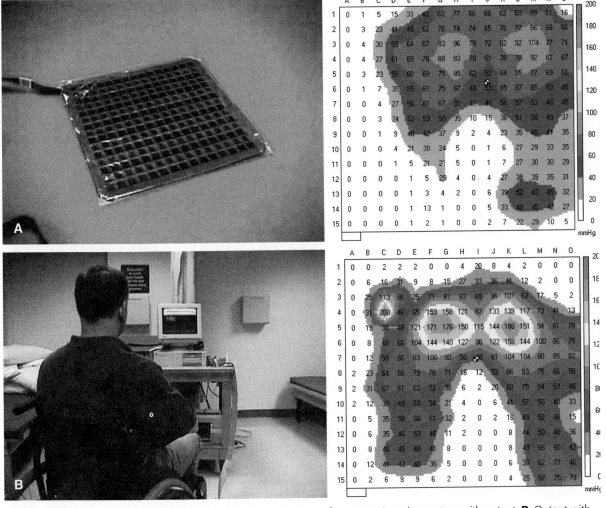

♦ **Figure 33-2** Pressure mapping system and outputs. **A,** General pressure mapping system with output. **B,** Output with symmetric sitting posture.

continued

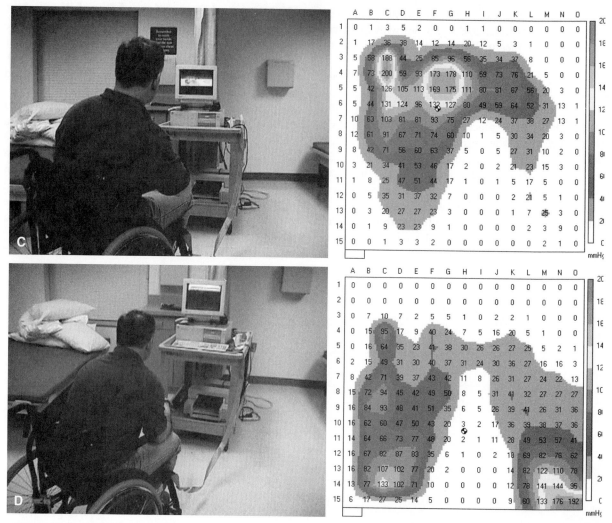

	A	B	C	D	E	F	G	H	I	J	K	L	M	N	O
1	0	1	3	5	2	0	0	1	1	0	0	0	0	0	0
2	1	17	36	38	14	12	14	20	12	5	3	1	0	0	0
3	5	58	188	44	25	85	96	56	35	34	37	8	0	0	0
4	7	73	200	59	93	173	178	110	59	73	76	21	5	0	0
5	5	42	126	105	113	169	175	111	80	81	67	56	20	3	0
6	5	44	130	124	96	132	127	80	49	59	64	52	31	13	1
7	10	63	103	81	81	93	75	27	12	24	37	38	27	13	1
8	12	61	91	67	71	74	60	10	1	5	30	34	20	3	0
9	8	42	71	56	60	63	37	5	0	5	27	31	10	2	0
10	3	21	34	41	53	46	17	2	0	2	21	23	15	3	0
11	1	8	25	47	51	44	17	1	0	1	5	17	5	0	0
12	0	5	35	31	37	32	7	0	0	0	2	21	5	1	0
13	0	3	20	27	27	23	3	0	0	0	1	7	25	3	0
14	0	1	9	23	23	9	1	0	0	0	0	2	3	9	0
15	0	0	1	3	3	2	0	0	0	0	0	0	2	1	0

	A	B	C	D	E	F	G	H	I	J	K	L	M	N	O
1	0	0	0	0	0	0	0	0	0	0	0	0	0	0	0
2	0	0	0	0	0	0	0	0	0	0	0	0	0	0	0
3	0	7	10	7	2	5	5	1	0	2	2	1	0	0	0
4	0	15	95	17	9	40	24	7	5	16	20	5	1	0	0
5	0	16	64	35	23	41	38	30	26	26	27	25	5	2	1
6	2	15	49	31	30	40	37	31	24	30	36	27	16	16	3
7	8	42	71	39	37	43		11	8	26	31	27	24	22	13
8	15	72	94	45	42	49	50	8	5	31	41	32	27	27	27
9	16	84	93	48	41	51	35	6	5	26	39	41	26	31	36
10	16	62	60	47	50	43	20	3	2	17	36	39	38	37	36
11	14	64	66	73	77	48	20	2	1	11	28	49	53	57	41
12	16	67	82	87	83	35	6	1	0	2	18	69	82	76	62
13	16	82	107	102	77	20	2	0	0	0	14	82	122	110	78
14	13	77	133	102	71	10	0	0	0	0	12	78	141	144	95
15	6	17	27	14	5	0	0	0	0	0	9	60	133	176	192

◆ **Figure 33-2, *cont'd***   Pressure mapping system and outputs. **C**, Output with shifting to one side in sitting. **D**, Output with shifting forward in sitting.

pressure relief in sitting. Skeletal asymmetries such as pelvic obliquity, hip dislocation, and scoliosis predispose children who sit in wheelchairs to pressure problems.

Pressure mapping devices (Fig. 33-2) have become highly sophisticated and are commonly used to study differences in pressure distribution in subjects with and without motor impairment, reduction of seat interface pressure using various seat surfaces, and prevention of decubiti. Adults without physical impairments display even pressure distribution from side to side and a biphasic pattern of pressure concentration with a posterior concentration on the ischial tuberosities and a second, but lesser, concentration on the distal thighs (Drummond et al., 1982). A similar biphasic pattern was found in adolescent boys; however, over a 3-hour period, pressure tended to be skewed slightly to one side or the other (Pate, 1988).

Patients with "unbalanced sitting" due to pelvic obliquity or scoliosis showed a pronounced shift of pressure laterally and often posteriorly, thereby severely loading one of the ischial tuberosities (Drummond et al., 1982).

For subjects without impairment, return to upright after a short period of recline in a wheelchair resulted in higher pressures and shear forces than in the original upright position (Gilsdorf et al., 1990). Leaning forward off the backrest returned the forces to initial values. Also, when the footrests were elevated, pressure under the ischial tuberosities was increased. There was no difference in pressure under the ischial tuberosities between upright sitting and 10° of recline in adults without impairment, but there was reduction of pressure in both positions when a lumbar support was added (Shields & Cook, 1988). The reclined position with lumbar support was recommended for patients with spinal cord injury because they slide or rotate off the lumbar support in upright position due to tight hamstrings or weak trunk musculature.

Magnetic resonance imaging can be used to evaluate soft tissue contours of the buttocks during loading. In a subject with paraplegia, less sitting pressure was required before soft tissue became compressed by a bony prominence, and there was increased stiffness and lateral shifting of the gluteal muscle mass (Reger et al., 1986). Foam cushions that were contoured to match the shape of the buttocks, as opposed to flat foam, improved the load transfer from buttocks to cushion because the total contact surface area was greater (Sprigle et al., 1990a). Foam stiffness was also important in determining the seat contours, with dense foam having less deflection under the load. When clients with spinal cord injury were seated on flat versus contoured foam cushions of varying stiffness, pressures were lower on the contoured cushions than on the flat cushions, and on the more compliant foam than on the stiffer foam (Sprigle et al., 1990b). The buttocks were encompassed more on the contoured and softer cushion with less tissue distortion. The authors cautioned that too soft a foam would deform too much and "bottom out" quickly. In contrast, when subjects with paraplegia sat with their trunks bent laterally, the mean pressure difference between the left and right ischial tuberosities was greater on a foam cushion than on a commercial air-bladder cushion (Koo et al., 1996).

Several studies have compared sitting pressures, skin temperature, and relative humidity in subjects seated on commercially available cushions (Garber & Dyerly, 1991; Palmieri et al., 1980; Seymour & Lacefield, 1985; Stewart et al., 1980). The findings indicate that no one cushion is effective for all clients and that a variety of cushion options are needed to meet individual needs. The subjects in most studies were adults with spinal cord injury; the unique needs of children, particularly those with severe pelvic and spinal deformity, as in myelodysplasia and CP, have not been studied.

ACTIVITY

Upper Extremity Control and Hand Function

Several authors have investigated the effect of seating configuration on upper body control and function. Wedging the seat did not improve hand function on a joystick-controlled targeting task in subjects with marked extensor spasticity (Seeger et al., 1984a), nor did it increase shoulder horizontal adduction movement time to trigger a switch in subjects with CP (Nwaobi et al., 1983). Movement time was faster with the hips in a 90°

position than in a wedged position, and slowest at a hip angle of 50°. When the hips were maintained at 90° of flexion but the entire system tilted posterior 15° or 30°, or anterior 5°, performance on the shoulder adduction task was best in the upright position and worst in the anterior position (Nwaobi, 1987).

Arm and hand function scores on a four-point rating scale were highest when seat angle was tilted anterior and children assumed a forward-leaning position described by Myhr and von Wendt (1991). In contrast, McClenaghan and associates (1992) reported that performance on six upper extremity tasks did not change appreciably for subjects with or without CP at seat angles of 0°, 5° anterior tilt, or 5° posterior tilt, possibly, as noted earlier, because of the very small change in seat angle. Reid (1996) reported that more than half of the subjects demonstrated faster and more accurate reaching movements when positioned in a saddle seat.

Oral-Motor, Speech, and Communication Functions

Very young children with impairments in multiple systems demonstrated improvements in oral-motor control during eating and drinking when positioned in individualized therapeutic seating devices (Hulme et al., 1987). No significant improvements were seen in self-feeding or independent drinking. Larnert and Ekberg (1995) used videofluoroscopy to examine swallowing in young children with CP with feeding difficulties. At 30° of recline, with the neck flexed, aspiration decreased in all five children, oral leak diminished in two children, and retention improved in one child compared with their typical upright eating position.

Spontaneous vocalizations in young children with spasticity or hypotonia increased after positioning in an adaptive seating system (Hulme et al., 1988). Vocalizations were measured from 3 months before to 6 months after use of the adaptive seating system. Increased frequency of speech sounds was found in seven children, and increased types of sounds were found in six. Bay (1991) studied a woman with spastic athetoid CP who activated her electronic communication device with a head-mounted light sensor. Her rate of head-controlled typing increased but her accuracy decreased when she was seated in her power wheelchair with lateral trunk supports and properly adjusted foot support, compared with seating in her manual wheelchair with no foot or trunk support and excessive seat height.

Mobility

Researchers have examined the effect of seating position on efficiency of manual wheelchair propulsion in adults

(Hughes et al., 1992; van der Woude et al., 1989). Altering seat height, seat inclination, or anterior-posterior orientation for individual subjects affected upper extremity movement patterns and wheeling efficiency. Wheeling performance was optimized by adjusting seating configurations in relation to the propulsion mechanism (hand-rims or lever), based on the functional characteristics of each user. The effect of customized seating systems on the ability of young children with physical impairments to learn self-wheeling has not been examined. Pope and colleagues (1994) included a description of improved power driving ability over a period of 3 years in their subjects, who used a forward-leaning sitting and mobility system, although descriptions were based on subjective assessment and lacked a control group.

PARTICIPATION

The assumption is often made that individuals who experience an increase in functional skills improve their ability to fill societal roles. Families reported positive changes in social participation after their children or adults received adaptive seating equipment that included wheelchairs, travel chairs, and strollers, with custom adaptations as needed (Hulme et al., 1983). The families of 41 individuals 1 to 67 years old who were unable to walk and had a developmental disability were surveyed. Families reported the following changes in motor behavior: increased ability to sit upright without leaning, more time spent in sitting and less time lying down, increased ability to grasp an object, and improved ability to eat with a spoon. Social behavior changes reported included an increased number of community places visited, more time during the day spent with someone else, and less time spent in the bedroom. Although there was no change in frequency of leaving the home, caregivers reported improved ease of taking the clients on outings.

Adults initiated interactions more often when the students were positioned in a wheelchair compared to positioning on the floor (McEwen, 1992). School-age children with profound multiple disabilities were positioned in a wheelchair, a sidelyer, and a freestyle position on a mat on the floor, and social-communicative interactions with classroom staff were measured. Adults initiated interactions more often when the students were in the wheelchair, whereas there was no difference in student initiations between the positions. For the lower-functioning group, the average duration of interaction during the structured session was higher in the freestyle position than in either of the other two positions, but there was no difference for the higher-functioning group.

SUMMARY ON EFFECTS OF ADAPTIVE SEATING

The variability in subject characteristics and responses support individualized decision making following the use of postural support system simulation. Research evidence suggests that therapeutic seating systems that provide external postural support improve pulmonary function in subjects with CP; reduce scoliosis when combined with a soft orthosis in subjects with muscular dystrophy; improve upper extremity function in subjects with CP; and improve oral-motor skills, vocalizations, and social interaction behaviors in subjects with multiple disabilities. More specifically, an upright orientation appears to correlate with decreased activity of extensor muscles in children with CP, improved pulmonary function in subjects with muscle weakness, improved upper extremity performance on a shoulder adduction task in subjects with CP, and an increase in adult-initiated interactions with students who have profound physical and cognitive impairments. Hip flexion greater than 90° did not reduce activity in extensor muscles, nor did it improve upper extremity function. For clients with severe impairments, effects of orientation in space and seat-to-back angles are more variable than for clients with mild-to-moderate impairments. This must be considered when assessing clients with severe impairments and supports the use of postural support system simulation.

The effects of sitting on an anterior tilted seat are inconclusive. Although anterior tilted seats appear to increase back extension and improve spinal alignment, it is unclear whether they improve stability or upper extremity function. Clinically, anterior tilted seats are used to encourage more "active sitting," with the goal of improving pelvic and spinal alignment for children with tight lower extremity musculature. A more vertical orientation of the pelvis when sitting on an anterior tilted seat may place the lumbar extensors at a better biomechanical advantage and reduce the need for the thoracic extensors to be excessively active for upper body flexion. Research is needed on the long-term effects of anterior tipped seats on performance and fatigue.

There is evidence that contoured cushions improve pressure distribution in subjects with spinal cord injury. Lumbar rolls tend to decrease pressure under the ischial tuberosities. The results with commercially available pressure relief cushions are variable, but of interest is the number of manufacturers that are adding blocks and foam pieces to provide custom-contouring of their products.

Much work remains to be done in defining the features and components of postural support systems that reduce impairment, improve function, and increase social participation of individuals with severe physical impairments. Consistent reporting of the specific disorders and severity of impairments in research reports is necessary. Even in studies involving subjects with similar conditions, results tend to be highly variable, indicating individualized responses. Reliable and valid clinical measures for evaluating the effectiveness of postural support systems such as seat interface pressure monitors and shape sensors must be developed and refined.

The impact of assistive technology clinics and programs on the cost of health care must be studied. Potentially, assistive technology can reduce costs of hospitalizations due to decubiti and corrective surgery. In some cases, the cost of assistive technology and vocational training may increase a client's employability but reduce his or her eligibility for Medicaid or other supplemental assistance. Comprehensive regional centers may be the most cost-effective way to deliver advanced technology to the greatest number of people; however, rural mobile vans may promote a broader range of access.

PRINCIPAL CONCEPTS IN THE PRESCRIPTION OF SEATING SYSTEMS

Assistive seating technology is evolving rapidly in many different regions of North America, creating a confusion of locally adopted language and terminology. RESNA has published a list of standardized seating terminology that is helpful in improving communication among research and service centers, clients, and funding sources (Medhat & Hobson, 1992). It is imperative that the team possess a strong knowledge base of what components will accomplish a child's and family's goals. If an inappropriate system is recommended, the child/user may lose function or experience secondary musculoskeletal impairment.

Examination and Evaluation

As part of the process of selection of a seating system, the physical therapist examines the child and evaluates findings. The physical therapist applies knowledge of anatomy, kinesiology, biomechanics, and principles of neuromuscular control of posture and function when examining the child. Letts (1991) and Myhr and von Wendt (1993) stressed the importance of thoroughly understanding and applying principles of biomechanics and movement to therapeutic seating. The child is examined in both supine and sitting. Range of motion, muscle tone, and muscle strength are examined. Anatomic linear measurements are taken. Precise measurement and documentation will help to determine the most

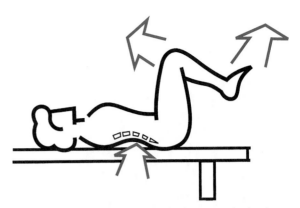

♦ **Figure 33-3**   The examiner must monitor the lumbar curve as the hips are flexed and the knees extended. *(Redrawn with permission from Bergen, AF, Presperin, J, & Tallman, T. Positioning for Function: Wheelchairs and Other Assistive Technologies. Valhalla, NY: Valhalla Rehabilitation Publications, 1990.)*

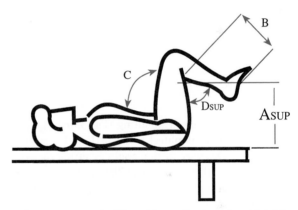

♦ **Figure 33-4**   Hip (C) and knee (D_{sup}) angles, thigh/hip length (A_{sup}) and calf length (B) are measured first in supine. *(Redrawn with permission from Bergen, AF, Presperin, J, & Tallman, T. Positioning for Function: Wheelchairs and Other Assistive Technologies. Valhalla, NY: Valhalla Rehabilitation Publications, 1990.)*

appropriate size and type of the seating system as well as assist in providing information needed for letters of medical justification to third-party payers. Additionally, good documentation over time provides valuable information regarding a child's growth and development.

Figures 33-3 to 33-6 illustrate the linear measurements needed to design and prescribe a well-fitting seating system. The following measurements are taken with the child positioned in supine (see Figs. 33-3 and 33-4): hip (C) and knee (D_{sup}) angles, thigh/hip length (A_{sup}), and calf length (B). Measurements in sitting are taken with the child sitting on a surface with a thin top and with feet supported, not dangling (Fig. 33-5). The following

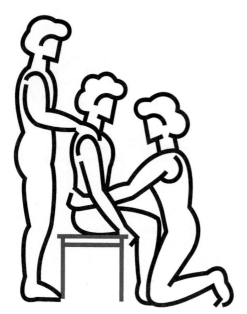

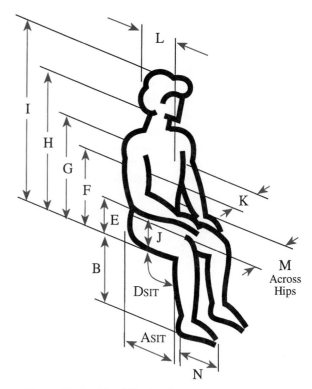

◆ **Figure 33-5**   Measurements in sitting must be taken with the client sitting on a surface with a thin top. This will allow the knees to flex as needed. *(Redrawn with permission from Bergen, AF, Presperin, J, & Tallman, T. Positioning for Function: Wheelchairs and Other Assistive Technologies. Valhalla, NY: Valhalla Rehabilitation Publications, 1990.)*

◆ **Figure 33-6**   The following figure measurements are added to those taken with the client in supine: A_{sit} (R & L), behind hips to popliteal fossa; right and left (R & L) popliteal fossa to heel; D_{sit}, knee flexion angle; E, sitting surface to pelvic crest; F, sitting surface to axilla; G, sitting surface to shoulder; H, sitting surface to occiput; I, sitting surface to crown of head; J, sitting surface to flexed elbow; K, width across trunk; L, depth of trunk; M, width across hips; N, heel to toe. *(Redrawn with permission from Bergen, AF, Presperin, J, & Tallman, T. Positioning for Function: Wheelchairs and Other Assistive Technologies. Valhalla, NY: Valhalla Rehabilitation Publications, 1990.)*

measurements are taken in sitting (Fig. 33-6): A_{sit} (R & L), behind hips to popliteal fossa; B (R & L), popliteal fossa to heel; D_{sit}, knee flexion angle; E, sitting surface to pelvic crest; F, sitting surface to axilla; G, sitting surface to shoulder; H, sitting surface to occiput; I, sitting surface to crown of head; J, sitting surface to hanging elbow; K, width across trunk; L, depth of trunk; M, width across hips; N, heel to toe.

Type of deformity and severity will influence the type of system and components chosen. A *flexible deformity*— one that can be manually corrected and maintained with a reasonable amount of force—can often be maintained in optimal alignment with the appropriate and balanced use of support components. Seating systems, however, are not intended to stretch tight musculature or correct bony deformity. Stretching invariably results in sacrifice of the optimal posture because the child will attempt to move and avoid the uncomfortable forces. *Fixed deformities*— those that are not correctable without an undue amount of force—and severe joint contractures must be accommodated in the seating system. Reduction of deformity is addressed through other interventions. Pharmacologic interventions or surgical intervention may be useful to achieve soft tissue relaxation and optimal positioning.

Range of motion measurements at the hips, knees, ankles, trunk, shoulders, elbows, and wrists/hands are

vital to the examination process. The seating system can accommodate or correct for range-of-motion losses and prevent future or further deformities from occurring. In the case of a fixed deformity, the seating system will accommodate and support the deformity. For instance, if a child is unable to be positioned with the hip flexed to 90°, the seat to back angle will be determined based on hip range of motion. In another scenario, if the child tends to scissor the lower extremities, but can achieve neutral hip alignment, the seating system can hold the hips in an abducted position, or positioning components can be added to the seat to prevent excessive adduction. Conversely, if the child has a tendency to maintain hips in extreme abduction, lateral supports can be used to position the lower extremities in a more neutral alignment. If the knees lack of range of motion, 60° hangers, instead of 90° hangers, may be used to accommodate for the loss of range. Additionally, the back cushion can support the trunk in neutral alignment or in an alternative posture if significant trunk asymmetries exist. Additional modifications or supports can be used to accommodate for lack of range of motion in the upper extremities.

The assessment of posture in a seating system begins with the pelvis and its relationship to its adjacent segments. The orientation and range of mobility of the pelvis in all three planes will determine the alignment and support needed at the trunk, head, and extremities. The effect of hip flexion and knee extension range of motion on the vertical orientation of the pelvis is among the most critical factors in selecting seating angles and components. If there are minimal contractures of the hamstrings, hip extensors, and hip flexors, the pelvis should retain a considerable amount of mobility, and vertical orientation of the pelvis and trunk is possible. If any or all of these muscles are tight, the pelvis may be fixed in either an anterior or a posterior tilt, or exhibit an obliquity, and the child will require a more individualized solution.

Pelvis alignment and an erect trunk are essential for optimal head control and arm and hand function. For many children, an erect trunk posture is achieved through neutral pelvic alignment. For children with severe scoliosis and pelvic obliquity, however, neutral alignment of the pelvis is not always possible and does not result in acceptable trunk and head alignment. In such cases, it is better to start with a relatively vertical head and level shoulders and allow the pelvis to be tilted and rotated.

In children at risk for skin breakdown due to pressure problems, measurement of seat and back interface pressures should be included in the examination process. Pressure mapping systems are increasingly common in the clinic for comparing pressures while seated on various cushions. Variable-tilt and variable-recline features of manual and power wheelchairs can provide another source of pressure relief throughout a long day of sitting for some children.

MATCHING THE SYSTEM TO THE CHILD'S NEEDS

Seating systems and extrinsic positional components typically are classified in three levels, planar or linear, contoured, and custom molded. The first and least intensive level is the *planar or linear system*, which consists of a flat seat and back (Fig. 33-7). Children with good postural stability and sitting balance, a minimum of

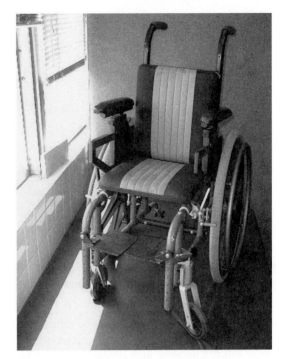

◆ **Figure 33-7**   Planar/linear seating system.

deformity, are most appropriate for this level of intervention. The seat and back consist of a solid base (plywood or plastic), covered by foam, and upholstered with vinyl or knit fabric. Linear trunk or pelvic supports may be added laterally. Many commercial variations are available, or they can be constructed in the clinic. This system is easily changed and adapted, and typically the least expensive.

The second level is the *generic contoured or modular system*, which provides external postural control by increasing the points of contact, especially laterally (Fig. 33-8). The seat and back surfaces are rounded by shaping layers of firm foam, air, or gel to correspond to the curves of the body. Contours also help distribute pressures more evenly. Contouring can range from simple to aggressive. A small amount of contouring can improve comfort and stability for many clients. A greater amount of contouring is often necessary for children with severe impairments. Many varieties are fabricated in the clinic of a solid base with varying densities and configurations of foam, or air, or gel materials to create the contours. This level of system can accommodate growth with modifications or adjustments to the positioning materials.

The third level is the *custom-molded system*. It provides an intimate fit by closely conforming to the shape of the child's body, thereby giving the most postural support

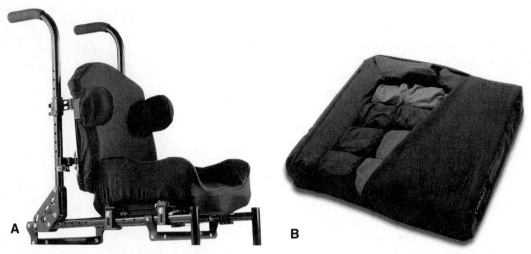

♦ **Figure 33-8**   Generic contour seating systems. **A**, Jay-fit adjustable contour system. **B**, ComforT cushion. (**A** *courtesy of Sunrise Medical;* **B** *courtesy of Otto Bock Health Care).*

(Fig. 33-9). Theoretically, when properly fabricated, the custom-molded system provides the greatest amount of pressure relief. The time and expense involved in the fabrication of custom-molded systems are considerable, and the molding process requires a great deal of skill. Production of the mold usually involves either a vacuum consolidation method or a chemical reaction of liquid foams injected into a special bag. Several varieties of custom-molded systems are available, including those that can be completed on site and those that are sent to a central fabrication center. Computer-aided design technology allows the clinician to bypass the making of molds by mapping and digitizing body shape data directly using an instrumented simulator. The information is then transferred via computer disk, fax, or modem to a computer-driven carving machine that produces the cushion. Custom-molded systems do not allow for growth and cannot be modified. Additionally, if a child is not positioned properly within the molded cushion, pressure spots can develop and cause breakdown of underlying soft tissue.

In summary, the general rule of thumb in selecting a system is that "less is better." If a child has no history of skin breakdown, can achieve independent pressure relief, and does not have significant positioning needs, a linear/planar seating system should be acceptable. However, if the child cannot maintain proper positioning with supports and has a history of skin breakdown, or is at risk for skin breakdown, a generic contour/modular seating system warrants consideration. Linear and generic contour systems can be changed and modified without great difficulty. The child with extensive positioning needs or who is high risk for skin breakdown may benefit from

a custom-molded seating system. The custom-molded systems are not adjustable or modifiable, so the clinicians must take into account growth and musculoskeletal changes that may occur. Often times a hybrid system is recommended. The hybrid seating system includes components from different categories; for instance, a planar seat with a generic contoured back, or a back that is custom molded exclusively along the paraspinal area and left flat on the periphery, which allows for the addition of adjustable lateral trunk supports.

PRESCRIPTION AND APPLICATION OF SEATING SYSTEMS

The scope of this chapter and the rapidly evolving nature of technology preclude a thorough discussion of all options and features of postural support systems. Many excellent resources provide detailed descriptions, problem-solving lists, and charts (Cook & Hussey, 1995, 2001; Galvin & Scherer, 1996; O'Sullivan & Schmitz, 2001). Regardless of the level of postural support required, there are several important considerations to keep in mind. In this section, some of the most salient points in the decision-making process are presented.

Seat Cushions

In most cases, the seat cushion is the most critical element of the seating system. The seat cushion will fall into the three previously mentioned categories: linear/planar, generic contour, or custom contour. The use of true planar seats is becoming less common because most therapists have found that a small amount of lateral contouring for even the highest-level sitter adds comfort

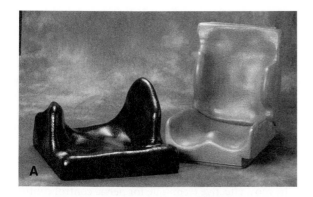

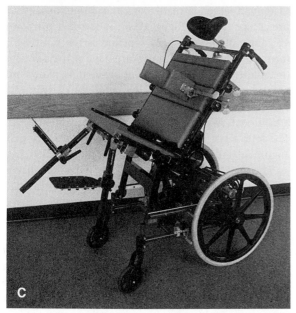

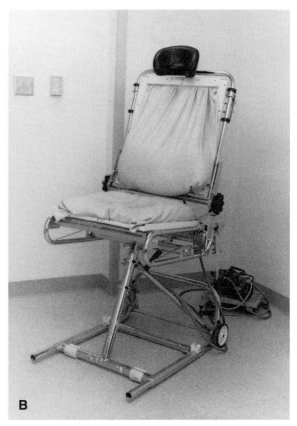

• **Figure 33-9**   Custom contoured seating systems. **A**, ProContour custom cushions. **B**, Commercially available seating simulator with adjustable angles shown with Contour-U (Invacare, Elyria, OH) vacuum-molding units for custom contoured seat and back inserts. **C**, Commercially available seating simulator with multiple adjustable components and angles. Shown mounted on a power mobility base that also allows assessment of driving ability and appropriate controls and switches. (**A** *courtesy of Otto Bock Health Care.*)

and stability (Bergen, 1992; Bergen et al., 1990). A number of commercially available air and gel pressure cushions have foam blocks and wedges to allow customization of cushion shape. Strategically placing commercial gel pads in a custom-made, contoured foam cushion can also supply that extra, critical amount of pressure relief needed by some children. In antithrust seats, a block of high-density foam placed just anterior to the ischial tuberosities prevents the pelvis from sliding forward and equalizes pressure distribution along the thighs (Siekman & Flanagan, 1983) (Fig. 33-10). Antithrust seats can be added to planar as well as contoured systems, but they are thought to work best with deep

lateral contours of the pelvis and lateral thigh supports (adductor pads).

Seat placement within the wheelchair frame is an important consideration. A thick cushion or inappropriate mounting hardware can place the seat too high, causing loss of independent transfers or wheeling, or can change the center of gravity to an unsafe position. Forward or backward placement, especially in very small children, can affect the knee angle required for foot placement on the footrests and can change the ease of wheeling by affecting access to the wheel rims or loading or unloading the front casters. For individuals who propel with their lower extremities, it is important to

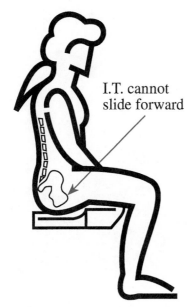

I.T. cannot
slide forward

♦ **Figure 33-10**   An antithrust seat can help hold the
pelvis back on the seat by blocking forward sliding of the
ischial tuberosities (I.T.). *(Redrawn with permission from
Bergen, AF, Presperin, J, & Tallman, T. Positioning for
Function: Wheelchairs and Other Assistive Technologies.
Valhalla, NY: Valhalla Rehabilitation Publications, 1990.)*

maintain a lower seat-to-floor height and a flat front edge
of the seat cushion. Often these individuals find it helpful
to relieve the pressure from the front edge of the seat to
allow full knee flexion without irritating the hamstrings.

Back Cushions

Back cushions also fall into three categories: linear/planar,
generic contour, and custom contoured. A back support
with a gently curved surface can improve lateral trunk
stability, posture, and comfort. Simple contouring and
lateral support can often be achieved within the integrity
of the back cushion by shaping the cushion. Many back
cushions are available with accompanying customized
support options. More aggressive contouring can be
achieved using blocks/wedges of high-density foam. A
custom-molded back should be used for children with
severe fixed spinal deformity. Some children who need
specific contact and support along the paraspinal muscles,
but are still growing, benefit from a hybrid back cushion.
The custom-molded back cushion contours along the
paraspinal region and flattens laterally. Linear lateral
trunk supports are then added to the contoured back. This
allows for growth and maintains support along the spine.
   Sagittal plane alignment of the spine has traditionally
been adjusted using lumbar rolls; however, control of
sagittal curves begins with the pelvis and sacrum rather

than the lumbar spine (Margolis, 1992; Margolis et al.,
1988). A "biangular back" has a vertical section behind
the pelvis, with the section above the pelvis angled back
a few degrees to encourage lumbar extension, or sacral
disks or pads can be added to the back surface. The child
must have sufficient range of motion and flexibility for
these adaptations to work. Over the long term, this type
of back cushion may increase lordosis, so it is imperative
to monitor spinal alignment.

Pelvic Stabilization

The most effective technique for pelvic control continues
to remain largely a matter of clinical opinion and user
preference (Reid & Rigby, 1996). A seat belt placed at a
45° angle at the seat-back junction is the most typical
form of pelvic stabilization. Placement of the belt across
the anterior thighs, just in front of the hips, allows more
natural active trunk and pelvic mobility (Bergen et al.,
1990). The pelvic positioning belt can use a two-point
attachment system or a four-point attachment system.
The four-point system allows for more control of pelvic
alignment and greater distribution of pressure.
   The subASIS bar is a form of rigid pelvic stabilization
consisting of a padded bar attached to plates lateral to
the pelvis (Margolis et al., 1988). The pelvis must be
maintained in a vertical orientation or the child will slide
under the bar. A less rigid variation is the semirigid pelvic
stabilizer (SRPS) (Carlson, 1987; Carlson & Grey, 1988)
(Fig. 33-11). Constructed of high-density foam mounted
on a reinforcing strip of thermoplastic splinting material,
the SRPS incorporates wedges that fit under the anterior
superior iliac spine while providing relief across the lower
abdomen. Like the subASIS bar, the SRPS provides direct
control of pelvis alignment, yet the angle of placement
can be varied, as with a seat belt, making it an option
for children with a mild fixed posterior pelvic tilt.
The flexibility of the SRPS may result in fewer pressure
problems than the subASIS bar, and it works especially
well for children who demonstrate a strong asymmetric
thrusting pattern.
   Dynamic pelvic stabilization uses individually
contoured pads that fit around the pelvis, with a pivot
mechanism allowing anterior-posterior tilting of the
pelvis without loss of stability (Noon et al., 1998).
Adjustments allow accommodation of deformity, control
of direction and amount of tilting, and a dynamic force to
return the pelvis to a neutral position.

Angles

There is no consensus as to the effects of seat and spatial
angles on alignment and function. Factors to consider in
determining seat angle include severity and nature of

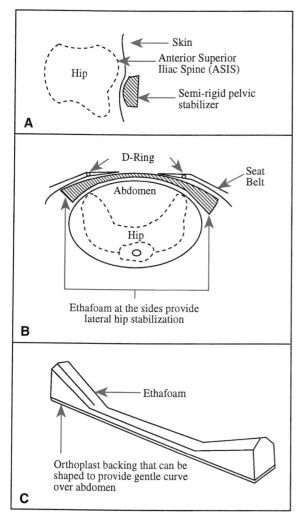

A

Skin
Anterior Superior
Iliac Spine (ASIS)
Hip
Semi-rigid pelvic
stabilizer

B

D-Ring
Seat
Belt
Abdomen
Hip
Ethafoam at the sides provide
lateral hip stabilization

C

Ethafoam
Orthoplast backing that can be
shaped to provide gentle curve
over abdomen

• **Figure 33-11**   Placement of the semirigid pelvic stabilizer from a side view (**A**) and from a top view (**B**). **C**, Detail of the stabilizer shape. *(Redrawn with permission from Carlson, SJ. The semi-rigid pelvic stabilizer for seating control. Assistive Devices Information Network Newsletter [University of Iowa, Iowa City, IA], 1[1]:2–3, 1987.)*

postural tone abnormalities, contractures, deformities; motor control of sitting; and design and purpose of the mobility base. Although the concept of upright 90-90-90 sitting, as previously discussed, is theoretically sound, it may not be an appropriate option for many children. Slight anterior wedging of the seat may improve head alignment or keep very young children from sliding. Opening the hip angle (tipping the front seat edge) may be necessary when hip extension contractures are present. Allowing the knees to flex reduces the rotation force on the pelvis, minimizing the effect of tight hamstrings.

A seat with an anterior tilt has potential benefits for children with hypoextensible lower extremity muscula-

ture but fair to good upper body control who "sacral sit" on a flat surface. A seat with an anterior tilt in a forward-lean position with a solid anterior chest support is also used for children with severe impairments. Good pelvic stabilization must be achieved to prevent sliding.

Variable seat-to-back angles allow adjustments of tilt and recline throughout the day. Tilt is useful for relief of pressure or relief of trunk or neck fatigue, and it provides a combination of active sitting and rest positions. When in a tilt system, the seat-to-back angle does not change. Recline is useful for relief of fatigue, for hip or back pain, and if catheterizations or other hygiene procedures must be performed in the chair. In a reclining seating system, the seat to back angle changes as the reclining position changes.

Dynamic or compliant seating systems are used for clients with severe and abrupt extensor spasms (Evans & Nelson, 1996; Orpwood, 1996). Often the severity of tone or spasms is exacerbated by the rigidity of a conventional system. Dynamic or compliant devices use hinges, pivot points, and springs to allow movement of the seat or back with the child and provide a gentle returning force. Clients who used these systems exhibited a decrease in the severity of spasms or fluctuating tone over a period of weeks as well as comfort, and ease of transfers were improved (Evans & Nelson, 1996; Orpwood, 1996)

Upholstery

Upholstery for the seat and back cushion can be made out of a variety of materials. When choosing a covering, consideration must be given to whether the child is incontinent, if the child is typically hot, and who will care for the coverings. Vinyl is a durable cushion covering; however, it can be hot and slippery and typically cannot be removed from the seating system. Synthetic knit fabrics with waterproof backing are also a popular choice of covering. They are less slippery, thus decreasing shear, and can be removable for easy cleaning. Ideally, a child should have at least two sets of cushion covers, thus allowing one to be laundered while using the other.

Front Riggings

Although a component of the mobility base, front riggings, or leg supports, are discussed in this section because of their direct influence on the entire seating system. Elevated leg rests are offset forward of the seat more than fixed leg rests and can contribute to forward sliding on the seat or poor positioning of the feet for weight bearing. Elevated leg rests should not be ordered unless specifically required. Choice of footrests on small, pediatric chairs can be especially difficult because they may interfere with caster action. Footplates that extend backward under the seat are helpful when clients have tight hamstrings. Footplates can be positioned parallel to the floor, or angled to match foot/ankle position. Shoe holders and foot straps hold the feet in the desired location to assist with lower body stability and weight bearing. For clients with deformity or limited joint movement, forcing the foot into neutral alignment on the footrest may impose undesirable stresses at the knees or hips (Bergen et al., 1990). Children who are able to make postural adjustments during weight shifting and actively place their feet should not have their feet constrained. If the child is able to transfer independently, learning to independently transfer, or assisted in a sit to stand transfer, the front riggings and footplates should swing out to the sides. The child whose seating system has tapered front riggings and a fixed footplate will transfer by either stepping over the footplates or stepping onto the footplates and then stepping down. Alternatively, children carefully lower themselves onto the footplate, and transfer from there.

Lateral and Medial Supports

Lateral trunk supports (or scoliosis pads) vary from simple, flat, padded blocks to contoured, wraparound supports. Swivel or swing-away mounting hardware allows the wraparound supports to fit properly, especially with varying seasonal clothing, and the child to transfer into and out of the seating system easily.

Contoured seats usually provide the most effective lateral thigh and pelvic support, as well as good pressure relief. Square or rectangular pads used as lateral thigh supports can maintain position of the legs and allow for growth. Medial thigh supports (abductor wedges or pommels) maintain hip alignment in neutral or slight abduction but do not stretch tight adductors or prevent forward sliding of the pelvis. Removable or swing-away pommels facilitate transfers and urinal or catheter use.

Anterior Supports

Anterior trunk supports are designed to maintain the spine erect and upright over the pelvis. Anterior support can be gained via an H or Y harness or anterior chest strap. Rigid shoulder retractors that project over the top of the backrest provide anterior shoulder control, but may be poorly tolerated. Butterfly-shaped straps should not be used as they present with extreme safety hazards. Padded axillary straps, sometimes known as Bobath straps or backback straps, also help maintain the trunk in an upright posture. They attach to the underside of the lateral thoracic support, are directed superiorly and medially over the front of the axilla, and attach at the top of the backrest, controlling shoulder protraction without

crossing the chest. Trefler and Angelo (1997) reported that the type of anterior chest supports used by children with CP did not influence performance on a switch activation task. They concluded that style of anterior chest support should be based on the child's preference.

Headrest

Facilitating good head position in children who have poor voluntary control is challenging. In children with limited postural control, poor head positioning can make an otherwise effective postural support system fail. On the other hand, barium swallow studies suggest that some clients with the most severe physical and cognitive impairments may need to adopt a forward-hanging head position to cope with increased oral secretions or reflux (Carlson & Ramsey, 1996). For such clients, supporting the head in a position that "looks good" may increase the risk of aspiration or choking (Carlson & Ramsey, 1996).

Support under the occiput provides better head support than a flat contact on the back of the head. Neck rings, two-step (with an occipital ledge), and contoured head supports are available in several options. Halos encircle the forehead and should always be used with caution, particularly during vehicular transport, because of the potential for neck injury. Static and dynamic forehead straps position and maintain the head secure on the headrest. Collars with a soft anterior chin support that are not attached to the wheelchair may be effective for the child who has constant neck flexion regardless of seating angles. Care must be taken that the head support does not unduly block the child's peripheral visual fields. Additionally, head supports can be the ideal mounting location for switches that control assistive technology or augmentative communication systems.

Upper Extremity Supports

Cutout trays are the most common type of upper extremity support and can be designed for a multitude of special purposes. Posterior elbow blocks help to reduce the tendency to retract the arms and maintain the upper extremities in a forward position. Clients with severe dystonia often prefer wrist or arm cuffs to reduce unwanted movement of one or both arms.

▌ WHEELED MOBILITY

The purpose of the mobility base is dependent on the child's level of function. For some, the primary purpose will be independent mobility, and the therapist/team must determine how best to achieve this. For others, the purpose of the base is to provide a means of being transported by a companion, and this must be accomplished in a comfortable and efficient manner. In either case, the base serves the additional role of supporting the seating system. Selection of a mobility base requires consideration of the seating system, the child's lifestyle, and the physical features of the environments in which the system will be used. Assessment for a new mobility base should ideally be done at the same time as assessment and simulation for the postural support system, because much of the same information regarding the child and the environment must be gathered.

RESEARCH ON MOBILITY

Excessive energy expenditure during locomotion is a common impairment of people with movement dysfunction. Persons with physical disability who walk with decreased speed and require an assistive device or who manually propel a wheelchair may prefer power mobility to reduce energy expenditure (Fisher & Gullickson, 1978). Children with CP were reported to walk at nearly half the velocity of children without disability and consume more oxygen per kilogram of body weight per minute when walking (Campbell & Ball, 1978). Buning and associates (2001) reported that individuals with severe mobility restrictions demonstrated a significant improvement in occupational performance, competence, adaptability, and self-esteem after transitioning to a power mobility device. Wheeled mobility is a more efficient mobility method than walking with braces and an assistive mobility device for children with myelomeningocele. Fifty percent of children with myelomeningocele who were ambulatory with braces stopped walking between ages 10 and 20 years (DeSouza & Carroll, 1976). Ambulation was 218% less energy efficient for children with myelomeningocele compared with children without disability. Children with muscle control at the L2 level or above expended energy equal to their maximal aerobic capacity when walking at slow speed, whereas children with muscle control at L3-L4 used 85% of their maximal aerobic capacity (Agre et al., 1987). In contrast, wheelchair propulsion required 42% less energy than crutch walking at the same speed. Oxygen consumption during wheelchair propulsion was only 9% greater than the oxygen consumption of children without disability during walking (Agre et al., 1987). Williams and associates (1983) also reported that during wheelchair propulsion energy expenditure and speed of mobility of children with myelomeningocele was efficient and fast as walking in children without disabilities. Fatigue associated with excessive energy expenditure during locomotion may adversely affect academic performance (Franks et al.,

1991). Academic performance (reading fluency, visual motor accuracy, and manual dexterity) was measured in three students attending middle school who alternately propelled their wheelchair or walked with assistive devices throughout the school day. Visual motor accuracy was significantly decreased for all three subjects when they walked. Manual dexterity decreased on days walked for one subject, and reading fluency did not change for any of the subjects.

Power mobility may increase social participation of children with CP who are unable to walk efficiency. Lepage and colleagues (1998) conducted a study of 98 children with all types of CP to determine the association between type of locomotion and the accomplishment of life habits, which included six activities of daily living and six social roles. Children who walked were reported to have fewer disruptions of life habits than children who used wheelchairs, with children who walked without assistive devices (walker, crutches, cane) reported to have the least disruption in four categories. The greatest disruption of life habits was found with children who used manual wheelchairs; children who used power wheelchairs showed somewhat less disruption in five of the life habit categories. Children using the manual wheelchair had more problems associated with CP such as visual and auditory impairments, epilepsy, and comprehension difficulties, which may contribute to why they did not use power mobility

Many factors affect the ability to manually propel a wheelchair, including physiologic capacities, such as strength and endurance, which are dependent on the user's diagnosis, age, sex, lifestyle, and build (Brubaker, 1986, 1988). The position of the individual within the wheelchair, particularly in relation to the handrims or other propulsion method, determines the mechanical advantage of the user to propel the chair. Wheelchair factors that affect mobility are rolling resistance, control, maneuverability, stability, and movement dynamics. These factors are dependent on the quality and construction of the wheelchair, such as weight, rigidity of the frame, wheel alignment, mass distribution, and suspension. Wheelchair propulsion in children with spinal cord injury was similar to that in a neurologically matched group of adults (Bednarczyk & Sanderson, 1994). The adults wheeled faster, but the children spent a similar proportion of the wheeling cycle in propulsion, and the angular changes in the kinematics of the elbow and shoulder over time were the same for both groups. Therefore, methods used to improve wheeling efficiency in adults may be applicable to children.

Self-mobility has important implications for development. The infant's experience with independent mobility impacts on perceptual, cognitive, emotional, and social processes (Kermoian, 1997). For children who lack mobility, early provision of mobility aids has the potential to enhance development of spatial, cognitive, affective, and social functions. Prone scooters, caster carts, and walkers are alternatives for some young children with functional upper extremities. For the child with more severe involvement, however, early power mobility offers the best choice and allows the child to increase his or her self-initiated movements during play (Deitz et al., 2002).

Historically, power mobility was considered a last option put off until children reached their teens, when all attempts at effective ambulation were exhausted. Power wheelchairs were considered too expensive and too difficult for young children to learn to drive, and walking was too important a goal to give up. Research does not support this perspective. Studies indicate that children as young as 24 months can successfully learn independent power mobility within a few weeks (Butler, 1986; Butler et al., 1983). Benefits attributed to the use of power mobility include an increase in self-initiated behaviors, including change in location, rate of interaction with objects, and frequency of communication (Berry et al., 1996; Butler, 1986). The benefits to social participation reported are increased peer interaction; increased interest in other forms of locomotion, including walking; increased family integration such as inclusion in outings; and decreased perception of helplessness by family members (Carlson & Myklebust, 2002; Schiaffino & Laux, 1986; Paulsson & Christoffersen, 1984; Verburg et al., 1984). Field (1999) concluded that the major issues affecting powered mobility performance are ability, technology features, environment, driving as an activity, and the interactions between these variables.

Instruction and training present an important consideration in making decisions about power mobility devices for children. Hasdai and colleagues (1998) used simulator programs to provide training to children and young adults ages 7 to 22. They determined that inexperienced drivers improved their overall driving performance after simulator training. The Internet is becoming a training site as well. The Oregon Research Institute has a public domain training program that is networked. A child can sign on to the site, chose the virtual reality device and environment, and race with other children on the network. The program records performance measures related to the child's driving ability. The virtual environment responds to the child's improving skills and the child is required to take interval skills assessments in order to continue using the program. The therapist and/or caregiver receive feedback about the child's performance.

The performance characteristics of the power base must be matched with the child's intended use, lifestyle, and comfort as part of the selection process. Deitz and colleagues (1991) studied the performance of children without disability on functional tasks while using four different power wheelchairs representing different designs, including a standard chair, a modular (all-terrain) base, a three-wheeled scooter, and the Turbo, a unique pediatric base with a power elevating seat (now called the Chairman, Jr by Permobil). Subjects were required to position themselves at a standard table, at a classroom desk, and at the blackboard. Access to the environment required the subjects to open a door, retrieve books from shelves, retrieve a book from the floor, turn on a water faucet, and turn on a light switch. Wheelchair maneuvering skills included U-turns, making left and right turns on a pathway, and speed and accuracy in straight driving. No chair was superior in all the tasks, although certain designs were advantageous for some tasks. The scooter and Turbo allowed positioning at the table and desk, respectively, whereas the other two bases did not. The Turbo offered the widest range of reaching; however, maneuverability was least for the Turbo and greatest for the conventional chair. When performance characteristics of conventional power chairs, all-terrain bases, three-wheelers, and children's all-terrain devices from six manufacturers were evaluated, results showed each chair to have advantages and disadvantages in straight driving speed, speed on a graded run with a 90° turn, curb jumps of varying thickness, and load pulling (Jones, 1988). An interdisciplinary U.S. Wheelchair Standards Committee, administered through RESNA and approved by the American National Standards Institute (ANSI), has completed a document on wheelchair standards. The standards represent a comprehensive approach to testing and disclosing information about wheelchairs. Manufacturers, suppliers, and consumers can use this information to improve their products, select chairs with the best performance for the cost, and identify chairs that meet specific performance needs. Thacker and colleagues (1994) have written a useful manual detailing the engineering and technical features of each component on the wheelchair, from frame construction, to caster bearings, to drive trains and batteries.

SELECTION OF A MOBILITY BASE

The goal in selecting a mobility base is to provide an appropriate means of getting from one location to another efficiently. It is inappropriate to require someone to rely on his or her everyday mobility for exercise.

Prohibiting the use of a manual wheelchair for a child with marginal ambulation, or that of a power wheelchair for a child with marginal manual wheelchair skills, places their functional and academic performance at risk due to excessive energy expenditure. A creative and structured fitness program is a more appropriate way of addressing strength and cardiovascular endurance goals.

It is generally agreed that the child's positioning needs are the most important factor when selecting a mobility system. At the same time, the design of the seating system should maximize potential for independent function in the wheelchair. This, in turn, influences chair modifications and the interface hardware needed. For example, if a 3-inch modular composite foam cushion is necessary for pressure relief, yet the child has short extremities as in myelodysplasia, both independent transfers and wheeling will be more difficult. A possible solution is to order a chair frame with a lower seat height and without upholstery so that drop brackets can be used to lower the cushion between the seat rails.

To assess driving skills and controller placement, seating simulators can be mounted on a power base. A remote, attendant-held control can override the user's control, ensuring safety and appropriate feedback during assessment and training. The child should be provided the opportunity to test a variety of bases with appropriately simulated postural support.

The first step in selecting a mobility base is to determine what type of functional mobility is desired. Three general types of mobility bases include companion chairs for dependent wheeling, standard manual wheelchairs, and power wheelchairs. Ideally, the selection is based on the potential level of independent mobility. Other considerations include methods of transportation, type of housing, availability of training or supervision, and availability of funding.

The second consideration is the style of the base. Within each type, there are several styles with different features and performance characteristics. Factors that influence this choice are the level and type of seating system required, the level of independence in other skills such as transfers and activities of daily living, the specific environments in which the chair will be used, the method of transportation, and the needs of caregivers.

The size of the mobility is based on the child's physical size, expected growth, the capability of the chair to accommodate growth, and the size and style of the seating system. Mobility bases designed for children are available in a variety of sizes and designs. The ability of mobility bases to expand and accommodate physical growth has improved as funding sources have demanded longer life from purchased items.

The final consideration is the model and manufacturer of the chair. Often the finer details of construction are important at this stage, such as the proportions of the chair, angles, orientations, adjustability of parts such as footrests and armrests, and swing-away, detachment, or folding mechanisms. Other important factors are performance characteristics, styling, comfort, durability, availability of parts, service record, and cost. Regional preferences for various models and manufacturers are evident across North America.

Companion Wheelchairs

Companion wheelchairs, transporter chairs, and dependent mobility bases (Fig. 33-12) are intended for individuals who will not need to access the wheels for independent mobility, including those with the most severe impairments and very young children. In other cases, this type of chair may be used as backup transportation for a child who ambulates or uses a power wheelchair. Many styles of companion wheelchairs exist, and occasionally manual wheelchairs are used as companion chairs. Companion chairs often include firm seats and backs and have a wide variety of positioning components as options. Alternatively, contoured or custom-molded seating systems can be fabricated and mounted on these frames. Some of these chairs can be used as vehicular transport seats and comply with federal safety standards. Others are designed for very young children and look and perform like a stroller.

When choosing a dependent mobility base, primary caregivers must be considered users as well as the child. Attention should be given to caregiver comfort and ease of use, including push handle height, rolling resistance, maneuverability, and ease of disassembly and transport. Parents of young children who are receiving their first mobility base and seating system may be very sensitive to the need for a wheelchair. Mobility bases that look like a stroller are popular and are often much less threatening. Some funding sources deny stroller bases because of their limitations in growth and ability to be adapted if the child's independent capabilities progress.

Manual tilt and recline features are incorporated into many companion chairs. A fixed angle of tilt or recline can be useful when designing the seating system for some clients. For others, the ability to vary the amount of tilt or recline throughout the day is critical for prevention of pressure sores, fatigue, and discomfort. New technology replaces the tilt system with a rotational system. The rotational system pivots around a single axis, reducing movement and shearing. The rotational system has a lower center of gravity, creating a more stable system when the child is not upright.

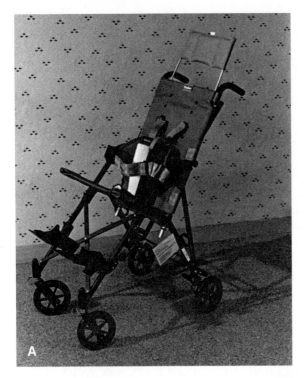

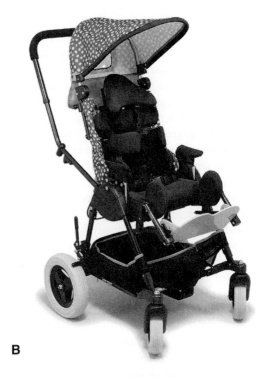

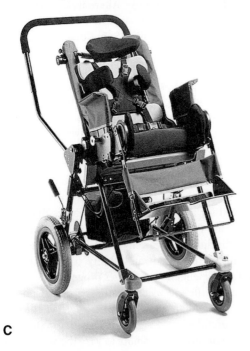

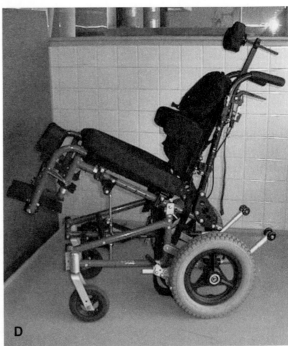

+ **Figure 33-12** Companion or transporter chairs. **A**, Collapsible stroller base. Stroller base with removable modular seating system Kid Kart XPress (**B**) and Kid Kart TLC (**C**). **D**, Manual wheelchair-style base with smaller rear wheels, stroller handles, and tilt mechanism. (**B** and **C** *courtesy of Sunrise Medical.*)

Manual Wheelchairs

The standard manual wheelchair has two large wheels, usually in back, for independent propulsion, and two small swiveling casters in front. Manual wheelchairs are often chosen as dependent mobility bases as well because of their ability to accept custom-designed seating systems, ease of use, and tilt and recline options (Fig. 33-13). For independent propellers, the 1980s and 1990s were the "new age" of manual wheelchairs when lightweight chairs and chairs designed for recreational use and athletic competition became widely available. Lightweight and durable metals and fabrics, alternative wheel placement, improved frame proportions and designs, adjustability, and adaptability to custom seating have all helped streamline the manual wheelchair to improve efficiency and control, ease of transfer, portability, and appearance. Lightweight chairs with the large wheels in front are much easier for young children to propel for short distances indoors. For the very active person, ultra-lightweight, high-performance chairs incorporate rigid frames and high-quality bearings for optimal performance. The serious athlete can find specialized designs dedicated to specific performance needs that barely resemble the traditional concept of a wheelchair.

One-arm-drive wheelchairs are designed for individuals with functional limitation in one arm that prevents bimanual propulsion (Fig. 33-14). The classic style is the

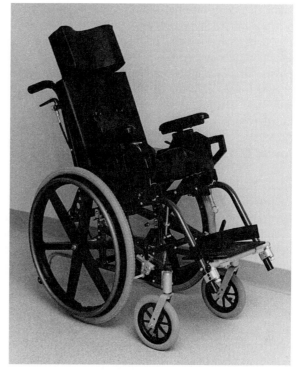

◆ **Figure 33-13**   Standard lightweight manual wheelchair with manual tilt mechanism, shown with a contoured seating system.

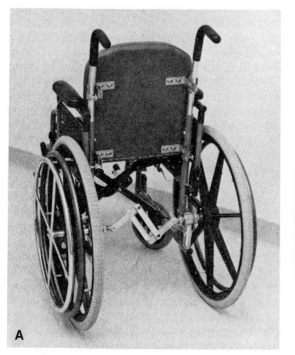

A

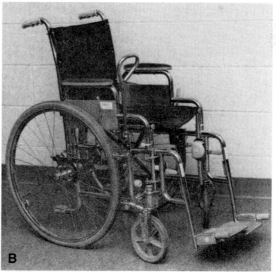

B

◆ **Figure 33-14**   One-arm drive manual wheelchair.

double-handrim on one side, with a linkage system to the other wheel. Styles that use a pumping action with a lever and ratchet system, although rarely used now, are generally easier and more efficient for both wheeling and steering but create more problems in dependent wheeling by caregivers. Operation of a one-arm-drive chair may exacerbate existing asymmetry in children with tonal disorders such as CP.

Power Mobility

Hays (1988) described four categories of function in children using power mobility. The first category includes children who do not walk or have a means of independent mobility other than use of a power device. The second category includes children with inefficient mobility, that is, they walk or use a manual wheelchair but with unacceptable functional speed or endurance. The third category includes children who have lost independent mobility through disease, brain injury, or spinal cord trauma. For this group, the developmental implications of independent mobility may be less important, but the acceptance of assisted mobility is a significant issue. The fourth category includes children

who require assisted mobility temporarily. This includes young children who are expected to walk as they get older, children who are recovering from surgery, and children who are recovering from an injury or trauma such as a head injury.

Advances in technology, over the past decade, have brought independent power mobility to a greater number of individuals with severe disabilities than ever before. A wide variety of power bases and options are available, with more reliable and precise controls than ever before possible. The three main types of power wheelchairs are the conventional design with integral seat and chassis (evolved from the traditional, tubular manual wheelchair frame), the powerbase or modular design with separate seat and chassis (often called an all-terrain wheelchair), and scooters with either three- or four-wheeled platforms (Fig. 33-15). Power chairs may be ordered with seats that tilt, backs that recline, units that recline and tilt, leg rests that elevate, and headrests that adjust, all with the touch of a switch. Manufacturers have responded to an increased demand for pediatric-sized power wheelchairs by producing wheelchairs that are lighter in weight, correctly proportioned for children, and have growth

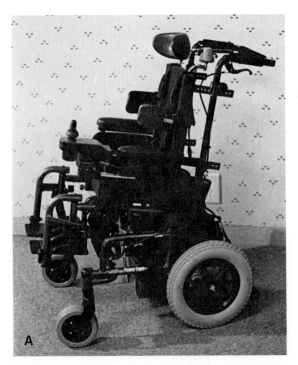

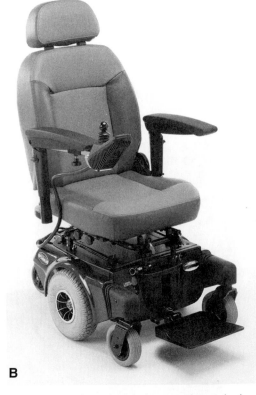

A   **B**

♦ **Figure 33-15** Power wheelchairs. **A**, Typical, pediatric-sized, rear-wheel, direct-drive model, shown with standard armrest-mounted proportional control. **B**, Freestyle midwheel drive power system. (**B** *courtesy of Sunrise Medical.*)

capabilities. Major advances in electronics have produced a greater variety of controls that are easier to access, more durable, and easier to adjust and customize. Power chairs are available in rear wheel, midwheel, or front wheel drive options. The rear wheel drive is the most common style. The front wheel drive allows the user a tighter turning radius.

The style of power mobility base chosen will depend in part on the child's upper body control. Scooters are steered using a tiller that requires good sitting balance and arm active range of motion. The control functions are usually mounted on the tiller and require a grip type action of the thumb or fingers. Jones (1990) described a range of scooters from "light duty mall crawlers to heavy duty barnyard rut jumpers." Scooters are easier to dismantle and transport in the trunk of a car and look least like a wheelchair. Although they remain popular among adults, funding is often denied based on their limited indoor mobility and poor vehicle tie-down capabilities. Manufacturers have responded by making them more rugged and suited to outdoor use. Whereas wheelchair bases are generally easy to adapt to a seating system, seating systems for scooters have limited adjustability and adaptability.

The conventional and powerbase designs offer the greatest range of seating and control options. The entire seating unit can be removed from the pedestal mount of the modular base. The traditional belt-driven chair is obsolete; the direct-drive motors improve power, as well as control in turning. Front-, mid-, and rear-wheel drive offer different advantages and disadvantages in stability while driving and stopping, stability during recline or tilt, maneuverability in tight spaces, and ability to climb curbs. The type of power wheelchair for a child must be as carefully selected as any other component of the wheelchair and seating system.

Power recline and power tilt capabilities offer excellent alternatives for children who require position changes throughout a long day of sitting to perform different functions or to prevent pain, fatigue, or pressure sores. The act of reclining, however, causes shearing of tissues due to the disproportionate movement between the child and the seating system. On returning to the upright position, most clients will have shifted position in the system, and the more complex the seating system, the more significant the effects. Power recliners are available in low-shear and zero-shear models to help address these problems. Power tilt in space models work well for children with severe hypertonia or contractures who cannot tolerate having the seat-to-back angle opened up or who, once having done so, cannot return to an upright position without significant sliding.

Controls for power wheelchairs are available in two basic types: proportional and latched. The former has a proportional relationship between movement of the joystick and speed of the chair or sharpness of turning, whereas the latter has an on/off relationship to chair movement. The proportional control is the standard joystick found on most power wheelchairs. It is customarily mounted on either armrest and will move in a 360° arc. The movement of the joystick controls the speed and the direction of the wheelchair. An alternative to the standard joystick is a remote proportional joystick that is smaller and more compact. This feature allows a great deal of flexibility for joystick placement, provided sturdy mounting hardware is used. Proportional joysticks are also available in short-throw models that require less movement and force for activation and in heavy-duty models that can withstand a great deal of force. Head control joysticks are available for some wheelchairs (Fig. 33-16).

A latched microswitch control system consists of four separate switches, with each switch controlling one

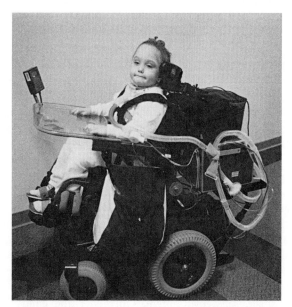

◆ **Figure 33-16** This child with a C4 spinal cord injury is learning to drive her power wheelchair with a proximity switch head array. The chair is equipped with power tilt for frequent pressure relief, low-shear power recline to allow catheterization procedures without a transfer, a swivel-mounted ventilator, and a suction machine tray that remains horizontal during tilt and recline. She is able to activate all driving and position functions, as well as access her computer, through the head array. The monitor to the right of her tray indicates which function mode she has chosen with the head switch.

direction—forward, reverse, left, and right. All four switches might be in one control box (resembling a standard proportional control) or assembled into a smaller, more compact, remote control. Microswitches are also available in heavy-duty and short-throw models, as are the proportional controls. Microswitches are somewhat more flexible for assessment purposes. For example, they may be separated and set up in arrays to evaluate head control, or each of the four switches may be positioned at different body sites. The wafer board and arm-slot control are examples of microswitch technology. Microswitch-driven chairs tend to be less precise and smooth while turning and changing directions because each direction is controlled by a separate switch.

With the recognition that age is no longer the determining factor in successful use of power mobility has come the need to define appropriate selection criteria. Schiaffino and Laux (1986) reported that children need a cognitive level of at least 2 years of age, although these children would take longer to train than children with cognitive skills at the 3-year level or above. More recently, transitional mobility programs are being developed for children as young as 12 to 14 months (Wright-Ott, 1997). Barnes (1991) described a "motoric language" needed to learn to drive a powered chair that includes relational vocabulary (in, on, under), substantive vocabulary (nouns), directionality (forward, backward, right, left), perceptual concepts (visual and auditory feedback with switch activation), spatial concepts (depth perception, location of self in an environment, and problem solving to avoid obstacles), and serial or sequential concepts (first, second; before, after).

An alternative perspective is that children may learn spatial relationships implicitly through training in a power device. Kangas (1997) provides a compelling argument for power mobility assessment for very young children based on the need for assistive mobility in any or all environments rather than "readiness for driving" skills. She suggests that the child be allowed to explore movement in the device over a period of many sessions, by first being restricted to a single turning direction in a small, safe environment. Only after the child has experienced moving, and stopping for the sake of being able to move again, has she experienced mobility, without regard for direction or purpose. This parallels the development of independent walking in toddlers. The child is never praised for "good driving" because this is meaningless to her. As the child's control over mobility expands, and the verbal labels for what she is doing are provided, the concepts described previously will develop. Power toys that are available at local toy stores make an excellent inexpensive alternative for power training of young children when the devices can be suitably adapted for seating and control.

Simulators have been proved to be successful train tools. Hasdai and colleagues (1998) found that inexperienced drivers given simulator driving experience improved their accuracy and performance. Newer virtual reality technology has allowed video gaming experiences to become wheelchair driver training experiences (Reid, 2002; Oregon Research Institute, 2003).

Oregon Research Institute/Applied Computer Simulation Labs has developed a virtual wheelchair mobility training course. Training environments were designed to help children learn to drive a powered wheelchair safely. Three-dimensional (3-D) computer gaming technology provides virtual reality environments in which students can practice driving with the use of an appropriately chosen joystick/input method. Additionally, data on the students driving performance are recorded. As the child's ability improves, the training environments become progressively more challenging. Internet connectivity allows the student to share training environments with others signed onto the system (Oregon Research Institute, 2003).

Galka and Lombard (1992) described functional criteria for safe driving, including the ability to turn the chair on and off, follow a straight course, turn both left and right, back the chair up, maneuver around objects and persons, and stop quickly. The "marginal driver" is one of any age who may show borderline cognitive or physical skills or whose visual-perceptual problems interfere with driving ability. With supervision, these individuals may do well driving in a very specific setting, such as their school, but are not successful in novel or unpredictable community settings. The value of a power chair in increasing self-esteem and promoting independence in specific skills must be carefully weighed against the expense and amount of training and supervision required.

Several practical considerations are unique to selection of power mobility. Building accessibility and space will affect where and how the device is used. Often the power chair is kept and maintained at school and a manual base is used at home. Care and maintenance of the power chair is more complex than for manual systems. Transportation is also a more complicated issue. Some school districts refuse to transport certain types of power wheelchairs, such as scooters. The family may need a van for transporting the chair, and a ramp or a lift may be required for loading and unloading. Funding options for more expensive power wheelchairs may be more restrictive. Usually, a backup manual chair is also required, especially during maintenance or repair of the power system. Responsibility for supervision, training, and routine wheelchair care should be determined prior to ordering the system.

The evaluation process for a power mobility system is often more complicated than for other types of wheelchairs. First, a variety of power bases should be available for trial and preferably with capabilities to adjust speed, acceleration, deceleration, turning speed, sensitivity, and tremor-dampening of the joystick. Children generally perform better in a pediatric-sized wheelchair rather than an adult-sized wheelchair. Because proper support is critical to performance in a power wheelchair, the therapist needs access to a variety of seating components, supports, and straps to provide the stability that is necessary to optimize the child's motor function for operating the controls. A variety of controls and mounting options should be available for trial. Evaluation may take place over a period of several days to weeks, and ideally in a variety of settings, especially for young and inexperienced drivers, who may require much practice with different options before reaching a final decision.

A standard proportional control mounted on the armrest should be the first option the therapist evaluates if a child is found to have reasonable upper extremity control. This is the simplest and least expensive control. If a more midline position of the joystick is desired, placement of the control bracket on the inside of the wheelchair armrest is relatively easy.

Site options for the control increase with the use of a remote joystick and the proper hardware. Some possibilities include center mounting of the joystick close to the user to compensate for decreased range of motion or strength, mounting the joystick at arm's length on top of a lap tray to provide support and increased stability when dyskinetic movements or fluctuating muscle tone is present, or mounting the joystick for chin or foot operation. For children with limited functional movements and site options, an integrated control permits operation not only of the wheelchair but also of other equipment such as a communication aid, electronic aid to daily living, or computer equipment.

TRANSPORTATION SAFETY

The U.S. society is generally mobile and on the go. This includes children and adults who use wheeled mobility. In recent years RESNA and ANSI have set federal standards for using wheelchairs within vehicle transportation. Best practice dictates that, when at all possible, wheelchair users should transfer out of their wheelchair and into an age- or weight-appropriate vehicle seat and occupant restraint system that meets all the federal safety standards. The wheelchair should be stored and secured within the vehicle to prevent it from becoming a harmful projectile.

If the occupant cannot transfer, a seating system is required that can be attached to a transit wheelchair frame. Transport wheelchairs meet ANSI/RESNA/WC19 standards, have been frontal crash tested, and have several advantageous features for use in vehicular transport compared with standard wheelchairs. A WC19 transport wheelchair can be secured at four identifiable and crash-tested sites located on the floor of the vehicle, in less than 10 seconds per site, from areas accessible from one side of the wheelchair in enclosed space. Transit wheelchairs have crashworthy frames, smooth hardware edges, improved battery retention, better accommodation of vehicle anchored belts, and proper instructions for use as a seat in a motor vehicle. It is imperative that the wheelchair and occupant face toward the front of the vehicle.

WC19 also set standards for lateral stability of a wheelchair in a forward-moving vehicle. This is due to the fact that wheelchair users are often injured when the wheelchair tips after a quick stop or sharp turn in a noncrash situation. Effective May 2002, regulations allow that a wheelchair occupant can use a crashworthy pelvic belt secured to the wheelchair frame, in which a separate vehicle-mounted shoulder belt could be inserted. This configuration may allow restraint systems to fit more securely.

If the occupant cannot transfer and cannot use the transport wheelchair, a wheelchair with a metal frame should be used with a Wheelchair Tiedown and Occupant Restraint System (WTORS). Restraint systems that meet WTORS standards will be labeled as SAE J2249. Four tie-down straps are attached to strong places on the wheelchair frame such as the welded frame joints. Attachment points should be as high as possible but below the seat surface. Rear tie down straps should maintain a 30° to 45° angle with the vehicle floor.

Wheelchair occupants should ride in an upright position with back reclined less than 30°. The headrest should be positioned to support the head and neck, and trays should be removed and secured.

The four-point tiedown system is considered as the universal system. When used properly, the four-point system is effective and affordable. Tiedown straps should meet SAE J2249 standards.

Just as the wheelchair frame needs to be secured to the vehicle, the occupant needs to be secured with crashworthy lap and shoulder safety belts. Standard positioning belts and harnesses are not meant to restrain an occupant in a vehicle crash. Currently most lap and shoulder belts anchor to the vehicle independent of the wheelchair user. Newer models of WC19 wheelchairs have crash for the occupant restraints mounted directly to the frame and allow the vehicle mounted shoulder belts to attach directly to the lap belt (Safe Transport Program, 2004).

EXAMINATION AND EVALUATION FOR ASSISTIVE TECHNOLOGY OTHER THAN SEATING AND MOBILITY

Assistive technologies offer children with motor or cognitive impairments an opportunity to participate more fully and become more independent in their daily lives. In addition to manual or powered mobility and specialized seating, these technologies include specialized switches, communication devices, computers, and electronic aids to daily living. Often the term *assistive technology* is used specifically to designate these latter four types of electric or electronic devices, although the Tech Act and RESNA include all forms of mobility, positioning, and related devices in the definition of assistive technology. The assessment and selection process for each of these types of assistive technology tends to be similar.

The physical therapist, as a member of the assistive technology team, is responsible for completing the physical skills examination needed for technology use. Before evaluation for use of assistive technology, a child who is nonambulatory should have a mobility device and be well positioned to minimize the effects of abnormal muscle tone, weakness, and pathologic movement patterns that interfere with controlled movement and function. Regardless of impairment or functional limitations, all children should be well positioned prior to completing an AT device evaluation. Proper positioning is essential for reducing fatigue, optimal control of head, trunk, and upper extremity movements, and selection of appropriate AT devices and services. A comprehensive physical examination includes range of motion, muscle strength, muscle tone, endurance, and gross and fine motor abilities. The therapist also examines righting and equilibrium reactions and notes the presence of primitive reflexes. These data provide the team with information concerning a child's functional motor abilities such as head and trunk control, the variety and quality of active movements, and the ability to isolate one movement from another. For successful technology use, these functional movements must be voluntary, reliable, repeatable, and in some cases sustainable. The movement patterns should not contribute to fatigue or pain, nor should they elicit pathologic reflexes or increase postural tone (Cook & Hussey, 1995; Dickey & Shealy, 1987; Stowers et al., 1987, O'Sullivan & Schmitz, 2001).

Collaboration among health professionals and agencies is vital to avoid duplication of services and unnecessary expense to families and third-party payers. Recent examinations by the child's physical therapist can be shared with a consulting assistive technology team. A detailed written report, a videotape or still pictures, a telemedicine videoconference, and participation of the child's physical therapist in the examination process are examples of different ways in which recommendations for positioning can be shared.

The physical therapist, along with the other team members, contributes information regarding the child's sensory, perceptual-motor, and cognitive abilities. Sensory skills needed for successful AT device use include visual and auditory discrimination and responses to tactile, kinesthetic, and proprioceptive input. Visual acuity allows a youngster to focus sharply on an image such as a switch, joystick, or computer screen, and visual accommodation allows the eyes to adjust to near and far objects. Limitations in visual field necessitate placement of controls or displays within the functional visual range of the child. Tracking is the ability to follow a moving object with the eyes, and scanning is when the eyes move to find an object, necessary skills for successful computer use. Hearing impairments compromise a child's ability to receive auditory information, as well as to produce and monitor speech output (Cook & Hussey, 2001). After members of the assistive technology team are aware of how a child processes sensory information, they are able to select devices that are highly motivating and ensure success. Children tend to learn to use devices that provide a variety of sensory cues more quickly than devices that do not. Auditory clicks or beeps, visual light displays, and tactile and proprioceptive cues such as textured or vibrating switches can be highly motivating.

Knowledge of a child's cognitive function and learning style are important for selection of appropriate access, feedback, application, and training with the various devices. During the assessment, the team directly observes a child's attention span; short-term memory; understanding of cause and effect; ability to follow directions, sequence, and problem solve; and intention and motivation for technology use (Swinth, 1996). Whenever possible, the child should participate in the decision-making process. This may be as simple as picking the color of his mobility device, cushion covers, or switches. In other words, the saying, "Nothing about me without me" (Vaccarella, 2001) should be heeded to by the team.

SWITCHES, CONTROLS, AND ACCESS SITES

Children with motor impairments may require special switches or controls to operate communication aids, computers, power wheelchairs, or electronic aids to daily living (EADLs). Switches are also called *control interfaces* and *input devices,* and practitioners who specialize in this area are referred to as *interface specialists.* Switch technology can help teach cause and effect, encourage independent play, promote group participation, and give a child control over a part of his or her environment. A child who does not have to depend on others is less likely to develop learned helplessness or disruptive behaviors (Angelo, 1997).

Typically an access site (a body part that can produce a consistent movement) is selected first and then the switch or control to operate a device is chosen. If a child has purposeful, controlled movement of any body part, the team can identify a suitable switch site. A variety of switches and controls are available from manufacturers who specialize in technologic aids for people with special needs. They vary in size, shape, cost, performance capabilities, and ways in which they are activated. Switches may be single (perform an on/off function), dual (perform on/off and a select function), or multiple (perform on/off and several functions). Examples of multiple-switch configurations are joysticks, wafer boards, slot controls, head arrays, and keyboards. Methods for activating switches include air pressure, light, magnetic fields, sound waves, and physical contact (Mann & Lane, 1995). Switches also have a wide array of activation modes including simultaneous, timed, latched, or proportional (Sullivan & Lewis, 2000).

As young as 6 months, children are capable of using hand or head switches for computer access (Sullivan & Lewis, 2000; Swinth et al., 1993). Using the hands to activate switches is the typical mode for most children; however, switches can be operated by other body parts such as the head, chin, tongue, eyebrows, elbows, or lower extremities. At times, children will require additional support or extension devices to use a switch or control such as a head or chin pointer, a mouth stick, finger or hand splints, styluses, mobile arm supports, or overhead slings (Fig. 33-17).

Some switches have been specially designed to use with a certain body part, such as an eyebrow switch, an eye blink switch, or a tongue touch keypad. Proximity switches will activate when a user gets near the switch, but actual physical contact is not required. A practical application of this technology is to imbed four proximity switches (one each for forward, reverse, right, and left) in an acrylic tray to operate a power wheelchair. Heavy-duty contact switches may be the most suitable choice for children with fluctuating muscle tone who have difficulty controlling the force of their movements, and tiny fiberoptic switches may be suitable for the user with very limited range and strength. At one spinal cord treatment facility, switch evaluations are performed at bedside as soon as the patient is stable. Functional movements are examined, including use of tongue, lips, eyes, eyelids, eyebrows, and jaw (Mitchell, 1995). Persons with high-level spinal cord injuries often use pneumatic breath control switches to operate assistive technology devices, and many find that integrated controls provide them with access to several types of technology.

An integrated control is one that controls several devices and may be the best choice for individuals who

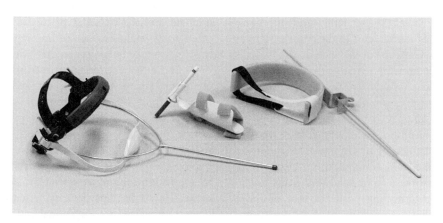

♦ **Figure 33-17** Devices for pointing or indicating that may be used with communication aids or electronic aids to daily living. *From left to right:* Chin pointer, thermoplastic hand splint with stylus, headstick.

use a variety of assistive technology devices. For example, a power wheelchair joystick can be designed as an integrated control that will also operate a communication device, computer equipment, or environmental controls. Guidelines to determine when an integrated control is the optimal choice include the following: when a user has a single reliable access site; if the access method is the same for all devices used; when speed, accuracy, or endurance is improved; and the child's or family's personal preference (Guerette & Sumi, 1994). There are also disadvantages to using integrated controls, including the higher cost of more sophisticated electronics required to perform several functions. Because the user is able to operate only one device at a time with the control, he or she will lose all functions if the controller breaks down and repairs are needed.

AUGMENTATIVE AND ALTERNATIVE COMMUNICATION

In addition to spoken or verbal output, communication includes body language, gestures, facial expressions, and written output. Speech impairments in children may occur as a result of congenital or acquired dysarthria, developmental apraxia, developmental aphasia, congenital anomalies, mental retardation, autism, or deafness (O'Sullivan & Schmitz, 2001). When the ability to communicate and interact is not functional, some form of augmentative or alternative communication (AAC) should be explored. *Augmentative communication* is any procedure or device that facilitates speech or spoken language. *Alternative communication* refers to the communication method used by a person without vocal ability (Accardo & Whitman, 2002). Ultimately, AAC should enable individuals to efficiently and effectively engage in a variety of interactions in their world (Galvin & Scherer, 1996). Users of AAC include individuals with cognitive limitations, individuals requiring written augmentation, and individuals with a temporary limitation in expression due to illness or injury.

The speech and language pathologist, along with the child and family members, assume the lead roles in identifying the best choice for an AAC system. In addition to contributing to the team examination and evaluation, the physical therapist plays an important ongoing role in the classroom in determining positions that optimize use of equipment for communication. Many classrooms contain a variety of chairs, corner chairs, prone or supine standers, and sidelyers, which typically require adjust-

ment or adaptation for a particular child. The physical therapist provides instruction to other team members in the proper use of positioning devices that enhance a child's communication. Therapists working in early intervention are in a unique position to influence development of effective communication skills in infants and young children. Attermeier (1987) encourages therapists to establish intervention goals that include developing head control, developing the ability to separate head and neck movements from eye movements, allowing the child to make choices, developing a method of indicating needs, and encouraging family members to talk to and read to their youngsters.

A number of techniques and devices for augmenting communication are available and classified as "high-tech" and "low-tech." Low-tech equipment includes devices that are powered by batteries or electricity or nothing at all. High-tech equipment includes devices with adapted computers and switching systems (O'Sullivan & Schmitz, 2001). Unaided techniques such as eye gaze, signing, or gesturing do not require external devices or equipment but rely on the child's ability to physically respond in some consistent manner. Aided techniques include the use of an external device, which may or may not be electronic. A communication sheet or notebook (with pictures, symbols, or words) is an example of a nonelectronic aid device.

Electronic communication aids offer a much greater range of capabilities and options for users, and as the capabilities of the devices increase, so do the costs. Simple devices may run less than $100; high-end devices cost several thousand dollars. One inexpensive aid is a tape recorder equipped with a loop tape message that repeats each time the switch is activated. This device may be a good starting place when assessing young children for augmentative communication because it is inexpensive and can be readily adapted with different switches mounted at various access sites. Some low-cost durable devices play a single message or series of messages, whereas others offer four, eight, or more messages. Generally, the messages can be quickly changed as desired.

At the other end of the spectrum are sophisticated, computer-driven AAC devices that allow a variety of input methods (direct, scanning, or coded), high-quality voice output, storage capability for vocabulary and phrases, printouts, and the capability to run a computer or EADL through the communication device (Fig. 33-18). Laptop computers with speech capabilities have multiple functions in addition to the ability to augment communication. Third-party payers may deny funding for laptops if they are viewed as educational equipment that should be provided by the student's local education agency. New devices are continually evolving that are more compact,

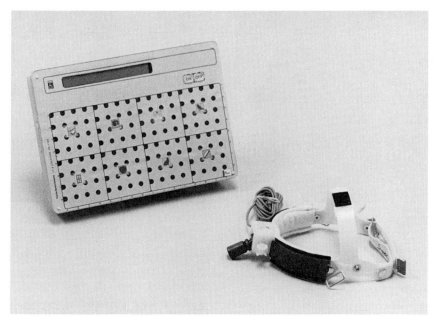

♦ **Figure 33-18**   This electronic communication device may be directly operated with an optical headpointer. Many other selection techniques are also possible, including row and column scanning, two-switch scanning, and joystick use.

durable, lighter in weight, and easier to transport. Operation and programming of newer AAC devices has simplified over time. Given the ever-expanding variety of AAC devices available, the assistive technology team should be able to identify a device that meets the motor and cognitive abilities of each child.

The input, or selection, method for AAC devices and computers typically includes direct select or scanning. Direct selection is faster and, thus, the preferred method to operate a communication system. Children with mild to moderate impairments often have sufficient motor control for direct selection. The child simply makes a choice from the options presented. For example, when a child touches a location on a communication device with a picture of a glass, the spoken response might be, "May I have a drink please?"

Children with severe motor impairment may need to rely on scanning to operate their AAC or computer. The device runs through a sequence of choices (usually rows, then columns), repeating the sequence until the user makes a selection. The scanning rate is adjustable, which allows beginners ample time to become familiar with the new equipment and to build confidence and accuracy before increasing the speed. In most cases the selection is made by using a special switch positioned to allow independent access. Examples include a pressure switch mounted on a laptray and activated with the touch of the hand, a lever switch positioned near the side of the head

and operated with lateral head movements, and a chin switch mounted on a collar and operated by flexion and extension movements of the head. Scanning can be both motorically and cognitively demanding for some users because they must be able to wait for the appropriate selection, activate the switch at the right moment, release the switch, and repeat these steps for the next selection.

COMPUTER TECHNOLOGY

Computers are typically used for word processing to compose and edit the written word, data collection and storage, graphics for drawing and publishing, communication via e-mail and the Internet, and various educational and recreational activities. A computer may be operated through a keyboard, the mouse, or both. Computers, as well as many computer-based devices such as communication aids, environmental controls, and power mobility controllers, are readily adaptable and can be customized as needed. Hundreds of products are commercially available to adapt a computer for an individual with special needs. This variety is important for users whose needs may change. Input to computers and communication devices can be direct or indirect (scanning or Morse code), with direct access being faster and generally more intuitive.

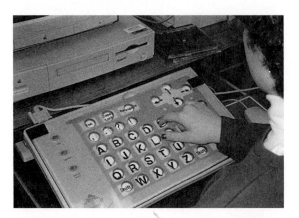

◆ **Figure 33-19** A keyshield or keyguard placed over a modified keyboard can eliminate unwanted keystrokes for individuals with poor fine motor control or accuracy.

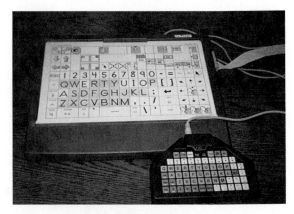

◆ **Figure 33-20** An expanded keyboard and a minikeyboard are examples of alternative keyboards.

KEYBOARD ADAPTATIONS AND ALTERNATIVES

In order to successfully access the computer, the child with a disability may require some customized accessing method to interface with the computer. These interfaces are often provided by additional software or additional hardware for the computer. A keyguard attached over a keyboard is used to prevent unwanted keystrokes when fine motor control or finger isolation is impaired (Fig. 33-19). Ergonomic keyboards or wrist-arm supports may be beneficial to a child requiring distal support or if tremor, pain, fatigue, or lack of endurance interferes with typing. Mobile arm supports and overhead slings also benefit users with muscle weakness. Software is available to decrease additional keystrokes with word prediction capabilities, minimize repetition of the same key, and allow activation of more than one key at a time.

Alternatives to the standard keyboard include minikeyboards, expanded keyboards, chord keyboards, and one-handed keyboards (Fig. 33-20). Minikeyboards are beneficial to children with muscular dystrophy who have accurate fine motor abilities but limited range of motion, decreased strength, or low endurance. Expanded or enlarged keyboards are helpful for children with poor coordination and difficulty isolating a finger. These keyboards have up to 128 pressure-sensitive areas referred to as keys, and because the number, size, shape, and location of these keys can be redefined, the possibilities for customization are numerous. For example, expanded keyboards could be set up to offer four choices with large contact areas, rather than 128 choices. A chord keyboard consists of an array of keys (typically 5 to 10, depending on the model) that are operated by pressing a predetermined combination of keys to type a character or symbol.

Court reporters use this type of technology. Chord keyboards are available in one-handed and two-handed models. Standard keyboards, minikeyboards, and enlarged keyboards may be set up in the typical *qwerty* (*typical keyboard*) pattern, in an *alphabetic* layout, or in a *frequency of use* layout. Dvorak keyboard patterns place frequently used keys near the home row and are available in one-handed or two-handed models (Anson, 1997; Cook & Hussey, 1995).

Touch screens may be attached to the computer monitor or used on a tabletop or wheelchair laptray. A touch screen is one example of a *concept keyboard,* which replaces the letters and numbers of a typical keyboard with pictures or symbols of the subject matter being taught. Because touch screens use direct selection, they tend to be less cognitively demanding, which may be important to children being introduced to computer technology (Cook & Hussey, 2001).

Children with visual impairments require technology specifically developed to meet their needs, such as software or hardware adaptations to provide auditory feedback, tactile keyboards, optical character recognition systems (screen readers that translate text to the spoken word), screen magnification systems, software that will enlarge the text on the screen up to 16 times, or Braille technology.

MOUSE ALTERNATIVES

Mouse functions include moving the cursor to a specific location on the screen, dragging a selected item to a different location on the screen, and clicking or double clicking to select items and functions. Modifications to the cursor such as enlarging it, changing its color, slowing it down, or giving it tails may make it easier for a child to locate the cursor on the computer screen. Keyboard functions using the arrow keys or the numeric keypad may assist a child who is unable to use a mouse effectively. Alternative mouse options are available, both on the general market and through manufacturers of special equipment, and include joysticks, trackballs, mouse pads, keypad mouse, and head-controlled mouse (Fig. 33-21). Therapists are encouraged to become familiar with commercially available input systems, as well as those developed for users with special needs, because they are often less expensive.

Virtual or on-screen keyboards display an image of a keyboard on the monitor, and the user moves the cursor to the desired key with a mouse, joystick, trackball, head-controlled mouse, or switch array. A selection is then made using a second switch or by dwelling on the key for a predetermined amount of time. On-screen keyboards with scanning programs are commonly used by children who rely on a single or dual switch to access assistive technology devices. Keyboard and mouse functions can also be achieved using light beams, infrared, ultrasonic, and speech recognition technology.

RATE ENHANCEMENT

Therapists are encouraged not only to become familiar with different access and input methods, but also to try them, because each access and input method requires different motor responses and cognitive processes. Consider that a trained typist without a disability is capable of transcribing text at an average of 100 words per minute. The same person typing, while composing text, averages 50 words per minute. Court reporters, using special chord keyboards, enter text at 150 words per minute. Contrast that with an average of 10 to 12 words per minute for a person typing with just one finger. The

person using scanning usually averages 3 to 5 words per minute (Cook & Hussey, 2001). Overall speed of production, although not an issue for all users, can become an issue for students in regular education who are expected to produce a similar amount of written output as their classmates. Productivity also becomes an issue during transition planning if prospective employment opportunities require a certain degree of proficiency in computer use.

When use of a computer or communication device is effortful and time consuming, use of macros, abbreviation expansion, or word prediction to enhance productivity should be investigated. Macro programs allow users to combine and automate tasks. Abbreviation expansion automatically types out an entire word or phrase when two or three letters have been typed. For example, a user can command the computer to type out "Physical Therapy" each time the user inputs the letters "PT." With word prediction software, the computer tries to predict what word is being typed after only two or three characters are entered. A numbered list of likely choices appears on the screen and the correct number is selected.

ELECTRONIC AIDS TO DAILY LIVING

An electronic aid to daily living (EADL), previously known as an environmental control unit (ECU), is a device or system of devices that allows the operation of electrical appliances or equipment in a variety of ways and places. Each of us encounters this technology on a daily basis in the form of energy- and time-saving devices such as electronic garage door openers, portable telephones, and remote controls for television and audio equipment. Many of these affordable, commercially available products require precise fine motor control, which precludes their use by children with motor dysfunction; however, a range of environmental control devices are available from manufacturers of equipment for children and adults with special needs. The purpose of an EADL is to apply technology to facilitate the user's control over the environment, to promote independent access to items required for daily living, and to improve the quality of life (MacNeil, 1998).

Control of the environment for a preschooler might include operating a blender with a head-activated switch to prepare treats at school or activating a pressure switch with the hand to operate a battery toy during free time (Fig. 33-22). An older child may use a headstick to operate the television remote control to select a channel, control the volume, and turn off the set when done.

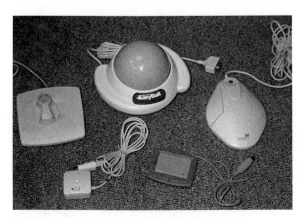

◆ **Figure 33-21**   Examples of mouse alternatives.

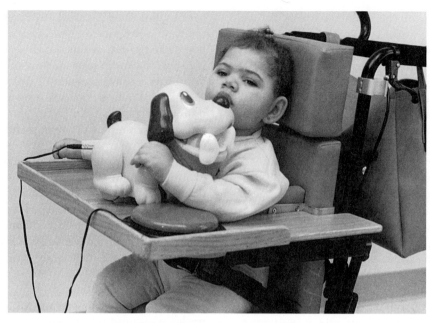

◆ **Figure 33-22** A large pressure switch can be used to activate a battery-operated toy placed on a laptray.

Adapted phone equipment can be programmed to store several numbers, automatically dial a number, and answer calls with the touch of a switch can allow a teenager access to important, age-appropriate socialization. These independent, functional activities help instill a sense of responsibility and independence from caregivers.

Benefits of EADLs for adults include increased personal satisfaction, increased participation in life activities, possible return to work, and possible reduction in cost for personal care attendants (Dickey & Shealy, 1987). The use of EADLs in one residential facility to operate televisions, radios, lights, tape recorders, and stereos reduced the amount of nursing care required by about 2 hours per day per participant (Symington et al., 1986). Both residents and nursing staff reported reduced frustration following introduction of EADLs. Persons with spinal cord injuries who used EADLs used the telephone more often, were more inclined to travel, and spent more time in educational pursuits than nonusers (Efthimiou et al., 1981). Radio use by elderly nursing home residents with mobility and fine motor impairments increased threefold compared with a control group once the participants were equipped with and trained in the use of remote devices to turn radios on and off (Mann, 1992).

An EADL generally includes three parts: the main control unit (central processing unit), the switch (transducer), and any devices (peripherals) to be controlled or activated. Most EADLs emit some type of tactile, visual, or auditory feedback that immediately indicates which function has been selected before the function is activated. Feedback can be an essential feature to the user with memory impairments and is helpful in initial assessment and training sessions with systems capable of multiple functions.

There are two basic types of EADLs: direct and remote. In a direct system, the devices to be controlled are plugged directly into the main control unit. In a remote system, the control unit acts as a transmitter, sending radio waves, ultrasonic signals, or infrared light beams to remote receivers, which, in turn, are connected to the devices to be activated. The remote system has the advantages of operating a number of devices or appliances from one location such as a wheelchair or bed and the absence of wires running from the unit to the device (Cook & Hussey, 2001).

Capabilities of systems vary from simply turning one device on and off to operating whole-house configurations and integrated computer workstations. Common functions include operation of a small electrical appliance, stereo, television, videocassette recorder, light fixture, door lock, intercom or call signal, electric bed, and telephone and computer equipment. EADLs can be activated through the wide variety of switches and controls described previously, through voice activation, or through the user's power wheelchair controller, electronic communication aid, or computer. Lange has produced a chart to assist practitioners in comparing the various features of popular EADLs that are commercially available (MacNeil, 1998). The chart includes input options; what type of equipment can be controlled; what devices the EADL will interface with, such as a computer or communication aid; whether battery backup is included; cost; and comments.

EFFECTS OF MANAGED CARE ON ACQUISITION OF ASSISTIVE TECHNOLOGY

State-funded Medicaid programs, traditionally a major source of funding for children with disabilities, have contracted much of their coverage to private managed care insurance organizations, which in many cases has affected accessibility to durable medical equipment and specialized devices (Carlson & Ramsey, 2000). Denials for requested items may increase, either because a narrower interpretation is used in determining medical necessity, or because nonstandard or customized items do not fit the billing codes. The time between the initial request and approval may be prolonged if the reviewers are less experienced in this specialized population and need more explanation, making repeated requests and justification necessary. Choice of products may be restricted because the amount that will be paid for a given item is often based on simpler adult equipment designs and do not cover the full cost of more expensive or more customized pediatric designs. The capitation rate paid to medical equipment suppliers is often inadequate to cover actual expenses, cutting their profit margins and making it difficult to provide and service sophisticated or customized equipment. In addition, many private insurance companies, as well as state-funded programs, have contracted with specific manufacturers to provide bulk orders of wheelchairs or other durable medical equipment, further restricting choice. Medical and equipment needs of individuals with disabilities are much higher than what many private companies anticipate. Some managed care companies have dropped contracts for state Medicaid patients, leaving those individuals with little or no choice of coverage, and often requiring a change of provider. In the next decade, we will face the dilemma of reconciling the huge variety of devices that can be designed and tailored for achieving independent function with the increasing restrictions in funding, choice, and accessibility.

SUMMARY

Assistive technology is a critical component of intervention for children who have impairments that limit their communication, mobility, and self-care. Assistive technology includes five major areas: alternative and augmentative communication, electronic activities of daily living, seating and positioning, wheeled mobility, and computer accessing. Current best practice involves a multidisciplinary, multilevel assessment involving the child and family. As a member of the team, the physical therapist should possess current knowledge of assistive technology, realizing that products are being improved and new technology developed. Sources of funding often must be identified. Assistive technology is federally mandated for children with disabilities under the age of 21 who need equipment to perform to their potential in school. Likewise, funding is available for adults who need devices to perform employment duties. Assistive technology must be monitored and needs reassessed as children grow and their physical and social environments change. The desired outcome is to select technology that optimizes the child's activity and participation in daily life. The potential impact of assistive technology on children's quality of life underlies the importance of evidence-based decision making that is individualized to the child, family, and environment.

CASE STUDIES

SCOTT

Scott was born in 1963 with spastic athetoid CP (Fig. 33-23). Scott is dependent on others for all personal care, including feeding, dressing, grooming, hygiene, toileting, transfers, and mobility, unless he is in his power wheelchair. Functional arm and hand usage is limited, with purposeful movement dominated by reflexive patterns and fluctuating tone. His speech is dysarthric, but his ability to communicate is excellent. Scott agreed to be featured in this chapter to provide a consumer's viewpoint of assistive technology. His words and thoughts (in italics) reflect many of the points made in this chapter regarding the need for team consultation, communication, respect for the client's opinion, customization of equipment and devices, and the revisions to equipment required over a lifetime.

Before passage of Public Law 94-142 in 1975, few local school districts were able or inclined to provide

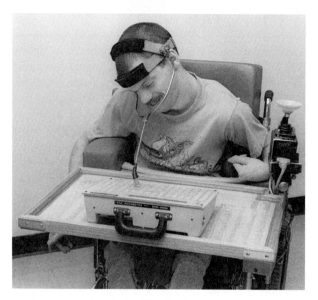

♦ **Figure 33-23**   Scott, sitting in his custom-molded seating system, mounted in his power wheelchair with swing-away chin control joystick. He is using his custom headstick to activate a Light Talker. His communication sheet, sealed in the frame on his laptray, is also visible.

educational services for children with severe physical disabilities. Scott's early education (from preschool in 1967 to junior high in 1975) was at a residential program at the University of Iowa. After he returned to his home school district, he continued to receive assistive technology services at the same facility, which was converted to a regional evaluation and consultation center.

In addition to classes, his early years were filled with individual therapy sessions, including speech, occupational, and physical therapy. A variety of assistive devices (called adaptive equipment at the time) were used over the years in Scott's therapeutic management, including Pope night splints; short leg braces; long leg braces with pelvic band; stand-up boxes; bilateral upper arm restraints; pelvic restraints; chest restraints; wooden armchairs; footboards with footstraps; cutout tables; various bowls, spoons, cups, and straws for feeding; communication boards; headsticks; electric typewriters with keyshield; and last, but not least, wheelchairs.

"*Manual wheelchairs…at first these required little or no adapting. As I got older, we tried one fancy chair I remember well. The back was in sections and could adjust to different positions. I remember about five people in the P.T. room working all day to adapt it to fit me.*" Wheelchairs were generally not adapted in the 1960s, and children relied on seat belts and pelvic or chest restraints; in some cases, their long leg braces locked in flexion at the hips and knees kept them safely in their chairs.

Records indicate that Scott was evaluated for his first seating system in 1973 and was provided with "*a wedged seat with 15° angle, a wedge between thighs, and a high back.*" His long leg braces were discontinued because the seating inserts were believed to provide adequate postural support for sitting. Over the next 20 years, Scott's seating systems changed from simple linear wood and foam inserts, to wood and foam with contouring, to orthotic molded inserts, to his currently used, custom-molded Contour-U (PinDot Products, Chicago, IL) seat and back cushions. Changes in his seating requirements closely paralleled changes in his musculoskeletal status over the years, which included slowly progressing kyphoscoliosis, hip flexion and adduction contractures, and knee flexion contractures.

Scott began using a headstick between 3 and 4 years of age for pointing and to manipulate objects in his environment. He soon developed proficiency with his headstick and eventually switched to a custom-made chin pointer style that he has had for over 15 years. "*I'm careful picking equipment out. I want the least amount of equipment on me as possible. This is so no more extra attention, looks, or glares come my way. However, I wear my headstick because it's my life. People see it before they see my face. But I think of it as a part of me. Once people get to know me, the headstick becomes less noticeable and everyone's happy.*"

While Scott was learning headstick skills, he was introduced to picture and word boards for communication. The combination of headstick skill plus his ability to spell and write to communicate progressed over the years, as did his selection and use of technology. "*Language boards/Touch Talkers…This has been a very 'lucky' area for me. I've had a word board ever since age 3. As I grew, so did my boards. My first try at a voice* [electronic device with voice output] *was a bomb! Other people were telling ME what I wanted! Finally, I took a stand and said 'No' to that device, and most people took that as my not wanting a 'voice.' That wasn't so, it was just too much work with a poor voice. I was saying, 'Let's wait.' My word board did fine back then. But as my life got busier, I had a greater need to communicate. I knew that was when I needed a voice output. The 1989 Touch Talker had a pretty good voice to it and so I fell in love with it. Now, with the Liberator* [a highly sophisticated AAC device from Prentke Romich Co., Shreve, OH, with voice or print output, ability to operate computers and EADLs, and ability to perform math and calculator functions], *I'm in heaven.*"

"*Power wheelchairs…I still remember my first electric chair. I had a big say in the driving method. Everyone was thinking 'headstick,' and I said, 'No, try my chin!' I was shocked at how well I could drive power chairs once the right method was found. Now better controls are coming out* so who knows what will be next." Scott received his first power wheelchair in 1981 and his second chair in 1988. *"My power wheelchair. It is my legs, my little home. I have everything in my backpack, it holds as much as a small house."* After fabrication and assembly of seating components, a custom swing-away mounting arm to hold the chin control was designed and fabricated by a rehabilitation engineer who worked closely with Scott to meet his needs. With this custom device, Scott is able to move the chin control into position for driving or swing it out of the way with his arm to access his communication equipment independently. Most important, the mounting hardware is sturdy, is durable, and does not slip out of alignment. The capability to customize cannot be overemphasized when providing technology for individuals with severe physical disabilities. One-of-a-kind designs and devices often provide the best solutions to technology puzzles. *"My chin control arm. It has no wires or batteries, it works off my power. Being homemade, it's made to last. My headstick is another good example."*

In the early years, much of Scott's therapeutic management and adaptive equipment reflected an attempt to intervene at the impairment level, such as by preventing contractures and increasing weight bearing with braces and standing boxes. Functional limitations were also addressed by providing alternatives to speech and walking, such as headsticks, communication boards, and wheelchairs. As Scott became older, it was evident that many of his impairments (scoliosis and contractures) needed to be accommodated, rather than corrected, to maximize function.

Now, as a young adult, Scott's priorities lie with minimizing his disabilities and increasing acceptance of his role in society. In 1995, he found a data entry position two mornings a week at a local law firm. About this time he also experienced weight loss secondary to lifelong oral-pharyngeal dysfunction with dysphagia. He subsequently developed a pressure sore over his right ischial tuberosity. A custom Silhouette seat was molded for Scott, which decreased sitting pressures, provided comfort, and promoted quick healing of the sore. He was then able to gradually increase his working hours to about 6 hours a day. Scott must carefully monitor how much income he earns to avoid reduction of his Medicaid entitlement. He continues to live in a group home with four other young men with physical disabilities and manages his personal life and affairs with the assistance of care attendants.

Technology has made a definite impact on Scott's life over the years. *"In general, special devices have changed my life in a good way. I'm doing more and more for myself. However, rapid changes in equipment design makes* knowing what to buy very hard." Future plans include working toward getting his own apartment with one or two hired personal care attendants and perhaps taking classes at the university or community college.

ANTHONY

Anthony is 11-year-old who attends fifth grade in a regular classroom at his local public school. He has CP, spastic quadriplegia. Anthony was born 8 weeks premature. He had periventricular leukomalacia and meningitis soon after birth. Anthony's father is a physical therapist and his mother works for the government.

Anthony received his first wheelchair at age 3. He initially used a linear seat and hybrid custom-molded back cushion with linear laterals on a power mobility system controlled with a joystick. It took him over 6 months to completely learn to drive the system. He currently uses a generically contoured seating system and a rear wheel drive power mobility system with a standard joystick. He also has a beach wheelchair that has a mesh seat and back, PVC tubing, and large rubber wheels that roll over the sand easily. The beach chair needs to be pushed by someone accompanying Anthony. He is transported to school on a bus that has been adapted to accommodate his wheelchair. Anthony uses a modified keyboard for his computer system to complete his class work in school and at home. He uses a low-tech page magnifier to help him read his textbooks. He does not use augmentative communication.

Anthony enjoys social activities typical of a fifth grader including the bowling team, religious education and participation as an alter server, computer games and hanging out with his friends, and horseback riding. His family drives a conversion van with a lift. When he grows up Anthony aspires to be a cowboy or a waiter!

REFERENCES

Agre, JC, Findley, TW, McNally, MC, Habeck, R, Leon, AS, Stradel, L, Birkebak, R, & Schmalz, R. Physical activity capacity in children with myelomeningocele. Archives of Physical Medicine and Rehabilitation, *68*:372–377, 1987.

American Physical Therapy Association. Guide to Practice Physical Therapist Practice. Alexandria, VA: APTA, 1999.

Anson, DK. Alternative Computer Access: A Guide to Selection. Philadelphia: FA Davis, 1997.

Arnold, RL. Safe transportation for persons with disabilities. Assistive Devices Information Network Newsletter (University of Iowa, Iowa City, IA), *2*(1):1–2, 1988.

Accardo, PJ, & Whitman, BY. Dictionary of Developmental Disabilities Terminology,- 2nd ed. Baltimore: Paul Brookes, 2002.

Attermeier, SM. Augmentative communication: An interdisciplinary challenge. Physical and Occupational Therapy in Pediatrics, *7*(2):3–11, 1987.

Bablich, K, Sochaniwskyj, A, & Koheil, R. Positional and electromyographic investigation of sitting posture of children with cerebral palsy (Abstract). Developmental Medicine and Child Neurology, 28(suppl 53):25, 1986.

Barnes, KH. Training young children for powered mobility. Developmental Disabilities Special Interest Section Newsletter (American Occupational Therapy Association, Rockville, MD), 14(2):1–2, 1991.

Bauer, AM, & Ulrich, ME. I've got a Palm in my pocket: Using handheld computers in an inclusive classroom. Teaching Exceptional Children, 35(2):18–22, 2002.

Bay, JL. Positioning for head control to access an augmentative communication machine. American Journal of Occupational Therapy, 45:544–549, 1991.

Bednarczyk, JH, & Sanderson, DJ. Kinematics of wheelchair propulsion in adults and children with spinal cord injury. Archives of Physical Medicine and Rehabilitation, 75:1327–1334, 1994.

Bergen, AF. Seating and positioning principles for the neurologically involved client. Presented at the American Physical Therapy Association Combined Sections Meeting, San Francisco, February 1992.

Bergen, AF, Presperin, J, & Tallman, T. Positioning for Function: Wheelchairs and Other Assistive Technologies. Valhalla, NY: Valhalla Rehabilitation Publications, 1990.

Berry, ET, McLaurin, SE, & Sparling, JW. Parent/caregiver perspectives on the use of power wheelchairs. Pediatric Physical Therapy, 8(4):146–150, 1996.

Brubaker, CE. Wheelchair prescription: An analysis of factors that affect mobility and performance. Journal of Rehabilitation Research and Development, 23(4):19–26, 1986.

Brubaker, CE. Manual mobility. Presented at the Fourth International Seating Symposium, Vancouver, BC, February 1988.

Bryant, L. Wheelchair standards ready to roll. TeamRehab Report, May–June 1991, pp. 44–45.

Buning, ME, Angelo, JA and Schmeler, MR. Occupational performance and the transition to powered mobility: A pilot study. American Journal of Occupational Therapy, 55(3):339–344, 2001.

Butler, C. Effects of powered mobility on self-initiated behaviors of very young children with locomotor disability. Developmental Medicine and Child Neurology, 28:325–332, 1986.

Butler, C, Okamoto, GA, & McKay, TM. Powered mobility for very young disabled children. Developmental Medicine and Child Neurology, 25:472–474, 1983.

Campbell, J, & Ball, J. Energetics of walking in cerebral palsy. Orthopedic Clinics of North America, 9:374–377, 1978.

Carlson, D, & Myklebust, J. Wheelchair use and social interaction. Topics in Spinal Cord Injury Rehabilitation, 7(3):28–46, 2002.

Carlson, JM, & Payette, M. Seating and spine support for boys with Duchenne muscular dystrophy. In Proceedings of the 8th Annual Conference on Rehabilitation Technology. Washington, DC: RESNA Press, 1985, pp. 36–38.

Carlson, SJ. The semi-rigid pelvic stabilizer for seating control. Assistive Devices Information Network Newsletter (University of Iowa, Iowa City, IA), 1(1):2–3, 1987.

Carlson, SJ, & Grey, TL. The semi-rigid pelvic stabilizer for seating control. Presented at the Fourth International Seating Symposium, Vancouver, BC, February 1988.

Carlson, SJ, & Ramsey, C. Assistive technology. In Campbell, SK, Vander Linden, DW, Palisano, RJ (Eds.). Physical Therapy for Children, 2nd ed. Philadelphia: WB Saunders, 2000.

Cook, A, & Hussey, SM. Assistive Technologies: Principles and Practice. St. Louis: Mosby, 1995.

Cook, A, & Hussey, SM. Assistive Technologies: Principles and Practice, 2nd ed. St. Louis: Mosby, 2001.

Crenshaw, RP, & Vistnes, LM. A decade of pressure sore research: 1977–1987. Journal of Rehabilitation Research and Development, 26:63–74, 1989.

Deitz, J, Jaffe, KM, Wolf, LS, Massagli, TL, & Anson, D. Pediatric power wheelchairs: Evaluation of function in the home and school environments. Assistive Technology, 3:24–31, 1991.

Deitz, J, Swinth, Y, & White, O. Powered mobility and preschoolers with complex developmental delays. American Journal of Occupational Therapy, 56(1):86–96, 2002.

DeSouza, LJ, & Carroll, N. Ambulation of the braced myelomeningocele patient. Journal of Bone and Joint Surgery (American), 58:1112–1118, 1976.

Dickey, R, & Shealy, SH. Using technology to control the environment. American Journal of Occupational Therapy, 41:717–721, 1987.

Dorman, SM. Assistive technology benefits for students with disabilities. The Journal of School Health, 68(3):120–123, 1998.

Drummond, DS, Narechania, RG, Rosenthal, AN, Breed, AL, Lange, TA, & Drummond, DK. A study of pressure distributions measured during balanced and unbalanced sitting. Journal of Bone and Joint Surgery (American), 64:1034–1039, 1982.

Efthimiou, MA, Gordon, WA, Sell, GH, & Stratford, C. Electronic assistive devices: Their impact on the quality of life of high-level quadriplegic persons. Archives of Physical Medicine and Rehabilitation, 62:131–134, 1981.

Evans, MA, & Nelson, WB. A dynamic solution to seating clients with fluctuating tone. In Proceedings of the 19th Annual Conference on Rehabilitation Technology. Arlington, VA: RESNA Press, 1996, pp. 189–190.

Fife, S, Roxborough, L, Cooper, D, & Steinke, T. Tonic electromyographic activity in seated subjects with spastic quadriplegia: A pilot study. Presented at the Fourth International Seating Symposium, Vancouver, BC, February 1988.

Fisher, SV, & Gullickson, G. Energy cost of ambulation in health and disability: A literature review. Archives of Physical Medicine and Rehabilitation, 59:124–133, 1978.

Franks, CA, Palisano, RJ, & Darbee, JC. The effect of walking with an assistive device and using a wheelchair on school performance in students with myelomeningocele. Physical Therapy, 71:570–579, 1991.

Galka, G, & Lombard, T. So...You're Considering Power Mobility. Iowa City, IA: Occupational Therapy Department, Division of Developmental Disabilities, University Hospital School, University of Iowa, 1992.

Galvin, JC, & Scherer, MJ. Evaluating, Selecting, and Using Appropriate Assistive Technology. Gaithersburg, MD: Aspen Publishers, 1996

Garber, SL, & Dyerly, LR. Wheelchair cushions for persons with spinal cord injury: An update. American Journal of Occupational Therapy, 45:550–554, 1991.

Gilsdorf, P, Patterson, R, Fisher, S, & Appel, N. Sitting forces and wheelchair mechanics. Journal of Rehabilitation Research and Development, 27:239–246, 1990.

Guerette, P, & Sumi, E. Integrating control of multiple assistive devices: A retrospective review. Assistive Technology, 6(1):67–76, 1994.

Hasdai A, Jessel, AS, & Weiss, PL. Use of computer simulator for training children with disabilities in the operation of a powered wheelchair. American Journal of Occupational Therapy, 52(3):215–220, 1998.

Hays, RM. Childhood motor impairments: Clinical overview and scope of the problem. Presented at the Fourth International Seating Symposium, Vancouver, BC, February 1988.

Hedman, G. Overview of rehabilitation technology. Physical and Occupational Therapy in Pediatrics, 10(2):1–10, 1990.

Hughes, CJ, Weimar, WH, Sheth, PN, & Brubaker, CE. Biomechanics of wheelchair propulsion as a function of seat position and user-to-chair interface. Archives of Physical Medicine and Rehabilitation, 73:263–269, 1992.

Hulme, JB, Bain, B, & Hardin, MA. The influence of adaptive seating devices on vocalization (Abstract). Developmental Medicine and Child Neurology, 30(suppl 57):35, 1988.

Hulme, JB, Shaver, J, Acher, S, Mullette, L, & Eggert, C. Effects of adaptive seating devices on the eating and drinking of children with multiple handicaps. American Journal of Occupational Therapy, 41:81–89, 1987.

Jones, CK. A sampler of available powered mobility bases: Hard facts and a little opinion. Presented at the Fourth International Seating Symposium, Vancouver, BC, February 1988.

Jones, CK. In search of power for the pediatric client. Physical and Occupational Therapy in Pediatrics, 10(2):47–68, 1990.

Kangas, KM. Seating, positioning, and physical access. Developmental Disabilities Special Interest Section Newsletter (American Occupational Therapy Association, Rockville, MD), 14(2):4, 1991.

Kangas, KM. Clinical assessment and training strategies for the child's mastery of independent powered mobility. In Furumasu, J (Ed.). Pediatric Powered Mobility: Developmental Perspectives, Technical Issues, Clinical Approaches. Arlington, VA: RESNA Press, 1997.

Kermoian, R. Locomotion experience and psychological development in infancy. In Furumasu, J (Ed.). Pediatric Powered Mobility: Developmental Perspectives, Technical Issues, Clinical Approaches. Arlington, VA: RESNA Press, 1997.

Koo, TK, Mak, AF, & Lee, YL. Posture effect on seating interface biomechanics: Comparison between two seating cushions. Archives of Physical Medicine and Rehabilitation, 77:40–47, 1996.

Lahm, EA, & Sizemore, L. Factors that influence assistive technology decision making. Journal of Special Education Technology, 17(1):15–26, 2002.

Langone, J, Malone, DM, & Kinsley, T. Technology solutions for young children with developmental concerns. Infants and Young Children, 4(11):65–78, 1999.

Larnert, G, & Ekberg, O. Positioning improves the oral and pharyngeal swallowing function in children with cerebral palsy. Acta Paediatrica, 84:689–692, 1995.

Lepage, C, Noreau, L, & Bernard, PM. Association between characteristics of locomotion and accomplishment of life habits in children with cerebral palsy. Physical Therapy, 78:458–469, 1998.

Letts, RM (Ed.). Principles of Seating the Disabled. Boca Raton, FL: CRC Press, 1991.

MacNeil, V. Electronic aids to daily living: A change for the better. TeamRehab Report, 9(11):53–56, 1998.

Mann, WC. Use of environmental control devices by elderly nursing home patients. Assistive Technology, 4(2):60–65, 1992.

Mann, WC, & Lane, JP. Assistive Technology for Persons with Disabilities, 2nd ed. Bethesda, MD: American Occupational Therapy Association, 1995.

Margolis, S. Lumbar support issues. Presented at the Eighth International Seating Symposium, Vancouver, BC, February 1992.

Margolis, SA, Wengert, ME, & Kolar, KA. The subASIS bar: No component is an island: A five-year retrospective. Presented at the Fourth International Seating Symposium, Vancouver, BC, February 1988.

McClenaghan, BA, Thombs, L, & Milner, M. Effects of seat-surface inclination on postural stability and function of the upper extremities of children with cerebral palsy. Developmental Medicine and Child Neurology, 34:40–48, 1992.

McEwen, IR. Assistive positioning as a control parameter of social-communicative interactions between students with profound multiple disabilities and classroom staff. Physical Therapy, 72:634–647, 1992.

Medhat, MA, & Hobson, DA. Standardization of Terminology and Descriptive Methods for Specialized Seating: A Reference Manual. Arlington, VA: RESNA Press, 1992.

Miedaner, JA. The effects of sitting positions on trunk extension for children with motor impairment. Pediatric Physical Therapy, 2:11–14, 1990.

Mitchell, CL. Switch access, environmental control and computer access: The evaluation process. Technology Special Interest Section Newsletter (American Occupational Therapy Association, Bethesda, MD), 5(1):3–4, 1995.

Monette M, Weiss-Lambrou, R, & Dansereau, J. In Search of a better understanding of wheelchair sitting comfort and discomfort. Proceedings of the RESNA conference, 1999, 218–220.

Myhr, U, & von Wendt, L. Improvement of functional sitting position for children with cerebral palsy. Developmental Medicine and Child Neurology, 33:246–256, 1991.

Myhr, U, & von Wendt, L. Influence of different sitting positions and abduction orthoses on leg muscle activity in children with cerebral palsy. Developmental Medicine and Child Neurology, 35:870–880, 1993.

Neilson, AR, Bardsley, GI, Rowley, DI, & Hogg, J. Measuring the effects of seating on people with profound and multiple disabilities—A preliminary study. Journal of Rehabiliation Research and Development, 38(2):201–213, 2001.

Noble-Jamieson, CM, Heckmatt, JZ, Dubowitz, V, & Silverman, M. Effects of posture and spinal bracing on respiratory function in neuromuscular disease. Archives of Disease in Childhood, 61:178–181, 1986.

Noon, JH, Chesney, DA, & Axelson, PW. Development of a dynamic pelvic stabilization system. In Proceedings of the 21st Annual Conference on Rehabilitation Engineering. Arlington, VA: RESNA Press, 1998, pp. 209–211.

Nwaobi, OM. Effects of body orientation in space on tonic muscle activity of patients with cerebral palsy. Developmental Medicine and Child Neurology, 28:41–44, 1986.

Nwaobi, OM. Seating orientations and upper extremity function in children with cerebral palsy. Physical Therapy, 67:1209–1212, 1987.

Nwaobi, OM, Brubaker, CE, Cusick, B, & Sussman, MD. Electromyographic investigation of extensor activity in cerebral-palsied children in different seating positions. Developmental Medicine and Child Neurology, 25:175–183, 1983.

Nwaobi, OM, & Cusick, B. The effect of hip flexion angle on the electrical activity of the hip adductors in cerebral palsied children. Unpublished report, 1980.

Nwaobi, OM, & Smith, PD. Effect of adaptive seating on pulmonary function of children with cerebral palsy. Developmental Medicine and Child Neurology, 28:351–354, 1986.

Oregon Research Institute, Applied Computer Simulation Labs, 2003; accessed at http://www.ori.org/~vr/.

Orpwood, R. A compliant seating system for a child with extensor spasms. In Proceedings of the 19th Annual Conference of Rehabilitation Engineering. Arlington, VA: RESNA Press, 1996, pp. 261–262.

O'Sullivan, SB, & Schmitz, T. Physical Rehabiliation: Assessment and Treatment, 4th ed. Philadelphia: FA Davis, 2001.

Parette, P, & McMahon, GA. What should we expect of assistive technology? Teaching Exceptional Children, 35(1):56–61, 2002.

Palmieri, VR, Haelen, GT, & Cochran, GV. Comparison of sitting pressures on wheelchair cushions as measured by air cell transducers and miniature electronic transducers. Bulletin of Prosthetic Research, 17(1):5–8, 1980.

Pate, G. Patterns of pressure during normal sitting. Presented at the Fourth International Seating Symposium, Vancouver, BC, February 1988.

Paulsson, K, & Christoffersen, M. Psychological aspects of technical aids: How does independent mobility affect the psychosocial and intellectual development of children with physical disabilities? In Proceedings of the 2nd International Conference on Rehabilitation Engineering. Washington, DC: RESNA Press, 1984.

Phillips, B, & Zhao, H. Predictors of assistive technology abandonment. Assistive Technology, 5:36–45, 1993.

Pope, PM, Bowes, CE, & Booth, E. Postural control in sitting the SAM system: Evaluation of use over three years. Developmental Medicine and Child Neurology, 36:241–252, 1994.

Reger, SI, Chung, KC, & Paling, M. Weightbearing tissue contour and deformation by magnetic resonance imaging. In Proceedings of the 9th Annual Conference on Rehabilitation Technology. Washington, DC: RESNA Press, 1986, pp. 387–389.

Reid, DT. The effects of the saddle seat on seated postural control and upper extremity movement in children with cerebral palsy. Developmental Medicine and Child Neurology, 38:805–815, 1996.

Reid, DT. Sitting Assessment for Children with Neuromotor Dysfunction: A Standardized Protocol for Describing Postural Control. San Antonio, TX: Therapy Skill Builders, 1997.

Reid, DT. The use of virtual reality to improve upper-extremity efficiency skills in children with cerebral palsy: a pilot study. Technology and Disability, 14(2):53–61, 2002.

Reid, DT, & Rigby, P. Towards improved anterior pelvic stabilization devices for paediatric wheelchair users with cerebral palsy. Canadian Journal of Rehabilitation, 9(3):147–157, 1996.

Reid, DT, & Sochaniwskyj, A. Effects of anterior-tipped seating on respiratory function of normal children and children with cerebral palsy. International Journal of Rehabilitation Research, 14:203–212, 1991.

Safe Transport for Children with Special Needs. Connecticut Children's Medical Center, Injury Prevention Center. www.ccmckids.org/training. Accessed 2004.

Schiaffino, S, & Laux, J. Prerequisite skills for the psychosocial impact of powered wheelchair mobility on young children with severe handicaps. Developmental Disabilities Special Interest Section Newsletter (American Occupational Therapy Association, Rockville, MD), 9(2):1, 3, 8, 1986.

Seeger, BR, Sutherland, AD, & Clark, MS. Orthotic management of scoliosis in Duchenne muscular dystrophy. Archives of Physical Medicine and Rehabilitation, 65:83–86, 1984.

Seymour, RJ, & Lacefield, WE. Wheelchair cushion effect on pressure and skin temperature. Archives of Physical Medicine and Rehabilitation, 66:103–108, 1985.

Shaw, G. Vehicular transport safety for the child with disabilities. American Journal of Occupational Therapy, 41:35–42, 1987.

Shields, RK, & Cook, TM. Effect of seat angle and lumbar support on seated buttock pressure. Physical Therapy, 68:1682–1686, 1988.

Siekman, AR, & Flanagan, K. The anti-thrust seat: A wheelchair insert for individuals with abnormal reflex patterns or other specialized problems. In Proceedings of the 8th Annual Conference on Rehabilitation Engineering. Washington, DC: RESNA Press, 1983, pp. 203–205.

Sprigle, S, Chung, KC, & Brubaker, CE. Factors affecting seat contour characteristics. Journal of Rehabilitation Research and Development, 27:127–134, 1990a.

Sprigle, S, Chung, KC, & Brubaker, CE. Reduction of sitting pressures with custom contoured cushions. Journal of Rehabilitation Research and Development, 27:135–140, 1990b.

Stewart, SFC, Palmieri, V, & Cochran, GVB. Wheelchair cushion effect on skin temperature, heat flux, and relative humidity. Archives of Physical Medicine and Rehabilitation, 61:229–233, 1980.

Stowers, S, Altheide, MR, & Shea, V. Motor assessment for unaided and aided augmentative communication. Physical and Occupational Therapy in Pediatrics, 7(2):61–77, 1987.

Swinth, Y, Anson, D, & Dietz, J. Single switch computer access for infants and toddlers. American Journal of Occupational Therapy, 47:1031–1038, 1993.

Sullivan, M, & Lewis, M. Assistive Technology for the very young: Creating responsive environments. Infants and Young Children, 12(4):34–52, 2000.

Symington, DC, Lywood, DW, Lawson, JS, & Maclean, J. Environmental control systems in chronic care hospitals and nursing homes. Archives of Physical Medicine and Rehabilitation, 67:322–325, 1986.

Thacker, JG, Sprigle, SH, & Morris, BO. Understanding the Technology When Selecting Wheelchairs. Arlington, VA: RESNA Press, 1994.

Trefler, E, & Angelo, J. Comparison of anterior trunk supports for children with cerebral palsy. Assistive Technology, 9(1):15–21, 1997.

Trefler, E, Hobson, DA, Taylor, SJ, Monahan, LC, & Shaw, CG. Seating and Mobility for Persons with Physical Disabilities. Tucson, AZ: Therapy Skill Builders, 1993.

Vaccarella, B. Finding our way through the maze of adaptive technology. Computers in Libraries, 21(9):44–47, 2001.

van der Woude, LHV, Veeger, DJ, Rozendal, RH, & Sargeant, TJ. Seat height in handrim wheelchair propulsion. Journal of Rehabilitation Research and Development, 26:31–50, 1989.

Verburg, G, Snell, E, Pilkington, M, & Milner, M. Effects of powered mobility on young handicapped children and their families. In Proceedings of the 2nd International Conference on Rehabilitation Engineering. Washington, DC: RESNA Press, 1984.

Washington K, Deitz JC, White OR, & Schwartz IS. The effects of a contoured foam seat on postural alignment and upper extremity function in infants with neuromotor impairment. Physical Therapy, 82(11):1064–1076, 2002.

Williams, LO, Anderson, AD, Campbell, J, Thomas, L, Feiwell, E, & Walker, JM. Energy cost of walking and of wheelchair propulsion by children with myelodysplasia: Comparison with normal children. Developmental Medicine and Child Neurology, 25:617–624, 1983.

World Health Organization: international classifications. www3.who.int/icf. Accessed July 2005.

Wright-Ott, C. The transitional powered mobility aid: A new concept and tool for early mobility. In Furumasu, J (Ed.). Pediatric Powered Mobility: Developmental Perspectives, Technical Issues, Clinical Approaches. Arlington, VA: RESNA Press, 1997.

∾

Chapter 34

The Burn Unit

Merilyn L. Moore
PT

Cynthia A. Robinson
PT, MS

Fires and burn injuries are the second leading cause of death in children (general trauma being the first). In 2000 Deitch reported that more than 1000 children under the age of 15 die in house fires each year, and about two thirds of them are under the age of 4. Additionally, 20,000 children require hospitalization out of the approximately 440,000 children who receive medical attention for burn injuries each year. Two thirds of these burn injuries in children are scalds secondary to household accidents or, less commonly, deliberate abuse. Reports of child abuse indicate that such injuries account for as many as 20% of burn unit pediatric admissions. Most of these injuries occur in children younger than 3 years of age and are scald or contact burns.

Great strides have been made in the management of thermal injuries, resulting in improvement in the survival rate of pediatric patients. In 1949, Bull and Squire reported a 50% mortality rate in children younger than 14 years of age with burns over 51% of the total body surface area. Forty-three years later Herndon and Rutan (1992a) reported a 50% mortality rate in children younger than 15 years of age with burns of greater than 95% of the total body surface area. Recent studies by Barrow and associates (2004) support correlations between demographics and inhalation injury on burn mortality rates (e.g., it may take longer to rescue someone from a multiple family dwelling, resulting in severe smoke inhalation). Children who sustain an inhalation injury are more likely to die as a result of their burn. It is also accepted that children younger than 4 years old are at greater risk for burn-related deaths because their skin is thin and can be deeply burned at low temperatures.

Treatment of children with burns is concerned not only with skin coverage and prevention of infection but also with psychologic and social outcomes. Pediatric burn survivors often must live with permanent disfigurement and physical disabilities. A study by Doctor and co-workers (1997) suggests that people who survive a severe burn experience a stable and relatively good health status after their injury. Their health status, however, remains worse than that of the general population. Furthermore, people who survive a major burn indicate that vocation and psychosocial function are often troublesome. The purpose of this chapter is to describe the pathophysiology and medical management of burns, identify impairments and potential functional limitations of the child with a burn, and discuss physical therapy interventions and resources associated with quality care in the burn unit.

CLASSIFICATION AND PATHOPHYSIOLOGY OF BURNS

Burn injuries occur when energy is transferred from a heat source to the body. If heat absorption exceeds heat dissipation, cellular temperature rises above the point at which cell survival is possible. Tissue damage begins at temperatures of 40°C and increases logarithmically as the temperature rises. At 45°C, denaturation of tissue proteins ensues and leads to cellular necrosis (Carvajal, 1990). The extent of injury is related to (1) heat intensity, (2) duration of the exposure, and (3) tissue conductance.

Burns may be categorized into four types, according to the primary mechanism of injury: thermal, radiation, electrical, or chemical. Thermal injuries include burns caused by contact with hot liquids (spills or immersion scalds), hot solid objects, or flames and make up approximately 95% of all burn injuries. Chemical and electrical injuries make up about 5% of burns treated at a regional burn center. Radiation injuries are extremely rare.

Burn injuries are classified as superficial, partial thickness, or full thickness according to the depth of tissue damage. Burn classification characteristics are depicted in Figure 34-1 and listed in Table 34-1. Deeper burns may at times extend into fascia, muscle, or bone. Burns involving tendon, muscle, or bone are most common on digits, hands, feet, and over bony prominences such as the iliac crest, patella, anterior tibia, and cranium, because these areas have only a thin covering of subcutaneous tissue.

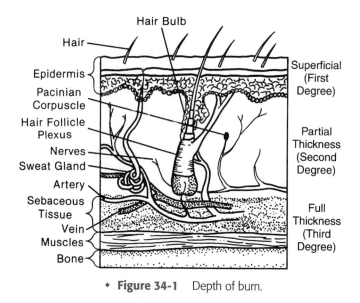

♦ **Figure 34-1**   Depth of burn.

| TABLE 34-1 | Classification of Burns | | | |

	SUPERFICIAL (FIRST DEGREE)	PARTIAL THICKNESS (SECOND DEGREE)		FULL THICKNESS (THIRD DEGREE)
		SUPERFICIAL	DEEP	
Depth	Superficial epidermis	Epidermis and a small part of the dermis	Epidermis and a deeper portion of the dermis	Total destruction of the epidermis and dermis; may involve deeper tissue (muscle or subcutaneous fat)
Sensation	Painful	Increased sensitivity to pain and temperature	Increased sensitivity to pain and temperature	No pain or temperature sensation present
Color	Bright red	Red	Marbled-white edematous appearance	White, brown-black charred appearance
Texture	Edematous	Normal or firm	Firm	Firm or leathery
Blisters	Some, blanches with pressure	Large, thick walled, will usually increase in size	Large, thick walled, will usually increase in size	None, or if present will not increase in size

Because skin varies in thickness in different parts of the body, application of the same intensity of heat for given periods of time results in different burn depth. Thus, in the young child in whom dermal papillae and appendages have yet to develop fully, deeper burns result from heat of the same intensity that produces a moderate partial-thickness burn in the adult. The skin is thickest on the back and on the palms of the hands and is thinnest on the inner arm. Burned parts involving the thickest areas of skin regenerate faster. Certain burn patterns are indicative of possible abuse, for example, burns of the buttocks, feet, and perineum when the backs of knees and anterior hip areas are not burned. This typically occurs when a child is placed in a tub of hot water. The child flexes into a protective position by curling up the knees and hips.

The extent of burn injury can be estimated in several ways. One approach is referred to as the "rule of nines," which divides the body surface into areas, each representing 9% or a multiple of 9% of body surface area. This method is particularly unreliable in children younger than 15 years of age because it underestimates burned areas of the head and neck and overestimates burned areas of the legs. Another method, the Berkow chart, recognizes that the proportion of body surface covering specific body parts changes with age. For example, the head and neck of an infant constitute 20% of the body surface compared with 9% in the adult. Major burn centers have developed electronic charting tools that can accurately calculate body surface area. Hospital personnel "draw" the burned areas on a computer image of the body. Based on the drawing, the computer calculates the area of partial thickness and deep burns.

Thermal destruction of the skin initiates a chain of physiologic changes in the local wound, as well as severe multiple systemic responses in almost all organ systems. The total amount of cell death and extracellular destruction is dependent on local chemical responses to the initial insult and on the systemic response to burn injury. Local responses include loss of the ability to regulate evaporative water loss, impairment of the body's first line of defense against infection, and the loss of massive amounts of body fluids through open wounds.

THE BURN UNIT AND TEAM APPROACH TO CARE

Appropriate treatment decisions can be made after calculation of the severity of the burn by following the American Burn Association treatment guidelines (http://www.ameriburn.org/BurnUnitReferral.pdf). Patients with minor burns may be treated as outpatients. Moderately severe uncomplicated burns may be treated in a community hospital by an experienced surgeon or physician. Burns that should be referred to a burn unit include larger partial-thickness burns (greater than 25% in adults or 20% in children); all full-thickness burns greater than 10%; burns of difficult areas such as the hands, face, eyes, ears, feet, and perineum; and burns with associated injuries, including inhalation or electrical injuries, fractures, or other trauma.

The burn unit is much like other intensive care units, but it also has unique characteristics. As in other units, it is a place characterized by high technology, specially trained staff, a team approach, and isolation, which may lead to a dehumanizing situation in which the patient is viewed in a fragmented and anatomic manner. The need for compassion, empathy, guidance, interest, and support is paramount. On the other hand, significant differences exist between the burn unit and other acute care units. The sights and smells characteristic of burn injury make for obvious differences from other emergency care settings. Isolation of both staff and patient from the outside world is often more pronounced in the burn unit, primarily because of fear of infection. There is the constant issue of pain management. Patients in burn centers stay longer than in other intensive care units, or indeed, any other hospital units. This results in a much more intense and prolonged patient-staff interaction.

A multidisciplinary team approach to burn care was developed in specialized burn treatment facilities established over the past 25 years. Presently, burn teams usually consist of physicians, nurse practitioners, nursing personnel, physical therapists, occupational therapists, nutritionists, social workers, psychiatrists or psychologists, child life specialists or recreation therapists, school teachers, and, when available, orthotists, prosthetists, and medical sculptors. All team members work together and each plays a key role. The team approach to burn management is based on a mutual respect and appreciation of each member's contribution to the overall care of the patient and a decision-making process that relies on the input of the child, family, and all professional team members. Discussions at burn team conferences not only lead to improved patient care, but also provide an opportunity for members to gain insights from the experiences of other team members who are caring for the same patient. Daily pressures the team must face include viewing mutilations and disfigurement, inflicting pain, dealing with emergency situations, and confronting death.

MEDICAL MANAGEMENT OF BURNS

When a child is admitted to the appropriate facility, an estimate of the depth and surface area of the burn and the child's overall condition is first made. These decisions determine the need for immediate lifesaving measures, such as endotracheal intubation, ventilatory support, and intravenous fluid therapy.

Shock is usual in children with burns affecting more than 12% of the surface area but can occur when the surface area is smaller if the burn is full thickness and when the child is younger than 1 year of age. An intravenous line and a urinary catheter are placed and fluid delivery is begun. Until the capillary leak stops, intravenous fluid therapy is necessary to maintain the circulation and perfusion of tissues. After fluid resuscitation has been started and a detailed history and physical examination completed, attention is directed to care of the burn.

Escharotomy, incision through the burn, may be necessary to relieve the pressure caused by progressive edema in the extremities or constriction of the trunk with circumferential deep burns. It is usually done when the tissue pressure exceeds 40 mm Hg. The incisions are made along the medial and lateral aspects of the limb. As the tissues are released, the subcutaneous fat bulges through the incision, tissue tension is relieved, and effective circulation is restored. Among patients with deep burns or high-voltage electrical injury involving muscle, fasciotomy may be necessary to relieve elevated pressure in fascial compartments unrelieved by simple escharotomy.

As soon as the patient's condition is stabilized, the wounds are assessed for the purpose of developing a plan for wound closure. Evaluation of the burn wound depth in pediatric patients is often difficult. A laser Doppler flowmeter with a temperature-controlled multichannel probe has been a useful tool for burn wound assessment in pediatric patients (Atiles et al., 1995). Necrotic tissue produced by the burn must be removed, either by daily mechanical debridement during wound care or, in deeper burns, by surgical excision either directly to fascia or tangentially (i.e., shaving sequential levels until viable tissue is exposed). Closure of deeper burns must be accomplished with autogenous split-thickness skin grafts.

Aggressive and thorough wound care is important to help delineate wounds before early surgical intervention, to protect and promote good granulation tissue until grafting, or to promote rapid healing in wounds that are healing without surgical intervention. There are three types of cleansing techniques: (1) local care of a particular wound or area (using a sterile container of water and cleansing agents at bedside or any convenient area); (2) spray hydrotherapy or nonsubmersion (using a shower head to allow the water to run intermittently over the burn wounds with the patient on a stretcher suspended over a tank or tub); and (3) submersion (submerging the patient or burned extremity in a tub or tank of water for up to 20 minutes). The choice depends on the depth of injury, extent and location of the wound, and medical condition of the patient.

Most burn wound protocols call for daily or twice daily dressing changes. Various topical burn creams and solutions are available. No single topical agent has been demonstrated to be universally effective for burn care. Each has advantages and disadvantages, and the effectiveness of a topical agent may decrease after time. Different agents may be used on the same patient either concurrently, on different burned areas, or sequentially as the wound and its bacterial flora change. Each topical agent is applied with gauze dressings (type used is need specific). Gauze should be wrapped distally to proximally on burned extremities, and burn surfaces should not be allowed to touch (e.g., fingers and toes should be wrapped separately, and burned ears should not touch the burned head). Such attention to detail helps prevent webbing caused by raw surfaces growing together. Wrapping digits individually also facilitates active and functional movements.

Excision of damaged tissue may be initiated a few days after the burn or as soon as the patient is hemodynamically stable and edema has decreased. An autograft is immediately placed, or a temporary biologic or synthetic dressing is used until autografting can be done in a subsequent operation. Surgical excision is advantageous in reducing complications from invasive burn wound sepsis and shortening the time period from injury to wound closure and hospital discharge.

Full-thickness wounds require skin grafts unless they are small in size. Wounds of partial-thickness depth that do not heal spontaneously within 21 days should also be closed with a skin graft to minimize the potential for hypertrophic scar formation. Split-thickness skin grafts are used almost exclusively. This implies that the grafts are cut through a partial thickness of depth of skin, leaving epidermal regenerative cells that allow re-epithelialization of the donor site. Full-thickness skin grafts and flaps are occasionally used in primary repair of specific burn wounds (e.g., very deep electrical burns) but are primarily used later in some reconstructive procedures. The full-thickness donor site must then be closed primarily or with a partial-thickness graft.

Skin grafts may be cut from virtually any area of the body except the face and hands. The foot as a skin donor source is generally impractical. The scalp is a superior donor site. It has excellent blood supply with deep, closely placed hair follicles that are able to effect re-epithelialization in 4 or 5 days. Regrowth of scalp hair hides the donor site. Donor sites of the torso and extremities heal more slowly. In the majority of instances, wounds of the hands, face, and neck take precedence for skin grafts. However, when there is limited donor skin, consideration must be given to covering larger areas to try to reduce the size of the wound to first preserve the patient's life. The next priority for skin grafts after the hands, face, and neck is the skin over joints.

Skin grafts must be undisturbed in order to adhere. Fibrin causes initial adherence. The cells of the graft are nourished by tissue fluid until inosculation (anastomosis) of blood vessels between the wound and the graft establishes a nutritive blood flow in the graft. Inosculation occurs in about 2 days. Joints must be held immobile until the take of the skin graft is ensured. Immobilization is usually accomplished by a splint or rarely by skeletal traction. In most cases there is enough tensile strength between the graft and the wound to permit active range of motion (ROM) on the fourth and certainly by the sixth day after skin grafting. Gentle passive ROM can be added on the sixth or seventh day.

Early massive excision of the burn wound has increased the median lethal dose to 98% of total body surface area burn but represents the problem of wound closure (Herndon & Rutan, 1992b). Autograft substitutes must be used for a large burn. Alternative methods of wound closure that are currently used include biologic dressings, biosynthetic dressings, artificial skin, and cultured skin.

Biologic dressings consist of viable or once-viable tissues that are used to temporarily cover wounds in place of either conventional dressings or leaving the wound exposed. Biologic dressings are intended to reduce the risk of wound infection and decrease fluid loss through the open wound. Commonly used materials are partial-thickness grafts from living or recently deceased humans (allografts) or partial-thickness skin grafts from pigs (xenografts). Biologic dressings, both viable and non-viable, can be used for short-term, several-day wound coverage. In a large burn, biologic dressings can be lifesaving by providing temporary wound closure until completion of autografting. They may also be effectively employed to protect wounds that have been covered by widely meshed graft. Used in this way, the wounds between the autografts are closed as well.

Growth factor technology and innovative combination wound dressings have been introduced in recent years, offering improved wound healing, function and cosmetic result. Skin substitutes and engineered tissue equivalents have changed the approach to wound coverage (Honari, 2004). Alternative wound closure options are summarized in Table 34-2. With new technologies and techniques, the practice of treating burn patients has become increasingly specialized. All clinical staff in a modern burn center must have a substantial base of knowledge and a familiarity with procedures that are virtually unique to the field. Therapy protocols, such as timing and amount of ROM exercise and mobilizing programs, are based on the type of wound closure technology being used, in addition to the patient's stage of healing.

PRIMARY PHYSICAL IMPAIRMENT

Partial-thickness burn injuries will heal by re-epithelializing. Regeneration of epithelial elements comes from the epithelial cells lining every hair follicle, sebaceous gland, and sweat gland. Healing of partial-thickness burns can take 14 days, but if the burn is sufficiently deep, these burns may take 21 days or more for complete healing. As the epithelium grows, the normal pigmentation gradually and progressively returns. As the regenerated epithelium differentiates and forms the keratin layer, the function of the skin in maintaining and conserving core body temperature is restored. Deep partial-thickness wounds that require more than 14 days to heal and wounds requiring skin grafting to achieve closure are at high risk for scar formation and resulting physical impairment.

BURN SCAR

Loss of capillary integrity is a pathophysiologic feature of burn injury that leads to edema formation. This results in the outpouring of protein-rich intravascular fluid into the interstitium. This process occurs at all areas of partial-thickness burns and at areas adjacent to full-thickness burns. As the patient voluntarily limits movement because of pain, and as a result of direct damage to the lymphatic system, this edema fluid accumulates and persists in tissue spaces around tendons, joints, and ligaments. If motion is not restored and edema reduced, new collagen fibers form in this protein-rich edema fluid and eventually organize into unyielding adhesions and thickened support structures whose normal elasticity is lost.

Healing of deep dermal wounds also results in the replacement of normal integument with a mass of meta-bolically highly active tissues lacking the normal architecture of the skin (Parks et al., 1977). Several different processes appear to be at work in the healing wound. These processes include the following: mass production of large amounts of fused, highly disorganized collagen;

TABLE 34-2	Alternative Wound Closure Options and Topical Agents

TYPE	DESCRIPTION	ADVANTAGES/INDICATIONS

Biologic
  Allograft
	Viable or once-viable tissue
	  Skin from living or recently deceased
	    human
		Used for short-term, several-day wound closure
		Tests bed for autograft preparedness. Covers, protects, facilitates healing of interstices in widely meshed autografts.

Xenograft	Pig skin	Left intact on partial-thickness scalds, it eliminates pain without impeding epithelialization.
Skin substitutes Integra (Johnson & Johnson, Arlington, TX)	Bilayered membrane system Bovine tendon collagen matrix attached to Silastic epidermal layer	Provides matrix for development of neodermis Provides wound coverage after excision of large burns. Needs only very thin (0.005 inch) skin graft for final autograft coverage. Results in minimal hypertrophic scarring or contracture.
Alloderm (LifeCell Corp, Branchburg, NJ)	Biologic dermal matrix processed from cadaver allograft	Serves as a scaffold for normal tissue regeneration. Requires concomitant placement of thin autografts.
Apligraf (Novartis International AG, Switzerland)	Dermal layer human fibroblasts in lattice of bovine collagen, epidermis of human keratinocytes	Viable bilayered skin equivalent for tissue regeneration.
OrCel (Ortec, New York, NY)	Human keratinocytes and dermal fibroblasts cultured in two separate layers into bovine collagen sponge	Matrix provides favorable environment for host cell migration, and contains cytokines and growth factors.
TransCyte (Smith & Nephew, Inc., Largo, FL)	Polymer membrane and neonatal human fibroblast cells on porcine dermal collagen silicone mesh	Forms a protective biologic barrier, removed as epithelialization occurs.
Biosynthetic Biobrane (Bertek Pharmaceuticals, Inc., Morgantown, WV)	Synthetic structure, biologic tissue added Knitted elastic flexible nylon fabric bonded to a thin Silastic membrane, both layers contain bovine collagen	Stimulates wound healing Allows wound exudates to pass through, and encourages adhesion to wound surface until epithelialization occurs underneath.
Calcium alginates	Mixed calcium/sodium salts of alginic acid (seaweed origin) create a hydrophilic gel on contact with wound exudate	Used for heavily exudative wounds to provide moist environment for healing.
Glucan 11 (Brennan Medical, St. Paul, MN)	Smooth gas-permeable layer and a mesh matrix containing beta-glucan (derived from oats)	Activates and stimulates macrophages. Becomes adherent, then lifts from healing wound.
Synthetic	Cellulose acetate or polyurethane products	Protects healing wounds
Petrolatum based	Adaptic (Johnson & Johnson, Arlington, TX), Aquaphor gauze, Aquaphor ointment – non-adherent (Smith & Nephew Healthcare Limited, UK)	Protects healing burns, grafts, and donor sites from desiccation and mechanical trauma.
Foam dressings	Lyofoam – soft, hydrophobic polyurethane foam sheets (Seton Healthcare Group, Oldham, UK)	Used to absorb exudates, for autodebridement, and to maintain moist environment → granulation tissue and epithelialization.
Polyurethane dressings	OpSite, Flexigrid, Tegaderm – thin polyurethane membrane coated with acrylic adhesive (Smith & Nephew Healthcare Limited, UK)	Permeable to water vapor and oxygen, impermeable to microorganisms. Used in minimally exudative superficial wounds.

TABLE 34-2	Alternative Wound Closure Options and Topical Agents—cont'd	

TYPE	DESCRIPTION	ADVANTAGES/INDICATIONS
Antimicrobial	Antibacterial ointments and creams	To prevent infection in burn wounds
Acticoat (Smith & Nephew, Inc., Largo, FL)	2 sheets of polyethylene mesh coated with ionic silver and a rayon/polyester core.	Provides broad-spectrum antimicrobial and bactericidal coverage. Dressing is left in place until wound heals.
Xeroform (Kendall Co, Mansfield, MA)	3% bismuth tribromophenate in petrolatum blend on fine-mesh gauze.	Antimicrobial dressing, nonabsorbent, used on burns, grafts and donor sites.
Petroleum- and mineral oil-based agents	Bacitracin, neomycin, polymyxin (Ben Venue Laboratories Inc., Bedford, OH)	Antibiotic topicals, nontoxic, are used for moisturizing.
	Mupirocin (GlaxoSmithKline, Research Triangle Park, NC)	Active against methicillin-resistant *Staphylococcus aureus*, oil-based.
	Mafenide acetate (Sulfamylon) (Bertek Pharmaceuticals, Inc., Morgantown, WV)	Mainly for short-term control of infection
	Silver nitrate	Painless hypotonic solution, stains black
	Silver sulfadiazine	Most commonly used burn cream or spray
	Cerium	Use in combination with silver sulfadiazine
	Nystatin	Antifungal to control candidal growth
Hypobaric	Vacuum assisted closure (VAC) – negative pressure	Stimulates granulation tissue and epidermal migration
VAC (Kinetics Concepts, Inc., San Antonio, TX)	Closed-cell polyurethane foam sponge, sealed with gas-permeable adhesive drape, and connected to a portable pump	Induces movement of blood, lymph, and interstitial fluid → reduces peripheral edema, bacterial load, and progression.

replacement of the normal dermal elastic ground substance with inelastic chondroitin sulfate A; involuntary contraction of myofibroblasts; and inflammatory response with increased vascularity and localized lymphedema.

The bonds between the twisted collagen and firm inelastic ground substance, coupled with the simultaneous contraction of the myofibroblasts, contribute to the "heaped up" appearance of the hypertrophic scar. In addition, voluntary contraction of underlying skeletal muscle reinforces the compaction of the collagen. The intensity and duration of the vascular response provides a visible clue to the likelihood of hypertrophic scarring and contracture formation (Larson et al., 1979). The hyperemia of the scar tissue signifies ongoing change within the closed wound. As long as hyperemia persists, scar maturation has not been completed and hypertrophy is a possibility. It has been long accepted that the darker a patient's skin, the more predisposed that patient is toward hypertrophic scarring. Also, children are more susceptible to hypertrophic scarring than adults (Sullivan, 1990). Current research indicates possible relationships between deep dermal burns and changes in other skin components, including fat cells, and an increase in nerve density within hypertrophic scar tissue (Liang et al., 2004).

The active phase of scarring gradually subsides and will usually be completed in 1.5 to 2 years after the burn. If appropriate measures are instituted during this active period, the scar tissue loses its redness and softens. Linares and co-workers (1973) have shown that "pressure induces loosening of collagen bundles and encourages parallel orientation of the collagen bundles to the skin surface with the disappearance of the dermal nodules." With the application of pressure there is a coincident restructuring of the collagen mass and a decrease in vascularity and cellularity. Larson and colleagues (1974) reported that at least 25 mm Hg pressure must be achieved to provide histologically and clinically significant pressure.

The position of comfort for most patients is that of flexion of the joints. Maintenance of a flexed posture permits new collagen fibers in the wound to fuse together, resulting in contracture formation. Eventually the scar will mature, becoming a solid mass of fused collagen with a Swiss-cheese appearance as a result of continuing reabsorption of the collagen. The contracture will remain because of fusion of some of the collagen fibers into the shortened position.

Additional impairments occur as a result of skin grafting required for full-thickness burns. When the skin is transplanted to the area of full-thickness burn, no hair follicles, sebaceous glands, or sweat glands are included. These specialized skin appendages will not redevelop. Without these, the grafted area has none of the normal body oils, resulting in excessively dry skin. The absence of sweat glands inhibits the ability to dissipate the core body temperature when it is too high. Patients who require extensive skin grafting must be cautioned about this problem and warned to avoid environments with high heat and humidity.

Regeneration of nerve endings into the burned areas likely accounts for patients' frequent reports of abnormal or odd sensations in their burn wounds. As the nerve endings grow through the areas of scar tissue, they frequently meet an obstruction that may cause an area of hypersensitivity. Hypersensitivity may also be the result of small neuromas occurring in scattered areas throughout the burned area. Scar formation is a natural sequela in the healing process of burned skin. It cannot be prevented, although current research suggests the potential for therapeutic use of interferons to downregulate collagen production and inhibit wound contraction (Ghahary et al., 1993; Nedelec et al., 1995). The subjective assessment of scar appearance is a widely used method in the evaluation of burn outcomes and the effectiveness of treatment. A numeric scar-rating scale has been developed and has proved to be a useful tool for the evaluation of scar surface, thickness, border height, and color differences between a scar and the adjacent normal skin (Yeong et al., 1997).

MUSCULOSKELETAL COMPLICATIONS

In addition to burn scarring, many musculoskeletal complications, including peripheral nerve involvement, exposed tendons and joints, heterotopic bone formation, and amputation, are associated with immobility and inactivity during the acute phase of burn rehabilitation. Peripheral nerve damage, occurring in 15% to 29% of patients, results from (1) electrical injury by passage of current through the nerve, (2) edema with elevated tissue pressure, (3) metabolic abnormalities and nutritional deficiencies, and (4) localized nerve compression or stretch injury from improper dressings or positioning.

The superficial location of the extensor tendons, intrinsic muscles, and joints, as well as the hand's specialized skin functions, make burns involving the hand particularly complex. Knowing where and how deep the burn is before initiating treatment in a healed hand are important. For example, at 4 weeks after burn, the wounds may be closed, but the fact that the terminal extensor tendon was damaged and weakened will not

be apparent. If a therapist were to initiate a vigorous splinting or exercise program to regain full distal interphalangeal (DIP) flexion without regard to the status of the tendon, a rupture or attenuation of the terminal extensor tendon might occur.

A burn of bone tissue is possible in severe thermal injuries. Necrosis of the periosteum and cortex can occur, especially in superficially located bone such as the skull, tibia, and olecranon process. The damaged bone is weakened and appropriate precautions must be observed related to this impaired strength. Exposed bone also presents a challenge for wound closure, as a bed of healthy tissue is needed for successful grafting.

Heterotopic bone formation around joints may cause a disabling complication in 2% to 3% of patients with burns who are hospitalized. Heterotopic bone formation is rare in children but may be evident in adolescents. The most common site of heterotopic ossification (HO) following burn injury is the elbow. The calcification is usually located posteriorly and medially with a bony bridge between the olecranon of the ulna and the medial epicondyle and intercondylar portion and posterior shaft of the humerus. Heterotopic bone disappears spontaneously in about one half of cases. If excision is indicated, heterotopic ossification usually does not re-form after removal, and functional and often full ROM is restored. Physical therapy intervention can be continued with caution in the presence of HO. The physical therapy goal is remobilization of the joint.

The patient with associated limb amputation presents a number of unique problems (Ward et al., 1990a), including intolerance of the stump to pressure or manipulation because of remaining open wounds, fragility of newly healed skin grafts, and wounds on other body surface areas. There is also an increased risk of developing joint contractures because of hypertrophic scarring and the inevitable loss of muscle strength from bed rest after surgery. Nevertheless, despite these problems, it appears that most patients with burns who require limb amputation can achieve successful prosthetic use (Ward et al., 1990b).

PHYSICAL THERAPY GOALS AND PROCEDURES

EXAMINATION, EVALUATION, AND PLAN OF CARE

The purposes of the therapist's initial examination and evaluation are to determine the child's status, identify the rehabilitation needs, and anticipate potential problems.

The first task is to ascertain the immediate postinjury status of the patient. The information necessary to make this determination includes an assessment of the circumstances of the injury; the duration, type, and extent of the burn; preexisting medical and rehabilitation problems; concurrent injuries; and ROM estimates. The developmental status of young children before the burn injury must be ascertained. Information on the level of achievement of school-age children, both physically and scholastically, should be obtained to set realistic functional outcomes.

The expected clinical course and approximate length of hospital stay should be estimated to anticipate potential emotional, physiologic, and rehabilitation problems. Identifying the rehabilitation needs of the child requires thorough evaluation of examination findings, as well as an understanding of the implications of different types of burns and their locations. For example, anticipated goals and outcomes will be achieved before the child's discharge home for burns that are likely to heal in 21 days. For deeper burns, whether or not the area is skin grafted, the child is likely to require outpatient physical therapy to ensure skin healing with minimal scarring and deformity. The child with a deep burn will require periodic team follow-up at the burn center in addition to outpatient physical therapy. Physical therapy examination in the postacute stage consists of the following assessments: burn scar (scar mobility, turgor, and texture), ROM of joints adjacent to burned areas, pain, gait, and functional ability. Goals of the therapy program at this stage are based on the child's status, the effectiveness of the treatment procedures performed during the acute care period or after previous reconstructive operations, and the compliance of patient and family. Goals must be discussed with the child who is old enough to understand and in every case with the family.

The advent of managed health care has contributed to changes in the role of the physical therapist. In recent years, the role of the physical therapist has expanded. In the past, the role of the physical therapist included examination and intervention to reduce impairments such as edema, scarring, joint contracture, and muscle weakness in order to restore function. The expanded role includes prevention of disability in home, school, and social settings; establishment of a time frame for attainment of goals and outcomes; documentation of goals and outcomes; education of managed care personnel, families, employers, case managers, and the medical team; and coordination of care.

The emphasis of physical therapy is on functional outcomes that prevent or reduce disability (Fletchall & Hickerson, 1997). Outcomes, therefore, should be client focused and important for function. Client-focused outcomes to prevent or reduce disability for children include ability to perform self-care and mobility and engage in age-appropriate roles within the family and during play and school. Establishment of functional outcomes for children who have difficulty communicating their needs and concerns can be challenging and is best performed within the context of family-centered care. Interviewing and clinical reasoning skills and the experience of the therapist are vital in evaluating the needs of a child and family and in determining outcomes that have a high probability of being achieved within a specific time frame.

The American Burn Association (1996) has published patient outcomes for the different phases of recovery (Staley & Richard, 1996). As part of this document, clinical indicators were established to assist service providers in evaluating patient progress in meeting desired outcomes. Having identified outcomes for burn care, the next step is the development of critical pathways that reflect best practice. Critical pathways can assist in identifying and quantifying differences between expected and actual outcomes. The functional-based outcomes that are the end points of a critical pathway are the focus of the rehabilitation program, including the following: examination, direct intervention, patient/client-related instruction and education, patient satisfaction, and cost containment. Program evaluation and clinical research are the means to evaluate the effectiveness of a critical pathway and to make modifications when necessary.

The elements of patient/client management in the Guide to Physical Therapist Practice (American Physical Therapy Association, 2001) describes a process for making clinical decisions for optimal intervention outcomes. Through the examination (history, systems review, and administration of tests and measures), the physical therapist identifies impairments, functional limitations, disabilities, or changes in physical function and health status to establish the prognosis (determination of the optimal level of improvement that might be attained and the amount of time required to reach that level) and to develop the plan of care (which specifies anticipated goals and desired outcomes, specific direct interventions, the frequency of visits, and criteria for discharge). The child, family, and caregivers participate by reporting activity performance and functional ability. The selection of examination procedures and the depth of the examination vary based on patient age; severity of the problem; stage of recovery; phase of rehabilitation; home, community, or work (job/school/play) situation; and other relevant factors. Examination procedures specific to a child with a burn include the following:

assessment of the burn, including bleeding, signs of infection, and exposed anatomic structures; assessment of wound tissue, including epithelium, granulation, mobility, necrosis, slough, texture, and turgor; assessment of activities and postures that aggravate the wound or scar; and assessment of scar tissue, including banding, pliability, sensation, texture, and pigmentation. Integumentary preferred practice patterns C, D, and E describe the elements of patient/client management for burns (American Physical Therapy Association, 2001).

Once the examination and evaluation are completed, an individualized plan of care is established in collaboration with the child, family, and other members of the burn care team. The plan of care includes the goals, outcomes, and procedural interventions. The plan is developed with the primary focus on prevention of deformities, and interventions vary with the stages of wound recovery. Throughout implementation, the plan of care is coordinated closely with interventions provided by other team members, because outcomes are multidisciplinary. Success depends not on an individual discipline but rather on the cooperation and knowledge of each team member.

Many patients hospitalized for care of burn injuries show transient psychologic distress independent of such factors as burn size and premorbid function. Patients with severe burns, resulting in extended hospitalization, are particularly vulnerable to development of psychologic distress. The repeated, intrusive, and aggressive nature of burn care, although necessary for survival, may contribute to feelings of loss of control. The symptoms seen in children include regression, anxiety, decreased physical activity, withdrawal, behavior problems, decreased social interaction and play, and other depressive symptoms. The child's psychologic status must be considered when developing the plan of care. The quota system (Ehde et al., 1998) has been shown to be an effective new approach to helplessness behaviors and depressive symptoms that develop in some patients with burn injuries. The quota system as described by Ehde and associates (1998) utilizes 80% of a patient's baseline behavior measures as an initial quota value. The behavioral quotas are increased systematically and gradually every day until goals are achieved.

The deforming effects of burn scar contractures can be decreased by use of the following procedural interventions: proper patient positioning and use of splints, ROM and graded resistive exercises, early ambulation, scar management techniques, and patient and family education regarding skin care and the rehabilitation program. Other modalities such as continuous passive motion, fluid therapy, and paraffin aid in increasing skin

pliability and desensitizing the healed burn area. The plan of care should also include play activities and training in functional activities to facilitate the development of coping behavior. The child should be allowed to perform as much self-care as is possible, depending on the stage of recovery. Participation in dressing changes, decision making when confronted with equal alternatives, and personal hygiene must be encouraged to give the child a sense of control. An overview of intervention options by body part burned is presented in Table 34-3.

POSITIONING AND SPLINTS

The goals of splinting and positioning in burn management include edema reduction, protection of weakened or exposed structures, preservation or restoration of ROM, and protection of new grafts. Interventions will vary based on location and depth of burn, stage of recovery, and individual needs of the child. Splinting and positioning interventions may include propping, static splints, dynamic splints, static-progressive splints, serial casting, and skeletal traction or fixators.

Proper positioning can help to reduce edema by utilizing the pull of gravity. Proper positioning, through propping or splinting, can help to maintain ROM and counteract contracture by placing the burned area in a lengthened position, thus maintaining proper flexibility of connective tissue and skin. Protective splints maintain slack on exposed tendons or ligaments until wound closure or until integrity of the structure is restored. New grafts are protected by immobilizing adjacent joints and applying gentle, direct pressure to the graft. Methods of positioning are illustrated in Figure 34-2.

Children usually have difficulty understanding the long-range benefits of splinting and positioning procedures and are therefore typically unable to maintain optimal positioning independently. A splint is the most appropriate and effective method for proper positioning, especially during unsupervised periods and during sleep, when positions that contribute to deformity are assumed. When the child is able to be active during the day, a night splint may be indicated to maintain ROM gained during the day. When voluntary movement is impaired, as in the presence of peripheral neuropathies, a splint must be worn continuously (except during physical therapy and wound care) to avoid joint contracture.

Factors to consider in a splint include construction, fit, application, and adjustability. A pliable, lightweight, low-heat thermoplastic material is desirable. Bulky dressings should be minimized because they interfere with the fit of the splint and compromise alignment. Splints must be checked at least once daily and necessary adjustments

TABLE 34-3   Burn Treatment Options by Body Part

INVOLVED AREA	EXERCISE	POSITIONING	SPLINTING	PRESSURE
Face, head	Massage, facial exercises, eye blinking, mouth opening, chewing, Therabite	No pillow, elevate head of bed	Nasal splints	Custom elastomer mask, custom fabric hood, chin strap, clear mask with silicone, silicone patches or tape
Neck	Neck ROM, shoulder wedge	No pillow, split mattress	Neck conformer, soft collar	Neck conformer, elastomer insert, silicone wrap
Axilla	Abduction/flexion exercises, overhead pulleys, finger ladder, wand exercises, wall weights, shoulder continuous passive motion	Arm trough, papoose, sheepskin slings, bedside table with pillows	Axillary conformer	Padded figure-of-eight wrap, clavicle strap, custom vest, inserts
Elbow	Wall weights, barbells, pronation exerciser	Extension, supination	Anterior conformer, cast	Tubigrip, custom sleeve, silicone sleeve
Wrist, hand	Hand exercises, gripping devices, hand CPM.	Elevation above heart, flexion wrap	Wrist cock-up splint, burn hand splint, flexion splint, pan extension splint	Coban, isotoner gloves, custom gloves, web spacers, silicone inserts
Trunk, buttock, hip	Ambulation, trunk stretches	Proning, no pillow under knees, specialty beds	T-shirt splint, hip spica splint, bivalved cast	Custom pantyhose, bicycle shorts, breastplate, silicone patches
Knee	Ambulation, exercise bike, knee CPM, stairs	No pillow under knees, prevent frog-lying	Knee conformer, knee immobilizer	Tubigrip, custom socks, leggings
Ankle, foot	Ambulation, ankle circles, toe stretches, stairs	Foam heel protectors	Posterior foot splint, derotational splint, Unna boot, toe flexion splint, burn shoe, cast.	Tubigrip, custom socks, toe web spacers, dorsal silicone inserts

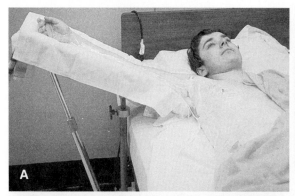

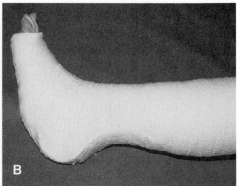

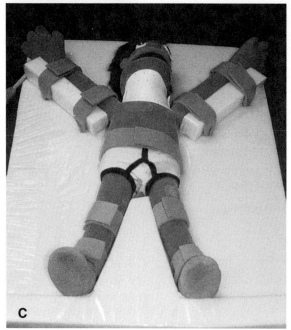

♦ **Figure 34-2** Positioning. Methods vary according to age and compliance of the patient. **A**, Teenager using arm trough attached to bed for axillary burn. **B**, Method of casting the foot used for infants and toddlers postoperatively. Note the bubble shape at the heel, where there is an air pocket, to eliminate pressure. **C**, Bernie the burn puppet demonstrating positioning in a foam papoose.

made. Pain, numbness, tingling, inflammation, or maceration of tissue indicates a poor-fitting or improperly applied splint, which can cause pressure necrosis of burned and unburned areas. Immediate adjustment is mandatory to prevent further damage. Examples of splints used for burns are illustrated in Figure 34-3.

During the emergent phase of burn recovery, the positioning plan involves elevation of burned extremities in order to facilitate edema reduction and protection of weakened or exposed structures. Pain and edema, rather than scarring, limit ROM during this stage of recovery. Positioning of the trunk and proximal extremities by propping on pillows, foam, and other objects may be adequate to maintain ROM. Proper positioning of the wrists, digits, and ankles typically requires splinting. A prefabricated ankle splint will likely be effective, but custom splinting of the wrist and hand is usually required. If the desired position is unable to be main-

tained with positioning, a splint should be fabricated. The positioning plan should be maintained at all times except during wound care and therapy sessions. Once burn resuscitation has been achieved and the patient is in the acute stage of recovery, the positioning plan will include maintaining gentle stretch to the burned skin. Passive and active ROM exercises will be initiated. If the patient is moving well and frequently throughout the day, in age-appropriate play/activity, positioning and splints are utilized at night and during daytime naps. For patients with deeper burns involving subdermal structures, or those with deep dermal burns who are unable to move sufficiently throughout the day, splints or positioning devices may need to be applied at all times except during wound care and therapy sessions. When skin grafts or biologic dressings are required, proper positioning contributes to good wound coverage. Splints and positioning devices used to immobilize skin grafts are

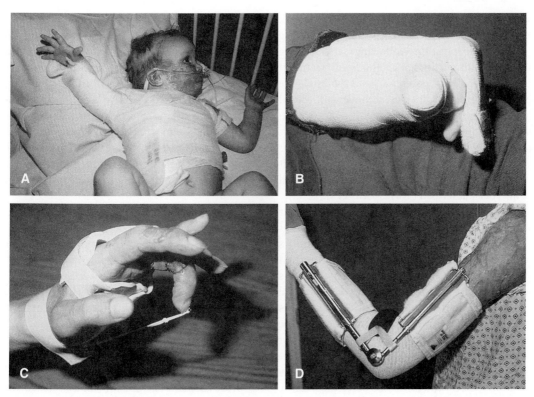

♦ **Figure 34-3**   Splints used for children with burns. **A**, Custom-molded axillary conformer. **B**, Casting the metacarpophalangeal joints into flexion. Note that this cast controls positioning of the first web space and allows for interphalangeal flexion of the fingers. **C**, Simple rubberband traction to provide gentle dynamic stretch to middle finger. **D**, Progressive stretch applied by dialing tension in this three-point elbow flexion Dyna splint.

typically kept in place at all times until the graft is deemed stable and ready for stretching, usually 5 to 7 days postoperatively. Most young children are able to continue moving and playing well, while the splint immobilizes the specific joint involved, as seen in the accompanying video clip.

Splints are also used to realign developing scar tissue or to stretch contracted skin. In these instances, they are applied at all times in order to apply a constant stretch or pressure. A series of positions should be designed for each involved joint, whereby the child alternates positions every 2 to 4 hours, because static positioning is not well tolerated.

Although the basic principles of splinting and scar contracture alignment must be adhered to for splints to be effective, therapists can be very creative with splint design. Recent publications illustrate modified and unusual designs for the neck (Foley et al., 2002; Serghiou, 2003), the axilla (Manigandan, 2003) and the hand (Van Straten, 2000).

Dynamic splints are the most effective method for reducing contractures involving the extensor surfaces of the wrist, hand, and posterior elbow. The proximity of the extensor tendons to the burned surface may result in scar adhesions forming around or attaching to the tendon. Dynamic splints that apply elastic tension in opposition to the contracture, but allow controlled resisted motion, facilitate excursion of the tendon through the scar formation. Application of constant tension is necessary to elongate tissue. These orthoses apply three-point pressure, are spring-loaded, and are designed to deliver a low-load, prolonged stretch to healing connective tissue. Dynamic orthoses, such as Dynasplint (Dynasplint Systems, Inc., Markham, Ontario) and JAS Systems (JAS, Effingham, IL), have been reported as effective in patients with burns. A dynamic elbow extension splint was reported as superior to a static splint when used to correct progressive loss of elbow ROM (Richard et al., 1995). Pediatric sizes are available.

Serial casting may be a successful alternative when low-force dynamic splints cannot be sized small enough for a child, when proper splint alignment cannot be maintained, or when patient compliance is unreliable. The goal in serial casting is gradual realignment of the collagen in a parallel and lengthened state by constant circumferential pressure from the cast. When casts are applied well and padded appropriately, there is little risk of pressure areas, because the casts are conforming and do not migrate position. Following serial casting for 7 days, the more traditional methods of treatment (paraffin, massage, ROM exercise, and splints) are continued to preserve the increased movement. Serial casting has been shown to be highly effective in increasing ROM of the burned foot (Ridgway et al., 1991; Johnson & Silverberg, 1995) and the burned hand (Harris et al., 1993). The fabrication and use of removable digit casts to improve ROM at the proximal interphalangeal joint have also been described (Torres-Gray et al., 1993).

Severe fixed ankle and foot deformities may occur when optimal positioning is not possible, such as when air-fluidized beds are used. The typical deformities include ankle plantar flexion and varus (equinovarus) and forefoot adduction and supination. External fixators have been introduced in burn management. A clinical report by Metzger and co-workers (1993) describes the use of Brooker and Hoffman fixators, which can be used to arrest further deformity but do not allow for correction, and Ilizarov fixators, which allow a multi-dimensional application of force to achieve anatomically correct positioning. The use of fixators, and the Ilizarov fixator in particular, is superior to splinting because of the propensity for formation of decubitus ulcers when rigid splints are used.

Clarke and colleagues (1990) noted that, in children, burns to the hand typically result from a different pattern of injury and respond differently to therapeutic intervention when compared with adults. Partial-thickness scald burns are most common in children. Children develop less stiffness in response to immobilization but tend to form more scar tissue compared with adults. Hand function therefore can be achieved in the majority of these cases. However, deep flame injuries to the hand present a challenge to the rehabilitation team. The hands of young children lack sufficient muscle strength to oppose the force of the contracting burn scar. The small size of their hands poses a challenge to splint fabrication. These potential problems can be managed with the full participation of the burn team, the child, and the family. Warden and associates (1993) demonstrated that individuals with severe hand burns necessitating partial joint amputation or individuals with exposed joints and tendons can achieve functional outcomes during the initial acute hospitalization when care is provided in a coordinated and efficient manner.

Splints may be used to reduce contracture and thereby preclude or minimize the need for extensive reconstructive surgery. Children who are developing contractures or scar bands over the volar aspect of the hand, wrist, elbow, posterior knee, or dorsum of the ankle and foot are fitted with conforming splints to oppose contracture formation by producing a softening and flattening effect on the scar band, which then allows increased skin excursion. Frequently, these splints are worn at night only, and the child is encouraged to move actively during the day. As ROM increases, the splint is remolded progressively until proper alignment of the part is achieved. The anterior surface of the neck is one area where a conforming splint worn at all times except for bath, meals, and exercise can be effective in maintaining ROM and skin contour.

EXERCISE AND ACTIVITIES

The child who has been burned tends to avoid movement, or, at best, moves rigidly and slowly. Structured exercise programs, therefore, are needed to prevent secondary complications. Although physical therapists have primary responsibility for implementation of these programs, optimal physical restoration will largely depend on the combined and concentrated efforts of all team members, the child, and the family.

Many factors influence the therapist's ability to provide adequate exercise for children with burn injuries. Pain, surgical procedures, wound complications, and the child's and the family's adjustment to the injury affect therapy. The therapist's skill in determining when to initiate exercise, choosing the type of exercise, and transferring of care to the child and family are important determinants of functional outcomes and the duration of the rehabilitation program.

Although children recovering from burns share common problems, the exercise program must be customized to each child's unique needs. Exercises for specific problems encountered by burn patients have been published (Richard & Staley, 1993). Therapists must be creative with exercises. Written instructions are necessary for parents to supervise young children and for older children to assume responsibility for their exercise program. Hayes-Lundy and associates (1993) performed a pilot study to test the usefulness of a computer-generated exercise program to create customized exercise programs for patients. Patients given computer-generated programs performed their exercises with an 88% success rate, compared with a 54% success rate for patients given handwritten programs. Several exercise software packages, such as Exercise Pro, are available commercially (BioEx Systems, Inc: www.bioexsystems.com).

Goals and the type of exercise needed for each stage of recovery are outlined in Table 34-4, and examples of exercises and activities are illustrated in Figure 34-4. The type and intensity of exercise are progressed according to

TABLE 34-4	**Exercise Goals for Each Stage of Recovery**	
STAGE	**EXERCISE GOALS**	**METHODS**
Emergent	Edema resolution, maintenance of joint mobility, prevention of respiratory complications	Slow gentle active or active-assistive ROM 2-4 times/day, PROM if patient unable to actively participate
Acute	Stretch healing skin, regain full joint ROM, preserve coordination of multiple joint movements, promote functional independence	ROM exercises, functional activities, ambulation
Postacute/rehabilitation	Increase joint ROM, prevent/correct contracture, strengthen and recondition, maximize functional abilities	ROM/ADL/ambulation programs, incorporating stretching, coordination, strengthening, endurance, and conditioning

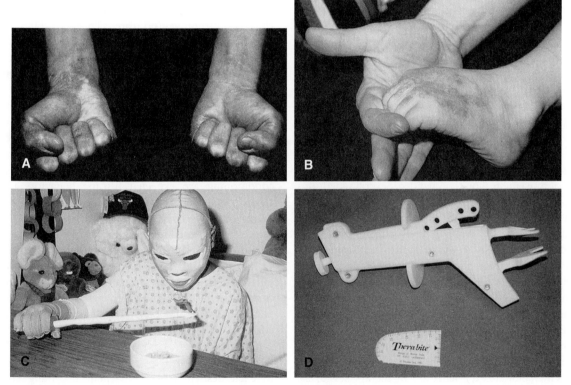

• **Figure 34-4**   Exercise and activity. **A**, Full active range of motion (ROM) of hands. Note that fingernails cannot be seen and the blanching of the skin over the proximal interphalangeal joints. **B**, Full passive flexion of the toes, in combination with ankle plantar flexion, indicating full extensibility of the healing skin. **C**, Everyday activities maintain mobility achieved by ROM exercises. This child has been given an extended-length spoon handle to accommodate the flexion deficit from heterotopic bone at the elbow. **D**, The Therabite jaw exerciser has proved to be effective in maintaining a stretch of the oral commissures in all directions. It can be patient controlled or fixed (shortened) and used as a static splint. The unit allows normal motion of the temporomandibular joint.

the child's recovery status. During the emergent or resuscitative period, emphasis of treatment is placed on passive range of motion (PROM), positioning, and splinting. However, if the child is alert, he or she may be able to engage in some movement activities such as bed mobility and positioning of extremities for dressing applications. ROM exercise is initiated for most patients as soon as adequate signs of burn shock resuscitation have been observed, generally within the first 24 to 72 hours after injury. Escharotomies do not preclude exercise. Exercises that would compromise or dislodge lines and airways are withheld, and emphasis is placed on positioning of the affected joints.

As the child makes the transition from the emergent phase to the acute phase of burn rehabilitation, the physical treatment program must also change to meet the patient's needs. The acute phase generally refers to the time period after emergent care through wound coverage, when the foundations of scarring are just beginning to form. Joint contracture is a major threat during this period.

Exercises are performed with each joint separately, then with all joints combined in a gentle sustained stretch that elongates the burned area. This is especially important when the burn crosses more than one joint. Richard and colleagues (1994, 1999) reported that a measurable amount of forearm skin movement occurs to permit wrist extension. In addition, the position of the elbow influences the amount of elongation of skin tissue necessary for wrist extension. Multiple vigorous repetitions of movement should be avoided. Several repetitions performed slowly with prolonged end-range hold are most effective. Active and active-assistive ROM with terminal stretch aids in maintaining joint mobility and tissue pliability, as well as minimizing loss of strength. In our experience, children will play while utilizing compensatory movements, but require intervention by a therapist to provide the amount of stretch needed to be effective in gaining ROM and function at joints limited by burn pain or developing scar tissue. Parents can be instructed to assist their child with ROM exercises, but may not be able to deal with the pain or sensation of stretching that it causes their child to experience during therapy sessions.

Burns around the mouth frequently result in contractures or microstomia. Over the years different orthoses have been used to stretch the mouth. In the past, the only true stretch achieved was horizontal. A device has been introduced that comfortably provides vertical and horizontal passive ROM and can be adapted and used by children who demonstrate fair to good compliance (Ridgway & Warden, 1995).

Compared with adults, children exhibit increased pain reactions during exercise, often owing to fear and apprehension. Coordinating administration of pain medications, and possibly antianxiolytics, with the nursing staff before exercise sessions greatly enhances the quality of exercise and amount of cooperation offered by the patient. It is also helpful for patient relaxation to initiate the exercise treatment with nonpainful or less painful exercises and gradually progress to the more painful exercises. Field (1995) reported that massage to non-burned areas results in lower anxiety and stress hormones and improved clinical course. Patients with burns who received massage before debridement demonstrated positive immediate and longer-term effects (Field et al., 1998). The positive effects may be attributable to reduction in pain, anger, and depression. Findings from a study by Hernandez-Reif in 2001 also support massage therapy in decreasing young children's distress responses to aversive procedures.

Various nonpharmacologic techniques have been developed and tested to promote the compliance of children during wound care (Thurber, 2000). These include provision of information, enhancement of predictability and control, provision of reinforcing distraction, promotion of self-mediated debridement, multimodal stress management, relaxation and bio-feedback, parent participation, and hypnosis. Overall, these techniques have been modestly effective in the reduction of pain behavior and in increasing cooperation of children. Complete reduction of distress may be impossible. Therefore, escape behavior and avoidance conditioning are expected. Escape behaviors include classic pain behaviors, such as yelling, whining, thrashing, questioning, swearing, and pleading. Avoidant behaviors that take place before wound care or therapy can also take many forms, usually some type of procrastination, such as distracting staff, suddenly becoming involved in unrelated activities, or spontaneous (perhaps fictitious) complaints of new ailments. The importance of pain management cannot be overemphasized. Any safe and effective method should be used.

Play and group activities are fun and allow children increased control. Play is perhaps the best method to elicit desired active movement in young children (Melchert-McKearnan et al., 2000). A report by Mahaney (1990) describes the loss of a severely burned child's ability to play and outlines the critical importance of play in the development of cognition, affectivity, and social learning (areas related to coping behavior). In addition, music therapy techniques employed during exercise sessions may provide an organizing structure within which rehabilitative and developmental gains can occur (Prensner, 2001). Use of empathy, empowerment of caregivers, modeling, and coaching techniques encourage a positive working alliance with caregivers and allows for successful transfer of the intervention to the family (Badger et al., 1993).

If pain control, relaxation, and exercise techniques have failed to maintain joint range, ROM exercise performed while the patient is under anesthesia is sometimes recommended to determine the extent of joint restriction and as an adjunct to routine exercise sessions. This procedure is beneficial in differentiating the underlying cause of ROM restrictions observed during interventions. In particular, it allows the therapist to determine if the child's pain, fear, apprehension, or manipulative behavior is interfering with achieving the goals of exercise sessions.

After grafting, exercise to the grafted area is discontinued for approximately 5 days to encourage incorporation of the graft into the wound bed. Proper patient positioning is stressed at this time. Exercise to joints proximal and distal to the grafted area might influence graft stability and therefore is contraindicated. Active and active-assistive ROM to all other nongrafted areas is continued. On removal of staples or sutures, if the graft appears stable, gentle active and active-assistive ROM exercise to the grafted area can be resumed with approval from the attending physician. It is recommended that the physical therapist observe dressing changes to identify areas of graft slough and possible tendon exposure.

It is typical that ROM decreases during the immobilization period after grafting. A general theory is that approximately 25% of the motion is lost during the postgraft stage. However, the patient who maintains essentially normal ROM during the pregrafting phase has a good prognosis to regain ROM. With most patients, full joint motion is expected 7 to 10 days after grafting.

As healing progresses, either spontaneously or after grafting, functional strengthening is introduced into the exercise program. Even if the child has open wounds and bandages, the therapist can apply minimal manual resistance. Resistance can be gently applied during isometric or isotonic muscle contraction. The postacute rehabilitative phase begins when the catabolic state reverses and there are few unhealed burn areas. This is the difficult and lengthy phase of wound contracture and hypertrophic scarring in which physical function and appearance can be altered significantly. A child who heals initially with full ROM has the potential to develop severe deformities during the postacute period as the healed skin matures and hypertrophic scarring develops. Sustained stretching is one of the most effective exercise techniques for lengthening bands of scar tissue and increasing ROM. Active-assistive ROM with the therapist applying mild manual stretching at the extremes of motion is well tolerated. Skin should be stretched to the point of blanching. Holding the stretch for 10 or 15 seconds is recommended at the terminal point of stretch as tolerated. Whenever possible, overall patterns of motion are emphasized because scar tissue may cause profound limitations of motion when multiple joints are involved. It is often helpful to simultaneously use deep tissue massage while stretching a tight scar band.

Coordinated movement is generally diminished after burn injury. It is essential that substitution patterns are identified and altered before they become habitual. Coordination exercises are extremely beneficial in eliminating the mechanical robot-like postures and movements frequently characteristic of patients with burns. In children, the application of neurodevelopmental treatment techniques provides a holistic means to address the goal of increased ROM by enhancing postural stability, mobility, and achievement of age-appropriate developmental milestones. By using this approach, Burne and colleagues (1993) have shown that therapeutic technique can be more easily incorporated into the child's home life through parent teaching, focusing on everyday activities, and consideration of the family's lifestyle.

Careful integration of physical conditioning as part of the postacute rehabilitation exercise program enhances the patient's activity and participation. When possible, conditioning exercise incorporates activities enjoyable to the child, such as bicycling, dancing, or swimming, and provides the child not only with a sense of physical well-being but also with an opportunity for social interaction. Moderate intensity progressive resistance and aerobic exercise conducted three times weekly for 1 hour in addition to standard therapy over 12 weeks has been shown to result in significant improvements in muscle mass, strength, and cardiovascular endurance (Cucuzzo, 2001). A recent clinical trial by Celis (2003) involving children with severe burns links exercise to a reduction in the number of surgeries for scar releases up to 2 years after the injury when compared with a control group. Subjects in the experimental group participated in a supervised exercise program of 60 to 90 minutes three times per week for 12 weeks. The exercise program included resistance and aerobic exercises performed at 70% to 85% maximal effort.

AMBULATION

The ability to move about has a significant impact on the restoration of independence. Children begin to ambulate as soon as their physical and medical condition warrants, usually by 48 to 72 hours after injury, when vital signs are stable and fluid resuscitation is complete. With proper precautions and necessary staff participation, children in the burn unit are assisted in ambulation to the limits of their physical endurance. Hollowed and associates (1993) have developed technical maneuvers and precautions for patients who are intubated to ensure safety during ambulation. Beginning ambulation while the patient is still intubated was effective in reducing pulmonary complications and has increased the survival rate in patients with acute burns from 88% to 95%. In difficult cases, use of a tilt table may be the only way to progress the child to weight bearing.

For nongrafted lower extremity burns, ambulation is initiated once the child is medically stable unless tendons or joint capsules are exposed, severe swelling or cellulitis is present, or the soles of the feet are severely burned. Mild to moderate burns of the feet do not preclude early ambulation. Dressings with extra padding and foam-soled slippers will protect the wounds and aid in reducing the discomfort of bearing weight. To avoid venous stasis in lower extremities and the resulting discomfort associated with upright positions, elastic bandages are applied from toe to groin before standing, and full weight bearing is encouraged. A figure-of-eight wrap is used, because this provides an even distribution of pressure and better support for the extremity than do spiral wraps.

Assistive devices such as walkers, crutches, and canes are not encouraged. A normal gait pattern is emphasized. However, young children often show regression in walking, particularly if they had been ambulating only a few weeks before the burn injury. Knowing what the child wants to play with or walk to may be the key to initiating ambulation. Toys such as tricycles can be great incentives.

When to initiate ambulation after grafting is controversial. A prospective study by Schmitt and associates (1991) indicated a significant reduction (mean of 4.1 days) in length of hospital stay for patients who ambulated on postoperative day 7 compared with patients who ambulated on postoperative day 11. Kowalske and colleagues (1993) reported no difference in graft take or time to complete wound closure following lower extremity skin grafting between early (postoperative day 3 or 4) and late (postoperative day 7, 8, or 9) ambulators. Increased skin graft loss was seen in patients whose physical conditions prohibited ambulation on the randomly assigned day.

The child with a less complicated burn can master the progression of walking with few problems. Dr. Paul Unna's "boot," a zinc oxide-calamine-gelatin bandage, has been marketed under various names such as Medicopaste (Graham-Field, Inc., Hauppage, NY 11788) and Primer (Glenwood, Inc., Tenafly, NJ 07670). It has been used with small wounds to allow patients to ambulate within 48 hours after grafting because of the adherent properties in securing the graft and the additional vascular support. Wells and co-workers (1995) demonstrated a mean reduction in hospital stay from 12.9 days to 1.4 days for a group of patients with uncomplicated noncircumferential lower extremity burns who were treated with split-thickness skin grafting and Unna paste. The Unna dressing has also proved effective in management of skin grafts to the hands of patients receiving outpatient services (Sanford & Gore, 1996).

PRESSURE GARMENTS AND INSERTS

Hypertrophic scarring remains a major problem for the recovering patient. The mainstay of treatment is controlled pressure to the involved areas using Coban or Ace bandages and presized or custom-fit elastic garments. Inserts of rubber, foam, or gel materials have been used to improve the response to pressure, particularly over concave surfaces. In the early 1970s, the use of pressure for the treatment of hypertrophic scars, keloids, and severe contractures became a standard of burn care. Use of controlled pressure originated and was promoted by the wound healing team of the Shriners Burns Institute at Galveston, Texas (Linares et al., 1993). Although the exact mechanism of action is unknown, pressure appears clinically to enhance the scar maturation process (Staley & Richard, 1997).

Based on the guidelines on the characteristics of burn treatment, the following features can help the therapist select methods of pressure: (1) healing time of the burn, (2) size of the unhealed areas, (3) fragility or condition of the healed skin, (4) location of the burn, and (5) treatment cost. Briefly, all patients whose burns require 14 to 21 days to heal and who have areas grafted with split-thickness grafts should have prophylactic pressure therapy. Pressure should be applied as early as possible. The type of pressure, however, will depend on the fragility of the newly healed skin and remaining open areas. Pressure therapy can be initiated during the acute phase of recovery using Ace wraps over bulky dressings, and progressing to Tubi-Grip when only thin dressings are required. Custom garments can be applied once the burn is 90% healed. This progression is necessary because new epithelium and grafts are susceptible to shearing. Lower extremity burns may require pressure not only to minimize scarring but also to minimize persistent edema and discoloration. Custom pressure garments are very expensive, so anticipated patient compliance should be carefully considered.

Signs that the pressure program has been successful can be seen as early as 24 to 48 hours after the initial application. Immediately after the removal of the garment,

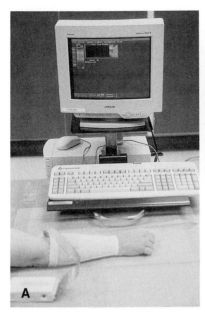
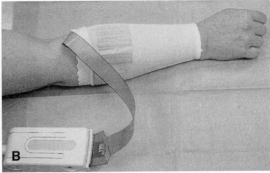

♦ **Figure 34-5**   Measuring pressure. **A**, The I-Scan system has been developed to accurately record the amount of pressure provided by garments and other pressure devices. **B**, The I-Scan sensor shown in place under a custom forearm sleeve.

evidence of effectiveness includes blanching of scar tissue, flattening of the scar, increased softness, decreased edema, minimal blistering, and no tingling or numbness. If any of these desirable effects are not observed, the therapist should evaluate the (1) fit of garment –(if the patient has gained or lost more than 10 pounds, this may be enough to decrease the pressure garment's effectiveness) and (2) condition of a garment –(the average life of custom pressure garments is 3 months). If the garment loses its stretch and does not cause blanching of the scar, it has lost its effectiveness; a new garment must be made. The amount of pressure being provided by the garment can be measured easily and accurately (Mann et al., 1997). The I-Scan system, shown in Figure 34-5, simplifies the accurate measurement of garment-scar interface pressure. Trouble spots receiving too much or too little pressure can be identified and altered.

When isolated areas of hypertrophy remain, sufficient pressure has not been applied. Areas where this commonly occurs include the sternum, face, volar aspect of the hand, angle of the mandible, web spaces, and across the flexor surface of the joint. To exert sufficient pressure on these areas, pressure garments frequently need to be supplemented by inserts (Fig. 34-6). Characteristics to be considered in choosing the composition of the insert include its texture, flexibility, compressibility, and ability to conform. The insert must be worn for the same amount of time as the pressure garment (23 hours per day) in order to be effective. A multidisciplinary team representing physical therapy, computer-aided design and computer-aided manufacturing (CAD/CAM), bio-

medical engineering, and prosthetics has advanced the method of developing total-contact burn masks by use of human body electronic imaging, computer graphics, and numerically controlled milling processes. High-resolution surface scanning and CAD/CAM have been used successfully to accurately fabricate face masks (Whitestone et al., 1995).

A thorough knowledge of the properties of the insert is required for decision making. No single material suffices for all situations. Many patients and therapists report difficulties when using silicone or other types of inserts under garments. The most common problems include irritation of skin from the pad, limited joint motion, sweating, annoying odor, and movement of the insert. One resourceful method used to apply a silicone elastomer pad beneath a pressure garment was described by Van den Kerckhove and colleagues (2001). Elastomer is molded on the patient between layers of Tubi-Grip. Another system for making a custom pocket has been described by Taylor (1993). Extra material in the form of a pocket can be stitched into the outer layer of the garment to keep an insert from shifting its position and to provide a soft, breathable, contact layer to the skin.

There is consensus in the literature that silicone pads are especially effective in diminishing the thickness of the scar. Some authors suggest that this happens only in the body areas where high pressure was maintained (Van den Kerckhove et al., 2001). Others have reported that silicone products induce a positive effect on burn scars without pressure (Davey, 1997). Good results can be obtained even with old scars.

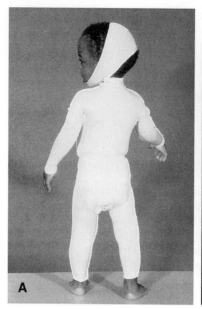
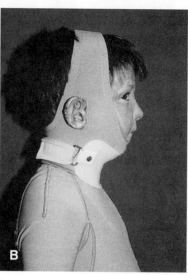

• **Figure 34-6**   Pressure garments. **A**, Interim pressure can be provided by soft fabric standard-sized garments. **B**, Custom-fit garments. Extra pressure is often needed to further enhance effectiveness of the garments, as illustrated by the silicone pad under the elastic vest and application of the conforming neck splint.

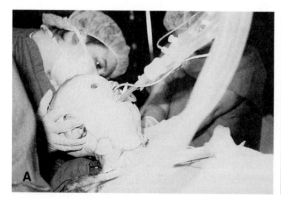
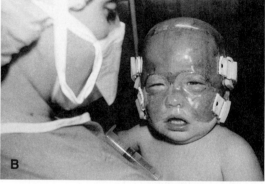

• **Figure 34-7**   Face mask. Because of the many concavities on the face, custom-molded face masks are needed to provide pressure to the entire surface. **A**, Custom-molded silicone elastomer face mask being applied in the operating room, immediately following skin grafting. It is held in place with a modified featureless fabric hood. **B**, For long-term pressure, hard, clear, molded face masks can be used if the patient is able to keep frequent appointments for adjustments and modifications.

The face is particularly difficult to fit for pressure garments and facemasks. Garments and facemasks such as those illustrated in Figure 34-7 require frequent monitoring and modification. Caution and close monitoring of face masks is essential, particularly when used in the young growing child. Two studies suggest serious complications in children with head and neck burns. Fricke and colleagues (1999) demonstrated changes in growth direction of the mandible and maxilla after consistent application of the total face mask. In addition, Chester and associates (1993) claim that the most common cause of obstructive sleep apnea is excessive pressure on the mandible by compression garments, particularly chin straps.

Compliance with wearing correctly applied pressure garments is crucial for effective scar control. External pressure support is prescribed to be worn 23 hours a day until the remodeling phase of healing is complete. Spurr and Shakespeare (1990) list the difficulties that arise with a pressure garment program. Pressure garments must be worn for up to 2 years. They are inconvenient for patients, and are relatively expensive. There is no guarantee that the child and parents will comply with the treatment recommendations. One study of adult patients reported that compliance with wearing pressure garments was less than 50% (Greenspan et al, 1993). Factors affecting compliance included patient perception of the burn and garment, understanding of the goals of the pressure program, psychosocial influences, garment-specific factors, and the level of functional independence related to the burn and garment use. Identification of factors that affect garment use is critical in formulating strategies to improve adherence.

Young children in diapers are difficult to fit with external vascular support garments. Soft diapers under a leotard decrease the amount of compression applied to buttock scars. While the healing wound, donor site, or graft remains active, the scar tissue remains painful or pruritic whenever the garment is removed. If the infant excoriates the scars when the garment is off, the scars become thicker and more painful. The discomfort of frequent diaper changes stresses parents, contributing to poor compliance with garment application. Various garments have been designed, such as detachable legs and an open crotch. The "brief" portion of the garment can be replaced without removing the stocking portions, and the open crotch allows ready diaper change without removing any portion of the garment. The introduction of colored pressure garments may increase social acceptance and contribute to better compliance (Thompson et al., 1992).

As scar tissue approaches maturity, the hyperemia fades and the scar flattens and becomes more pliable and soft. When these qualities persist for several weeks after removal of the pressure garments, the scar tissue is mature, and the garments and inserts may then be discontinued.

OTHER MODALITIES

Numerous modalities, each having a specific physiologic effect, are available in rehabilitation. In the author's experience, the only one shown to be consistently affordable and effective in burn scar management is paraffin. The combination of paraffin and sustained stretch usually is introduced late in the acute phase of rehabilitation after major healing has occurred, and it is generally continued throughout the patient's rehabilitation. The use of paraffin is particularly indicated when a painful and contracting scar limits joint ROM. The superficial heat and lubrication reduce scar pain and improve scar extensibility. The paraffin mixture is used when it reaches a temperature of 46°C to 48°C or when a light skim covers the top of the mixture. Caution is suggested for

newly healed scar tissue, which will blister easily if the standard paraffin bath temperature is used. Pouring or patting of the paraffin is done after the patient is positioned with the affected part in a sustained maximum stretch. The treatment time is 20 to 30 minutes. In the authors' experience, patients report decreased joint pain, and objective measurements show a 5° to 10° increase in ROM after paraffin treatment. When paraffin is used in combination with massage, sustained stretching, and functional activity, the patient can frequently maintain ROM gains until the next therapy session.

FAMILY EDUCATION

It is crucial that the child's family understand the daily care that will be required at home. There may be extensive technical and medical information for parents to absorb, and it is best if the family begins early in the child's hospitalization to be instructed in all aspects of care and to ask questions, discuss treatments, and watch demonstrations. Some centers have found it helpful to create manuals to be reviewed with family members before discharge (Bochke, 1993; Reed & Heinle, 1993). In this way parents have a chance to absorb written material and to practice the child's care under supervision of the health care providers before discharge. Thus, when they arrive home with the child, they will feel more confident about their ability to carry out the required therapy. Special patient and family problems such as illiteracy, low learning levels, fluency in English, and deafness have also been addressed with customized guides, including pictorial guides, laminated flip charts, card file systems, audiotapes, videotapes, and photographic guides (Walling et al., 1993).

INDIRECT SERVICES

Indirect services such as management, supervision, quality assurance, consultation, and research are also important components of the physical therapist's role in burn care. Management is concerned with the delivery of effective care in a cost-efficient manner. Managed health care systems have affected burn care. Clients with managed health care insurance have experienced a lack of reimbursement for rehabilitation when functional outcomes are not achieved (Fletchall & Hickerson, 1997). Therapists must develop the ability to communicate and present data illustrating how therapy relates to costs, goals, outcomes, and time frames. Anticipating and developing rationales for burn rehabilitation can facilitate reimbursement, minimize delay between inpatient and outpatient therapy programs, and ensure optimal outcomes. The quality and appropriateness of physical therapy services are monitored through the use of quality assurance programs, including participation in accreditation procedures. Technologic advances in the treatment of burn injuries offer ongoing opportunities for collaborative research to improve the quality of care of the child with burn injuries.

OUTPATIENT THERAPY AND FOLLOW-UP

Perhaps the most difficult problem that a therapist faces during home care is the tendency for the child to manipulate his or her parents and thereby fail to carry out the prescribed home program. This is particularly true if the parents feel guilty about the burn accident. Some children take advantage of feelings of guilt or sympathy and will resist therapy at home, even if they were cooperative while in the hospital. In conjunction with this, some parents also perceive their child to have more problems than the child or his or her teacher reports. Results of a study by Meyer and associates (1994) suggest that troubled parents may overestimate the difficulties of their child. Shelby and associates (1993) have identified additional family factors. Parents of children who sustained burns reported more depression and anxiety than spouses of adults who were burned. Higher somatic symptom reporting was associated with fewer social resources, higher anxiety, and depression. Lower somatic symptoms were seen in parents reporting high hardiness, esteem, and perceived family social support.

Most children continue to require daily intervention provided by a physical therapist after they make the transition into postacute rehabilitation, although therapy services should serve a secondary role. Housinger and co-workers (1992) demonstrated that the success of pediatric outpatient rehabilitation is dependent on the dedicated effort of parents. Duration of sessions varies according to parent involvement and the child's tolerance. Moderate to major burns require anywhere from 1 to 5 hours of treatment per day, including rest periods. As the child demonstrates increased independence and goals are achieved, sessions are reduced to two to three times per week and eventually to weekly rechecks. Although therapy is demanding and crucial during this time, children should also be allowed time for other activities to make the transition to home, school, and community. Reybons (1992) stresses that leisure and recreation activities provide an opportunity to reestablish control over leisure time.

After discharge from the burn unit, settings for postacute rehabilitation are highly variable. In acute hospitals, the patient may continue to be seen in outpatient therapy settings. Burn centers sometimes transfer daily therapy care of children who travel great distances to a community hospital and then follow the patient periodically in an outpatient burn clinic. Some burn centers have rehabilitation beds or step-down units that continue medical care until the patient and family are ready for discharge to home. Other centers have transitional units, in which children and their families assume responsibility for care in a protective environment (Daugherty et al., 1993). Children with complex injuries, amputations, large body surface area burns, or neurologic involvement may need several months in a designated rehabilitation center.

In most cases it is desirable for the child to return to the burn facility for follow-up outpatient clinic visits. Frequent checkups will allow the burn team to monitor the child's progress and adherence to the therapy program, and to progress the plan of care when appropriate. The checkups enable the staff to detect any problems that may develop and to recommend changes to the therapy program as necessary. The burn team can answer questions for the child and family, such as those regarding skin care as healing occurs. Common problems addressed in follow-up clinics include skin breakdown, maceration, dryness, itch, sun intolerance, and impaired thermoregulation. Other issues that are addressed include physical activity level, continued use and fit of pressure garments and splints, maturation of scars, application of cosmetics, and plans for further surgical procedures. If the family does not live near the primary care facility, local follow-up care can be arranged. In all cases, however, family members should be encouraged to contact the burn unit staff when they have concerns or questions. With open communication, the development of secondary complications is minimized.

CHRONIC FUNCTIONAL LIMITATIONS

Persistent cutaneous inflexibility may result in tightening of underlying muscles, tendons, ligaments, joint capsules, and fascia. Chronic limitation of motion, therefore, may continue to affect the physical ability of a child and become more noticeable with growth. Functional outcomes that are also aesthetically pleasing may be more difficult to achieve in children compared with adults. Reconstructive procedures are often required after growth spurts and until bony growth is complete (Dado & Angelats, 1990). The child will require further intervention by the physical therapist after each reconstructive procedure for management of the new grafts.

The incidence of surgical release of contractures is higher in children than in adults, even though burn wound size may be similar. The hand and the central body regions (head, neck, and axilla) are likely to have the highest incidence of contracture formation. Central body region contractures, plus contractures at sites that had been previously fascially excised, have the poorest outcome after surgical reconstruction. It has been common practice to delay reconstructive surgery, when possible, until the burn scars have matured. However, early contracture release can be successfully performed in patients with severe contractures that limit function.

Potential impairments for each body area are listed in Table 34-5. Surgical and rehabilitative goals for correction of chronic impairments vary according to the age and stated needs of each child. Consideration of length, sensation, mobility, stability, strength, and, to a lesser extent, appearance dictate the reconstructive needs. The emphasis on function versus appearance is different for children of each age group. One of the more challenging areas requiring reconstruction after burn injury is the neck. Perineal contractures are also a frequent problem in the pediatric population. Pisarski and co-workers (1994) list several procedures for correction but report a high recurrence rate (46%), even with postoperative pressure garments, splints, and exercise.

In one study, the health care worker's perception of burn scars was compared with that of the patient (Prothman et al., 1993). Of scar variables, including color, texture, dryness, lack of hair, lack of stretch, wrinkles,

TABLE 34-5   Potential Impairments

BODY AREA	IMPAIRMENT
Face	Facial disfigurement (contractures of eyelids, nose, mouth, ears, and adjacent facial skin)
	Inability to close eyes
	Loss of facial expression
	Teeth malalignment
	Drooling and inability to close lips
	Lower lip eversion
Neck	Loss of normal cervical spine ROM
	Limited visual fields
	Difficulties with anesthesia due to decreased neck ROM
Trunk	Protraction of shoulders
	Kyphosis
	Functional scoliosis
	Decreased respiratory function
	Breast entrapment
	Peroneal banding
Axilla	Type 1: either anterior or posterior contracture
	Type 2: anterior and posterior contracture with sparing of dome
	Type 3: anterior and posterior contracture and axillary dome
Hands	Metacarpophalangeal extension deformities
	Wrist extension deformities
	Proximal interphalangeal flexion deformities
	Interdigital web contractures
	Clawing of fourth and fifth digits
	Thumb contractures (adduction, opposition, flexion, and extension)
Arms and legs	Antecubital banding and flexion
	Posterior popliteal banding and flexion
	Anterior hip banding and flexion
	Medial and lateral malleolar scarring
Foot and ankle	Hyperextension of metatarsophalangeal joints
	Equinovarus
	Cavus foot
	Rocker-bottom deformity

height, and mesh appearance, only interrater scores for vascularity correlated positively with patient scores for scar appearance. Patients most often stated that nothing bothered them about the scar. However, when problems were reported, the scar variables that were most unattractive to the patient were often different from those that bothered the staff. This must be considered when planning reconstructive surgery.

Older children appear to have a much more difficult time accepting the residual scar. When faced with the burden of coping with disfigurement resulting from a burn injury, the adolescent's sense of self-esteem may be diminished. Providing adolescents the opportunity to learn makeup techniques that lessen the impact of their scars is an effective intervention for enhancing self-perception and their perception of how others view them. This was demonstrated in a study of 115 patients attending reconstructive makeup clinics (Beattie et al., 1993).

ASSESSMENT OF PERFORMANCE IN LIFE ROLES

The ultimate goal of a comprehensive program is to assure that children with severe burns heal sufficiently to regain their potential for productive and satisfying lives. The road to recovery is long and complex, requiring meticulous medical and social management after discharge from acute care. The "wellness" of a child and success of intervention should be measured from multiple perspectives, including physical, emotional, and social outcomes. Assessment of these outcomes should take into account factors related to the burn itself, such as severity, as well as adaptations to the consequences of the burn. Successful return to school is an essential part of the "return-to-wellness" process and should be regarded as an important outcome measure.

The barriers to successful recovery for a child with a severe burn can be considered using the International Classification of Functioning, Disability, and Health (ICF) (Pidcock et al., 2003). In regard to body function and structures, minimizing the extent and severity of contractures is a primary goal. Length of initial hospitalization; the number of skin graft procedures; the number of joint surface areas requiring skin grafting; the percent of hospitalization spent in intensive care; septic or bacteremic bouts; and ventilator dependence are factors that may affect the extent and severity of burn-related contractures including the number and complexity of reconstructive surgeries undertaken to improve joint mobility.

Suboptimal management of contractures results in activity limitations and participation restrictions. Poor problem solving, inadequate compensatory strategies and increased anxiety with physical demands are personal factors that contribute to activity limitations and participation restrictions. Limitations in self-care, mobility, and fine motor skills can restrict social interaction, learning, and leisure pursuits at school and in the community. Extending care across multiple levels, including support in the educational system through the provision of therapeutic services to ensure success in school, may help address problems at this level.

Other factors may influence the child's return to school and potential for future employment. These factors include preinjury status and the need for long-term and periodic treatment. Physical therapists, as part of the burn team, are often involved in the return-to-school process. The physical therapist may provide school personnel with information regarding the child's current abilities and provide recommendations to school therapists and physical educators. Therapists may also participate in preparing the teachers and students for the child's abilities and needs (by means of individualized videotapes and, when necessary, on-site school visits). School reintegration programs have been developed to enhance a positive sense of self-worth in a child who has been burned. The premise of these programs is that cognitive and affective education about children with burns will diminish the anxiety of the child with a burn, the child's family, faculty and staff of the school, and the students. Five principles guide school reentry programs: (1) preparation begins as soon as possible, (2) planning includes the patient and family, (3) each program is individualized, (4) each patient is encouraged to return to school quickly after hospital discharge, and (5) burn team professionals remain available for consultation to the school (Blakeney, 1995). The student who has sustained a burn injury, the school's personnel, and the student's peer groups benefit from a school reentry program. Concrete, factual information about the burn injury helps open lines of communication between the returning student and peers. The concerns and expectations of school personnel are addressed (Bishop & Gilinsky, 1995).

Research on psychologic adjustment of children following severe burns is encouraging. Blakeney and associates (1993) concluded that following severe burns (affecting >80% of total body surface area), children develop positive feelings about themselves and appear no more troubled than a comparable group of children without burns. The impact on the families, however, was significant and must be considered in the rehabilitation process. A recent follow-up study of 101 young adults with major burn injury during childhood indicates that most are progressing satisfactorily in the domains of education, occupation, and serial relationships (Meyer et al., 2004). Although most children do not have significant psychologic problems despite visible sequelae of their burn injuries, the burn team should carefully observe and inquire about child and family distress and provide support and guidance.

SUMMARY

Physical therapy for children with burns should begin at the time of injury and may extend for several years beyond the initial hospitalization. There is no single best physical therapy intervention for children with burns. Each child has unique problems, and specific procedures and techniques are incorporated into an individualized rehabilitation program developed by the team, the child, and the family. The recovery process is long and often complicated, but successful rehabilitation, based on a comprehensive psychologic, social, and physical view of the child, is extremely gratifying.

REFERENCES

American Burn Association, Committee on the Organization and Delivery of Burn Care. Burn care outcomes and clinical indicators. Journal of Burn Care and Rehabilitation, 17(2):17A–39A, 1996.

American Physical Therapy Association. Guide to Physical Therapy Practice. Physical Therapy, 81(1):S587–S655, 2001.

Atiles, L, Mileski, W, Spann, K, Purdue, G, Hunt, J, & Baxter, C. Early assessment of pediatric burn wounds by laser Doppler flowmetry. Journal of Burn Care and Rehabilitation, 16(6):596–601, 1995.

Badger, K, Gaboury, T, & Warden, GD. A collaborative effort: Music therapy and occupational/physical therapy in pediatric burn rehabilitation. Poster presented at the meeting of the American Burn Association, Cincinnati, March 1993.

Barrow, RE, Spies, M, Barrow, LN, & Herndon, DN. Influence of demographics and inhalation injury on burn mortality in children. Burns, 30:72–77, 2004.

Beattie, DM, Chedekel, DS, & Krawczyk, T. Utilization of a reconstructive makeup clinic for self-image enhancement in burned adolescents. Paper presented at the meeting of the American Burn Association, Cincinnati, March 1993.

Bishop, B, & Gilinsky, V. School reentry for the patient with burn injuries: Video and/or on-site intervention. Journal of Burn Care and Rehabilitation, 16(4):455–457, 1995.

Blakeney, P. School reintegration. Journal of Burn Care and Rehabilitation, 16(2):180–187, 1995.

Blakeney, P, Meyer, W, Moore, P, Murphy, L, Robson, M, & Herndon, D. Psychosocial sequelae of pediatric burns involving 80% or greater total body surface area. Journal of Burn Care and Rehabilitation, 14(6):684–689, 1993.

Bochke, I, Frauenfeld, A, Hartlieb, D, Zwicker, M, & Inkson, T. Patient and family education in burn care: Development of a series of teaching books by a multidisciplinary team. Poster presented at the meeting of the American Burn Association, Cincinnati, March 1993.

Burne, BA, Hackencamp, TB, Pfabe-Wiggans, S, & Sprecht, D. The application of neurodevelopmental treatment in pediatric burns. Poster presented at the meeting of the American Burn Association, Cincinnati, March 1993.

Carvajal, HF. Burns in children and adolescents: Initial management as the first step in successful rehabilitation. Pediatrician, 17:237–243, 1990.

Celis, MM, Suman, OE, Huang, TT, Yen, P, & Herndon, DN. Effect of a supervised exercise and physiotherapy program on surgical intervention in children with thermal injury. Journal of Burn Care and Rehabilitation, 24(1):57–61, 2003.

Chester, CH, Candlish, S, & Zuker, RM. Prevention of obstructive sleep apnea in children with burns of the head and neck. Paper presented at the meeting of the American Burn Association, Cincinnati, March 1993.

Clarke, HM, Wittpenn, GP, McLeod, AME, Candlish, SE, Guernsey, CJ, Weleff, DK, & Zuker, RM. Acute management of pediatric hand burns. Hand Clinics, 6:221–232, 1990.

Cucuzzo, NA, Ferrando, A, & Herndon, DN. The effects of exercise programming vs. traditional outpatient therapy in the rehabilitation of severely burned children. Journal of Burn Care and Rehabilitation, 22(3):214–220, 2001.

Dado, DV, & Angelats, J. Management of burns of the hands in children. Hand Clinics, 6:711–721, 1990.

Daugherty, MB, DeSerna, C, Barthel, P, & Warden, GD. Moving patients and families toward independence: Establishing a transitional unit. Poster presented at the meeting of the American Burn Association, Cincinnati, March 1993.

Davey, RB. The use of contact media for burn scar hypertrophy. Journal of Wound Care, 6(2):80–82, 1997.

Deitch, EA, & Rutan, RL. The challenges of children: The first 48 hours. Journal of Burn Care and Rehabilitation, 21(5):424–430, 2000.

Doctor, JN, Patterson, DR, & Mann, R. Health outcome for burn survivors. Journal of Burn Care and Rehabilitation, 18(6):490–495, 1997.

Ehde, DM, Patterson, DR, & Fordyce, WE. The quota system in burn rehabilitation. Journal of Burn Care and Rehabilitation, 19(5):436–440, 1998.

Field, T. Massage therapy for infants and children. Journal of Developmental and Behavioral Pediatrics, 16(2):105–111, 1995.

Field, T, Peck, M, Krugman, S, Tuchel, T, Schanberg, S, Kuhn, C, & Burman, T. Burn injuries benefit from massage therapy. Journal of Burn Care and Rehabilitation, 19(3):241–244, 1998.

Fletchall, S, & Hickerson, WL. Managed health care: Therapist responsibilities. Journal of Burn Care and Rehabilitation, 18(1):61–63, 1997.

Foley, KH, Doyle, B, Paradise, P, Parry, I, Palmieri, T, & Greenhalgh, DG. Use of an improved Watusi collar to manage pediatric neck burn contractures. Journal of Burn Care and Rehabilitation, 23(3):221–226, 2002.

Fricke, NB, Omnell, ML, Dutcher, KA, Hollender, LG, & Engrav, LH. Skeletal and dental disturbances in children after facial burns and pressure garment use: A 4-year follow-up. Journal of Burn Care and Rehabilitation, 20(3):239–249, 1999.

Ghahary, A, Shen, YJ, Scott, PG, Gong, Y, & Tredget, EE. Enhanced expression of mRNA for transforming growth factor-beta, type I and type III procollagen in human post-burn hypertrophic scar tissues. Journal of Laboratory Clinical Medicine, 122(4):465–473, 1993.

Greenspan, B, Johnson, J, Gorga, D, Goodwin, CW, & Naglet, W. Compliance with pressure garment use in burn survivors. Paper presented at the meeting of the American Burn Association, Cincinnati, March 1993.

Harris, LD, Hatler, B, Adams, S, Gilliam, KS, & Helm, P. Serial casting and its efficacy in the treatment of the burned hand. Paper presented at the meeting of the American Burn Association, Cincinnati, March 1993.

Hayes-Lundy, C, Ward, S, Mills, P, & Same, J. Use of computer-generated exercise programs to augment therapy programs. Poster presented at the meeting of the American Burn Association, Cincinnati, March 1993.

Hernandez-Reif, M, Field, T, Largie, S, Hart, S, Redzepi, M, Nierenberg, B, & Peck, TM. Childrens' distress during burn treatment is reduced by massage therapy. Journal of Burn Care and Rehabilitation, 22(2):191–195, 2001.

Herndon, DN, & Rutan, RL. Have we improved burn care? In Carlson, RW, & Reines, HD (Eds.). Critical Care State of the Art, Vol. 13. Anaheim, CA: Society of Critical Care Medicine, 1992a, pp. 389–406.

Herndon, DN, & Rutan, RL. Use of dermal templates and cultured cells for permanent skin replacement. Wounds, 4(2):50–53, 1992b.

Hollowed, KA, Gunde, MA, Lewis, MS, & Jordon, MH. Ambulation of intubated burn patients. Poster presented at the meeting of the American Burn Association, Cincinnati, March 1993.

Honari, SH. Topical therapies and antimicrobials in the management of burn wounds. Critical Care Nursing Clinics of North America, 16:1–11, 2004.

Housinger, T, Mortess, C, Dinkler, T, & Warden, GD. Outpatient therapy: Its efficacy in pediatric burns. Paper presented at the meeting of the American Burn Association, Salt Lake City, April 1992.

Johnson, J, & Silverberg, R. Serial casting of the lower extremity to correct contractures during the acute phase of burn care. Physical Therapy, 75(8):767–768, 1995.

Kowalske, K, Purdue, G, Hunt, J, & Helm, P. Early ambulation following skin grafting of lower extremity burns: A randomized controlled trial. Paper presented at the meeting of the American Burn Association, Cincinnati, March 1993.

Larson, DL, Abston, S, Willis, B, Linares, HA, Dobrkovsky, M, Evans, EB, & Lewis, SR. Contracture and scar formation in the burn patient. Clinics in Plastic Surgery, 1:653, 1974.

Larson, DL, Huang, T, Dobrkovsky, M, Bauer, PS, & Parks, DH. Prevention and treatment of scar contracture. In Artz, CP, Moncrief, JA, & Pruitt, B (Eds.). Burns: A Team Approach. Philadelphia: WB Saunders, 1979, pp. 466–491.

Liang, Z, Engrav, LH, Muangman, P, Muffley, LA, Zhu, KQ, Carrougher, GJ, Underwood, RA, & Gibran, NS. Nerve quantification in female red Duroc pig (FRDP) scar compared to human hypertrophic scar. Burns, 30:57–64, 2004.

Linares, HA, Kischer, CW, Dobrkovsky, M, & Larson, DL. On the origin of the hypertrophic scar. Journal of Trauma, 13:70–75, 1973.

Linares, HA, Larson, DL, & Willis-Galstaum, BA. Historical notes on the use of pressure in the treatment of hypertrophic scars or keloids. Burns, 19:17–21, 1993.

Mahaney, NB. Restoration of play in a severely burned three-year-old child. Journal of Burn Care and Rehabilitation, 11:57–63, 1990.

Manigandan, C, Gupta, AK, Venugopal, K, Ninan, S, & Cherian, RE. A multi-purpose, self-adjustable aeroplane splint for the splinting of axillary burns. Burns, 29(3):276–279, 2003.

Mann, R, Yeong, EK, Moore, ML, & Engrav, LH. A new tool to measure pressure under burn garments. Journal of Burn Care and Rehabilitation, 18(2):160–163, 1997.

Melchert-McKearnan, K, Deitz, J, Engel, JM, & White, O. Children with burn injuries: purposeful activity versus rote exercise. American Journal of Occupational Therapy, 54(4):381–390, 2000.

Metzger, DJ, Cioffi, WG, Martin, S, McManus, WF, & Pruitt, BA. Ilizarov technique in the management of joint deformity in thermally injured patients. Paper presented at the meeting of the American Burn Association, Cincinnati, March 1993.

Meyer, W, Blakeney, P, Moore, P, Murphy, L, Robson, M, & Herndon, D. Parental well-being and behavioral adjustment of pediatric survivors of burns. Journal of Burn Care and Rehabilitation, 15(1):62–68, 1994.

Meyer, WJ, Blakeney, P, Russell, W, Thomas, C, Robert, R, Berninger, F, & Holzer, C. Psychological problems reported by young adults who were burned as children. Journal of Burn Care and Rehabilitation, 25(1):98–106, 2004.

Nedelec, B, Shen, YJ, Ghahary, A, Scott, PG, & Tredget, EE. The effect of interferon alpha 2b on the expression of cytoskeletal proteins in an in vitro model of wound contraction. Journal of Laboratory Clinical Medicine, 126(5):474–484, 1995.

Parks, DH, Bauer, PS, & Larson, DL. Late problems in burns. Clinics in Plastic Surgery, 4:547, 1977.

Pidcock, FS, Fauerbach, JA, Ober, M, & Carney, J. The rehabilitation/school matrix: a model for accommodating the non-compliant child with severe burns. Journal of Burn Care and Rehabilitation, 24(5):342–346, 2003.

Pisarski, GP, Greenhalgh, DG, & Warden, GD. The management of perineal contractures in children with burns. Journal of Burn Care and Rehabilitation, 15(3):256–259, 1994.

Prensner, JD, Yowler, CJ, Smith, LF, Steele, AL, & Fratianne, RB. Music therapy for assistance with pain and anxiety management in burn treatment. Journal of Burn Care and Rehabilitation, 22(1):83–88, 2001.

Prothman, J, Engrav, L, & Cain, V. Evaluating appearance of burn scars: Patient vs. health care worker perceptions. Paper presented at the meeting of the American Burn Association, Cincinnati, March 1993.

Reed, L, & Heinle, J. Meeting the challenge of education for a diversified patient population in a burn treatment center: Design of 2 patient handbooks. Poster presented at the meeting of the American Burn Association, Cincinnati, March 1993.

Reybons, MD. Community re-entry and leisure: Reuniting a lifestyle with a burn survivor. Progress Report, 4(3):20–22, 1992.

Richard, R, DerSarkisian, D, Miller, SF, Johnson, RM, & Staley, M. Directional variance in skin movement. Journal of Burn Care and Rehabilitation, 20(3):259–264, 1999.

Richard, R, Ford, J, Miller, SF, & Staley, M. Photographic measurement of volar forearm skin movement with wrist extension: The influence of elbow position. Journal of Burn Care and Rehabilitation, 15(1):58–61, 1994.

Richard, R, Shanesy, CP, III, & Miller, SF. Dynamic versus static splints: A prospective case for sustained stress. Journal of Burn Care and Rehabilitation, 16(3):284–287, 1995.

Richard, RL, Staley, MF, Miller, SF, Warden, GD, & Finley, RK, Jr. Biomechanical basis for physical management of burn patients. Poster presented at the meeting of the American Burn Association, Cincinnati, March 1993.

Ridgway, CL, Daugherty, MB, & Warden, GD. Serial casting as a technique to correct burn scar contractures. Journal of Burn Care and Rehabilitation, 12:67–72, 1991.

Ridgway, CL, & Warden, GD. Evaluation of a vertical mouth stretching orthosis: Two case reports. Journal of Burn Care and Rehabilitation, 16(1):74–78, 1995.

Sanford, S, & Gore, D. Unna's boot dressings facilitate outpatient skin grafting of hands. Journal of Burn Care and Rehabilitation, 17(4):323–326, 1996.

Schmitt, MA, French, L, & Kalil, ET. How soon is safe? Ambulation of the patient with burns after lower-extremity skin grafting. Journal of Burn Care and Rehabilitation, 12:33–37, 1991.

Serghiou, MA, McLaughlin, A, & Herndon, DN. Alternative splinting methods for the prevention and correction of burn scar torticollis. Journal of Burn Care and Rehabilitation, 24(5):336–340, 2003.

Shelby, J, Groussman, M, Addison, C, Burgess, Y, Sullivan, J, & Saffie, J. Stress resiliency in close relatives of thermally injured patients. Paper presented at the meeting of the American Burn Association, Cincinnati, March 1993.

Spurr, ED, & Shakespeare, PG. Incidence of hypertrophic scarring in burn-injured children. Burns, *16*:179–181, 1990.

Staley, M, & Richard, R. Critical pathways to enhance the rehabilitation of patients with burns. Journal of Burn Care and Rehabilitation, *17*(6):S12–S14, 1996.

Staley, MJ, & Richard, RL. Use of pressure to treat hypertrophic burn scars. Advances in Wound Care, *10*(3):44–46, 1997.

Sullivan, T. Rating the burn scar. Journal of Burn Care and Rehabilitation, *11*:256–260, 1990.

Taylor, A. Pockets stitched into external vascular supports improve management of hypertrophic scars. Poster presented at the meeting of the American Burn Association, Cincinnati, March 1993.

Thompson, R, Summers, S, Dobbs, R, & Wheeler, T. Color-pressure garments: Perceptions from the public. Paper presented at the meeting of the American Burn Association, Salt Lake City, April 1992.

Thurber, CA, Martin-Herz, SP, & Patterson, DR. Psychological principles of burn wound pain in children I: Theoretical framework. Journal of Burn Care and Rehabilitation, *21*(4):376–387, 2000.

Torres-Gray, D, Johnson, J, Greenspan, B, Goodwin, CW, & Naglet, W. The fabrication and use of removable digit casts to improve range of motion at the proximal interphalangeal joint. Poster presented at the meeting of the American Burn Association, Cincinnati, March 1993.

Van den Kerckhove, E, Stappaerts, K, Boeckx, W, Van den Hof, B, Monstrey, S, Van den Kelen, A, & De Cubber, J. Silicones in the rehabilitation of burns: a review and overview. Burns, *27*(3):205–214, 2001.

Van Straten, O, & Sagi, A. "Supersplint": A new dynamic combination splint for the burned hand. Journal of Burn Care and Rehabilitation, *21*(1):71–73, 2000.

Walling, S, Walling, R, & Warden, GD. The development of home program instructional guides to accommodate the special needs of patients and families. Poster presented at the meeting of the American Burn Association, Cincinnati, March 1993.

Ward, RS, Hayes-Lundy, C, Schnebly, WA, Reddy, R, & Saffle, JR. Rehabilitation of burn patients with concomitant limb amputation: Case reports. Burns, *16*(5):390–392, 1990a.

Ward, RS, Hayes-Lundy, C, Schnebly, WA, & Saffle, JR. Prosthetic use in patients with burns and associated limb amputations. Journal of Burn Care and Rehabilitation, *11*:361–364, 1990b.

Warden, GD, Lang, D, & Housinger, TA. Management of pediatric hand burns with tendon, joint and bone injury. Paper presented at the meeting of the American Burn Association, Cincinnati, March 1993.

Wells, NJ, Boyle, JC, Snelling, CF, & Carr, NJ. Lower extremity burns and Unna paste: Can we decrease health care costs without compromising patient care? Canadian Journal of Surgery, *38*(6):533–536, 1995.

Whitestone, JJ, Richard, RL, Slemker, TC, Ause-Ellias, KL, & Miller, SF. Fabrication of total-contact burn masks by use of human body topography and computer-aided design and manufacturing. Journal of Burn Care and Rehabilitation, *16*(5):543–547, 1995.

Yeong, EK, Mann, R, Engrav, LH, Goldberg, M, Cain, V, Costa, B, Moore, M, Nakamura, D, & Lee, J. Improved burn scar assessment with use of a new scar-rating scale. Journal of Burn Care and Rehabilitation, *18*(4):353–355, 1997.

Chapter 35

THE SPECIAL CARE NURSERY

LINDA KAHN-D'ANGEL
PT, ScD

RACHEL A. UNANUE ROSE
PT, PhD, PCS

This chapter describes the history and organization of the special care nursery and discusses which neonates and infants are at risk for central nervous system (CNS) dysfunction or developmental delay. A theoretic basis for physical therapy examination, evaluation, prognosis, and interventions for infants in the special care nursery is presented and recommendations are provided for clinical practice. The gestational and pathophysiologic conditions considered in this chapter are prematurity, hypoxic-ischemic encephalopathy, fetal alcohol syndrome, fetal abstinence syndrome, exposure to human immunodeficiency virus (HIV) infection, neonatal seizures, birth injuries related to the CNS, and spina bifida. The follow-up of infants after discharge from the special care nursery is addressed, and two case histories illustrate and integrate the material presented in this chapter.

HISTORY OF THE SPECIAL CARE NURSERY

Modern neonatal care was born with the development of the first incubator by Couveuse in France in 1880 (Hodgman, 1985). The first text on the premature infant, *The Nursling,* authored by Budin, a student of Couveuse, was published in 1900. Dr. Martin Couney, who was one of Budin's students, used these principles of treatment for the premature infant, and in a bizarre entrepreneurial twist, exhibited them to the public for a fee (Silverman, 1979). The main principles of neonatal care were support of body temperature, control of nosocomial infection, minimal handling, and provision of special nursing care. Interestingly, nurseries were quiet, and lights were dimmed at night. Dr. Julius Hess attended this exhibition in Chicago and applied these principles in the late 1940s. Dr. Hess achieved a neonatal mortality rate for preterm infants of 20%, which was respectable for the time. In response to the increased survival rate of premature infants reported by Hess, these principles of care spread across the United States.

During the 1950s, a number of cities developed centers for the care of premature infants and a number of states developed maternal mortality committees that gathered data to be used as a basis for planning activities directed at preventing maternal death. During the 1960s, Arizona, Massachusetts, and Wisconsin promulgated standards for maternity units and developed regional perinatal care centers. Reports from these three states and several professional organizations, including the American Medical Association, the American College of Obstetricians and Gynecologists, the American Academy of Pediatrics, and the Academy of Family Physicians, stimulated the development of the regional organization of perinatal services (Fanaroff & Graven, 1992).

By the late 1960s, full-term infants with health complications were also being treated in the neonatal nursery. Advances in microlaboratory techniques for biochemical determinations from minute quantities of blood and the development of miniaturized monitoring equipment, ventilatory support systems, and means to conserve body heat improved the care of the neonate with serious illness (Fanaroff & Graven, 1992). Expansion of neonatal pharmacology, widespread use of phototherapy for management of hyperbilirubinemia, and methods of delivery of high-caloric solutions parenterally when oral feeding was not possible also improved the chances for survival of the very sick neonate. In 1975, the emergence of the new subspecialties of neonatology and perinatology provided specialists in the field of caring for infants in the high-technology nursery.

During the past two decades there has been considerable progress in the treatment of neonates and children with critical illnesses. For example, there has been an increase in the survival rate of infants born at 23 to 25 weeks of gestational age from 27% in 1984 to 1989 to 42% in 1990 to 1995, with most of the increase in disability being mild (Emsley et al., 1998). The improvement in survival and quality of life for these patients resulted from nationwide development of regional neonatal intensive care units (NICUs) in which an organized, highly specialized, multidisciplinary approach became the standard of care. The number of neonates needing close supervision and expert cardiorespiratory and metabolic support is large enough to make such units an essential component of a perinatal health care delivery system (Sarnaik & Preston, 1985). The increase in the number of NICUs resulted in a significant drop in neonatal and perinatal mortality rates of low birth weight (LBW) infants (Lubchenco et al., 1974; McDonald, 1981; Teberg et al., 1977). By 1996, the survival rate of extremely low birth weight (ELBW) infants (750–1000 g) had increased to 86% and the survival rate of infants who weighed 500 to 750 g at birth was 54%, which are in stark contrast to the 10% survival rate in 1960 for infants with birth weights of 750 to 1000 g (Lemons and Stevenson and Wright, 1998). Currently, there are 700 NICUs in the United States, which is a 30-fold to 40-fold increase since the 1960s. Long-term outcome of the very low birth weight (VLBW) infant, however, came under scrutiny with the suspicion that the typical nursery stay of several weeks may have a significantly detrimental effect on later behavioral performance (Hodgman, 1985). Research ensued on the effects of different sensory input during the NICU stay and the concept of neonatal care facilitating optimal development was born (Als, 1986; Als et al., 1986, 1994; Glass et al., 1985; Hilton, 1987).

ORGANIZATION OF PERINATAL SERVICES

Special care units are designed to meet a wide range of special needs, from the monitoring of apparently well infants at risk of serious illness to the intensive treatment of infants with acute illness. This range of services

Box 35-1	In-Hospital Perinatal Services

Basic Care: Surveillance and care of all patients admitted to obstetric service with triage to identify high-risk patients.

Specialty Care: Care of high-risk mothers and fetuses. Stabilization of ill newborns prior to transfer. Care of preterm infants with birth weight of 1500 g or more.

Subspecialty Care: Provision of comprehensive perinatal services for mothers and neonates of all risk categories. Research and educational support. Analysis and evaluation of regional data. Initial evaluation of new high-risk technologies.

Adapted from American Academy of Pediatrics, American College of Obstetricians and Gynecologists. Guidelines for Perinatal Care. 4th ed. Elk Grove Village, IL, Washington, DC: American Academy of Pediatrics, American College of Obstetricians and Gynecologists; 1997.

requires that the special care nursery be arranged for graduated care to meet the diverse and changing needs of infants (Whaley & Wong, 1991). Because it was not economically feasible for every hospital to have the personnel and technology to care for neonates with complex needs, these services were originally organized on a regional basis. Recent efforts to contain the cost of health care has led to deregionalization in many areas, and blurring of differences in levels of care. Levels of care are currently described by the American Academy of Pediatrics (1997) as Level I Basic Care, Level II Specialty Care, and Level III Subspecialty Care (Box 35-1). A broad-based Committee on Perinatal Health recently concluded that a strong focus of perinatal care is preventive health care, education, and counseling (Bagwell & Armstrong, 1998).

THE NEONATAL INTENSIVE CARE UNIT ENVIRONMENT

NICUs were designed to decrease neonatal morbidity and mortality rates. In an attempt to meet this goal, the NICU provides the neonate with a habitat for growth starkly different from the intrauterine environment. The NICU is a busy, often crowded place, where the atmosphere is frequently high pressure (Pelletier & Palmeri, 1985). The intrauterine environment is replaced by bright lights, high noise levels, and the intrusive medical procedures characteristic of high-technology treatment (Campbell, 1986; Gottfried, 1985). Each tiny baby lies in an incubator, an open warmer, or a crib, surrounded by and connected to ventilators and monitors, including heart, apnea, and oxygen monitors and infusion pumps (Fig. 35-1). The incubator is often surrounded by equipment including phototherapy lights; diagnostic transilluminators; and portable radiographic, electroencephalographic, and ultrasonographic units. The amount and complexity of the equipment can be overwhelming to parents and families.

Lighting

Typically, the ambient illumination within the NICU consists of daylight and artificial fluorescent lighting (Moseley et al., 1988). The American Academy of Pediatrics recommends a minimum light intensity of 100 foot-candles at the infant's level for adequate visualization by staff (Weibley, 1989). This same level of illumination may contribute to retinopathy of prematurity (ROP) (Glass et al., 1985; Kretzer & Hittner, 1986). No diurnal rhythmicity of light exists in the NICU, which some investigators believe may interfere with the infant's development of normal biologic rhythms. Glass and colleagues (1985) studied the effects of draping sunglass-filtering material over the incubators. They found that there was a significant increase in ROP in the infants in incubators without the filtering material, especially in the infants who weighed less than 1000 g. As a result of this study, an editorial in the journal that published the study recommended immediate diurnal cycling and dimming of lights (Weibley, 1989). Subsequent studies have not replicated these findings (Phelps & Watts, 2001).

Sound

Sound levels within the incubator have been found to be significantly higher than those measured outside (Kent et al., 2002). In the intrauterine environment, auditory stimuli include sound levels at about 85 dB consisting of rhythmic swooshing and bubbling sounds punctuated by the steady pulse of the maternal heartbeat (Gottfried, 1985; Gottfried & Hodgman, 1984). In the NICU the infant is surrounded by noise on a level comparable with that of auto traffic and, at times, heavy machinery. High noise levels are present from trash receptacles, addressograph machines, centrifuges, telephones, and monitor alarms (Hilton, 1987). About 80% of these peak sounds are human related including opening and closing doors, banging the incubator hood, and tearing and opening bags (Chen & Chang, 2001). These harsh sounds can cause some infants to become hypoxic as part of a startle

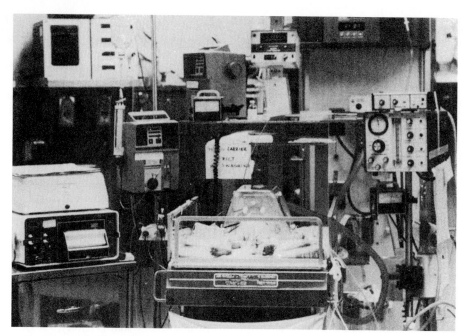

◆ **Figure 35-1**   Infant surrounded by typical NICU equipment. *(From Crane, L. Physical therapy for the neonate with respiratory disease. In Irwin, S, & Tecklin, JS [Eds]. Cardiopulmonary Physical Therapy, 2nd ed. St. Louis: Mosby, 1990, p. 400.)*

response (Thomas, 1989). The environment inside the incubator is characterized by continuous white noise. Harsh mechanical noises penetrate clearly, but speech sounds are indistinct and deflected (Newman, 1981). This lack of distinctness and the deflection of speech sounds may have negative effects on later interactive behavior if the infant learns to look away from the speaker to locate him or her. Drugs commonly used in the nursery are known from animal studies to potentiate noise-induced hearing loss (American Academy of Pediatrics, 1997; Perlstein, 1992). The American Academy of Pediatrics has recommended that noise levels be reduced to less than 70 dB, manufacturers of incubators reduce the noise levels of motors below 58 dB, and physicians limit the use of ototoxic drugs in neonates (Peabody & Lewis, 1985; Perlstein, 1992). Auditory evoked potential tests are typically done in every nursery before a neonate is discharged to establish risk for hearing loss. The American Academy of Pediatrics Committee on Environmental Health has issued recommendations for noise in the environment and its effects on the fetus and newborn, including the infant in the special care nursery. Acoustic foam placed in the corners of the incubator and change in staff behavior decreased noise level (Johnson, 2001; Philbin & Gray, 2002).

Medical Procedures

In the NICU, the infant is placed on a flat mattress and is exposed to a dry, cool, air-filled environment. In the uterine environment the 28- to 32-week fetus sleeps 80% of the time. In contrast, premature infants were found to be disturbed an average of 23 times in 24 hours (Altmier et al., 1999). Tactile input often heralds medical or technical events and causes sustained arousal, which exacts a physiologic toll on the infant. Unable to make sense of life-sustaining efforts, the infant begins to respond negatively to touch (Gottfried & Hodgman, 1984).

DEVELOPMENTAL CARE AND THE SPECIAL CARE NURSERY

In view of the research cited in the preceding sections about the iatrogenic effects of neonatal intensive care, and the shifting of emphasis from survival to the prevention and amelioration of the complications of prematurity, Als and co-workers (1986) have developed the concept of individualized, comprehensive, family-focused, developmentally supportive care for infants in the special care nursery. A growing body of literature supports this type of care (Als, 1986; Als et al., 1986, 1994; Buehler et al., 1995; Byers, 2003; Fleisher et al., 1995; Mouradian & Als, 1994; Parker et al., 1992). Whether or not this specific approach is used, more special care nursery staff members are incorporating a developmentally supportive environment and interventions such as diurnal light cycles; clustering care; specific rest time;

interventions, including sponge baths, as needed rather than on a schedule; skin-to-skin contact, including "kangaroo" care; presentation of organizing environmental input such as music; the scent of the mother on clothing; odor of milk on the pacifier; single room care; and co-bedding of multiple-birth neonates (Bosque et al., 1995; delEstard & Lennox, 1995; Standley & Moore, 1995; Tessier et al., 1998). Research on these methods has shown improvement in such dependent variables as weight gain, days on ventilator, oxygen saturation, number of days in the hospital, infant state, and neuromotor behavior, nonnutritive sucking during gavage feeding, perceptual and cognitive abilities, and parenting process (Brown & Taquino, 2001; Bingham et al., 2003, delEstard & Lennox, 1995; Feldman et al., 2002; Mouradian & Als, 1994; Mueller, 1996).

DEFINING THE AT-RISK INFANT

The meaning of the designation "high-risk infant" differs according to the area of expertise of the professional using the term. The neonatologist defines *risk* as related to morbidity or mortality, whereas psychologists, physical therapists, occupational therapists, and speech therapists may define the *at-risk infant* as one who has a high probability of manifesting developmental delay as a result of exposure to any one of a number of medical factors (Rossetti, 1986; Wilhelm, 1991). High-risk infants are classified according to birth weight, gestational age, and pathophysiologic problems (Whaley & Wong, 1991). Problems related to physiologic status are closely associated with the maturity of the infant and hypoxic episodes during the perinatal period, as well as with fetal exposure to alcohol and drugs and with HIV infection and environmental factors.

PREMATURITY AND LOW BIRTH WEIGHT

Infants born prematurely or who are small for gestational age (SGA) are divided into three major categories: LBW, from 1501 to 2500 g; VLBW, below 1501 g; and ELBW, below 1000 g. Preterm delivery occurs in 8% to 10% of all live births in the United States in spite of current therapies to halt and prevent such deliveries (Harmon & Kenner, 1998). Approximately 75% to 80% of all neonatal morbidity and deaths is due to premature birth. More than 40,000 VLBW infants are born each year, and half of neonatal deaths occur in VLBW infants (Semmler, 1989).

These high-risk infants are a heterogeneous group, including infants born preterm (less than 37 weeks of gestation) and those born at term but of reduced weight (Kleigman, 1992).

Black mothers are two to three times more likely than white mothers to deliver VLBW infants (Iyasu & Tomashek, 2002). Causes for LBW and preterm delivery for blacks include racial differences in maternal medical care, stress, and lack of social support. VLBW infants have an increased incidence of neurologic sequelae, delayed development, and lower intellectual and language abilities (Teberg, 1977; Volpe, 1995).

There have been several optimistic reports of prematurity prevention programs that include assessment of prenatal risk, weekly educational interventions, enhanced nutritional support, referral to a perinatologist when necessary, and pH self-measurements. These programs have shown a reduction in NICU admissions and preterm deliveries (Fangman et al., 1994; Joffe et al., 1995; Novy et al., 1995; Saling, 1997).

SGA infants are those whose birth weights are below the 10th percentile of published norms or whose ponderal index (ratio of birth weight to the cube root of the infant's length at birth) is low (Als et al., 1976). Term SGA infants demonstrate developmental problems such as behavioral and learning disorders, and preterm SGA infants may have an even greater prevalence of abnormal developmental problems than term SGA neonates (Kahn-D'Angelo, 1987).

The Clinical Assessment of Gestational Age in the Newborn Infant, developed by Dubowitz and colleagues (1970), is the test most often used by physicians and nurses to assess gestational age. The determination of gestational age is crucial for infants in the special care nursery to interpret neurologic and behavioral findings relative to the correct gestational age. This test includes 10 neurologic and reflex items and 11 external or superficial criteria that are scored on a four-point scale. The accuracy of gestational age is determined within 2 weeks on each assessment with a 95% confidence level. This test was standardized on 167 infants whose mothers were sure of the date of their last menstrual period. It has been used in the assessment of growth in early infancy and, in conjunction with the neurologic examination, to assess differences in development between twins, preterm infants with intraventricular hemorrhage (IVH) and the effects of eclampsia, placental abruption, and intrauterine growth retardation (Francis et al., 1987). Ballard and associates (1991) developed a simplified Dubowitz Newborn Maturity Rating to assess neonates from 20 to 44 weeks of age. Gestational age is also determined by ultrasound, measurements, and amniotic fluid analysis (Kenner &

Lott, 2003). Although gestational age is usually determined by physicians or nurses, the physical therapist should be familiar with the Clinical Assessment of Gestational Age in the Newborn Infant and how gestational age is determined.

MEDICAL COMPLICATIONS AND TREATMENT IN PREMATURITY

PULMONARY COMPLICATIONS

Respiratory Distress Syndrome

Respiratory distress syndrome (RDS), or hyaline membrane disease, is the most common single cause of respiratory distress in neonates. The principal factors in the pathophysiology of RDS are pulmonary immaturity and deficiency of surfactant. Prematurity, low birth weight, low Apgar score at 1 and 5 minutes, maternal age over 34 years, and neonatal transport have been reported as risk factors for RDS (Rubaltelli et al., 1998; Shlossman et al., 1997). Low surfactant production results in increased surface tension, alveolar collapse, diffuse atelectasis, and decreased lung compliance. These factors cause an increase in pulmonary artery pressure that leads to extrapulmonary right-to-left shunting of blood and ventilation-perfusion mismatching (Carlo & Chatburn, 1988; Sweeney & Swanson, 2001; Walsh et al., 1988). Infants with RDS also demonstrate higher heart rates and reduced heart rate variability compared with full-term neonates, indicating that premature birth has an influence on cardiac function for up to 6 months after birth (Henslee et al., 1997).

Prophylactic use of corticosteroids such as dexamethasone and hydrocortisone to accelerate lung development prior to preterm birth are effective in preventing RDS and neonatal death (Crowley, 2002). Intervention for infants with RDS depends on the severity of the disorder and includes oxygen supplementation, assisted ventilation, surfactant administration, and extracorporeal membrane oxygenation (ECMO). Prophylactic surfactant administration of intubated infants younger than 30 weeks of gestational age correlated with an initial improvement in respiratory status and a decrease in the incidence of RDS, pneumothorax, bronchopulmonary dysplasia (BPD), and death (Soll, 2002). Early administration of multiple doses of natural or synthetic surfactant extract results in improved clinical outcome and appears to be the most effective method of administration. When a choice of natural or synthetic surfactant is available, natural surfactant shows greater early improvement in requirement for ventilatory support (Soll, 2002; Yost & Soll,

2002). Continuous distending-pressure ventilators, either positive or negative pressure, are used in the management of RDS. The positive-pressure ventilator is used more often; the negative-pressure ventilator assists ventilation by creating a negative pressure around the thorax and abdomen. Nasal and nasopharyngeal prongs are used for these ventilators (Crane, 1990). (See Chapter 26 for a more detailed description of ventilators.)

Permissive hypercapnia is an experimental ventilatory strategy for acute respiratory failure in which lungs are ventilated with a low inspiratory volume and pressure with the goal being minimization of lung damage during mechanical ventilation (Bigatello et al, 2001). Partial liquid ventilation or perfluorocarbon-associated gas exchange has been used experimentally in conjunction with surfactant administration and has resulted in improved clinical course in a small sample of infants with severe respiratory distress syndrome (Leach et al., 1996). It has been suggested that this technology will provide a strong addition to available treatments for preterm infants and that there will be a resultant decrease in barotrauma and in BPD (Donovan et al., 1998; Vals-I-Soler et al., 2001).

The prognosis of infants with RDS varies with the severity of the original disease (Carlo & Chatburn, 1988). The mortality rate is about 10%, and RDS is the leading cause of neonatal death and morbidity. Infants who do not require assisted ventilation recover without sequelae, but the clinical course of the very immature infant may be complicated by air leaks in the lungs and BPD. Infants who survive severe RDS often require frequent hospitalization for upper respiratory tract infections and have an increased incidence of neurologic sequelae.

ECMO is a technique of cardiopulmonary bypass modified from techniques developed for open-heart surgery that are used to support heart and lung function (for review of ECMO and implications for pediatric physical therapy, see Caron & Berlandi, 1997, and Pax Lowes & Palisano, 1995). In newborns with acute respiratory failure, the immature lungs are allowed to rest and recover to avoid the damaging effects of artificial ventilation. Because of the need for systemic administration of heparin and the resultant risk of systemic and intracranial hemorrhage, ECMO is reserved for use with infants who are at least 34 weeks of gestational age, weigh more than 2000 g, have no evidence of intracranial bleeding, required less than 10 days of assisted ventilation, and have reversible lung disease (Stork, 1992). ECMO is now used with considerable frequency in support of neonates with severe but reversible respiratory failure, including complicating meconium aspiration, congenital diaphragmatic hernia, sepsis, persistent fetal circulation,

RDS, and BPD (Hibbs, 2001; Martin & Fanaroff, 1992). High-frequency oscillatory ventilation has been used as a bridge from ECMO to conventional ventilation in cases in which conventional ventilation was not initially successful (Schexnayder et al., 1995).

Bronchopulmonary Dysplasia and Chronic Lung Disease of Infancy

Bronchopulmonary dysplasia (BPD) and chronic lung disease of infancy (CLD) are two chronic pulmonary conditions that are caused by incomplete or abnormal repair of lung disease during the neonatal period (Ho, 2002). Infants are diagnosed with BPD when they are 28 days chronologic age and continue to require supplemental oxygen; have an abnormal physical examination with tachypnea, wheezes, and retractions; and have an abnormal chest radiograph (Farrell & Fiascone 1997). CLD is diagnosed at 36 weeks' postmenstrual age, if there is a continued need for supplemental oxygen, abnormal physical examination, and abnormal chest radiograph. The overall incidence varies from 13% to 69% of infants weighing less than 1500 g and requiring ventilation, depending on diagnostic criteria and the neonatal population being studied (Mitchell, 1996). Boys are at greater risk for developing CLDs, perhaps due to a lag of 1 to 2.5 weeks in pulmonary and cerebral maturation in boys (Lauterback et al., 2001).

Pathophysiologic features of BPD include interstitial fibrosis resulting from absorption of intra-alveolar exudate by the alveolar wall during the resolution of RDS. Alveolar collapse may cause parts of the lung to become airless and solid. These nonaerated regions form scars of condensed lung tissue and become fibrotic. Mucosa of the bronchioles becomes dysplastic and inflamed, and there is hypertrophy of the smooth muscle of bronchioles and arterioles. Pulmonary function testing reveals severe maldistribution of ventilation in these infants. They have increased airway resistance, decreased dynamic compliance, and a large increase in the work of breathing.

Prematurity, barotrauma from high pressures used in assisted ventilation, and pulmonary oxygen toxicity are accepted as key causal components of BPD (Bancalari, 1992). Also, the endotracheal tube itself hinders drainage of tracheal secretions and increases both dead space and resistance to airflow. Other factors that may contribute to the pathogenesis of BPD are infection, pulmonary edema resulting from a patent ductus arteriosus or excessive fluid administration, and increased airway resistance. Immaturity of the pulmonary antioxidant systems and neutrophil-generated lung damage are two of the multiple factors associated with the etiology of both BPD and CHD (Ho, 2002; Mitchell, 1996). A genetic disposi-

tion to the development has been proposed due to a greater risk of BPD in families with a strong family history of asthma.

Treatment strategies for BPD are aimed at preventing or inhibiting the events that trigger the cascade of pathogenic mechanisms (Goetzman, 1986). These strategies include prevention of premature birth; surfactant replacement therapy; prevention of barotrauma, by using mechanical ventilation for as short a period as is possible, and volutrauma; minimizing oxygen toxicity and increasing antioxidant defenses; control of infection; anti-inflammatory therapy; use of bronchodilators and preventing pulmonary edema by fluid restriction (Ho, 2002). The use of positive end-expiratory pressure during mechanical ventilation, permissive hypercapnia, nasal continuous positive airway pressure, and superoxide dismutase enzymes as an antioxidant are currently under investigation for treatment of BPD and CLD (Ho, 2002).

Because infants with BPD are prone to developing cor pulmonale, congestive heart failure, and pulmonary edema, chronic diuretic therapy is instituted. The infant or child with BPD must also be closely monitored for infections, especially those caused by bacteria and fungi. Steroids are used to decrease inflammatory responses and improve lung functions through reduction in pulmonary edema, bronchial edema, and bronchospasm (Kenner, 1998). Other treatments for bronchospasm include inhaled bronchodilator and theophylline therapy (Bancalari, 1992; Davis et al., 1990). Stimulus reduction is also recommended in the nursing care of the infant with BPD (Kenner, 1998).

The incidence of developmental disability, such as mental retardation and cerebral palsy, in infants and children with BPD has been reported to be 29% to 34% (Robertson et al., 1991; Vidyasagar, 1985; Vohr et al., 1991). The important predictors for these disabilities are intracranial hemorrhage and periventricular echodensity, rather than severity of the BPD (Luchi et al., 1991). Transient neuromotor delays have been documented for infants with BPD because of prolonged periods of increased work of breathing, frequent infections, and recurrent hospitalizations (Mitchell, 1996).

NEUROLOGIC COMPLICATIONS

Periventricular Leukomalacia

Periventricular leukomalacia (PVL) is a symmetric, non-hemorrhagic, ischemic lesion to the brain of the premature infant (Volpe, 2001). It involves a characteristic distribution of necrosis of white matter dorsal and lateral to the external angles of the lateral ventricles. The area

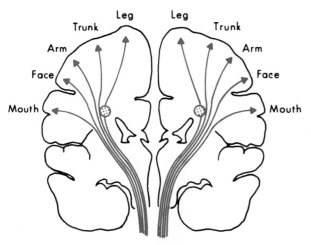

◆ **Figure 35-2** Diagram of corticospinal tracts. Dotted circular areas indicate periventricular leukomalacia that would be expected to affect descending fibers for control of the lower extremity. *(From Volpe, JJ. Neurology of the Newborn, 2nd ed. Philadelphia: WB Saunders, 1987, p. 314.)*

affected includes the white matter through which long descending motor tracts travel to the spinal cord from the motor cortex. Because the motor tracts involved in the control of leg movements are closest to the ventricles, and therefore more likely to be damaged, spastic diplegia is the most common clinical sequela (Fig. 35-2). If the lesion extends laterally, the arms may be involved, with resulting spastic quadriplegia. Visual deficits may also result from damage to the optic radiations (Catto-Smith et al., 1985; Papile, 1997).

The incidence of white matter damage in premature infants increases with decreased gestational age. The lesion is caused by a reduction in cerebral blood flow in the highly vulnerable periventricular region of the brain where the arterial "end zones" of the middle, posterior, and anterior cerebral arteries meet and is often associated with intraventricular hemorrhage (IVH) (Volpe, 2001). Decreased cerebral blood flow leads to an increase in ischemia and a decrease in antioxidant defenses. The resulting generation of free oxygen radicals and glutamate toxicity are factors that contribute to periventricular leukomalacia. Systemic hypotension associated with a difficult resuscitation at birth and ECMO may be causal factors. Patent ductus arteriosus and severe apneic spells are other contributing factors, particularly after the first week of life (McMenamin et al., 1984; Sweeney & Swanson, 2001; Volpe 2001).

Serial ultrasonography, computed tomography, magnetic resonance imaging, and positron emission tomography are useful diagnostic tools for periventricular leukomalacia (Mizuguchi & Takashima, 2002; Sinha et al.,

1990; Volpe 2000). White matter echodensities and echolucencies on high-resolution cranial ultrasonography are predictive of neurologic sequelae associated with cerebral palsy (Leviton & Paneth, 1990; Miller & Murray, 1992). Serial ultrasonographic studies are important because the evolution of periventricular echodensity is related to prognosis. Early periventricular echodensity that resolves during the first weeks of life is not correlated with childhood disability; development of cysts as a result of dissolution of brain tissue secondary to infarction, however, are correlated with cerebral palsy and cognitive deficits (Mantovani & Powers, 1991). Cerebral palsy occurs in more than 90% of infants who develop bilateral cysts larger than 3 mm in diameter in the parietal or occipital areas. Magnetic resonance imaging (MRI) is more sensitive and specific to detection of PVL; however, use with infants who require monitoring equipment is contraindicated (Volpe, 2001).

The basic elements of medical management of PVL include prevention of intrauterine asphyxia, maintenance of adequate ventilation and perfusion, avoidance of systemic hypotension, and control of seizures (Volpe, 2001). Prevention of intrauterine asphyxia includes identification of high-risk pregnancies, fetal monitoring, fetal blood sampling, and cesarean section as indicated. Maintenance of adequate ventilation includes avoiding common causes of hypoxemia such as inappropriate feeding, inserting or removing ventilator connections, painful procedures and examinations, handling, and excessive noise. Adequate perfusion can be maintained with appropriate treatment if the infant exhibits apnea and severe bradycardia. Methods for prevention of systemic hypotension include proper handling, use of volume-expanding medications, treatment of pneumothorax, and abrupt closure of patent ductus arteriosus. Treatment for neonatal seizures includes phenobarbital and calcium-channel blockers, free radical scavengers such as allopurinol, and maternal use of magnesium sulfate as a neuroprotective agent (Volpe, 2001).

Germinal Matrix-Intraventricular Hemorrhage and Periventricular Hemorrhage

Germinal matrix-intraventricular hemorrhage (GM-IVH) is the most common type of neonatal intracranial hemorrhage and is characteristic of the premature infant of less than 32 weeks of gestational age and weighing less than 1500 g. GM-IVH typically occurs in preterm infants with RDS requiring ventilation. An inverse relationship exists between gestational age and incidence of GM-IVH. The average incidence has been reported at 15% in preterm infants who are in the aforementioned categories

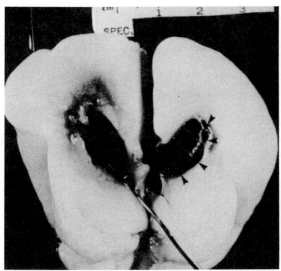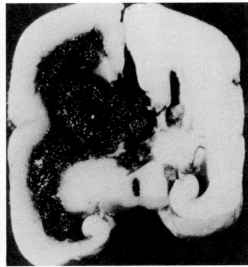

• **Figure 35-3**   Coronal section of the cerebrum showing intraventricular hemorrhage. *(From Volpe, JJ. Neurology of the Newborn, 2nd ed. Philadelphia: WB Saunders, 1987, p. 314.)*

for gestational age and weight (Volpe, 2001). Most hemorrhages occur within the first 2 postnatal days, and 90% occur within 72 hours of birth (Papile, 1997; Volpe, 2001). This lesion involves bleeding into the subependymal germinal matrix, which is a gelatinous area that contains a rich vascular network supplied mainly by Heubner's artery, a branch of the anterior cerebral artery; branches of the middle cerebral artery, and internal carotid. This matrix is prominent from 26 to 34 weeks of gestation and is usually gone by term. The vessels that traverse the matrix are primitive in appearance, with a single layer of endothelium without smooth muscle, elastin, or collagen, and the area is devoid of supportive stroma. The site of origin of hemorrhage is from these primitive capillaries. In a small number of preterm infants, hemorrhage may occur from the choroid plexus or roof of the fourth ventricle (Fig. 35-3). GM-IVH pathogenesis includes fluctuating cerebral blood flow, a decrease followed by an increase in cerebral blood flow, an increase in cerebral venous pressure, and platelet and coagulation disturbance (Volpe, 2001).

Neuropathologic complications of IVH are hydrocephalus, germinal matrix destruction, cyst formation, and accompanying hypoxic-ischemic lesions. A four-level grading scale based on ultrasound scan has been developed by Papile to classify hemorrhages (Papile et al., 1983). Grade I is an isolated germinal matrix hemorrhage. Grade II is an IVH with normal-sized ventricles that occurs when hemorrhage in the subependymal germinal matrix ruptures through the ependyma into the

lateral ventricles. Grade III includes an IVH with acute ventricular dilation, and grade IV involves a hemorrhage into the periventricular white matter.

It has recently been shown that the cause of periventricular hemorrhage is not a simple extension of blood into the cerebral white matter from the germinal matrix, but that the lesion is a hemorrhagic venous infarction with the major cause being obstruction of blood flow in the terminal vein caused by GM-IVH (Volpe, 2001). Periventricular hemorrhagic infarction is most often unilateral or markedly asymmetric, and grossly hemorrhagic. Accompanying lesions include periventricular leukomalacia, pontine neuronal necrosis, and hydrocephalus. Catastrophic IVH is the least common and occurs in infants with severe hemorrhaging. Volpe (2001) describes three IVH syndromes: catastrophic, saltatory, and clinically silent. Clinical correlates for the catastrophic IVH include coma, respiratory abnormalities, generalized tonic seizures, decerebrate posturing, eyes fixed to vestibular stimulation, and flaccid quadriparesis. Presenting signs of the saltatory syndrome include an alteration in level of consciousness, decrease in quantity and quality of spontaneous and elicited movement, hypotonia, and eye abnormalities such as downward vertical drift. These neurologic signs are subtle and often difficult to detect in early weeks of life via clinical examination. A more sensitive finding is an unexplained fall in hematocrit.

Serial portable cranial sonography is the procedure of choice in the diagnosis, identification, grading, and timing of GM-IVH because of high-resolution imaging, portable instrumentation, lack of ionizing radiation, and relative affordability (Papile, 1997; Volpe, 2001). Computed tomography scanning is useful for identification of complicating lesions such as posterior fossa lesions, subdural hemorrhage, and parenchymal abnormalities. Lumbar puncture findings for IVH include a high number of red blood cells and increased protein content, which both correlate with the severity of the hemorrhage. MRI provides excellent imaging of IVH and parenchymal details but requires transport, and absence of metallic monitoring equipment (Volpe, 2001). Dubowitz and Dubowitz (1981a, 1981b) have noted that a tight popliteal angle (130° or less in infants up to 31 weeks of gestation and 110° or less at 32 to 35 weeks of gestation) is a sign of IVH.

Methods to prevent IVH include measures to prevent premature birth, transport in utero and prenatal administration of corticosteroid to women at risk for preterm birth (Volpe, 2001; Crowley, 2002). Treatment includes support of cerebral perfusion by maintaining arterial blood pressure and avoidance of cerebral hemodynamic disturbances caused by rapid volume expansion, pneumothorax, increased arterial blood pressure, and hypoxemia. Serial ultrasound scans to monitor ventricular size and ventriculostomy or shunting for hydrocephalus are also important treatment components (Volpe, 2001). Prophylactic measures include transport of the infant in utero to a level III nursery, limiting handling, optimal management of labor and delivery, cesarean section before active phase of labor, and medications such as phenobarbital, indomethacin, and ethamsylate (to reduce capillary bleeding). Vitamins E and K are currently under investigation to reduce capillary bleeding. When hemorrhage has occurred, medical management includes maintenance of cerebral perfusion through control of blood pressure and decrease in intracranial pressure through lumbar puncture and ventricular drainage.

Short-term outcome of the infant with GM-IVH is correlated with the severity of the hemorrhage, but long-term outcome depends on the degree of associated parenchymal injury (Volpe, 2001). Volpe reported that for neonates with parenchymal injury greater than 1 cm, the mortality rate was 59% and the rate of major neurologic sequelae such as spastic hemiparesis or asymmetric spastic quadriplegia was 87%. In addition, 73% of the survivors had cognitive impairments. The risk of major neurologic disability in LBW preterm infants increases with each higher grade of IVH (McMenamin et al., 1984). The incidences of neurologic sequelae for grades I, II, and III are 5%, 15%, and 35%, respectively (Volpe, 2001).

HYPOXIC-ISCHEMIC ENCEPHALOPATHY

Hypoxic-ischemic encephalopathy (HIE) is the major perinatal cause of neurologic morbidity in both the premature and full-term infant (Vannucci, 1997). Perinatal asphyxia results in hypoxemia (reduced amount of oxygen in the blood) and ischemia, with ischemia being the most important form of oxygen deprivation. The period of reperfusion is when many of the complications that affect the metabolism, function, and structure of the brain occur. The relative importance of antepartum, intrapartum, and postnatal hypoxic-ischemic insults is difficult to determine. Major signs of HIE include seizures and abnormalities in state of consciousness, tone, posture, reflexes (especially disturbed suck, swallow, gag, and tongue movements), respiratory pattern, and autonomic function. Conditions associated with increased risk for fetal asphyxia are altered placental exchange, reduced maternal blood flow to the placenta, and decreased maternal oxygen saturation. Altered placental exchange may result from abruption, placenta previa, postmaturity, prolapsed umbilical cord, umbilical cord around the neck, and placental insufficiency. Maternal hypotension may reduce the blood flow to the placenta, and maternal hypoventilation, hypoxia, or cardiopulmonary disease may decrease maternal oxygenation. Intrapartum insults include those related to traumatic delivery, prolonged labor, and acute placental or cord problems. Prolonged partial asphyxia from any cause sets into motion a spiral of cytotoxic edema, with impaired cerebral blood flow, which leads to cerebral necrosis or ulegyria (Fig. 35-4). Infants with HIE commonly have disturbances of pulmonary, cardiovascular, hepatic, and renal functions.

Therapeutic care of an infant at risk for development of HIE includes careful monitoring by serial neurologic assessments, detection of reduced cerebral perfusion pressure, and assessment of the structural status of brain with computed tomography, ultrasound, magnetic resonance imaging, magnetic resonance spectroscopy, technetium scan, and electroencephalography or evoked potential tests (Volpe, 2001). Treatment principles include prevention of intrauterine asphyxia; maintenance of adequate ventilation, perfusion, and blood glucose levels; and control of seizures and brain swelling.

Preventive measures for intrauterine asphyxia include antepartum assessment and identification of the high-risk pregnancy, electronic fetal monitoring, fetal blood sampling, and cesarean section when necessary. Maintenance of adequate oxygenation is essential to prevent

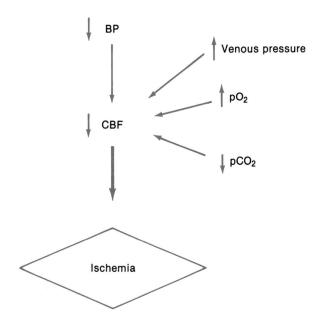

+ **Figure 35-4**   Model for production of cerebral edema. Decreased blood pressure (BP) leads to decreased cerebral blood flow (CBF) and ischemia. *(From Campbell, SK: Clinical decision making: Management of the neonate with movement dysfunction. In Wolf, SL [Ed.]. Clinical Decision Making in Physical Therapy. Philadelphia: FA Davis, 1985, p. 299.)*

additional injury. Volume expansion with the use of drugs to increase blood pressure (pressor agents) is used to maintain cerebral blood flow. Partial exchange transfusion may be done if the infant's hematocrit is low to decrease hyperviscosity and enhance tissue oxygenation. Sodium bicarbonate and glucose are administered to treat severe, persistent metabolic acidosis and hypoglycemia, respectively. The use of barbiturates is being studied because they reduce the energy requirements of the brain and have been shown to decrease intracranial pressure in adults. Phenobarbital is the drug of choice for seizure control, with lorazepam as adjunctive therapy.

Sarnat and Sarnat (1976) identified three stages of encephalopathy after asphyxia. Stage 1 lasts less than 24 hours and is characterized by hyperalertness, low-threshold Moro and stretch reflexes, and normal muscle tone and electroencephalogram. The duration for stage 2 is approximately 5 days; clinical signs include lethargy, mild hypotonia, strong distal flexion, hyperactive stretch reflexes, weak suck and Moro reflexes, strong tonic neck reflex, and multifocal seizures. Stage 3 is stupor, which lasts from a few hours to 4 weeks, with flaccidity alternating with decerebrate posturing, absent reflexes, response only to strong noxious stimuli, occasional seizures, and an isopotential electroencephalogram.

When the infant with hypoxic-ischemic insult has a normal neurologic examination by 1 week of age, sequelae are minimal. Those who continue to have an abnormal neurologic examination by 3 weeks of age, however, are at risk of developing major neurologic sequelae (Harper & Yoon, 1987). The neurologic sequelae of HIE include motor deficits with or without mental retardation, seizures, or both. Neuropathologic classifications of HIE include selective neuronal necrosis, periventricular leukomalacia, parasagittal cerebral injury, and focal ischemic brain necrosis (Volpe, 2001).

SELECTIVE NEURONAL NECROSIS

Selective neuronal necrosis, the most common type of HIE, is the death of neurons in a widespread but characteristic pattern and commonly accompanies the other manifestations of HIE. The major sites of neuronal necrosis include the hippocampus of the cerebral cortex and parts of the diencephalon, basal ganglia, pons, medulla, cerebellum, thalamus, brainstem, and spinal cord (Cabanas et al., 1991) (Box 35-2, Table 35-1, and Fig. 35-5). Topography is related to the severity and duration of the HIE and the gestational age of the infant or fetus (Volpe, 2001). The pathogenesis of selective neuronal necrosis includes regional vascular factors because neuronal injury is more marked in vascular border zones, regional metabolic factors, and the regional distribution of glutamate receptors, particularly the NMDA type (Volpe, 2001). Clinical findings include stupor, coma, seizures, hypotonia, and problems in ocular, sucking, and tongue movements. Long-term sequelae include cognitive impairment, spastic quadriparesis, seizure disorder, ataxia, bulbar and pseudobulbar palsy, hyperactivity, impaired attention, and atonic quadriparesis.

Status marmoratus is neuronal loss, gliosis, and hypermyelinization of the basal ganglia and thalamus. Impairments are not fully manifested until the latter part of the first year of life, although injury occurs in the perinatal period (Volpe, 2001). The pathogenesis of this lesion is related primarily to glutamate-induced neuronal death, as well as regional circulatory and metabolic factors (Volpe, 2001). Neonatal findings are unknown at this time, but long-term clinical sequelae include choreoathetosis, cognitive impairment, and spastic quadriplegia.

PARASAGITTAL CEREBRAL INJURY

Parasagittal cerebral injury results in a lesion of the cerebral cortex and subcortical white matter. This injury is usually bilateral and symmetric, with the parietal-occipital regions most affected (Volpe, 2001). The areas of

Box 35-2 **Selective Neuronal Necrosis in Neonatal Hypoxic-Ischemic Encephalopathy—Major Sites**

Cerebral cortex —hippocampus, supralimbic cortex
Diencephalon —thalamus, hypothalamus, and lateral geniculate body
Basal ganglia —caudate, putamen, and globus pallidus
Midbrain —inferior colliculus, oculomotor and trochlear nuclei, red nucleus, substantia nigra, and reticular formation

Pons —motor nuclei of trigeminal and facial nerves; dorsal, ventral cochlear nuclei; reticular formation; and pontine nuclei
Medulla —dorsal motor nucleus of vagus nerve, nucleus ambiguus, inferior olivary nuclei, cuneate and gracilis nuclei
Cerebellum —Purkinje cells, dentate, and other roof nuclei

From Volpe, JJ. Neurology of the Newborn, 2nd ed. Philadelphia: WB Saunders, 1987, p. 213.

TABLE 35-1 **Sites of Particular Predilection for Apparent Hypoxic-Ischemic Selective Neuronal Injury in Premature and Term Newborns***

BRAIN REGION	PREMATURE	TERM
Cerebral neocortex		+[†]
Hippocampus		
Sommer's sector		+
Subiculum	+	
Basal ganglia/thalamus	=[†]	=
Brainstem		
Cranial nerve nuclei	=	=
Pons (ventral)	+	
Inferior olivary nuclei	+	
Cerebellum		
Purkinje cells		+
Internal granule cells	+	
Spinal cord		
Anterior horn cells (alone)		+
Infarction (including anterior horn cells)	+	

*See text for references.
[†]+, Relatively more common in term versus premature newborn (or vice versa); =, equally common in term and premature newborns.

necrosis are the border zones between the end fields of the major cerebral arteries. Clinical signs in the neonatal period include proximal limb weakness, especially in the upper extremities. Long-term sequelae include spastic quadriparesis and specific intellectual deficits such as delay in development of language, visuospatial abilities, or both.

FOCAL ISCHEMIC BRAIN NECROSIS AND CAVITATION

The category of focal ischemic brain necrosis includes large, localized areas of neuronal death in the distribution of single or multiple major blood vessels in the cerebral cortex and subcortical white matter. Most of these lesions are unilateral and involve the middle cerebral artery. The focal ischemic brain necrosis occurs perinatally as the result of cerebrovascular insufficiency secondary to malformation of vessels, arterial obstruction due to thrombi or emboli, or systemic circulatory insufficiency near the end of the second trimester. Resolution of neuronal necrosis results in the formation of cavities. Neurologic features during the neonatal period include hemiparesis, quadriparesis, and stereotyped and non-habituating reflex responses. This lesion results in spastic

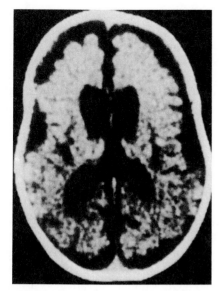

♦ **Figure 35-5** Computed tomography scan of selective cortical neuronal necrosis of a 4-week-old infant who experienced severe perinatal asphyxia. Note cortical atrophy and white matter injury. *(From Volpe, JJ. Neurology of the Newborn, 2nd ed. Philadelphia: WB Saunders, 1987, p. 245.)*

hemiparesis in the case of a limited focal lesion, mental retardation, and seizure disorder (Volpe, 2001).

NECROTIZING ENTEROCOLITIS

Necrotizing enterocolitis (NEC) is an acute inflammatory disease of the bowel that occurs most frequently during the first 6 weeks of life in premature infants weighing less than 2000 g (Whaley & Wong, 1991). Although the precise cause of the disease is not known, several factors appear to play a role in the pathogenesis of NEC. These factors include intestinal ischemia, infectious agents and toxins, and enteral formula alimentation (McElhinney et al., 2000; McGuire & Antony, 2003). Diminished blood supply results in death of mucosal cells lining the bowel wall, decreasing secretion of lubricating mucus. The thin bowel wall becomes susceptible to proteolytic enzymes, swells, breaks down and is permeable to exotoxins. Gas-forming bacteria invade the damaged area to produce pneumatosis intestinalis, air in the submucosal or sub-serosal surfaces of the bowel (Hockenberry et al., 2003).

Diagnosis is made by physical examination, laboratory studies, and radiography. Vomiting, abdominal distention, bloody stools, retention of stools, lethargy, decreased urine output, and alterations in respiratory status are signs of NEC (Dolgin et al., 1998; Hockenberry et al., 2003). Medical care of infants with NEC includes parenteral alimentation, gastric suction, and administration of broad-spectrum antibiotics (Cressinger et al., 1992). Laboratory findings include anemia, leukopenia, and electrolyte imbalance. Breath hydrogen measurements have been found to be 99% effective in detecting absence of the disease and are suggested as an aid to diagnosis of NEC (Cheu et al., 1989). Abdominal radiographs are performed every 6 to 8 hours to detect progressive intestinal obstruction or possible perforation.

Preventive treatment includes withholding oral feedings for at least 24 to 48 hours from infants who suffered birth asphyxia. Breast milk is the preferred enteral nutrient because it allows for passive immunity (Hockenberry et al., 2003). Kamitsuka and associates (2000) reported that implementation of a standard feeding protocol in infants weighing 1250 to 2500 g and who are less than 35 weeks' gestation reduced the occurrence of NEC by 24%. Medical treatment of confirmed NEC includes discontinuation of all oral feedings, abdominal decompression via nasogastric suction, administration of intravenous antibiotics, and correction of fluid and electrolyte imbalances (Hockenberry et al., 2003). Surgical intervention is indicated when there is radiographic evidence of fixed, dilated intestinal loops accompanied by intestinal distention (Cressinger et al., 1992). Surgical procedures include intestinal decompression by nasogastric tube placement or gastrostomy, resection of necrotic bowel, and diversion of the proximal fecal stream by ileostomy, jejunostomy, or colostomy. Although enterostomy is a lifesaving procedure, it has been reported to be a major cause of morbidity (O'Connor & Swain, 1998).

NEC is the most common cause of death in neonates undergoing surgery and is the most frequent and lethal gastrointestinal disease of premature infants (Nadler et al., 2001). Factors that are predictive of poor outcome include prior enteral feeding, PDA, indomethacin use, and perforation (Wang et al., 2002). Mortality rates in the 1990s (9% to 28%) are considerably lower that the rates reported in the 1960s and 1970s (24% to 65%) (Kenner & Lott, 2003). The average mortality rate after surgery is 30% to 40%. Stricture formation, which is abnormal narrowing of the intestines, occurs in 25% to 35% of the survivors of medical or surgical treatment and causes failure to thrive, feeding abnormalities, diarrhea, or bowel obstruction (Cressinger et al., 1992).

RETINOPATHY OF PREMATURITY

Retinopathy of prematurity (ROP) is a lesion caused by an ischemic event that interferes with the development of retinal blood vessels. Cessation of this normal retinal angiogenesis is followed by hyperpoliferative neovascular response to retinal ischemia. Subsequently, there is vascular proliferation of retinal capillaries into the hypoxic area. New vessels proliferate toward the lens, and the aqueous humor and then the vitreous humor become turbid. The retina becomes edematous, and hemorrhages separate the retina from its attachment (Phelps, 1992). The outcome of the disease ranges from normal vision to total loss of vision if there is advanced scarring from the retina to the lens resulting in retinal detachment (Whaley & Wong, 1991). ROP was called retrolental fibroplasia in the early 1940s and was virtually eliminated with the severe restriction of oxygen use between 1950 and 1970. The condition has recurred as one of the major causes of disability in preterm infants as a result of the increased survival of VLBW infants. The incidence of ROP increases with lower gestational age, lower birth weight, and BPD (Holmstrom et al., 1998).

The pathogenesis of ROP is abnormal angiogenesis (development of the blood vessels) in the retina. Vascular endothelial growth factor (VEGF) seems to play a key role in the normal and abnormal angiogenesis. The VEGF gene is responsive to oxygen tension. Hypoxia stimulates VEGF transcription and hyperoxia decreases VEGF transcription. When oxygen is administered to premature infants, relatively hyperoxic conditions occur and VEGF levels decrease. Supplemental oxygen supports the avascular retina, but as oxygen is weaned the retina becomes ischemic. This ischemia stimulates VEGF transcription and angiogenesis resumes often in an uncontrolled hyperproliferative manner (Holstrom et al., 1998).

The severity of ROP is classified in five stages (Stout & Stout, 2003). In stage 1 there is a visible line of demarcation between posterior vascularized retina and the anterior avascular retina. In stage 2 pathologic neovascularization is confined to the retina that appears as a ridge at the vascular/avascular junction. Stage 3 includes new vascularization and migration into the vitreous gel. Stage 4 is defined by a subtotal retinal detachment. Stage 5 is complete retinal detachment.

Hyperoxia, shock, asphyxia, hypothermia, vitamin E deficiency, and light exposure have been implicated as possible pathogenic factors (Kretzer & Hittner, 1986). Antenatal dexamethasone administration appears to be associated with a decreased incidence of development of ROP of stage 2 or higher (Higgins et al., 1998). Light reduction was not shown to be effective in altering the incidence of ROP (Reynolds et al., 1998).

Prevention and treatment include oxygen administration at PaO$_2$ between 50 and 70 mm Hg and administration of vitamin A (which is still under investigation) (Darlow & Graham, 2002). All premature infants given supplemental oxygen are at risk for ROP and should be screened. Guidelines approved by the American Academy of Pediatrics include two screening examinations 4 to 6 weeks after birth or within 31 to 33 weeks postconceptual age, whichever is later. Subsequent intervals for examination are based on initial findings (Stout & Stout, 2003). A study conducted in Sweden recommended that screening criterion be lowered to 31 weeks or less to identify infants with severe ROP (Larsson & Holmstrom, 2002). Surgical intervention can be divided into two overlapping objectives: treatment of neovascular process with retinal cryotherapy and surgical intervention for retinal detachment (laser photocoagulation, cryotherapy, vitrectomy, and scleral buckling) (Stout & Stout 2003; Kretzer & Hittner, 1986). Supplemental oxygen with target oxygen saturation of 99% with Po$_2$ of no higher than 100 mm Hg was associated with regression of prethreshold ROP, without appearing to arrest retinal vascular maturation (Gaynon et al., 1997). Implementation of an oxygen management policy that included strict guidelines for increasing and weaning of Fio$_2$ (fraction of inspired oxygen), monitoring of oxygen saturation parameters in delivery room, in-house transport, and hospitalization for infants 500 to 1500 g birth weight resulted in a decreased incidence of ROP stages 3 to 4 and decreased the need for laser treatment (Chow et al., 2003). Surgical outcome ranges from complete recovery or mild myopia to blindness, depending on the extent of the disease.

HYPERBILIRUBINEMIA

Hyperbilirubinemia, or physiologic jaundice, is the accumulation of excessive amounts of bilirubin in the blood. Bilirubin is one of the breakdown products of hemoglobin from red blood cells. This condition is seen commonly in premature infants who have immature hepatic functions, an increased hemolysis of red blood cells as a result of high concentrations of circulating red blood cells, a shorter life span of red blood cells, and possible polycythemia from birth injuries (Hockenberry et al., 2003). The primary goal in treatment of hyperbilirubinemia is the prevention of kernicterus, which is the deposition of unconjugated bilirubin in the brain, especially in the basal ganglia and hippocampus. LBW infants of less than 2000 g receive phototherapy at 24 hours of life for 96 hours, regardless of bilirubin concentration. Phototherapy is administered by placing 8 to 10 fluorescent lamps 12 to 16 inches above the infant (Gartner & Lee, 1992). The infant is positioned in an open radiant warmer or incubator and the eyes are shielded to avoid retinal damage. Studies show that on/off cycles of more than 1 hour are as effective as continuous treatment. Infants who received traditional phototherapy for 23 hours and kangaroo care (skin to skin contact with parent) with fiberoptic panel held against their back showed comparable declines in bilirubin levels (Ludington-Hoe & Swinth, 2001). A technique of fiberoptic phototherapy uses light from a halogen lamp transmitted through a fiberoptic bundle to a blanket that is wrapped around the infant (Biliblanket) (Gartner & Lee, 1992).

If phototherapy is not effective in reducing the total serum bilirubin concentrations to acceptable levels, or if there is a rapidly rising bilirubin level, exchange transfusion is done (Shaw, 1998). In this technique, approximately 85% of the infant's red blood cells are replaced. Care must be taken so as not to disrupt cerebral blood flow and intracranial pressure (Volpe, 2001). Initial human trials have shown beneficial effects of metalloporphyrins such as tin (Sn) mesoporphyrin and tin protoporphyrin used as prophylaxis and treatment to reduce hyperbilirubinemia. These substances are inhibitors of heme oxygenase, which is an enzyme in the synthesis of bilirubin that limits the rate of degradation of heme to bile (Gartner & Lee, 1992; Kenner & Lott, 2003). Infants with severe hyperbilirubinemia unresponsive to phototherapy whose parents are Jehovah's Witnesses and rejected exchange transfusion have been successfully treated with Sn-mesoporphyrin (Kappas et al., 2001). Less frequently used therapy is enterohepatic circulation enhancement by administration of agar that binds to bilirubin in the intestine, inhibits resorption, and promotes excretion. Conjugation of bilirubin has been induced as a side effect of phenobarbital (Volpe, 2001).

NEONATAL SEIZURES

Seizures are the most frequent and distinct neurologic signs that occur in the neonatal period (Volpe, 2001; Brann & Wiznitzer, 1992). Seizures are the most frequent overt sign of neurologic disorders (Volpe, 2001). HIE, low birth weight, low gestational age, jaundice during the last 3 days, maternal disease in the last 2 years before pregnancy, intrapartum fever, jaundice during the first 3 days of life, and the need for cardiopulmonary resuscitation are related to neonatal seizures (Arpino et al., 2001; Lieberman et al., 2000). Most seizures occur between the second and fifth days of life, and 85% occur in the first 15 days of life with a sharply increased incidence in infants less than 1500 g. A seizure during the neonatal period is a medical emergency, because it may indicate a life-threatening disease or disorder that can produce immediate and irreversible brain damage. Repeated neonatal seizures may also result in decreased DNA content and brain cell number. The causes of neonatal seizures include hypoxic-ischemic encephalopathy secondary to perinatal asphyxia, intracranial hemorrhage, hypoglycemia, hypocalcemia, intracranial infection, developmental defects, and drug withdrawal (Volpe, 2001).

Clinical manifestations of seizures in neonates differ greatly from those in older infants and children because of the immaturity of the brain. Clinical signs in the neonate include facial, oral, lingual, and ocular movements and autonomic manifestations such as apnea and changes in blood pressure, heart rate, and pupil size (Box 35-3). Abnormal movements and alteration of tone in the trunk and extremities, including rowing and bicycling movements, are also clinical signs of neonatal seizure (Mizrahi & Kellaway, 1987). Symptoms of seizures in premature infants include staring, nystagmus, apnea, hiccough, and chewing, ocular, and pedaling movements (Volpe, 2001). Treatment includes administration of anticonvulsants such as phenobarbital, phenytoin, and diazepam to control seizures and intravenous glucose for hypoglycemia.

Approximately 25% to 35% of all infants with neonatal seizures later exhibit cognitive impairment, motor impairment, or both. Seizures that occur in conjunction with perinatal asphyxia, severe IVH, intracranial infection, and prematurity with prolonged hypoglycemia have poor prognoses, with possible permanent neurologic sequelae

Box 35-3	Characteristics of Subtle Seizures in Premature and Full-Term Infants
Ocular-tonic horizontal deviation of eyes (jerking) and sustained eye opening with ocular fixation Eyelid blinking or fluttering	Sucking, smacking, drooling, and other oral-buccal-lingual movements "Swimming," "rowing," and "pedaling" movements Apneic spell

From Volpe, JJ. Neurology of the Newborn, 2nd ed. Philadelphia: WB Saunders, 1987, p. 134.

such as cerebral palsy or cognitive impairment. Seizures that occur with subarachnoid hemorrhage without asphyxia or as a result of metabolic disorders have good prognoses if treatment begins early (Volpe, 2001).

FETAL ALCOHOL SYNDROME

Chronic alcohol exposure in utero may result in a multitude of symptoms at birth, including withdrawal symptoms of irritability, tremors, apnea, and seizures (Volpe, 2001; West et al., 1998). When severe, phenobarbital or paregoric (morphine) may be used to control withdrawal symptoms (Harper & Yoon, 1987). Alcohol rapidly crosses the placenta and the blood-brain barrier of the fetus, and there is a dose-dependent relationship between maternal alcohol intake in the first weeks of pregnancy and the occurrence of features of the fetal alcohol syndrome (FAS).

The full manifestation of FAS, one of the most common causes of mental retardation in the world, is characterized by a triad of symptoms composed of growth deficiency; cardiac defects; and CNS disturbance, such as microcephaly, mental retardation, and dysmorphology (including facial, genital, and joint abnormalities) (Barbour, 1990; Volpe, 2001). The severity of cognitive disability is correlated with the severity of dysmorphic features. Prenatal exposure to alcohol causes deficits in all domains of adaptive functioning including problems with socialization behavior of young children (Whaley et al., 2001).

In utero alcohol exposure is related to a wide continuum of effects ranging from full FAS to partial FAS, also referred to as fetal alcohol effects, to more subtle effects, such as neurologic disorders without dysmorphology (Scott et al., 1991). These subtle neurologic effects include hyperactivity, delayed language development, fine and gross motor problems, slowed reaction time, and problems with judgment and comprehension (Autti-Ramo & Granström, 1991; Scott et al., 1991). The Institute of Medicine has recently proposed the terms alcohol-related neurodevelopmental disorder (ARND) and alcohol-related birth defects (ARBD) to replace FAE (fetal alcohol effects) and FAS in describing conditions in which there is a history of maternal alcohol exposure and an outcome that confirms effects of such exposure (American Academy of Pediatrics, 2000). Long-term effects of prenatal alcohol exposure include deficits in several areas of intellectual functioning, including information processing, short-term memory, encoding, and preacademic skills (Coles et al., 1991; Little et al., 1989). Streissguth (1986) reported

that 24% of children born to binge drinkers and 15% born to nonbinge drinkers were receiving special education services at 7.5 years of age. In addition to cognitive deficits, behavioral and communication problems lead to maladaptive social functioning, including impulsive behavior, anxiety, and dysphoria (Volpe, 2001).

NEONATAL ABSTINENCE SYNDROME

Maternal use of narcotics during pregnancy leads to the development of dependency on that drug by the fetus. The most commonly used drugs are heroin, methadone, and cocaine, and there is often maternal use of several drugs during pregnancy (Finnegan, 1988; Kenner & Lott, 2003). Women who use cocaine during pregnancy receive less prenatal care and are more likely to smoke, consume alcohol, be malnourished, and be exposed to sexually transmitted diseases (Tronick & Beeghly, 1999). The fetus experiences withdrawal or neonatal abstinence syndrome (NAS) when the mother is withdrawn from her drug or drugs or when the fetus is delivered (D'Apolito & Hepworth, 2001). The onset of withdrawal symptoms usually occurs within the first 72 hours after birth. (D'Apolito & Hepworth, 2001). Symptoms of withdrawal include neurologic, gastrointestinal, and respiratory signs as well as autonomic dysfunction (Kenner & Lott, 2003). Neurologic symptoms include signs of CNS excitability such as hyperactivity, irritability, tremors, seizures, apnea, increased muscle tone, inability to sleep, hyperactive deep tendon reflexes, and poor coordination. Gastrointestinal symptoms include hyperactive sucking soon after birth and then disorganized, ineffective sucking of reduced rate and pressure that is poorly coordinated with swallowing. Respiratory signs in NAS include tachypnea, irregular respirations, rhinorrhea, stuffy nose, nasal flaring, chest retractions, intermittent cyanosis, and apnea. Regurgitation and/or aspiration may occur. Signs of autonomic dysfunction include frequent sneezing, yawning, mottling of the skin, excessive tearing and generalized sweating, and shrill crying (Dixon, 1989; Hayford et al., 1988; Volpe, 2001, Kenner & Lott, 2003).

Premature delivery, meconium aspiration, low birth weight, small for gestational age, decreased head circumference, and abruptio placentae are common complications of labor and delivery (Chasnoff, 1988; Handler et al., 1991; Kenner & Lott, 2003). Disturbances in the behavioral organization and interactive abilities of these neonates make early bonding and attachment difficult (Hume et al., 1989). Follow-up studies indicate growth retardation, long-term intellectual impairment, and learning difficulties such as problems with sustained attention and with processing in the visual modality in children exposed to drugs in utero (Bauman & Levine, 1986; Coles, et al., 2002) and problems in adaptive and social functioning (Whaley et al., 2001; Free et al., 1990; Hume et al., 1989; Lewis et al., 1989; Davis & Templer, 1988). Treatment of NAS includes pharmacologic therapy for narcotic withdrawal, but infants exposed to only cocaine do not usually require such treatment (Askin & Diehl-Jones, 2001). Reducing environmental stimulation and using techniques such as swaddling and flexed positioning are effective strategies for calming infants experiencing CNS irritation (Askin & Diehl-Jones, 2001). Small, frequent feedings and additional calories may be needed.

EXPOSURE TO HUMAN IMMUNODEFICIENCY VIRUS

The risk of infants born to women with a positive HIV titer developing HIV infection was estimated to be 10% to 40% in 1995 (Volpe, 2001). Wortley and associates (2001) reported that with good prenatal surveillance for HIV with use of ZDV, only 8% of children exposed to HIV in utero were infected. Isolation is not necessary for the neonate exposed to HIV. An infant born to an HIV-positive mother should not be breastfed, as breast milk is a vehicle for transmission of the virus between mother and infant. Using virologic techniques such as HIV culture, polymerase chain reaction, and immune complex-dissociation, diagnosis of HIV infection can be made in almost 50% of infants at birth and 95% or more of infants by 1 to 3 months of age. Infection early in fetal development may lead to microcephaly, cerebral atrophy, basal ganglia and white matter calcification, calcific vasculopathy of the CNS, spinal cord myelin loss, and facial anomalies (Volpe, 2001). Infants exposed to HIV should be monitored for signs of infection, such as failure to thrive, weight loss, temperature instability, and diarrhea, and assessed for opportunistic infections, such as herpes simplex virus infection, cytomegalovirus infection, lymphoid interstitial pneumonia, and viral, fungal, or protozoal infections. Breastfeeding should not occur because of transmission of the virus and cytomegalovirus (Pursell, 1998; Mussi-Pinhata et al., 1998). Because neonates with HIV infection are usually asymptomatic, they are not admitted to the NICU unless there are problems unrelated to HIV. It should be noted, however, that infants who were seropositive exhibited significantly lower scores on the Bayley Scales of Infant Development than infants who were seronegative (Aylward et al., 1992).

BIRTH INJURIES RELATED TO THE NERVOUS SYSTEM

Birth injuries are those sustained during labor and delivery and represent an important cause of neonatal morbidity (Mangurten, 1992). The most common traumatic lesions related to the nervous system include caput succedaneum, linear skull fracture, and brachial plexus palsy.

CAPUT SUCCEDANEUM

Caput succedaneum or molding is hemorrhagic edema caused by compression of a portion of the scalp from the pressure of the uterus or vaginal wall during a vertex delivery. Incidence is 20% to 40% of deliveries by vacuum extraction (Volpe, 2000). The clinical manifestation is a soft swelling usually a few millimeters thick. The edema is external to the periosteum and crosses suture lines. The lesion steadily resolves over the first days of life, and no intervention is necessary.

LINEAR SKULL FRACTURE

Linear skull fractures are relatively common in newborns and are caused by direct compression of the head during a prolonged labor and delivery and use of forceps during delivery. Uncomplicated linear skull fractures are diagnosed by radiographs and require no treatment. However, the fracture should alert the physician to the remote possibility of a more serious intracranial traumatic lesion (Volpe, 2001).

BIRTH BRACHIAL PLEXUS PALSY

Birth brachial plexus palsy (BBPP) is a paralysis or weakness involving the muscles of the upper extremity after mechanical trauma to the spinal roots of the fifth cervical (C5) through the first thoracic (T1) nerves during birth. Brachial plexus palsies are classified into three types: Erb's (73% to 86%), or upper arm, paralysis (involving C5 and C6); Klumpke's (less than 1%), or lower arm, paralysis (involving C8 and T1); and Erb-Klumpke (20%), or whole arm, paralysis (Dodds & Wolfe, 2000). Most cases of brachial plexus palsy follow a prolonged and difficult labor. The infant is often of high birth weight, sedated, and hypotonic, rendering the arm vulnerable to separation of bony segments, overstretching, and soft tissue injury (Mangurten, 1992; Scoles, 1992; Shepherd, 1991). Traction on the shoulder during delivery of the head in a breech presentation, and lateral traction of the head and neck while delivering the

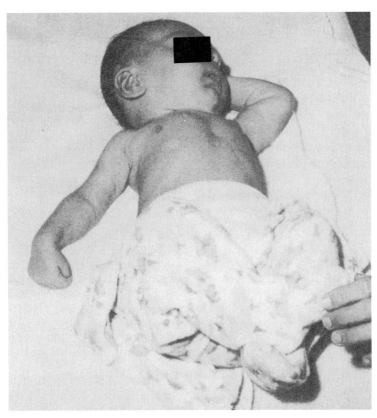

◆ **Figure 35-6**   Four-week-old infant with partial paralysis of right arm as a result of brachial plexus injury. *(From Shepherd, RB. Brachial plexus injury. In Campbell, SK [Ed.]. Pediatric Neurologic Physical Therapy. New York: Churchill Livingstone, 1991, p. 107.)*

shoulders in a vertex presentation, can injure the C5 and C6 roots. More forceful traction may result in paralysis of the whole arm. Forceful elevation and abduction of the arm, stretching the lower plexus under and against the coracoid process of the scapula, may be the cause of the less common lower palsy. The birth trauma that injures the brachial plexus may also be associated with other lesions. Associated lesions may include injury to the facial nerve, fractures of the clavicle or humerus, subluxation of the shoulder, torticollis, or a hemiparalysis of the diaphragm by injuring the phrenic nerve at C4. The position of the arm and direction of forces that are applied are related to the injury (Jennett et al., 2002). It has been proposed that intrauterine fetal maladaptation is the cause of some neonatal brachial injuries with disuse osteoporosis as evidence (Jennett & Tarby, 2001).

In most infants with brachial plexus injury, the nerve sheath is torn and the nerve fibers are compressed by hemorrhage and edema. Clinical manifestations include a characteristic arm position of adduction, internal rotation with extension of the elbow, pronation of the forearm, and flexion of the wrist (Fig. 35-6). Passive

abduction results in the arm falling limply. The Moro, biceps, and radial reflexes are absent; grasp is intact. Electromyography is used to detect a decrease in micropotential and signs of denervation. Magnetic resonance imaging can detect avulsions of the roots. Real-time ultrasound can be used to determine if the diaphragm is involved, which can occur with Erb's palsy (Volpe, 2001).

Treatment of brachial plexus injury includes rest for 7 to 10 days after injury to allow hemorrhage and edema to decrease. During this time, partial immobilization is accomplished by positioning the limb gently across the upper abdomen (Volpe, 2001). Physical therapy and occupational therapy begin after the initial period of immobilization and are important interventions throughout all phases of treatment of BBPP (Nelson, 2000). The goals of therapy intervention is to maintain range of motion (ROM) by gentle passive exercising, to stimulate muscle function as neural regeneration occurs, and to encourage active movement (Fig. 35-7) (see Shepherd, 1991, for a comprehensive physical therapy assessment and treatment plan). Splinting is controversial, and continuous splinting in the "Statue of

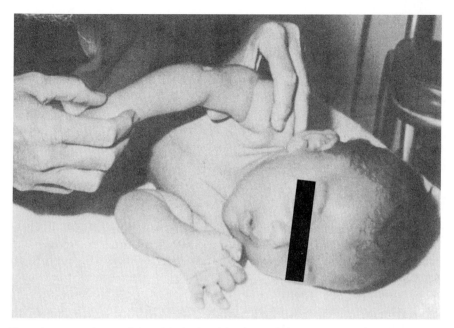

♦ **Figure 35-7**   Therapist attempting to elicit activity in the deltoid muscle by encouraging hand-to-face movement. *(From Shepherd, RB. Brachial plexus injury. In Campbell, SK [Ed.]. Pediatric Neurologic Physical Therapy. New York: Churchill Livingstone, 1991, p. 112.)*

Liberty" splint is no longer recommended because it results in formation of abduction contractures and subsequent hypermobility of the shoulder. Intermittent splinting of the wrist and stabilization of the fingers are recommendations for lower arm palsy (Volpe, 2001; Mangurten, 1992). If improvement in active movement is not noted within the first few months, electromyography and nerve conduction studies are performed to determine the extent of damage, to follow recovery, and to determine if microsurgical repair is needed. Surgery is usually done at 3 to 6 months (Dodds & Wolfe, 2000).

Botulinum toxin injections into the antagonists of paralyzed muscles have been used in young children with brachial plexus injury to increase range of motion, decrease contractures, and improve body scheme (Desiato & Risina, 2001). It has been proposed that developmental dyspraxia may occur because of neonatal brachial plexus injury and resultant lack of, or inappropriate use of, the extremity (Rapalino & Levine, 2000; Brown et al., 2000).

▌SPINA BIFIDA

Spina bifida includes a continuum of congenital anomalies of the spine that range from failure of fusion of the posterior vertebral arch or arches to open spinal defects such as myelomeningocele (Edwards & Derechin,

1988) (see Chapter 25 for a full discussion of myelodysplasia). Approximately 80% of all lesions in infants with myelomeningocele occur in the lumbar area, which may reflect the fact that this is the last region of the neural tube to close (Volpe, 2001; Noetzel, 1989). Prenatal diagnosis of neural tube defects is based on levels of alpha-fetoprotein in maternal serum at 14 to 16 weeks, ultrasound, and acetylcholinesterase (AChE) assays. The sensitivity of AChE combined with real-time ultrasound in detecting neural tube deficits approaches 100% (Volpe, 2001). When an open defect is present, early closure of the back lesion is performed during the first 24 to 48 hours after birth to prevent infections such as meningitis or ventriculitis and to prevent trauma to the exposed tissue and stretching of the other nerve roots, which can lead to a loss of motor function. If prophylactic antibiotics are administered from 24 hours of life until surgery, infection rates are low. The most prudent course seems to be prompt closure after rational decision making by the parents and physicians (Volpe, 2001). The objective of sac closure is to replace the neural tissue into the vertebral canal, cover the spinal defect, and achieve a flat and watertight closure of the sac (Huttenlocher, 1987). An exciting new option is open fetal surgical repair of myelomeningocele at 20 to 26 weeks' gestational age with subsequent cesarean section delivery. The goals of open fetal surgical repair are to decrease trauma to the neural tissue, the need for shunting for hydrocephalus, musculoskeletal deformity, and correction of Arnold-Chiari syndrome with the overall goal of improvement in neurologic function (Hedrick & Crombleholme, 2001).

Hydrocephalus is a common complication of myelodysplasia. The incidence of hydrocephalus varies according to the site of the lesion (Noetzel, 1989; Volpe, 2001). With lesions involving the thoracolumbar, lumbar, or lumbosacral areas, the incidence of hydrocephalus is approximately 90%. With occipital, cervical, thoracic, or sacral lesions, the incidence of hydrocephalus is 60%. Ventriculoperitoneal shunting is performed when there are clinical or diagnostic signs of hydrocephalus. Clinical signs include full anterior fontanel and split cranial sutures. Hydrocephalus is most commonly associated with overt clinical signs 2 to 3 weeks after birth. Serial computed tomography and ultrasonography are tools used to diagnose hydrocephalus.

Physical therapy examination of the neonate with myelodysplasia in the special care nursery may be done before or after closure of the back, or both before and after. This assessment is important to evaluate skeletal alignment, range of motion, motor and sensory function, reflex development, and behavioral organization. The neonate with myelomeningocele may have joint deformities as the result of imbalance of muscle action and positioning in utero. Positioning may also help improve or maintain skeletal alignment, such as prone positioning to maintain hip joint range of motion and encourage development of the extensor muscles. Side lying can be used to encourage a symmetric posture. The supine position should be avoided because of the effects of gravity. Splinting or serial casting may also be used to improve skeletal alignment (Schneider et al., 1995).

Examination of range of motion (ROM) in the newborn with spina bifida is indicated to identify impairments and, if necessary, to take advantage of the neonatal period of hyperplasticity of ligaments, resulting from transplacental transfer of relaxin and estrogen from the mother (Hensinger, 1977; Sweeney & Swanson, 2001). The therapist must be aware of normal neonatal physiologic flexion of the hips and knees and the possibility of hip dislocation. Because of the latter, it is recommended that hip adduction be tested only to the neutral position. Limitations in ROM are not an indication for aggressive stretching. ROM exercises should be performed slowly and gently to avoid fractures of paralyzed lower extremities. Common limitations in muscle extensibility for neonates with spina bifida include tightness of hip flexors, hip adductors, and dorsiflexors or evertors of the ankle (Mazur & Menelaus, 1991; Tappit-Emas, 1999). ROM exercises should be done with hands placed close to the joint being moved with a

brief hold at the end of the range preventing unnecessary stress to soft tissue and joint structures (Tappit-Emas, 1999).

Muscle testing is performed by the physical therapist to determine the level of muscle innervation. Obviously, conventional methods of muscle testing are not appropriate for the neonate. Schneider and associates (1995) offer some strategies for eliciting muscle contraction that include carefully considering the state of the infant, tickling, holding the extremities in positions such as hip and knee flexion, and holding a limb in an antigravity position to stimulate the infant to move or hold a limb. Movements of the extremities may be observed, and contractions may be palpated. Gentle resistance may be given to elicit a stronger response (Tappit-Emas, 1999). Muscle strength may be graded as present, absent, or trace. Repeated assessment is recommended to obtain as accurate a picture as possible of muscle function.

Sensory testing should be performed when the neonate is in a quiet, awake state in order to determine the level of sensation. The skin is stroked with a pin or other sharp object to determine the neonate's reaction to pain, such as facial grimacing. The therapist begins at the anal area, the lowest sacral innervation level, and strokes across the buttocks, down the posterior thigh and leg, up the anterior surface of the leg and thigh, and across the abdominal musculature to determine reaction to pain (Schneider et al., 1995). The neonate's response should be recorded for each dermatome.

The physical therapist may also include reflex and behavioral testing such as the Brazelton Neonatal Behavioral Assessment Scale in the evaluation of the neonate with spina bifida (Brazelton & Nugent, 1995). The purpose of this part of the assessment is to evaluate reflex activity such as sucking and swallowing and to determine the current status of the infant's organization of physiologic response to stress, state control, motor control, and social interaction (Schneider et al., 1995). The physical therapist notes the neonate's strengths as well as the problems the neonate is having. Repeated behavioral testing may help monitor progress in organization and reflect recovery. When performing a reflex or behavioral assessment, it is important to ascertain whether the neonate's performance is affected by CNS-depressant drugs.

Intermittent taping, positioning, ROM exercising, and splinting are techniques used by the physical therapist to treat joint deformities. Intermittent taping is more adaptable to the nursery setting and is reported to be more effective than ROM exercises to improve mobility (Sweeney & Swanson, 2001). A thorough knowledge of arthrokinematic principles and techniques is necessary to position the joint in a corrected position before taping. An external skin protection solution is applied under the tape, and an adhesive removal solution is used when the tape is removed. The therapist who performs taping must carefully observe skin condition and vascular tolerance when developing a taping schedule. Taping schedules begin with 1 hour and increase by 1 hour as tolerated.

PAIN

The neonate's ability to perceive pain has become a focus of both clinical and research attention (Pigeon et al., 1989). Previously, it was assumed that the neonate's nervous system functioned at a decorticate level, with insufficient myelinization of pain tracts and centers to perceive, feel, or remember pain (Franck, 1987; Shiao et al., 1987; Whaley & Wong, 1997). Increased knowledge of the capabilities of the newborn brain and advances in neonatal pharmacology have fostered a concern for the importance of protecting the neonate from stresses in the NICU environment. Evidence exists that pain pathways, cortical and subcortical centers of pain perception, and neurochemical systems associated with pain transmission are intact and functional in the prematurely born neonate. Slow conduction speed is the result of less myelinization, but it is balanced by shorter interneuronal distances traveled by painful nerve impulses and the fact that most nociceptive impulses are transmitted by non-myelinated C fibers (Anand & Hickey, 1987). However, the endorphin system, which mediates analgesia, may not be completely functional, leaving the preterm infant more sensitive to pain than term or older infants (Stevens & Franck, 1995). Infants may feel pain even more intensely than adults because of the immaturity of descending inhibition pathways in the spinal cord (Fitzgerald & Beggs, 2001; Anand, 1998; Franck, 1992). Early damage in infancy can lead to prolonged structural and functional alterations in pain pathways such as lower threshold and hypersensitivity that may persist into adult life (Fitzgerald & Beggs, 2001).

Although it is difficult to assess pain in the neonate, the physical therapist working in the special care nursery should be aware of the methods used to assess pain and be able to perform the nonpharmacologic procedures to alleviate pain. Both physiologic and behavioral responses of the neonate to nociceptive or painful stimuli have been identified. Physiologic manifestations of pain include increased heart rate, heart rate variability, blood pressure, and respirations, with evidence of decreased oxygenation. Skin color and character when pain is present include pallor or flushing, diaphoresis, and palmar sweating.

Other indicators of pain are increased muscle tone, dilated pupils, and laboratory evidence of metabolic or endocrine changes (Chiswick, 2000). Neonatal behavioral responses to nociceptive input include sustained and intense crying; facial expression of grimaces, furrowed brow, quivering chin, or eyes tightly closed; motor behavior such as limb withdrawal, thrashing, rigidity, flaccidity, fist clenching, finger splaying and limb extension; and changes in state (Granau et al., 2000; Pigeon et al., 1989). An infant may, however, be experiencing pain when lying quietly with closed eyes (Shapiro, 1989).

Several neonatal pain measures have been developed, including the Neonatal Facial Coding System (Gruneau et al., 1990; Gruneau & Craig, 1987); the Neonatal Infant Pain Scale (Barrier et al., 1989); the Modified Behavioral Pain Scale (Taddio et al., 1995); and the Premature Infant Pain Profile (Stevens & Franck, 1995).

Nonpharmacologic methods to alleviate pain include decreasing stimulation, swaddling, nonnutritive sucking, tactile comfort measures, rocking, containment, and music (Abad et al., 1996; Burke et al., 1995; Franck, 1987; Whaley & Wong, 1997). Preterm neonates showed a significantly lower mean heart rate, shorter crying time, and shorter mean sleep disruption after heel stick with facilitated tucking (containing the infant with hands softly holding the infant's extremities in soft flexion) than without (Corff et al., 1995). Morphine, fentanyl, and topical mixture of a local anesthetic cream (EMLA) are the most commonly used analgesics in the NICU (Stevens & Franck, 1995).

FAMILY RESPONSE TO PREMATURE BIRTH

Although medical interventions are critical to the survival of the premature infant, there is an increased awareness of the importance of recognizing the needs of families and providing supports. Taking on the parenting role is a major life task that is greatly complicated by the crisis of a critically ill newborn. Families react to this crisis in different and individual ways. Common emotions include anxiety, guilt, fear, resentment, feelings of inadequacy, and anger (Berns & Brown, 1998). In addition, the high-tech NICU environment is unfamiliar, frightening, and stressful for parents and can interfere with parent-infant interaction (Miles, 1989; Sheilds-Poe & Pinelli, 1997; Ward, 1999; Willis, 1991). Als (1992) proposed that the normal emotional preparation for parenting is interrupted by preterm birth. The desynchronization of emotional unpreparedness compounded by fear for the life of the infant often leads parents to experience feelings of helplessness, anger, grief, and sometimes prolonged depression. These experiences pose significant barriers to regaining confidence in oneself and daring to become invested in and committed to the infant. The costs to the other family members also must be considered. Als and colleagues (1992) suggest that goals for developmental care in the special care nursery include the following: (1) supporting parents as active partners; (2) helping parents learn how to observe their infant's stress and comfort signs; (3) assisting parents to develop competence in helping their infant to self-comfort, regulate, and organize behavior; and (4) reinforcing parents' feelings of their importance and effectiveness in caring for their infant. Parent education focusing on behavioral cues, handling, and positioning to improve parent handling and caregiving abilities is recommended as a goal of physical therapy (Unanue, 2002).

Although the NICU experience can pose a barrier to parent confidence, parents have rated themselves high in their abilities to perform caregiving activities and their understanding of information provided to them (Unanue, 2002; White et al., 2000). Parents should progress in the care of their infant at their own pace. Sources of formal support include staff, counseling, and parent group meetings. Coordination of care and parent education and support are essential at transfer and discharge time. Several studies report benefits of both hospital and home-based family-centered intervention after discharge (Cusson & Lee, 1993).

THEORETIC FRAMEWORK FOR NEONATAL PHYSICAL THERAPY

The theoretic basis for neonatal physical therapy may be conceptualized from general and specific frameworks. The model of the International Classification of Functioning, Disability, and Health (ICF) (World Health Organization, 2001) provides a standard language and framework for describing components of health and health-related states. High-risk neonates frequently demonstrate impairments in muscle tone, range of motion, sensory organization, and postural reactions. Limitations in activity may include problems in respiration, feeding, visual and auditory responsiveness, and motor abilities, such as head control and movement of hands to mouth. The interaction between impairments and activity limitations may contribute to restrictions in parent-infant interaction (participation). In the ICF model, the person and environment are contextual factors that influence body functions and structure, activity, and participation. Personal factors include an infant's health complications and temperament. Environmental factors include lighting and noise in special care nursery and family support. The examples provided potentially impact on all three components of health including heart rate, respiratory rate, oxygen saturation, feeding, and parent-infant interaction.

The purpose of the physical therapy examination and evaluation is to identify the presence of and risk for impairment, activity limitations and participation restrictions and contextual factors that may increase risk and determine appropriate interventions. Physical therapy intervention focuses on the needs of both the family and infant. Intervention includes handling, positioning, state transitions, and self-calming. In addition, as the infant approaches term age, developmental skills may be added to the intervention program. Another important focus of physical therapy intervention in the NICU is parent support and education. Parent education may include teaching parents about behavioral cues and how to identify their baby's cues, proper positioning and handling, and developmental activities to perform with their baby. Another role of the physical therapist is to determine the needs of the infants once discharged home. Infants may need to transition to community services such as an early intervention program or they may need to be followed through the NICU follow-up clinic on a consultation basis.

The American Physical Therapy Association, Section on Pediatrics has published guidelines for physical therapy practice in the NICU (Sweeney et al., 1999). These guidelines provide the physical therapist with a structure for clinical training, an algorithm for decision making, and clinical competencies based on roles, proficiencies, and knowledge areas. The NICU guidelines propose a theoretic framework based on the dynamic systems, the enablement and disablement model such as the ICF, preventive care, and family-centered care. The concepts within this framework optimize the functional posture and movement in infants to promote development. In the dynamic systems, all systems interact to produce a response (Thelan & Smith, 1994). When applying this concept to the NICU, the infant's biologic make-up, the sociocultural and physical environments, and the task interact to influence the function of the neonate.

Sweeney and Swanson (2001) have also described a theoretic framework specific to neonatal physical therapy that incorporates concepts of dynamic systems, neonatal behavioral organization, and crisis intervention. Neonatal behavioral organization concepts of this model are those proposed in the synactive model of behavioral organization (Als, 1986). This model describes how newborn infants interact with the environment through five behavioral systems: autonomic, motor, state, attentional, and self-regulatory. The five systems are in continuous interaction with one another (synactive). The synactive model is useful when trying to determine the risk-benefit ratio for intervention, including the tolerance of a neonate to developmental examination and procedural interventions. For example, a neonate who reacts to examination procedures with autonomic and visceral stress signals such as gagging, tremors, or irregular respirations is demonstrating physiologic instability. These reactions indicate a higher risk than benefit from this developmental assessment. The neonate who reacts to the same assessment with smooth respirations, pink color, well-regulated tone, and smooth movements is tolerating the procedure with a beneficial interaction of subsystems. Determination of the risk-benefit ratio and tolerance of the neonate to developmental assessment and intervention is an important part of the theoretic framework proposed by Sweeney and Swanson (2001).

Physical therapists who work in special care nurseries should base their intervention strategies on current knowledge of neonatal development and intervention (Fetters, 1986). Models that address characteristics of the infant and the environment, such as the ICF and synactive model, provide a theoretic framework for the development of guidelines for intervention in the NICU. These models also allow for generation of hypotheses that may be examined through clinical research.

The physical therapist experienced in neonatal care has much to offer as a member of a developmental team in coordination of care, sharing information and providing instruction to families, prevention of impairments, and sensorimotor development. It has been recommended that physical therapists working in the NICU complete continuing education in neonatal medicine, fetal development, assessment and development in early infancy, parental education, early intervention, and interdisciplinary interaction in the specialized setting of the special care nursery (Campbell, 1985; Sweeney et al., 1999; Sweeney & Swanson, 2001). Knowledge of current theories of motor control and early motor learning is also beneficial. Other recommendations include a supervised preceptorship in an NICU, which may include training in the use of neonatal assessments such as the Neonatal Individualized Developmental Care and Assessment Program (NIDCAP) (Als, 1984) and the Neonatal Behavioral Assessment Scale (NBAS)

(Brazelton, 1984). These assessments are discussed in the section on developmental physical therapy examination.

PULMONARY FUNCTION

Examination of pulmonary function in the infant requiring special care includes observation, inspection, and auscultation (Crane, 1995; Parker, 1985). Percussion is generally not appropriate for small infants (Crane, 1995). Observation and inspection include assessing signs of respiratory distress, chest configuration, skin color, breathing patterns, coughing, and sneezing. Signs of respiratory distress include retractions, nasal flaring, expiratory grunting, inspiratory stridor, use of accessory respiratory muscles (manifested by head bobbing), and bulging of intercostal muscles during expiration (Fig. 35-8) (Crane, 1995). Abnormal chest configurations include barrel-shaped chest and pectus excavatum. Cyanosis around the lips and mouth is a significant sign of hypoxemia (Crane, 1995).

Irregularity of respiration is normal in a neonate, and respiratory rates should be counted over a period of 60 seconds to account for this (Crane, 1995). The auscultation of an infant is an inexact procedure because of the thin chest wall, proximity of structures, and easy transmission of sounds (Fig. 35-9). This is also confounded by mechanical ventilation. During auscultation, the therapist is listening for normal, abnormal, and adventitious breath sounds. In infants, the specific location of the sound does not always correlate with the underlying lung segment. For this reason, auscultatory findings must be correlated with radiologic evidence. Palpation of the mediastinum and the trachea in the suprasternal notch is performed to ascertain if there is subcutaneous emphysema, edema, or rib fracture (Crane, 1995, 1987, 1986).

Positioning is indicated to enhance ventilation-perfusion ratios and to drain bronchopulmonary segments. Advantages of the prone position include improving oxygenation, lung compliance, state of alertness, and vital signs, whereas the primary advantage of the semierect position is to improve oxygenation (Crane, 1995; Martin et al., 1979; Wagoman et al., 1979). Positioning for postural drainage may need to be modified because of precautions and contraindications to certain positions in the neonate (Table 35-2). For example, the prone position is contraindicated by an untreated tension pneumothorax, and the head-down Trendelenburg position is contraindicated when there is an IVH of grades III and IV, acute congestive heart failure, or cor pulmonale (Crane, 1995).

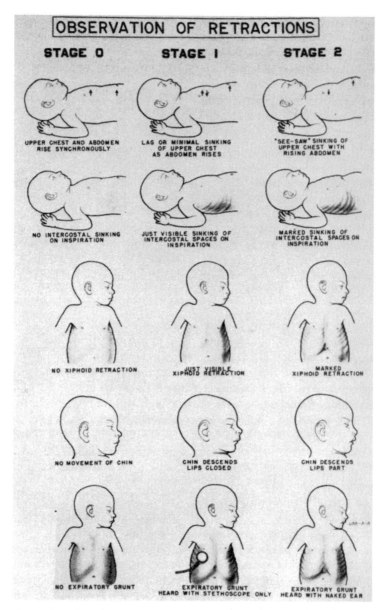

◆ **Figure 35-8** Observation and scoring of respiratory retractions. *(From Silverman, WA, & Andersen, DH. Controlled clinical trial of water mist on obstructive respiratory signs: Death rate among premature infants. Pediatrics, 17:1–10, 1956.)*

DEVELOPMENTAL EXAMINATION AND EVALUATION

The purposes of the developmental physical therapy examination and evaluation are to identify the following: (1) impairments in body function and structure that require intervention; (2) methods of positioning and handling; and (3) how to adapt the environment to optimize development. Based on examination findings, the physical therapist also evaluates the risk for activity limitations in development and parent-infant interaction. During examination procedures, the therapist must be aware of signs that the infant is undergoing stress, such as hypoxemia, excessive increase in heart rate, gagging, choking, and gasping. The therapist may need several brief sessions to fully assess the infant who is medically fragile (Sweeney, 1986). If the infant is too fragile for physical handling, observation of postures and spontaneous motor behavior may be useful.

Tests and measures appropriate for the premature infant include the Neurologic Assessment of the Preterm

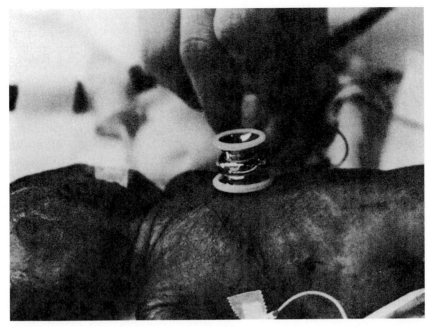

• **Figure 35-9**   Auscultation of infant's lungs with neonatal stethoscope. *(From Crane, L. Physical therapy for the neonate with respiratory disease. In Irwin, S, & Tecklin, JS [Eds.]. Cardiopulmonary Physical Therapy, 2nd ed. St. Louis: Mosby, 1990, p. 402.)*

TABLE 35-2	Precautions and Contraindications for Postural Drainage in a Neonate	
POSITION	**PRECAUTION**	**CONTRAINDICATION**
Prone	Umbilical arterial catheter Continuous positive airway pressure in nose Excessive abdominal distention Abdominal incision Anterior chest tube	Untreated tension pneumothorax
Trendelenburg position (head down)	Distended abdomen SEH/IVH* (grades I and II) Chronic congestive heart failure or cor pulmonale Persistent fetal circulation Cardiac dysrhythmias Apnea and bradycardia Infant exhibiting signs of acute respiratory distress Hydrocephalus Less than 28 weeks of gestational age	Untreated tension pneumothorax Recent tracheoesophageal fistula repair Recent eye or intracranial surgery Intraventricular hemorrhage (grades III and IV) Acute congestive heart failure or cor pulmonale

From Crane, L. Physical therapy for the neonate with respiratory disease. In Irwin, S, & Tecklin, JS (Eds.), Cardiopulmonary Physical Therapy, 2nd ed. St. Louis: Mosby, 1990, p. 406.
*Subependymal hemorrhage/intraventricular hemorrhage.

and Full-Term Newborn Infant (Dubowitz & Dubowitz, 1981a, 1981b), the Neonatal Individualized Developmental Care and Assessment Program (NIDCAP) (Als, 1984), and the Test of Infant Motor Performance (TIMP) (Campbell et al., 2001). Tests and measures designed for at-risk full-term infants include the Morgan Neonatal Neurobehavioral Examination (Morgan et al., 1988).

Observation of movement is an important component of the physical therapist's examination and is included in many of the standardized assessments. The assessment of spontaneous movement in infants can identify infants who require early intervention services. Prechtl and colleagues observed videotaped assessments of movement in both preterm and full-term infants in order to identify infants in need of early intervention services (Prechtl et al., 1997). The presence of fidgety movements was a good indicator of normal neurologic outcome; abnormal and absent fidgety movements were indicative of poor outcome (Prechtl et al., 1997). Kakebeeke and colleagues (1997) developed a 10-point scale to rate the fluency and spatiotemporal variability of arm and leg movements and sequencing of general movement patterns. Significant differences were found for these three movement quality parameters among term, low-risk preterm, and high-risk preterm infants.

NEUROLOGIC ASSESSMENT OF THE PRETERM AND FULL-TERM NEWBORN INFANT

The Neurologic Assessment of the Preterm and Full-Term Newborn Infant is a systematic, quickly administered, neurologic and neurobehavioral assessment developed by Dubowitz and Dubowitz (1981a, 1981b; Dubowitz, 1988). The test was developed to document changes in neonatal behavior in the preterm infant after birth, to compare preterm neonates with full-term neonates, to detect deviations in neurologic signs, and to document patterns of resolution in neurologic deficits (Sweeney, 1986). The test includes multiple neurobehavioral items of the Brazelton NBAS (Brazelton, 1984) using the six behavioral states. The neurobehavioral items include habituation to light and sound while sleeping, auditory and visual orientation responses, quality and duration of alertness, defensive reaction to cloth over face, peak of excitement, irritability, and consolability. The 15 neurologic items were taken from the Clinical Assessment of Gestational Age by Dubowitz and colleagues (1970), the Neurologic Examination of the Newborn (Prechtl & Beintema, 1964), and the neurologic examination of the full-term infant and the abnormal inventory protocol by Saint-Anne Dargassies (1977). The

Neurologic Assessment of the Preterm and Full-Term Newborn Infant was tested on more than 500 infants during a 2-year period. The test takes 15 minutes or less to administer. Scoring is done by looking at patterns of response rather than by determining a summary or total score.

In a prospective study of the predictive validity of the Neurologic Assessment of the Preterm and Full-Term Newborn Infant, Dubowitz and colleagues (1984) found that 91% of premature infants who were classified as normal at 40 weeks of gestation were normal according to detailed neurologic assessment and the Griffiths Mental Development Scale at 1 year. Sixty-five percent of infants classified as abnormal at 40 weeks of gestation, including those with cerebral palsy, dystonia, global delays, clumsiness, and hearing or visual deficit, were considered abnormal at 1 year.

Although reliability has not been determined, this examination has great potential for physical therapists who work in the NICU because of its brief administration time and systematic method of recording. Caution must be used when administering this assessment because it has been documented that medically stable preterm infants demonstrated an increase in heart rate during and after this examination (Sweeney, 1986).

NEONATAL INDIVIDUALIZED DEVELOPMENTAL CARE AND ASSESSMENT PROGRAM

The NIDCAP was developed to provide developmental observation and assessment training for neonatal health care professionals and includes Naturalistic Observation of Newborn Activity (Als, 1984). This involves systematic observation—without the observer manipulating or interacting—of the preterm or full-term infant in the nursery or at home during caregiving and handling. The NIDCAP is scored by observation and, therefore, is appropriate for infants who are unable to tolerate handling. A behavior observation checklist based on the concepts of the Assessment of Preterm Infant Behavior (APIB) (Als et al., 1982) includes environmental characteristics such as light, sound, and positioning apparatus. The self-regulatory ability of the infant is recorded, with some of the signs of stress being irregular respirations, color other than pink, tremors, startles and twitches, and visceral signs, including spitting up, gagging, hiccoughing, grunting, and gasping. Other signs of stress that can be recorded include flaccidity, frequent extensor movements of extremities, arching, tongue thrusts, finger splaying and fisting, fussing, yawning, and eye averting. Physiologic signs include heart rate below

120 or above 160 beats per minute, respiratory rate below 40 or above 60, and transcutaneous PO_2 below 55 mm Hg or above 80 mm Hg. Suggestions for caregiving modifications that may reduce stress for the infant are developed from the summary. The physical therapist can share this information with the NICU team and provide suggestions for modifying the environment and caregiving activities. These suggestions may pertain to lighting, noise level, activity level, bedding, aids to self-regulation, interaction, timing of manipulations, and facilitation of transitions from one activity to another. A list of training centers may be obtained from the National NIDCAP Center, 320 Longwood Ave., Boston, MA 02115.

TEST OF INFANT MOTOR PERFORMANCE

The TIMP is the first test designed specifically for use by physical and occupational therapists (see Chapter 1) to assess the functional motor performance of infants from 32 weeks' postconceptional age to 4 months post term (Campbell et al., 2001). The construct of the TIMP is postural alignment and selective control necessary for functional movements in early infancy. Items from the TIMP were adapted from neurologic and developmental tests by Brazelton (1984), Dubowitz and Dubowitz (1981b), and Amiel-Tison and Grenier (1986). The scoring scales and additional items were developed by Campbell and colleagues (1995). The TIMP requires approximately 25 to 45 minutes for administration and scoring (Campbell & Hedeker, 2001). Spontaneous and elicited movements are assessed with separate subscales. The Observed Scale consists of dichotomously scored behaviors that reflect the infant's spontaneous attempts to orient the body, to selectively move individual body segments, and to perform qualitative movements such as ballistic or oscillating movements (Campbell et al., 1995). Examples of observed behaviors include individual finger and ankle movements, reaching, and aligning the head in midline while supine. The Elicited Scale items are scored on a five-, six-, or seven-point hierarchic scale (Campbell, 1999a). Elicited behaviors reflect the infant's response to positioning and handling in a variety of spatial orientations and to visual and auditory stimuli. Examples include rolling prone with head righting when the leg is rotated across the body and turning the head to follow a visual stimulus or to search for a sound in prone.

The TIMP is a valid and reliable assessment for infants up to 4 months post term (Campbell, 1999a; Campbell et al., 1995; Campbell & Kolobe, 2000). Test-retest reliability is good across the age range of the TIMP (r = 0.89) (Campbell, 1999a). Construct validity of the TIMP has been established, specifically the ability of the TIMP to discriminate on the basis of both medical complications and maturation (Campbell et al., 1995; Campbell & Hedeker, 2001). Scores on the TIMP increase with increasing postconceptional age. Infants with medical complications have lower scores than healthy infants of the same age (Campbell et al., 1995). In addition, the TIMP can discriminate among infants at risk for motor delays (Campbell & Hedeker, 2001). A study has also been performed that looks at the relationship between environmental demands placed on infants during caregiving activities, including play, and the demands placed on the infant during the administration of the Elicited Scale items of the TIMP (Murney & Campbell, 1998). During caregiving activities, approximately 50% of the demands placed on the infants corresponded to items on the TIMP. In addition, 98% of the TIMP Elicited Scale items corresponded to observed environmental demands (Murney & Campbell, 1998). These findings suggest that TIMP items are representative of typical environmental demands, lending further support to the construct validity of the TIMP. In addition to construct validity, concurrent validity of the TIMP has also been examined (Campbell & Kolobe, 2000). The TIMP and Alberta Infant Motor Scales (AIMS) have similarities in their items. When scoring the same infants at 3 months of age, the TIMP and AIMS identify a similar group of infants with low motor performance. These findings support the concept of concurrent validity (Campbell & Kolobe, 2000).

The TIMP has also been examined for predictive validity (Campbell et al., 2002; Flegel & Kolobe, 2002). TIMP scores within the first 3 months predict AIMS scores at 6, 9, and 12 months. The greatest predictive validity is between the 3-month TIMP scores and the 12-month scores on the AIMS (Campbell et al., 2002). The TIMP can be used for early identification of very young infants at risk for poor motor performance (Barbosa et al., 2003; Campbell et al., 2002; Flegel & Kolobe, 2002). The TIMP scores identified delayed functional motor performance in children later diagnosed with cerebral palsy as early as 3 months of age (Barbosa et al., 2003).

The TIMP is currently being normed. Normative data is currently being collected on the TIMP. Although normative data are not available, data are available for typical performance on the TIMP for the different age ranges. Until norms are available, these scores can be used to identify infants who may benefit from early intervention (Campbell, 1999b). The TIMP is a useful tool with preterm and high-risk infants. Time may be a factor with infants who are not able to tolerate more than 15 to 20 minutes of handling. Making sure the infant is in the optimal state and administering each item only once can reduce the amount of time needed to perform the TIMP.

MORGAN NEONATAL NEUROBEHAVIORAL EXAMINATION

The Morgan Neonatal Neurobehavioral Examination (NNE) was designed to quantify the neurobehavioral abilities of infants between 37 and 40 weeks of conceptional age (Morgan et al., 1988). The authors stated that a quantitative rather than a qualitative assessment would be valuable in identification of infants at risk for developmental disabilities and would also provide a research tool for evaluating early intervention protocols. The test was constructed from items taken from the work of Brazelton (1984) and Dubowitz and Dubowitz (1981a). The 27 assessment items are organized into sections on tone and motor patterns, primitive reflexes, and behavioral responses. Interestingly, the response decrement items of the Brazelton scale were not included because the authors believed that high-risk infants must habituate themselves to noxious sounds and lights because they are continuously exposed to them in an NICU. A three-point scoring system is used for each item, with the highest total score being 81 and the lowest possible score being 27.

The NNE was standardized on 54 healthy full-term infants at 2 days of age and on 298 high-risk infants at 37 to 40 weeks of conceptional age (gestational age at birth plus chronologic age) or at discharge, whichever came first. Scores fell into three clusters for the high-risk infants, which correlated with conceptional age and not with severity of illness or gestational age at birth. These clusters represented performance at greater than 36 weeks, 32 to 36 weeks, and less than 32 weeks of gestational age. This suggests that the NNE reflects gestational maturation and quantitatively represents neurobehavioral status. Intertester reliability is reported as 88% agreement by item and 95% agreement by total score (Morgan et al., 1988). Lee and colleagues (1989) reported that the NNE can be used to predict motor outcome for high-risk infants born at or below 1500 g or between 37 and 42 weeks of gestation.

Although not widely used, the Morgan NNE provides the therapist useful information about the infant's motor response, reflexes, and behavior. The assessment does not require much time, an advantage for infants who do not tolerate handling well. Although the NNE can be used to predict motor outcome for high-risk infants born at or below 1500 g or between 37 and 42 weeks' gestation, scoring is based on the development of healthy full-term infants, not infants born at high risk or prematurely.

ORAL-MOTOR EXAMINATION

Oral-motor examination is another competency of the neonatal therapist. Two useful measures are the Neonatal Oral-Motor Assessment Scale (NOMAS) (Braun & Palmer, 1985/1986), which has been updated (Gaebler & Hanzlik, 1996), and the Nursing Child Assessment Feeding Scale (NCAFS) (Barnard & Eyres, 1979). The NOMAS measures components of nutritive and non-nutritive sucking. Variables assessed during sucking include rate, rhythmicity, jaw excursion, tongue configuration, and tongue movement. A pilot study determined cutoff scores for oral-motor disorganization and dysfunction. The NCAFS assesses parent-infant feeding interaction and evaluates responsiveness of parents to their infant's cues, signs of distress, and social interaction during feeding.

There are also instruments to study the pressure generated by each suck and the length of sucking bursts such as the Kron Nutritive Sucking Apparatus (Medoff-Cooper & Gennaro, 1996) and the Actifier (Finan & Barlow, 1996), which can also be used as a method for stimulation of intraoral tissue in neonates.

HIGH-RISK PROFILES

Examination and evaluation may lead to identification of the infant as having one of three basic high-risk profiles described by Sweeney and Swanson (2001). Although not all neonates fit the behaviors described in the high-risk profiles, the profiles address the need for individualized levels of stimulation and approaches to the management of infants with abnormal tone and movement (Sweeney & Swanson, 2001). The profiles represent the extremes in sensorimotor and interactional behavior. The profiles identify impairments in muscle tone, behavioral characteristics, and interactional styles associated with motor status, and therefore, have implications for the development of individualized goals, outcomes, and intervention strategies.

The infant who is irritable and hypertonic is often in a state of overstimulation, with poor self-quieting abilities. These infants have a low tolerance for handling and position changes. Extensor patterns of posture and movement predominate, with limited antigravity flexion. Movement is disorganized and tremulous, with poor midline orientation. Feeding is difficult as a result of increased tone in the oral musculature. Visual tracking is also difficult.

The infant who is hypotonic and lethargic is often difficult to arouse even at feeding time. Crying is weak and of short duration. Hypotonicity is noted in the trunk, intercostal, and neck accessory musculature, with decreased respiratory capacity. An infant who fits this profile demonstrates paucity of movement, weak and uncoordinated sucking, and poor interactive capability.

Infants who are hypotonic and lethargic mold themselves to the arm's of the person holding them and use contact with the surface for stabilization.

The infant who is disorganized demonstrates fluctuating tone and movement and is easily overstimulated. An infant who fits this profile remains passive when left alone but responds well to swaddling. When calm, the infant interacts and feeds well; but when distracted and overstimulated, the infant becomes hypertonic and irritable.

DEVELOPMENTAL INTERVENTIONS

Neonatal physical therapy is a subspecialty of pediatric physical therapy that emerged in the mid-1970s (Sweeney & Chandler, 1990). As specialists in the NICU, it is important to know the evidence guiding and supporting our practice. Several studies have shown support for developmental intervention in the NICU. Scarr-Salapatek and Williams (1973) reported greater developmental progress at 4 weeks and 12 months in infants who received developmental intervention that included visual, tactile, and kinesthetic stimulation in the nursery. Leib and associates (1980) reported that an intervention program consisting of visual, tactile, kinesthetic, and auditory stimulation enhanced the quality of development for high-risk preterm infants. In addition, Field and co-workers (1986) demonstrated that preterm infants benefited from a program of tactile and kinesthetic stimulation in the NICU. Parker and colleagues (1992) reported the positive benefits of a developmental intervention program in the NICU for infants of mothers of low socioeconomic status. Als and co-workers (1994) have also demonstrated the positive effects of individualized developmentally supportive care. Although physical therapists were not involved in these studies, the interventions are those typically performed during physical therapy intervention in the NICU.

Although there is evidence to support developmental interventions for preterm infants in the NICU, stimulation in the form of tactile, kinesthetic, visual, and auditory stimulation has the potential to be harmful. Physical therapists, therefore, must carefully monitor infants during intervention. Monitoring includes oxygen saturation, heart rate, respiratory rate, and identification of behavioral signs indicating stress. Careful monitoring of infants during intervention is essential to avoid potentially adverse physiologic effects.

The goals of physical therapy for neonates may include reduction or prevention of impairments in muscle tone, ROM, postural adaptation, and control of extremity movements. Outcomes include improved regulation and organization of motor behavior, interactions with caregivers and the environment, and family interaction (Campbell, 1985; Sweeney & Swanson, 1990). Parents, primary nurses, and other caregivers should be involved in the development of goals and outcomes and coordination of the care plan. Strategies for both direct intervention and consultation include modification of the environment, positioning, promotion of efficient movement, and modulation of sensory input (e.g., oral-motor stimulation, hydrotherapy, and the use of water mattresses). Parent education and support regarding the development and input appropriate for neonates is an important aspect of intervention (Gottwald & Thurman, 1990).

The design for a care plan should be individualized based on infant and caregiver needs. Factors to consider include the infant's postconceptional age, physiologic abilities, and behavioral abilities. These individualized care plans should include the provision of social interaction stimuli during alert periods, avoidance of handling during quiet sleep periods, and immediate termination or alteration of stimulation producing avoidance responses (Campbell, 1985). Avoidance responses include vomiting, sneezing, coughing, hiccoughing, gagging, sighing, respiratory changes, and changes in tone (Als, 1986). While the neonate is in the NICU, the environment should be modified to avoid overstimulation by excessive light, noise, or physical handling (Avery & Glass, 1989; Field, 1990). Caregivers should provide tactile and kinesthetic stimuli that are contingent on the neonate's responses to alleviate stress, if possible, or to help the infant prepare for, or adapt to, stress-producing stimuli.

POSITIONING

Positioning has already been mentioned in relation to improving oxygenation. Positioning is also important to promote state organization, stimulate the flexed midline positions typical of the full-term infant, and maintain ROM (Sweeney & Swanson, 2001). The premature infant does not have the opportunity to develop physiologic flexion and may demonstrate hypotonia (Fig. 35-10). The preterm infant must also contend with ventilatory and infusion equipment, which often exaggerates extension of the neck, trunk, and extremities. Hypotonic extended limbs may also be fixed to padded boards to protect intravenous lines (Fetters, 1986). Prolonged hyperextension may lead to neck extensor muscle contracture (Sweeney & Swanson, 2001) (Fig. 35-11).

The prone position, with the head in midline and elevation of the head at 30°, has the beneficial effects of

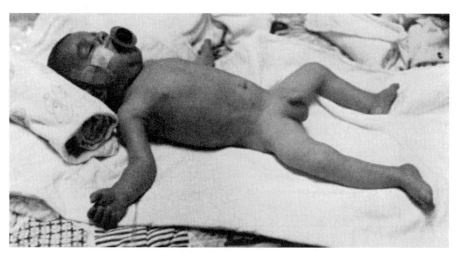

◆ **Figure 35-10** Characteristic hypotonic posture with minimal movement against gravity in a premature infant at 4 months of age. *(From Sweeney, JK, & Swanson, MW. At-risk neonates and infants: NICU management and follow-ups. In Umphred, DA [Ed.]. Neurological Rehabilitation, 2nd ed. St. Louis: Mosby, 1990, p. 218.)*

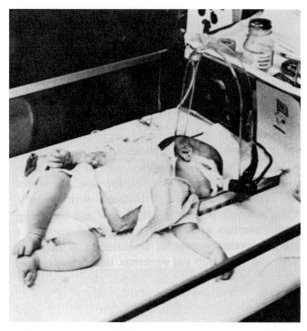

◆ **Figure 35-11** Neck hyperextension posture exaggerated by position of the endotracheal tube. *(From Sweeney, JK, & Swanson, MW. At-risk neonates and infants: NICU management and follow-ups. In Umphred, DA [Ed.]. Neurological Rehabilitation, 2nd ed. St. Louis: Mosby, 1990, p. 201.)*

decreasing intracranial pressure, gastroesophageal reflux, and aspiration and increasing stomach emptying (Semmler, 1989; Wolfson et al., 1992). Many different methods are used for placing the infant in prone and side-lying positions, including blanket or diaper rolls, sandbags, customized foam inserts, buntings, and nests (Creger & Browne, 1995; Semmler, 1989; Sweeney & Swanson, 2001) (Figs. 35-12 through 35-14). The desired posture includes neck flexion or chin tucking, trunk flexion, shoulder protraction, posterior pelvic tilt, and symmetric flexion of legs. When supine positioning is used, the head is positioned in midline and blanket rolls may be placed along the infant's sides and under the shoulder girdle for support, as well as under the knees. Supported semierect positions while the infant is swaddled may also be beneficial to elicit the alert state, head righting, and visual and auditory tracking.

Hammocks and water mattresses are also used in conjunction with positioning. Supine positioning in a hammock has been shown to be associated with a higher neuromuscular maturity score on the Assessment of Maturity Scale (Ballard, 1979) and a more relaxed state as shown by lower heart rate and respiratory rate (Keller et al., 2003). Water mattresses are soft, and the surface intermittently oscillates, providing gentle vestibular and proprioceptive stimulation. Water mattresses have proved effective in decreasing apnea, reducing position-induced head flattening, and improving skin conditions (Deiriggi, 1990; Piecuch, 1988; Sweeney & Swanson, 2001; Taylor & Dalbec, 1989). Positions should be changed throughout the day, especially for infants with respiratory problems involving increased secretions (Crane, 1987).

SENSORIMOTOR STIMULATION

Physical therapy intervention includes appropriate interaction with the neonate, which involves sensory

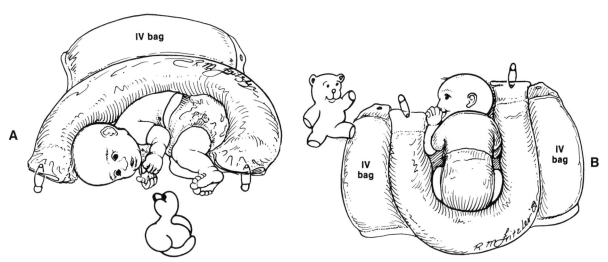

⬥ **Figure 35-12**   Positioning in flexion using a long blanket roll reinforced by a sand or intravenous bag. *(From Sweeney, JK, & Swanson, MW. At-risk neonates and infants: NICU management and follow-ups. In Umphred, DA [Ed.]. Neurological Rehabilitation, 2nd ed. St. Louis: Mosby, 1990, p. 201.)*

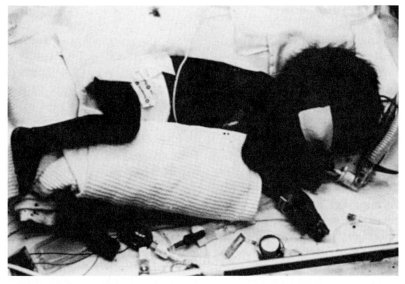

⬥ **Figure 35-13**   Side-lying positioning to reduce extension posturing. *(From Sweeney, JK, & Swanson, MW. At-risk neonates and infants: NICU management and follow-ups. In Umphred, DA [Ed.]. Neurological Rehabilitation, 2nd ed. St. Louis: Mosby, 1990, p. 200.)*

input. Psychologists and nurses have studied the effect of supplemental stimulation on weight gain, visual responsiveness, growth, development, and sensorimotor functions (Fetters, 1986; Field, 1980; Heriza, 1989; Mueller, 1996). Most of these studies have involved the relatively healthy premature infant weighing more than 1000 g at birth. Little research has been published on the effects of supplemental stimulation of the sicker, VLBW, or asphyxiated newborn (Campbell, 1985). The majority of supplemental stimulation studies used predetermined,

packaged, nonindividualized treatments (Harris et al., 1988). In a few studies, sensory stimulation interventions have been individualized and based on behavioral cues from the infant (Heriza, 1989; Als, 1986; Fetters, 1986). Mueller (1996) has published an integrated review of research on multimodal stimulation of premature infants. Interestingly, she included developmental care as one type of multimodal stimulation. In this context, sensorimotor stimulation would include any sensory input, such as the visual input of the therapist's face,

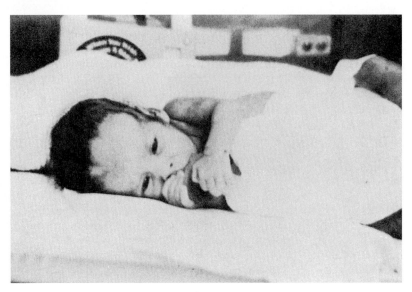

• **Figure 35-14**   Use of anterior roll and pacifier promotes flexed position. *(From Sweeney, JK, & Swanson, MW. At-risk neonates and infants: NICU management and follow-ups. In Umphred, DA [Ed.]. Neurological Rehabilitation, 2nd ed. St. Louis: Mosby, 1990, p. 200.)*

tactile input, physical handling, positioning, offering visual or auditory stimuli, and social interaction.

The purposes of providing contingent sensorimotor stimulation to infants in the NICU include improving behavioral organization, promoting integration of the sensory systems, enhancing development of motor and interactive abilities, and supporting parent-infant attachment. Sensory input must be provided in a graded manner that is contingent on the infant's behavioral cues. Gradual introduction of unimodal sensory stimulation may be necessary at first to allow the infant to maintain physiologic and state control. Once the infant is able to maintain state control, multimodal stimuli may be used.

Techniques to aid the infant's state organization, self-consolation, and orienting include encasement (gentle tactile contact with infant's head or soles of feet in a gently flexed position), swaddling, and firm tactile input to the soles of the feet. Constant vigilance must be practiced to weigh the costs and benefits of any intervention. The therapist must be constantly aware of changes in heart rate, blood pressure, and oxygen levels, as well as state control or organization changes during and after intervention.

Using the high-risk infant assessment profiles of Sweeney and Swanson (2001) as a point of reference, it is obvious that strategies of intervention should be individualized. The infant who is lethargic and hypotonic needs stimulation to reach the alert state and facilitation of proximal neck and trunk musculature, whereas the infant who is irritable and hypertonic needs calming to the alert state and inhibition of increased tone.

Als (1986) found that infants who were dependent on a respirator and at high risk for BPD improved self-regulation capabilities after a series of procedures were implemented. These procedures included inhibition through firm tactile input to the soles of the feet, encasement of the infant's trunk and back of the head in the caregiver's hand, the tactile input of a finger to squeeze or suck, and nonnutritive sucking of a finger or a "suckel" (something for the infant to suck on). By contrast, sensory inputs such as rocking, stroking, and talking were not well tolerated by infants.

Methods of calming an infant who is irritable and hypertonic include swaddling, that is, wrapping the infant in a blanket or using a bunting. If swaddling is done with flexed, midline extremity positioning, there may be facilitation of flexor tone, increased hand-to-mouth awareness, and decreased jittery and disorganized movements. Vestibular stimulation in a horizontal position with the infant swaddled has a calming effect.

Procedures used to promote an alert state include positioning in supported sitting, swaddling, and using a bunting or tactile containment. In the infant who is more robust, carefully graded, arrhythmic vestibular input, such as quick rocking in the upright position, and light touch may be used for state arousal. Once the alert state is reached and maintained, sensory input such as visual or auditory stimuli may be added one at a time and modified as indicated by the infant's response.

Visual stimuli include the therapist's face, a black-and-white bull's-eye target, and a red ball. Auditory stimuli include classical instrumental music, calling the infant's name, and a soft rattle (Burke et al., 1995; Collins & Kuck, 1991). Once the infant can maintain an alert state and can fixate on an object, visual tracking may be attempted.

Early movement experiences such as hand-to-mouth contact, shoulder protraction and retraction, pelvic tilt, movement of extremities against gravity, and holding of the head in midline may also be facilitated (Campbell, 1985). Hand-to-hand, hand-to-knee, and hand-to-foot activities are encouraged to provide tactile stimulation and flexion input.

ORAL-MOTOR THERAPY

The infant in the special care nursery often exhibits feeding difficulties related to neurologic immaturity, abnormal muscle tone, depressed oral reflexes, or prolonged use of endotracheal tubes for mechanical ventilation (Sweeney & Swanson, 2001). Decreased tongue mobility, tongue thrusting, poor seal on nipple due to weak lip closure, weak sucking, or hypersensitivity of the oral area may also have a negative impact on feeding (Semmler, 1989).

Nonnutritive sucking should be encouraged early with the immediate aim of self-consolation and the long-term goal of normal oral-motor development (Gaebler & Hanzlik, 1996; Pickler et al., 1996). Achieving a quiet alert state and positioning the infant in supported sitting with semiflexion of the neck may also enhance feeding behavior. Methods of tactile stimulation of facial muscles and intraoral structure and external support to the infants' cheeks have been described and have resulted in weight gain and decreased hospital stay for infants in level II special care (Anderson, 1986; Gaebler & Hanzlik, 1996; Harris, 1986; Sweeney & Swanson, 2001). Waber and colleagues (1998) reported that once infants were able to breastfeed or bottle feed, they fed on demand rather than on a schedule, showed more feeding cues, and had a shorter hospital stay.

FAMILY-CENTERED CARE

Family-centered care is a concept of service delivery to infants and their families (Rosenbaum et al., 1998). Using a family-centered approach to care recognizes the family as a constant in the infant's life and recognizes the individual strengths and needs of each family. The concept of family-centered care involves the parents in the decision-making process and promotes collaboration

between the physical therapist and parents (Dunst et al., 1991; Harrison, 1993; Johnson, 1990; Rosenbaum et al., 1998; Shelton & Stepaneck, 1995). In the NICU, the health care team includes the parents as active members. Each family has unique strengths and needs that the physical therapist must recognize and integrate into the interventions in order to provide the family as well as the infant with the necessary services. Using a family-centered approach to intervention, physical therapists should provide parents with information both specific to their infant and general information about development. Parents who are provided information using a family-centered approach display improvements in their care-giving abilities compared to parents who only receive general information on development (Unanue, 2002).

DEVELOPMENTAL FOLLOW-UP AFTER DISCHARGE FROM THE SPECIAL CARE NURSERY

Infants who are discharged home from the NICU or special care nursery often need early intervention services. As part of the Individuals with Disabilities Education Improvement Act of 2004 (Public Law 108-446), infants and toddlers under the age of 3 are provided services under Part C. Part C provides developmental services to meet the needs of the infant; however, developmental follow-up of infants after discharge varies from state to state and with the particular problems or risk factors of each infant. Primary care is usually provided by a pediatrician in private practice, through a hospital, or through a community-based clinic. An interdisciplinary program such as an early intervention program also provides assessment, monitoring, and direct intervention, as well as a support group for parents (Hack, 1992; Leonard, 1988). As part of early intervention services under Part C, each infant must have a comprehensive individualized family service plan (IFSP) which is developed by the team. In keeping with family-centered care, the parent is an active member of the team developing the IFSP. Because many early intervention programs have waiting lists for physical therapy and occupational therapy, services initially may be provided by the community visiting nurse association or other home care agencies.

Physical therapists working with families and infants in the NICU have a role in the transition of infants and families to early intervention services. The physical therapist needs to communicate with the therapist or agency providing services to that infant and family. Although the ideal situation would be for the early intervention team to meet with the family and therapists providing services in the NICU, this is not realistic for providers who live a distance from the NICU. In this case, the physical therapist must provide the community therapist with as much information as possible regarding current interventions. In some areas, physical therapists working in home care agencies are not pediatric therapists and require information and guidance from the hospital-based staff.

Level III nurseries typically have a developmental follow-up clinic for high-risk infants. Clinics vary in staffing and their criteria for follow-up care. Factors such as birth weight, gestational age, Apgar scores, time on a ventilator, IVH, seizures, and environmental factors such as maternal drug or alcohol use are useful criteria. Results of developmental assessments administered at the follow-up clinic are useful in determining whether specialized therapy services are necessary beyond the provision of general recommendations for development and parent education. Specialized referral for nutrition, audiology, and ophthalmology also is made when necessary.

The physical therapist has a role in the follow-up care of infants as a member of an early intervention program, a visiting nurse association, or a follow-up clinic. As a team member, the therapist plays an important role in the examination and monitoring of sensorimotor development and pulmonary function in order to prevent or decrease the risk of impairment or functional limitation and provide parent education and anticipatory guidance (Platzker et al., 1988; Resnick et al., 1987; Rothberg, 1991; Thom, 1988). Interventions such as positioning, sensory stimulation, and facilitation of movement are also provided when necessary. The physical therapist also assists families in coordination of care and initiates referrals to other professionals and community agencies when appropriate.

The following two hypothetical case histories serve as examples of the neonates seen in the special care nursery and illustrate their physical therapy examination, evaluation, and intervention. Several other excellent case histories have been published (Campbell, 1999b; Sweeney & Swanson, 2001).

▌SUMMARY

The special care nursery is a specialized setting for providing high technologic medical interventions to newborn infants who are unable to sustain basic physiologic processes secondary to premature birth or other neonatal complications. Provision of services to infants and families in the special care nursery is a subspecialty area of pediatric physical therapist practice. Knowledge of fetal and infant development, medical complications, and competency in monitoring vital signs and behaviors are essential for providing therapy services in the special care nursery. The examination and evaluation process includes issues identified by families and members of the team and observation of how the infant is positioned and responds to caregiving procedures. Standardized tests and measures are useful in evaluation of infant development and identification of areas of need. Depending on an infant's needs and ability to tolerate sensory stimulation and movement, interventions may include positioning, strategies to minimize physiologic stress, and sensorimotor development. Prevention of musculoskeletal impairments is an important outcome of intervention. Communication and coordination of care with team members, families, and external agencies such as early intervention providers are important components of intervention. Perhaps, the most important role of the physical therapist is education and instruction of family members in the infant's behavioral cues and responses and handling and caring for the infant in anticipation of transition to home.

After discharge, an important role of the physical therapist in high-risk follow-up clinics is to monitor infant motor development, address family information needs and concerns, and coordinate care with community service providers.

CASE STUDIES

TOMMY

Tommy was born at 24 weeks' gestational age and had a birth weight of 525 g (1.16 lb). His mother is 25 years old. Her pregnancy was complicated by severe preeclampsia and excessive weight gain during the last month of pregnancy. Tommy was blue and limp at birth with Apgar scores of 2 at 1 minute and 4 at 5 minutes. He received bag/mask ventilation and was intubated in the delivery room. Tommy was mechanically ventilated for 9 weeks. He required multiple attempts to wean him from the ventilator. Tommy remained on supplemental oxygen via nasal cannula after his extubation. Tommy's hospital course was complicated by severe BPD, a grade II IVH revealed by head ultrasound on day of life 7, a patent ductus arteriosus treated with indomethacin, and hyperbilirubinemia.

Tommy was referred to physical therapy at 6 weeks of life (30 weeks' postconceptional age). Practice Pattern 5C: Impaired Motor Function and Sensory Integrity Associated with Nonprogressive Disorders of the Central Nervous System — Congenital Origin or Acquired in Infancy or Childhood (American Physical Therapy Association, 2001) was used to guide the physical therapy examination, evaluation, and intervention. The physical therapist reviewed Tommy's history through a chart review and spoke with his primary nurse. His nurse reported that Tommy was irritable and felt very stiff when moving his extremities. The physical therapist observed Tommy during routine nursing care using the Neonatal Individualized Developmental Care and Assessment Program (Als, 1984). He demonstrated a low tolerance to handling and position changes and was frequently overstimulated. Tommy's stress signs included irregular respirations, increased heart rate, startling, grunting, and straightening extremities with tension. He displayed few approach and calming behaviors. Tommy was difficult to calm, but would eventually calm with a pacifier and swaddling. During the observation, Tommy was not able to transition to or maintain an awake alert state. With handling, he frequently was asleep or in a cry state, but did not transition to an alert state even for a brief period of time.

During the physical therapy examination, the physical therapist noted poor midline orientation, limited anti-gravity movement, and increased tone in his extremities. Tommy displayed postures and movements that were predominantly into extension, tremulous, and disorganized. His upper extremities were frequently in a position of scapular retraction with shoulder abduction and external rotation with elbow flexion. He displayed a head preference to the right with tightness noted in left neck rotation. Tommy demonstrated impaired visual tracking. When presented with a visual stimulus, Tommy displayed an increase in stress signs. He was not able to maintain an alert state. With any type of handling, Tommy quickly transitioned to a cry state. He required frequent breaks and consoling by the therapist during the examination. Calming Tommy was difficult, but he would eventually calm with containment and his pacifier.

As part of the test and measures in the ongoing physical therapy examination, the physical therapist performed the Test of Infant Motor Performance (TIMP) when Tommy reached 34 weeks' postconceptional age (PCA) and had been extubated for 1 week. The TIMP was chosen because (1) the test is appropriate for use from 32 weeks' PCA until 4 months post term; (2) it is a valid and reliable test; (3) the TIMP discriminates infants with various risks for delays; and (4) the TIMP can identify very young infants at risk for poor motor performance. Tommy scored a 40. Based on the suggested ranges for performance on the TIMP, Tommy scored below average for an infant at 34 weeks' PCA (Campbell, 1999b). Tommy's performance on the TIMP showed poor visual tracking, poor response to an auditory stimuli, poor head control, trunk hyperextension, and asymmetries between the right and left side when rolling was facilitated from both the arms and legs. Tommy only transitioned to brief alert states during the testing and required frequent rest breaks to calm.

Tommy's mother does not visit the NICU very often. She lives 3 hours away and relies on others for transportation to the hospital. She is not able to stay close to the hospital because she has two other children and Tommy's father is not involved. She went back to work shortly after Tommy's birth in order to be off when he is discharged home. She is afraid of losing her job if she takes time off because the health insurance for Tommy and his siblings is through her employer. His mother tries to come on weekends when other family members are able to watch her other children and she can get a ride to the hospital. She feels very torn between being at the hospital and working and being home for her other children. She is very interested in learning about Tommy and how she can best care for him. Because Tommy's mother was not present during the physical therapy examination, the physical therapist called his mother to discuss the purpose of physical therapy intervention and to determine what her goals and needs were. The physical therapist also arranged to meet with Tommy's mother on the weekend when she is at the hospital. The physical therapist leaves weekly notes at bedside for Tommy's mother, including activities she can do while visiting.

Using a family-centered approach, the physical therapist developed a plan of care for Tommy that included handling tolerance, positioning, state transitions, gentle neck ROM, and parent education. When developing the plan, the physical therapist took into account Tommy's mother's goals and needs that were discussed over the phone. Physical therapy was provided three to five times a week to Tommy's tolerance for the duration of his hospital stay. Goals for Tommy included the following: (1) maintenance of an alert state during physical therapy intervention with increasing duration throughout his stay; (2) visual fixing and tracking to both the left and right; (3) auditory tracking; (4) increasing antigravity movements into flexion; (5) ability to self-calm; (6) increasing head control in prone, supine, and supported sitting; (7) midline orientation; (8) decreasing tightness in his neck; and (7) mother's independence in reading Tommy's behavioral cues and understanding appropriate developmental activities.

Physical therapy intervention included positioning to increase flexion in Tommy's extremities and to provide midline orientation. This was achieved through swaddling or using rolls under Tommy's legs and alongside his arms and head. Interventions to increase handling tolerance and state transitions included swaddling, containment, and gentle rocking or patting. Once Tommy was able to maintain an alert state for brief periods, unimodal stimulation such as an adult's face or voice was initiated to engage visual and auditory tracking. The therapist also performed gentle ROM to Tommy's neck to decrease the tightness on his left side as a result of his right-sided head preference. Self-calming was also a focus of intervention. This was achieved through facilitated hands to midline and hands to mouth. As Tommy tolerance for handling and position changes improved, the therapist also began to work on developmental activities such as increasing head control in prone, supine, and supported sitting. The physical therapist constantly monitored Tommy's physiologic and state responses to her interaction with him.

The physical therapist communicated on a daily basis with Tommy's nurse. She also posted signs at Tommy's bedside for his mother, as well as for the nurses in the evenings. On a weekly basis, the physical therapist updated his progress and added to the activities Tommy's mother could do while she was visiting. The physical therapist met with his mother on several Saturdays when she was able to get a ride to the hospital for the weekend. Tommy's mother was concerned with her abilities to identify when Tommy was overstimulated, how to calm him, and how to position him in bed correctly. The therapist was able to teach Tommy's mother how to identify Tommy's behavioral cues, help Tommy to calm himself, and properly position Tommy to provide flexion and midline orientation. The therapist also instructed mom in developmental activities that she could do with Tommy while she visited. The physical therapist recommended several books for Tommy's mother to read, including the book by Klein and Ganon (1998). The information provided to Tommy's mother was modified at each meeting to accommodate for her needs and goals as she became more comfortable with reading behavioral cues, calming, and positioning.

Tommy was ready for discharge from the hospital at 40 weeks' PCA. At this time, Tommy was reassessed using the TIMP. His TIMP score was 61. Based on the suggested ranges for performance on the TIMP, Tommy again scored below average for an infant at 40 weeks' PCA, although overall he had shown improvements in his score (Campbell, 1999b). At discharge, Tommy had achieved many of his goals. He was visually tracking left and right approximately 30°. He would turn his head right and left in response to auditory stimuli. Tommy moved his extremities in small ranges against gravity. His movements continued to be jerky. Tommy was able to bring his hands to midline and to mouth. He no longer had a head preference to the right and did not have tightness in his neck ROM. He was easily consoled with rocking, gentle patting, hands to mouth, and sucking on a pacifier. Tommy was able to consistently clear his face in prone and was beginning to make attempts at head control while in supported sitting. Tommy's mother was able to read his behavioral signs and respond appropriately to them. She felt comfortable taking him home. As part of the discharge plan, the physical therapist referred Tommy to a local home health agency and an early intervention program close to his house. The physical therapist contacted the social worker within the NICU to arrange for the physical therapy services that Tommy would need at home. Tommy was also to return to the NICU follow-up clinic, which included physical, occupational, and speech therapy.

SUSAN

Susan was born at full term and her birth weight was 3300 g (7.26 lb). Her mother is 32 years old; her pregnancy was uncomplicated. Susan was born with the cord wrapped around her neck and was blue and limp. Her Apgar scores were 2 at 1 minute and 6 at 5 minutes. She received bag/mask ventilation, but did not require intubation in the delivery room. Shortly after her transfer to the NICU, Susan began having seizures with associated decreases in respiratory rate requiring bagging. On neurologic examination, Susan had absent suck and gag reflexes and was slow to respond to stimuli.

Susan was referred for a physical therapy examination on day 2 of life. The physical therapist used Practice Pattern 5C: Impaired Motor Function and Sensory Integrity Associated with Nonprogressive Disorders of the Central Nervous System — Congenital Origin or Acquired in Infancy or Childhood (American Physical Therapy Association, 2001) to guide her examination, evaluation, and intervention. The physical therapist reviewed Susan's medical history during the chart review and spoke to nursing about any concerns noted during routine caregiving activities. The physical therapist observed Susan before, during, and after a routine nursing activity using the Neonatal Individualized Developmental Care and Assessment Program (NIDCAP) (Als, 1984). Susan demonstrated poor handling tolerance with an increase in stress signs. Stress signs included a decrease in respiratory rate, startles, arching, and cry. Susan also demonstrated an inability to maintain an awake state and poor state transitions. She quickly transitioned from being lethargic to a hyperalert state to cry without any intervening quiet alert states. In addition, Susan was not able to calm herself by using self-regulatory behaviors such as hand to mouth, hands to midline, and sucking.

A family-focused approach to physical therapy was used in the NICU. This approach incorporates the family's goals and needs into the care plan. As part of this, the physical therapist spoke with Susan's parents, explaining the role of the physical therapist in Susan's care. Both parents appeared very interested in Susan, although they did voice concerns about her poor handling tolerance and sudden changes from being asleep to crying. Both parents were interested in activities they could do with Susan and appropriate methods to calm her down.

As part of the examination process, the physical therapist performed the Morgan Neonatal Neurobehavioral Examination (NNE) (Morgan et al., 1988). The NNE was chosen because (1) it has been standardized on full-term and high-risk infants; (2) it is quick and easy to administer; and (3) the items include muscle tone and motor patterns, reflexes, and behavioral responses. Susan demonstrated low tone, poor head and trunk control, weak suck, and delayed or absent reflexes. Susan received a total score of 60 on the test. This indicates that she was performing below that of typical full-term infants.

In addition to administering the NNE, the therapist observed Susan's postures, movements, state control, and interactive behaviors. Susan's strengths included brief response to voice and calming with tight swaddling and rocking. Susan did not have any limitations in ROM in her arms or legs. When Susan did move her arms and legs, she was able to move them in very global patterns through her available range. When supine, Susan postured with her lower extremities in a frog-leg position and her upper extremities abducted and externally rotated. Susan was either lethargic with eyes closed or crying during the examination and was very difficult to console. The therapist also noted that Susan was unable to bring her hands to midline or to mouth. She displayed minimal movements of the arms and legs. Movements were jerky and into extension. Susan did not focus on or track objects left or right.

The physical therapist developed a plan of care for Susan that included positioning, handling tolerance, and sensory stimulation. Physical therapy was provided three to five times a week to Susan's tolerance or up to 30 minutes. This episode of care was for the duration of Susan's stay in the hospital. As part of the care plan, positioning was done to encourage midline and symmetry, to bring her shoulders forward (prevent abduction and external rotation), and to promote hip flexion with neutral rotation. Pictures of side-lying, supine, and prone positions were posted at bedside for both nursing and the family.

Handling tolerance was increased using swaddling with gentle sensory stimulation such as rocking. As handling tolerance increased, Susan transitioned to a cry state less often. With this decrease in crying, the therapist worked on state transitions to an awake, alert state. Along with the development of handling tolerance, the therapist worked on self-calming behaviors such as hands to midline and hands to mouth. Slowly, visual stimulation was brought into the plan to work on fixing and following.

The physical therapist wrote specific outcomes to guide her physical therapy intervention with Susan. These goals focused on the limitations that were noted during Susan's evaluation. The goals included the following: (1) transitions to a quiet alert state and maintenance of this state for increasing periods of time; (2) ability to briefly self-calm using hands to mouth, holding onto clothes, or sucking on hand or pacifier; (3) visual fixing on an object for a brief time with increasing duration over time; (4) developmental activities such as lifting head to clear face in prone or briefly (1 to 2 seconds) holding head vertical in midline in supported sitting; and (5) parents independent in caring for her physical needs at home. Although the therapist wrote five outcomes for Susan, they were not all addressed within each session.

Weekly updates were posted at the bedside for both parents with activities to improve response to handling, improve self-calming, and encourage an alert state. Susan's mother visited daily. The physical therapist included Susan's mother in all treatment sessions in which she was present. This was at least once or twice per week. The physical therapist explained all activities during Susan's treatment session. In addition, the therapist actively involved Susan's mother in handling and self-calming activities. All activities discussed and demonstrated during a treatment session with Susan's mother were written down and pictures included for the mother's reference. The therapist also communicated with nursing daily. The physical therapist requested a referral for occupational therapy to work on oral-motor skills. The therapist reexamined Susan weekly to update her plan of care. The therapist was involved in her discharge planning, which included a referral to an early intervention program, as well as the hospital's NICU follow-up clinic.

After discharge from the NICU, Susan showed improvements, achieving several of her outcomes. Her parents were independent in her caregiving and felt very comfortable with the activities the therapist gave them. Susan was tolerating handling for longer periods of time, approximately 15 to 20 minutes. She was able to transition to a quiet alert state for a brief period of time, up to 5 minutes. She still was easily overstimulated, which caused her to transition to a cry state and decreased her handling tolerance. She began fixing on stationary objects, such as a black-and-white picture. She did not follow objects left or right. In addition, Susan inconsistently cleared her face while prone, continued to have a complete head lag with pull-to-sit, and did not make attempts to maintain her head vertically in midline while in supported sitting. Susan began receiving home physical therapy through a local early intervention program with frequent visits to the follow-up clinic for monitoring of her progress.

REFERENCES

Abad, F, Diaz, NM, Domenech, E, Robayna, M, & Rico, J. Oral sweet solution reduces pain-related behavior in preterm infants. Acta Paediatrica, 85:854–858, 1996.

Als, H. Neonatal Individualized Developmental Care and Assessment Program (NIDCAP). Boston: Children's Hospital, 1984.

Als, H. A synactive model of neonatal behavioral organization: Framework for the assessment of neurobehavioral development in the premature infant and for support of infants and parents in the neonatal intensive care environment. Physical and Occupational Therapy in Pediatrics, 6(3/4):3–54, 1986.

Als, H. Individualized, family-focused developmental care for the very low-birth weight preterm infant in the NICU. In Friedman, SL, & Sigman, MD (Eds.). The Psychological Development of Low Birth-weight Children, Advances in Applied Developmental Psychology, Vol 6. Norwood NJ: Ablex Publishing, 1992.

Als, H, Lawhon, G, Brown, E, Gives, R, Duffy, F, McAnulty, G, & Blickman, J. Individualized behavioral and environmental care for the very low birth weight preterm infant at high risk for broncho-pulmonary dysplasia: Neonatal intensive care unit and developmental outcome. Pediatrics, 78:1123–1132, 1986.

Als, H, Lawhon, G, Duffy, H, McAnulty, G, Gibes-Grossman, R, & Blickman, G. Individualized developmental care for the very low-birth-weight preterm infant. Journal of the American Medical Association, 272:853–858, 1994.

Als, H, Lester, BM, Tronick, E, & Brazelton, TB. Towards a research instrument for the assessment of preterm infants' behavior (APIB). In Fitzgerald, HE, & Yosman, MW (Eds.). Theory and Research in Behavioral Pediatrics, Vol. 1. New York: Plenum Press, 1982, pp. 35–63.

Als, H, Tronick, E, Adamson, L, & Brazelton, TB. The behavior of the full-term yet underweight newborn infant. Developmental Medicine and Child Neurology, 18:590–602, 1976.

Altmier L. Value study. Neonatal Network, 18(4):35–38, 1999.

American Academy of Pediatrics. Noise: A hazard for the fetus and newborn. Pediatrics, 100:724–727, 1997.

American Academy of Pediatrics, Committee on Substance Abuse and Committee on Children with Disabilities: Fetal alcohol syndrome and alcohol-related neurodevelopmental disorders. Pediatrics, 106(2):358–361, 2000a.

American Academy of Pediatrics: Serving the family from birth to the medical home: Newborn screening: A blueprint for the future. Pediatrics, 106(2 pt 2):389–427, 2000b.

American Physical Therapy Association. Guide to Physical Therapist Practice, 2nd ed. Physical Therapy, 81(1):347–364, 2001.

Amiel-Tison, C, & Grenier, A. Neurological Assessment During the First Year of Life. New York, New York: Oxford University Press, 1986.

Anand, KJ. Clinical importance of pain and stress in preterm neonates. Biology of the Neonate, 73:1–9, 1998.

Anand, KJ, & Hickey, P. Pain and its effects in the human neonate and fetus. New England Journal of Medicine, 317:1321–1329, 1987.

Anderson, J. Sensory intervention with the preterm infant in the neonatal intensive care unit. American Journal of Occupational Therapy, 40(1):19–26, 1986.

Arpino, C, Domizio, D, Carrieri MP, Brescianini, DS, Sabatin, MG & Curatolo, P. Prenatal and perinatal determinants of neonatal seizures occurring in the first week of life. Journal of Child Neurology, 9:651–656, 2001.

Askin, DF, & Diehl-Jones, B. Cocaine; effects of in utero exposure on the fetus and neonate. Journal of Perinatal and Neonatal Nursing, 14(4):83–102, 2001.

Autti-Ramo, I, & Granström, ML. The effect of intrauterine alcohol exposition in various durations on early cognitive development. Neuropediatrics, 22:203–210, 1991.

Avery, GB, & Glass, P. The gentle nursery: Developmental intervention in the NICU. Journal of Perinatology, 9(2):204–206, 1989.

Aylward, EH, Butz, AM, Hutton, N, Joyner, ML, & Vogelhut, JW. Cognitive and motor development in infants at risk for human immunodeficiency virus. American Journal of Diseases of Children, 146:218–222, 1992.

Bagwell, G, & Armstrong, V. Regionalization of care. In Kenner, C, Lott, J, & Flandermeyer, A (Eds.). Comprehensive Neonatal Nursing: A Physiologic Perspective. Philadelphia: WB Saunders, 1998, pp. 144–151.

Ballard, JL, Kazmaier, KN, & Driver, M. A simplified score for assessment of fetal maturation of newly born infants. Journal of Pediatrics, 95:769–774, 1979.

Ballard JL, Khoury JC, & Wedig K. New Ballard Score, expanding to include extremely premature infants. Journal of Pediatrics, 119:417–423, 1991.

Bancalari, E. Neonatal chronic lung disease. In Fanaroff, AA, & Martin, RJ (Eds.). Neonatal-Perinatal Medicine: Diseases of the Fetus and Infant. St. Louis: Mosby, 1992, pp. 861–875.

Barbosa, VM, Campbell, SK, Sheftel, D, Singh, J, & Beligere, N. Longitudinal performance of infant with cerebral palsy on the Test of Infant Motor Performance and on the Alberta Infant Motor Scale. Physical and Occupational Therapy in Pediatrics, 23(3):7–29, 2003.

Barbour, BG. Alcohol and pregnancy. Journal of Nurse-Midwifery, 35(2):78–85, 1990.

Barnard, KE, & Eyres, SJ. Feeding scale. In Child Health Assessment (DHEW Publication No. HRA 79-25). Hyattsville, MD: US Department of Health, Education, and Welfare, Health Resources Administration, Bureau of Health Manpower, Division of Nursing, 1979.

Barrier G, Attia, J, Mayer, MN, Amiel-Tison, CL, & Shnider, SM. Measurement of postoperative pain and narcotic administration in infants using a new clinical scoring system. Intensive Care Medicine, 15:S37–S39, 1989.

Bauman, P, & Levine, S. The development of children of drug addicts. International Journal of Addiction, 21(8):849–863, 1986.

Berns, S, & Brown, L. The changing family. In Kenner, C, Lott, J, & Flandermeyer, A (Eds.). Comprehensive Neonatal Nursing: Physiologic Perspectives. Philadelphia: WB Saunders, 1998, pp. 61–68.

Bigatello, LM, Patroniti, N, & Sangalli, F. Permissive hypercapnia. Current Opinion in Critical Care, 7(1):34–40, 2001.

Bingham PM, Abassi, S, Sivieri, E. A pilot study of milk odor effect on nonnutritive sucking by premature newborns. Archives of Pediatrics and Adolescent Medicine, 157(1):72–75, 2003.

Bosque, E, Brady, J, Affonso, D, & Wahlberg, V. Physiologic measures of kangaroo versus incubator care in a tertiary-level nursery. Journal of Obstetric, Gynecologic, and Neonatal Nursing, 24:219–226, 1995.

Brann, AW, Jr, & Wiznitzer, M. Seizures. In Fanaroff, AA, & Martin, RJ (Eds.). Neonatal-Perinatal Medicine: Diseases of the Fetus and Infant. St. Louis: Mosby, 1992, pp. 729–733.

Braun, MA, & Palmer, MM. A pilot study of oral-motor dysfunction in "at-risk" infants. Physical and Occupational Therapy in Pediatrics, 5(4):13–25, Winter 1985/1986.

Brazelton, TB. Neonatal Behavioral Assessment Scale, 3rd ed. Clinics in Developmental Medicine, Philadelphia: JB Lippincott, 1995.

Brown, P, & Taquino, LT. Designing and delivering neonatal care in single rooms. Journal of Pernatal Nursing, 15(1):68–83, 2001.

Brown, T, Cupido, C, Scarfone, H, Pape, K, Galea, V, & McComas, A. Developmental apraxia arising from neonatal brachial plexus palsy. Neurology, 55(1):24–30, 2000.

Buehler, D, Als, H, Duffy, F, McAnulty, G, & Liederman, J. Effectiveness of individualized developmental care for low-risk preterm infants: Behavioral and electrophysiologic evidence. Pediatrics, 96:923–932, 1995.

Burke, M, Walsh, J, Oehler, J, & Gingras, J. Music therapy following suctioning: Four case studies. Neonatal Network: Journal of Neonatal Nursing, 14:41–49, 1995.

Byers, JF. Components of developmental care and the evidence for their use in the NICU. American Journal of Maternal Child Nursing, 28(3):174–180, 2003.

Cabanas, F, Pellicer, A, Perez-Higueras, A, Garcia-Alix, A, Roche, C, & Quero, J. Ultrasonographic findings in thalamus and basal ganglia in term asphyxiated infants. Pediatric Neurology, 7:211–215, 1991.

Campbell, SK. Clinical decision making: Management of the neonate with movement dysfunction. In Wolf, SL (Ed.). Clinical Decision Making in Physical Therapy. Philadelphia: FA Davis, 1985, pp. 295–324.

Campbell, SK. Organizational and educational considerations in creating an environment to promote optimal development of high-risk neonates. Physical and Occupational Therapy in Pediatrics, 6 (3/4):191–204, 1986.

Campbell, SK. Test-retest reliability of the Test of Infant Motor Performance. Pediatric Physical Therapy, 11:60–66, 1999a.

Campbell, SK. The infant at risk for developmental disability. In Campbell, S.K. (Ed.). Decision Making in Pediatric Neurologic Physical Therapy. New York: Churchill Livingstone, 1999b, pp. 260–332.

Campbell, SK, Kolobe, THA, Osten, ET, Lenke, M, & Girolami, GL. Construct validity of the Test of Infant Motor Performance. Physical Therapy, 75:585–596, 1995.

Campbell, SK, & Kolobe, THA. Concurrent validity of the Test of Infant Motor Performance with the Alberta Infant Motor Scale. Pediatric Physical Therapy, 12:2–9, 2000.

Campbell, SK, & Hedeker, D. Validity of the Test of Infant Motor Performance for discriminating among infants with varying risk for poor motor outcome. Journal of Pediatrics, 139:546–551, 2001.

Campbell, SK: The Test of Infant Motor Performance. Chicago: Infant Motor Performance Scales, 2001.

Campbell, SK, Kolobe, THA, Wright, BD, & Linacre, JM. Validity of the Test of Infant Motor Performance for prediction of 6-, 9- and 12-month scores on the Alberta Infant Motor Scale. Developmental Medicine & Child Neurology, 44:263–272, 2002.

Carlo, WA, & Chatburn, RL. Assisted ventilation of the newborn. In Carlo, WA, & Chatburn, RL (Eds.). Neonatal Respiratory Care. Chicago: YearBook, 1988, pp. 320–346.

Caron, E, & Berlandi, J. Extracorporeal membrane oxygenation. Advances and Emerging Topics in Perioperative Pediatric Nursing, 32:125–140, 1997.

Catto-Smith, AG, Yu, VYH, Bajuk, B, Orgill, AA, & Astbury, J. Effect of neonatal periventricular haemorrhage on neurodevelopmental outcome. Archives of Disease in Childhood, 60:8–11, 1985.

Chasnoff, IJ. Drug use in pregnancy: Parameters of risk. Pediatric Clinics of North America, 35:1403–1412, 1988.

Chen, HF, & Chang YJ. Noise distribution of an incubator with nebulizer at neonatal intensive care unit in southern Taiwan. Journal of Nursing Research, 9(3):25–31, 2002.

Cheu, HW, Brown, DR, & Rowe, M. Breath hydrogen excretion as a screening test for the early diagnosis of necrotizing enterocolitis. American Journal of Diseases of Children, 143:156–159, 1989.

Chiswick, M. Assessment of pain in neonates. Lancet, 355(9197):6–9, 2000.

Chow, LC, Wright, KW, & Sola, A. Can changes in clinical practice decrease the incidence of severe retinopathy of prematurity in very low birth weight infants? Pediatrics, 111(2):339–345, 2003.

Coles, CD, Brown, RT, Smith, IE, Platzman, KA, Erickson, S, & Falek, A. Effects of prenatal alcohol exposure at school age. Neurotoxicology and Teratology, 13:357–367, 1991.

Coles, CD, Platzman, KA, Lynch ME, & Freides D. Auditory and visual sustained attention in adolescents prenatally exposed to alcohol. Alcoholism: Clinical and Experimental Research, 26(2):263–271, 2002.

Collins, SK, & Kuck, K. Music therapy in the neonatal intensive care unit. Neonatal Network, 9(6):23–26, 1991.

Corff, K, Seideman, R, Venkataraman, P, Lutes, L, & Yates, B. Facilitated tucking: A nonpharmacologic comfort measure for pain in preterm neonates. Journal of Gynecologic and Neonatal Nursing, 24:143–147, 1995.

Crane, LD. Cardiorespiratory management of the high-risk neonate: Implications for developmental therapists. Physical and Occupational Therapy in Pediatrics, 6(3/4):255–282, 1986.

Crane, LD. The neonate and child. In Frownfelter, DL (Ed.). Chest Physical Therapy and Pulmonary Rehabilitation, 2nd ed. Chicago: YearBook, 1987, pp. 666–698.

Crane, LD. Physical therapy for the neonate with respiratory disease. In Irwin, S, & Tecklin, JS (Eds.). Cardiopulmonary Physical Therapy, 2nd ed. St. Louis: Mosby, 1990, pp. 486–515.

Crane, LD. Physical therapy for the neonate with respiratory disease. In Irwin, S, & Tecklin, JS (Eds.). Cardiopulmonary Physical Therapy, 3rd ed. St. Louis: Mosby, 1995, pp. 486–515.

Creger, PJ, & Browne, JV. Developmental Interventions for Preterm and High-Risk Infants. Tucson, AZ: Therapy Skill Builders, 1995, pp. 97–144.

Cressinger, KD, Ryckman, FC, Flake, AW, & Balistreri, WF. Necrotizing enterocolitis. In Fanaroff, AA, & Martin, RJ (Eds.). Neonatal-Perinatal Medicine: Diseases of the Fetus and Infant. St. Louis: Mosby, 1992, pp. 1068–1074.

Crowley, P. Prophylactic corticosteroids for preterm birth. Cochrane Library (Oxford). CD000065, 2002.

Cusson, R, & Lee, A. Parental interventions and the development of the preterm infant. Journal of Gynecologic and Neonatal Nursing, 23:60–68, 1993.

D'Apolito, K, & Hepworth, JT. Prominence of withdrawal symptoms in polydrug-exposed infants. Journal of Perinatal and Neonatal Nursing, 14(4):46–60, 2001.

Darlow, BA, & Graham, PJ. Vitamin A supplementation for preventing morbidity and mortality in very low birthweight infants. Chichester, UK: John Wiley & Sons, Ltd.: The Cochrane Database of Systematic Reviews 2002, Issue 4.

Davis, DD, & Templer, DI. Neurobehavioral functioning in children exposed to narcotics in utero. Addictive Behaviors, *13*:275–283, 1988.

Davis, JM, Sinkin, RA, & Aranda, JV. Drug therapy for bronchopulmonary dysplasia. Pediatric Pulmonology, *8*:117–125, 1990.

Dean, E. The intensive care unit: Principles and practice of physical therapy. In Frownfelter, DL (Ed.). Chest Physical Therapy and Pulmonary Rehabilitation. Chicago: YearBook, 1987, pp. 377–442.

Deiriggi, PM. Effects of waterbed flotation on indicators of energy expenditure in preterm infants. Nursing Research, *39*:140–146, 1990.

delEstard, K, & Lennox, K. Developmental care: Making your NICU a gentler place. Canadian Nurse, *2*:23–26, 1995.

Desiato, MT, & Risina, B. The role of botulinum toxin in the neurorehabilitation of young patients with brachial plexus birth palsy. Pediatric Rehabilitation, *4*(1):29–36, 2001.

Dixon, SD. Effects of transplacental exposure to cocaine and methamphetamine on the neonate (specialty conference). Western Journal of Medicine, *150*:436–442, 1989.

Dodds, SD, & Wolfe, SW. Perinatal brachial plexus palsy. Current Opinions in Pediatrics, *12*:40–47, 2000.

Dolgin, SE, Shlasko, E, Levitt, MA, Hong, AR, Brillhart, S, Rynkowski, M, & Holzman, I. Alterations in respiratory status: Early signs of necrotizing enterocolitis. Journal of Pediatric Surgery, *33*:856–858, 1998.

Donovan, E, Schwartz, J, & Moles, L. New technologies applied to the management of respiratory dysfunction. In Kenner, C, Lott, J, & Flandermeyer, A (Eds.). Comprehensive Neonatal Nursing: Physiologic Perspectives. Philadelphia: WB Saunders, 1998, pp. 268–289.

Dubowitz, L. Neurologic assessment. In Ballard, RA (Ed.). Pediatric Care of the ICN Graduate. Philadelphia: WB Saunders, 1988, pp. 59–85.

Dubowitz, L, & Dubowitz, V. The Neurological Assessment of the Preterm and Full-Term Newborn Infant. London: Heinemann, 1981a.

Dubowitz, L, & Dubowitz, V. The neurological assessment of the preterm and full-term newborn infant. Clinics in Developmental Medicine, No. 79. Philadelphia: JB Lippincott, 1981b.

Dubowitz, L, Dubowitz, V, & Goldberg, C. Clinical assessment of gestational age in the newborn infant. Journal of Pediatrics, *77*:1–10, 1970.

Dubowitz, L, Dubowitz, V, Palmer, PG, Miller, G, Fawer, CL, & Levene, MI. Correlation of neurologic assessment in the preterm newborn infant with outcome at 1 year. Journal of Pediatrics, *105*:452–456, 1984.

Dunst, CJ, Johanson, C, Trivette, SM, & Hamby, D. Family-oriented early intervention policies and practices: Family-centered or not? Exceptional Parent, *58*:115–126, 1991.

Edwards, MSB, & Derechin, ME. Neurosurgical problems in the infant. In Ballard, RA (Ed.). Pediatric Care of the ICN Graduate. Philadelphia: WB Saunders, 1988, pp. 196–204.

Emsley, HC, Wardle, SP, Sims, DG, Chiswick, ML, & Souza, SW. Increased survival and deteriorating developmental outcome in 23 to 25 week old gestation infants, 1990–4 compared with 1984–9. Archives of Disease in Childhood (Fetal and Neonatal Edition), *78*:99–104, 1998.

Fanaroff, AA, & Graven, SN. Perinatal services and resources. In Fanaroff, AA, & Martin, RJ (Eds.). Neonatal-Perinatal Medicine: Diseases of the Fetus and Infant. St. Louis: Mosby, 1992, pp. 12–21.

Fangman, JJ, Marj, PM, Pratt, L, & Conway, KK. Prematurity prevention programs: An analysis of successes and failures. American Journal of Obstetrics and Gynecology, *170*:744–750, 1994.

Farrell, PA, & Fiascone, JM. Bronchopulmonary dysplasia in 1990's:

A review for the pediatrician. Current Problems in Pediatrics, *27*:129–163, 1997.

Feldman, R, Eidelman, AI, Sirota, L, & Weller, A. Comparison of skin-skin (kangaroo) and traditional care: Parenting outcomes and preterm infant development. Pediatrics, *110*(Pt 1):16–26, 2002.

Fetters, L. Sensorimotor management of the high-risk neonate. Physical and Occupational Therapy in Pediatrics, *6*(3/4):217–230, 1986.

Field, T. Alleviating stress in newborn infants in the intensive care unit. Clinics in Perinatology, *17*(1):1–9, 1990.

Field, TM, Schanberg, SM, Scafidi, F, Bauer, CR, Vega-Lahr, N, Garcia, R, Nystrom, J, & Kuhn, CM. Tactile/kinesthetic stimulation effects on preterm neonates. Pediatrics, *77*(5):654–658, 1986.

Finan, DS, & Barlow, S. The actifier: A device for neurophysiological studies of orofacial control in human infants. Journal of Speech and Hearing Research, *39*:833–838, 1996.

Finnegan, L. Management of maternal and neonatal substance abuse problems. National Institute on Drug Abuse Research Monograph Series, *90*:177–189, 1988.

Fiterman, C. Physical therapy in the NICU. In Connolly, BH, & Montgomery, PC (Eds.). Therapeutic Exercise in Developmental Disabilities. Chattanooga, TN: Chattanooga Corporation, 1987, pp. 29–41.

Fitzgerald, M, & Beggs, S. The Neurobiology of Pain: Developmental Aspects. The Neuroscientist, *7*(3):246–257, 2001.

Flegel, J, & Kolobe, THA. Predictive validity of the Test of Infant Motor Performance as measured by the Bruininks-Oseretsky Test of Motor Proficiency at school age. Physical Therapy, *82*(8):762–771, 2002.

Fleisher, B, VandenBerg, K, Constantinou, J, Heller, C, Benitz, W, Johnson, A, Rosenthal, A, & Stevenson, D. Individualized developmental care for very-low-birth-weight premature infants. Clinical Pediatrics, *34*:523–529, 1995.

Francis, PL, Self, PA, & Horowitz, FD. The behavioral assessment of the neonate: An overview. In Osofsky, JD (Ed.). Handbook of Infant Development, 2nd ed. New York: Wiley, 1987, pp. 723–779.

Franck, LS. A national survey of the assessment and treatment of pain and agitation in the neonatal intensive care unit. Journal of Gynecological and Neonatal Nursing, Nov/Dec 1987, pp. 387–393.

Franck, LS. The influence of sociopolitical, scientific, and technological forces on the study and treatment of neonatal pain. Advanced Nursing Science, *15*:11–12, 1992.

Free, T, Russell, F, Mills, B, & Hathaway, D. A descriptive study of infants and toddlers exposed prenatally to substance abuse. Maternal Child Nursing, *15*:245–249, 1990.

Gaebler, C, & Hanzlik, R. The effects of prefeeding stimulation program on preterm infants. American Journal of Occupational Therapy, *50*:184–192, 1996.

Gartner, LM, & Lee, KS. Unconjugated hyperbilirubinemia. In Fanaroff, AA, & Martin, RJ (Eds.). Neonatal-Perinatal Medicine: Diseases of the Fetus and Infant. St. Louis: Mosby, 1992, pp. 1075–1103.

Gaynon, MW, Stevenson, DK, Sunshine P, Fleisher, BE, & Landers, MB. Supplemental oxygen may decrease progression of prethreshold disease to threshold retinopathy of prematurity. Journal of Perinatology, *17*:434–438, 1997.

Glass, P, Avery, GB, Siva Subramanian, KN, Keys, MP, Sostek, AM, & Friendly, DS. Effect of bright light in the hospital nursery on the incidence of retinopathy of prematurity. New England Journal of Medicine, *313*:401–404, 1985.

Goetzman, BW. Understanding bronchopulmonary dysplasia. American Journal of Diseases of Children, *140*:332–334, 1986.

Gottfried, AW. Environment of newborn infants in special care units. In Gottfried, AW, & Gaiter, JL (Eds.). Infant Stress Under Intensive Care. Baltimore: University Park Press, 1985, pp. 23–54.

Gottfried, AW, & Hodgman, J. How intensive is newborn intensive care? An environmental analysis. Pediatrics, 74:292–294, 1984.

Gottwald, SR, & Thurman, SK. Parent-infant interaction in neonatal intensive care units: Implications for research and service delivery. Infants and Young Children, 2(3):1–9, 1990.

Grunau, E, Holsti, L, Whitfield, M, & Ling, E. Are twitches, startles, and body movements pain indicators in extremely low birth weight infants? Clinical Journal of Pain, 16:37–45, 2000.

Gruneau, RVE, & Craig, KD. Pain expression in neonates: Facial action and cry. Pain, 28:395–410, 1987.

Gruneau, RVE, Johnston, CC, & Craig, KD. Neonatal facial and cry responses to invasive and non-invasive procedures. Pain, 42:295–305, 1990.

Guidelines for Perinatal Care, 4th ed. Elk Grove Village, IL, and Washington, DC: American Academy of Pediatrics and American College of Obstetricians and Gynecologists, 1997, pp. 4–6.

Hack, M. Follow-up for high-risk neonates. In Fanaroff, AA, & Martin, RJ (Eds.). Neonatal-Perinatal Medicine: Diseases of the Fetus and Infant. St. Louis: Mosby, 1992, pp. 753–758.

Handler, A, Kistin, N, & Davis, F. Cocaine use during pregnancy: Perinatal outcomes. American Journal of Epidemiology, 133:818–825, 1991.

Harmon, J, & Kenner, C. High-risk pregnancy. In Kenner, C, Lott, J, & Flandermeyer, A (Eds.). Comprehensive Neonatal Nursing: Physiologic Perspective. Philadelphia: WB Saunders, 1998, pp. 144–151.

Harper, RG, & Yoon, JJ. Handbook of Neonatalogy, 2nd ed. Chicago: YearBook, 1987.

Harris, MB. Oral-motor management of the high-risk neonate. Physical and Occupational Therapy in Pediatrics, 6(3/4):231–254, 1986.

Harris, SR, Atwater, SW, & Crowe, TK. Accepted and controversial neuromotor therapies for infants at high risk for cerebral palsy. Journal of Perinatology, 8:3–12, 1988.

Harrison, H. The principles of family-centered neonatal care. Pediatrics, 92:643–650, 1993.

Hayford, SM, Epps, RP, & Dahl-Regis, M. Behavior and development patterns in children born to heroin-addicted and methadone-addicted mothers. Journal of the National Medical Association, 80:1197–1200, 1988.

Hedrick, H, & Crombleholme, T. Current status of fetal surgery: After nearly a quarter century of research, fetal surgery has emerged as an accepted therapy. Contemporary Obstetrics and Gynecology, 46(12):42–57, 2001.

Hensinger, RN. Orthopedic problems of the shoulder and neck. Pediatric Clinics of North America, 24:889, 1977.

Henslee, JA, Schechtman, VL, Lee, MY, & Harper, RM. Developmental patterns of heart rate and variability in prematurely-born infants with apnea of prematurity. Early Human Development, 47:35–50, 1997.

Heriza, CB. The neonate with cerebral palsy. In Scully, R, & Barnes, ML (Eds.). Physical Therapy. Philadelphia: JB Lippincott, 1989, pp. 1238–1257.

Hibbs A, Evans JR, Gerdes, M, & Hunter, JV. Outcome of infants who receive extracorporeal membrane oxygenation therapy. Journal of Pediatric Surgery, 36(10):1479–1484, 2001.

Higgins, RD, Mendelsohn, AL, DeFeo, MJ, Ucsel, R, & Hendricks-Munoz, KD. Antenatal dexamethasone and decreased severity of retinopathy of prematurity. Archives of Ophthalmology, 116:601–605, 1998.

Hilton, A. The hospital racket: How noisy is your unit? American Journal of Nursing, 87:59–61, 1987.

Ho, YL: Bronchopulmonary dysplasia and chronic lung disease of infancy: Strategies for prevention and management. Annals of the Academy of Medicine, Singapore, 31(1):119–130, 2002.

Hockenberry, M, Wilson, D, Winklestein, M, & Kline, N (Eds.). Wong's Nursing Care of Infants and Children. St. Louis: Mosby, 2003.

Hodgman, JE. Introduction. In Gottfried, AW, & Gaiter, JL (Eds.). Infant Stress Under Intensive Care. Baltimore: University Park Press, 1985, pp. 1–6.

Holmstrom, G, Broberger, U, & Thomassen, P. Neonatal risk factors for retinopathy—A population-based study. Acta Ophthalmologica Scandinavica, 76:204–207, 1998.

Hume, RF, Jr, O'Donnell, KJ, Stanger, CL, Killam, AP, & Gingras, JL. In utero cocaine exposure. Observations of fetal behavioral state may predict neonatal outcome. American Journal of Obstetrics and Gynecology, 161:685–690, 1989.

Huttenlocher, PR. The nervous system. In Behrman RE, Vaughn, VC, & Nelson, WE (Eds.). Nelson Textbook of Pediatrics, 13th ed. Philadelphia: WB Saunders, 1987, pp. 1274–1330.

Iyasu, S, & Tomashek, K. Infant mortality and low birth weight among black and white infants — United States, 1980–2000. Morbidity and Mortality Weekly Report, 5I(27):589–593, July 12, 2002.

Jennett, RJ, & Tarby, TJ. Disuse osteoporosis as evidence of brachial-plexus palsy due to intrauterine fetal maladaptation. American Journal of Obstetrics and Gynecology, 1:236–237, 2001.

Jennett, RJ, Tarby, TJ, & Krauss RL. Erb's palsy contrasted with Klumpke's and total palsy: Different mechanisms are involved. American Journal of Obstetrics and Gynecology, 6:1216–1219, 2002.

Joffe, GM, Symonds, R, Alverson, D, & Chilton, L. The effect of comprehensive prematurity prevention program on the number of admissions to the neonatal intensive care unit. Journal of Perinatology, 15:305–309, 1995.

Johnson, AN. Neonatal response to control of noise inside the incubator. Pediatric Nursing, 27(6):600–605, 2001.

Johnson, BH. The changing role of the families in health care. Children's Health Care, 19:234–241, 1990.

Kahn-D'Angelo, L. Is the small for gestational age, term infant at risk for developmental delay? Physical and Occupational Therapy in Pediatrics, 7(3):69–73, 1987.

Kakebeeke, TH, Von Siebenthal, K, & Largo, LH. Differences in movement quality at term among preterm and term infants. Biology of the Neonate, 71(6):367–378, 1997.

Kamitsuka, MD, Horton, MK, & Williams, MA: The incidence of necrotizing enterocolitis after introducing standarized feeding schedules for infants between 1250 and 2500 grams and less than 35 weeks gestation. Pediatrics, 105(2):378–384, 2000.

Kappas, A, Drummond, GS, Munson, DP, & Marshall, JR. Sn-Meso-porphyrin interdiction of severe hyperbilirubinemia in Jehovah's Witness newborns as an alternative to exchange transfusion. Pediatrics, 108(6):1374–1377, 2001.

Keller, A, Arbel, N, Merlob, P, & Davidson, S. Neurobehavioral and autonomic effects of hammock positioning in infants with very low birth weight. Pediatric Physical Therapy, 15:3–7, 2003.

Kennell, JH, & Klaus, MH. Care of the parents. In Carlo, WA, & Chatburn, RL (Eds.). Neonatal Respiratory Care. Chicago: YearBook, 1988, pp. 212–235.

Kenner, C. Complications of respiratory management. In Kenner, C, Lott, J, & Flandermeyer, A (Eds.). Comprehensive Neonatal Nursing: A Physiologic Perspective. Philadelphia: WB Saunders, 1998, pp. 290–305.

Kenner, C, & Lott, J: Comprehensive Neonatal Nursing: A Physiologic Perspective, 3rd ed. St. Louis: WB Saunders, 2003.

Kent, W, Tan, A, Clarke, M, & Bardell, T. Excessive noise level in the neonatal ICU: Potential effects on auditory system development. Journal of Otolaryngology, 3(6):355–360, 2002.

Kingham, JD. Classification of retinopathy of prematurity. In McPherson, AR, Hittner, HM, & Kretzer, FL (Eds.). Retinopathy and Prematurity. Toronto: BC Decker, 1986, pp. 17–26.

Kleigman, R. Bioethics of the mother, fetus and newborn. In Fanaroff, AA, & Martin, RJ (Eds.). Neonatal-Perinatal Medicine: Diseases of the Fetus and Infant. St. Louis: Mosby, 1992, pp. 22–35.

Klein, AH, & Ganon, JA. Caring for Your Premature Baby A Complete Resource for Parents. New York: Harper Perennial, 1998.

Kretzer, FL, & Hittner, HM. Human retinal development: Relationship to the pathogenesis of retinopathy of prematurity. In McPherson, AR, Hittner, HM, & Kretzer, FL (Eds.). Retinopathy and Prematurity. Toronto: BC Decker, 1986, pp. 27–52.

Larrson, E, & Holmstrom, G. Screening for retinopathy of prematurity: evaluation and modification of guidelines. British Journal of Ophthalmology, 86(12):1399–402, 2002.

Lauterback, MD, Raz, S, & Sander, CJ. Neonatal hypoxic risk in preterm birth infants: The influence of sex and severity of respiratory distress on cognitive recovery. Neuropsychology, 15(3):411–420, 2001.

Lee, VL, Morgan, A, & Ling, W. Predictability for the Neonatal Neurobehavioral Examination at 6 and 18 months corrected age. Physical Therapy, 69:362, 1989.

Leib, SA, Benfield, G, & Guidubaldi, J. Effects of early intervention and stimulation on the preterm infant. Pediatrics, 66 (1):83–90, 1980.

Leonard, CH. High-risk infant follow-up programs. In Ballard, RA (Ed.). Pediatric Care of the ICN Graduate. Philadelphia: WB Saunders, 1988, pp. 17–23.

Leviton, A, & Paneth, N. White matter damage in preterm newborns: An epidemiologic perspective. Early Human Development, 24:1–22, 1990.

Lewis, KD, Bennett, B, & Schmeder, NH. The care of infants menaced by cocaine abuse. Maternal Child Nursing, 14:324–329, 1989.

Lieberman, E, Lang, J, Richardson, DK, Frigoletto, FD, Heffner, LJ, & Cohen, J. Intrapartum maternal fever and neonatal outcome. Pediatrics, 105(1 part 1):8–13,2000.

Little, RE, Anderson, KW, Ervin, CH, Worthington-Roberts, B, & Clarren, SK. Maternal alcohol use during breast-feeding and infant mental and motor development at one year. New England Journal of Medicine, 321:425–430, 1989.

Lubchenco, LO, Bard, H, Goldman, AL, Coyer, WE, McIntyre, C, & Smith, DM. Newborn intensive care and long-term prognosis. Developmental Medicine and Child Neurology, 16:421–431, 1974.

Luchi, JM, Bennett, FC, & Jackson, JC. Predictors of neurodevelopmental outcome following bronchopulmonary dysplasia. American Journal of Diseases of Children, 145:813–817, 1991.

Ludington-Hoe, SM, & Swinth, JY. Kangaroo mother care during phototherapy: effect on bilirubin profile. Neonatal Network, 20(5):41–48, 2001.

Mangurten, HH. Birth injuries. In Fanaroff, AA, & Martin, RJ (Eds.). Neonatal-Perinatal Medicine: Diseases of the Fetus and Infant. St. Louis: Mosby, 1992, pp. 346–371.

Mantovani, JF, & Powers, J. Brain injury in premature infants: Patterns on cranial ultrasound, their relationship to outcome, and the role of developmental intervention in the NICU. Infants and Young Children, 4(2):20–32, 1991.

Martin, RJ, & Fanaroff, AA. The respiratory distress syndrome and its management. In Fanaroff, AA, & Martin, RJ (Eds.). Neonatal-Perinatal Medicine: Diseases of the Fetus and Infant. St. Louis: Mosby, 1992, pp. 810–819.

Martin, RJ, Herrell, N, Rubin, D, & Fanaroff, A. Effect of supine and prone positions on arterial oxygen tension in the preterm infant. Pediatrics, 63:528–531, 1979.

Mazur, JM, & Menelaus, MB. Neurologic status of spina bifida patients and the orthopedic surgeon. Clinical Orthopedics, 264:54–64, 1991.

McDonald, AD. Survival and handicap in infants of very low birthweight. Lancet, 2:194–198, 1981.

McElhinney, DB, Hedrick, H, Bush, DM, & Pereia, GR. Necrotizing enterocolitis in neonates with congenital heart disease: Risk factors and outcomes. Pediatrics, 106(5):1080–1087, 2000.

McGuire, W, & Anthony, MY. Donor milk versus formula for preventing necrotising enterocolitis in preterm infants: Systemic review. Archives of Disease in Childhood: Fetal Neonatal Education, 88(1): F11–4, 2003.

McMenamin, JB, Shackelford, GD, & Volpe, JJ. Outcome of neonatal intraventricular hemorrhage with periventricular echodense lesions. Annals of Neurology, 15:285–290, 1984.

Medoff-Cooper, B, & Gennaro, S. Prediction of developmental outcomes of infants of very low birth weight. Nursing Research, 45(5):291–296, 1996.

Miles, MS. Parents of critically ill premature infants: Sources of stress. Infants & Young Children, 12(3): 69–74, 1989.

Miller, MJ, & Murrary, GS. Noninvasive diagnostic techniques. In Fanaroff, AA, & Martin, RJ (Eds.). Neonatal-Perinatal Medicine: Diseases of the Fetus and Infant. St. Louis: Mosby, 1992, pp. 700–702.

Mitchell, S. Infants with bronchopulmonary dysplasia: A developmental perspective. Journal of Pediatric Nursing, 11:145–151, 1996.

Mizrahi, EM, & Kellaway, P. Characterization and classification of neonatal seizures. Neurology, 37:1837–1844, 1987.

Mizuguchi, M, & Takashima, S. Imaging and pathology in pediatric neurological disorders. Neuropathology, 22:85–89, 2002.

Morgan, AM, Koch, U, Lee, V, & Aldag, J. Neonatal Neurobehavioral Examination. Physical Therapy, 68:1352–1358, 1988.

Moseley, MJ, Thompson, JR, Levene, MI, & Fielder, AR. Effects of nursery illumination on frequency of eyelid opening and state in preterm neonates. Early Human Development, 18:13–26, 1988.

Mouradian, L, & Als, H. The influence of neonatal intensive care unit caregiving practices on motor functioning of preterm infants. America Journal of Occupational Therapy, 48:527–533, 1994.

Mueller, C. Multidisciplinary research of multimodal stimulation of premature infants: An integrated review of the literature. Maternal-Child Nursing Journal, 24:18–31, 1996.

Murney, ME, & Campbell, S. The ecological relevance of the Test of Infant Motor Performance Elicited Scale items. Physical Therapy, 78:479–489, 1998.

Mussi-Pinhata, MM, Yamamoto, AY, Figueredo, LT, Cervi, MC, & Duarte G. Congenital and perinatal cytomegalovirus infection in infants born to mothers infected with human immunodeficiency virus. Journal of Pediatrics, 132(2):285–290, 1998.

Nadler, EP, Upperman, JS, & Ford, HR. Controversies in the management of necrotizing enterocolitis. Surgical Infection, 2(2):113–119, 2001.

Nelson, MR. Birth brachial plexus. Physical Medicine and Rehabilitation: State of the Art Reviews, 14(2):237–246, 2000.

Newman, LF. Social and sensory environment of low birth weight infants in a special care nursery. Journal of Nervous and Mental Disease, 169:448–455, 1981.

Noetzel, MJ. Myelomeningocele: Current concepts of management. Clinics in Perinatology, 16:311–329, 1989.

Northway, WH, Jr, Moss, RB, Carlisle, KB, Parker, BR, Popp, RL, Pitlick, PT, Eichler, I, Lamm, RL, & Brown, BW, Jr. Late pulmonary sequelae of bronchopulmonary dysplasia. New England Journal of Medicine, 323:1793–1799, 1990.

Novy, MJ, McGregor, J, & Iams, JD. New perspectives on the prevention of extreme prematurity. Clinical Obstetrics and Gynecology, 38:790–808, 1995.

O'Connor, A, & Sawin, RS. High morbidity of enterostomy and its closure in premature infants with necrotizing enterocolitis. Archives of Surgery, 133:875–880, 1998.

Papile, LA. Periventricular-intraventricular hemorrhage. In Fanaroff, AA, & Martin, RJ (Eds.). Neonatal-Perinatal Medicine: Diseases of the Fetus and Infant. St. Louis: Mosby, 1997, pp. 891–899.

Papile, L, Munsick-Bruno, G, & Schaefer, A. Relationship of cerebral intraventricular hemorrhage and early childhood neurological handicaps. Journal of Pediatrics, 193:273–277, 1983.

Parker, A. Chest physiotherapy in the neonatal intensive care unit. Physiotherapy, 71(2):63–65, 1985.

Parker, S, Zahr, L, Cole, J, & Brecht ML. Outcome after developmental intervention in the neonatal intensive care unit for mothers of preterm infants with low socioeconomic status. Journal of Pediatrics, 120:780–785, 1992.

Pax Lowes, L, & Palisano, RJ. Review of medical and developmental outcome of neonates who received extracorporeal membrane oxygenation. Pediatric Physical Therapy, 7:215–221, 1995.

Peabody, JL, & Lewis, K. Consequences of newborn intensive care. In Gottfried, AW, & Gaiter, JL (Eds.). Infant Stress Under Intensive Care. Baltimore: University Park Press, 1985, pp. 199–226.

Pelletier, JM, & Palmeri, A. High risk infants. In Clark, PN, & Allen, AS (Eds.). Occupational Therapy for Children. St. Louis: Mosby, 1985, pp. 292–311.

Perlstein, PH. Physical environment. In Fanaroff, AA, & Martin, RJ (Eds.). Neonatal-Perinatal Medicine: Diseases of the Fetus and Infant. St. Louis: Mosby, 1992, pp. 401–419.

Phelps, DL. Retinopathy of prematurity. In Fanaroff, AA, & Martin, RJ (Eds.). Neonatal-Perinatal Medicine: Diseases of the Fetus and Infant. St. Louis: Mosby, 1992, pp. 1391–1395.

Phelps, DL, & Watts, JL. Early light reduction for preventing retinopathy of prematurity in very low birth weight infants. Chichester, UK: John Wiley & Sons, Ltd: The Cochrane Database of Systematic Reviews 2002, Issue 1.

Philbin, MK, & Gray, L. Changing levels of quiet in an intensive care nursery. Journal of Perinatology, 22(6):455–460, 2002.

Pickler, RH, Frankel, HB, Walsh, KM, & Thompson, NM. Effects on nonnutritive sucking on behavioral organization and feeding performance in preterm infants. Nursing Research, 45:132–135, 1996.

Piecuch, R. Cosmetics: Skin scars, and residual traces of the ICN. In Ballard, RA (Ed.). Pediatric Care of the ICN Graduate. Philadelphia: WB Saunders, 1988, pp. 50–56.

Pigeon, HM, McGrath, PJ, Lawrence, J, & MacMurray, SB. Nurses' perceptions of pain in the neonatal intensive care unit. Journal of Pain Symptom Management, 4:179–183, 1989.

Platzker, ACG, Lew, CD, Cohen, SR, Thompson, J, Ward, SLD, & Keens, TG. Home care of infants with chronic lung disease. In Ballard, RA (Ed.). Pediatric Care of the ICN Graduate. Philadelphia: WB Saunders, 1988, pp. 289–294.

Prechtl, H, & Beintema, D. The Neurological Examination of the Newborn Infant. Clinics in Developmental Medicine, No. 12. London: Heinemann Educational Books, 1964.

Prechtl, H, Einspieler, C, Cioni, G, Bos, AF, Ferrari, F, & Sontheimer, D. An early marker for neurological deficits after perinatal brain lesions. Lancet, 349:1361–1363, 1997.

Public Law 108-446, Individuals with Disabilities Education Improvement Act of 2004.

Pursell, E. The diagnosis, transmission and prevention of HIV-1 in the infant under 18 months of age. Journal of Clinical Nursing, 7(4):297–306, 1998.

Rapalino, OA, & Levine, DN. Developmental apraxia arising from neonatal brachial plexus palsy. Neurology, 55(11):1761, 2000.

Resnick, MB, Eyler, FD, Nelson, RM, Eitzman, DV, & Bucciarelli, RL. Developmental intervention for low birth weight infants: Improved early developmental outcome. Pediatrics, 80:68–74, 1987.

Reynolds, JD, Hardy, RJ, Spencer, R, van Heuven, WA, & Fiedler, AR. Lack of efficacy of light reduction in preventing retinopathy of prematurity. Light reduction in retinopathy of prematurity cooperative group. New England Journal of Medicine, 338:1572–1576, 1998.

Robertson, CM, Etches, PC, Goldson, E, & Kyle, JM. Eight-year school performance, neurodevelopmental, and growth outcome of neonates with bronchopulmonary dysplasia: A comparative study. Pediatrics, 89:365–372, 1991.

Rosenbaum, P, King, S, Law, M, King, G, & Evans, J. Family-centered services: A conceptual framework and research review. In Law, M (Ed.). Family-Centered Assessment and Intervention in Pediatric Rehabilitation. New York: The Haworth Press, 1998, pp. 1–20.

Rossetti, LM. High-Risk Infants: Identification, Assessment, and Intervention. Boston: Little, Brown, 1986.

Rothberg, AD, Goodman, M, Jacklin, LA, & Cooper, PA. Six-year follow-up of early physiotherapy intervention in very low birth weight infants. Pediatrics, 88:547–552, 1991.

Rubaltelli, F, Bonafe, L, Tangucci, M, Spagnolo, A, & Dani, C. Epidemiology of neonatal acute respiratory disorders. A multicenter study on incidence and fatality rates of neonatal acute respiratory disorders according to gestational age, maternal age, pregnancy complications and type of delivery. Italian Group of Neonatal Pneumology. Biology of the Neonate, 74:7–15, 1998.

Saint-Anne Dargassies, S. Neurological Development in the Full-Term and Premature Neonate. New York: Excerpta Medica, 1977.

Saling, E. Prevention of prematurity. A review of our activities during the last 25 years. Journal of Perinatal Medicine, 25:406–417, 1997.

Sarnaik, AP, & Preston, G. The organization of a pediatric critical care service. In Vidyasagar, D, & Sarnaik, AP (Eds.). Neonatal and Pediatric Intensive Care. Littleton, MA: PSG, 1985, pp. 339–344.

Sarnat, HB, & Sarnat, MS. Neonatal encephalopathy following fetal distress: A clinical and electroencephalographic study. Archives of Neurology, 33:696, 1976.

Scarr-Salapatek, S, & Williams, ML. The effects of early stimulation on low-birth-weight infants. Child Development, 44:94–101, 1973.

Schexnayder, SM, Torres, A, Binns, M, Anders, M, & Heulitt, MJ. High frequency oscillatory ventilation as a bridge from extracorporeal membrane oxygenation in pediatric respiratory failure. Respiratory Care, 40:44–47, 1995.

Schneider, JW, Krosschell, K, & Gabriel, KL. Congenital spinal cord injury. In Umphred, DA (Ed.). Neurological Rehabilitation, 3rd ed. St. Louis: Mosby, 1995, pp. 454–483.

Scoles, PV. Neonatal musculoskeletal disorders. In Fanaroff, AA, & Martin, RJ (Eds.). Neonatal-Perinatal Medicine: Diseases of the Fetus and Infant. St. Louis: Mosby, 1992, pp. 1396–1403.

Scott, KG, Urbano, JC, & Boussy, CA. Long-term psychoeducational outcome of prenatal substance exposure. Seminars in Perinatology, 15:317–323, 1991.

Semmler, CJ. A Guide to Care and Management of Very Low Birth Weight Infants: A Team Approach. Tucson, AZ: Therapy Skill Builders, 1989.

Shapiro, C. Pain in the neonate: Assessment and intervention. Neonatal Network, 8(1):7–21, 1989.

Shaw, N. Assessment and management of hematologic dysfunction. In Kenner, C, Lott, J, & Flandermeyer, A (Eds.). Comprehensive Neonatal Nursing: A Physiologic Perspective. Philadelphia: WB Saunders, 1998, pp. 520–563.

Shelton, TL, & Stepanek, JS. Excerpts from family-centered care for children needing specialized health and developmental services. Pediatric Nursing, 21:362–364, 1995.

Shepherd, RB. Brachial plexus injury. In Campbell, SK (Ed.). Pediatric

Neurologic Physical Therapy, 2nd ed. New York: Churchill Livingstone, 1991, pp. 101–130.

Shiao, SPK, Chang, Y, Lannon, H, & Yarandi, H. Meta-analysis of the effects on nonnutritive sucking on heart rate and peripheral oxygenation: Research from the past 30 years. Issues in Comprehensive Pediatric Nursing, 20:11–24, 1997.

Shields-Poe, D, & Pinelli, J. Variables associated with parental stress in neonatal intensive care units. Neonatal Network, 16:29–37, 1997.

Shlossman, PA, Manley, JS, Sciscione, AC, & Colmorgen, GH. An analysis of neonatal morbidity and mortality in maternal (in utero) and neonatal transports at 24–34 weeks gestation. American Journal of Perinatology, 14:449–456, 1997.

Silverman, WA. Incubator-baby side shows. Pediatrics, 64:127–141, 1979.

Sinha, SK, D'Souza, SW, Rivlin, E, & Chiswick, ML. Ischaemic brain lesions diagnosed at birth in preterm infants: Clinical events and developmental outcome. Archives of Disease in Childhood, 65:1017–1020, 1990.

Soll, RF. Synthetic surfactant for respiratory distress syndrome in preterm infants. The Cochrane Library (Oxford), CD 001149, 2002.

Standley, J, & Moore, R. Therapeutic effects of music and mother's voice on premature infants. Pediatric Nursing, 21:509–512, 1995.

Stevens, B, & Franck, L. Special needs of preterm infants in the management of pain and discomfort. Journal of Gynecologic and Neonatal Nursing, 24:856–861, 1995.

Stork, EK. Extracorporeal membrane oxygenation. In Fanaroff, AA, & Martin, RJ (Eds.). Neonatal-Perinatal Medicine: Diseases of the Fetus and Infant. St. Louis: Mosby, 1992, pp. 876–882.

Stout, AU, & Stout, T. Retinopathy of prematurity. Pediatric Clinics of North America, 50:77–87, 2003.

Streissguth, AP. The behavioral teratology of alcohol: Performance, behavioral, and intellectual deficits in prenatally exposed children. In West, JR (Ed.). Alcohol and Brain Development. New York: Oxford University Press, 1986, pp. 3–44.

Sweeney, JK. Physiologic adaptation of neonates to neurological assessment. Physical and Occupational Therapy in Pediatrics, 6(3/4):155–170, 1986.

Sweeney, JK, & Swanson, MW. Low birth weight infants: Neonatal care and follow-up. In Umphred, DA (Ed.). Neurological Rehabilitation, 4th ed. St. Louis: Mosby, 2001, pp. 203–258.

Sweeney, JK, Heriza, CB, Reilly, MA, Smith, C, & VanSant, AF. Practice guidelines for the physical therapist in the neonatal intensive care unit (NICU). Pediatric Physical Therapy, 11:119–132, 1999.

Sweeney, JK, & Chandler, LS. Neonatal physical therapy: Medical risks and professional education. Infants and Young Children, 2(3):59–68, 1990.

Taddio, A, Nulman, I, Koren, BS, Stevens, B, & Koren, G. A revised measure of acute pain in infants. Journal of Pain and Symptom Management, 6:456–463, 1995.

Tappit-Emas, E. Spina bifida. In Tecklin, JS (Ed.). Pediatric Physical Therapy, 3rd ed. Philadelphia: Lippincott/Williams & Wilkins, 1999, pp. 163–222.

Taylor, KJ, & Dalbec, S. Use of a pressure-reducing cushion in a neonatal setting. Journal of Enterostomal Therapy, 16:137–138, 1989.

Teberg, A, Hodgman, JE, Wu, PYK, & Spears, RL. Recent improvements in outcome for the small premature infant. Clinical Pediatrics, 16:307–313, 1977.

Tessier, R, Cristo, M, Velez, S, Giron, M, & De-Calume, ZF. Kangaroo mother care and the bonding hypothesis. Pediatrics, 102:e17, 1998.

Thelan, E, & Smith, LB. A Dynamic Systems Approach to the Development of Cognition and Action. Cambridge, Massachusetts: The MIT Press, 1994.

Thom, VA. Physical therapy: Follow-up of the special-care infant. In Ballard, RA (Ed.). Pediatric Care of the ICN Graduate. Philadelphia: WB Saunders, 1988, pp. 86–93.

Thomas, KA. How the NICU environment sounds to a preterm infant. Maternal Child Nursing, 14:249–251, 1989.

Tronick, EZ, & Beeghly, M. Prenatal cocaine exposure, child development, and the compromising effects of cumulative risk. Clinics in Perinatology, 26(1):151–171, 1999.

Unanue, RA. The effect of parent education on the motor performance of premature infants and parent caregiving abilities. Unpublished doctoral dissertation, MCP Hahnemann University, Philadelphia, 2002.

Valls-I-Soler, A, Alvarez, FJ, & Gastiasoro, E. Liquid ventilation: From experimental to clinical application. Biology of the Neonate, 80(Suppl 1):29–33, 2001.

Vannucci, R. Hypoxia-Ischemia: Clinical aspects. In Fanaroff, AA, & Martin, RJ (Eds.). Neonatal-Perinatal Medicine: Diseases of the Fetus and Infant. St. Louis: Mosby, 1997, pp. 856–876.

Vidyasagar, D. The organization of a neonatal intensive care unit. In Vidyasagar, D, & Sarnaik, AP (Eds.). Neonatal and Pediatric Intensive Care. Littleton, MA: Publishing Sciences Group, 1985, pp. 344–347.

Vohr, BR, Coll, CG, Lobato, D, Yunis, KA, O'Dea, C, & Oh, W. Neurodevelopmental and medical status of low-birthweight survivors of bronchopulmonary dysplasia at 10 to 12 years of age. Developmental Medicine and Child Neurology, 33:690–697, 1991.

Volpe, JJ. Brain injury in the premature infant: Neuropathology, clinical aspects, and pathogenesis. MRDD Research Review, 3:3–12, 1997.

Volpe, JJ. Neurologic outcome of prematurity. Archives of Neurology, 55:297–300, 1998.

Volpe, JJ. (Ed.). Neurology of the Newborn, 2nd ed. Philadelphia: WB Saunders, 1987.

Volpe, JJ. (Ed.). Neurology of the Newborn, 4th ed. Philadelphia: WB Saunders, 2001.

Waber, B, Hubler, EG, & Padden, ML. Clinical observations. A comparison of outcomes in demand versus schedule formula-fed premature infants. Nutrition in Clinical Practice, 13:132–135, 1998.

Wagoman, MJ, Shutack, JG, & Moomjian, AS. Improved oxygenation and lung compliance with prone positioning of neonates. Journal of Pediatrics, 94:787–791, 1979.

Walsh, MC, Carlo, WA, & Miller, MJ. Respiratory diseases of the newborn. In Carlo, WA, & Chatburn, RL (Eds.). Neonatal Respiratory Care. Chicago: YearBook, 1988, pp. 260–288.

Wang, YH, Su, BH, Wu, SF, Chen, AC, & Lin, TW. Clinical analysis of necrotizing enterocolitis with intestinal perforation in premature infants. Acta Paediatrics Taiwan, 43(4):199–203, 2002.

Ward, KG. A TEAM approach to NICU care. RN, 62:47–49, 1999.

Weibley, TT. Inside the incubator. Maternal Child Nursing, 14:96–100, 1989.

West, JR, Perrotta, DM, & Erickson, CK. Fetal alcohol syndrome: A review for Texas physicians. Texas Medicine, 94:61–67, 1998.

Whaley, LF, & Wong, DL. Nursing Care of Infants and Children, 4th ed. St. Louis: Mosby, 1991.

Whaley, SE, O'Connor, MJ, & Gunderson, B. Comparison of the adaptive functioning of children prenatally exposed to alcohol to a nonexposed clinical sample. Alcoholism: Clinical and Experimental Research, 25(7):1018–1024, 2001.

White, JC, Smith, MM, Lowman, DK, Reidy, TG, Murphy, SM., & Lane, SJ. Parent support of feeding in the neonatal intensive care unit: Perspectives of parents and occupational therapists. Physical and Occupational Therapy in Pediatrics, 19:111–126, 2000.

Wilhelm, IJ. The neurologically suspect neonate. In Campbell, SK (Ed.). Pediatric Neurologic Physical Therapy, 2nd ed. New York: Churchill Livingstone, 1991, pp. 67–100.

Willis, WO. Parental perspectives on the system of care for low birth weight infants. Infants & Young Children, 3:v–x, 1991.

Wolfson, MR, Jackson, JC, DeLemos, R, & Fuhrman, BP. Partial liquid ventilation with perflubron in premature infants with severe respiratory distress syndrome. The LiquiVent Study Group. New England Journal of Medicine, 335:761–767, 1996.

Wolfson, MR, Greenspan, JS, Deoras, KS, Allen, JL, & Shaffer, TH. Effect of position on the mechanical interaction between the rib cage and abdomen in preterm infants. Journal of Applied Physiology, 72:1032–1038, 1992.

World Health Organization. International Classification of Functioning, Disability, and Health: ICF. Geneva: World Health Organization, 2001, pp. 3–25.

Wortley, PM , Lindegren, ML, & Fleming, PL. Successful implementation of perinatal HIV prevention guidelines. Morbidity and Mortality Weekly Review, 50(RR06):15–28, 2001.

Yeh, TF, Lilien, LD, Leu, ST, & Pildes, RS. Increased O_2 consumption and energy loss in premature infants following medical care procedures. Biology of the Neonate, 46:157–162, 1984.

Yost, CC, & Soll, RF. Early versus delayed selective surfactant treatment for neonatal respiratory distress syndrome. The Cochrane Library (Oxford), CD001456, 2002.

Chapter 36

PRIVATE PRACTICE PEDIATRIC PHYSICAL THERAPY: A QUEST FOR INDEPENDENCE AND SUCCESS

VENITA S. LOVELACE-CHANDLER
PT, PhD, PCS

BENJAMIN R. LOVELACE-CHANDLER
PT, PhD, PCS

The first edition of this text (Campbell, 1994) described the health care climate of the 1960s and 1970s, when many physical therapists were opposed to the private enterprise arena and when private practice therapists were described in unprofessional terms

(Guglielmo, 1988). The changes of the 1980s and early 1990s resulted in a strong, independent private sector that had been accepted as an ideal rather than an abomination in physical therapy (Carlson, 1987). Since that time, a profession has been defined by autonomy, public image, and income more than specialty or discipline (Wood, 1986), and society's value of a professional service has been judged by the extent of private practice (Cooper, 1982). The continued growth in support of private practice is evidenced by the activities of the American Physical Therapy Association (APTA). In 2001 and 2002, articles supporting private practice were published in *PT Magazine*, a publication of the APTA (Johnson, 2002; Smith, 2001; Wilson, 2002), and beginning in September 2003 and continuing into 2004, a series of articles to assist the private practitioner were published (Connell, 2003; Farmer, 2004; Ries, 2004; Wilson, 2004). The growth of private practice has been slow and may have hindered the development of professionalism within physical therapy. The APTA has launched multiple initiatives to increase professionalism and the perception of physical therapy as a doctoring profession. Support of private practice appears to be important to the professional organization as a whole.

The issue of slow growth in private practice may be of particular concern to pediatric services because the number of physical therapists limiting their private practices to pediatrics, although unknown, is perceived to be extremely small. Of 1609 respondents to a 1992 survey on private practice (Private Practice Section, 1992), only 26.6% indicated that pediatric services were among the services offered by their practices. Furthermore, 10 of 13 clinical service areas were predicted to expand in private practice to a greater extent than pediatric services, with only cardiopulmonary and mental health services predicted to have less growth. The 1996 survey on private practice (Private Practice Section, 1996) did not seek information relative to type of service. Membership in the Private Practice Section (PPS) of APTA at that time was approximately 3600, having decreased from approximately 4300 in 1992. In December 1998, PPS membership was below 3000. The trend appears to have reversed, and the 2004 membership statistics (Private Practice Section, 2004) indicate that the membership has grown to 3673.

Pediatric private practice may still be quite limited. Approximately 17% of members responded to the latest PPS Membership Survey, and 74% of those respondents listed their primary practice area as orthopedics (Private Practice Section, 2004). Only 1.2% of respondents listed their primary specialty as pediatrics, and only 2.4% indicated that pediatrics was a secondary specialty. Less than 1% of respondents indicated that they held a special certification in pediatrics. Although the question asked in 1992 seeking information about the inclusion of pediatric services among offered services has not been repeated in subsequent surveys, the responses do not appear to indicate a growth in pediatric private practice, and in fact, the number of practitioners in pediatric private practice appears to have decreased.

The motivators for establishing a private practice include greater patient contact, larger income, independence, autonomy, fulfilling community or client needs, and prestige (Cole, 1986; Smoyak, 1986; Wood, 1986, Wilson, 2002). Pediatric physical therapists should be interested in pursuing these goals. Our experience in pediatric private practice was initiated with motivations for independence in decision making and the desire to reduce the length of the chain of command. Each of us had held more than one employed physical therapy administrative position, yet neither of us had been satisfied with the control that existed at that level of authority. In every instance, a higher administrator determined staffing patterns, equipment purchases, funding for continuing education, and often the types and amount of physical therapy services to be offered. Frequently, services were selected for productivity rather than to address the best interests of clients or families, and rates were established to recover costs elsewhere in the institution rather than to reflect the costs of providing physical therapy. Often, we were thwarted in efforts to design services that were based on our philosophy of best practice.

In 1982, one of us was in an employed administrative position experiencing these negative factors when the decision was made to begin a private practice. The practice was established as a sole proprietorship with the therapist/owner who provided treatment and a spouse/therapist who volunteered as business manager, bookkeeper, and billing specialist. We selected a sole proprietorship, the legal title for a business with one owner (Gwinn, 2002), because the organizational structure is simple, the paperwork is minimal, and governmental restrictions are few. For example, our practice was opened by merely ordering business cards.

In our case, the spouse was satisfied in an employed position and provided financial security during the first 2 years of the practice, including health, dental, and life insurance. The spouse had 2 years of experience as an insurance filing clerk and the willingness to work part time for the practice. With sufficient resources and the desire to be independent in professional practice, the business was established and flourished. Even during difficult periods, the owner experienced enormous control, independence, and job satisfaction, and both of us were delighted with the financial gain, which exceeded expectations.

More physical therapists must seek the private practice setting if increased recognition as a profession is to be achieved, and pediatric physical therapists must be among those practitioners who accept the risks and rewards that accompany private practice. A paucity of material related to pediatric private practice is available and may help to explain the small number of pediatric private practitioners. This chapter is written for the physical therapist who may be considering developing a pediatric private practice or for the student who may wish to learn about a possible work setting, that of the full-time independent pediatric practitioner. The purposes of this chapter are to (1) define the private practitioner, including characteristics and responsibilities; (2) provide information on risk management concepts for establishing and maintaining a private practice; (3) present current trends in private practice; and (4) provide insight into the uniqueness of a pediatric private practice through a description of one experience.

Most published research and information on topics related to private practice are specific to adults. In this chapter, information from other professions and adult services has been extrapolated for application to pediatric physical therapy, and no evidence can be offered for the appropriateness of this extrapolation. We hope that the chapter will provide informative reading and direction for the pediatric physical therapist beginning a private practice and will allow the reader to avoid many of the mistakes and problems of our early years. A revelation to us in preparing this chapter was the quantity of information available to the therapist interested in private practice relative to how little we knew as beginners. Our intent is for the entrepreneurial pediatric therapist or student to be encouraged and to use the information of this chapter in a quest for the independence and success available in private practice.

THE PRIVATE PRACTITIONER

HISTORY AND DEFINITION

Although the origin of physical therapy private practice is difficult to ascertain, evidence exists that a few therapists were engaged in such practices in the 1950s and that these therapists exchanged information regarding the private practice setting during a meeting at the 1954 Annual Conference of the APTA (Dicus, 1991). In 1955, the APTA responded to a request from private practice therapists by establishing a steering committee to make recommendations on the advisability of creating a Self-Employed Section. The committee members perceived defining who constituted a self-employed therapist as one of the most difficult problems in the development of the section. Dicus (1991) noted that this difficulty in clearly delineating the private practitioner resulted in such problems as uncertainty regarding the philosophy of the section, a lack of common ground among members, diversity in educational needs, and misunderstanding of governmental regulations. The problems persisted during the section's formative years and during the evolution into the current PPS (renamed in 1975) (Reuss, 1991). In 1996, the section's board recommended a name change to the Section on Business Practice (PPS Impact, 1997). At the PPS General Business Meeting, members voted to retain the existing name. The 1996 survey (Private Practice Section, 1996) indicated a discrepancy regarding future focus of the PPS. Several members wanted to welcome corporation members, but the majority of respondents looked to the section to protect the interests of PT-owned independent practices (Valente, 1996). The 2004 survey (Private Practice Section, 2004) revealed that 88% of the respondents were owners or partners in a private practice.

Frazian (1985) noted that the definition of private practice is still disputed. Between the staff therapist, employed by an institution, and the independent therapist, owner of a practice or corporation, are innumerable therapists who are establishing lifestyles and professional private practices to meet the needs of society and themselves. Examples of the variety of private practices include performing a few hours of home health care services in addition to a full-time employed position, working part time in an employed position and part time as owner of a practice, and providing numerous hours

through several contractual arrangements. Contracting denotes assuming responsibility for providing clinical services in a particular setting for a fixed payment (Bernstein, 1986). Contractors are self-employed and have differing financial processes in regard to income tax, Social Security tax, and retirement funds, but little difference may be noted in the actual provision of clinical services by employees or contractors. A 2003 article (Connell) on starting a private practice suggests that one way to acquire the knowledge essential to private practice is to become an independent contractor and bill by the hour or by the appointment.

Although Brown (1992) questions the use of the term *private practice* and alludes to every physical therapist as an independent practitioner with a high level of decision-making ability and professionalism, the guidelines in this chapter are directed to a very specific practitioner whom we have defined as follows: *The private practice physical therapist has autonomy, uses minimal bureaucracy, practices according to professional values, and takes risks to achieve financial and professional independence and success.*

Autonomy

A frequent misconception is that any therapist contracting for services is a private practitioner (Faust & Meaker, 1991). Private practice is more than having a contract with an agency or a facility. The first requirement of self-employment is the ability to function in an autonomous manner as a businessperson. When one giant corporation enters into a business relationship with another corporation, autonomous practice is absent, and this arrangement is no more a private practice than the per diem therapist who engages in a contractual relationship with a large health care institution. Selker (1995) cautions that a managed health care system has goals that are increasingly determined by managerial issues rather than the issues of an autonomous practitioner. He asks whether autonomy needs to be shared. A hybrid model has been suggested for persons who want to own a practice but are concerned about solo responsibilities (Connell, 2003). Companies offer physical therapists a practice, but the corporation retains a majority share of ownership. The therapist has an assured paycheck, and the corporation assumes responsibility for insurance and some business decisions. The practitioner may be rewarded for growth, but disadvantages of this model include corporation approval for some decisions, thereby reducing autonomy. The financial income may be limited related to the percentage of ownership, and options for exiting the business in a beneficial manner may be minimal.

Pediatric physical therapists must be willing to assume autonomy in managing the practice, designing and offering services, implementing marketing strategies, billing for services, establishing relationships with children and families, and consulting with other professionals and agencies, but these practitioners may need to be flexible in sharing autonomy in order to maintain business success.

Minimal Bureaucracy

Private practice is characterized by low levels of internal bureaucracy as opposed to the management style of a typical corporation (Faust & Meaker, 1991). Private practitioners are free to choose a streamlined bookkeeping system and may have less paperwork than that required by agencies. Within the boundaries established by licensure laws, the rules and standards for continuing education, promotion, supervision and delegation, and collegial consultation can be established without approval from other administrative bodies. Decisions regarding equipment purchases, budgeting, and secretarial support are made by the owner, often the sole practitioner, but may in larger practices include input from other appropriate employees. Pediatric therapists must be willing to exercise independent decision making and must understand that supervisors, department directors, and administrators are usually not available to assist (or resist) the private practitioner's decisions. Olsen (1999) suggests that private practitioners are leaders in new delivery models because of the ability to quickly respond to changing needs.

Professional Practice

Professional values and norms direct the behavior of the private practice organization. Corporations, including health agencies, often use marketing forces and business perspectives to determine organizational structure and behavior. Although knowledge and use of business principles are essential to survival in private practice, the services must be offered in a manner in which professional standards are paramount and supersede financial considerations. Wood (1986) suggests that private practice is more a philosophy than a work setting and that professional success can be achieved without financial success, but we believe that financial success in private practice cannot be achieved without quality services. The pediatric physical therapist in private practice will find that the business will be successful only when professionalism and quality coexist with financial concerns to offer the consumer a service worth purchasing. The *Guide to Physical Therapist Practice* (American Physical Therapy Association, 2001) is essential for the pediatric therapist.

The *Guide* describes the elements of accepted practice, standardizes practice terminology, and provides preferred practice patterns. The practice patterns are based on expert opinion and describe acceptable intervention strategies and procedures (Hack, 1998).

Professionalism has been identified as critical to physical therapy in achieving status as a doctoring profession. In 2002, the APTA held a consensus conference to determine the core values of the profession and the indicators (judgments, decisions, attitudes, and behaviors) of those values (Bezner, 2004). Seven core values are described as essential to professionalism: accountability, altruism, compassion/caring, excellence, integrity, professional duty, and social responsibility. Definitions and indicators for each core value are provided to assist practitioners in decision making in daily practice.

Risk Taking

The great risks involved in initiating a private practice, including costs, the potential for mistakes, and competing with physicians or others in the marketplace have been cited by several authors (Cole, 1986; Flower, 1986; Kooper & Sullivan, 1986; McClain et al., 1992; Olsen, 1999; Parish, 1986; Walker, 1977; Wood, 1986; Woody, 1986). Many practicing therapists are not interested in management and avoid the business responsibilities and attention to detail required in private practice (Deaton, 1992b; Walker, 1977). Many small businesses with marketable services or products fail because the initial financial resources are exhausted before income can be produced (Walker, 1977) or because business responsibilities have been mismanaged.

One characteristic of private practice is the personal assumption of risk and the realization that service delivery within private enterprise carries the opportunity to fail (Wood, 1986). Areas of potential risk include financial, professional, personal relationships, and legal aspects. Pediatric private practitioners must have sufficient general knowledge of business management to understand basic principles and to seek qualified counsel when needed. Although many risks will be present at the onset of the practice, additional risks are associated with expansion of an established practice, whether the expansion involves purchasing equipment, hiring additional personnel, or changing office space (Cole, 1986). Three important considerations before starting a private practice are that (1) risk taking involves the possibility of either negative or positive outcome; (2) risk management fosters positive outcome and allows entering risky situations with hope as opposed to avoiding risky situations for fear of negative results; and (3) methods for minimizing risks have been identified and are available for use by new private practitioners (McFadden & Hanschu, 1985).

Baskin (1997) describes starting a practice in 1992 when many private practitioners were joining corporations or closing practices. He indicates 4 years later that private practice gives the therapist the highest level of accountability and that the greatest risks result in the largest rewards. One private practitioner indicated an appreciation that her own productivity resulted in her financial survival (Wilson, 2002). Pediatric physical therapists still have options for initiating private practices, but consideration of risk factors must be paramount.

PERSONAL AND PROFESSIONAL CHARACTERISTICS

Although Walker (1977) advocates that only experienced physical therapists should consider entering private practice, a setting he considers unsuited for the novice, physical therapy will not achieve increased recognition as a profession until more practitioners seek the private practice setting. New graduates and other therapists may enter this arena if personal characteristics and professional skills are compatible with private practice. The person drawn to private practice is attracted primarily by the opportunity to be self-governed and by the desire to be one's own boss (Cole, 1986; Wilson, 2002). The private practitioner is focused on self-control, independence, self-governance, and diversity of tasks. Expertise or specialization is necessary to the success of a practice. Wood (1986) offers the following two very direct statements that should be carefully considered by the therapist interested in private practice: "If you don't have anything to market, stay out of the marketplace" (p. 6), and "It is impossible to be too blunt with yourself when assessing your skills and expertise" (p. 7).

Walker (1977) suggests that the physical therapist in private practice must possess the following seven traits:

1. The therapist needs good physical and mental health to sustain the long hours and work stress. Good health helps to maintain coping mechanisms and manage the interference with routine often associated with a new private practice.
2. The ability to develop strong relationships with clients, physicians, and other health care personnel is essential to the business aspects of the practice, and the ability to maintain a supportive relationship with family and friends is essential to personal well-being.
3. Self-discipline, including adherence to a self-imposed schedule, timely devotion to business details, and self-initiation skills, is crucial to the private practitioner. The therapist who functions best when responsible for someone else's schedule and goals should remain in an employed position.
4. An interest in business management and such subjects as accounting, bookkeeping, and economics is necessary for financial success. The ability to handle personal finances and to promptly manage personal bank accounts, tax files, real estate issues, insurance coverage and claims, and savings accounts might provide insight into the probability of successful business management.
5. Good oral and written communication skills are important to successful interaction with clients, physicians, third-party payers, and other health care personnel. Private practitioners must be comfortable with face-to-face professional contacts with the intent of securing referrals, with technical report writing to enhance reimbursement, and with difficult situations such as collecting payment from clients.
6. Professional training and experience must be adequate for the services to be marketed. Self-advancement and self-directed learning are essential to building a successful private practice.
7. Dedication and determination to address the problems as well as the promises of a private practice are necessary for successful risk management.

Olsen (1999) suggests that private practice enhances leadership traits because the owner has the opportunity to establish circumstances and to hire staff members appropriate to the leadership style of the owner. The private practitioner facilitates interrelationships, identifies opportunities, and becomes a leader of staff.

The Committee on Private Practice of the American Speech-Language-Hearing Association (ASHA) (1991) provides 13 personal characteristics that should be considered when initiating a private practice: necessary experience, an established reputation, good clinical skills, an affinity for the work, willingness and ability to work long hours for a few years, handling a challenge, learning what is not known, acceptance of no or low income for a period of time, desire for a private practice, family support, stress management, strong self-image, and a network or support system. Physical therapy private practitioners also will find these characteristics to be essential.

Cole (1986), writing about speech-language pathology and audiology but offering advice applicable to any private practitioner, cautions that individuals should examine their professional practice attitudes and personal characteristics in relation to the roles that must be assumed as business owner, manager, and clinician. The business aspects of owning and managing a private practice are often shocking to therapists who consider their work as a service to be given to clients. Therapists must be willing to regard services as a product to be sold for a profit but realize that most of the time and energy for the first year or more will be devoted to building the practice without experiencing any profit.

All health care professionals who engage in private practice probably do so for similar professional reasons. Smoyak (1986) noted that private practice offers psychiatric nurses the advantages of maximal autonomy for patients and professionals with little bureaucratic red tape and interference with professional judgment. The author offers the following comment:

> Patients, if they can afford it or have insurance that will allow it, can freely select the practitioner of their choice, using such criteria as age, sex, race, credentials, style, location, availability, cost, educational background, and recommendation of others. Theoretically, this freedom to select the therapist may increase the probability that the treatment will be helpful. Similarly, therapists' freedom to concentrate on specific treatments and kinds of patients should enhance their clinical skills. A fee-for-service system, with practitioners earning income by hours spent in treating patients, tends to maximize productivity and minimize time spent on paperwork, meetings, and other non-revenue producing functions (Smoyak, 1986, p. 22).

Parsons (1986) refers to private practitioners as "heroes" and "politicians" who develop expertise through limiting practice to a specialty area and letting others know about their expertise through marketing. The individual practitioner is able to use the expertise in a practice area for visibility and clarity about capabilities and limitations. For example, the practice may be limited to a specific age range, such as infants and toddlers, preschoolers, or adolescents, or to a diagnostic category, such as developmental disabilities or orthopedics. The therapist should learn how services are perceived by different segments of the community where the practice will be established and market services that address consumer needs. The ability to develop referral sources depends on others' perceptions of the therapist's competence, which is influenced by professional visibility and charisma. Building a caseload requires offering unique services, accepting third-party payment, providing flexible scheduling, meeting with physicians and other health care professionals, being competent, giving speeches, meeting local health needs, cultivating personal referral sources, and achieving professional visibility. Speaking to community groups, giving workshops, publishing, and participating in professional activities increase visibility. In our practice, free services were provided to clients who had no funding in order to establish relationships with physicians who were sending referrals to pediatric centers that required reimbursement. Calling the physicians regarding client issues, writing thorough reports, and providing follow-up letters to referral sources were practices that contributed to the rapid expansion of our referral base. After only 1 month, client referrals were sufficient to meet operating costs of the practice and to provide a very minimal salary.

Glinn (2002) suggests that many seemingly outstanding therapists have mediocre practices while many seemingly mediocre therapists have substantial income, a possible symbol of an outstanding practice. He states that ability, access, and atmosphere are each equally important to a successful practice. Ability includes business, clinical, and marketing skills. Access includes availability and ease of scheduling appointments, accepting contracts, membership provider panels and network memberships, and the location of the practice. Atmosphere provides a positive experience and the tone for the practice culture. Atmosphere is a strong internal marketing tool accomplished by cleanliness, congeniality, professionalism, and team eagerness exhibited by talented people willing to realize their potential. Pediatric private practitioners will want atmospheres that are comfortable for children and their families.

The Small Business Administration (SBA) is a federal funding entity that provides support to owners of small businesses. The mission of the SBA is to strengthen the economy by assisting and protecting the interests of small business. The website of the SBA (www.sba.gov) provides a variety of materials related to starting and managing a business. The site suggests that necessary skills include a working knowledge of basic record keeping; financial management; personnel management; market analysis; breakeven analysis; product or service knowledge; federal, state, and local taxes; legal structure; and communication skills. Of these basic skills, the typical therapist will possess service knowledge and communication skills. The SBA website can be used to obtain information to develop the other needed skills. For example the financing information includes details on financing basics, estimating costs, finding capital, personal versus business financing, applying for a loan, startup costs, and financial statements. The SBA has links to other helpful sites including to a free online course for small business owners. The topics covered in the course are comprehensive, and the course includes quizzes and feedback.

Deaton (1992a), a frequent speaker at the annual meetings of the PPS, has complimented physical therapists in private practice. He indicated the respect he had for the education and body of knowledge of physical therapy. As new graduates, therapists enter a complex health care system with a maze of administrative, reimbursement, social, and clinical issues. Therapists survive the maze, providing quality services to clients with a wide range of impairments and functional limitations. As if this feat were not enough, an increasing number of therapists decide to enter the private enterprise arena. The skills required to be a successful business owner are not possessed (or even known).

Deaton's description certainly fit our business adventure. The owner and spouse possessed several but not all of the professional characteristics recommended as essential. Clinical skills in the area of pediatrics were varied and advanced. We both had 11 years of pediatric experience, master's degrees that included coursework in pediatric physical therapy, doctoral degrees in health education, and certification in specific clinical techniques such as neurodevelopmental treatment. The owner had administrative experience from serving as a physical therapy department director in an outpatient pediatric physical therapy center, as director of physical therapy at a residential facility for 1200 clients with developmental disabilities, and as the director of rehabilitation at an urban children's medical center. An interest in business management, accounting, bookkeeping, and economics was absolutely lacking, and the business aspects of owning and managing the practice were shocking to us. We were anxious to implement our philosophy of care and anticipated the outstanding services that we would offer children and families, but we never considered cash flow problems, third-party payers who provided reimbursement but only after months of delay, families who received payment from third-party payers and spent the funds on personal expenditures, parents who were offended when asked for payment, and funding agencies who refused to reimburse for outpatient services provided by a private practitioner in an office or home when identical outpatient services were reimbursable if provided in a hospital or center by the same practitioner.

The spouse had 2 years of experience in insurance processing, and all billing was done in evening hours. For the first 12 years, only one client who was expected to pay failed to do so. Our collection rate was incredible, but the toll on personal lives, marriage, and children cannot be overestimated. If we had been aware of the business aspects of private practice and our obvious deficiencies in management, the practice would still have been initiated, but we would have sought assistance from others earlier and would not have considered ourselves as failures because of the reimbursement, tax, accounting, and record-keeping problems. Physical therapists who desire to enter private practice in pediatrics must develop business skills or purchase business services from others if professional and personal satisfaction is to be optimal. Prior authorization in order to receive reimbursement for services became a factor during the last several years of our practice. Most reimbursement issues were between our corporation and third-party payers. Families were rarely involved in the reimbursement process except occasionally to advocate with their reimbursement entity if payment for services was being denied.

Jayaratne and colleagues (1991) found that although the need for a continuous supply of clients and concerns over the business aspects of a private practice may produce stress in social workers, the private practice setting created less strain than agency settings. Social workers in private practice reported fewer psychologic and health strains, higher levels of performance, and better feelings about their life circumstances. These authors suggested that individuals who seek private practice may differ from employed individuals by being healthier from the beginning, having characteristics that foster health, serving kinds of clients that produce less stress in the practitioner, or experiencing different psychosocial aspects of business in the private practice arena. We believe that the private practice environment has afforded more happiness and better mental health for the owner than any previous employed position. The spouse has been able to experience many of the rewards of the practice through a sense of accomplishment, less marital stress, and greater financial gains.

PERSONAL AND PROFESSIONAL RESPONSIBILITIES

Standards of practice, preferred practice patterns, and statements of ethical principles and conduct have been developed by the APTA (2000a, 2000b, 2001a, 2001b, 2002, 2003). Although these standards and statements apply universally to members of that association and may be adopted by nonmember physical therapists and physical therapist assistants, ethical behavior is situational, and specific circumstances may determine the manner in which the ethical principles are applied. We have perceived that employed therapists have greater ethical expectations of private practitioners than of themselves or other employed therapists. Flower (1986) determined that speech-language pathologists and audiologists perceive private practice as entailing unique ethical considerations and responsibilities that are more challenging than the ethical concerns of employed therapists, suggesting that increased expectations for private practitioners are not unique to the profession of physical therapy. He suggests that although private practitioners may engage in unethical practices such as treating clients with dubious prognoses, maintaining clients endlessly in treatment programs, making recommendations without regard for economic impact, and failing to obtain informed consent, employed therapists commit the same unprofessional behaviors. Ethical considerations remain similar regardless of the delivery system, and personal and professional responsibilities for quality services at reasonable cost are not limited to the private practice environment.

Wood (1986) notes that certain aspects of professional morality underlie the spirit of ethical principles and that these aspects include responsibility, integrity, and competence. Institutions frequently provide administrative leadership that reduces individual professional responsibility, or at least perceived responsibility, and institutions are able to compensate for limited professional competence in one practitioner through supervision by or use of other practitioners. In institutions, several therapists may collaborate on difficult ethical decisions and produce a superior decision, but poor ethical decisions by one therapist may also be concealed and the therapist protected by other staff members. Concerns regarding ethical practice should be heeded by physical therapists because sheltering and protection are not usually available to private practitioners in any profession.

Flower (1986) suggests six areas of frequent ethical dilemmas for private practitioners that, if monitored appropriately, produce ethical practices: professional competence (practitioner and employees), confidentiality and informed consent, fees and financial activities, marketing and advertisement, relationships, and product recommendation and dispensing. The reader is referred to Flower's work for a comprehensive discussion of each area. The new core values defined for the profession of physical therapy apply to all members of the APTA and not only to private practitioners (Bezner, 2004). We suggest that the pediatric physical therapist in private practice may ethically provide services to any patient unless a misfit exists between the patient's needs and the therapist's skills. A sole practitioner may be more limited in treatment strategies than therapists in a hospital or group practice. A practitioner should seek advice or make referral to another therapist if other strategies are warranted. Private practitioners are cautioned that pride, an unwillingness to limit a practice, and fear of economic loss may prevent admission of shortcomings.

The Code of Ethics of the APTA (2000a) and the guides for conduct (APTA, 2000b, 2001a, 2002) are valuable resources for all private practitioners. Additionally, the Section on Pediatrics of the APTA offers documents to assist pediatric practitioners in offering ethical and appropriate services (Scull & Deitz, 1989; Task Force on Early Intervention, 1991; Sweeney et al., 1999). Both the Section on Pediatrics and PPS provide sources for articles, commentaries, and other information of value to private practitioners through such publications as *Pediatric Physical Therapy* and *PPS Impact*. Adhering to the regulations regarding state licensure and pursuing development through continuing education will assist in maintaining ethical and competent practice.

The SBA suggests developing a company ethics policy. Ethics originates at the top of an organization, and owners of private practices should establish a well-defined ethics policy and the related standards of conduct to increase employee morale and commitment that may lead to higher profits, as well. Profits should not be the motivating factor, and the policy should help define how the practice relates to society and helps to fulfill the greater good. The ethics policy will be a reflection of the important values of the practice.

RISK MANAGEMENT IN ESTABLISHING A PRIVATE PRACTICE

Walker (1977) notes that no clear-cut "how to" methods exist for establishing a professional office, but several considerations and procedures are recommended. Knowledge of the process might lessen the mistakes, risks, and costs, thereby increasing the rewards for the pediatric therapist beginning a private practice. Sims (1992) suggests identifying and building the practice desired by the individual therapist, not the practice everyone else thinks should be built. Pediatric private practitioners must determine the ages and types of disabilities of children for whom services will be provided. A subspecialty practice within the broader pediatric specialty may be appropriate.

STARTING A PRACTICE

As mentioned previously, the APTA now views private practice as important to the development of professionalism. Smith (2001) provides a compendium of resources provided by the APTA to help private practitioners state a practice. The appendix provides a listing of website resources available through the APTA. The sites provide information on starting and running a practice, managing personnel, the women's initiative program, general practice policies, and print materials available from the APTA. The APTA also offers benefits to members that may be of particular value to private practitioners. Health, life, disability, and liability insurance; credit card programs; equipment leasing programs; investment and retirement planning programs; and mentors/consultants may be accessed through the APTA. The Consulting Service allows members to be linked with qualified consultants at competitive rates (Wilson, 2002). The consultants have experience in a variety of practice management issues and provide personalized guidance. The APTA Risk Management and Member Benefit Services Department can help the private practitioners decide what type of business plan is needed and the appropriate legal structure.

Both the Private Practice Section and the Section on Health Policy and Administration provide resources and information helpful to starting a private practice. The PPS provides discounts on business services and insurance programs (Wilson, 2002). The Annual Conference of the PPS provides extensive educational workshops, and the annual PPS survey seeks topics and services desired by members. The Member Mentor Program allows member private practitioners to strengthen private practice by mentoring less experienced members who have questions or concerns about starting or managing a practice. Excellent webcasts with informative topics are available to members, and numerous books and other printed resources may be obtained from the Section (see information in Appendix 1). The Section on Health Policy and Administration website has information for all types of administrators, including private practitioners. Members have access to a listserve for the exchange of ideas and information. The International Private Practitioners Association (linked from the PPS website) is an organization serving private practitioners across the world and is associated with the World Confederation of Physical Therapy.

Niche practices are increasingly prevalent and have been suggested as a method for maintaining a private practice as reimbursement policies affect fiscal security (Huelskamp, 1997). A niche market may be a narrowly focused effort, a place or use that is unique, or a small area of specialization. Remember that the practitioner must possess the skills and expertise for the planned practice and that a niche in the marketplace must exist if success is to be obtained. Glinn (2002) suggests that most niche practices are not successful because practitioners fail to examine four internal marketing barometers and fail to make a marketing plan. The first three barometers are the no show/cancellation rate, the percent of repeat customers, and patient satisfaction survey measurements. Number of no shows should never exceed cancellations,

and both together should average less than 10% of the practice. If the practice is over 5 years old, he suggests that 10% should be former patients returning for additional care. Ninety percent of your patients (or in the case of pediatric practice, the parents) should express satisfaction on a survey. Glinn (2002) states that the first three barometers should be measured and stabilized first. Then the fourth barometer, the percentage of total patients/clients choosing to purchase a cash-based service, should be measured. The target for cash-based patients/clients should be 10%, and services that focus on fitness and aftercare should be the easiest to market. Cash-based services indicate that your practice has been identified as needed by the patient/family, and that the patient/family has become aware of your services. His examples of niche practices are for adult clients/patients. We suggest the following possibilities for niche practices for the pediatric private practitioner: hippotherapy, aquatics, dance or performing arts, sports for the young athlete or for the athlete with disability, fitness or obesity reduction, and practices limited to a specific philosophy of care such as neurodevelopmental treatment or sensory integration. Limiting practices to serving certain populations of patients might allow for more depth of interventions, and some possible populations are children with autism spectrum disorder, cerebral palsy, or cognitive impairment. Some families might be interested in cash-based group services in which the cost of care is distributed among several participants. Practices limited to meeting the health care needs and philosophy of a particular ethnic group might be successful in locations with large minority populations who feel uncomfortable in majority-oriented environments.

The SBA suggests that owners considering a niche practice should conduct a market survey and use the results to determine the niche areas already served by competitors. A table or graph can be developed to illustrate where an opening might exist for the proposed service. The owner should seek the configuration that ensures the least direct competition with other owners, or in this case, with other private practitioners or facilities.

Our practice was envisioned as an office-based practice that would provide services for young children with developmental disabilities, probably from birth to 12 years of age. The office practice never flourished as well as desired, and in the early years, few infants and toddlers were referred. A niche in the marketplace did not exist for office services for young children because most families could obtain this type of physical therapy service from a variety of outpatient treatment centers that also provided social services, educational classes for preschoolers, and other therapies. Our business became particularly successful because services were provided at schools, child care centers, or client homes as was necessary to provide ecologically based services to children. Our niche in the marketplace developed by addressing special situations such as contracting with school districts to relieve the shortage of school-based therapists, serving the children of working parents in the everyday environment of the child, providing treatment to clients receiving educational services at home, and traveling to the homes of families without transportation or to small, nearby towns where several families resided but where no services were available.

During the first 2 years, our practice was not the business we had envisioned, but autonomy, low bureaucracy, and our philosophy of care were present. Within a few years, the practice was shaped into the desired business, but even during the early years, the practice was limited to clients younger than 21 years of age. The owner declined adult clients, even though numerous referrals were received for adults with neuromuscular involvement. Continued success has been the result of blending the wishes of the owner with the needs in the marketplace.

SELECTING A LEGAL STRUCTURE

Every business organization must have a legal structure (Hampton, 1986). Numerous potential legal structures exist and should be considered by the therapist initiating a private practice. The tax obligations, financial advantages, applicable laws and liabilities, and employer and employee benefits for each legal entity are determined by federal and state regulations. An attorney and an accountant, both with expertise in small businesses, should be consulted to determine the legal form most appropriate for the planned practice and before changes are made in the legal structure of an existing practice. The county clerk and the state licensing board can provide information about the legal forms available in a specific geographic location (ASHA, 1991). Generally, an individual practice consists of a single therapist providing services for a fee through a small business, an associate private practice consists of professional and technical staff members employed and directed by one therapist, and a partnership has two or more co-owners (McClain et al., 1992). The specific legal form for each of these organizational patterns may vary. For example, a single practitioner may be a sole proprietor or the owner of a corporation.

The four common and most appropriate legal structures for a professional practice are sole proprietorship, partnership, corporation, and limited liability company (LLC) (Gwinn, 2002). As indicated previously, the sole proprietorship is the simplest form of legal structure.

Additionally, this form is used by more than half of all business organizations, and almost half of all sole proprietorships are service organizations (Hampton, 1986). The sole proprietorship is easy and inexpensive to begin and the easiest to dissolve (Gwinn, 2002). The owner has complete control over the entire practice, including profits, as long as the business follows legal guidelines. The most important disadvantage of a sole proprietorship is personal liability. The owner and the business are viewed as one entity under the law. The business debt becomes the sole proprietor's debt. This type of practice is difficult to expand, and recruitment of other therapists may be difficult because they have no possibilities for partial ownership.

Partnerships have two or more owners who enter into business together (Hampton, 1986). This legal structure is almost as simple as a sole proprietorship, but the profit, responsibilities, and liabilities are divided between the co-owners (Gwinn, 2002). Parish (1986) notes that a partnership is similar to a marriage and that this form of legal structure requires partners who are personally compatible and possess complementary abilities. One partner must have controlling interest in the business, or final decisions may be difficult to achieve. If the partnership is split equally among partners, disputes are resolved only by compromise or defeat. When disputes cannot be resolved, dissolution of the partnership may be required and also may be similar to a marriage that ends in divorce. A buy-sell agreement established at the initiation of the partnership indicates the mechanism for dissolving the partnership by allowing one partner to buy the percentage of the business held by other partners or to sell the partner's percentage to other partners or someone else. Gwinn (2002) adds that the method for admitting new partners must be determined at the outset as well. He still considers partnerships to have advantages and suggests that partners may be able to offer more variety of services because of the varying expertise of the co-owners. The SBA suggests that partnership agreements are helpful in solving disputes, but responsibilities still exist for the business actions of either partner. The partnership agreement should include such information as the type of business, the equity of each partner, the duration of partnership, the restrictions of expenditures, and the settlement in case of death.

Corporations form the most complex type of legal structure, and the use of an attorney is highly recommended by the SBA. The corporation is a legal entity, and the owner who incorporates a company becomes an employee of the corporation. High income levels may indicate the need for a corporate structure to maximize tax benefits (Sullivan, 1986). Two variations of the corporation are the S corporation and the C corporation (Gwinn, 2002). In a C corporation, taxes are paid on the profits of the corporation, and shareholders pay taxes on their profits as well. An S corporation does not tax dividends in the same manner but requires more shareholders. These structures work well for a large practice, but the laws regarding corporations change periodically and are complex. Legal counsel must be ongoing. A corporation separates business debts from personal finances and can serve to protect personal assets. This type of legal structure is enduring because ownership transfers more easily. Costs of incorporating a business vary according to the geographic location and the type of corporate structure (Sullivan, 1986). The SBA notes that a small, closely held corporation can operate informally and may not need regular board of directors' meetings and annual stockholders' meetings. However, record keeping is still required, and officers of a corporation with stockholders can be liable to stockholders for improper actions.

A limited liability company, or LLC, has the ease and tax benefits of sole proprietorships or partnerships but the protection of a corporation (Gwinn, 2002). Fewer shareholders are required, but the business must be registered like a corporation. These legal structures are ideally designed for private practices, but still require legal consultation.

For 6 years, our business was operated as a sole proprietorship, but we incorporated the practice during the seventh year. A lawyer advised that incorporation would assist in several of the tax complications relating to contracting with other therapists and would provide better liability protection for the owner. In a sole proprietorship, our home and cars could be taken to settle a business debt in the event of litigation, and we believed that our personal assets had to be safe from the liabilities of the business. The private practice pediatric therapist should seek advice from a lawyer, a tax consultant, and a financial advisor to determine the most suitable organizational structure for the proposed practice.

Hampton (1986) suggests that the private practitioner will have the final decision regarding the legal structure of the business and that the decision will be based on personal or professional needs. In our experience, we did not have the expertise to determine the best legal structure and were forced to rely on an accountant we trusted. Our accountant has changed the type of corporation once since we incorporated to better reflect the financial status of our business. Parish (1986) warns that the complexity of the tax structure for corporations requires that accountants and attorneys will be needed for the foreseeable future. We are unable to intelligently read our incorporation documents or our corporate tax forms even though the spouse had tax preparation experience

and filed all tax documents for the sole proprietorship without assistance from an accountant. We accept the premise that changes in the practice in subsequent years and changes in tax law may require adjustment in the legal structure of the business. Periodic review of the status of any pediatric private practice is recommended.

DEVELOPING A BUSINESS PLAN

A business plan is the key to obtaining financing and to business success and should be developed as soon as the type of practice has been determined (Sims, 1992). A fundamental task in business planning is to set goals and objectives for development of the practice. Formulating strategies and establishing alternative courses of action to achieve the goals must be accomplished and must include the financial, physical, and human resources necessary for goal attainment (Dillon & Duke, 1991). The SBA provides a business plan outline for a typical business consisting of an introduction, a marketing statement, a financial management statement, an operations description, and concluding statements. The introduction should give a detailed description of your practice and the goals, discuss the ownership and legal structure, list the skills and experience of the owner(s), and discuss the advantages of your practice over competitors. The marketing portion of the plan should discuss the services to be offered, the demand for services, the size of the anticipated market, the planned advertisement, and the pricing strategies. The financial management portion of the plan should explain the source and amount of initial capital, the monthly operating budget for the first year, the expected cash flow, the breakeven point, the personal method of compensation, and the maintenance of accounting records. Alternative proposals for anticipated problems should be included. The operations portion of the plan should explain daily management, discuss personnel plans, and discuss insurance, lease, or other necessary agreements. Concluding statements for the business plan will summarize the business goals and express commitment to your business.

A business plan is a form of self-education that should be developed by the private practitioner. Olsen (1999) suggests that the business plan determines the strategic direction for the practice. In addition to the previously described steps, Olsen recommends preparing a cover letter and an executive summary. Both the SBA and Olsen suggest that business associates, family, mentors, lawyers, and friends should review the business plan. The owner will learn from the process of explaining and justifying the business plan. The PPS views the business plan as among the most important steps in having a successful practice. Members are offered the opportunity to earn a certificate in business planning in collaboration with a university.

PLANNING FOR FINANCIAL RESOURCES

The financial aspects of the business plan include the initial or start-up costs for the entire practice (Sims, 1992). All expected expenses should be arranged within a monthly, quarterly, and yearly spending budget. Projected revenues for the practice should be compiled using the same time periods. Reviewing the finances and writing a short narrative on how the pediatric practice fits into the physical therapy market in the projected area will prepare the therapist to discuss the plan with other persons. Bankers, accountants, and businesspersons are able to review the feasibility of the plan. Two forms of the financial plan might be designed (Driskell, 1988). The short form should be designed to provide the lender an overview of the business. The long form complements the short form by providing detailed information to allow the practitioner to answer all questions. The two forms have the same format, but more detail is included in the longer form. The lender will need information on physical therapy in general, licensure and legal considerations, and the growth of physical therapy services. Include the types of services you will offer, referral sources, the available market, and information on your education and work experience. Provide the same information for other staff you intend to use. Explain how the loan will be used and the proposed method of repayment.

Professional assistance is recommended when designing the financial plan. Aydelotte and associates (1988) inferred that nurse entrepreneurs in private practice who sought assistance from sources other than nurses made higher incomes than nurses who sought assistance from other nurses when initially establishing a practice. These authors suggested that further research is needed to determine if assistance from sources other than nurses leads to higher income levels for private practice nurses. However, the inference is sufficient to suggest that expertise in business is critical to accurate development of a financially sound business plan and that physical therapists may not possess the knowledge necessary for financial planning for a pediatric private practice. We suggest that new practitioners seek sufficient advice to minimize financial risks.

Therapists with a written plan and an understanding of the financial risk should apply for the needed capital from a bank. Aydelotte and associates (1988) found that nurses who used sources of venture capital other than personal savings received higher gross income than nurses who used individual savings. No explanation was offered by the authors, but the possibility exists that true entrepreneurial ventures and subsequent income might be restricted if only existing savings are considered in planning. However, the loan application for a novice businessperson may be denied by the bank, and the plan and presentation may need to be adjusted before proceeding to the next bank (Sims, 1992). The banker may want a financial projection for 1 to 5 years, which is a difficult task for many new private practitioners. Nevertheless, adequately capitalizing for the needs of the practice at the beginning and adhering to a budget will minimize financial pressures (Walker, 1977).

Money must flow into the practice if the business is to continue. The business plan should include obtaining enough income to cover salaries for 4 to 6 months. The bank will assist in establishing a line of credit so that only the amount of money needed for expenses will be borrowed. The base of referrals is the financial foundation to a practice, and time will be required to establish a referral base in a community. Be innovative in marketing the services of the practice, and do not rely on referrals from one or two sources to maintain the practice. A maximum of 5% of referrals from any one source will avoid financial pressures should the source terminate referrals. Initially, the private practitioner may need to accept referrals from any source, but the goal of diversity among referral sources should be sought as the practice develops (Sims, 1992).

While speaking to a group of students regarding private practice, Finch (1982) remarked that if he terminated his practice of approximately 15 years, he could still receive an income for 2 to 3 years from his outstanding accounts. Cash flow may be very slow in the initial stages of a practice, and numerous accounts will require several months or more for collection. The SBA provides information to help the private practitioner distinguish cash, cash flow, accounts receivable, profit, and property. A cash flow statement should be utilized to determine operating cash flow, investing cash flow, financing cash flow, and positive or negative cash flow. Historical cash flow statements may be used to manage future cash flow. We experienced very minimal cash flow for the first 2 years of the practice, and accounts receivables mounted. Accounts receivables averaged $125,000 to $150,000 when the practice employed numerous therapists. A major third-party payer once delayed payment of a large account for 3 years. We have found that many insurance companies will require numerous requests before payment is sent. Learn how to bill and collect for your services by recognizing what different insurance companies require for claim submission, as well as what each will pay when billed. Learn about the possibility of using a universal billing form. Suggestions for improving cash flow include collecting co-pays promptly, having credit card terminals, providing patients with an estimate of costs per visit, collecting payment for supplies for home use, reviewing charges against scheduled visits to minimize missed billing opportunities, developing relationships with insurance companies, establishing a line of credit, and negotiating payment terms with suppliers (Farmer, 2004)

Medicaid is a federally funded program administered by a state agency to provide reimbursement for medical services for low-income clients and includes physical therapy services. Many pediatric clients will have Medicaid funding, and billing for these clients can be accomplished through electronic billing on a computer. The state provides the necessary software and in-service training on electronic billing, and this method is superior in processing and collection. Information on Medicaid can be obtained through the Centers for Medicare and Medicaid Services (CMS). Presently, insurance companies accept electronic billing but also seek copies of all intervention documentation. We do not find the electronic billing process helpful with most private insurance companies.

Our practice was opened with no established referral base. Miraculously, four clients were referred after contact with pediatricians and orthopedic surgeons and formed the income source for the first few weeks. The owner moonlighted on weekends at a general hospital to pay the costs of the business for the first 4 months. Contracts with school districts and other agencies were negotiated, and additional clients were referred to the office. Several contracts with state-supported centers for children with developmental disabilities have been available at various times. These centers desire their own employees but contract with the practice when necessary. Most of our client base for several years has been for individual care.

The determination of fees to be charged for services may be simple or complex. The fee schedule may be based on the general fee structure of other service providers in the geographic area, but if the private practitioner has lower overhead costs than agencies or other providers, the fees may be appropriately lower. Major insurance companies will have established "usual and customary" rates, and payment for pediatric physical therapy services will be based on those rates regardless of the established fees of the practice. Practitioners should charge only for services rendered, should establish fees commensurate with the costs of providing the services, should disclose the schedule of fees, and should learn to discuss fees with potential clients or their caretakers (Bernstein, 1986).

PLANNING FOR PHYSICAL RESOURCES

Office space is an important consideration when preparing the business plan. The space should meet the needs of both clients and staff and provide for the placement of needed equipment so that an efficient flow can occur (Sims, 1992). Walker (1977) suggests listing space and utility requirements and drawing a tentative floor plan before shopping for office space. He notes that the needs of the practice will change and growth should be anticipated. An office might be considered a luxury at first but will become a necessity as the practice grows. A waiting area is nonproductive space but will be necessary to meet the needs of clients and families. Restrooms also are a necessity, and local and state codes may determine whether employees and clients may use the same restroom facilities and whether the space may be used by both genders. Remember to note parking and accessibility needs when planning or selecting space. Water supply, storage closets and cabinets, cleaning and maintenance, utility costs, convenience for the targeted market, and the option to extend the lease are other important considerations in acquiring space. Ries (2004) notes that most private practitioners will need to rent, rather than own, space.

We chose to rent a two-room office with a 3-year lease. The rent was satisfactory and the location was one of convenience to the owner's home, but no market survey or other consideration was given to the location as a marketing tool to acquire clients. No lawyer reviewed the lease, and although the specifics of the lease were adequate, the time frame proved too long for our needs. We were unaware of the advice to allow for growth, and we desired larger space before the lease expired. Luckily, the company that held the lease was able to offer us an office with more space at a nearby location. Because the move was profitable for the company, we were allowed to terminate the first lease with no penalty.

Although individual treatment areas provide privacy for clients and diversity of design to meet specific client needs, the requirements for additional electrical wiring, ventilation, lighting, decorating, and equipment increase costs. If the tentative floor plan is drawn to scale and incorporates the planned use of the space for ambulation, exercise, play, or other activities, the practitioner should be able to identify space requirements. A realtor will be helpful in locating suitable space, in negotiating the price, and in arranging for structural changes in the space if warranted for the practice, and a lawyer should review the lease.

Some practitioners interested in private practice will find themselves in an employed position with a contract that prohibits competing with the employer in a certain geographic area or for a specific period of time following employment. This restriction may limit the choice of locations. Burch and Iglarsh (1988) suggest that at least 5 miles and probably 7.5 to 10 miles should exist between the practice location and other competitors and that this distance usually satisfies legal issues regarding competition clauses. Pediatric therapists with no legal encumbrances to geographic location will want to consider the distance between the private practice and other pediatric service providers. Pediatric therapists, however, may have a smaller percentage of a market area as potential clients than other specialists and may need to draw from a larger geographic base. The uniqueness of the private practice environment may allow competition with other pediatric service providers.

Our practice was initiated in a city with a population of approximately 200,000 persons and with two established pediatric outpatient agencies and a children's hospital that provided outpatient services. At the time we established the service, no other pediatric private practices existed, but we were not certain that a city of that size could support a practice limited to pediatrics. As indicated previously, we had to revise our practice goals to accommodate the marketplace, but the practice was very successful. Over the next several years, numerous physical therapists engaged in pediatric private practice and occupational therapists also established practices limited to pediatrics. Although we have changed locations several times since the practice began, the market for our practice was the entire city, surrounding smaller towns, and a few sites in other areas of the state. The last office was located in close proximity to several pediatric physician offices, but these offices did not form a strong referral base for the practice. Proximity to other providers and to a physician referral base are suggestions for the locations of adult practices in larger cities or states, but we are unable to determine if these suggestions apply to pediatric practices.

Equipment needs include both office equipment and physical therapy equipment. Office equipment may cost up to $10,000 (Sims, 1992), and estimates for physical therapy equipment offered to us by private practitioners engaged in orthopedic practice varied from $100,000 to $300,000. Pediatric private practitioners are able to initiate a practice with much less funding. The specific disabilities of the clients who will be served will influence the selection of physical therapy equipment, but an office that provides play-based therapy for clients who are developmentally challenged might require only mats, therapeutic balls, bolsters, mirrors, toys, stairs, vestibular swings, and a standing/ambulation area. Bernstein (1986) notes that crayons, dolls, blocks, and brand-name toys may serve the needs of younger children, but games and more sophisticated entertainment are required for older children.

Our initial office was very modest with minimal furniture and office equipment. The treatment room consisted of a mat placed on the floor, a large wall mirror, and numerous toys. The initial cost for these items was only several hundred dollars. A later office contained a large, carpeted treatment room with floor mat, therapeutic balls, bolsters, shelves, and toys. One small treatment room contained a floor mat, a large mirror, shelves, and toys, and the other small treatment room contained a platform mat and large mirror. The hall and large treatment room provided space for walking, as did the outdoor sidewalk and lawn areas in good weather. The waiting room was very small. The casting room contained a sink and cabinets; the billing office had a desk, desk chair, side chair, telephone, and computer; and the staff office contained several desk areas, a reception area with a window opening into the waiting room, telephone, lamp, computer, typewriter, copier, and other office equipment. Although the equipment assets of the practice now total several thousand dollars, these assets were obtained over several years. The typical pediatric physical therapy practice will never experience equipment costs in the hundred thousand dollar range.

PLANNING FOR HUMAN RESOURCES

A practitioner may employ other therapists and staff or contract for other services if needed. The solo practitioner will have difficulty attending continuing education programs, taking vacation time, or using sick leave unless help is available. Burch and Iglarsh (1988) recommend finding a therapist who can be trusted with the practice to offer relief to the solo practitioner. Employing or contracting with other therapists and support staff requires an understanding of laws and regulations for personnel. The services of the lawyer and tax consultant for the practice can be used to determine the best plan for obtaining the services of other persons.

Planning for needed support staff must be as deliberate as planning for other aspects of the business (Sims, 1992). Office staff must have the equipment necessary to accomplish the required tasks, must be clearly informed of the job responsibilities, and must be given time to learn the equipment and the management systems for the practice. Some practices use a medical billing and collecting firm to manage accounts receivable if the staff does not have expertise in billing.

An administrative assistant may provide the expertise in business management not typically possessed by the physical therapist owner. Private practices have differing needs, and the administrative assistant may be an on-the-job trained office manager or a certified public accountant and financial planner (Wilson, 1992). The owner must determine the needs of the practice, seek an administrative assistant with the skills necessary to meet needs, and relinquish the responsibilities and tasks to the administrative assistant. The administrative assistant may have responsibility for any task that is not directly treatment related, but all administrative assistants should have experience with preparation and collection of accounts receivable. Lynch (1992) suggests that the administrative assistant should mirror the practitioner/owner in personality, image, competence, and commitment. The PPS has supported the development of the Private Practice Physical Therapy Administrative Assistants group, which has bylaws and publishes a newsletter. This group meets at annual meetings of the PPS and provides excellent information and support for administrative assistants and private practitioners.

Salaries for yourself and other staff, if employed, are the major expense of a service business. A friend with a long-standing adult orthopedic private practice suggested establishing a 3-year goal for the owner to reach the salary that was abandoned to start the practice. The first-year salary for the owner for our practice was set at $15,000, the amount necessary to supplement the spouse's salary for our personal expenses. As previously noted, the spouse provided billing services, and no additional staff were employed. The telephone answering machine served as receptionist when a client was being treated. All bills and the salary as established were paid, and the net loss for the first year was $97.00. During the second year, an additional therapist was hired as an independent contractor, and the salary available to the owner exceeded the salary originally determined to be the 3-year goal. The salary level for the owner grew at a rapid rate, and competitive salaries were soon offered to therapists employed by the practice.

As a practice grows, a decision will have to be made on whether to keep the practice small or to allow growth and to offer exclusively physical therapy services or to expand into other services. During the first 10-year period, our practice expanded to include 14 physical therapists, 1

full-time and 1 part-time secretary, and 1 administrative assistant. In retrospect, the administrative assistant should have been employed earlier and responsibilities for billing should have been delegated from the beginning. Several sources offer suggestions for recruiting and retaining quality staff in a physical therapy private practice (Deaton & Gutterud, 1992; McNeil, 1990, 1991). Hiring additional therapists or staff may be expensive and may not translate into greater profit. Private practitioners may wish to consider alternative compensation strategies such as profit sharing, paying by the visit, or employing part-time therapists to keep expenses consistent with income.

RISK MANAGEMENT IN MAINTAINING A PRIVATE PRACTICE

Resource development and availability are important aspects of the business plan. As the practice matures, the practitioner will need to continually assess the strengths and weaknesses of the practice, take advantage of change, and exhibit management control (Dillon & Duke, 1991). Management control involves using resources in an effective manner to accomplish the goals and objectives of the practice. Dillon and Duke (1991) suggest the use of critical success factors, the crucial components of a business, to achieve success. The owner should identify the specific key components and measure performance by focusing on these components through information gathering and reporting. Deaton (1992a) noted that therapists in private practice often use computer programs to collect and produce lengthy reports that do not highlight the crucial components of the business. For example, information on the number of units of service for each referring physician would not be useful in a practice in which the therapists determine the frequency and type of treatment procedures to be provided. Information on the number of units of service generated each month would be useful in determining peak service months and in planning for vacations and staffing.

Dillon and Duke (1991) provide several questions that may assist the owner in identifying the critical success factors for the practice. Measurable indicators for each critical success factor must be determined and used for management control. Indicators should allow comparison to a desired level of performance, use staff input to enhance compliance and cooperation, be reliable, provide timely information, and allow for simple identification of problem areas.

We did not employ risk management concepts using critical success factors or any other type of control processes when the business was initiated, nor for the first several years. Experience in accounts receivable collection enhanced success, but luck was a primary factor in maintaining the practice. Eventually, we realized the need to gather information on the number of patients treated in each facility and at the office; the collection rate for different insurance companies; the cost of each employee, including vacation time, sick time, and continuing education time and expenses; the revenue generated by each employee; and the cost of supplies and casting materials. We perceived this information as comprising the critical success factors for our business, and as control over these crucial components was established and maintained, the profit for the practice increased significantly. As when planning a practice, the financial, physical, and human resources should be considered in maintaining a successful practice.

MAINTAINING FINANCIAL RESOURCES

Efficient collection of outstanding accounts and determination of when to refer an account to an attorney or a collection agency for assistance in bringing the account current are important but difficult tasks. As previously mentioned, many accounts will be outstanding for lengthy periods of time. Prompt and consistent billing of new charges and reminders of outstanding charges will allow for continual collections after the first year or so of practice. The owner must establish standards by which credit is extended to clients and by which sufficient information is obtained to enable collection of an account should delinquency occur. In addition to the demographic information obtained from clients at the initiation of treatment, the owner or staff member responsible for billing should find out where the individual responsible for payment of the charges is employed and where banking is done. If possible, a copy of the bank account number should be obtained by copying one of the checks (Merry, 1992), and the insurance card should be copied. Merry (1992) provides suggestions on contracts with clients, collecting debt, terminating services for clients with delinquent accounts, and using an attorney to collect accounts. He notes that failure to implement and follow collection practices will be costly to a private practice. Newell (1988) provides samples of a payment policy statement, a reminder letter, and a final notice letter, as well as suggestions for collecting accounts by telephone.

We require the party responsible for payment to authorize payment of benefits to the practice (Fig. 36-1). This policy necessitates that all billing be done by the practice rather than having clients submit claim forms,

but we are comfortable with the collection rate obtained through the use of assignment of benefits to the practice. Occasionally, an insurance company will reimburse the client for services. If an authorization for payment to the practice is on file, however, the insurance company will pay the practice and assume responsibility for recovery of the payment from the client.

Financial resources may be compromised by unethical staff. Deaton (1992a) asked a large audience of private practice physical therapists to indicate the incidence of stealing by staff. Over 50% of the practitioners indicated that staff had taken funds from the practice. In our practice, we believe that billing specialists managed to divert several thousand dollars into personal accounts on two separate occasions. Staff members are able to bill for relatives who never received services and for fictitious clients using a false address. A second bank account may be established for deposits. The owner may never know that the false billing has occurred. An accountant will be able to assist in planning to prevent stealing and in designing safeguards for the owner who is not competent in the business aspects of the practice.

Ball and Lindquist (1998) report that government and law enforcement agencies are intensely scrutinizing health care practices. They suggest developing and implementing a compliance program with internal policies consistent with the business and with the law. The compliance program will allow identification of potentially volatile situations and avoid activities that could expose you to charges of fraud.

Many pediatric therapists will find that current laws and regulations ensure services to infants and toddlers through mechanisms funded by the state, and that referral source will form a substantial portion of the revenue for a practice. We experienced a severe cash flow problem in the tenth year of business when low state revenues jeopardized funding for Medicaid. Very quickly, the state owed more than $100,000, and the business experienced the only true threat to continuation. The funds were eventually paid in full, but we learned that a successful business could be at risk if a major funding source was eliminated.

Likewise, if the business continues to grow, cash flow problems will recur. Employees will often be paid several months before the funds generated by the employees are received. Each owner will have to determine the desire for growth and the tolerance for cash flow difficulties. An established practice will be able to maintain an ongoing line of credit with the bank and to pay bills and employees while experiencing growth. Dobrin (1991) cautions that approval for a loan may be difficult if the client base is not evident.

CLIENT:	ADDRESS:	PHONE #:	SS #:	DATE OF BIRTH:	SEX: Male ____ Female ____	DIAGNOSIS:		
PHYSICIAN:	PHYSICIAN'S ADDRESS:	PHYSICIAN'S PHONE #:	PARENT'S NAMES and SS #: Father: SS#: Mother: SS #:	PARENT'S ADDRESS:	PARENT'S PHONE #: Home: Work:			
INSURANCE INFO: Primary Insurance Company:	Employer:	Employee:	ID #:	Group #:	OTHER INSURANCE: Secondary Insurance Company:	Employer:	Employee:	ID #:

ASSIGNMENT OF BENEFITS

I authorize payment of medical benefits be paid directly for services rendered.

_____
Signature

AUTHORIZATION FOR TREATMENT

I authorize treatment be given as ordered by my physician.

_____
Signature

AUTHORIZATION TO RELEASE MEDICAL INFORMATION

I authorize release of any medical information to another physician or insurance company to assist in treatment or claim processing.

_____
Signature

• **Figure 36-1**   Example of a client information sheet and assignment form for a private practice.

Fonte (1998) and Cohen (1998) have suggested strategies to avoid the influence of managed care on financial resources. Many adult practices are becoming cash-only practices or are accepting only clients with private-pay insurers. Pediatric therapists will need to monitor the environment to determine if these strategies can be successful for pediatric clients.

MAINTAINING PHYSICAL RESOURCES

Although physical resources, particularly office space and location, may change with growth of the practice, few pediatric physical therapists will have yearly purchases of expensive equipment, as is the case for therapists engaged in practice areas using ever-advancing, high-technology equipment. In our practice, the purchase of tests and measures, electrotherapy equipment, casting supplies, and equipment for ambulation have resulted in expenditures in the area of physical resources. Mats, therapeutic balls and bolsters, and equipment for therapists who provide services outside the office have been purchased. Much of the initial equipment was used for 20 or more years of practice, and few major equipment expenses have occurred. Toys and expendable play supplies represent the largest portion of expenses for the practice beyond salaries, health insurance, mileage reimbursement, and continuing education.

MAINTAINING HUMAN RESOURCES

A challenge for private practitioners is attracting and retaining qualified physical therapists (Deaton & Gutterud, 1992). In 1990, McNeil suggested that the gap between supply and demand was still increasing at an intimidating rate and that private practices experience employee turnover of up to 40% annually. New and experienced therapists and assistants are seeking the best employment offer, and owners must offer a salary and benefit package that is competitive (Deaton & Gutterud, 1992). An increase in the number of schools, the number of graduates, and the number of graduates interested in pediatrics has occurred in the last several years, and we find filling positions much easier. McNeil (1990) notes that role modeling, having a defined philosophy of management, gaining credibility with employees, and offering opportunities for growth and development are some key points in reducing turnover in physical therapy private practices. In order to retain the best possible employees, we believe that we must adhere to good management practices regardless of the availability of practitioners.

Most of the therapists and physical therapist assistants in our practice work in relative isolation, meeting only weekly for a staff conference or for supervisory sessions between therapists and assistants. This isolation is common in private practice but presents a particular challenge for pediatric therapists who are accustomed to center-based practices. New graduates in our practice have had fewer adjustment difficulties than experienced therapists, and this phenomenon was a surprise to the owner, who was hesitant to employ new graduates in a private practice with so many isolated activities. One explanation for the success with new graduates may be that educational programs are preparing graduates for diverse practice environments. All the new graduates employed in recent years have held the professional master or doctor of physical therapy degree. In 2002, the PPS launched an educational initiative to encourage students to enter private practice (Porterfield, 2002). Educational programs for physical therapists were asked to allow a PPS member to speak to students and to include private practice content in curricula. This initiative may increase the pool of new graduates prepared for private practice. In our environment, new graduates receive orientation and mentoring on a planned basis, and all therapists and assistants have access to their co-workers by telephone. Social activities are included in the weekly staff meetings to promote a sense of belonging and collegiality.

Student affiliation agreements may be maintained with physical therapist assistant and physical therapist educational programs. We found that students could participate in all aspects of the practice and serve as a source for recruitment, as well as motivators for the staff. Students often provide in-service presentations and perform unique projects that stimulate therapists, assistants, and clients.

Continued education and opportunities for growth are of primary importance in our practice. Information regarding specialized skills, such as inhibitive casting or family-guided services, is shared freely among practitioners either through consultation or in-service education. The practice supports graduate or other formal education experiences. Tuition reimbursement is available to therapists and physical therapist assistants who seek further academic education. Achievement of specialization is fostered, and therapists in addition to the owner and co-therapist have become certified pediatric specialists.

Attracting therapists willing to travel to multiple locations, including some potentially unsafe home environments, was also a challenge for our practice.

We have attempted to balance this challenge with the practical benefit of reimbursing mileage costs and with philosophic advantages. Each therapist is offered the opportunity to provide services within a philosophy of private practice including maximal autonomy, self-governance, reduced bureaucracy, and independence in exercising professional judgment. Each assistant is afforded similar opportunity within the constraints of supervision and delegation. The result has been a good retention rate.

Between 1982 and 1998, our practice grew to more than 40 employees, including occupational therapists, speech-language pathologists, audiologists, a nurse, and four separate offices. The state Medicaid funding changes of 1998 and managed care payers forced the need to downsize the practice and salaries (which were highly competitive) or increase the productivity of each employee. Several therapists matured into practitioners who were willing to take risks in their own private practices rather than take potential decreases in salary, and left the practice. Our success in getting these practitioners to adopt the philosophy of private practice resulted in an eventual loss to the practice and increased competition as new practices developed. A common discussion at meetings of the PPS is that good employees must be made partners or they will eventually become competitors. We have chosen to remain as owners without partners and accept the risks that are inevitable with that decision. As we aged, we were content with a smaller practice meeting our philosophical perspectives.

TRENDS IN PRIVATE PRACTICE

Issues identified by the Private Practice Section of the APTA as potentially harmful to private practitioners include the rapid growth of non–physical therapist corporate-owned practices and cost-containment measures that provide inequitable constraints on physical therapists. The PPS has acknowledged that physical therapists need to take a proactive stance in addressing these issues. The 2004 PPS Member Survey (Private Practice Section) demonstrated that members were very interested in legislative advocacy, reimbursement, legal issues, direct access, physician-owned practices, and practice management. Pediatric physical therapy is not exempt from these concerns, and many pediatric therapists are not reimbursed for services or are reimbursed at a lower rate if services are provided in a private practice setting rather than in a hospital or rehabilitation center.

The Section on Pediatrics of the APTA has recognized some movement toward private practice among section members. The movement appears to be primarily for increased autonomy and because of disenchantment with practice settings in which pediatric therapists perceive themselves as "revenue generators" for a facility rather than as caregivers for clients (Dasch & Finney, 1991).

Current trends indicate the need for physical therapists to move into environments such as health maintenance organizations, preferred provider arrangements, and point-of-service plans and less often into individual practice settings. One projection is that physical therapist–owned practices using a group mode will be more common as the base for practice than the solo mode (Moffat, 1991). Faust and Meaker (1991) suggest that a group private practice can have the three key elements: (1) high autonomy, (2) strong professional identity, and (3) low bureaucracy. These authors note that therapists tend to distance themselves from the important topics of reimbursement, business, and administration. Group practice might allow several therapists to combine resources to address these business needs and to meet the essential practice roles of clinical services, management, administration, and professional activities.

Moffat (1991) also recommends using the skills of the physical therapist assistant to complement practice and to free therapists to maximize their own skills. Assistants have traditionally been encouraged to seek general hospital experiences (Infante et al., 1976; Larson & Davis, 1975; Physical Therapy Assistant Program, 1975). Settings providing specialized health care have been suggested as appropriate for employment of the assistant (Lovelace-Chandler & Lovelace-Chandler, 1979).

Our philosophy includes the belief that some components of interventions may be performed by physical therapist assistants. Tasks related to treatment are delegated only after a therapist performs the initial examination, establishes a care plan, and implements the plan to determine response. We have identified factors, including individual patients' differences, unique circumstances, individual assistants' competencies, and acute or severe problems that might restrict the delegation of tasks (Lovelace-Chandler & Lovelace-Chandler, 1979). We also have suggested how to develop a job description for the physical therapist assistant, determine the skills of an assistant, and provide education or remediation if skills are lacking. We have experienced a general reluctance on the part of pediatric physical therapists to use the skills of the physical therapist assistant. The pediatric therapist in private practice must recognize that effective use of assistants is essential to providing high-quality services at the lowest cost.

One of the most significant recent trends in private practice is the support of the APTA and the development of numerous resources for practitioners. Private practice appears to have been embraced as an essential practice arena and as important to the development of professionalism in a doctoring profession.

THE UNIQUE PHILOSOPHY OF PEDIATRIC PHYSICAL THERAPY

Any practitioner considering a private practice limited to pediatric physical therapy must be cognizant of the uniqueness of pediatrics as a specialty. Cherry (1991) has summarized the philosophy, the scientific components, and the quantitative and qualitative differences that must be considered in selecting treatment techniques that meet the needs of children. Albeit evolved from the philosophy and techniques of the wider field of physical therapy, pediatric physical therapy is distinguished by a distinct philosophy. Inherent in this philosophy are the beliefs that a child is viewed as a whole person existing in the context of the family and with natural ecologic settings that the developmental characteristics of children require unique knowledge of existing and future development, and that children require advocacy.

The natural ecologic settings for children are the home and school (Cherry, 1991). Other common settings include child care centers, churches or other religious environments, and settings where leisure activities are enjoyed. Therapists in private practice must be willing to provide services within natural settings, using the natural activities of the settings as the intervention strategies. Private practitioners must accept family members, in addition to the child, as clients with wishes and needs, and be responsive to those wishes and needs. Otherwise services will be sought from facilities or practitioners who identify and implement family goals. Family-focused therapy became prominent in the United States after the passage of Public Law 99-457, and the private practitioner has numerous resources available to assist in service design using family theory (see Chapter 31).

Developmental science, pediatric medical pathology, examination, and management of children with developmental disabilities form the scientific bases of pediatric physical therapy. Intervention strategies and procedures for children may be adapted from adult treatment or may be specific to the young client (Cherry, 1991). Private practitioners wishing to offer services to children must possess the unique knowledge and skills necessary for the practice of pediatrics.

RECOMMENDATIONS FOR BEST PRACTICE

The following recommendations summarize our beliefs regarding best practice in private practice physical therapy. We have not always followed these recommendations, but the business would probably have been more successful if we had done so. You will be able to determine which recommendations meet your philosophy of care and your needs regarding the financial, physical, and human resources of the practice.

1. Possess advanced skill in the specialty area of pediatrics. Although recognized specialization such as that awarded by the American Board of Physical Therapy Specialists (ABPTS) should not be a requirement for initiating a pediatric practice, any clinician who is not acquiring the skills essential to that credential should not be in pediatric private practice.
2. Gain knowledge of all appropriate laws, regulations, policies, and position statements that affect pediatric physical therapy. Federal laws have greatly influenced the practice of pediatric physical therapy in recent years, and state laws and regulations determine which pediatric therapy services are allowable and will be reimbursed. State and city laws and regulations affect the operation of the business.
3. Have persons with business skills available to the practice. The owner/therapist does not need to have knowledge of accounting, taxes, bookkeeping, and management, but this knowledge must be accessible to the business through the use of lawyers, accountants, bankers, and billing specialists. Business sense is required to achieve business cents (translate: dollars).
4. Provide services that are needed in the marketplace. The trends in health care cost containment and private practice service provision will increase competition among health care providers. Pediatric therapists must be responsive to the needs and wants of clients and families.
5. Identify the quantity of services you can provide. Do not exceed that quantity, or quality will suffer.
6. Design the appropriate practice setting. If an office practice is used, the space and decor should reflect the clients you serve. Employ staff that support your philosophy and image.
7. Purchase the proper supplies. Experienced pediatric therapists will know that diapers, tissues, crayons, toys, games, holiday decorations, and

stickers are more important purchases than massage lotion. Vendors who serve practices for adults may not be able to recommend the correct supplies for new pediatric practitioners.

8. Know how to interact and play with the clients you serve. New graduates may not have knowledge of play activities commensurate with their knowledge of therapeutic techniques. Seek continuing education or consultation for areas of service provision in which you are lacking.

9. Understand the ecologically appropriate environments for children. The work of children is their play, and children function within the context of family life, preschool, or school. Design the practice to fit into the lives of children and families.

10. Offer family-guided physical therapy in the private enterprise arena. Understand the context of the family and the advocacy role of the family. Develop cultural competence for the families you serve. Learn about the language, food, holiday, religious, childrearing, and discipline preferences of your clients. Accept the closeness you will develop with families and children. In private practice, professional distance is reduced. Demonstrate affection or even love for your clients. Aloofness and professional demeanor are inconsistent with the intimacy found in most private practices.

SUMMARY

The pediatric physical therapist in private practice has autonomy, uses professional values, and takes risks with a minimum of bureaucracy to achieve independence and success. The roles of owner, business manager, and clinician must coexist, and the private practitioner must seek services from such resources as accountants, bankers, lawyers, realtors, and other therapists to augment the knowledge and skills required for private practice. Personal and professional characteristics and responsibilities have been suggested by numerous authors, and possession or development of these attributes will diminish risk and liability. A private practice is established and maintained through selection of an appropriate legal structure and consideration of the necessary financial, physical, and human resources. Societal trends offer private practitioners the opportunity for creative business activities when services are envisioned through the unique philosophy of pediatric physical therapy and with regard for best practices. The APTA has embraced the concept of private practice, and professionalism

in pediatric physical therapy will be enhanced as an increased number of therapists enter the private practice arena.

REFERENCES

American Physical Therapy Association. Code of Ethics. Alexandria, VA: APTA, 2000a.

American Physical Therapy Association. Standards of Ethical Conduct for the Physical Therapist Assistant. Alexandria, VA: APTA, 2000b.

American Physical Therapy Association. Guide for Conduct of the Affiliate Member. Alexandria, VA: APTA, 2001a.

American Physical Therapy Association. Guide for Professional Conduct. Alexandria, VA: APTA, 2002.

American Physical Therapy Association. Guide to Physical Therapist Practice. Physical Therapy, 77:1163–1650, 2001b.

American Physical Therapy Association. Standards of Practice for Physical Therapy and the Criteria. Alexandria, VA: APTA, 2003.

American Speech-Language-Hearing Association. Considerations for establishing a private practice in audiology and/or speech-language pathology. ASHA, 33(suppl 3):10–21, 1991.

Aydelotte, MK, Hardy, MA, & Hope, KL. Nurses in Private Practice: Characteristics, Organizational Arrangements, and Reimbursement Policy. Kansas City, MO: American Nurses' Foundation, 1988.

Ball, JA, & Lindquist, SC. Searching for fraud: Will your practice be the next target? Advance for Directors in Rehabilitation, 7(8):43–44, 1998.

Baskin, W. Making a move. Advance for Directors in Rehabilitation, 6(8):37, 39, 1997.

Bernstein, DK. Part-time private practice in speech-language pathology and audiology. In Butler, KG (Ed.). Prospering in Private Practice: A Handbook for Speech-Language Pathology and Audiology. Gaithersburg, MD: Aspen, 1986, pp. 13–46.

Bezner, J. Getting to the core of professionalism. PT Magazine, 12(1):25–27, 2004.

Brown, S. Sorry—I'm not in private practice. Clinical Management, 12(1):14–15, 1992.

Burch, EA, & Iglarsh, A. A conversation about starting a private practice. Physical Therapy Today, 11(4):37–42, 1988.

Campbell, SK. Physical Therapy for Children. Philadelphia: WB Saunders, 1994.

Carlson, T. Tom Carlson, 1987 Robert G. Dicus award winner. Whirlpool, 10:35–37, 1987.

Cherry, DB. Pediatric physical therapy: Philosophy, science, and techniques. Pediatric Physical Therapy, 3(2):70–75, 1991.

Cohen, RS. Running a cash-only practice: Tips to keep the minnows swimming upstream. Advance for Directors in Rehabilitation, 7(5):57–58, 63, 1998.

Cole, PR. Private practice: Personal prerequisites and potential. In Butler, KG (Ed.). Prospering in Private Practice: A Handbook for Speech-Language Pathology and Audiology. Gaithersburg, MD: Aspen, 1986, pp. 3–11.

Connell, M. Focus on private practice: Should you start a practice from scratch or purchase one? PT Magazine, 11(9):52–54, 2003.

Cooper, E. The state of the profession and what to do about it. ASHA, 24:931–936, 1982.

Dasch, D, & Finney, M. The future and specialty practice. Clinical Management, 11(6):26–33, 1991.

Deaton, WC. Do you know where your practice is tonight? Paper presented at the 1992 Private Practice Section Annual Conference and Exposition, Dallas, TX, November 11–15, 1992a.

Deaton, WC. Running your practice by the numbers. Physical Therapy Today, 15(2):31–35, 1992b.

Deaton, WC, & Gutterud, SR. Attracting and retaining quality staff: Using fringe benefits and incentive compensation. Physical Therapy Today, 15(3):44–47, 1992.

Dicus, RG. Origins of the self-employed section. Physical Therapy Today, 14(4):19–20, 22, 1991.

Dillon, RD, & Duke, PJ. Planning for success. Clinical Management, 11(5):28–32, 1991.

Dobrin, J. Private practice: Big, small, or not at all. Physical Therapy Today, 14(3):52, 54, 56, 1991.

Driskell, C. Planning for success: Developing a business plan to secure financing. Physical Therapy Today, 11(1):40–41, 1988.

Farmer, J. Improving cash flow for the private practitioner. PT Magazine, 12(4):60–62, 2004.

Faust, L, & Meaker, MK. Private practice occupational therapy in the skilled nursing facility: Creative alliance or mutual exploitation? American Journal of Occupational Therapy, 45:621–627, 1991.

Finch, J. Private Practice Physical Therapy: Presentation for Physical Therapy Students. Conway, AR, 1982.

Flower, RM. Ethical concerns in private practice. In Butler, KG (Ed.). Prospering in Private Practice: A Handbook for Speech-Language Pathology and Audiology. Gaithersburg, MD: Aspen, 1986, pp. 101–123.

Fonte, AM, & Boutique PT: How to succeed without managed care. Advance for Directors in Rehabilitation, 7(11):51–52, 1998.

Frazian, BW. Tidal surge and private practice: The historic eighties. In Cromwell, FS (Ed.). Private Practice in Occupational Therapy. New York: Haworth Press, 1985, pp. 7–13.

Glinn, JE. The balanced physical therapy private practice. PPS Impact, October, 2002.

Guglielmo, FX. The 1988 Robert G. Dicus award recipient. Physical Therapy Today, 11(4):18–24, 1988.

Gwinn, B. Choose a legal practice structure. PPS Impact, February, 2002.

Hack, LM. History, purpose, and structure of part two: Preferred practice patterns. PT Magazine, 6(6):72–79, 1998.

Hampton, D. Establishing and equipping an audiology private practice. In Butler, KG (Ed.). Prospering in Private Practice: A Handbook for Speech-Language Pathology and Audiology. Gaithersburg, MD: Aspen, 1986, pp. 135–148.

Huelskamp, S. Finding your niche: Niche marketing—An answer to staying competitive. Advance for Directors in Rehabilitation, 6(3):37, 39, 1997.

Infante, MS, Speranza, KA, & Gillespie, PW. An interdisciplinary approach to the education of health professional students. Journal of Allied Health, 5(4):13–22, 1976.

Jayaratne, S, Davis-Sacks, ML, & Chess, WA. Private practice may be good for your health and well-being. Social Work, 36(3):224–229, 1991.

Johnson, LH. A place of their own: Women PTs who own their own businesses. PT Magazine, 10(9):42–45, 2002.

Kooper, JD, & Sullivan, CA. Professional liability: Management and prevention. In Butler, KG (Ed.). Prospering in Private Practice: A Handbook for Speech-Language Pathology and Audiology. Gaithersburg, MD: Aspen, 1986, pp. 59–79.

Larson, CW, & Davis, ER. Following up the physical therapist assistant graduate: A curriculum evaluation process. Physical Therapy, 55:601–606, 1975.

Lovelace-Chandler, V, & Lovelace-Chandler, B. Employment of physical therapist assistants in a residential state school. Physical Therapy, 59(10):1243–1246, 1979.

Lynch, R. Selection of an administrative assistant. Physical Therapy Today, 15(2):50–51, 1992.

McClain, L, McKinney, J, & Ralston, J. Occupational therapists in private practice. American Journal of Occupational Therapy, 46:613–618, 1992.

McFadden, SM, & Hanschu, B. Risk taking in occupational therapy. In Cromwell, FS (Ed.). Private Practice in Occupational Therapy. New York: Haworth Press, 1985, pp. 3–6.

McNeil, LL. The people part of practice management. Physical Therapy Today, 13(1):34–35, 37–38, 40, 1990.

McNeil, LL. Employee turnover: Do we have a problem? Physical Therapy Today, 14(3):57–60, 1991.

Merry, TR. Ten commonly asked questions in dealing with accounts receivable: What every private practice owner would like to ignore but can't. Physical Therapy Today, 15(1): 59–62, 64–65, 1992.

Moffat, M. Beyond 2000: Who will you be? Clinical Management, 11(6):8–9, 1991.

Newell, D. Collecting accounts receivable by telephone. Physical Therapy Today, 11(2):28–31, 1988.

Olsen, D. Entrepreneurship: Ownership and private practice physical therapy. In Nosse, LJ, Friberg, DG, & Kovacek, PR. Managerial and Supervisory Principles for Physical Therapists. Baltimore: Williams & Wilkins, 1999, pp. 278–298.

Parish, R. Constraints and commitments: An introduction to the financial aspects of private practice. In Butler, KG (Ed.). Prospering in Private Practice: A Handbook for Speech Language Pathology and Audiology. Gaithersburg, MD: Aspen, 1986, pp. 81–99.

Parsons, L. Planning and initiating a private practice in nursing psychotherapy. In Durham, JD, & Hardin, SB (Eds.). The Nurse Psychotherapist in Private Practice. New York: Springer, 1986, pp. 75–86.

Physical Therapy Assistant Program. Physical therapy assistant program evaluation. Charlotte, NC: Central Piedmont Community College, 1975.

Porterfield, J. PPS launches new educational initiative. PPS Impact, October, 2002.

Private Practice Section. 1992 profile of a private practice physical therapist. Physical Therapy Today, 15(3):60–69, 1992.

Private Practice Section. 1996 Member Needs and Assessment Survey. Washington, DC: PPS, APTA, 1996.

Private Practice Section. PPS Membership Votes to Retain Section Name and Mission Statement. PPS Impact, February 1997.

Private Practice Section. Member Survey, January 2004. Washington, DC: PPS, APTA, 2004.

Reuss, R. The maturation of the private practice section. Physical Therapy Today, 14(4):24–26, 28–32, 34–36, 38–48, 1991.

Ries, E. Capital advice for the private practitioner. PT Magazine, 12(3):42–44, 2004.

Scull, S, & Deitz, J. Competencies for the physical therapist in the neonatal intensive care unit (NICU). Pediatric Physical Therapy, 1(1):11–14, 1989.

Selker, LG. Human resources in physical therapy: Opportunities for service in a rapidly changing health system. Physical Therapy, 75(1):31–37, 1995.

Sims, D. Wishing you continued success. Physical Therapy Today, 15(1):7–11, 1992.

Smith, LC. Starting a PT practice: A compendium of resources. PT Magazine, 9(4):62–66, 2001.

Smoyak, SA. The nurse psychotherapist as unique practitioner. In Durham, JD, & Hardin, SB (Eds.). The Nurse Psychotherapist in Private Practice. New York: Springer, 1986, pp. 21–23.

Sullivan, CA. Business and management aspects of private practice in speech-language pathology and audiology. In Butler, KG (Ed.). Prospering in Private Practice: A Handbook for Speech-Language

Pathology and Audiology. Gaithersburg, MD: Aspen, 1986, pp. 149–165.

Sweeney, JK, Heriza, CB, Reilly, MA, Smith, C, & VanSant, AF. Practice guidelines for the physical therapist in the neonatal intensive care unit (NICU). Pediatric Physical Therapy, 11(3):119–132, 1999.

Task Force on Early Intervention, Section on Pediatrics, APTA. Competencies for physical therapists in early intervention. Pediatric Physical Therapy, 3(2):77–80, 1991.

Valente, CM. Member needs and assessment survey results. PPS Impact, June, 1996.

Walker, RC. Over My Shoulder: Reflections on Beginning a Private Practice in Physical Therapy. Cedar Rapids, IA: RC Walker, 1977.

Wilson, FD. Administrative assistants: What role should they play? Physical Therapy Today, 15(2):47–49, 1992.

Wilson, M. Private practice management. PT Magazine, 10(12):30–34, 2002.

Wilson, M. Practice valuation: What's the bottom line? PT Magazine, 12(1):52–53, 2004.

Wood, ML. Private Practice in Communication Disorders. Boston: College-Hill, 1986.

Woody, RH. Legal issues for private practitioners in speech language pathology and audiology. In Butler, KG (Ed.). Prospering in Private Practice: A Handbook for Speech-Language Pathology and Audiology. Gaithersburg, MD: Aspen 1986, pp. 47–57.

※

MEDICOLEGAL ISSUES IN THE UNITED STATES

WENDY E. PHILLIPS
PT, MS, PhD

MICHAEL L. SPOTTS
JD

▮ OVERVIEW

The implementation of federal legislation along with increased litigation related to patient care and outcome in a rapidly evolving medical system increases the likelihood of an interaction between pediatric physical therapists and the legal system. A conceptual understanding of public laws, such as the Individuals with Disabilities Education Act (IDEA) (Public Law 105-17) and the Americans with Disabilities Act (ADA) (Public Law 101-336), is required of the physical therapist providing services to children and adolescents with disabilities and their families. Similarly, familiarity with the litigation process, such as medical malpractice and petitions for the determination of appropriate medical treatment, is useful.

The purpose of this chapter is to provide an overview of IDEA, the ADA, and the process of litigation as it pertains to pediatric patients, using case histories as examples. The physical therapist's responsibility in reporting cases of child abuse and neglect is also included along with related ethical issues. The clinical implications of the federal legislation discussed in this chapter are described in several chapters of this book, particularly Chapter 30 (The Environment and Intervention), Chapter 31 (Early Intervention Services), and Chapter 32 (The Educational Environment).

INDIVIDUALS WITH DISABILITIES EDUCATION ACT

The Individuals with Disabilities Education Act is a federal law passed in 1975 (Public Law 94-142), reauthorized in 1990 (Public Law 101-476), and amended in 1997 (Public Law 105-17). It mandates that all children receive a free, appropriate public education regardless of the level or severity of their disability. It provides funds to assist states in the education of students with disabilities and requires that states ensure that students with special needs receive an individualized education program. The individualized education program is based on the student's unique needs and provided in the least restrictive environment possible. IDEA provides guidelines for determining what related services are necessary. This chapter reviews those sections of the law that are particularly relevant to physical therapy.

AMERICANS WITH DISABILITIES ACT

In an attempt to rectify past discrimination against individuals with physical and mental disabilities related to housing, employment, and other areas, the ADA (Public Law 101-336) was enacted. Although the ADA may appear to be related to adults with disabilities, various provisions are directly or indirectly applicable to families who have children with disabilities. Aspects of the law that are particularly relevant to children and families will be discussed in this chapter.

For example, parents are protected from discrimination with respect to employment hiring practices based on their status as parents of a child with a disability. The act ensures that a parent cannot be denied health insurance for the family because of the child's condition. These and other provisions of the act that may affect children and families served by physical therapists are discussed.

CHILD ABUSE AND NEGLECT

Although laws with respect to child abuse and neglect vary in the United States from state to state, their purpose is consistent: to protect children whose health and welfare are adversely affected and further threatened by the conduct of those responsible for their care and protection. The law dictates that certain persons, including hospital or medical personnel, report all suspected cases of abuse and neglect to the appropriate state agency. Failure to report a suspected case of abuse or neglect results in a misdemeanor charge.

Physical abuse, sexual abuse, and neglect are all conditions that by law must be reported. Child and adult behaviors associated with physical and sexual abuse may not be easily identified by the physical therapist. For example, the behaviors associated with child sexual abuse, including enuresis, nightmares, a decline in academic performance, secretiveness, and helpless behavior,

may not routinely be identified as possibly related to suspected child sexual abuse. This section includes a description of child and adult behavior that may be associated with abuse, as well as a general protocol for the documentation and reporting of suspected abuse. Appropriate referrals to other professionals in situations of suspected abuse are also considered.

LITIGATION

Although litigation is an unsavory topic to many pediatric physical therapists, it has become common in the United States health care system. As the number of lawsuits increases, so does the probability that the pediatric physical therapist's documentation may be subpoenaed for use in court. There are various reasons for an emphasis on objective and comprehensive documentation, including determination of need for services, child's areas of strength and limitations, and evaluation of the effectiveness of intervention. When records may be reviewed or interpreted by persons who do not share the physical therapist's vocabulary and who are not familiar with procedural interventions, use of objective data and valid tests and measures is essential. With the use of a case history format, this chapter considers the usefulness and relevance of various types of documentation and includes a situation in which the physical therapist's documentation was important in determining the outcome of the case.

MEDICAL TECHNOLOGY

Technologic advances in medical treatment have increased the rate of survival of infants and children who are medically fragile. Increasingly, differences of opinion among medical professionals or between parents and medical professionals regarding the choice of treatment and the continuation or deceleration of medical support have been decided in the courts. The child's present functional status and prognosis for motor function may be considerations in the determination of a plan of appropriate medical care. Prognosis may be estimated by the physician, psychologist, or physical therapist based on research evidence and personal experience.

Formulation of a functional prognosis for a child with a central nervous system deficit or congenital anomaly may not be a familiar task for the pediatric physical therapist. Should an opinion be requested, the pediatric physical therapist will require skills, including the ability to draw from past experience with similar cases and from the results of outcome-focused research studies, and in the presentation of the results of the examination, which may include the use of standardized measures. A case history is presented in this chapter as an illustration.

A related issue involves the pediatric physical therapist's ability to identify any personal values and beliefs that may affect objectivity in the formulation of an opinion regarding a child's functional abilities and outcome. Consideration of the relationship between belief systems and decision making, as well as the influence of the therapist's ethical standards, is included in this chapter.

INDIVIDUALS WITH DISABILITIES EDUCATION ACT

BACKGROUND AND PURPOSE

The purpose of the Individuals with Disabilities Education Act is to ensure that all children with disabilities have access to free and appropriate educational services. This includes special educational services and related services that meet each child's unique needs. Physical therapy is a primary service for children in early intervention (birth to age 3) and a related service for students in elementary through secondary education programs. Depending on state policy, physical therapy may be a primary or related service for children 3 to 5 years of age in preschool. The act seeks to protect the rights of children and their parents while assisting states and localities in providing education for all children with disabilities. IDEA attempts to ensure the effectiveness of efforts to educate children with disabilities. The focus of this section of the chapter is to summarize the Individuals with Disabilities Education Act Amendments of 1997 (Public Law 105-17) that are particularly relevant to physical therapy.

The purposes for the 1997 amendments are as follows [20 USC 14319(b)]:

1. Develop and implement a statewide comprehensive, coordinated multidisciplinary interagency system that provides early intervention services for infants and toddlers with disabilities and their families
2. Facilitate the coordination of payments for early intervention services from federal, state, and local and private sources (including public and private insurance coverage)
3. Enhance the capacity to provide quality early intervention services and expand and improve existing early intervention services being provided to infants and toddlers with disabilities and their families

4. Encourage states to expand opportunities for children under 3 years of age who would be at risk for having substantial developmental delay if they did not receive early intervention services

The background section of the amendments, based on a review of research, lists ways that programs providing special education services for children may be further strengthened and improved. Those suggestions include supporting the role of parents and ensuring that families have the opportunity to participate in their children's education, providing special education and related services in the regular classroom, and supporting high-quality professional development for all personnel.

Additionally, the issue of the effect of the changing cultural demographics on the educational environment of children with disabilities is raised. The rate of population increase for groups of people who are considered "minorities" in the United States is greater than that for white Americans. For example, it has been predicted that between 2000 and 2020, the rate in the population for white Americans will actually decrease by 4.4% while the rate of increase for racial and ethnic minorities will be much higher: 15% for Hispanics, 13.5% for African Americans, and 5.4% for Asians. By the year 2040, the population of the United States is expected to be 391 million and nearly 1 of every 3 people will be African-American, Hispanic, Asian-American, or American Indian.

The effect of population changes on public school systems is noted. Children from cultural groups that are considered minorities in the United States make up the majority of students in urban school systems. For example, in 2000 percentages of children from minority groups in public schools were 84% in Miami, 89% in Chicago, 78% in Philadelphia, 84% in Baltimore, 88% in Houston, and 88% in Los Angeles.

Many of these children have limited proficiency for communication in English, are more likely to be referred to special education services, and are more likely to drop out of school than white students. The number of teachers from "minority" cultural groups is also disproportionately low. Possible interventions to consider evolving student needs are addressed among funding priorities and a protocol for nondiscriminatory procedures to be used in testing and evaluation.

SERVICES FOR INFANTS AND TODDLERS

Title I of IDEA relates to delivery of early intervention services, including physical therapy, to children younger than 3 years of age. Important definitions include the following:

1. At risk infant or toddler:
   The term "at risk infant or toddler" means an individual under 3 years of age who would be at risk of experiencing a substantial developmental delay if early intervention services were not provided to the individual.
2. Council:
   The term "council" means a state interagency coordinating council established under section 1441 of this title.
3. Developmental delay:
   The term "developmental delay" when used with respect to an individual residing in a State, has the meaning given such term by the State under section 1435 (a) (1) of this title.
4. Early intervention services:
   The term "early intervention services" means developmental services that:
   A. are provided under public supervision;
   B. are provided at no cost except where Federal or State law provides for a system of payments by families, including a schedule of sliding fees;
   C. are designed to meet the developmental needs of an infant or toddler with a disability in any one or more of the following areas:
      i.   physical development
      ii. cognitive development
      iii. communication development
      iv. social or emotional development
      v.   adaptive development
   D. meet the standards of the State in which they are provided, including the requirements of this subchapter;
   E. include:
      i.   family training, counseling, and home visits;
      ii.   special instruction;
      iii. speech-language pathology and audiology services;
      iv.   occupational therapy;
      v.   physical therapy;
      vi.   psychological services;
      vii. service coordination services;
      viii. vision services;
      ix.   assistive technology devices and assistive technology;
      x.   transportation and related costs that are necessary to enable an infant or toddler and the infant's or toddler's family to receive another service described in this paragraph;
   F. are provided by qualified personnel, including:
      i.   special educators
      ii.   speech-language pathologists and audiologists
      iii. occupational therapists
      iv.   physical therapists
      v.   psychologists
      vi.   social workers
      vii. nurses

      viii. nutritionists
      ix.   family therapists
      x.   orientation and mobility specialists
      xi.   pediatricians and other physicians
   G. to the maximum extent appropriate, are provided in natural environments, including the home, and community settings in which children without disabilities participate; and
   H. are provided in conformity with an individualized family service plan adopted in accordance with section 1436 of this title.
5. Infant or toddler with a disability:
   The term "infant or toddler with a disability":
   A. means an individual under 3 years of age who needs early intervention services because the individual:
      i.   is experiencing developmental delays, as measured by appropriate diagnostic instruments and procedures in one or more of the areas including cognitive development, physical development, communication development, social or emotional development, and adaptive development; or
      ii. has a diagnosed physical or mental condition which has a high probability of resulting in developmental delay; and
   B. may also include at a state's discretion, at risk infants and toddlers.

   20 USC §§ 1432 et seq.

The inclusion of physical therapy as an early intervention service is related to the identification of physical development, including gross motor skill development, as one of the areas in which an infant with disabilities may receive intervention. Physical therapists are the professionals who are best qualified to examine and provide services to children with disabilities affecting motor development and their families.

IDEA identifies a wide range of professionals who provide coordinated services in partnership with an infant or toddler and her or his family. The physical therapist who works in early intervention will need to develop a style of interaction and communication that allows him or her to work with families and other members of the multidisciplinary team to best address the infant's or toddler's and family's needs. In early childhood, areas of development are interrelated, and children may not require direct services from all members of the team. Pediatric physical therapists, therefore, may need to broaden their skills in order to provide support in areas of development not ordinarily considered their areas of expertise (see Chapters 30 and 31).

Individual state policy on the magnitude of delay that will allow an infant or toddler to qualify to receive early intervention services will influence the physical therapist's plans for examination. Pediatric physical therapists should be sure the tests and measures they use are easily interpreted in light of the state's definition of developmental delay. For example, if delay is defined by the state in terms of standard deviations below the mean for age, the pediatric physical therapist will need to use an instrument on which performance scores may be presented as standard deviations varying around the mean score for the child's age.

AMENDMENTS RELATED TO THE INDIVIDUAL EDUCATIONAL PLAN

IDEA guarantees a free, appropriate public education to children with disabilities, 3 to 21 years old, including children who have previously been suspended from school. A system for locating children with disabilities who live in the state and offering such students special education services is outlined in the revision. The requirement for an individual educational plan (IEP) as the document that guides the child's participation in special education programs is stated.

Parents, regular and special education teachers, and, when appropriate, the child with a disability are identified as members of the IEP team. Although the physical therapist is not required to attend the IEP meeting, participation is encouraged when physical therapy will be included in the IEP or when there are issues regarding the need for physical therapy. The physical therapist may also be included on the IEP team at the request of a parent or other members of the team because of his or her knowledge or special expertise regarding the student.

Children with disabilities are to receive their education in the same environment as children who are not disabled to the maximum extent that is appropriate. A child should be removed from the regular education environment only when the nature or severity of a child's disability does not allow participation in regular classes, even if supplementary aids and special education services are offered.

The IDEA amendments of 1997 gives states the authority to refer children with disabilities to a private school or facility if a free, appropriate public education is not otherwise available. This referral must be in conformance with the IEP, and the private school or facility must provide special education services. The child will attend the private school or facility at no cost to the parents. The school or facility must meet the state educational agency's and the local educational agency's standards and requirements. The child in a private education setting has all the rights of a child with a disability who is served by a public agency.

If a child with a disability is placed in a private school or facility by the parents, the public agency is not required to pay for the child's education at the private school or facility. The public agency, however, must make services available to the child. Children with disabilities who attend private schools are to receive special education and related services in accordance with an IEP. Services may be provided on the premises of private and parochial schools.

An emphasis of the IDEA amendments on providing the opportunity for children with disabilities to receive their education in regular education settings will influence the contexts in which pediatric physical therapists practice. In the past, pediatric physical therapists working in school systems have practiced in schools where the majority of students had disabilities. In accordance with IDEA, physical therapists will work primarily in settings that are inclusive of all students. Children with disabilities are likely to receive services in private, parochial, and public school settings (see Chapter 32).

The emphasis on including children with disabilities in the general education curriculum in their neighborhood school has direct implications for the provision of physical therapy services. A therapist's caseload may involve students from several schools, necessitating time for travel between schools. Therapy goals focus not only on a child's ability to function independently within the physical structure of the school, but also on learning motor skills necessary to participate in activities that are part of the general education curriculum. Therapists will plan therapeutic activities using materials that are readily available in schools or easily transported to a student's school. Coordination, communication, and consultation with teachers and other school personnel are important roles of the physical therapist in the educational setting.

EVALUATION

The 1997 amendments to IDEA include guidelines for all personnel involved in the evaluation of children with disabilities. The term *evaluation* as used in federal laws is similar to *examination* as defined in the *Guide to Physical Therapist Practice* (American Physical Therapy Association, 1997). Following the guidelines established by the IDEA ensures that the physical therapist will evaluate an infant, toddler, or student in an appropriate manner consistent with standards for best practice.

The IDEA amendment requires the following:

1. The person performing an evaluation will use a variety of tests and measures to gather information relevant to a child's function and development, including information provided by the parent, that

may assist in determining whether the child qualifies for services, and the child's IEP, including information related to a child's ability to participate in the general curriculum or, for preschool children, to participate in appropriate activities.

2. The person performing an evaluation will not use the results of any single test or measure as the sole criterion for determining whether a child qualifies for services or for determining an appropriate educational program for the child. The IEP must not only state goals the team is trying to achieve but also the child's current level of function.

3. The person performing an evaluation will use technically sound instruments that may assess the relative contribution of cognitive and behavioral factors, in addition to physical or developmental factors.

Additionally, there are requirements to help prevent discrimination against children from varied cultural backgrounds during the evaluation process. Specifically, the amendment requires that

A. tests and other materials used to evaluate a child are:
   i. selected and administered so as not to be discriminatory on a racial or cultural basis; and
   ii. provided and administered in the child's native language or other mode of communication, unless it is clearly not feasible to do so; and
B. standardized tests that are given to the child:
   i. have been validated for the specific purpose for which they are used;
   ii. are administered by trained and knowledgeable personnel; and
   iii. are administered in accordance with any instructions provided by the authors of the tests;
C. the child is assessed in all areas of suspected disability; and
D. the tests and measures used provide relevant information that assists persons in determining the educational needs of the child.

Title 20, USC § 1414(b)

Eligibility determination is to be made by a team of qualified professionals, which may include the physical therapist. The team must be sure that a child is not determined to have a disability solely because of a lack of proper educational instruction or because of limited English proficiency. Eligibility determination must take into consideration existing evaluation data, classroom-based observations, teacher and related service provider observations, and input from the child's parents. The IEP should be explained to the parents in their native language.

Nondiscriminatory Procedures

In addition to federal requirements, each state must include procedural safeguards to ensure that testing and evaluation materials and procedures are not racially or culturally discriminatory. The parent must be fully informed of all information relevant to the evaluation in his or her native language. The evaluation materials or procedures shall be provided and administered in the child's native language or mode of communication, unless it is clearly not feasible. No single procedure should be the sole criterion for determination of an appropriate educational program for a child.

In accordance with the guidelines for evaluation outlined in the revision, physical therapists must carefully consider selection of tests and evaluation procedures. In order for findings to be valid, a child must be evaluated using tests or measures that have been standardized or normed on children of the same cultural group and economic level.

Consideration of the child's developmental experiences and culture is essential when deciding on the appropriate tests given the diverse cultural backgrounds of today's student population. The physical therapist must be sure that assumptions about the developmental experiences of the child being evaluated are accurate. For example, authors of a test may assume that preschool-age children have had experiences on riding toys and that riding a tricycle will be a familiar experience for a 3-year-old child. The performance of a child who has recently immigrated to the United States from a Southeast Asian refugee camp and has never ridden on a tricycle cannot be considered a valid indicator of gross motor and coordination skills. Similarly, if a test item is based on the assumption that preschool-age children have experience eating with a spoon, administration of the item to a child from a family that uses bread held in the fingers to scoop and eat food may not be valid.

The IDEA amendments require that no one instrument or score be used alone to determine eligibility and that observation of the child's functioning in the school environment be included as part of the evaluation. The use of information and data from multiple sources (child, teacher, parent, direct observation) will help the physical therapist consider various aspects of the child's functional abilities in the evaluation process and will decrease the possibility that the therapist will make erroneous conclusions concerning the child's true abilities.

STATE ADVISORY PANEL

Each state shall establish a state advisory panel on the education of children with disabilities. The function of the advisory panel is to advise the state educational agency of needs within the state in education of children with disabilities. The advisory panel is to comment on promulgated rules and policies with regard to children with disabilities and assist the state in developing and reporting information to the federal government. The governor or other authorized state official appoints the members of the advisory panel. The advisory panel must be composed of persons involved in or concerned with the education of children with disabilities. The membership must include at least one person representative of each of the following groups:

> Individuals with disabilities
> Teachers of children with disabilities
> Parents of children with disabilities
> State and local education officials
> Special education program administrators

The majority of the advisory panel should be individuals with disabilities or parents of children with disabilities.

PERSONNEL STANDARDS

Physical therapists are identified in the IDEA as professionals who are appropriate to work with infants, toddlers, and children with disabilities. Each state is required to establish standards to ensure that personnel have the necessary qualifications and are adequately prepared. Personnel preparation standards are based on the highest requirements in the state applicable to the profession or discipline in which a person is providing special education or related services. This ensures that physical therapy services are provided by or under the direction of licensed physical therapists. A role of the state advisory panel is to ensure that problems with the provision of special educational services are identified and corrected.

CASE STUDY

JACQUELINE

Jacqueline is a 3-year-old girl who is a student in a self-contained special education class in a school that is about a 30-minute drive from her home. Jacqueline's parents requested that she attend her neighborhood school with her sister so that the two girls could go to school together. Jacqueline's family is Mexican and Spanish is spoken at home. Preschool is the only setting where Jacqueline is spoken to in English.

As the school prepared to decide about the parents' request, Jacqueline underwent testing aimed at determining her levels of function. Jacqueline was determined to have significant limitations in her language and cognitive skills. When questioned at the IEP meeting, the teacher and speech pathologist revealed that all testing had been done in English. This was assumed to be appropriate because Jacqueline's placement was in a classroom of English-speaking teachers and students. Based on the evaluation findings, the director of special education recommended against Jacqueline's placement in her neighborhood school.

Response

This scenario brings to light two issues. The first is the parents' desire to have Jacqueline attend her neighborhood school. The requirement of the IDEA is that children with disabilities be placed in the least restrictive environment (LRE). Unless the IEP requires some other arrangement, the child should be educated in the school that she would attend if she did not have a disability (CFR 42 300.522 E). When the LRE is at issue, the school district bears the burden of proving compliance with the least restrictive environment requirement of the IDEA (*Oberti v. Board of Education of the Borough of Clementes School District*).

The second issue to be considered is the way this evaluation was conducted. English is not Jacqueline's first language. Evaluations and tests used to assess a child must be selected and administered so as not to be discriminatory on racial or cultural bias. School systems must ensure that children's tests are provided and administered in the child's native language or another method of communication unless it is clearly not feasible to do so. The materials and procedures used to assess a child with limited English proficiency are selected and administered to ensure that they measure the extent to which the child has a disability and needs special education services rather than measuring the child's English proficiency (42 CFR § 300.532).

Finally, the United States Commission on Civil Rights recognizes that children from minority populations may be overrepresented in special education classes in some jurisdictions. If a therapist suspects this is the case, the Commission on Civil Rights should be contacted.

Outcome

Following action by an attorney representing Jacqueline's family, evaluation of Jacqueline's cognitive and language skills was repeated with services of a translator. The translator worked with the teacher and speech and language pathologist. The evaluation was done in Jacqueline's home where her mother felt that she was more comfortable and communicated most effectively. Based on the results, Jacqueline was placed in her neighborhood school in a regular 4-year-old pre-kindergarten classroom. Jacqueline's regular education teacher also had a background in special education. A full-time aide, fluent in Spanish, was assigned to the classroom and her primary responsibility was the support of Jacqueline and one other student. Jacqueline received physical, occupational, and speech therapy services from itinerant therapists who visited Jacqueline's neighborhood school.

Early Intervention Fiscal Crisis

In 2004, Georgia's Medicaid department experienced a financial crisis related to a shortfall in projected tax collections and the technical failures and errors made by a subcontractor responsible for paying therapists' and other providers' claims. The errors resulted in overpayment in the form of estimated claims payments.

In an attempt to avoid a complete collapse of the payment system, the state decided to require the payment of a premium for Medicaid insurance offered to families of children with disabilities participating in the Katie Beckett program. The Katie Beckett program provides supplementary Medicaid coverage to families who have private health insurance that is deemed inadequate for the costs of medical care for their medically fragile children. Physical therapists working by contract with early intervention programs are reimbursed by a combination of private insurance and Medicaid payments for children participating in the Katie Beckett program.

In March, parents of children participating in the Katie Beckett program were ordered to send copies of their 2003 income tax returns and were given as little as 2 weeks' notice, so that the state could determine the amount of their required premium. Premium payments were to begin in 2004, and the failure to pay the premium would result in the discontinuation of the child's Medicaid insurance. No state legislative changes accompanied this decision and the related requests.

Response

Medicaid has been extended through the implementation of the Katie Beckett program. The program is a special eligibility process that allows certain children with long-term disabilities or complex medical needs to obtain a Medicaid card. To qualify, a child must meet the following criteria:

Younger than 19 years old and living at home.
Determined to be disabled by the standards of the Social Security Act.
Requires a level of care at home that is typically provided in a hospital or nursing facility.
Can be provided safe and appropriate care in the family home.
The child as an individual does not have income of assets in excess of the current standard for a child living in an institution.
The cost of services for the child's home does not exceed the cost Medicaid would pay if the child were in an institution.

If the Katie Beckett application is approved, the child receives a Medicaid card that can be used to pay for services and equipment allowed under the Medicaid program.

In this case, because only the child's income and resources are used to determine financial eligibility it is difficult for the state to charge or increase premiums for Medicaid insurance. The parents' or guardians' income cannot be considered, therefore there must be a change (increase) in the *child's* income for a premium to be considered.

Outcome

The proposed creation of policy that required the payment of Medicaid premiums based the parents' income was deemed not to be legal and was abandoned.

When the state Medicaid system was unable to increase available funds by collecting premiums from families enrolled in the Katie Beckett program, the number of allowable physical, occupational, and speech therapy visits allowed per month was reduced by 50%. The Medicaid program outlined a process for applying for an exemption to the reduced number of visits allowed per month, but these prior approval requests were summarily denied.

Children participating in the early intervention program were receiving services, as outlined in their family's Individualized Family Services Plan. Many children's plans indicated a frequency of physical therapy services of two visits per week, which exceeded the new number of allowable visits per month (five).

The state responded by suggesting that physical therapists continue providing services at the frequency outlined in the IFSP, and to request an exemption and authorization for the two visits per week outlined in the IFSP, at least until the current IFSP expired. If denied, the state stated in a memo that the counties would "try" to reimburse the therapists for services that Medicaid denied.

Response

The state attempted to cut services after the attempt to collect premiums from families enrolled in the Katie Beckett program failed. However the IFSP required more frequent service and the only way the IFSP could be altered is if there was a change in the child's condition or at an IFSP meeting with the parents' involvement and agreement to decrease the frequency of therapy services.

Because Medicaid has changed the number of visits it will reimburse, but the IFSP requires more frequent visits, the argument can be made that the child has become ineligible for Medicaid coverage for the sessions recommended in the IFSP that are in excess of the new Medicaid guidelines. Because the county is the payer of last resort, the county is obligated to pay for these visits for the remainder of the period of the current IFSP.

AMERICANS WITH DISABILITIES ACT

Although the Americans with Disabilities Act is frequently considered to be most closely related to employment and public access for individuals with disabilities, sections of the law are particularly relevant to families of children with disabilities. The purpose of this section is to summarize portions of this law that are useful to physical therapists in their role as advocates for families of children with disabilities. Illustrative case examples are included.

EMPLOYMENT

The ADA prevents an employer from denying an employment opportunity or benefit because of an individual's association with a person who has a disability. The law protects a parent from being denied a job because she or he has a child with a disability. An employer cannot assume that because an employee is the parent of a child with a disability, the employee may be unavailable or unreliable with respect to job requirements.

The law also prohibits discrimination related to health insurance benefits that are offered as a fringe benefit of employment. An employer cannot deny an applicant a job or refuse to hire a parent of a child with a disability because the employer anticipates an increase in insurance costs, nor can an employer subject an employee who has a child with a disability to different terms or conditions of insurance. Although the parent of a child with a disability is protected from discrimination in the areas of hiring

and insurance, the employer is not obligated to modify work schedules to accommodate child care.

The ADA also protects parents from discrimination related to association with other individuals with disabilities or to working with organizations associated with persons with disabilities. For example, a parent who does volunteer work for a service organization for acquired immunodeficiency syndrome cannot be discriminated against in employment opportunities or in benefits of employment such as health insurance.

ENFORCEMENT PROVISIONS

Parents who believe that they have been discriminated against in relation to hiring or insurance can file a charge with the United States Department of Justice. Parents may also file a charge if they believe that retaliation has occurred as a result of filing a charge or opposing a discriminatory practice.

The Department of Justice investigates charges of discrimination. If the Department of Justice believes that discrimination has occurred, an attempt at resolution will be made. If conciliation fails, the Department of Justice will file suit or issue a "right to sue" letter to the person who filed the charge. Remedies for violations of the ADA related to employment include hiring, reinstatement, promotion, the payment of back pay and front pay, and restoration of benefits, including health insurance.

The ADA covers all activities of state and local governments regardless of the government entity's size or receipt of federal funding. The act requires that state and local governments give people with disabilities an equal opportunity to benefit from all of their programs, services, courts, and activities (e.g., public education, employment, transportation, recreation, health care, social services, courts, voting, and town meetings).

Complaints of ADA violations may be filed with the Department of Justice within 180 days of the date of discrimination. In certain situations, cases may be referred to a mediation program sponsored by the Department of Justice. The Department of Justice may bring a lawsuit when it has investigated a matter and has been unable to resolve violations.

TRANSPORTATION

The ADA protects individuals with disabilities from discrimination with respect to participation in any public services, programs, or activities. Public transportation, including buses and rapid rail systems, is included under the rubric of "public services." According to the law, new buses and rail cars purchased after July 26, 1990, as well as stations constructed after this date, must be accessible to individuals with disabilities who may require wheelchairs or other assistive devices for mobility or who may have a visual impairment.

Public transportation services for individuals with disabilities must be available on a schedule that is comparable to that provided for persons without a disability. Available transportation may include transportation that is accessible to a person who does or does not require a wheelchair lift for transportation. The law provides for assistance with transportation to regular public transportation stops for those who are unable to reach these stops without assistance. The law also provides for transportation of an accompanying assistant for the individual with a disability as long as the assistant's seat is not needed for another person with a disability.

Parents of children with disabilities who live in areas served by public transportation should expect increased availability of accessible transportation services. Bus service, for example, should be available on the same schedule as service for persons without a disability. Public transportation service may also become available at a family's residence, should a child be unable to get to a regular transportation stop independently. On intercity and commuter rail systems, at least one rail car per train must be accessible to individuals with disabilities.

PHYSICAL STRUCTURES

The ADA also protects individuals with disabilities from discrimination related to limited access to public accommodations. Public accommodations may include hotels, restaurants, food and retail stores, and shopping malls. Recreational facilities, such as amusement parks, zoos, and museums, are also included. Educational facilities, such as nurseries, elementary or secondary schools, and public and private undergraduate and graduate colleges and universities, must be accessible.

State and local governments are required to follow specific architectural standards in the new construction and alteration of their buildings. They also must relocate programs or otherwise provide access in inaccessible older buildings and communicate effectively with people who have hearing, vision, or speech disabilities. Public entities are not required to make modifications that would involve undue financial and administrative burdens. They are required to make reasonable modifications to policies, practices, and procedures where necessary to avoid discrimination, unless they can demonstrate that doing so would fundamentally alter the nature of the service, program, or activity being provided.

Families of children with disabilities may expect greater access to structures in their communities related to education, shopping, and recreation. Greater access for persons who require assistance or devices for mobility should facilitate the integration of these individuals into all areas of the community.

CASE STUDY

ANNA

Ms. Jones is the single parent of Anna, a child with Down syndrome. Ms. Jones is a licensed ultrasound technologist and worked until the birth of her daughter. She planned to return to work 3 months after her daughter's birth; however, because of the medical complications Anna experienced, Ms. Jones decided to remain at home, forfeiting her past position. By the time Anna was 8 months old, she was doing well medically, and Ms. Jones applied for a job with a small, private company that contracted out ultrasonography services to local hospitals and physicians' offices.

During the employment interview, the personnel director commented favorably on Ms. Jones' excellent work record and references from her past employer. He inquired regarding the reason that Ms. Jones decided not to return to her old position. When Ms. Jones related the circumstances of her daughter's birth and disability, the tone of the interview changed. The personnel director questioned Ms. Jones regarding her ability to meet her daughter's medical needs and the demands of a full-time job and interjected his personal experience with a family in his neighborhood who had a child with a disability. In that family, the mother's decision to remain at home was considered a necessity.

Ms. Jones believed when she left the interview that she would probably not be offered the job. Her suspicion was confirmed when she received a letter stating that the job was offered to another qualified applicant. Ms. Jones was puzzled when the company continued to advertise the position. She contacted the personnel director again and was able to convince him of her ability to handle both the job and the care of her daughter. After considerable negotiation, she was offered the position under the stipulation that she accept a lower amount of health insurance coverage than the company's other employees and pay a slightly higher rate. Ms. Jones questioned the personnel manager's right to make such an offer and wondered if she should seek the opinion of an employment rights specialist.

Response

Ms. Jones should seek the opinion of an employment rights specialist. Under the employment component of the ADA, the actions of this employer are illegal. In a hiring situation, it is illegal even to consider a dependent with a disability. This act attempts to level the playing field for parents of children with disabilities. Questions as to the health of dependent children are not related to the job and, therefore, are prohibited under ADA.

Second, Ms. Jones is entitled to the same benefits as the company's other employees. It is illegal under ADA to require Ms. Jones to contribute more for health insurance or to provide her with less coverage. The employer cannot pass the extra cost of the insurance on to the parent.

CHILD ABUSE AND NEGLECT

The subject of child abuse and neglect is discussed more openly and freely than in the past. A possibly related phenomenon is the increase in the number of reported cases of child abuse (De Jong et al., 1983; Hampton & Newberger, 1985). Because physical therapists may provide services to children who are at risk for or have experienced abuse or neglect, a review of the signs of abuse and the physical therapist's responsibility with respect to reporting suspected abuse is provided in this section.

NEGLECT

Child abuse and neglect are defined by the Child Abuse Prevention and Treatment Act of 1974 as "the physical or mental injury, sexual abuse, negligent treatment or maltreatment of a child under the age of eighteen by a person who is responsible for the child's welfare under circumstances which indicate that the child's health and welfare are harmed or threatened hereby" (Public Law 93-247, p. 247). Child abuse and neglect may occur in various forms, including, but not limited to, severe physical injury that may be fatal or life-threatening.

Neglect occurs when a child's basic needs are not being met by an adult who is responsible for the child's well-being. Neglectful situations may involve inadequate or unstable shelter or inadequate or inappropriate nutrition. Neglect may also occur related to lack of needed medical or dental care. Concerning medical neglect, the physical therapist may be the member of the health care team who observes and documents a pattern of missed appointments or noncompliance with instructions that results in deterioration in the child's status. In such a situation, the physical therapist is responsible for reporting the suspected neglect to the proper authorities.

A difficulty in the determination of neglect is related to willfulness. Neglect need not be a willful act on the part of the adult responsible (Newberger et al., 1987). Neglect may be related to a parent's inability to meet a child's needs because of extreme environmental stresses or may be related to a parent's limited knowledge concerning appropriate stimulation and behavior management for children.

Neglect that is not willful may be distressing to report from the physical therapist's perspective. Filing a report may be associated with blaming the parents for the child's situation. An important consideration in a case of nonwillful neglect is the ultimate effect on the child: If the child is not thriving because nutritional, medical, or other physical or emotional needs are not being met, intervention is needed. Examples of situations in which neglect may be present are listed in Box 37-1.

PHYSICAL ABUSE

The symptoms associated with physical abuse have been collectively termed the *battered child syndrome* (Kempe et al., 1962). Associated physical injuries may be detected

---

Box 37-1	Signs and Situations Associated with Child Neglect

Evidence of poor nutrition	Lack of compliance with medical or therapy
Reports of hunger	appointments
Nutritionally inadequate diet	Excessive cancellations
Evidence of poor hygiene	Frequent "no shows"
Soiled clothing	Lack of follow-through with home program
Soiled skin, body odors	instructions, resulting in a decline in the child's
Skin breakdown in diaper area	status
Dental caries	

Box 37-2	**Signs and Symptoms of Physical Abuse: Battered Child Syndrome**
Bony fractures	Welts
Soft tissue injuries	Internal injuries
Burns	Contusions
Hematomas	

by a child's pediatrician, an emergency department physician, or a school nurse. The physical manifestations include injury to bone and soft tissue, as well as affective changes. Signs and symptoms associated with the battered child syndrome are listed in Box 37-2.

Because a child's clothing is sometimes removed during physical therapy provided in a clinic setting, signs of physical abuse may be more readily and naturally observed than in other settings, such as the school classroom. When symptoms are observed, the suspected abuse must be reported to the proper authorities. The fact that symptoms commonly associated with abuse may also be related to other medical conditions or common childhood accidents deserves careful consideration. A differential diagnosis can be made only by a physician. Questionable symptoms require further investigation by a physician.

SEXUAL ABUSE

The signs of sexual abuse that may be observed by the pediatric physical therapist are likely to be manifested behaviorally. Psychosomatic or behavioral illnesses, behavioral alterations, and acting-out behaviors may accompany sexual child abuse (Gommes-Schwartz et al., 1985). Somatization, or the expression of emotional conflicts as symptoms of physical illness, frequently occurs in association with sexual child abuse (Rosenfeld, 1982; Rosenfeld & Sarles, 1986). The occurrence of behavioral disorders such as anorexia nervosa, bulimia, enuresis, or encopresis may signal sexual abuse. Abdominal pain without an organic cause is an example of a psychosomatic problem that may be associated with sexual abuse. Behavioral changes such as an alteration in school performance, atypical shyness, and extroverted or hostile behavior may be associated with sexual abuse (Rosenfeld, 1982; Rosenfeld & Sarles, 1987).

Psychosomatic and behavioral problems, however, may be associated with problems other than sexual abuse, and such symptoms and signs require further evaluation by a professional such as a medical social worker, psychologist, or physician. Sexual acting-out behavior, sexual

aggression toward other children, or an overly sophisticated knowledge of sexual activities and practice are salient signs of sexual abuse.

Child sexual abuse accommodation syndrome (Summitt, 1982) describes the behaviors associated with a child's attempt to adapt to sexual abuse that occur over time. As a young child attempts to cope with feelings of disbelief, rejection, helplessness, and self-blame associated with victimization by sexual abuse, long-lasting behavioral changes may be noted. Secrecy; helplessness; entrapment and accommodation; delayed, conflicted, and unconvincing disclosure of incidents; and retraction of reported abuse are all behaviors associated with child sexual abuse accommodation syndrome.

A physical therapist who observes a child behaving in a manner that may be associated with ongoing sexual abuse should give such behavior careful consideration. Secrecy regarding relationships with certain adults or conflicting reports about incidents that are suspicious may be indicators of a child's victimization by sexual abuse. A physical therapist who suspects sexual abuse may work together with a social worker, psychologist, or physician to further evaluate the child's situation and make necessary reports to the appropriate authorities.

LEGAL OBLIGATION TO REPORT

A review of state laws in various geographic regions of the United States reveals that health care professionals, including physical therapists, are unequivocally required to immediately report suspected child abuse to the proper agency (III Illinois Annotated Statutes; Official Code of Georgia, Annotated). Each state or county has an established protocol for the reporting of suspected abuse. Protocols describe the routing of reports of abuse, the consideration of factors in the determination of the child's risk status, and a plan for removal from the home, if necessary (California Penal Code). Protocols are available for examination through county departments of family and children's services and agencies such as state councils on child abuse.

Failure to report suspected child abuse is a misdemeanor in most states. Associated penalties include monetary fines, imprisonment, or both. Failure to report suspected abuse may also result in the revocation or suspension of a professional license or the denial of licensure renewal.

Many state statutes protect an individual who reports suspected abuse from civil action related to a lack of substantiation of the report (Official Code of Georgia, Annotated). Such a statute frees the individual making the report from undue concern over retaliation on the part of the accused party should the report be unconfirmed. State statutes also address the situation in which individuals knowingly make false reports of abuse (23 Illinois Annotated Statutes). A consideration of the repercussions for failure to report suspected abuse reflects the seriousness of this crime and its effect on children.

If abuse is suspected, the physical therapist should call the proper authorities immediately. Delaying a call could place a child at further risk. The physical therapist does not need to know for certain that abuse or neglect has occurred to make a report. The therapist need only suspect that there is a risk that abuse or neglect may occur to make a report.

The physical therapist should not investigate the circumstances for child abuse. The responsibility for investigation rests with the proper authorities. Any investigation by persons other than a child protection worker or a police officer may prejudice efforts to protect the child.

The following case history taken from the experience of one of the authors illustrates issues related to the reporting of suspected child abuse by health care professionals in general and by pediatric physical therapists specifically.

CASE STUDY

JERRY

Amy, a pediatric physical therapist working in an early intervention program, makes routine home visits to infants and their families. A considerable proportion of Amy's caseload is with families who are indigent. One of Amy's patients is Jerry, an 18-month-old infant with spina bifida. Jerry's defect is at the upper thoracic level of his spine. Jerry demonstrates some functional use of his upper extremities but no volitional movement in his lower extremities.

Jerry lives with his parents, Mr. and Mrs. Smith, and two older siblings. Mrs. Smith was in junior high school when her eldest child was born. She is now 18 years old. Mrs. Smith has attempted to complete her high school education, but her course work has been interrupted by Jerry's frequent hospitalizations. In a conversation with Amy, Mrs. Smith related that she does not receive much support from Mr. Smith, who believes that Jerry will somehow eventually recover from his disability. She also told Amy about Mr. Smith's history of substance abuse and her own history of having been abused during her childhood. At the present time, Mrs. Smith appears listless, and Amy believes that Mrs. Smith is depressed.

On her visits to Jerry's house, Amy has been concerned about Jerry's care. He is not usually bathed and dressed by the time she visits at 1 o'clock in the afternoon. His diaper is usually wet, and his pajamas smell of urine. He often acts hungry and weak. Mrs. Smith frequently reports that she has fed Jerry "a few bites from her own plate," but not a full meal of his own.

One occasion when Amy worked with Jerry in his own bedroom, she noticed that one of the railings of his crib was missing, leaving an open space. Amy was also concerned because on one of her visit days, she had met Mrs. Smith walking home from the store and Mrs. Smith reported that Jerry was not at home and said that Amy should not come in. Amy believed that she had heard Jerry's voice inside the home.

During Amy's most recent visit to Jerry's home, she discovered a small decubitus ulcer forming in the sacral region of Jerry's spine. Amy was concerned about Jerry's health and safety but at the same time did not want to blame Mrs. Smith. Amy believed that Mrs. Smith was probably doing the best she could, considering her depression, her lack of resources, and lack of support from Jerry's father. Amy decided that she needed to try to determine her responsibility in informing an outside agency about her concerns for Jerry's welfare.

Response

The state laws usually require that all cases of suspected abuse and neglect be reported immediately to the proper authorities. The key word here is "suspected" abuse and neglect. The law does not require a case of neglect to be proved before being reported. It requires that any information that would tend to indicate that a child is abused or neglected be reported.

It is important that the physical therapist document specific findings and report a case to the authorities. Many states make failure to report a case of suspected abuse or neglect a misdemeanor punishable by up to 12 months in jail.

LITIGATION

Although litigation is an area in which physical therapists may not wish to be involved, issues related to medical malpractice are permeating all areas of the health care system. Medically related lawsuits are increasing rapidly in our society. Physical therapists must be aware of the process of litigation and of how they may willingly or unwillingly be involved. In this section, issues relevant to litigation are presented from an attorney's perspective to make the pediatric physical therapist aware of how components of practice, such as medical documentation, fit in the scheme of medically related litigation.

O'Sullivan (1975) has outlined the process for review of the medical record in preparation for the presentation of a medical malpractice case in court. Consistency in chart records is considered to be a primary point of evaluation of a medical record. A medical record should, according to O'Sullivan, be straightforward and flow smoothly from beginning to end. Chart records should be consistent. Inconsistencies in charting are "red flags" for further scrutiny by the attorney involved. Among noted inconsistencies are discrepancy between diagnoses and selected therapy or intervention and chronologic inconsistencies between objective findings and corresponding changes in intervention. Improper use of forms and improper reporting of information or incidents to authorities are also examples of inconsistencies. Even the smallest of inconsistencies are considered relevant, particularly to the attorney whose client alleges hospital liability or negligence on the part of the health care provider.

Progress notes should include documentation of changes in patient status. Notes are expected to include changes in symptoms, complaints, objective signs, and the results of tests that contribute to the understanding of the diagnosed condition. When progress notes are complete, "there is no reason to evaluate other records" (O'Sullivan, 1975, p. 125).

Documentation serves as the interface between the physical therapist and the attorney in legal cases. Clear, objective, and accurate documentation is an essential component of quality treatment, regardless of whether it is ever evaluated by an attorney or outside party. However, in the event that records are subpoenaed, organized, clear, and objective records will serve both to protect the physical therapist from liability and to provide an accurate account of the status and progress of the patient.

When a medical record may be evaluated by an outside party who is not an expert in the characteristics and usual physical therapy interventions for a child with a specific developmental disability, documentation such as progress notes or evaluations should be written in terms that are understandable and meaningful to individuals who are not physical therapists and who are not familiar with a particular approach or theoretic orientation.

Therapists must document change objectively and clearly so that findings are understood by people not familiar with the child's health condition. The use of norm-referenced, standardized measures may provide data concerning a child's motor performance in comparison with peers that is easily understood by others and useful for assessment and possibly documentation of change.

MEDICAL TECHNOLOGY

Another potential interface between physical therapists and the legal system involves children who are dependent on medical technology for survival. As medical technology has become more sophisticated, the ability to support children whose illnesses or injuries would, in other times, have been fatal has increased (see Chapter 26).

The point at which the continuation of technologic life support compromises the quality of a child's life is not easily determined. Because individual physicians, health care professionals, and families differ in their beliefs about issues related to quality of life and preservation of life, differences of opinion exist regarding the extent to which technologic life-support measures should be employed. At times, disagreements between parents and physicians and other members of the health care team, such as nurses and social workers, have been so extreme that decisions regarding the appropriateness of medical interventions have been made by the court system (National Center for State Courts, 1991).

One of the considerations in the determination of whether technologic life support should continue for a particular child may be the child's prognosis with respect to the expected future level of functioning. Although physicians have formulated prognoses for children in court cases in the past, it is not unlikely that the physical therapist may be asked to contribute a clinical opinion regarding a child's developmental outcome. The following case study provides an example of a physical therapist's involvement in a health care team decision regarding the continuation of technologic life support for an infant. Although this particular case was not decided in court, it is representative of the type of situation in which pediatric physical therapists may increasingly be involved.

CASE STUDY

KENNY

Kenny is an infant born at 23 to 24 weeks' gestational age at a birth weight of 770 g. Kenny's mother is a single parent who received no prenatal care. His father was involved in an emotional relationship with his mother; however, their relationship was physically abusive. One child previously was removed from the home by the Department of Family and Children's Services.

Kenny experienced multiple neonatal complications, including necrotizing enterocolitis, severe broncho-pulmonary dysplasia, and several unsuccessful attempts to permanently wean him from ventilator support. Kenny's other medical complications include metabolic bone disease, intrahepatic cholestasis, and multiple bouts of sepsis. He also experienced a grade III intraventricular hemorrhage. His head circumference is significantly less than would be expected for his age and other anthropometric measurements, probably as a result of cerebral atrophy.

At 10 months chronologic age, Kenny's physical therapist, Sharon, estimated Kenny's level of motor functioning to be at 1 month. At this time, he began to experience a slow deterioration of his cardiopulmonary system, including congestive heart failure. Related to the deterioration of his health status, Sharon reported that it was difficult to follow through with the physical therapy intervention plan because the infant was frequently too ill to tolerate being handled and moved. He was infrequently alert and did not demonstrate visual observation of faces or other interactive behavior. Active movements were athetoid in quality. Just before a significant decline in his status, including congestive heart failure, Kenny experienced a few days in which he was able to tolerate being placed on a mat and handled.

Subsequently, Kenny experienced a decline in his status and was reintubated and ventilated. Kenny's primary physician, a pediatric intensive care specialist, and other members of Kenny's health care team began to consider the appropriateness of the repeated intubation and ventilation and other technologic support measures. Kenny's mother frequently inquired about his prognosis and level of functioning and was willing to consider a deceleration in his care. Kenny's father, however, was not in agreement with such a plan.

Kenny's doctor approached Sharon with questions about Kenny's current level of motor functioning and his expected outcome in future years should the infant's medical condition become more stable. In light of this request, the therapist was asked for information on Kenny's present status and prognosis for future level of functioning.

Response

In a situation such as Kenny's, the physical therapist, Sharon, could integrate information from a variety of sources in the formulation of her opinion. She could use her own clinical judgment, based on experience with other infants who had similar characteristic motor patterns and shared a similar medical history. Fortunately, Sharon had several years of pediatric experience with toddlers and older children in addition to her work in a neonatal intensive care unit. In this case, Kenny's lack of behavioral interaction, severely delayed motor skills, and athetoid movements were considered in the formulation of Sharon's opinion.

Sharon also considered the results of outcome research studies on infants who experienced some of the same neonatal complications that Kenny experienced. In her review of outcome studies, Sharon found that grade III intracranial hemorrhage and cerebral atrophy were associated with a poor neurodevelopmental outcome. Based on assessment and observations, past experience with infants whose motor abilities were similar to Kenny's, and a review of the literature concerning neuro-developmental outcome, Sharon was able to formulate an opinion regarding Kenny's developmental prognosis. Sharon expected that Kenny would have lifelong motor impairments and severe limitations in mobility and self-care.

Because Kenny died before the issues related to technologic support were resolved, this case did not reach the court system. Nevertheless, Sharon's strategy for the formulation of an opinion could have been used in a legal case. Sharon's use of her past experience together with a review of the outcome literature helped her to formulate an opinion. Although not used in this instance, results of a norm-referenced standardized measure of motor development would also have been helpful.

Ethical Concerns

Although not a consideration in this case, the formulation of an opinion about Kenny might have presented an ethical dilemma for Sharon. For example, if Sharon's personal beliefs regarding the continuation or removal of technologic support for critically ill patients had not been congruent with that of the family and other members of the health care team, the formulation of an opinion might have been difficult. Health care professionals' personal beliefs regarding the sources of health improvement in their patients are as likely to contribute to the clinical decision-making formulation as is past experience or a review of the literature.

In the development of their measurement tool, the Child Health Improvement Locus of Control scales, DeVellis and colleagues (1985) considered the relation between parental beliefs and behavior associated with their child's illness. The Child Health Improvement Locus of Control scales assess parental beliefs related to the source of control over a child's recovery and outcome. Research using the Child Health Improvement Locus of Control scales demonstrated that parents may ascribe different amounts of responsibility for child health improvement to factors such as the child himself or herself, health care professionals, parents, chance, or divine influence as determinants of their child's recovery (DeVellis et al., 1985). For example, whereas one parent may believe that professionals are primarily responsible for their child's recovery, another may attribute recovery to divine intervention or to chance.

Health care professionals, like parents, may attribute health improvement in infants and children to various factors. Health care professionals' locus of control with respect to health improvement in children may influence their decision making in cases such as Kenny's. For example, had Sharon attributed an improvement in Kenny's health to divine influence and had another member of the team attributed Kenny's improvement to intervention by professionals, Sharon's clinical opinion would have been influenced by factors related to her own belief system that were different from those of her colleague.

Although not often acknowledged, a physical therapist's belief system may influence decision making or may be a source of personal stress when it is not congruent with that of other members of the health care team. Identification of the therapist's own beliefs with respect to locus of control for health improvement in children and identification of how beliefs may influence decision making increase the objectivity of clinical decision making and the formation of opinions related to expected outcomes for children.

SUMMARY

As pediatric practice has evolved, physical therapists have assumed more responsibility for decision making and a larger role in communication and coordination of care.

Knowledge of public laws, such as the Individuals with Disabilities Education Act (IDEA) (Public Law 105-17), the Individuals with Disabilities Education Improvement Act (IDEIA) (Public Law 108-446), and the Americans with Disabilities Act (ADA) (Public Law 101-336), is required of the physical therapist providing services to children and adolescents with disabilities and their families. Knowledge of federal and state mandates is particularly important for therapists working in early intervention or the public school system to ensure practice is in compliance with public law and effectively support families in advocating for their children's needs. Contemporary practice also requires familiarity with the litigation process, such as medical malpractice and petitions for the determination of appropriate medical treatment. Physical therapists also have a responsibility in reporting cases of child abuse and neglect. Legal and ethical issues that pediatric physical therapists encounter are presented using a case history format to facilitate application to clinical practice.

REFERENCES

American Physical Therapy Association. Guide to Physical Therapist Practice. Physical Therapy, 77:1163–1650, 1997.

California Penal Code, Section 11166 (G).

De Jong, AR, Hervada, AR, & Emmett, GA. Epidemiological variations in childhood sexual abuse. Child Abuse and Neglect, 7:155–162, 1983.

DeVellis, SR, DeVellis, SBM, Revcki, DA, Lurie, SJ, Runyan, DIC, & Bristol, M. Development and validation of the Child Health Improvement Locus of Control (CHILC) scales. Journal of Social and Clinical Psychology, 3:307–324, 1985.

Gommes-Schwartz, B, Horowitz, JM, & Sauzier, M. Severity of emotional distress among sexually abused preschool, school aged and adolescent children. Hospital Community Psychiatry, 11:503–508, 1985.

Hampton, RH, & Newberger, EH. Child abuse incidence and reporting by hospitals: Significance of severity, class and race. American Journal of Public Health, 75:56–64, 1985.

23 Illinois Annotated Statutes. 2053, Sec. 4.

III Illinois Annotated Statutes. 4267-0.

Kempe, CH, Silverman, FW, Steele, BF, Droegemueller, W, & Silver, HK. The battered child syndrome. Journal of the American Medical Association, 181:17–24, 1962.

National Center for State Courts. Guidelines for state court decision making in authorizing or withholding life-sustaining medical treatment, Vol. 18, No. 10. Williamsburg, VA: National Center for State Courts, 1991, pp. 253–275.

Newberger, EH, Hyde, JN, Jr, Holter, JC, & Rosenfeld, A. Child abuse and neglect. In Hoekelman, RA, Blatman, S, Friedman, SB, Nelson, NM, & Seidel, HM (Eds.). Primary Pediatric Care. St. Louis: Mosby, 1987, pp. 629–638.

Official Code of Georgia, Annotated. Title 19, Chapter 7, 5(2)F.

O'Sullivan, DD. Evaluation of the medical record. Medicine Trial Technique Quarterly. Chicago: Callaghan, 1975.

Public Law 93-247, Child Abuse Prevention and Treatment Act of 1974, 42 USCS 5101–5106.

Public Law 94-142, Education of All Handicapped Children Act (1975), 20 USCS 1400.

Public Law 99-457, Education of the Handicapped Act Amendments of 1986, 20 USCS 1400.

Public Law 101-336, Americans with Disabilities Act (1990), 42 USCS 12102.

Public Law 101-476, Individuals with Disabilities Education Act Amendments of 1990, 20 USCS 1400.

Public Law 102-119, Individuals with Disabilities Education Act Amendments of 1991, 105 Stat. 587-608.

Public Law 105-17, Individuals with Disabilities Education Act Amendments of 1997, 111 Stat. 37-157.

Rosenfeld, A. Sexual abuse of children: Personal and professional responses. In Newberger, E (Ed.). Child Abuse. Boston: Little, Brown, 1982, pp. 57–74.

Rosenfeld, A, & Sarles, RM. Sexual misuse of children. In Hoekelman, RA, Blatman, S, Friedman, SB, Nelson, NM, & Seidel, HM (Eds.). Primary Pediatric Care. St. Louis: Mosby, 1986, pp. 642–651.

Summit, RC. The child sexual abuse accommodation syndrome. Child Abuse and Neglect, 7:177–193, 1982.

INDEX

Atrovent. *See* Ipratropium.
ATS. *See* Assistive technology supplier.
Attachment issues after open-heart surgery, 897, 899
Attentional ability in brain injury, 717, 721
Attention-deficit hyperactivity disorder, 560, 569, 576
Attribution theory of social support, 921
Auditory evoked response, 715
Augmented feedback, 148–149
Augmented or alternative communication, 1014–1015, 1015f
Auscultation
   in asthma, 869t
   in cystic fibrosis, 829, 831
   in premature infant, 1075, 1076f, 1077f
   in preparticipation examination, 520
Authority, self-determination and, 612b
Autism, federal definition of, 959b
Autogenic drainage for cystic fibrosis, 824, 838
Autograft for burn injury, 1029
Autonomic dysreflexia after spinal cord injury, 687
Autonomy in private practice, 1101
Autosomal dominant disorders, 239–240
   achondroplasia, 504
   neurofibromatosis 1, 239–240
   osteogenesis imperfecta, 402, 403t
   tuberous sclerosis complex, 240, 240t
Autosomal recessive disorders, 240–241, 242t
   congenital muscular dystrophy, 435
   cystic fibrosis, 819
   osteogenesis imperfecta, 402, 403t
Autosomal trisomies, 229–231
   Down syndrome, 229f, 229–231, 230t
   trisomy 13, 231
   trisomy 18, 231
Avascular necrosis
   developmental dysplasia of hip and, 493, 494
   metatarsal epiphysis and, 542–543
   slipped capital femoral epiphysis and, 500–501
   sports-related injury and, 539
Average feedback, 149
AVN. *See* Avascular necrosis.
Avoidant behavior in burn injury intervention, 1040
Avulsion fracture, 532
   of elbow, 536
   of hip, 539, 539f
   of tibial insertion, 540
Axilla, burn injury of, 1035t
   potential impairments associated with, 1047t
Axis
   ossification of, 338
   thigh-foot, 485
Axon
   motor, 191–192
   spinal cord injury and, 684
Axonotmesis, 667
Azithromycin, 825
Azmacort. *See* Triamcinolone.

B

Back cushion, 1000
   upholstery for, 1001
Back injury, sports-related, 534–535
Back pain, 503
   in adults with cerebral palsy, 651
   in scoliosis, 347
   in spondylolisthesis, 352
Back sleeping in infant, 38
Backback straps, 1002
Baclofen for cerebral palsy-associated spasticity, 647
Bacterial infection
   in cystic fibrosis, 823
      sputum culture of, 828–829

in osteomyelitis, 496–497
   in septic arthritis, 497
BAER. *See* Brainstem auditory evoked response.
Balance
   in brain injury, 720
   in hemophilia, 331
   in spinal cord injury, 691, 691f
Ball therapy, 839, 839f
Bandwidth corrective feedback, 149
Barbiturates use by athletes, 523
Barlow maneuver, 492, 492f
Barotrauma, bronchopulmonary dysplasia and, 1059
Basal ganglia, neuronal necrosis of, 1063, 1063b, 1064t
Baseball injuries, 533, 535, 536
Baseline variables in positive pressure ventilation, 799t
Basic perinatal care, 1055b
Bathing of infant with osteogenesis imperfecta, 408
Battered child syndrome, 1133, 1133b
Battle v. Commonwealth of Pennsylvania, 962
Bayley Scales of Infant Development, 67
   in brain injury, 721
   in cerebral palsy, 628
   after open-heart surgery, 898
   in osteogenesis imperfecta, 407
BBPP. *See* Birth brachial plexus palsy.
Bear-walking, 53, 56f
Becker muscular dystrophy, 423t, 434–435
Beclomethasone, 855t
Beclovent, 855t
Bed
   mobility in
      following scoliosis surgery, 346
      after spinal cord injury, 688t, 695
   power-controlled, 434
Behavior
   adaptive in cognitive impairment, 599
   associated with effective interviewing, 941
   in burn injury intervention, 1040
   creative, 138
   culture and, 923
   in McGraw's theory of motor development, 40
   sexual abuse and, 1134
Behavioral objectives in intervention outcomes evaluation, 23
   in cognitive impairment, 608–609
Behavioral programming intervention in cognitive impairment, 606–607
Behavioral theory of motor development, 35t, 36
Behavioral therapy, cognitive, 305
Beliefs
   categorical, 923
   compensatory, 923
   of parents, 918–919
   perspectivistic, 923
Berkow chart, 1027
Beta blockers use by athletes, 523
Bilateral hold of two objects, 56, 58f
Bilirubin, jaundice and, 1066–1067
Bill of rights for communication, 608, 609f
Biochemical genetic disorders, 241, 242t
Bioelectric impedance analysis, 276
Biofeedback
   in cerebral palsy, 647–648
   in juvenile rheumatoid arthritis, 305, 307
   in myelodysplasia, 775
Biologic dressing for burn injury, 1029, 1030t
   positioning and splinting and, 1036
Biomechanical factors
   in gait development, 162–167
      at 3 to 3.5 years, 167, 167f
      at 6 to 7 years, 167
      at 9 to 15 months, 165–166
      at 18 to 24 months, 166f, 166–167
      birth to age 9 months, 163–165, 164f

in locomotion development, 96
   in motor development, 92–93
   in seating system prescription assessment, 995, 995f, 996f
Biopsy
   chorionic villus
      in cystic fibrosis, 822
      in osteogenesis imperfecta, 406
   muscle
      in arthrogryposis multiplex congenita, 382
      in spinal muscular atrophy, 438–439
Biphasic positive airway pressure, 842
Birth brachial plexus palsy, 1069–1070, 1070f, 1071f
Birth history in torsional conditions, 482
Birth injury
   brachial plexus, 665–680. *See Also* Brachial plexus injury.
   related to nervous system, 1069–1070, 1070f, 1071f
Birth weight
   brachial plexus injury and, 665–666
   low, 1057
      asthma and, 853
      cerebral palsy and, 626–627
Bisphosphonates, 404
Bladder, neurogenic in myelodysplasia, 753
Blalock-Taussig shunt, 885, 887, 888
Bleeding. *See* Hemorrhage.
Blindness
   in athlete, 544, 545
   federal definition of, 959b
Blocked task sequencing, 145
Blood flow
   cerebral, developmental coordination disorders and, 562
   exercise and, 262t
   training and, 279t
Blood gas analysis, 828
Blood lactate level, exercise and, 260, 262t
Blood pressure
   exercise and, 260, 262t
   normal values of, 805b
   in preparticipation examination, 520
Blount's disease, 490–491
BMD. *See* Becker muscular dystrophy.
BMI. *See* Body mass index.
Bobath strap, 1002
Body alignment in cerebral palsy, 640
Body composition
   in myelodysplasia, 765–766
   physical fitness and, 258t, 276–278
   sports preparticipation examination and, 522–523
Body fat
   assessment of in preparticipation examination, 522
   body composition and, 277
   gait development and, 163
Body functions in International Classification of Functioning, Disability and Health, 11, 12f
Body mass
   development of locomotion and, 96
   gait development and
      birth to age 9 months, 163
      18 to 24 months, 166
   postural control and, 92
Body mass index assessment in preparticipation examination, 522
Body structures in International Classification of Functioning, Disability and Health, 11, 12f
Body water, total, 276, 277
Body weight
   assessment of in preparticipation examination, 522
   bone mass and strength and, 204

S